AMERICA'S
TOP DOCTORS®
A CASTLE CONNOLLY GUIDE

8th Edition

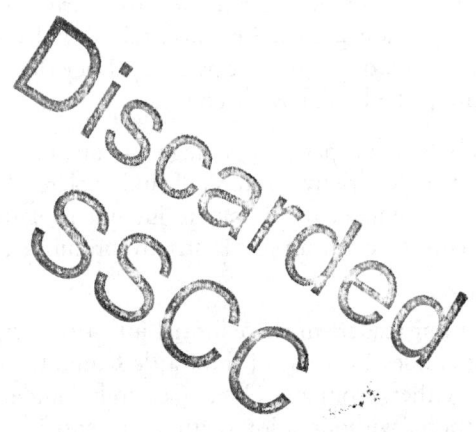
America's trusted source for identifying Top Doctors

For more information, please contact:

Castle Connolly Medical Ltd., 42 West 24th St, New York, New York 10010
212-367-8400x10
E-mail: info@castleconnolly.com
Web site: http://www.castleconnolly.com.

Library of Congress Control Number: 2008936744

| ISBN | 1-883769-98-1; | 978-1-883769-98-7 | (paperback) |
| ISBN | 1-883769-97-3; | 978-1-883769-97-0 | (hardcover) |

Printed in the United States of America

Table of Contents

Table of Contents

Table of Contents

Table of Contents

Table of Contents

Table of Contents

Table of Contents

Table of Contents

Table of Contents

Table of Contents

America's Top Doctors® 8th Edition

Table of Contents

Table of Contents

Table of Contents

Table of Contents

Appendices

Indices

About The Publishers

John K. Castle has spent much of the last three decades involved with healthcare institutions and issues. Mr. Castle served as Chairman of the Board of New York Medical College for eleven years, an institution where he served on the Board of Trustees for twenty-two years.

Mr. Castle has been extensively involved in other healthcare and voluntary activities as well. He served for five years as a public commissioner on the Joint Commission on Accreditation of Healthcare Organizations (JCAHO), the body which accredits most public and private hospitals throughout the United States. Mr. Castle has also served as a trustee of five different hospitals in the metropolitan New York region, including New York-Presbyterian Hospital, where he continues to serve.

Mr. Castle is also the Chairman of the Columbia Presbyterian Science Advisory Council and a Director of the Whitehead Institute for Biomedical Research. He is a Fellow of The New York Academy of Medicine and has served as a Trustee of the Academy. He is Chairman of the United Hospital Fund of New York's Capital Campaign. He continues as Director Emeritus of the United Hospital Fund. He is a Life Member of the MIT Corporation, the governing body of the Massachusetts Institute of Technology.

Mr. Castle is the Chairman and Co-Publisher of Castle Connolly Medical Ltd. and affiliated companies which publish *Castle Connolly America's Top Doctors® 8th Edition*; *Castle Connolly Top Doctors: New York Metro Area* and other books to help people find the best healthcare.

John J. Connolly, Ed.D. is the President & CEO of Castle Connolly Medical Ltd., and is the nation's foremost authority on identifying top physicians. Dr. Connolly's experience in healthcare is extensive.

For more than a decade he served as President of New York Medical College, the nation's second largest private medical college. He is a Fellow of the New York Academy of Medicine, a Fellow of the New York Academy of Sciences, a Director of the New York Business Group on Health, a member of the President's Council of the United Hospital Fund, and a member of the Board of Advisors of Funding First, a Lasker Foundation initiative. Dr. Connolly has served as a trustee of two hospitals and as Chairman of the Board of one. He is extensively involved in healthcare and community activities and has served on a number of voluntary and corporate boards including the Board of the American Lyme Disease Foundation, of which he is a founder and past chairman, and the Board of Advisors of the Whitehead Institute for Biomedical Research. He is also a Director and Chairman of the Professional Examination Service. He holds a Bachelor of Science degree from Worcester State College, a Master's degree from the University of Connecticut, and a Doctor of Education degree in College and University Administration from Teacher's College, Columbia University.

Dr. Connolly has appeared on or been interviewed by over 100 television and radio stations nationwide including *"Good Morning America"* (ABC-TV), *"The Today Show"* (NBC-TV), *"20/20"* (ABC-TV), *"48 Hours"* (CBS-TV), *"Fox Cable News"* (national), *"Morning News"* (CNN) and *"Weekend Today in New York"* (WNBC-TV). The *New York Times*, the *Chicago Tribune*, the *Daily News* (New York), the *Boston Herald* and other newspapers, as well as many national and regional magazines, have featured Castle Connolly Guides and/or Dr. Connolly in stories.

Foreword

The challenge of finding the best healthcare is a formidable one for most Americans and for others who seek medical care in the United States. While this country offers the best medical care in the world, many people are overwhelmed by its complexity and bureaucracy.

While most of us are fortunate and never need to venture beyond our local communities to find medical specialists able to meet our healthcare needs, the needs of many patients cannot be met in their local areas. For them, the search for the top specialists can be as important as life itself!

This great nation is fortunate in possessing some of the world's leading medical centers and specialty hospitals where cutting edge research is conducted and innovative new therapies are practiced daily. These health centers employ and train many of the world's most skilled physicians. The organization which I formerly headed, the Association of Academic Health Centers, serves as a forum of exchange for these centers of medical excellence and, therefore, I know them well. However, I also know well the difficulty and challenges that patients and their families face in identifying and locating the tremendous wealth of medical talent and dedication that lies within the walls of these outstanding facilities.

Castle Connolly Medical Ltd. has dedicated extensive time and resources to identify-ing the best healthcare this nation has to offer. They have done this not to serve physicians or hospitals, but to serve healthcare consumers. Their efforts will be vital and important resources to Americans and others who seek the best medical care available in this country—wherever it is being practiced.

Roger Bulger, M.D.
Former President, Association of Academic Health Centers (AAHC)
Washington DC

Introduction

There are times in life when the nature of a disease or medical condition that afflicts you or a loved one warrants identifying the top doctor—the very best specialist anywhere in the nation—to diagnose or treat that particular medical problem. At times like these, you need Castle Connolly **America's Top Doctors**®, the national guide designed to assist you under just these circumstances.

While the overall quality of medical care throughout the United States is generally of very high quality and in many places is superb, there are still those rare, complex or extremely difficult problems that demand resources beyond the ordinary or that require talents that are exceptional.

This guide identifies those top medical specialists throughout the country who possess the skill and experience to address these problems. Top specialists who provide excellent care tend to be located predominantly, although not exclusively, at major medical centers, specialty hospitals and leading teaching hospitals. These exceptional physicians are acknowledged as such by their peers and are recognized for their expertise by the medical profession.

The top specialists we have identified are not the only excellent physicians who are caring for patients in this nation. Since there are more than 720,000 doctors in the United States, we cannot identify every top specialist. Therefore, we have included narrative to assist those using this guide who may not find the specialist they need within its listings. Clearly, there are many primary care physicians and other well-trained specialists in communities and hospitals throughout the United States.

Most physicians in this guide are board certified not only in a specialty, but also in a subspecialty or in multiple subspecialties. Board or subspecialty certification alone, however, does not distinguish them from excellent specialists at hospitals in your community, many of whom are also board certified in both a specialty and a subspecialty.

However, the majority of physicians included in this guide have trained at the top medical centers under medical pioneers who possess state-of-the-art knowledge in a specific disease or problem and have often devised new techniques and therapeutic approaches, many of which are life-saving procedures or cures. These doctors most often practice their science and art at leading hospitals and, more specifically, in programs at hospitals that are recognized for their excellence in a given field. Many others have been trained at leading centers in other nations since the U.S. is not alone in pioneering new medical knowledge, although its position as the leader in "high-tech" medicine is generally acknowledged.

Another major characteristic distinguishing the majority of physicians in this guide from those at local hospitals is their continued focus and training. Rather than practicing at a community hospital (or even at a leading regional hospital) and developing a general, broad-based practice, these physicians continued their training in a particular disease, syndrome or subspecialty to such a degree that they developed extensive knowledge and unique skills in treating that particular problem.

Often that focused, advanced training is accompanied by active involvement in clinical research. This is an additional reason why the physicians listed in this guide are located at only a few hundred of the more than six thousand hospitals in the United States. It is difficult, although not impossible, to conduct important clinical research in isolation or without an environment supportive of research. It takes time, money, residents, research associates, technicians, equipment and more to produce significant clinical research. Certainly there have been individuals who have made important and lasting contributions to research with little or none of this support, but those instances are rare. Today, for the most part, major advances in medicine occur in the labs and on the floors of major medical centers and specialty hospitals, in medical schools and in clinical labs created and financed for that purpose by commercial enterprises.

How Physicians Were Selected For Inclusion In This Guide

The basis of the Castle Connolly selection process is peer nomination. In some ways, this resembles an enhancement of the process in which a personal physician provides a patient with a referral to another physician for a particular problem. However, if the recommendation of one doctor is good, the recommendation of many doctors is even better. So, we ask many doctors for their recommendations; in fact, more than 230,000 doctors were surveyed during our first effort at building this database.

How do we accomplish this enormous task? Over the years, the Castle Connolly physician-led research team developed its extensive database of physicians across the nation through periodic mail, telephone and email surveys. This cumulative database is systematically maintained and continuously updated. Surveyed physicians nominate top doctors in both their own and related specialties – especially those to whom they would refer their own patients. Each year this database is supplemented by further mail surveys and telephone interviews with leaders in the various medical specialties and leading physicians at major medical centers. In our research for the first edition of this guide, online surveys also were conducted with members of Physicians' Online (POL), the country's largest community of physicians connected through the Internet.

To augment our large mail, telephone and online samplings, additional surveys are conducted among the following carefully selected groups: directors of graduate medical programs; directors of clinical services at member hospitals of the Council of Teaching Hospitals (COTH); board members of medical specialty academies, associations and societies; and deans and chairs of departments at medical schools.

Building on years of prior research, thousands of top doctors included in earlier editions of our guides, as well as a random sample of physicians not listed, are invited to offer their nominations for Castle Connolly *America's Top Doctors*®.

Over 25,000 physicians have been nominated through this process. Extensive biographical forms were sent to those physicians most frequently nominated for completion. After careful review of their professional backgrounds, the Castle Connolly research staff conducted further research to check disciplinary and license histories.

The result is a carefully researched and highly selective list of the top specialists in the nation. This select group of physicians, identified through our extensive research process, constitutes a list of physicians recognized by their peers for their excellence in providing care for specific diseases and problems.

Undoubtedly, there will be comments that we have missed some fine doctors who should be included. That is inevitable, since this guide is designed to identify only those doctors noted for excellence in diagnosing or treating a specific problem or disease.

We do not intentionally include physicians simply because they have important titles. While a position as a chief of service or a department head at a teaching hospital is an important post, such positions are achieved through a combination of many talents including administrative skills, seniority and factors that are not as important for inclusion in this guide as is skill in clinical care. The same is true of leaders of county medical societies, professional associations or even specialty groups. While these are significant positions and acknowledge a leadership among peers, these titles are not essential to clinical skill recognition.

The same perspective applies to research expertise. Many physicians listed in the Guide are engaged in clinical research and make significant contributions to their fields, with some devoting a substantial portion of their time to research. However, we avoided including those physicians who solely conduct research and who do not provide patient care.

The result of this extensive research effort is a list of outstanding, highly skilled physicians who are recognized as among the best in their specialties and in the nation; a list which consumers/patients can use to find the very best specialists to meet their particular needs.

Lastly, this book differs from the regional Castle Connolly Guides in two important ways. First, Castle Connolly *America's Top Doctors* **8th Edition** is national, not regional, in scope. Second, the regional Guides are based on the generally accurate premise that healthcare is local and most people find their healthcare where they live and work. However, Castle Connolly *America's* **Top Doctors** **8th Edition** is designed to meet the needs of those people who cannot find the right specialists locally but who can and will travel anywhere in the country to be cared for by a top specialist at an outstanding hospital. This guide will assist readers in that important search and, for that reason, does not include primary care physicians.

Using This Guide To Find Top Specialists

This guide is organized and planned to be as user-friendly as possible. Still, as with anything as complex as medical specialties, subspecialties and the myriad of diseases and problems that specialists treat, there needs to be a system to organize the physicians' names, the diseases and problems they manage and their special expertise.

To organize the specialists in this guide, we have followed the American Board of Medical Specialties (ABMS) format. The ABMS is the authoritative body for the recognition of medical specialties. Without the ABMS as the official controlling body there would be hundreds of unregulated medical specialties.

The ABMS recognizes twenty-five specialties and more than ninety subspecialties. The listing of ABMS specialties and subspecialties can be found in Appendix A. In addition to ABMS recognized specialties, there are at least one hundred other groups calling themselves "medical specialists" that are not recognized by the ABMS. Some of these groups are working toward recognition and have exams and other standards for membership. Others are organizations of physicians interested in a particular problem or area of medicine that exist to exchange information but have no intention of seeking ABMS recognition. Some groups calling themselves "boards" really have little authority or meaningful standards. Thus, while a physician may state he/she is, for example, a specialist in cosmetic surgery, there is no ABMS recognized specialty by that name. Therefore, you have no idea whether this physician has any special training and expertise or is simply trying to recruit paying patients to a lucrative aspect of surgical practice.

You can get information on a doctor's credentials from the doctor, from the doctor's hospital (Medical Affairs Office) or from your health plan if a doctor is in the network. You can also get this information from numerous Web sites, including www.castleconnolly.com. You can check on a physician's board certification by calling the ABMS at (866) 275-2267 or by logging on to its Web site at www.abms.org.

If you seek a particular type of specialist or subspecialist, turn to the section of this guide covering that medical specialty or subspecialty. There you will be able to further restrict your search to a specific geographic region or, if you prefer, to search throughout the nation.

Using This Guide To Find Top Specialists

To make your search easier, we have organized the specialties and subspecialties into the following regions: New England, Mid Atlantic, Midwest, Southeast, Southwest, Great Plains and Mountains, and West Coast and Pacific. To find an outstanding cardiologist in St. Louis, for example, look under Cardiovascular Disease and then under the Midwest region. (See Page 39 for geographical regions and states.)

A second way to use this guide is to look at the Special Expertise Index, which lists the areas of special expertise of included physicians. This list of special expertise indicates more than 2,000 medical topics including diseases, therapeutic approaches and techniques. You can look up the particular disease, problem or technique you are interested in and locate a physician in that manner. We assume that many people using this guide will know what their particular problem is and will begin their exploration with this index. However, we encourage you to read the entire text since it will help you to better understand how to find the right physician for yourself or a family member, especially if one is not found in this guide.

Choosing An Appropriate Specialist

It may seem that choosing the correct specialist to treat a particular medical problem is simply a matter of finding a top doctor in a specific medical specialty. For treatment of a problem with your vision, you would choose an ophthalmologist. A skin or hair problem would require treatment by a dermatologist and a broken bone would need the care of an orthopaedic surgeon.

Sometimes, however, the type of specialist needed may not be obvious. For example, back surgery may be performed by either an orthopaedic surgeon or a neurosurgeon. Different aspects of sports medicine, as another example, are practiced by orthopaedic surgeons who treat sports-related injuries in both adults and children, pediatricians who treat only children or internists and family practitioners whose focus is on prevention of injuries.

In some cases, several specialists with expertise in different areas of medical practice all become involved in treating the same patient's health problem. For example, a person with diabetes might need care from an endocrinologist, a cardiologist and an ophthalmologist. In other situations, doctors trained in different specialties may use varied approaches or differing therapies to manage a disease or condition. Such is the case, for example, with prostate cancer: a patient could be treated by a urologist, a medical oncologist, or a radiation oncologist. The urologist might provide the patient with a surgical treatment option, while the medical oncologist would treat the patient with chemotherapy and the radiotherapist would use radiation therapy and/or radioactive seed implantation. All approaches could be successful, or one might be preferable to another, depending on the patient and his condition. Therefore, a wise patient will thoroughly explore all options before making a choice.

America's Top Doctors® 8th Edition

Finding the right specialist is also important in terms of the quality of your care. For example, many orthopaedic surgeons will operate on hands, but it is clearly preferable to have someone trained and certified specifically in hand surgery (a subspecialty of both orthopaedic surgery and plastic surgery) to perform that delicate surgery. Similarly, a dermatologist may indicate that his/her practice includes cosmetic surgery; however, there is no approved ABMS dermatology subspecialty or fellowship training in cosmetic surgery. While many dermatologists do pursue additional training in cosmetic surgery, it should be understood that dermatologic practice is limited to cutaneous procedures ranging from the removal of skin tumors to laser resurfacing. On the other hand, some board certified otolaryngologists have additional training that enables them to perform cosmetic surgery procedures on the head and neck.

Choosing the right type of specialist is as important as selecting the right doctor. For example, the diagnosis of melanoma, a very serious, potentially life threatening form of skin cancer, is missed in many cases. Therefore, if you have a skin lesion that might possibly be melanoma, you should be certain that the pathologist reading your slides is board certified in the subspecialty of dermatopathology.

These examples illustrate this important principle: always seek the best healthcare. Look for the best-trained doctors, not those who simply can do the job. That doesn't mean that you need to consult a doctor listed in this guide every time you have a health problem. It does mean you should be certain that the physicians who care for you, whether in your community or at a world-class medical center, are trained appropriately and are qualified to provide the care you require. Remember, when it comes to healthcare no one wants second best!

Given this complexity, how do you find the right specialist to provide your care? The first and most important person to look to for guidance is your primary care physician. He/she will assess your medical condition, determine the appropriate type of specialist to recommend and perhaps refer you to a specific doctor or doctors. You should always ask your primary care physician why a particular specialist is being recommended, since that specialist may be a colleague in your doctor's medical group or may be the only (or the most conveniently located) specialist of the type in your health plan. Ask how well your primary care physician knows the specialist, whether they have a long-standing professional relationship and if other patients referred to the specialist had successful outcomes. Be sure to ask for several recommendations, if possible, to provide you with some choice among specialists.

If you do not have a primary care doctor, try to learn as much as you can about your medical problem and the type of specialist best suited to treat it. However, keep in mind that many diseases or conditions present with symptoms that often are indistinguishable from those of other diseases or conditions, making them difficult to diagnose precisely even for physicians armed with the results of diagnostic tests.

Using This Guide To Find Top Specialists

Judging The Qualifications Of A Physician

The specialists listed in Castle Connolly *America's Top Doctors* ® are clearly among the best in the nation and have been identified through a rigorous research process and thorough screening by the Castle Connolly research team. Through our extensive surveys and research we have done much of the work in finding a top referral specialist for you. But how do you judge the qualifications of a physician who may not be listed in this Guide? If you are trying to find a specialist on your own, how should you go about it? How can you tell when a physician has the appropriate training in a specialty and how do you distinguish what is meaningful and what is not from among all those plaques and certificates on a doctor's wall?

The following pages will outline that process for you. In fact, what is written here reflects much of the logic that underlies the selection of physicians for this book.

The following material will help you not only in finding a top specialist in this Guide, but it also should be helpful to you in choosing among the many specialists, primary care doctors and other physicians that you will need to consult throughout your life.

The reality is that few of us see only one doctor in our lifetime. Each of us may be cared for by a primary care physician, an ophthalmologist, an orthopaedic surgeon, a dermatologist, a surgeon or a number of other specialists. The choices can be many and they can be among the most important choices that we make in our lives.

Education

Your review of your prospective doctor's education and training should begin with medical school. While you may feel that the institution at which someone earned a bachelor's degree could be an indication of the quality of the doctor, most people in the medical field do not believe it plays a major role. A degree from a highly selective undergraduate college or university will help an aspiring doctor gain admission to a medical school, but once there, all students are peers. However, the information on undergraduate colleges, if important to you, is available in *The Official ABMS Directory of Board Certified Medical Specialists*® and other medical directories.

American medical schools are highly standardized, at least in terms of basic quality. A group known as the Liaison Committee for Medical Education (LCME) accredits all U.S. medical schools that grant medical degrees (MDs) and osteopathic degrees (DOs). Most also are accredited by the appropriate state agency, if one exists, and by regional accrediting agencies that accredit colleges and universities of all kinds.

Furthermore, U.S. medical schools have universally high standards for admission, including success on the undergraduate level and on the Medical College Admissions Tests (MCATs). Although frequently criticized for being slow to change and for training too many specialists, the system of medical education in the United States has insured high quality in medical practice. One recent positive change is a strong effort in most medical schools to diversify the composition of the student body. While these schools have been less successful in enrolling racial minorities, the number of women in U.S. medical schools has increased to the point that women now make up about 50 percent of most classes. In certain specialties preferred by women medical graduates (pediatrics, for example) it is possible that in coming years the majority of specialists will be female.

Most doctors practicing in the United States are graduates of U.S. medical schools, but there are two other groups of doctors who make up a relatively small portion of the total physician population. They are (1) foreign nationals who graduated from foreign schools and (2) U.S. nationals who graduated from foreign schools. (Canadian medical schools are not considered foreign).

Foreign Medical Graduates

Foreign medical schools vary greatly in quality. Even some of the oldest and finest European schools have become virtually "open door," with huge numbers of unscreened students making teaching and learning difficult. Others are excellent and provided the model for our system of medical education.

The fact that someone graduated from a foreign school does not mean that he/she is a poor doctor. Foreign schools, like U.S. schools, produce good doctors and poor doctors. Foreign medical graduates must pass the same exam taken by U.S. graduates for licensure, but the failure rate for foreign graduates is significantly higher. In the first year of using the new United States Medical Licensing Exam (USMLE), 93 percent of U.S. medical school graduates passed Step II, the clinical exam, as compared with 39 percent of the foreign graduates. It is clear that the quality of foreign schools, if not individual doctors, is not the same as U.S. medical schools, at least as measured by our standards. Nonetheless, many communities and patients have been well served by foreign medical graduates practicing in this country—often in areas where it has been difficult to attract graduates of American schools.

In addition, many foreign medical schools and their teaching hospitals are world renowned for their leadership in medical care, research and teaching and many of the technologies and techniques we utilize in the U.S. today have been developed and perfected in foreign countries.

Residency

Most doctors practicing today have at least three years of postgraduate training (following the MD or DO) in an approved residency program. This not only is an important step in the process of becoming a competent doctor, but it is also a requirement for board (specialty) certification. Most people assume that a prospective doctor needs to complete a three-year residency program to obtain a medical license. That is not an accurate assumption! New York State, for example, requires only one postgraduate year. However, since all approved residencies last at least three years and some, such as those in neurosurgery, general surgery, orthopaedic surgery and urology, may extend for five or more years, it is important to know the details of a doctor's training. Licensure alone is not enough of a basis upon which to make a decision.

Without undertaking extensive and detailed research on every residency program, the best assessment you can make of a doctor's residency program is to see if it took place in a large medical center whose name you recognize. The more prestigious institutions tend to attract the best medical students, sometimes regardless of the quality of the individual residency program. If in doubt about a doctor's training, ask the doctor if the residency he/she completed was in the specialty of the practice; if not, ask why not.

It is also important to be certain that a doctor completed a residency that has been approved by the appropriate governing board of the specialty, such as the American Board of Surgery, the American Board of Radiology, or the American Osteopathic Board of Pediatrics. These board groups are listed in Appendix A. If you are really concerned about a doctor's training, you should call the hospital that offered the residency and ask if the residency program was approved by the appropriate specialty group. If still in doubt, consult the publication *Directory of Graduate Medical Education Programs*, often called the "green book," found in medical school or hospital libraries, which lists all approved residencies.

Board Certification

With an MD or DO degree and a license, an individual may practice in any medical specialty with or without additional training. For example, doctors with a license but no special training may call themselves cardiologists, pediatricians or gynecologists. This is why board certification is such an important factor. The American Board of Medical Specialties (ABMS) recognizes 25 specialties and more than 90 subspecialties. Visit www.abms.org or call 866-275-2267 for more information. Eighteen boards certify in 106 specialties under the aegis of the American Osteopathic Association (AOA). Visit www.osteopathic.org or call 800-621-1773 for more information. Doctors who have qualified for such specialization are called board certified; they have completed an approved residency and passed the board's exam. (See Appendix A for the approved ABMS and AOA lists). While many doctors who are not board certified do call themselves "specialists," board certification is the best standard by which to measure competence and training. Throughout this Guide a description of each specialty and subspecialty is provided as an introduction to the listing of physicians in that specialty.

You can be confident that doctors who are board certified have, at a minimum, the proper training in their specialty and have demonstrated their proficiency through supervision and testing. While there are many non-board certified doctors who are highly competent, it is more difficult to assess the level of their training. While board certification alone does not guarantee competence, it is a standard that reflects successful completion of an appropriate training program. If it is impossible to find a doctor in your area who is board certified in a particular subspecialty, for example, geriatric medicine or sports medicine, at least be certain the physician is board certified in a related specialty such as internal medicine or orthopaedic surgery.

Board certified doctors are referred to as Diplomates of the Board. Some of the colleges of medical specialties (e.g., the American College of Radiology, the American College of Surgeons) have multiple levels of recognition. The first is basic membership and the second, more prestigious and difficult to obtain, is status as a Fellow. Fellowship status in the colleges is meaningful and is based on experience, professional achievement and recognition by one's peers, including extensive experience in patient care. It should be viewed as a significant professional qualification.

Board Eligibility

Many doctors who have been more recently trained are waiting to take the boards. They are sometimes described as "board eligible," a common term that the ABMS advocates abandoning because of its ambiguity. Board eligible means that the doctor has completed an approved residency and is qualified to sit for the related board's exam.

Each member board of the ABMS has its own policy regarding the use and recognition of the board eligible term. Therefore, the description "board eligible" should not be viewed as a genuine qualification, especially if a doctor has been out of medical school long enough to have taken the certification exam. To the boards, a doctor is either board certified or not. Furthermore, most of the specialty boards permit unlimited attempts to pass the exam and, in some cases, doctors who have failed the exam twice or even ten times continue to call themselves board eligible. In osteopathic medicine, the board eligible status is recognized only for the first six years after completion of a residency.

Using This Guide To Find Top Specialists

In addition to the approved lists of specialties and subspecialties of the ABMS and AOA, there are a wide variety of other doctors and groups of doctors who call themselves specialists. At present there are at least 100 such groups called "self-designated medical specialties." They range from doctors who are working to create a recognized body of knowledge and subspecialty training to less formal groups interested in a particular approach to the practice of medicine. These groups may or may not have standards for membership. There is no way to determine the true extent of their members' training and neither the ABMS or the AOA recognizes them. While you should be cautious of doctors who claim they are specialists in these areas, many do have advanced training and the groups at least offer a listing of people interested in a particular approach to medical care. Rely on board certification to assure yourself of basic competence, and use membership in one of these groups to indicate strong interest and possible additional training in a particular aspect of medicine. A list of these self-designated medical specialties may be found in Appendix B.

Recertification

A relatively new focus of the specialty boards is the area of recertification. Until recently, board certification lasted for an unlimited time. Now, almost all the boards have put time limits on the certification period. For example, in Internal Medicine and Anesthesiology, the time limit is ten years; in Family Practice, six, and under some circumstances, seven years. These more stringent standards reflect an increasing emphasis on recertification by both the medical boards and state agencies responsible for licensing doctors.

Since the policies of the boards vary widely, it is a good procedure to ask a doctor if certification was awarded and when. If the date was seven to ten years ago, ask if he/she has been recertified. Unfortunately, many boards permit "grandfathering," whereby already certified doctors do not have to be recertified, and recertification requirements apply only to newly certified doctors. Appendix A contains a list of the names and addresses of the boards and the certification period for each board specialty. Even if recertification is not required, it is good professional practice for doctors to undertake the process. It assures you, the patient, that they are attempting to stay current.

Many states have a continuing medical education requirement for doctors. These states typically require a minimum number of continuing medical education (CME) credits for a doctor to maintain a medical license. Seven states require 150 CME credits over a three-year period. Osteopathic doctors are required to take 120 hours of CME credits within three years to maintain certification.

Fellowships

The purpose of a fellowship is to provide advanced training in the clinical techniques and research of a particular specialty. Fellowships usually, but not always, are designed to lead to board certification in a subspecialty such as cardiology, which is a subspecialty of internal medicine. Many physicians listed in this Guide have had fellowship training. In the U.S. there are a variety of fellowship programs available to doctors, which fall into two broad categories: approved and unapproved. Approved fellowships are those that are approved by the appropriate medical specialty board (e.g., the American Board of Radiology) and lead to subspecialty certificates. Fellowship programs that are unapproved are often in the same areas of training as those that are approved, but they do not lead to subspecialty certificates. Unfortunately, all too often, an unapproved fellowship exists only to provide relatively inexpensive labor for the research and/or patient care activities of a clinical department in a medical school or hospital. In such cases, the learning that takes place is secondary and may be a good deal less than in an approved fellowship. On the other hand, any fellowship is better than none at all and some unapproved fellowships have that status for a valid reason that should not reflect negatively on the program. For example, the fellowship may have been recently created, with approval being sought. To check that a fellowship is an approved one, call the hospital where the training took place or call the medical board for that specialty.

Some physicians may have completed more than one fellowship and may be boarded in two or more subspecialties. Also, some physicians may pursue fellowship training and subspecialty certification, but then choose to practice in their primary field of certification. For example, a doctor who is board certified in internal medicine also may have obtained board certification in cardiology, but may choose to practice primarily internal medicine rather than cardiology. For the most part, the physicians in this Guide practice in their subspecialties.

Professional Reputation

There are doctors who meet every professional standard on paper, but who are simply not good doctors. In all probability the medical community has ascertained that and, while the individual may still practice medicine, his/her reputation will reflect that collective assessment. There are also doctors who are outstanding leaders in their fields because of research or professional activities but who are not particularly strong, or perhaps even active, in patient care. It is important to distinguish that kind of professional reputation from a reputation as a competent, caring doctor in delivering patient care, or in the case of this Guide, as an outstanding practitioner in a given specialty.

Using This Guide To Find Top Specialists

Hospital Appointment

Most doctors are on the medical staff of one or more hospitals and are known as "attendings;" some are not. If a doctor does not have admitting privileges or is not on the attending staff of a hospital, you may wish to consider choosing a different doctor. It can be very difficult to ascertain whether or not the lack of hospital appointment is for a good reason. For example, it is understandable that some doctors who are raising families or heading toward retirement choose not to meet the demands (meetings, committees, etc.) of being an attending. However, if you need care in a hospital, the lack of such an appointment means that another doctor will have to oversee that care. In some specialties, such as dermatology and psychiatry, doctors may conduct their entire practice in the office and a hospital appointment is not as essential, or as good a criterion for assessment, as in other specialties.

While mistakes are made, most hospitals are quite careful about admissions to their medical staffs. The best hospitals are highly selective, so a degree of screening (or "credentialing") has been done for you. In other words, the best doctors practice at the best hospitals. Since caring for a patient in a hospital is often a team effort involving a number of specialists, the reputation of the hospital to which the doctor admits patients carries special weight. Hospital medical staffs review their colleagues' credentials and authorize performance of specific procedures. In addition, they typically review and reappoint their medical staff every two or three years. In effect, this is an additional screening to protect patients. It is especially true of hospitals that have what are known as closed staffs, where it is impossible to obtain admitting privileges unless there is a vacancy that the administration and medical staff deem necessary to fill. If you are having a surgical procedure and are concerned about the doctor's skill or experience, it may be worthwhile to call the Medical Affairs office at the doctor's hospital to see if he/she is authorized to perform that procedure in that hospital.

The reasons for a hospital's selectivity are easy to understand: no hospital wishes to expose itself to liability and every hospital wants to have the best reputation possible in order to attract patients. Obviously, the quality of the medical staff is immensely important in creating that reputation.

Physicians listed in this guide are primarily on the staffs of major medical centers, usually teaching hospitals, and leading specialty hospitals, e.g. children's, cancer, heart, psychiatric, etc. There are many excellent physicians on the staffs of community hospitals that call themselves "medical centers," but they are not physicians who typically attract complex cases and referrals from outside their area.

To learn about a hospital visit its website. It is also useful to review a hospital's accreditation status under the Joint Commission on the Accreditation of Healthcare Organizations at www.JCAHO.com. A new website created by the federal government, www.hospitalcompare.com, offers some measures of comparative hospital quality and may be of interest as well.

A last and very important reason why a hospital appointment is an essential requirement in your choice of doctor is that some states permit doctors to practice without malpractice insurance. If you are injured as a result of a doctor's poor care, you could be without recourse. However, few hospitals permit doctors to practice in them unless they carry malpractice insurance. This not only protects the hospital, but the patient as well.

Medical School Faculty Appointment

Many doctors have appointments on the faculties of medical schools. There is a range of categories from "straight" appointments, meaning full-time appointment as professor, associate professor, assistant professor or instructor, to clinical ranks that may reflect lesser degrees of involvement in teaching or research. If someone carries what is known as a straight academic rank (i.e. "professor of surgery," without clinical in the title), this usually means that the individual is engaged full-time in medical school research, teaching activities and patient care. The title "clinical professor of surgery" usually indicates a less direct involvement in medical school activities such as teaching and research.

Doctors who are full-time academicians may be in the forefront of new techniques and research, but they are not necessarily better doctors. Nonetheless, you would be assured that they have the support of other faculty, residents and medical students.

When you are seeking a subspecialist, a doctor's relationship to a medical school becomes more meaningful since medical school faculties tend to be made up of subspecialists. You are less likely to find large numbers of general or primary care practitioners engaged full-time on a medical school faculty. The newest approaches and techniques in medicine, for the most part, are explored and developed by medical school faculties in their laboratories and clinical practice settings. This is where they practice their subspecialties, as well as teach and conduct research. Such leading specialists are not necessarily better doctors than community doctors; rather, they are trained to provide a different kind of medical care. Obviously the type of medical care users of this guide are seeking is that different kind of care available primarily from top subspecialists at leading hospitals and medical centers.

Medical Society Membership

Most medical society memberships sound very prestigious and some are; however, there are many societies that are not selective and which virtually any doctor can join. In addition, membership in many of the more prestigious societies is based on research and publication or on leadership in the field and may have little to do with direct patient care. While it is clearly an honor to be invited to join these groups, membership may be less than helpful in discerning whether a doctor can deliver the excellent clinical care you require.

Using This Guide To Find Top Specialists

Experience

Experience is difficult to assess. Obviously, in most cases, an older doctor has more experience; on the other hand, a younger doctor has been more recently immersed in the challenge of medical school, residency, or even a fellowship, and may be the most up-to-date. If a doctor is board certified, you may assume that assures at least a minimal amount of experience, but since it could be as little as a year, check the date of graduation from medical school or completion of residency to know precisely how long a doctor has been in practice.

There is a good deal of evidence that there is a positive relationship between quantity of experience and quality of care. It may be that, the more a doctor performs a procedure, the better he/she becomes at it. That is why it is important to ask a doctor about his or her experience with the procedure that you need. Does the doctor see and treat similar cases every day, every week or only rarely? Of course, with some rare diseases, rarely is the only possible answer, but it is relative frequency that is critical. Major metropolitan areas, especially New York and San Francisco, became leaders in the treatment of AIDS because of the number of patients seen in those metropolitan areas. Doctors in the suburbs of New York City (especially in New York's Westchester, Nassau and Suffolk counties) and in Fairfield County, Connecticut became leaders in the research and treatment of Lyme disease because that region is the epicenter of the disease.

In some states, data is available on volume or numbers of certain procedures performed at hospitals. For this information in New York you can call the Center for Medical Consumers, a non-profit advocacy organization, or visit its web site at www.medicalconsumers.org. For volume and outcome information in other states, visit the web site of Health Care Choices at www.healthcarechoices.org. The federal government has posted outcome data for hospitals, but for a limited number of procedures, on a website www.healthcarecompare.com. There is a good deal of controversy, however, on the validity and usefulness of such data. Opponents cite the fact that some of the data is produced from Medicare patient records only and, thus, is based solely on an elderly population that does not represent the total activity of a hospital or doctor. Proponents of the use of such volume data agree that it is not perfect, but suggest it can be one useful criterion in selecting the best places to receive care for these specific problems

The one type of experience you should specifically want to know about is that dealing with any special procedure, particularly a surgical one, that has recently been developed and introduced into practice. For example, in the 1980's many doctors using laparoscopic cholecystectomy, a then new surgical technique for removing gallbladders, experienced a high percentage of problems because they were not properly trained. This prompted the American Board of Surgery to announce new standards for the training of surgeons using this technique. Do not hesitate to ask about your doctor's training in a procedure and how frequently and with what degree of success he/she has performed it. Practice may not lead to perfection, but it does improve skills and enhance the probability of success.

In some cases, relatively young doctors have recently completed residency or fellowship training under recognized leaders who have developed new approaches or techniques for dealing with a particular problem. They may have learned the new techniques from their mentors and may be far ahead of the field (and ahead of more senior and distinguished colleagues) in using those approaches. So age and experience must be considered and weighed along with other factors when choosing a physician.

Second Opinions

Second opinions are a valuable medical tool, too infrequently used in many instances and overused in others. Clearly, you do not want to seek another doctor's opinion on every ailment or problem that you face, but a second opinion should be pursued in the following situations:

• before major surgery

• if the diagnosis is serious or life threatening

• if a rare disease is diagnosed

• if a diagnosis is uncertain

• if the number of tests or procedures recommended might be excessive

• if a test result has serious implications (e.g., a positive Pap smear)

• if the treatment suggested is risky or expensive

• if you are uncomfortable with the diagnosis and/or treatment

• if a course of treatment is not successful

• if you question your doctor's competence

• if your insurance company requires it

Most doctors will be supportive if you request a second opinion and many will recommend it. In many cases, insurance companies will pay for second opinions, but check ahead of time to make sure your insurance plan does cover them. In an HMO you may have to be more assertive because one way HMOs control costs is by limiting second opinions. Often, the opinion of a second doctor will confirm the opinion of the first, but the reassurance may be worth the time and extra cost. On the other hand, if the second opinion differs from the first, you have two alternatives: seek the opinion of a third doctor, or educate yourself as much as possible by talking to both doctors, reading up on the problem, and trusting your instincts about which diagnosis is correct.

Using This Guide To Find Top Specialists

Office And Practice Arrangements

Although clearly not as important as training or reputation, a specialist's office and practice arrangements often are of significance to patients. Practice arrangements include office hours, office location, billing procedures and accessibility among the many factors that result in how well the office is run.

Some specialists only will see new patients who are referred to them by another doctor. Therefore, you may need to have your treating physician contact the specialist's office to arrange for your initial visit. Your health plan may also require that your primary care doctor provide a referral.

If English is not your first language, it may be advisable to determine whether someone in the specialist's office speaks your primary language or if a translator can be present during appointments. This will ease communication and assure that all questions, responses and instructions are understood.

Accessibility of the specialist's office may be a concern if you are wheelchair-bound, are elderly or cannot climb stairs or negotiate narrow corridors. Convenient parking may also be important to you.

Other arrangements that may need to be made in advance of your first visit or discussed with the specialist's office staff concern payment. You may wish to ask the following:

- Does the specialist accept your health insurance coverage?

- Is the specialist within your plan's network and will you need to pay a co-payment? Or, is the specialist out-of-network and will you have to pay for your care out-of-pocket, meet a deductible or submit a form for reimbursement?

- Are credit cards an acceptable mode of payment?

- Does the specialist accept Medicare, Medicaid or no-fault insurance? Does the specialist treat workers' compensation cases?

- If you are a non-resident of the United States, will you need to arrange for the transfer or exchange of currency to pay the specialist's fee?

When you are choosing a top specialist, these issues may be of lesser or greater importance, depending on the problem and type of care warranted. If you are traveling a great distance to have a specific procedure performed by a top specialist at a major medical center, continuing long-term monitoring or follow-up care by that physician may not be required or may not be feasible and such things as office practice arrangements are of less importance. On the other hand, if you have a chronic problem that needs to be monitored with follow-up care provided by the same top specialist, then such issues as accessibility of the doctor's office, appointment hours, waiting times and courtesy and professionalism of the staff become more significant.

Personal Chemistry

One element of the doctor-patient relationship that we stress in our guides is chemistry between doctor and patient, a part of which is often referred to as a doctor's "bedside manner." While this factor is of major import in a long-term relationship such as one you would have with your primary care physician, it is of less importance when you see a specialist only once or twice. However, since many people using this book may have chronic conditions that require ongoing care, it is important to give the matter some consideration.

It is vital that there is a sense of mutual trust and respect between patient and doctor; a judgment that individuals must make for themselves. Among the many talented doctors listed in this guide, there are very likely some to whom you would relate well and others with whom you may not feel as comfortable.

Patients prefer doctors who listen, demonstrate concern, are responsive to patient needs and spend sufficient time with them. The qualities of physicians in this regard, even the excellent ones in this guide, vary immensely.

You, the patient, are the only one who can assess these qualities because individuals react differently to various personalities. It is important for you to carefully judge your feelings towards a physician, especially if you are embarking on a long-term relationship. You should feel you can be open, trusting and responsive to your physician and that your relationship will be a positive one. Otherwise, find another doctor, since not doing so could adversely affect your care.

Once you have used this guide to identify the top specialist(s) best suited to treat your condition, there is much you can do to maximize the value of your first visit.

Maximizing Your First Appointment With A Top Doctor

After your research is done and you've secured an appointment for an initial consultation with a top doctor known for his/her expertise in the diagnosis or treatment of your particular medical condition, what should you do?

Whether your visit to the specialist's office is a car ride or a plane trip away, there undoubtedly will be arrangements to make before your appointment. You may have to take time off from work, arrange for childcare while you are away and make travel plans and hotel reservations, but there are a number of other important steps to take to assure that you and the specialist make the best use of the time you spend together.

Have you done everything you can to prepare yourself and the specialist for the consultation? The following checklist will help you maximize the value of your visit to the specialist and will go a long way toward focusing you on the task at hand—getting the best advice or treatment for your health problem from one of the top doctors in the medical specialty related to your condition.

Gathering The Facts
- Does the specialist have all the information needed to make a diagnosis of or treatment plan for your condition?

- Have your medical records, test results and X-rays been sent ahead of time to allow for their review by the specialist in advance of your first appointment?

- Have you written out your medical history, including that of your siblings, parents and grandparents, emphasizing the particular problem for which you are visiting this specialist?

- Are you prepared with a written list of questions?

- Do you understand the answers?

A specialist becoming newly involved in your care needs to learn as much as possible about the state of your health in a very limited time. Since top doctors are extremely busy people with many demands on their time, you should make certain that all relevant records and case summaries are obtained and sent to the specialist well in advance of your appointment.

Obtaining Your Records

All healthcare providers, including hospitals, doctors and their staffs, are under legal obligation to maintain the privacy of your medical records. In order to obtain release of those records, you must make a request in writing. If you need to obtain records from a number of providers, you should write one clear and concise letter authorizing release of your records and including your name, address, telephone number, date of birth, identification number and any other identifying information such as a hospital chart number. You then can make photocopies of this letter, but be sure to sign and date each copy as if it were an original. You also may want to specifically name those test results (e.g., pathology slides) or X-ray films (not just written reports or summaries) that must be included in addition to making a general request for your records. It's also a good idea to indicate the date of your appointment so the office staff can respond in a timely manner.

Although state laws require the timely release of medical records, hospital medical records departments and doctors' offices often take several weeks to pull and review patient charts and get them in the mail either to you or to another doctor. In addition to written authorization, you may be asked to pay the costs involved in copying your records, test results and X-ray films because many doctors' offices will not release the originals. Consider placing a call in advance to determine the procedure for releasing your records, how long you can expect it to take and the costs involved so that you can save time by including payment with your release authorization letter. Be sure to allow sufficient time in advance of your consultation appointment for your request to be processed. Since you often must wait several weeks for an appointment with a specialist, allow at least that amount of time to obtain your records.

Even after making your written requests, you should follow up each letter with a telephone call to be sure that your records actually are sent. You should not assume that your request for records will be promptly fulfilled by an often overburdened, although well-intentioned, office staff.

Remember, the more information the specialist has about your condition, the fewer repeat or additional tests or procedures you will need to undergo, the lower the costs of your consultation and, most important, the more expeditiously the specialist will be able to render an opinion.

The Facts And Only The Facts

Be thorough and organized in documenting your personal and familial medical histories, the medications you take and in relaying information about your condition. Even seemingly minor bits of information may provide subtle clues to the nature of your medical problem and the optimal way in which to treat it. It's also advisable to bring a list with you of names, addresses and telephone numbers of all physicians who have cared for you, especially those you have seen regarding your current medical problem.

Even though thoroughness is essential to presenting a clear picture of your medical condition, bear in mind that the specialist needs to get to your core health concerns as quickly as possible. Therefore, if you have a complex medical history, you may want to ask your current doctors to provide treatment summaries in addition to copies of your medical records. Hospital records should include your admission history and physical exam, dictated consultation and operation notes and discharge summaries for all hospitalizations. You may also be able to get a cumulative lab and X-ray summary for your hospital stays.

Unlike X-rays, which can be copied at reasonable cost, original pathology slides must be transported by mail or hand-carried. Your specialist may wish to have the pathologist with whom he/she works speak directly with the pathologist who initially interpreted your slides as part of the process of evaluating your case.

Being Prepared

You are likely to be a bit nervous when you meet with the specialist you have chosen. Anxiety about your health and concern about your future care may cause you to forget information you should provide or miss hearing or understanding important information that the specialist communicates. Therefore, you may want to write down all relevant information so that you do not leave out anything of importance when you meet with the specialist or complete forms in the office. You also may want to write out your questions in advance so you don't forget anything.

To avoid leaving out important details of your condition or past treatment, prepare a concise, chronological summary before your consultation takes place. You may wish to type it and provide a copy to the specialist for inclusion in your chart. Highlight major medical results or significant events in the course of an illness or treatment if these will enlighten the doctor about your condition. Your personal perspective on the state of your health is vital to a full understanding of your medical problem.

It is possible that the specialist will use language that you do not understand or may speak quickly assuming certain knowledge on your part about your condition or its treatment. Don't hesitate to ask for clarification as often or repeatedly as you may need to in order to fully comprehend what you are being told. If you are concerned that you may forget what the doctor tells you, ask the doctor's permission to take notes or ask if you might bring along a tape recorder so you can later replay what was said, especially any instructions you are given. You may prefer to bring along a relative or close friend to serve as a "second set of ears," but, again, seek the doctor's permission to do so in advance of your appointment.

Following this process will assure that you and the specialist you are consulting get the most from your appointment. After all, you both have the same goal: restoring you to optimal health and well being.

What To Do If You Can't Get An Appointment

At times it may be difficult, perhaps even impossible, to secure an appointment with the specific specialist you have identified. There are a number of reasons why this may occur. For example, the specialist may not be taking any new patients or may have such a busy schedule that it takes several weeks or months to get an appointment. He/she may only see patients during very limited hours because of teaching, research or other responsibilities or currently may have other limitations related to the acceptance of new patients.

However, bear in mind that the doctors in this guide are the leaders in their specialties and therefore they work with and train the very best and brightest in their specialties. So, if you are unable to consult with a particular doctor, consider making an appointment with one of his/her outstanding colleagues. You can do this by asking a member of the doctor's office staff to refer you to an associate who is a member of the practice group or to another excellent physician who is specially trained to address your particular medical issue.

You can be comfortable knowing that you will receive high quality care from another specialist who practices in the same top setting.

Utilizing Special Resources

The following information on special resources has been included to meet the needs of healthcare consumers who have extraordinarily difficult or unique health problems, and have been unable to identify the resources to address their problems. These patients and their doctors may need to search for very new, cutting-edge, perhaps even experimental and not yet approved therapies. In such cases the search may lead to clinical trials; tests of new drugs and new medical devices or innovative therapeutic approaches. Fortunately, these situations are rare, but when they do occur, they are critical.

In addition to the outstanding private and public hospitals recognized in this guide, the U.S. government maintains its own unique, expert source of patient care and clinical research at the National Institutes of Health (NIH). In fact, the NIH operates its own hospital at which the care provided is usually related to clinical studies its researchers are undertaking.

In addition to those at the NIH, clinical trials also are conducted at leading medical centers and other organizations throughout the country. These facilities may be testing a new drug therapy, a new use for an existing medication or a medical device to deal with a problem that is not being resolved through the use of more traditional approaches.

This section will guide you in utilizing these special resources.

The Clinical Trial As A Treatment Option

For some patients the best medical treatment may only be available through clinical trials (also called treatment studies), which are designed to develop improved ways to use current medical treatments or to find new medical treatments by studying their effects on humans. Treatments are studied to determine if they are safe, effective and better treatments than conventional or standard therapies. Only if they meet all three of these criteria are they made available to the general public.

Many people are frightened by the term "clinical trial" because it conveys the notion of being a "guinea pig" in an experiment. Contrary to popular belief, however, most new treatments are extensively studied by scientists in the laboratory before they are ever tested by physicians in clinical settings. Among the factors that keep patients from participating in clinical trials are: lack of awareness about clinical trials as a treatment option; fear of side effects or adverse reactions to treatment; refusal of insurance companies to pay for experimental treatments; failure of a physician to inform the patient about clinical trials; difficulty finding suitable clinical trials; unavailability of clinical trials for certain medical problems; distance of the patient from major medical centers conducting clinical trials; disruption of personal and family life; and the decision to stop medical treatment altogether.

Despite these and other obstacles, many people do seek out clinical trials. One of the most pressing reasons to participate is the opportunity to obtain treatment that might not be available otherwise. New medical treatments can offer participants hope for a cure, an extended lifespan, or an improvement in how they feel. Some participants also take comfort in knowing that others may benefit from their contribution to medical knowledge.

Deciding if a clinical trial is the right treatment option for you is no simple matter. Certainly, you will want to talk about it with your doctor(s) and other professionals involved in your care, as well as with family members and friends. But in order to fully benefit from what others have to say — based on either their professional knowledge or personal experience — you need to understand exactly what a clinical trial is and what your role as a volunteer will be.

Understanding Clinical Trials

Clinical trials are conducted for just about every medical condition, including life-threatening diseases such as AIDS or cancer; chronic illnesses such as diabetes and asthma; psychiatric disorders such as depression or anxiety; behavioral problems such as smoking and substance abuse; and even common ailments such as hair loss and acne. Chances are, there is at least one trial (and probably more) that may be appropriate for you.

With more than 100 different types of cancer, it is understandable that a large number of clinical trials are cancer-related. Extensive information about clinical trials for cancer can be found on www.cancer.gov, the Web site of the National Cancer Institute (NCI). NCI is part of the NIH. CenterWatch, an online clinical trials listing service, identifies over 14,000 clinical trials that are actively recruiting patients. Veritas Medicine, another useful online organization, allows individuals to perform personalized searches of its clinical trials database. See Appendix D for "Selected Resources" for more information on clinical trials.

Most clinical trials study new medical treatments, combinations of treatments, or improvements in conventional treatments using drugs, surgery and other medical procedures, medical devices, radiation or other therapies. Newer types of clinical trials, called screening or prevention trials, study how to prevent the incidence or recurrence of disease through the use of medicines, vitamins, minerals or other supplements; and how to screen for disease, especially in its early stages. Another type of trial studies how to improve the quality of life for patients, including both their physical and emotional well-being.

Clinical trials are sponsored both by the federal government (through the National Institutes of Health, the National Cancer Institute and many others) and by private industry through pharmaceutical and biotechnology companies, and through healthcare institutions (hospitals or health maintenance organizations) and community-based physician-investigators. The National Cancer Institute sponsors clinical trials at more than 1000 sites in the United States. Trials are carried out in major medical research centers such as teaching hospitals as well as in community hospitals, specialized medical clinics (for example, those for the treatment of AIDS or Alzheimer's disease) and in doctors' offices.

Though clinical trials often involve hospitalized patients, a fair number of trials are conducted on an outpatient basis. Many trials are part of a cooperative network which may include as few as one or two sites or hundreds of locations, although one center generally assumes responsibility for overall coordination of the research. More than 45 research-oriented institutions, recognized for their scientific excellence, have been designated by the NCI as comprehensive or clinical cancer centers. See Appendix D "Selected Resources" to find out how to locate these centers.

Clinical research is based on a protocol (established rules or procedures) describing who will be studied, how and when medications, procedures and/or treatments will be administered and how long the study will last. Trials that are conducted simultaneously at different sites use the same protocol to ensure that all patients are treated identically and all data are collected uniformly so that study findings can be compared.

Clinical trials generally are conducted in three phases, as outlined in the study protocol. The first phase begins testing of the treatment on a small group of human subjects after rigorous and successful animal testing has been concluded. The interim phase varies, but usually involves a broader test group and is designed to further evaluate the treatment's safety and more accurately determine appropriate dosage, application methods and side effects. In some trials there may be a fourth phase, conducted after the treatment is in widespread use, to monitor the results of long-term use and the occurrence of any serious side effects.

Some clinical trials test one treatment on one group of subjects, while others compare two or more groups of subjects. In such comparison studies participants are divided into two groups: the control group that receives the standard treatment and the experimental or treatment group which receives the new treatment. For example, the control group may undergo a surgical procedure while the experimental or treatment group undergoes a surgical procedure plus radiation to determine which treatment modality is more effective. To ensure that patient characteristics do not unduly influence the study findings, patients may be randomly assigned to either the control or the experimental group, meaning that each patient's assignment is based purely on chance. In cases in which a standard treatment does not exist for a particular disease, the experimental group of patients receives the new treatment and the control group receives no treatment at all, or receives a placebo, an inactive medicine or procedure that has no treatment value and is sometimes called a "dummy" pill or a "sugar" pill. It is important to keep in mind that patients are never put into a control group without any treatment if there is a known treatment that could help them. Also, whether a patient is receiving an investigational drug or a placebo, he/she receives the same level and quality of medical care as those receiving the investigational treatment.

Questions to ask your doctor and the trial's research team if you are considering participating in a clinical trial:

- Who is sponsoring the trial?

- How many patients will be involved?

- Will the trial be testing a single treatment or a combination of treatments?

- Will there be one treatment group or more than one treatment group?

- If more than one treatment group, how are patients assigned to each group?

- Has this treatment been studied in previous clinical trials? What were the findings?

Protecting the Rights of Participants

The safety of those who participate in clinical trials is a serious matter and is the number one priority of medical investigators. All clinical research, regardless of type of sponsorship, is guided by the same ethical and legal codes that govern the medical profession and the practice of medicine. Most clinical research is federally funded or federally regulated (at least in part) with built-in safeguards for patients. According to federal government regulations (and some state laws), every clinical trial in the United States must be approved and monitored by an Institutional Review Board (IRB), which is an independent committee of physicians, statisticians, community advocates and others (representing at least five distinct disciplines) to ensure that the protocol is being followed.

Government regulations require researchers to fully inform participants about all aspects of a clinical trial before they agree to participate through a process called informed consent. To be sure that you understand your role in a clinical trial, you should jot down any questions beforehand so as not to forget them. You should also consider bringing along a friend or family member for support and additional input, and perhaps even tape recording the conversation (after asking permission to do so) to make sure you do not forget or misunderstand anything. Each participant in a clinical trial must be given a written consent form, which should be available in English and other languages. The consent form explains the following:

- Why the research is being done.

- What the researchers hope to accomplish.

- What types of treatment interventions (and other tests or procedures) will be performed.

- How long the study will continue.

- What the expected benefits and the possible risks are.

- What other treatments are available.

- What costs will be covered by the study, by the patient or by third-party payers such as Medicare, Medicaid or private insurance.

Patients also are informed that they may leave the trial, or exclude themselves from any part of it, at any time. Informed consent means exactly what the term implies: you agree to join a clinical trial only after you completely understand exactly what your participation will involve for the duration of the study. By law, each patient must be provided with a copy of the signed consent form, which also must include the name and telephone number of a contact person for questions or additional information. Informed consent is a continuous process, so do not hesitate to ask questions before, during or after the trial.

The investigators must protect the privacy of each participant in a clinical trial by ensuring that all medical records are kept confidential except for inspection by the sponsoring agency, the Food and Drug Administration and other agencies involved in regulating the drug or treatment, and all data are collected anonymously by assigning a numeric code or initials to each individual.

During the course of the trial, participants are regularly seen by members of the research team to monitor their health and well-being. Participants also should be responsible for their own health by following the treatment plan (such as taking the proper dosage of medications on time), keeping all scheduled visits and informing members of the healthcare team about any symptoms that occur. If during the course of the trial, the treatment proves to be ineffective or harmful, the patient is free to leave the study and still obtain conventional care. Conversely, as soon as there is evidence that one treatment modality is better than another, all patients in the trial are given the benefit of the new information.

Questions to ask the sponsors about your rights as a participant in a clinical trial:

- Who is responsible for approving and monitoring this research? Is there an IRB?

- Who informs me about the trial process? Do I sign a consent form? Will I receive a copy?

- May I leave the trial at any time? Have previous patients dropped out? Why?

- Whom do I contact if I am experiencing any difficulty with this trial?

Enrolling In Clinical Trials

Each clinical trial has its own guidelines, called eligibility criteria, for determining who can participate. Treatment studies recruit participants who have a disease or other medical condition, while screening and prevention studies generally recruit healthy volunteers. Inclusion criteria (those that allow you to participate in a study) and exclusion criteria (those that keep you from participating in a study) ensure that the study will answer the research questions posed in the research protocol while maintaining the safety of participants. The disease being studied is a primary factor in selecting suitable patients, but other factors such as the patient's gender, age, treatment history and other diagnosed medical conditions may also be important. Unfortunately, eligibility also may depend upon ability to pay. Many health plans do not cover all of the costs associated with clinical trials because they define these trials as experimental procedures. However, trials sometimes pay volunteers for their time and/or reimburse them for travel, childcare, meals and lodging.

To prevent people who qualify from being excluded from clinical trials for financial reasons, agencies such as the National Cancer Institute are working with health plans to find solutions and a growing number of states require insurance companies to pay for all routine patient care costs in cancer trials. To encourage more senior citizens to participate in cancer trials, Medicare plans to revise its payment policy to cover those trials.

When choosing a clinical trial you should determine the factors that are most important to you. For instance, patients generally prefer to participate in trials near their homes so that they can maintain their usual day-to-day activities, be surrounded by family and friends and avoid travel and lodging costs. If travel or temporary location becomes necessary, try to find a trial site that is near to some family member or friend or one that is in a locale similar to your own city or town. Many organizations, such as the National Cancer Institute, will work with patients and their families to identify support networks for them wherever they participate.

Questions to ask the trial's sponsor about eligibility criteria:

- What are the inclusion and exclusion criteria for the clinical trial(s) I am considering?

- How can I improve my chances of being accepted?
  Can I change my health plan to one that will cover the trial's costs?
  Can I relocate to another city or state?

- If I am not eligible for one trial, what other trials are being conducted for my condition?

- Will I be paid for my time or reimbursed for my out-of-pocket expenses?

Participating In A Clinical Trial

Clinical trials are conducted by a research team led by a principal investigator (usually a physician) and are comprised of physicians, nurses and other health professionals such as social workers, psychologists and nutritionists. As a participant you may be required to commit a fair amount of time to a clinical trial, often more than with standard treatment. Initially, you will probably be given a physical examination and asked for your medical history. During the trial, you will have regular or periodic visits to the trial site which may include diagnostic and laboratory tests. You also may be asked to follow fixed schedules for medications and other interventions and to keep detailed records of your symptoms and health condition. Generally, clinical trials last from six to twenty-six weeks, though some (called maintenance trials) can last up to a year to determine if a treatment will prevent the relapse of a medical condition.

Participants in clinical trials should remain under the care of their regular physician(s) since clinical trials tend to provide short-term treatment for a specific medical condition and do not generally provide comprehensive primary care. In fact, some trials require that a patient's regular physician sign a consent form before the patient is enrolled. In addition, your regular physician can collaborate with the research team to make sure there are no adverse reactions between your other medications or treatments and the investigational treatment.

Questions to ask the research team or your physician about your role in a clinical trial:

- Who are the members of the health team?
  Who will be in charge of my care?

- How long will the trial last?

- How does treatment in the trial compare with or differ from the standard treatment?

- Will I be hospitalized? How often? For how long a period of time?

- What will occur during each visit?
  What treatments or procedures will I be given?

- Will I still be able to see my regular physician(s)?
  Will my doctor and the research team collaborate?

- Can I be put in touch with other patients who have participated in this trial?

Weighing The Benefits And Risks Of A Clinical Trial

If you are considering participation in a clinical trial, you need to consider the medical, emotional and financial ramifications of participation. Of course, the obvious benefit of a clinical trial is the chance that a new treatment may improve your health and prognosis. You will have access to drugs and other medical interventions before they are widely available to the public and you will obtain expert and specialized medical care at leading healthcare facilities. Many patients receive an added psychological benefit by taking an active role in their treatment.

It is important to bear in mind that some medical interventions used in clinical trials may carry potential risks depending upon the type of treatment and the patient's condition. While many side effects or adverse reactions are temporary (such as hair loss and nausea caused by some anti-cancer drugs), other more serious reactions can be permanent and even life-threatening (for example, heart, liver or kidney damage).

Deciding whether or not to participate in a clinical trial is often a matter of determining if the trial's potential benefits outweigh its possible risks. This is a highly personal decision that may be difficult to make in situations involving experimental treatment in which limited medical information may be available.

Questions to ask the research team about the benefits and risks of a clinical trial:

- What other treatment option(s) do I have at this time?
  Is there any chance that a more promising treatment may be available soon?

- What are the short and long-term benefits and risks as compared with standard treatment?

- Will I experience any known side effects or adverse reactions?
  Will these be temporary, long-term or permanent?
  Relatively minor or perhaps life-threatening?

- If I am harmed in any way by the new treatment, what other treatments will I be entitled to?
  Who will pay for subsequent treatment?

Getting Information On Clinical Trials

The more information you have about a clinical trial, the easier it will be to make a decision about whether or not it is right for you, and the more confident you will be that you made an appropriate decision. In addition to the "Selected Resources" appendix in this guide, the staff at your local public library, community hospital, or major medical center can assist you in locating the information you need from books, consumer organizations and on the Internet.

Learning About The National Institutes Of Health(NIH)

The National Institutes of Health (NIH) comprise one of the world's leading medical research centers and the Federal government's principal agency for biomedical research. An agency of the United States Department of Health, United States Public Health Service, NIH encompasses 25 separate institutions and centers with its main campus located in Bethesda, Maryland. Research is also conducted at several field units across the country and abroad.

Patient Care At The NIH

The Warren Grant Magnuson Clinical Center, NIH's principal medical research center and hospital located in Bethesda, Maryland, provides medical care only to patients participating in clinical research programs. Two categories of patients participate in the Clinical Center studies: children and adults who wish to improve their own health, such as those with newly diagnosed medical problems, ongoing medical problems or family history of disease; and healthy volunteers wishing to advance knowledge about the causes, progress and treatment of disease. The patient's case must fit into an ongoing NIH research project for which the patient has the precise kind or stage of illness under investigation. General diagnostic and treatment services common to community hospitals are not available.

The Magnuson Clinical Center is the world's largest biomedical research hospital and ambulatory care facility, housing 1,600 laboratories conducting basic and clinical research. There are 1,200 tenured physicians, dentists and researchers on staff along with 660 nurses and 570 allied healthcare professionals (dieticians, imaging technologists, medical technologists, medical records and clerical staff, pharmacists and therapists).

The Center's hospital is specially designed for medical research and accommodates 540 carefully selected patients who are participating in clinical research programs. Its 350-bed facility has 24 inpatient care units to which 7,000 patients are admitted annually. The Center also has an Ambulatory Care Research Facility (ACRF) that serves 68,000 outpatient visits each year. A new facility, called the Mark O. Hatfield Clinical Research Center, which began accepting patients in early 2005, has 242 beds for inpatient care and 90 day-hospital stations for outpatient care. The Mark O. Hatfield Center carries out the latest biomedical research that results in new forms of disease diagnosis, prevention and treatment, which is then incorporated into improved methods of patient care.

This is a fine example of Translational Medicine where excellent research discoveries are translated into new and improved methods of clinical treatment. In other words, the laboratory discoveries are brought to the bedside.

The Clinical Center also maintains a Children's Inn for pediatric outpatients and their families. This family-centered residence operates 24 hours a day, 7 days a week, 365 days a year.

In an effort to bring clinical research to the community, NIH supports approximately 80 General Clinical Research Centers (GCRCs) around the country, located within hospitals of major academic medical centers.

It is important to note that, as part of the federal government, the Warren Grant Magnuson Clinical Center provides treatment in clinical trials at no cost to its patients. In some cases, patients receive a stipend to help cover the costs of traveling to Bethesda for treatment and follow-up care. Travel costs for the initial screening visit, however, are not covered.

Areas Of Clinical Study At The NIH

At the Magnuson Clinical Center alone, NIH physician-scientists conduct nearly 1,000 studies each year. Among the areas of study are cancer and related diseases.

Not all of these clinical areas are under investigation at any given time, however. The Patient Recruitment and Public Liaison Office (PRPL) at the NIH Clinical Center assists patients, their families and their physicians in obtaining information about participation in NIH clinical trials. Trained nurses are available to answer questions about the research programs and admission procedures.

Cancer Care At The Warren Grant Magnuson Clinical Center

The National Cancer Institute (NCI) is the largest of the biomedical research institutes and centers at NIH. There, clinical studies are designed to evaluate new and promising ways to prevent, detect, diagnose and treat cancer. The Warren Grant Magnuson Clinical Center provides a separate outpatient division for cancer patients and also has several designated inpatient units.

If you are interested in entering a cancer study at the Magnuson Clinical Center (or at the General Clinical Research Centers), you should first discuss treatment options with a physician. As a general rule, patients interested in participating in clinical studies must be referred by a physician. However, in some instances, self-referral may be permitted.

Patients with medical problems other than cancer or healthy volunteers who wish to participate in a clinical study should contact the particular NIH institute responsible for the clinical area involved.

Cancer Care At The NCI Clinical Centers And Comprehensive Cancer Centers

You may also obtain clinical oncology services (education, screening, diagnosis or treatment) or participate in clinical trials at one of the 22 Cancer Centers or 39 Comprehensive Cancer Centers designated by the NCI for their scientific excellence and extensive resources devoted to cancer and cancer-related problems. Centers are located in 32 states, with the majority of sites in California, New York and Pennsylvania. You can find out about clinical trials at the NCI-designated centers by contacting NCI's Clinical Studies Support Center (CSSC) or by calling each center directly. Information about other cancer-related services at these centers also may be obtained from the center itself. For more information, you can visit the National Cancer Institute's website at www.cancer.gov.

How To Use This Guide

Locating A Specialist

This guide is organized to make finding the right specialists for you or your loved ones as simple as possible. Physicians' biographies are presented by specialty and are organized by geographic region within each specialty or subspecialty. Thus, you may search for a particular type of specialist or subspecialist in one or more regions or throughout the nation.

A second way to locate the right specialist is to use the **"Special Expertise Index"** beginning on page 1163. This index is organized according to diseases, conditions and procedures or techniques. For example, you can locate a top specialist for diabetes or for Mohs' surgery by looking for those terms in the **"Special Expertise Index."**

If you already know a specialist's name, you can find his/her listing by using the **"Alphabetical Listing of Doctors"** beginning on page 1249.

SAMPLE PHYSICIAN LISTING

Smith, John MD [Ped] - **Spec Exp:** Asthma Allergy; **Hospital:** Children's Hosp (page 120);
      Name [Specialty]   Special Expertise(s)   Admitting Hospital & Hospital
                                                     Information Page

Address: 300 Ridge Road Boston, MA 12345; **Phone:** (617) 555-2343; **Board Cert:** Ped 75;
           Office Address   Office Phone   Board Certification(s)

Med School: Harvard Med Sch 70; **Resid:** Ped, Children's Hosp 73;
           Medical School   Residency(ies)

Fellow: AM, Children's Hosp 74; **Fac Appt:** Assoc Prof Ped, The Med Sch
           Fellowship(s)   Faculty Appointment

How To Use This Guide

Geographic Regions And States

To assist you in using Castle Connolly *America's Top Doctors*® in the most efficient and effective manner, the Guide is divided into seven geographic regions. This will help you to locate a specialist in your local or neighboring region. For example, if you live in Mississippi in the Southeast region and you are willing and able to travel to Louisiana in the Southwest region to consult with a specialist in neurology, you can review just those two regions, under the section headed "NEUROLOGY." However, if you prefer to review the information on neurologists throughout the country, you can search the entire neurology section. Or, you can consult the "SPECIAL EXPERTISE INDEX" in the back of this Guide and choose a neurologist who has specific expertise to meet your particular needs.

The geographic regions are as follows:

New England

Mid Atlantic

Southeast

Midwest

Great Plains and Mountains

Southwest

West Coast and Pacific

The states that are included in each region are listed on the following page and a map of the regions is also provided. Please note that not all regions are represented in all specialties. For example, in "Geriatric Psychiatry" there are no listings in the Southwest region.

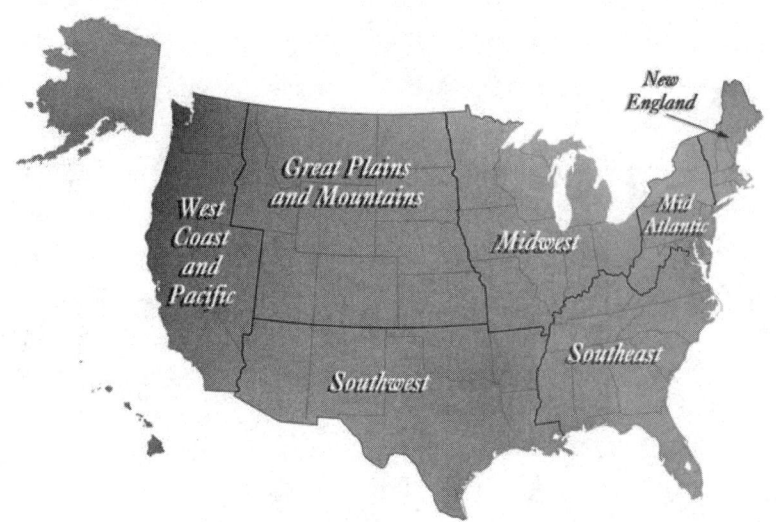

West Coast and Pacific:
Alaska
California
Hawaii
Nevada
Oregon
Washington

Great Plains and Mountains:
Colorado
Idaho
Kansas
Montana
Nebraska
North Dakota
South Dakota
Utah
Wyoming

Southwest:
Arizona
Arkansas
Louisiana
New Mexico
Oklahoma
Texas

Midwest:
Illinois
Indiana
Iowa
Michigan
Minnesota
Missouri
Ohio
Wisconsin

New England:
Connecticut
Maine
Massachusetts
New Hampshire
Rhode Island
Vermont

Mid Atlantic:
Delaware
Maryland
New Jersey
New York
Pennsylvania
Washington, DC
West Virginia

Southeast:
Alabama
Florida
Georgia
Kentucky
Mississippi
North Carolina
South Carolina
Tennessee
Virginia

Medical Specialties

In the pages that follow, each list of doctors in a medical specialty or subspecialty is preceded by a brief description of that specialty (or subspecialty) and the training required for board certification.

Critical Care Medicine has been excluded because in emergency situations there is neither time nor opportunity for choice. A number of other specialities not relevant to most patients (e.g., Forensic Psychiatry) have not been included as well.

The following descriptions of medical specialties and subspecialties were provided by the American Board of Medical Specialties (ABMS), an organization comprised of the 24 medical specialty boards that provide certification in 25 medical specialties. A complete listing of all specialists certified by the ABMS can be found in *The Official ABMS Directory of Board Certified Medical Specialists*, and is published by *Marquis Who's Who*. It is available (either in a multi-volume directory or on CD-ROM) in most public libraries, hospital libraries, university libraries and medical libraries. The ABMS also operates a toll-free phone line at 1-866-275-2267 and a website at www.abms.org to verify the certification status of individual doctors.

The following important policy statement, approved by the ABMS Assembly on March 19, 1987, remains valid.

The Purpose Of Certification

The intent of the certification process, as defined by the member boards of the American Board of Medical Specialties, is to provide assurance to the public that a certified medical specialist has successfully completed an approved educational program and an evaluation, including an examination process designed to assess the knowledge, experience and skills requisite to the provision of high quality patient care in that specialty.

Medical Specialties

Medical Specialty and Subspecialty Descriptions and Abbreviations

The following medical specialties and subspecialties are indicated in the doctors' listings by their abbreviations. Specialties are indicated in bold, subspecialties in italics, and the four primary care specialties in bold capitals. To review the official American Board of Medical Specialties (ABMS) organization of specialties, refer to Appendix A.

Addiction Psychiatry   *AdP*

Deals with habitual psychological and physiological dependence on a substance or practice which is beyond voluntary control.

Adolescent Medicine   *AM*

Involves the primary care treatment of adolescents and young adults.

Allergy & Immunology   **A&I**

Diagnosis and treatment of allergies, asthma, and skin problems such as hives and contact dermatitis.

Anesthesiology   **Anes**

Provides pain relief in maintenance or restoration of a stable condition during and following an operation. Anesthesiologists also diagnose and treat acute and long standing pain problems.

Cardiac Electrophysiology (Clinical)   *CE*

Involves complicated technical procedures to evaluate heart rhythms and determine appropriate treatment for them.

Cardiovascular Disease   *Cv*

Involves the diagnosis and treatment of disorders of the heart, lungs, and blood vessels.

Child & Adolescent Psychiatry   *ChAP*

Deals with the diagnosis and treatment of mental diseases in children and adolescents.

Child Neurology   *ChiN*

Diagnosis and medical treatment of disorders of the brain, spinal cord, and nervous system in children.

Clinical Genetics   **CG**

Deals with identifying the genetic causes of inherited diseases and ailments and preventing, when possible, their occurrence.

Colon and Rectal Surgery   **CRS**

Surgical treatment of diseases of the intestinal tract, colon and rectum, anal canal, and perianal area.

Critical Care Medicine   *CCM*

Involves diagnosing and taking immediate action to prevent death or further injury of a patient. Examples of critical injuries include shock, heart attack, drug overdose, and massive bleeding.

Dermatology
Diagnosis and treatment of benign and malignant disorders of the skin, mouth, external genitalia, hair and nails, as well as a number of sexually transmitted diseases.

D

Diagnostic Radiology
Involves the study of all modalities of radiant energy in medical diagnoses and therapeutic procedures utilizing radiologic guidance.

DR

Endocrinology, Diabetes & Metabolism
Involves the study and treatment of patients suffering from hormonal and chemical disorders.

EDM

FAMILY MEDICINE
Deals with and oversees the total healthcare of individual patients and their family members. Family practitioners are more common in rural areas and may perform procedures more commonly performed by specialists (e.g., minor surgery).

FP

Forensic Psychiatry
Concerns the evaluation of certain diagnostic groups of patients that include those with sexual disorders, antisocial personality disorders, paranoid disorders, and addictive disorders.

FPsy

Gastroenterology
The study, diagnosis and treatment of diseases of the digestive organs including the stomach, bowels, liver, and gallbladder.

Ge

Geriatric Medicine
Deals with diseases of the elderly and the problems associated with aging.

Ger

Geriatric Psychiatry
Involves the diagnosis, prevention, and treatment of mental illness in the elderly.

GerPsy

Gynecologic Oncology
Deals with cancers of the female genital tract and reproductive systems.

GO

Hand Surgery
Involves the treatment of injury to the hand through surgical techniques.

HS

Hematology
Involves the diagnosis and treatment of diseases and disorders of the blood, bone marrow, spleen, and lymph glands.

Hem

Infectious Disease
The study and treatment of diseases caused by a bacterium, virus, fungus, or animal parasite.

Inf

INTERNAL MEDICINE
Diagnosis and nonsurgical treatment of diseases, especially those of adults. Internists may act as primary care specialists, highly trained family doctors, or they may subspecialize in specialties such as cardiology or nephrology.

IM

Maternal & Fetal Medicine
Involves the care of women with high-risk pregnancies and their unborn fetuses.

MF

Medical Specialties

Medical Oncology   *Onc*
Refers to the study and treatment of tumors and other cancers.

Neonatal-Perinatal Medicine   *NP*
Involves the diagnosis and treatments of infants prior to, during, and one month beyond birth.

Nephrology   *Nep*
Concerned with disorders of the kidneys, high blood pressure, fluid and mineral balance, dialysis of body wastes when the kidneys do not function, and consultation with surgeons about kidney transplantation.

Neurological Surgery   **NS**
Involves surgery of the brain, spinal cord, and nervous system.

Neurology   **N**
Diagnosis and medical treatment of disorders of the brain, spinal cord, and nervous system.

Neuroradiology   *NRad*
Involves the utilization of imaging procedures during diagnosis as they relate to the brain, spine and spinal cord, head, neck, and organs of special sense in adults and children.

Nuclear Medicine   **NuM**
Evaluation of the functions of all the organs in the body and treatment of thyroid disease, benign and malignant tumors, and radiation exposure through the use of radioactive substances.

Nuclear Radiology   *NR*
Involves the use of radioactive substances to diagnose and treat certain functions and diseases of the body.

OBSTETRICS & GYNECOLOGY   **ObG**
Deals with the medical aspects of and intervention in pregnancy and labor and the overall health of the female reproductive system.

Occupational Medicine   *OM*
Concentrates on the effect of the work environment on the health of employees.

Ophthalmology   **Oph**
Diagnosis and treatment of diseases of and injuries to the eye.

Orthopaedic Surgery   **OrS**
Involves operations to correct injuries which interfere with the form and function of the extremities, spine, and associated structures.

Otolaryngology   **Oto**
Explores and treats diseases in the interrelated areas of the ears, nose and throat.

Otology/Neurotology   *ON*
Concentrates on the management, prevention, cure and care of patients with diseases of the ear and temporal bone, including disorders of hearing and balance.

Pain Medicine   PM

Involves providing a high level of care for patients experiencing problems with acute or chronic pain in both hospital and ambulatory settings.

Pediatric Cardiology   PCd

Involves the diagnosis and treatment of heart disease in children.

Pediatric Critical Care Medicine   PCCM

Involves the care of children who are victims of life threatening disorders such as severe accidents, shock, and diabetes acidosis.

Pediatric Dermatology   PD

Diagnosis and treatment of benign and malignant disorders of the skin, mouth, external genitalia, hair and nails in children.

Pediatric Endocrinology   PEn

Involves the study and treatment of children with hormonal and chemical disorders.

Pediatric Gastroenterology   PGe

The study, diagnosis, and treatment of diseases of the digestive tract in children.

Pediatric Hematology-Oncology   PHO

The study and treatment of cancers of the blood and blood-forming parts of the body in children.

Pediatric Infectious Disease   PInf

The study and treatment of diseases caused by a virus, bacterium, fungus, or animal parasite in children.

Pediatric Nephrology   PNep

Deals with the diagnosis and treatment of disorders of the kidneys in children.

Pediatric Otolaryngology   POto

Involves the diagnosis and treatment of disorders of the ear, nose, and throat which affect children.

Pediatric Pulmonology   PPul

Involves the diagnosis and treatment of diseases of the chest, lungs, and chest tissue in children.

Pediatric Radiology   PR

Involves diagnostic imaging as it pertains to the newborn, infant, child, and adolescent.

Pediatric Rheumatology   PRhu

Involves the treatment of diseases of the joints and connective tissues in children.

Pediatric Surgery   PS

Treatment of disease, injury, or deformity in children through surgical techniques.

PEDIATRICS   **Ped**

Diagnosis and treatment of diseases of childhood and monitoring of the growth, development, and well-being of preadolescents.

Medical Specialties

Physical Medicine & Rehabilitation   **PMR**

The use of physical therapy and physical agents such as water, heat, light electricity, and mechanical manipulations in the diagnosis, treatment, and prevention of disease and body disorders.

Plastic Surgery   **PlS**

Involves reconstructive and cosmetic surgery of the face and other body parts.

Preventive Medicine   **PrM**

A specialty focusing on the prevention of illness and on the health of groups rather than individuals.

Psychiatry   **Psyc**

Examination, treatment, and prevention of mental illness through the use of psychoanalysis and/or drugs.

Public Health & General Preventive Medicine   *PHGPM*

Involves the investigation of the causes of epidemic disease and the prevention of a wide variety of acute and chronic illness.

Pulmonary Disease   *Pul*

Involves the diagnosis and treatment of diseases of the chest, lungs, and airways.

Radiation Oncology   *RadRo*

Involves the use of radiant energy and isotopes in the study and treatment of disease, especially malignant cancer.

Reproductive Endocrinology   *RE*

Deals with the endocrine system (including the pituitary, thyroid, parathyroid, adrenal glands, placenta, ovaries, and testes) and how its failure relates to infertility.

Rheumatology   *Rhu*

Involves the treatment of diseases of the joints, muscles, bones and associated structures.

Sleep Medicine   *Sleep Med*

Involves the investigation and treatment of patients with sleep disorders.

Spinal Cord Injury Medicine   *SpCdInj*

Involves the prevention, diagnosis, treatment and management of traumatic spinal cord injuries.

Sports Medicine   *SM*

Refers to the practice of an orthopaedist or other physician who specializes in injuries to the bone or other soft tissues (muscles, tendons, ligaments) caused by participation in athletic activity.

Surgery   **S**

Treatment of disease, injury, and deformity by surgical procedures.

Surgery of the Hand   *SHd*

Involves providing appropriate care for all structures in the upper extremity directly affecting the hand and wrist function.

Surgical Critical Care   *SCC*

Involves specialized care in the management of the critically ill patient, particularly the trauma victim and postoperative patient in the emergency department, intensive care unit, trauma unit, burn unit, and other similar settings.

Thoracic Surgery (includes open heart surgery)   **TS**

Involves surgery on the heart, lungs, and chest area.

Urology   **U**

Diagnosis and treatment of diseases of the genitals in men and disorders of the urinary tract and bladder in both men and women.

Vascular & Interventional Radiology   *VIR*

Involves diagnosing and treating diseases by percutaneous methods guided by various radiologic imaging modalities.

Vascular Surgery   *VascS*

Involves the operative treatment of disorders of the blood vessels excluding those to the heart, lungs, or brain.

The Training Of A Specialist

Excerpted from "Which Medical Specialist For You?" American Board of Medical Specialties, Evanston, IL, Revised 2000

Everyone knows that a "medical doctor" is a physician who has had years of training to understand the diagnosis, treatment and prevention of disease. The basic training for a physician specialist includes four years of premedical education in a college or university, four years of medical school, and after receiving the M.D. degree, at least three years of specialty training under supervision (called a "residency"). Training in subspecialties can take an additional one to three years.

Some specialists are primary care doctors such as family physicians, general internists and general pediatricians. Other specialists concentrate on certain body systems, specific age groups, or complex scientific techniques developed to diagnose or treat certain types of disorders. Specialties in medicine developed because of the rapidly expanding body of knowledge about health and illness and the constantly evolving new treatment techniques for disease.

A subspecialist is a physician who has completed training in a general medical specialty and then takes additional training in a more specific area of that specialty called a subspecialty. This training increases the depth of knowledge and expertise of the specialist in that particular field. For example, cardiology is a subspecialty of internal medicine, pediatric surgery is a subspecialty of surgery and pediatrics, and child and adolescent psychiatry is a subspecialty of psychiatry. The training of a subspecialist within a specialty requires an additional one or more years of full-time education.

The training, or residency, of a specialist begins after the doctor has received the M.D. degree from a medical school. Resident physicians dedicate themselves for three to seven years to full-time experience in hospital and/or ambulatory care settings, caring for patients under the supervision of experienced specialists. Educational conferences and research experience are often part of that training. In years past, the first year of post-medical school training was called an internship, but is now called residency.

The Training Of A Specialist

Licensure

The legal privilege to practice medicine is governed by state law and is not designed to recognize the knowledge and skills of a trained specialist. A physician is licensed to practice general medicine and surgery by a state board of medical examiners after passing a state or national licensure examination. Each state or territory has its own procedures to license physicians and sets the general standards for all physicians in that state or territory.

Who Credentials A Specialist And Subspecialist?

Specialty boards certify physicians as having met certain published standards. There are 24 specialty boards that are recognized by the American Board of Medical Specialties (ABMS) and the American Medical Association (AMA). All of the specialties and subspecialties recognized by the ABMS and the AMA are listed in the brief descriptions that follow. Remember, a subspecialist first must be trained and certified as a specialist.

In order to be certified as a medical specialist by one of these recognized boards a physician must complete certain requirements. Generally, these include:

1 Completion of a course of study leading to the M.D. or D.O. (Doctor of Osteopathy) degree from a recognized school of medicine.

2 Completion of three to seven years of full-time training in an accredited residency program designed to train specialists in the field.

3 Many specialty boards require assessments and documentation of individual performance from the residency training director, or from the chief of service in the hospital where the specialist has practiced.

4 All of the ABMS Member Boards require that a person seeking certification have an unrestricted license to practice medicine in order to take the certification examination.

5 Finally, each candidate for certification must pass a written examination given by the specialty board. Fifteen of the 24 specialty boards also require an oral examination conducted by senior specialists in that field. Candidates who have passed the exams and other requirements are then given the status of "Diplomate" and are certified as specialists. A similar process is followed for specialists who want to become subspecialists.

All of the ABMS Member Boards now, or will soon, issue only time-limited certificates which are valid for six to ten years. In order to retain certification, diplomates must become "recertified," and must periodically go through an additional process involving continuing education in the specialty, review of credentials and further examination. Boards that may not yet require recertification have provided voluntary recertification with similar requirements.

America's Top Doctors® 8th Edition

How To Determine If A Physician Is A Certified Specialist

Certified specialists are listed in *The Official ABMS Directory of Board Certified Medical Specialists* published by *Marquis Who's Who*. The ABMS Directory can be found in most public libraries, hospital libraries, university libraries and medical libraries, and is also available on CD-ROM. Alternatively, you could ask for that information from your county medical society, the American Board of Medical Specialties, or one of the specialty boards.

The ABMS operates a toll free number (1-866-275-2267) to verify the certification status of individual physicians. Additionally, information about the ABMS organization and links to an electronic directory of certified specialists can be accessed through the ABMS Web site at www.abms.org.

Almost all board certified specialists also are members of their medical specialty societies. These societies are dedicated to furthering standards, practice and professional and public education within individual medical specialties. Some, such as the American College of Surgeons and the American College of Obstetricians and Gynecologists, require board certification for full membership. A physician who has attained full membership is called a "Fellow" of the society and is entitled to use this designation in all formal communications such as certificates, publications, business cards, stationery and signage. Thus, "John Doe, M.D., F.A.C.S." (Fellow of the American College of Surgeons) is a board certified surgeon. Similarly, F.A.A.D. (Fellow of the American Academy of Dermatology) following the M.D. or D.O. in a physician's title would likely indicate board certification in that specialty.

The Partnership For Excellence Program

Among the more than 6,000 acute care and specialty hospitals in the United States, many have extraordinary capabilities for superior patient care. These hospitals, renowned for their use of state-of-the-art equipment and up-to-the-minute technology, also attract outstanding physicians and other healthcare professionals. Many of their physicians are among those in the listings in this Guide.

To assist you in your search for top specialists and to supplement the information contained in the physician listings that follow, we invited a select group of these fine institutions to profile their services, special programs and centers of excellence in the *Partnership for Excellence* program. This special section contains pages sponsored by the included hospitals. This paid sponsorship program is totally separate from the physician selection process, which is based upon nominations by physicians a completely independent review by our physician led research team.

The *Partnership for Excellence* program provides an overview of the programs and services offered by the included hospitals with information related to their accreditation and sponsorship. Most also provide their physician referral numbers, should you wish to ask the hospitals for recommendations of doctors not listed in Castle Connolly *America's Top Doctors*® 8th Edition.

In addition to the *Partnership for Excellence* program, profiled hospitals were also invited to highlight their special programs or services that focus on a particular disease or medical condition. These can be found in the "Centers of Excellence" sections that are interspersed throughout this book following the medical specialties and/or subspecialties to which they relate. Sponsored pages in the centers of excellence sections reflect the depth of commitment of these hospitals, which provide the staff, resources and financial support necessary to develop these special programs.

By visiting our website **www.CastleConnolly.com**, you may also link to the websites of these outstanding hospitals for even more detailed information on their cancer programs. We believe you will find this informaton helpful in your search for the best healthcare—from both physicians and hospitals—through out the United States!

Participating Hospitals

- Bascom Palmer Eye Institute

- Cleveland Clinic

- Continuum Health Partners

- Fox Chase Cancer Center

- Hospital for Special Surgery

- Hospital of the University of Pennsylvania - UPHS

- The Johns Hopkins Hospital

- Lenox Hill Hospital

- Maimonides Medical Center

- Mount Sinai Medical Center

- New York Eye & Ear Infirmary

- New York-Presbyterian Hospital

- NYU Cancer Institute

- NYU Langone Medical Center

- NYU Hospital for Joint Diseases

- Rusk Institute of Rehabilitation Medicine

- St. Francis Hospital -The Heart Center

- Wake Forest University Baptist Medical Center

America's Top Doctors® 8th Edition

Bascom Palmer
EYE INSTITUTE
UNIVERSITY OF MIAMI HEALTH SYSTEM

www.bascompalmer.org
800-329-7000

Miami:
900 NW 17th Street, Miami, FL 33136 • 305-326-6000
Palm Beach Gardens:
7101 Fairway Drive, Palm Beach Gardens, FL 33418 • 561-515-1500
Naples:
311 9th Street North, Naples, FL 34102 • 239-659-3937
Plantation:
1000 South Pine Island Road, Plantation, FL 33324 • 954-465-2700

Bascom Palmer Specialists in Miami, Palm Beach Gardens, Naples and Plantation, Florida

INTERNATIONALLY ACCLAIMED

Bascom Palmer Eye Institute is committed to the protection and preservation of the treasured gift of sight. The Institute's full-time faculty of internationally-respected physicians and scientists are skilled in every ophthalmic subspecialty. Bascom Palmer Eye Institute, which serves as the Department of Ophthalmology for the University of Miami Miller School of Medicine in Miami, Florida, is recognized as one of the world's finest and most progressive centers for ophthalmic care, research and education.

BASCOM PALMER EYE INSTITUTE EARNS TOP RATINGS

Bascom Palmer Eye Institute continues to be ranked the nation's best ophthalmic hospital by board-certified ophthalmologists from across the United States. In 2008, Bascom Palmer was named the #1 eye hospital in the United States by *U.S. News & World Report* for the fifth year in a row. Bascom Palmer has also received the #1 ranking for its Clinical (Patient Care) and Residency programs by *Ophthalmology Times*, which annually ranks the top ophthalmology programs in the United States.

BASCOM PALMER RESEARCHERS ADVANCE OPHTHALMIC CARE AND TREATMENT

Consistent with its mission to resolve diseases and disorders of the eye, the physicians and scientists of Bascom Palmer Eye Institute develop new theories, therapeutic techniques and surgical instruments. Many of the institute's innovations have advanced the course of ophthalmic practices worldwide, including:

- Discovering a new treatment for wet macular degeneration and introducing the use of bevacizumab (Avastin) as a remarkable breakthrough therapy.
- Alerting ophthalmologists around the world of fungal infections affecting contact lens users, significantly reducing the number of new infections
- Performing the first successful vitreous surgery – and inventing miniature surgical instrumentation required for this procedure.
- Unraveling the mystery of normal tension glaucoma.
- Establishing predictive tests and new treatments for complicated retinal detachments.

Bascom Palmer Eye Institute has four convenient Florida locations: In Miami, Palm Beach Gardens, Naples, and Plantation. Each of the Institute's 55 internationally respected clinical faculty members specialize in a specific area of ophthalmology and all are board-certified by the American Board of Ophthalmology. In addition to providing care to more than 200,000 patients annually, all clinical faculty members have research and teaching responsibilities at the University of Miami Miller School of Medicine.

TO SCHEDULE AN APPOINTMENT PLEASE CALL
1-800-329-7000
www.bascompalmer.org

Cleveland Clinic

Hospital Overview

One of the largest and busiest health centers in America. Number one in heart care. National leaders in urology, rheumatology and digestive diseases. Treating all illnesses and disorders of the body. Second opinions a specialty.

"Better care of the sick, investigation of their problems and further education of those who serve."

General Overview

Founded in 1921, Cleveland Clinic is a 1,000-staffed-bed hospital that integrates clinical and hospital care with research and education in a private, non-profit group practice. This group practice model provides an environment that allows our physicians to stay at the cutting edge of medical technology. They pool their expertise and their wisdom for the benefit of the patient and the community.

Vital Statistics

In 2007, more than 1,800 full-time physicians and scientists, representing 120 medical specialties and subspecialties, provided for 3 million outpatient visits, 53,000 hospital admissions and 74,000 surgeries for patients from throughout the United States and more than 80 countries.

One of America's Best

In 2008, Cleveland Clinic was ranked one of the top 4 hospitals in America in the *U.S.News & World Report* annual "America's Best Hospitals" survey. In cardiology and cardiac surgery, we lead the nation. Our heart program has been ranked number one in America for 14 years in a row. Cleveland Clinic's Urology, Rheumatology and Digestive Disease programs are ranked second in the nation. Additional specialties rated among America's best include Cancer, Endocrinology, Geriatric Care, Gynecology, Nephrology, Neurology and Neurological Surgery, Ophthalmology, Orthopaedics, Otolaryngology, Psychiatry and Pulmonary.

"Patients First"

"Patients First" is the guiding principle of Cleveland Clinic. It declares the primacy of patient care, patient comfort and patient communication in every activity we undertake. It affirms the importance of research and education for their contributions to clinical medicine and the improvement of patient care. At the same time, "Patients First" demands a relentless focus on measurable quality. By setting standards, collecting data and analyzing the results, Cleveland Clinic puts patients first through improved outcomes and better service, providing a healthier future for all.

Global Patient Services

Global Patient Services is a full-service department dedicated to meeting the needs of both our out-of-state and international patients. The National Center and the International Center, which make up Global Patient Services, provide personalized concierge programs and services to welcome patients and add to their comfort before, during and after their stay.

For more information about Cleveland Clinic, to schedule a second opinion or to learn about assistance for out-of-town patients, call 800.890.2467 or visit www.clevelandclinic.org/topdocs.

Cleveland Clinic | 9500 Euclid Avenue / AC311 | Cleveland OH 44195

Beth Israel   **Roosevelt Hospital**   **St. Luke's Hospital**   **Long Island College Hospital**   **NY Eye & Ear Infirmary**

Phone (800) 420 – 4004   www.chpnyc.org

Sponsorship: Voluntary Not-for-profit   **Beds:** 2,727 certified beds
Accreditation: Joint Commission of Accreditation of Healthcare Organizations (JCAHO), Accreditation Council for Graduate Medical Education, Medical Society of New York, in conjunction with the Accreditation Council for Continuing Medical Education

A STRONG PARTNERSHIP WITH A PROUD HERITAGE
Continuum Health Partners is a partnership of six venerable health care providers: Beth Israel Medical Center-Milton and Carroll Petrie Division, Beth Israel Medical Center-Kings Highway Division, St. Luke's Hospital, Roosevelt Hospital, Long Island College Hospital of Brooklyn, and The New York Eye and Ear Infirmary. Each of the six partner institutions was established more than a century ago by individuals committed to improving health and health care in their communities. Today, the system represents over 4,000 physicians and dentists and is superbly equipped to respond to the health care needs of the populations we serve. Continuum providers also see patients in group and private practice settings and in ambulatory centers in New York City and Westchester County.

LOCATIONS
Continuum Health Partners has campuses throughout Manhattan and Brooklyn. Beth Israel Medical Center has two divisions: the Milton and Caroll Petrie Division on the East Side, and the Kings Highway Division in Brooklyn. The Phillips Ambulatory Care Center, a state-of-art outpatient center, is located at Union Square. St. Luke's Hospital is in Morningside Heights and Roosevelt Hospital is in the Columbus Circle and Lincoln Center neighborhoods on the West Side. Long Island College Hospital of Brooklyn is located in the Brooklyn Heights/Cobble Hill section of Brooklyn. The New York Eye and Ear Infirmary is located on Second Avenue and 14th street.

ACADEMIC AFFILIATIONS
Beth Israel Medical Center is the University Hospital and Manhattan Campus for the Albert Einstein College of Medicine. St. Luke's-Roosevelt Hospital Center is an Academic Affiliate of Columbia University College of Physicians and Surgeons. Long Island College Hospital of Brooklyn is the primary teaching affiliate of the SUNY-Health Science Center in Brooklyn. The New York Eye and Ear Infirmary is the primary teaching center of the New York Medical College and affiliated teaching hospitals in the areas of ophthalmology and otolaryngology.

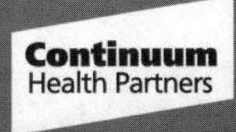

Continuum
Health Partners

For a referral to a great doctor in your neighborhood, call (800) 420-4004. Our Physician Referral Service can help you find a primary care physician or specialist affiliated with Beth Israel, St. Luke's, Roosevelt, Long Island College Hospital, or The New York Eye and Ear Infirmary. Visit our Website at www.chpnyc.org

FOX CHASE
CANCER CENTER

333 Cottman Avenue
Philadelphia, PA 19111-2497
Phone: 1-888-FOX CHASE • Fax: 215-728-270
www.fccc.edu

Sponsorship	Independent Nonprofit
Beds	100 licensed beds
Accreditation	The Joint Commission; American Hospital Association; American Colleg of Surgeons Commission on Cancer; College of American Pathology; American College of Radiology

U.S. News & World Report consistently ranks Fox Chase Cancer Center among the nation's best. Fox Chase is also the first hospital in Pennsylvania and the nation's first cancer hospital to earn the Magn Award for Nursing Excellence from the American Nurses Credentialing Center.

Overview
Fox Chase Cancer Center was founded in 1904 in Philadelphia as the nation's first cancer hospital. In 1974, Fox Chase became one of the first institutions designated as a National Cancer Institute Comprehensive Cancer Center. The mission of Fox Chase is to reduce the burden of human cancer through the highest-quality programs in basic, clinical, population and translational research; pro- grams of prevention, detection and treatment of cancer; and community outreach.

- Fox Chase's 100-bed hospital is one of the few in the country devoted entirely to adult cancer car
- Annual hospital admissions exceed 4,100 and outpatient visits to physicians total more than 71,500 a year.
- Fox Chase's board-certified specialists are recognized nationally and internationally in medical, radiation and surgical oncology, diagnostic imaging, diagnostic pathology, pain management, oncology nursing and oncology social work.
- The staff provides a coordinated approach to meet the treatment needs of each patient. Special multidisciplinary centers provide consultations and treatment recommendations for specific types of cancer.
- The nursing staff of specially trained oncology nurses provides one of the best nurse-to-patient ratios in the area.
- Fox Chase investigators have received numerous awards and honors, including Nobel Prizes in medicine and chemistry; a Kyoto Prize, a Lasker Clinical Research Award, memberships in the National Academy of Sciences and General Motors Cancer Research Foundation Prizes.
- Fox Chase is a founding member of the National Comprehensive Cancer Network, an alliance of the nation's leading academic cancer centers, and the hub of Fox Chase Cancer Center Partners, a select group of more than 25 community hospitals with Fox Chase-affiliated cancer programs.

For more about Fox Chase physicians and services, visit our web site, www.fccc.edu, or call 1-888-FOX CHASE.

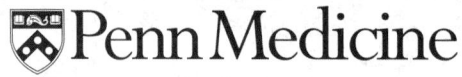

OVERVIEW

For more than two centuries, Penn physicians and scientists have been committed to the highest standards of patient care, education and research. Our commitment has been recognized by our peers and by others throughout the greater Philadelphia region and across the nation.

Penn Medicine ranks second nationally in special grant funding from the National Institutes of Health, with several departments ranking first nationally. Overall, Penn has more individual departments ranked in the top five than any other academic medical center. *U.S.News* also consistently ranks the University of Pennsylvania Schools of Medicine and Nursing among the nation's best.

We Are Medicine

Our physicians and scientists are united in the health system's mission to expand the frontiers of medicine through new discoveries in the detection, treatment and prevention of human disease. Because we develop and test new treatments through clinical trials, our patients gain access to the very latest advances and future generations will benefit from the work we do today.

Penn continues to lead the way in discovering new treatment methods for diseases once considered incurable, including groundbreaking research in cancer, cardiac, neurosciences, orthopaedics, genetics and imaging. Over the past 30 years, Penn physicians and scientists have participated in many important discoveries, including:

- The first general vaccine against pneumonia.

- The introduction of total intravenous feeding.

- The development of cognitive therapy.

- The development of magnetic resonance imaging and other imaging technologies.

- The discovery of the Philadelphia chromosome, which revolutionized cancer research by making the connection between genetic abnormalities and cancer.

- The development of a cure for atrial fibrillation.

- Pioneering new procedures in robotic-assisted surgery.

Locations

Patients are seen at:

- Hospital of the University of Pennsylvania
- Penn Presbyterian Medical Center
- Pennsylvania Hospital
- Penn Medicine at Cherry Hi
- Penn Medicine at Radnor
- Penn Medicine at Rittenhous
- PennCare, our primary care physician network, provides services in the local communities in Bucks, Ches Delaware, Montgomery and Philadelphia counties in Pennsylvania and in Souther New Jersey.
- Hospice and home care serv are provided by Penn Home Care and Hospice Services.

On the Web

Visit pennhealth.com for the latest patient education with explanation of surgical procedures and follow-up care screening tools, drug interactio and descriptions as well as an encyclopedia of health information.

To learn more about Penn physicians or services, call 1-800-789-PENN or visit pennhealth.com

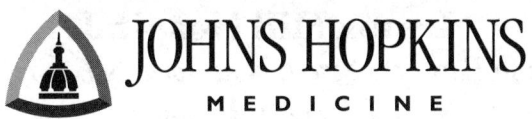

JOHNS HOPKINS
MEDICINE

600 North Wolfe Street, Baltimore Maryland 21287
www.hopkinsmedicine.org

Johns Hopkins Medicine unites physicians and scientists of the Johns Hopkins University School of Medicine with the organizations, health professionals and facilities of the Johns Hopkins Health System, including the world-renowned Johns Hopkins Hospital. All share a single mission: to improve the health of the community and the world by setting the standard of excellence in medical education, research and clinical care.

We heal. Ranked as America's top hospital year after year by *U.S. News & World Report*, The Johns Hopkins Hospital and its related facilities serve as beacons of hope for thousands of patients in our community, in our nation and throughout the world.

We discover. Research is the foundation of clinical care. Johns Hopkins physicians and researchers consistently receive more research grants from the National Institutes of Health than faculty at any other institution. Johns Hopkins has been home to three Nobel laureates, 11 Lasker awardees, 12 National Academy of Sciences members and 32 members of the Institute of Medicine.

We teach. The Johns Hopkins University School of Medicine educates and trains medical students, graduate students and postdoctoral fellows from around the world.

Our Centers of Excellence include
- Asthma & Allergy Center
- Brady Urologic Institute
- Children's Center
- Sidney Kimmel Comprehensive Cancer Center
- Comprehensive Transplant Center
- Heart Institute
- Institute of Basic Biomedical Sciences
- Solomon H. Snyder Department of Neuroscience
- McKusick-Nathans Institute for Genetic Medicine
- Wilmer Eye Institute

The Marburg Pavilion, a special group of patient rooms offering five-star hotel-like accommodations and amenities, is available at The Johns Hopkins Hospital. An executive physical program also is available that offers comprehensive and expedited examinations.

To find a physician or make an appointment at Johns Hopkins, call 410-955-5464 in Baltimore. For calls outside Baltimore, call 410-735-4872. For calls outside the United States, call +01-410-955-8032.

Lenox Hill Hospital
100 East 77th Street, New York, NY 10075
Tel: 212-434-2000
www.lenoxhillhospital.org

Beds: 652
Sponsorship: Voluntary Not-for-Profit
Accreditation: Joint Commission, College of American Pathologists, American Association of Blood Banks, Accreditation Council for Graduate Medical Education, Accreditation Council for Continuing Medical Education, Commission on Accreditation of Allied Health Education Programs, American College of Radiology

GENERAL PROFILE
Lenox Hill Hospital is a 652-bed, fully accredited, acute care hospital with a national reputation for providing the highest quality care, training new physicians, and contributing to progress in research. Recognized nationally as a leader in cardiac care, orthopedics and maternal/child health, the Hospital also offers a wide range of services in radiology, and medical and surgical specialties.

MEDICAL STAFF AND TEACHING PROGRAMS
Lenox Hill Hospital's 1,400 physicians have national and international reputations in their fields. The Hospital independently sponsors 16 accredited residency and fellowship programs.

CENTERS OF EXCELLENCE
LENOX HILL HEART AND VASCULAR INSTITUTE OF NEW YORK (LHHVI)
Lenox Hill Hospital is five-star rated for coronary interventional procedures, cardiology care, and treatment of heart attack and heart failure by HealthGrades, and was the recipient of the 2008 HealthGrades Cardiac Care Excellence Award. For the fifth year in a row, Lenox Hill Hospital was ranked among the Top 5% in the Nation for coronary interventions. In 2008, LHHVI was ranked #25 nationally in Heart and Heart Surgery by U.S. News & World Report. This is in keeping with a tradition of excellence begun in 1938, when Lenox Hill Hospital cardiologists performed the first angiogram in the U.S. In 1978, Hospital cardiologists performed the first ever coronary angioplasty. In 1991, they implanted one of the first coronary stents in NYC, and in 1994 performed the nation's first minimally invasive direct coronary artery bypass surgery.

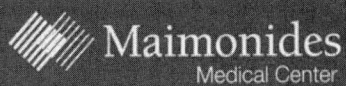

Sponsorship:	Voluntary, Not-for-Profit
Beds:	705 acute, 70 psychiatric
Accreditation:	The Joint Commission
	American College of Surgeons
	American Council of Graduate Medical Education (ACGME)

Maimonides Medical Center is among the largest independent teaching hospitals in the US, and trains more than 450 medical and surgical residents each year. Widely recognized for major achievements in medical technology and patient safety, Maimonides is a conductor of clinical trials for new treatments and therapies, and cited for clinical excellence by numerous health care evaluation services.

CENTERS OF EXCELLENCE

Cancer Center
Maimonides Cancer Center offers a fully integrated approach that includes prevention, screening, diagnostics, treatment, palliative care and clinical research. Staffed by leading physicians, nurses and social workers, the Center provides compassionate, patient-centered, state-of-the-art care.

Cardiac Institute
Renowned for its Catheterization Lab and pioneering new surgical procedures, the Institute includes an electrophysiology (EP) lab, two ICUs, Chest Pain Observation Unit, Advanced Cardiac Care Unit, Congestive Heart Failure program and Atrial Fibrillation Center.

Stroke Center
The Stroke Center at Maimonides is ranked among the best in the nation. It is currently the site of clinical trials for new stroke medications, medical devices and protocols. The Center is one of the few that provides interventional neuroradiology techniques to remove stroke-causing blood clots without surgery.

Infants & Children's Hospital
The Maimonides Infants & Children's Hospital, one of only four accredited children's hospitals in NYC includes comprehensive inpatient services and more than 30 pediatric subspecialties. The Hospital also has a Child Life Program, Pediatric ICU, Neonatal ICU, and Pediatric ER.

Vascular Institute
The Vascular Institute at Maimonides provides comprehensive diagnostic, clinical, and vascular surgical services for patients with circulatory complications. The Vascular Institute is one of only five centers in New York certified to train vascular surgeons.

Stella & Joseph Payson Birthing Center
Maimonides is ranked among the best in the nation for maternity care by HealthGrades and delivers more babies than any other hospital in New York State. The Payson Birthing Center offers a home-like setting with advanced technology that includes a perinatal testing center.

Geriatrics Program
Maimonides serves one of the oldest populations in New York City, with one in ten patients over the age of 85. The Geriatrics Program is fully equipped to meet the special needs of seniors and encompasses inpatient and outpatient services.

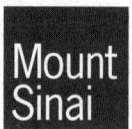
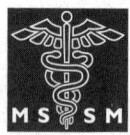

THE MOUNT SINAI MEDICAL CENTER
One Gustave L. Levy Place
Fifth Avenue and 100th Street
New York, NY 10029-6574
Physician Referral: 1-800-MD-SINAI (637-4624)
www.mountsinai.org

MOUNT SINAI
SCHOOL OF
MEDICINE

Sponsorship: Voluntary Not-for-Profit
Beds: 1,171
Accreditation: Joint Commission on Accreditation of Healthcare Organizations (JCAHO);
Commission for Accreditation of Rehabilitation Facilities (CARF);
Magnet Award for Nursing Excellence

The Mount Sinai Medical Center, located on the Upper East Side in New York City, consists of The Mount Sinai Hospital, a tertiary and quaternary care facility known for excellence in patient care, and Mount Sinai School of Medicine, a leader in medical research and in the education of tomorrow's physicians by internationally known faculty. Mount Sinai has been ranked in eleven specialties in the 2008 *U.S. News & World Report* publication of *America's Best Hospitals* with seven specialties ranking in the top twenty. Founded in 1852, The Mount Sinai Hospital is one of the oldest voluntary teaching hospitals in the nation. Today the patients of Mount Sinai benefit from teams of physicians and scientists who work together to rapidly translate laboratory research into new patient treatments. Many of the groundbreaking approaches that result from these collaborations are initially available at only a handful of facilities in the nation—some, only at Mount Sinai. These advances make Mount Sinai the first choice for patients with complex medical and surgical needs.

Mount Sinai Heart, under the direction of Valentin Fuster, MD, PhD, combines Mount Sinai's world-class resources with innovative thinking, creative programs, and an unwavering commitment to the prevention and treatment of cardiovascular disease. Capitalizing on the talent and expertise of internationally renowned Mount Sinai physicians David Adams, MD; Michael Marin, MD; Samin Sharma, MD; Eric Rose, MD; and a host of other highly regarded cardiac surgeons, interventionalists, and cardiologists, Mount Sinai Heart provides an integrated approach to clinical care utilizing basic and clinical research. With the rapid translation of innovative research concepts into improved preventive, diagnostic, and therapeutic care, patients receive multidisciplinary treatment of unprecedented quality.

The Multidisciplinary Head and Neck Cancer Center, under the leadership of Eric Genden, MD, FACS, provides each patient with a team of nationally recognized physicians and surgeons who work together to provide state-of-the-art curative management of tumors of the oral cavity, larynx, skull base, and thyroid gland.

The Recanati/Miller Transplantation Institute is recognized as a national leader in organ transplantation and is one the few institutes in the country to provide combined organ transplantation. Renowned for its long-term experience in the field, The Mount Sinai Hospital was the site of the first liver transplant in New York State.

Minimally Invasive Surgery at Mount Sinai continues to be at the forefront of providing advanced procedures using state-of-the-art instruments. We provide specialized and unique expertise in the use of minimally invasive procedures in addition to traditional surgery options.

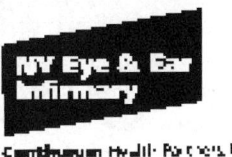

NY Eye & Ear Infirmary

Continuum Health Partners, Inc.

THE NEW YORK EYE AND EAR INFIRMARY

310 East 14th Street
New York, New York 10003
Tel. 212.979.4000   Fax. 212.228.0664
www.nyee.edu

BEDS:	69; Operating Rooms: 17; Surgical Cases: 25,000+ a year
Sponsorship:	Voluntary Not-for-Profit
Accreditation:	The Joint Commission
	College of American Pathologists

GENERAL OVERVIEW

The New York Eye and Ear Infirmary is one of the world's leading facilities for the diagnosis and treatment of diseases of the eyes, ears, nose, throat and related conditions. Founded in 1820, it is the first and most historic specialty hospital in the nation, as well as one of the busiest.

ACADEMIC AND CLINICAL AFFILIATIONS

A voluntary, not-for-profit institution, the Infirmary is a member of Continuum Health Partners, Inc. and an affiliated teaching hospital of New York Medical College. There are highly regarded residency programs in ophthalmology and otolaryngology, plus some two dozen post-graduate fellowship positions.

THE MEDICAL STAFF

The Medical Staff includes more than 500 board-certified attending physicians and surgeons throughout the metropolitan area. Many are renowned for their breakthrough research introducing widely practiced techniques.

SPECIALTIES

Ophthalmology: Within this area are subspecialties of cataract, glaucoma, retina, cornea and external disease, ocular plastic surgery, pediatric ophthalmology and strabismus, neuro-ophthalmology. ocular tumor and uveitis. Laser, photography, fluorescein angiography and electrophysiological testing are among the most advanced services available anywhere.

Otolaryngology: The department is in the forefront of treatment modalities using highly sophisticated endoscopic and laser equipment. Subspecialties include rhinology, laryngology, head & neck surgery, otology/neurotology, facial plastic surgery, pediatric otolaryngology, audiology, speech therapy and hearing aid dispensing.

Plastic & Reconstructive Surgery: Microsurgical capabilities and premium patient accommodations provide an optimum environment for facial plasty, liposuction and repair of defects from disease or trauma.

RELATED SERVICES

New York Eye Trauma Center: An advanced program for emergency treatment of eye injuries, it also is the Eye Injury Registry of New York State and leading collector of data which will help develop preventative strategies.

Ambulatory Surgery: A comprehensive Ambulatory Surgery Center is designed to expedite admission testing, pre-op preparation and post-op recovery in an efficient and comfortable setting.

Pediatric Specialty Care: Services of eye and ear, nose and throat specialists are coordinated with other professional and support staff especially sensitive to the youngest patients.

RESEARCH AND EDUCATION

The New York Eye and Ear Infirmary is a national and international leader in research in its specialties, achieving many "firsts" in successful surgical procedures and medical treatments. Laboratories include Cell Culture, Ocular Imaging, and Microsurgical Education. Over a hundred studies and clinical trials are currently being conducted.

Physician Referral: Call 1.800.449.HOPE (4673)

NewYork-Presbyterian
The University Hospital of Columbia and Cornell

Affiliated with Columbia University College of Physicians and Surgeons and Weill Medical College of Cornell University

NewYork-Presbyterian Hospital
Weill Cornell Medical Center
525 East 68th Street
New York, NY 10021

NewYork-Presbyterian Hospital
Columbia University Medical Center
622 West 168th Street
New York, NY 10032

Sponsorship: Voluntary Not-for-Profit
Beds: 2,335
Accreditation: Joint Commission on Accreditation of Healthcare Organizations (JCAHO), Commission on Accreditation of Rehabilitation Facilities (CARF) and College of American Pathologists (CAP)

The *U.S. News & World Report* has ranked NewYork-Presbyterian Hospital higher in more specialties than any other hospital in the New York area. NewYork-Presbyterian Hospital was named to the *Honor Roll of America's Best Hospitals.*

OVERVIEW:

NewYork-Presbyterian Hospital is the largest hospital in New York and one of the most comprehensive health-care institutions in the world with 5,500 physicians, approximately 96,000 discharges and nearly 1 million out-patient visits annually, and with its affiliated medical schools, more than $330 million in research support.

AMONG ITS RENOWNED CENTERS OF EXCELLENCE ARE:

Morgan Stanley Children's Hospital and the Komansky Center for Children's Health – One of the largest, most comprehensive children's hospitals in the world providing highly sophisticated pediatric medical, surgical and intensive care, including a pediatric cardiovascular center, in a compassionate environment.

NewYork-Presbyterian Cancer Centers – Coordinated, multidisciplinary care and the latest therapeutic options and clinical trials available for all types of cancer.

NewYork-Presbyterian Heart – Expert diagnostic capabilities and medical and surgical innovations for simple to complex heart conditions.

NewYork-Presbyterian Neuroscience Centers – Latest research, diagnosis and treatment capabilities in Alzheimer's disease, Multiple Sclerosis, Parkinson's disease, aneurysms, epilepsy, brain tumors, stokes and other neurological disorders.

NewYork-Presbyterian Psychiatry – World-renowned center of excellence in psychiatric treatment, research and education.

NewYork-Presbyterian Transplant Institute – Adult and pediatric heart, liver, and kidney and adult pancreas and lung transplantation and cutting-edge research.

NewYork-Presbyterian Vascular Care Center – Comprehensive and integrated preventive, diagnostic and treatment program for diverse problems related to arteries and veins throughout the body.

NewYork-Presbyterian Digestive Disease Services – Expert capabilities in the broad range of conditions that affect the organs as well as other components of the digestive system.

William Randolph Hearst Burn Center – Largest and busiest burn center in the nation which also conducts research to improve survival and enhance quality of life for burn victims.

In addition, the Hospital offers extraordinary expertise, comprehensive programs and specialized resources in the fields of AIDS, Complementary Medicine, Gene Therapy, Reproductive Medicine and Infertility, Trauma Center and Women's Health Care.

ACADEMIC AFFILIATIONS:

NewYork-Presbyterian is the only hospital in the world affiliated with two Ivy League medical schools; The Joan and Sanford I Weill Medical College of Cornell University and the Columbia University College of Physicians and Surgeons.

Physician Referral: To find a NewYork-Presbyterian Hospital affiliated physician to meet your needs, call toll free 1-877-NYP-WELL (1-877-697-9355) or visit our website at www.nyp.org

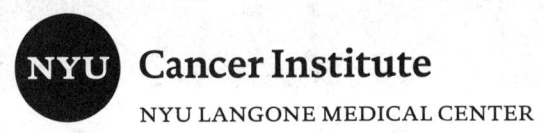

Cancer Institute
NYU LANGONE MEDICAL CENTER

NYU Clinical Cancer Center
160 East 34th Street
New York, New York 10016
www.nyuci.org/atcd

NYU Langone Medical Center
550 First Avenue
(at 31st Street)
New York, New York 10016
www.nyumc.org/atcd

Stephen D. Hassenfeld Children's Center for Cancer and Blood Disorders
160 East 32nd Street
New York, New York 10016
www.nyumc.org/hassenfeld

A Collaborative Approach
The NYU Cancer Institute, an NCI designated center, is a "matrix cancer center" without walls operating within the larger NYU Langone Medical Center. With over 175 members and a research funding base of over $81 million, this structure strengthens our capabilities to forge collaborations across medical and scientific disciplines, which translates to comprehensive care for our patients and discoveries that will influence the future of this disease.

Renowned Expertise
Team members' compassion and expertise help patients better manage the symptoms of their disease as well as their special needs. Our highly skilled Magnet™ nursing team not only plays a pivotal role in coordinating direct patient care, but is also a source of invaluable patient education.

A Patient-Focused Setting
The NYU Clinical Cancer Center, with over 70 faculty members from various disciplines at the New York University School of Medicine, is the principal outpatient facility of the Cancer Institute and serves as home for our patients and their caregivers. The center and its multidisciplinary team of experts provide access to the latest treatment options and clinical trials along with a variety of programs in cancer prevention, screening, diagnostics, genetic counseling, and supportive services. When it comes to kids and cancer, the Stephen D. Hassenfeld Children's Center for Cancer and Blood Disorders offers not just innovation but insight. As a leading member of the NCI-sponsored Children's Oncology Group, our physicians are known for developing new ways to treat childhood cancer. Our affiliation with Bellevue Hospital, the oldest public hospital in the country, affords clinically distinctive opportunities to learn and care for patients with cancer by observing its presentation and behavior in a variety of patient groups.

A LEADER IN PATIENT CARE

NYU Langone Medical Center is one of the nation's leading academic medical centers, combining excellence in patient care, research and medical education. A not-for-profit institution, NYU Langone Medical Center includes Tisch Hospital, a voluntary 705-bed tertiary care facility serving more than 32,000 inpatients annually, and the Rusk Institute of Rehabilitation Medicine which has 174 beds and serves 2,000 inpatients and more than 74,000 outpatients annually and the Hospital for Joint Disease, which has 200 beds and is one of the nation's premier hospitals for treating orthopaedic and rheumatological disorders.

A DISTINGUISHED FACULTY

NYU Langone Medical Center has approximately 4,000 faculty members at Tisch Hospital, Rusk Institute, Hospital for Joint Diseases, Bellevue Hospital Center - one of the largest and oldest municipal hospitals in North America and an affiliate of NYU Langone Medical Center - and in the Veterans Administration system. Many faculty members have distinguished national and international reputations.

A LEADER IN EDUCATION

NYU School of Medicine enrolls more than 714 students and has over 1123 resident physicians and fellows who are graduates of the nation's finest medical schools. NYU School of Medicine offers a robust research and educational experience, providing residency training programs in virtually every medical specialty. The rich environment of research and training is translated into leading-edge care at our hospitals.

SPECIAL PROGRAMS

Cancer

Understanding Cancer. And you. The National Cancer Institute (NCI)—designated NYU Cancer Institute provides access to the latest research, treatment options, technology, clinical trials and a variety of programs in cancer prevention, education, screening, diagnostics, genetic counseling and supportive services. Its multidisciplinary team of experts may offer surgical, radiation, chemotherapeutic, biologic and/or investigational therapies designed to address each individual's specific type of cancer and situation.

Cardiac Surgery

NYU Langone Medical Center's cardiovascular surgeons are leaders in the development of minimally invasive techniques for heart valve and bypass surgery, which are significantly less painful and require a much shorter recovery period. More minimally invasive cardiac surgeries have been performed at Tisch than at any other hospital in the world.

Cardiology

A complete range of services is available, including non-invasive cardiology services, cardiac stress testing, and the full range of diagnostic and interventional procedures in cardiac catheterization and electrophysiology. The Pediatric Cardiology Program provides comprehensive care to children who have congenital or acquired heart diseases. The Joan and Joel Smilow Cardiac Prevention and Rehabilitation Center provides an array of services for people at risk for heart disease and those recovering from cardiac surgery.

Epilepsy

The Comprehensive Epilepsy Center for treatment of adults and children is the largest facility of its kind on the east coast. The Center's unique team approach includes evaluations conducted jointly by epileptologists, neuropsychologists and neurosurgeons, as well as diagnostic studies and therapies for seizure control.

Neurosurgery

The interdisciplinary team of physicians, nurses, and allied healthcare professionals is prepared to diagnose and treat the total spectrum of neurological problems. With an approach that blends compassionate care, support for families, and advanced technology, these healthcare professionals continue to bring new hope for recovery to patients with brain tumors, arteriovenous malformations, and functional brain disorders such as Parkinson's disease and epilepsy.

Obstetrics

NYU Langone Medical Center offers unparalleled diagnostic techniques and surgical & Gynecology innovations to treat women of all ages, with world-class expertise in infertility treatment and management of high-risk pregnancies.

Orthopaedics

With a wide range of services and specialty programs, the Department of Orthopaedic Surgery at NYU Hospital for Joint Diseases caters to the unique treatment needs of today's patients. Our expert physicians combine their experience and research with the latest technology to provide personalized care of bone and joint problems that affect our patients' comfort and ability to function.

Otolaryngology

The Department of Otolaryngology is one of the premier Otolaryngology-Head and Neck Surgery programs in the country, delivering state of the art patient care, performing innovative research, and providing superb training in Otolaryngology and its subspecialties.

Pain Management

The Pain Management Center team works closely with a broad range of specialists to provide highly individualized care for each patient. Acute cancer and chronic pain management services are among the Center's specialties.

Reconstructive Survery

The Institute of Reconstructive Plastic Surgery is the largest facility of its kind Plastic Surgery in the world, performing 1,500 operations a year and treating problems ranging from severe deformities stemming from congenital birth defects, to injuries and burns. Its staff has pioneered techniques in craniofacial surgery, microsurgery, hand surgery, breast reconstruction, and aesthetic surgery.

Skin Diseases

The Charles C. Harris Skin and Cancer Unit is an internationally-acclaimed center for the treatment of serious and rare skin diseases. It also provides regular outpatient services in specialty clinics for a wide range of common skin problems. Surgery Leading the nation in advancement of minimally invasive procedures and surgical techniques.

Surgery

The Department of Surgery is highly regarded and nationally recognized. Our faculty includes world-renowned members that are recognized for their work, their leadership positions in both regional and national surgical societies, and for upholding the department's goal of developing leaders in clinical surgery while providing the optimal academic surgical environment for patients, residents and staff

Transplant

The Mary Lea Johnson Richards Organ Transplant Center is one of the nation's leading centers for liver, kidney, and pancreas transplants including a living donor program. Its clinical team is one of the most experienced in the world, with some of the best patient and graft survival statistics in the nation.

Urology

NYU Langone Medical Center's urologists are leaders in treating prostate disorders, including prostate cancer, as well as many other male and female urological problems. They helped pioneer minimally invasive surgical techniques to preserve a man's sexual function after surgery, and they were leaders in clinical trials of Viagra.

REHABILITATION MEDICINE

Founded by Dr. Howard A. Rusk in 1948, the Rusk Institute of Rehabilitation Medicine is the world's first and one of the largest university centers for the treatment of adults and children with disabilities. The Rusk Institute has been ranked the #1 rehabilitation medicine center in the New York area by the U.S.News & World Report's annual "Best Hospitals" survey for the last nineteen years.

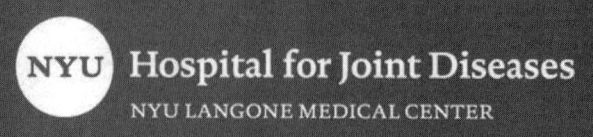

NYU Hospital for Joint Diseases
NYU LANGONE MEDICAL CENTER

301 East 17th Stree
(at Second Avenue
New York, NY 1000
212-598-6000 FAX: 212-260-120
www.nyuhjd.or

Sponsorship:	NYU Langone Medical Center
Beds:	190
Accreditation:	Joint Commission on Accreditation of Healthcare Organizations (JCAHO), Commission of Accreditation for Rehabilitation Facilities (CARF)

PROFILE
NYU Hospital for Joint Diseases is one of the nation's leading orthopaedic, rheumatologic, rehabilitation and
neurologic specialty sites dedicated to the prevention and treatment of neuromusculoskeletal diseases. NYUHJD is a voluntary, not-for-profit teaching institution and is part of NYU Medical Center.

MEDICAL STAFF
NYU Hospital for Joint Diseases has over 500 board certified members of the attending medical staff specializing in orthopaedics, rheumatology, rehabilitation medicine, neurology and anesthesiology.

TEACHING PROGRAMS
NYUHJD sponsors a fully accredited five-year orthopaedic surgery residency program with twelve residents each year. In addition, seven different fellowships are offered in the subspecialty areas of orthopaedics including hand, foot and ankle, spine, sports medicine, shoulder, and total joint replacement..

SPECIAL PROGRAMS
Orthopaedic Surgery: Arthritis and Joint Replacement Center, The Spine Center, Arthroscopic Surgery, Pediatric Orthopaedics, Bone Tumors and Orthopaedic Oncology, Foot and Ankle Surgery, Hand Surgery, Limb Lengthening and Bone Growth, Occupational and Industrial Orthopaedic Care, Sports Medicine, Shoulder and Elbow Service, Center for Neuromuscular and Developmental Disorders, Diabetes Foot and Ankle Center, The Harkness Center for Dance Injuries, and an Orthopaedic Urgent Care Center.

Division of Rheumatology: Center for Arthritis & Autoimmunity and the Peter D. Seligman Center for Advanced Therapeutics. Rheumatoid Arthritis, Osteoarthritis, Psoriatic Arthritis, Lupus, Osteoporosis, Fibromyalgia, Scleroderma, Sjogren's Syndrome.

Rehabilitation Medicine: The Rusk Institute of Rehabilitation Medicine at 17th Street offers comprehensive inpatient (orthopaedic and neurological rehabilitation, pain management) and outpatient rehabilitation services at NYUHJD and other locations.

Additional Programs: Orthopaedic Neurology, Initiative for Women with Disabilities, Multiple Sclerosis, Neuroimmunology, Neurosurgery, Comprehensive Pain Treatment Center, Clinical Neurophysiology, Movement Disorders, Infusion Center, and Neurorehabilitation.

OTHER SERVICES
Managed Care Plans: NYU Hospital for Joint Diseases participates in over 44 managed care plans covering approximately 100 different products (i.e., HMO, POS, PPO, Medicare, Medicaid, etc.).

Physician Referral NYUHJD offers a free telephone physician referral service, Monday-Friday, 8:30 am to 6:00 pm. The physician referral service can be reached at 1-888-HJD-DOCS (1-888-453-3627)

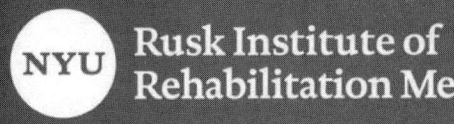

St. Francis Hospital The Heart Center®
100 Port Washington Blvd.
Roslyn, New York 11576
www.stfrancisheartcenter.com
(516) 562-6000   1-888-HEARTNY

St. Francis Hospital, The Heart Center® is New York State's only specialty designated cardiac center, offering one of the leading cardiac care programs in the nation. Founded in 1922 by the Franciscan Missionaries of Mary, the Hospital is recognized as an innovator in the delivery of specialized cardiovascular services in an environment where excellence and compassion are emphasized. St. Francis also offers a superb program in non-cardiac surgery, including some of the most advanced technology and minimally invasive techniques available for vascular, prostate, ear-nose-throat (ENT), and orthopedic surgery.

Cardiac Diagnostics and Treatment
St. Francis Hospital performs more cardiac procedures than any other hospital in New York State and has been consistently recognized for its outstanding quality of care. In 2008, St. Francis Hospital was ranked as one of America's best hospitals by *U.S. News & World Report*.

Cardiac surgery: In 2007, 1,549 open-heart surgeries were performed at St. Francis Hospital. The Hospital's eight cardiothoracic surgeons have the combined experience of over 20,000 open-heart procedures in the last 10 years alone and are experts in all types of heart surgery, from conventional, open-heart bypass to off-pump coronary artery bypass (OPCAB) to the newest, minimally invasive valve procedures, including surgical techniques designed to treat certain cardiac arrhythmias or irregular heart rhythms.

Cardiac catheterization: In 2007, St. Francis interventional cardiologists performed 8,284 cardiac catheterizations and 3,121 percutaneous coronary interventions (angioplasty and insertion of stents). According to the most recent report by the Department of Health, St. Francis had the highest three-year caseload in New York State. The Hospital is also recognized as one of the East Coast's highest volume centers for catheter-based techniques to close atrial septal defects (ASDs) and patent foramen ovale (PFO).

Arrhythmia and Pacemaker Center: St. Francis has a leading national program for pacemaker implantation and the diagnosis and treatment of cardiac rhythm abnormalities. The Center has unparalleled expertise in radiofrequency cardiac ablation, including treatment of atrial fibrillation.

Research and Technology: At the St. Francis Cardiac Research Institute, a team of world-renowned researchers is working with the latest non-invasive imaging technology, including advanced techniques and world class expertise in cardiac CT angiography, cardiac magnetic resonance imaging and three-dimensional echocardiography. This multimodality approach to investigating the heart's function and disease processes is aimed at improving methods of diagnosing heart disease.

Prevention and Education
St. Francis Hospital's satellite campus, The DeMatteis Center for Cardiac Research and Education, in Greenvale, New York, is one of the few freestanding campuses in the U.S. dedicated to the prevention of heart disease. It is the site of community health lectures, as well as the largest medically staffed cardiac fitness and rehabilitation program on Long Island.

Physician referral: **1-888-HEARTNY**
Sponsorship: Voluntary not-for-profit
Beds: 308
Accreditation: Awarded accreditation from the Joint Commission:
                 A member of Catholic Health Services of Long Island

Wake Forest University Baptist
MEDICAL CENTER ®

Medical Center Boulevard • Winston-Salem, NC 27157
PAL® (Physician-to-physician calls) 1-800-277-7654
Health On-Call® (Patient access) 1-800-446-2255
www.wfubmc.edu • www.brennerchildrens.org • www.besthealth.com

OVERVIEW

Wake Forest University Baptist Medical Center encompasses **Wake Forest University School of Medicine**, whose reputation attracts some of the nation's top doctors to its Wake Forest University Physicians faculty practice, and **North Carolina Baptist Hospital**, a nationally ranked, academic tertiary care facility. Internationally known for state-of-the-art treatment and technology, research leadership and teaching excellence, Wake Forest University Baptist Medical Center is ranked a top hospital by *U.S.News & World Report* (since 1993). More than 550 physicians offer preventive and highly specialized care.

COMPREHENSIVE SPECIALTY CENTERS AND SERVICES

Brenner Children's Hospital . . . the highest levels of neonatal and pediatric care in a state-of-the-art setting; **Heart Center** . . . groundbreaking research, technology and treatment, region's only transplant service; **Comprehensive Cancer Center of WFU** . . . NCI-designated for research, advanced technologies, treatments such as Gamma Knife, Intensity Modulated Radiation Therapy; **Neurosciences** . . . Stroke, ALS, Epilepsy, and Brain Tumor Centers, expertise in deep brain stimulation for Parkinson's; the region's most comprehensive, advanced service in **Digestive Health, Orthopaedics, Otolaryngology, Urology.**

RESEARCH EXCELLENCE

Wake Forest Baptist has more than 1,000 research and clinical trials under way, and a new Translational Science Institute is accelerating discovery that will benefit patients. At the **Wake Forest Institute for Regenerative Medicine**, doctors are applying tissue engineering to build more than 20 organs and tissues and have successfully implanted human, laboratory-grown bladders. The **Center for Human Genomics** is advancing knowledge of gene-based therapies for cardiovascular and pulmonary diseases, prostate cancer and diabetes. The **Brain Tumor Center** is at the forefront of molecular medicine therapies and radiation-induced brain injury research. The **Center for Biomolecular Imaging** is creating new ways to view the brain, heart and cancers.

TECHNOLOGY LEADERSHIP

Committed to serving our patients with "tomorrow's medicine" today, Wake Forest Baptist is home to one of North America's first **Integrated Brachytherapy Units**, a faster, extremely precise cancer treatment using radioactive seed implants . . . one of the nation's first **Bioanatomic Imaging and Treatment Programs**, allowing for new levels of accuracy in tumor identification and treatment . . . North Carolina's only **MEG** (magnetoencephalography), brain-function imaging that enables highly precise neurosurgical planning . . . N.C.'s first **Gamma Knife**, the gold standard for non-invasive brain surgeries.

OUTSTANDING CARE

WFUBMC is the **top consumer choice** in its area for health care, according to National Research Corp. surveys. **Patient satisfaction** scores are among the highest in the nation as compared to its peer group, according to Press Ganey. **Outstanding nursing** earned Wake Forest Baptist one of the nation's first 15 Magnet Awards for nursing excellence, awarded by the American Nurses Credentialing Center.

To make an appointment or find a specialist at Wake Forest University Baptist Medical Center, call Health On-Call® at **1-800-446-2255**.

KNOWLEDGE MAKES ALL THE DIFFERENCE.

Physician Listings

Adolescent Medicine
a subspecialty of Pediatrics

An internist or pediatrician who specializes in adolescent medicine is a multidiciplinary healthcare specialist trained in the unique physical, psychological and social characteristics of adolescents, their healthcare problems and needs.

Training Required: Three years in internal medicine OR three years in pediatrics *plus* additional training and examination for certification in adolescent medicine

ADOLESCENT MEDICINE

New England

Emans, Sarah Jean H MD [AM] - **Spec Exp:** Pediatric Gynecology; Adolescent Gynecology; **Hospital:** Children's Hospital - Boston; **Address:** Childrens Hosp, Dept Adolescent Med, 300 Longwood Ave, Boston, MA 02115-5724; **Phone:** 617-355-7181; **Board Cert:** Pediatrics 1993; Adolescent Medicine 2002; **Med School:** Harvard Med Sch 1970; **Resid:** Pediatrics, Chldns Hosp 1973; **Fellow:** Adolescent Medicine, Chldns Hosp 1974; **Fac Appt:** Prof Ped, Harvard Med Sch

Mid Atlantic

Diaz, Angela MD [AM] - **Spec Exp:** Adolescent Gynecology; Abuse/Neglect; **Hospital:** Mount Sinai Med Ctr (page 64); **Address:** 320 E 94th St Fl 2, New York, NY 10128-5604; **Phone:** 212-423-2900; **Board Cert:** Pediatrics 1987; Adolescent Medicine 2004; **Med School:** Columbia P&S 1981; **Resid:** Pediatrics, Mt Sinai Med Ctr 1984; **Fellow:** Adolescent Medicine, Mt Sinai Med Ctr 1985; **Fac Appt:** Prof Ped, Mount Sinai Sch Med

Murray, Pamela J MD [AM] - **Spec Exp:** Adolescent Gynecology; **Hospital:** Chldns Hosp of Pittsburgh - UPMC; **Address:** Children's Hosp Pittsburgh, Addolescent Medicine, 3705 Fifth Ave at DeSoto St, Pittsburgh, PA 15213; **Phone:** 412-692-8504; **Board Cert:** Pediatrics 1983; Adolescent Medicine 2002; **Med School:** Med Coll PA 1978; **Resid:** Pediatrics, Children's Hosp 1981; **Fellow:** Public Health, Univ New South Wales 1987; **Fac Appt:** Assoc Prof Ped, Univ Pittsburgh

Rudy, Bret J MD [AM] - **Spec Exp:** HIV in Adolescents; AIDS/HIV; **Hospital:** Chldns Hosp of Philadelphia, The; **Address:** Children's Hosp of Philadelphia, 3535 Market St, Ste 1517, Philadelphia, PA 19104; **Phone:** 215-590-1468; **Board Cert:** Pediatrics 1998; Adolescent Medicine 2001; **Med School:** Univ Pittsburgh 1985; **Resid:** Pediatrics, Chldns Hosp of Philadelphia 1989; **Fellow:** Immunology, Chldns Hosp of Philadelphia 1991

Southeast

Ford, Carol Ann MD [AM] - **Hospital:** Univ NC Hosps; **Address:** UNC-Chapel Hill, Dept Ped Adol Med, 231 Mac Nider Bldg Ave, Box 7225, Chapel Hill, NC 27599-7225; **Phone:** 919-966-2504; **Board Cert:** Internal Medicine 1987; Pediatrics 1998; Adolescent Medicine 1994; **Med School:** Univ Fla Coll Med 1983; **Resid:** Internal Medicine, North Carolina Meml Hosp 1987; Pediatrics, North Carolina Meml Hosp 1987; **Fellow:** Adolescent Medicine, UCSF Med Ctr 1995; **Fac Appt:** Asst Prof Ped, Univ NC Sch Med

Midwest

Fortenberry, J Dennis MD [AM] - **Spec Exp:** Sexually Transmitted Diseases; **Hospital:** Riley Hosp for Children; **Address:** Indiana Univ - Adolescent Medicine, 410 W 10th, rm 1001, Indianapolis, IN 46202; **Phone:** 317-274-8812; **Board Cert:** Internal Medicine 1983; Adolescent Medicine 2004; **Med School:** Univ Okla Coll Med 1979; **Resid:** Internal Medicine, Univ OK Hlth Sci Ctr 1982; **Fellow:** Adolescent Medicine, Univ OK Hlth Sci Ctr 1983; **Fac Appt:** Prof Med, Indiana Univ

Kokotailo, Patricia K MD [AM] - **Spec Exp:** Adolescent Gynecology; Substance Abuse; **Hospital:** Univ WI Hosp & Clins; **Address:** Univ Wisc Chldns Hosp, Dept Peds-Adol Med, 2800 University Ave, Ste 200, Madison, WI 53705; **Phone:** 608-263-6421; **Board Cert:** Pediatrics 1987; Adolescent Medicine 2002; **Med School:** Northwestern Univ 1982; **Resid:** Pediatrics, Johns Hopkins Hosp 1985; **Fellow:** Adolescent Medicine, Johns Hopkins Hosp 1989; **Fac Appt:** Prof Ped, Univ Wisc

Great Plains and Mountains

Kaplan, David W MD [AM] - **Spec Exp:** Eating Disorders; Depression; Headache; **Hospital:** Chldn's Hosp - Aurora, The; **Address:** Chldns Hosp, 13123 E 16th Ave, Box B025, Aurora, CO 80045; **Phone:** 720-777-6131; **Board Cert:** Pediatrics 1975; Public Health & Genl Preventive Med 1980; Adolescent Medicine 2002; **Med School:** Case West Res Univ 1970; **Resid:** Pediatrics, Univ Colorado Med Ctr 1972; Pediatrics, Chldns Hosp Med Ctr 1975; **Fellow:** Public Health & Genl Preventive Med, Harvard Sch Pub Hlth 1976; **Fac Appt:** Prof Ped, Univ Colorado

Southwest

Bermudez, Ovidio B MD [AM] - **Spec Exp:** Eating Disorders; Obesity; **Hospital:** Laureate Psyc Clinic & Hosp; **Address:** Eating Disorders Clinic, 6655 S Yale Ave, Tulsa, OK 74136; **Phone:** 918-491-3702; **Board Cert:** Pediatrics 2005; Adolescent Medicine 2002; **Med School:** Dominican Republic 1985; **Resid:** Pediatrics, Med Coll Penn 1988; **Fellow:** Adolescent Medicine, Univ Alabama 1990; **Fac Appt:** Clin Prof Ped, Univ Okla Coll Med

West Coast and Pacific

Anderson, Martin M MD [AM] - **Hospital:** Ronald Reagan UCLA Med Ctr; **Address:** UCLA Med Ctr, Dept Pediatrics, 10833 Le Conte Ave, 12-476 MDcc, Los Angeles, CA 90095; **Phone:** 310-825-9346; **Board Cert:** Pediatrics 1986; Adolescent Medicine 2002; **Med School:** UC Davis 1980; **Resid:** Pediatrics, Mott Chldns Hosp 1983; **Fellow:** Adolescent Medicine, UCSF Med Ctr 1986; **Fac Appt:** Prof Ped, UCLA

Irwin Jr, Charles E MD [AM] - **Spec Exp:** Eating Disorders; Adolescent Gynecology; **Hospital:** UCSF Med Ctr; **Address:** UCSF Chldns Hosp, 400 Parnassus Ave Fl 2, Box 0503, San Francisco, CA 94143; **Phone:** 415-353-2002; **Board Cert:** Pediatrics 1993; Adolescent Medicine 2002; **Med School:** UCSF 1971; **Resid:** Pediatrics, UCSF Med Ctr 1974; **Fellow:** Adolescent Medicine, UCSF Med Ctr 1977; **Fac Appt:** Prof Ped, UCSF

MacKenzie, Richard G MD [AM] - **Spec Exp:** Eating Disorders; Menstrual Disorders; **Hospital:** Chldns Hosp - Los Angeles; **Address:** 5000 Sunset Blvd, Fl 4, Los Angeles, CA 90027-5861; **Phone:** 323-361-2112; **Med School:** McGill Univ 1966; **Resid:** Internal Medicine, Royal Victoria Hosp-Montreal 1969; **Fellow:** Adolescent Medicine, Chidrens Hosp 1970; **Fac Appt:** Assoc Prof Ped, USC Sch Med

Morris, Robert E MD [AM] - **Spec Exp:** Chronic Illness; Teen Behavior Evaluation-High Risk; Juvenile Correctional Health Care; **Hospital:** Santa Monica - UCLA Med Ctr, Ronald Reagan UCLA Med Ctr; **Address:** UCLA Sch Med, Dept Peds, 10833 Le Conte Ave, Los Angeles, CA 90095-1752; **Phone:** 310-825-9346; **Board Cert:** Pediatrics 1986; Adolescent Medicine 2005; **Med School:** Temple Univ 1971; **Resid:** Pediatrics, Univ Wash 1974; Pediatric Gastroenterology, UCLA Med Ctr 1982; **Fac Appt:** Prof Ped, UCLA

Allergy & Immunology

An allergist-immunologist is trained in evaluation, physical and laboratory diagnosis and management of disorders involving the immune system. Selected examples of such conditions include asthma, anaphylaxis, rhinitis, eczema and adverse reactions to drugs, foods and insect stings as well as immune deficiency diseases (both acquired and congenital), defects in host defense and problems related to autoimmune disease, organ transplantation or malignancies of the immune system. As our understanding of the immune system develops, the scope of this specialty is widening.

Training programs are available at some medical centers to provide individuals with expertise in both allergy/immunology and adult rheumatology, or in both allergy/immunology and pediatric pulmonology. Such individuals are candidates for dual certification.

Training Required: Two years in allergy/immunology OR prior certification in internal medicine or pediatrics *plus* additional training and examination

ALLERGY & IMMUNOLOGY

New England

MacLean, James A MD [A&I] - **Spec Exp:** Asthma; Allergy; Urticaria; **Hospital:** Mass Genl Hosp, N Shore Med Ctr - Salem Hosp; **Address:** Mass General Hosp, 55 Fruit St, Cox 201, Boston, MA 02114-2621; **Phone:** 617-726-3850; **Board Cert:** Internal Medicine 1988; Allergy & Immunology 1991; **Med School:** McGill Univ 1985; **Resid:** Internal Medicine, Royal Victoria Hosp 1989; **Fellow:** Allergy & Immunology, Mass Genl Hosp 1991; Immunopathology, Mass Genl Hosp 1994; **Fac Appt:** Asst Prof A&I, Harvard Med Sch

Umetsu, Dale T MD/PhD [A&I] - **Spec Exp:** Asthma; Immune Deficiency; Eczema; **Hospital:** Children's Hospital - Boston; **Address:** Div Immunology, Children's Hosp, 1 Blackfan Cir, Karp Labs, rm 10127, Boston, MA 02115; **Phone:** 617-919-2439; **Board Cert:** Pediatrics 1984; Allergy & Immunology 1985; **Med School:** NYU Sch Med 1979; **Resid:** Pediatrics, Chldns Hosp 1982; **Fellow:** Allergy & Immunology, Chldns Hosp 1984; **Fac Appt:** Prof Ped, Harvard Med Sch

Wong, Johnson T MD [A&I] - **Spec Exp:** Asthma; Rhinosinusitis; Urticaria; Food Allergy; **Hospital:** Mass Genl Hosp, Newton - Wellesley Hosp; **Address:** 8 Hawthorne Pl, Ste 104, Boston, MA 02114; **Phone:** 617-742-5730; **Board Cert:** Internal Medicine 1983; Allergy & Immunology 1985; **Med School:** UCSF 1980; **Resid:** Internal Medicine, UCLA-Wadsworth VA Hosp 1983; **Fellow:** Allergy & Immunology, Mass Genl Hosp 1986; **Fac Appt:** Asst Prof Med, Harvard Med Sch

Mid Atlantic

Buchbinder, Ellen MD [A&I] - **Spec Exp:** Asthma; Allergy; Rhinitis; Sinusitis; **Hospital:** Mount Sinai Med Ctr (page 64); **Address:** 111B E 88th St, New York, NY 10128; **Phone:** 212-410-3246; **Board Cert:** Internal Medicine 1981; Allergy & Immunology 1983; **Med School:** Tulane Univ 1978; **Resid:** Internal Medicine, New England Deaconess Hosp 1981; **Fellow:** Allergy & Immunology, Mass Genl Hosp 1983; **Fac Appt:** Asst Clin Prof Med, Mount Sinai Sch Med

Chandler, Michael MD [A&I] - **Spec Exp:** Asthma; Sinus Disorders; Airway Disorders; **Hospital:** Lenox Hill Hosp (page 62), Mount Sinai Med Ctr (page 64); **Address:** 115 E 61st St Fl 12, New York, NY 10021-8183; **Phone:** 212-486-6715; **Board Cert:** Internal Medicine 1984; Allergy & Immunology 1987; **Med School:** Wayne State Univ 1981; **Resid:** Internal Medicine, Northwestern Meml Hosp 1984; **Fellow:** Allergy & Immunology, Northwestern Meml Hosp 1986; **Fac Appt:** Asst Clin Prof Med, Mount Sinai Sch Med

Cohn, John R MD [A&I] - **Spec Exp:** Asthma; Allergic Rhinitis; Voice Disorders & Allergies; **Hospital:** Thomas Jefferson Univ Hosp; **Address:** 1015 Chestnut St, Ste 1300, Philadelphia, PA 19107; **Phone:** 215-923-7685; **Board Cert:** Internal Medicine 1979; Allergy & Immunology 1981; Pulmonary Disease 1982; **Med School:** Thomas Jefferson Univ 1976; **Resid:** Internal Medicine, Thomas Jefferson Univ Hosp 1979; **Fellow:** Allergy & Immunology, Duke Univ Med Ctr 1982; Pulmonary Disease, Duke Univ Med Ctr 1982; **Fac Appt:** Clin Prof Med, Thomas Jefferson Univ

Cunningham-Rundles, Charlotte MD/PhD [A&I] - **Spec Exp:** Immunotherapy; Immunodeficiency Disorders; **Hospital:** Mount Sinai Med Ctr (page 64); **Address:** 5 E 98th St, New York, NY 10029; **Phone:** 212-659-9268; **Board Cert:** Internal Medicine 1972; **Med School:** Columbia P&S 1969; **Resid:** Internal Medicine, Bellevue Hosp Ctr 1972; **Fellow:** Allergy & Immunology, NYU Med Ctr 1974; **Fac Appt:** Prof Med, Mount Sinai Sch Med

Ein, Daniel MD [A&I] - **Spec Exp:** Asthma & Allergy; Sinus Disorders; Chemical Exposure; Immune Deficiency; **Hospital:** G Washington Univ Hosp; **Address:** 2150 Pennsylvania Ave NW, Ste G400, Washington, DC 20037; **Phone:** 202-741-2770; **Board Cert:** Internal Medicine 1980; Allergy & Immunology 1989; **Med School:** Albert Einstein Coll Med 1964; **Resid:** Internal Medicine, Mass Genl Hosp 1969; **Fellow:** Immunology, Natl Cancer Inst 1968; **Fac Appt:** Clin Prof Med, Geo Wash Univ

Fishman, Henry J MD [A&I] - **Spec Exp:** Asthma & Allergy; Chemical Exposure; **Hospital:** G Washington Univ Hosp; **Address:** 2141 K St NW, Ste 206, Washington, DC 20037; **Phone:** 202-833-3500; **Board Cert:** Internal Medicine 1982; Allergy & Immunology 1985; **Med School:** Univ Rochester 1979; **Resid:** Internal Medicine, Geo Wash Med Ctr 1982; **Fellow:** Allergy & Immunology, Georgetown Univ Hosp 1984; **Fac Appt:** Asst Clin Prof Med, Georgetown Univ

Kaliner, Michael A MD [A&I] - **Spec Exp:** Asthma & Allergy; Sinusitis; Rhinitis; **Address:** Institute for Asthma and Allergy, 5454 Wisconsin Ave, Ste 700, Chevy Chase, MD 20815; **Phone:** 301-986-9262; **Board Cert:** Internal Medicine 1974; Allergy & Immunology 1993; **Med School:** Univ MD Sch Med 1967; **Resid:** Internal Medicine, UCSF Med Ctr 1970; **Fellow:** Allergy & Immunology, Harvard Univ 1973; **Fac Appt:** Clin Prof Med, Geo Wash Univ

Levinson, Arnold MD [A&I] - **Spec Exp:** Autoimmune Disease; Immune Deficiency; Allergy; **Hospital:** Hosp Univ Penn - UPHS (page 60); **Address:** Hosp Univ Penn, Div A&I, 39th and Market St, Mutch Bldg Fl 5, Philadelphia, PA 19104; **Phone:** 215-662-2425; **Board Cert:** Internal Medicine 1972; Allergy & Immunology 1975; **Med School:** Univ MD Sch Med 1969; **Resid:** Internal Medicine, Baltimore City Hosps 1971; Immunology, Hosp Univ Penn 1972; **Fellow:** Clinical Immunology, UCSF Med Ctr 1973; Allergy & Immunology, Hosp Univ Penn 1975; **Fac Appt:** Prof Med, Univ Pennsylvania

Mazza, David S MD [A&I] - **Spec Exp:** Asthma; Sinus Disorders; Eczema; **Hospital:** St Luke's - Roosevelt Hosp Ctr - Roosevelt Div (page 57), St Vincent Cath Med Ctrs - Manhattan; **Address:** 7 Lexington Ave, Ste 3, New York, NY 10010-5517; **Phone:** 212-677-7170; **Board Cert:** Pediatrics 1983; Allergy & Immunology 1999; **Med School:** Univ VT Coll Med 1977; **Resid:** Pediatrics, NYU-Bellevue Hosp 1980; **Fellow:** Pediatrics, Bellevue Hosp 1982; Allergy & Immunology, St Luke's-Roosevelt Hosp Ctr 1989; **Fac Appt:** Assoc Prof Ped, Columbia P&S

Metcalfe, Dean D MD [A&I] - **Spec Exp:** Mast Cell Diseases; Food Allergy; **Hospital:** Natl Inst of Hlth - Clin Ctr; **Address:** Natl Inst Allergy & Infectious Disease, Allergic Disease Lab, 10 Center Drive Bldg 10 - rm 11C205, Bethesda, MD 20892-1881; **Phone:** 301-496-2165; **Board Cert:** Internal Medicine 1975; Allergy & Immunology 1977; Rheumatology 1980; **Med School:** Univ Tenn Coll Med, Memphis 1972; **Resid:** Internal Medicine, Univ Mich Hosps 1974; Allergy & Immunology, Natl Inst Allergy & Infectious Dis-NIH 1977; **Fellow:** Rheumatology, Peter Bent Brigham Hosp 1979

Reisman, Robert E MD [A&I] - **Spec Exp:** Anaphylaxis; Asthma; Insect Allergies; **Hospital:** Buffalo General Hosp, Women's & Chldn's Hosp of Buffalo, The; **Address:** Buffalo Medical Group, 295 Essjay Rd, Williamsville, NY 14221-8216; **Phone:** 716-630-1130; **Board Cert:** Internal Medicine 1969; Allergy & Immunology 1972; **Med School:** SUNY Buffalo 1956; **Resid:** Internal Medicine, Buffalo Genl Hosp 1959; **Fellow:** Allergy & Immunology, Buffalo Genl Hosp 1961; **Fac Appt:** Clin Prof Med, SUNY Buffalo

Shepherd, Gillian M MD [A&I] - **Spec Exp:** Food & Drug Allergy; Rhinosinusitis & Asthma; Urticaria; Insect Allergies; **Hospital:** NY-Presby Hosp/Weill Cornell (page 66), Meml Sloan-Kettering Cancer Ctr; **Address:** 235 E 67th St, Ste 203, New York, NY 10021-6040; **Phone:** 212-288-9300; **Board Cert:** Internal Medicine 1979; Allergy & Immunology 1981; **Med School:** NY Med Coll 1976; **Resid:** Internal Medicine, Lenox Hill Hosp 1979; **Fellow:** Allergy & Immunology, New York Hosp-Cornell 1981; **Fac Appt:** Assoc Clin Prof Med, Cornell Univ-Weill Med Coll

Allergy & Immunology

Slankard, Marjorie MD [A&I] - **Spec Exp:** Rhinitis; Asthma; Sinusitis; Food Allergy; **Hospital:** NY-Presby Hosp/Columbia (page 66), Valley Hosp; **Address:** 16 E 60th St, Ste 321, New York, NY 10022-1002; **Phone:** 212-326-8410; **Board Cert:** Internal Medicine 1974; Allergy & Immunology 1977; **Med School:** Univ MO-Columbia Sch Med 1971; **Resid:** Internal Medicine, New York Hosp 1974; Internal Medicine, Rockefeller Univ Hosp 1974; **Fellow:** Immunology, New York Hosp-Cornell 1976; Immunology, Mount Sinai Med Ctr 1980; **Fac Appt:** Clin Prof Med, Columbia P&S

Strober, Warren MD [A&I] - **Spec Exp:** Immune Deficiency; Inflammatory Bowel Disease/Crohn's; **Hospital:** Natl Inst of Hlth - Clin Ctr; **Address:** NIH-Laboratory of Clinical Investigation, Bldg 10-CRC, rm 5-3940, Bethesda, MD 20892-1890; **Phone:** 301-496-6810; **Board Cert:** Internal Medicine 1974; Allergy & Immunology 1977; **Med School:** Univ Rochester 1962; **Resid:** Internal Medicine, Strong Meml Hosp 1964; Allergy & Immunology, Natl Inst Hlth 1972

Southeast

Benenati, Susan V MD [A&I] - **Spec Exp:** Asthma; Latex Allergy; Sinus Disorders; **Hospital:** Baptist Hosp of Miami, South Miami Hosp; **Address:** 7000 SW 62nd Ave, Ste 510, South Miami, FL 33143-4721; **Phone:** 305-665-1623; **Board Cert:** Internal Medicine 1988; Allergy & Immunology 1999; **Med School:** Univ S Fla Coll Med 1984; **Resid:** Internal Medicine, Indiana Univ Med Ctr 1988; **Fellow:** Allergy & Immunology, Johns Hopkins Hosp 1990

Bonner, James R MD [A&I] - **Spec Exp:** Asthma; Urticaria; Sinusitis; **Hospital:** Univ of Ala Hosp at Birmingham; **Address:** Univ Alabama Hosp, Allergy/Immunology, 2000 Sixth Ave S, Birmingham, AL 35233-2110; **Phone:** 205-801-8100; **Board Cert:** Internal Medicine 1974; Infectious Disease 1976; Allergy & Immunology 1979; **Med School:** Univ Mich Med Sch 1971; **Resid:** Internal Medicine, Univ Ala Med Ctr 1974; **Fellow:** Allergy & Immunology, Univ Ala Med Ctr 1977; **Fac Appt:** Prof Med, Univ Ala

deShazo, Richard D MD [A&I] - **Spec Exp:** Immunodeficiency Disorders; Allergy; Rheumatology; **Hospital:** Univ Hosps & Clins - Jackson, Baptist Hosp - Jackson; **Address:** Univ Mississippi Med Ctr, Dept Med, 2500 N State St, Jackson, MS 39216; **Phone:** 601-984-5600; **Board Cert:** Internal Medicine 1974; Allergy & Immunology 1977; Rheumatology 1982; Geriatric Medicine 2005; **Med School:** Univ Ala 1971; **Resid:** Internal Medicine, Walter Reed Genl Hosp 1974; **Fellow:** Microbiology, Walter Reed Army Inst Rsch 1975; Clinical Immunology, Walter Reed Genl Hosp 1977; **Fac Appt:** Prof Med, Univ Miss

Fox, Roger W MD [A&I] - **Spec Exp:** Asthma; Rhinosinusitis; Urticaria; **Hospital:** University Comm Hosp, Tampa Genl Hosp; **Address:** 13801 Bruce B Downs Blvd, Ste 502, Tampa, FL 33613; **Phone:** 813-971-9743; **Board Cert:** Internal Medicine 1978; Allergy & Immunology 1981; **Med School:** St Louis Univ 1975; **Resid:** Internal Medicine, Univ S Florida Affil Hosps 1978; **Fellow:** Allergy & Immunology, Univ S Florida Affil Hosps 1980; **Fac Appt:** Assoc Prof Med, Univ S Fla Coll Med

Friedman, Stuart A MD [A&I] - **Spec Exp:** Asthma; Sinus Disorders; Allergy; **Hospital:** Boca Raton Comm Hosp, Delray Med Ctr; **Address:** 5162 Linton Blvd, Ste 201, Delray Beach, FL 33484-6567; **Phone:** 561-495-2580; **Board Cert:** Internal Medicine 1980; Allergy & Immunology 1983; **Med School:** Spain 1976; **Resid:** Internal Medicine, Winthrop Univ Hosp 1980; **Fellow:** Immunology, Univ Cincinnati Med Ctr 1982; **Fac Appt:** Asst Clin Prof Med, Univ Miami Sch Med

Gluck, Joan MD [A&I] - **Spec Exp:** Asthma in Pregnancy; Asthma & Allergy; Food Allergy; **Hospital:** Baptist Hosp of Miami, South Miami Hosp; **Address:** 9035 Sunset Drive, Ste 202, Miami, FL 33173; **Phone:** 305-279-3366; **Med School:** NYU Sch Med 1972; **Resid:** Pediatrics, Jackson Meml Hosp 1974; **Fellow:** Allergy & Immunology, Jackson Meml Hosp 1976

America's Top Doctors® 8th Edition

Ledford, Dennis K MD [A&I] - **Spec Exp:** Asthma; **Hospital:** University Comm Hosp, Tampa Genl Hosp; **Address:** Univ So Florida Coll Med, Dept Allergy & Immunology, 13801 Bruce B Downs Blvd, Ste 502, Tampa, FL 33613-4745; **Phone:** 813-971-9743; **Board Cert:** Internal Medicine 1980; Rheumatology 1984; Allergy & Immunology 1985; Clinical & Laboratory Immunology 1986; **Med School:** Univ Tenn Coll Med, Memphis 1976; **Resid:** Internal Medicine, City of Memphis Hosp 1980; **Fellow:** Rheumatology, NYU Hosp-Bellevue 1982; Allergy & Immunology, Univ S Florida Coll Med 1985; **Fac Appt:** Assoc Prof A&I, Univ S Fla Coll Med

Lieberman, Phillip L MD [A&I] - **Spec Exp:** Asthma; Rhinitis; Anaphylaxis; **Hospital:** Baptist Memorial Hospital - Memphis, Methodist Univ Hosp - Memphis; **Address:** 7205 Wolf River Blvd, Ste 200, Germantown, TN 38138; **Phone:** 901-757-6100; **Board Cert:** Internal Medicine 1970; Allergy & Immunology 2003; **Med School:** Univ Tenn Coll Med, Memphis 1965; **Resid:** Internal Medicine, Memphis City Hosps 1969; **Fellow:** Allergy & Immunology, Northwestern Univ 1971; **Fac Appt:** Clin Prof A&I, Univ Tenn Coll Med, Memphis

Lockey, Richard F MD [A&I] - **Spec Exp:** Immune Deficiency; Asthma; Rhinitis; **Hospital:** University Comm Hosp, Tampa Genl Hosp; **Address:** 13801 Bruce B Downs Blvd, Ste 502, Tampa, FL 33613-3946; **Phone:** 813-971-9743; **Board Cert:** Internal Medicine 1970; Allergy & Immunology 1974; **Med School:** Temple Univ 1965; **Resid:** Internal Medicine, Univ Mich Hosp 1968; **Fellow:** Allergy & Immunology, Univ Mich Hosp 1970; **Fac Appt:** Prof Med, Univ S Fla Coll Med

Pacin, Michael P MD [A&I] - **Spec Exp:** Insect Allergies; Asthma; Rhinitis; **Hospital:** Baptist Hosp of Miami, South Miami Hosp; **Address:** 9035 Sunset Drive, Ste 202, Miami, FL 33173; **Phone:** 305-279-3366; **Board Cert:** Internal Medicine 1974; Allergy & Immunology 1979; **Med School:** Washington Univ, St Louis 1969; **Resid:** Internal Medicine, Jewish Hosp 1971; Internal Medicine, Jackson Meml Hosp 1972; **Fellow:** Allergy & Immunology, Long Beach VA Hosp 1974

Stein, Mark R MD [A&I] - **Spec Exp:** Asthma; Immune Deficiency; Gastroesophageal Reflux Disease (GERD); **Hospital:** Good Sam Med Ctr - W Palm Beach, Palm Beach Gardens Med Ctr; **Address:** 840 US Hwy 1, Ste 235, North Palm Beach, FL 33408-3835; **Phone:** 561-626-2006; **Board Cert:** Internal Medicine 1975; Allergy & Immunology 1977; **Med School:** Jefferson Med Coll 1968; **Resid:** Internal Medicine, Letterman Army Med Ctr 1975; **Fellow:** Allergy & Immunology, Fitzsimmons Army Med Ctr 1977

Sullivan, Timothy J MD [A&I] - **Spec Exp:** Drug Allergy; Anaphylaxis; Asthma; **Hospital:** Northside Hosp, St Joseph's Hosp - Atlanta; **Address:** 5555 Peachtree Dunwoody Rd, Ste 125, Atlanta, GA 30342; **Phone:** 404-255-2918; **Board Cert:** Allergy & Immunology 1979; **Med School:** Univ Miami Sch Med 1966; **Resid:** Internal Medicine, Barnes Hosp 1971; **Fellow:** Allergy & Immunology, Barnes Hosp 1973

Midwest

Baker Jr, James Russell MD [A&I] - **Spec Exp:** Immune Deficiency-Thyroid; **Hospital:** Univ Michigan Hlth Sys; **Address:** UM Allergy Specialty Clinic, 24 Frank Lloyd Wright Drive, Ste H-2100, P.O.Box 442, Ann Arbor, MI 48106; **Phone:** 734-647-2777; **Board Cert:** Internal Medicine 1981; Allergy & Immunology 1983; Clinical & Laboratory Immunology 1986; **Med School:** Loyola Univ-Stritch Sch Med 1978; **Resid:** Internal Medicine, Walter Reed Army Med Ctr 1981; **Fellow:** Allergy & Immunology, Walter Reed Army Med Ctr/NIAID 1984; **Fac Appt:** Prof A&I, Univ Mich Med Sch

Allergy & Immunology

Berger, Melvin MD/PhD [A&I] - **Spec Exp:** Immune Deficiency; Asthma & Allergy; **Hospital:** Rainbow Babies & Chldns Hosp, Univ Hosps Case Med Ctr; **Address:** Pediatric Immunology, 11100 Euclid Ave, MC 6008B, Cleveland, OH 44106-1736; **Phone:** 216-844-3237; **Board Cert:** Pediatrics 1981; Allergy & Immunology 1981; **Med School:** Case West Res Univ 1976; **Resid:** Pediatrics, Chldns Hosp Med Ctr 1978; **Fellow:** Allergy & Immunology, Natl Inst Allergy & Infect Dis (NIH) 1981; **Fac Appt:** Prof Ped, Case West Res Univ

Busse, William MD [A&I] - **Spec Exp:** Asthma; Autoimmune Disease; Rhinitis; **Hospital:** Univ WI Hosp & Clins; **Address:** 600 Highland Ave, rm B6-242, Madison, WI 53792; **Phone:** 608-263-6180; **Board Cert:** Internal Medicine 1972; Allergy & Immunology 1974; **Med School:** Univ Wisc 1966; **Resid:** Internal Medicine, Cincinnati Genl Hosp 1968; Internal Medicine, Cincinnati Genl Hosp 1971; **Fellow:** Allergy & Immunology, Univ Wisconsin 1973; **Fac Appt:** Prof Med, Univ Wisc

Gewurz, Anita T MD [A&I] - **Spec Exp:** Immune Deficiency; Asthma; **Hospital:** Rush Univ Med Ctr; **Address:** Univ Consultants, 1725 W Harrison St, Ste 117, Chicago, IL 60612; **Phone:** 312-942-6296; **Board Cert:** Pediatrics 1976; Allergy & Immunology 1977; **Med School:** Albany Med Coll 1970; **Resid:** Pediatrics, Univ Illinois Med Ctr 1973; Allergy & Immunology, Rush-Presby-St Lukes Hosp 1976; **Fellow:** Allergy & Immunology, Grant Hosp 1977; Allergy & Immunology, Northwestern Univ Med Sch 1985; **Fac Appt:** Prof Med, Rush Med Coll

Grammer, Leslie C MD [A&I] - **Spec Exp:** Asthma; Sinusitis; Drug Allergy; **Hospital:** Northwestern Meml Hosp, Rehab Inst - Chicago; **Address:** Northwestern Med Faculty Fdn-Amb Care Ctr, 675 N St Clair, Fl 18 - Ste 18-250, Chicago, IL 60611-5975; **Phone:** 312-695-8624; **Board Cert:** Internal Medicine 1979; Allergy & Immunology 1981; Clinical & Laboratory Immunology 1986; Occupational Medicine 1989; **Med School:** Northwestern Univ 1976; **Resid:** Internal Medicine, Northwestern Meml Hosp 1979; **Fellow:** Allergy & Immunology, Northwestern Univ 1981; **Fac Appt:** Prof Med, Northwestern Univ

Greenberger, Paul A MD [A&I] - **Spec Exp:** Asthma; Anaphylaxis; Drug Allergy; **Hospital:** Northwestern Meml Hosp, Jesse A Brown VA Med Ctr; **Address:** Northwestern Medical Faculty Fdn, Ambulatory Care Center, 675 N St Clair Fl 18 - Ste 18-250, Chicago, IL 60611; **Phone:** 312-695-8624; **Board Cert:** Internal Medicine 1976; Allergy & Immunology 1979; Diagnostic Lab Immunology 1986; **Med School:** Indiana Univ 1973; **Resid:** Internal Medicine, Jewish Hosp 1976; **Fellow:** Allergy & Immunology, Northwestern Meml Hosp 1978; **Fac Appt:** Prof Med, Northwestern Univ

Korenblat, Phillip E MD [A&I] - **Spec Exp:** Allergy; Asthma; Anaphylaxis; **Hospital:** Barnes-Jewish Hosp, Missouri Baptist Med Ctr; **Address:** 1040 N Mason Rd, Ste 115, St Louis, MO 63141-6361; **Phone:** 314-542-0606; **Board Cert:** Internal Medicine 1971; Allergy & Immunology 1974; **Med School:** Univ Ark 1960; **Resid:** Internal Medicine, Jewish Hosp 1965; **Fellow:** Allergy & Immunology, Scripps Clin Rsch Fdn 1966; **Fac Appt:** Clin Prof Med, Washington Univ, St Louis

Routes, John M MD [A&I] - **Spec Exp:** Immunodeficiency Disorders; Asthma; Allergy; **Hospital:** Chldns Hosp - Wisconsin; **Address:** Children's Hosp Wisconsin, 9000 W Wisconsin Ave, Ste 440, Milwaukee, WI 53226; **Phone:** 414-266-6840; **Board Cert:** Internal Medicine 1984; Allergy & Immunology 1987; **Med School:** Indiana Univ 1981; **Resid:** Internal Medicine, Univ Utah Affil Hosps 1984; **Fellow:** Allergy & Immunology, Natl Jewish Hosp 1989; Infectious Disease, Natl Jewish Hosp 1990; **Fac Appt:** Prof Ped, Univ Colorado

Sanders, Georgiana MD [A&I] - **Spec Exp:** Asthma; Food Allergy & Eczema; Rhinitis; **Hospital:** Univ Michigan Hlth Sys, St Joseph Med Ctr; **Address:** Domino's Farms Allergy Specialy Clin, 24 Frank Lloyd Wright Dr, Ste H-2100, PO Box 442, Ann Arbor, MI 48106; **Phone:** 734-936-5634; **Board Cert:** Pediatrics 1982; Allergy & Immunology 1985; **Med School:** Univ Cincinnati 1975; **Resid:** Pediatrics, Children's Hosp Mich 1978; Pediatrics, Boston City Hospi 1979; **Fellow:** Allergy & Immunology, Univ of Michigan Hosp 1984; **Fac Appt:** Asst Clin Prof Med, Univ Mich Med Sch

America's Top Doctors® 8th Edition

Ten, Rosa Maria MD/PhD [A&I] - **Spec Exp:** Immune Deficiency; Asthma; **Hospital:** Riley Hosp for Children; **Address:** Riley Hosp for Children, 702 Barnhill Drive, rm 4270, Indianapolis, IN 46202-5225; **Phone:** 317-274-7208; **Board Cert:** Allergy & Immunology 1997; **Med School:** Spain 1982; **Resid:** Internal Medicine, Mayo Clinic 1994; **Fellow:** Immunology, Inst Pasteur 1991; Allergy & Immunology, Mayo Clinic 1996; **Fac Appt:** Assoc Prof Ped, Indiana Univ

Wood, John A MD [A&I] - **Spec Exp:** Asthma; **Hospital:** St Luke's Hosp - Chesterfield, MO; **Address:** 224 S Woodsmill Rd, Ste 500S, Chesterfield, MO 63017; **Phone:** 314-878-6260; **Board Cert:** Internal Medicine 1972; Pulmonary Disease 1978; Allergy & Immunology 1979; **Med School:** Univ Okla Coll Med 1968; **Resid:** Internal Medicine, Univ Hosp 1970; Internal Medicine, Barnes Hosp-Wash Univ Sch Med 1971; **Fellow:** Pulmonary Disease, Wash Univ Sch Med 1977; Allergy & Immunology, Wash Univ Sch Med 1977; **Fac Appt:** Asst Prof Med, Washington Univ, St Louis

Southwest

Freeman, Theodore M MD [A&I] - **Spec Exp:** Insect Allergies; Asthma; Rhinitis; **Hospital:** SW TX Meth Hosp; **Address:** 8285 Fredericksberg Rd, San Antonio, TX 78229; **Phone:** 210-614-3923; **Board Cert:** Internal Medicine 1983; Allergy & Immunology 1987; Clinical & Laboratory Immunology 1988; **Med School:** Univ S Fla Coll Med 1980; **Resid:** Internal Medicine, Keesler Med Ctr 1983; **Fellow:** Allergy & Immunology, Wilford Hall Med Ctr 1986; Diagnostic Lab Immunology, Mass Genl Hosp 1987; **Fac Appt:** Assoc Prof Med, Uniformed Srvs Univ, Bethesda

Gruchalla, Rebecca S MD/PhD [A&I] - **Spec Exp:** Asthma & Allergy; Drug Allergy; **Hospital:** UT Southwestern Med Ctr - Dallas, Chldns Med Ctr of Dallas; **Address:** Univ Tex SW, Div A&I, 5323 Harry Hines Blvd, Dallas, TX 75390-8859; **Phone:** 214-645-2866; **Board Cert:** Internal Medicine 1988; Allergy & Immunology 2001; **Med School:** Univ Tex SW, Dallas 1985; **Resid:** Internal Medicine, Hosp Univ Penn 1988; **Fellow:** Allergy & Immunology, Univ Tex SW Med Ctr 1990; **Fac Appt:** Assoc Prof Med, Univ Tex SW, Dallas

Lewis, John C MD [A&I] - **Spec Exp:** Autoimmune Disease; **Hospital:** Mayo Clinic - Scottsdale; **Address:** Mayo Clinic, Div Allergy & Immunology, 13400 E Shea Blvd, ALRG-2B, Scottsdale, AZ 85259-5404; **Phone:** 480-301-8227; **Board Cert:** Internal Medicine 1985; Allergy & Immunology 2001; **Med School:** Loyola Univ-Stritch Sch Med 1982; **Resid:** Internal Medicine, Wilford Hall USAF Med Ctr 1985; **Fellow:** Allergy & Immunology, Mayo Clinic 1990; **Fac Appt:** Prof Med, Mayo Med Sch

Schubert, Mark S MD/PhD [A&I] - **Spec Exp:** Asthma & Allergy; Sinus Disorders; Immunodeficiency Disorders; **Hospital:** Banner Good Samaritan Regl Med Ctr - Phoenix, St Joseph's Hosp & Med Ctr - Phoenix; **Address:** Asthma Allergy Clinic, 300 W Clarendon Rd, Ste 120, Phoenix, AZ 85013-2517; **Phone:** 602-277-3337; **Board Cert:** Internal Medicine 1987; Allergy & Immunology 1999; **Med School:** Univ Ariz Coll Med 1983; **Resid:** Neurological Surgery, Barrow Neurological Inst 1985; Internal Medicine, Good Samaritan Med Ctr 1987; **Fellow:** Allergy Immunology & Rheumatology, Stanford Univ Med Ctr 1989; **Fac Appt:** Assoc Clin Prof Med, Univ Ariz Coll Med

West Coast and Pacific

Altman, Leonard C MD [A&I] - **Spec Exp:** Urticaria; Asthma; Sinusitis; Allergy; **Hospital:** Univ Wash Med Ctr, Chldns Hosp and Regl Med Ctr - Seattle; **Address:** 4540 Sand Point Way NE, Ste 200, Seattle, WA 98105-3941; **Phone:** 206-527-1200; **Board Cert:** Internal Medicine 1975; Allergy & Immunology 1979; **Med School:** Harvard Med Sch 1969; **Resid:** Internal Medicine, Univ Wash Affil Hosps 1971; **Fellow:** Allergy & Immunology, Natl Inst Hlth 1974; **Fac Appt:** Clin Prof Med, Univ Wash

Allergy & Immunology

Henderson Jr, William R MD [A&I] - **Spec Exp:** Asthma; Allergic Rhinitis; Allergic Diseases; **Hospital:** Univ Wash Med Ctr; **Address:** 815 Mercer St, Ste 254, Seattle, WA 98109; **Phone:** 206-543-3780; **Board Cert:** Internal Medicine 1976; Allergy & Immunology 1979; **Med School:** UCSF 1973; **Resid:** Internal Medicine, Stanford Med Ctr 1975; Internal Medicine, Natl Inst Hlth 1976; **Fellow:** Allergy & Immunology, Natl Inst Hlth 1978; **Fac Appt:** Prof Med, Univ Wash

Meltzer, Eli MD [A&I] - **Spec Exp:** Asthma & Allergy; Sinus Disorders; **Hospital:** Rady Children's Hosp - San Diego, Sharp Meml Hosp; **Address:** Allergy & Asthma Medical & Research Ctr, 9610 Granite Ridge Drive, Ste B, San Diego, CA 92123-2661; **Phone:** 858-292-1144; **Board Cert:** Pediatrics 1969; Allergy & Immunology 1972; **Med School:** Jefferson Med Coll 1964; **Resid:** Pediatrics, St Christophers Hosp for Chld 1967; **Fellow:** Pediatric Allergy & Immunology, National Jewish Hosp 1969; **Fac Appt:** Clin Prof Ped, UCSD

Montanaro, Anthony MD [A&I] - **Spec Exp:** Asthma; Allergy; Anaphylaxis; Immunodeficiency Disorders; **Hospital:** OR Hlth & Sci Univ; **Address:** OHSU Div Allergy & Clin Immunology, 3181 SW Sam Jackson Park Rd, MC OP-34, Portland, OR 97239-2098; **Phone:** 503-494-4300; **Board Cert:** Internal Medicine 1981; Allergy & Immunology 1993; Rheumatology 1984; **Med School:** Univ Wash 1978; **Resid:** Internal Medicine, Mercy Med Ctr 1981; **Fellow:** Allergy Immunology & Rheumatology, Oregon Hlth Sci Univ 1983; **Fac Appt:** Prof Med, Oregon Hlth Sci Univ

Ostrom, Nancy K MD [A&I] - **Spec Exp:** Asthma & Allergy; **Hospital:** Rady Children's Hosp - San Diego; **Address:** 9610 Granite Ridge Drive, Ste B, San Diego, CA 92123; **Phone:** 858-292-1144; **Board Cert:** Pediatrics 1984; Allergy & Immunology 1987; **Med School:** Mayo Med Sch 1980; **Resid:** Pediatrics, Mayo Clinic 1983; **Fellow:** Allergy & Immunology, Mayo Clinic 1985; **Fac Appt:** Assoc Clin Prof Ped, UCSD

Tamaroff, Marc A MD [A&I] - **Spec Exp:** Sinus Disorders; Asthma; Rhinitis; **Hospital:** Long Beach Meml Med Ctr, Lakewood Reg Med Ctr; **Address:** 3816 Woodruff Ave, Ste 209, Long Beach, CA 90808-2145; **Phone:** 562-496-4749; **Board Cert:** Internal Medicine 1979; Allergy & Immunology 1983; **Med School:** Univ Ariz Coll Med 1974; **Resid:** Internal Medicine, St Mary Med Ctr 1977; **Fellow:** Allergy & Immunology, UCLA Med Ctr 1979; **Fac Appt:** Assoc Clin Prof Med, UCLA

Wasserman, Stephen MD [A&I] - **Spec Exp:** Asthma; Rhinitis; Sinus Disorders; Urticaria; **Hospital:** UCSD Med Ctr; **Address:** UCSD, MC 0637, Stein Bldg-rm 244, 9500 Gilman Drive, La Jolla, CA 92093-0637; **Phone:** 858-822-4261; **Board Cert:** Internal Medicine 1973; Allergy & Immunology 1975; **Med School:** UCLA 1968; **Resid:** Internal Medicine, Peter Bent Brigham Hosp 1970; **Fellow:** Allergy & Immunology, R Breck-PB Brigham Hosp 1974; **Fac Appt:** Prof Med, UCSD

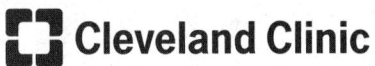

Cleveland Clinic

Pulmonary, Allergy and Critical Care Medicine

The Section of Allergy/Immunology at Cleveland Clinic is one of the largest allergy and immunology groups in the United States with a national reputation for excellence. Patients have access not only to state-of-the-art medical therapies but also to investigational protocols. From 2003 to 2007, more than 135,000 skin tests were safely performed to identify inhalant, food, drug or venom allergy.

Allergy/immunology diagnosis and treatment takes place in a multidisciplinary fashion that includes close coordination with specialists in other areas.

Asthma

We provide state-of-the-art management for patients whose asthma is not well controlled. This includes assessments of coexisting conditions that make asthma difficult to treat or unresponsive to standard treatment. We offer new medications that may not be available in primary care settings and interventions that may not be provided by asthma specialists in the community.

Aspirin Sensitivity and Desensitization

Individuals who are sensitive to aspirin often experience respiratory reactions, including wheezing, shortness of breath, or skin reactions, such as hives or swelling. We offer a special desensitization program for aspirin-sensitive patients who have respiratory reactions but require aspirin for cardiovascular or rheumatic conditions. This procedure, available at only a few centers in the United States, can permit such patients to take aspirin safely.

Areas of Expertise

- Asthma
- Rhinitis, allergic and non-allergic
- Sinusitis
- Chronic cough
- Aspirin sensitivity
- Urticaria/angioedema
- Atopic dermatitis

- Adverse reactions to medicine, food and bee stings
- Anaphylaxis
- Systemic mastocytosis
- Immunodeficiency

For more information about the Cleveland Clinic Department of Pulmonary, Allergy and Critical Care Medicine, to schedule a second opinion or to learn about assistance for out-of-town patients, call 800.890.2467 or visit www. clevelandclinic.org/allergytopdocs.

Department of Pulmonology, Allergy and Critical Care Medicine
9500 Euclid Avenue / AC311 | Cleveland OH 44195

Cardiovascular Disease
a subspecialty of Internal Medicine

Cardiovascular Disease: An internist specializing in diseases of the heart, lungs and blood vessels and manages complex cardiac conditions such as heart attacks and life-threatening, abnormal heartbeat rhythms.

Cardiac Electrophysiology: A field of special interest within the subspecialty of cardiovascular disease which involves intricate technical procedures to evaluate heart rhythms and determine appropriate treatment for them.

Interventional Cardiology: An area of medicine within the subspecialty of cardiology which uses specialized imaging and other diagnostic techniques to evaluate blood flow and pressure in the coronary arteries and chambers of the heart, and uses technical procedures and medications to treat abnormalities that impair the function of the heart.

Training Required: Three years in internal medicine *plus* additional training and examination for certification in cardiovascular disease, clinical electrophysiology or interventional cardiology

CARDIOVASCULAR DISEASE

New England

Balady, Gary MD [Cv] - **Spec Exp:** Preventive Cardiology; **Hospital:** Boston Med Ctr; **Address:** Boston Med Ctr, Dept Cardiology, 88 East Newton St, Bldg C8, Boston, MA 02118; **Phone:** 617-638-7490; **Board Cert:** Internal Medicine 1982; Cardiovascular Disease 1985; **Med School:** UMDNJ-Rutgers Med Sch 1979; **Resid:** Internal Medicine, Boston Univ Med Ctr 1982; **Fellow:** Cardiovascular Disease, Boston Univ Med Ctr 1985; **Fac Appt:** Prof Med, Boston Univ

Baughman, Kenneth MD [Cv] - **Spec Exp:** Congestive Heart Failure; Cardiomyopathy; **Hospital:** Brigham & Women's Hosp; **Address:** Brigham & Womens Hosp, Shapiro Cardiovascular Ctr, 75 Francis St, Office 05-154, Boston, MA 02115; **Phone:** 857-307-1964; **Board Cert:** Internal Medicine 1975; Cardiovascular Disease 1979; **Med School:** Univ MO-Columbia Sch Med 1972; **Resid:** Internal Medicine, Johns Hopkins Hosp 1977; **Fellow:** Cardiovascular Disease, Mass Genl Hosp 1979; **Fac Appt:** Prof Med, Harvard Med Sch

Cabin, Henry S MD [Cv] - **Spec Exp:** Interventional Cardiology; Cardiac Catheterization; **Hospital:** Yale-New Haven Hosp; **Address:** 333 Cedar St, PO Box 208017, New Haven, CT 06520-8017; **Phone:** 203-785-4129; **Board Cert:** Internal Medicine 1978; Cardiovascular Disease 1983; Interventional Cardiology 2000; **Med School:** Yale Univ 1975; **Resid:** Internal Medicine, Yale-New Haven Hosp 1978; **Fellow:** Internal Medicine, Natl Heart Lung and Blood Inst 1981; Cardiovascular Disease, Yale New Haven Hosp 1982; **Fac Appt:** Prof Med, Yale Univ

Hutter Jr, Adolph M MD [Cv] - **Hospital:** Mass Genl Hosp; **Address:** 55 Fruit St, Yawkey Ctr, rm 5B, Boston, MA 02114-3139; **Phone:** 617-726-2884; **Board Cert:** Internal Medicine 1969; Cardiovascular Disease 1971; **Med School:** Univ Wisc 1963; **Resid:** Internal Medicine, Strong Meml Hosp 1968; **Fellow:** Cardiovascular Disease, Mass Genl Hosp 1970; **Fac Appt:** Prof Med, Harvard Med Sch

Johnson, Paula A MD [Cv] - **Spec Exp:** Heart Disease in Women; Preventive Cardiology; Congestive Heart Failure; **Hospital:** Brigham & Women's Hosp; **Address:** Brigham & Womens Hosp, 75 Francis St, PB5-534, Boston, MA 02115; **Phone:** 617-732-4837; **Board Cert:** Internal Medicine 1988; Cardiovascular Disease 2001; **Med School:** Harvard Med Sch 1985; **Resid:** Internal Medicine, Brigham & Womens Hosp 1988; **Fellow:** Cardiovascular Disease, Brigham & Womens Hosp 1991; **Fac Appt:** Assoc Prof Med, Harvard Med Sch

Kirshenbaum, James M MD [Cv] - **Spec Exp:** Cardiac Catheterization; Coronary Artery Disease; Congestive Heart Failure; **Hospital:** Brigham & Women's Hosp; **Address:** Brigham & Womens Hosp, Div Cardiology, 75 Francis St, Boston, MA 02115-6110; **Phone:** 857-307-1967; **Board Cert:** Internal Medicine 1982; Cardiovascular Disease 1985; Interventional Cardiology 1999; **Med School:** Harvard Med Sch 1979; **Resid:** Internal Medicine, Peter Bent Brigham Hosp 1982; **Fellow:** Cardiovascular Disease, Brigham & Womens Hosp 1985; **Fac Appt:** Assoc Prof Med, Harvard Med Sch

Konstam, Marvin A MD [Cv] - **Spec Exp:** Transplant Medicine-Heart; Heart Failure; Coronary Angioplasty/Stents; **Hospital:** Tufts Med Ctr, Beth Israel Deaconess Med Ctr - Boston; **Address:** New England Med Ctr, Div Cardiology, 750 Washington St, Box 108, Boston, MA 02111; **Phone:** 617-636-6293; **Board Cert:** Internal Medicine 1979; Cardiovascular Disease 1981; Diagnostic Radiology 1980; **Med School:** Columbia P&S 1975; **Resid:** Diagnostic Radiology, Mass Genl Hosp 1978; Internal Medicine, Mass Genl Hosp 1979; **Fellow:** Cardiovascular Disease, Brigham & Women's Hosp 1981; **Fac Appt:** Prof Med, Tufts Univ

Liang, Bruce T MD [Cv] - **Spec Exp:** Ischemic Heart Disease; Congestive Heart Failure; **Hospital:** Univ of Conn Hlth Ctr, John Dempsey Hosp; **Address:** Univ Connecticut Health Ctr, Cardiopulmonary & Hypertension Service, 263 Farmington Ave, Farmington, CT 06030-2202; **Phone:** 860-679-3343; **Board Cert:** Internal Medicine 1985; Cardiovascular Disease 1987; **Med School:** Harvard Med Sch 1982; **Resid:** Internal Medicine, Hosp Univ Penn 1985; **Fellow:** Cardiovascular Disease, Brigham & Womens Hosp 1987; **Fac Appt:** Prof Med, Univ Conn

Libby, Peter MD [Cv] - **Spec Exp:** Preventive Cardiology; Coronary Artery Disease; Cholesterol/Lipid Disorders; **Hospital:** Brigham & Women's Hosp; **Address:** Brigham & Women's Hosp, Cardiovasc Div, 75 Francis St, Boston, MA 02115-5822; **Phone:** 617-732-8086; **Board Cert:** Internal Medicine 1976; Cardiovascular Disease 1981; **Med School:** UCSD 1973; **Resid:** Internal Medicine, Peter Bent Brigham Hosp 1976; **Fellow:** Physiology, Harvard Med Sch 1979; Cardiovascular Disease, Brigham & Woman's Hosp 1980; **Fac Appt:** Prof Med, Harvard Med Sch

Loscalzo, Joseph MD/PhD [Cv] - **Spec Exp:** Coronary Artery Disease; Peripheral Vascular Disease; **Hospital:** Brigham & Women's Hosp; **Address:** Brigham & Women's Hosp, Div Cardiology, 75 Francis St, Boston, MA 02115; **Phone:** 617-732-6340; **Board Cert:** Internal Medicine 1981; Cardiovascular Disease 1983; **Med School:** Univ Pennsylvania 1978; **Resid:** Internal Medicine, Peter Bent Brigham Hosp 1981; **Fellow:** Cardiovascular Disease, Brigham & Women's Hosp 1983; **Fac Appt:** Prof Med, Harvard Med Sch

Manning, Warren MD [Cv] - **Spec Exp:** Heart Valve Disease; Echocardiography; **Hospital:** Beth Israel Deaconess Med Ctr - Boston; **Address:** BIDMC, Dept Non-Invasive Cardiology, 330 Brookline Ave, Boston, MA 02215-5400; **Phone:** 617-667-2192; **Board Cert:** Internal Medicine 1986; Cardiovascular Disease 1989; **Med School:** Harvard Med Sch 1983; **Resid:** Internal Medicine, Beth Israel Hosp 1986; **Fellow:** Cardiovascular Disease, Beth Israel Hosp 1989; **Fac Appt:** Prof Med, Harvard Med Sch

O'Gara, Patrick T MD [Cv] - **Spec Exp:** Heart Valve Disease; Coronary Artery Disease; Aortic Diseases & Dissection; **Hospital:** Brigham & Women's Hosp; **Address:** Brigham & Womens Hosp, Cardiovascular Div, 75 Francis St, Boston, MA 02115-6106; **Phone:** 857-307-1990; **Board Cert:** Internal Medicine 1981; Cardiovascular Disease 1983; **Med School:** Northwestern Univ 1978; **Resid:** Internal Medicine, Mass Genl Hosp 1981; **Fellow:** Cardiovascular Disease, Mass Genl Hosp 1983; **Fac Appt:** Assoc Prof Med, Harvard Med Sch

Palacios, Igor F MD [Cv] - **Spec Exp:** Interventional Cardiology; **Hospital:** Mass Genl Hosp; **Address:** Mass Genl Hosp, Cardiac Unit, 55 Fruit St, GRB 800, Boston, MA 02114; **Phone:** 617-726-8424; **Board Cert:** Internal Medicine 1979; Cardiovascular Disease 1981; Interventional Cardiology 1999; **Med School:** Venezuela 1969; **Resid:** Cardiovascular Disease, Hosp Univ de Caracas 1973; **Fellow:** Cardiovascular Disease, Mass Genl Hosp-Harvard 1980; **Fac Appt:** Assoc Prof Med, Harvard Med Sch

Pfeffer, Marc Alan MD [Cv] - **Hospital:** Brigham & Women's Hosp; **Address:** Brigham & Women's Hospital, 75 Francis St, Boston, MA 02115; **Phone:** 617-732-5681; **Board Cert:** Internal Medicine 1979; Cardiovascular Disease 1981; **Med School:** Univ Okla Coll Med 1976; **Resid:** Internal Medicine, Peter Bent Brigham Hosp 1979; **Fellow:** Cardiovascular Disease, Peter Bent Brigham Hosp 1980; **Fac Appt:** Prof Med, Harvard Med Sch

Phillips, Robert A MD/PhD [Cv] - **Spec Exp:** Hypertension; Coronary Artery Disease; Heart Valve Disease; **Hospital:** UMass Memorial Med Ctr; **Address:** U Mass Memorial, 55 Lake Ave North, S3-866, Worcester, MA 01655; **Phone:** 508-856-3452; **Board Cert:** Internal Medicine 1983; Cardiovascular Disease 1985; **Med School:** Mount Sinai Sch Med 1980; **Resid:** Internal Medicine, Columbia Presby Med Ctr 1983; **Fellow:** Cardiovascular Disease, Mount Sinai Med Ctr 1985; Hypertension, Mount Sinai Med Ctr 1986; **Fac Appt:** Prof Med, Univ Mass Sch Med

Cardiovascular Disease

Ridker, Paul M MD [Cv] - **Spec Exp:** Coronary Artery Disease; Preventive Cardiology; Cholesterol/Lipid Disorders; **Hospital:** Brigham & Women's Hosp; **Address:** Brigham & Women's Hospital, Div Preventive Medicine, 640 Center St, Jamaica Plains, MA 02130; **Phone:** 617-983-4100; **Board Cert:** Internal Medicine 1989; **Med School:** Harvard Med Sch 1986; **Resid:** Internal Medicine, Brigham & Women's Hosp 1989; **Fellow:** Cardiovascular Disease, Brigham & Women's Hosp 1991; **Fac Appt:** Assoc Prof Med, Harvard Med Sch

Roberts, Barbara H MD [Cv] - **Spec Exp:** Heart Disease in Women; Preventive Cardiology; **Hospital:** Miriam Hosp; **Address:** The Miriam Hosp - Women's Cardiac Ctr, 164 Summit Ave, Fain Hlth Ctrs Fl 2, Providence, RI 02906; **Phone:** 401-793-7870; **Board Cert:** Internal Medicine 1975; Cardiovascular Disease 1975; **Med School:** Case West Res Univ 1968; **Resid:** Internal Medicine, Yale-New Haven Hosp 1971; **Fellow:** Cardiovascular Disease, PB Brigham Hosp-Harvard 1975; **Fac Appt:** Assoc Clin Prof Med, Brown Univ

Simons, Michael MD [Cv] - **Spec Exp:** Ischemic Heart Disease; Nuclear Cardiology; **Hospital:** Yale-New Haven Hosp; **Address:** 333 Cedar St, New Haven, CT 06520; **Phone:** 203-785-4114; **Board Cert:** Internal Medicine 1987; Cardiovascular Disease 2001; **Med School:** Yale Univ 1984; **Resid:** Internal Medicine, New England Med Ctr 1986; **Fellow:** Cardiology Research, Natl Inst Hlth 1989; Cardiovascular Disease, Beth Israel Hosp 1991; **Fac Appt:** Prof Med, Dartmouth Med Sch

Stevenson, Lynne W MD [Cv] - **Spec Exp:** Heart Failure; Cardiomyopathy; Transplant Medicine-Heart; **Hospital:** Brigham & Women's Hosp; **Address:** Brigham & Women's Hospital, 75 Francis St, Boston, MA 02115; **Phone:** 857-307-4000; **Board Cert:** Internal Medicine 1982; Cardiovascular Disease 1985; **Med School:** Stanford Univ 1979; **Resid:** Internal Medicine, UCLA Med Ctr 1982; **Fellow:** Cardiovascular Disease, UCLA Med Ctr 1984; **Fac Appt:** Assoc Prof Med, Harvard Med Sch

Zaret, Barry L MD [Cv] - **Spec Exp:** Nuclear Cardiology; Heart Failure; Coronary Artery Disease; **Hospital:** Yale-New Haven Hosp; **Address:** 333 Cedar St, 3-FMP, New Haven, CT 06520-8017; **Phone:** 203-785-4127; **Board Cert:** Internal Medicine 1973; Cardiovascular Disease 1973; **Med School:** NYU Sch Med 1966; **Resid:** Internal Medicine, Bellevue Hosp Ctr 1969; **Fellow:** Cardiovascular Disease, Johns Hopkins Hosp 1971; **Fac Appt:** Prof Med, Yale Univ

Zusman, Randall M MD [Cv] - **Spec Exp:** Hypertension; **Hospital:** Mass Genl Hosp; **Address:** Massachusettes Hospital, Yawkey Ctr, 55 Fruit St, Ste 5928, Boston, MA 02114; **Phone:** 617-726-7790; **Board Cert:** Internal Medicine 1976; Cardiovascular Disease 1983; **Med School:** Yale Univ 1973; **Resid:** Internal Medicine, Mass General Hosp 1978; Internal Medicine, Natl Heart, Lung, & Blood Inst (NHBLI) 1977; **Fellow:** Cardiovascular Disease, Mass General Hosp 1979; **Fac Appt:** Assoc Prof Med, Harvard Med Sch

Mid Atlantic

Blumenthal, David S MD [Cv] - **Spec Exp:** Heart Valve Disease; Preventive Cardiology; Coronary Artery Disease; Atherosclerosis; **Hospital:** NY-Presby Hosp/Weill Cornell (page 66); **Address:** 407 E 70th St, Fl 1, New York, NY 10021-5302; **Phone:** 212-861-3222; **Board Cert:** Internal Medicine 1978; Cardiovascular Disease 1981; **Med School:** Cornell Univ-Weill Med Coll 1975; **Resid:** Internal Medicine, New York Hosp 1978; Internal Medicine, New York Hosp 1981; **Fellow:** Cardiovascular Disease, Johns Hopkins Hosp 1980; **Fac Appt:** Clin Prof Med, Cornell Univ-Weill Med Coll

America's Top Doctors® 8th Edition

Blumenthal, Roger S MD [Cv] - **Spec Exp:** Preventive Cardiology; Hypertension; Cardiovascular Disease/Young Adult; **Hospital:** Johns Hopkins Hosp - Baltimore (page 61); **Address:** Johns Hopkins Hospital, Div Cardiology, 600 N Wolfe St Blalock Bldg - rm 524C, Baltimore, MD 21287; **Phone:** 410-955-7376; **Board Cert:** Internal Medicine 1988; Cardiovascular Disease 2003; **Med School:** Cornell Univ-Weill Med Coll 1985; **Resid:** Internal Medicine, Johns Hopkins Hosp 1988; **Fellow:** Cardiovascular Disease, Johns Hopkins Hosp 1992; **Fac Appt:** Assoc Prof Med, Johns Hopkins Univ

Borer, Jeffrey MD [Cv] - **Spec Exp:** Heart Valve Disease; Heart Failure; Nuclear Cardiology; **Hospital:** NY-Presby Hosp/Weill Cornell (page 66); **Address:** NY Presby Hosp, Gilman Inst Heart Dis, 525 E 68th St, Box 118, New York, NY 10065-4870; **Phone:** 212-746-4646; **Board Cert:** Internal Medicine 1973; Cardiovascular Disease 1975; **Med School:** Cornell Univ-Weill Med Coll 1969; **Resid:** Internal Medicine, Mass Genl Hosp 1971; **Fellow:** Cardiovascular Disease, Natl Heart, Lung & Blood Inst 1974; Cardiovascular Disease, Guy's Hosp 1975; **Fac Appt:** Prof Med, Cornell Univ-Weill Med Coll

Bove, Alfred A MD/PhD [Cv] - **Spec Exp:** Diving Medicine; Heart Failure; Sports Medicine; **Hospital:** Temple Univ Hosp; **Address:** Temple Univ Hosp, Div Cardiology, 3401 N Broad St, Parkinson Pavillon, Philadelphia, PA 19140; **Phone:** 215-707-5757; **Board Cert:** Internal Medicine 1971; Cardiovascular Disease 1983; Undersea & Hyperbaric Medicine 2000; **Med School:** Temple Univ 1966; **Resid:** Internal Medicine, Temple Univ Hosp 1970; **Fellow:** Physiology, Temple Univ Hosp 1970; Physiology, Mayo Clinic 1971; **Fac Appt:** Prof Emeritus Med, Temple Univ

Brozena, Susan C MD [Cv] - **Spec Exp:** Transplant Medicine-Heart; Congestive Heart Failure; Heart Disease in Women; **Hospital:** Hosp Univ Penn - UPHS (page 60); **Address:** Hosp Univ Penn, Div Cardiovascular Med, 3400 Spruce St, 6 Penn Tower, Philadelphia, PA 19104-4283; **Phone:** 215-615-0800; **Board Cert:** Internal Medicine 1984; Cardiovascular Disease 1987; **Med School:** Temple Univ 1981; **Resid:** Internal Medicine, Temple Univ Hosp 1984; **Fellow:** Cardiovascular Disease, Temple Univ Hosp 1986; **Fac Appt:** Assoc Prof Med, Univ Pennsylvania

Cohen, Howard A MD [Cv] - **Spec Exp:** Interventional Cardiology; Carotid Artery Stent Placement; **Hospital:** Lenox Hill Hosp (page 62); **Address:** Lenox Hill Hospital, Interventional Cardiology, 130 E 77th St Fl 9, New York, NY 10021; **Phone:** 212-434-6401; **Board Cert:** Internal Medicine 1976; Cardiovascular Disease 1977; **Med School:** NYU Sch Med 1970; **Resid:** Internal Medicine, Bellevue Hosp Ctr 1974; **Fellow:** Cardiovascular Disease, Johns Hopkins Hosp 1976

Coppola, John T MD [Cv] - **Spec Exp:** Cardiac Catheterization; Angioplasty; **Hospital:** St Vincent Cath Med Ctrs - Manhattan; **Address:** 275 7th Ave Fl 3, New York, NY 10001; **Phone:** 646-660-9999; **Board Cert:** Internal Medicine 1981; Cardiovascular Disease 1983; Interventional Cardiology 1999; **Med School:** NY Med Coll 1978; **Resid:** Internal Medicine, St Vincent Catholic Med Ctr 1981; **Fellow:** Cardiovascular Disease, St Vincent Catholic Med Ctr 1983

Devereux, Richard B MD [Cv] - **Spec Exp:** Marfan's Syndrome; **Hospital:** NY-Presby Hosp/Weill Cornell (page 66); **Address:** 525 E 68th St, rm K-415, New York, NY 10021-4870; **Phone:** 212-746-4655; **Board Cert:** Internal Medicine 1974; Cardiovascular Disease 1977; **Med School:** Univ Pennsylvania 1971; **Resid:** Internal Medicine, New York Hosp 1974; **Fellow:** Cardiovascular Disease, Hosp Univ Penn 1976; **Fac Appt:** Prof Med, Cornell Univ-Weill Med Coll

Edmundowicz, Daniel MD [Cv] - **Spec Exp:** Preventive Cardiology; Cholesterol/Lipid Disorders; **Hospital:** UPMC Presby, Pittsburgh, Magee-Womens Hosp - UPMC; **Address:** Cardiovascular Inst at Univ Center, 120 Lytton Ave, Ste 302, Pittsburgh, PA 15213; **Phone:** 412-802-3010; **Board Cert:** Internal Medicine 2005; Cardiovascular Disease 1998; **Med School:** Hahnemann Univ 1990; **Resid:** Internal Medicine, Temple Univ Hosp 1993; **Fellow:** Cardiovascular Disease, Univ Pittsburgh Med Ctr 1996; **Fac Appt:** Assoc Prof Med, Univ Pittsburgh

Cardiovascular Disease

Eisen, Howard J MD [Cv] - **Spec Exp:** Transplant Medicine-Heart; Congestive Heart Failure; **Hospital:** Hahnemann Univ Hosp; **Address:** Drexel Univ Coll Med, Div Cardiology, 245 N 15th St, MS 1012, Philadelphia, PA 19102; **Phone:** 215-762-3829; **Board Cert:** Internal Medicine 1984; Cardiovascular Disease 1987; **Med School:** Univ Pennsylvania 1981; **Resid:** Internal Medicine, Hosp Univ Penn 1984; **Fellow:** Cardiovascular Disease, Barnes Jewish Hosp 1987; **Fac Appt:** Prof Med, Drexel Univ Coll Med

Follansbee, William P MD [Cv] - **Spec Exp:** Nuclear Cardiology; **Hospital:** UPMC Presby, Pittsburgh; **Address:** UPMC Cardiovascular Inst, 200 Lothrop St, Ste 5B, Pittsburgh, PA 15213; **Phone:** 412-647-3437; **Board Cert:** Internal Medicine 1977; Cardiovascular Disease 1981; **Med School:** Univ Pennsylvania 1974; **Resid:** Internal Medicine, Hosp Univ Penn 1979; **Fellow:** Cardiovascular Disease, Hosp Univ Penn 1978; **Fac Appt:** Prof Med, Univ Pittsburgh

Friedman, Sanford MD [Cv] - **Spec Exp:** Preventive Cardiology; **Hospital:** Mount Sinai Med Ctr (page 64); **Address:** 103 E 81st St, New York, NY 10028; **Phone:** 212-988-3772; **Board Cert:** Internal Medicine 1980; Cardiovascular Disease 1977; **Med School:** Tufts Univ 1971; **Resid:** Internal Medicine, Mt Sinai Med Ctr 1974; **Fellow:** Cardiovascular Disease, Mt Sinai Med Ctr 1976; **Fac Appt:** Assoc Clin Prof Med, Mount Sinai Sch Med

Fuster, Valentin MD/PhD [Cv] - **Spec Exp:** Coronary Artery Disease; Heart Valve Disease; Congenital Heart Disease; Atherosclerosis; **Hospital:** Mount Sinai Med Ctr (page 64); **Address:** One Gustave L Levy Pl, Box 1030, New York, NY 10029-6500; **Phone:** 212-241-7911; **Board Cert:** Internal Medicine 1976; Cardiovascular Disease 1977; **Med School:** Spain 1967; **Resid:** Internal Medicine, Mayo Clinic 1972; Cardiovascular Disease, Mayo Clinic 1974; **Fellow:** Cardiovascular Disease, Univ Edinburgh 1971; **Fac Appt:** Prof Med, Mount Sinai Sch Med

Gliklich, Jerry MD [Cv] - **Spec Exp:** Heart Valve Disease; Arrhythmias; **Hospital:** NY-Presby Hosp/Columbia (page 66); **Address:** 161 Fort Washington Ave, Ste 535, New York, NY 10032-3713; **Phone:** 212-305-5588; **Board Cert:** Internal Medicine 1978; Cardiovascular Disease 1981; **Med School:** Columbia P&S 1975; **Resid:** Internal Medicine, New York Hosp 1978; **Fellow:** Cardiovascular Disease, Columbia-Presby Med Ctr 1981; **Fac Appt:** Clin Prof Med, Columbia P&S

Gottdiener, John S MD [Cv] - **Spec Exp:** Echocardiography; **Hospital:** Univ of MD Med Sys; **Address:** 22 S Greene St, rm S3B08, Baltimore, MD 21201; **Phone:** 410-328-6190; **Board Cert:** Internal Medicine 1975; Cardiovascular Disease 1979; **Med School:** Georgetown Univ 1970; **Resid:** Internal Medicine, Univ NC Hosp 1972; **Fellow:** Cardiovascular Disease, Georgetown Univ Hosp 1976; **Fac Appt:** Prof Med, Univ MD Sch Med

Gottlieb, Stephen Scott MD [Cv] - **Spec Exp:** Heart Failure; Transplant Medicine-Heart; **Hospital:** Univ of MD Med Sys; **Address:** Univ Maryland Med Ctr, Cardiology, 22 S Greene St, rm S3B08, Baltimore, MD 21201; **Phone:** 410-328-8788; **Board Cert:** Internal Medicine 1984; Cardiovascular Disease 1987; **Med School:** Brown Univ 1981; **Resid:** Internal Medicine, Univ Chicago Hosps 1984; **Fellow:** Cardiovascular Disease, Mt Sinai Hosp 1985; **Fac Appt:** Prof Med, Univ MD Sch Med

Greenberg, Mark MD [Cv] - **Spec Exp:** Interventional Cardiology; Cardiac Catheterization; Cardiac Consultation; Heart Valve Disease; **Hospital:** Montefiore Med Ctr; **Address:** 111 E 210th St, Division of Cardiology, Bronx, NY 10467; **Phone:** 718-920-4212; **Board Cert:** Internal Medicine 1973; Cardiovascular Disease 1979; Interventional Cardiology 1999; **Med School:** Univ IL Coll Med 1973; **Resid:** Internal Medicine, Montefiore Hosp Med Ctr 1976; **Fellow:** Cardiovascular Disease, Montefiore Hosp Med Ctr 1978; **Fac Appt:** Clin Prof Med, Albert Einstein Coll Med

Halperin, Jonathan L MD [Cv] - **Spec Exp:** Peripheral Vascular Disease; Atrial Fibrillation; **Hospital:** Mount Sinai Med Ctr (page 64); **Address:** 1190 5th Ave, New York, NY 10029; **Phone:** 212-241-7243; **Board Cert:** Internal Medicine 1980; Cardiovascular Disease 1981; **Med School:** Boston Univ 1975; **Resid:** Internal Medicine, Mass Genl Hosp 1977; **Fellow:** Vascular Medicine, Boston Univ Med Ctr 1978; Cardiovascular Disease, Boston Univ Med Ctr 1980; **Fac Appt:** Prof Med, Mount Sinai Sch Med

Herling, Irving M MD [Cv] - **Spec Exp:** Cholesterol/Lipid Disorders; Preventive Cardiology; **Hospital:** Hosp Univ Penn - UPHS (page 60); **Address:** Hosp Univ Penn, Div Cardiology, 3400 Spruce St, Ste 800 Penn Tower, Philadelphia, PA 19104; **Phone:** 215-662-6020; **Board Cert:** Internal Medicine 1977; Cardiovascular Disease 1979; **Med School:** Univ Pennsylvania 1974; **Resid:** Internal Medicine, Hosp Univ Penn 1977; **Fellow:** Cardiovascular Disease, Hosp Univ Penn 1979; **Fac Appt:** Assoc Prof Med, Univ Pennsylvania

Inra, Lawrence A MD [Cv] - **Spec Exp:** Coronary Artery Disease; Heart Valve Disease; Cholesterol/Lipid Disorders; Hypertension; **Hospital:** NY-Presby Hosp/Weill Cornell (page 66), Hosp For Special Surgery (page 59); **Address:** 407 E 70th St, New York, NY 10021; **Phone:** 212-249-1011; **Board Cert:** Internal Medicine 1979; Cardiovascular Disease 1981; **Med School:** Johns Hopkins Univ 1976; **Resid:** Internal Medicine, New York Hosp 1979; **Fellow:** Cardiovascular Disease, Mount Sinai Hosp 1981; **Fac Appt:** Assoc Prof Med, Cornell Univ-Weill Med Coll

Kostis, John B MD [Cv] - **Spec Exp:** Hypertension; Coronary Artery Disease; Cholesterol/Lipid Disorders; **Hospital:** Robert Wood Johnson Univ Hosp - New Brunswick; **Address:** UMDNJ-Robert Wood Johnson Med School, 1 Robert Wood Johnson Pl, Box 19, New Brunswick, NJ 08903-0019; **Phone:** 732-235-7685; **Board Cert:** Internal Medicine 1973; Cardiovascular Disease 1973; **Med School:** Greece 1960; **Resid:** Internal Medicine, Evanglismos Hosp 1964; Internal Medicine, Cumberland Med Ctr 1967; **Fellow:** Cardiovascular Disease, Philadelphia Genl Hosp 1969; **Fac Appt:** Prof Med, UMDNJ-RW Johnson Med Sch

Mather, Paul MD [Cv] - **Spec Exp:** Heart Failure; Transplant Medicine-Heart; **Hospital:** Thomas Jefferson Univ Hosp; **Address:** 925 Chesnut St, Mezzanine, Philadelphia, PA 19107; **Board Cert:** Internal Medicine 2002; Cardiovascular Disease 1995; **Med School:** Temple Univ 1988; **Resid:** Internal Medicine, Temple Univ 1991; **Fellow:** Cardiovascular Disease, Temple Univ 1994; **Fac Appt:** Assoc Prof Med, Temple Univ

Meller, Jose MD [Cv] - **Spec Exp:** Cardiac Catheterization; Hypertension; Angioplasty; **Hospital:** Mount Sinai Med Ctr (page 64); **Address:** 103 E 81st St, New York, NY 10028; **Phone:** 212-988-3772; **Board Cert:** Internal Medicine 1973; Cardiovascular Disease 1975; **Med School:** Chile 1969; **Resid:** Internal Medicine, Elmhurst Hosp 1971; Internal Medicine, Mt Sinai Med Ctr 1972; **Fellow:** Cardiovascular Disease, Mt Sinai Med Ctr 1974; **Fac Appt:** Prof Med, Mount Sinai Sch Med

Mosca, Lori J MD/PhD [Cv] - **Spec Exp:** Preventive Cardiology; **Hospital:** NY-Presby Hosp/Columbia (page 66); **Address:** NY Presby Med Ctr, Div Preventive Cardiology, 622 W 168th St, PH10-203D, New York, NY 10032; **Phone:** 212-305-4866; **Board Cert:** Internal Medicine 1989; **Med School:** SUNY Upstate Med Univ 1984; **Resid:** Internal Medicine, SUNYHealth Sci Ctr 1987; **Fellow:** Cardiovascular Disease, Columbia Presby Med Ctr 1991; Epidemiology, Columbia Presby Med Ctr 1992; **Fac Appt:** Assoc Prof Med, Columbia P&S

Cardiovascular Disease

Naccarelli, Gerald V MD [Cv] - **Spec Exp:** Cardiac Electrophysiology; Pacemakers; Arrhythmias; **Hospital:** Penn State Milton S Hershey Med Ctr; **Address:** Heart & Vascular Institute, 500 University Drive, rm H1511, PO Box 850, MC HO47, Hershey, PA 17033; **Phone:** 717-531-3907; **Board Cert:** Internal Medicine 1979; Cardiovascular Disease 1981; **Med School:** Penn State Univ-Hershey Med Ctr 1976; **Resid:** Internal Medicine, NC Bapt Hosp 1978; Internal Medicine, Hershey Med Ctr 1979; **Fellow:** Cardiovascular Disease, Indiana Univ Med Ctr 1982; **Fac Appt:** Prof Med, Penn State Univ-Hershey Med Ctr

Parrillo, Joseph E MD [Cv] - **Spec Exp:** Septic Shock; Cardiogenic shock; Heart Failure; **Hospital:** Cooper Univ Hosp; **Address:** Cooper Medical Ctr, Div Cardiology, 1 Cooper Plaza, Dorrance Bldg, Ste D384, Camden, NJ 08103; **Phone:** 856-342-8349; **Board Cert:** Internal Medicine 1975; Allergy & Immunology 1977; Cardiovascular Disease 1981; Critical Care Medicine 2005; **Med School:** Cornell Univ-Weill Med Coll 1972; **Resid:** Internal Medicine, Mass General Hosp 1975; Allergy & Immunology, NIH 1978; **Fellow:** Cardiovascular Disease, Mass General Hosp 1980; **Fac Appt:** Prof Med, UMDNJ-RW Johnson Med Sch

Plehn, Jonathan MD [Cv] - **Spec Exp:** Echocardiography; Congestive Heart Failure; Heart Valve Disease; **Hospital:** Natl Naval Med Ctr, Natl Inst of Hlth - Clin Ctr; **Address:** Natl Naval Med Ctr, Div of Cardiology, 8901 Wisconsin Ave, Bethesda, MD 20889; **Phone:** 301-295-4484; **Board Cert:** Internal Medicine 1981; Cardiovascular Disease 1983; **Med School:** NYU Sch Med 1977; **Resid:** Internal Medicine, Montefiore Hosp 1980; Cardiovascular Disease, Montefiore Hosp 1981; **Fellow:** Cardiovascular Disease, Rush Presby-St Lukes Hosp 1983

Poon, Michael MD [Cv] - **Spec Exp:** Coronary Artery Disease; Pulmonary Hypertension; Cardiac CT Angiography; Cardiac Imaging; **Hospital:** Mount Sinai Med Ctr (page 64), Beth Israel Med Ctr - Petrie Division (page 57); **Address:** 80 Bowery St, rm 502, New York, NY 10013; **Phone:** 917-254-4088; **Board Cert:** Cardiovascular Disease 1997; **Med School:** Mount Sinai Sch Med 1987; **Resid:** Internal Medicine, Mount Sinai Med Ctr 1991; **Fellow:** Cardiovascular Disease, Mount Sinai Med Ctr 1993; **Fac Appt:** Assoc Prof Med, Mount Sinai Sch Med

Reis, Steven E MD [Cv] - **Spec Exp:** Heart Disease in Women; Congestive Heart Failure; Syndrome X; Preventive Cardiology; **Hospital:** UPMC Presby, Pittsburgh, Magee-Womens Hosp - UPMC; **Address:** UPMC Cardiovascular Inst at Univ Ctr, 120 Lytton Ave, Ste 100B, Pittsburgh, PA 15213; **Phone:** 412-802-3000; **Board Cert:** Internal Medicine 2000; Cardiovascular Disease 2000; **Med School:** Harvard Med Sch 1987; **Resid:** Internal Medicine, Brigham & Womens Hosp 1990; **Fellow:** Cardiovascular Disease, Johns Hopkins Hosp 1994; **Fac Appt:** Assoc Prof Med, Univ Pittsburgh

Sacchi, Terrence J MD [Cv] - **Spec Exp:** Arrhythmias; Cardiac Catheterization; Coronary Angioplasty/Stents; **Hospital:** New York Methodist Hosp; **Address:** 506 6th St, Brooklyn, NY 11215; **Phone:** 718-780-7830; **Board Cert:** Internal Medicine 1979; Cardiovascular Disease 1981; Interventional Cardiology 1999; **Med School:** Albany Med Coll 1976; **Resid:** Internal Medicine, St Vincents Hosp 1979; **Fellow:** Cardiovascular Disease, Georgetown Univ Hosp 1981; Interventional Cardiology, Mercy Hospital 1986; **Fac Appt:** Assoc Clin Prof Med, SUNY Downstate

Saunders, Elijah MD [Cv] - **Spec Exp:** Hypertension-Complex; Coronary Disease in Black Populations; **Hospital:** Univ of MD Med Sys; **Address:** Univ MD Med Sch, Div Hypertension, 419 W Redwood St, Ste 620, Baltimore, MD 21201; **Phone:** 410-328-4366; **Med School:** Univ MD Sch Med 1960; **Resid:** Internal Medicine, Univ Maryland Med Ctr; **Fellow:** Cardiovascular Disease, Univ Maryland Med Ctr; **Fac Appt:** Prof Med, Univ MD Sch Med

Schulman, Steven P MD [Cv] - **Hospital:** Johns Hopkins Hosp - Baltimore (page 61); **Address:** 600 N Wolfe St, Carnegie 568, Baltimore, MD 21287; **Phone:** 410-955-7378; **Board Cert:** Internal Medicine 1986; Cardiovascular Disease 1989; **Med School:** Johns Hopkins Univ 1981; **Resid:** Internal Medicine, Johns Hopkins Hosp 1984; **Fellow:** Cardiovascular Disease, Johns Hopkins Hosp 1988; **Fac Appt:** Assoc Prof Med, Johns Hopkins Univ

Schwartz, Allan MD [Cv] - **Spec Exp:** Interventional Cardiology; Cardiac Catheterization; Mitral Valve Disease; **Hospital:** NY-Presby Hosp/Columbia (page 66); **Address:** 161 Ft Washington Ave, Ste 551, New York, NY 10032-3713; **Phone:** 212-305-5367; **Board Cert:** Internal Medicine 1977; Cardiovascular Disease 1979; **Med School:** Columbia P&S 1974; **Resid:** Internal Medicine, Columbia-Presby Med Ctr 1976; **Fellow:** Cardiovascular Disease, Mass Genl Hosp 1978; **Fac Appt:** Clin Prof Med, Columbia P&S

Schwartz, William MD [Cv] - **Spec Exp:** Coronary Artery Disease; Cardiac Catheterization; Congestive Heart Failure; **Hospital:** Lenox Hill Hosp (page 62), Mount Sinai Med Ctr (page 64); **Address:** 150 E 77th St, Ste 1E, Broadway Cardiopulmonary, New York, NY 10021; **Phone:** 212-439-6000; **Board Cert:** Internal Medicine 1978; Cardiovascular Disease 1981; **Med School:** Albert Einstein Coll Med 1975; **Resid:** Internal Medicine, Bronx Municipal Hosp 1978; **Fellow:** Cardiovascular Disease, Bronx Municipal Hosp 1979

Shlofmitz, Richard A MD [Cv] - **Spec Exp:** Interventional Cardiology; Cardiac Catheterization; **Hospital:** St Francis Hosp - The Heart Ctr (page 72); **Address:** 100 Port Washington Blvd, Ste 105, Roslyn, NY 11576-1353; **Phone:** 516-390-9640; **Board Cert:** Internal Medicine 1984; Cardiovascular Disease 1987; **Med School:** NYU Sch Med 1980; **Resid:** Internal Medicine, North Shore Univ Hosp 1984; **Fellow:** Cardiovascular Disease, Columbia Presby Med Ctr 1987

Smart, Frank W MD [Cv] - **Spec Exp:** Congestive Heart Failure; Transplant Medicine-Heart; Ventricular Assist Device (LVAD); **Hospital:** Morristown Mem Hosp, Overlook Hosp; **Address:** Morristown Meml Hosp, Dept Cardiology, 100 Madison Ave, Box 5, Morristown, NJ 07962; **Phone:** 973-971-4179; **Board Cert:** Internal Medicine 1988; Cardiovascular Disease 2001; **Med School:** Louisiana State U, New Orleans 1985; **Resid:** Internal Medicine, Ochsner Fdn Hosp 1988; **Fellow:** Cardiovascular Disease, Baylor Coll Med 1991

Steingart, Richard MD [Cv] - **Spec Exp:** Heart Failure; Nuclear Cardiology; Heart Disease in Cancer Patients; **Hospital:** Meml Sloan-Kettering Cancer Ctr; **Address:** 1275 York Avenue, New York, NY 10065; **Phone:** 800-525-2225; **Board Cert:** Internal Medicine 1977; Cardiovascular Disease 1979; **Med School:** Mount Sinai Sch Med 1974; **Resid:** Internal Medicine, Yale-New Haven Hosp 1977; **Fellow:** Cardiovascular Disease, Mt Sinai Med Ctr 1979; **Fac Appt:** Prof Med, Cornell Univ-Weill Med Coll

Tenenbaum, Joseph MD [Cv] - **Spec Exp:** Heart Valve Disease; Coronary Artery Disease; Atrial Fibrillation; **Hospital:** NY-Presby Hosp/Columbia (page 66); **Address:** 161 Ft Washington Ave, Ste 535, Irving Pavilion, New York, NY 10032-3713; **Phone:** 212-305-5288; **Board Cert:** Internal Medicine 1977; Cardiovascular Disease 1979; **Med School:** Harvard Med Sch 1974; **Resid:** Internal Medicine, Columbia-Presby Med Ctr 1977; **Fellow:** Cardiovascular Disease, Mt Sinai Hosp 1979; **Fac Appt:** Clin Prof Med, Columbia P&S

Waxman, Harvey L MD [Cv] - **Spec Exp:** Arrhythmias; Cardiac Catheterization; Heart Valve Disease; **Hospital:** Penn Presby Med Ctr - UPHS (page 60); **Address:** Penn Presby Med Ctr, Philadelphia Heart Institute, 39th & Market Sts, 4PHI, Philadelphia, PA 19104; **Phone:** 215-662-9000; **Board Cert:** Internal Medicine 1977; Cardiovascular Disease 1979; Cardiac Electrophysiology 2002; **Med School:** Mount Sinai Sch Med 1974; **Resid:** Internal Medicine, Bellevue Hosp 1977; **Fellow:** Cardiovascular Disease, Jackson Meml Hosp 1979; Cardiac Electrophysiology, Hosp Univ Penn 1980; **Fac Appt:** Clin Prof Med, Univ Pennsylvania

Webb, Gary D MD [Cv] - **Spec Exp:** Congenital Heart Disease-Adult; **Hospital:** Hosp Univ Penn - UPHS (page 60); **Address:** Philadelphia Adult Congenital Heart Ctr, 3400 Spruce St, Penn Tower Fl 6, Philadelphia, PA 19104; **Phone:** 215-615-3388; **Board Cert:** Internal Medicine ; Cardiovascular Disease ; **Med School:** McGill Univ 1967; **Resid:** Internal Medicine, Royal Victoria Hosp 1972; **Fellow:** Cardiovascular Disease, Toronto Genl Hosp 1974

Cardiovascular Disease

Weitz, Howard H MD [Cv] - **Spec Exp:** Preventive Cardiology; **Hospital:** Thomas Jefferson Univ Hosp; **Address:** Jefferson Heart Institute, 925 Chestnut St, Mezzanine Level, Philadelphia, PA 19107; **Phone:** 215-955-4194; **Board Cert:** Internal Medicine 1981; Cardiovascular Disease 1985; **Med School:** Thomas Jefferson Univ 1978; **Resid:** Internal Medicine, Thos Jefferson Univ Hosp 1982; **Fellow:** Cardiovascular Disease, Thos Jefferson Univ Hosp 1984; **Fac Appt:** Prof Med, Thomas Jefferson Univ

Southeast

Bashore, Thomas M MD [Cv] - **Spec Exp:** Heart Valve Disease; Pulmonary Hypertension; Congenital Heart Disease-Adult; **Hospital:** Duke Univ Med Ctr; **Address:** Duke Univ Med Ctr, PO Box 3012, Durham, NC 27710-0001; **Phone:** 919-684-2407; **Board Cert:** Internal Medicine 1975; Cardiovascular Disease 1977; **Med School:** Ohio State Univ 1972; **Resid:** Internal Medicine, NC Meml Hosp 1975; **Fellow:** Cardiovascular Disease, Duke Univ Med Ctr 1977; **Fac Appt:** Prof Med, Duke Univ

Bass, Theodore A MD [Cv] - **Spec Exp:** Interventional Cardiology; **Hospital:** Shands Jacksonville; **Address:** Health Science Center/Jacksonville, 655 W 8th St ACC Bldg Fl 5, Jacksonville, FL 32209; **Phone:** 904-244-2655; **Board Cert:** Internal Medicine 1979; Cardiovascular Disease 1981; Interventional Cardiology 2001; **Med School:** Brown Univ 1976; **Resid:** Internal Medicine, Mayo Clinic 1979; **Fellow:** Cardiovascular Disease, University Hosp 1981; **Fac Appt:** Prof Med, Univ Fla Coll Med

Beller, George A MD [Cv] - **Spec Exp:** Coronary Artery Disease; Nuclear Cardiology; **Hospital:** Univ Virginia Med Ctr; **Address:** UVA Hlth Systems, Cardiology Dept, Box 800158, Charlottesville, VA 22908-0158; **Phone:** 434-924-2134; **Board Cert:** Internal Medicine 1971; Cardiovascular Disease 1977; **Med School:** Univ VA Sch Med 1966; **Resid:** Internal Medicine, Univ Wisconsin Hosps 1968; Cardiovascular Disease, Boston City Hosp 1970; **Fellow:** Cardiovascular Disease, Mass Genl Hosp 1974; **Fac Appt:** Prof Med, Univ VA Sch Med

Borzak, Steven MD [Cv] - **Spec Exp:** Coronary Artery Disease; Arrhythmias; Heart Failure; Cholesterol/Lipid Disorders; **Hospital:** JFK Med Ctr - Atlantis, Bethesda Memorial Hosp; **Address:** 110 JFK Drive, Ste 110, Atlantis, FL 33462-1146; **Phone:** 561-641-9541; **Board Cert:** Internal Medicine 1987; Cardiovascular Disease 2001; **Med School:** Univ IL Coll Med 1984; **Resid:** Internal Medicine, Michael Reese Hosp 1988; **Fellow:** Cardiovascular Disease, Brigham & Womens Hosp 1991; **Fac Appt:** Prof Med, Nova SE Univ, Coll Osteo Med

Bourge, Robert C MD [Cv] - **Spec Exp:** Heart Failure; Transplant Medicine-Heart; Pulmonary Hypertension; **Hospital:** Univ of Ala Hosp at Birmingham; **Address:** UAB Div Cardiovascular Disease, 311 THT, 1900 University Blvd, Birmingham, AL 35294-0001; **Phone:** 205-934-3624; **Board Cert:** Internal Medicine 1982; Cardiovascular Disease 1985; Nuclear Medicine 1987; **Med School:** Louisiana State U, New Orleans 1979; **Resid:** Internal Medicine, Univ Alabama Hosps 1982; Nuclear Medicine, Univ Alabama Hosps 1985; **Fellow:** Cardiovascular Disease, Univ Alabama Hosps 1984; **Fac Appt:** Prof Med, Univ Ala

Byrd III, Benjamin F MD [Cv] - **Spec Exp:** Congenital Heart Disease; Echocardiography; **Hospital:** Vanderbilt Univ Med Ctr; **Address:** Vanderbilt Heart Inst, 1215 21st Ave, MCE S Tower, Ste 5209, Nashville, TN 37232; **Phone:** 615-322-2318; **Board Cert:** Internal Medicine 1981; Cardiovascular Disease 1983; **Med School:** Vanderbilt Univ 1977; **Resid:** Psychiatry, Harvard Univ 1979; Internal Medicine, Vanderbilt Univ Hosp 1981; **Fellow:** Cardiovascular Disease, Vanderbilt Univ Hosp 1983; Cardiovascular Disease, UCSF 1984; **Fac Appt:** Assoc Prof Med, Vanderbilt Univ

Califf, Robert M MD [Cv] - **Spec Exp:** Coronary Artery Disease; Cholesterol/Lipid Disorders; Heart Failure; **Hospital:** Duke Univ Med Ctr; **Address:** 2400 Pratt St, Ste 0311, Durham, NC 27705; **Phone:** 919-681-5816; **Board Cert:** Internal Medicine 1984; Cardiovascular Disease 1985; **Med School:** Duke Univ 1978; **Resid:** Internal Medicine, UCSF Med Ctr 1980; **Fellow:** Cardiovascular Disease, Duke Univ Med Ctr 1983; **Fac Appt:** Prof Med, Duke Univ

Chizner, Michael A MD [Cv] - **Hospital:** Broward General Med Ctr, Imperial Point Med Ctr; **Address:** 1625 SE 3rd Ave, Ste 300, Fort Lauderdale, FL 33316; **Phone:** 954-355-5001; **Board Cert:** Internal Medicine 1977; Cardiovascular Disease 1979; **Med School:** Cornell Univ-Weill Med Coll 1974; **Resid:** Internal Medicine, New York Hosp 1976; **Fellow:** Cardiovascular Disease, Georgetown Affil Hosps 1979; **Fac Appt:** Clin Prof Med, Univ Miami Sch Med

Clements Jr, Stephen MD [Cv] - **Spec Exp:** Cardiac Catheterization; Echocardiography; **Hospital:** Emory Univ Hosp; **Address:** Emory Clinic, 1365 Clifton Rd NE Bldg A, Atlanta, GA 30322; **Phone:** 404-778-3468; **Board Cert:** Internal Medicine 1971; Cardiovascular Disease 1975; **Med School:** Med Coll GA 1966; **Resid:** Internal Medicine, Grady Meml Hosp 1970; **Fellow:** Cardiovascular Disease, Emory Univ Hosp 1971; **Fac Appt:** Prof Med, Emory Univ

Douglas Jr, John S MD [Cv] - **Spec Exp:** Interventional Cardiology; Cardiac Catheterization; Coronary Artery Disease; **Hospital:** Emory Univ Hosp; **Address:** Emory Univ Hosp, 1364 Clifton Rd, rm F606, Atlanta, GA 30322; **Phone:** 404-727-7040; **Board Cert:** Internal Medicine 1972; Cardiovascular Disease 1975; Interventional Cardiology 1999; **Med School:** Washington Univ, St Louis 1967; **Resid:** Internal Medicine, NC Memorial Hosp 1969; Internal Medicine, Grady Memorial Hosp 1972; **Fellow:** Cardiovascular Disease, Emory Affil Hosps 1974; **Fac Appt:** Prof Med, Emory Univ

Gandy Jr, Winston MD [Cv] - **Spec Exp:** Echocardiography; Invasive Cardiology; **Hospital:** Piedmont Hosp; **Address:** Atlanta Cardiology Group, 95 Collier Rd, Ste 5015, Atlanta, GA 30309; **Phone:** 404-605-5100; **Board Cert:** Internal Medicine 1989; Cardiovascular Disease 2002; **Med School:** Howard Univ 1986; **Resid:** Internal Medicine, Emory Univ 1989; **Fellow:** Cardiovascular Disease, Univ Alabama 1992

Hare, Joshua M MD [Cv] - **Spec Exp:** Heart Failure; Stem Cell Therapy in Heart Failure; **Hospital:** Univ of Miami Hosp & Clins/Sylvester Comp Canc Ctr; **Address:** University of Miami, Miller School, 1120 NW 14th St, Ste 1124, Miami, FL 33136; **Phone:** 305-243-1998; **Board Cert:** Cardiovascular Disease 2006; **Med School:** Johns Hopkins Univ 1988; **Resid:** Internal Medicine, Johns Hopkins Hosp 1991; **Fellow:** Cardiovascular Disease, Brigham & Women's Hosp 1993

Harrison, John K MD [Cv] - **Spec Exp:** Interventional Cardiology; Heart Valve Disease; **Hospital:** Duke Univ Med Ctr; **Address:** Duke Univ Med Ctr, PO Box 3331, Durham, NC 27710; **Phone:** 919-681-3763; **Board Cert:** Internal Medicine 1988; Cardiovascular Disease 2001; Interventional Cardiology 2003; **Med School:** NYU Sch Med 1984; **Resid:** Internal Medicine, Johns Hopkins Hosp 1987; **Fellow:** Cardiovascular Disease, Duke Univ Med Ctr 1990; **Fac Appt:** Prof Med, Duke Univ

Iskandrian, Ami E MD [Cv] - **Spec Exp:** Nuclear Cardiology; Coronary Artery Disease; Heart Valve Disease; **Hospital:** Univ of Ala Hosp at Birmingham; **Address:** Univ Alabama Birmingham, 311 LHRB, 1900 University Blvd, Birmingham, AL 35294; **Phone:** 205-934-0545; **Board Cert:** Internal Medicine 1974; Cardiovascular Disease 1975; **Med School:** Iraq 1965; **Resid:** Internal Medicine, Univ Baghdad Affil Hosp 1971; Internal Medicine, Hahnemann Univ Hosp 1973; **Fellow:** Cardiovascular Disease, Hahnemann Univ Hosp 1975; **Fac Appt:** Prof Med, Univ Ala

Cardiovascular Disease

Linton, MacRae F MD [Cv] - **Spec Exp:** Cholesterol/Lipid Disorders; Preventive Cardiology; **Hospital:** Vanderbilt Univ Med Ctr; **Address:** Vanderbilt Heart Inst, 1215 21st Ave, MCE S Tower, Ste 2509, Nashville, TN 37232-8802; **Phone:** 615-322-2318; **Board Cert:** Internal Medicine 1988; **Med School:** Univ Tenn Coll Med, Memphis 1985; **Resid:** Internal Medicine, Vanderbilt Univ Med Ctr 1988; **Fellow:** Endocrinology, UCSF Med Ctr 1991; **Fac Appt:** Prof Med, Vanderbilt Univ

Miller, D Douglas MD [Cv] - **Spec Exp:** Heart Disease in Women; Nuclear Cardiology; **Hospital:** Med Coll of GA Hosp and Clin; **Address:** Medical Coll Georgia, 1120 15th St, rm AA152, Augusta, GA 30912-4750; **Phone:** 706-721-2426; **Med School:** McGill Univ 1978; **Resid:** Internal Medicine, Montreal Genl Hosp 1981; Cardiovascular Disease, Montreal Heart Inst 1982; **Fellow:** Cardiovascular Disease, Emory Univ 1984; Nuclear Cardiology, Mass Genl Hosp-Harvard 1986; **Fac Appt:** Prof Med, St Louis Univ

Myerburg, Robert MD [Cv] - **Spec Exp:** Cardiac Electrophysiology; Arrhythmias; Pacemakers; Heart Attack; **Hospital:** Jackson Meml Hosp; **Address:** Univ Miami School Med, Div Cardiology, PO Box 016960 (D-39), Miami, FL 33101-6960; **Phone:** 305-585-5523; **Board Cert:** Internal Medicine 1968; Cardiovascular Disease 1970; **Med School:** Univ MD Sch Med 1961; **Resid:** Internal Medicine, Charity Hosp 1966; **Fellow:** Cardiovascular Disease, Grady Meml Hosp 1968; Cardiac Electrophysiology, Columbia P&S 1970; **Fac Appt:** Prof Med, Univ Miami Sch Med

Nocero Jr, Michael A MD [Cv] - **Spec Exp:** Nuclear Cardiology; **Hospital:** Florida Hosp - Orlando; **Address:** 1745 N Mills Ave, Orlando, FL 32803; **Phone:** 407-841-7151; **Board Cert:** Internal Medicine 1972; Cardiovascular Disease 1976; **Med School:** NYU Sch Med 1966; **Resid:** Internal Medicine, Bellevue Hosp Ctr NYU 1971; **Fellow:** Cardiovascular Disease, Bellevue Hosp Ctr NYU 1973

O'Neill, William W MD [Cv] - **Spec Exp:** Interventional Cardiology; Heart Valve Disease; **Hospital:** Univ of Miami Hosp & Clins/Sylvester Comp Canc Ctr; **Address:** Univ Miami Dept Medicine, 1600 NW 10 Ave, R-MSB 1122A, Miami, FL 33136; **Phone:** 305-243-9483; **Board Cert:** Internal Medicine 1980; Cardiovascular Disease 1983; Interventional Cardiology 1999; **Med School:** Wayne State Univ 1977; **Resid:** Internal Medicine, Wayne State Univ Affil Hosps 1980; **Fellow:** Cardiovascular Disease, Univ Mich Med Ctr 1982; **Fac Appt:** Prof Med, Univ Miami Sch Med

Oparil, Suzanne MD [Cv] - **Spec Exp:** Hypertension; Heart Disease in Women; **Hospital:** Univ of Ala Hosp at Birmingham; **Address:** Hypertension Program, 115 Comm Hlth Service Bldg, 933 19th St S, Birmingham, AL 35294; **Phone:** 205-934-9281; **Board Cert:** Internal Medicine 1970; **Med School:** Columbia P&S 1965; **Resid:** Internal Medicine, Columbia Presby Med Ctr 1967; Internal Medicine, Mass Genl Hosp 1968; **Fellow:** Cardiovascular Disease, Mass Genl Hosp 1971; **Fac Appt:** Prof Med, Univ Ala

Pepine, Carl J MD [Cv] - **Spec Exp:** Coronary Artery Disease; Hypertension; Heart Disease in Women; **Hospital:** Shands at Univ of FL; **Address:** Univ Florida, Div Cardiovascular Med, 1600 SW Archer Rd, Box 100277, Gainesville, FL 32610-0277; **Phone:** 352-846-0620; **Board Cert:** Internal Medicine 1971; Cardiovascular Disease 1973; **Med School:** UMDNJ-NJ Med Sch, Newark 1966; **Resid:** Internal Medicine, Jefferson Univ Hosp 1968; Internal Medicine, Naval Hosp-Thomas Jefferson Univ 1969; **Fellow:** Cardiovascular Disease, Naval Hosp-Thomas Jeff Univ 1971; **Fac Appt:** Prof Med, Univ Fla Coll Med

Phillips III, Harry R MD [Cv] - **Spec Exp:** Angioplasty; Cardiac Catheterization; **Hospital:** Duke Univ Med Ctr; **Address:** Duke Univ Med Ctr, Box 3126, Durham, NC 27710; **Phone:** 919-681-4804; **Board Cert:** Internal Medicine 1978; Cardiovascular Disease 1979; Interventional Cardiology 2001; **Med School:** Duke Univ 1975; **Resid:** Internal Medicine, Mass General Hosp 1977; **Fellow:** Cardiovascular Disease, Mass General Hosp 1979

　　　　　　　　　　　　　　　　　　　　America's Top Doctors® 8th Edition

Powers, Eric R MD [Cv] - **Spec Exp:** Heart Valve Disease; Interventional Cardiology; Coronary Artery Disease; **Hospital:** MUSC Med Ctr; **Address:** MUSC Heart & Vascular Ctr, 25 Courtenay Drive, ART 7052, MSC 592, Charleston, SC 29425-5920; **Phone:** 843-792-1152; **Board Cert:** Internal Medicine 1977; Cardiovascular Disease 1979; Interventional Cardiology 2000; **Med School:** Harvard Med Sch 1974; **Resid:** Internal Medicine, Mass Genl Hosp 1976; **Fellow:** Cardiovascular Disease, Mass Genl Hosp 1979; **Fac Appt:** Prof Med, Med Univ SC

Rogers, Joseph MD [Cv] - **Spec Exp:** Congestive Heart Failure; Transplant Medicine-Heart; **Hospital:** Duke Univ Med Ctr; **Address:** DUMC, Box 3034, Durham, NC 27710; **Phone:** 919-681-3398; **Board Cert:** Internal Medicine 1991; Cardiovascular Disease 1995; **Med School:** Univ Nebr Coll Med 1988; **Resid:** Internal Medicine, Univ Nebraska Med Ctr 1991; **Fellow:** Cardiovascular Disease, Wash Univ Med Ctr 1995; **Fac Appt:** Assoc Prof Med, Duke Univ

Smith Jr, Sidney C MD [Cv] - **Spec Exp:** Cholesterol/Lipid Disorders; Coronary Artery Disease; Invasive Cardiology; **Hospital:** Univ NC Hosps; **Address:** UNC Div Cardiology, Burnett Womack Bldg Fl 6th, 099 Manning Dr, CB 7075, Chapel Hill, NC 27599; **Phone:** 919-966-7244; **Board Cert:** Internal Medicine 1972; Cardiovascular Disease 1973; **Med School:** Yale Univ 1967; **Resid:** Internal Medicine, Peter Bent Brigham Hosp 1969; **Fellow:** Cardiovascular Disease, Peter Bent Brigham Hosp 1971; Research, Harvard Med Sch 1971; **Fac Appt:** Prof Med, Univ NC Sch Med

Vaughan, Douglas E MD [Cv] - **Spec Exp:** Bleeding/Coagulation Disorders; Cholesterol/Lipid Disorders; **Hospital:** Vanderbilt Univ Med Ctr; **Address:** Vanderbilt Heart Inst, 1215 21st Ave S, MCE-Ste 5209, South Tower, Nashville, TN 37232; **Phone:** 615-322-2318; **Board Cert:** Internal Medicine 1984; Cardiovascular Disease 1987; **Med School:** Univ Tex SW, Dallas 1980; **Resid:** Internal Medicine, Parkland Meml Hosp 1984; **Fellow:** Cardiovascular Disease, Brigham & Womens Hosp 1987; **Fac Appt:** Prof Med, Vanderbilt Univ

Vetrovec, George MD [Cv] - **Spec Exp:** Interventional Cardiology; **Hospital:** Med Coll of VA Hosp; **Address:** 1200 E Broad St, rm 607, Box 980036, West Hospital, Richmond, VA 23298; **Phone:** 804-628-1215; **Board Cert:** Internal Medicine 1974; Cardiovascular Disease 1977; Interventional Cardiology 1999; **Med School:** Univ VA Sch Med 1970; **Resid:** Internal Medicine, Med Coll Virginia Hosp 1974; **Fellow:** Cardiovascular Disease, Med Coll Virginia Hosp 1976; **Fac Appt:** Prof Med, Med Coll VA

Vignola, Paul MD [Cv] - **Spec Exp:** Interventional Cardiology; **Hospital:** Mount Sinai Med Ctr - Miami; **Address:** Mt Sinai Med Ctr, Greenspan Pavilion, 4300 Alton Rd, Ste 2110, Miami Beach, FL 33140-2800; **Phone:** 305-674-2780; **Board Cert:** Internal Medicine 1974; Cardiovascular Disease 1977; Cardiac Electrophysiology 1999; **Med School:** Yale Univ 1971; **Resid:** Internal Medicine, Yale-New Haven Hosp 1974; **Fellow:** Cardiovascular Disease, Mass Genl Hospital-Harvard 1976; **Fac Appt:** Assoc Clin Prof Med, Univ Miami Sch Med

Midwest

Armstrong, William F MD [Cv] - **Spec Exp:** Echocardiography; Cardiac Consultation; **Hospital:** Univ Michigan Hlth Sys; **Address:** 1500 E Med Ctr Drive, rm L3119, Women's/0273, Ann Arbor, MI 48109; **Phone:** 734-647-7321; **Board Cert:** Internal Medicine 1979; Cardiovascular Disease 1981; **Med School:** Med Coll VA 1976; **Resid:** Internal Medicine, Med Coll Va Hosp 1979; **Fellow:** Cardiovascular Disease, Indiana Univ Hosp 1982; **Fac Appt:** Prof Med, Univ Mich Med Sch

Cardiovascular Disease

Bonow, Robert O MD [Cv] - **Spec Exp:** Heart Valve Disease; Coronary Artery Disease; Cardiomyopathy; **Hospital:** Northwestern Meml Hosp; **Address:** Northwestern Cardiovascular Inst, 675 N St Clair St, Galter 19-100, Chicago, IL 60611; **Phone:** 312-695-4965; **Board Cert:** Internal Medicine 1976; Cardiovascular Disease 1981; **Med School:** Univ Pennsylvania 1973; **Resid:** Internal Medicine, Hosp Univ Penn 1976; **Fellow:** Cardiovascular Disease, NIH-NHLBI 1979; **Fac Appt:** Prof Med, Northwestern Univ

Braverman, Alan C MD [Cv] - **Spec Exp:** Marfan's Syndrome; Aortic Diseases & Dissection; **Hospital:** Barnes-Jewish Hosp; **Address:** Wash Univ Med Sch, Div Cardiovascular Disease, 660 S Euclid Ave, Box 8086, St Louis, MO 63110; **Phone:** 314-362-1291; **Board Cert:** Internal Medicine 1988; Cardiovascular Disease 2001; **Med School:** Univ MO-Kansas City 1985; **Resid:** Internal Medicine, Brigham & Womens Hosp 1991; **Fellow:** Cardiovascular Disease, Brigham & Womens Hosp/Harvard 1990; **Fac Appt:** Prof Med, Washington Univ, St Louis

Burket, Mark W MD [Cv] - **Spec Exp:** Peripheral Vascular Disease; Coronary Artery Disease; Percutaneous Vascular Interventions; **Hospital:** Univ of Toledo Med Ctr; **Address:** 3000 Arlington Ave, Ste 1192, Toledo, OH 43614; **Phone:** 419-383-3697; **Board Cert:** Internal Medicine 1982; Cardiovascular Disease 1985; Interventional Cardiology 1999; **Med School:** Ohio State Univ 1979; **Resid:** Internal Medicine, Ohio State Univ 1982; **Fellow:** Cardiovascular Disease, Med Coll Ohio 1985; **Fac Appt:** Prof Med, Med Univ Ohio at Toledo

Cerqueira, Manuel MD [Cv] - **Spec Exp:** Cardiac Imaging; Nuclear Cardiology; **Hospital:** Cleveland Clin Fdn (page 56); **Address:** Cleveland Clinic, 9500 Euclid Ave, MC GB3, Cleveland, OH 44195; **Phone:** 216-444-2665; **Board Cert:** Internal Medicine 1981; Nuclear Medicine 1984; Cardiovascular Disease 1989; **Med School:** NYU Sch Med 1976; **Resid:** Internal Medicine, Bellevue Hosp Ctr 1980; Cardiovascular Disease, Yale-New Haven Hosp 1982; **Fellow:** Nuclear Medicine, Yale-New Haven Hosp 1983; **Fac Appt:** Prof Med, Cleveland Cl Coll Med/Case West Res

Chaitman, Bernard R MD [Cv] - **Spec Exp:** Nuclear Cardiology; Echocardiography; **Hospital:** St Louis Univ Hosp; **Address:** Univ Club Tower, 1034 S Brentwood Blvd, Ste 1550, St Louis, MO 63117; **Phone:** 314-725-4668; **Board Cert:** Internal Medicine 1973; Cardiovascular Disease 1975; **Med School:** McGill Univ 1969; **Resid:** Internal Medicine, Royal Victoria Hosp 1972; **Fellow:** Cardiovascular Disease, Univ Oregon Hosps 1974; Cardiovascular Disease, Univ of Montreal 1975; **Fac Appt:** Prof Med, St Louis Univ

Connolly, Heidi M MD [Cv] - **Spec Exp:** Congenital Heart Disease; Carcinoid Heart Disease; Heart Disease in Pregnancy; **Hospital:** Mayo Med Ctr & Clin - Rochester; **Address:** Mayo Clinic, 200 First St SW, Gonda 6-207, Rochester, MN 55905; **Phone:** 507-284-1226; **Board Cert:** Internal Medicine 1989; Cardiovascular Disease 2001; **Med School:** Ireland 1986; **Resid:** Internal Medicine, Mayo Clinic 1989; **Fellow:** Cardiovascular Disease, Mayo Clinic 1991; **Fac Appt:** Assoc Prof Med, Mayo Med Sch

Cooper, Christopher MD [Cv] - **Spec Exp:** Renal Artery Revascularization; Interventional Cardiology; **Hospital:** Univ of Toledo Med Ctr; **Address:** University of Toledo, Cardiovascular Medicine, 3000 Arlington Ave, Ste 1192, Toledo, OH 43614-2595; **Phone:** 419-383-3963; **Board Cert:** Internal Medicine 2004; Cardiovascular Disease 2005; Interventional Cardiology 1999; **Med School:** Univ Cincinnati 1988; **Resid:** Internal Medicine, Brigham & Womens Hosp 1991; **Fellow:** Cardiovascular Disease, Brigham & Women's Hosp-Harvard Med Sch 1994; **Fac Appt:** Prof Med, Med Univ Ohio at Toledo

America's Top Doctors® 8th Edition

Eagle, Kim A MD [Cv] - **Spec Exp:** Aortic Diseases & Dissection; Acute Coronary Syndromes; Heart Attack; Peripheral Vascular Disease; **Hospital:** Univ Michigan Hlth Sys; **Address:** Dominos Farms, 24 Frank Lloyd Wright Drive, Ann Arbor, MI 48106-0363; **Phone:** 734-998-7400; **Board Cert:** Internal Medicine 1982; Cardiovascular Disease 1987; **Med School:** Tufts Univ 1979; **Resid:** Internal Medicine, Yale New Haven Hosp 1983; **Fellow:** Cardiovascular Disease, Mass Genl Hosp-Harvard 1986; **Fac Appt:** Asst Prof Med, Univ Mich Med Sch

Geltman, Edward M MD [Cv] - **Spec Exp:** Congestive Heart Failure; Transplant Medicine-Heart; Invasive Cardiology; **Hospital:** Barnes-Jewish Hosp; **Address:** Washington Univ Sch of Med, Cardiovascular Div, 660 S Euclid Ave, Box 8086, St Louis, MO 63110; **Phone:** 314-362-1291; **Board Cert:** Internal Medicine 1974; Cardiovascular Disease 1979; **Med School:** NYU Sch Med 1971; **Resid:** Internal Medicine, Bellevue Hosp 1974; **Fellow:** Cardiovascular Disease, Barnes Jewish Hosp 1978; **Fac Appt:** Prof Med, Washington Univ, St Louis

Gibbons, Raymond J MD [Cv] - **Spec Exp:** Nuclear Cardiology; Heart Attack; **Hospital:** Mayo Med Ctr & Clin - Rochester; **Address:** Mayo Clinic, Div Cardiovascular Disease, 200 First St SW, Rochester, MN 55905; **Phone:** 507-284-2541; **Board Cert:** Internal Medicine 1979; Cardiovascular Disease 1981; **Med School:** Harvard Med Sch 1976; **Resid:** Internal Medicine, Mass Genl Hosp 1978; **Fellow:** Cardiovascular Disease, Duke Univ Med Ctr 1981; **Fac Appt:** Prof Med, Mayo Med Sch

Grubb, Blair P MD [Cv] - **Spec Exp:** Autonomic Disorders; Cardiac Electrophysiology; **Hospital:** Univ of Toledo Med Ctr, St Vincent's Mercy Med Ctr - Toledo; **Address:** Med Univ Ohio - Cardiology Clinic, 3000 Arlington Ave, Toledo, OH 43614-2598; **Phone:** 419-383-3963; **Board Cert:** Internal Medicine 1985; Cardiovascular Disease 1987; **Med School:** Dominican Republic 1980; **Resid:** Internal Medicine, Grtr Baltimore Med Ctr 1985; **Fellow:** Cardiovascular Disease, MS Hershey Med Ctr/Penn State 1987; Cardiac Electrophysiology, MS Hershey Med Ctr/Penn State 1988; **Fac Appt:** Prof Med, Univ SD Sch Med

Hauptman, Paul J MD [Cv] - **Spec Exp:** Heart Failure; **Hospital:** St Louis Univ Hosp; **Address:** SLUCare Cardiology, University Club Tower, 1034 S Brentwood Blvd, Ste 1120, Saint Louis, MO 63117; **Phone:** 314-977-4663; **Board Cert:** Cardiovascular Disease 2003; **Med School:** Cornell Univ 1987; **Resid:** Internal Medicine, Brigham & Womens Hosp 1990; **Fellow:** Cardiovascular Disease, Mt Sinai Hosp 1992; Cardiovascular Disease, Brigham & Womens Hosp 1993; **Fac Appt:** Prof Med, St Louis Univ

Hayes, Sharonne N MD [Cv] - **Spec Exp:** Heart Disease in Women; Preventive Cardiology; Cholesterol/Lipid Disorders; Echocardiography; **Hospital:** Mayo Med Ctr & Clin - Rochester; **Address:** Mayo Clinic Women's Heart Clinic, 200 First St SW Gonda 5 Bldg - rm 368, Rochester, MN 55905; **Phone:** 507-538-6309; **Board Cert:** Internal Medicine 1986; Cardiovascular Disease 1989; **Med School:** Northwestern Univ 1983; **Resid:** Internal Medicine, Mayo Clinic 1986; **Fellow:** Cardiovascular Research, Mayo Clinic 1987; Cardiovascular Disease, Mayo Clinic 1990; **Fac Appt:** Assoc Prof Med, Mayo Med Sch

Heroux, Alain MD [Cv] - **Spec Exp:** Transplant Medicine-Heart; Heart Failure; **Hospital:** Loyola Univ Med Ctr; **Address:** 2160 S 1st Ave Bldg 111 - rm 1110, Maywood, IL 60153; **Phone:** 708-327-2738; **Med School:** Canada 1981; **Resid:** Internal Medicine, Laval Univ Med Ctr 1985; Cardiovascular Disease, Royal Victory Hosp 1987; **Fellow:** Univ Virginia Med Coll 1989; **Fac Appt:** Asst Prof Med, Rush Med Coll

Cardiovascular Disease

Jaffe, Allan S MD [Cv] - **Spec Exp:** Ischemic Heart Disease; Heart Disease & Depression; **Hospital:** Mayo Med Ctr & Clin - Rochester; **Address:** Mayo Clinic, Div Cardiovascular Disease, 200 First St SW, Gonda 5-468, Rochester, MN 55905; **Phone:** 507-284-3680; **Board Cert:** Internal Medicine 1976; Cardiovascular Disease 1979; **Med School:** Univ MD Sch Med 1973; **Resid:** Internal Medicine, Barnes Hosp 1975; Internal Medicine, Wash Univ 1976; **Fellow:** Cardiovascular Disease, Barnes Hosp 1978; **Fac Appt:** Prof Med, Mayo Med Sch

Johnson, Maryl R MD [Cv] - **Spec Exp:** Congestive Heart Failure; Transplant Medicine-Heart; **Hospital:** Univ WI Hosp & Clins; **Address:** Univ Wisconsin Hosp/Clinics - Cardiology, 600 Highland Ave, Madison, WI 53792-0001; **Phone:** 608-263-0080; **Board Cert:** Internal Medicine 1981; Cardiovascular Disease 1983; **Med School:** Univ Iowa Coll Med 1977; **Resid:** Internal Medicine, Univ Iowa Hosp 1981; **Fellow:** Cardiovascular Disease, Univ Iowa Hosp 1982; **Fac Appt:** Prof Med, Univ Wisc

Kereiakes, Dean J MD [Cv] - **Spec Exp:** Coronary Angioplasty/Stents; Cardiomyopathy; Congestive Heart Failure; **Hospital:** Christ Hospital; **Address:** 2123 Auburn Ave, Ste 136, Cincinnati, OH 45219-2966; **Phone:** 513-721-8881; **Board Cert:** Internal Medicine 1981; Cardiovascular Disease 1985; **Med School:** Univ Cincinnati 1978; **Resid:** Internal Medicine, UCSF Med Ctr 1982; Internal Medicine, Mass Genl Hosp 1981; **Fellow:** Cardiovascular Disease, UCSF 1984; Coronary Angioplasty, Sequoia Hospital 1984; **Fac Appt:** Clin Prof Med, Ohio State Univ

Klein, Lloyd W MD [Cv] - **Spec Exp:** Coronary Artery Disease; Angiography-Coronary; Interventional Cardiology; **Hospital:** Gottlieb Meml Hosp, Rush Univ Med Ctr; **Address:** Clinical Cardiology Assocs, 675 W North Ave, POB Bldg Fl 2 - Ste 202, Melrose Park, IL 60160; **Phone:** 708-681-7862; **Board Cert:** Internal Medicine 1980; Cardiovascular Disease 1983; Interventional Cardiology 1999; **Med School:** Univ Cincinnati 1977; **Resid:** Internal Medicine, Montefiore Med Ctr 1980; **Fellow:** Cardiovascular Disease, Mt Sinai Hosp 1982; **Fac Appt:** Prof Med, Rush Med Coll

Mehlman, David J MD [Cv] - **Spec Exp:** Echocardiography; Heart Valve Disease; Coronary Artery Disease; **Hospital:** Northwestern Meml Hosp; **Address:** Northwestern Cardiovascular Inst, 675 N St Clair St, Galter Bldg Fl 19 - Ste 100, Chicago, IL 60611; **Phone:** 312-695-4965; **Board Cert:** Internal Medicine 1976; Cardiovascular Disease 1979; **Med School:** Johns Hopkins Univ 1973; **Resid:** Internal Medicine, Johns Hopkins Hosp 1976; **Fellow:** Cardiovascular Disease, Univ Chicago Hosps 1978; **Fac Appt:** Assoc Prof Med, Northwestern Univ

Moran, John F MD [Cv] - **Spec Exp:** Coronary Artery Disease; Congestive Heart Failure; Cholesterol/Lipid Disorders; **Hospital:** Loyola Univ Med Ctr; **Address:** 2160 S 1st Ave, Bldg 110 - Ste 6210, Maywood, IL 60153; **Phone:** 708-327-2784; **Board Cert:** Internal Medicine 1971; Cardiovascular Disease 1973; **Med School:** Loyola Univ-Stritch Sch Med 1964; **Resid:** Internal Medicine, Univ Illinois Hosps 1967; **Fellow:** Cardiovascular Disease, Univ Chicago Hosps 1969; **Fac Appt:** Prof Med, Loyola Univ-Stritch Sch Med

Nemickas, Rimgaudas MD [Cv] - **Spec Exp:** Coronary Artery Disease; Heart Valve Disease; Cholesterol/Lipid Disorders; **Hospital:** Adv Illinois Masonic Med Ctr, Holy Cross Hosp - Chicago; **Address:** 4901 W 79th St, Ste 7, Burbank, IL 60459; **Phone:** 708-233-5630; **Board Cert:** Internal Medicine 1969; Cardiovascular Disease 1973; **Med School:** Loyola Univ-Stritch Sch Med 1961; **Resid:** Internal Medicine, Univ Illinois Hosp 1967; **Fellow:** Cardiovascular Disease, Cook County Hosp 1963; Cardiovascular Disease, Univ Chicago Hosps 1969; **Fac Appt:** Clin Prof Med, Loyola Univ-Stritch Sch Med

Nishimura, Rick A MD [Cv] - **Spec Exp:** Echocardiography; Cardiomyopathy; Pericardial Disease; **Hospital:** Mayo Med Ctr & Clin - Rochester, St Mary's Hosp - Rochester; **Address:** Mayo Clinic, 200 First St SW Gonda 5 Bldg - rm 368, Rochester, MN 55905; **Phone:** 507-284-8342; **Board Cert:** Internal Medicine 1981; Cardiovascular Disease 1983; **Med School:** Rush Med Coll 1978; **Resid:** Internal Medicine, Mayo Clinic 1980; **Fellow:** Cardiovascular Disease, Mayo Clinic 1983; **Fac Appt:** Prof Med, Mayo Med Sch

Nissen, Steven E MD [Cv] - **Spec Exp:** Cholesterol/Lipid Disorders; Intravascular Ultrasound; Coronary Intensive Care; **Hospital:** Cleveland Clin Fdn (page 56); **Address:** 9500 Euclid Ave, MC F15, Ave, Cleveland, OH 44195; **Phone:** 216-445-6852; **Board Cert:** Internal Medicine 1981; Cardiovascular Disease 1983; **Med School:** Univ Mich Med Sch 1978; **Resid:** Internal Medicine, UC Davis Medical Ctr 1981; **Fellow:** Cardiovascular Disease, Univ Kentucky-Chandler Med Ctr 1983; **Fac Appt:** Prof Med, Cleveland Cl Coll Med/Case West Res

Rahko, Peter S MD [Cv] - **Spec Exp:** Congestive Heart Failure; Heart Valve Disease; Echocardiography; **Hospital:** Univ WI Hosp & Clins, Meriter Hosp; **Address:** 600 Highland Ave, rm G7-343 CSC, MC 3248, Madison, WI 53792-3248; **Phone:** 608-263-1530; **Board Cert:** Internal Medicine 1982; Cardiovascular Disease 1985; **Med School:** Univ Minn 1979; **Resid:** Internal Medicine, Indiana Univ Med Ctr 1982; **Fellow:** Cardiovascular Disease, Univ Pittsburgh 1985; **Fac Appt:** Assoc Prof Med, Univ Wisc

Reiss, Craig MD [Cv] - **Spec Exp:** Ischemic Heart Disease; Heart Valve Disease; Preventive Cardiology; Cardiomyopathy; **Hospital:** Barnes-Jewish Hosp, Barnes-Jewish West County Hosp; **Address:** Wash Univ Med Sch, Div Cardiovascular Disease, 660 S Euclid Ave, Box 8086, St Louis, MO 63110; **Phone:** 314-362-1291; **Board Cert:** Internal Medicine 1986; Cardiovascular Disease 1989; **Med School:** Univ MO-Kansas City 1983; **Resid:** Internal Medicine, Brigham & Women's Hosp 1989; **Fellow:** Cardiovascular Disease, Brigham & Women's Hosp 1988; **Fac Appt:** Assoc Prof Med, Washington Univ, St Louis

Rich, Stuart MD [Cv] - **Spec Exp:** Pulmonary Hypertension; Heart Failure; **Hospital:** Univ of Chicago Hosps; **Address:** 5841 S Maryland Ave, MC 2016, Chicago, IL 60637; **Phone:** 773-702-5589; **Board Cert:** Internal Medicine 1978; Cardiovascular Disease 1981; **Med School:** Loyola Univ-Stritch Sch Med 1974; **Resid:** Internal Medicine, Barnes-Jewish Hosp 1978; **Fellow:** Cardiovascular Disease, Univ Chicago 1980; **Fac Appt:** Prof Med, Rush Med Coll

Rosenbush, Stuart W MD [Cv] - **Spec Exp:** Cardiac Catheterization; Coronary Angioplasty/Stents; Heart Failure; Coronary Artery Disease; **Hospital:** Rush Univ Med Ctr; **Address:** Assocs In Cardiology Ltd, 1725 W Harrison St, Ste 1138, Chicago, IL 60612-3835; **Phone:** 312-563-3233; **Board Cert:** Internal Medicine 1979; Cardiovascular Disease 1981; Interventional Cardiology 2000; **Med School:** Univ IL Coll Med 1976; **Resid:** Internal Medicine, Michael Reese Hosp 1979; **Fellow:** Cardiovascular Disease, Rush Presby-St Lukes Med Ctr 1981; **Fac Appt:** Asst Prof Med, Rush Med Coll

Safian, Robert D MD [Cv] - **Spec Exp:** Interventional Cardiology; **Hospital:** William Beaumont Hosp; **Address:** Beaumont Heart Ctr, 3601 W 13 Mile Rd Fl 3, Royal Oak, MI 48073; **Phone:** 248-898-4163; **Board Cert:** Internal Medicine 1983; Cardiovascular Disease 1987; Interventional Cardiology 1999; **Med School:** Univ Fla Coll Med 1979; **Resid:** Pathology, Univ Miami Med Ctr 1981; Internal Medicine, UCSD Med Ctr 1983; **Fellow:** Cardiovascular Disease, Beth Israel Hosp-Harvard 1987

Cardiovascular Disease

Sanborn, Timothy MD [Cv] - **Spec Exp:** Interventional Cardiology; Gene Therapy-Cardiac Angiogenesis; Heart Valve Disease; Carotid Artery Stent Placement; **Hospital:** Evanston Hosp, Glenbrook Hosp; **Address:** 2650 Ridge Ave, Walgreen Bldg Fl 3, Evanston, IL 60201; **Phone:** 847-570-2250; **Board Cert:** Internal Medicine 1980; Cardiovascular Disease 2003; Interventional Cardiology 1999; **Med School:** Northwestern Univ 1977; **Resid:** Internal Medicine, Boston City Hosp 1980; **Fellow:** Cardiovascular Disease, Boston Univ Med Ctr 1983; **Fac Appt:** Prof Med, Northwestern Univ

Seward, James B MD [Cv] - **Spec Exp:** Pediatric Cardiology; Echocardiography; **Hospital:** Mayo Med Ctr & Clin - Rochester, St Mary's Hosp - Rochester; **Address:** Mayo Clinic, Div Cardiovasc Disease, 200 First St SW, Rochester, MN 55905; **Phone:** 507-284-3581; **Board Cert:** Internal Medicine 1974; Cardiovascular Disease 1975; **Med School:** Univ Mich Med Sch 1968; **Resid:** Internal Medicine, Boston City Hosp 1971; Internal Medicine, Mayo Clinic 1972; **Fellow:** Cardiovascular Disease, Mayo Clinic 1975; **Fac Appt:** Prof Ped, Mayo Med Sch

Shapiro, Jerrold MD [Cv] - **Spec Exp:** Echocardiography; Preventive Cardiology; **Hospital:** Swedish Covenant Hosp; **Address:** 4801 W Peterson Ave, Ste 610, Chicago, IL 60646-5713; **Phone:** 773-283-5900; **Board Cert:** Internal Medicine 1976; Cardiovascular Disease 1977; **Med School:** Univ IL Coll Med 1968; **Resid:** Internal Medicine, Ill Masonic Med Ctr 1972; **Fellow:** Cardiovascular Disease, Northwestern Meml Hosp 1974

Sorrentino, Matthew MD [Cv] - **Spec Exp:** Preventive Cardiology; Hypertension; **Hospital:** Univ of Chicago Hosps; **Address:** 5841 S Maryland Ave, MC 6080, Chicago, IL 60637; **Phone:** 773-702-9461; **Board Cert:** Internal Medicine 1987; Cardiovascular Disease 2001; **Med School:** Univ Chicago-Pritzker Sch Med 1984; **Resid:** Internal Medicine, Univ Chicago Hosps 1989; **Fellow:** Cardiovascular Disease, Univ Chicago Hosps 1991; **Fac Appt:** Assoc Prof Med, Univ Chicago-Pritzker Sch Med

Stein, James H MD [Cv] - **Spec Exp:** Preventive Cardiology; Echocardiography; Cholesterol/Lipid Disorders; **Hospital:** Univ WI Hosp & Clins; **Address:** Univ WI Hosp, Clinic Sci Center, 600 Highland Ave, Ste G7341, MC 3248, Madison, WI 53792; **Phone:** 608-263-9648; **Board Cert:** Internal Medicine 2003; Cardiovascular Disease 1997; **Med School:** Yale Univ 1990; **Resid:** Internal Medicine, Univ Chicago Hosps 1993; **Fellow:** Cardiovascular Disease, Rush-Presby St Lukes Med Ctr 1996; **Fac Appt:** Prof Med, Univ Wisc

Stewart, William J MD [Cv] - **Spec Exp:** Heart Valve Disease; Echocardiography; **Hospital:** Cleveland Clin Fdn (page 56); **Address:** Div Cardiovascular Medicine, 9500 Euclid Ave, MC F15, Cleveland, OH 44195; **Phone:** 216-444-5923; **Board Cert:** Internal Medicine 1980; Cardiovascular Disease 1983; **Med School:** Univ Cincinnati 1977; **Resid:** Internal Medicine, Univ Mich Hosp 1980; **Fellow:** Cardiovascular Disease, Boston Univ Med Ctr 1982; Cardiovascular Disease, Mass Genl Hosp 1984; **Fac Appt:** Assoc Prof Med, Cleveland Cl Coll Med/Case West Res

Volgman, Annabelle S MD [Cv] - **Spec Exp:** Heart Disease in Women; Arrhythmias; Atrial Fibrillation; Preventive Cardiology; **Hospital:** Rush Univ Med Ctr; **Address:** Rush Heart Ctr for Women, 1725 W Harrison St, Ste 1159, Chicago, IL 60612; **Phone:** 312-942-5020; **Board Cert:** Cardiovascular Disease 2006; **Med School:** Columbia P&S 1984; **Resid:** Internal Medicine, Univ Chicago Hosps 1987; **Fellow:** Cardiovascular Disease, Northwestern Meml Hosp 1989; Cardiac Electrophysiology, Northwestern Meml Hosp 1990; **Fac Appt:** Assoc Prof Med, Rush Med Coll

von der Lohe, Elisabeth MD [Cv] - **Spec Exp:** Heart Disease in Women; Interventional Cardiology; **Hospital:** Indiana Univ Hosp, Methodist Hosp - Indianapolis; **Address:** Krannert Inst Cardiology, Womens Heart Clinic, 1800 N Capital Blvd, Ste E400, Indianapolis, IN 46202; **Phone:** 317-962-0561; **Board Cert:** Internal Medicine 2000; Cardiovascular Disease 2001; Interventional Cardiology 2003; **Med School:** Germany 1978; **Resid:** Internal Medicine, Marien Hosp 1981; **Fellow:** Cardiovascular Disease, Klinikum Aachen 1986; **Fac Appt:** Prof Med, Indiana Univ

America's Top Doctors® 8th Edition

Wagoner, Lynne E MD [Cv] - **Spec Exp:** Congestive Heart Failure; Heart Disease in Women; Transplant Medicine-Heart; **Hospital:** Univ Hosp - Cincinnati, Christ Hospital; **Address:** 2123 Auburn Ave, Ste 624, Cincinnati, OH 45219; **Phone:** 513-751-4222; **Board Cert:** Internal Medicine 1989; Cardiovascular Disease 2003; **Med School:** E Carolina Univ 1986; **Resid:** Internal Medicine, Pitt Co Meml Hosp 1989; **Fellow:** Cardiovascular Disease, Univ Utah 1994; **Fac Appt:** Assoc Prof Med, Univ Cincinnati

Walsh, Mary N MD [Cv] - **Spec Exp:** Heart Disease in Women; Nuclear Cardiology; Congestive Heart Failure; **Hospital:** St Vincent Hosp & Hlth Svcs - Indianapolis; **Address:** Indiana Heart Inst, 8333 Naab Rd, Ste 400, Indianapolis, IN 46260; **Phone:** 317-338-6666; **Board Cert:** Internal Medicine 1986; Cardiovascular Disease 2001; **Med School:** Univ Minn 1983; **Resid:** Internal Medicine, Univ Tex SW Med Ctr 1986; **Fellow:** Cardiovascular Disease, Wash Univ 1989; **Fac Appt:** Asst Clin Prof Med, Indiana Univ

Weaver, W Douglas MD [Cv] - **Spec Exp:** Heart Attack; Angioplasty; Cholesterol/Lipid Disorders; **Hospital:** Henry Ford Hosp; **Address:** Henry Ford Hosp, 2799 W Grand Blvd, Cardiology K-14, Detroit, MI 48202-2689; **Phone:** 313-916-4420; **Board Cert:** Internal Medicine 1974; Cardiovascular Disease 1977; **Med School:** Tufts Univ 1971; **Resid:** Internal Medicine, Univ Wash Hosps 1974; **Fellow:** Cardiovascular Disease, Univ Wash Hosps 1976

Williams, Kim A MD [Cv] - **Spec Exp:** Nuclear Cardiology; Coronary Artery Disease; **Hospital:** Univ of Chicago Hosps; **Address:** 5758 S Maryland Ave, MC 9015, Chicago, IL 60637; **Phone:** 773-702-9461; **Board Cert:** Internal Medicine 1982; Cardiovascular Disease 1985; Nuclear Medicine 1986; **Med School:** Univ Chicago-Pritzker Sch Med 1979; **Resid:** Internal Medicine, Emory Univ 1982; **Fellow:** Cardiovascular Disease, Univ Chicago 1984; Nuclear Medicine, Univ Chicago 1986; **Fac Appt:** Assoc Prof Med, Univ Chicago-Pritzker Sch Med

Young, James B MD [Cv] - **Spec Exp:** Transplant Medicine-Heart; Heart Failure; **Hospital:** Cleveland Clin Fdn (page 56); **Address:** 9500 Euclid Ave, MC T13, Cleveland, OH 44195; **Phone:** 216-444-2270; **Board Cert:** Internal Medicine 1977; Cardiovascular Disease 1979; **Med School:** Baylor Coll Med 1974; **Resid:** Internal Medicine, Baylor Affil Hosp 1977; Internal Medicine, Methodist Hosp 1980; **Fellow:** Cardiovascular Disease, Baylor Affl Hosp 1979; **Fac Appt:** Prof Med, Cleveland Cl Coll Med/Case West Res

Great Plains and Mountains

Anderson, Jeffrey L MD [Cv] - **Spec Exp:** Arrhythmias; Cholesterol/Lipid Disorders; Cardiac MRI; **Hospital:** LDS Hosp, Salt Lake Regional Med Ctr; **Address:** Intermountain Med Ctr, 5121 S Cottonwood St, Salt Lake City, UT 84107; **Phone:** 801-507-4757; **Board Cert:** Internal Medicine 1975; Cardiovascular Disease 1979; Cardiac Electrophysiology 2002; **Med School:** Harvard Med Sch 1972; **Resid:** Internal Medicine, Mass Genl Hosp 1974; **Fellow:** Research, Natl Inst Hlth 1976; Cardiovascular Disease, Stanford Univ Med Ctr 1978; **Fac Appt:** Prof Med, Univ Utah

Benjamin, Ivor J MD [Cv] - **Spec Exp:** Arrhythmias; Cardiomyopathy; **Hospital:** Univ Utah Hosps and Clins; **Address:** Univ UT Health Sci Ctr, Div Cardiology, 30 N 1900 E, rm 4A100, Salt Lake City, UT 84132; **Phone:** 801-581-7715; **Board Cert:** Internal Medicine 1985; Cardiovascular Disease 1989; **Med School:** Johns Hopkins Univ 1982; **Resid:** Internal Medicine, Yale-New Haven Hosp 1985; **Fellow:** Cardiology Research, Yale-New Haven Hosp 1988; Echocardiography, Michael Reese Hosp 1989; **Fac Appt:** Prof Med, Univ Utah

Cardiovascular Disease

Lindenfeld, JoAnn MD [Cv] - **Spec Exp:** Congestive Heart Failure; Transplant Medicine-Heart; Heart Disease in Women; **Hospital:** Univ Colorado Hosp; **Address:** Univ Colorado Hlth Sci Ctr, 12602 E 16th Ave, Box B-120, Aurora, CO 80045; **Phone:** 720-848-2258; **Board Cert:** Internal Medicine 1976; Cardiovascular Disease 1979; **Med School:** Univ Mich Med Sch 1973; **Resid:** Internal Medicine, UCSD Med Ctr 1977; **Fellow:** Cardiovascular Disease, Univ Tex Hlth Sci Ctr 1979; **Fac Appt:** Prof Med, Univ Colorado

Southwest

Carabello, Blase A MD [Cv] - **Spec Exp:** Heart Valve Disease; **Hospital:** DeBakey VA Med Ctr-Houston; **Address:** Houston VA Medical Ctr, 2002 Holcombe Blvd, MS 111MCL, Houston, TX 77030; **Phone:** 713-794-7070; **Board Cert:** Internal Medicine 1977; Cardiovascular Disease 1979; **Med School:** Temple Univ 1973; **Resid:** Internal Medicine, Mass General Hosp 1976; **Fellow:** Cardiovascular Disease, Peter Bent Brigham Hosp 1978; **Fac Appt:** Prof Med, Baylor Coll Med

Freeman, Gregory L MD [Cv] - **Spec Exp:** Interventional Cardiology; Angioplasty; **Hospital:** Univ Hlth Sys - Univ Hosp (San Antonio, TX); **Address:** Cardiology Clinical Associates, 4411 Medical Drive, Ste 300, San Antonio, TX 78229; **Phone:** 210-614-5400; **Board Cert:** Internal Medicine 1979; Cardiovascular Disease 1983; **Med School:** Loyola Univ-Stritch Sch Med 1976; **Resid:** Internal Medicine, Cook County Hosp 1979; **Fellow:** Cardiovascular Disease, Loyola Univ Med Ctr 1981; Research, UCSD Sch Med 1983; **Fac Appt:** Prof Med, Univ Tex, San Antonio

Gould, K Lance MD [Cv] - **Spec Exp:** Preventive Cardiology; PET Imaging; Cholesterol/Lipid Disorders; **Hospital:** Meml Hermann Hosp - Texas Med Ctr; **Address:** Univ Texas - PET Imaging Ctr, 6431 Fannin, Rm 4.256 MSB, Houston, TX 77030-1501; **Phone:** 713-500-6611; **Med School:** Case West Res Univ 1964; **Resid:** Internal Medicine, Univ Wash Med Ctr 1967; Cardiovascular Disease, Univ Wash Med Ctr 1964; **Fellow:** Cardiovascular Disease, Univ Wash Med Ctr 1971; **Fac Appt:** Prof Med, Univ Tex, Houston

Krajcer, Zvonimir MD [Cv] - **Spec Exp:** Peripheral Vascular Disease; **Hospital:** St Luke's Episcopal Hosp - Houston; **Address:** 6624 Fannin St, Ste 2780, Houston, TX 77030; **Phone:** 713-791-4158; **Board Cert:** Internal Medicine 1975; Cardiovascular Disease 1977; **Med School:** Slovenia 1970; **Resid:** Internal Medicine, Northwestern Medical Ctr 1974; **Fellow:** Cardiovascular Disease, St Luke's Episcopal Hosp 1977; **Fac Appt:** Clin Prof Med, Baylor Coll Med

Massin, Edward Krauss MD [Cv] - **Spec Exp:** Congestive Heart Failure; Transplant Medicine-Heart; Coronary Artery Disease; **Hospital:** St Luke's Episcopal Hosp - Houston; **Address:** Cardiology Consultants Houston, 6624 Fannin St, Ste 2310, Houston, TX 77030-2335; **Phone:** 713-796-2668; **Board Cert:** Internal Medicine 1973; Cardiovascular Disease 1973; **Med School:** Washington Univ, St Louis 1965; **Resid:** Internal Medicine, Barnes Hosp 1967; **Fellow:** Cardiovascular Disease, Univ Colo Med Ctr 1971; **Fac Appt:** Clin Prof Med, Baylor Coll Med

McPherson, David D MD [Cv] - **Spec Exp:** Echocardiography; Congenital Heart Disease-Adult; Heart Valve Disease; **Hospital:** Univ Hlth Sys - Univ Hosp (San Antonio, TX); **Address:** 6431 Fannin, Houston, TX 77030; **Phone:** 713-500-6553; **Board Cert:** Internal Medicine 2005; Cardiovascular Disease 1997; **Med School:** Univ Alberta 1978; **Resid:** Internal Medicine, Dalhousie Univ 1981; **Fellow:** Cardiovascular Disease, Dalhousie Univ 1983; Cardiovascular Disease, Iowa Univ Med 1984; **Fac Appt:** Prof Med, Northwestern Univ

America's Top Doctors® 8th Edition

Nagueh, Sherif F MD [Cv] - **Spec Exp:** Echocardiography; Heart Failure; **Hospital:** Methodist Hosp - Houston; **Address:** Methodist DeBakey Heart & Vascular Ctr, 6550 Fannin, Ste 1901, Smith Tower, Houston, TX 77030; **Phone:** 713-441-1100; **Board Cert:** Internal Medicine 2003; Cardiovascular Disease 2007; **Med School:** Egypt 1986; **Resid:** Internal Medicine, Baylor Coll Med 1993; **Fellow:** Cardiovascular Disease, Baylor Coll Med 1996; **Fac Appt:** Prof Med, Cornell Univ-Weill Med Coll

Quinones, Miguel A MD [Cv] - **Spec Exp:** Echocardiography; Heart Valve Disease; **Hospital:** Methodist Hosp - Houston; **Address:** Methodist DeBakey Cardiology Assocs, 6550 Fannin St Smith Bldg - rm 1901, Houston, TX 77030; **Phone:** 713-441-1100; **Board Cert:** Internal Medicine 1972; Cardiovascular Disease 1974; **Med School:** Puerto Rico 1968; **Resid:** Internal Medicine, Harlem Hosp 1971; **Fellow:** Cardiovascular Disease, Baylor Coll Med 1974; **Fac Appt:** Prof Med, Univ Tex, Houston

Ramee, Stephen Robert MD [Cv] - **Spec Exp:** Angiography-Coronary; Interventional Cardiology; **Hospital:** Ochsner Fdn Hosp; **Address:** Ochsner Clinic, Cath Lab, 1514 Jefferson Hwy, New Orleans, LA 70121; **Phone:** 504-842-3724; **Board Cert:** Internal Medicine 1983; Cardiovascular Disease 1985; Interventional Cardiology 1999; **Med School:** Geo Wash Univ 1980; **Resid:** Internal Medicine, Letterman Army Med Ctr 1983; **Fellow:** Cardiovascular Disease, Letterman Army Med Ctr 1985

Tajik, A Jamil MD [Cv] - **Spec Exp:** Echocardiography; Heart Valve Disease; **Hospital:** Mayo Clinic - Scottsdale; **Address:** 13400 E Shea Blvd, Scottsdale, AZ 85259; **Phone:** 480-301-4876; **Board Cert:** Internal Medicine 1973; Cardiovascular Disease 1973; **Med School:** Pakistan 1965; **Resid:** Internal Medicine, Mayo Clinic 1970; **Fellow:** Cardiovascular Disease, Mayo Clinic 1972

Thames, Marc D MD [Cv] - **Spec Exp:** Coronary Artery Disease; Congestive Heart Failure; **Hospital:** Scottsdale Hlthcare - Shea; **Address:** Cardiovascular Consultants, 3805 E Bell Rd, Ste 3100, Phoenix, AZ 85032-3356; **Phone:** 602-867-8644; **Board Cert:** Internal Medicine 1974; Cardiovascular Disease 1979; **Med School:** Med Coll VA 1970; **Resid:** Internal Medicine, Peter Bent Brigham Hosp 1974; **Fellow:** Cardiology Research, Peter Bent Brigham Hosp 1975; Cardiovascular Disease, Mayo Clinic 1977

Wilansky, Susan MD [Cv] - **Spec Exp:** Heart Disease in Women; Heart Disease in Pregnancy; Echocardiography; **Hospital:** Mayo Clinic - Scottsdale; **Address:** Mayo Clinic, Dept Cardiology, 13400 E Shea Blvd, Scottsdale, AZ 85259; **Phone:** 480-301-8200; **Board Cert:** Cardiovascular Disease 1989; **Med School:** McMaster Univ 1979; **Resid:** Internal Medicine, Univ Toronto Hosp 1983; **Fellow:** Cardiovascular Disease, Univ Toronto Hosp 1985; Echocardiography, Univ Toronto Hosp 1986; **Fac Appt:** Assoc Prof Med, Mayo Med Sch

Willerson, James T MD [Cv] - **Spec Exp:** Ischemic Heart Disease; Stem Cell Therapy in Heart Failure; **Hospital:** St Luke's Episcopal Hosp - Houston; **Address:** 7000 Fannin St, Ste 1700, Houston, TX 77030; **Phone:** 832-355-3942; **Board Cert:** Internal Medicine 1972; Cardiovascular Disease 1974; **Med School:** Baylor Coll Med 1965; **Resid:** Internal Medicine, Mass Genl Hosp 1967; **Fellow:** Cardiovascular Disease, Mass Genl Hosp 1967; **Fac Appt:** Prof Med, Univ Tex, Houston

Zoghbi, William A MD [Cv] - **Spec Exp:** Echocardiography; **Hospital:** Methodist Hosp - Houston; **Address:** SM-677 6550 Fannin, Houston, TX 77030; **Phone:** 713-790-4342; **Board Cert:** Internal Medicine 1982; Cardiovascular Disease 1985; **Med School:** Meharry Med Coll 1979; **Resid:** Internal Medicine, Baylor Coll Affil Hosps 1982; **Fellow:** Cardiovascular Disease, Baylor Coll Med 1985

Cardiovascular Disease

West Coast and Pacific

Bairey-Merz, C Noel MD [Cv] - **Spec Exp:** Preventive Cardiology; Heart Disease in Women; **Hospital:** Cedars-Sinai Med Ctr; **Address:** Cedars-Sinai Women's Hlth Program, 444 S San Vicente Blvd, Ste 600, Los Angeles, CA 90048; **Phone:** 310-423-9680; **Board Cert:** Internal Medicine 1984; Cardiovascular Disease 1987; **Med School:** Harvard Med Sch 1981; **Resid:** Internal Medicine, UCSF Med Ctr 1984; **Fellow:** Cardiovascular Disease, Cedars-Sinai Med Ctr 1986; **Fac Appt:** Assoc Clin Prof Med, UCLA

Brindis, Ralph G MD [Cv] - **Spec Exp:** Acute Coronary Syndromes; Interventional Cardiology; **Hospital:** Kaiser Permanente Oakland Med Ctr, Alta Bates Summit Med Ctr - Summit Campus; **Address:** Hospital Bldg Fl 2, 280 W MacArthur Blvd, Oakland, CA 94611; **Phone:** 510-752-6424; **Board Cert:** Internal Medicine 1980; Cardiovascular Disease 1983; Interventional Cardiology 1999; **Med School:** Emory Univ 1977; **Resid:** Internal Medicine, Herbert C Moffitt Hosp 1980; Internal Medicine, Fort Miley VA Hosp 1981; **Fellow:** Cardiovascular Disease, Herbert C Moffitt Hosp 1983; **Fac Appt:** Prof Med, UCSF

Budoff, Matthew J MD [Cv] - **Spec Exp:** Cholesterol/Lipid Disorders; Coronary Artery Disease; Cardiac Imaging; **Hospital:** LAC - Harbor - UCLA Med Ctr; **Address:** 1124 W Carson St, Torrance, CA 90502; **Phone:** 310-222-4107; **Board Cert:** Internal Medicine 2003; Cardiovascular Disease 1997; **Med School:** Geo Wash Univ 1990; **Resid:** Internal Medicine, UCLA/Harbor Med Ctr 1993; **Fellow:** Cardiovascular Disease, UCLA/Harbor Med Ctr 1997; **Fac Appt:** Assoc Prof Med, UCLA

Chatterjee, Kanu MD [Cv] - **Spec Exp:** Coronary Artery Disease; Congestive Heart Failure; **Hospital:** UCSF Med Ctr; **Address:** 1182 Moffitt Hospital, 505 Parnassus Ave, Box 0124, San Francisco, CA 94143-0327; **Phone:** 415-476-1326; **Board Cert:** Internal Medicine 1973; Cardiovascular Disease 1975; **Med School:** India 1956; **Resid:** Internal Medicine, Coventry & Warwickshire Hosps 1966; **Fellow:** Cardiovascular Disease, St George's Hosp 1969; Research, Brompton Hosp 1971; **Fac Appt:** Prof Med, UCSF

Dichek, David A MD [Cv] - **Spec Exp:** Gene Therapy; Atherosclerosis; **Hospital:** Univ Wash Med Ctr; **Address:** University of Washington, Dept Cardiology, 1959 NE Pacific St, Box 357710, Seattle, WA 98195; **Phone:** 206-598-4300; **Board Cert:** Internal Medicine 1987; Cardiovascular Disease 2004; **Med School:** UCLA 1984; **Resid:** Internal Medicine, Mass Genl Hosp 1987; **Fellow:** Cardiovascular Disease, NIH/Johns Hopkins Hosp 1992; **Fac Appt:** Prof Med, Univ Wash

Elkayam, Uri MD [Cv] - **Spec Exp:** Congestive Heart Failure; Heart Disease in Pregnancy; Heart Valve Disease; **Hospital:** LAC & USC Med Ctr, USC Univ Hosp - R K Eamer Med Plz; **Address:** LAC & USC Med Ctr, Div Cardiology, 1200 N State St, rm 7621, Los Angeles, CA 90033; **Phone:** 323-226-7541; **Board Cert:** Internal Medicine 1989; **Med School:** Israel 1973; **Resid:** Internal Medicine, Ichilov Hosp 1976; **Fellow:** Cardiovascular Disease, Albert Einstein Hosp 1978; Cardiovascular Disease, Cedars Sinai Med Ctr 1979; **Fac Appt:** Prof Med, USC Sch Med

Fishbein, Daniel P MD [Cv] - **Spec Exp:** Congestive Heart Failure; Transplant Medicine-Heart; **Hospital:** Univ Wash Med Ctr; **Address:** Univ Wash, Div Cardiology, 1959 NE Pacific St, Box 356422, Seattle, WA 98195-6422; **Phone:** 206-221-4507; **Board Cert:** Internal Medicine 1983; Cardiovascular Disease 1987; **Med School:** Albert Einstein Coll Med 1980; **Resid:** Internal Medicine, Univ Wash Med Ctr 1983; **Fellow:** Cardiovascular Disease, Univ Wash Med Ctr 1987; Interventional Cardiology, Univ Wash Med Ctr 1989; **Fac Appt:** Assoc Prof Med, Univ Wash

Fonarow, Gregg C MD [Cv] - **Spec Exp:** Preventive Cardiology; Heart Failure; Cardiomyopathy; Cholesterol/Lipid Disorders; **Hospital:** Ronald Reagan UCLA Med Ctr; **Address:** 200 UCLA Medical Plaza, Ste 224, Los Angeles, CA 90095; **Phone:** 310-825-8816; **Board Cert:** Cardiovascular Disease 2003; **Med School:** UCLA 1987; **Resid:** Internal Medicine, UCLA Med Ctr 1990; **Fellow:** Cardiovascular Disease, UCLA Med Ctr 1993; **Fac Appt:** Prof Med, UCLA

Hunt, Sharon Ann MD [Cv] - **Spec Exp:** Transplant Medicine-Heart; **Hospital:** Stanford Univ Med Ctr; **Address:** 300 Pasteur Drive CVRB 265 Bldg, Stanford, CA 94305; **Phone:** 650-498-6605; **Board Cert:** Internal Medicine 1977; Cardiovascular Disease 1979; **Med School:** Stanford Univ 1972; **Resid:** Internal Medicine, Stanford Univ Hosp 1974; **Fellow:** Cardiovascular Disease, Stanford Univ Hosp 1976; **Fac Appt:** Prof Med, Stanford Univ

Johnson, Allen D MD [Cv] - **Spec Exp:** Coronary Artery Disease; Heart Valve Disease; Congenital Heart Disease-Adult; Congestive Heart Failure; **Hospital:** Scripps Green Hosp; **Address:** Scripps Clinic-Torrey Pines, 10666 N Torrey Pines Rd, rm SW206, La Jolla, CA 92037; **Phone:** 858-554-8836; **Board Cert:** Internal Medicine 1973; Cardiovascular Disease 1973; **Med School:** Johns Hopkins Univ 1965; **Resid:** Internal Medicine, Johns Hopkins Hosp 1969; **Fellow:** Cardiovascular Disease, UCSD Med Ctr 1972; **Fac Appt:** Clin Prof Med, Univ SD Sch Med

Judelson, Debra R MD [Cv] - **Spec Exp:** Hypertension; Cholesterol/Lipid Disorders; Heart Disease in Women; **Hospital:** Cedars-Sinai Med Ctr, Brotman Med Ctr; **Address:** Women's Heart Institute, Cardiovascular Med Group Southern CA, 414 N Camden Drive, Ste 1100, Beverly Hills, CA 90210-4532; **Phone:** 310-278-3400 x155; **Board Cert:** Internal Medicine 1979; Cardiovascular Disease 1981; **Med School:** Harvard Med Sch 1976; **Resid:** Internal Medicine, Kaiser Foundation Hosp 1979; **Fellow:** Cardiovascular Disease, Kaiser Foundation Hosp 1981

Kaul, Sanjiv MD [Cv] - **Spec Exp:** Cardiac Imaging; Echocardiography; **Hospital:** OR Hlth & Sci Univ; **Address:** OHSU Cardiovascular Med, 3181 SW Sam Jackson Park Rd, MC UHN62, Portland, OR 97239; **Phone:** 503-494-8750; **Board Cert:** Internal Medicine 1980; Cardiovascular Disease 1983; **Med School:** India 1975; **Resid:** Internal Medicine, Univ Vermont Med Ctr 1980; Cardiovascular Disease, Wadsworth VA Hosp-UCLA 1982; **Fellow:** Cardiovascular Disease, Mass Genl Hosp 1984; **Fac Appt:** Prof Med, Oregon Hlth Sci Univ

Kobashigawa, Jon Akira MD [Cv] - **Spec Exp:** Transplant Medicine-Heart; **Hospital:** Ronald Reagan UCLA Med Ctr; **Address:** 100 UCLA Med Plaza, Ste 630, Los Angeles, CA 90095-6988; **Phone:** 310-794-1200; **Board Cert:** Internal Medicine 1983; Cardiovascular Disease 1987; **Med School:** Mount Sinai Sch Med 1980; **Resid:** Internal Medicine, UCLA Med Ctr 1983; **Fellow:** Cardiovascular Disease, UCLA Med Ctr 1986; **Fac Appt:** Clin Prof Med, UCLA

Lewis, Sandra J MD [Cv] - **Spec Exp:** Heart Disease in Women; Preventive Cardiology; Congestive Heart Failure; **Hospital:** Legacy Good Samaritan Hosp and Med Ctr, Legacy Emanuel Hospitals; **Address:** Portland Cardiovascular Inst, 2222 NW Lovejoy St, Ste 606, Portland, OR 97210; **Phone:** 503-229-7554; **Board Cert:** Internal Medicine 1980; Cardiovascular Disease 1985; **Med School:** Stanford Univ 1977; **Resid:** Internal Medicine, Stanford Univ Med Ctr 1980; **Fellow:** Cardiovascular Disease, Stanford Univ 1983; **Fac Appt:** Assoc Clin Prof Med, Oregon Hlth Sci Univ

Redberg, Rita F MD [Cv] - **Spec Exp:** Echocardiography; Heart Disease in Women; Preventive Cardiology; **Hospital:** UCSF Med Ctr; **Address:** UCSF Cardiology, 350 Parnassus Ave, Ste 300, San Francisco, CA 94143; **Phone:** 415-353-2873; **Board Cert:** Internal Medicine 1985; Cardiovascular Disease 1989; **Med School:** Univ Pennsylvania 1982; **Resid:** Internal Medicine, Columbia-Presby Med Ctr 1985; **Fellow:** Cardiovascular Disease, Columbia-Presby Med Ctr 1988; **Fac Appt:** Prof Med, UCSF

Cardiovascular Disease

Schnittger, Ingela MD [Cv] - **Spec Exp:** Cardiovascular Imaging; Cardiac Imaging; **Hospital:** Stanford Univ Med Ctr; **Address:** 300 Pasteur Drive, rm H2157, Stanford, CA 94305-5233; **Phone:** 650-723-5196; **Board Cert:** Internal Medicine 1980; Cardiovascular Disease 1983; **Med School:** Sweden 1975; **Resid:** Internal Medicine, Stanford Univ Hosp 1980; **Fellow:** Cardiovascular Disease, Stanford Univ Hosp 1983; **Fac Appt:** Assoc Prof Med, Stanford Univ

Shah, Prediman K MD [Cv] - **Spec Exp:** Coronary Artery Disease; Cholesterol/Lipid Disorders; **Hospital:** Cedars-Sinai Med Ctr; **Address:** Cedars-Sinai Med Ctr, 8700 Beverly Blvd, Ste 5531, Los Angeles, CA 90048-1865; **Phone:** 310-423-3884; **Board Cert:** Internal Medicine 1975; Cardiovascular Disease 1977; **Med School:** India 1969; **Resid:** Internal Medicine, All India Inst Med Scis 1971; Internal Medicine, Montefiore Hosp 1974; **Fellow:** Cardiovascular Disease, Montefiore Hosp 1976; **Fac Appt:** Prof Med, UCLA

CARDIAC ELECTROPHYSIOLOGY

New England

Batsford, William P MD [CE] - **Spec Exp:** Arrhythmias; **Hospital:** Yale-New Haven Hosp; **Address:** Yale Univ School Medicine, Section Cardiovascular Medicine, 333 Cedar St, 3 FMP, Box 208017, New Haven, CT 06520-8017; **Phone:** 203-785-4126; **Board Cert:** Internal Medicine 1972; Cardiovascular Disease 1977; **Med School:** Albany Med Coll 1969; **Resid:** Internal Medicine, Hosp Univ Penn 1972; **Fac Appt:** Prof Med, Yale Univ

Buxton, Alfred E MD [CE] - **Spec Exp:** Arrhythmias; **Hospital:** Rhode Island Hosp; **Address:** 2 Dudley St, Ste 360, Providence, RI 02905; **Phone:** 401-444-3020; **Board Cert:** Internal Medicine 1977; Cardiovascular Disease 1981; Cardiac Electrophysiology 2002; **Med School:** Univ Pennsylvania 1973; **Resid:** Internal Medicine, Hosp Univ Penn 1977; **Fac Appt:** Prof Med, Brown Univ

Epstein, Laurence M MD [CE] - **Spec Exp:** Arrhythmias; **Hospital:** Brigham & Women's Hosp; **Address:** Brigham & Women's Hosp, Cardiology, 75 Francis St, Boston, MA 02115; **Phone:** 857-307-1945; **Board Cert:** Internal Medicine 1989; Cardiovascular Disease 2001; Cardiac Electrophysiology 2002; **Med School:** Univ Chicago-Pritzker Sch Med 1985; **Resid:** Internal Medicine, UCSF Med Ctr 1989; **Fellow:** Cardiovascular Disease, Hosp U Penn 1991; Cardiac Electrophysiology, UCSF Med Ctr 1992; **Fac Appt:** Assoc Prof Med, Harvard Med Sch

Josephson, Mark Eric MD [CE] - **Spec Exp:** Arrhythmias; **Hospital:** Beth Israel Deaconess Med Ctr - Boston; **Address:** 185 Pilgrim Rd, Baker 4 Cardiology, Boston, MA 02215; **Phone:** 617-667-8800; **Board Cert:** Internal Medicine 1973; Cardiovascular Disease 1975; Cardiac Electrophysiology 2002; **Med School:** Columbia P&S 1969; **Resid:** Internal Medicine, Mt Sinai Med Ctr 1971; **Fellow:** Cardiovascular Disease, Hosp Univ Penn 1975; **Fac Appt:** Prof Med, Harvard Med Sch

Ruskin, Jeremy N MD [CE] - **Spec Exp:** Arrhythmias; **Hospital:** Mass Genl Hosp; **Address:** Mass General Hosp, Arrhythmia Service, 55 Fruit St, Boston, MA 02114; **Phone:** 617-726-8514; **Board Cert:** Internal Medicine 1974; Cardiovascular Disease 1975; Cardiac Electrophysiology 2003; **Med School:** Harvard Med Sch 1971; **Resid:** Internal Medicine, Beth Israel Hosp 1974; Cardiovascular Disease, Mass Genl Hosp 1977; **Fac Appt:** Assoc Prof Med, Harvard Med Sch

Stevenson, William G MD [CE] - **Spec Exp:** Arrhythmias; **Hospital:** Brigham & Women's Hosp; **Address:** Brigham & Womens Hosp, Cardiology, 75 Francis St, Boston, MA 02115; **Phone:** 857-307-1948; **Board Cert:** Internal Medicine 1982; Cardiovascular Disease 1985; Cardiac Electrophysiology 2005; **Med School:** Tulane Univ 1979; **Resid:** Internal Medicine, UCLA Med Ctr 1982; **Fellow:** Cardiovascular Disease, UCLA Med Ctr 1984; Cardiac Electrophysiology, UCLA Med Ctr 1985; **Fac Appt:** Prof Med, Harvard Med Sch

Mid Atlantic

Callans, David J MD [CE] - **Spec Exp:** Arrhythmias; Pacemakers; **Hospital:** Hosp Univ Penn - UPHS (page 60); **Address:** Penn Cardiac Care at Hosp U Penn, 3400 Spruce St Founders Bldg Fl 9, Philadelphia, PA 19104; **Phone:** 215-662-6052; **Board Cert:** Internal Medicine 1989; Cardiovascular Disease 2005; Cardiac Electrophysiology 2005; **Med School:** Johns Hopkins Univ 1986; **Resid:** Internal Medicine, Hosp U Penn 1989; Cardiovascular Disease, Hosp U Penn 1999; **Fac Appt:** Prof Med, Univ Pennsylvania

Chinitz, Larry MD [CE] - **Spec Exp:** Arrhythmias; Pacemakers; Defibrillators; Atrial Fibrillation; **Hospital:** NYU Med Ctr (page 68); **Address:** 403 E 34th St Fl 2, New York, NY 10016-6402; **Phone:** 212-263-7149; **Board Cert:** Internal Medicine 1982; Cardiovascular Disease 1985; Cardiac Electrophysiology 1998; **Med School:** NYU Sch Med 1979; **Resid:** Internal Medicine, Bellevue Hosp 1983; **Fellow:** Cardiovascular Disease, NYU Med Ctr/Bellevue 1985; Cardiac Electrophysiology, Montefiore/NYU 1985; **Fac Appt:** Assoc Prof Med, NYU Sch Med

Cohen, Martin B MD [CE] - **Spec Exp:** Interventional Cardiology; Pacemakers; Defibrillators; **Hospital:** Westchester Med Ctr; **Address:** 19 Bradhurst Ave, Ste 700, Hawthorne, NY 10532-2140; **Phone:** 914-593-7800; **Board Cert:** Internal Medicine 1983; Cardiovascular Disease 1985; Cardiac Electrophysiology 2006; Interventional Cardiology 2004; **Med School:** SUNY Downstate 1980; **Resid:** Internal Medicine, Univ Hosp 1983; **Fellow:** Cardiovascular Disease, Univ Hosp 1985; Interventional Cardiology, Westchester Co Med Ctr 1986; **Fac Appt:** Assoc Clin Prof Med, NY Med Coll

Gomes, J Anthony MD [CE] - **Spec Exp:** Arrhythmias; Heart Attack; Atrial Fibrillation; Pacemakers; **Hospital:** Mount Sinai Med Ctr (page 64); **Address:** Mount Sinai Medical Ctr, One Gustave L Levy Pl, Box 1054, New York, NY 10029-6500; **Phone:** 212-241-7272; **Board Cert:** Internal Medicine 1974; Cardiovascular Disease 1975; **Med School:** India 1970; **Resid:** Internal Medicine, Mt Sinai Med Ctr 1973; **Fellow:** Cardiovascular Disease, Mt Sinai Med Ctr 1975; **Fac Appt:** Prof Med, Mount Sinai Sch Med

Lerman, Bruce MD [CE] - **Spec Exp:** Catheter Ablation; Defibrillators; Arrhythmias; **Hospital:** NY-Presby Hosp/Weill Cornell (page 66); **Address:** NY Weill Cornell Med Ctr, 520 E 70th St, Starr 4, New York, NY 10021-9800; **Phone:** 212-746-2169; **Board Cert:** Internal Medicine 1980; Cardiovascular Disease 1985; Cardiac Electrophysiology 2002; **Med School:** Loyola Univ-Stritch Sch Med 1977; **Resid:** Internal Medicine, Northwestern Univ Hosp 1980; Internal Medicine, Univ Michigan Med Ctr 1981; **Fellow:** Cardiovascular Disease, Hosp Univ Penn 1982; Cardiovascular Disease, Johns Hopkins Hosp 1983; **Fac Appt:** Prof Med, Cornell Univ-Weill Med Coll

Levine, Joseph H MD [CE] - **Spec Exp:** Arrhythmias; Sudden Death Prevention; Catheter Ablation; Pacemakers; **Hospital:** St Francis Hosp - The Heart Ctr (page 72), Good Samaritan Hosp Med Ctr - West Islip; **Address:** 100 Port Washington Blvd, Roslyn, NY 11576; **Phone:** 516-622-1011; **Board Cert:** Internal Medicine 1983; Cardiovascular Disease 1987; Cardiac Electrophysiology 2003; **Med School:** Univ Rochester 1980; **Resid:** Internal Medicine, Yale-New Haven Hosp 1983; **Fellow:** Cardiovascular Disease, Johns Hopkins Hosp 1986; Cardiac Electrophysiology, Hosp Univ Penn 1986

Cardiac Electrophysiology

Marchlinski, Francis E MD [CE] - **Spec Exp:** Pacemakers; Arrhythmias; **Hospital:** Hosp Univ Penn - UPHS (page 60), Penn Presby Med Ctr - UPHS (page 60); **Address:** Hosp University Penn, Div Cardiology, 3400 Spruce St Founders Bldg Fl 9, Philadelphia, PA 19104-4206; **Phone:** 215-662-6005; **Board Cert:** Internal Medicine 1979; Cardiovascular Disease 1981; Cardiac Electrophysiology 2002; **Med School:** Univ Pennsylvania 1976; **Resid:** Internal Medicine, Hosp Univ Penn 1979; **Fellow:** Cardiovascular Disease, Hosp Univ Penn 1982; **Fac Appt:** Prof Med, Univ Pennsylvania

Southeast

Curtis, Anne B MD [CE] - **Spec Exp:** Pacemakers; Arrhythmias; Defibrillators; **Hospital:** Tampa Genl Hosp, VA Hosp - Tampa; **Address:** S Tampa Ctr for Advanced Health Care, 2A Columbia Drive Fl 3, Tampa, FL 33606; **Phone:** 813-259-0600; **Board Cert:** Internal Medicine 1982; Cardiovascular Disease 1985; Cardiac Electrophysiology 2002; **Med School:** Columbia P&S 1979; **Resid:** Internal Medicine, Columbia- Presby Hosp 1982; **Fellow:** Cardiovascular Disease, Duke Univ Med Ctr 1986; **Fac Appt:** Prof Med, Univ S Fla Coll Med

Del Negro, Albert A MD [CE] - **Spec Exp:** Arrhythmias; **Hospital:** Inova Fairfax Hosp, Inova Alexandria Hosp; **Address:** 3020 Hamaker Ct, Ste 401, Fairfax, VA 22031; **Phone:** 703-849-0770; **Board Cert:** Internal Medicine 1979; Cardiovascular Disease 1981; **Med School:** Georgetown Univ 1969; **Resid:** Internal Medicine, DC Genl Hosp 1972; **Fellow:** Cardiovascular Disease, Georgetown Univ Med Ctr 1973; Cardiovascular Disease, VA Med Ctr 1974; **Fac Appt:** Asst Clin Prof Med, Georgetown Univ

DiMarco, John P MD/PhD [CE] - **Spec Exp:** Arrhythmias; Pacemakers; Defibrillators; **Hospital:** Univ Virginia Med Ctr; **Address:** Univ Virginia Hlth Scis Ctr, PO Box 800158, Charlottesville, VA 22908-0158; **Phone:** 434-924-2031; **Board Cert:** Internal Medicine 1978; Cardiovascular Disease 1981; Cardiac Electrophysiology 2005; **Med School:** Case West Res Univ 1975; **Resid:** Internal Medicine, Mass Genl Hosp 1977; Critical Care Medicine, Case West Res Univ 1978; **Fellow:** Cardiovascular Disease, Mass Genl Hosp 1980; Cardiac Electrophysiology, Mass Genl Hosp 1981; **Fac Appt:** Prof Med, Univ VA Sch Med

Ellenbogen, Kenneth A MD [CE] - **Spec Exp:** Arrhythmias; Pacemakers; Defibrillators; **Hospital:** Med Coll of VA Hosp, Henrico Doctors Hosp; **Address:** Med Coll VA/ Electrophysiology, PO Box 980053, Richmond, VA 23298; **Phone:** 804-828-7565; **Board Cert:** Internal Medicine 1983; Cardiovascular Disease 1985; Cardiac Electrophysiology 2005; **Med School:** Johns Hopkins Univ 1980; **Resid:** Internal Medicine, Johns Hopkins Hosp 1983; **Fellow:** Cardiovascular Disease, Duke Univ Med Ctr 1986; **Fac Appt:** Assoc Prof Med, Med Coll VA

Epstein, Andrew Ernest MD [CE] - **Spec Exp:** Arrhythmias; Defibrillators; Catheter Ablation; **Hospital:** Univ of Ala Hosp at Birmingham; **Address:** UAB Div Cardiovascular Disease, 321 THT, 1530 3rd Ave South, Birmingham, AL 35294-0006; **Phone:** 205-934-7114; **Board Cert:** Internal Medicine 1980; Cardiovascular Disease 1983; Cardiac Electrophysiology 2006; **Med School:** Univ Rochester 1977; **Resid:** Internal Medicine, Barnes Hosp 1980; **Fellow:** Cardiovascular Disease, Univ Ala Hosp 1982; **Fac Appt:** Prof Med, Univ Ala

Interian Jr, Alberto MD [CE] - **Hospital:** Mercy Hosp, Jackson Meml Hosp; **Address:** Mercy Hospital, 3641 S Miami Ave, Bayside Bavillion Bldg, Miami, FL 33136; **Phone:** 305-285-2685; **Board Cert:** Internal Medicine 1985; Cardiovascular Disease 1987; Cardiac Electrophysiology 2000; **Med School:** Univ Miami Sch Med 1982; **Resid:** Internal Medicine, Univ Miami Hosps 1985; **Fellow:** Cardiovascular Disease, Univ Miami Hosps 1988; **Fac Appt:** Prof Med, Univ Miami Sch Med

Kay, G Neal MD [CE] - **Spec Exp:** Arrhythmias; Pacemakers; **Hospital:** Univ of Ala Hosp at Birmingham; **Address:** UAB, Div Cardiovascular Disease, 321-J THT, 1530 3rd Ave South, Birmingham, AL 35294; **Phone:** 205-934-1335; **Board Cert:** Internal Medicine 1983; Cardiovascular Disease 1989; Cardiac Electrophysiology 2006; **Med School:** Univ Mich Med Sch 1979; **Resid:** Internal Medicine, Univ Alabama Hosp 1983; **Fellow:** Cardiovascular Disease, Duke Univ Med Ctr 1986; **Fac Appt:** Prof Med, Univ Ala

Sorrentino, Robert A MD [CE] - **Spec Exp:** Arrhythmias; Defibrillators; Pacemakers; Heart Failure; **Hospital:** Med Coll of GA Hosp and Clin; **Address:** Medical College of Georgia, 1120 15th St BBR Bldg - rm 6518, Augusta, GA 30912-0004; **Phone:** 706-721-4997; **Board Cert:** Internal Medicine 1988; Cardiovascular Disease 2002; Cardiac Electrophysiology 2008; **Med School:** Albany Med Coll 1985; **Resid:** Internal Medicine, Duke Univ Med Ctr 1988; **Fellow:** Cardiovascular Disease, Duke Univ Med Ctr 1991; **Fac Appt:** Prof Med, Med Coll GA

Midwest

Anderson, Mark E MD/PhD [CE] - **Spec Exp:** Arrhythmias; **Hospital:** Univ Iowa Hosp & Clinics; **Address:** Univ Iowa-Carver College Medicine, 200 Hawkins Dr, E315, GH, Iowa City, IA 52242-1081; **Phone:** 319-353-7101; **Board Cert:** Internal Medicine 2005; Cardiovascular Disease 2005; **Med School:** Univ Minn 1989; **Resid:** Internal Medicine, Stanford Univ Med Ctr 1991; **Fellow:** Cardiovascular Disease, Stanford Univ Sch Med 1994; Cardiac Electrophysiology, Stanford Univ Sch Med 1996; **Fac Appt:** Prof Med, Univ Iowa Coll Med

Hammill, Stephen C MD [CE] - **Spec Exp:** Pacemakers; Arrhythmias; **Hospital:** Mayo Med Ctr & Clin - Rochester; **Address:** Mayo Clinic, 200 First St SW, Rochester, MN 55905; **Phone:** 507-284-4888; **Board Cert:** Internal Medicine 1978; Cardiovascular Disease 1981; Cardiac Electrophysiology 2005; **Med School:** Univ Colorado 1974; **Resid:** Internal Medicine, Univ Colo Hlth Sci Ctr 1977; **Fellow:** Cardiovascular Disease, Duke Univ Med Ctr 1981; **Fac Appt:** Prof Med, Mayo Med Sch

Hayes, David L MD [CE] - **Spec Exp:** Pacemakers; **Hospital:** Mayo Med Ctr & Clin - Rochester; **Address:** Mayo Clinic, 200 1st St SW Gonda 5 Bldg - rm 200, Rochester, MN 55905; **Phone:** 507-284-3684; **Board Cert:** Internal Medicine 1980; Cardiovascular Disease 1981; **Med School:** Univ MO-Kansas City 1977; **Resid:** Internal Medicine, Mayo Clinic 1980; **Fellow:** Cardiovascular Disease, Mayo Clinic 1982; **Fac Appt:** Prof Med, Mayo Med Sch

Lindsay, Bruce MD [CE] - **Spec Exp:** Arrhythmias; **Hospital:** Barnes-Jewish Hosp; **Address:** Cleveland Clinic Main Campus, MC F15, 9500 Euclid Ave, Cleveland, OH 44195; **Phone:** 216-444-4293; **Board Cert:** Internal Medicine 1980; Cardiovascular Disease 1987; Cardiac Electrophysiology 2002; **Med School:** Jefferson Med Coll 1976; **Resid:** Internal Medicine, Univ Michigan Medical Ctr 1980; **Fellow:** Cardiovascular Disease, Barnes-Jewish Hosp 1985; **Fac Appt:** Assoc Prof Med, Univ Wash

Morady, Fred MD [CE] - **Spec Exp:** Arrhythmias; WPW Syndrome; **Hospital:** Univ Michigan Hlth Sys; **Address:** Specialty Electrophysiology, 1500 E Med Ctr Drive, 2394 CVC/5853, Ann Arbor, MI 48109; **Phone:** 734-647-7321; **Board Cert:** Internal Medicine 1978; Cardiovascular Disease 1981; Cardiac Electrophysiology 2005; **Med School:** UCSF 1975; **Resid:** Internal Medicine, UCSF Med Ctr 1978; **Fellow:** Cardiovascular Disease, UCSF Med Ctr 1980; **Fac Appt:** Prof Med, Univ Mich Med Sch

Cardiac Electrophysiology

Prystowsky, Eric N MD [CE] - **Spec Exp:** Arrhythmias; Catheter Ablation; Atrial Fibrillation; **Hospital:** St Vincent Hosp & Hlth Svcs - Indianapolis; **Address:** 8333 Naab Rd, Ste 400, Indianapolis, IN 46260; **Phone:** 317-338-6024; **Board Cert:** Internal Medicine 1976; Cardiovascular Disease 1979; Cardiac Electrophysiology 2006; **Med School:** Mount Sinai Sch Med 1973; **Resid:** Internal Medicine, Mt Sinai Hosp 1976; **Fellow:** Cardiovascular Disease, Duke Univ Med Ctr 1979; **Fac Appt:** Prof Med, Duke Univ

Schuger, Claudio D MD [CE] - **Spec Exp:** Arrhythmias; Defibrillators; **Hospital:** Henry Ford Hosp; **Address:** Henry Ford Hosp, Div Cardiology, 2799 W Grand Blvd, Detroit, MI 48202; **Phone:** 313-916-2417; **Board Cert:** Cardiac Electrophysiology 1998; Cardiovascular Disease 2007; **Med School:** Argentina 1977; **Resid:** Internal Medicine, Hacarmel Hosp 1982; Cardiovascular Disease, Hacarmel Hosp 1982; **Fellow:** Cardiovascular Disease, Bikur Cholim Hosp 1985; Cardiac Electrophysiology, Harper Hosp-Wayne State Univ 1990; **Fac Appt:** Assoc Prof Med, Wayne State Univ

Tchou, Patrick J MD [CE] - **Spec Exp:** Arrhythmias; **Hospital:** Cleveland Clin Fdn (page 56); **Address:** Dept Cardiology, 9500 Euclid Ave, MC F15, Cleveland, OH 44195; **Phone:** 216-444-6792; **Board Cert:** Internal Medicine 1982; Cardiovascular Disease 1985; Cardiac Electrophysiology 2002; **Med School:** Case West Res Univ 1979; **Resid:** Internal Medicine, Metro Genl Hosp 1982; **Fellow:** Cardiovascular Disease, Metro Genl Hosp 1984; Cardiac Electrophysiology, Mt Sinai Med Ctr 1985; **Fac Appt:** Prof Med, Ohio State Univ

Waldo, Albert MD [CE] - **Spec Exp:** Arrhythmias; Syncope; Atrial Fibrillation; **Hospital:** Univ Hosps Case Med Ctr; **Address:** Univ Hosps Case Med Ctr-Cardiology, 11100 Euclid Ave, MS LKS-5038, Cleveland, OH 44106-1736; **Phone:** 216-844-7690; **Board Cert:** Internal Medicine 1971; Cardiovascular Disease 1975; **Med School:** SUNY Downstate 1962; **Resid:** Internal Medicine, Baltimore City Hosp 1965; Internal Medicine, Kings Co Hosp 1966; **Fellow:** Cardiovascular Disease, Columbia Presby Med Ctr 1968; Cardiac Electrophysiology, Columbia Presby Med Ctr 1969; **Fac Appt:** Prof Med, Case West Res Univ

Wilber, David James MD [CE] - **Spec Exp:** Atrial Fibrillation; Catheter Ablation; Sudden Death Prevention; **Hospital:** Loyola Univ Med Ctr; **Address:** Loyola Univ Med Ctr, Cardiovascular Inst, 2160 S First Ave Bldg 110 - rm 6232, Maywood, IL 60153; **Phone:** 708-216-2642; **Board Cert:** Internal Medicine 1980; Cardiovascular Disease 1985; Cardiac Electrophysiology 2002; **Med School:** Northwestern Univ 1977; **Resid:** Internal Medicine, Northwestern Meml Hosp 1980; **Fellow:** Cardiovascular Disease, Univ Mich Med Sch 1984; Cardiac Electrophysiology, Mass Genl Hosp 1986; **Fac Appt:** Prof Med, Loyola Univ-Stritch Sch Med

Great Plains and Mountains

Lewkowiez, Laurent MD [CE] - **Spec Exp:** Arrhythmias; Ventricular Tachycardia Ablation; Atrial Fibrillation; **Hospital:** Denver Health Med Ctr; **Address:** Denver Health Med Ctr, Div Cardiology, 777 Bannock St, Denver, CO 80204; **Phone:** 303-436-5499; **Board Cert:** Cardiovascular Disease 2000; Cardiac Electrophysiology 2003; **Med School:** Univ SC Sch Med 1992; **Resid:** Internal Medicine, Univ Colorado Hlth Sci Ctr 1996; **Fellow:** Nuclear Cardiology, Univ Colorado Hlth Sci Ctr 1998; Cardiac Electrophysiology, Univ Colorado Hlth Sci Ctr 2001; **Fac Appt:** Asst Prof Med, Univ Colorado

West Coast and Pacific

Cannom, David S MD [CE] - **Spec Exp:** Arrhythmias; **Hospital:** Good Samaritan Hosp - Los Angeles; **Address:** 1245 Wilshire Blvd, Ste 703, Los Angeles, CA 90017-4806; **Phone:** 213-977-0419; **Board Cert:** Internal Medicine 1980; Cardiovascular Disease 1975; **Med School:** Univ Minn 1967; **Resid:** Internal Medicine, Yale-New Haven Hosp 1969; **Fellow:** Cardiovascular Disease, Stanford Unv 1973; **Fac Appt:** Clin Prof Med, UCLA

Gang, Eli Shimshon MD [CE] - **Spec Exp:** Arrhythmias; **Hospital:** Cedars-Sinai Med Ctr, Brotman Med Ctr; **Address:** 414 N Camden Drive, Ste 1100, Beverly Hills, CA 90210; **Phone:** 310-278-3400; **Board Cert:** Internal Medicine 1978; Cardiovascular Disease 1981; **Med School:** Columbia P&S 1975; **Resid:** Internal Medicine, Roosevelt Hosp 1978; **Fellow:** Cardiovascular Disease, Columbia Presby Hosp 1979; **Fac Appt:** Clin Prof Med, UCLA

Swerdlow, Charles D MD [CE] - **Spec Exp:** Defibrillators; Arrhythmias; **Hospital:** Cedars-Sinai Med Ctr; **Address:** 8635 W 3rd St, Ste 1190W, Los Angeles, CA 90048-6101; **Phone:** 310-652-4600; **Board Cert:** Internal Medicine 1979; Cardiovascular Disease 1981; Cardiac Electrophysiology 2004; **Med School:** Harvard Med Sch 1976; **Resid:** Internal Medicine, LA Co-Harbor Genl Hosp 1979; **Fellow:** Cardiovascular Disease, Stanford Univ Med Ctr 1981; **Fac Appt:** Clin Prof Med, UCLA

INTERVENTIONAL CARDIOLOGY

New England

Diver, Daniel J MD [IC] - **Spec Exp:** Angioplasty; Coronary Artery Disease; **Hospital:** St Francis Hosp & Med Ctr; **Address:** St Francis Hosp - Div Cardiology, 114 Woodland St, Hartford, CT 06105; **Phone:** 860-714-4019; **Board Cert:** Internal Medicine 1984; Cardiovascular Disease 1989; Interventional Cardiology 1999; **Med School:** Johns Hopkins Univ 1981; **Resid:** Internal Medicine, Johns Hopkins Hosp 1984; **Fellow:** Cardiovascular Disease, Beth Israel Hosp/Harvard 1987; **Fac Appt:** Prof Med, Univ Conn

Jacobs, Alice K MD [IC] - **Spec Exp:** Cardiac Catheterization; Heart Disease in Women; Interventional Cardiology; **Hospital:** Boston Med Ctr; **Address:** Boston Univ Med Ctr, Dept Cardiology, 88 E Newton St, rm C822, Boston, MA 02118; **Phone:** 617-638-8707; **Board Cert:** Internal Medicine 1978; Endocrinology 1979; Cardiovascular Disease 1985; Interventional Cardiology 1999; **Med School:** St Louis Univ 1975; **Resid:** Internal Medicine, St Louis Univ Hosp 1977; **Fellow:** Endocrinology, UCSD Med Ctr 1980; Cardiovascular Disease, Boston Univ Med Ctr 1982; **Fac Appt:** Prof Med, Boston Univ

Laham, Roger MD [IC] - **Spec Exp:** Angioplasty; **Hospital:** Beth Israel Deaconess Med Ctr - Boston; **Address:** Beth Israel Deaconess Med Ctr, 185 Pilgrim Rd, Baker 4, Boston, MA 02215; **Phone:** 617-667-8800; **Board Cert:** Internal Medicine 2004; Cardiovascular Disease 2005; Interventional Cardiology 1999; **Med School:** Amer Univ Beirut 1989; **Resid:** Internal Medicine, Duke Univ Med Ctr 1992; **Fellow:** Cardiovascular Disease, Harvard Med Sch 1995; **Fac Appt:** Assoc Prof Med, Harvard Med Sch

Interventional Cardiology

Williams, David O MD [IC] - **Hospital:** Rhode Island Hosp; **Address:** Rhode Island Hosp, Div Cardiology, 593 Eddy St, rm APC 814, Providence, RI 02903; **Phone:** 401-444-4581; **Board Cert:** Internal Medicine 1972; Cardiovascular Disease 1975; Interventional Cardiology 1999; **Med School:** Hahnemann Univ 1969; **Resid:** Internal Medicine, Hahnemann Univ Hosp 1972; **Fellow:** Cardiovascular Disease, UC Davis Med Ctr 1974; **Fac Appt:** Prof Med, Brown Univ

Mid Atlantic

Herrmann, Howard C MD [IC] - **Spec Exp:** Cardiac Catheterization; Angioplasty & Stent Placement; Heart Valve Disease; Atrial Septal Defect Closure; **Hospital:** Hosp Univ Penn - UPHS (page 60), Penn Presby Med Ctr - UPHS (page 60); **Address:** Hosp Univ Penn, Div Cardiovascular Med, 3400 Spruce St, 9.120 Founders Bldg, Philadelphia, PA 19104-4283; **Phone:** 215-662-2180; **Board Cert:** Internal Medicine 1984; Cardiovascular Disease 1987; Interventional Cardiology 1999; **Med School:** Harvard Med Sch 1981; **Resid:** Internal Medicine, Mass General Hosp 1984; **Fellow:** Cardiovascular Disease, Mass General Hosp 1987; **Fac Appt:** Prof Med, Univ Pennsylvania

Leon, Martin MD [IC] - **Hospital:** NY-Presby Hosp/Columbia (page 66); **Address:** 161 Ft Washington Ave Fl 5, New York, NY 10032; **Phone:** 212-305-7060; **Board Cert:** Internal Medicine 1979; Cardiovascular Disease 1983; Interventional Cardiology 1999; **Med School:** Yale Univ 1975; **Resid:** Internal Medicine, Yale-New Haven Hosp 1978; **Fellow:** Cardiovascular Disease, Yale-New Haven Hosp 1980

Moses, Jeffrey W MD [IC] - **Spec Exp:** Angiography-Coronary; Angioplasty & Stent Placement; Heart Valve Disease; **Hospital:** NY-Presby Hosp/Columbia (page 66); **Address:** 161 Fort Washington Fl 5, New York, NY 10032; **Phone:** 212-305-7060; **Board Cert:** Internal Medicine 1977; Cardiovascular Disease 1981; Interventional Cardiology 1999; **Med School:** Univ Pennsylvania 1974; **Resid:** Internal Medicine, Presby Univ Med Ctr 1977; **Fellow:** Cardiovascular Disease, Presby Univ Penn Med Ctr 1980

Petrossian, George A MD [IC] - **Spec Exp:** Carotid Artery Stent Placement; Peripheral Vascular Disease; Coronary Angioplasty/Stents; Renovascular Disease; **Hospital:** St Francis Hosp - The Heart Ctr (page 72), South Nassau Comm Hosp; **Address:** New York Cardiology Group, 1405 Old Northern Blvd, Roslyn, NY 11576-1353; **Phone:** 516-484-6777; **Board Cert:** Internal Medicine 1986; Cardiovascular Disease 1989; Interventional Cardiology 2000; **Med School:** Mount Sinai Sch Med 1983; **Resid:** Internal Medicine, Columbia-Presby Med Ctr 1987; **Fellow:** Cardiovascular Disease, Columbia -Presby Med Ctr 1989; Interventional Cardiology, Mass Genl Hosp 1990

Pichard, Augusto MD [IC] - **Spec Exp:** Angioplasty & Stent Placement; Cardiac Catheterization; **Hospital:** Washington Hosp Ctr; **Address:** 110 Irving St NW, Ste 4B1, Washington, DC 20010; **Phone:** 202-877-5975; **Board Cert:** Internal Medicine 1975; Cardiovascular Disease 1977; Interventional Cardiology 1999; **Med School:** Chile 1969; **Resid:** Internal Medicine, Univ Chile 1970; Internal Medicine, Catholic Univ 1971; **Fellow:** Cardiovascular Disease, Cleveland Clinic 1973; **Fac Appt:** Clin Prof Med, Geo Wash Univ

Reiner, Jonathan S MD [IC] - **Spec Exp:** Angioplasty & Stent Placement; **Hospital:** G Washington Univ Hosp; **Address:** MFA, Dept Cardiology, 2150 Pennsylvania Ave NW, Washington, DC 20037; **Phone:** 202-741-3333; **Board Cert:** Internal Medicine 1989; Cardiovascular Disease 2004; Interventional Cardiology 1999; **Med School:** Georgetown Univ 1986; **Resid:** Internal Medicine, North Shore Univ Hosp 1989; **Fellow:** Cardiovascular Disease, George Wash Univ Sch Med 1993; **Fac Appt:** Asst Prof Med, Geo Wash Univ

Resar, Jon R MD [IC] - **Spec Exp:** Percutaneous Coronary Intervention; Percutaneous Valvulo-plasty; Percutaneous ASD/PFO closure; **Hospital:** Johns Hopkins Hosp - Baltimore (page 61); **Address:** Johns Hopkins Hosp, Dept Cardiology, 600 N Wolfe St, Blalock 524, Baltimore, MD 21287; **Phone:** 410-614-1132; **Board Cert:** Internal Medicine 1988; Cardiovascular Disease 2000; Interventional Cardiology 1999; **Med School:** Med Coll Wisc 1985; **Resid:** Internal Medicine, Johns Hopkins Hosp 1988; **Fellow:** Cardiovascular Disease, Johns Hopkins Hosp 1990; Interventional Cardiology, Johns Hopkins Hosp; **Fac Appt:** Assoc Prof Med, Johns Hopkins Univ

Roubin, Gary MD/PhD [IC] - **Spec Exp:** Coronary Angioplasty/Stents; Carotid Artery Stent Placement; Peripheral Vascular Disease; **Hospital:** Lenox Hill Hosp (page 62); **Address:** 130 E 77th St Fl 9th, New York, NY 10021; **Phone:** 212-434-2606; **Med School:** Australia 1975; **Resid:** Internal Medicine, Royal Prince Albert Hosp 1979; Cardiovascular Disease, Hallstrom Inst of Cardiology 1981; **Fellow:** Cardiology Research, Natl Heart Fdn 1983; Interventional Cardiology, Emory Univ 1985; **Fac Appt:** Clin Prof Med, NYU Sch Med

Shani, Jacob MD [IC] - **Spec Exp:** Cardiac Catheterization; Angioplasty & Stent Placement; Percutaneous Valvuloplasty; **Hospital:** Maimonides Med Ctr (page 63); **Address:** Maimonides Med Ctr, Cardiac Cath Lab, 4802 10th Ave, Brooklyn, NY 11219-2844; **Phone:** 718-283-7480; **Board Cert:** Internal Medicine 1981; Cardiovascular Disease 1983; Interventional Cardiology 1999; **Med School:** Israel 1977; **Resid:** Internal Medicine, Maimonides Med Ctr 1981; **Fellow:** Cardiovascular Disease, Beth Israel Hosp 1983; **Fac Appt:** Prof Med, Mount Sinai Sch Med

Shorofsky, Stephen R MD/PhD [IC] - **Spec Exp:** Arrhythmias; **Hospital:** Univ of MD Med Sys; **Address:** Univ Maryland Med Ctr, Div Cardiology, 22 S Greene St, rm N3W77, Baltimore, MD 21201; **Phone:** 410-328-6056; **Board Cert:** Internal Medicine 1988; Cardiovascular Disease 2001; Cardiac Electrophysiology 2004; **Med School:** Univ Chicago-Pritzker Sch Med 1985; **Resid:** Internal Medicine, Univ Chicago Hosps 1988; **Fellow:** Cardiovascular Disease, Univ Chicago Hosps 1991; **Fac Appt:** Assoc Prof Med, Univ MD Sch Med

Stone, Gregg W MD [IC] - **Spec Exp:** Angioplasty & Stent Placement; Coronary Artery Disease; **Hospital:** NY-Presby Hosp/Columbia (page 66); **Address:** Columbia Univ Med Ctr, 161 Fort Washington Ave Fl 5, New York, NY 10032; **Phone:** 212-851-9304; **Board Cert:** Internal Medicine 1985; Cardiovascular Disease 1987; Interventional Cardiology 1999; **Med School:** Johns Hopkins Univ 1982; **Resid:** Internal Medicine, NY Hosp-Cornell Medical Ctr 1985; **Fellow:** Cardiovascular Disease, Cedars-Sinai Medical Ctr 1988; Coronary Angioplasty, Mid-America Heart Inst 1989

Southeast

Applegate, Robert J MD [IC] - **Spec Exp:** Cardiac Catheterization; Angioplasty; **Hospital:** Wake Forest Univ Baptist Med Ctr (page 73); **Address:** Wake Forest Univ Baptist Med Ctr, Div Cardio, Medical Center Blvd, Winston-Salem, NC 27157-1045; **Phone:** 336-716-6674; **Board Cert:** Internal Medicine 1983; Cardiovascular Disease 1987; Interventional Cardiology 1999; **Med School:** Univ VA Sch Med 1980; **Resid:** Internal Medicine, Oregon Hlth Sci Univ Hosp 1983; **Fellow:** Pharmacology, Univ Texas Hlth Sci Ctr 1984; Cardiovascular Disease, Univ Texas Hlth Sci Ctr 1986; **Fac Appt:** Prof Med, Wake Forest Univ

Khawaja, Shazib N MD [IC] - **Spec Exp:** Peripheral Vascular Disease; Vascular Medicine; Echocardiography; Nuclear Cardiology; **Hospital:** Tanner Med Ctr; **Address:** 100 Professional Park, Ste 310, Carrollton, GA 30117; **Phone:** 770-836-9326; **Board Cert:** Internal Medicine 1998; Cardiovascular Disease 2001; Interventional Cardiology 2003; Vascular Medicine 2007; **Med School:** Univ S Ala Coll Med 1995; **Resid:** Internal Medicine, Albany Med Ctr 1998; **Fellow:** Cardiovascular Disease, Dartmouth Hitchcock Med Ctr 2000; Interventional Cardiology, Univ Minnesota Med Ctr 2002; **Fac Appt:** Asst Clin Prof Med, Univ S Ala Coll Med

Interventional Cardiology

Margolis, James MD [IC] - **Spec Exp:** Cardiac Catheterization; Invasive Cardiology; Angioplasty; **Hospital:** Univ of Miami Hosp, Baptist Hosp of Miami; **Address:** Miami Intl Cardiac Consultants, 3801 Biscayne Blvd Fl 3, Miami, FL 33137; **Phone:** 305-571-0620; **Board Cert:** Internal Medicine 1973; Cardiovascular Disease 1975; Interventional Cardiology 1999; **Med School:** Univ IL Coll Med 1968; **Resid:** Internal Medicine, Barnes Hosp 1972; **Fellow:** Cardiovascular Disease, Duke Med Ctr 1974; **Fac Appt:** Clin Prof Med, Univ Miami Sch Med

Matar, Fadi MD [IC] - **Spec Exp:** Angioplasty; **Hospital:** Tampa Genl Hosp, St Joseph's Hosp - Tampa; **Address:** 509 S Armenia Ave, Ste 200, Tampa, FL 33609; **Phone:** 813-353-1515; **Board Cert:** Interventional Cardiology 1999; Cardiovascular Disease 2007; **Med School:** Amer Univ Beirut 1987; **Resid:** Internal Medicine, Maryland Genl Hosp 1990; **Fellow:** Cardiovascular Disease, Wash Hosp Ctr 1994; **Fac Appt:** Asst Prof Med, Univ S Fla Coll Med

Morris, Douglas MD [IC] - **Spec Exp:** Interventional Cardiology; **Hospital:** Emory Univ Hosp, Crawford Long Hosp of Emory Univ; **Address:** Heart Center, 1365 Clifton Rd NE A Bldg - Ste A2205, Atlanta, GA 30322; **Phone:** 404-778-5310; **Board Cert:** Internal Medicine 1973; Cardiovascular Disease 1975; Interventional Cardiology 1999; **Med School:** Baylor Coll Med 1968; **Resid:** Internal Medicine, Vanderbilt Univ Med Ctr 1970; Internal Medicine, Vanderbilt Univ Med Ctr 1973; **Fellow:** Cardiovascular Disease, Emory Univ Hosps 1975; **Fac Appt:** Prof Med, Emory Univ

Midwest

Ellis, Stephen G MD [IC] - **Spec Exp:** Angioplasty & Stent Placement; Angiogenesis; **Hospital:** Cleveland Clin Fdn (page 56); **Address:** Cleveland Clinic, Div Cardiovasc Med, 9500 Euclid Ave, Desk F25, Cleveland, OH 44195; **Phone:** 216-445-6712; **Board Cert:** Internal Medicine 1981; Cardiovascular Disease 1985; Interventional Cardiology 1999; **Med School:** UCLA 1978; **Resid:** Internal Medicine, Cedars-Sinai Med Ctr 1981; **Fellow:** Cardiovascular Disease, Stanford Univ Med Ctr 1985; Interventional Cardiology, Emory Univ Hosp 1986; **Fac Appt:** Prof Med, Cleveland Cl Coll Med/Case West Res

Feldman, Ted E MD [IC] - **Spec Exp:** Angioplasty; **Hospital:** Evanston Hosp; **Address:** ENH Med Group, Cardiology, 2650 Ridge Ave Walgreen Bldg Fl 3, Evanston, IL 60201; **Phone:** 847-570-2250; **Board Cert:** Internal Medicine 1981; Cardiovascular Disease 1985; Interventional Cardiology 1999; **Med School:** Indiana Univ 1978; **Resid:** Internal Medicine, Rush-Presby-St Lukes Hosp 1982; **Fellow:** Cardiovascular Disease, Univ Chicago 1985; **Fac Appt:** Prof Med, Northwestern Univ

Henry, Timothy D MD [IC] - **Spec Exp:** Acute Coronary Syndromes; Angiogenesis; **Hospital:** Abbott - Northwestern Hosp; **Address:** Minneapolis Heart Inst, 920 E 28th St, Ste 40, Minneapolis, MN 55407; **Phone:** 612-863-3900; **Board Cert:** Internal Medicine 1985; Cardiovascular Disease 1989; Interventional Cardiology 2000; **Med School:** UCSF 1982; **Resid:** Internal Medicine, Univ Colorado Hosp 1985; **Fellow:** Cardiovascular Disease, Univ Minnesota 1990; Interventional Cardiology, Univ Minnesota 1991; **Fac Appt:** Assoc Prof Med, Univ Minn

Holmes Jr, David R MD [IC] - **Spec Exp:** Heart Attack; Acute Coronary Syndromes; Angioplasty & Restenosis; **Hospital:** Mayo Med Ctr & Clin - Rochester; **Address:** Mayo Clinic, Div Cardiovasc Dis, 200 First St SW, Rochester, MN 55905; **Phone:** 507-255-2504; **Board Cert:** Internal Medicine 1974; Cardiovascular Disease 1977; Interventional Cardiology 1999; **Med School:** Med Coll Wisc 1971; **Resid:** Internal Medicine, Mayo Clinic 1974; **Fellow:** Cardiovascular Disease, Mayo Clinic 1977; **Fac Appt:** Prof Med, Mayo Med Sch

Losordo, Douglas W MD [IC] - **Spec Exp:** Stem Cell Therapy in Heart Failure; Angiogenesis; Angioplasty & Stent Placement; Heart Attack; **Hospital:** Northwestern Meml Hosp; **Address:** 675 N St Clair St, Galter Bldg Fl 11 - Ste 240, Chicago, IL 60611; **Phone:** 312-695-0072; **Board Cert:** Internal Medicine 1986; Cardiovascular Disease 1989; Interventional Cardiology 2002; **Med School:** Univ VT Coll Med 1983; **Resid:** Internal Medicine, St Elizabeth's Med Ctr 1986; **Fellow:** Cardiovascular Disease, St Elizabeth's Med Ctr 1989; **Fac Appt:** Prof Med, Northwestern Univ-Feinberg Sch Med

Schreiber, Theodore L MD [IC] - **Spec Exp:** Coronary Angioplasty/Stents; Carotid Artery Disease; **Hospital:** Harper Univ Hosp; **Address:** Harper University Hospital, 3990 John R St, Webber Bldg - Ste 9370, Detroit, MI 48201; **Phone:** 313-745-7025; **Board Cert:** Internal Medicine 1981; Cardiovascular Disease 1983; Interventional Cardiology 2000; **Med School:** Cornell Univ-Weill Med Coll 1978; **Resid:** Internal Medicine, New Yok Hosp-Cornell Med Ctr 1981; **Fellow:** Cardiovascular Disease, NY Hosp-Cornell Med Ctr 1983; **Fac Appt:** Assoc Prof Med, Wayne State Univ

Whitlow, Patrick MD [IC] - **Spec Exp:** Cardiac Catheterization; **Hospital:** Cleveland Clin Fdn (page 56); **Address:** Dept Cardiology, 9500 Euclid Ave, Desk F25, Cleveland, OH 44195; **Phone:** 216-444-1746; **Board Cert:** Internal Medicine 1979; Cardiovascular Disease 1981; Interventional Cardiology 1999; **Med School:** Duke Univ 1976; **Resid:** Internal Medicine, Parkland Meml Hosp 1979; **Fellow:** Cardiovascular Disease, Univ Alabama Hosp 1981

Southwest

Bailey, Steven R MD [IC] - **Spec Exp:** Coronary Artery Disease; Coronary Angioplasty/Stents; **Hospital:** Univ Hlth Sys - Univ Hosp (San Antonio, TX); **Address:** 7703 Floyd Curl Drive, MC 7872, San Antonio, TX 78229-3900; **Phone:** 210-567-4601; **Board Cert:** Internal Medicine 1981; Cardiovascular Disease 1983; Interventional Cardiology 1999; **Med School:** Oregon Hlth Sci Univ 1978; **Resid:** Internal Medicine, Fitzsimmons AMC 1981; **Fellow:** Cardiovascular Disease, Fitzsimmons AMC 1983; **Fac Appt:** Prof Med, Univ Tex, San Antonio

Kleiman, Neal Stephen MD [IC] - **Spec Exp:** Angioplasty; **Hospital:** Methodist Hosp - Houston; **Address:** 6550 Fannin, Smith Tower St, Ste 1901, Houston, TX 77030; **Phone:** 713-441-1100; **Board Cert:** Internal Medicine 1984; Cardiovascular Disease 1987; Interventional Cardiology 1999; **Med School:** Columbia P&S 1981; **Resid:** Internal Medicine, Baylor Coll Med 1984; **Fellow:** Interventional Cardiology, Baylor Coll Med 1987; **Fac Appt:** Assoc Prof Med, Baylor Coll Med

Perin, Emerson C MD [IC] - **Spec Exp:** Stem Cell Therapy in Heart Failure; Angiogenesis; **Hospital:** St Luke's Episcopal Hosp - Houston; **Address:** Southwest Cardiology Consultants, 6624 Fannin St, Ste 2220, St Lukes Medical Tower Fl 22, Houston, TX 77030-2334; **Phone:** 713-791-9400; **Board Cert:** Internal Medicine 1988; Interventional Cardiology 1999; **Med School:** Brazil 1983; **Resid:** Internal Medicine, Jackson Meml Hosp 1988; **Fellow:** Cardiovascular Disease, St Luke's Episcopal Hosp 1991; **Fac Appt:** Asst Prof Med, Baylor Coll Med

Smalling, Richard Warren MD/PhD [IC] - **Spec Exp:** Coronary Artery Disease; Peripheral Vascular Disease; Heart Valve Disease; Congenital Heart Disease; **Hospital:** Meml Hermann Hosp - Texas Med Ctr; **Address:** 6431 Fannin St, MS 1246, Houston, TX 77030-1501; **Phone:** 713-500-6559; **Board Cert:** Internal Medicine 1978; Cardiovascular Disease 1981; Interventional Cardiology 1999; **Med School:** Univ Tex, Houston 1975; **Resid:** Internal Medicine, UCSD Med Ctr 1978; **Fellow:** Cardiovascular Disease, UCSD Med Ctr 1980; **Fac Appt:** Prof Med, Univ Tex, Houston

Interventional Cardiology

West Coast and Pacific

Buchbinder, Maurice MD [IC] - **Spec Exp:** Cardiac Catheterization; Peripheral Vascular Disease; **Hospital:** Scripps Meml Hosp - La Jolla; **Address:** 9834 Genesee Ave, Ste 310, La Jolla, CA 92037; **Phone:** 858-625-4488; **Board Cert:** Internal Medicine 1981; Cardiovascular Disease 1983; **Med School:** Canada 1978; **Resid:** Internal Medicine, Jewish Genl Hosp 1980; Internal Medicine, Stanford Univ Hosp 1982; **Fellow:** Cardiovascular Disease, Stanford Univ Hosp 1983

Teirstein, Paul S MD [IC] - **Spec Exp:** Coronary Angioplasty/Stents; Coronary Radiation Therapy; **Hospital:** Scripps Green Hosp; **Address:** Scripps Clinic, 10666 N Torrey Pines Rd, Mail Drop S1056, La Jolla, CA 92037; **Phone:** 858-554-9905; **Board Cert:** Internal Medicine 1983; Cardiovascular Disease 1987; Interventional Cardiology 1999; **Med School:** Mount Sinai Sch Med 1980; **Resid:** Internal Medicine, Brigham & Womens Hosp 1983; **Fellow:** Cardiovascular Disease, Stanford Univ 1986; Interventional Cardiology, Mid-Amer Heart Inst 1987

Yeung, Alan MD [IC] - **Spec Exp:** Mitral Valve Disease; Coronary Artery Disease; **Hospital:** Stanford Univ Med Ctr; **Address:** Stanford Univ Medical Ctr, Dept Interventional Cardiology, 300 Pasteur Drive, rm H2103, MC 5218, Stanford, CA 94305-5218; **Phone:** 650-723-0180; **Board Cert:** Internal Medicine 1987; Cardiovascular Disease 1989; Interventional Cardiology 2000; **Med School:** Harvard Med Sch 1984; **Resid:** Internal Medicine, Mass General Hosp 1987; **Fellow:** Cardiovascular Disease, Brigham & Women's Hosp 1990; **Fac Appt:** Prof Med, Stanford Univ

America's Top Doctors® 8th Edition

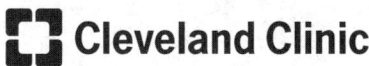 **Cleveland Clinic**

Heart and Vascular Institute

America's Best Care

Cleveland Clinic's Heart and Vascular Institute is one of the largest and most experienced cardiovascular specialty groups in the world, providing patients with expert medical management and a full range of therapies. Our areas of expertise combine research, education and clinical practice to provide innovative and scientifically based treatments for cardiovascular disease. *U.S.News & World Report* has ranked the Cleveland Clinic best in the nation for heart care every year since 1995.

Patients come to the Heart and Vascular Institute from every state in the country and from around the world. In 2007, our staff recorded 290,000 patient visits, completed more than 13,000 procedures and performed more than 3,400 open heart surgeries. This experience, along with our outcomes, distinguishes the Cleveland Clinic Heart and Vascular Institute from all other institutions.

Clinical Trials and Research

Our Heart and Vascular Institute is a recognized leader in multicenter and international trials. An outstanding clinical infrastructure and strong commitment to basic science allow Cleveland Clinic to remain on the cutting edge of treatment and research in cardiovascular disease. More than 200 clinical research projects and trials currently are under way here, ranging from basic cellular research to the development of a new artificial heart. Cleveland Clinic researchers have recently made history with their confirmation of a specific gene identified as a cause of human coronary heart disease.

New Home to the Heart and Vascular Institute

The #1 heart program in America now has a new home in the Sydell and Arnold Miller Family Pavilion. The one million-square-foot building, the country's largest single-use facility for heart and vascular care, features 16 state-of-the-art operating rooms, 12 new catheterization labs, eight electrophysiology labs and four dedicated intensive care units.

This patient-centered facility also features private patient rooms, comfortable accommodations for family members, a light-filled central lobby and an extraordinary rooftop plaza, making the building as beautiful as it is efficient.

History of Innovations

Cleveland Clinic doctors have helped define the modern era of cardiovascular care, having pioneered coronary angiography and saphenous vein bypass surgery. Today, our staff continues this proud tradition of innovation and discovery to shape the future of the field.

For more information about the Cleveland Clinic Heart and Vascular Institute, to schedule a second opinion or to learn about assistance for out-of-town patients, call 800.890.2467 or visit www.clevelandclinic.org/hearttopdocs.

Heart and Vascular Institute | 9500 Euclid Avenue / AC311 | Cleveland OH 44195

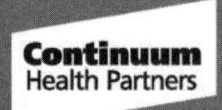

Beth Israel Medical Center
Roosevelt Hospital
St. Luke's Hospital
Long Island College Hospital of Brooklyn

Cardiac Services

(800) 420-4004

Continuum Health Partners offers outstanding cardiac programs at its member hospitals—Beth Israel Medical Center, Roosevelt Hospital, St. Luke's Hospital and Long Island College Hospital of Brooklyn—with a constant dedication to clinical excellence.

The Continuum hospitals offer the full array of clinical expertise needed to diagnose and treat the many conditions that can affect the heart, including coronary artery disease, heart valve insufficiencies, congenital and non-congenital structural abnormalities, hypertension, heart failure, heart rhythm abnormalities and hypertrophic cardiomyopathy.

We are strong believers in prevention and early detection, and our experts provide complete cardiac diagnostic testing, utilizing state-of-the-art echocardiography, nuclear and non-nuclear stress testing, angiography, PET scanning and more. We also offer programs for coronary artery disease prevention, smoking cessation, treatment centers for obesity and diabetes, and complementary techniques for relaxation and stress reduction, such as massage therapy and therapeutic touch.

Our state-of-the-art cardiac catheterization labs are available around the clock for emergency cardiac cases—when every minute counts—offering life-saving angioplasty to patients arriving in our emergency departments with acute heart attack conditions.

Our cardiac surgery outcomes have been recognized by the New York State Department of Health as having some of the lowest mortality rates in New York City, and our programs have maintained a consistent level of performance since their inception.

Some of the unique features in the cardiac programs at the Continuum hospitals include robotic surgical capabilities for minimally invasive cardiac surgery, a nationally recognized arrhythmia service, a 64-slice CT scanner used to rapidly perform non-invasive cardiac angiograms, minimally invasive radial artery harvesting for bypass surgery, nationally and internationally recognized experts in multiple areas of cardiac care, and a commitment to research to find the cures of tomorrow.

Beth Israel   Roosevelt Hospital   St. Luke's Hospital   Long Island College Hospital   NY Eye & Ear Infirmary

PENN CARDIAC CARE

Penn Cardiac Care combines the renowned expertise of its researchers, clinicians and educators to provide the best patient care and services. Our team offers patients the highest level of cardiac care, with access to the expertise, resources and research available only from Penn.

Penn's heart specialists are experts in preventing, diagnosing and treating routine and complex conditions related to the heart, including but not limited to:

- Blocked heart arteries
- Congenital heart defects
- Heart failure
- Heart palpitations
- High blood pressure
- High cholesterol
- Valve disease
- Vascular disease

World-Class Heart Care

Penn is recognized as one of the nation's leading heart programs with expertise in heart failure and transplantation, thoracic aortic surgery, mitral valve repair and replacement, endovascular stent graft repair, cardiac electrophysioiogy, interventional cardiology and preventive cardiology.

Opening in 2009, the **Penn Heart and Vascular Center** at the Perelman Center for Advanced Medicine will provide patients an integrated array of medical, diagnostic, and surgical services to manage and treat heart disease.

State-Of-The-Art Technology And Research

- Penn is among the few surgical institutions in the nation with a fully incorporated research facility, ensuring the future progress of cardiovascular research.
- Pioneering the most advanced techniques and devices, such as ablation therapy for atrial fibrillation.

- Offering a full-range of surgical options including minimally invasive robotic, off-pump, port access, and bloodless techniques.
- Conducting numerous clinical studies, such as mechanical assist devices and percutaneous approaches to treating valvular and structural heart disease.
- Serving as the lead national site for several trials, including endovascular stent graft repair for thoracic aortic aneurysms.
- Implanting the first temporary total artificial heart in the region, Penn continues to bring a new generation of ventricular assist devices to the treatment of late-stage heart failure.

Regional Referral Center

Penn Cardiac Care provides comprehensive care for patients with heart failure, offering more treatment options than ever before. Cutting-edge therapy for heart failure includes:

- Drug therapy
- Pacemakers
- Implantable cardioverter defibrillators (ICDs)
- Ablative therapy
- Coronary artery bypass grafting (CABG)
- Heart valve repair or replacement
- Ventricular assist devices (VADs)
- Heart transplantation

Penn is among the nation's top 5 adult heart transplant centers, performing more adult heart transplants than all other Philadelphia area hospitals combined.

The Penn Thoracic Aortic Surgery Program is the first comprehensive program of its kind in the region to treat thoracic aortic diseases, including aneurysms and dissections.

Nationally Recognized Expertise

Penn's doctors have been recognized for excellence in cardiology and cardiothoracic services:

- Penn Cardiac Care at the Hospital of the University of Pennsylvania is ranked 12th in the nation, and best in the Philadelphia region, for heart care and heart surgery by *U.S.News & World Report*'s 2008 Best Hospitals ranking.
- Penn Presbyterian Medical Center was among *Thomson's* "100 Top Cardiovascular Hospitals" for five years in a row.
- *Best Doctors in America*® lists more doctors from the University of Pennsylvania Health System than any other health system in the Philadelphia region.
- The Hospital of the University of Pennsylvania and Penn Presbyterian are recognized by Independence Blue Cross as "Centers of Blue Distinction" for excellence in quality standards and patient care.

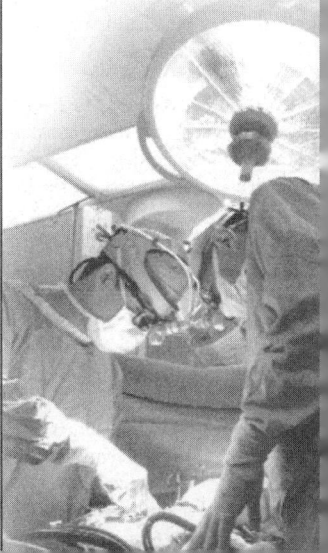

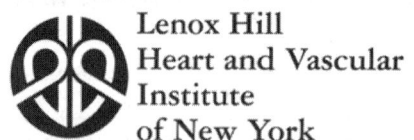

Lenox Hill Heart and Vascular Institute of New York

Lenox Hill Hospital
100 East 77th Street, New York, NY 10075
Tel: 212-434-2000
www.lenoxhillhospital.org

SETTING THE WORLD STANDARD FOR COMPLEX CARDIAC CARE

The Lenox Hill Heart and Vascular Institute is among the leading cardiovascular care programs nationwide. From diagnosis to treatment and recovery, the Institute provides comprehensive care through its distinguished team of cardiologists, interventional cardiologists, electrophysiologists, cardiothoracic and vascular surgeons, and radiologists.

DEPTH OF EXPERIENCE

Lenox Hill Hospital has been a leader in cardiovascular care for decades, developing groundbreaking techniques to minimize heart damage and speed recovery:

- 1938 — Lenox Hill Hospital cardiologists performed first angiogram in U.S.
- 1978 — first coronary angioplasty in the U.S. performed at Lenox Hill Hospital
- 1991 — Lenox Hill Hospital doctors implanted first coronary stent in NYC
- 1994 — Lenox Hill Hospital surgeons introduced minimally invasive direct coronary artery bypass surgery to nation
- 2003 — First FDA approved drug coated stent in the nation was implanted at Lenox Hill Hospital in a procedure our doctors now perform over 3,000 times each year
- 2004 — Largest carotid stent program in U.S.
- 2005 — Largest minimally invasive heart assist program in tri-state area; second largest nationally
- 2008 — Ranked #25 nationally among top hospitals in Heart and Heart Surgery by U.S. News & World Report
- 2008— Recipient of the HealthGrades Cardiac Care Excellence Award
- 2008—Ranked among Top 5% in the Nation by HealthGrades for Coronary Interventions five years in a row
- 2008—First 256 Slice Computer Tomographic (CT) Scanner in the Northeastern U.S., and only one of three in the country, was installed at Lenox Hill Hospital

A WIDE RANGE OF TREATMENTS

Physicians at the Institute constantly seek to broaden the understanding of heart and vascular disease and expand the boundaries of care through research and clinical trials. The interventional cardiology team is recognized for leadership in the use of angioplasty to clear clogged arteries. The endovascular specialists are involved in groundbreaking research involving the use of carotid stents to provide lower-risk treatment of arterial blockages without surgery, and also perform minimally invasive procedures to treat complex abdominal aneurysms. The Institute's cardiothoracic surgeons are pioneers in "beating heart" surgery, and the use of robotics and minimally invasive procedures including coronary bypass, valve repair, atrial fibrillation surgery, and heart failure surgery. Surgeons specializing in vascular surgery perform surgery on the aorta, and the carotid and lower extremity arteries, including aneurysms. The Institute's electrophysiology specialists perform diagnostic, treatment and curative procedures for abnormal heart rhythms.

2008 was a year of particular distinction for Lenox Hill Hospital. Lenox Hill Hospital was the recipient of the 2008 HealthGrades Cardiac Care Excellence Award, and ranked among the Top 5% in the nation for Coronary Interventions for the fifth year in a row. LHH was also five-star rated for coronary interventional procedures, cardiology care, and treatment of heart attack and heart failure by HealthGrades. The first 256 Slice Computer Tomographic (CT) Scanner in the Northeastern United States was installed at LHH, making it the one of only three hospitals in the country to acquire this advanced cardiovascular imaging system. Images from the scanner show the coronary arteries with extreme clarity making it easier to detect and treat structural heart disease, peripheral vascular disease, and carotid artery disease.

TIME IS MUSCLE

It's a fact. The faster a person is treated for a heart attack, the greater the chances of saving precious heart muscle and making a full recovery. That's why doctors say "time is muscle."

Today, using the most advanced technologies and sophisticated emergency communications from our ambulance directly to our cardiologists, Lenox Hill Hospital doctors have drastically reduced the time it takes for a heart attack patient to get lifesaving treatment. After all, time is muscle – and you know how important that is.

Maimonides Medical Center
MAIMONIDES CARDIAC INSTITUTE

4802 Tenth Avenue • Brooklyn, New York 11219
Phone: (800) 682-5558/(718) 283-8902 • Fax: (718) 635-7505
http://www.maimonidesmed.org

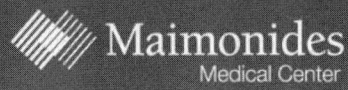

Maimonides
Medical Center

Having pioneered numerous heart care innovations through the years, the Cardiac Institute offers a rapidly growing number of diagnostic studies and therapeutic treatments, procedures and surgeries. Ranked by the Centers for Medicare and Medicaid Services as one of the only three hospitals in the country to achieve excellent ratings in both heart attack and heart failure patient outcomes.

Cardiology
Among the most published and respected in the field, the Maimonides cardiology team continuously sets higher standards for patient care. Edgar Lichstein, MD, Chair of Medicine, has been chief investigator of NIH-sponsored cardiac drug trials, and our Congestive Heart Failure (CHF) Program is cited as the best in the Northeast.

Interventional Cardiology
Led by Cardiac Institute Chairman Jacob Shani, MD, drug-eluting stents were trialed here and numerous therapeutic devices were developed and implemented. Our Electrophysiology Lab has a superb record of achievement in diagnosing and treating arrhythmias. A close collaboration with the Department of Emergency Medicine ensures that chest pain patients are evaluated immediately and that interventional procedures are used to stop heart attacks in progress whenever necessary.

Cardiothoracic Surgery
The Maimonides Cardiothoracic Surgery program has an illustrious history, setting the national standard for advances in service. Under the direction of Stephen Lahey, MD, minimally invasive and robotic heart surgeries are offered in state-of-the-art facilities. In collaboration with Electrophysiology, Cardiothoracic Surgery has established an Atrial Fibrillation Center of Excellence. Maimonides provides one of the most prestigious cardiothoracic residency programs in the US.

Historic Moments
• In 1967, the first successful human heart transplant in the nation was performed at Maimonides.
• The intra-aortic balloon pump was developed here in 1970.
• Surgical techniques that protect the spine during cardiothoracic surgery were perfected here in 1982.
• Revolutionary cardiac catheterization devices invented here in 1992 and 1997.
• Maimonides was the first hospital in US to implement fully automatic external cardiac defibrillators in 2001.

Physicians at Maimonides are among the ten percent in the US who use computers to enter patient orders, thereby reducing the risk of errors, increasing efficiency, and speeding the healing process. Maimonides has appeared on the American Hospital Association's "Most Wired" and "Most Wireless" lists more often than any other healthcare institution in the metropolitan area. Advanced technology allows our doctors to focus more attention on caring for their patients.

Maimonides Medical Center – Passionate about medicine, compassionate about people.

www.maimonidesmed.org/cardiac

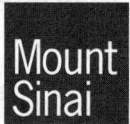 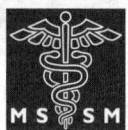

THE MOUNT SINAI MEDICAL CENTE
MOUNT SINAI HEART—CARDIOVASCULAR HEALT
One Gustave L. Levy Plac
Fifth Avenue and 100th Stree
New York, NY 10029-657
Physician Referral: 1-800-MD-SINAI (637-462‹
www.mountsinai.or

MOUNT SINAI
SCHOOL OF
MEDICINE

At Mount Sinai Heart, we take both a personal and a global view of cardiovascular health. Our system of integrated care combines the world's most accomplished physicians, research scientists, and educators with innovative thinking, creative programs, and an unwavering commitment to the prevention and treatment of cardiovascular disease. With access to the latest discoveries and the most experienced minds, our doctors bring a diversity of views to ensure that patients receive the perfect treatments for their individual needs. The rapid translation of innovative research concepts into prevention, diagnosis, and therapy means that patients receive multidisciplinary treatment of unprecedented quality. Our programs span the care of patients from the earliest stages of life—our pediatric cardiologists can detect cardiac disease in the unborn fetus—well into the advanced elderly years through specialized geriatric cardiology.

In addition to consultative cardiology, cardiac catheterization, heart and lung transplantation, cardiovascular surgery, heart failure, pulmonary hypertension, lipid management, and hypertension, we specialize in the following areas:

- *Noninvasive diagnostic imaging* – leading techniques for echocardiography, nuclear cardiology, PET, CT, and MRI technology;

- *Coronary artery disease* – ranked the New York State's safest center for patients undergoing coronary angioplasty and other catheter-based interventions;

- *Cardiac rhythm disturbances* – expert management of all aspects of heart rhythm disorders, such as atrial fibrillation and tachycardias, and implantable devices such as pacemakers and defibrillators;

- *Valvular heart disease* – a wide range of medical and surgical options, including a leading program for valve repair and long-term follow-up care;

- *Aortic diseases* – pioneering techniques for stent-graft repair of thoracic and abdominal aortic aneurysms and for surgical correction of the most complex aortic pathology;

- *Congenital heart disease* – specialists in pediatric cardiology and experts in minimally invasive approaches to the correction of congenital heart defects in children and adults;

- *Cardiac failure and transplantation* – a multidisciplinary team approach to comprehensive, compassionate care for patients with the most advanced forms of heart failure and cardiomyopathy;

- *Comprehensive cardiac disease prevention and rehabilitation* – a unique synergism that provides unparalleled patient care while yielding breakthroughs in the prevention and treatment of cardiovascular disease;

- *Vascular medicine and surgery* – noninvasive diagnostic procedures and an interdisciplinary approach to disease management, from medical, surgical, catheter-based, and gene therapy techniques for arterial obstruction, limb salvage, venous, and lymphatic diseases.

Mount Sinai's Cardiac Catheterization Laboratories offer leading-edge technologies of all kinds to study the heart with the greatest precision available, including diagnostic angiography, angioplasty, and biopsy We are pioneering genetic techniques to grow new vessels in patients with diseased arteries and to help damaged heart muscle repair itself.

LEADING SURGEONS, INNOVATIVE TREATMENT Under the creative direction of internationally renowned cardiologist Valentin Fuster, MD, PhD, Mount Sinai is recognized worldwide for expertise in evaluating, managing, and preventing cardiovascular disease through the integration of patient care, education, and research. Mount Sinai Heart encompasses the Zena and Michael A. Wiener Cardiovascular Institute and the Marie-Josée and Henry R. Kravis Center for Cardiovascular Health at The Mount Sinai Medical Center, preeminent resources for the study and treatment of heart and blood vessel diseases. The cardiac conditions treated at Mount Sinai Heart include: arrhythmia (including atrial fibrillation, pacemakers, defibrillators, and other implanted devices coronary artery disease, hear attack and angina, heart failure and transplantation, hyperlipidemia (cholesterol), hypertension, mitral valve prolapse, myocarditis, pericardial disease, aortic diseases, peripheral vascular disease and intermittent claudication, pulmonary hypertension, and valvular heart disease.

NYU Cardiac and Vascular Institute
NYU LANGONE MEDICAL CENTER

550 First Avenue (at 31St Street)
New York, NY 10016
Physician Referral:
(888)7-NYU-MED (888-769-8633)
www.nyumc.org

Collaboration with the NYU Cardiac & Vascular Institute brings care full circle.

The skilled, world-class heart and vascular specialists at the NYU Cardiac & Vascular Institute (CVI) never take any patient with cardiovascular disease for granted. Each case is unique. The philosophy has made the NYU CVI a leader in developing new techniques for repairing heart valves, curing heart rhythm disorders, treating aortic disease and developing care plans for congestive heart failure. Our cardiac and vascular physicians work collaboratively with the cardiac rehabilitation team to move patients seamlessly from treatment into the recovery and maintenance phase of their care. Other programs such as weight management, smoking cessation and diabetic management focus on prevention. It is total patient experience at NYU that has resulted in so many successes for patients of all ages with cardiovascular hear disease.

Cardiology
NYU's Division of Cardiology is a world-renowned leader in cardiovascular biomedical research. Patient care and education, with a longstanding tradition of educating and training some of the brightest and most promising physicians and researchers of the future. Members of the Division of Cardiology are devoted to providing evidence-based, state-of-the-art, compassionate healthcare. Our clinicians and researchers are advancing the field of cardiovascular medicine, and contribute to the reputation of NYU as comprehensive cardiovascular center of excellence.

Cardiac Surgery
NYU's Cardiac surgeons are internationally recognized for pioneering mitral valve repair and minimally invasive cardiac surgery. Our team has performed mote than 3,000 minimally invasive valve repairs and replacements, changing the standard of care fore heart surgery and dramatically improving results. NYU's surgeons are widely known for expert care of elderly and high-risk patients, using new technology and less invasive techniques to improve results and lowest risks. This expertise is shared with other surgeons from around the world, who come to NYU to study with the cardiac surgical team.

Vascular Surgery
With decades of expertise treating thousands of patients with conditions ranging from life-threatening issues of arterial aneurysms to deep vein thrombosis, as well as carotid stenosis and limb salvage, the Division of Vascular and Endovascular Surgery offers expert patient care with emphasis on minimally invasive diagnostic and treatment approaches. Traditionally cosmetic procedures such as treatment of varicose and spider veins, are performed at the NYU Vein Center with comprehensive, medical approach. Our vascular surgeons are part of the teaching team for NYU School of Medicine and are training the next generation of physicians through a top vascular surgery fellowship program. The Division also holds training courses in minimally invasive vein surgery, endovascular aortic surgery, thoracic aneurysm correction, and abdominal aneurysm interventions for practicing surgeons throughout the world.

Cardiac Catheterization Lab
At the leading edge of interventional cardiology, the Cardiac Catheterization Lab at NYU continues to set the standard for catheter-based diagnosis and evaluation of cardiac health. Located at Tisch Hospital, the Cath Lab provides a full range of procedures to evaluate how well the heart muscle and valves are working; to detect and measure any narrowing in the coronary arteries; and to recommend appropriate treatment as needed. Our lab is defined by its comprehensive, evidence-based approach to the care of each individual patient.

Cardiac Rehabilitation Center
Rehabilitation is a necessary for the cardiac patients who have undergone heart procedures. With distinguishes cardiac rehab at NYU Medical Center is its individualized patient care. At the Cardiac Rehab Center, physical rehabilitation takes place in a state-of-the-art facility, where patients work on building both aerobic capacity and strength. Our Cardiac Rehab team works closely with cardiologists, physiatrists, nurses, physical and occupational therapists, psychologists, social workers, exercise physiologists, nutritionists and other healthcare professionals to help patients return, rehabilitated, to their everyday lives.

NYU Langone Medical Center

550 First Avenue (at 31St Street)
New York, NY 10016
Physician Referral:
(888)7-NYU-MED (888-769-8633)
www.nyumc.org

ADULT CARDIOVASCULAR SERVICES

MINIMALLY INVASIVE CARDIAC SURGERY

NYU Langone Medical Center's physician-scientists have been at the forefront of innovation in modem cardiovascular medicine for more than a half-century. In recent years, cardiothoracic surgeons at NYU have pioneered minimally invasive cardiac surgery, dramatically improving treatment of the most common forms of heart disease. More minimally invasive cardiac surgeries have been performed at NYU than at any other hospital in the world.

With the development of minimally invasive technology, surgeons achieve results that are comparable or even superior to those obtained via traditional open-chest surgery. Procedures such as coronary artery bypass grafting (CABG) and mitral valve repair or replacement (MVR) are now performed through a single small incision between the ribs. This approach not only lowers the risk of complications, such as bleeding and infei l Bn, but also reduces postoperative pain and scarring, speeds the recovery process, and helps patients resume their normal lives in record time.

THE CARDIAC CATHETERIZATION LABORATORY
AND ELECTROPIIYSIOLOGY PROGRAM

At the cutting edge of interventional cardiology, the Cardiac Catheterization Laboratory at NYU continues to set the standard of care for catheter-based diagnosis and evaluation of cardiac health. Located at Tisch Hospital, and integrated with the newly opened Blechman CV Center, the Cath Lab provides a full range of procedures to evaluate how well the heart muscle and valves are working, whether the heart is beating at regular intervals, detect and measure any narrowing in the coronary arteries, and recommend appropriate treatment if needed.

THE CARDIAC REHABILITATION CENTER

Follow-up care for cardiac patients is all about rehabilitation. What distinguishes cardiac rehab at NYU Langone Medical Center is its quality of organization, rigorousness, and individualized patient care. At the Cardiac Rehab Center, physical rehabilitation takes place in a state- of-the-art gym, replete with spectacular views of the river and the Manhattan skyline. Patients work out to build both aerobic capacity and strength, and are fully supervised to maximize safety. Patient care at the Rehab Center is premised on the powerful idea that it takes a "village" to treat a patient. At NYU, that village is a team of cardiologists, physiatrists, nurses, physical and occupational therapists, psychologists, social workers, exercise physiologists, nutritionists, and other healthcare professionals. The goal is to return patients to their normal lives, rehabilitated and ready to meet the challenges of the world.

St. Francis Hospital The Heart Center®
100 Port Washington Blvd.
Roslyn, New York 11576
www.stfrancisheartcenter.com
(516) 562-6000   1-888-HEARTNY

Non-Invasive Cardiac Imaging
Using the latest in non-invasive cardiac imaging technology, St. Francis Hospital's physicians have immediate access to information regarding blood flow, heart muscle strength, anatomy, and coronary artery blockages that allows them to more effectively guide a patient's course of treatment.

Among the most recent advances in St. Francis Hospital's range of services are:

Coronary CT Angiography
St. Francis Hospital was the first hospital on Long Island to offer Multidetector Computed Tomography (MDCT) for non-invasive coronary artery imaging and helped pioneer a new Cardiac Imaging Specialist network which has exclusive rights to perform MDCT for several leading health insurers. This technology provides previously unobtainable non-invasive visualization of the coronary arteries and plaque buildup in the walls of the arteries.

Cardiac MRI
The only center on Long Island with world-class expertise in cardiac MRI, St. Francis Hospital has the ability to non-invasively evaluate heart anatomy, function, scarring, blood flow and inflammation using advanced techniques on two state-of-the-art scanners. Cardiac MRI allows physicians to evaluate effects of heart attack, effects of coronary artery blockages and the causes of heart failure to determine whether or not patients will benefit from heart surgery or other therapies. World-renowned cardiac MRI authority Nathaniel Reichek, M.D., leads St. Francis Hospital's clinical and research applications with cardiac MRI.

Three-Dimensional Echocardiography
St. Francis Hospital is an internationally recognized leader in three-dimensional echocardiography for quantifying the effects of heart disease and the leading center in the New York metropolitan area in this field. By creating three-dimensional reconstructions of the heart and blood flow within it, this technology provides diagnostic information that far surpasses that available with conventional echocardiography in many patients.

Nuclear Imaging
Nuclear imaging, which involves the injection of nuclear isotopes and continuous imaging by a gamma camera that circles the patient's body, improves the accuracy of stress testing. St. Francis Hospital offers the latest advances in nuclear cardiology, such as single-photon emission computed tomography with CT image correction (SPECT/CT). The nuclear cardiology laboratory at St. Francis Hospital is also a leader in developing new types of computer analysis to improve the value of SPECT imaging, and was among the first facilities in the U.S. to receive accreditation from The Intersocietal Commission for the Accreditation of Nuclear Medicine Laboratories. In 2009, St. Francis will become the only Long Island hospital offering cardiac positron emission tomography with CT, or PET/CT, a new advanced approach which can further enhance diagnostic assessment and clinical decision making.

Non-Invasive Imaging at St. Francis Hospital
Non-invasive imaging services at St. Francis Hospital include:
- multidetector computed tomographic coronary angiography
- cardiac MRI
- SPECT/CT nuclear imaging
- transesophageal echocardiography
- three-dimensional echocardiography
- Stress testing with nuclear, echocardiographic or MRI imaging

St. Francis Hospital's cutting-edge non-invasive imaging technology is also being applied in its research programs on cardiovascular disease. Applying its depth of experience with various imaging modalities, the Hospital has launched a multi-disciplinary effort at its St. Francis Cardiac Research Institute to improve methods for the diagnosis and treatment of cardiac disease. Past research efforts at the Hospital include The St. Francis Heart Study—the largest study on coronary risk factors to be conducted at any single center—which supported the use of CT scanning for atherosclerotic plaque detection as a tool for cardiac risk evaluation.

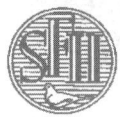

St. Francis Hospital The Heart Center®

100 Port Washington Blvd.
Roslyn, New York 11576
www.stfrancisheartcenter.com
(516) 562-6000   1-888-HEARTNY

A Leader in Cardiac Care

St. Francis Hospital, The Heart Center® is New York State's only specialty designated cardiac center and is the busiest heart center in the Northeast. Located in Roslyn, New York, on Long Island's North Shore, St. Francis Hospital has been ranked among the best hospitals in the United States by *U.S. News & World Report* in heart and heart surgery, digestive disorders and geriatrics.

St. Francis:

• Performs more open-heart surgeries and cardiac interventional procedures than any other hospital in New York State

• Offers innovative approaches to cardiac surgery, including minimally invasive procedures and off-pump coronary artery bypass surgery, designed to minimize trauma and reduce surgical complications

• Performs one of the region's highest volumes of catheter-based techniques to close atrial septal defects (ASDs) and patent foramen ovale (PFO)

• Operates a nationally recognized Arrhythmia and Pacemaker Center staffed with electrophysiologists with over a decade of experience in radiofrequency ablation, a permanent cure for certain arrhythmias, including atrial fibrillation

• Maintains a high volume center for the implantation of cardiac pacemakers and defibrillators

• Offers the only world-class program in cardiac imaging that fully integrates all technologies including advanced methods in cardiac MRI, coronary CT angiography and three-dimensional echocardiography

• Has received the Magnet Award for excellence in nursing services

• Is a premier center for clinical trials and studies of the application of image-guided methods of diagnosis and treatment of heart disease

St. Francis Hospital has near-perfect patient satisfaction ratings, with over 99 percent of patients saying they would recommend the Hospital to family and friends.

"Our large cardiac caseload and our growing research program put us in an excellent position to introduce new techniques that can benefit thousands of people in need each year."

–Alan D. Guerci,M.D.
President and Chief Executive Officer
St. Francis Hospital, The Heart Center®

Child Neurology
a subspecialty of Neurology

A neurologist specializes in the diagnosis and treatment of all types of disease or impaired function of the brain, spinal cord, peripheral nerves, muscles and autonomic nervous system, as well as the blood vessels that relate to these structures. A child neurologist has special skills in the diagnosis and management of neurologic disorders of the neonatal period, infancy, early childhood and adolescence.

Training Required: Four years

CHILD NEUROLOGY

New England

Darras, Basil T MD [ChiN] - **Spec Exp:** Neuromuscular Disorders; Cerebral Palsy; **Hospital:** Children's Hospital - Boston; **Address:** 300 Longwood Ave, Childrens Hosp, Neurology, Fegan 11, Boston, MA 02115; **Phone:** 617-355-8235; **Board Cert:** Pediatrics 1988; Child Neurology 1992; Clinical Genetics 1987; **Med School:** Greece 1977; **Resid:** Pediatrics, Nassau County Med Ctr 1982; Child Neurology, Tufts-New England Med Ctr 1985; **Fellow:** Clinical Genetics, Yale Univ Sch Med 1988; **Fac Appt:** Prof N, Harvard Med Sch

Holmes, Gregory L MD [ChiN] - **Spec Exp:** Epilepsy/Seizure Disorders; **Hospital:** Dartmouth - Hitchcock Med Ctr; **Address:** Dartmouth-Hitchcock Med Ctr, Dept Neurology, 1 Medical Center Drive, Lebanon, NH 03756; **Phone:** 603-650-8586; **Board Cert:** Pediatrics 1979; Neurology 1980; **Med School:** Univ VA Sch Med 1974; **Resid:** Pediatrics, Yale-New Haven Hosp 1976; **Fellow:** Pediatric Neurology, Univ Virginia 1979; **Fac Appt:** Prof N, Dartmouth Med Sch

Mandelbaum, David E MD/PhD [ChiN] - **Spec Exp:** Epilepsy/Seizure Disorders; Brain Tumors-Pediatric; Neonatal Neurology; Autism; **Hospital:** Rhode Island Hosp, Women & Infants Hosp of RI; **Address:** Dept of Neurology, 110 Lockwood St, Ste 342, Providence, RI 02903; **Phone:** 401-444-5685; **Board Cert:** Child Neurology 1987; Pediatrics 1987; Clinical Neurophysiology 2003; Neurodevelopmental Disabilities 2001; **Med School:** Columbia P&S 1980; **Resid:** Pediatrics, Yale-New Haven Hosp 1982; Neurology, Neuro Inst-Columbia 1983; **Fellow:** Child Neurology, Neuro Inst-Columbia 1985; **Fac Appt:** Prof Ped, Brown Univ

Novotny, Edward MD [ChiN] - **Spec Exp:** Epilepsy/Seizure Disorders; Neurologic Imaging; Neurophysiology-Pediatric; **Hospital:** Yale-New Haven Hosp; **Address:** Dept of Pediatrics, Yale Sch of Med, PO Box 208064, New Haven, CT 06520-8064; **Phone:** 203-785-5730; **Board Cert:** Pediatrics 1986; Child Neurology 1986; Clinical Neurophysiology 2004; **Med School:** St Louis Univ 1979; **Resid:** Pediatrics, Univ CA Daivs Med Ctr 1981; Neurology, Stanford Univ Med Ctr 1984; **Fellow:** Epilepsy, Stanford Univ Med Ctr 1986; Magnetic Resonance Imaging, Yale Univ 1989; **Fac Appt:** Assoc Prof Ped, Yale Univ

Pomeroy, Scott L MD/PhD [ChiN] - **Spec Exp:** Neuro-Oncology; Brain Tumors; **Hospital:** Children's Hospital - Boston, Dana-Farber Cancer Inst; **Address:** Chldns Hosp, Dept Neurology-Fegan 11, 300 Longwood Ave, Boston, MA 02115; **Phone:** 617-355-6386; **Board Cert:** Pediatrics 2003; Child Neurology 1988; **Med School:** Univ Conn 1982; **Resid:** Pediatrics, Chldns Hosp 1984; Neurology, Barnes Hosp/Washington Univ 1985; **Fellow:** Pediatric Neurology, St Louis Chldns Hosp 1987; Neurological Biology, Washington Univ 1989; **Fac Appt:** Prof N, Harvard Med Sch

Sahin, Mustafa MD/PhD [ChiN] - **Spec Exp:** Tuberous Sclerosis; **Hospital:** Children's Hospital - Boston; **Address:** Childrens Hospital Boston, 300 Longwood Ave, Fegan 11, Boston, MA 02115; **Phone:** 617-355-2711; **Board Cert:** Child Neurology 2001; **Med School:** Yale Univ 1995; **Resid:** Pediatrics, Chldns Hosp 1997; Child Neurology, Chldns Hosp 2000; **Fac Appt:** Asst Prof N, Harvard Med Sch

Shaywitz, Bennett A MD [ChiN] - **Spec Exp:** Learning Disorders; Dyslexia; Headache; **Hospital:** Yale-New Haven Hosp; **Address:** Yale Univ Sch Med, Dept Peds, 333 Cedar St, Box 208064, New Haven, CT 06520-8064; **Phone:** 203-785-4641; **Board Cert:** Pediatrics 1968; Child Neurology 1973; **Med School:** Washington Univ, St Louis 1963; **Resid:** Pediatrics, Bronx Muni Hosp Ctr 1967; **Fellow:** Child Neurology, Albert Einstein Coll Med 1970; **Fac Appt:** Prof Ped, Yale Univ

Volpe, Joseph J MD [ChiN] - **Spec Exp:** Neonatal Neurology; Cerebral Palsy; **Hospital:** Children's Hospital - Boston, Mass Genl Hosp; **Address:** 300 Longwood Ave, Fegan 11, Boston, MA 02115-5724; **Phone:** 617-355-6388; **Board Cert:** Pediatrics 1970; Child Neurology 1974; **Med School:** Harvard Med Sch 1964; **Resid:** Pediatrics, Mass Genl Hosp 1966; Neurology, Mass Genl Hosp 1971; **Fellow:** Research, Natl Inst Child Hlth Human Dev 1968; **Fac Appt:** Prof N, Harvard Med Sch

Mid Atlantic

Allen, Jeffrey MD [ChiN] - **Spec Exp:** Neuro-Oncology; Brain Tumors; **Hospital:** NYU Med Ctr (page 68); **Address:** Hassenfeld Childrens Ctr, 160 E 32nd St, New York, NY 10016; **Phone:** 212-263-6725; **Board Cert:** Child Neurology 1977; **Med School:** Harvard Med Sch 1969; **Resid:** Pediatrics, Montreal Chldns Hosp 1973; Pediatric Neurology, Montreal Neur Inst/McGill 1976; **Fac Appt:** Prof Ped, NYU Sch Med

Crawford, Thomas O MD [ChiN] - **Spec Exp:** Neuromuscular Disorders; Muscular Dystrophy; Ataxia Telangiectasia; **Hospital:** Johns Hopkins Hosp - Baltimore (page 61); **Address:** Pediatric Neurology, 200 N Wolfe St, Ste 2158, Baltimore, MD 21287; **Phone:** 410-955-4259; **Board Cert:** Pediatrics 1986; Child Neurology 1990; Clinical Neurophysiology 1997; **Med School:** USC Sch Med 1980; **Resid:** Pediatrics, LAC-USC Med Ctr 1984; Child Neurology, Childrens Hosp 1987; **Fellow:** Neuromuscular Medicine, Johns Hopkins Hosp 1988; **Fac Appt:** Assoc Prof N, Johns Hopkins Univ

De Vivo, Darryl C MD [ChiN] - **Spec Exp:** Metabolic Disorders; Neuromuscular Disorders; Spinal Muscular Atrophy (SMA); **Hospital:** NY-Presby Hosp/Columbia (page 66); **Address:** Neurological Institute, 710 W 168th St, rm 201, New York, NY 10032; **Phone:** 212-305-5244; **Board Cert:** Child Neurology 1972; **Med School:** Univ VA Sch Med 1964; **Resid:** Pediatrics, Mass Genl Hosp 1966; Neurology, Mass Genl Hosp 1967; **Fellow:** Neurology, Natl Inst Hlth 1969; Child Neurology, Children's Hosp 1970; **Fac Appt:** Prof N, Columbia P&S

Duffner, Patricia K MD [ChiN] - **Spec Exp:** Brain Tumors; Krabbe Disease; Cancer Survivors-Late Effects of Therapy; **Hospital:** Women's & Chldn's Hosp of Buffalo, The; **Address:** Women & Childrens Hosp, Dept Neurology, 219 Bryant St, Buffalo, NY 14222-2006; **Phone:** 716-878-7819; **Board Cert:** Pediatrics 1977; Child Neurology 1979; **Med School:** SUNY Buffalo 1972; **Resid:** Pediatrics, Buffalo Chldns Hosp 1975; **Fellow:** Child Neurology, SUNY Buffalo-Buffalo Chldns Hosp 1978; **Fac Appt:** Prof N, SUNY Buffalo

Eviatar, Lydia MD [ChiN] - **Spec Exp:** Headache; Balance Disorders; Tourette's Syndrome; Cerebral Palsy; **Hospital:** Schneider Chldn's Hosp, Blythedale Children's Hosp; **Address:** 410 Lakeville Rd, Ste 105, New Hyde Park, NY 11040-1433; **Phone:** 516-465-5255; **Board Cert:** Pediatrics 1968; Child Neurology 1977; **Med School:** Israel 1961; **Resid:** Pediatrics, Tel Hashomer Hosp 1966; **Fellow:** Child Neurology, UCLA Med Ctr 1967; Neurology, UCLA Med Ctr 1969; **Fac Appt:** Prof N, Albert Einstein Coll Med

Maytal, Joseph MD [ChiN] - **Spec Exp:** Epilepsy/Seizure Disorders; Migraine; **Hospital:** Schneider Chldn's Hosp; **Address:** Dept Pediatric Neurology, Schneider Children's Hospital, 410 Lakeville Rd, Ste 105, New Hyde Park, NY 11042; **Phone:** 516-465-5255; **Board Cert:** Pediatrics 1986; Child Neurology 1988; **Med School:** Israel 1979; **Resid:** Pediatrics, Brookdale Hosp 1983; Child Neurology, Montefiore Med Ctr 1986; **Fellow:** Neurological Physiology, Albert Einstein Med Coll 1987; **Fac Appt:** Clin Prof N, Albert Einstein Coll Med

Child Neurology

Packer, Roger MD [ChiN] - **Spec Exp:** Brain Tumors; Neurofibromatosis; **Hospital:** Chldns Natl Med Ctr; **Address:** Chldns Natl Med Ctr, Dept Neurology, 111 Michigan Ave NW, Washington, DC 20010-2978; **Phone:** 202-476-2120; **Board Cert:** Child Neurology 1982; Pediatrics 1982; **Med School:** Northwestern Univ 1976; **Resid:** Pediatrics, Chldns Med Ctr 1978; Neurology, Chldns Hosp-Univ Penn 1981; **Fac Appt:** Prof N, Geo Wash Univ

Phillips, Peter C MD [ChiN] - **Spec Exp:** Brain Tumors; Neuro-Oncology; **Hospital:** Chldns Hosp of Philadelphia, The; **Address:** Childrens Hosp Philadelphia, 34th St & Civic Center Blvd, Philadelphia, PA 19104; **Phone:** 215-590-5188; **Board Cert:** Pediatrics 1985; Child Neurology 1986; **Med School:** Univ Conn 1978; **Resid:** Pediatrics, Chldns Hosp 1980; Pediatric Neurology, Neuro Inst 1983; **Fellow:** Neuro-Oncology, Meml Sloan Kettering Hosp 1986; **Fac Appt:** Prof N, Univ Pennsylvania

Shinnar, Shlomo MD/PhD [ChiN] - **Spec Exp:** Epilepsy/Seizure Disorders; Headache; **Hospital:** Montefiore Med Ctr; **Address:** Montefiore Medical Ctr, Children's Hospital, 111 E 210th St Fl 4, Bronx, NY 10467-2401; **Phone:** 718-920-4378; **Board Cert:** Neurology 1984; Pediatrics 1984; Clinical Neurophysiology 2005; **Med School:** Albert Einstein Coll Med 1978; **Resid:** Pediatrics, Johns Hopkins Hosp 1980; Neurology, Johns Hopkins Hosp 1983; **Fac Appt:** Prof N, Albert Einstein Coll Med

Southeast

Fenichel, Gerald M MD [ChiN] - **Spec Exp:** Neuromuscular Disorders; Muscular Dystrophy; **Hospital:** Vanderbilt Univ Med Ctr, Vanderbilt Children's Hosp; **Address:** Vanderbilt Childrens Hosp, Dept Neurology, 2200 Childrens Way, DOT, rm 11244, Nashville, TN 37232-9559; **Phone:** 615-936-5536; **Board Cert:** Neurology 1966; Child Neurology 1968; **Med School:** Yale Univ 1959; **Resid:** Neurology, Natl Inst Neuro Disorders-NIH 1963; Neurology, Yale-New Haven Hosp 1964; **Fac Appt:** Prof N, Vanderbilt Univ

Greenwood, Robert S MD [ChiN] - **Spec Exp:** Neurofibromatosis; Epilepsy; **Hospital:** Univ NC Hosps; **Address:** 101 Manning Drive, Chapel Hill, NC 27599; **Phone:** 919-966-1401; **Board Cert:** Pediatrics 1974; Child Neurology 1979; **Med School:** Univ Tex Med Br, Galveston 1968; **Resid:** Pediatrics, Chldns Hosp 1971; Child Neurology, Chldns Hosp 1975; **Fellow:** Child Neurology, Chldns Hosp 1977; **Fac Appt:** Prof N, Univ NC Sch Med

Lavenstein, Bennett L MD [ChiN] - **Spec Exp:** Movement Disorders; Neuromuscular Disorders; **Hospital:** Chldns Natl Med Ctr, Inova Fairfax Hosp for Chldn; **Address:** 8501 Arlington Blvd, Fairfax, VA 22031; **Phone:** 571-226-8368; **Board Cert:** Pediatrics 1977; Child Neurology 1979; **Med School:** Univ MD Sch Med 1974; **Resid:** Pediatrics, Univ of MD Hlth System 1977; Neurology, Georgetown Univ Hosp 1979; **Fellow:** Neuromuscular Medicine, Natl Inst Hlth; **Fac Appt:** Assoc Clin Prof N, Univ VA Sch Med

Wheless, James W MD [ChiN] - **Spec Exp:** Epilepsy/Seizure Disorders; **Hospital:** Le Bonheur Chldns Med Ctr, St Jude Children's Research Hosp; **Address:** 777 Washington Ave, Ste 240, Memphis, TN 38105; **Phone:** 901-287-5060; **Board Cert:** Pediatrics 1987; Child Neurology 1989; **Med School:** Univ Okla Coll Med 1982; **Resid:** Pediatrics, Univ Oklahoma Med Ctr 1985; **Fellow:** Pediatric Neurology, Children's Meml Hosp 1988; Epilepsy, Med Coll Georgia 1989; **Fac Appt:** Prof N, Univ Tenn Coll Med, Memphis

Midwest

Brunstrom, Janice MD [ChiN] - **Spec Exp:** Cerebral Palsy; **Hospital:** St Louis Chldns Hosp; **Address:** Washington Univ Sch Med, Dept Ped Neuro, 660 S Euclid Ave, Box 8111, St Louis, MO 63110; **Phone:** 314-454-6120; **Board Cert:** Pediatrics 2003; Child Neurology 2005; **Med School:** Med Coll VA 1987; **Resid:** Neurology, St Louis Chldns Hosp 1989; Neurology, Barnes Jewish Hosp 1990; **Fellow:** Child Neurology, St Louis Chldns Hosp 1995; **Fac Appt:** Asst Prof N, Washington Univ, St Louis

Charnas, Lawrence R MD/PhD [ChiN] - **Spec Exp:** Pediatric Neurology; Genetic Disorders-Nervous System; Neurofibromatosis; **Hospital:** Univ Minn Med Ctr, Fairview - Univ Campus; **Address:** Pediatric Clinical Neuroscience, 420 Delaware St SE, MMC 486, Minneapolis, MN 55455; **Phone:** 612-625-7466; **Board Cert:** Neurology 1986; Clinical Genetics 1990; Clinical Biochemical Genetics 1990; Child Neurology 1999; **Med School:** Univ Pennsylvania 1981; **Resid:** Neurology, Johns Hopkins Hosp 1985; **Fellow:** Genetics, NIH 1989; Child Neurology, Univ Minn Hosps & Clinics 1998; **Fac Appt:** Assoc Prof N, Univ Minn

Cohen, Bruce H MD [ChiN] - **Spec Exp:** Brain Tumors; Epilepsy; Neurometabolic Disorders; Pain Management; **Hospital:** Cleveland Clin Fdn (page 56); **Address:** Cleveland Clinic, 9500 Euclid Ave, Desk S71, Cleveland, OH 44195; **Phone:** 216-444-9182; **Board Cert:** Pediatrics 2004; Child Neurology 1990; **Med School:** Albert Einstein Coll Med 1982; **Resid:** Pediatrics, Chldns Hosp 1984; Child Neurology, Neurologic Inst-Columbia 1987; **Fellow:** Pediatric Neuro-Oncology, Chldns Hosp 1989

Edgar, Terence MD [ChiN] - **Spec Exp:** Neuromuscular Disorders; Cerebral Palsy; Epilepsy; **Hospital:** St Vincent Hosp - Green Bay, Aurora Sinai Med Ctr; **Address:** Prevea Health, 1821 S Webster Fl 3rd, Green Bay, WI 54301; **Phone:** 920-272-1270; **Board Cert:** Pediatrics 2003; Child Neurology 1997; **Med School:** South Africa 1984; **Resid:** Pediatrics, Univ Wisconsin Hosp & Clin 1995; **Fellow:** Pediatrics, Univ Wisconsin Hosp & Clin 1993; Child Neurology, Univ Wisconsin Hosp & Clin 1996; **Fac Appt:** Assoc Prof N, Univ Wisc

Epstein, Leon G MD [ChiN] - **Spec Exp:** AIDS/HIV; **Hospital:** Children's Mem Hosp; **Address:** Chldns Meml Hosp, Div Neurology, 2300 Childrens Plaza, Box 51, Chicago, IL 60614; **Phone:** 773-880-4352; **Board Cert:** Child Neurology 1979; **Med School:** Wayne State Univ 1973; **Resid:** Neurology, St Josephs Mercy Hosp 1974; Neurology, Univ Arizona Med Ctr 1976; **Fellow:** Neurology, Columbia Presby Med Ctr 1978; **Fac Appt:** Prof Ped, Northwestern Univ

Kotagal, Suresh MD [ChiN] - **Spec Exp:** Sleep Disorders/Apnea; **Hospital:** Mayo Med Ctr & Clin - Rochester, St Mary's Hosp - Rochester; **Address:** Mayo Clinic, 200 First St SW, Rochester, MN 55905-0002; **Phone:** 507-266-0774; **Board Cert:** Pediatrics 1979; Child Neurology 1982; **Med School:** India 1974; **Resid:** Child Neurology, Chldns Hosp Mich 1976; Pediatrics, St Louis Univ 1979; **Fellow:** Sleep Medicine, Stanford Univ 1982; **Fac Appt:** Prof N, Mayo Med Sch

Kovnar, Edward H MD [ChiN] - **Spec Exp:** Epilepsy/Seizure Disorders; Neurophysiology; Developmental Disorders; **Hospital:** Chldns Hosp - Wisconsin; **Address:** Advanced Healthcare, SC, 3003 W Good Hope Rd, Milwaukee, WI 53209-0996; **Phone:** 414-352-8828; **Board Cert:** Pediatrics 1984; Child Neurology 1984; Neurodevelopmental Disabilities 2005; **Med School:** Washington Univ, St Louis 1977; **Resid:** Pediatrics, Chldns Hosp 1979; Neurology, Barnes Hosp 1980; **Fellow:** Pediatric Neurology, Chldns Hosp 1982; Clinical Neurophysiology, Chldns Hosp 1991

Noetzel, Michael MD [ChiN] - **Spec Exp:** Cerebral Palsy; Brain Injury; Movement Disorders; **Hospital:** St Louis Chldns Hosp; **Address:** 660 S Euclid Ave, Box 8111, St Louis, MO 63110; **Phone:** 314-454-6120; **Board Cert:** Child Neurology 1984; Pediatrics 1984; **Med School:** Univ VA Sch Med 1977; **Resid:** Pediatrics, St Louis Chldns Hosp 1979; Neurology, Barnes Hosp 1980; **Fellow:** Child Neurology, St Louis Chldns Hosp 1982; **Fac Appt:** Prof Ped, Washington Univ, St Louis

Child Neurology

Nordli Jr, Douglas R MD [ChiN] - **Spec Exp:** Epilepsy; Rasmussen's Syndrome; **Hospital:** Children's Mem Hosp; **Address:** Children's Memorial Hospital, Epilepsy Ctr, 2300 Children's Plaza, Box 29, Chicago, IL 60614-3394; **Phone:** 773-883-6159; **Board Cert:** Child Neurology 1990; Clinical Neurophysiology 1997; **Med School:** Columbia P&S 1984; **Resid:** Pediatrics, Babies Hosp 1986; Child Neurology, Neuro Inst/Columbia-Presby Med Ctr 1989; **Fellow:** Clinical Neurophysiology, Neuro Inst/Columbia-Presby Med Ctr 1990; **Fac Appt:** Assoc Prof N, Northwestern Univ

Patterson, Marc MD [ChiN] - **Spec Exp:** Neurogenetics; Developmental Delay; Metabolic Disorders; **Hospital:** Mayo Med Ctr & Clin - Rochester; **Address:** Mayo Clinic, Dept Neurology, 200 First St SW, Rochester, MN 55905; **Phone:** 507-284-9974; **Board Cert:** Child Neurology 2004; Neurodevelopmental Disabilities 2001; **Med School:** Australia 1981; **Resid:** Neurology, Univ Queenland 1988; Child Neurology, Mayo Clinic 1990; **Fellow:** Metabolic Neurology, Natl Inst Health 1992; Pediatrics, Mayo Cilnic 1993; **Fac Appt:** Prof N, Mayo Med Sch

Wiznitzer, Max MD [ChiN] - **Hospital:** Rainbow Babies & Chldns Hosp; **Address:** Rainbow Babies & Chldns Hosp, 11100 Euclid Ave, Ste 585, MS RBC6090, Cleveland, OH 44106; **Phone:** 216-844-3691; **Board Cert:** Pediatrics 1982; Child Neurology 1986; Neurodevelopmental Disabilities 2004; **Med School:** Northwestern Univ 1977; **Resid:** Pediatrics, Chldns Hosp Med Ctr 1980; **Fellow:** Developmental-Behavioral Pediatrics, Cincinnati Med Ctr 1981; Pediatric Neurology, Chldns Hosp 1984; **Fac Appt:** Assoc Prof Ped, Case West Res Univ

Wyllie, Elaine MD [ChiN] - **Spec Exp:** Epilepsy/Seizure Disorders; **Hospital:** Cleveland Clin Fdn (page 56); **Address:** Div Ped Neurology, 9500 Euclid Ave, Desk S51, Cleveland, OH 44195; **Phone:** 216-444-2095; **Board Cert:** Pediatrics 1982; Child Neurology 1986; **Med School:** Indiana Univ 1978; **Resid:** Pediatrics, Indiana Univ Med Ctr 1980; Pediatrics, Case West Med Ctr 1981; **Fellow:** Child Neurology, Cleveland Clinic 1984; Clinical Neurophysiology, Cleveland Clinic 1985

Great Plains and Mountains

Bale Jr, James F MD [ChiN] - **Spec Exp:** Infections-Neurologic; Infections-Congenital; **Hospital:** Primary Children's Med Ctr, Univ Utah Hosps and Clins; **Address:** Primary Chldns Med Ctr, Ped Res Office, 100 N Mario Capecchi Drive, Salt Lake City, UT 84113; **Phone:** 801-587-7575; **Board Cert:** Pediatrics 2002; Child Neurology 1982; **Med School:** Univ Mich Med Sch 1975; **Resid:** Pediatrics, Univ Utah Hosps 1977; Neurology, Univ Utah Hosps 1980; **Fellow:** Infectious Disease, Univ Utah 1981; Neurovirology, UCSF-VA Med Ctr 1982; **Fac Appt:** Prof N, Univ Utah

Southwest

Fishman, Marvin A MD [ChiN] - **Spec Exp:** Seizure Disorders; Epilepsy/Seizure Disorders; Headache; **Hospital:** Texas Chldns Hosp - Houston; **Address:** 6621 Fannin CC1250, Houston, TX 77030; **Phone:** 832-822-5046; **Board Cert:** Pediatrics 1966; Child Neurology 1972; Neurodevelopmental Disabilities 2001; **Med School:** Univ IL Coll Med 1961; **Resid:** Pediatrics, Michael Reese Hosp 1964; Child Neurology, Mass Genl Hosp 1967; **Fellow:** Child Neurology, Chldns Hosp 1969; **Fac Appt:** Prof Ped, Baylor Coll Med

Iannaccone, Susan T MD [ChiN] - **Spec Exp:** Neuromuscular Disorders; **Hospital:** Chldns Med Ctr of Dallas, UT Southwestern Med Ctr - Dallas; **Address:** Division of Pediatric Neurology, Ambulatory Care Pavilion in Dallas, 2350 Stemmons Frwy., Ste 5074, Dallas, TX 75207; **Phone:** 214-456-2768; **Board Cert:** Pediatrics 1975; Child Neurology 1976; **Med School:** SUNY Hlth Sci Ctr 1969; **Resid:** Pediatrics, St Louis Chldns Hosp 1972; Neurology, Strong Meml Hosp 1975; **Fellow:** Neurology, Strong Meml Hosp 1975

Riviello Jr, James J MD [ChiN] - **Spec Exp:** Epilepsy/Seizure Disorders; Epilepsy in Tuberous Sclerosis; **Hospital:** Texas Chldns Hosp - Houston; **Address:** 6701 Fannin Fl 9, Dept Neurology, Houston, TX 77030; **Phone:** 832-822-1750; **Board Cert:** Pediatrics 1984; Child Neurology 1985; Clinical Neurophysiology 2006; **Med School:** Tulane Univ 1978; **Resid:** Pediatrics, St Christopher Hosp Chldn 1981; Neurology, Temple Univ Hosp 1982; **Fellow:** Pediatric Neurology, St Christopher Hosp Chldn 1983; **Fac Appt:** Prof N, Baylor Coll Med

Sharp, Gregory B MD [ChiN] - **Spec Exp:** Epilepsy; **Hospital:** UAMS Med Ctr, Arkansas Chldns Hosp; **Address:** 800 Marshall St, Ste 512-15, Little Rock, AR 72202; **Phone:** 501-364-1100; **Board Cert:** Pediatrics 2004; Child Neurology 1993; **Med School:** Univ Ark 1984; **Resid:** Pediatrics, Univ Ark Chldns Hosp 1987; **Fellow:** Pediatric Neurology, Mayo Clinic 1990; **Fac Appt:** Asst Prof Ped, Univ Ark

West Coast and Pacific

Ashwal, Stephen MD [ChiN] - **Spec Exp:** Metabolic Disorders; **Hospital:** Loma Linda Univ Med Ctr; **Address:** Pediatric Neurosciences Ctr, 2195 Club Center Drive, Ste A, San Bernadino, CA 92408; **Phone:** 909-835-1810; **Board Cert:** Pediatrics 1975; Child Neurology 1978; **Med School:** NYU Sch Med 1970; **Resid:** Pediatrics, Bellevue Hosp 1973; **Fellow:** Child Neurology, Univ Minn Med Ctr 1976; **Fac Appt:** Prof Ped, Loma Linda Univ

Ferriero, Donna MD [ChiN] - **Spec Exp:** Neuroendocrinology; **Hospital:** UCSF Med Ctr; **Address:** UCSF, Box 0410, 350 Parnassus Ave, Ste 609, San Francisco, CA 94143-0663; **Phone:** 415-353-2525; **Board Cert:** Pediatrics 1986; Child Neurology 1987; **Med School:** UCSF 1979; **Resid:** Pediatrics, Mass Genl Hosp 1982; Child Neurology, UCSF Med Ctr 1985; **Fellow:** Neurological Endocrinology, UCSF Med Ctr 1987; **Fac Appt:** Prof N, UCSF

Fisher, Paul G MD [ChiN] - **Spec Exp:** Neuro-Oncology; Brain Tumors; **Hospital:** Lucile Packard Chldns Hosp/Stanford Univ Med Ctr; **Address:** Stanford Cancer Ctr-Dept Neurology, 875 Blake Wilbur Drive, rm 2220, Stanford, CA 94305; **Phone:** 650-725-8630; **Board Cert:** Pediatrics 1995; Child Neurology 1998; **Med School:** UCSF 1989; **Resid:** Pediatrics, Johns Hopkins Univ Hosp 1991; Neurology, Johns Hopkins Univ Hosp 1994; **Fellow:** Neuro-Oncology, Children's Hosp 1994; **Fac Appt:** Assoc Prof Ped, Stanford Univ

Haas, Richard H MD [ChiN] - **Spec Exp:** Mitochondrial Disorders; Neurometabolic Disorders; **Hospital:** UCSD Med Ctr, Rady Children's Hosp - San Diego; **Address:** UCSD Sch Med, Div Ped Neuro, 9500 Gilman Drive, MC 0935, La Jolla, CA 92093-0935; **Phone:** 858-822-6700; **Board Cert:** Child Neurology 1983; Pediatrics 1985; **Med School:** England 1972; **Resid:** Pediatrics, Univ London 1979; Child Neurology, Univ Colo Hlth Sci Ctr 1981; **Fellow:** Biochemical Mental Retardation, Univ Colo Hlth Sci Ctr 1981; **Fac Appt:** Prof Ped, UCSD

Lott, Ira T MD [ChiN] - **Spec Exp:** Down Syndrome; **Hospital:** UC Irvine Med Ctr, Chldns Hosp Orange Co - CHOC; **Address:** UC Irvine Med Ctr, Dept Ped Neur, 101 City Drive S, Orange, CA 92868; **Phone:** 714-532-7554; **Board Cert:** Pediatrics 1975; Child Neurology 1977; **Med School:** Ohio State Univ 1967; **Resid:** Pediatrics, Mass Genl Hosp 1969; **Fellow:** Research, Natl Inst Hlth 1971; Neurology, Harvard-Mass Genl Hosp 1974; **Fac Appt:** Prof N, UC Irvine

Mitchell, Wendy G MD [ChiN] - **Spec Exp:** Epilepsy/Seizure Disorders; Opsoclonus-Ataxia in Children; **Hospital:** Chldns Hosp - Los Angeles; **Address:** Chldns Hosp Los Angeles, Dept Neuro, 4650 Sunset Blvd, Box 82, Los Angeles, CA 90027-6062; **Phone:** 323-361-2498; **Board Cert:** Pediatrics 1978; Child Neurology 1983; **Med School:** UCSF 1973; **Resid:** Pediatrics, Moffit Hosp-UCSF 1975; Child Neurology, Univ North Carolina 1981; **Fellow:** Behavioral Pediatrics, Mt Zion Hosp 1976; Univ North Carolina 1978; **Fac Appt:** Prof N, USC Sch Med

Child Neurology

Roddy, Sarah M MD [ChiN] - **Spec Exp:** Tourette's Syndrome; **Hospital:** Loma Linda Chldns Hosp; **Address:** Pediatric Neuroscience Center, 2195 Club Center Drive, Ste A, San Bernadino, CA 92408; **Phone:** 909-835-1810; **Board Cert:** Child Neurology 1987; Pediatrics 1987; **Med School:** Loma Linda Univ 1980; **Resid:** Pediatrics, Loma Linda Univ Med Ctr 1983; **Fellow:** Pediatric Neurology, Loma Linda Univ Med Ctr 1986; **Fac Appt:** Assoc Prof N, Loma Linda Univ

Rosser, Tena L MD [ChiN] - **Spec Exp:** Neurocutaneous Disorders; Neurofibromatosis; Tuberous Sclerosis; **Hospital:** Chldns Hosp - Los Angeles; **Address:** Chldns Hosp Los Angeles, Dept Neurology, 4650 Sunset Blvd, #82, Los Angeles, CA 90027; **Phone:** 323-361-2471; **Board Cert:** Pediatrics 1999; Child Neurology 2003; **Med School:** Univ NC Sch Med 1996; **Resid:** Pediatrics, Chldns Natl Med Ctr 1999; **Fellow:** Child Neurology, Chldns Natl Med Ctr 2003; **Fac Appt:** Asst Prof N, USC-Keck School of Medicine

Sankar, Raman MD/PhD [ChiN] - **Spec Exp:** Epilepsy/Seizure Disorders; Headache; Migraine; **Hospital:** Mattel Chldns Hosp at UCLA, Ronald Reagan UCLA Med Ctr; **Address:** UCLA Sch Med-Div Ped Neurology, 22-474 MDCC, Box 951752, Los Angeles, CA 90095-1752; **Phone:** 310-825-6196; **Board Cert:** Child Neurology 2005; **Med School:** Tulane Univ 1986; **Resid:** Pediatrics, Chldns Hosp 1988; Neurology, UCLA Med Ctr 1989; **Fellow:** Child Neurology, UCLA Med Ctr 1991; **Fac Appt:** Prof Ped, UCLA

Shields, William Donald MD [ChiN] - **Spec Exp:** Epilepsy/Seizure Disorders; **Hospital:** Ronald Reagan UCLA Med Ctr; **Address:** UCLA Med Ctr, Dept Ped Neurology, 10833 Le Conte Ave, Los Angeles, CA 90095-1752; **Phone:** 310-825-6196; **Board Cert:** Child Neurology 1977; Pediatrics 1978; **Med School:** Univ Utah 1971; **Resid:** Pediatrics, USC Med Ctr 1973; Neurology, Univ Utah Med Ctr 1976; **Fac Appt:** Prof Ped, UCLA

Trauner, Doris A MD [ChiN] - **Spec Exp:** Autism; Speech Disorders; **Hospital:** Rady Children's Hosp - San Diego; **Address:** UCSD Med Ctr, Div Ped Neurology, 9500 Gilman Drive, Dept 0935, La Jolla, CA 92093-0935; **Phone:** 858-966-5819; **Board Cert:** Pediatrics 1978; Child Neurology 1979; Neurodevelopmental Disabilities 2001; **Med School:** Med Coll VA 1972; **Resid:** Pediatrics, UCSD Med Ctr 1974; Neurology, UCSD Med Ctr 1975; **Fellow:** Child Neurology, Univ Chicago 1977; **Fac Appt:** Prof Ped, UCSD

Clinical Genetics

A specialist trained in diagnostic and therapeutic procedures for patients with genetically-linked diseases. This specialist uses modern cytogenetic, radiologic and biochemical testing to assist in specialized genetic counseling, implements needed therapeutic interventions and provides prevention through prenatal diagnosis.

A clinical geneticist demonstrates competence in providing comprehensive diagnostic, management and counseling services for genetic disorders.

A medical geneticist plans and coordinates large scale screening programs for inborn errors of metabolism, hemoglobinopathies, chromosome abnormalities and neural tube defects.

Training Required: Two or four years

CLINICAL GENETICS

New England

Bale, Allen E MD [CG] - **Spec Exp:** Cancer Genetics; **Hospital:** Yale-New Haven Hosp; **Address:** Yale Genetics, 20 York St, West Pavilion Fl 2, New Haven, CT 06519; **Phone:** 203-785-5745; **Board Cert:** Internal Medicine 1983; Clinical Genetics 1987; Clinical Molecular Genetics 2006; **Med School:** Univ Mass Sch Med 1979; **Resid:** Internal Medicine, Western Penn Hosp 1983; **Fellow:** Medical Genetics, NIH 1987; **Fac Appt:** Assoc Prof CG, Yale Univ

Bianchi, Diana MD [CG] - **Spec Exp:** Twin to Twin Transfusion Syndrome (TTTS); Fetal Abnormalities; **Hospital:** Tufts Med Ctr; **Address:** New Engl Med Ctr/Div Med Genetics, 800 Washington St, Box 394, Boston, MA 02111; **Phone:** 617-636-1468; **Board Cert:** Pediatrics 1985; Clinical Genetics 1987; Neonatal-Perinatal Medicine 1987; **Med School:** Stanford Univ 1980; **Resid:** Pediatrics, Childrens Hosp 1983; **Fellow:** Neonatology, Childrens Hosp 1986; Clinical Genetics, Harvard Med Sch 1987; **Fac Appt:** Prof Ped, Tufts Univ

Holmes, Lewis B MD [CG] - **Spec Exp:** Birth Defects; Inherited Disorders; Prenatal Diagnosis; **Hospital:** Mass Genl Hosp; **Address:** Mass Genl Hosp, Dept Pediatrics, 175 Cambridge St Fl 5 - rm 504, Boston, MA 02114; **Phone:** 617-726-1742; **Board Cert:** Pediatrics 1968; Clinical Genetics 1982; **Med School:** Duke Univ 1963; **Resid:** Pediatrics, Mass Genl Hosp 1965; **Fellow:** Pediatric Endocrinology, Mass Genl Hosp 1966; **Fac Appt:** Prof Ped, Harvard Med Sch

Mahoney, Maurice J MD [CG] - **Spec Exp:** Fetal Therapy; Prenatal Diagnosis; **Hospital:** Yale-New Haven Hosp; **Address:** Yale Genetics Consultation Serv, 333 Cedar St, rm WWW330, New Haven, CT 06520-8005; **Phone:** 203-785-2661; **Board Cert:** Pediatrics 1967; Clinical Genetics 1982; Clinical Biochemical Genetics 1982; **Med School:** Univ Pittsburgh 1962; **Resid:** Pediatrics, Johns Hopkins Hosp 1965; Pediatrics, Childrens Hosp 1966; **Fellow:** Clinical Genetics, Yale Univ Sch Med 1970; **Fac Appt:** Prof CG, Yale Univ

Seashore, Margretta MD [CG] - **Spec Exp:** Inherited Metabolic Disorders; **Hospital:** Yale-New Haven Hosp; **Address:** Yale Univ Sch Med, Dept Genetics, 333 Cedar St, rm 305, Box 208005, New Haven, CT 06520-8005; **Phone:** 203-785-2660; **Board Cert:** Pediatrics 1970; Clinical Biochemical Genetics 1982; Clinical Genetics 1982; **Med School:** Yale Univ 1965; **Resid:** Pediatrics, Yale-New Haven Hosp 1968; **Fellow:** Clinical Genetics, Yale-New Haven Hosp 1970; **Fac Appt:** Prof CG, Yale Univ

Mid Atlantic

Anyane-Yeboa, Kwame MD [CG] - **Spec Exp:** Dysmorphology; Prenatal Diagnosis; **Hospital:** NYPresby-Morgan Stanley Children's Hosp (page 66), St Luke's - Roosevelt Hosp Ctr - Roosevelt Div (page 57); **Address:** Morgan Stanley Children's Hospital of NY, 3959 Broadway Fl 6N - rm 601A, New York, NY 10032; **Phone:** 212-305-6731; **Board Cert:** Pediatrics 1979; Clinical Genetics 1982; **Med School:** Ghana 1972; **Resid:** Pediatrics, Harlem Hosp 1977; **Fellow:** Clinical Genetics, Babies Hosp-Columbia Presby 1980; **Fac Appt:** Assoc Prof Ped, Columbia P&S

Bialer, Martin G MD/PhD [CG] - **Spec Exp:** Marfan's Syndrome; Neurofibromatosis; Metabolic Genetic Disorders; **Hospital:** Schneider Chldn's Hosp, Long Island Jewish Med Ctr; **Address:** 1554 Northern Blvd, Ste 204, Manhasset, NY 11030; **Phone:** 516-365-3996; **Board Cert:** Clinical Genetics 1990; Clinical Biochemical Genetics 1990; Clinical Molecular Genetics 1990; Pediatrics 1987; **Med School:** Med Univ SC 1983; **Resid:** Pediatrics, N Shore Univ Hosp 1986; **Fellow:** Clinical Genetics, Univ VA Hlth Sci Ctr 1989; **Fac Appt:** Clin Prof Ped, NYU Sch Med

Davis, Jessica G MD [CG] - **Spec Exp:** Marfan's Syndrome; Mental Retardation; Neurofibromatosis; Ehlers-Danlos Syndrome; **Hospital:** NY-Presby Hosp/Weill Cornell (page 66), Hosp For Special Surgery (page 59); **Address:** 525 E 68th St, Box 128, New York, NY 10021-4870; **Phone:** 212-746-1496; **Board Cert:** Clinical Genetics 1984; **Med School:** Columbia P&S 1959; **Resid:** Pediatrics, St Luke's Hosp 1962; Clinical Genetics, Albert Einstein Coll Med 1965; **Fellow:** Cytogenetics, Albert Einstein Coll Med 1966; Pediatrics, Albert Einstein Col Med 1968; **Fac Appt:** Assoc Clin Prof Ped, Cornell Univ-Weill Med Coll

Desnick, Robert J MD/PhD [CG] - **Spec Exp:** Inherited Metabolic Disorders; Fabry's Disease; Gaucher Disease; Porphyria; **Hospital:** Mount Sinai Med Ctr (page 64), Elmhurst Hosp Ctr; **Address:** Mt Sinai Sch Med, Box 1498, Fifth Ave @ 100th St, New York, NY 10029; **Phone:** 212-241-6947; **Board Cert:** Clinical Genetics 1982; Clinical Molecular Genetics 1999; Clinical Biochemical Genetics 1982; **Med School:** Univ Minn 1971; **Resid:** Pediatrics, Univ Minn Hosps 1973; **Fac Appt:** Prof CG, Mount Sinai Sch Med

Desposito, Franklin MD [CG] - **Spec Exp:** Birth Defects; Genetic Disorders; **Hospital:** UMDNJ-Univ Hosp-Newark; **Address:** 90 Bergen St, Ste 5400, Newark, NJ 07103; **Phone:** 973-972-3300; **Board Cert:** Pediatrics 1986; Clinical Genetics 1982; Clinical Cytogenetics 1990; Clinical Molecular Genetics 2006; **Med School:** Ros Franklin Univ/Chicago Med Sch 1957; **Resid:** Pediatrics, Long Island Jewish Hosp 1961; **Fellow:** Hematology, Univ Wisc Sch Med 1963; **Fac Appt:** Prof Ped, UMDNJ-NJ Med Sch, Newark

Driscoll, Deborah A MD [CG] - **Spec Exp:** Prenatal Genetic Diagnosis; Fetal Abnormalities; Adolescent Gynecology; **Hospital:** Hosp Univ Penn - UPHS (page 60); **Address:** Chldns Hosp of Philadelphia, Clin Genetics Ctr, 34th St and Civic Ctr Blvd, rm 9S20, Philadelphia, PA 19104; **Phone:** 215-662-3232; **Board Cert:** Obstetrics & Gynecology 2005; Clinical Genetics 1990; Clinical Molecular Genetics 1993; **Med School:** NYU Sch Med 1983; **Resid:** Obstetrics & Gynecology, Hosp Univ Penn 1987; **Fellow:** Clinical Genetics, Hosp Univ Penn 1989; **Fac Appt:** Assoc Prof ObG, Univ Pennsylvania

Marion, Robert MD [CG] - **Spec Exp:** Spina Bifida; Williams Syndrome; Marfan's Syndrome; Down Syndrome; **Hospital:** Montefiore Med Ctr, Blythedale Children's Hosp; **Address:** Montefiore Med Ctr, Dept Pediatrics, 111 E 210th St, Bronx, NY 10467-2401; **Phone:** 718-741-2323; **Board Cert:** Pediatrics 1985; Clinical Genetics 1987; **Med School:** Albert Einstein Coll Med 1979; **Resid:** Pediatrics, Montefiore Med Ctr 1982; **Fellow:** Clinical Genetics, Montefiore Med Ctr 1984; **Fac Appt:** Prof Ped, Albert Einstein Coll Med

Ostrer, Harry MD [CG] - **Spec Exp:** Genetic Disorders; Hereditary Cancer; **Hospital:** NYU Med Ctr (page 68); **Address:** NYU Medical Ctr, 550 1st Ave, rm MSB136, New York, NY 10016; **Phone:** 212-263-5746; **Board Cert:** Clinical Genetics 1984; Pediatrics 1985; Clinical Cytogenetics 1990; Clinical Molecular Genetics 2004; **Med School:** Columbia P&S 1976; **Resid:** Pediatrics, Johns Hopkins Hosp 1978; Clinical Genetics, Natl Inst Health 1981; **Fellow:** Molecular Genetics, Johns Hopkins Hosp 1983; **Fac Appt:** Prof Ped, NYU Sch Med

Pyeritz, Reed E MD/PhD [CG] - **Spec Exp:** Marfan's Syndrome; Hereditary Hemorrhagic Telangiectasia; Inherited Disorders; **Hospital:** Hosp Univ Penn - UPHS (page 60), Chldns Hosp of Philadelphia, The; **Address:** Univ Penn, Div Medical Genetics, 3400 Spruce St, 538 Maloney Bldg, Philadelphia, PA 19104; **Phone:** 215-662-4740; **Board Cert:** Internal Medicine 1978; Clinical Genetics 2004; **Med School:** Harvard Med Sch 1975; **Resid:** Internal Medicine, Peter Bent Brigham Hosp 1977; Clinical Genetics, Johns Hopkins Hosp 1978; **Fac Appt:** Prof Med, Univ Pennsylvania

Clinical Genetics

Rosenbaum, Kenneth MD [CG] - **Spec Exp:** Birth Defects; **Hospital:** Chldns Natl Med Ctr; **Address:** Chldns Natl Med Ctr, Dept Med Genetics, 111 Michigan Ave NW, rm 1950, Washington, DC 20010; **Phone:** 202-476-2187; **Board Cert:** Pediatrics 1976; Clinical Genetics 1982; Clinical Cytogenetics 1982; **Med School:** Univ Louisville Sch Med 1971; **Resid:** Pediatrics, Childrens Natl Med Ctr 1974; **Fellow:** Clinical Genetics, Johns Hopkins Hosp 1977; **Fac Appt:** Assoc Prof Ped, Geo Wash Univ

Shapiro, Lawrence R MD [CG] - **Spec Exp:** Dysmorphology; Prenatal Diagnosis; Hereditary Cancer; Developmental Disorders; **Hospital:** Westchester Med Ctr; **Address:** Regional Med Genetics Ctr, 19 Bradhurst Ave, Ste 1600, Hawthorne, NY 10532-2140; **Phone:** 914-593-8900; **Board Cert:** Pediatrics 1967; Clinical Genetics 1982; Clinical Cytogenetics 1982; **Med School:** NYU Sch Med 1962; **Resid:** Pediatrics, Chldns Hosp 1964; Pediatrics, Bellevue Hosp 1965; **Fellow:** Clinical Genetics, Mount Sinai Med Ctr 1968; **Fac Appt:** Prof Ped, NY Med Coll

Zackai, Elaine MD [CG] - **Spec Exp:** Craniosynostosis; Cytogenetic Disorders; **Hospital:** Chldns Hosp of Philadelphia, The; **Address:** Childrens Hosp Philadelphia, Dept Clinical Genetics, 34th St & Civic Center Blvd, rm 2NE004, Philadelphia, PA 19104; **Phone:** 215-590-2920; **Board Cert:** Pediatrics 1977; Clinical Genetics 1982; Clinical Cytogenetics 1982; **Med School:** NYU Med 1968; **Resid:** Pediatrics, Chldns Hosp 1970; **Fellow:** Clinical Genetics, Chldns Hosp 1971; Clinical Genetics, Yale Univ Med Sch 1972; **Fac Appt:** Prof Ped, Univ Pennsylvania

Southeast

Driscoll, Daniel J MD/PhD [CG] - **Spec Exp:** Prader-Willi Syndrome; Obesity; Angelman Syndrome; **Hospital:** Shands at Univ of FL; **Address:** Univ Florida-Pediatric Genetics, 1600 SW Archer Rd, Box 100296, Gainesville, FL 32610-0296; **Phone:** 352-392-4104; **Board Cert:** Pediatrics 1987; Clinical Genetics 1990; Clinical Cytogenetics 1990; **Med School:** Albany Med Coll 1983; **Resid:** Pediatrics, Johns Hopkins Hosp 1986; **Fellow:** Clinical Genetics, Johns Hopkins Hosp 1989; **Fac Appt:** Prof Ped, Univ Fla Coll Med

Fernhoff, Paul M MD [CG] - **Spec Exp:** Birth Defects; Metabolic Genetic Disorders; **Hospital:** Chldns Hlthcare Atlanta - Scottish Rite, Emory Univ Hosp; **Address:** Emory Univ Sch Med, Div Med Genetics, 2165 N Decatur Rd, Decatur, GA 30033-5307; **Phone:** 404-778-8500; **Board Cert:** Pediatrics 1976; Clinical Genetics 1982; **Med School:** Jefferson Med Coll 1971; **Resid:** Pediatrics, Children's Hosp 1974; **Fellow:** Clinical Genetics, Emory Univ Hosp 1979; **Fac Appt:** Assoc Prof Ped, Emory Univ

Korf, Bruce R MD/PhD [CG] - **Spec Exp:** Inherited Disorders; Neuro-Genetics; Neurofibromatosis; **Hospital:** Univ of Ala Hosp at Birmingham; **Address:** Univ Alabama Birmingham-KAUL 230, 720 20th St S, Birmingham, AL 35294-0024; **Phone:** 205-934-9411; **Board Cert:** Clinical Genetics 1984; Child Neurology 1986; Pediatrics 1988; Clinical Molecular Genetics 2006; **Med School:** Cornell Univ-Weill Med Coll 1980; **Resid:** Pediatrics, Chldns Hosp 1982; Child Neurology, Chldns Hosp 1985; **Fellow:** Clinical Genetics, Chldns Hosp 1985; **Fac Appt:** Prof CG, Univ Ala

Saul, Robert MD [CG] - **Spec Exp:** Birth Defects; Neurofibromatosis; **Hospital:** Self Regional Healthcare; **Address:** Greenwood Genetic Ctr, 101 Gregor Mendel Cir, Greenwood, SC 29646-2307; **Phone:** 864-941-8100; **Board Cert:** Pediatrics 1981; Clinical Genetics 1982; **Med School:** Univ Colorado 1976; **Resid:** Pediatrics, Duke Med Ctr 1979; **Fellow:** Clinical Genetics, Greenwood Genetics Ctr 1981; **Fac Appt:** Clin Prof Ped, Univ SC Sch Med

Stevenson, Roger E MD [CG] - **Spec Exp:** Birth Defects; Mental Retardation; **Hospital:** Self Regional Healthcare; **Address:** Greenwood Genetic Ctr, 101 Gregor Mendel Circle, Greenwood, SC 29646; **Phone:** 864-941-8100; **Board Cert:** Pediatrics 1971; Clinical Genetics 1982; Clinical Cytogenetics 1984; **Med School:** Wake Forest Univ 1966; **Resid:** Pediatrics, Johns Hopkins Hosp 1969; **Fellow:** Clinical Genetics, Johns Hopkins Hosp 1972

Sutphen, Rebecca MD [CG] - **Spec Exp:** Genetic Disorders; Hereditary Cancer; Cancer Risk Assessment; **Hospital:** H Lee Moffitt Cancer Ctr & Research Inst; **Address:** Lifetime Cancer Screening, H Lee Moffitt Cancer Ctr, 4117 E Fowler Ave, Tampa, FL 33617; **Phone:** 813-745-5739; **Board Cert:** Pediatrics 2001; Clinical Cytogenetics 2007; Clinical Genetics 2007; Clinical Molecular Genetics 2007; **Med School:** Temple Univ 1990; **Resid:** Pediatrics, All Children's Hosp 1993; **Fellow:** Clinical Genetics, Univ S Fla Coll Med 1995; **Fac Appt:** Assoc Prof CG, Univ S Fla Coll Med

Midwest

Burton, Barbara MD [CG] - **Spec Exp:** Marfan's Syndrome; Phenylketonuria (PKU); Lysosomal Diseases; **Hospital:** Children's Mem Hosp; **Address:** Chldns Meml Hosp, Dept Genetics, 2300 Children's Plaza, Box 59, Chicago, IL 60614-3363; **Phone:** 773-880-4462; **Board Cert:** Pediatrics 1978; Clinical Genetics 1982; Clinical Biochemical Genetics 1982; **Med School:** Northwestern Univ 1973; **Resid:** Pediatrics, Chldns Meml Hosp 1975; **Fellow:** Clinical Genetics, Chldns Meml Hosp 1977; **Fac Appt:** Prof Ped, Northwestern Univ

Charrow, Joel MD [CG] - **Spec Exp:** Biochemical Genetics; Lysosomal Diseases; Neurofibromatosis; **Hospital:** Children's Mem Hosp; **Address:** Chldns Meml Hosp-Div Genetics, 2300 Chldn Plaza, MS 59, Chicago, IL 60614-3318; **Phone:** 773-880-4462; **Board Cert:** Pediatrics 1980; Clinical Genetics 1982; Clinical Biochemical Genetics 1987; **Med School:** Mount Sinai Sch Med 1976; **Resid:** Pediatrics, Chldns Meml Hosp 1979; **Fellow:** Clinical Genetics, Chldns Meml Hosp-Northwestern Univ 1981; **Fac Appt:** Prof Ped, Northwestern Univ

Elias, Sherman MD [CG] - **Spec Exp:** Prenatal Diagnosis; Reproductive Genetics; **Hospital:** Northwestern Meml Hosp; **Address:** 675 N St Claire, Chicago, IL 60611-3095; **Phone:** 312-472-3636; **Board Cert:** Obstetrics & Gynecology 1996; Clinical Genetics 2004; **Med School:** Univ KY Coll Med 1972; **Resid:** Obstetrics & Gynecology, Michael Reese Hosp 1973; Obstetrics & Gynecology, Univ Louisville Hosp 1976; **Fellow:** Clinical Genetics, Yale Univ 1975; Clinical Genetics, Northwestern Univ 1978; **Fac Appt:** Prof ObG, Northwestern Univ

Pergament, Eugene MD/PhD [CG] - **Spec Exp:** Prenatal Genetic Diagnosis; Down Syndrome; Genetic Preimplantation Diagnosis; **Hospital:** Northwestern Meml Hosp; **Address:** 680 N Lake Shore Drive, Ste 1230, Chicago, IL 60611; **Phone:** 312-981-4360; **Board Cert:** Clinical Genetics 1982; Clinical Cytogenetics 1984; **Med School:** Univ Chicago-Pritzker Sch Med 1970; **Resid:** Pediatrics, Univ Chicago 1972; **Fac Appt:** Prof ObG, Northwestern Univ

Saal, Howard M MD [CG] - **Spec Exp:** Craniofacial Disorders; Cleft Palate/Lip; Neurofibromatosis; **Hospital:** Cincinnati Chldns Hosp Med Ctr; **Address:** Chldns Hosp Med Ctr, Div Human Genetics, 3333 Burnet Ave Bldg E5 - rm 5430, MC 4006, Cincinnati, OH 45229-3039; **Phone:** 513-636-4760; **Board Cert:** Clinical Genetics 1984; Clinical Cytogenetics 1984; Pediatrics 1985; **Med School:** Wayne State Univ 1979; **Resid:** Pediatrics, Univ Conn Hlth Ctr 1982; **Fellow:** Medical Genetics, Univ Washington 1984; **Fac Appt:** Prof Ped, Univ Cincinnati

Clinical Genetics

Weaver, David D MD [CG] - **Spec Exp:** Bone Disorders-Inherited; Genetic Disorders; Inherited Disorders; Birth Defects; **Hospital:** Riley Hosp for Children, Indiana Univ Hosp; **Address:** 975 W Walnut St IB Bldg - Ste 130, Indianapolis, IN 46202-5251; **Phone:** 317-274-1057; **Board Cert:** Pediatrics 1978; Clinical Genetics 1982; **Med School:** Oregon Hlth Sci Univ 1966; **Resid:** Pediatrics, Oregon Hlth Scis Univ Sch Med 1972; **Fellow:** Clinical Genetics, Univ Washington Sch Med 1974; Metabolic Diseases, Oregon Health Scis Med Ctr 1976; **Fac Appt:** Prof Emeritus CG, Indiana Univ

Whelan, Alison MD [CG] - **Spec Exp:** Gynecologic Cancer Risk; Colon & Rectal Cancer Risk; Hereditary Cancer; **Hospital:** Barnes-Jewish Hosp, St Louis Chldns Hosp; **Address:** Washington Univ Sch Med, 660 S Euclid Ave, Campus Box 8073, St Louis, MO 63110; **Phone:** 314-454-6093; **Board Cert:** Internal Medicine 1989; Clinical Genetics 2007; **Med School:** Washington Univ, St Louis 1986; **Resid:** Internal Medicine, Barnes Hosp 1989; Pediatrics, Wash Univ Sch Med 1994; **Fellow:** Research, Wash Univ Sch Med 1991; Clinical Genetics, Wash Univ Sch Med 1994; **Fac Appt:** Prof Med, Washington Univ, St Louis

Great Plains and Mountains

Carey, John C MD [CG] - **Spec Exp:** Neurofibromatosis; Birth Defects; Hearing Loss; **Hospital:** Primary Children's Med Ctr, Univ Utah Hosps and Clins; **Address:** Univ Utah Med Ctr-Div of Med Gen, 50 N Med Drive Bldg SOM - rm 2C412, Salt Lake City, UT 84132; **Phone:** 801-581-8943; **Board Cert:** Pediatrics 1979; Clinical Genetics 1982; **Med School:** Georgetown Univ 1972; **Resid:** Pediatrics, UCSF Med Ctr 1975; **Fellow:** Clinical Genetics, UCSF Med Ctr 1979; **Fac Appt:** Prof Ped, Univ Utah

Hoyme, H Eugene MD [CG] - **Spec Exp:** Fetal Alcohol Syndrome; Cytogenetic Disorders; Dysmorphology; **Hospital:** Sanford Health SD; **Address:** PO Box 5039, 1305 W 18th St, Sioux Falls, SD 57717-5039; **Phone:** 605-333-6447; **Board Cert:** Pediatrics 1980; Clinical Genetics 1984; Clinical Cytogenetics 1987; **Med School:** Univ Chicago-Pritzker Sch Med 1976; **Resid:** Pediatrics, UCSD Med Ctr 1979; **Fellow:** Dysmorphology, UCSD Med Ctr 1981; **Fac Appt:** Prof Ped, Univ SD Sch Med

Southwest

Beaudet, Arthur L MD [CG] - **Spec Exp:** Genetic Biochemical Disorders; **Hospital:** Texas Chldns Hosp - Houston; **Address:** Texas Children's Hosp, 6621 Fannin St, MC CC1560, Houston, TX 77030; **Phone:** 832-822-4280; **Board Cert:** Pediatrics 1973; Clinical Genetics 1982; Clinical Biochemical Genetics 1982; Clinical Molecular Genetics 2004; **Med School:** Yale Univ 1967; **Resid:** Pediatrics, Johns Hopkins Hosp 1969; **Fellow:** Biochemical Genetics, Natl Inst Hlth 1971; **Fac Appt:** Prof CG, Baylor Coll Med

Craigen, William MD [CG] - **Spec Exp:** Biochemical Genetics; Mitochondrial Disorders; **Hospital:** Texas Chldns Hosp - Houston, Ben Taub Genl Hosp; **Address:** Texas Children's Hosp, 6621 Fannin St, MC CC1560, Houston, TX 77030; **Phone:** 832-822-4280; **Board Cert:** Pediatrics 1992; Clinical Genetics 1993; Clinical Biochemical Genetics 1993; **Med School:** Baylor Coll Med 1988; **Resid:** Pediatrics, Baylor Coll Med 1990; Pediatrics, Baylor Coll Med 1992; **Fellow:** Clinical Genetics, Baylor Coll Med 1990; **Fac Appt:** Assoc Prof CG, Baylor Coll Med

Cunniff, Christopher M MD [CG] - **Spec Exp:** Birth Defects; **Hospital:** Univ Med Ctr - Tucson; **Address:** Univ Ariz Coll Med, Dept Ped Genetics, 1501 N Campbell Ave, Tucson, AZ 85724; **Phone:** 520-626-5175; **Board Cert:** Pediatrics 2003; Clinical Genetics 1990; **Med School:** Univ Ala 1984; **Resid:** Pediatrics, MC Hosp Vermont 1987; **Fellow:** Dysmorphology, UCSD 1989; **Fac Appt:** Assoc Prof Ped, Univ Ariz Coll Med

Mulvihill, John J MD [CG] - **Spec Exp:** Genetic Disorders; Neurofibromatosis; Fertility in Cancer Survivors; **Hospital:** Chldns Hosp OU Med Ctr; **Address:** Childrens Hosp, 940 NE 13th St, rm 2B2418, Oklahoma City, OK 73104; **Phone:** 405-271-8685; **Board Cert:** Pediatrics 1975; Clinical Genetics 1982; **Med School:** Univ Wash 1969; **Resid:** Pediatrics, Johns Hopkins Hosp 1974; **Fellow:** Research, NCI-Natl Inst Hlth 1972; **Fac Appt:** Prof CG, Univ Okla Coll Med

Northrup, Hope MD [CG] - **Spec Exp:** Biochemical Genetics; Neuro-Genetics; Dysmorphology; **Hospital:** Meml Hermann Hosp - Texas Med Ctr, LBJ General Hosp; **Address:** Univ TX Med Sch, Dept Peds-Div Med Genetics, rm MSB-3.144, Box 20708, Houston, TX 77225-0708; **Phone:** 713-500-5760; **Board Cert:** Pediatrics 1988; Clinical Genetics 1990; Clinical Biochemical Genetics 1990; **Med School:** Med Univ SC 1983; **Resid:** Pediatrics, Chldns Med Ctr-Univ Tex SW 1986; **Fellow:** Clinical Genetics, Inst Molec Gene-Baylor Coll Med 1989; **Fac Appt:** Prof Ped, Univ Tex, Houston

West Coast and Pacific

Boles, Richard G MD [CG] - **Spec Exp:** Mitochondrial Disorders; Vomiting-Cyclic; **Hospital:** Chldns Hosp - Los Angeles; **Address:** 4650 Sunset Blvd, MS 90, Los Angeles, CA 90027; **Phone:** 323-361-2178; **Board Cert:** Clinical Genetics 2006; Clinical Biochemical Genetics 2006; Pediatrics 2002; **Med School:** UCLA 1987; **Resid:** Pediatrics, Harbor-UCLA Med Ctr 1990; **Fellow:** Genetics and Metabolism, Yale Univ Sch Med 1993; **Fac Appt:** Assoc Prof Ped, USC Sch Med

Cassidy, Suzanne MD [CG] - **Spec Exp:** Prader-Willi Syndrome; Connective Tissue Disorders; Neurocutaneous Disorders; **Hospital:** UCSF Med Ctr; **Address:** 533 Parnassus Ave, rm U-100A, Box 0706, San Francisco, CA 94143; **Phone:** 415-476-2757; **Board Cert:** Pediatrics 1982; Clinical Genetics 1983; **Med School:** Vanderbilt Univ 1976; **Resid:** Pediatrics, Univ Wash Affil Prgms 1979; **Fellow:** Clinical Genetics, Univ Wash 1981; **Fac Appt:** Prof Ped, UC Irvine

Cederbaum, Stephen D MD [CG] - **Spec Exp:** Inborn Errors of Metabolism; **Hospital:** Ronald Reagan UCLA Med Ctr; **Address:** 635 Charles E Young Drive S, rm 347, Los Angeles, CA 90095-7332; **Phone:** 310-825-0402; **Board Cert:** Clinical Genetics 1982; Clinical Biochemical Genetics 1982; **Med School:** NYU Sch Med 1964; **Resid:** Internal Medicine, Barnes Hosp 1966; **Fellow:** Clinical Genetics, Univ Wash 1970; **Fac Appt:** Prof Ped, UCLA

Curry, Cynthia J MD [CG] - **Hospital:** Chldns Hosp Central California, Comm Med Ctr - Fresno; **Address:** Genetic Medicine Central California, 351 E Barstow, Ste 106, Fresno, CA 93710-6073; **Phone:** 559-227-4472; **Board Cert:** Pediatrics 1973; Clinical Genetics 1982; **Med School:** Yale Univ 1967; **Resid:** Pediatrics, Univ Wash Orth Chldns Hosp 1969; Pediatrics, Univ Minn Hosp 1970; **Fellow:** Dysmorphology, UCSF Med Ctr 1976; **Fac Appt:** Prof CG, UCSF

Falk, Rena MD [CG] - **Spec Exp:** Prenatal Diagnosis; Mental Retardation; Prenatal Genetic Diagnosis; **Hospital:** Cedars-Sinai Med Ctr; **Address:** 8700 Beverly Blvd, MOT West 1150, Los Angeles, CA 90048; **Phone:** 310-423-9914; **Board Cert:** Pediatrics 1976; Clinical Genetics 1982; Clinical Cytogenetics 1984; **Med School:** UCLA 1971; **Resid:** Pediatrics, Cedars-Sinai Med Ctr 1973; **Fellow:** Clinical Genetics, UCLA Med Schl 1975; UCLA 1977; **Fac Appt:** Prof Ped, UCLA

Graham Jr, John M MD [CG] - **Spec Exp:** Dysmorphology; Craniofacial Disorders; Mental Retardation; **Hospital:** Cedars-Sinai Med Ctr; **Address:** 8700 Beverly Blvd, MOT West 1150, Los Angeles, CA 90048; **Phone:** 310-423-9914; **Board Cert:** Pediatrics 1982; Clinical Genetics 1982; **Med School:** Med Univ SC 1975; **Resid:** Pediatrics, Boston Chldns Hosp-Harvard 1977; **Fellow:** Developmental-Behavioral Pediatrics, Boston Chldns Hosp 1978; Dysmorphology, Univ Wash 1980; **Fac Appt:** Prof Ped, UCLA

Clinical Genetics

Grody, Wayne W MD/PhD [CG] - **Spec Exp:** Genetic Disorders; Hereditary Cancer; **Hospital:** Ronald Reagan UCLA Med Ctr; **Address:** UCLA School Medicine, Division of Genetic Molecular Pathology, 10833 Le Conte Ave, #37-121CHS Ave, Los Angeles, CA 90095-1732; **Phone:** 310-825-5648; **Board Cert:** Clinical Genetics 1990; Anatomic & Clinical Pathology 1987; Clinical Biochemical Genetics 1990; Molecular Genetic Pathology 2001; **Med School:** Baylor Coll Med 1977; **Resid:** Pathology, UCLA Med Ctr 1986; **Fellow:** Clinical Genetics, UCLA Med Ctr 1987; **Fac Appt:** Prof CG, UCLA

Hudgins, Louanne MD [CG] - **Spec Exp:** Congenital Anomalies-Limb; **Hospital:** Stanford Univ Med Ctr; **Address:** Stanford Univ Med Ctr, Dept Pediatrics-Medical Genetics, 300 Pasteur Drive, rm H315, Stanford, CA 94305; **Phone:** 650-723-6858; **Board Cert:** Pediatrics 2004; Clinical Genetics 2006; **Med School:** Univ Kans 1984; **Resid:** Pediatrics, Univ Conn Hlth Ctr 1987; **Fellow:** Clinical Genetics, Univ Conn Hlth Ctr 1990; **Fac Appt:** Assoc Prof Ped, Stanford Univ

Jonas, Adam J MD [CG] - **Spec Exp:** Biochemical Genetics; Inherited Disorders; **Hospital:** LAC - Harbor - UCLA Med Ctr; **Address:** Harbor-UCLA Med Ctr, Div Med Genetics, 1000 W Carson St, Box 17, Torrance, CA 90509-2910; **Phone:** 310-222-2301; **Board Cert:** Pediatrics 1982; Clinical Biochemical Genetics 1987; Clinical Genetics 1990; **Med School:** UCSD 1976; **Resid:** Pediatrics, Chldns Ortho Hosp 1978; Pediatrics, Univ Hosp 1979; **Fellow:** Genetics and Metabolism, UCSD Sch Med 1982; **Fac Appt:** Prof Ped, UCLA

Jones, Marilyn MD [CG] - **Spec Exp:** Dysmorphology; Craniofacial Disorders; **Hospital:** Rady Children's Hosp - San Diego, UCSD Med Ctr; **Address:** 3020 Children's Way, MC 5031, San Diego, CA 92123-2746; **Phone:** 858-966-5840; **Board Cert:** Pediatrics 1979; Clinical Genetics 1982; **Med School:** Columbia P&S 1974; **Resid:** Internal Medicine, UCSD Med Ctr 1977; Pediatrics, UCSD Med Ctr 1978; **Fellow:** Dysmorphology, UCSD Med Ctr 1979

Morris, Colleen A MD [CG] - **Spec Exp:** Williams Syndrome; Inherited Disorders; Fetal Alcohol Syndrome; **Hospital:** Univ Med Ctr - Las Vegas; **Address:** Univ Nevada Sch Medicine, Dept Pediatrics/Genetics, 2040 W Charleston Blvd, Ste 401, Las Vegas, NV 89102; **Phone:** 702-671-2200; **Board Cert:** Pediatrics 1986; Clinical Genetics 1987; **Med School:** Loyola Univ-Stritch Sch Med 1981; **Resid:** Pediatrics, Phoenix Hosp 1984; **Fellow:** Clinical Genetics, Univ Utah Sch Med 1986; **Fac Appt:** Prof Ped, Univ Nevada

Nussbaum, Robert MD [CG] - **Spec Exp:** Genetic Disorders; **Hospital:** UCSF Med Ctr; **Address:** Institute of Human Genetics, 513 Parnassus Ave, rm HSE901E, San Francisco, CA 94143-0794; **Phone:** 415-476-1127; **Board Cert:** Internal Medicine 1978; Clinical Genetics 1982; Clinical Molecular Genetics 2004; **Med School:** Harvard Med Sch 1975; **Resid:** Internal Medicine, Barnes Hosp 1978; **Fellow:** Clinical Genetics, Baylor Univ 1983

Pagon, Roberta A MD [CG] - **Spec Exp:** Eye Diseases-Hereditary; Sexual Differentiation Disorders; **Hospital:** Chldns Hosp and Regl Med Ctr - Seattle; **Address:** Chldns Hosp Med Ctr, 4800 Sand Point Way, Box 5371, Seattle, WA 98105; **Phone:** 206-987-2056; **Board Cert:** Pediatrics 1978; Clinical Genetics 1982; **Med School:** Harvard Med Sch 1972; **Resid:** Pediatrics, Univ Wash Affil Hosp 1975; **Fellow:** Clinical Genetics, Univ Wash 1979; **Fac Appt:** Prof Ped, Univ Wash

Randolph, Linda MD [CG] - **Spec Exp:** Dysmorphology; Neurocutaneous Disorders; Prenatal Diagnosis; **Hospital:** Chldns Hosp - Los Angeles; **Address:** 4650 Sunset Blvd, MS 90, Los Angeles, CA 90027; **Phone:** 323-669-2178; **Board Cert:** Pediatrics 1987; Clinical Genetics 1987; Clinical Cytogenetics 1990; **Med School:** Geo Wash Univ 1982; **Resid:** Pediatrics, Chldns Natl Med Ctr 1985; **Fellow:** Clinical Molecular Genetics, Harbor-UCLA Med Ctr 1989; **Fac Appt:** Asst Prof Ped, USC-Keck School of Medicine

Rimoin, David L MD/PhD [CG] - **Spec Exp:** Skeletal Dysplasia; Marfan's Syndrome; Birth Defects; **Hospital:** Cedars-Sinai Med Ctr; **Address:** 8700 Beverly Blvd, MOT West 1150, Los Angeles, CA 90048; **Phone:** 310-423-9914; **Board Cert:** Internal Medicine 1968; Clinical Genetics 1984; **Med School:** McGill Univ 1961; **Resid:** Internal Medicine, Royal Victoria Hosp 1963; Internal Medicine, Johns Hopkins Hosp 1964; **Fellow:** Clinical Genetics, Johns Hopkins Hosp 1967; **Fac Appt:** Prof Ped, UCLA

Seaver, Laurie H MD [CG] - **Spec Exp:** Birth Defects; Fetal Alcohol Syndrome; Dysmorphology; **Hospital:** Kapiolani Med Ctr for Women & Chldn, Queen's Med Ctr - Honolulu; **Address:** Hawaii Community Genetics, 1441 Kapiolani Blvd, Ste 1800, Honolulu, HI 96814; **Phone:** 808-973-3403; **Board Cert:** Pediatrics 2005; Clinical Genetics 2006; **Med School:** Univ Ariz Coll Med 1987; **Resid:** Pediatrics, Univ Ariz 1990; **Fellow:** Clinical Genetics, Univ Ariz Coll Med 1993

Weitzel, Jeffrey N MD [CG] - **Spec Exp:** Breast Cancer; Ovarian Cancer; Hereditary Cancer; **Hospital:** City of Hope Natl Med Ctr & Beckman Rsch; **Address:** City of Hope Cancer Ctr, 1500 E Duarte Rd, Duarte, CA 91010; **Phone:** 626-256-8662; **Board Cert:** Internal Medicine 1986; Medical Oncology 1989; Clinical Genetics 1996; **Med School:** Univ Minn 1983; **Resid:** Internal Medicine, Univ Minn Hosps 1986; Hematology, Hammersmith Hosp 1987; **Fellow:** Hematology & Oncology, Tufts -New England Med Ctr 1992; Clinical Genetics, Tufts-New England Med Ctr 1996; **Fac Appt:** Assoc Clin Prof Med, USC Sch Med

Wilcox, William MD [CG] - **Spec Exp:** Inborn Errors of Metabolism; Skeletal Dysplasia; **Hospital:** Cedars-Sinai Med Ctr; **Address:** Cedars Sinai Med Ctr, Dept Med Genetics, 8700 Beverly Blvd, Ste SSB 122, Los Angeles, CA 90048; **Phone:** 310-423-9914; **Board Cert:** Clinical Genetics 2006; Clinical Biochemical Genetics 2007; Clinical Molecular Genetics 2007; **Med School:** UCLA 1988; **Resid:** Pediatrics, UCLA Med Ctr 1991; **Fellow:** Clinical Genetics, Cedars-Sinai Med Ctr 1994; **Fac Appt:** Prof Ped, UCLA

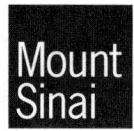
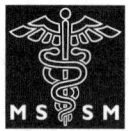

Mount Sinai

M S S M

MOUNT SINAI
SCHOOL OF
MEDICINE

THE MOUNT SINAI MEDICAL CENTE
GENETICS AND GENOMIC SCIENCE
One Gustave L. Levy Pla
Fifth Avenue and 100th Stre
New York, NY 10029-65
Physician Referral: 1-800-MD-SINAI (637-462
www.mountsinai.o

The Department of Genetics and Genomic Sciences at The Mount Sinai Medical Center is one of the largest medical genetics units in the nation, providing expert diagnostic, therapeutic, and counseling services for patients and families with genetic disorders, birth defects, and pregnancy loss. The department performs sophisticated diagnostic tests in its state-of-the-art DNA, biochemical, and cytogenetics laboratories.

The Department has more than fifty internationally recognized physician and scientist faculty members, ten experienced genetic counselors, and a full support and research staff of more than 150 people who provide expert clinical services.

Programs and services offered by the Department include:
• Comprehensive genetic diagnostic and counseling services
• Clinical and laboratory evaluation of patients with genetic disorders, birth defects, and reproductive loss
• Genetic Screening Program
• Prenatal Diagnostic Services
• Cancer Genetic Counseling Program
• The Center for Jewish Genetic Disease (the first such center in the world)
• Program for Inherited Metabolic Diseases
• The Comprehensive Gaucher Disease Treatment Program
• The International Center for Fabry Disease
• The International Center for Types A and B Niemann-Pick Disease

GROUNDBREAKING RESEARCH AND NEW FORMS OF TREATMENT
Almost everyone has a disease or condition that runs in their family. In fact, there are more than 10,000 known genetic disorders, and current research is identifying the genetic susceptibilities or predispositior for many common diseases and cancers. Moving toward this goal, the Department of Genetics and Genomic Sciences at Mount Sinai is performing research to develop new and improved methods for the diagnosis, prevention, and treatment of rare and common diseases. The Human Genome Project and advances in gene therapy and stem cell biology have accelerated this research.

ADVANCES IN DIAGNOSIS AND DISEASE TREATMENT
In the past several years, Mount Sinai researchers have had remarkable success in identifying the genes responsible for genetic diseases and in developing new treatments for two inherited disorders. The following are some examples and results of this important work:

• Research pioneered by the Department of Genetics and Genomic Sciences resulted in the developmen of a safe and effective, FDA-approved treatment for Fabry disease, an inherited metabolic disorder tha results in kidney failure, heart disease, stroke, and premature death.

• Departmental faculty have developed a treatment for Niemann-Pick Type B disease, a hereditary disorder that results in death in childhood or early adulthood.

• We have identified the genes responsible for several diseases, including a debilitating juvenile arthritis syndrome. The identification of this gene may lead to greater understanding and new treatments for arthritis. We have also recently identified a gene linked to prostate cancer.

• Our researchers have identified three genes causing Noonan syndrome, a common genetic disorder th causes congenital heart defects. Affected families can now receive early diagnosis and prevention.

NYU Langone Medical Center

550 First Avenue (at 31St Street)
New York, NY 10016
Physician Referral:
(888)7-NYU-MED (888-769-8633)
www.nyumc.org

CLINICAL GENETICS

The Clinical Genetics Program at NYU Langone Medical Center offers a comprehensive program of genetic evaluation, counseling, and testing, supported by vital, ongoing research efforts and active treatment protocols. Our integrated team approach includes centralized, easy access to medical geneticists and genetic counselors. We are nationally known for groundbreaking work identifying genetic markers for breast, colorectal, ovarian, and prostate cancer, and assessing cancer risks.

BREAST AND OVARIAN CANCER - a leading participant in the New York Breast Cancer Study and the National Ovarian Cancer Early Detection Program; latest blood test can help identify early indications of ovarian cancer

COLORECTAL CANCER - diagnostic evaluations followed by tests for identifying high-risk individuals.

PROSTATE CANCER - the latest research and ongoing protocols.

EARLY DETECTION - in the absence of a targeted test we provide screening tests to identify high-risk patients in need of follow-up care.

COUNSELING - personalized, confidential insight into matters related to prevention, surveillance, and early diagnosis and treatment in a non-judgmental

Specialists at the NCI-designated NYU Cancer Institute seek to enhance and coordinate the extensive resources of NYU Medical Center to optimize research, treatment, and the ultimate control of cancer.

Our NYU Clinical Center is located at 160 East 34th Street. This sate-of-the-are 13-level, 85,000-square-foot building serves as "home base" for patients, by providing the latest cancer prevention, screening, diagnostic treatment, genetic counseling, and support services in one central location. The NYU Clinical Cancer Center stands to dramatically improve the lives of people with cancer. As part of NYU Langone Medical Center, patients can access a variety of other noncancer services throughout the institution.

Colon & Rectal Surgery

A colon and rectal surgeon is trained to diagnose and treat various diseases of the intestinal tract, colon, rectum, anal canal and perianal area by medical and surgical means. This specialist also deals with other organs and tissues (such as the liver and gallbladder) involved with primary
intestinal disease.

Colon and rectal surgeons have the expertise to diagnose and often manage anorectal conditions such as hemorrhoids, fissures (painful tears in the anal lining), abscesses and fistulae (infections located around the anus and rectum) in the office setting. They also treat problems of the intestine and colon and perform endoscopic procedures to evaluate and treat problems such as cancer, polyps (precancerous growths) and inflammatory conditions.

Training Required: Six years (including general surgery)

COLON & RECTAL SURGERY

New England

Bleday, Ronald MD [CRS] - **Spec Exp:** Colon & Rectal Cancer; **Hospital:** Brigham & Women's Hosp, Dana-Farber Cancer Inst; **Address:** Brigham & Women's Hosp, Dept Genl Surg, 75 Francis St, ASB II, Boston, MA 02115; **Phone:** 617-732-8460; **Board Cert:** Surgery 1999; Colon & Rectal Surgery 2003; **Med School:** McGill Univ 1982; **Resid:** Surgery, Rhode Island Hosp 1989; Surgical Oncology, Brigham & Womens Hosp 1986; **Fellow:** Endoscopy, Mass Genl Hosp 1990; Colon & Rectal Surgery, Univ Minn 1991; **Fac Appt:** Assoc Prof S, Harvard Med Sch

Harnsberger, Jeffrey R MD [CRS] - **Spec Exp:** Inflammatory Bowel Disease; Colon & Rectal Cancer; **Hospital:** Dartmouth - Hitchcock Med Ctr, Elliot Hosp; **Address:** Dartmouth-Hitchcock Manchester, 100 Hitchcock Way, Manchester, NH 03104; **Phone:** 603-695-2840; **Board Cert:** Surgery 2001; Colon & Rectal Surgery 2005; **Med School:** Med Coll OH 1987; **Resid:** Surgery, Dartmouth-Hitchcock Med Ctr 1992; **Fellow:** Colon & Rectal Surgery, St Louis Univ Med Ctr 1993; **Fac Appt:** Asst Prof S, Dartmouth Med Sch

Hyman, Neil H MD [CRS] - **Spec Exp:** Inflammatory Bowel Disease; Colon & Rectal Cancer; **Hospital:** FAHC - Med Ctr Campus; **Address:** Fletcher Allen Hospital, 111 Colchester Ave, Burlington, VT 05401; **Phone:** 802-847-3339; **Board Cert:** Surgery 1998; Colon & Rectal Surgery 2003; **Med School:** Univ VT Coll Med 1984; **Resid:** Surgery, Mt Sinai Med Ctr 1989; **Fellow:** Colon & Rectal Surgery, Cleveland Clinic 1990; **Fac Appt:** Prof S, Univ VT Coll Med

Longo, Walter E MD [CRS] - **Spec Exp:** Colon & Rectal Cancer; Gastrointestinal Surgery; Inflammatory Bowel Disease; **Hospital:** Yale-New Haven Hosp; **Address:** Yale Univ School Medicine, Dept Surgery/Gastroenterology, Box 208062, New Haven, CT 06520-8062; **Phone:** 203-785-2616; **Board Cert:** Surgery 2001; Colon & Rectal Surgery 2006; **Med School:** NY Med Coll 1984; **Resid:** Surgery, Yale-New Haven Hosp 1990; **Fellow:** Research, Yale-New Haven Hosp 1988; Colon & Rectal Surgery, Cleveland Clinic 1991; **Fac Appt:** Prof S, Yale Univ

Nagle, Deborah A MD [CRS] - **Hospital:** Beth Israel Deaconess Med Ctr - Boston; **Address:** Beth Israel Deaconess Med Ctr, 330 Brookline Ave Stoneman Bldg - rm 932, Boston, MA 02215; **Phone:** 617-667-4159; **Board Cert:** Colon & Rectal Surgery 2006; Surgery 2004; **Med School:** Thomas Jefferson Univ 1988; **Resid:** Surgery, Thos Jefferson U Hosp 1993; Colon & Rectal Surgery, Thos Jefferson U Hosp 1994

Roberts, Patricia L MD [CRS] - **Spec Exp:** Diverticulitis; Colon & Rectal Cancer; Inflammatory Bowel Disease; **Hospital:** Lahey Clin; **Address:** 41 Mall Rd, Burlington, MA 01805; **Phone:** 781-744-8243; **Board Cert:** Surgery 1996; Colon & Rectal Surgery 2003; **Med School:** Boston Univ 1981; **Resid:** Surgery, Boston City Hosp 1986; **Fellow:** Colon & Rectal Surgery, Lahey Clinic 1988; **Fac Appt:** Assoc Prof S, Tufts Univ

Schoetz, David MD [CRS] - **Spec Exp:** Inflammatory Bowel Disease/Crohn's; Colon & Rectal Cancer; Incontinence-Fecal; Anorectal Disorders; **Hospital:** Lahey Clin; **Address:** Lahey Clinic Med Ctr, Dept Colon & Rectal Surg, 41 Mall Rd, Burlington, MA 01805-0001; **Phone:** 781-744-8889; **Board Cert:** Surgery 2001; Colon & Rectal Surgery 1983; **Med School:** Med Coll Wisc 1974; **Resid:** Surgery, Boston Univ Med Ctr 1981; Internal Medicine, St Mary's Hospital 1977; **Fellow:** Colon & Rectal Surgery, Lahey Clin Med Ctr 1982; **Fac Appt:** Prof S, Tufts Univ

Shellito, Paul C MD [CRS] - **Spec Exp:** Colon & Rectal Cancer; Ulcerative Colitis; Anorectal Disorders; **Hospital:** Mass Genl Hosp; **Address:** 15 Parkman St, Ste 460, Boston, MA 02114-3117; **Phone:** 617-724-0365; **Board Cert:** Surgery 2002; Colon & Rectal Surgery 1994; **Med School:** Harvard Med Sch 1977; **Resid:** Surgery, Mass Genl Hosp 1983; Surgery, Auckland Univ Med Sch 1981; **Fellow:** Colon & Rectal Surgery, Univ Minn 1985; **Fac Appt:** Asst Prof S, Harvard Med Sch

Mid Atlantic

Caushaj, Fillor Philip MD [CRS] - **Spec Exp:** Colon & Rectal Cancer; Inflammatory Bowel Disease; Laparoscopic Surgery; **Hospital:** Western Penn Hosp; **Address:** 4815 Liberty Ave, Ste GR-59, Mellon Pavilion, Pittsburgh, PA 15224-2156; **Phone:** 412-578-1425; **Board Cert:** Colon & Rectal Surgery 1986; Surgery 2004; **Med School:** Johns Hopkins Univ 1979; **Resid:** Surgery, Columbia-Presby Med Ctr 1984; **Fellow:** Colon & Rectal Surgery, Lahey Clinic 1985; **Fac Appt:** Prof S, Temple Univ

Eisenstat, Theodore E MD [CRS] - **Spec Exp:** Colon & Rectal Cancer; Inflammatory Bowel Disease; Anorectal Disorders; Hemorrhoids; **Hospital:** Robert Wood Johnson Univ Hosp - New Brunswick, JFK Med Ctr - Edison; **Address:** 3900 Park Ave, Ste 101, Edison, NJ 08820-3032; **Phone:** 732-494-6640; **Board Cert:** Surgery 1974; Colon & Rectal Surgery 1994; **Med School:** NY Med Coll 1968; **Resid:** Surgery, Thomas Jefferson Univ Hosp 1971; Surgery, Pennsylvania Hosp 1973; **Fellow:** Colon & Rectal Surgery, Muhlenberg Med Ctr 1978; **Fac Appt:** Clin Prof S, UMDNJ-RW Johnson Med Sch

Fry, Robert D MD [CRS] - **Spec Exp:** Colon & Rectal Cancer; Inflammatory Bowel Disease/Crohn's; Anal Cancer; **Hospital:** Pennsylvania Hosp (page 60), Hosp Univ Penn - UPHS (page 60); **Address:** Pennsylvania Hospital, Div Colon & Rectal Surgery, 700 Spruce St, Ste 305, Philadelphia, PA 19106-4023; **Phone:** 215-829-5333; **Board Cert:** Surgery 2006; Colon & Rectal Surgery 1998; **Med School:** Washington Univ, St Louis 1972; **Resid:** Surgery, Barnes Jewish Hosp 1977; **Fellow:** Colon & Rectal Surgery, Cleveland Clinic 1978; **Fac Appt:** Prof S, Univ Pennsylvania

Gingold, Bruce S MD [CRS] - **Spec Exp:** Colostomy Avoidance; Inflammatory Bowel Disease/Crohn's; Anorectal Disorders; Colon & Rectal Cancer; **Hospital:** St Vincent Cath Med Ctrs - Manhattan; **Address:** 36 7th Ave, Ste 522, New York, NY 10011-6600; **Phone:** 212-675-2997; **Board Cert:** Colon & Rectal Surgery 1976; Surgery 1977; **Med School:** Jefferson Med Coll 1970; **Resid:** Surgery, St Vincent's Hosp & Med Ctr 1975; **Fellow:** Colon & Rectal Surgery, Cleveland Clinic 1976; **Fac Appt:** Assoc Clin Prof S, NY Med Coll

Goldstein, Scott D MD [CRS] - **Spec Exp:** Colon & Rectal Cancer; Inflammatory Bowel Disease; Laparoscopic Surgery; **Hospital:** Thomas Jefferson Univ Hosp; **Address:** 1100 Walnut St, Ste 702, Philadelphia, PA 19107; **Phone:** 215-955-5869; **Board Cert:** Colon & Rectal Surgery 1997; **Med School:** SUNY Upstate Med Univ 1978; **Resid:** Surgery, Lenox Hill Hosp 1983; Colon & Rectal Surgery, UMDNJ Med Ctr 1984; **Fac Appt:** Assoc Prof S, Thomas Jefferson Univ

Gorfine, Stephen MD [CRS] - **Spec Exp:** Anal Disorders & Reconstruction; Hemorrhoids; Rectal Cancer; Anal Cancer; **Hospital:** Mount Sinai Med Ctr (page 64), Lenox Hill Hosp (page 62); **Address:** 25 E 69th St, New York, NY 10021-4925; **Phone:** 212-517-8600; **Board Cert:** Internal Medicine 1981; Surgery 1996; Colon & Rectal Surgery 1988; **Med School:** Univ Mass Sch Med 1978; **Resid:** Internal Medicine, Mount Sinai Hosp 1981; Surgery, Mount Sinai Hosp 1985; **Fellow:** Colon & Rectal Surgery, Ferguson Hosp 1987; **Fac Appt:** Clin Prof S, Mount Sinai Sch Med

Colon & Rectal Surgery

Guillem, Jose MD [CRS] - **Spec Exp:** Colon & Rectal Cancer; Rectal Cancer/Sphincter Preservation; Colon & Rectal Cancer-Familial Polyposis; Peritoneal Mucinous Carcinomatosis; **Hospital:** Meml Sloan-Kettering Cancer Ctr; **Address:** 1275 York Avenue, New York, NY 10065; **Phone:** 800-525-2225; **Board Cert:** Colon & Rectal Surgery 2005; Surgery 2004; **Med School:** Yale Univ 1983; **Resid:** Surgery, Columbia-Presby Med Ctr 1990; **Fellow:** Colon & Rectal Surgery, Lahey Clinic 1991; **Fac Appt:** Prof CRS, Cornell Univ-Weill Med Coll

Medich, David MD [CRS] - **Spec Exp:** Colon & Rectal Cancer; Ulcerative Colitis; Inflammatory Bowel Disease/Crohn's; **Hospital:** Allegheny General Hosp; **Address:** Allegheny General Hosp, South Tower, 320 E North Ave Fl 5, Pittsburgh, PA 15212; **Phone:** 412-359-3901; **Board Cert:** Surgery 2004; Colon & Rectal Surgery 2006; **Med School:** Ohio State Univ 1987; **Resid:** Surgery, Univ Pittsburgh Med Ctr 1990; **Fellow:** Research, Univ Pittsburgh 1993; Colon & Rectal Surgery, Cleveland Clin Fdn 1994; **Fac Appt:** Assoc Prof CRS, Drexel Univ Coll Med

Milsom, Jeffrey W MD [CRS] - **Spec Exp:** Inflammatory Bowel Disease; Laparoscopic Surgery; Colon & Rectal Cancer; Crohn's Disease; **Hospital:** NY-Presby Hosp/Weill Cornell (page 66); **Address:** NY Cornell Med Ctr, Div Colorectal Surgery, 1315 York Ave Fl 2, New York, NY 10065-5304; **Phone:** 212-746-6030; **Board Cert:** Colon & Rectal Surgery 1986; **Med School:** Univ Pittsburgh 1979; **Resid:** Surgery, Roosevelt Hosp 1981; Surgery, Univ Virginia Med Ctr 1984; **Fellow:** Colon & Rectal Surgery, Ferguson Hosp 1985; **Fac Appt:** Prof S, Cornell Univ-Weill Med Coll

Read, Thomas E MD [CRS] - **Spec Exp:** Colon & Rectal Cancer; Inflammatory Bowel Disease; Laparoscopic Surgery; **Hospital:** Western Penn Hosp; **Address:** 4815 Liberty Ave, Ste GR-59, Mellon Pavilion, Pittsburgh, PA 15224; **Phone:** 412-578-1425; **Board Cert:** Surgery 2005; Colon & Rectal Surgery 2006; **Med School:** UCSF 1988; **Resid:** Surgery, UCSF Med Ctr 1995; **Fellow:** Colon & Rectal Surgery, Lahey Clinic 1996; **Fac Appt:** Assoc Prof S, Temple Univ

Rombeau, John L MD [CRS] - **Spec Exp:** Colon & Rectal Cancer; Inflammatory Bowel Disease/Crohn's; Ulcerative Colitis; Rectal Cancer/Sphincter Preservation; **Hospital:** Temple Univ Hosp; **Address:** Department of Surgery, 3401 N Broad St, Parkinson Pavilion Fl 4, Philadelphia, PA 19104-5103; **Phone:** 215-707-3133; **Board Cert:** Colon & Rectal Surgery 1977; **Med School:** Loma Linda Univ 1967; **Resid:** Surgery, Good Samaritan Hosp 1971; Surgery, LAC-USC Med Ctr 1975; **Fellow:** Colon & Rectal Surgery, Cleveland Clinic 1976; **Fac Appt:** Prof S, Temple Univ

Steinhagen, Randolph MD [CRS] - **Spec Exp:** Colostomy Avoidance; Colon & Rectal Cancer; Inflammatory Bowel Disease/Crohn's; **Hospital:** Mount Sinai Med Ctr (page 64); **Address:** Div Colon & Rectal Surgery, 5 E 98th St Fl 14, Box 1259, New York, NY 10029-6501; **Phone:** 212-241-3547; **Board Cert:** Surgery 2002; Colon & Rectal Surgery 1985; **Med School:** Wayne State Univ 1977; **Resid:** Surgery, Mount Sinai Hosp 1982; **Fellow:** Colon & Rectal Surgery, Cleveland Clinic 1983; **Fac Appt:** Assoc Prof S, Mount Sinai Sch Med

Whelan, Richard L MD [CRS] - **Spec Exp:** Laparoscopic Surgery; Colon & Rectal Cancer; **Hospital:** NY-Presby Hosp/Columbia (page 66); **Address:** 161 Ft Washington Ave, rm 817, New York, NY 10032; **Phone:** 212-342-1155; **Board Cert:** Surgery 1997; Colon & Rectal Surgery 1989; **Med School:** Columbia P&S 1982; **Resid:** Surgery, Columbia Presby Hosp 1987; **Fellow:** Colon & Rectal Surgery, Univ Minn Med Ctr 1988; **Fac Appt:** Assoc Clin Prof S, Columbia P&S

Wong, W Douglas MD [CRS] - **Spec Exp:** Rectal Cancer/Sphincter Preservation; Colon & Rectal Cancer; Anal Disorders & Reconstruction; **Hospital:** Meml Sloan-Kettering Cancer Ctr; **Address:** 1275 York Avenue, New York, NY 10065; **Phone:** 800-525-2225; **Board Cert:** Surgery 1997; Colon & Rectal Surgery 2004; **Med School:** Univ Manitoba 1972; **Resid:** Surgery, Univ Manitoba Hosp 1977; **Fellow:** Colon & Rectal Surgery, Univ Minn Med Ctr 1984; **Fac Appt:** Prof S, Cornell Univ-Weill Med Coll

Southeast

Galandiuk, Susan MD [CRS] - **Spec Exp:** Colon & Rectal Cancer; Inflammatory Bowel Disease/Crohn's; **Hospital:** Univ of Louisville Hosp, Norton Hosp; **Address:** 601 S Floyd St, Ste 700, Louisville, KY 40202; **Phone:** 502-583-8303; **Board Cert:** Surgery 1998; Colon & Rectal Surgery 1999; **Med School:** Germany 1982; **Resid:** Surgery, Cleveland Clinic Fdtn 1988; **Fellow:** Research, Univ Louisville Hosp 1989; Colon & Rectal Surgery, Mayo Clinic 1990; **Fac Appt:** Prof CRS, Univ Louisville Sch Med

Golub, Richard MD [CRS] - **Spec Exp:** Colon & Rectal Cancer; Laparoscopic Surgery; Hemorrhoids; **Hospital:** Sarasota Meml Hosp, Doctors Hosp - Sarasota; **Address:** Sarasota Memorial Hospital, 3333 Cattlemen Rd, Ste 206, Sarasota, FL 34232; **Phone:** 941-341-0042; **Board Cert:** Surgery 2000; Colon & Rectal Surgery 2003; **Med School:** Albert Einstein Coll Med 1984; **Resid:** Surgery, Univ Hosp Stony Brook 1990; **Fellow:** Colon & Rectal Surgery, Grant Medical Center 1991

Hartmann, Rene MD [CRS] - **Spec Exp:** Laparoscopic Surgery; Rectovaginal Fistula; Colon Cancer; Inflammatory Bowel Disease; **Hospital:** Mercy Hosp, Baptist Hosp of Miami; **Address:** Mercy Hospital, 3661 S Miami Ave, Ste 301, Miami, FL 33133; **Phone:** 305-285-2787; **Board Cert:** Colon & Rectal Surgery 1994; **Med School:** Venezuela 1971; **Resid:** Surgery, Jackson Meml Hosp 1976; Surgery, Orange Meml Hosp 1977; **Fellow:** Colon & Rectal Surgery, Grant Hosp 1978; **Fac Appt:** Assoc Clin Prof S, Univ Miami Sch Med

Mantyh, Christopher MD [CRS] - **Spec Exp:** Inflammatory Bowel Disease; Colon & Rectal Cancer & Surgery; Rectal Cancer/Sphincter Preservation; Incontinence-Fecal; **Hospital:** Duke Univ Med Ctr; **Address:** Duke Univ Med Ctr, Box 3117, Durham, NC 27710; **Phone:** 919-681-3977; **Board Cert:** Colon & Rectal Surgery 2000; Surgery 1999; **Med School:** Univ Wisc 1991; **Resid:** Surgery, Duke Univ Med Ctr 1998; **Fellow:** Colon & Rectal Surgery, Cleveland Clinic 1999

Marcet, Jorge MD [CRS] - **Spec Exp:** Colon & Rectal Cancer; **Hospital:** H Lee Moffitt Cancer Ctr & Research Inst, Tampa Genl Hosp; **Address:** H Lee Moffitt Cancer Ctr, Ste F145, Box 1289, Tampa, FL 33601; **Phone:** 813-844-4545; **Board Cert:** Colon & Rectal Surgery 2003; Surgery 2001; **Med School:** Cornell Univ-Weill Med Coll 1985; **Resid:** Surgery, St Luke's-Roosevelt Med Ctr 1990; **Fellow:** Colon & Rectal Surgery, Columbia Presby Med Ctr 1990; Colon & Rectal Surgery, St Luke's-Roosevelt Med Ctr 1991; **Fac Appt:** Assoc Prof S, Univ S Fla Coll Med

Nogueras, Juan J MD [CRS] - **Spec Exp:** Colon & Rectal Cancer; Inflammatory Bowel Disease/Crohn's; Incontinence-Fecal; **Hospital:** Cleveland Clin - Weston; **Address:** Cleveland Clinic, Dept Colorectal Surgery, 2950 Cleveland Clinic Blvd, Weston, FL 33331; **Phone:** 954-659-5251; **Board Cert:** Surgery 1997; Colon & Rectal Surgery 2003; **Med School:** Jefferson Med Coll 1982; **Resid:** Surgery, Columbia Presby Med Ctr 1987; **Fellow:** Colon & Rectal Surgery, Univ Minn Med Ctr 1991

Vernava III, Anthony M MD [CRS] - **Spec Exp:** Colon & Rectal Cancer; Incontinence-Fecal; Inflammatory Bowel Disease; **Hospital:** Physicians Regl Med Ctr; **Address:** Medical Surgical Specialists, 6101 Pine Ridge Rd, Naples, FL 34119; **Phone:** 239-348-4000; **Board Cert:** Surgery 1997; Colon & Rectal Surgery 1989; **Med School:** St Louis Univ 1982; **Resid:** Surgery, St Louis Univ Med Ctr 1988; Colon & Rectal Surgery, Univ Minnesota Med Ctr 1989; **Fellow:** Colon & Rectal Surgery, St Marks Hosp 1990

Wexner, Steven MD [CRS] - **Spec Exp:** Colon & Rectal Cancer; Inflammatory Bowel Disease/Crohn's; Laparoscopic Surgery; **Hospital:** Cleveland Clin - Weston; **Address:** 2950 Cleveland Clinic Blvd, Weston, FL 33331-3609; **Phone:** 954-659-5278; **Board Cert:** Surgery 2005; Colon & Rectal Surgery 2006; **Med School:** Cornell Univ-Weill Med Coll 1982; **Resid:** Surgery, Roosevelt Hosp 1987; **Fellow:** Colon & Rectal Surgery, Univ Minn 1988; **Fac Appt:** Prof S, Cleveland Cl Coll Med/Case West Res

Colon & Rectal Surgery

Midwest

Abcarian, Herand MD [CRS] - **Spec Exp:** Rectal Cancer/Sphincter Preservation; Inflammatory Bowel Disease; Anorectal Disorders; Incontinence-Fecal; **Hospital:** Univ of IL Med Ctr at Chicago, Gottlieb Meml Hosp; **Address:** 675 W North Ave, Ste 406, Melrose Park, IL 60160; **Phone:** 708-450-5075; **Board Cert:** Surgery 1972; Colon & Rectal Surgery 1972; **Med School:** Iran 1965; **Resid:** Surgery, Cook County Hosp 1971; Colon & Rectal Surgery, Cook County Hosp 1972; **Fac Appt:** Prof S, Univ IL Coll Med

Delaney, Conor P MD/PhD [CRS] - **Spec Exp:** Laparoscopic Surgery; Colon & Rectal Cancer; Inflammatory Bowel Disease/Crohn's; **Hospital:** Univ Hosps Case Med Ctr; **Address:** 11100 Euclid Ave, MS 5047, Cleveland, OH 44106-5047; **Phone:** 216-844-8087; **Board Cert:** Surgery 1998; Colon & Rectal Surgery 1998; **Med School:** Ireland 1989; **Resid:** Surgery, Univ Hosp 1993; Surgery, Univ Hosp 1999; **Fellow:** Research, Univ of Pittsburgh 1995; Colon & Rectal Surgery, Cleveland Clinic 2000; **Fac Appt:** Prof S, Cleveland Cl Coll Med/Case West Res

Fleshman, James MD [CRS] - **Spec Exp:** Colon & Rectal Cancer; Laparoscopic Surgery; Inflammatory Bowel Disease; **Hospital:** Barnes-Jewish Hosp, Barnes-Jewish West County Hosp; **Address:** Wash Univ Sch Med, Div Col Rectal Surgery, 660 S Euclid Ave, Box 8109, St Louis, MO 63110; **Phone:** 314-454-7177; **Board Cert:** Colon & Rectal Surgery 1988; Surgery 1996; **Med School:** Washington Univ, St Louis 1980; **Resid:** Surgery, Jewish Hospital 1986; **Fellow:** Colon & Rectal Surgery, Univ Toronto 1987; **Fac Appt:** Prof S, Washington Univ, St Louis

Foley, Eugene F MD [CRS] - **Spec Exp:** Colon & Rectal Cancer; Ulcerative Colitis; **Hospital:** Univ WI Hosp & Clins; **Address:** Univ WI Hosp & Clins, 600 Highland Ave, Madison, WI 53792-7375; **Phone:** 608-263-7502; **Board Cert:** Surgery 2003; Colon & Rectal Surgery 2005; **Med School:** Harvard Med Sch 1985; **Resid:** Surgery, New England Deaconess Hosp 1991; **Fellow:** Colon & Rectal Surgery, Lahey Clinic 1993; **Fac Appt:** Prof S, Univ Wisc

Kodner, Ira J MD [CRS] - **Spec Exp:** Colon & Rectal Cancer; Inflammatory Bowel Disease/Crohn's; Laparoscopic Surgery; **Hospital:** Barnes-Jewish Hosp; **Address:** Wash Univ Sch Med, Div Col Rectal Surgery, 660 S Euclid Ave, Box 8109, St Louis, MO 63110; **Phone:** 314-454-7177; **Board Cert:** Surgery 1975; Colon & Rectal Surgery 1975; **Med School:** Washington Univ, St Louis 1967; **Resid:** Surgery, Barnes-Jewish Hosp 1974; **Fellow:** Colon & Rectal Surgery, Cleveland Clinic 1975; **Fac Appt:** Prof S, Washington Univ, St Louis

Lavery, Ian C MD [CRS] - **Spec Exp:** Colon & Rectal Cancer; Inflammatory Bowel Disease; Pediatric Gastrointestinal Surgery; **Hospital:** Cleveland Clin Fdn (page 56); **Address:** 9500 Euclid Ave, Desk A30, Cleveland, OH 44195; **Phone:** 216-444-6930; **Board Cert:** Colon & Rectal Surgery 1998; **Med School:** Australia 1967; **Resid:** Surgery, Princess Alexandra Hosp 1974; Colon & Rectal Surgery, Cleveland Clinic 1977; **Fac Appt:** Prof S, Case West Res Univ

Lowry, Ann C MD [CRS] - **Spec Exp:** Anal Sphincter Repair; Rectovaginal Fistula; Inflammatory Bowel Disease; **Hospital:** Abbott - Northwestern Hosp, Fairview Southdale Hosp; **Address:** 6363 France Ave S, Ste 212, Edina, MN 55435; **Phone:** 651-312-1700; **Board Cert:** Colon & Rectal Surgery 1988; **Med School:** Tufts Univ 1977; **Resid:** Surgery, New Eng Med Ctr Hosps 1982; **Fellow:** Colon & Rectal Surgery, Univ Minn Affil Hosps 1987; **Fac Appt:** Clin Prof S, Univ Minn

Madoff, Robert D MD [CRS] - **Spec Exp:** Colon & Rectal Cancer; Inflammatory Bowel Disease; Incontinence/Pelvic Floor Disorders; **Hospital:** Univ Minn Med Ctr, Fairview - Univ Campus; **Address:** 516 Delaware St SE, Phillips-Wangensteen Bldg, MMC 88, Minneapolis, MN 55455; **Phone:** 612-624-9708; **Board Cert:** Surgery 1995; Colon & Rectal Surgery 2002; **Med School:** Columbia P&S 1979; **Resid:** Surgery, Univ Minn Hosps 1987; **Fellow:** Colon & Rectal Surgery, Univ Minn Hosps 1988; **Fac Appt:** Prof S, Univ Minn

Nelson, Heidi MD [CRS] - **Spec Exp:** Colon & Rectal Cancer; Gastrointestinal Cancer; **Hospital:** Mayo Med Ctr & Clin - Rochester, Rochester Methodist Hosp; **Address:** Mayo Clinic, Gonda 9 South, 200 First St SW, Rochester, MN 55905; **Phone:** 507-284-3329; **Board Cert:** Surgery 1995; Colon & Rectal Surgery 1989; **Med School:** Univ Wash 1981; **Resid:** Surgery, Oregon Hlth Sci Univ Hosp 1987; Colon & Rectal Surgery, Oregon Hlth Sci Univ Hosp 1985; **Fellow:** Colon & Rectal Surgery, Mayo Clinic 1988; **Fac Appt:** Prof S, Mayo Med Sch

Pemberton, John MD [CRS] - **Spec Exp:** Inflammatory Bowel Disease/Crohn's; Colon & Rectal Cancer; **Hospital:** St Mary's Hosp - Rochester, Rochester Methodist Hosp; **Address:** Mayo Clinic, Div Colon & Rectal Surg, 200 First St SW, Gonda 9-S, Rochester, MN 55905; **Phone:** 507-284-2359; **Board Cert:** Surgery 2001; Colon & Rectal Surgery 1985; **Med School:** Tulane Univ 1976; **Resid:** Surgery, Mayo Clinic 1983; **Fellow:** Colon & Rectal Surgery, Mayo Clinic 1984; **Fac Appt:** Prof S, Mayo Med Sch

Rafferty, Janice F MD [CRS] - **Spec Exp:** Colon & Rectal Cancer; Ulcerative Colitis; Crohn's Disease; Anal Disorders & Reconstruction; **Hospital:** Univ Hosp - Cincinnati; **Address:** U of Cincinnati, Colon & Rectal Surgery, 2123 Auburn Ave, Ste 524, Cincinnati, OH 45219; **Phone:** 513-929-0104; **Board Cert:** Colon & Rectal Surgery 2008; Surgery 2004; **Med School:** Ohio State Univ 1988; **Resid:** Surgery, Univ CincinnatiHosp 1995; Colon & Rectal Surgery, Barnes Jewish Hosp 1996; **Fac Appt:** Assoc Prof S, Univ Cincinnati

Rothenberger, David A MD [CRS] - **Spec Exp:** Colon & Rectal Cancer; **Hospital:** Univ Minn Med Ctr, Fairview - Univ Campus; **Address:** Univ Minnesota Med Ctr, Dept Surg, 420 Delaware St SE, MMC 195, Minneapolis, MN 55455; **Phone:** 612-625-3660; **Board Cert:** Colon & Rectal Surgery 2005; **Med School:** Tufts Univ 1973; **Resid:** Surgery, St Paul-Ramsey Med Ctr 1978; **Fellow:** Colon & Rectal Surgery, Univ Minnesota Hosps 1979; **Fac Appt:** Prof S, Univ Minn

Saclarides, Theodore J MD [CRS] - **Spec Exp:** Rectal Cancer/Sphincter Preservation; Incontinence-Fecal; Inflammatory Bowel Disease; **Hospital:** Rush Univ Med Ctr, Rush N Shore Med Ctr; **Address:** University Surgeons, 1725 W Harrison St, Ste 810, Chicago, IL 60612-3832; **Phone:** 312-942-6543; **Board Cert:** Surgery 1996; Colon & Rectal Surgery 1989; **Med School:** Univ Miami Sch Med 1982; **Resid:** Surgery, Rush Presby-St Luke's Hosp 1987; **Fellow:** Colon & Rectal Surgery, Mayo Clinic 1988; **Fac Appt:** Prof S, Rush Med Coll

Senagore, Anthony MD [CRS] - **Spec Exp:** Laparoscopic Surgery; Colon & Rectal Cancer; Anorectal Disorders; Inflammatory Bowel Disease/Crohn's; **Hospital:** Spectrum Hlth Blodgett Campus; **Address:** Spectrum Health, 100 Michigan St NE, MC 005, Grand Rapids, MI 49503; **Phone:** 616-391-2467; **Board Cert:** Surgery 1995; Colon & Rectal Surgery 2001; **Med School:** Mich State Univ 1981; **Resid:** Surgery, Butterworth Hosp 1987; Colon & Rectal Surgery, Ferguson Hosp 1989; **Fac Appt:** Prof S, Med Univ Ohio at Toledo

Stryker, Steven J MD [CRS] - **Spec Exp:** Colon & Rectal Cancer; Inflammatory Bowel Disease; Laparoscopic Surgery; **Hospital:** Northwestern Meml Hosp; **Address:** 676 N Saint Clair St, Ste 1525A, Chicago, IL 60611-2862; **Phone:** 312-943-5427; **Board Cert:** Surgery 2004; Colon & Rectal Surgery 1986; **Med School:** Northwestern Univ 1978; **Resid:** Surgery, Northwestern Meml Hosp 1983; **Fellow:** Colon & Rectal Surgery, Mayo Clinic 1985; **Fac Appt:** Clin Prof S, Northwestern Univ

Wolff, Bruce G MD [CRS] - **Spec Exp:** Inflammatory Bowel Disease; Crohn's Disease; Colon & Rectal Cancer; **Hospital:** Mayo Med Ctr & Clin - Rochester; **Address:** Mayo Clinic, Gonda 9 South, 200 First St SW, Rochester, MN 55905; **Phone:** 507-284-3329; **Board Cert:** Surgery 2000; Colon & Rectal Surgery 2001; **Med School:** Duke Univ 1973; **Resid:** Surgery, NY Hosp-Cornell Med Ctr 1981; **Fellow:** Colon & Rectal Surgery, Mayo Clinic 1982; **Fac Appt:** Prof S, Mayo Med Sch

Colon & Rectal Surgery

Great Plains and Mountains

Thorson, Alan G MD [CRS] - **Spec Exp:** Colon & Rectal Cancer; Laparoscopic Surgery; Incontinence-Fecal; **Hospital:** Nebraska Meth Hosp, Archbishop Bergan Mercy Med Ctr; **Address:** 9850 Nicholas St, Ste 100, Omaha, NE 68114-2191; **Phone:** 402-343-1122; **Board Cert:** Colon & Rectal Surgery 1999; **Med School:** Univ Nebr Coll Med 1979; **Resid:** Surgery, Univ Nebraska 1984; Colon & Rectal Surgery, Univ Minn 1985; **Fac Appt:** Assoc Clin Prof S, Creighton Univ

Southwest

Adkins, Terrance P MD [CRS] - **Spec Exp:** Colon & Rectal Cancer; Inflammatory Bowel Disease; **Hospital:** Tucson Med Ctr; **Address:** Southwestern Surgery Assoc, 1951 N Wilmot Rd Bldg 2, Tucson, AZ 85712; **Phone:** 520-795-5845; **Board Cert:** Surgery 2001; Colon & Rectal Surgery 2004; **Med School:** Univ Tex SW, Dallas 1985; **Resid:** Surgery, Univ Utah Med Ctr 1991; **Fellow:** Colon & Rectal Surgery, Univ Texas Med Ctr 1992; **Fac Appt:** Asst Clin Prof S, Univ Ariz Coll Med

Bailey, Harold R MD [CRS] - **Spec Exp:** Rectal Cancer/Sphincter Preservation; Inflammatory Bowel Disease; Incontinence-Fecal; Endometriosis-Intestine; **Hospital:** Methodist Hosp - Houston, St Luke's Episcopal Hosp - Houston; **Address:** Colon & Rectal Clinic, Smith Twr, 6550 Fannin St, Ste 2307, Houston, TX 77030-2717; **Phone:** 713-790-9250; **Board Cert:** Surgery 1974; Colon & Rectal Surgery 2004; **Med School:** Univ Tex SW, Dallas 1968; **Resid:** Surgery, Hermann Hosp-Univ Tex Med Sch 1973; **Fellow:** Colon & Rectal Surgery, Ferguson-Droste Hosp 1974; **Fac Appt:** Clin Prof S, Univ Tex, Houston

Beck, David E MD [CRS] - **Spec Exp:** Colon & Rectal Cancer; Minimally Invasive Surgery; Inflammatory Bowel Disease; **Hospital:** Ochsner Fdn Hosp, Summit Hosp-Baton Rouge; **Address:** Ochsner Clinic Fdn, Colorectal Surgery, 1514 Jefferson Hwy, 4th Fl, rm 04 East, New Orleans, LA 70121-2429; **Phone:** 504-842-4060; **Board Cert:** Colon & Rectal Surgery 1987; **Med School:** Univ Miami Sch Med 1979; **Resid:** Surgery, Wilford Hall USAF Med Ctr 1984; **Fellow:** Colon & Rectal Surgery, Cleveland Clinic Fdn 1986; **Fac Appt:** Assoc Clin Prof S, Louisiana State U, New Orleans

Efron, Jonathan E MD [CRS] - **Spec Exp:** Colon & Rectal Cancer; Incontinence-Fecal; Inflammatory Bowel Disease; Anorectal Disorders; **Hospital:** Mayo Clinic - Scottsdale; **Address:** Mayo Clinic, Concourse B, 13400 E Shea Blvd, Scottsdale, AZ 85259; **Phone:** 480-342-2697; **Board Cert:** Surgery 1999; Colon & Rectal Surgery 2000; **Med School:** Univ MD Sch Med 1993; **Resid:** Surgery, LIJ Medical Ctr 1999; **Fellow:** Colon & Rectal Surgery, Cleveland Clinic 2000; Research, Cleveland Clinic 2001; **Fac Appt:** Assoc Prof S, Mayo Med Sch

Heppell, Jacques P MD [CRS] - **Spec Exp:** Colon & Rectal Cancer; Inflammatory Bowel Disease; Anorectal Disorders; **Hospital:** Mayo Clinic - Phoenix; **Address:** Mayo Clinic, ATTN: GENS/CB/Distribution 13, 5777 E Mayo Blvd, Phoenix, AZ 85054; **Phone:** 480-342-2697; **Board Cert:** Surgery 2004; Colon & Rectal Surgery 1995; **Med School:** Univ Montreal 1974; **Resid:** Surgery, Univ Montreal Med Ctr 1979; **Fellow:** Colon & Rectal Surgery, Mayo Clinic 1983; **Fac Appt:** Prof S, Mayo Med Sch

Huber Jr, Philip J MD [CRS] - **Spec Exp:** Colon & Rectal Cancer; Inflammatory Bowel Disease; **Hospital:** Med City Dallas Hosp, Presby Hosp of Dallas; **Address:** 7777 Forest Lane, Ste C-760, Dallas, TX 75230; **Phone:** 972-566-8039; **Board Cert:** Surgery 1997; Colon & Rectal Surgery 1993; **Med School:** Columbia P&S 1972; **Resid:** Surgery, Parkland Hosp 1977; Colon & Rectal Surgery, Presby Hosp 1978

West Coast and Pacific

Beart Jr, Robert W MD [CRS] - **Spec Exp:** Colon & Rectal Cancer; Inflammatory Bowel Disease/Crohn's; **Hospital:** USC Norris Comp Cancer Ctr, USC Univ Hosp - R K Eamer Med Plz; **Address:** USC Comprehensive Cancer Center, Topping Tower Suite 7418, 1441 Eastlake Ave, Los Angeles, CA 90033; **Phone:** 323-865-3690; **Board Cert:** Surgery 1993; Colon & Rectal Surgery 1995; **Med School:** Harvard Med Sch 1971; **Resid:** Surgery, Univ Colo Med Ctr 1976; Colon & Rectal Surgery, Mayo Clinic 1978; **Fellow:** Transplant Surgery, Univ Colo Med Ctr 1975; **Fac Appt:** Prof S, USC Sch Med

Chiu, Yanek S MD [CRS] - **Hospital:** CA Pacific Med Ctr - Pacific Campus; **Address:** 3838 California St, Ste 616, San Francisco, CA 94118; **Phone:** 415-668-0411; **Board Cert:** Colon & Rectal Surgery 1997; **Med School:** Boston Univ 1971; **Resid:** Surgery, Boston Med Ctr 1976; **Fellow:** Colon & Rectal Surgery, Mayo Clinic 1978; **Fac Appt:** Assoc Clin Prof CRS, UCSF

Coutsoftides, Theodore MD [CRS] - **Spec Exp:** Laparoscopic Surgery; Inflammatory Bowel Disease; Anal Sphincter Repair; **Hospital:** St Joseph's Hosp - Orange; **Address:** 1310 W Stewart Drive, Ste 605, Orange, CA 92868-3857; **Phone:** 714-532-2544; **Board Cert:** Colon & Rectal Surgery 1977; **Med School:** Israel 1970; **Resid:** Surgery, Cleveland Clinic 1973; Surgery, Royal Victoria Hosp 1976; **Fellow:** Colon & Rectal Surgery, Cleveland Clinic 1977; **Fac Appt:** Assoc Prof S, UC Irvine

Stamos, Michael J MD [CRS] - **Spec Exp:** Rectal Cancer/Sphincter Preservation; Laparoscopic Surgery; Inflammatory Bowel Disease; Colon & Rectal Cancer; **Hospital:** UC Irvine Med Ctr; **Address:** UC Irvine Med Ctr, Div Colon & Rectal Surg, 333 City Blvd W, Ste 850, Orange, CA 92868-2993; **Phone:** 888-717-4463; **Board Cert:** Surgery 2000; Colon & Rectal Surgery 2003; **Med School:** Case West Res Univ 1985; **Resid:** Surgery, Jackson Meml Hosp 1990; Colon & Rectal Surgery, Ochsner Clinic 1991; **Fac Appt:** Prof S, UC Irvine

Welton, Mark L MD [CRS] - **Spec Exp:** Ulcerative Colitis; Crohn's Disease; Colon & Rectal Cancer; Anal Cancer; **Hospital:** Stanford Univ Med Ctr; **Address:** Stanford Univ - Colon & Rectal Surgery, 300 Pasteur Drive, rm H 3680, Stanford, CA 94305-5655; **Phone:** 650-723-5461; **Board Cert:** Surgery 2000; Colon & Rectal Surgery 2005; **Med School:** UCLA 1984; **Resid:** Surgery, UCLA Med Ctr 1992; **Fellow:** Colon & Rectal Surgery, Barnes Jewish Hosp 1993; **Fac Appt:** Assoc Prof S, Stanford Univ

Wong, Ronald J MD [CRS] - **Spec Exp:** Laparoscopic Surgery; **Hospital:** Queen's Med Ctr - Honolulu; **Address:** Queen's Physicians' Office Bldg 1, 1380 Lusitana St, Ste 614, Honolulu, HI 96813; **Phone:** 808-524-1856; **Board Cert:** Surgery 1997; **Med School:** Univ Hawaii JA Burns Sch Med 1981; **Resid:** Surgery, Univ Hawaii 1985; Surgery, Catholic Med Ctr 1987; **Fellow:** Colon & Rectal Surgery, Suburban Hosp 1989; Research, Cornell Univ Med Ctr 1988; **Fac Appt:** Clin Prof S, Univ Hawaii JA Burns Sch Med

Worsey, M Jonathan MD [CRS] - **Spec Exp:** Colon & Rectal Cancer; Inflammatory Bowel Disease; **Hospital:** Scripps Meml Hosp - La Jolla; **Address:** Advanced Surgical Associates, 9834 Genesee Ave, Ste 201, La Jolla, CA 92037; **Phone:** 858-558-2272; **Board Cert:** Surgery 1998; Colon & Rectal Surgery 1999; **Med School:** England 1985; **Resid:** Surgery, Bristol Royal Infirm & Royal Gwent Hosp 1989; Surgery, Univ Pittsburgh Med Ctr 1997; **Fellow:** Colon & Rectal Surgery, Cleveland Clinic 1998

NYU Langone Medical Center

550 First Avenue (at 31St Street
New York, NY 1001
Physician Referra
(888)7-NYU-MED (888-769-8633
www.nyumc.or

COLON AND RECTAL SURGERY

The gastrointestinal surgery program is a division of the Department of Surgery, whose surgeons perform over 5,000 outpatient and inpatient procedures each year using laser, laparoscopic, endoscopic, and other minimally invasive techniques. It maintains a nationally-regarded residency training program in Surgery through the NYU School of Medicine. Candidates for gastrointestinal surgery receive same-day care that includes imaging, radiation, and nutritional support.

The program provides an integrated team approach based on communication between surgeons and caregivers. The result is cancer care in a lull service environment that offers a complete, patient-centered approach.

Virtual colonoscopies — a noninvasive method of cancer screening that uses the same techniques as a CT scan

Laparoscopic techniques — surgeons use tiny incisions to remove a segment of the colon; this dramatically speeds recovery and reduces the need for pain medication

Liver lesions — these are effectively treated using painless radiofrequency ablation

Dermatology

A dermatologist is trained to diagnose and treat pediatric and adult patients with benign and malignant disorders of the skin, mouth, external genitalia, hair and nails, as well as a number of sexually transmitted diseases. The dermatologist may have additional training and experience in the diagnosis and treatment of skin cancers, melanomas, moles and other tumors of the skin, the management of contact dermatitis and other allergic and nonallergic skin disorders, and in the recognition of the skin manifestations of systemic (including internal malignancy) and infectious diseases. Dermatologists may have special training in dermatopathology and in the surgical techniques used in dermatology. They also have expertise in the management of cosmetic disorders of the skin such as hair loss and scars, and the skin changes associated with aging.

Training Required: Four years.

Certification in the following subspecialties requires additional training and examination.

Dermatopathology: A dermatopathologist has the expertise to diagnose and monitor diseases of the skin including infectious, immunologic, degenerative and neoplastic diseases. This entails the examination and interpretation of specially prepared tissue sections, cellular scrapings and smears of skin lesions by means of routine and special (electron and fluorescent) microscopes.

Pediatric Dermatology: A dermatologist trained to diagnose and treat pediatric patients with dermatologic diseases.

DERMATOLOGY

New England

Anderson, Richard Rox MD [D] - **Spec Exp:** Cosmetic Dermatology; **Hospital:** Mass Genl Hosp; **Address:** Dermatology Laser Center, 50 Staniford St, Ste 250, Boston, MA 02114; **Phone:** 617-724-6960; **Board Cert:** Dermatology 2001; **Med School:** Harvard Med Sch 1984; **Resid:** Dermatology, Mass Genl Hosp 1991; **Fellow:** Dermatologic Research, Mass Genl Hosp 1988; **Fac Appt:** Assoc Prof D, Harvard Med Sch

Arndt, Kenneth MD [D] - **Spec Exp:** Skin Laser Surgery; Cosmetic Dermatology; **Hospital:** Beth Israel Deaconess Med Ctr - Boston, New England Bapt Hosp; **Address:** Skincare Phys of Chestnut Hill, 1244 Boylston St, Ste 302, Chestnut Hill, MA 02467; **Phone:** 617-731-1600; **Board Cert:** Dermatology 1966; **Med School:** Yale Univ 1961; **Resid:** Dermatology, Mass Genl Hosp 1965; **Fellow:** Dermatology, Harvard Med Sch 1965; **Fac Appt:** Clin Prof D, Harvard Med Sch

Del Giudice, Stephen M MD [D] - **Spec Exp:** Skin Cancer; Phototherapy; Psoriasis; Acne; **Hospital:** Concord Hospital; **Address:** Dartmouth Hitchcock Concord-Dermatology, 253 Pleasant St, Concord, NH 03301; **Phone:** 603-226-6119; **Board Cert:** Dermatology 1987; **Med School:** Tufts Univ 1981; **Resid:** Dermatology, Yale-New Haven Hosp 1987

Dover, Jeffrey MD [D] - **Spec Exp:** Cosmetic Dermatology; **Hospital:** Beth Israel Deaconess Med Ctr - Boston, New England Bapt Hosp; **Address:** 1244 Boylston St, Ste 302, Chesnut Hill, MA 02467; **Phone:** 617-731-1600; **Board Cert:** Dermatology 1985; **Med School:** Univ Ottawa 1981; **Resid:** Dermatology, Univ Toronto 1984; Dermatology, St Johns Hosp 1985; **Fellow:** Dermatology, Mass Genl Hosp-Harvard 1987; **Fac Appt:** Assoc Prof D, Dartmouth Med Sch

Edelson, Richard L MD [D] - **Spec Exp:** Cutaneous Lymphoma; Immune Deficiency-Skin Disorders; **Hospital:** Yale-New Haven Hosp; **Address:** 2 Church St S, Ste 305, New Haven, CT 06519; **Phone:** 203-789-1249; **Board Cert:** Dermatology 1977; **Med School:** Yale Univ 1970; **Resid:** Dermatology, Mass Genl Hosp 1972; Dermatology, Natl Inst Hlth 1975; **Fac Appt:** Prof D, Yale Univ

Falanga, Vincent MD [D] - **Spec Exp:** Wound Healing/Care; Collagen Vascular Diseases; Scleroderma; **Hospital:** Roger Williams Hosp; **Address:** Roger Williams Med Ctr, Dept Dermatology, 50 Maude St Elmhurst Bldg, Providence, RI 02908; **Phone:** 401-456-2521; **Board Cert:** Internal Medicine 1980; Dermatology 1982; **Med School:** Harvard Med Sch 1977; **Resid:** Internal Medicine, Univ Miami 1980; **Fellow:** Dermatology, Univ Penn 1982; **Fac Appt:** Prof D, Boston Univ

Fewkes, Jessica L MD [D] - **Spec Exp:** Mohs' Surgery; Skin Cancer-Head & Neck; Melanoma-Head & Neck; **Hospital:** Mass Eye & Ear Infirmary, Mass Genl Hosp; **Address:** Mass Eye & Ear Infirmary, 243 Charles St Fl 9, Boston, MA 02114; **Phone:** 617-573-3789; **Board Cert:** Dermatology 1982; **Med School:** UCSF 1978; **Resid:** Dermatology, Mass General Hosp 1982; **Fellow:** Chemosurgery, Duke Univ Med Ctr 1983; **Fac Appt:** Asst Prof D, Harvard Med Sch

Gilchrest, Barbara MD [D] - **Spec Exp:** Photoaging; Melanoma; Skin Cancer; **Hospital:** Boston Med Ctr; **Address:** 609 Albany St Bldg J - Ste 507, Boston, MA 02118-2394; **Phone:** 617-638-7420; **Board Cert:** Internal Medicine 1975; Dermatology 1978; **Med School:** Harvard Med Sch 1971; **Resid:** Internal Medicine, Boston City Hosp 1973; Dermatology, Harvard Med Sch 1976; **Fellow:** Photo Biology, Harvard Med Sch 1975; **Fac Appt:** Prof D, Boston Univ

Gottlieb, Alice MD/PhD [D] - **Spec Exp:** Psoriasis; Psoriatic Arthritis; Eczema; **Hospital:** Tufts Med Ctr; **Address:** 800 Washington St, Box 114, Boston, MA 02111; **Phone:** 617-636-5370; **Board Cert:** Internal Medicine 1982; Dermatology 2001; Rheumatology 1984; **Med School:** Cornell Univ-Weill Med Coll 1980; **Resid:** Internal Medicine, New York Hosp 1982; Dermatology, New York Hosp 1993; **Fellow:** Rheumatology, Hosp Special Surgery 1984; **Fac Appt:** Prof Med, Tufts Univ

Kane, Kay S MD [D] - **Spec Exp:** Pediatric Dermatology; **Hospital:** Children's Hospital - Boston; **Address:** Children's Hospital Boston, Dermatology Program, Fegan-6, 300 Longwood Ave, Boston, MA 02115; **Phone:** 617-355-6117; **Board Cert:** Dermatology 2005; **Med School:** Harvard Med Sch 1993; **Resid:** Dermatology, Mass General Hosp 1997; **Fac Appt:** Prof D, Harvard Med Sch

Kupper, Thomas S MD [D] - **Spec Exp:** Melanoma; Cutaneous Lymphoma; Skin Cancer; **Hospital:** Brigham & Women's Hosp, Dana-Farber Cancer Inst; **Address:** Brigham & Women's Hosp, Dept Dermatology, 77 Avenue Louis Pasteur, Ste 671, Boston, MA 02115; **Phone:** 617-525-5550; **Board Cert:** Dermatology 1989; **Med School:** Yale Univ 1981; **Resid:** Surgery, Yale-New Haven Hosp 1983; Dermatology, Yale-New Haven Hosp 1989; **Fac Appt:** Prof D, Harvard Med Sch

Leffell, David J MD [D] - **Spec Exp:** Mohs' Surgery; Melanoma; Skin Cancer; Skin Laser Surgery; **Hospital:** Yale-New Haven Hosp; **Address:** New Haven Hosp-Dept Dermatology, 40 Temple St, Ste 5A, PO Box 208059, New Haven, CT 06520; **Phone:** 203-785-3466; **Board Cert:** Internal Medicine 1984; Dermatology 1987; **Med School:** McGill Univ 1981; **Resid:** Internal Medicine, New York Hosp 1984; Dermatology, Yale-New Haven Hosp 1986; **Fellow:** Dermatology, Yale-New Haven Hosp 1987; Dermatologic Surgery, Univ Michigan Med Ctr 1988; **Fac Appt:** Prof D, Yale Univ

Maloney, Mary MD [D] - **Spec Exp:** Mohs' Surgery; Skin Laser Surgery; **Hospital:** UMass Memorial Med Ctr; **Address:** Univ Mass Med Ctr, Dept Derm, 281 Lincoln St Fl 4, Worcester, MA 01605-2138; **Phone:** 508-334-5962; **Board Cert:** Dermatology 1982; **Med School:** Univ VT Coll Med 1977; **Resid:** Internal Medicine, Hartford Hospital 1979; Dermatology, Dartmouth-Hitchcock Med Ctr 1982; **Fellow:** Dermatologic Surgery, UCSF Med Ctr 1983; **Fac Appt:** Prof D, Univ Mass Sch Med

McDonald, Charles J MD [D] - **Spec Exp:** Cutaneous Lymphoma; Autoimmune Disease; Melanoma; Psoriasis; **Hospital:** Rhode Island Hosp; **Address:** Rhode Island Hosp, Dept Dermatology, 593 Eddy St, APC-10, Providence, RI 02903-4923; **Phone:** 401-444-7959; **Board Cert:** Dermatology 1966; **Med School:** Howard Univ 1960; **Resid:** Internal Medicine, Hosp St Raphael 1963; Dermatology, Yale New Haven Hosp 1965; **Fellow:** Clinical Oncology, Yale New Haven Hosp 1966; **Fac Appt:** Prof D, Brown Univ

Mihm Jr, Martin C MD [D] - **Spec Exp:** Melanoma; Vascular Birthmarks; Dermatopathology; **Hospital:** Mass Genl Hosp; **Address:** Mass General Hosp, 55 Fruit St, Warren Bldg 825, Boston, MA 02114-2926; **Phone:** 617-724-1350; **Board Cert:** Dermatology 1969; Dermatopathology 1974; Anatomic Pathology 1974; **Med School:** Univ Pittsburgh 1961; **Resid:** Internal Medicine, Mt Sinai Hosp 1964; Dermatology, Mass Genl Hosp 1967; **Fellow:** Anatomic Pathology, Mass Genl Hosp 1972; **Fac Appt:** Clin Prof Path, Harvard Med Sch

Neel, Victor A MD/PhD [D] - **Spec Exp:** Mohs' Surgery; Skin Cancer; **Hospital:** Mass Genl Hosp; **Address:** 50 Staniford St, Ste 270, Boston, MA 02114; **Phone:** 617-726-1869; **Board Cert:** Dermatology 2000; **Med School:** Cornell Univ-Weill Med Coll 1995; **Resid:** Pediatrics, Rhode Island Hosp 1997; Dermatology, Rhode Island Hosp 2000; **Fellow:** Mohs Surgery, UCLA Med Ctr 2001

Dermatology

Olbricht, Suzanne M MD [D] - **Spec Exp:** Skin Cancer; Mohs' Surgery; **Hospital:** Lahey Clin; **Address:** Lahey Clinic, 41 Mall Rd, Burlington, MA 01805; **Phone:** 781-744-8348; **Board Cert:** Dermatology 1983; Internal Medicine 1979; **Med School:** Baylor Coll Med 1976; **Resid:** Internal Medicine, Mass General Hosp 1979; Dermatology, Mass General Hosp 1983; **Fellow:** Mohs Surgery, Mass General Hosp 1991; **Fac Appt:** Assoc Prof D, Harvard Med Sch

Sober, Arthur MD [D] - **Spec Exp:** Melanoma; Skin Cancer; **Hospital:** Mass Genl Hosp; **Address:** Mass General Hospital, 50 Staniford St, Ste 200, Boston, MA 02114; **Phone:** 617-726-2914; **Board Cert:** Dermatology 1975; Internal Medicine 1974; **Med School:** Geo Wash Univ 1968; **Resid:** Internal Medicine, Beth Israel Hosp 1970; Dermatology, Mass General Hosp 1974; **Fellow:** Immunology, Peter Bent Brigham Hosp 1976; **Fac Appt:** Prof D, Harvard Med Sch

Mid Atlantic

Alster, Tina MD [D] - **Spec Exp:** Cosmetic Dermatology; Scar Revision; Hemangiomas/Birthmarks; **Hospital:** Georgetown Univ Hosp; **Address:** 1430 K St NW Fl 2, Washington, DC 20005; **Phone:** 202-628-8855; **Board Cert:** Dermatology 1990; **Med School:** Duke Univ 1986; **Resid:** Dermatology, Yale Univ 1989; **Fellow:** Dermatologic Laser Surgery, Boston Univ Hosp 1990; **Fac Appt:** Clin Prof D, Georgetown Univ

Anhalt, Grant J MD [D] - **Spec Exp:** Blistering Diseases; Pemphigus; Autoimmune Disease; **Hospital:** Johns Hopkins Hosp - Baltimore (page 61); **Address:** 7401 Osler Drive, Ste 107, Towson, MD 21204; **Phone:** 410-321-5900; **Board Cert:** Dermatology 1980; Clinical & Laboratory Dematologic Immunology 1987; **Med School:** Canada 1975; **Resid:** Internal Medicine, Hlth Scis Ctr 1977; Dermatology, Univ Mich Med Ctr 1980; **Fellow:** Immunology, Univ Mich Med Ctr 1981; **Fac Appt:** Prof D, Johns Hopkins Univ

Bernstein, Robert M MD [D] - **Spec Exp:** Hair Restoration/Transplant; **Hospital:** NY-Presby Hosp/Columbia (page 66); **Address:** 110 E 55th St, New York, NY 10022; **Phone:** 212-826-2400; **Board Cert:** Dermatology 1982; Hair Restoration Surgery 1998; **Med School:** UMDNJ-NJ Med Sch, Newark 1978; **Resid:** Dermatology, Albert Einstein Med Ctr 1982; **Fac Appt:** Clin Prof D, Columbia P&S

Bickers, David MD [D] - **Spec Exp:** Skin Cancer; Photodynamic Therapy; Psoriasis; Phototherapy; **Hospital:** NY-Presby Hosp/Columbia (page 66); **Address:** 16 E 60th St, Ste 300, New York, NY 10022-1002; **Phone:** 212-326-8465; **Board Cert:** Dermatology 1974; **Med School:** Univ VA Sch Med 1967; **Resid:** Dermatology, NYU Med Ctr 1973; **Fellow:** Pharmacology, Rockefeller Univ Hosp 1974; **Fac Appt:** Prof D, Columbia P&S

Brandt, Fredric S MD [D] - **Spec Exp:** Botox Therapy; Cosmetic Dermatology; **Address:** Laser & Skin Surgery Ctr, 317 E 34th St Fl 6, New York, NY 10016; **Phone:** 212-889-7096; **Board Cert:** Internal Medicine 1978; Dermatology 1981; **Med School:** Hahnemann Univ 1975; **Resid:** Internal Medicine, VA Hosp 1981; Dermatology, Univ Miami Hosps 1983

Braun III, Martin MD [D] - **Spec Exp:** Mohs' Surgery; Skin Cancer; **Hospital:** G Washington Univ Hosp; **Address:** 2112 F St NW, Ste 701, Washington, DC 20037; **Phone:** 202-293-7618; **Board Cert:** Dermatology 1977; Dermatopathology 1982; **Med School:** Univ MD Sch Med 1970; **Resid:** Dermatology, Univ Mich Med Ctr 1976; **Fellow:** Mohs Surgery, Precept w/ Dr Frederic Mohs 1975; **Fac Appt:** Clin Prof D, Geo Wash Univ

Brodland, David MD [D] - **Spec Exp:** Mohs' Surgery; Skin Cancer; Reconstructive Surgery-Skin; **Hospital:** UPMC Shadyside, Jefferson Hosp - Pittsburgh; **Address:** South Hills Med Bldg, 575 Coal Valley Rd, Ste 360, Clairton, PA 15025; **Phone:** 412-466-9400; **Board Cert:** Dermatology 1989; **Med School:** Southern IL Univ 1985; **Resid:** Dermatology, Mayo Grad Sch Med 1989; **Fellow:** Mohs Surgery, John A Zitelli MD 1990; **Fac Appt:** Asst Clin Prof D, Univ Pittsburgh

Bystryn, Jean Claude MD [D] - **Spec Exp:** Melanoma; Blistering Diseases; Skin Cancer; Hair loss; **Hospital:** NYU Med Ctr (page 68); **Address:** 530 1st Ave, Ste 7F, New York, NY 10016; **Phone:** 212-889-3846; **Board Cert:** Dermatology 1970; Clinical & Laboratory Dermatologic Immunology 1985; **Med School:** NYU Sch Med 1962; **Resid:** Internal Medicine, Montefiore Hosp 1964; Dermatology, NYU Med Ctr 1969; **Fellow:** Immunology, New York Univ 1972; **Fac Appt:** Prof D, NYU Sch Med

Cotsarelis, George MD [D] - **Spec Exp:** Hair loss; Scalp Disorders; Hair Restoration/Transplant; **Hospital:** Hosp Univ Penn - UPHS (page 60); **Address:** Penn Medicine at Radnor, Dermatology, 250 King of Prussia Rd, Radnor, PA 19087; **Phone:** 610-902-2400; **Board Cert:** Dermatology 2001; **Med School:** Univ Pennsylvania 1987; **Resid:** Dermatology, Hosp Univ Penn 1992; **Fellow:** Dermatology, Hosp Univ Penn; **Fac Appt:** Asst Prof D, Univ Pennsylvania

Deleo, Vincent A MD [D] - **Spec Exp:** Photosensitive Skin Diseases; Contact Dermatitis; Facial Rejuvenation; Eczema; **Hospital:** St Luke's - Roosevelt Hosp Ctr - Roosevelt Div (page 57), Beth Israel Med Ctr - Petrie Division (page 57); **Address:** 425 W 59th St, Ste 5C, New York, NY 10019-1104; **Phone:** 212-523-6003; **Board Cert:** Dermatology 1976; **Med School:** Louisiana State U, New Orleans 1969; **Resid:** Dermatology, Columbia-Presby Med Ctr 1976; **Fac Appt:** Assoc Prof D, Columbia P&S

Dzubow, Leonard MD [D] - **Spec Exp:** Mohs' Surgery; Skin Cancer; **Address:** 101 Chesley Drive, Media, PA 19063; **Phone:** 484-621-0082; **Board Cert:** Internal Medicine 1978; Dermatology 1980; **Med School:** Univ Pennsylvania 1975; **Resid:** Internal Medicine, Hosp Univ Penn 1978; Dermatology, NYU-Skin Cancer Unit 1980; **Fellow:** Mohs Surgery, NYU-Skin Cancer Unit 1981; **Fac Appt:** Prof D, Univ Pennsylvania

Franks Jr, Andrew G MD [D] - **Spec Exp:** Lupus/SLE; Raynaud's Disease; Scleroderma; **Hospital:** NYU Med Ctr (page 68), Lenox Hill Hosp (page 62); **Address:** 60 Gramercy Park N, Ste 1N, New York, NY 10010-5429; **Phone:** 212-475-2312; **Board Cert:** Internal Medicine 1975; Dermatology 1977; Rheumatology 1978; **Med School:** NYU Sch Med 1971; **Resid:** Internal Medicine, Beth Israel Med Ctr 1974; Dermatology, Columbia-Presby Med Ctr 1975; **Fellow:** Rheumatology, Columbia-Presby Med Ctr 1977; **Fac Appt:** Prof D, NYU Sch Med

Geronemus, Roy MD [D] - **Spec Exp:** Skin Laser Surgery; Cosmetic Dermatology; Mohs' Surgery; Skin Cancer; **Hospital:** NYU Med Ctr (page 68), New York Eye & Ear Infirm (page 65); **Address:** 317 E 34 St, Ste 11N, New York, NY 10016-4974; **Phone:** 212-686-7306; **Board Cert:** Dermatology 1983; **Med School:** Univ Miami Sch Med 1979; **Resid:** Dermatology, NYU-Skin Cancer Unit 1983; **Fellow:** Mohs Surgery, NYU-Skin Cancer Unit 1984; **Fac Appt:** Clin Prof D, NYU Sch Med

Gordon, Marsha MD [D] - **Spec Exp:** Cosmetic Dermatology; Botox Therapy; Aging Skin; Skin Cancer; **Hospital:** Mount Sinai Med Ctr (page 64); **Address:** 5 E 98th St Fl 5, New York, NY 10029-6501; **Phone:** 212-241-9728; **Board Cert:** Dermatology 1988; **Med School:** Univ Pennsylvania 1984; **Resid:** Dermatology, Mount Sinai Hosp 1988; **Fac Appt:** Clin Prof D, Mount Sinai Sch Med

Dermatology

Granstein, Richard D MD [D] - **Spec Exp:** Autoimmune Disease; Skin Cancer; Psoriasis; **Hospital:** NY-Presby Hosp/Weill Cornell (page 66); **Address:** 1305 York Ave Fl 9, New York, NY 10021; **Phone:** 646-962-7546; **Board Cert:** Dermatology 1983; Clinical & Laboratory Dermatologic Immunology 1985; **Med School:** UCLA 1978; **Resid:** Dermatology, Mass Genl Hosp 1981; **Fellow:** Research, Natl Cancer Inst 1982; Dermatology, Mass Genl Hosp 1983; **Fac Appt:** Prof D, Cornell Univ-Weill Med Coll

Grossman, Melanie MD [D] - **Spec Exp:** Skin Laser Surgery; Tattoo Removal; Laser Resurfacing; Facial Rejuvenation; **Hospital:** NY-Presby Hosp/Columbia (page 66); **Address:** 161 Madison Ave, Ste 4NW, New York, NY 10016-5405; **Phone:** 212-725-8600; **Board Cert:** Dermatology 1999; **Med School:** NYU Sch Med 1988; **Resid:** Internal Medicine, Yale-New Haven Hosp 1989; Dermatology, Columbia-Presby Med Ctr 1992; **Fellow:** Laser Surgery, Mass Genl Hosp 1995; **Fac Appt:** Asst Clin Prof D, Columbia P&S

Halpern, Allan C MD [D] - **Spec Exp:** Skin Cancer; Melanoma; Melanoma Early Detection/Prevention; **Hospital:** Meml Sloan-Kettering Cancer Ctr; **Address:** 1275 York Avenue, New York, NY 10065; **Phone:** 800-525-2225; **Board Cert:** Internal Medicine 1984; Dermatology 1988; **Med School:** Albert Einstein Coll Med 1981; **Resid:** Internal Medicine, Montefiore Hosp 1985; Dermatology, Hosp Univ Penn 1989; **Fellow:** Epidemiology, Hosp Univ Penn 1989; **Fac Appt:** Assoc Prof Med, Cornell Univ-Weill Med Coll

James, William D MD [D] - **Spec Exp:** Contact Dermatitis; Acne; Rosacea; **Hospital:** Hosp Univ Penn - UPHS (page 60); **Address:** Univ Penn Dept Dermatology, 3600 Spruce St, 2 Maloney, Philadelphia, PA 19104; **Phone:** 215-662-4282; **Board Cert:** Dermatology 1981; Diagnostic Lab Immunology 1985; **Med School:** Indiana Univ 1975; **Resid:** Dermatology, Letterman Army Med Ctr 1981; **Fac Appt:** Prof D, Univ Pennsylvania

Katz, Stephen MD [D] - **Spec Exp:** Immune Deficiency-Skin Disorders; **Hospital:** Natl Inst of Hlth - Clin Ctr; **Address:** NIH-Dermatology Branch, 31 Center Drive, MSC 2350, Bldg 31 - rm 4C32, Bethesda, MD 20892; **Phone:** 301-496-2481; **Board Cert:** Dermatology 1971; Clinical & Laboratory Dermatologic Immunology 1985; **Med School:** Tulane Univ 1966; **Resid:** Dermatology, Jackson Meml Hosp 1970; **Fellow:** Research 1974

Kriegel, David MD [D] - **Spec Exp:** Mohs' Surgery; Botox Therapy; Skin Laser Surgery; Cosmetic Dermatology; **Hospital:** Mount Sinai Med Ctr (page 64); **Address:** 250 W 57th St, Ste 825, New York, NY 10107-0809; **Phone:** 212-489-6669; **Board Cert:** Dermatology 2003; **Med School:** Boston Univ 1987; **Resid:** Dermatology, New England Med Ctr 1991; **Fellow:** Mohs Surgery, Stony Brook Univ Hosp 1993; **Fac Appt:** Assoc Prof D, Mount Sinai Sch Med

Lebwohl, Mark MD [D] - **Spec Exp:** Skin Cancer; Cutaneous Lymphoma; Psoriasis; Pseudoxanthoma Elasticum; **Hospital:** Mount Sinai Med Ctr (page 64); **Address:** 5 E 98th St Fl 5, New York, NY 10029-6501; **Phone:** 212-241-9728; **Board Cert:** Internal Medicine 1981; Dermatology 1983; **Med School:** Harvard Med Sch 1978; **Resid:** Internal Medicine, Mount Sinai Hosp 1981; **Fellow:** Dermatology, Mount Sinai Hosp 1983; **Fac Appt:** Prof D, Mount Sinai Sch Med

Lessin, Stuart R MD [D] - **Spec Exp:** Melanoma; Skin Cancer; Cutaneous Lymphoma; Melanoma Risk Assessment; **Hospital:** Fox Chase Cancer Ctr (page 58); **Address:** Fox Chase Cancer Ctr, Dept Dermatology, 333 Cottman Ave, Philadelphia, PA 19111; **Phone:** 215-728-2570; **Board Cert:** Dermatology 1986; **Med School:** Temple Univ 1982; **Resid:** Dermatology, Hosp Univ Penn 1986; **Fellow:** Molecular Biology, Wistar Inst 1987; **Fac Appt:** Prof D, Temple Univ

America's Top Doctors® 8th Edition

Miller, Stanley J MD [D] - **Spec Exp:** Skin Cancer; Mohs' Surgery; Melanoma; **Hospital:** Johns Hopkins Hosp - Baltimore (page 61); **Address:** Charles Towson Bldg, 1104 Kenilworth Drive, Ste 201, Towson, MD 21204; **Phone:** 443-279-0340; **Board Cert:** Dermatology 1989; **Med School:** Univ VT Coll Med 1984; **Resid:** Dermatology, UCSD Med Ctr 1989; **Fellow:** Dermatologic Surgery, Univ Penn 1991; **Fac Appt:** Prof D, Johns Hopkins Univ

Nigra, Thomas P MD [D] - **Spec Exp:** Hair loss; Psoriasis; Skin Cancer; Vitiligo; **Hospital:** Washington Hosp Ctr; **Address:** Dermatology Assocs, 110 Irving St NW, 2B44, Washington, DC 20010; **Phone:** 202-877-6227; **Board Cert:** Dermatology 1973; **Med School:** Univ Pennsylvania 1967; **Resid:** Dermatology, Mass Genl Hosp 1973; Dermatology, Natl Insts of Health 1971; **Fac Appt:** Clin Prof D, Geo Wash Univ

Orlow, Seth MD/PhD [D] - **Spec Exp:** Pediatric Dermatology; Hemangiomas/Birthmarks; Psoriasis/Eczema; **Hospital:** NYU Med Ctr (page 68); **Address:** 530 1st Ave, Ste 7R, New York, NY 10016-6402; **Phone:** 212-263-5889; **Board Cert:** Dermatology 1990; Pediatric Dermatology 2004; **Med School:** Albert Einstein Coll Med 1986; **Resid:** Pediatrics, Mt Sinai Hosp 1987; Dermatology, Yale-New Haven Hosp 1989; **Fellow:** Dermatology, Yale-New Haven Hosp 1990; **Fac Appt:** Prof D, NYU Sch Med

Ramsay, David L MD [D] - **Spec Exp:** Cutaneous Lymphoma; Skin Cancer; **Hospital:** NYU Med Ctr (page 68); **Address:** 530 1st Ave, Ste 7G, New York, NY 10016-6402; **Phone:** 212-683-6283; **Board Cert:** Dermatology 1974; **Med School:** Indiana Univ 1969; **Resid:** Dermatology, New York Univ Med Ctr 1973; **Fellow:** Dermatology, Univ Ill Hosp 1973; **Fac Appt:** Clin Prof D, NYU Sch Med

Rigel, Darrell S MD [D] - **Spec Exp:** Melanoma; Skin Cancer; Cosmetic Dermatology; **Hospital:** NYU Med Ctr (page 68), Mount Sinai Med Ctr (page 64); **Address:** 35 E 35th Street, Ste 208, New York, NY 10016-3823; **Phone:** 212-684-5964; **Board Cert:** Dermatology 1983; **Med School:** Geo Wash Univ 1978; **Resid:** Dermatology, NYU Med Ctr 1982; **Fellow:** Dermatologic Surgery, NYU Med Ctr 1983; **Fac Appt:** Clin Prof D, NYU Sch Med

Robins, Perry MD [D] - **Spec Exp:** Mohs' Surgery; Skin Cancer; Melanoma; **Hospital:** NYU Med Ctr (page 68), Bellevue Hosp Ctr; **Address:** 625 Park Ave, New York, NY 10065; **Phone:** 212-263-7222; **Med School:** Germany 1961; **Resid:** Dermatology, VA Med Ctr 1964; **Fellow:** Dermatology, NYU Med Ctr 1967; **Fac Appt:** Prof D, NYU Sch Med

Rook, Alain H MD [D] - **Spec Exp:** Cutaneous Lymphoma; Immune Deficiency-Skin Disorders; Mycosis Fungoides; **Hospital:** Hosp Univ Penn - UPHS (page 60); **Address:** Hosp Univ Penn, Dept Dermatology, 3400 Spruce St Maloney Bldg Fl 2nd, Philadelphia, PA 19104; **Phone:** 215-662-7610; **Board Cert:** Internal Medicine 1979; Nephrology 1980; Dermatology 2001; **Med School:** Univ Mich Med Sch 1975; **Resid:** Internal Medicine, McGill Univ Med Ctr 1977; Dermatology, Hosp Univ Penn 1989; **Fellow:** Nephrology, McGill Univ Med Ctr 1979; Immunology, NIH 1986; **Fac Appt:** Prof D, Univ Pennsylvania

Schultz, Neal MD [D] - **Spec Exp:** Cosmetic Dermatology; Skin Cancer; Skin Laser Surgery; Tattoo Removal; **Hospital:** Mount Sinai Med Ctr (page 64), Lenox Hill Hosp (page 62); **Address:** 1130 Park Ave, New York, NY 10128; **Phone:** 212-369-9600; **Board Cert:** Dermatology 1978; **Med School:** Columbia P&S 1973; **Resid:** Internal Medicine, Mount Sinai Hosp 1975; Dermatology, Mount Sinai Hosp 1978; **Fac Appt:** Asst Clin Prof D, Mount Sinai Sch Med

Shalita, Alan MD [D] - **Spec Exp:** Acne; Rosacea; **Hospital:** SUNY Downstate Med Ctr, Kings County Hosp Ctr; **Address:** SUNY Downstate Med Ctr, 450 Clarkson Ave, Dermatology, Box 46, Brooklyn, NY 11203-2012; **Phone:** 718-270-1230; **Board Cert:** Dermatology 1971; **Med School:** Wake Forest Univ 1964; **Resid:** Dermatology, NYU Med Ctr 1970; **Fellow:** Dermatologic Research, NYU Med Ctr 1973; **Fac Appt:** Prof D, SUNY Downstate

Dermatology

Shupack, Jerome L MD [D] - **Spec Exp:** Rare Skin Disorders; Psoriasis; Geriatric Dermatology; **Hospital:** NYU Med Ctr (page 68); **Address:** 530 1st Ave, New York, NY 10016-6402; **Phone:** 212-263-7344; **Board Cert:** Dermatology 1970; **Med School:** Columbia P&S 1963; **Resid:** Internal Medicine, Mt Sinai Hosp 1965; Dermatology, NYU Med Ctr 1970; **Fac Appt:** Prof D, NYU Sch Med

Soter, Nicholas A MD [D] - **Spec Exp:** Urticaria; Psoriasis; Vasculitis; **Hospital:** NYU Med Ctr (page 68); **Address:** 530 1st Ave, Ste 7R, New York, NY 10016-6402; **Phone:** 212-263-5889; **Board Cert:** Dermatology 1970; Diagnostic Lab Immunology 1985; **Med School:** Univ Tex SW, Dallas 1965; **Resid:** Dermatology, Baylor Med Ctr 1968; Dermatology, Mass Genl Hosp 1969; **Fellow:** Immunology, Harvard 1973; **Fac Appt:** Prof D, NYU Sch Med

Stanley, John R MD [D] - **Spec Exp:** Blistering Diseases; Pemphigus; **Hospital:** Hosp Univ Penn - UPHS (page 60); **Address:** Univ of Pennsylvania, Dept Dermatology, 3400 Spruce St, 2 Rhoads Pavilion, Philadelphia, PA 19104; **Phone:** 215-662-2737; **Board Cert:** Dermatology 1978; Clinical & Laboratory Dematologic Immunology 1985; **Med School:** Harvard Med Sch 1974; **Resid:** Dermatology, NYU Med Ctr 1978; **Fac Appt:** Prof D, Univ Pennsylvania

Werth, Victoria P MD [D] - **Spec Exp:** Autoimmune Disease; Lupus/SLE; Connective Tissue Disorders; Blistering Diseases; **Hospital:** Hosp Univ Penn - UPHS (page 60); **Address:** Univ Penn Health Services, 3600 Spruce St, 2 Rhoads Pavilion, Philadelphia, PA 19104; **Phone:** 215-662-2737; **Board Cert:** Internal Medicine 1983; Dermatology 1986; Diagnostic Lab Immunology 1989; **Med School:** Johns Hopkins Univ 1980; **Resid:** Internal Medicine, Northwestern Meml Hosp 1983; Dermatology, NYU Med Ctr 1986; **Fellow:** Immunological Dermatology, NYU Sch Med 1988; **Fac Appt:** Assoc Prof D, Univ Pennsylvania

Yan, Albert C MD [D] - **Spec Exp:** Pediatric Dermatology; **Hospital:** Chldns Hosp of Philadelphia, The; **Address:** Children's Hosp of Philadelphia, Dept Dermatology, 34th & Civic Ctr Blvd, Philadelphia, PA 19104; **Phone:** 215-590-2169; **Board Cert:** Dermatology 1999; Pediatrics 2004; Pediatric Dermatology 2004; **Med School:** Univ Pennsylvania 1993; **Resid:** Pediatrics, Children's Hosp 1996; Dermatology, Hosp U Penn 1999; **Fac Appt:** Asst Prof D, Univ Pennsylvania

Zitelli, John MD [D] - **Spec Exp:** Mohs' Surgery; Skin Cancer; Melanoma; **Hospital:** UPMC Shadyside, Jefferson Hosp - Pittsburgh; **Address:** Shadyside Med Ctr, 5200 Centre Ave, Ste 303, Pittsburgh, PA 15232-1312; **Phone:** 412-681-9400; **Board Cert:** Dermatology 1980; **Med School:** Univ Pittsburgh 1976; **Resid:** Dermatology, Univ Hlth Ctr Hosp 1979; **Fellow:** Mohs Surgery, Univ Wisconsin 1980; **Fac Appt:** Assoc Clin Prof D, Univ Pittsburgh

Southeast

Amonette, Rex A MD [D] - **Spec Exp:** Skin Cancer; Mohs' Surgery; **Hospital:** Methodist Univ Hosp - Memphis, Baptist Memorial Hospital - Memphis; **Address:** Memphis Dermatology Clinic, 1455 Union Ave, Memphis, TN 38104-6727; **Phone:** 901-726-6655; **Board Cert:** Dermatology 1974; **Med School:** Univ Ark 1966; **Resid:** Dermatology, Univ Tenn Med Ctr 1971; **Fellow:** Mohs Surgery, NYU Med Ctr 1972; **Fac Appt:** Clin Prof D, Univ Tenn Coll Med, Memphis

Brody, Harold J MD [D] - **Spec Exp:** Cosmetic Dermatology; Cosmetic Surgery; **Hospital:** Crawford Long Hosp of Emory Univ; **Address:** 1218 W Paces Ferry Rd NE, Ste 200, Atlanta, GA 30327; **Phone:** 404-525-7409; **Board Cert:** Dermatology 1978; **Med School:** Med Univ SC 1974; **Resid:** Dermatology, Emory Affil Hosps 1978; **Fac Appt:** Clin Prof D, Emory Univ

Burton III, Claude S MD [D] - **Spec Exp:** Leg Ulcers; Wound Healing/Care; Hemangiomas; **Hospital:** Duke Univ Med Ctr; **Address:** DUMC, Box 3511, Durham, NC 27710; **Phone:** 919-684-3432; **Board Cert:** Internal Medicine 1982; Dermatology 1984; **Med School:** Duke Univ 1979; **Resid:** Internal Medicine, Duke Univ Med Ctr 1982; Dermatology, Duke Univ Med Ctr 1984; **Fac Appt:** Assoc Prof Med, Duke Univ

Callen, Jeffrey P MD [D] - **Spec Exp:** Lupus/SLE; Dermatomyositis; Vasculitis; **Hospital:** Univ of Louisville Hosp, Jewish Hosp HlthCre Svcs Inc; **Address:** 310 E Broadway, Ste 200, Louisville, KY 40202; **Phone:** 502-583-1749; **Board Cert:** Internal Medicine 1975; Dermatology 1999; **Med School:** Univ Mich Med Sch 1972; **Resid:** Internal Medicine, Univ Mich Med Ctr 1975; Dermatology, Univ Mich Med Ctr 1977; **Fac Appt:** Prof Med, Univ Louisville Sch Med

Camisa, Charles MD [D] - **Spec Exp:** Psoriasis; Oral Dermatology; Lichen Planus; **Hospital:** Physicians Regl Med Ctr; **Address:** 6101 Pine Ridge Rd, Naples, FL 34119; **Phone:** 239-348-4335; **Board Cert:** Dermatology 1981; Clinical & Laboratory Dematologic Immunology 1987; **Med School:** Mount Sinai Sch Med 1977; **Resid:** Dermatology, NYU Med Ctr 1981; **Fac Appt:** Assoc Prof D, Univ S Fla Coll Med

Cohen, Bernard H MD [D] - **Spec Exp:** Hair Restoration/Transplant; **Hospital:** Jackson Meml Hosp; **Address:** 4425 Ponce de Leon Blvd, Ste 230, Coral Gables, FL 33146; **Phone:** 305-476-9544; **Board Cert:** Dermatology 1972; **Med School:** Columbia P&S 1967; **Resid:** Dermatology, NYU Med Ctr 1971; **Fac Appt:** Clin Prof D, Univ Miami Sch Med

Cook, Jonathan L MD [D] - **Spec Exp:** Skin Cancer; Mohs' Surgery; Reconstructive Surgery-Skin; Laser Surgery; **Hospital:** Duke Univ Med Ctr; **Address:** Duke Univ Med Ctr, Box 3915, Durham, NC 27710; **Phone:** 919-684-6805; **Board Cert:** Dermatology 2005; **Med School:** Med Univ SC 1992; **Resid:** Dermatology, Emory Univ Hosp 1996; **Fellow:** Dermatologic Surgery, Hosp Univ Penn 1997; **Fac Appt:** Prof D, Duke Univ

Eichler, Craig J MD [D] - **Spec Exp:** Skin Cancer; Dermatologic Surgery; **Hospital:** Physicians Regl Med Ctr; **Address:** 6101 Pine Ridge Rd, Naples, FL 34119-3900; **Phone:** 239-348-4335; **Board Cert:** Dermatology 2003; **Med School:** Univ Fla Coll Med 1989; **Resid:** Dermatology, Univ Texas Med Branch 1993

Elmets, Craig A MD [D] - **Spec Exp:** Psoriasis/Eczema; Phototherapy; Skin Cancer; Photodynamic Therapy; **Hospital:** Univ of Ala Hosp at Birmingham, VA Med Ctr; **Address:** Univ of Alabama-Birmingham-Derm Dept, 1530 Third Ave S, EFH 414, Birmingham, AL 35294; **Phone:** 205-996-7546; **Board Cert:** Dermatology 1980; Internal Medicine 1978; Clinical & Laboratory Dematologic Immunology 1989; **Med School:** Univ Iowa Coll Med 1975; **Resid:** Internal Medicine, Kansas Med Ctr 1978; Dermatology, Univ Iowa Hosps 1980; **Fellow:** Immunological Dermatology, Univ Texas Hlth Sci Ctr 1982; **Fac Appt:** Prof D, Univ Ala

Fenske, Neil A MD [D] - **Spec Exp:** Skin Cancer; Melanoma; Psoriasis; **Hospital:** H Lee Moffitt Cancer Ctr & Research Inst, Tampa Genl Hosp; **Address:** 12901 Bruce B Downs Blvd, MDC-79, Tampa, FL 33612-4742; **Phone:** 813-974-2920; **Board Cert:** Dermatology 1977; Dermatopathology 1984; **Med School:** St Louis Univ 1973; **Resid:** Dermatology, Wisconsin Hlth Sci Ctr 1977; **Fac Appt:** Prof Med, Univ S Fla Coll Med

Flowers, Franklin P MD [D] - **Spec Exp:** Mohs' Surgery; Dermatopathology; **Hospital:** Shands at Univ of FL; **Address:** Shands Healthcare, PO Box 100383, Gainesville, FL 32610-0383; **Phone:** 352-265-8001; **Board Cert:** Dermatology 1976; Dermatopathology 1981; **Med School:** Univ Fla Coll Med 1971; **Resid:** Dermatology, Ohio State Univ 1975; **Fellow:** Mohs Surgery, Univ Alabama 1993; **Fac Appt:** Prof Med, Univ Fla Coll Med

Dermatology

Garrett, Algin MD [D] - **Spec Exp:** Skin Cancer; Mohs' Surgery; **Hospital:** Med Coll of VA Hosp; **Address:** Stonypoint Medical Park, 9000 Stonypoint Pkwy Fl 2, Richmond, VA 23235; **Phone:** 804-560-8919; **Board Cert:** Dermatology 1983; **Med School:** Penn State Univ-Hershey Med Ctr 1978; **Resid:** Internal Medicine, VA Med Ctr 1980; Dermatology, Med Col VA 1983; **Fellow:** Mohs Surgery, Cleveland Clinic Found 1988; **Fac Appt:** Prof D, Va Commonwealth Univ Sch Med

Green, Howard A MD [D] - **Spec Exp:** Mohs' Surgery; Skin Cancer; **Hospital:** St Mary's Med Ctr - W Palm Bch, JFK Med Ctr - Atlantis; **Address:** 120 Butler St, Ste A, West Palm Beach, FL 33407-6106; **Phone:** 561-659-1510; **Board Cert:** Internal Medicine 1988; Dermatology 2004; **Med School:** Boston Univ 1985; **Resid:** Internal Medicine, Jefferson Univ Hosp 1988; Dermatology, Harvard Affil Hosps 1992; **Fellow:** Mohs Surgery, Boston Univ Med Ctr 1993

Grichnik, James M MD/PhD [D] - **Spec Exp:** Melanoma; Skin Cancer; **Hospital:** Duke Univ Med Ctr; **Address:** Duke Univ Med Ctr, Dept Medicine/Dermatology, Box 3135, Durham, NC 27710; **Phone:** 919-684-3270; **Board Cert:** Dermatology 2003; **Med School:** Harvard Med Sch 1990; **Resid:** Dermatology, Duke Univ Med Ctr 1994; **Fac Appt:** Assoc Prof D, Duke Univ

Johr, Robert MD [D] - **Spec Exp:** Pigmented Lesions; Melanoma; Pediatric Dermatology; **Hospital:** Univ of Miami Hosp & Clins/Sylvester Comp Canc Ctr, Boca Raton Comm Hosp; **Address:** 1050 NW 15th St, Ste 201A, Boca Raton, FL 33486-1341; **Phone:** 561-368-4545; **Board Cert:** Dermatology 1981; **Med School:** Mexico 1975; **Resid:** Dermatology, Roswell Park Cancer Ctr 1977; Dermatology, Metro Med Ctr/Case Western Reserve 1979; **Fac Appt:** Clin Prof D, Univ Miami Sch Med

Jorizzo, Joseph L MD [D] - **Spec Exp:** Rheumatologic Dermatology; Immune Deficiency-Skin Disorders; **Hospital:** Wake Forest Univ Baptist Med Ctr (page 73); **Address:** Wake Forest Univ Sch Med, Dept Derm, Med Ctr Blvd, Winston-Salem, NC 27157-0001; **Phone:** 336-716-3926; **Board Cert:** Dermatology 1979; **Med School:** Boston Univ 1975; **Resid:** Dermatology, Univ North Carolina Hosps 1979; **Fellow:** Dermatology, Dermatology Inst 1980; **Fac Appt:** Prof D, Wake Forest Univ

Kirsner, Robert S MD/PhD [D] - **Spec Exp:** Wound Healing/Care; Leg Ulcers; **Hospital:** Univ of Miami Hosp, Jackson Meml Hosp; **Address:** Univ Miami, Dept Dermatology, 1444 NW 9th Ave, Miami, FL 33136-1406; **Phone:** 305-243-6704; **Board Cert:** Dermatology 2005; **Med School:** Univ Miami Sch Med 1988; **Resid:** Internal Medicine, Jackson Meml Hosp 1990; Dermatology, Jackson Meml Hosp 1995; **Fellow:** Wound Healing, Univ Miami 1992; **Fac Appt:** Prof D, Univ Miami Sch Med

Leshin, Barry MD [D] - **Spec Exp:** Skin Cancer; Mohs' Surgery; **Address:** 125 Sunnynoll Ct, Ste 100, Winston-Salem, NC 27106; **Phone:** 336-724-2434; **Board Cert:** Dermatology 1985; **Med School:** Univ Tex, Houston 1981; **Resid:** Dermatology, Univ Iowa Hosp 1985; **Fellow:** Dermatologic Surgery, Univ Iowa Hosp 1986; **Fac Appt:** Clin Prof PlS, Wake Forest Univ

Olsen, Elise A MD [D] - **Spec Exp:** Hair loss; Hirsutism; Cutaneous Lymphoma; **Hospital:** Duke Univ Med Ctr; **Address:** Duke Univ Med Ctr, Box 3294, Durham, NC 27710; **Phone:** 919-684-3432; **Board Cert:** Dermatology 1983; **Med School:** Baylor Coll Med 1978; **Resid:** Internal Medicine, Univ NC Meml Hosp 1980; Dermatology, Duke Univ Med Ctr 1983; **Fac Appt:** Prof D, Duke Univ

Sherertz, Elizabeth F MD [D] - **Spec Exp:** Eczema; Contact Dermatitis; Occupational Skin Diseases; **Address:** 1400 West Gate Ctr Drive, Ste 200, Winston-Salem, NC 27103; **Phone:** 336-774-8636; **Board Cert:** Dermatology 1982; **Med School:** Univ VA Sch Med 1978; **Resid:** Dermatology, Duke Univ Med Ctr 1982; **Fac Appt:** Clin Prof D, Wake Forest Univ

America's Top Doctors® 8th Edition

Sobel, Stuart MD [D] - **Spec Exp:** Skin Cancer; Cosmetic Dermatology; **Hospital:** Meml Regl Hosp, Joe Di Maggio Chldns Hosp; **Address:** 4340 Sheridan St, Ste 101, Hollywood, FL 33021-3511; **Phone:** 954-983-5533; **Board Cert:** Dermatology 1977; **Med School:** Tufts Univ 1972; **Resid:** Dermatology, Mt Sinai Hosp 1976

Sokoloff, Daniel O MD [D] - **Spec Exp:** Skin Cancer; Cosmetic Dermatology; **Hospital:** St Mary's Med Ctr - W Palm Bch, Good Sam Med Ctr - W Palm Beach; **Address:** Palm Beach Dermatology, 1000 45th St, Ste 1, West Palm Beach, FL 33407-2416; **Phone:** 561-863-1000; **Board Cert:** Dermatology 1982; **Med School:** Geo Wash Univ 1977; **Resid:** Dermatology, Baylor Coll Med 1982

Thiers, Bruce H MD [D] - **Spec Exp:** Cutaneous Lymphoma; Skin Cancer; Psoriasis; **Hospital:** MUSC Med Ctr; **Address:** MUSC Dept Dermatology, 135 Rutledge Ave Fl 11, Box 250578, Charleston, SC 29425; **Phone:** 843-792-5858; **Board Cert:** Dermatology 1978; **Med School:** SUNY Buffalo 1974; **Resid:** Dermatology, SUNY Buffalo Med Ctr 1978; **Fac Appt:** Prof D, Med Univ SC

Midwest

Bailin, Philip L MD [D] - **Spec Exp:** Mohs' Surgery; Skin Laser Surgery; Skin Cancer; **Hospital:** Cleveland Clin Fdn (page 56); **Address:** Cleveland Clinic, Dept Dermatology, 9500 Euclid Ave, Desk A61, Cleveland, OH 44195-5032; **Phone:** 216-444-2115; **Board Cert:** Dermatology 1975; **Med School:** Northwestern Univ 1968; **Resid:** Dermatology, Cleveland Clin Fdn 1974; **Fellow:** Dermatopathology, Armed Forces Inst Pathology 1975; Mohs Surgery, Univ Wisc Hosp & Clin

Cornelius, Lynn A MD [D] - **Spec Exp:** Melanoma; **Hospital:** Barnes-Jewish Hosp, St Louis Chldns Hosp; **Address:** Washington Univ Dept Dermatology, 660 S Euclid, Box 8123, St Louis, MO 63110; **Phone:** 314-362-2643; **Board Cert:** Dermatology 1989; **Med School:** Univ MO-Columbia Sch Med 1984; **Resid:** Dermatology, Barnes Jewish Hosp-Wash Univ 1989; **Fellow:** Immunological Dermatology, Emory Univ Med Ctr 1992; **Fac Appt:** Assoc Prof D, Washington Univ, St Louis

Fivenson, David MD [D] - **Spec Exp:** Blistering Diseases; Wound Healing/Care; Lupus/SLE; **Hospital:** St Joseph Mercy Hosp - Ann Arbor; **Address:** 3001 Miller Rd, Ann Arbor, MI 48103; **Phone:** 734-222-9630; **Board Cert:** Dermatology 1989; Clinical & Laboratory Dematologic Immunology 1991; **Med School:** Univ Mich Med Sch 1984; **Resid:** Dermatology, Univ Cincinnati Med Ctr 1989; **Fellow:** Immunological Dermatology, UCSD Med Ctr 1986

Garden, Jerome M MD [D] - **Spec Exp:** Skin Laser Surgery; Facial Rejuvenation; Vascular Birthmarks; Botox Therapy; **Hospital:** Northwestern Meml Hosp, Children's Mem Hosp; **Address:** 150 E Huron St, Ste 1200, Chicago, IL 60611-2946; **Phone:** 312-280-0890; **Board Cert:** Dermatology 1984; **Med School:** Northwestern Univ 1980; **Resid:** Internal Medicine, Northwestern Univ 1981; Dermatology, Northwestern Univ 1984; **Fac Appt:** Prof D, Northwestern Univ

Hanke, C William MD [D] - **Spec Exp:** Mohs' Surgery; Skin Laser Surgery; Cosmetic Dermatology; Photodynamic Therapy; **Hospital:** St Vincent Carmel Hosp, Clarian Hlth Ptrs; **Address:** Laser & Skin Surgery Ctr of Indiana, 13450 N Meridian St, Ste 355, Carmel, IN 46032-1486; **Phone:** 317-582-8484; **Board Cert:** Dermatology 1978; Dermatopathology 1982; **Med School:** Univ Iowa Coll Med 1971; **Resid:** Dermatology, Cleveland Clinic 1978; Dermatopathology, Indiana Univ 1982; **Fellow:** Cutaneous Oncology, Cleveland Clinic 1979; **Fac Appt:** Clin Prof D, Indiana Univ

Dermatology

Hruza, George J MD [D] - **Spec Exp:** Skin Laser Surgery; Mohs' Surgery; Cosmetic Surgery; **Hospital:** St Luke's Hosp - Chesterfield, MO, St Louis Univ Hosp; **Address:** Laser & Derm Surg Ctr, 14377 Woodlake Drive, Ste 111, St Louis, MO 63017-5735; **Phone:** 314-878-3839; **Board Cert:** Dermatology 1986; **Med School:** NYU Sch Med 1982; **Resid:** Dermatology, NYU Med Ctr-Skin Cancer Unit 1986; **Fellow:** Laser Surgery, Mass Genl Hosp-Harvard 1987; Surgery, Univ Wisc 1988; **Fac Appt:** Assoc Clin Prof D, St Louis Univ

Johnson, Timothy M MD [D] - **Spec Exp:** Melanoma; Mohs' Surgery; **Hospital:** Univ Michigan Hlth Sys; **Address:** Univ Michigan Dermatology, 1910 Taubman Ctr, 1500 E Medical Center Drive, Ann Arbor, MI 48109-5314; **Phone:** 734-936-4190; **Board Cert:** Dermatology 1988; **Med School:** Univ Tex, Houston 1984; **Resid:** Dermatology, Univ Texas Med Ctr 1988; **Fellow:** Cutaneous Oncology, Univ Mich Med Ctr 1989; Mohs Surgery, Univ Oregon Hlth Sci Ctr 1990; **Fac Appt:** Prof D, Univ Mich Med Sch

Lim, Henry W MD [D] - **Spec Exp:** Phototherapy; Vitiligo; Cutaneous Lymphoma; Skin Cancer; **Hospital:** Henry Ford Hosp; **Address:** Henry Ford Hosp, Dept Derm, 3031 W Grand Blvd, Ste 800, Detroit, MI 48202-3141; **Phone:** 313-916-4060; **Board Cert:** Dermatology 2005; Clinical & Laboratory Dematologic Immunology 1985; **Med School:** SUNY Downstate 1975; **Resid:** Dermatology, NYU Med Ctr 1979; **Fellow:** Immunological Dermatology, NYU Med Ctr 1980; **Fac Appt:** Prof Path, Wayne State Univ

Lowe, Lori MD [D] - **Spec Exp:** Dermatopathology; Skin Cancer; **Hospital:** Univ Michigan Hlth Sys; **Address:** Univ Michigan Dept Pathology, 1301 Catherine Rd, M3261-Med Sci I, Ann Arbor, MI 48109-0602; **Phone:** 734-764-4460; **Board Cert:** Dermatology 1990; Dermatopathology 1991; **Med School:** Univ Tex, Houston 1985; **Resid:** Dermatology, Univ Tex Hlth Sci Ctr 1990; **Fellow:** Dermatopathology, Univ Colo Hlth Sci Ctr 1991; **Fac Appt:** Prof D, Univ Mich Med Sch

Lucky, Anne W MD [D] - **Spec Exp:** Pediatric Dermatology; Acne; **Hospital:** Cincinnati Chldns Hosp Med Ctr; **Address:** Derm Assocs Cincinnati, 7691 Five Mile Rd, Cincinnati, OH 45230; **Phone:** 513-232-3332; **Board Cert:** Pediatrics 1975; Pediatric Endocrinology 1978; Dermatology 1981; Pediatric Dermatology 2004; **Med School:** Yale Univ 1970; **Resid:** Pediatrics, Boston Chldns Hosp 1973; Dermatology, Yale-New Haven Hosp 1981; **Fellow:** Pediatric Endocrinology, Natl Inst Hlth 1976; **Fac Appt:** Prof D, Univ Cincinnati

Neuburg, Marcelle MD [D] - **Spec Exp:** Mohs' Surgery; Skin Cancer; Pigmented Lesions; **Hospital:** Froedtert Meml Lutheran Hosp; **Address:** Med Coll Wisconsin, Dept Dermatology, 9200 W Wisconsin Ave, Milwaukee, WI 53226; **Phone:** 414-805-5300; **Board Cert:** Internal Medicine 1985; Dermatology 1988; **Med School:** Oregon Hlth Sci Univ 1982; **Resid:** Internal Medicine, Georgetown Univ Hosp 1985; Dermatology, Boston Univ Sch Med Ctr 1988; **Fellow:** Mohs Surgery, Tufts New England Med Ctr 1990; **Fac Appt:** Prof D, Med Coll Wisc

Otley, Clark C MD [D] - **Spec Exp:** Mohs' Surgery; Skin Cancer; Skin Cancer in Transplant Patients; Dermatologic Surgery; **Hospital:** Mayo Med Ctr & Clin - Rochester; **Address:** Mayo Clinic, 200 First St SW, Rochester, MN 55905; **Phone:** 507-284-3579; **Board Cert:** Dermatology 2004; **Med School:** Duke Univ 1991; **Resid:** Dermatology, Mass Genl Hosp 1995; **Fellow:** Dermatologic Surgery, Mayo Clinic 1996; **Fac Appt:** Assoc Prof D, Mayo Med Sch

Paller, Amy S MD [D] - **Spec Exp:** Genetic Disorders-Skin; Immune Deficiency-Skin Disorders; Atopic Dermatitis; Pediatric Dermatology; **Hospital:** Children's Mem Hosp; **Address:** 676 N St Clair St, Chicago, IL 60611-2997; **Phone:** 773-327-3446; **Board Cert:** Pediatrics 1982; Pediatric Dermatology 2004; Dermatology 2007; **Med School:** Stanford Univ 1978; **Resid:** Pediatrics, Chldns Meml Hosp 1981; Dermatology, Northwestern Meml Hosp 1983; **Fellow:** Research, Univ NC Hosp 1984; **Fac Appt:** Prof D, Northwestern Univ

America's Top Doctors® 8th Edition

Treadwell, Patricia MD [D] - **Spec Exp:** Pediatric Dermatology; Vascular Birthmarks; **Hospital:** Riley Hosp for Children, Wishard Hlth Srvs; **Address:** 1001 W 10th St Bryce Bldg, Fl 2 - rm B2100, Indianapolis, IN 46202; **Phone:** 317-630-7396; **Board Cert:** Pediatrics 1982; Dermatology 1983; **Med School:** Cornell Univ-Weill Med Coll 1977; **Resid:** Pediatrics, James Whitcomb Riley Hosp 1980; Dermatology, Indiana Univ Med Ctr 1983; **Fac Appt:** Prof D, Indiana Univ

Voorhees, John MD [D] - **Spec Exp:** Psoriasis; Photoaging; **Hospital:** Univ Michigan Hlth Sys; **Address:** Univ Michigan, Dept Dermatology, 1500 E Med Ctr Drive, rm 1910 Taubman Ctr, Ann Arbor, MI 48109-5314; **Phone:** 734-936-4054; **Board Cert:** Dermatology 1970; **Med School:** Univ Mich Med Sch 1963; **Resid:** Dermatology, Univ Mich Hosp 1969; **Fac Appt:** Prof D, Univ Mich Med Sch

Wheeland, Ronald MD [D] - **Spec Exp:** Skin Laser Surgery; Mohs' Surgery; Cosmetic Dermatology; **Hospital:** Univ of Missouri Hosp & Clins; **Address:** Univ Missouri, Dept Dermatology, One Hospital Drive, Columbia, MO 65212; **Phone:** 573-882-1429; **Board Cert:** Dermatology 1977; Dermatopathology 1978; **Med School:** Univ Ariz Coll Med 1973; **Resid:** Dermatology, Univ Ok Hlth Sci Ctr 1977; **Fellow:** Dermatopathology, Univ Ok Hlth Sci Ctr 1978; Dermatologic Surgery, Cleveland Clin Fnd 1984; **Fac Appt:** Prof D, Univ MO-Columbia Sch Med

Wood, Gary S MD [D] - **Spec Exp:** Cutaneous Lymphoma; Melanoma; Skin Cancer; **Hospital:** Univ WI Hosp & Clins, VA Hospital, Madison; **Address:** Univ Wisconsin Health, Dept Dermatology, 1 S Park St Fl 7, Madison, WI 53715-1375; **Phone:** 608-287-2620; **Board Cert:** Anatomic Pathology 1983; Dermatology 1986; Dermatopathology 1987; **Med School:** Univ IL Coll Med 1979; **Resid:** Anatomic Pathology, Stanford Univ Med Ctr 1983; Dermatology, Stanford Univ Med Ctr 1985; **Fellow:** Immunopathology, Stanford Univ Med Ctr 1981; **Fac Appt:** Prof D, Univ Wisc

Zelickson, Brian D MD [D] - **Spec Exp:** Skin Laser Surgery; **Hospital:** Abbott - Northwestern Hosp, Fairview Southdale Hosp; **Address:** 825 Nicollet Mall, Med Arts Bldg - Ste 1002, Minneapolis, MN 55402; **Phone:** 612-338-0711; **Board Cert:** Dermatology 1999; **Med School:** Mayo Med Sch 1986; **Resid:** Dermatology, Mayo Clinic 1990; **Fac Appt:** Asst Prof D, Univ Minn

Great Plains and Mountains

Belsito, Donald V MD [D] - **Spec Exp:** Contact Dermatitis; Cutaneous Lymphoma; Immune Deficiency-Skin Disorders; Skin Cancer; **Hospital:** Univ of Kansas Hosp; **Address:** American Dermatology Assocs, 6333 Long Ave, Shawnee, KS 66216; **Phone:** 913-631-6330; **Board Cert:** Internal Medicine 1979; Dermatology 1983; Clinical & Laboratory Dematologic Immunology 1985; **Med School:** Cornell Univ-Weill Med Coll 1976; **Resid:** Internal Medicine, Case West Res Univ Hosps 1979; Dermatology, NYU Med Ctr 1982

Bowen, Glen M MD [D] - **Spec Exp:** Melanoma; Cutaneous Lymphoma; Clinical Trials; Mohs' Surgery; **Hospital:** Univ Utah Hosps and Clins, Cottonwood Hosp & Med Ctr; **Address:** Huntsman Cancer Inst, 500 N Medical Drive, 4B454-SOM, Salt Lake City, UT 84132; **Phone:** 801-585-0197; **Board Cert:** Dermatology 1995; **Med School:** Univ Utah 1990; **Resid:** Dermatology, Univ Michigan Med Ctr 1993; **Fellow:** Immunological Dermatology, Univ Michigan Med Ctr 1995; Mohs Surgery, Univ Utah 2001; **Fac Appt:** Assoc Prof D, Univ Utah

Krueger, Gerald MD [D] - **Spec Exp:** Psoriasis; **Hospital:** Univ Utah Hosps and Clins; **Address:** Univ Utah Hlth Sci Ctr, Dept Derm, 30 N 1900 E, Ste 4A330, Salt Lake City, UT 84132; **Phone:** 801-581-6465; **Board Cert:** Dermatology 1973; **Med School:** Loma Linda Univ 1966; **Resid:** Dermatology, Univ Colorado Med Ctr 1972; **Fac Appt:** Prof D, Univ Utah

Dermatology

Southwest

Butler, David F MD [D] - **Spec Exp:** Skin Cancer; **Hospital:** Scott & White Mem Hosp; **Address:** Scott White Meml Hosp, Dept Dermatology, 409 W Adams St, Temple, TX 76501; **Phone:** 254-742-3724; **Board Cert:** Dermatology 1985; **Med School:** Univ Tex Med Br, Galveston 1980; **Resid:** Dermatology, Walter Reed Army Med Ctr 1985; **Fac Appt:** Assoc Prof D, Texas Tech Univ

Carney, John M MD [D] - **Spec Exp:** Mohs' Surgery; Skin Cancer; **Hospital:** UAMS Med Ctr; **Address:** Southwest Med Arts Bldg, 11321 Interstate 30, Ste 201, Little Rock, AR 72209; **Phone:** 501-455-4700; **Board Cert:** Dermatology 1984; **Med School:** Northwestern Univ 1979; **Resid:** Dermatology, Univ Hosps 1984; **Fellow:** Physiology, Harvard Med Sch 1985; Dermatologic Surgery, Univ Tenn Med Ctr 1986

Cockerell, Clay J MD [D] - **Spec Exp:** Dermatopathology; **Hospital:** UT Southwestern Med Ctr - Dallas; **Address:** Dermatopath Labs, 2330 Butler St, Ste 115, Dallas, TX 75235; **Phone:** 214-638-2222; **Board Cert:** Dermatology 1999; Dermatopathology 1986; **Med School:** Baylor Coll Med 1981; **Resid:** Dermatology, NYU Med Ctr 1985; **Fellow:** Dermatopathology, NYU Med Ctr 1986; **Fac Appt:** Prof DP, Univ Tex SW, Dallas

Duvic, Madeleine MD [D] - **Spec Exp:** Cutaneous Lymphoma; Skin Cancer; Alopecia Areata; **Hospital:** UT MD Anderson Cancer Ctr; **Address:** MD Anderson Cancer Ctr, Dept Dermatology, 1515 Holcombe Blvd, Unit 434, Houston, TX 77030; **Phone:** 713-745-1113; **Board Cert:** Dermatology 1981; Internal Medicine 1982; **Med School:** Duke Univ 1977; **Resid:** Dermatology, Duke Univ Med Ctr 1980; Internal Medicine, Duke Univ Med Ctr 1982; **Fellow:** Geriatric Medicine, Duke Univ Med Ctr 1984; **Fac Appt:** Prof D, Univ Tex, Houston

Hansen, Ronald C MD [D] - **Spec Exp:** Pediatric Dermatology; **Hospital:** Phoenix Children's Hosp; **Address:** Phoenix Childrens Hosp, Dept Dermatology, 1920 E Cambridge Ave, Ste E200, Phoenix, AZ 85006; **Phone:** 602-546-0895; **Board Cert:** Pediatrics 1974; Dermatology 1980; **Med School:** Univ Iowa Coll Med 1968; **Resid:** Pediatrics, Childrens Hosp 1970; Pediatrics, Stanford Univ Med Ctr 1972; **Fellow:** Dermatology, Univ Medical Ctr 1980; **Fac Appt:** Prof D, Univ Ariz Coll Med

Levy, Moise L MD [D] - **Spec Exp:** Pediatric Dermatology; Vascular Malformations; **Hospital:** Children's Hospital - Austin; **Address:** 1301 Barbara Jordan Blvd, Austin, TX 78723; **Phone:** 512-628-1920; **Board Cert:** Pediatrics 1985; Dermatology 1986; **Med School:** Univ Tex, Houston 1979; **Resid:** Pediatrics, Univ Tex Affil Hosp 1983; Dermatology, Baylor Coll Med 1986; **Fac Appt:** Prof D, Baylor Coll Med

Menter, M Alan MD [D] - **Spec Exp:** Psoriasis; Cosmetic Dermatology; **Hospital:** Baylor Univ Medical Ctr; **Address:** 3900 Junius St, Ste 145, Dallas, TX 75246; **Phone:** 972-386-7546 x400; **Board Cert:** Dermatology 1978; **Med School:** South Africa 1966; **Resid:** Dermatology, Pretoria Genl Hosp 1971; Dermatology, Guys Hosp 1972; **Fellow:** Dermatology, St Johns Hosp 1973; Dermatology, Univ Texas SW 1979; **Fac Appt:** Clin Prof D, Univ Tex SW, Dallas

Orengo, Ida F MD [D] - **Spec Exp:** Melanoma; Mohs' Surgery; **Hospital:** St Luke's Episcopal Hosp - Houston, DeBakey VA Med Ctr-Houston; **Address:** Baylor College of Medicine, 6620 Main St, Ste 1425, Houston, TX 77030; **Phone:** 713-798-6925; **Board Cert:** Dermatology 2001; **Med School:** Harvard Med Sch 1988; **Resid:** Dermatology, Baylor Coll Med 1991; **Fac Appt:** Assoc Prof D, Baylor Coll Med

Sontheimer, Richard D MD [D] - **Spec Exp:** Immune Deficiency-Skin Disorders; Lupus/SLE; **Hospital:** OU Med Ctr, VA Med Ctr - Oklahoma City; **Address:** 619 NE 13th St, Oklahoma City, OK 73104; **Phone:** 405-271-6110; **Board Cert:** Internal Medicine 1976; Dermatology 1979; Clinical & Laboratory Dematologic Immunology 1985; **Med School:** Univ Tex SW, Dallas 1972; **Resid:** Internal Medicine, Univ Utah Affil Hosps 1976; Dermatology, Parkland Meml Hosp 1979; **Fellow:** Research, Southwestern Med Sch 1978; **Fac Appt:** Prof D, Univ Iowa Coll Med

Taylor, R Stan MD [D] - **Spec Exp:** Mohs' Surgery; Melanoma; Skin Cancer; **Hospital:** UT Southwestern Med Ctr - Dallas, Parkland Meml Hosp - Dallas; **Address:** Univ Tex SW Med Sch, Dept Derm, 5323 Harry Hines Blvd, MC 9192, Dallas, TX 75390-7208; **Phone:** 214-645-8950; **Board Cert:** Dermatology 1989; **Med School:** Univ Tex Med Br, Galveston 1985; **Resid:** Dermatology, Univ Mich Med Ctr 1989; **Fellow:** Immunological Dermatology, Univ Mich 1990; Mohs Surgery, Oregon Hlth Sci Univ 1991; **Fac Appt:** Prof D, Univ Tex SW, Dallas

West Coast and Pacific

Bennett, Richard G MD [D] - **Spec Exp:** Mohs' Surgery; Skin Cancer; **Hospital:** Ronald Reagan UCLA Med Ctr, USC Univ Hosp - R K Eamer Med Plz; **Address:** 1301 20th St Ste 570 Bldg, Santa Monica, CA 90404-2080; **Phone:** 310-315-0171; **Board Cert:** Dermatology 1975; **Med School:** Case West Res Univ 1970; **Resid:** Dermatology, Hosp Univ Penn 1974; **Fellow:** Chemosurgery, NYU Med Ctr 1977; **Fac Appt:** Clin Prof D, UCLA

Berg, Daniel MD [D] - **Spec Exp:** Skin Cancer; Mohs' Surgery; Skin Laser Surgery; Cosmetic Dermatology; **Hospital:** Univ Wash Med Ctr; **Address:** 4225 Roosevelt Way NE, Seattle, WA 98105; **Phone:** 206-598-6647; **Board Cert:** Dermatology 1999; **Med School:** Univ Toronto 1985; **Resid:** Internal Medicine, Sunnybrook Med Ctr 1988; Dermatology, Duke Univ Med Ctr 1991; **Fellow:** Dermatologic Surgery, Univ Toronto 1992; Dermatologic Surgery, Univ British Columbia 1994; **Fac Appt:** Prof D, Univ Wash

Eichenfield, Lawrence F MD [D] - **Spec Exp:** Eczema; Acne; Vascular Birthmarks; Pediatric Dermatology; **Hospital:** Rady Children's Hosp - San Diego, UCSD Med Ctr; **Address:** Chldns Hosp, Ped & Adolescent Dermatology, 8010 Frost St, Ste 602, San Diego, CA 92123-4204; **Phone:** 858-966-6795; **Board Cert:** Dermatology 1999; Pediatric Dermatology 2004; **Med School:** Mount Sinai Sch Med 1984; **Resid:** Pediatrics, Chldns Hosp 1987; Dermatology, Hosp Univ Penn 1991; **Fac Appt:** Prof Ped, UCSD

Fitzpatrick, Richard E MD [D] - **Spec Exp:** Cosmetic Dermatology; Skin Laser Surgery-Resurfacing; Hair Restoration/Transplant; **Hospital:** Scripps Meml Hosp - La Jolla; **Address:** 9850 Genesee St, Ste 480, La Jolla, CA 90237; **Phone:** 858-452-2066; **Board Cert:** Dermatology 2003; **Med School:** Emory Univ 1970; **Resid:** Dermatology, UCLA Med Ctr 1978; **Fac Appt:** Assoc Clin Prof D, UCSD

Frieden, Ilona J MD [D] - **Spec Exp:** Pediatric Dermatology; Vascular Birthmarks; Hemangiomas; **Hospital:** UCSF - Mt Zion Med Ctr; **Address:** UCSF, Dept Dermatology, 1701 Divisadero St, Fl 3, Box 0316, San Francisco, CA 94115-0316; **Phone:** 415-353-7800; **Board Cert:** Dermatology 2005; Pediatrics 1983; Pediatric Dermatology 2004; **Med School:** UCSF 1977; **Resid:** Pediatrics, UCSF Med Ctr 1980; Dermatology, UCSF Med Ctr 1983; **Fac Appt:** Clin Prof D, UCSF

Glogau, Richard G MD [D] - **Spec Exp:** Cosmetic Dermatology; Skin Laser Surgery; Mohs' Surgery; Botox Therapy; **Hospital:** UCSF Med Ctr; **Address:** 350 Parnassus Ave, Ste 400, San Francisco, CA 94117; **Phone:** 415-564-1261; **Board Cert:** Dermatology 1978; Dermatopathology 1982; **Med School:** Harvard Med Sch 1973; **Resid:** Dermatology, UCSF Med Ctr 1977; **Fellow:** Chemosurgery, UCSF Med Ctr 1978; **Fac Appt:** Clin Prof D, UCSF

Dermatology

Greenway, Hubert T MD [D] - **Spec Exp:** Skin Cancer; Mohs' Surgery; Melanoma; **Hospital:** Scripps Green Hosp; **Address:** Scripps Clinic, Dept Mohs' Surgery, 10666 N Torrey Pines Rd, MS 112A, La Jolla, CA 92037; **Phone:** 858-554-8646; **Board Cert:** Dermatology 1982; **Med School:** Med Coll GA 1974; **Resid:** Dermatology, Naval Hosp 1982; **Fellow:** Mohs Surgery, Univ Wisconsin Med Ctr 1981

Grimes, Pearl E MD [D] - **Spec Exp:** Pigmented Lesions; Ethnic Skin Disorders; **Hospital:** Ronald Reagan UCLA Med Ctr; **Address:** 5670 Wilshire Blvd, Ste 650, Los Angeles, CA 90036; **Phone:** 323-467-4389; **Board Cert:** Dermatology 1979; **Med School:** Washington Univ, St Louis 1974; **Resid:** Dermatology, Howard Univ 1979; **Fac Appt:** Clin Prof D, UCLA

Hanifin, Jon M MD [D] - **Spec Exp:** Atopic Dermatitis; **Hospital:** OR Hlth & Sci Univ; **Address:** Oregon Hlth & Sci Univ, Dept Derm, 3303 SW Bond Ave, MC CH16D, Portland, OR 97239; **Phone:** 503-418-3376; **Board Cert:** Dermatology 1970; **Med School:** Univ Wisc 1965; **Resid:** Dermatology, UCSF Med Ctr 1969; **Fac Appt:** Prof D, Oregon Hlth Sci Univ

Kilmer, Suzanne L MD [D] - **Spec Exp:** Skin Laser Surgery-Resurfacing; Facial Rejuvenation; Cosmetic Dermatology; **Hospital:** Mercy General Hosp - Sacramento; **Address:** The Laser & Skin Surgery Center, 3835 J St, Sacramento, CA 95816-5520; **Phone:** 916-456-0400; **Board Cert:** Dermatology 1999; **Med School:** UC Davis 1987; **Resid:** Dermatology, UC Davis Med Ctr 1991; **Fellow:** Laser Surgery, Mass Genl Hosp 1992; **Fac Appt:** Asst Clin Prof D, UC Davis

Kim, Youn-Hee MD [D] - **Spec Exp:** Cutaneous Lymphoma; Skin Cancer; **Hospital:** Stanford Univ Med Ctr; **Address:** 900 Blake Wilbur Drive, rm W0010, MC 5334, Stanford Univ Med Ctr, Dept Dermatology, Stanford, CA 94305-5334; **Phone:** 650-723-6316; **Board Cert:** Dermatology 1989; **Med School:** Stanford Univ 1984; **Resid:** Dermatology, Metropolitan Hospital 1989

Klein, Arnold W MD [D] - **Spec Exp:** Cosmetic Dermatology; Botox Therapy; **Hospital:** Ronald Reagan UCLA Med Ctr, Cedars-Sinai Med Ctr; **Address:** 435 N Roxbury Dr, Ste 204, Beverly Hills, CA 90210-5027; **Phone:** 310-275-5136; **Board Cert:** Dermatology 1976; **Med School:** Univ Pennsylvania 1971; **Resid:** Dermatology, Hosp Univ Penn 1973; Dermatology, UCLA Med Ctr 1975; **Fac Appt:** Prof D, UCLA

Koo, John Ying Ming MD [D] - **Spec Exp:** Psoriasis/Eczema; Photosensitive Skin Diseases; Psychodermatology; **Hospital:** UCSF Med Ctr; **Address:** Psoriasis Day Treatment Ctr, 515 Spruce St, San Francisco, CA 94118; **Phone:** 415-476-4701; **Board Cert:** Dermatology 1988; Psychiatry 1988; **Med School:** Harvard Med Sch 1981; **Resid:** Psychiatry, UCLA Neur Psyc Inst 1985; Dermatology, UCSF Med Ctr 1988; **Fac Appt:** Prof D, UCSF

Lask, Gary P MD [D] - **Spec Exp:** Skin Laser Surgery-Resurfacing; Cosmetic Dermatology; **Hospital:** Ronald Reagan UCLA Med Ctr; **Address:** 16260 Ventura Blvd, Ste 530, Encino, CA 91436; **Phone:** 818-788-4022; **Board Cert:** Dermatology 1983; **Med School:** Mexico 1977; **Resid:** Dermatology, Martin Luther King Jr Hosp 1983; **Fac Appt:** Clin Prof D, UCLA

Rubin, Mark G MD [D] - **Spec Exp:** Skin Laser Surgery; Cosmetic Dermatology; **Hospital:** UCSD Med Ctr; **Address:** 153 S Lasky Drive, Ste 1, Beverly Hills, CA 90212; **Phone:** 310-556-0119; **Board Cert:** Dermatology 1985; **Med School:** Jefferson Med Coll 1981; **Resid:** Dermatology, Henry Ford Hosp 1985; **Fac Appt:** Assoc Prof D, UCSD

Swanson, Neil MD [D] - **Spec Exp:** Skin Cancer; Cosmetic Dermatology; **Hospital:** OR Hlth & Sci Univ, VA Medical Center - Portland; **Address:** Oregon HSU, Center for Health & Healing, 3303 SW Bond Ave, CH16D, Portland, OR 97239; **Phone:** 503-418-3376; **Board Cert:** Dermatology 1980; **Med School:** Univ Rochester 1976; **Resid:** Dermatology, Univ Michigan Med Ctr 1979; **Fellow:** Dermatology, UCSF Med Ctr 1980; **Fac Appt:** Prof D, Oregon Hlth Sci Univ

America's Top Doctors® 8th Edition

Swetter, Susan M MD [D] - **Spec Exp:** Melanoma; Melanoma Early Detection/Prevention; Skin Cancer; **Hospital:** Stanford Univ Med Ctr, VA Hlth Care Sys - Palo Alto; **Address:** Stanford Univ Med Ctr, Dept Dermatology, 900 Blake Wilbur Dr, W0069, MC 5334, Stanford, CA 94305; **Phone:** 650-723-0119; **Board Cert:** Dermatology 2001; **Med School:** Univ Pennsylvania 1990; **Resid:** Dermatology, Stanford Univ Med Ctr 1994; **Fac Appt:** Assoc Prof D, Stanford Univ

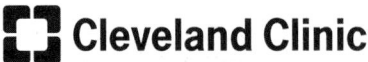 **Cleveland Clinic**

Dermatology

Cleveland Clinic Department of Dermatology, part of the Dermatology and Plastic Surgery Institute offers a full array of subspecialized care for adult and pediatric patients. Our physicians diagnose and treat all disorders of the skin, hair and nails, whether primary or related to an underlying systemic illness, including industrial-related conditions.

Dermatologic Surgery

The department offers a full range of procedures in the subspecialty area of dermatologic surgery. These include Mohs micrographic surgery for high-risk skin cancers (including local tissue reconstruction), laser surgery, chemical peels, soft tissue augmentation, botox injections, hair transplant and liposuction. Additionally, our Cutaneous Care Center provides outpatient treatment, rather than hospitalization, for patients with extensive, severe or chronic skin diseases utilizing phototherapy and excimer laser treatment.

Staff dermatologists and residents are involved in research, either institutionally or through industrial support of clinical trials.

Cleveland Clinic dermatologists offer expert diagnostic and management options including:

- Skin Cancer and Mohs Surgery
- Psoriasis
- Varicose Veins and Spider Veins
- Phototherapy
- Pediatric Dermatology
- Industrial Dermatology
- Cosmetic Dermatology
- Laser Surgery

For more information about the Cleveland Clinic Department of Dermatology, to schedule a second opinion or to learn about assistance for out-of-town patients, call 800.890.2467 or visit www.clevelandclinic.org/dermtopdocs.

Department of Dermatology
9500 Euclid Avenue / AC311 | Cleveland OH 44195

NYU Langone Medical Center

550 First Avenue (at 31St Street)
New York, NY 10016
Physician Referral:
(888)7-NYU-MED (888-769-8633)
www.nyumc.org

DERMATOLOGY
State-of-the-Art Care of Skin Problems

With a history dating back to 1882, the Ronald O. Perelman Department of Dermatology at NYU Langone Medical Center is recognized nationally and internationally as a leader in dermatology. Through the Charles C. Harris Skin and Cancer Pavilion, in the offices of Dermatologic Associates, and in the general and specialty clinics at affiliated hospital facilities, the staff members of the Department provide primary and consultative dermatologic care for over 100,000 ambulatory and hospitalized patients yearly. In addition, faculty members of the Department conduct major research projects aimed at the most significant dermatologic problems of our day including major efforts aimed at prevention, detection and therapy of melanoma and other skin cancers.

The expertise of NYU Medical Center's dermatologists encompasses all facets of medical, surgical, pediatric and cosmetic dermatology, including diseases of the hair, nails, and mucous membranes. Laser surgery is performed for a wide variety of skin and hair problems, and Mohs micrographic surgery and is available for skin cancers. Dermatologists at NYU Medical Center work closely with researchers trying to better understand and help alleviate dermatologic conditions, so their care of even the most common dermatological problems such as acne, eczema, psoriasis, and warts takes advantage of the most up-to-date breakthroughs in medicine and science. Research in the Department is carried out in a variety of settings, and the Department of Dermatology's Cutaneous Biology Research Program encompasses an entire floor of the new Smilow Translational Research Building.

Research for the purpose of discovering the causes of and developing new treatments for skin diseases goes hand in hand with patient care and teaching. The Department conducts a strong and diversified research program in the basic and applied sciences, studying fundamental processes which have a bearing on clinical practice, as well as new and different methods of therapy. Over 25 members of the fulltime faculty are engaged in laboratory and clinical research and active participation in their research projects forms an integral part of the educational program for the many young dermatologists trained in the Department.

Areas of Basic and Clinical Research

AIDS: Kaposi's sarcoma and skin infections

Bullous Diseases: Pemphigus and bullous pemphigoid

Congenital and Genetic Skin Siseases

Contact Dermatitis and Occupational Dermatitis

Dermatopharmacology: clinical trials of the latest therapeutic agents and diagnostic devices

Dermatopathology: study of the microscopic diagnosis of skin disease

Pediatric Dermatology: Hemangiomas, eczema, psoriasis, birthmarks

Epithelial Biology: Psoriasis and Ichthyosis

Allergic Diseases: Hives and Vaculitis

Viral Diseases: AIDS and Herpes

Laser: Birthmarks, skin tumors, pigmentary disorders

Mycology: Superficial and deep fungal infections

Oncology: Melanoma, basal cells carcinoma, squamous cell carcinoma, cutaneous lymphoma

Photomedicine: Psoriasis, vitiligo Surgery: cosmetic and cancer surgery

Hair: Alopecia and Hirsutism

Endocrinology, Diabetes & Metabolism
a subspecialty of Internal Medicine

An internist who concentrates on disorders of the internal (endocrine) glands such as the thyroid and adrenal glands. This specialist also deals with disorders such as diabetes, metabolic and nutritional disorders, pituitary diseases, menstrual and sexual problems.

Training Required: Three years in internal medicine *plus* additional training and examination for certification in endocrinology, diabetes and metabolism.

Endocrinology, Diabetes & Metabolism

ENDOCRINOLOGY, DIABETES & METABOLISM

New England

Abrahamson, Martin J MD [EDM] - **Spec Exp:** Diabetes; **Hospital:** Beth Israel Deaconess Med Ctr - Boston; **Address:** Joslin Diabetes Clinic, 1 Joslin Pl, Boston, MA 02215; **Phone:** 617-732-2501; **Board Cert:** Internal Medicine 2005; Endocrinology, Diabetes & Metabolism 2005; **Med School:** South Africa 1977; **Resid:** Internal Medicine, Groote Schuuer Hosp-Univ Cape Town 1983; **Fellow:** Endocrinology, Diabetes & Metabolism, Groote Schuuer Hosp-Univ Cape Town 1985; Research, Univ Cape Town 1987; **Fac Appt:** Assoc Prof Med, Harvard Med Sch

Axelrod, Lloyd MD [EDM] - **Spec Exp:** Diabetes; Geriatric Endocrinology; **Hospital:** Mass Genl Hosp; **Address:** 50 Stanford St Fl 3 - Ste 340, Boston, MA 02114; **Phone:** 617-726-8722; **Board Cert:** Internal Medicine 1973; Endocrinology, Diabetes & Metabolism 1973; **Med School:** Harvard Med Sch 1967; **Resid:** Internal Medicine, Peter Bent Brigham Hosp 1969; Internal Medicine, Mass Genl Hosp 1971; **Fellow:** Endocrinology, Diabetes & Metabolism, Peter Bent Brigham Hosp 1970; Endocrinology, Diabetes & Metabolism, Mass Genl Hosp 1972; **Fac Appt:** Assoc Prof Med, Harvard Med Sch

Beaser, Richard S MD [EDM] - **Spec Exp:** Diabetes; **Hospital:** Beth Israel Deaconess Med Ctr - Boston; **Address:** Joslin Clinic, 1 Joslin Pl, Boston, MA 02215; **Phone:** 617-732-2665; **Board Cert:** Internal Medicine 1980; **Med School:** Boston Univ 1977; **Resid:** Internal Medicine, Mass Med Ctr 1980; **Fellow:** Endocrinology, Diabetes & Metabolism, Joslin Clinic 1981; **Fac Appt:** Assoc Clin Prof Med, Harvard Med Sch

Biller, Beverly M K MD [EDM] - **Spec Exp:** Pituitary Disorders; Cushing's Syndrome; Acromegaly; **Hospital:** Mass Genl Hosp; **Address:** Neuroendocrine Clinic Center, Zero Emerson Pl, Ste 112, Boston, MA 02114-3117; **Phone:** 617-726-3870; **Board Cert:** Internal Medicine 1986; Endocrinology 1989; **Med School:** Univ Okla Coll Med 1983; **Resid:** Internal Medicine, Beth Israel Deaconness Hosp 1986; **Fellow:** Endocrinology, Diabetes & Metabolism, Mass Genl Hosp 1989; **Fac Appt:** Assoc Prof Med, Harvard Med Sch

Comi, Richard J MD [EDM] - **Spec Exp:** Diabetes; Hypoglycemia; Thyroid Disorders; Pituitary Disorders; **Hospital:** Dartmouth - Hitchcock Med Ctr; **Address:** Dartmouth-Hitchcock Med Ctr, Endocrinology, One Medical Ctr Drive, Lebanon, NH 03756; **Phone:** 603-650-8630; **Board Cert:** Internal Medicine 1983; Endocrinology 1987; **Med School:** Harvard Med Sch 1980; **Resid:** Internal Medicine, Mass Genl Hosp 1983; **Fellow:** Endocrinology & Diabetes, Natl Inst Hlth 1986

Daniels, Gilbert MD [EDM] - **Spec Exp:** Thyroid Disorders; Parathyroid Disease; Adrenal Disorders; **Hospital:** Mass Genl Hosp; **Address:** 15 Parkman St, Bldg WACC - Ste 730, Boston, MA 02114; **Phone:** 617-726-8430; **Board Cert:** Internal Medicine 1972; Endocrinology, Diabetes & Metabolism 1975; **Med School:** Harvard Med Sch 1966; **Resid:** Internal Medicine, Mass Genl Hosp 1972; **Fellow:** Biochemistry, Natl Inst Hlth 1970; Endocrinology, Diabetes & Metabolism, UCSF Med Ctr 1971; **Fac Appt:** Prof Med, Harvard Med Sch

Godine, John E MD/PhD [EDM] - **Spec Exp:** Diabetes; **Hospital:** Mass Genl Hosp; **Address:** 50 Staniford St Fl 3 - Ste 340, Boston, MA 02114; **Phone:** 617-726-8722; **Board Cert:** Internal Medicine 1979; Endocrinology, Diabetes & Metabolism 1981; **Med School:** Harvard Med Sch 1976; **Resid:** Internal Medicine, Mass Genl Hosp 1978; **Fellow:** Endocrinology, Diabetes & Metabolism, Mass Genl Hosp 1981; **Fac Appt:** Asst Prof Med, Harvard Med Sch

Inzucchi, Silvio E MD [EDM] - **Spec Exp:** Diabetes; Pituitary Disorders; Growth Hormone Disorder-Adult; Cholesterol/Lipid Disorders; **Hospital:** Yale-New Haven Hosp; **Address:** Yale Univ Sch Med, Div Endocrinology, Box 208020, New Haven, CT 06520-8020; **Phone:** 203-737-1932; **Board Cert:** Internal Medicine 1988; Endocrinology, Diabetes & Metabolism 2006; **Med School:** Harvard Med Sch 1985; **Resid:** Internal Medicine, Yale-New Haven Hosp 1988; **Fellow:** Endocrinology, Diabetes & Metabolism, Yale-New Haven Hosp 1994; **Fac Appt:** Prof Med, Yale Univ

Kahn, Barbara B MD [EDM] - **Spec Exp:** Obesity; Nutrition; **Hospital:** Beth Israel Deaconess Med Ctr - Boston; **Address:** Beth Israel Deaconess Medical Ctr, 330 Brookline Ave, rm RN380-6, Boston, MA 02215; **Phone:** 617-667-2151; **Board Cert:** Internal Medicine 1980; Endocrinology, Diabetes & Metabolism 1985; **Med School:** Stanford Univ 1977; **Resid:** Internal Medicine, UC Davis Med Ctr 1980; **Fellow:** Endocrinology, Diabetes & Metabolism, Natl Inst Hlth 1982; **Fac Appt:** Prof Med, Harvard Med Sch

Klibanski, Anne MD [EDM] - **Spec Exp:** Pituitary Disorders; Prolactin Disorders; Acromegaly; **Hospital:** Mass Genl Hosp; **Address:** Neuroendocrine Clinic Ctr, Zero Emerson Pl, Ste 112, Boston, MA 02114; **Phone:** 617-726-7948; **Board Cert:** Internal Medicine 1978; Endocrinology, Diabetes & Metabolism 1981; **Med School:** NYU Sch Med 1975; **Resid:** Internal Medicine, Bellevue Hosp Ctr 1978; **Fellow:** Endocrinology, Mass Genl Hosp 1981; **Fac Appt:** Prof Med, Harvard Med Sch

LeBoff, Meryl S MD [EDM] - **Spec Exp:** Osteoporosis; Metabolic Bone Disease; **Hospital:** Brigham & Women's Hosp; **Address:** 221 Longwood Ave, Boston, MA 02115; **Phone:** 617-732-5666; **Board Cert:** Internal Medicine 1979; Endocrinology, Diabetes & Metabolism 1981; **Med School:** UMDNJ-NJ Med Sch, Newark 1975; **Resid:** Internal Medicine, USC Med Ctr 1979; **Fellow:** Endocrinology, Brigham & Womens Hosp 1982; **Fac Appt:** Assoc Prof Med, Harvard Med Sch

Lechan, Ronald MD/PhD [EDM] - **Spec Exp:** Pituitary Disorders; Hypothalamic Dysfunction; Islet Cell Tumors; **Hospital:** Tufts Med Ctr; **Address:** New England Med Ctr, 750 Washington St, Box 268, Boston, MA 02111; **Phone:** 617-636-5689; **Board Cert:** Internal Medicine 1979; Endocrinology, Diabetes & Metabolism 1981; **Med School:** Univ VT Coll Med 1976; **Resid:** Internal Medicine, Beth Israel Hosp 1978; **Fellow:** Endocrinology, Diabetes & Metabolism, Tufts-New England Med Ctr 1981; **Fac Appt:** Prof Med, Tufts Univ

Levine, Robert A MD [EDM] - **Spec Exp:** Thyroid Cancer; Growth/Development Disorders; Metabolic Bone Disease; Thyroid Disorders; **Hospital:** St Joseph Hosp; **Address:** Thyroid Center of New Hampshire, 5 Coliseum Ave, Nashua, NH 03060; **Phone:** 603-881-7141; **Board Cert:** Internal Medicine 1984; Endocrinology, Diabetes & Metabolism 1987; **Med School:** Univ Conn 1981; **Resid:** Internal Medicine, Mt Auburn Hosp 1984; **Fellow:** Endocrinology, Yale Univ 1987

Seely, Ellen Wells MD [EDM] - **Spec Exp:** Pregnancy & Endocrine Disorders; Diabetes in Pregnancy; Diabetes in Women; Thyroid Disorders in Pregnancy; **Hospital:** Brigham & Women's Hosp; **Address:** Brigham & Womens Hosp, Endocrine Div, 221 Longwood Ave, rm 277, Boston, MA 02115-5804; **Phone:** 617-732-5661; **Board Cert:** Internal Medicine 1984; Endocrinology, Diabetes & Metabolism 1987; **Med School:** Columbia P&S 1981; **Resid:** Internal Medicine, Brigham & Womens Hosp 1984; **Fellow:** Endocrinology, Diabetes & Metabolism, Brigham & Womens Hosp 1987; **Fac Appt:** Assoc Prof Med, Harvard Med Sch

Sherwin, Robert MD [EDM] - **Spec Exp:** Diabetes; **Hospital:** Yale-New Haven Hosp; **Address:** Yale Univ Sch Med, Sect Endocrinology, 333 Cedar St, Box 208020, New Haven, CT 06520-8020; **Phone:** 203-785-4183; **Board Cert:** Internal Medicine 1972; **Med School:** Albert Einstein Coll Med 1967; **Resid:** Internal Medicine, Mt Sinai Hosp 1969; Internal Medicine, Mt Sinai Hosp 1972; **Fellow:** Metabolism, Yale-New Haven Hosp 1973; **Fac Appt:** Prof Med, Yale Univ

Endocrinology, Diabetes & Metabolism

Mid Atlantic

Ball, Douglas W MD [EDM] - **Spec Exp:** Thyroid Cancer; **Hospital:** Johns Hopkins Hosp - Baltimore (page 61); **Address:** Sidney Kimmel Cancer Ctr, 1830 E Monument St, Ste 333, Baltimore, MD 21287; **Phone:** 410-955-8964; **Board Cert:** Internal Medicine 1987; **Med School:** Geo Wash Univ 1984; **Resid:** Internal Medicine, Univ Pittsburgh 1987; **Fellow:** Endocrinology, Diabetes & Metabolism, Johns Hopkins Hosp 1991; **Fac Appt:** Assoc Prof Med, Johns Hopkins Univ

Bergman, Donald MD [EDM] - **Spec Exp:** Osteoporosis; Thyroid Disorders; Calcium Disorders; **Hospital:** Mount Sinai Med Ctr (page 64); **Address:** 1199 Park Ave, Ste 1F, New York, NY 10128; **Phone:** 212-876-7333; **Board Cert:** Internal Medicine 1975; Endocrinology, Diabetes & Metabolism 1977; **Med School:** Jefferson Med Coll 1971; **Resid:** Obstetrics & Gynecology, Mount Sinai Hosp 1972; Internal Medicine, Mount Sinai Hosp 1975; **Fellow:** Endocrinology, Diabetes & Metabolism, Mount Sinai Hosp 1977; **Fac Appt:** Clin Prof Med, Mount Sinai Sch Med

Bilezikian, John P MD [EDM] - **Spec Exp:** Osteoporosis; Bone Disorders-Metabolic; Parathyroid Disease; **Hospital:** NY-Presby Hosp/Columbia (page 66); **Address:** Columbia Med Ctr, Metabolic Bone Diseases, Harkness Pavilion, 180 Ft Washington Ave Fl 9 - Ste 904, New York, NY 10032; **Phone:** 212-305-2663; **Board Cert:** Internal Medicine 1975; Endocrinology, Diabetes & Metabolism 1977; **Med School:** Columbia P&S 1969; **Resid:** Internal Medicine, Columbia-Presby Hosp 1975; **Fellow:** Endocrinology, Diabetes & Metabolism, Natl Inst Health 1977; **Fac Appt:** Prof Med, Columbia P&S

Blum, Conrad B MD [EDM] - **Spec Exp:** Cholesterol/Lipid Disorders; Thyroid Disorders; Diabetes; **Hospital:** NY-Presby Hosp/Columbia (page 66); **Address:** 16 E 60th St, Ste 320, New York, NY 10022-1002; **Phone:** 212-326-8421; **Board Cert:** Internal Medicine 1976; Endocrinology, Diabetes & Metabolism 1977; **Med School:** Northwestern Univ 1971; **Resid:** Internal Medicine, Brigham Hosp 1976; **Fellow:** Endocrinology, Diabetes & Metabolism, Northwestern Univ Med Sch 1977; **Fac Appt:** Clin Prof Med, Columbia P&S

Bockman, Richard MD/PhD [EDM] - **Spec Exp:** Bone Disorders-Metabolic; Osteoporosis; Thyroid Disorders; **Hospital:** Hosp For Special Surgery (page 59), NY-Presby Hosp/Weill Cornell (page 66); **Address:** 519 E 72nd St, New York, NY 10021; **Phone:** 212-606-1458; **Board Cert:** Internal Medicine 1975; **Med School:** Yale Univ 1968; **Resid:** Internal Medicine, NYU Med Ctr 1975; **Fellow:** Internal Medicine, NY-Cornell Med Ctr 1973; **Fac Appt:** Prof Med, Cornell Univ-Weill Med Coll

Calvi, Laura MD [EDM] - **Spec Exp:** Osteoporosis; Parathyroid Disease; **Hospital:** Univ of Rochester Strong Meml Hosp; **Address:** 601 Elmwood Ave, Box 693, Rochester, NY 14642; **Phone:** 585-275-2901; **Board Cert:** Internal Medicine 1998; Endocrinology, Diabetes & Metabolism 2000; **Med School:** Harvard Med Sch 1995; **Resid:** Internal Medicine, Mass Genl Hosp 1998; **Fac Appt:** Asst Prof Med, Univ Rochester

Cooper, David S MD [EDM] - **Spec Exp:** Thyroid Disorders; **Hospital:** Johns Hopkins Hosp - Baltimore (page 61); **Address:** Div Endocrinology & Metabolism, 1830 E Monument St, Ste 333, Baltimore, MD 21287; **Phone:** 410-955-3663; **Board Cert:** Internal Medicine 1987; Endocrinology, Diabetes & Metabolism 1979; **Med School:** Tufts Univ 1973; **Resid:** Internal Medicine, Barnes Hosp 1976; **Fellow:** Endocrinology, Mass Genl Hosp 1978; **Fac Appt:** Prof Med, Johns Hopkins Univ

Davies, Terry MD [EDM] - **Spec Exp:** Thyroid Disorders in Pregnancy; Graves' Disease; Hashimoto's Disease; Thyroid Cancer; **Hospital:** Mount Sinai Med Ctr (page 64), VA Med Ctr - Manhattan; **Address:** 5 E 98th St, Box 1055, New York, NY 10029-6500; **Phone:** 212-241-7975; **Med School:** England 1971; **Resid:** Internal Medicine, Univ Newcastle 1975; **Fellow:** Endocrinology, Diabetes & Metabolism, Univ Newcastle 1977; Endocrinology, Diabetes & Metabolism, Natl Inst Hlth 1979; **Fac Appt:** Prof Med, Mount Sinai Sch Med

Dobs, Adrian S MD [EDM] - **Spec Exp:** Hormonal Disorders; Hypogonadism-Male; Metabolic Disorders; Complementary Medicine; **Hospital:** Johns Hopkins Hosp - Baltimore (page 61); **Address:** Johns Hopkins Hosp, 1830 E Monument St, Fl 3 - Ste 328, Baltimore, MD 21287; **Phone:** 410-955-2130; **Board Cert:** Internal Medicine 1981; Endocrinology 1987; **Med School:** Albany Med Coll 1978; **Resid:** Internal Medicine, Montefiore Hosp 1982; **Fellow:** Endocrinology, Johns Hopkins Hosp 1984; **Fac Appt:** Prof Med, Johns Hopkins Univ

Felig, Philip MD [EDM] - **Spec Exp:** Diabetes; Thyroid Disorders; Osteoporosis; **Hospital:** Lenox Hill Hosp (page 62), Beth Israel Med Ctr - Petrie Division (page 57); **Address:** 1056 5th Ave, New York, NY 10028-0112; **Phone:** 212-534-5900; **Board Cert:** Internal Medicine 1968; **Med School:** Yale Univ 1961; **Resid:** Internal Medicine, Yale-New Haven Hosp 1967; **Fellow:** Endocrinology, Diabetes & Metabolism, Peter Bent Brigham Hosp 1969

Fleischer, Norman MD [EDM] - **Spec Exp:** Thyroid Disorders; Adrenal Disorders; Pituitary Disorders; **Hospital:** Montefiore Med Ctr - Weiler-Einstein Div; **Address:** 1575 Blondell Ave, Ste 200, Bronx, NY 10461-2601; **Phone:** 866-633-8253; **Board Cert:** Internal Medicine 1968; Endocrinology, Diabetes & Metabolism 1973; **Med School:** Vanderbilt Univ 1961; **Resid:** Internal Medicine, Bronx Muni Hosp Ctr 1964; **Fellow:** Endocrinology, Diabetes & Metabolism, Vanderbilt Univ 1966; **Fac Appt:** Prof Med, Albert Einstein Coll Med

Greene, Loren Wissner MD [EDM] - **Spec Exp:** Thyroid Disorders; Osteoporosis; Pituitary Disorders; Diabetes; **Hospital:** NYU Med Ctr (page 68), NY Downtown Hosp; **Address:** 530 1st Ave, Ste 4B, New York, NY 10016-6402; **Phone:** 212-263-7449; **Board Cert:** Internal Medicine 1978; Endocrinology, Diabetes & Metabolism 1981; **Med School:** NYU Sch Med 1975; **Resid:** Internal Medicine, Bellevue Hosp Ctr-NYU 1978; **Fellow:** Endocrinology, Bellevue Hosp Ctr-NYU 1980; **Fac Appt:** Assoc Clin Prof Med, NYU Sch Med

Greenspan, Susan L MD [EDM] - **Spec Exp:** Osteoporosis; **Hospital:** UPMC Presby, Pittsburgh; **Address:** Univ Pittsburgh, Osteoporosis Ctr, 3471 Fifth Ave, Kaufmann Bldg - Ste 1110, Pittsburgh, PA 15213; **Phone:** 412-692-2472; **Board Cert:** Internal Medicine 1982; Endocrinology, Diabetes & Metabolism 1987; Geriatric Medicine 1998; **Med School:** Harvard Med Sch 1979; **Resid:** Internal Medicine, Beth Israel Hosp 1982; **Fellow:** Endocrinology, Mass Genl Hosp 1985; **Fac Appt:** Prof Med, Univ Pittsburgh

Jacobs, Thomas MD [EDM] - **Spec Exp:** Adrenal Disorders; Pituitary Disorders; Calcium Disorders; **Hospital:** NY-Presby Hosp/Columbia (page 66); **Address:** 161 Fort Washington Ave, rm 210, New York, NY 10032-3713; **Phone:** 212-305-5578; **Board Cert:** Internal Medicine 1973; Endocrinology, Diabetes & Metabolism 1975; **Med School:** Johns Hopkins Univ 1968; **Resid:** Internal Medicine, Columbia Presby Hosp 1973; **Fellow:** Endocrinology, Diabetes & Metabolism, Univ Wash Med Ctr 1975; **Fac Appt:** Clin Prof Med, Columbia P&S

Kleinberg, David MD [EDM] - **Spec Exp:** Neuroendocrinology; Pituitary Disorders; **Hospital:** NYU Med Ctr (page 68); **Address:** 530 1st Ave, Ste 4C, New York, NY 10016; **Phone:** 212-263-6772; **Board Cert:** Internal Medicine 1972; Endocrinology 1975; **Med School:** Univ Miami Sch Med 1966; **Resid:** Internal Medicine, Maimonides Med Ctr 1968; Internal Medicine, Columbia-Presby Med Ctr 1971; **Fellow:** Endocrinology, Diabetes & Metabolism, Columbia-Presby Med Ctr 1970; **Fac Appt:** Prof Med, NYU Sch Med

Korytkowski, Mary T MD [EDM] - **Spec Exp:** Diabetes; Polycystic Ovarian Syndrome; Thyroid Disorders; Diabetic Vascular Disease; **Hospital:** UPMC Presby, Pittsburgh; **Address:** Center for Diabetes & Endocrinology, 3601 Fifth Ave, Falk Med Bldg, Ste 562, Pittsburgh, PA 15213-3403; **Phone:** 412-586-9714; **Board Cert:** Internal Medicine 1985; Endocrinology 1989; **Med School:** Univ NC Sch Med 1982; **Resid:** Internal Medicine, Francis Scott Key Med Ctr 1985; **Fellow:** Endocrinology, Diabetes & Metabolism, Sinai Hosp/Johns Hopkins Hosp 1988; **Fac Appt:** Prof Med, Univ Pittsburgh

Endocrinology, Diabetes & Metabolism

Ladenson, Paul W MD [EDM] - **Spec Exp:** Thyroid Disorders; Thyroid Cancer; **Hospital:** Johns Hopkins Hosp - Baltimore (page 61); **Address:** Johns Hopkins-Div Endocrinology & Metabolism, 1830 E Monument St, rm 333, Baltimore, MD 21287; **Phone:** 410-955-3663; **Board Cert:** Internal Medicine 1978; Endocrinology, Diabetes & Metabolism 1981; **Med School:** Harvard Med Sch 1975; **Resid:** Internal Medicine, Mass Genl Hosp 1978; **Fellow:** Endocrinology, Diabetes & Metabolism, Mass Genl Hosp 1980; **Fac Appt:** Prof Med, Johns Hopkins Univ

Mahler, Richard J MD [EDM] - **Spec Exp:** Thyroid Disorders; Diabetes; **Hospital:** NY-Presby Hosp/Weill Cornell (page 66); **Address:** 220 E 69th St, New York, NY 10021-5737; **Phone:** 212-879-4073; **Board Cert:** Internal Medicine 1987; **Med School:** NY Med Coll 1959; **Resid:** Internal Medicine, NY Med-Metro Med 1962; Endocrinology, Diabetes & Metabolism, NY Med Coll 1963; **Fellow:** Endocrinology, Diabetes & Metabolism, Univ Durham/Univ New Castle 1964; **Fac Appt:** Assoc Clin Prof Med, Cornell Univ-Weill Med Coll

Mandel, Susan J MD [EDM] - **Spec Exp:** Thyroid Disorders; Calcium Disorders; **Hospital:** Hosp Univ Penn - UPHS (page 60); **Address:** Hosp Univ Penn, Div Endocrinology, 3400 Spruce St, 1 Maloney, Philadelphia, PA 19104; **Phone:** 215-662-2300; **Board Cert:** Internal Medicine 1989; Endocrinology 2001; **Med School:** Columbia P&S 1986; **Resid:** Internal Medicine, Columbia Presby Med Ctr 1989; **Fellow:** Endocrinology, Brigham & Womens Hosp 1992; **Fac Appt:** Assoc Prof Med, Univ Pennsylvania

McConnell, Robert John MD [EDM] - **Spec Exp:** Thyroid Disorders; Thyroid Ultrasound; **Hospital:** NY-Presby Hosp/Columbia (page 66); **Address:** 161 Fort Washington Ave, Ste 210, New York, NY 10032-3713; **Phone:** 212-305-5579; **Board Cert:** Internal Medicine 1978; Endocrinology, Diabetes & Metabolism 1981; **Med School:** Columbia P&S 1973; **Resid:** Internal Medicine, Barnes Hosp 1975; **Fellow:** Endocrinology, Diabetes & Metabolism, Columbia-Presby Hosp 1978; **Fac Appt:** Prof Med, Columbia P&S

Mersey, James H MD [EDM] - **Spec Exp:** Diabetes; **Hospital:** Greater Baltimore Med Ctr, St Joseph Med Ctr; **Address:** 6535 N Charles St, Ste 400, Towson, MD 21204; **Phone:** 410-828-7417; **Board Cert:** Internal Medicine 1975; Endocrinology, Diabetes & Metabolism 1977; **Med School:** Johns Hopkins Univ 1972; **Resid:** Internal Medicine, Johns Hopkins Hosp 1977; **Fellow:** Endocrinology, Diabetes & Metabolism, Peter Bent Brigham Hosp 1976; **Fac Appt:** Asst Prof Med, Johns Hopkins Univ

Roberts, Michelle M MD [EDM] - **Spec Exp:** Osteoporosis; Diabetes; **Hospital:** UPMC Presby, Pittsburgh; **Address:** Falk Medical Bldg, 3601 Fifth Ave, Ste 3B, Pittsburgh, PA 15213; **Phone:** 412-586-9714; **Board Cert:** Internal Medicine 1986; Endocrinology, Diabetes & Metabolism 1989; **Med School:** Duke Univ 1983; **Resid:** Internal Medicine, Univ Pittsburgh Med Ctr 1986; **Fellow:** Endocrinology, Diabetes & Metabolism, Univ Pittsburgh Med Ctr 1989; **Fac Appt:** Assoc Clin Prof Med, Univ Pittsburgh

Saudek, Christopher D MD [EDM] - **Spec Exp:** Diabetes; **Hospital:** Johns Hopkins Hosp - Baltimore (page 61); **Address:** 600 N Wolfe St, Osler 575, Baltimore, MD 21287; **Phone:** 410-955-2132; **Board Cert:** Internal Medicine 1972; **Med School:** Cornell Univ-Weill Med Coll 1967; **Resid:** Internal Medicine, Presby-St Lukes Hosp 1969; Internal Medicine, Boston City Hosp 1970; **Fellow:** Endocrinology, Diabetes & Metabolism, Thorndale Lab-Harvard 1972; **Fac Appt:** Prof Med, Johns Hopkins Univ

Schwartz, Stanley S MD [EDM] - **Spec Exp:** Diabetes; **Hospital:** Hosp Univ Penn - UPHS (page 60); **Address:** Hosp Univ Penn, EDM Div, 3400 Spruce St, 9-Penn Twr, Philadelphia, PA 19104; **Phone:** 215-662-2518; **Board Cert:** Internal Medicine 1976; Endocrinology, Diabetes & Metabolism 1979; **Med School:** Univ Chicago-Pritzker Sch Med 1973; **Resid:** Internal Medicine, Hosp Univ Penn 1976; **Fellow:** Endocrinology, Diabetes & Metabolism, Univ Chicago Hosps 1978; **Fac Appt:** Assoc Clin Prof Med, Univ Pennsylvania

America's Top Doctors® 8th Edition

Shuldiner, Alan R MD [EDM] - **Spec Exp:** Diabetes; Eating Disorders/Obesity; **Hospital:** Univ of MD Med Sys; **Address:** Univ MD Sch Med, Div Endocrinology, 660 W Redwood St, rm HH-494, Baltimore, MD 21201; **Phone:** 410-706-1623; **Board Cert:** Internal Medicine 1988; Endocrinology 1989; **Med School:** Harvard Med Sch 1984; **Resid:** Internal Medicine, Columbia-Presby Hosp 1986; **Fellow:** Endocrinology, Diabetes & Metabolism, Natl Inst Hlth 1990; **Fac Appt:** Prof Med, Univ MD Sch Med

Siris, Ethel MD [EDM] - **Spec Exp:** Osteoporosis; Paget's Disease of Bone; Bone Disorders-Metabolic; **Hospital:** NY-Presby Hosp/Columbia (page 66); **Address:** 180 Ft Washington Ave, Harkness Bldg - Ste 904, New York, NY 10032-3710; **Phone:** 212-305-9531; **Board Cert:** Internal Medicine 1974; Endocrinology, Diabetes & Metabolism 1977; **Med School:** Columbia P&S 1971; **Resid:** Internal Medicine, Columbia-Presby Med Ctr 1974; **Fellow:** Endocrinology, Diabetes & Metabolism, Natl Inst Hlth 1976; Endocrinology, Diabetes & Metabolism, Columbia-Presby Med Ctr 1977; **Fac Appt:** Prof Med, Columbia P&S

Snyder, Peter J MD [EDM] - **Spec Exp:** Pituitary Tumors; Reproductive Endocrinology-Male; **Hospital:** Hosp Univ Penn - UPHS (page 60); **Address:** Univ Pennsylvania Med Group, 3400 Spruce St, Philadelphia, PA 19104; **Phone:** 215-898-0208; **Board Cert:** Internal Medicine 1972; Endocrinology, Diabetes & Metabolism 1972; **Med School:** Harvard Med Sch 1965; **Resid:** Internal Medicine, Beth Israel Hosp 1967; Internal Medicine, Beth Israel Hosp 1970; **Fellow:** Endocrinology, Diabetes & Metabolism, Hosp Univ Penn 1971; **Fac Appt:** Prof Med, Univ Pennsylvania

Surks, Martin MD [EDM] - **Spec Exp:** Thyroid Disorders; **Hospital:** Montefiore Med Ctr, N Central Bronx Hosp; **Address:** 3400 Bainbridge Ave Fl 2, Bronx, NY 10467; **Phone:** 866-633-8255; **Board Cert:** Internal Medicine 1967; Endocrinology, Diabetes & Metabolism 1977; **Med School:** NYU Sch Med 1960; **Resid:** Internal Medicine, Montefiore Hosp Med Ctr 1962; Internal Medicine, VA Hosp 1964; **Fellow:** Research, Natl Inst Arthritis-Metabolic Disease 1964; **Fac Appt:** Prof Med, Albert Einstein Coll Med

Tuttle, R Michael MD [EDM] - **Spec Exp:** Thyroid Cancer; **Hospital:** Meml Sloan-Kettering Cancer Ctr; **Address:** 1275 York Avenue, New York, NY 10065; **Phone:** 800-525-2225; **Board Cert:** Endocrinology, Diabetes & Metabolism 2004; **Med School:** Univ Louisville Sch Med 1987; **Resid:** Internal Medicine, DD Eisenhower Army Med Ctr 1990; **Fellow:** Endocrinology, Diabetes & Metabolism, Madigan Army Med Ctr 1993; **Fac Appt:** Assoc Prof Med, Cornell Univ-Weill Med Coll

Wartofsky, Leonard MD [EDM] - **Spec Exp:** Thyroid Cancer; Thyroid Disorders; **Hospital:** Washington Hosp Ctr; **Address:** 110 Irving St NW, Ste 2A62, Washington, DC 20010-2975; **Phone:** 202-877-3109; **Board Cert:** Internal Medicine 1971; Endocrinology, Diabetes & Metabolism 1972; **Med School:** Geo Wash Univ 1964; **Resid:** Internal Medicine, Barnes Jewish Hosp 1966; Internal Medicine, Montefiore Med Ctr 1967; **Fellow:** Endocrinology, Diabetes & Metabolism, Boston City Hosp 1969; **Fac Appt:** Prof Med, Georgetown Univ

Young, Iven MD [EDM] - **Spec Exp:** Thyroid Disorders; Osteoporosis; Pituitary Disorders; **Hospital:** St Vincent Cath Med Ctrs - Manhattan; **Address:** 130 W 12th St, Ste 7D, New York, NY 10011-8250; **Phone:** 212-675-9332; **Board Cert:** Internal Medicine 1966; Endocrinology, Diabetes & Metabolism 1973; **Med School:** NYU Sch Med 1959; **Resid:** Internal Medicine, VA Med Ctr 1963; **Fellow:** Endocrinology, NYU Med Ctr 1966; **Fac Appt:** Assoc Clin Prof Med, NY Med Coll

Endocrinology, Diabetes & Metabolism

Southeast

Ain, Kenneth B MD [EDM] - **Spec Exp:** Thyroid Cancer; Thyroid Disorders; **Hospital:** Univ of Kentucky Chandler Hosp, VA Med Ctr - Lexington; **Address:** Markey Cancer Center, 800 Rose St, rm CC455, Lexington, KY 40536-0001; **Phone:** 859-323-3778; **Board Cert:** Internal Medicine 1984; Endocrinology, Diabetes & Metabolism 1987; **Med School:** Brown Univ 1981; **Resid:** Internal Medicine, Hahnemann Univ 1984; **Fellow:** Endocrinology, Univ Chicago 1986; Thyroid Oncology, NIDDK, Natl Inst Hlth 1990; **Fac Appt:** Prof Med, Univ KY Coll Med

Barrett, Eugene J MD [EDM] - **Spec Exp:** Diabetes; Cholesterol/Lipid Disorders; **Hospital:** Univ Virginia Med Ctr; **Address:** Univ Virginia, Div Endocrinology, PO Box 801410, Charlottesville, VA 22908; **Phone:** 434-924-1175; **Board Cert:** Internal Medicine 1978; Endocrinology, Diabetes & Metabolism 1995; **Med School:** Univ Rochester 1975; **Resid:** Internal Medicine, Strong Meml Hosp 1977; **Fellow:** Endocrinology, Diabetes & Metabolism, Yale Univ 1980; **Fac Appt:** Prof Med, Univ VA Sch Med

Bell, David S H MD [EDM] - **Spec Exp:** Diabetes; Diabetes-Insulin Pump Therapy; Diabetic Vascular Diaease; **Hospital:** Univ of Ala Hosp at Birmingham; **Address:** 1020 26th St S, Birmingham, AL 35205; **Phone:** 205-933-2667; **Board Cert:** Internal Medicine 1987; Endocrinology, Diabetes & Metabolism 1981; **Med School:** Ireland 1970; **Resid:** Internal Medicine, Royal Victoria Hosp 1973; Endocrinology, Diabetes & Metabolism, Univ Saskatchewan Hosp 1975; **Fellow:** Endocrinology, Diabetes & Metabolism, Greater Baltimore Med Ctr 1976; **Fac Appt:** Prof Med, Univ Ala

Clore, John MD [EDM] - **Spec Exp:** Diabetes; Hypoglycemia; **Hospital:** Med Coll of VA Hosp; **Address:** PO Box 980155, Richmond, VA 23298; **Phone:** 804-828-2161; **Board Cert:** Internal Medicine 1985; Endocrinology, Diabetes & Metabolism 1989; **Med School:** Med Coll VA 1982; **Resid:** Internal Medicine, Med Coll Virginia 1985; **Fellow:** Endocrinology, Diabetes & Metabolism, Med Coll Virginia 1988; **Fac Appt:** Assoc Prof Med, Va Commonwealth Univ Sch Med

Dalkin, Alan Craig MD [EDM] - **Spec Exp:** Bone Disorders-Metabolic; Osteoporosis; **Hospital:** Univ Virginia Med Ctr; **Address:** Univ VA Hlth Sys, Div Endocrinology, PO Box 801412, Charlottesville, VA 22908; **Phone:** 434-243-2603; **Board Cert:** Internal Medicine 1987; Endocrinology 1989; **Med School:** Univ Mich Med Sch 1984; **Resid:** Internal Medicine, Univ Chicago Hosps 1987; **Fellow:** Endocrinology, Diabetes & Metabolism, Univ Mich Med Ctr 1990; **Fac Appt:** Assoc Prof Med, Univ VA Sch Med

Earp III, H Shelton MD [EDM] - **Spec Exp:** Cancer-Hormonal Influences; **Hospital:** Univ NC Hosps; **Address:** UNC Lineberger Comprehensive Cancer Center, 450 West Drive, Fl 1 - rm 10-012, Chapel Hill, NC 27599; **Phone:** 919-966-3036; **Board Cert:** Internal Medicine 1976; Endocrinology, Diabetes & Metabolism 1977; **Med School:** Univ NC Sch Med 1970; **Resid:** Internal Medicine, NC Memorial Hosp 1975; **Fellow:** Endocrinology, Diabetes & Metabolism, Univ North Carolina Hosp 1977; **Fac Appt:** Prof Med, Univ NC Sch Med

Feinglos, Mark MD [EDM] - **Spec Exp:** Diabetes; Thyroid Disorders; **Hospital:** Duke Univ Med Ctr; **Address:** Duke Univ Med Ctr, Box 3921, Durham, NC 27710-0001; **Phone:** 919-684-4005; **Board Cert:** Internal Medicine 1976; Endocrinology, Diabetes & Metabolism 1977; **Med School:** McGill Univ 1973; **Resid:** Internal Medicine, Duke Univ Med Ctr 1975; **Fellow:** Endocrinology, Diabetes & Metabolism, Duke Univ Med Ctr 1977; **Fac Appt:** Prof Med, Duke Univ

Koch, Christian A MD [EDM] - **Spec Exp:** Endocrine Cancers; Thyroid Cancer; Growth Hormone Disorder-Adult; Hypertension; **Hospital:** Univ Hosps & Clins - Jackson; **Address:** 2500 N State St, Jackson, MS 39216; **Phone:** 601-984-5525; **Board Cert:** Internal Medicine 1999; Endocrinology, Diabetes & Metabolism 2000; **Med School:** Germany 1991; **Resid:** Internal Medicine, Ohio State Univ Hosp 1997; **Fellow:** Endocrinology, Natl Inst Hlth 2001; **Fac Appt:** Prof Med, Univ Miss

Marshall, John C MD/PhD [EDM] - **Spec Exp:** Pituitary Disorders; Neuroendocrinology; Polycystic Ovarian Syndrome; **Hospital:** Univ Virginia Med Ctr; **Address:** Univ VA Hlth System, Hospital Dr, Box 800612, Charlottesville, VA 22908-0001; **Phone:** 434-924-2431; **Board Cert:** Internal Medicine 1978; Endocrinology, Diabetes & Metabolism 1981; **Med School:** England 1965; **Resid:** Neurology, Natl Hosp Queen Square 1968; Cardiovascular Disease, Natl Heart Hosp 1969; **Fellow:** Endocrinology, Diabetes & Metabolism, Hammersmith Hosp 1972; Endocrinology, Diabetes & Metabolism, UCLA 1974; **Fac Appt:** Prof Med, Univ VA Sch Med

Nestler, John E MD [EDM] - **Spec Exp:** Polycystic Ovarian Syndrome; Diabetes; **Hospital:** Med Coll of VA Hosp; **Address:** Med Coll Va, Div Endocrinology, Box 980111, Richmond, VA 23298-0111; **Phone:** 804-828-2161; **Board Cert:** Internal Medicine 1982; Endocrinology 1985; **Med School:** Univ Pennsylvania 1979; **Resid:** Internal Medicine, Med Coll Virginia 1983; **Fellow:** Endocrinology, Hosp Univ Penn 1985; **Fac Appt:** Prof Med, Med Coll VA

Ontjes, David A MD [EDM] - **Spec Exp:** Osteoporosis; Thyroid Disorders; Adrenal Disorders; Pituitary Disorders; **Hospital:** Univ NC Hosps; **Address:** UNC-Chapel Hill, 257 MacNider Bldg, Chapel Hill, NC 27599-7527; **Phone:** 919-966-3336; **Board Cert:** Internal Medicine 1980; Endocrinology, Diabetes & Metabolism 1972; **Med School:** Harvard Med Sch 1964; **Resid:** Internal Medicine, Boston City Hosp 1966; **Fac Appt:** Prof Med, Univ NC Sch Med

Ovalle, Fernando MD [EDM] - **Spec Exp:** Diabetes; Polycystic Ovarian Syndrome; Hypoglycemia; **Hospital:** Univ of Ala Hosp at Birmingham; **Address:** UAB Sch Med, 510 20th St S FOT Bldg Fl 7 - Ste 702, Birmingham, AL 35294; **Phone:** 205-975-2422; **Board Cert:** Endocrinology, Diabetes & Metabolism 1997; **Med School:** Mexico 1989; **Resid:** Internal Medicine, Henry Ford Hosp 1995; **Fellow:** Endocrinology, Diabetes & Metabolism, Barnes Jewish Hosp 1997; **Fac Appt:** Assoc Prof Med, Univ Ala

Powers, Alvin C MD [EDM] - **Spec Exp:** Diabetes; Thyroid Disorders; **Hospital:** Vanderbilt Univ Med Ctr; **Address:** Vanderbilt Univ Med Ctr, Div Endocrinology, 2213 Garland Ave, MRB#4, Nashville, TN 37232-0475; **Phone:** 615-936-1653; **Board Cert:** Internal Medicine 1982; Endocrinology, Diabetes & Metabolism 1985; **Med School:** Univ Tenn Coll Med, Memphis 1979; **Resid:** Internal Medicine, Duke Univ Med Ctr 1982; **Fellow:** Endocrinology, Diabetes & Metabolism, Joslin Diabetes Ctr 1983; Endocrinology, Diabetes & Metabolism, Mass Genl Hosp 1985; **Fac Appt:** Prof Med, Vanderbilt Univ

Quinn, Suzanne L MD [EDM] - **Hospital:** Shands at Univ of FL, Malcolm Randall VA Med Ctr; **Address:** Shands Univ Florida, Dept Endocrinology, 2000 SW Archer Rd, Gainesville, FL 32610; **Phone:** 352-265-8230; **Board Cert:** Internal Medicine 1988; Endocrinology, Diabetes & Metabolism 2003; **Med School:** Univ Fla Coll Med 1985; **Resid:** Internal Medicine, Univ Fla Coll Med 1988; **Fellow:** Endocrinology, Diabetes & Metabolism, Univ Fla Coll Med 1992; **Fac Appt:** Assoc Prof Med, Univ Fla Coll Med

Skyler, Jay S MD [EDM] - **Spec Exp:** Diabetes; **Hospital:** Jackson Meml Hosp, Univ of Miami Hosp & Clins/Sylvester Comp Canc Ctr; **Address:** Diabetes Research Inst, 1450 NW 10th Ave, Ste 3054, Miami, FL 33136; **Phone:** 305-243-6146; **Board Cert:** Internal Medicine 1972; Endocrinology, Diabetes & Metabolism 1973; **Med School:** Jefferson Med Coll 1969; **Resid:** Internal Medicine, Duke Univ Med Ctr 1971; **Fellow:** Endocrinology, Diabetes & Metabolism, Duke Univ Med Ctr 1973; **Fac Appt:** Prof Med, Univ Miami Sch Med

Vance, Mary Lee MD [EDM] - **Spec Exp:** Pituitary Disorders; Adrenal Disorders; **Hospital:** Univ Virginia Med Ctr; **Address:** Univ Virginia Hlth Sys, PO Box 800601, Charlottesville, VA 22908-0601; **Phone:** 434-924-2284; **Board Cert:** Internal Medicine 1980; **Med School:** Louisiana State U, New Orleans 1977; **Resid:** Internal Medicine, Baylor Univ Med Ctr 1980; **Fellow:** Endocrinology, Univ Virginia Med Ctr 1983; **Fac Appt:** Prof Med, Univ VA Sch Med

Endocrinology, Diabetes & Metabolism

Weissman, Peter MD [EDM] - **Spec Exp:** Diabetes; **Hospital:** Baptist Hosp of Miami; **Address:** 7867 N Kendall Drive, Ste 80, Miami, FL 33156; **Phone:** 305-595-0777; **Board Cert:** Internal Medicine 1972; Endocrinology, Diabetes & Metabolism 1972; **Med School:** NYU Sch Med 1966; **Resid:** Internal Medicine, Barnes Hosp/Wash Univ 1968; **Fellow:** Geriatric Medicine, Gerontology Rsch Ctr 1970; Endocrinology, Diabetes & Metabolism, Univ Mich Hosp 1972; **Fac Appt:** Assoc Clin Prof Med, Univ Miami Sch Med

Midwest

Bahn, Rebecca S MD [EDM] - **Spec Exp:** Graves' Disease; Graves' Disease-Eye; **Hospital:** Mayo Med Ctr & Clin - Rochester; **Address:** Mayo Clinic, Div Endocrinology, 200 First St SW, Rochester, MN 55905; **Phone:** 507-284-1600; **Board Cert:** Internal Medicine 1985; Endocrinology, Diabetes & Metabolism 1987; **Med School:** Mayo Med Sch 1981; **Resid:** Internal Medicine, Mayo Clinic 1984; **Fellow:** Endocrinology, Diabetes & Metabolism, Mayo Clinic 1986; **Fac Appt:** Prof Med, Mayo Med Sch

Brennan, Michael D MD [EDM] - **Spec Exp:** Thyroid Disorders; Diabetes; **Hospital:** Mayo Med Ctr & Clin - Rochester; **Address:** Mayo Clinic, Div Endocrinology, 200 First St SW, Rochester, MN 55905; **Phone:** 507-266-5247; **Board Cert:** Internal Medicine 1975; Endocrinology, Diabetes & Metabolism 1977; **Med School:** Ireland 1969; **Resid:** Internal Medicine, Mayo Clinic 1975; Internal Medicine, Henry Ford Hosp 1972; **Fellow:** Endocrinology, Diabetes & Metabolism, Mayo Clinic 1977; **Fac Appt:** Assoc Prof Med, Mayo Med Sch

Clutter, William E MD [EDM] - **Spec Exp:** Endocrine Cancers; Calcium Disorders; Metabolic Bone Disease; **Hospital:** Barnes-Jewish Hosp, Washington Univ Med Ctr; **Address:** Washington Univ, Dept Internal Medicine, 4921 Parkview Pl Fl 5 - Ste C, St Louis, MO 63110; **Phone:** 314-362-3500; **Board Cert:** Internal Medicine 1978; Endocrinology, Diabetes & Metabolism 1981; **Med School:** Ohio State Univ 1975; **Resid:** Internal Medicine, Barnes Jewish Hosp 1978; **Fellow:** Endocrinology, Diabetes & Metabolism, Barnes Jewish Hosp 1980; **Fac Appt:** Prof Med, Washington Univ, St Louis

Cryer, Philip E MD [EDM] - **Spec Exp:** Diabetes; Hypoglycemia; **Hospital:** Barnes-Jewish Hosp, St Louis Chldns Hosp; **Address:** Wash Univ Sch Med, Div Endo, Metab & Lipid Rsch, 660 S Euclid Ave, Box 8127, St Louis, MO 63110-1093; **Phone:** 314-362-7635; **Board Cert:** Internal Medicine 1972; Endocrinology, Diabetes & Metabolism 1972; **Med School:** Northwestern Univ 1965; **Resid:** Internal Medicine, Barnes Jewish Hosp 1972; **Fellow:** Endocrinology, Diabetes & Metabolism, Wash Univ Sch Med 1968; **Fac Appt:** Prof Med, Washington Univ, St Louis

Econs, Michael J MD [EDM] - **Spec Exp:** Osteoporosis; Paget's Disease of Bone; Metabolic Bone Disease; **Hospital:** Indiana Univ Hosp; **Address:** 541 N Clinical Dr, CL 459, Indianapolis, IN 46202; **Phone:** 317-274-1339; **Board Cert:** Internal Medicine 1986; Endocrinology, Diabetes & Metabolism 1989; **Med School:** UCSF 1983; **Resid:** Internal Medicine, Univ Maryland Hosp 1986; **Fellow:** Endocrinology, Duke Univ Med Ctr 1989; **Fac Appt:** Prof Med, Indiana Univ

Ehrmann, David A MD [EDM] - **Spec Exp:** Polycystic Ovarian Syndrome; Diabetes; **Hospital:** Univ of Chicago Hosps; **Address:** Univ Chicago, Div Endocrinology, 5758 S Maryland Ave, Ste 5A, MC 1027, Chicago, IL 60637; **Phone:** 773-702-6138; **Board Cert:** Internal Medicine 1985; Endocrinology, Diabetes & Metabolism 1987; **Med School:** Univ Mich Med Sch 1982; **Resid:** Internal Medicine, Univ Mich Med Ctr 1985; **Fellow:** Endocrinology, Diabetes & Metabolism, Univ Chicago Hosps 1987; **Fac Appt:** Assoc Prof Med, Univ Chicago-Pritzker Sch Med

Emanuele, Mary Ann MD [EDM] - **Spec Exp:** Diabetes; **Hospital:** Loyola Univ Med Ctr; **Address:** Loyola Univ Med Ctr, Dept Endocrinology, 2160 S 1st Ave Bldg 54 - rm 137A, Maywood, IL 60153-3304; **Phone:** 708-216-0160; **Board Cert:** Internal Medicine 1978; Endocrinology, Diabetes & Metabolism 1983; **Med School:** Loyola Univ-Stritch Sch Med 1975; **Resid:** Internal Medicine, Univ Hawaii Med Ctr 1978; **Fellow:** Endocrinology, Edward Hines Jr VA Hosp 1980; **Fac Appt:** Prof Med, Loyola Univ-Stritch Sch Med

Emanuele, Nicholas V MD [EDM] - **Hospital:** Hines VA Hosp; **Address:** Hines VA Hosp Bldg 200 - rm 1426, PO Box 5000, Hines, IL 60141; **Phone:** 708-202-8387 x21415; **Board Cert:** Internal Medicine 1975; Endocrinology 1979; **Med School:** Northwestern Univ 1967; **Resid:** Internal Medicine, Hines VA Hosp 1974; **Fellow:** Endocrinology, Northwestern Univ 1976

Herman, William H MD [EDM] - **Spec Exp:** Diabetes; Diabetes in Pregnancy; **Hospital:** Univ Michigan Hlth Sys; **Address:** A Alfred Taubman Health Care Ctr, 1500 E Medical Ctr Dr, 3920 TC, SPC5334, Ann Arbor, MI 48109-0354; **Phone:** 734-647-5922; **Board Cert:** Internal Medicine 1982; Endocrinology, Diabetes & Metabolism 1989; **Med School:** Boston Univ 1979; **Resid:** Internal Medicine, Univ Mich Med Ctr 1982; Preventive Medicine, Ctrs Dis Control 1985; **Fellow:** Endocrinology, Diabetes & Metabolism, Univ Mich Med Ctr 1988; **Fac Appt:** Prof Med, Univ Mich Med Sch

Hoogwerf, Byron J MD [EDM] - **Spec Exp:** Diabetes; Cholesterol/Lipid Disorders; Clinical Trials; Preventive Cardiology; **Hospital:** Cleveland Clin Fdn (page 56); **Address:** Cleveland Clinic, Div Endocrinology, 9500 Euclid Ave, Desk A-53, Cleveland, OH 44195-0001; **Phone:** 216-444-8347; **Board Cert:** Internal Medicine 1978; Endocrinology, Diabetes & Metabolism 1981; **Med School:** Univ Minn 1971; **Resid:** Internal Medicine, Hennepin Co Med Ctr 1978; **Fellow:** Endocrinology, Diabetes & Metabolism, Univ Minn Hosps 1981; **Fac Appt:** Prof Med, Ohio State Univ

Jensen, Michael D MD [EDM] - **Spec Exp:** Eating Disorders/Obesity; Nutrition; **Hospital:** Mayo Med Ctr & Clin - Rochester; **Address:** Mayo Clinic, Div Endocrinology, 200 First St SW, Rochester, MN 55905; **Phone:** 507-284-2462; **Board Cert:** Internal Medicine 1982; Endocrinology, Diabetes & Metabolism 1985; **Med School:** Univ MO-Kansas City 1979; **Resid:** Internal Medicine, Mayo Clinic 1982; **Fellow:** Endocrinology, Diabetes & Metabolism, Mayo Clinic 1985; **Fac Appt:** Prof Med, Mayo Med Sch

Khosla, Sundeep MD [EDM] - **Spec Exp:** Osteoporosis; Bone Disorders-Metabolic; **Hospital:** Mayo Med Ctr & Clin - Rochester; **Address:** Mayo Clinic, Div Endocrinology, 200 First St SW, Rochester, MN 55905; **Phone:** 507-284-1600; **Board Cert:** Internal Medicine 1985; Endocrinology 1987; **Med School:** Harvard Med Sch 1982; **Resid:** Internal Medicine, Mass Genl Hosp 1985; **Fellow:** Endocrinology, Diabetes & Metabolism, Mass Genl Hosp 1988; **Fac Appt:** Asst Prof Med, Mayo Med Sch

Kloos, Richard MD [EDM] - **Spec Exp:** Thyroid Cancer; **Hospital:** Ohio St Univ Med Ctr; **Address:** 446 McCampbell Hall, 1581 Dodd Drive, Columbus, OH 43210; **Phone:** 614-292-3800; **Board Cert:** Nuclear Medicine 2005; Internal Medicine 2002; Endocrinology, Diabetes & Metabolism 2005; **Med School:** Case West Res Univ 1989; **Resid:** Internal Medicine, MetroHealth MC 1992; **Fellow:** Endocrinology, Diabetes & Metabolism, Univ Michigan 1995; Nuclear Medicine, Univ Michigan 1996; **Fac Appt:** Assoc Prof Med, Ohio State Univ

Kopp, Peter A MD [EDM] - **Spec Exp:** Thyroid Cancer; Pituitary Disorders; Parathyroid Disease; Diabetes; **Hospital:** Northwestern Meml Hosp; **Address:** Northwestern Meml Hospital, 675 N St Clair St, Ste 14-100, Chicago, IL 60611; **Phone:** 312-695-7970; **Board Cert:** Internal Medicine 2003; Endocrinology, Diabetes & Metabolism 2004; **Med School:** Switzerland 1985; **Resid:** Internal Medicine, Regl Hosp 1992; Endocrinology, Diabetes & Metabolism, Univ Berne 1990; **Fellow:** Endocrinology, Diabetes & Metabolism, Northwestern Univ Hosp 1997; **Fac Appt:** Assoc Prof Med, Northwestern Univ-Feinberg Sch Med

Endocrinology, Diabetes & Metabolism

Licata, Angelo A MD [EDM] - **Spec Exp:** Bone Disorders-Metabolic; Osteoporosis; Calcium Disorders; **Hospital:** Cleveland Clin Fdn (page 56); **Address:** Div Endocrinology, 9500 Euclid Ave, Desk A53, Cleveland, OH 44195; **Phone:** 216-444-6248; **Board Cert:** Internal Medicine 1983; **Med School:** Univ Rochester 1973; **Resid:** Internal Medicine, Washington Univ Hosp 1974; Internal Medicine, Georgetown Univ Hosp 1978; **Fellow:** Endocrinology, Diabetes & Metabolism, Natl Inst Hlth 1976; **Fac Appt:** Asst Clin Prof Med, Case West Res Univ

Mazzone, Theodore MD [EDM] - **Spec Exp:** Cholesterol/Lipid Disorders; Diabetes; **Hospital:** Univ of IL Med Ctr at Chicago; **Address:** Univ Illinois Chicago, Div Diabetes & Metabolism, 1819 W Polk St, Chicago, IL 60612-7333; **Phone:** 312-355-4426; **Board Cert:** Internal Medicine 1980; Endocrinology, Diabetes & Metabolism 1983; **Med School:** Northwestern Univ 1977; **Resid:** Internal Medicine, UCLA Med Ctr 1980; **Fellow:** Endocrinology, Diabetes & Metabolism, Univ Wash Med Ctr 1983; **Fac Appt:** Prof Med, Univ IL Coll Med

McGill, Janet B MD [EDM] - **Spec Exp:** Diabetes; **Hospital:** Barnes-Jewish Hosp; **Address:** 4921 Parkview Pl, Box 8127, St Louis, MO 63110-1010; **Phone:** 314-747-7300; **Board Cert:** Internal Medicine 1983; Endocrinology, Diabetes & Metabolism 1987; **Med School:** Mich State Univ 1979; **Resid:** Internal Medicine, William Beaumont Hosp 1984; Endocrinology, Diabetes & Metabolism, William Beaumont Hosp 1985; **Fellow:** Diabetes, Washington Univ 1987; **Fac Appt:** Assoc Prof Med, Washington Univ, St Louis

McMahon, M Molly MD [EDM] - **Spec Exp:** Nutrition; Diabetes; **Hospital:** Mayo Med Ctr & Clin - Rochester; **Address:** Mayo Clinic, Div Endocrinology, 200 First St SW, Rochester, MN 55905; **Phone:** 507-284-2463; **Board Cert:** Internal Medicine 1985; Endocrinology, Diabetes & Metabolism 1987; **Med School:** Univ Wisc 1981; **Resid:** Internal Medicine, Med Coll Wisc 1984; **Fellow:** Endocrinology, Diabetes & Metabolism, Mayo Clinic 1987; Nutrition, New Eng Deaconess Hosp 1988

Polonsky, Kenneth S MD [EDM] - **Spec Exp:** Diabetes; **Hospital:** Barnes-Jewish Hosp; **Address:** Wash Univ School Medicine, Div Endo, Metab, & Lipid Rsch, 660 S Euclid Ave, Campus Box 8066, St Louis, MO 63110-1010; **Phone:** 314-362-8061; **Board Cert:** Internal Medicine 1978; **Med School:** South Africa 1973; **Resid:** Internal Medicine, Michael Reese Hosp & Med Ctr 1976; Internal Medicine, VA Hosp 1976; **Fellow:** Internal Medicine, Univ Chicago 1978; **Fac Appt:** Prof Med, Washington Univ, St Louis

Rizza, Robert Alan MD [EDM] - **Spec Exp:** Diabetes; Cholesterol/Lipid Disorders; **Hospital:** St Mary's Hosp - Rochester, Rochester Methodist Hosp; **Address:** Mayo Clinic - Div Endo, 200 First St SW, Fl W18B, Rochester, MN 55905-0002; **Phone:** 507-284-1600; **Board Cert:** Internal Medicine 1976; Endocrinology, Diabetes & Metabolism 1979; **Med School:** Univ Fla Coll Med 1971; **Resid:** Internal Medicine, Johns Hopkins Hosp 1973; **Fellow:** Endocrinology, Mayo Clinic 1979; **Fac Appt:** Prof Med, Mayo Med Sch

Semenkovich, Clay F MD [EDM] - **Spec Exp:** Cholesterol/Lipid Disorders; Diabetes; Endocrinology; **Hospital:** Barnes-Jewish Hosp; **Address:** Wash Univ Sch Med, Div Endo, Metab & Lipid Rsch, 660 S Euclid Ave, Box 8127, St Louis, MO 63110; **Phone:** 314-362-7617; **Board Cert:** Internal Medicine 1984; Endocrinology, Diabetes & Metabolism 1987; **Med School:** Washington Univ, St Louis 1981; **Resid:** Internal Medicine, Barnes Hosp 1984; **Fellow:** Endocrinology, Diabetes & Metabolism, Wash Univ 1986; **Fac Appt:** Prof Med, Washington Univ, St Louis

Service, Frederick J MD/PhD [EDM] - **Spec Exp:** Hypoglycemia; Diabetes; **Hospital:** Mayo Med Ctr & Clin - Rochester; **Address:** Mayo Clinic, Div Endocrinology, 200 First St SW, Rochester, MN 55905-0001; **Phone:** 507-284-5643; **Board Cert:** Internal Medicine 1977; Endocrinology, Diabetes & Metabolism 1972; **Med School:** McGill Univ 1962; **Resid:** Internal Medicine, Royal Victoria Hosp 1965; **Fellow:** Endocrinology, Diabetes & Metabolism, Mayo Grad Sch 1969; **Fac Appt:** Prof Med, Mayo Med Sch

America's Top Doctors® 8th Edition

Sowers, James R MD [EDM] - **Spec Exp:** Diabetes; Hypertension; Cholesterol/Lipid Disorders; **Hospital:** Univ of Missouri Hosp & Clins; **Address:** UMC, Dept Internal Med, One Hospital Drive, rm D109, Columbia, MO 65212; **Phone:** 573-882-2573; **Board Cert:** Internal Medicine 1974; Endocrinology, Diabetes & Metabolism 1977; **Med School:** Univ MO-Columbia Sch Med 1971; **Resid:** Internal Medicine, St Johns Mercy Med Ctr 1974; **Fellow:** Endocrinology, Wadsworth VA Hosp Ctr-UCLA 1976; **Fac Appt:** Prof Med, Univ MO-Columbia Sch Med

Veldhuis, Johannes D MD [EDM] - **Spec Exp:** Reproductive Endocrinology; Pituitary Disorders; Adrenal Disorders; Hypogonadism; **Hospital:** Mayo Med Ctr & Clin - Rochester; **Address:** Mayo Clinic, Div Endocrinology, 200 First St Sw, Joseph 5-194, Rochester, MN 55905; **Phone:** 507-284-3915; **Board Cert:** Internal Medicine 1977; Endocrinology 1979; **Med School:** Penn State Univ-Hershey Med Ctr 1974; **Resid:** Internal Medicine, Mayo Grad Sch Med 1977; **Fellow:** Endocrinology, Diabetes & Metabolism, Penn State Univ Hosp 1978; **Fac Appt:** Prof Med, Mayo Med Sch

Watts, Nelson B MD [EDM] - **Spec Exp:** Osteoporosis; Metabolic Bone Disease; Paget's Disease of Bone; **Hospital:** Univ Hosp - Cincinnati; **Address:** Univ Bone Health & Osteoporosis Ctr, 222 Piedmont Ave, Ste 6300, Cincinnati, OH 45219; **Phone:** 513-475-7400; **Board Cert:** Internal Medicine 1972; Endocrinology, Diabetes & Metabolism 1985; **Med School:** Univ NC Sch Med 1969; **Resid:** Internal Medicine, Charlotte Meml Hosp 1972; **Fellow:** Endocrinology, Diabetes & Metabolism, NC Meml Hosp 1971; **Fac Appt:** Prof Med, Univ Cincinnati

Werner, Phillip L MD [EDM] - **Spec Exp:** Diabetes; **Hospital:** Adv Luth Genl Hosp; **Address:** 1775 Ballard Rd, Nesset Pavilion, Park Ridge, IL 60068; **Phone:** 847-318-2400; **Board Cert:** Internal Medicine 1975; Endocrinology 1977; **Med School:** Univ IL Coll Med 1972; **Resid:** Internal Medicine, Univ Illinois Affl Hosp 1975; **Fellow:** Endocrinology, Diabetes & Metabolism, Univ Wash 1977; **Fac Appt:** Prof Med, Ros Franklin Univ/Chicago Med Sch

Great Plains and Mountains

Eckel, Robert H MD [EDM] - **Spec Exp:** Cholesterol/Lipid Disorders; Eating Disorders/Obesity; Diabetes; **Hospital:** Univ Colorado Hosp; **Address:** Univ Colorado Hlth Scis Ctr, PO Box 6510, MS F732, Aurora, CO 80045; **Phone:** 720-848-2650; **Board Cert:** Internal Medicine 1976; Endocrinology, Diabetes & Metabolism 1979; **Med School:** Univ Cincinnati 1973; **Resid:** Internal Medicine, Univ Wisconsin Hosps 1976; **Fellow:** Endocrinology, Diabetes & Metabolism, Univ Washington 1979; **Fac Appt:** Prof Med, Univ Colorado

Recker, Robert Roy MD [EDM] - **Spec Exp:** Osteoporosis; Diabetes; Endocrinology; **Hospital:** Creighton Univ Med Ctr, VA Medical Ctr - Omaha; **Address:** Creighton Univ Osteoporosis, Div Endocrinology, 601 N 30th St, Ste 4820, Omaha, NE 68131; **Phone:** 402-280-4470; **Board Cert:** Internal Medicine 1971; **Med School:** Creighton Univ 1963; **Resid:** Internal Medicine, Creighton Affil Hosps 1969; **Fellow:** Endocrinology, Diabetes & Metabolism, Creighton Univ 1971; **Fac Appt:** Prof Med, Creighton Univ

Ridgway, E Chester MD [EDM] - **Spec Exp:** Thyroid Cancer; Thyroid Disorders; Pituitary Disorders; **Hospital:** Univ Colorado Hosp, VA Med Ctr; **Address:** UCHSC at Fitzsimons, Endocrinology, 1635 N Ursula St, Box 6510, MS F732, Aurora, CO 80045; **Phone:** 720-848-2650; **Board Cert:** Internal Medicine 1972; Endocrinology 1973; **Med School:** Univ Colorado 1968; **Resid:** Internal Medicine, Mass Genl Hosp 1970; **Fellow:** Endocrinology, Mass Genl Hosp 1972; **Fac Appt:** Prof Med, Univ Colorado

Endocrinology, Diabetes & Metabolism

Southwest

Cunningham, Glenn R MD [EDM] - **Spec Exp:** Diabetes; Hypogonadism; Erectile Dysfunction; **Hospital:** St Luke's Episcopal Hosp - Houston; **Address:** 6624 Fannin St, Ste 1180, Houston, TX 77030; **Phone:** 832-355-7208; **Board Cert:** Internal Medicine 1972; Endocrinology, Diabetes & Metabolism 1972; **Med School:** Univ Okla Coll Med 1966; **Resid:** Internal Medicine, Duke Univ Med Ctr 1970; **Fellow:** Endocrinology, Duke Univ Med Ctr 1971; **Fac Appt:** Prof Med, Baylor Coll Med

Lavis, Victor Ralph MD [EDM] - **Spec Exp:** Diabetes; **Hospital:** UT MD Anderson Cancer Ctr, Meml Hermann Hosp - Texas Med Ctr; **Address:** MD Anderson Cancer Ctr, 1515 Holcombe Blvd, Ste 435, Houston, TX 77050; **Phone:** 713-792-2841; **Board Cert:** Internal Medicine 1969; Endocrinology, Diabetes & Metabolism 1998; **Med School:** Stanford Univ 1962; **Resid:** Internal Medicine, Boston Cty Hosp 1964; Internal Medicine, UCLA Med Ctr 1967; **Fellow:** Endocrinology, Diabetes & Metabolism, Univ Washington 1970; **Fac Appt:** Prof Med, Univ Tex, Houston

Raskin, Philip MD [EDM] - **Spec Exp:** Diabetes; **Hospital:** Parkland Meml Hosp - Dallas, UT Southwestern Med Ctr - Dallas; **Address:** Univ Tex SW Med Ctr, 5323 Harry Hines Blvd, Ste G5.238, Dallas, TX 75390-8858; **Phone:** 214-645-2800; **Board Cert:** Internal Medicine 1972; Endocrinology 1973; **Med School:** Univ Pittsburgh 1966; **Resid:** Internal Medicine, Hlth Ctr Hosps-Univ Pittsburgh 1968; **Fellow:** Endocrinology, Diabetes & Metabolism, UT SW Med Sch 1972; **Fac Appt:** Prof Med, Univ Tex SW, Dallas

Reasner II, Charles A MD [EDM] - **Spec Exp:** Thyroid Disorders; **Hospital:** Univ Hlth Sys - Univ Hosp (San Antonio, TX); **Address:** Texas Diabetes Inst, 701 S Zarzamora St, MS 12-5, San Antonio, TX 78207; **Phone:** 210-358-7402; **Board Cert:** Internal Medicine 1983; Endocrinology 1985; **Med School:** Loma Linda Univ 1979; **Resid:** Internal Medicine, USAF Med Ctr 1983; **Fellow:** Endocrinology, Diabetes & Metabolism, Wilford Hall Med Ctr 1985; **Fac Appt:** Assoc Prof Med, Univ Tex, San Antonio

Robbins, Richard MD [EDM] - **Spec Exp:** Thyroid Cancer; Pituitary Tumors; Pituitary Disorders; **Hospital:** Methodist Hosp - Houston; **Address:** The Methodist Hosp, 6550 Fannin St, Ste 1001, Houston, TX 77030; **Phone:** 713-441-6640; **Board Cert:** Internal Medicine 1978; Endocrinology, Diabetes & Metabolism 1983; **Med School:** Creighton Univ 1975; **Resid:** Internal Medicine, New York Hosp-Cornell Med Ctr 1978; **Fellow:** Endocrinology, New England Med Ctr 1981; **Fac Appt:** Prof Med, Cornell Univ-Weill Med Coll

Rubenfeld, Sheldon MD [EDM] - **Spec Exp:** Thyroid Cancer; Thyroid Disorders; Diabetes; **Hospital:** St Luke's Episcopal Hosp - Houston, Methodist Hosp - Houston; **Address:** 7515 S Main St, Ste 690, Houston, TX 77030; **Phone:** 713-795-5750; **Board Cert:** Internal Medicine 1976; Endocrinology, Diabetes & Metabolism 1979; **Med School:** Georgetown Univ 1971; **Resid:** Internal Medicine, Baylor Affil Hosps 1976; **Fellow:** Endocrinology, Baylor Affil Hosps 1978; **Fac Appt:** Clin Prof Med, Baylor Coll Med

Sherman, Steven I MD [EDM] - **Spec Exp:** Thyroid Cancer; Endocrine Cancers; **Hospital:** UT MD Anderson Cancer Ctr; **Address:** MD Anderson Cancer Ctr, 1515 Holcombe Blvd, Unit 435, Houston, TX 77030; **Phone:** 713-792-2840; **Board Cert:** Internal Medicine 1988; Endocrinology, Diabetes & Metabolism 2007; **Med School:** Johns Hopkins Univ 1985; **Resid:** Internal Medicine, Johns Hopkins Hosp 1988; **Fellow:** Endocrinology, Diabetes & Metabolism, Johns Hopkins Hosp 1991

Waguespack, Steven G MD [EDM] - **Spec Exp:** Thyroid Cancer; Pituitary Tumors; Adrenal Tumors & Disorders; **Hospital:** UT MD Anderson Cancer Ctr; **Address:** MD Anderson Cancer Ctr, Dept Endocrine Neoplasia, 1400 Holcombe Blvd, Unit 435, Houston, TX 77030; **Phone:** 713-563-4400; **Board Cert:** Internal Medicine 1998; Endocrinology, Diabetes & Metabolism 2002; Pediatric Endocrinology 2003; **Med School:** Univ Tex, Houston 1994; **Resid:** Internal Medicine & Pediatrics, Indiana Univ Hosp 1998; **Fellow:** Endocrinology, Indiana Univ Hosp 2002; **Fac Appt:** Assoc Prof Med, Univ Tex, Houston

West Coast and Pacific

Berkson, Richard A MD [EDM] - **Spec Exp:** Diabetes; Thyroid Disorders; **Hospital:** St Mary Med Ctr - Long Beach, CA, Long Beach Meml Med Ctr; **Address:** 1868 Pacific Ave, Long Beach, CA 90806-6113; **Phone:** 562-595-4718; **Board Cert:** Internal Medicine 1975; Endocrinology, Diabetes & Metabolism 1977; **Med School:** SUNY Buffalo 1972; **Resid:** Internal Medicine, SUNY Buffalo Affil Hosp 1975; **Fellow:** Endocrinology, Diabetes & Metabolism, Joslin Clinic 1976; Endocrinology, Diabetes & Metabolism, UCLA Med Ctr 1977; **Fac Appt:** Assoc Clin Prof Med, UCLA

Braunstein, Glenn D MD [EDM] - **Spec Exp:** Hormonal Disorders; **Hospital:** Cedars-Sinai Med Ctr; **Address:** Cedars Sinai Med Ctr, 8700 Beverly Blvd, Ste 2119, Los Angeles, CA 90048; **Phone:** 310-423-5140; **Board Cert:** Internal Medicine 1973; Endocrinology, Diabetes & Metabolism 1975; **Med School:** UCSF 1968; **Resid:** Internal Medicine, Peter Bent Bringham Hosp 1970; Endocrinology, Diabetes & Metabolism, Natl Inst Hlth-NICHHD 1972; **Fellow:** Endocrinology, Diabetes & Metabolism, LA Co Harbor Genl Hosp 1973; **Fac Appt:** Prof Med, UCLA

Chopra, Inder J MD [EDM] - **Spec Exp:** Thyroid Disorders; Endocrine Disorders; **Hospital:** Ronald Reagan UCLA Med Ctr; **Address:** UCLA Sch Med, Div Endocrinology, 900 Veteran Ave, Ste 24-130, Los Angeles, CA 90095-7073; **Phone:** 310-825-2346; **Board Cert:** Internal Medicine 1972; Endocrinology, Diabetes & Metabolism 1973; **Med School:** India 1961; **Resid:** Internal Medicine, All India Inst Med Sci 1965; Internal Medicine, Queens Med Ctr 1968; **Fellow:** Endocrinology, Diabetes & Metabolism, LAC-Harbor-UCLA Med Ctr 1971; **Fac Appt:** Prof Med, UCLA

Darwin, Christine H MD [EDM] - **Spec Exp:** Pituitary Tumors; Diabetes; **Hospital:** Ronald Reagan UCLA Med Ctr; **Address:** 200 UCLA Medical Plaza, Ste 365A, Box 951693, Los Angeles, CA 90095-7065; **Phone:** 310-794-5584; **Board Cert:** Geriatric Medicine 1994; Endocrinology, Diabetes & Metabolism 1997; **Med School:** India 1980; **Resid:** Internal Medicine, UC Irvine Med Ctr 1987; **Fellow:** Endocrinology, VA Hosp 1988; Endocrinology, USC Med Ctr 1993; **Fac Appt:** Assoc Prof Med, UCLA

Fitzgerald, Paul A MD [EDM] - **Spec Exp:** Diabetes; Thyroid Cancer; Pituitary Tumors; Thyroid Disorders; **Hospital:** UCSF Med Ctr; **Address:** 350 Parnassus Ave, Ste 710, San Francisco, CA 94117; **Phone:** 415-665-1136; **Board Cert:** Internal Medicine 1975; Endocrinology, Diabetes & Metabolism 1981; **Med School:** Jefferson Med Coll 1972; **Resid:** Internal Medicine, Presby Med Ctr-Univ Colo 1975; **Fellow:** Endocrinology, Diabetes & Metabolism, UCSF Med Ctr 1978; **Fac Appt:** Clin Prof Med, UCSF

Heber, David MD [EDM] - **Spec Exp:** Nutrition & Cancer Prevention; Nutrition & Disease Prevention/Control; Nutrition & Obesity; **Hospital:** Ronald Reagan UCLA Med Ctr; **Address:** 900 Veteran Ave, Rm 12-217, UCLA Center for Human Nutrition, Los Angeles, CA 90095-1742; **Phone:** 310-206-1987; **Board Cert:** Internal Medicine 1976; Endocrinology, Diabetes & Metabolism 1977; **Med School:** Harvard Med Sch 1973; **Resid:** Internal Medicine, LA Co Harbor Genl Hosp 1975; **Fellow:** Endocrinology, Diabetes & Metabolism, LA Co Harbor Genl Hosp 1978; **Fac Appt:** Prof Med, UCLA

Endocrinology, Diabetes & Metabolism

Hirsch, Irl B MD [EDM] - **Spec Exp:** Diabetes; **Hospital:** Univ Wash Med Ctr; **Address:** Univ Wash Med Ctr, Diabetes Care Ctr, 4225 Roosevelt Way NE, Ste 101, Seattle, WA 98105; **Phone:** 206-548-4882; **Board Cert:** Internal Medicine 1987; Endocrinology, Diabetes & Metabolism 1989; **Med School:** Univ MO-Columbia Sch Med 1984; **Resid:** Internal Medicine, Mt Sinai Med Ctr 1987; **Fellow:** Metabolism, Washington Univ Sch Med 1989; **Fac Appt:** Prof Med, Univ Wash

Hoffman, Andrew R MD [EDM] - **Spec Exp:** Pituitary Disorders; Pituitary Tumors; Neuroendocrinology; **Hospital:** Stanford Univ Med Ctr, VA Hlth Care Sys - Palo Alto; **Address:** 300 Pastur Drive Boswell Bldg - rm A-175, Stanford, CA 94305; **Phone:** 650-723-6961; **Board Cert:** Internal Medicine 1979; Endocrinology 1981; **Med School:** Stanford Univ 1976; **Resid:** Internal Medicine, Mass Genl Hosp 1978; **Fellow:** Pharmacology, Mass Genl Hosp 1980; Endocrinology, Diabetes & Metabolism, Mass Genl Hosp 1982; **Fac Appt:** Prof Med, Stanford Univ

Hsueh, Willa Ann MD [EDM] - **Spec Exp:** Diabetes; Hypertension; **Hospital:** Ronald Reagan UCLA Med Ctr; **Address:** 900 Veteran Ave, Ste 24-130, Los Angeles, CA 90095; **Phone:** 310-794-5403; **Board Cert:** Internal Medicine 1976; Endocrinology, Diabetes & Metabolism 1977; **Med School:** Ohio State Univ 1973; **Resid:** Internal Medicine, Johns Hopkins Hosp 1975; **Fellow:** Endocrinology, Diabetes & Metabolism, Johns Hopkins Hosp 1976; **Fac Appt:** Prof Med, UCLA

Ipp, Eli MD [EDM] - **Spec Exp:** Diabetes; **Hospital:** LAC - Harbor - UCLA Med Ctr; **Address:** 21840 S Normandy Ave, Ste 700, Torrance, CA 90502; **Phone:** 310-222-5101; **Board Cert:** Internal Medicine 1979; Endocrinology, Diabetes & Metabolism 1981; **Med School:** South Africa 1968; **Resid:** Internal Medicine, Tel Hashomer Hosp 1974; **Fellow:** Endocrinology, Diabetes & Metabolism, Univ Tex SW Med Ctr 1978; **Fac Appt:** Prof Med, UCLA

Kamdar, Vikram V MD [EDM] - **Spec Exp:** Diabetes; Diabetic Leg/Foot; Thyroid Disorders; **Hospital:** Santa Monica - UCLA Med Ctr, Ronald Reagan UCLA Med Ctr; **Address:** 1801 Wilshire Blvd, Ste 100, Santa Monica, CA 90403; **Phone:** 310-828-7172; **Board Cert:** Internal Medicine 1978; Endocrinology, Diabetes & Metabolism 1979; **Med School:** India 1971; **Resid:** Internal Medicine, Lemuel Shattuck Hosp 1972; Endocrinology, Diabetes & Metabolism, Cedars-Sinai Med Ctr 1977; **Fellow:** Endocrinology, Diabetes & Metabolism, LA Co-USC Med Ctr 1975; **Fac Appt:** Assoc Clin Prof Med, UCLA

Kandeel, Fouad MD/PhD [EDM] - **Spec Exp:** Thyroid Cancer; Endocrine Cancers; Neuroendocrinology; **Hospital:** City of Hope Natl Med Ctr & Beckman Rsch; **Address:** City of Hope, Diabetes Department, 1500 E Duarte Rd, Duarte, CA 91010; **Phone:** 626-256-4673 x62251; **Med School:** Egypt 1969; **Fac Appt:** Assoc Clin Prof Med, UCLA

Melmed, Shlomo MD [EDM] - **Spec Exp:** Pituitary Tumors; Acromegaly; Pituitary Disorders; **Hospital:** Cedars-Sinai Med Ctr; **Address:** Cedars Sinai Med Ctr, 8700 Beverly Blvd, Ste 2015, Los Angeles, CA 90048; **Phone:** 310-423-4691; **Board Cert:** Internal Medicine 1979; Endocrinology, Diabetes & Metabolism 1983; **Med School:** South Africa 1970; **Resid:** Internal Medicine, Sheba Med Ctr 1976; **Fellow:** Endocrinology, Diabetes & Metabolism, Wadsworth VA Hosp 1980; **Fac Appt:** Prof Med, UCLA

Orwoll, Eric S MD [EDM] - **Spec Exp:** Osteoporosis; Osteoporosis in Men; **Hospital:** OR Hlth & Sci Univ; **Address:** Oregon Hlth & Sci Univ, Bone/Mineral Unit, 3181 SW Sam Jackson Park Rd, MC PPV05, Portland, OR 97239; **Phone:** 503-494-3273; **Board Cert:** Internal Medicine 1977; Endocrinology, Diabetes & Metabolism 1979; **Med School:** Univ MD Sch Med 1974; **Resid:** Internal Medicine, Providence Med Ctr 1977; **Fellow:** Endocrinology, Diabetes & Metabolism, Univ Oregon Hlth Sci Ctr 1979; **Fac Appt:** Prof Med, Oregon Hlth Sci Univ

Riddle, Matthew C MD [EDM] - **Spec Exp:** Diabetes; Clinical Trials; **Hospital:** OR Hlth & Sci Univ; **Address:** Oregon Hlth & Sci Univ, Div Endo, 3181 SW Sam Jackson Park Rd, MC L-345, Portland, OR 97239-3011; **Phone:** 503-494-3273; **Board Cert:** Internal Medicine 1972; Endocrinology, Diabetes & Metabolism 1972; **Med School:** Harvard Med Sch 1964; **Resid:** Internal Medicine, Rush-Presby-St Lukes Hosp 1969; **Fellow:** Endocrinology, Diabetes & Metabolism, Rush Presby-St Lukes Hosp 1971; Endocrinology, Diabetes & Metabolism, Univ Washington 1973; **Fac Appt:** Prof Med, Oregon Hlth Sci Univ

Singer, Peter A MD [EDM] - **Spec Exp:** Thyroid Disorders; **Hospital:** USC Univ Hosp - R K Eamer Med Plz; **Address:** 1520 San Pablo St Fl 1 - Ste 1000, Los Angeles, CA 90033; **Phone:** 323-442-5100; **Board Cert:** Internal Medicine 1972; Endocrinology, Diabetes & Metabolism 1973; **Med School:** UCSF 1965; **Resid:** Internal Medicine, LAC-USC Med Ctr 1971; **Fellow:** Endocrinology, Diabetes & Metabolism, LAC-USC Med Ctr 1973; **Fac Appt:** Clin Prof Med, USC Sch Med

Swerdloff, Ronald S MD [EDM] - **Spec Exp:** Reproductive Endocrinology-Male; Pituitary Disorders; **Hospital:** LAC - Harbor - UCLA Med Ctr; **Address:** 1000 W Carson St, Box 446, Torrance, CA 90509-2910; **Phone:** 310-222-1867; **Board Cert:** Internal Medicine 1968; Endocrinology 1972; **Med School:** UCSF 1962; **Resid:** Internal Medicine, Univ Washington Hosp 1964; Endocrinology, Diabetes & Metabolism, NIH Gerontology Branch 1966; **Fellow:** Endocrinology, Diabetes & Metabolism, Harbor-UCLA Med Ctr 1969; **Fac Appt:** Prof Med, UCLA

Woeber, Kenneth A MD [EDM] - **Spec Exp:** Thyroid Disorders; **Hospital:** UCSF Med Ctr; **Address:** 2200 Post St, rm C-432, Box 1640, San Francisco, CA 94143; **Phone:** 415-885-7574; **Board Cert:** Internal Medicine 1980; Endocrinology, Diabetes & Metabolism 1973; **Med School:** South Africa 1957; **Resid:** Internal Medicine, Jackson Meml Hosp 1962; **Fellow:** Endocrinology, Diabetes & Metabolism, Harvard/Boston City Hosp 1964; **Fac Appt:** Prof Med, UCSF

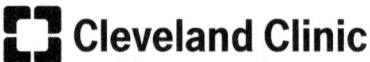 **Cleveland Clinic**

Endocrinology, Diabetes and Metabolism

Cleveland Clinic Department of Endocrinology treats patients in all the major disease categories such as diabetes, thyroid disorders, sexual hormone disorders, metabolism, pituitary disorders and more. In addition, the department has several specialty clinics dedicated to:

- Cardiovascular risk reduction
- Type 1 Diabetes
- Pituitary
- Thyroid
- Transition Clinic (Pediatrics to Adult)
- Intensive Diabetic Care- DM2 Clinic

Patients with difficult-to-control diabetes or high risk patients with diabetes (i.e. diabetics who recently experienced a heart attack or underwent bypass surgery) can be treated at the Diabetes Mellitus Disease Management (DM2) Clinic for seamless, intensive management of their disease. The goal is to stabilize patients within six months, and return them back to their primary care providers within twelve months.

Thyroid Biopsy
The department has been a leader in incorporating fine needle aspirations and ultrasounds into the realm of endocrinology. Our fellowship program was one of the first in the nation to train fellows in ultrasound-guided biopsy techniques of the thyroid.

Pituitary Clinic
Pituitary care at Cleveland Clinic is a collaborative approach between endocrinologists, neurosurgeons and radiation oncologists, resulting in national recognition. Cleveland Clinic is one of the top centers in the U.S. for volume of pituitary surgeries at an institution.

Center for Osteoporosis and Metabolic Bone Disease
A joint effort between the Departments of Endocrinology and Rheumatology, the Center for Osteoporosis and Metabolic Bone Disease is devoted to the evaluation and treatment of patients with osteoporosis and other forms of diseases that affect bones. The Center's goal is to evaluate patients at an early stage to prevent complications and treat patients at the earliest possible stage to prevent additional disease manifestations.

For more information about the Cleveland Clinic Department of Endocrinology, Diabetes and Metabolism, to schedule a second opinion or to learn about assistance for out-of-town patients, call call 800.890.2467 or visit www.clevelandclinic.org/endotopdocs.

Department of Endocrinology, Diabetes and Metabolism
9500 Euclid Avenue / AC311 | Cleveland OH 44195

Gastroenterology
a subspecialty of Internal Medicine

An internist who specializes in diagnosis and treatment of diseases of the digestive organs including the stomach, bowels, liver and gallbladder. This specialist treats conditions such as abdominal pain, ulcers, diarrhea, cancer and jaundice and performs complex diagnostic and therapeutic procedures using endoscopes to see internal organs.

Training Required: Three years in internal medicine *plus* additional training and examination for certification in gastroenterology.

GASTROENTEROLOGY

New England

Carr-Locke, David L MD [Ge] - **Spec Exp:** Pancreatic/Biliary Endoscopy (ERCP); Pancreatic & Biliary Disease; Endoscopy; **Hospital:** Brigham & Women's Hosp; **Address:** Brigham & Women's Hosp-Endoscopy Ctr, 45 Francis St, Boston, MA 02115-6106; **Phone:** 617-732-7414; **Board Cert:** Internal Medicine 1974; **Med School:** England 1972; **Resid:** Obstetrics & Gynecology, Orsett Hosp 1974; Internal Medicine, Leicester Hosp 1976; **Fellow:** Gastroenterology, Leicester Hosp 1978; Research, New Eng Baptist Hosp 1979; **Fac Appt:** Assoc Prof Med, Harvard Med Sch

Dienstag, Jules L MD [Ge] - **Spec Exp:** Liver Disease; Hepatitis; Transplant Medicine-Liver; **Hospital:** Mass Genl Hosp; **Address:** Mass Genl Hosp, GI Unit, 55 Fruit St Warren Bldg Fl 10, Boston, MA 02114-2622; **Phone:** 617-724-7562; **Board Cert:** Internal Medicine 1975; **Med School:** Columbia P&S 1972; **Resid:** Internal Medicine, Univ Chicago-Billings Hosp 1974; **Fellow:** Infectious Disease, Natl Inst Hlth 1976; Gastroenterology, Mass Genl Hosp 1978; **Fac Appt:** Prof Med, Harvard Med Sch

Friedman, Lawrence S MD [Ge] - **Spec Exp:** Liver Disease; **Hospital:** Newton - Wellesley Hosp, Mass Genl Hosp; **Address:** Newton-Wellesley Hospital, Dept Medicine, 2014 Washington St, Newton, MA 02462; **Phone:** 617-243-5480; **Board Cert:** Internal Medicine 1981; Gastroenterology 2005; **Med School:** Johns Hopkins Univ 1978; **Resid:** Internal Medicine, Johns Hopkins Hosp 1981; **Fellow:** Gastroenterology, Mass Genl Hosp 1984; **Fac Appt:** Prof Med, Harvard Med Sch

Levine, Joel B MD [Ge] - **Spec Exp:** Colon & Rectal Cancer Detection; Colonoscopy; Gastroesophageal Reflux Disease (GERD); **Hospital:** Univ of Conn Hlth Ctr, John Dempsey Hosp; **Address:** Univ Connecticut Health Center, Colon Cancer Prevention Program, 263 Farmington Ave, Farmington, CT 06030-2813; **Phone:** 860-679-4567; **Board Cert:** Internal Medicine 1973; Gastroenterology 1977; **Med School:** SUNY Downstate 1969; **Resid:** Internal Medicine, Univ Chicago Hosps 1971; Internal Medicine, Mass Genl Hosp 1974; **Fellow:** Gastroenterology, Mass Genl Hosp 1977; **Fac Appt:** Prof Med, Univ Conn

Mason, Joel B MD [Ge] - **Spec Exp:** Nutrition in Acute Illness; Nutrition in Bowel Disorders; Nutrition & Cancer Prevention; **Hospital:** Tufts Med Ctr; **Address:** Tupper Research Institute, 8, Box 239, 15 Kneeland St, Boston, MA 02111; **Phone:** 617-636-7754; **Board Cert:** Internal Medicine 1984; Gastroenterology 1987; **Med School:** Univ Chicago-Pritzker Sch Med 1981; **Resid:** Internal Medicine, Univ Iowa Hosps 1984; **Fellow:** Gastroenterology, Univ Chicago Hosps 1986; Nutrition, Univ Chicago Hosps 1986; **Fac Appt:** Assoc Prof Med, Tufts Univ

Rothstein, Richard I MD [Ge] - **Spec Exp:** Gastroesophageal Reflux Disease (GERD); Swallowing Disorders; Barrett's Esophagus; Endoscopy; **Hospital:** Dartmouth - Hitchcock Med Ctr; **Address:** Dartmouth-Hitchcock Medical Center, Div Gastroenterology, 1 Medical Center Drive, Lebanon, NH 03756; **Phone:** 603-650-8343; **Board Cert:** Internal Medicine 1983; Gastroenterology 1987; **Med School:** Boston Univ 1980; **Resid:** Internal Medicine, Univ Mass Med Ctr 1983; **Fellow:** Gastroenterology, Dartmouth-Hitchcock Med Ctr 1985; **Fac Appt:** Prof Med, Dartmouth Med Sch

Wolfe, M Michael MD [Ge] - **Hospital:** Boston Med Ctr; **Address:** 650 Albany St, Ste 504, Boston, MA 02118; **Phone:** 617-638-7440; **Board Cert:** Internal Medicine 1979; Gastroenterology 1981; **Med School:** Ohio State Univ 1976; **Resid:** Internal Medicine, Med Coll Penn Hosp 1979; **Fellow:** Gastroenterology, Univ Florida Hosps 1982; **Fac Appt:** Prof Med, Boston Univ

Mid Atlantic

Albert, Michael B MD [Ge] - **Spec Exp:** Inflammatory Bowel Disease; Ulcerative Colitis; **Hospital:** G Washington Univ Hosp; **Address:** 2141 K St NW, Ste 208, Washington, DC 20037; **Phone:** 202-223-5544; **Board Cert:** Internal Medicine 1985; Gastroenterology 1987; **Med School:** Johns Hopkins Univ 1982; **Resid:** Internal Medicine, Mayo Clinic 1984; Internal Medicine, Duke Univ Med Ctr 1985; **Fellow:** Gastroenterology, G Washington Univ Med Ctr 1987; **Fac Appt:** Prof Med, Geo Wash Univ

Aronchick, Craig A MD [Ge] - **Spec Exp:** Barrett's Esophagus; Pancreatic/Biliary Endoscopy (ERCP); **Hospital:** Pennsylvania Hosp (page 60); **Address:** 230 W Washington Square, Farm Journal Bldg, Fl 4, Philadelphia, PA 19106; **Phone:** 215-829-3561; **Board Cert:** Internal Medicine 1981; Gastroenterology 1983; **Med School:** Temple Univ 1978; **Resid:** Internal Medicine, Temple Univ Hosp 1981; **Fellow:** Gastroenterology, Hosp Univ Penn 1983; **Fac Appt:** Assoc Clin Prof Med, Univ Pennsylvania

Bayless, Theodore MD [Ge] - **Spec Exp:** Inflammatory Bowel Disease/Crohn's; Ulcerative Colitis; Malabsorption Syndrome; **Hospital:** Johns Hopkins Hosp - Baltimore (page 61); **Address:** 600 N Wolfe St, Blalock Bldg - Ste 461, C/O Johns Hopkins Hosp, Baltimore, MD 21287-0005; **Phone:** 410-955-4166; **Board Cert:** Internal Medicine 1966; **Med School:** Ros Franklin Univ/Chicago Med Sch 1957; **Resid:** Internal Medicine, Cornell-Bellevue Hosp 1958; Internal Medicine, Meml Sloan Kettering Hosp 1960; **Fellow:** Gastroenterology, Johns Hopkins Hosp 1962; **Fac Appt:** Prof Med, Johns Hopkins Univ

Bodenheimer Jr, Henry C MD [Ge] - **Spec Exp:** Hepatitis; Transplant Medicine-Liver; Liver & Biliary Disease; **Hospital:** Beth Israel Med Ctr - Petrie Division (page 57); **Address:** Beth Israel Med Ctr, Div Digestive Diseases, 1st Ave @ 16th St, New York, NY 10003; **Phone:** 212-420-4015; **Board Cert:** Internal Medicine 1978; Gastroenterology 1981; Transplant Hepatology 2006; **Med School:** Tufts Univ 1975; **Resid:** Internal Medicine, Mount Sinai Hosp 1978; **Fellow:** Gastroenterology, Mount Sinai Hosp 1979; Gastroenterology, Rhode Island Hosp 1981; **Fac Appt:** Prof Med, Albert Einstein Coll Med

Borum, Marie L MD [Ge] - **Spec Exp:** Colonoscopy; AIDS/HIV-Gastrointestinal Complications; Women's Health; Liver Disease; **Hospital:** G Washington Univ Hosp; **Address:** MFA Dept Medicine, 2150 Pennsylvania Ave NW, Ste 3-410, Washington, DC 20037; **Phone:** 202-741-3333; **Board Cert:** Internal Medicine 1988; Gastroenterology 2001; **Med School:** UMDNJ-Rutgers Med Sch 1985; **Resid:** Internal Medicine, G Washington Univ Med Ctr 1988; **Fellow:** Gastroenterology, G Washington Univ Med Ctr 1991; **Fac Appt:** Prof Med, Geo Wash Univ

Brandt, Lawrence MD [Ge] - **Spec Exp:** Geriatric Gastroenterology; Inflammatory Bowel Disease; **Hospital:** Montefiore Med Ctr; **Address:** 3400 Bainbridge Ave Fl 2, Bronx, NY 10467-2401; **Phone:** 866-633-8255; **Board Cert:** Internal Medicine 1972; Gastroenterology 1975; **Med School:** SUNY Downstate 1968; **Resid:** Internal Medicine, Mount Sinai Hosp 1972; **Fellow:** Gastroenterology, Mount Sinai Hosp 1972; **Fac Appt:** Prof Med, Albert Einstein Coll Med

Canto, Marcia MD [Ge] - **Spec Exp:** Endoscopy; Endoscopic Ultrasound; Pancreatic Cancer-Early Detection; **Hospital:** Johns Hopkins Hosp - Baltimore (page 61); **Address:** Dept of Med, Gastroenterology, 1830 E Monument St, rm 426, Baltimore, MD 21205; **Phone:** 410-614-5388; **Board Cert:** Internal Medicine 1989; **Med School:** Philippines 1985; **Resid:** Internal Medicine, SUNY Hlth Sci Ctr 1991; **Fellow:** Gastroenterology, SUNY Hlth Sci Ctr 1993; **Fac Appt:** Assoc Prof Med, Johns Hopkins Univ

Gastroenterology

Cohen, Jonathan MD [Ge] - **Spec Exp:** Pancreatic/Biliary Endoscopy (ERCP); Pancreatic Disease; Liver Disease; Colonoscopy; **Hospital:** NYU Med Ctr (page 68); **Address:** 232 E 30th St, New York, NY 10016-8202; **Phone:** 212-889-5544; **Board Cert:** Internal Medicine 1993; Gastroenterology 1995; **Med School:** Harvard Med Sch 1990; **Resid:** Internal Medicine, Beth Israel Hosp 1993; **Fellow:** Gastroenterology, UCLA Med Ctr 1995; Endoscopy, Wellesley Hosp 1995; **Fac Appt:** Clin Prof Med, NYU Sch Med

Cohen, Lawrence B MD [Ge] - **Spec Exp:** Gastroesophageal Reflux Disease (GERD); Esophageal Disorders; Colon & Rectal Cancer; **Hospital:** Mount Sinai Med Ctr (page 64); **Address:** 311 E 79th St, Ste 2A, New York, NY 10021-0903; **Phone:** 212-996-6633; **Board Cert:** Internal Medicine 1981; Gastroenterology 1983; **Med School:** Hahnemann Univ 1978; **Resid:** Internal Medicine, Mount Sinai Hosp 1981; **Fellow:** Gastroenterology, Mount Sinai Hosp 1983; **Fac Appt:** Assoc Clin Prof Med, Mount Sinai Sch Med

Dieterich, Douglas MD [Ge] - **Spec Exp:** Hepatitis; AIDS/HIV-Gastrointestinal Complications; Liver Disease; Endoscopy; **Hospital:** Mount Sinai Med Ctr (page 64), NYU Med Ctr (page 68); **Address:** 5 E 98th St Fl 11, New York, NY 10029; **Phone:** 212-241-7270; **Board Cert:** Internal Medicine 1981; Gastroenterology 1987; **Med School:** NYU Sch Med 1978; **Resid:** Internal Medicine, Bellevue Hosp Ctr-NYU 1981; **Fellow:** Gastroenterology, Bellevue Hosp Ctr-NYU 1983; **Fac Appt:** Prof Med, Mount Sinai Sch Med

DiMarino, Anthony J MD [Ge] - **Spec Exp:** Celiac Disease; Gastroesophageal Reflux Disease (GERD); Ulcerative Colitis; Irritable Bowel Syndrome; **Hospital:** Thomas Jefferson Univ Hosp; **Address:** T Jefferson Univ, Div Gastroenterology, 132 S 10th St, Ste 480, Philadelphia, PA 19107; **Phone:** 215-955-2728; **Board Cert:** Internal Medicine 1977; Gastroenterology 1972; **Med School:** Hahnemann Univ 1968; **Resid:** Internal Medicine, Hahnemann Univ Hosp 1970; Internal Medicine, Hosp Univ Penn 1971; **Fellow:** Gastroenterology, Hosp Univ Penn 1973; **Fac Appt:** Prof Med, Thomas Jefferson Univ

Farmer, Richard G MD [Ge] - **Spec Exp:** Inflammatory Bowel Disease/Crohn's; **Hospital:** Univ of Rochester Strong Meml Hosp; **Address:** Univ Rochester Med Ctr, 601 Elmwood Ave, Box 646, Rochester, NY 14642; **Phone:** 585-275-7432; **Board Cert:** Internal Medicine 1963; Gastroenterology 1968; **Med School:** Univ MD Sch Med 1956; **Resid:** Internal Medicine, Mayo Clinic 1960; **Fellow:** Gastroenterology, Mayo Clinic 1960; **Fac Appt:** Prof Med, Univ Rochester

Fisher, Robert S MD [Ge] - **Spec Exp:** Gastrointestinal Motility Disorders; **Hospital:** Temple Univ Hosp; **Address:** 3401 N Broad St, Philadelphia, PA 19140; **Board Cert:** Internal Medicine 1971; Gastroenterology 1973; **Med School:** Univ Pennsylvania 1964; **Resid:** Internal Medicine, Temple Univ Med Ctr 1970; **Fellow:** Gastroenterology, Hosp Univ Penn 1972; **Fac Appt:** Prof Med, Temple Univ

Freiman, Hal MD [Ge] - **Spec Exp:** Gastroesophageal Reflux Disease (GERD); Biliary Disease; Pancreatic/Biliary Endoscopy (ERCP); Hepatitis; **Hospital:** St Vincent Cath Med Ctrs - Manhattan; **Address:** 59 W 12th St, Ste 1D, New York, NY 10011-8520; **Phone:** 212-206-0074; **Board Cert:** Internal Medicine 1981; Gastroenterology 1983; **Med School:** Albany Med Coll 1978; **Resid:** Internal Medicine, St Vincent's Hosp 1981; **Fellow:** Gastroenterology, Westchester Co Med Ctr 1983; **Fac Appt:** Asst Clin Prof Med, NY Med Coll

Gerdes, Hans MD [Ge] - **Spec Exp:** Endoscopy; Endoscopic Ultrasound; Barrett's Esophagus; Gastrointestinal Cancer; **Hospital:** Meml Sloan-Kettering Cancer Ctr; **Address:** 1275 York Avenue, New York, NY 10065; **Phone:** 800-525-2225; **Board Cert:** Internal Medicine 1987; Gastroenterology 1989; **Med School:** Cornell Univ-Weill Med Coll 1983; **Resid:** Internal Medicine, New York Hosp 1986; **Fellow:** Gastroenterology, Meml Sloan Kettering Cancer Ctr 1989

America's Top Doctors® 8th Edition

Ginsberg, Gregory G MD [Ge] - **Spec Exp:** Pancreatic/Biliary Endoscopy (ERCP); Endoscopy; Endoscopic Ultrasound; **Hospital:** Hosp Univ Penn - UPHS (page 60); **Address:** Clinical Practices of U Pennsylvania, 3400 Spruce St 3 Dulles Bldg, Philadelphia, PA 19104; **Phone:** 215-349-8222; **Board Cert:** Internal Medicine 2000; Gastroenterology 2000; **Med School:** Jefferson Med Coll 1987; **Resid:** Internal Medicine, Georgetown Univ Med Ctr 1990; **Fellow:** Gastroenterology, Georgetown Univ Med Ctr 1992; **Fac Appt:** Prof Med, Univ Pennsylvania

Goggins, Michael MD [Ge] - **Spec Exp:** Pancreatic Cancer-Early Detection; **Hospital:** Johns Hopkins Hosp - Baltimore (page 61); **Address:** Johns Hopkins Univ Sch Med, 1550 Orleans St, CRB-2 St, rm 342, Baltimore, MD 21231; **Phone:** 410-955-3511; **Med School:** Ireland 1988; **Resid:** Internal Medicine, St Jame's Hosp 1990; **Fellow:** Gastroenterology, St Jame's Hosp 1992; **Fac Appt:** Assoc Prof Med, Johns Hopkins Univ

Green, Peter MD [Ge] - **Spec Exp:** Celiac Disease; Endoscopy; Colonoscopy; Malabsorption Syndrome; **Hospital:** NY-Presby Hosp/Columbia (page 66); **Address:** Celiac Disease Ctr, Harkness Bldg, 180 Fort Washington Ave, rm 956, New York, NY 10032-3713; **Phone:** 212-305-5590; **Med School:** Australia 1970; **Resid:** Internal Medicine, North Shore Med Ctr 1974; **Fellow:** Gastroenterology, North Shore Med Ctr 1976; Gastroenterology, Beth Israel Hosp 1977; **Fac Appt:** Clin Prof Med, Columbia P&S

Greenwald, Bruce D MD [Ge] - **Spec Exp:** Endoscopic Ultrasound; Barrett's Esophagus; Esophageal Cancer; Clinical Trials; **Hospital:** Univ of MD Med Sys; **Address:** Univ of Maryland Hosp, Gastroenterology, 22 S Greene St Fl 3 - rm N3W62, Baltimore, MD 21201-1544; **Phone:** 410-328-5780; **Board Cert:** Internal Medicine 2000; Gastroenterology 2000; **Med School:** Univ MD Sch Med 1987; **Resid:** Internal Medicine, Univ of Virginia Hosp 1990; **Fellow:** Gastroenterology, Univ of Maryland Hosp 1992; **Fac Appt:** Assoc Prof Med, Univ MD Sch Med

Haber, Gregory B MD [Ge] - **Spec Exp:** Endoscopy; Pancreatic/Biliary Endoscopy (ERCP); **Hospital:** Lenox Hill Hosp (page 62); **Address:** 100 E 77th St, New York, NY 10075; **Phone:** 212-434-6279; **Med School:** Univ Toronto 1970; **Resid:** Internal Medicine, Univ Toronto Med Ctr 1975; **Fellow:** Gastroenterology, Univ Toronto Med Ctr 1978

Haluszka, Oleh MD [Ge] - **Spec Exp:** Pancreatic/Biliary Endoscopy (ERCP); Gastrointestinal Cancer; Endoscopic Ultrasound; Endoscopy; **Hospital:** Fox Chase Cancer Ctr (page 58); **Address:** Fox Chase Cancer Ctr, 333 Cottman Ave, Ste C307, Philadelphia, PA 19111; **Phone:** 215-214-1424; **Board Cert:** Internal Medicine 1987; Gastroenterology 2001; **Med School:** Uniformed Srvs Univ, Bethesda 1982; **Resid:** Internal Medicine, US Naval Hosp 1987; **Fellow:** Gastroenterology, US Naval Hosp 1990; Endoscopy, Med Coll Wisconsin 1993; **Fac Appt:** Assoc Clin Prof Med, Temple Univ

Hoops, Timothy C MD [Ge] - **Spec Exp:** Esophageal Disorders; Endoscopy; Colonoscopy; **Hospital:** Penn Presby Med Ctr - UPHS (page 60); **Address:** Penn Presbyterian Medical Ctr, 51 N 39th St, Ste 218, Philadelphia, PA 19104; **Phone:** 215-662-8900; **Board Cert:** Internal Medicine 1984; Gastroenterology 1987; **Med School:** Univ IL Coll Med 1981; **Resid:** Internal Medicine, U Colorado Hlth Sci Ctr 1984; **Fellow:** Gastroenterology, U Colorado Hlth Sci Ctr 1986; **Fac Appt:** Assoc Clin Prof Med, Univ Pennsylvania

Itzkowitz, Steven H MD [Ge] - **Spec Exp:** Colon & Rectal Cancer; Colon & Rectal Cancer Detection; Inflammatory Bowel Disease; **Hospital:** Mount Sinai Med Ctr (page 64); **Address:** 5 E 98th St, Box 1625, New York, NY 10029-6501; **Phone:** 212-241-4299; **Board Cert:** Internal Medicine 1982; Gastroenterology 1985; **Med School:** Mount Sinai Sch Med 1979; **Resid:** Internal Medicine, Bellevue Hosp/NYU Med Ctr 1982; **Fellow:** Gastroenterology, UCSF Med Ctr 1984; **Fac Appt:** Prof Med, Mount Sinai Sch Med

Gastroenterology

Jacobson, Ira MD [Ge] - **Spec Exp:** Liver Disease; Pancreatic/Biliary Endoscopy (ERCP); Colonoscopy; Hepatitis; **Hospital:** NY-Presby Hosp/Weill Cornell (page 66); **Address:** 1305 York Ave, Fl 4, New York, NY 10021-5016; **Phone:** 646-962-4040; **Board Cert:** Internal Medicine 1982; Gastroenterology 1985; Transplant Hepatology 2006; **Med School:** Columbia P&S 1979; **Resid:** Internal Medicine, UCSF Med Ctr 1982; **Fellow:** Gastroenterology, Mass Genl Hosp 1984; **Fac Appt:** Prof Med, Cornell Univ-Weill Med Coll

Kalloo, Anthony N MD [Ge] - **Spec Exp:** Endoscopy; Pancreatic Disease; **Hospital:** Johns Hopkins Hosp - Baltimore (page 61); **Address:** Cancer Research Bldg II, 1550 Orleans St, 1-M12, Baltimore, MD 21231; **Phone:** 410-955-9697; **Board Cert:** Internal Medicine 1985; Gastroenterology 1987; **Med School:** Jamaica 1979; **Resid:** Internal Medicine, Howard Univ Hosp 1985; **Fellow:** Gastroenterology, VA Med Ctr/Georgetown Univ Hosp 1987; **Fac Appt:** Assoc Prof Med, Johns Hopkins Univ

Kantsevoy, Sergey V MD/PhD [Ge] - **Spec Exp:** Pancreatic Disease; Endoscopic Ultrasound; Pancreatic/Biliary Endoscopy (ERCP); **Hospital:** Johns Hopkins Hosp - Baltimore (page 61); **Address:** Johns Hopkins Gastroenterology, 1830 E Monument St, rm 426, Baltimore, MD 21287; **Phone:** 410-614-6798; **Board Cert:** Internal Medicine 1997; Gastroenterology 2000; **Med School:** Russia 1983; **Resid:** Internal Medicine, Bronx-Lebanon Hosp Ctr 1995; Internal Medicine, Washington Hosp Ctr 1997; **Fellow:** Gastroenterology, Johns Hopkins Hosp 2000; **Fac Appt:** Asst Prof Med, Johns Hopkins Univ

Katz, Philip O MD [Ge] - **Spec Exp:** Gastroesophageal Reflux Disease (GERD); Swallowing Disorders; Barrett's Esophagus; Esophageal Disorders; **Hospital:** Albert Einstein Med Ctr; **Address:** 5501 Old York Rd, Klein Bldg - Ste 363, Philadelphia, PA 19141; **Phone:** 215-456-8210; **Board Cert:** Internal Medicine 1981; Gastroenterology 1987; **Med School:** Bowman Gray 1978; **Resid:** Internal Medicine, NC Baptist Hosp 1981; **Fellow:** Gastroenterology, NC Baptist Hosp 1986; **Fac Appt:** Clin Prof Med, Thomas Jefferson Univ

Kochman, Michael L MD [Ge] - **Spec Exp:** Endoscopy; Pancreatic/Biliary Endoscopy (ERCP); Gastrointestinal Cancer; **Hospital:** Hosp Univ Penn - UPHS (page 60); **Address:** Hosp Univ Penn, Div Gastroenterology, 3400 Spruce St, 3 Dulles, Philadelphia, PA 19104-4206; **Phone:** 215-349-8222; **Board Cert:** Internal Medicine 1989; Gastroenterology 2003; **Med School:** Univ IL Coll Med 1986; **Resid:** Internal Medicine, Univ Illinois Med Ctr 1990; **Fellow:** Gastroenterology, Univ Michigan Med Ctr 1993; **Fac Appt:** Prof Med, Univ Pennsylvania

Korsten, Mark A MD [Ge] - **Spec Exp:** Constipation; Gastrointestinal Motility Disorders; Spinal Cord Injury & Colonic Motility; Liver Disease; **Hospital:** Mount Sinai Med Ctr (page 64), VA Med Ctr - Bronx; **Address:** 130 W Kingsbridge Rd, Bronx, NY 10468-3904; **Phone:** 718-584-9000 x6753; **Board Cert:** Internal Medicine 1973; Gastroenterology 1975; **Med School:** Yale Univ 1970; **Resid:** Internal Medicine, Mt Sinai Hosp 1973; **Fellow:** Gastroenterology, Mt Sinai Hosp 1975; **Fac Appt:** Prof Med, Mount Sinai Sch Med

Kotler, Donald P MD [Ge] - **Spec Exp:** Esophageal Disorders; Nutrition & AIDS; **Hospital:** St Luke's - Roosevelt Hosp Ctr - St Luke's Hosp (page 57); **Address:** 1111 Amsterdam Ave, SR 12, New York, NY 10025; **Phone:** 212-523-3670; **Board Cert:** Internal Medicine 1976; Gastroenterology 1979; **Med School:** Albert Einstein Coll Med 1973; **Resid:** Internal Medicine, Jacobi Med Ctr 1976; **Fellow:** Gastroenterology, Hosp Univ Penn 1978; **Fac Appt:** Assoc Prof Med, Columbia P&S

Kowalski, Thomas E MD [Ge] - **Spec Exp:** Pancreatic Disease; Biliary Disease; Pancreatic/Biliary Endoscopy (ERCP); Endoscopic Ultrasound; **Hospital:** Thomas Jefferson Univ Hosp; **Address:** 132 S 10th St Main Bldg - Ste 480, Philadelphia, PA 19107; **Phone:** 215-955-9936; **Board Cert:** Internal Medicine 2003; Gastroenterology 2003; **Med School:** SUNY Buffalo 1988; **Resid:** Internal Medicine, Johns Hopkins Hosp 1991; **Fellow:** Gastroenterology, Hosp Univ Penn 1993; Advanced Endoscopy, Hosp Univ Penn 1994; **Fac Appt:** Asst Prof Med, Thomas Jefferson Univ

Kurtz, Robert C MD [Ge] - **Spec Exp:** Gastrointestinal Cancer; Pancreatic Cancer; Endoscopy; Nutrition & Cancer Prevention/Control; **Hospital:** Meml Sloan-Kettering Cancer Ctr; **Address:** 1275 York Avenue, New York, NY 10065; **Phone:** 800-525-2225; **Board Cert:** Internal Medicine 1971; Gastroenterology 1977; **Med School:** Jefferson Med Coll 1968; **Resid:** Internal Medicine, NY Hosp/Meml Sloan Kettering Cancer Ctr 1971; **Fellow:** Gastroenterology, Meml Sloan Kettering Cancer Ctr 1973; **Fac Appt:** Prof Med, Cornell Univ-Weill Med Coll

Lebwohl, Oscar MD [Ge] - **Spec Exp:** Endoscopy; Inflammatory Bowel Disease/Crohn's; Ulcerative Colitis; **Hospital:** NY-Presby Hosp/Columbia (page 66); **Address:** 161 Fort Washington Ave, rm 420, New York, NY 10032-3713; **Phone:** 212-305-5363; **Board Cert:** Internal Medicine 1975; Gastroenterology 1977; **Med School:** Harvard Med Sch 1972; **Resid:** Internal Medicine, Mt Sinai Med Ctr 1975; **Fellow:** Gastroenterology, Columbia-Presby Med Ctr 1976; Hepatology, Mt Sinai Med Ctr 1977; **Fac Appt:** Clin Prof Med, Columbia P&S

Lewis, Blair MD [Ge] - **Spec Exp:** Endoscopy; Capsule Endoscopy; **Hospital:** Mount Sinai Med Ctr (page 64); **Address:** 1067 5th Ave, New York, NY 10128-0101; **Phone:** 212-369-6600; **Board Cert:** Internal Medicine 1985; Gastroenterology 1987; **Med School:** Albert Einstein Coll Med 1982; **Resid:** Internal Medicine, Montefiore Hosp Med Ctr 1985; **Fellow:** Gastroenterology, Mount Sinai Med Ctr 1987; **Fac Appt:** Clin Prof Med, Mount Sinai Sch Med

Lichtenstein, Gary R MD [Ge] - **Spec Exp:** Inflammatory Bowel Disease; **Hospital:** Hosp Univ Penn - UPHS (page 60); **Address:** Univ Penn, Div Gastroenterology, 3400 Spruce St, 3 Ravdin Bldg, Philadelphia, PA 19104-4283; **Phone:** 215-349-8222; **Board Cert:** Internal Medicine 1987; Gastroenterology 1989; **Med School:** Mount Sinai Sch Med 1984; **Resid:** Internal Medicine, Duke Univ Med Ctr 1987; **Fellow:** Gastroenterology, Hosp Univ Penn 1990; **Fac Appt:** Assoc Prof Med, Univ Pennsylvania

Lightdale, Charles MD [Ge] - **Spec Exp:** Barrett's Esophagus; Gastrointestinal Cancer; Endoscopic Ultrasound; **Hospital:** NY-Presby Hosp/Columbia (page 66); **Address:** Columbia-Presby Med Ctr, Irving Pavilion, 161 Fort Washington Ave, rm 812, New York, NY 10032-3713; **Phone:** 212-305-3423; **Board Cert:** Internal Medicine 1972; Gastroenterology 1973; **Med School:** Columbia P&S 1966; **Resid:** Internal Medicine, Yale-New Haven Hosp 1968; Internal Medicine, NY Hosp-Cornell 1969; **Fellow:** Gastroenterology, NY Hosp-Cornell 1973; **Fac Appt:** Prof Med, Columbia P&S

Lipshutz, William H MD [Ge] - **Spec Exp:** Inflammatory Bowel Disease/Crohn's; Colonoscopy; Esophageal Disorders; Gastroesophageal Reflux Disease (GERD); **Hospital:** Pennsylvania Hosp (page 60); **Address:** 230 W Washington Sq, Farm Journal Bldg, Fl 4, Philadelphia, PA 19106; **Phone:** 215-829-3561; **Board Cert:** Internal Medicine 1972; Gastroenterology 1973; **Med School:** Univ Pennsylvania 1967; **Resid:** Internal Medicine, Pennsylvania Hosp 1972; **Fellow:** Gastroenterology, Hosp Univ Penn 1971; **Fac Appt:** Clin Prof Med, Univ Pennsylvania

Magun, Arthur MD [Ge] - **Spec Exp:** Hepatitis; Ulcerative Colitis; Endoscopy; Inflammatory Bowel Disease/Crohn's; **Hospital:** NY-Presby Hosp/Columbia (page 66); **Address:** 161 Fort Washington Ave, rm 338, New York, NY 10032-3713; **Phone:** 212-305-5287; **Board Cert:** Internal Medicine 1980; Gastroenterology 1983; **Med School:** Mount Sinai Sch Med 1977; **Resid:** Internal Medicine, Columbia-Presby Med Ctr 1980; **Fellow:** Gastroenterology, Columbia-Presby Med Ctr 1983; **Fac Appt:** Clin Prof Med, Columbia P&S

Markowitz, David MD [Ge] - **Spec Exp:** Gastroesophageal Reflux Disease (GERD); Esophageal Disorders; Endoscopy; **Hospital:** NY-Presby Hosp/Columbia (page 66); **Address:** 161 Ft Washington Ave, Ste 853, New York, NY 10032; **Phone:** 212-305-1024; **Board Cert:** Internal Medicine 1988; Gastroenterology 2001; **Med School:** Columbia P&S 1985; **Resid:** Internal Medicine, Columbia-Presby Hosp 1988; **Fellow:** Gastroenterology, Columbia-Presby Hosp 1991; **Fac Appt:** Asst Clin Prof Med, Columbia P&S

Gastroenterology

Mayer, Lloyd MD [Ge] - **Spec Exp:** Inflammatory Bowel Disease/Crohn's; Ulcerative Colitis; **Hospital:** Mount Sinai Med Ctr (page 64); **Address:** 1425 Madison Ave, rm 11-20, Box 1089, New York, NY 10029; **Phone:** 212-659-9266; **Board Cert:** Internal Medicine 1979; Gastroenterology 1981; **Med School:** Mount Sinai Sch Med 1976; **Resid:** Internal Medicine, Bellevue Hosp 1979; **Fellow:** Gastroenterology, Mount Sinai Hosp 1981; **Fac Appt:** Prof Med, Mount Sinai Sch Med

Metz, David C MD [Ge] - **Spec Exp:** Peptic Acid Disorders; Neuroendocrine Tumors; Gastroesophageal Reflux Disease (GERD); Gastrointestinal Motility Disorders; **Hospital:** Hosp Univ Penn - UPHS (page 60); **Address:** Hosp Univ Penn, Div Gastroenterology, 3400 Spruce St, 3 Ravdin, Philadelphia, PA 19104; **Phone:** 215-662-4279; **Board Cert:** Internal Medicine 1989; Gastroenterology 2001; **Med School:** South Africa 1982; **Resid:** Internal Medicine, Albert Einstein Med Ctr 1988; **Fellow:** Gastroenterology, Natl Inst Hlth 1991; **Fac Appt:** Prof Med, Univ Pennsylvania

Miskovitz, Paul MD [Ge] - **Spec Exp:** Endoscopy; Liver Disease; **Hospital:** NY-Presby Hosp/Weill Cornell (page 66); **Address:** 635 Madison Ave Fl 17, New York, NY 10022; **Phone:** 212-717-4966; **Board Cert:** Internal Medicine 1978; Gastroenterology 1981; **Med School:** Cornell Univ-Weill Med Coll 1975; **Resid:** Internal Medicine, NY Hosp 1978; **Fellow:** Gastroenterology, NY Hosp 1980; **Fac Appt:** Clin Prof Med, Cornell Univ-Weill Med Coll

Pochapin, Mark B MD [Ge] - **Spec Exp:** Pancreatic Cancer; Endoscopic Ultrasound; Colon & Rectal Cancer Detection; Diarrheal Diseases; **Hospital:** NY-Presby Hosp/Weill Cornell (page 66); **Address:** The Jay Monahan Ctr for GI Hlth, 1315 York Ave, New York, NY 10021; **Phone:** 212-746-4014; **Board Cert:** Gastroenterology 2004; **Med School:** Cornell Univ-Weill Med Coll 1988; **Resid:** Internal Medicine, NY Hosp-Cornell Med Ctr 1991; **Fellow:** Gastroenterology, Montefiore Med Ctr 1993; **Fac Appt:** Assoc Clin Prof Med, Cornell Univ-Weill Med Coll

Ravich, William J MD [Ge] - **Spec Exp:** Swallowing Disorders; Gastroesophageal Reflux Disease (GERD); Barrett's Esophagus; **Hospital:** Johns Hopkins Hosp - Baltimore (page 61), Greater Baltimore Med Ctr; **Address:** 10751 Falls Rd, Ste 401, Lutherville, MD 21093; **Phone:** 410-616-2840; **Board Cert:** Internal Medicine 1978; Gastroenterology 1981; **Med School:** Ros Franklin Univ/Chicago Med Sch 1975; **Resid:** Internal Medicine, Montefiore Hosp 1978; **Fellow:** Gastroenterology, Johns Hopkins Hosp 1981; **Fac Appt:** Assoc Prof Med, Johns Hopkins Univ

Reddy, K Rajender MD [Ge] - **Spec Exp:** Liver Disease; Hepatitis; Transplant Medicine-Liver; **Hospital:** Hosp Univ Penn - UPHS (page 60); **Address:** Hosp Univ Penn, Div Gastroenterology, 3 Dulles, 3400 Spruce St, Philadelphia, PA 19104; **Phone:** 215-349-8222; **Board Cert:** Internal Medicine 1980; Gastroenterology 1983; Transplant Hepatology 2006; **Med School:** India 1972; **Resid:** Internal Medicine, NY Med Coll Hosps 1980; **Fellow:** Gastroenterology, E Tenn State Univ 1982; Hepatology, Univ Miami Hosps 1983; **Fac Appt:** Prof Med, Univ Pennsylvania

Reynolds, James C MD [Ge] - **Spec Exp:** Gastroesophageal Reflux Disease (GERD); Gastrointestinal Motility Disorders; Barrett's Esophagus; **Hospital:** Hahnemann Univ Hosp; **Address:** Drexel Gastroenterology Assocs, 219 N Broad St Fl 5, Philadelphia, PA 19107; **Phone:** 215-965-6000; **Board Cert:** Internal Medicine 1980; Gastroenterology 1985; **Med School:** Univ Fla Coll Med 1977; **Resid:** Internal Medicine, New York Hosp 1980; **Fellow:** Gastroenterology, Univ Penn 1983; **Fac Appt:** Prof Med, Drexel Univ Coll Med

Richter, Joel E MD [Ge] - **Spec Exp:** Gastroesophageal Reflux Disease (GERD); Esophageal Disorders; **Hospital:** Temple Univ Hosp; **Address:** Temple Univ Hospital, Parkinson Pavilion, 3401 N Broad St, Fl 8 - Ste 801, Philadelphia, PA 19140; **Phone:** 215-707-5069; **Board Cert:** Internal Medicine 1978; Gastroenterology 1981; **Med School:** Univ Tex SW, Dallas 1975; **Resid:** Internal Medicine, Natl Naval Med Ctr 1978; **Fellow:** Gastroenterology, Natl Naval Med Ctr 1980; **Fac Appt:** Prof Med, Temple Univ

Sachar, David MD [Ge] - **Spec Exp:** Inflammatory Bowel Disease-Consult; **Hospital:** Mount Sinai Med Ctr (page 64); **Address:** 5 E 98th St Fl 11, New York, NY 10029; **Phone:** 212-241-4299; **Board Cert:** Internal Medicine 1969; Gastroenterology 1972; **Med School:** Harvard Med Sch 1963; **Resid:** Internal Medicine, Beth Israel Hosp 1965; Internal Medicine, Beth Israel Hosp 1968; **Fellow:** Gastroenterology, Mount Sinai Hosp 1970; **Fac Appt:** Clin Prof Med, Mount Sinai Sch Med

Schiano, Thomas D MD [Ge] - **Spec Exp:** Liver Disease; Transplant Medicine-Liver; Liver Failure; **Hospital:** Mount Sinai Med Ctr (page 64); **Address:** Mount Sinai Medical Ctr, One Gustave L Levy Pl, Box 1104, New York, NY 10029; **Phone:** 212-241-0034; **Board Cert:** Internal Medicine 2000; Gastroenterology 2005; Transplant Hepatology 2006; **Med School:** Mexico 1987; **Resid:** Internal Medicine, Maimonides Med Ctr 1991; Gastroenterology, Temple Univ 1992; **Fellow:** Nutrition, Meml Sloan-Kettering Cancer Ctr 1993; Hepatology, Mt Sinai Med Ctr 1995; **Fac Appt:** Assoc Prof Med, Mount Sinai Sch Med

Shike, Moshe MD [Ge] - **Spec Exp:** Gastrointestinal Cancer; Nutrition & Cancer Prevention; Endoscopy; **Hospital:** Meml Sloan-Kettering Cancer Ctr, NY-Presby Hosp/Weill Cornell (page 66); **Address:** 1275 York Avenue, New York, NY 10065; **Phone:** 800-525-2225; **Board Cert:** Internal Medicine 1977; Gastroenterology 1981; **Med School:** Israel 1975; **Resid:** Internal Medicine, Mt Auburn Hosp 1977; **Fellow:** Gastroenterology, Toronto Genl Hosp 1981; **Fac Appt:** Prof Med, Cornell Univ-Weill Med Coll

Tobias, Hillel MD [Ge] - **Spec Exp:** Liver Disease; Hepatitis B & C; Liver & Biliary Disease; **Hospital:** NYU Med Ctr (page 68); **Address:** 232 E 30th St, New York, NY 10016-8202; **Phone:** 212-889-5544; **Board Cert:** Internal Medicine 1967; Gastroenterology 1979; **Med School:** Washington Univ, St Louis 1960; **Resid:** Internal Medicine, Bellevue Hosp 1963; **Fellow:** Hepatology, Royal Free Hosp 1965; Hepatology, Mount Sinai Hosp 1967; **Fac Appt:** Prof Med, NYU Sch Med

Waye, Jerome MD [Ge] - **Spec Exp:** Endoscopy; Colon Cancer; Colonoscopy; **Hospital:** Mount Sinai Med Ctr (page 64), Lenox Hill Hosp (page 62); **Address:** 650 Park Ave, New York, NY 10021-6115; **Phone:** 212-439-7779; **Board Cert:** Internal Medicine 1965; Gastroenterology 1970; **Med School:** Boston Univ 1958; **Resid:** Internal Medicine, Mount Sinai Hosp 1961; **Fellow:** Gastroenterology, Mount Sinai Hosp 1962; **Fac Appt:** Clin Prof Med, Mount Sinai Sch Med

Whitcomb, David C MD/PhD [Ge] - **Spec Exp:** Pancreatic Disease; **Hospital:** UPMC Presby, Pittsburgh; **Address:** Digestive Disorders Center, 200 Lothrop St, Mezz 2-C Wing PUH, Pittsburgh, PA 15213; **Phone:** 412-647-8666; **Board Cert:** Internal Medicine 1989; Gastroenterology 1991; **Med School:** Ohio State Univ 1985; **Resid:** Internal Medicine, Duke Univ Med Ctr 1988; **Fellow:** Gastroenterology, Duke Univ Med Ctr 1991; **Fac Appt:** Prof Med, Univ Pittsburgh

Winawer, Sidney J MD [Ge] - **Spec Exp:** Colonoscopy; Colon Cancer; Cancer Prevention; **Hospital:** Meml Sloan-Kettering Cancer Ctr; **Address:** 1275 York Avenue, New York, NY 10065; **Phone:** 800-525-2225; **Board Cert:** Internal Medicine 1965; Gastroenterology 1973; **Med School:** SUNY Downstate 1956; **Resid:** Internal Medicine, VA Hosp 1961; Internal Medicine, Maimonides Hosp 1962; **Fellow:** Gastroenterology, Boston City Hosp 1964; **Fac Appt:** Prof Med, Cornell Univ-Weill Med Coll

Gastroenterology

Southeast

Abreu, Maria T MD [Ge] - **Spec Exp:** Inflammatory Bowel Disease/Crohn's; Ulcerative Colitis; **Hospital:** Univ of Miami Hosp; **Address:** Univ Miami Miller Sch Med, PO Box 016960 (D-49), Miami, FL 33101; **Phone:** 305-243-8644; **Board Cert:** Gastroenterology 2005; **Med School:** Univ Miami Sch Med 1990; **Resid:** Internal Medicine, Brigham & Women's Hosp 1992; **Fellow:** Gastroenterology, UCLA Med Ctr 1995; **Fac Appt:** Prof Med, Univ Miami Sch Med

Barkin, Jamie S MD [Ge] - **Spec Exp:** Pancreatic & Biliary Disease; Gastrointestinal Cancer; Endoscopy; **Hospital:** Mount Sinai Med Ctr - Miami, Univ of Miami Hosp & Clins/Sylvester Comp Canc Ctr; **Address:** Mount Sinai Medical Center, Gumenick Bldg, 4300 Alton Rd, Ste 2522, Miami Beach, FL 33140-2800; **Phone:** 305-674-2240; **Board Cert:** Internal Medicine 1973; Gastroenterology 1975; **Med School:** Univ Miami Sch Med 1970; **Resid:** Internal Medicine, Univ Miami Hosp 1973; **Fellow:** Gastroenterology, Univ Miami Hosp 1975; **Fac Appt:** Prof Med, Univ Miami Sch Med

Bloomer, Joseph R MD [Ge] - **Spec Exp:** Porphyria; Liver Disease; Transplant Medicine-Liver; **Hospital:** Univ of Ala Hosp at Birmingham; **Address:** UAB, Division Gastroenterology, 1918 University Blvd, 395 MCLM, Birmingham, AL 35294-0005; **Phone:** 205-975-9699; **Board Cert:** Internal Medicine 1972; **Med School:** Case West Res Univ 1966; **Resid:** Internal Medicine, UCSF Med Ctr 1968; **Fellow:** Hepatology, Yale Univ 1972; **Fac Appt:** Prof Med, Univ Ala

Boyce Jr, H Worth MD [Ge] - **Spec Exp:** Esophageal Disorders; Barrett's Esophagus; Esophageal Cancer; **Hospital:** H Lee Moffitt Cancer Ctr & Research Inst, Tampa Genl Hosp; **Address:** Ctr for Swallowing Disorders, 12901 Bruce B Downs Blvd, MDC 72, Tampa, FL 33612-4742; **Phone:** 813-974-3374; **Board Cert:** Internal Medicine 1977; Gastroenterology 1965; **Med School:** Wake Forest Univ 1955; **Resid:** Internal Medicine, Brooke Army Hosp 1959; Gastroenterology, Brooke Army Hosp 1960; **Fac Appt:** Prof Med, Univ S Fla Coll Med

Brazer, Scott R MD [Ge] - **Spec Exp:** Gastroesophageal Reflux Disease (GERD); Chest Pain-Non Cardiac; Colonoscopy; **Hospital:** Univ NC Hosps; **Address:** 249 E Highway 54, Ste 200, Durham, NC 27713; **Phone:** 919-806-8322; **Board Cert:** Internal Medicine 1984; Gastroenterology 1987; **Med School:** Case West Res Univ 1981; **Resid:** Internal Medicine, Duke Univ Med Ctr 1984; Internal Medicine, Duke Univ Med Ctr 1988; **Fellow:** Gastroenterology, Duke Univ 1987

Castell, Donald O MD [Ge] - **Spec Exp:** Esophageal Disorders; Gastroesophageal Reflux Disease (GERD); Gastrointestinal Motility Disorders; **Hospital:** MUSC Med Ctr; **Address:** MUSC Digestive Disease Ctr, 96 Jonathan Lucas St, Box 250327, Charleston, SC 29425; **Phone:** 843-792-7522; **Board Cert:** Internal Medicine 1977; Gastroenterology 1970; **Med School:** Geo Wash Univ 1960; **Resid:** Internal Medicine, US Naval Hosp 1965; **Fellow:** Gastroenterology, Tufts Univ 1969; **Fac Appt:** Prof Med, Univ SC Sch Med

Cominelli, Fabio MD/PhD [Ge] - **Spec Exp:** Inflammatory Bowel Disease/Crohn's; Ulcerative Colitis; **Hospital:** Univ Virginia Med Ctr; **Address:** Univ VA Hlth Sys, Div Gastroenterology, PO Box 800708, Charlottesville, VA 22908; **Phone:** 434-243-6400; **Med School:** Italy 1983; **Resid:** Gastroenterology, Careggi Hosp-Univ Italy 1986; **Fellow:** Gastroenterology, Harbor-UCLA Med Ctr 1989; **Fac Appt:** Prof Med, Univ VA Sch Med

Cotton, Peter MD [Ge] - **Spec Exp:** Pancreatic Disease; Biliary Disease; Pancreatic/Biliary Endoscopy (ERCP); **Hospital:** MUSC Med Ctr; **Address:** MUSC, Digestive Disease Center - 210 CSB, 96 Jonathan Lucas St, Box 250327, Charleston, SC 29425; **Phone:** 843-792-6865; **Med School:** England 1963; **Resid:** Internal Medicine, St Thomas' Hosp 1970; Gastroenterology, St Thomas' Hosp 1973; **Fac Appt:** Prof Med, Med Univ SC

America's Top Doctors® 8th Edition

DeVault, Kenneth MD [Ge] - **Spec Exp:** Gastroesophageal Reflux Disease (GERD); **Hospital:** Mayo - Jacksonville, St Luke's Hosp - Jacksonville; **Address:** Mayo Clinic, Davis Bldg, 6th Fl, 4500 San Pablo Rd S, Jacksonville, FL 32224-1865; **Phone:** 904-953-2254; **Board Cert:** Internal Medicine 1989; Gastroenterology 2003; **Med School:** Bowman Gray 1986; **Resid:** Internal Medicine, Vanderbilt Univ Med Ctr 1989; **Fellow:** Gastroenterology, T Jefferson Univ Med Ctr 1992; **Fac Appt:** Prof Med, Mayo Med Sch

Drossman, Douglas A MD [Ge] - **Spec Exp:** Gastrointestinal Motility Disorders; Pain-Abdominal/Functional; Gastrointestinal Functional Disorders; **Hospital:** Univ NC Hosps; **Address:** Univ NC, Div Digestive Diseases, 4150 Bio Informatics Bldg, Campus Box 7080, Chapel Hill, NC 27599-7080; **Phone:** 919-966-0141; **Board Cert:** Internal Medicine 1973; Gastroenterology 1979; **Med School:** Albert Einstein Coll Med 1970; **Resid:** Internal Medicine, NC Meml Hosp 1972; Internal Medicine, Bellevue Hosp Ctr-NYU 1973; **Fellow:** Psychiatry, Univ Rochester 1976; Gastroenterology, NC Meml Hosp-UNC 1978; **Fac Appt:** Prof Med, Univ NC Sch Med

Eloubeidi, Mohamad A MD [Ge] - **Spec Exp:** Gastrointestinal Cancer; Colon & Rectal Cancer; Pancreatic Cancer; Endoscopic Ultrasound; **Hospital:** Univ of Ala Hosp at Birmingham; **Address:** 1530 3rd Ave S, Ste LHRB-406, Birmingham, AL 35294-0007; **Phone:** 205-934-7955; **Board Cert:** Gastroenterology 2000; **Med School:** Lebanon 1993; **Resid:** Internal Medicine, Duke Univ Med Ctr 1996; **Fellow:** Gastroenterology, Duke Univ Med Ctr 1999; Advanced Endoscopy, Med Univ South Carolina 2000; **Fac Appt:** Assoc Prof Med, Univ Ala

Fallon, Michael B MD [Ge] - **Spec Exp:** Liver Disease; Hepatitis C; **Hospital:** Univ of Ala Hosp at Birmingham; **Address:** UAB, Div Gastroenterology, 1530 S 3rd Ave, MCLM 290, Birmingham, AL 35294; **Phone:** 205-975-5676; **Board Cert:** Internal Medicine 1988; Gastroenterology 2001; **Med School:** Univ VA Sch Med 1984; **Resid:** Internal Medicine, Yale-New Haven Hosp 1988; **Fellow:** Gastroenterology, Yale-New Haven Hosp 1990; **Fac Appt:** Assoc Prof Med, Univ Ala

Forsmark, Christopher MD [Ge] - **Spec Exp:** AIDS/HIV-Gastrointestinal Complications; Colonoscopy; Pancreatic Disease; Pancreatic/Biliary Endoscopy (ERCP); **Hospital:** Shands at Univ of FL; **Address:** University of Florida, 1600 SW Archer Rd, Box 100214, Gainesville, FL 32610; **Phone:** 352-392-2877; **Board Cert:** Internal Medicine 1986; Gastroenterology 1989; **Med School:** Johns Hopkins Univ 1983; **Resid:** Internal Medicine, UCSF Med Ctr 1987; **Fellow:** Gastroenterology, USCF Med Ctr 1990; **Fac Appt:** Prof Med, Univ Fla Coll Med

Hawes, Robert H MD [Ge] - **Spec Exp:** Endoscopic Ultrasound; Pancreatic/Biliary Endoscopy (ERCP); Pancreatic Disease; **Hospital:** MUSC Med Ctr; **Address:** 96 Jonathan Lucas St, Ste 210, Box 250327, Charleston, SC 29425; **Phone:** 843-792-7896; **Board Cert:** Internal Medicine 1985; Gastroenterology 1987; **Med School:** Indiana Univ 1980; **Fac Appt:** Prof Med, Med Univ SC

Hoffman, Brenda J MD [Ge] - **Spec Exp:** Liver & Biliary Disease; Endoscopic Ultrasound; Gastrointestinal Cancer; Colon & Rectal Cancer-Familial Polyposis; **Hospital:** MUSC Med Ctr; **Address:** MUSC Digestive Disease Center, 25 Courteney Drive, rm MS7100A, MSC290, Charleston, SC 29425; **Phone:** 843-792-6999; **Board Cert:** Internal Medicine 1986; Gastroenterology 1989; **Med School:** Univ KY Coll Med 1983; **Resid:** Internal Medicine, MUSC Med Ctr 1987; **Fellow:** Gastroenterology, MUSC Med Ctr 1989; **Fac Appt:** Prof Med, Univ SC Sch Med

Lambiase, Louis MD [Ge] - **Spec Exp:** Pancreatic Disease; Endoscopic Ultrasound; **Hospital:** Shands Jacksonville, Naval Hosp - Jacksonville; **Address:** 4555 Emerson Expressway Fl 3 - Ste 300, Jacksonville, FL 32207; **Phone:** 904-633-0797; **Board Cert:** Internal Medicine 2002; Gastroenterology 2003; **Med School:** Univ Miami Sch Med 1987; **Resid:** Internal Medicine, Univ Pittsburgh-Presby/ VA Hosps 1990; **Fellow:** Gastroenterology, Univ Fla Coll Med 1993; **Fac Appt:** Assoc Prof Med, Univ Fla Coll Med

Gastroenterology

Liddle, Rodger A MD [Ge] - **Spec Exp:** Inflammatory Bowel Disease; Pancreatic Disease; Hormone Secreting Tumors; **Hospital:** Duke Univ Med Ctr, VA Med Ctr - Durham; **Address:** Duke Univ Med Ctr, Div Gastroenterology, Box 3913, Durham, NC 27710; **Phone:** 919-681-6380; **Board Cert:** Internal Medicine 1981; Gastroenterology 1983; **Med School:** Vanderbilt Univ 1978; **Resid:** Internal Medicine, UCSF Med Ctr 1981; **Fellow:** Gastroenterology, UCSF Med Ctr 1984; **Fac Appt:** Prof Med, Duke Univ

Lind, Christopher D MD [Ge] - **Spec Exp:** Gastroesophageal Reflux Disease (GERD); Swallowing Disorders; Biliary Disease; **Hospital:** Vanderbilt Univ Med Ctr; **Address:** Vanderbilt Univ Med Ctr, Div GI, 1660 TVC GI Clinic, Nashville, TN 37232-5280; **Phone:** 615-322-0128; **Board Cert:** Internal Medicine 1984; Gastroenterology 1987; **Med School:** Vanderbilt Univ 1981; **Resid:** Internal Medicine, Univ Virginia Hosps 1985; **Fellow:** Gastroenterology, Shands/Univ Florida 1986; Gastroenterology, Univ Virginia Hosps 1988; **Fac Appt:** Prof Med, Vanderbilt Univ

Martin, Paul MD [Ge] - **Spec Exp:** Liver Disease; Hepatitis; Transplant Medicine-Liver; **Hospital:** Univ of Miami Hosp, Jackson Meml Hosp; **Address:** Schiff Liver Inst/Ctr for Liver Diseases, 1500 NW 12 Ave, Jackson Medical Tower E-1101, Miami, FL 33136; **Phone:** 305-243-4615; **Board Cert:** Internal Medicine 1984; Gastroenterology 1987; Transplant Hepatology 2006; **Med School:** Ireland 1978; **Resid:** Internal Medicine, St Vincent's Hosp 1982; Internal Medicine, Univ Alberta 1984; **Fellow:** Gastroenterology, Queen Univ 1986; Hepatology, Natl Inst Hlth 1989; **Fac Appt:** Prof Med, Univ Miami Sch Med

Mertz, Howard MD [Ge] - **Spec Exp:** Irritable Bowel Syndrome; Endoscopic Ultrasound; Inflammatory Bowel Disease; **Hospital:** Saint Thomas Hosp - Nashville; **Address:** 4230 Harding Rd, Ste 309W, Nashville, TN 37205; **Phone:** 615-383-0165; **Board Cert:** Internal Medicine 1989; Gastroenterology 2002; **Med School:** Baylor Coll Med 1986; **Resid:** Internal Medicine, Johns Hopkins Hosp 1989; **Fellow:** Gastroenterology, UCLA Med Ctr 1991; **Fac Appt:** Assoc Prof Med, Vanderbilt Univ

Plevy, Scott MD [Ge] - **Spec Exp:** Inflammatory Bowel Disease; **Hospital:** Univ NC Hosps; **Address:** 4100 Bioinformatics Bldg, 130 Mason Farm Rd, Chapel Hill, NC 27599; **Phone:** 919-966-6000; **Board Cert:** Internal Medicine 1991; Gastroenterology 1993; **Med School:** Columbia P&S 1988; **Resid:** Internal Medicine, Brigham-Womens Hosp 1991; **Fellow:** Gastroenterology, Univ of California 1992; Inflammatory Bowel Disease, Cedars-Sinai Med CTR 1994; **Fac Appt:** Assoc Prof Med, Univ NC Sch Med

Raiford, David S MD [Ge] - **Spec Exp:** Autoimmune Liver Disease; Steatohepatitis; Liver Disease; Transplant Medicine-Liver; **Hospital:** Vanderbilt Univ Med Ctr; **Address:** Vanderbilt Hepatology, 1660 The Vanderbilt Clinic, Nashville, TN 37232-5280; **Phone:** 615-322-0128; **Board Cert:** Internal Medicine 1989; Gastroenterology 2001; **Med School:** Johns Hopkins Univ 1985; **Resid:** Internal Medicine, Johns Hopkins Hosp 1988; **Fellow:** Hepatology, Johns Hopkins Hosp 1991; **Fac Appt:** Prof Med, Vanderbilt Univ

Sartor, R Balfour MD [Ge] - **Spec Exp:** Inflammatory Bowel Disease; **Hospital:** Univ NC Hosps; **Address:** Univ NC Sch Med, Div Gastroenterology/Hepatology, Biomolecular Bldg- rm 7309, Box 7032, Chapel Hill, NC 27599-7032; **Phone:** 919-966-6000; **Board Cert:** Internal Medicine 1978; Gastroenterology 1981; **Med School:** Baylor Coll Med 1974; **Resid:** Internal Medicine, Baylor Affil Hosp 1977; **Fellow:** Gastroenterology, Univ NC Hosps 1981; **Fac Appt:** Prof Med, Univ NC Sch Med

America's Top Doctors® 8th Edition

Schiff, Eugene MD [Ge] - **Spec Exp:** Hepatitis C; Liver Disease; **Hospital:** Univ of Miami Hosp, Jackson Meml Hosp; **Address:** Sylvester Cancer Ctr, 1500 NW 12th Ave, Miami, FL 33136; **Phone:** 305-243-5787; **Board Cert:** Internal Medicine 1980; Gastroenterology 1972; **Med School:** Columbia P&S 1962; **Resid:** Internal Medicine, Cincinnati Genl Hosp 1964; Internal Medicine, Parkland Meml Hosp 1967; **Fellow:** Gastroenterology, Univ Tex SW Med Ctr 1969; **Fac Appt:** Prof Med, Univ Miami Sch Med

Scudera, Peter MD [Ge] - **Spec Exp:** Transplant Medicine-Liver; Pancreatic/Biliary Endoscopy (ERCP); Hepatitis C; **Hospital:** Inova Fair Oaks Hosp, Inova Fairfax Hosp; **Address:** 3700 Joseph Siewick Dr, Ste 308, Fairfax, VA 22033; **Phone:** 703-716-8700; **Board Cert:** Internal Medicine 1987; Gastroenterology 1989; **Med School:** Cornell Univ-Weill Med Coll 1984; **Resid:** Internal Medicine, New York Hosp 1987; **Fellow:** Gastroenterology, New York Hosp-Cornell 1989

Seidner, Douglas L MD [Ge] - **Spec Exp:** Nutrition; Inflammatory Bowel Disease; Endoscopy; **Hospital:** Vanderbilt Univ Med Ctr; **Address:** Vanderbilt Center for Human Nutrition, 1211 21st Ave S, 514 Medical Arts Building, Nashville, TN 37232; **Phone:** 615-936-1288; **Board Cert:** Internal Medicine 1986; Gastroenterology 2000; **Med School:** SUNY Upstate Med Univ 1983; **Resid:** Internal Medicine, Beth Israel Deaconess Med Ctr 1986; **Fellow:** Nutrition & Metabolism, Beth Israel Deaconess Med Ctr 1987; Gastroenterology, George Washington Univ Med Ctr 1989

Shiffman, Mitchell MD [Ge] - **Spec Exp:** Transplant Medicine-Liver; Hepatitis C; Liver Disease; **Hospital:** Med Coll of VA Hosp; **Address:** VCU Health Systems, Hepatology Section, Box 980341, Richmond, VA 23298-0341; **Phone:** 804-828-4060; **Board Cert:** Internal Medicine 1986; Gastroenterology 1989; **Med School:** SUNY Upstate Med Univ 1983; **Resid:** Internal Medicine, Med Coll Va Hosp 1986; **Fellow:** Gastroenterology, Med Coll Va Hosp 1988; **Fac Appt:** Prof Med, Med Coll VA

Toskes, Phillip MD [Ge] - **Spec Exp:** Nutrition; Malabsorption Syndrome; Pancreatic Disease; **Hospital:** Shands at Univ of FL; **Address:** Univ Florida, Div Gastroenterolgy, P.O. Box 100214, Gainesville, FL 32610-0214; **Phone:** 352-392-2877; **Board Cert:** Internal Medicine 1970; Gastroenterology 1973; **Med School:** Univ MD Sch Med 1965; **Resid:** Internal Medicine, Univ Maryland Hosp 1968; **Fellow:** Gastroenterology, Hosp Univ Penn 1970; **Fac Appt:** Prof Med, Univ Fla Coll Med

Vaezi, Michael F MD/PhD [Ge] - **Spec Exp:** Gastroesophageal Reflux Disease (GERD); Esophageal Disorders; **Hospital:** Vanderbilt Univ Med Ctr; **Address:** 1301 Medical Center Drive, Ste 1660, Nashville, TN 37232; **Phone:** 615-322-0128; **Board Cert:** Internal Medicine 2007; Gastroenterology 1999; **Med School:** Univ Ala 1992; **Resid:** Internal Medicine, Univ AL-Birmingham Med Ctr 1995; **Fellow:** Gastroenterology, Cleveland Clinic 1996; **Fac Appt:** Prof Med, Vanderbilt Univ

Wilcox, C Mel MD [Ge] - **Spec Exp:** AIDS/HIV-Gastrointestinal Complications; Endoscopy; Pancreatic & Biliary Disease; **Hospital:** Univ of Ala Hosp at Birmingham; **Address:** UAB-Div Gastroenterology, 703 S 19th St, ZRB 633, Birmingham, AL 35294-0007; **Phone:** 205-975-4958; **Board Cert:** Internal Medicine 1986; Gastroenterology 2007; **Med School:** Med Coll GA 1983; **Resid:** Internal Medicine, Univ Alabama Hosps 1986; **Fellow:** Gastroenterology, UCSF 1990; **Fac Appt:** Prof Med, Univ Ala

217

Gastroenterology

Midwest

Achkar, Edgar MD [Ge] - **Spec Exp:** Esophageal Disorders; Gastrointestinal Motility Disorders; **Hospital:** Cleveland Clin Fdn (page 56); **Address:** 9500 Euclid Ave, Desk A31, Cleveland, OH 44195; **Phone:** 216-444-6523; **Board Cert:** Internal Medicine 1978; Gastroenterology 1979; **Med School:** Lebanon 1964; **Resid:** Internal Medicine, Lahey Clin 1967; **Fellow:** Gastroenterology, Lahey Clin 1968; Gastroenterology, Clevland Clin 1969; **Fac Appt:** Prof Med, Cleveland Cl Coll Med/Case West Res

Bacon, Bruce MD [Ge] - **Spec Exp:** Hepatitis C; Hepatic Iron Metabolism; Liver Disease; **Hospital:** St Louis Univ Hosp, SSM St Mary's Hlth Ctr - St Louis; **Address:** 3660 Vista Ave, Ste 308, St Louis, MO 63110-2540; **Phone:** 314-977-6150; **Board Cert:** Internal Medicine 1978; Gastroenterology 1983; Transplant Hepatology 2006; **Med School:** Case West Res Univ 1975; **Resid:** Internal Medicine, Metro Genl Hosp 1979; **Fellow:** Gastroenterology, Metro Genl Hosp 1982; **Fac Appt:** Prof Med, St Louis Univ

Baron, Todd H MD [Ge] - **Spec Exp:** Endoscopy; Pancreatic/Biliary Endoscopy (ERCP); **Hospital:** Mayo Med Ctr & Clin - Rochester; **Address:** Mayo Clinic, 200 First St SW, Charleton 8, Rochester, MN 55905; **Phone:** 507-266-6931; **Board Cert:** Internal Medicine 1989; Gastroenterology 2003; **Med School:** Univ Fla Coll Med 1986; **Resid:** Internal Medicine, Univ Alabama Med Ctr 1990; **Fellow:** Gastroenterology, Univ Alabama Med Ctr 1993; **Fac Appt:** Assoc Prof Med, Univ Ariz Coll Med

Brown, Kimberly A MD [Ge] - **Spec Exp:** Liver Disease; Transplant Medicine-Liver; Hepatitis C; Liver Cancer; **Hospital:** Henry Ford Hosp; **Address:** Henry Ford Hosp, Dept Gastroenterology, 2799 W Grand Blvd Bldg K Fl 7, Detroit, MI 48202-2608; **Phone:** 313-916-8632; **Board Cert:** Internal Medicine 1988; Gastroenterology 2002; Transplant Hepatology 2006; **Med School:** Wayne State Univ 1985; **Resid:** Internal Medicine, Univ Michigan Med Ctr 1989; **Fellow:** Gastroenterology, Univ Michigan Med Ctr 1992

Chari, Suresh T MD [Ge] - **Spec Exp:** Pancreatic Disease; **Hospital:** Mayo Med Ctr & Clin - Rochester; **Address:** Mayo Clinic, 200 First St SW Mayo Bldg Fl 9, Rochester, MN 55905; **Phone:** 507-266-4347; **Board Cert:** Gastroenterology 1999; **Med School:** India 1982; **Resid:** Internal Medicine, Univ Arizona Hlth Sci Ctr 1996; **Fellow:** Gastroenterology, Mayo Clinic 1999; **Fac Appt:** Prof Med, Mayo Med Sch

Craig, Robert M MD [Ge] - **Spec Exp:** Inflammatory Bowel Disease/Crohn's; Liver Disease; Swallowing Disorders; Diarrheal Diseases; **Hospital:** Northwestern Meml Hosp; **Address:** 233 E Erie St, Ste 206, Chicago, IL 60611-5938; **Phone:** 312-908-9644; **Board Cert:** Internal Medicine 1972; Gastroenterology 1975; **Med School:** Northwestern Univ 1967; **Resid:** Internal Medicine, VA Rsch Hosp 1969; Internal Medicine, VA Rsch Hosp 1972; **Fellow:** Gastroenterology, Northwestern Meml Hosp 1974; **Fac Appt:** Prof Med, Northwestern Univ

Crippin, Jeffrey S MD [Ge] - **Spec Exp:** Transplant Medicine-Liver; Liver Disease; Liver Failure; Gastrointestinal Cancer; **Hospital:** Barnes-Jewish Hosp; **Address:** Barnes Jewish Hosp, Div Gastroenterology, 660 S Euclid Ave Campus Box 8124, St Louis, MO 63110; **Phone:** 314-454-8160; **Board Cert:** Internal Medicine 1987; Gastroenterology 2001; Transplant Hepatology 2006; **Med School:** Univ Kans 1984; **Resid:** Internal Medicine, Kansas Univ Med Ctr 1988; **Fellow:** Gastroenterology, Mayo Clinic 1991; **Fac Appt:** Assoc Prof Med, Washington Univ, St Louis

Di Bisceglie, Adrian M MD [Ge] - **Spec Exp:** Hepatitis C; Hepatitis; Liver Cancer; **Hospital:** St Louis Univ Hosp; **Address:** St Louis Univ Hosp, Dept. Gastroenterology, 3635 Vista Ave, PO Box 15250, St Louis, MO 63110-0250; **Phone:** 314-577-8764; **Board Cert:** Internal Medicine 2002; Gastroenterology 2002; **Med School:** South Africa 1977; **Resid:** Internal Medicine, Baragwanath Hosp 1984; **Fellow:** Hepatology, Natl Inst Hlth 1988; **Fac Appt:** Prof Med, St Louis Univ

Edmundowicz, Steven A MD [Ge] - **Spec Exp:** Endoscopy; Biliary Disease; Pancreatic Disease; **Hospital:** Barnes-Jewish Hosp; **Address:** Washington Univ Sch Med, Div Gastroenterology, 660 S Euclid Ave, Box 8124, St Louis, MO 63110; **Phone:** 314-747-2066; **Board Cert:** Internal Medicine 1986; Gastroenterology 1989; **Med School:** Jefferson Med Coll 1983; **Resid:** Internal Medicine, Barnes Hosp 1986; **Fellow:** Gastroenterology, Barnes Hosp/Wash Univ 1989; **Fac Appt:** Assoc Prof Med, Washington Univ, St Louis

Elliott, David MD [Ge] - **Spec Exp:** Celiac Disease; Inflammatory Bowel Disease/Crohn's; Intestinal Parasites; **Hospital:** Univ Iowa Hosp & Clinics; **Address:** Univ Iowa Hosp, Digestive Disease, 200 Hawkins Drive, rm 4611-JCP, Iowa City, IA 52242; **Phone:** 319-356-4060; **Board Cert:** Internal Medicine 1991; Gastroenterology 1993; **Med School:** Wayne State Univ 1988; **Resid:** Internal Medicine, Johns Hopkins Hosp 1991; **Fellow:** Gastroenterology, Univ Iowa Hosps 1993; **Fac Appt:** Assoc Prof Med, Univ Iowa Coll Med

Elta, Grace H MD [Ge] - **Spec Exp:** Biliary Disease; **Hospital:** Univ Michigan Hlth Sys; **Address:** Univ Michigan Health System, 1500 E Medical Ctr Drive, 3912 Taubman Center, Ann Arbor, MI 48109-0362; **Phone:** 888-229-7408; **Board Cert:** Internal Medicine 1980; Gastroenterology 1983; **Med School:** Univ Mich Med Sch 1977; **Resid:** Internal Medicine, New England Med Ctr 1980; **Fellow:** Gastroenterology, New England Med Ctr 1982; **Fac Appt:** Prof Med, Univ Mich Med Sch

Goldberg, Michael J MD [Ge] - **Spec Exp:** Colon Cancer; Inflammatory Bowel Disease; Pancreatic & Biliary Disease; Pancreatic/Biliary Endoscopy (ERCP); **Hospital:** Evanston Hosp, Glenbrook Hosp; **Address:** 2650 Ridge Ave, Ste G-208, Evanston, IL 60201; **Phone:** 847-657-1900; **Board Cert:** Internal Medicine 1978; Gastroenterology 1981; **Med School:** Univ IL Coll Med 1975; **Resid:** Internal Medicine, Univ Illinois Hosp 1978; **Fellow:** Gastroenterology, Tufts-New England Med Ctr 1980; **Fac Appt:** Assoc Clin Prof Med, Northwestern Univ

Gostout, Christopher MD [Ge] - **Spec Exp:** Gastroscopy; Endoscopy; **Hospital:** Mayo Med Ctr & Clin - Rochester; **Address:** Mayo Clinic, Div GI, 200 First St SW Mayo Bldg Fl 9, Rochester, MN 55905; **Phone:** 507-266-6932; **Board Cert:** Internal Medicine 1979; Gastroenterology 1981; **Med School:** SUNY Downstate 1976; **Resid:** Internal Medicine, Mayo Clinic 1979; **Fellow:** Gastroenterology, Mayo Clinic 1981

Hanauer, Stephen B MD [Ge] - **Spec Exp:** Inflammatory Bowel Disease; Crohn's Disease; Ulcerative Colitis; Clinical Trials; **Hospital:** Univ of Chicago Hosps; **Address:** Univ Chicago Hosps, 5841 S Maryland Ave, MC 4076, Chicago, IL 60637-1426; **Phone:** 773-702-1466; **Board Cert:** Internal Medicine 1980; Gastroenterology 1983; **Med School:** Univ IL Coll Med 1977; **Resid:** Internal Medicine, Univ Chicago Hosps 1980; **Fellow:** Gastroenterology, Univ Chicago Hosps 1982; **Fac Appt:** Prof Med, Univ Chicago-Pritzker Sch Med

Jensen, Donald M MD [Ge] - **Spec Exp:** Transplant Medicine-Liver; Hepatitis C; Liver & Biliary Disease; Liver Cancer; **Hospital:** Univ of Chicago Hosps; **Address:** Univ of Chicago, Ctr for Liver Disease, 5841 S Maryland Ave, MC 7120, Chicago, IL 60637; **Phone:** 773-702-2300; **Board Cert:** Internal Medicine 1975; Gastroenterology 1981; **Med School:** Univ IL Coll Med 1972; **Resid:** Internal Medicine, Rush Presby St Lukes Hosp 1975; Gastroenterology, Rush Presby St Lukes Hosp 1976; **Fellow:** Gastroenterology, King's College Hosp 1978; **Fac Appt:** Prof Med, Univ Chicago-Pritzker Sch Med

Kahrilas, Peter J MD [Ge] - **Spec Exp:** Esophageal Disorders; Swallowing Disorders; **Hospital:** Northwestern Meml Hosp; **Address:** 675 N St Clair, Fl 17 - Ste 250, Chicago, IL 60611; **Phone:** 312-695-0606; **Board Cert:** Internal Medicine 1982; Gastroenterology 1987; **Med School:** Univ Rochester 1979; **Resid:** Internal Medicine, Univ Hosp 1982; **Fellow:** Gastroenterology, Northwestern Univ 1984; Research, Med Coll Wisconsin 1986; **Fac Appt:** Prof Med, Northwestern Univ

Gastroenterology

Konicek, Frank J MD [Ge] - **Spec Exp:** Endoscopy; Inflammatory Bowel Disease/Crohn's; Pancreatic Disease; Liver Disease; **Hospital:** Swedish Covenant Hosp, Adv Illinois Masonic Med Ctr; **Address:** 3004 N Ashland Ave, Chicago, IL 60657-3012; **Phone:** 773-871-4600; **Board Cert:** Internal Medicine 1977; Gastroenterology 1975; **Med School:** Loyola Univ-Stritch Sch Med 1963; **Resid:** Internal Medicine, St Francis Hosp 1965; Internal Medicine, Hines VA Hosp 1969; **Fellow:** Gastroenterology, Hines VA Hosp 1971; **Fac Appt:** Clin Prof Med, Loyola Univ-Stritch Sch Med

Kwo, Paul Y MD [Ge] - **Spec Exp:** Hepatitis B & C; Transplant Medicine-Liver; **Hospital:** Indiana Univ Hosp; **Address:** 975 W Walnut St, IB327, Indianapolis, IN 46202-5181; **Phone:** 317-274-3090; **Board Cert:** Gastroenterology 2005; Transplant Hepatology 2006; **Med School:** Wayne State Univ 1988; **Resid:** Internal Medicine, Univ Maryland Med Ctr 1991; **Fellow:** Gastroenterology, Mayo Clinic 1995; **Fac Appt:** Clin Prof Med, Indiana Univ

La Russo, Nicholas F MD [Ge] - **Spec Exp:** Transplant Medicine-Liver; Liver & Biliary Disease; **Hospital:** Mayo Med Ctr & Clin - Rochester; **Address:** Mayo Clinic, Div Gastroenterology, 200 First St SW, Rochester, MN 55905-0001; **Phone:** 507-284-2141; **Board Cert:** Internal Medicine 1972; Gastroenterology 1979; **Med School:** NY Med Coll 1969; **Resid:** Internal Medicine, Mayo Clinic 1972; **Fellow:** Gastroenterology, Mayo Clinic 1975; **Fac Appt:** Prof Med, Mayo Med Sch

Lashner, Bret A MD [Ge] - **Spec Exp:** Inflammatory Bowel Disease; **Hospital:** Cleveland Clin Fdn (page 56); **Address:** 9500 Euclid Ave, Desk A30, Cleveland, OH 44195; **Phone:** 216-444-6524; **Board Cert:** Internal Medicine 1983; Gastroenterology 1985; **Med School:** NYU Sch Med 1980; **Resid:** Internal Medicine, Temple Univ Hosp 1983; **Fellow:** Gastroenterology, Univ Chicago Hosps 1986; **Fac Appt:** Assoc Prof Med, Case West Res Univ

Lindor, Keith MD [Ge] - **Spec Exp:** Liver Disease; Biliary Disease; **Hospital:** Mayo Med Ctr & Clin - Rochester; **Address:** Mayo Clinic, Div Gastroenterology, 200 First St SW, Rochester, MN 55905; **Phone:** 507-284-4313; **Board Cert:** Internal Medicine 1983; Gastroenterology 1987; **Med School:** Mayo Med Sch 1979; **Resid:** Internal Medicine, N Carolina Baptist Hosp 1982; **Fellow:** Gastroenterology, Mayo Clinic 1986; **Fac Appt:** Prof Med, Mayo Med Sch

Lucey, Michael R MD [Ge] - **Spec Exp:** Liver Disease; Transplant Medicine-Liver; **Hospital:** Univ WI Hosp & Clins; **Address:** Univ Wisc Hosps & Clins, 600 Highland Ave, H6-516 CSC, Madison, WI 53792; **Phone:** 608-263-7322; **Board Cert:** Internal Medicine 2001; Gastroenterology 2001; Transplant Hepatology 2006; **Med School:** Ireland 1980; **Resid:** Internal Medicine, Fed Dublin Vol Hosps 1979; Gastroenterology, St Bartholomews Hosp/Kings Coll Hosp 1985; **Fellow:** Gastroenterology, Univ Michigan Med Ctr 1987; **Fac Appt:** Prof Med, Univ Wisc

Luxon, Bruce MD/PhD [Ge] - **Spec Exp:** Liver Disease; Hepatitis C; Autoimmune Liver Disease; **Hospital:** Univ Iowa Hosp & Clinics; **Address:** 4607 JCP UIHC, 200 Hawkins Drive, Iowa City, IA 52242; **Phone:** 319-356-4060; **Board Cert:** Internal Medicine 1989; Gastroenterology 2001; **Med School:** Univ MO-Columbia Sch Med 1985; **Resid:** Internal Medicine, Univ MO-Columbia Sch Med 1989; **Fellow:** Gastroenterology, UCSF Med Ctr 1992; **Fac Appt:** Prof Med, St Louis Univ

Meiselman, Mick S MD [Ge] - **Spec Exp:** Colonoscopy; Pancreatic & Biliary Disease; Gastroesophageal Reflux Disease (GERD); **Hospital:** Evanston Hosp, Glenbrook Hosp; **Address:** 506 Green Bay Rd, Kenilworth, IL 60043-1002; **Phone:** 847-256-3495; **Board Cert:** Internal Medicine 1982; Gastroenterology 1985; **Med School:** Northwestern Univ 1979; **Resid:** Internal Medicine, Cedars-Sinai/UCLA 1982; **Fellow:** Gastroenterology, UCSF Med Ctr 1984; **Fac Appt:** Assoc Clin Prof Med, Northwestern Univ

Murray, Joseph A MD [Ge] - **Spec Exp:** Celiac Disease; Esophageal Disorders; **Hospital:** Mayo Med Ctr & Clin - Rochester; **Address:** Mayo Clinic, Div Gastroenterology, 200 First St SW, Rochester, MN 55905; **Phone:** 507-284-2631; **Board Cert:** Internal Medicine 1999; Gastroenterology 2000; **Med School:** Ireland 1983; **Resid:** Internal Medicine, St Laurences Hosp 1986; Gastroenterology, Beaumont Hosp 1988; **Fellow:** Gastroenterology, Univ Iowa Hosps & Clins 1990; **Fac Appt:** Prof Med, Mayo Med Sch

O'Brien, John J MD [Ge] - **Spec Exp:** Esophageal Disorders; Liver Disease; **Hospital:** Providence Hosp - Southfield; **Address:** Providence Hosp, 16001 W 9 Mile Rd, Southfield, MI 48075; **Phone:** 248-849-3152; **Board Cert:** Internal Medicine 1988; Gastroenterology 2005; **Med School:** Univ MO-Columbia Sch Med 1981; **Resid:** Internal Medicine, St Lukes Hosp 1984; Gastroenterology, Univ KY Med Ctr 1986; **Fellow:** Gastroenterology, Johns Hopkins Hosp 1989; **Fac Appt:** Prof Med, Univ Mich Med Sch

Owyang, Chung MD [Ge] - **Spec Exp:** Gastrointestinal Motility Disorders; Digestive Disorders; **Hospital:** Univ Michigan Hlth Sys; **Address:** Univ Mich, Div Gastroenterology, 1500 E Med Ctr Dr, Rm 3912 Taubman Ctr, Ann Arbor, MI 48109-0362; **Phone:** 734-936-4785; **Board Cert:** Internal Medicine 1976; Gastroenterology 1981; **Med School:** McGill Univ 1972; **Resid:** Internal Medicine, Montreal Genl Hosp 1975; **Fellow:** Gastroenterology, Mayo Grad Med Sch 1978; **Fac Appt:** Prof Med, Univ Mich Med Sch

Rao, Satish S C MD [Ge] - **Spec Exp:** Constipation; Incontinence-Fecal; Chest Pain-Non Cardiac; **Hospital:** Univ Iowa Hosp & Clinics; **Address:** Univ Iowa Hosp & Clinics, Div Gastro, 200 Hawkins Drive, rm 4612 JCP, Iowa City, IA 52242; **Phone:** 319-353-6602; **Board Cert:** Internal Medicine 1996; Gastroenterology 1998; **Med School:** India 1978; **Resid:** Internal Medicine, Sunderland Hosps 1982; Internal Medicine, York Dist Hosp 1984; **Fellow:** Royal Hallamshire Hosp 1986; Gastroenterology, Royal Liverpool Hosp 1988; **Fac Appt:** Prof Med, Univ Iowa Coll Med

Reichelderfer, Mark MD [Ge] - **Spec Exp:** Endoscopy; Inflammatory Bowel Disease; **Hospital:** Univ WI Hosp & Clins; **Address:** 600 Highland Ave, H6/516, Madison, WI 53792-5124; **Phone:** 608-263-8094; **Board Cert:** Internal Medicine 1977; Gastroenterology 1979; **Med School:** Columbia P&S 1974; **Resid:** Internal Medicine, Mary Imogene Bassett Hosp 1977; **Fellow:** Gastroenterology, Univ Wisc Hosps & Clin 1979; **Fac Appt:** Prof Med, Univ Wisc

Rex, Douglas K MD [Ge] - **Spec Exp:** Endoscopy; Endoscopic Ultrasound; **Hospital:** Indiana Univ Hosp; **Address:** 550 N University Blvd, Ste 4100, Indianapolis, IN 46202; **Phone:** 317-278-9763; **Board Cert:** Internal Medicine 1985; Gastroenterology 1987; **Med School:** Indiana Univ 1980; **Resid:** Internal Medicine, Indiana Univ Med Ctr 1982; Internal Medicine, Indiana Univ Hosp 1985; **Fellow:** Gastroenterology, Indiana Univ Med Ctr 1984; **Fac Appt:** Prof Med, Indiana Univ

Sandborn, William J MD [Ge] - **Spec Exp:** Inflammatory Bowel Disease/Crohn's; Ulcerative Colitis; Crohn's Disease; **Hospital:** Mayo Med Ctr & Clin - Rochester; **Address:** Mayo Clinic, Div GI, 200 First St SW, Rochester, MN 55905; **Phone:** 507-284-0959; **Board Cert:** Gastroenterology 2003; Gastroenterology 2003; **Med School:** Loma Linda Univ 1987; **Resid:** Internal Medicine, Loma Linda Univ 1990; **Fellow:** Gastroenterology, Mayo Clinic 1993; **Fac Appt:** Assoc Prof Med, Mayo Med Sch

Schulze, Konrad S MD [Ge] - **Spec Exp:** Gastroesophageal Reflux Disease (GERD); Peptic Acid Disorders; Gastroparesis; **Hospital:** Univ Iowa Hosp & Clinics; **Address:** UIHC, Dept Gastroenterology, 200 Hawkins Drive, rm 4551B JCP, Iowa City, IA 52242; **Phone:** 319-356-4060; **Board Cert:** Internal Medicine 1987; Gastroenterology 1975; **Med School:** Germany 1968; **Resid:** Psychiatry, Boston City Hosp 1971; Internal Medicine, Montreal Genl Hosp 1974; **Fellow:** Gastroenterology, Univ Iowa 1977; **Fac Appt:** Prof Med, Univ Iowa Coll Med

Gastroenterology

Semrad, Carol E MD [Ge] - **Spec Exp:** Celiac Disease; Diarrheal Diseases; Malabsorption Syndrome; Nutrition; **Hospital:** Univ of Chicago Hosps; **Address:** 5841 S Maryland Ave, MC 4080.S401, Chicago, IL 60637; **Phone:** 773-702-6921; **Board Cert:** Internal Medicine 1985; Gastroenterology 1987; **Med School:** Columbia P&S 1982; **Resid:** Internal Medicine, Columbia-Presby Med Ctr 1985; **Fellow:** Gastroenterology, Columbia-Presby Med Ctr 1986; **Fac Appt:** Assoc Prof Med, Univ Chicago-Pritzker Sch Med

Shaker, Reza MD [Ge] - **Spec Exp:** Swallowing Disorders; Gastrointestinal Motility Disorders; Gastroesophageal Reflux Disease (GERD); Pancreatic/Biliary Endoscopy (ERCP); **Hospital:** Froedtert Meml Lutheran Hosp; **Address:** Med Coll Wisconsin/Gastroenterology, 9200 W Wisconsin Ave, rm E4510, Milwaukee, WI 53226; **Phone:** 414-456-6840; **Med School:** Iran 1975; **Resid:** Internal Medicine, Kingsbrook Jewish Med Ctr 1985; **Fellow:** Gastroenterology, Med Coll Wisconsin 1988; **Fac Appt:** Prof Med, Univ Wisc

Sherman, Stuart MD [Ge] - **Spec Exp:** Pancreatic & Biliary Disease; Endoscopy; Pancreatic/Biliary Endoscopy (ERCP); **Hospital:** Indiana Univ Hosp; **Address:** Indiana Univ Medical Ctr, 550 N University Blvd, Ste 4100, Indianapolis, IN 46202; **Phone:** 317-274-0925; **Board Cert:** Internal Medicine 1985; Gastroenterology 1989; **Med School:** Washington Univ, St Louis 1982; **Resid:** Internal Medicine, Presby Univ Hosp 1985; **Fellow:** Gastroenterology, UCLA Med Ctr 1989; **Fac Appt:** Clin Prof Med, Indiana Univ

Silverman, William B MD [Ge] - **Spec Exp:** Pancreatic/Biliary Endoscopy (ERCP); **Hospital:** Univ Iowa Hosp & Clinics; **Address:** UIHC, Div GI/Hepatology, 200 Hawkins Drive, rm 4551B JCP, Iowa City, IA 52242; **Phone:** 319-356-4060; **Board Cert:** Internal Medicine 1988; Gastroenterology 2008; **Med School:** Belgium 1984; **Resid:** Internal Medicine, Lutheran General Hosp 1987; **Fellow:** Gastroenterology, Case Western Res Univ 1989; Gastroenterology, Indiana Univ Hosp 1990; **Fac Appt:** Prof Med, Univ Iowa Coll Med

Tremaine, William J MD [Ge] - **Spec Exp:** Inflammatory Bowel Disease/Crohn's; Ulcerative Colitis; Irritable Bowel Syndrome; **Hospital:** Mayo Med Ctr & Clin - Rochester, St Mary's Hosp - Rochester; **Address:** Mayo Clinic, Div Gastroenterology, 200 First St SW, Rochester, MN 55905-0002; **Phone:** 507-284-2468; **Board Cert:** Internal Medicine 1979; Gastroenterology 1981; **Med School:** Univ Miss 1976; **Resid:** Internal Medicine, Mayo Clinic 1980; **Fellow:** Gastroenterology, Mayo Clinic 1981; **Fac Appt:** Prof Med, Mayo Med Sch

Van Thiel, David H MD [Ge] - **Spec Exp:** Transplant Medicine-Liver; Hepatitis; Liver Disease; **Hospital:** Rush Univ Med Ctr; **Address:** Rush Univ Hepatologists, 1725 W Harrison Rd, Ste 158, Chicago, IL 60612; **Phone:** 312-942-8910; **Board Cert:** Internal Medicine 1972; Gastroenterology 1975; **Med School:** UCLA 1967; **Resid:** Internal Medicine, NY Hosp 1969; Internal Medicine, Univ Hosp 1972; **Fellow:** Gastroenterology, Univ Hosp 1974; Research, NIH 1976; **Fac Appt:** Prof Med, Loyola Univ-Stritch Sch Med

Vege, Santhi S MD [Ge] - **Spec Exp:** Pancreatic Disease; **Hospital:** Mayo Med Ctr & Clin - Rochester; **Address:** Mayo Clinic, 200 First St SW Gonda Bldg Fl 9, Rochester, MN 55905; **Phone:** 507-284-2478; **Board Cert:** Internal Medicine 2007; **Med School:** India 1975; **Resid:** Internal Medicine, Govt Genl Hosp 1978; Internal Medicine, Mayo Clinic 1997; **Fellow:** Gastroenterology, Post Grad Inst 1981; Gastroenterology, Mayo Clinic 1998; **Fac Appt:** Prof Med, Mayo Med Sch

Wald, Arnold MD [Ge] - **Spec Exp:** Constipation; Gastrointestinal Motility Disorders; Irritable Bowel Syndrome; **Hospital:** Univ WI Hosp & Clins; **Address:** Univ Wisconsin Hosp & Clinics, 600 Highland Ave, H6/516 CSC, Madison, WI 57392-2451; **Phone:** 608-263-1995; **Board Cert:** Internal Medicine 1972; Gastroenterology 1975; **Med School:** SUNY Downstate 1968; **Resid:** Internal Medicine, SUNY - Downstate Med Ctr 1971; **Fellow:** Gastroenterology, Johns Hopkins Hosp 1975; **Fac Appt:** Prof Med, Univ Wisc

Waxman, Irving MD [Ge] - **Spec Exp:** Gastrointestinal Cancer; Pancreatic Cancer; Endoscopy; **Hospital:** Univ of Chicago Hosps; **Address:** University of Chicago Hospitals, 5758 S Maryland Ave, MC 9028, Chicago, IL 60637; **Phone:** 773-702-1459; **Board Cert:** Internal Medicine 1988; Gastroenterology 2003; **Med School:** Mexico 1985; **Resid:** Internal Medicine, New England Deaconess Hosp 1988; **Fellow:** Gastroenterology, Georgetown Univ Med Ctr 1991; Endoscopy, Univ Academic Med Ctr 1991; **Fac Appt:** Prof Med, Univ Chicago-Pritzker Sch Med

Wiesner, Russell MD [Ge] - **Spec Exp:** Transplant Medicine-Liver; **Hospital:** Mayo Med Ctr & Clin - Rochester; **Address:** Mayo Clinic, Div GI, 200 First St SW, Rochester, MN 55905; **Phone:** 507-284-8714; **Board Cert:** Internal Medicine 1978; Gastroenterology 1981; **Med School:** Med Coll Wisc 1975; **Resid:** Internal Medicine, Mayo Clinic 1978

Winans, Charles S MD [Ge] - **Spec Exp:** Esophageal Disorders; Gastroesophageal Reflux Disease (GERD); Swallowing Disorders; **Hospital:** Univ of Chicago Hosps; **Address:** 5841 S Maryland Ave, MC 4076, Chicago, IL 60637-1426; **Phone:** 773-834-4180; **Board Cert:** Internal Medicine 1968; Gastroenterology 1970; **Med School:** Case West Res Univ 1961; **Resid:** Internal Medicine, Univ Hosp 1964; **Fellow:** Gastroenterology, Boston Univ Med Ctr 1966; **Fac Appt:** Prof Med, Univ Chicago-Pritzker Sch Med

Great Plains and Mountains

Bjorkman, David MD [Ge] - **Spec Exp:** Peptic Acid Disorders; Endoscopy; **Hospital:** Univ Utah Hosps and Clins; **Address:** 30 N 1900 East, 1900 E, Salt Lake City, UT 84132; **Phone:** 801-581-6436; **Board Cert:** Internal Medicine 1983; Gastroenterology 1985; **Med School:** Univ Utah 1980; **Resid:** Internal Medicine, Brigham & Women's Harvard 1983; **Fellow:** Gastroenterology, Brigham & Women's Harvard 1985; **Fac Appt:** Prof Med, Univ Utah

Burt, Randall W MD [Ge] - **Spec Exp:** Colon Cancer; Colon & Rectal Cancer-Familial Polyposis; **Hospital:** Univ Utah Hosps and Clins; **Address:** Huntsman Cancer Institute, 2000 Circle of Hope, Salt Lake City, UT 84112; **Phone:** 801-585-3281; **Board Cert:** Internal Medicine 1977; Gastroenterology 1979; **Med School:** Univ Utah 1974; **Resid:** Internal Medicine, Barnes Hosp 1977; **Fellow:** Gastroenterology, Univ Utah Med Ctr 1979; **Fac Appt:** Prof Med, Univ Utah

Everson, Gregory T MD [Ge] - **Spec Exp:** Liver Disease; Hepatitis; Transplant Medicine-Liver; **Hospital:** Univ Colorado Hosp; **Address:** Univ Colorado Hlth Sci Ctr, Div Hepatology, 4200 E 9th Ave, Box B154, Denver, CO 80262; **Phone:** 720-848-2245; **Board Cert:** Internal Medicine 1979; Gastroenterology 1983; **Med School:** Cornell Univ-Weill Med Coll 1976; **Resid:** Internal Medicine, Creighton Univ Med Ctr 1979; **Fellow:** Gastroenterology, Univ Colorado Health Sci Ctr 1982; **Fac Appt:** Prof Med, Univ Colorado

Fang, John C MD [Ge] - **Spec Exp:** Endoscopy; Esophageal Disorders; Irritable Bowel Syndrome; Barrett's Esophagus; **Hospital:** Univ Utah Hosps and Clins; **Address:** 1525 W 2100 S, Salt Lake City, UT 84119; **Phone:** 801-213-9900; **Board Cert:** Gastroenterology 1998; **Med School:** Washington Univ, St Louis 1989; **Resid:** Internal Medicine, Temple Univ Hosp 1992; **Fellow:** Gastroenterology, Univ VA Hlth Sci Ctr 1995; **Fac Appt:** Assoc Prof Med, Univ Utah

Hunter, Ellen B MD [Ge] - **Spec Exp:** Hepatitis; **Hospital:** St. Luke's Reg Med Ctr - Boise; **Address:** 425 W Vannock St, Boise, ID 83702; **Phone:** 208-343-6458; **Board Cert:** Internal Medicine 1986; Gastroenterology 1989; **Med School:** Georgetown Univ 1983; **Resid:** Internal Medicine, Vanderbilt Univ Med Ctr 1986; **Fellow:** Gastroenterology, Mayo Clinic 1989

Gastroenterology

Sorrell, Michael MD [Ge] - **Spec Exp:** Transplant Medicine-Liver; Hepatitis; Liver Tumors; Liver Disease; **Hospital:** Nebraska Med Ctr; **Address:** 983285 Nebraska Medical Ctr, Omaha, NE 68198-3285; **Phone:** 402-559-7912; **Board Cert:** Internal Medicine 1972; **Med School:** Univ Nebr Coll Med 1959; **Resid:** Internal Medicine, Univ Nebraska Hosp 1968; Gastroenterology, Univ Nebraska Hosp 1969; **Fellow:** Hepatology, New Jersey Coll Med 1971; **Fac Appt:** Prof Med, Univ Nebr Coll Med

Southwest

Anderson, Karl MD [Ge] - **Spec Exp:** Porphyria; Liver Disease; **Hospital:** UT Med Br Hosp at Galveston; **Address:** Univ Tex Med Branch, 700 Harborside Dr, Galveston, TX 77555-1109; **Phone:** 409-747-7500; **Board Cert:** Internal Medicine 1972; Gastroenterology 1972; **Med School:** Johns Hopkins Univ 1965; **Resid:** Internal Medicine, Vanderbilt Univ Hosp 1967; Internal Medicine, New York Hosp-Cornell Med Ctr 1968; **Fellow:** Gastroenterology, New York Hosp-Cornell Med Ctr 1970; **Fac Appt:** Prof Med, Univ Tex Med Br, Galveston

Balart, Luis A MD [Ge] - **Spec Exp:** Hepatitis C; **Hospital:** Tulane Univ Hosp & Clin; **Address:** 1415 Tulane Ave, New Orleans, LA 70112; **Phone:** 504-988-5800; **Board Cert:** Internal Medicine 1976; Gastroenterology 1981; **Med School:** Cuba 1973; **Resid:** Internal Medicine, Naval Regl Med Ctr 1976; **Fac Appt:** Assoc Clin Prof Med, Louisiana State U, New Orleans

Boland, C Richard MD [Ge] - **Spec Exp:** Colon & Rectal Cancer Detection; Cancer Genetics; **Hospital:** Baylor Univ Medical Ctr; **Address:** GI Cancer Research Lab H-250, 3500 Gaston Ave, Dallas, TX 75246; **Phone:** 214-820-2692; **Board Cert:** Internal Medicine 1978; Gastroenterology 1981; **Med School:** Yale Univ 1973; **Resid:** Internal Medicine, USPHS Hosp 1978; **Fellow:** Gastroenterology, UCSF Med Ctr 1981; **Fac Appt:** Clin Prof Med, Univ Tex SW, Dallas

Boyer, Thomas D MD [Ge] - **Spec Exp:** Liver Disease; Hepatitis; Transplant Medicine-Liver; **Hospital:** Univ Med Ctr - Tucson; **Address:** Arizona Liver Institute, 1501 N Campbell Ave, Box 245136, Tucson, AZ 85724; **Phone:** 520-626-5952; **Board Cert:** Internal Medicine 1975; Gastroenterology 1977; **Med School:** USC Sch Med 1969; **Resid:** Internal Medicine, LAC-USC Med Ctr 1974; **Fellow:** Hepatology, John Wesley Co Hosp-USC Med Ctr 1976; **Fac Appt:** Prof Med, Univ Ariz Coll Med

Brady III, Charles E MD [Ge] - **Spec Exp:** Esophageal Disorders; **Hospital:** Univ Hlth Sys - Univ Hosp (San Antonio, TX); **Address:** Univ Tex Hlth Sci Ctr, Div GI, 7703 Floyd Curl Drive, MC 7878, San Antonio, TX 78229-3900; **Phone:** 210-567-4879; **Board Cert:** Internal Medicine 1974; Gastroenterology 1977; **Med School:** Med Coll VA 1971; **Resid:** Internal Medicine, Wilford Hall Med Ctr 1974; **Fellow:** Gastroenterology, Univ Tex 1976; **Fac Appt:** Assoc Prof Med, Univ Tex, San Antonio

Bresalier, Robert MD [Ge] - **Spec Exp:** Gastrointestinal Cancer; Peptic Acid Disorders; **Hospital:** UT MD Anderson Cancer Ctr; **Address:** MD Anderson Canc Ctr, GI Med & Nutrition, 1515 Holcombe Blvd - Unit 436, Houston, TX 77030-4009; **Phone:** 713-745-4340; **Board Cert:** Internal Medicine 1981; Gastroenterology 1983; **Med School:** Univ Chicago-Pritzker Sch Med 1978; **Resid:** Internal Medicine, Barnes Hosp-Washington Univ 1981; **Fellow:** Gastroenterology, UCSF Med Ctr 1983; **Fac Appt:** Prof Med, Univ Tex, Houston

Cunningham, John T MD [Ge] - **Spec Exp:** Biliary Disease; Pancreatic Disease; **Hospital:** Univ Med Ctr - Tucson; **Address:** Univ Medical Ctr, Div Gastroenterology, 1501 N Campbell Ave, PO Box 245028, Tucson, AZ 85724-5028; **Phone:** 520-626-6119; **Board Cert:** Internal Medicine 1975; Gastroenterology 1977; **Med School:** Med Coll VA 1970; **Resid:** Internal Medicine, Med Univ S Carolina 1975; **Fellow:** Gastroenterology, Med Univ S Carolina 1977; **Fac Appt:** Prof Med, Univ Ariz Coll Med

Das, Ananya MD [Ge] - **Spec Exp:** Endoscopy; Endoscopic Ultrasound; Pancreatic/Biliary Endoscopy (ERCP); **Hospital:** Mayo Clinic - Scottsdale; **Address:** Mayo Clinic, Div Gastroenterology, 13400 E Shea Blvd, Scottsdale, AZ 85259; **Phone:** 480-301-6990; **Board Cert:** Gastroenterology 1998; **Med School:** India 1987; **Resid:** Internal Medicine, SUNY Hlth Sci Ctr 1996; **Fellow:** Gastroenterology, Cleveland Clinic 1998; Endoscopy, Cleveland Clinic 2000; **Fac Appt:** Assoc Prof Med, Mayo Med Sch

Davis, Gary L MD [Ge] - **Spec Exp:** Liver Disease; Hepatitis; Transplant Medicine-Liver; **Hospital:** Baylor Univ Medical Ctr; **Address:** 3500 Gaston Ave, 4 Roberts, Transplant Services Department, Dallas, TX 75246; **Phone:** 214-820-8500; **Board Cert:** Internal Medicine 1979; Gastroenterology 1983; **Med School:** Univ Minn 1976; **Resid:** Internal Medicine, Mayo Clinic 1979; **Fellow:** Gastroenterology, Mayo Clinic 1981; Hepatology, Natl Inst Hlth 1984; **Fac Appt:** Prof Med, Baylor Coll Med

Feldman, Mark MD [Ge] - **Spec Exp:** Peptic Acid Disorders-Consultation; **Hospital:** Presby Hosp of Dallas; **Address:** 8200 Walnut Hill Ln, Dept Internal Med, Dallas, TX 75231; **Phone:** 214-345-7881; **Board Cert:** Internal Medicine 1976; Gastroenterology 1989; **Med School:** Temple Univ 1972; **Resid:** Internal Medicine, Temple Univ 1977; **Fellow:** Gastroenterology, Univ SW Texas 1976; **Fac Appt:** Prof Med, Univ Tex SW, Dallas

Fleischer, David MD [Ge] - **Spec Exp:** Barrett's Esophagus; Esophageal Cancer; **Hospital:** Mayo Clinic - Scottsdale; **Address:** Mayo Clinic - Scottsdale, 13400 E Shea Blvd, Div Gastroenterology 2A, Scottsdale, AZ 85259; **Phone:** 480-301-8484; **Board Cert:** Internal Medicine 1975; Gastroenterology 1977; **Med School:** Vanderbilt Univ 1970; **Resid:** Internal Medicine, Metro General Hosp 1975; **Fellow:** Gastroenterology, LA Co Harbor-UCLA Med Ctr 1977; **Fac Appt:** Prof Med, Mayo Med Sch

Galati, Joseph Steven MD [Ge] - **Spec Exp:** Liver Disease; Transplant Medicine-Liver; Hepatitis C; **Hospital:** St Luke's Episcopal Hosp - Houston, Meml Hermann Hosp - Texas Med Ctr; **Address:** 6624 Fannin St, Ste 1990, Houston, TX 77030; **Phone:** 713-794-0700; **Board Cert:** Gastroenterology 2005; **Med School:** Grenada 1987; **Resid:** Internal Medicine, SUNY Hlth Sci Ctr-Kings Co Hosp 1991; **Fellow:** Gastroenterology, Univ Nebraska 1994; **Fac Appt:** Asst Prof Med, Univ Tex, Houston

Glombicki, Alan Paul MD [Ge] - **Spec Exp:** Hepatitis; Transplant Medicine-Liver; Digestive Disorders; **Hospital:** St Luke's Episcopal Hosp - Houston, Meml Hermann Hosp - Texas Med Ctr; **Address:** 7737 SW Freeway, Ste 840, Houston, TX 77074; **Phone:** 713-777-2555; **Board Cert:** Internal Medicine 1986; Gastroenterology 1987; **Med School:** Univ IL Coll Med 1981; **Resid:** Internal Medicine, Baylor Coll Med 1984; Hepatology, Baylor Coll Med 1987; **Fellow:** Gastroenterology, Baylor Coll Med 1986; **Fac Appt:** Asst Clin Prof Med, Univ Tex, Houston

Hodges, David S MD [Ge] - **Spec Exp:** Inflammatory Bowel Disease/Crohn's; Irritable Bowel Syndrome; Gastrointestinal Functional Disorders; **Hospital:** Univ Med Ctr - Lubbock; **Address:** Tex Tech Med Ctr, Dept Int Med, 3601 4th St, MC 9410, Lubbock, TX 79430; **Phone:** 806-743-3150; **Board Cert:** Internal Medicine 1986; Gastroenterology 1989; **Med School:** Texas Tech Univ 1983; **Resid:** Internal Medicine, Lubbock Genl Hosp 1986; **Fellow:** Gastroenterology, Lubbock Genl Hosp 1989; **Fac Appt:** Assoc Prof Med, Texas Tech Univ

Olden, Kevin W MD [Ge] - **Spec Exp:** Psychiatry in Gastrointestinal Illness; Pain-Abdominal/Functional; Vomiting-Chronic; **Hospital:** UAMS Med Ctr; **Address:** Univ Arkansas, Dept Medicine, 4301 W Markham, Slot 567, Little Rock, AR 72205; **Phone:** 501-686-8000; **Board Cert:** Internal Medicine 1982; Gastroenterology 1989; Psychiatry 2002; Addiction Psychiatry 2002; **Med School:** SUNY Downstate 1976; **Resid:** Internal Medicine, UCLA Med Ctr 1979; Psychiatry, Mass Genl Hosp 1981; **Fellow:** Addiction Psychiatry, Stanford Univ Med Ctr 1983; Endoscopy, VA Med Ctr 1989; **Fac Appt:** Prof Med, Univ Ark

Gastroenterology

Pasricha, Pankaj MD [Ge] - **Spec Exp:** Swallowing Disorders-Botox Therapy; Gastrointestinal Motility Disorders; Pancreatic Disease; **Hospital:** UT Med Br Hosp at Galveston; **Address:** Univ Texas Medical Branch, 301 University Blvd, 4.106 McCullough Bldg, Galveston, TX 77555-0764; **Phone:** 409-772-5615; **Board Cert:** Internal Medicine 1988; Gastroenterology 2006; **Med School:** India 1983; **Resid:** Internal Medicine, DC Genl Hosp 1988; **Fellow:** Pulmonary Disease, New England Med Ctr 1990; Gastroenterology, Johns Hopkins Hosp 1992; **Fac Appt:** Prof Med, Univ Tex Med Br, Galveston

Speeg, Kermit V MD/PhD [Ge] - **Spec Exp:** Transplant Medicine-Liver; **Hospital:** Univ Hlth Sys - Univ Hosp (San Antonio, TX); **Address:** Univ Tex Hlth Sci Ctr, Div GI, 7703 Floyd Curl Drive, MC 7878, San Antonio, TX 78229-3900; **Phone:** 210-567-4879; **Board Cert:** Internal Medicine 1976; **Med School:** Univ Tex SW, Dallas 1972; **Resid:** Internal Medicine, Vanderbilt Univ Hosp 1974; **Fellow:** Gastroenterology, Vanderbilt Univ Hosp 1977; **Fac Appt:** Prof Med, Univ Tex, San Antonio

Vierling, John M MD [Ge] - **Spec Exp:** Liver Disease; Transplant Medicine-Liver; Autoimmune Liver Disease; Hepatitis; **Hospital:** St Luke's Episcopal Hosp - Houston; **Address:** Dept of Med, Baylor College of Med, 1709 Dryden, Ste 500, Houston, TX 77030; **Phone:** 713-798-8070; **Board Cert:** Internal Medicine 1975; Gastroenterology 1979; **Med School:** Stanford Univ 1972; **Resid:** Internal Medicine, Strong Meml Hosp 1974; Hepatology, Natl Inst Hlth 1977; **Fellow:** Gastroenterology, UCSF Med Ctr 1978; **Fac Appt:** Prof Med, Baylor Coll Med

West Coast and Pacific

Cello, John P MD [Ge] - **Spec Exp:** Endoscopy; Colonoscopy; Capsule Endoscopy; Pancreatic/Biliary Endoscopy (ERCP); **Hospital:** San Francisco Genl Hosp, UCSF Med Ctr; **Address:** San Francisco Genl Hosp-Univ California, 1001 Potrero Ave, Ste NH3D, San Francisco, CA 94110; **Phone:** 415-206-4746; **Board Cert:** Internal Medicine 1972; Gastroenterology 1977; **Med School:** Harvard Med Sch 1969; **Resid:** Internal Medicine, Peter Bent Brigham Hosp 1972; **Fellow:** Gastroenterology, UCSF Med Ctr 1977; **Fac Appt:** Prof Med, UCSF

Chang, Kenneth J MD [Ge] - **Spec Exp:** Gastrointestinal Cancer; Endoscopic Ultrasound; **Hospital:** UC Irvine Med Ctr; **Address:** UC Irvine Medical Ctr, 101 The City Drive 22C Bldg - rm 99, Orange, CA 92868; **Phone:** 714-456-6187; **Board Cert:** Internal Medicine 1988; Gastroenterology 2001; **Med School:** Brown Univ 1985; **Resid:** Internal Medicine, Rhode Island Hosp 1988; **Fellow:** Gastroenterology, UC-Irvine Med Ctr 1990

Ellis, Jonathan C MD [Ge] - **Spec Exp:** Colonoscopy; Endoscopy; Inflammatory Bowel Disease; **Hospital:** Cedars-Sinai Med Ctr; **Address:** 9090 Wilshire Blvd, Ste 101, Beverly Hills, CA 90211; **Phone:** 310-550-0400; **Board Cert:** Internal Medicine 1985; Gastroenterology 1989; **Med School:** Stanford Univ 1982; **Resid:** Internal Medicine, Cedars Sinai Med Ctr 1986; **Fellow:** Gastroenterology, UCLA 1988; **Fac Appt:** Assoc Prof Med, UCLA

Fennerty, Brian MD [Ge] - **Spec Exp:** Gastroesophageal Reflux Disease (GERD); **Hospital:** OR Hlth & Sci Univ; **Address:** Digestive Hlth, Ctr for Hlth & Healing, 3303 SW Bond Ave Fl 6, Portland, OR 97239; **Phone:** 503-494-4373; **Board Cert:** Internal Medicine 1984; Gastroenterology 1989; **Med School:** Creighton Univ 1980; **Resid:** Internal Medicine, Naval Hospital; **Fellow:** Gastroenterology, Arizona Hlth Sci Ctr; **Fac Appt:** Prof Med, Oregon Hlth Sci Univ

Gerson, Lauren Battat MD [Ge] - **Spec Exp:** Gastroesophageal Reflux Disease (GERD); Barrett's Esophagus; Esophageal Disorders; Capsule Endoscopy; **Hospital:** Stanford Univ Med Ctr; **Address:** Stanford Univ Med Ctr, Gastroenterology, 300 Pasteur Drive, rm A149, MC 5202, Stanford, CA 94305; **Phone:** 650-723-1380; **Board Cert:** Gastroenterology 1993; **Med School:** SUNY Buffalo 1990; **Resid:** Internal Medicine, California Pacific Med Ctr 1993; **Fellow:** Gastroenterology, Stanford Univ Med Ctr 1995; **Fac Appt:** Assoc Prof Med, Stanford Univ

Gish, Robert MD [Ge] - **Spec Exp:** Liver Cancer; Transplant Medicine-Liver; Hepatitis; Clinical Trials; **Hospital:** CA Pacific Med Ctr - Pacific Campus; **Address:** 2340 Clay St Fl 3, San Francisco, CA 94115; **Phone:** 415-600-1020; **Board Cert:** Internal Medicine 1984; Gastroenterology 1987; **Med School:** Univ Kans 1980; **Resid:** Internal Medicine, UCSD Med Ctr 1983; **Fellow:** Gastroenterology, UCLA Med Ctr 1988; **Fac Appt:** Assoc Clin Prof Med, UCSF

Han, Steven-Huy B MD [Ge] - **Spec Exp:** Transplant Medicine-Liver; Hepatitis B & C; Liver Disease; **Hospital:** Ronald Reagan UCLA Med Ctr; **Address:** UCLA Medical Ctr, 200 UCLA Medical Plaza, Ste 214, Los Angeles, CA 90095; **Phone:** 310-794-7788; **Board Cert:** Gastroenterology 1998; Transplant Hepatology 2007; **Med School:** Albany Med Coll 1990; **Resid:** Internal Medicine, Santa Clara Valley Med Ctr 1993; **Fellow:** Gastroenterology, USC Med Ctr 1996; Hepatology, UCLA Med Ctr 1996; **Fac Appt:** Assoc Prof Med, UCLA

Hillebrand, Donald J MD [Ge] - **Spec Exp:** Transplant Medicine-Liver; Liver Failure; **Hospital:** Scripps Green Hosp; **Address:** Scripps Green Hospital, 10666 N Torrey Pines Rd, MC 203N, La Jolla, CA 92037; **Phone:** 858-554-8055; **Board Cert:** Internal Medicine 2004; Gastroenterology 2006; Transplant Hepatology 2006; **Med School:** Univ Iowa Coll Med 1990; **Resid:** Internal Medicine, Univ Iowa Hosps 1993; **Fellow:** Gastroenterology, Univ Iowa Hosps 1994

Kimmey, Michael B MD [Ge] - **Spec Exp:** Pancreatic/Biliary Endoscopy (ERCP); Endoscopy; Endoscopic Ultrasound; **Hospital:** St Joseph Med Ctr - Tacoma, Tacoma Genl Hosp; **Address:** 1112 6th Ave, Ste 200, Tacoma, WA 98405; **Phone:** 253-272-8664; **Board Cert:** Internal Medicine 1982; Gastroenterology 1987; **Med School:** Washington Univ, St Louis 1979; **Resid:** Internal Medicine, Univ Wash Med Ctr 1982; **Fellow:** Gastroenterology, Univ Wash Med Ctr 1987; **Fac Appt:** Clin Prof Med, Univ Wash

Kozarek, Richard MD [Ge] - **Spec Exp:** Pancreatic/Biliary Endoscopy (ERCP); Inflammatory Bowel Disease; Pancreatic Disease; **Hospital:** Virginia Mason Med Ctr, Swedish Med Ctr - Seattle; **Address:** 1100 9th Ave, Seattle, WA 98101-2756; **Phone:** 206-223-6934; **Board Cert:** Internal Medicine 1977; Gastroenterology 1979; **Med School:** Univ Wisc 1973; **Resid:** Internal Medicine, Good Samaritan Hosp 1976; **Fellow:** Gastroenterology, Univ Arizona/ VA Hosp 1978; **Fac Appt:** Clin Prof Med, Univ Wash

Ostroff, James MD [Ge] - **Spec Exp:** Pancreatic/Biliary Endoscopy (ERCP); Colonoscopy; **Hospital:** UCSF Med Ctr, UCSF - Mt Zion Med Ctr; **Address:** 350 Parnassus Ave, Ste 410, San Francisco, CA 94117-3608; **Phone:** 415-502-2112; **Board Cert:** Internal Medicine 1980; Gastroenterology 1983; **Med School:** Cornell Univ-Weill Med Coll 1977; **Resid:** Internal Medicine, NY Hosp-Cornell Med Ctr 1980; **Fellow:** Gastroenterology, UCSF Hosps 1982; **Fac Appt:** Prof Med, UCSF

Poordad, Fred F MD [Ge] - **Spec Exp:** Liver Disease; Hepatitis B & C; Transplant Medicine-Liver; **Hospital:** Cedars-Sinai Med Ctr; **Address:** Cedars Sinai Medical Ctr, Liver Diseases, West Tower, 8635 W 3rd St, Ste 590, Los Angeles, CA 90048; **Phone:** 310-423-2641; **Board Cert:** Gastroenterology 2005; Transplant Hepatology 2006; **Med School:** Canada 1990; **Resid:** Internal Medicine, St Thomas Med Ctr/Ohio State Univ Med Ctr 1993; **Fellow:** Gastroenterology, Univ S Carolina Med Ctr 1995; Hepatology, Johns Hopkins Hosp 2005; **Fac Appt:** Assoc Prof Med, UCLA-David Geffen Sch Med

Roth, Bennett E MD [Ge] - **Spec Exp:** Gastroesophageal Reflux Disease (GERD); Inflammatory Bowel Disease/Crohn's; Irritable Bowel Syndrome; **Hospital:** Ronald Reagan UCLA Med Ctr; **Address:** 200 UCLA Med Plaza, Ste 365A, Los Angeles, CA 90095; **Phone:** 310-825-1597; **Board Cert:** Internal Medicine 1972; Gastroenterology 1975; **Med School:** Hahnemann Univ 1968; **Resid:** Internal Medicine, Hosp Univ Penn 1971; **Fellow:** Gastroenterology, UCLA Med Ctr 1974; **Fac Appt:** Prof Med, UCLA

Gastroenterology

Surawicz, Christina MD [Ge] - **Spec Exp:** Clostridium Difficile Disease; Infectious Diarrhea; **Hospital:** Harborview Med Ctr, Univ Wash Med Ctr; **Address:** 325 9th Ave, Box 359773, Seattle, WA 98104-2420; **Phone:** 206-731-5021; **Board Cert:** Internal Medicine 1976; Gastroenterology 1979; **Med School:** Univ KY Coll Med 1973; **Resid:** Internal Medicine, Univ Washington Med Ctr 1976; **Fellow:** Gastroenterology, Univ Washington Med Ctr 1979; **Fac Appt:** Prof Med, Univ Wash

Targan, Stephan R MD [Ge] - **Spec Exp:** Inflammatory Bowel Disease; Crohn's Disease; **Hospital:** Cedars-Sinai Med Ctr; **Address:** Cedars-Sinai IBD Ctr, 8730 Alden Drive, Ste 2E, Los Angeles, CA 90048; **Phone:** 310-423-4100; **Board Cert:** Internal Medicine 1974; Infectious Disease 1976; Gastroenterology 1979; **Med School:** Johns Hopkins Univ 1971; **Resid:** Internal Medicine, Harbor-UCLA Med Ctr 1976; **Fellow:** Infectious Disease, Harbor-UCLA Med Ctr 1976; Gastroenterology, UCLA Med Ctr 1978; **Fac Appt:** Prof Med, UCLA

America's Top Doctors® 8th Edition

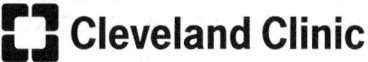 **Cleveland Clinic**

Digestive Disease Institute

A National Leader in Digestive Disease

Cleveland Clinic Digestive Disease Institute is one of the largest in the country and the first to fully integrate its departments of Colorectal Surgery, Gastroenterology & Hepatology, Hepatic-pancreatic-biliary and Transplant Surgery, and Nutrition Services. Combining these disciplines in one location facilitates unprecedented patient care, multidisciplinary education and collaborative research.

Cleveland Clinic colorectal surgeons have performed over 2,100 laparoscopic intestinal resections and currently average eight to ten cases each week, which demonstrates their leadership in performing minimally invasive intestinal surgery. Although colon surgery is one of the more difficult procedures to perform laparoscopically, the latest research suggests that laparoscopic surgery – even for colorectal cancer – offers an equally good outcome as open surgery when performed by experienced surgeons.

Additionally, the Digestive Disease Institute is a recognized leader in many areas, including pelvic pouch procedures. Digestive Disease Institute surgeons have performed more than 3,700 pelvic pouch procedures and are the established leaders in pouch salvage. Furthermore, a comprehensive Functional Bowel Disorder Center has three surgeons dedicated to the subspecialty of rectal function and fecal incontinence. Over the years, the staff of the Digestive Disease Institute has pioneered many new technologies and procedures for treating digestive disorders, and has developed key specialties in:

- Colon & Rectal Cancer
- Crohn's & Ulcerative Colitis
- Ostomy Avoidance
- Familial Adenomatous Polyposis
- Diverticulitis
- Laparoscopic Surgery
- Anorectal Disease (Fistulas, Hemorrhoids)
- Functional Bowel Disorders/Incontinence
- Enterostomal Therapy/Ostomy Reversal
- Hepatobiliary Surgery
- Liver Transplant
- Pancreatic Disease

- Therapeutic Endoscopy
- Esophageal Disorders
- Liver Disease
- Deep Enteroscopy
- Capsule Endoscopy
- Abdominal Fistulas
- Nutrition Therapy
- IBD/Pouchitis
- Clinical Trials

Cleveland Clinic Digestive Disease Institute is ranked #2 in the nation by *U.S.News and World Report's* 2008 "America's Best Hospitals" Survey.

For more information about Cleveland Clinic Digestive Disease Institute, or to schedule a second opinion or learn about assistance for out-of-state patients, call 800.890.2467 or visit www.clevelandclinic.org/gastrotopdocs.

Digestive Disease Institute
Cleveland Clinic | 9500 Euclid Avenue / AC311 | Cleveland OH 44195

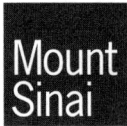
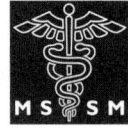

MOUNT SINAI
SCHOOL OF
MEDICINE

THE MOUNT SINAI MEDICAL CENTER
GASTROINTESTINAL AND SURGICAL SPECIALTIES

One Gustave L. Levy Place
Fifth Avenue and 100th Street
New York, NY 10029-6574
Physician Referral: 1-800-MD-SINAI (637-4624)
www.mountsinai.org

Mount Sinai's *Divisions of Gastroenterology, Colon and Rectal Surgery, Liver Diseases,* and *Pediatric Gastroenterology, Nutrition, and Liver Diseases* are renowned for their delivery of patient care, research, and education in diseases of the gastrointestinal (GI) tract. In 2000, the National Institutes of Health (NIH) recognized the importance of Mount Sinai as a research center with a grant for GI/Liver fellowship training. Mount Sinai is the only medical school in New York City to earn this prestigious award.

Division of Gastroenterology

Successes within the Division include breakthroughs in the medical and surgical management of inflammatory bowel disease (IBD), ulcerative colitis, and Crohn's disease. Mount Sinai spearheaded novel therapies for treating severe IBD and helped establish the role of colonoscopy for preventing colon cancer by removing precancerous polyps. More recent innovations include employing a tiny camera within a swallowable capsule to capture images in the stomach and intestines. Mount Sinai's Small Intestine Transplantation Program is one of only four such programs in the nation. Mount Sinai's IBD Center, Women's GI Health Center, and GI Cancer Center offer patients the latest comprehensive, interdisciplinary care, newer agents through clinical trials, and services such as psychologists and nutritionists.

Division of Colon and Rectal Surgery

Mount Sinai surgeons have a distinguished history in the surgical treatment of gastrointestinal disorders, and surgeons in the Division continue that tradition today, focusing on surgical therapies for all diseases involving the colon, rectum, and anus. With special expertise in the treatment of Crohn's disease (which was first described at Mount Sinai in 1932), ulcerative colitis, colon and rectal cancer, and diverticulitis, we specialize in the newer techniques of rectal surgery with special emphasis on colostomy avoidance. The newest minimally invasive techniques are offered as well as other cutting-edge technologies for the treatment of such disorders as hemorrhoids, fistulas, and rectal tumors.

Division of Liver Diseases

Mount Sinai has a long history of outstanding clinical care and scientific investigation, with a tradition of excellence in several clinical areas, including liver transplantation; diagnosis and treatment of viral hepatitis; treatment of scarring, or fibrosis; management of primary biliary cirrhosis, an autoimmune disease of bile ducts; treatment of liver cancer; and diagnosis and treatment of genetic liver diseases, including Wilson's disease (copper overload) and hemachromatosis (iron overload). With a steadily growing research budget, Mount Sinai carries out a diverse portfolio of research projects.

Division of Pediatric Gastroenterology, Nutrition, and Liver Diseases

The Division provides consultative services and treatment for the full range of children's digestive and nutritional diseases. The Children's IBD Center is the only multidisciplinary center for pediatric patients with Crohn's disease and ulcerative colitis in the New York metropolitan area and receives referrals from across the country. The Transplant Program is one of the largest in the nation and was the first program in New York to perform liver transplants and, later, small bowel transplants. The Division is active in clinical research in IBD, focusing on issues of genetic factors, psychosocial interactions, and drug trials. Several NIH grants support research in the areas of biliary atresia, bile salt absorption, and outcome analysis in children with liver failure.

Mount Sinai provides a comprehensive center, uniting the medical disciplines of gastroenterology and its related surgical specialties, as well as an array of minimally invasive surgical programs. The center houses renowned programs for the treatment of IBD and colorectal diseases, as well as Reconstructive and Laparoscopic Surgery Programs through the Division of Laparoscopic Surgery, which is internationally known for pioneering a number of minimally invasive procedures for the treatment of Crohn's disease and ulcerative colitis.

NewYork-Presbyterian

The University Hospital of Columbia and Cornell

NewYork-Presbyterian Digestive Disease Services

Affiliated with Columbia University College of Physicians and Surgeons and Weill Medical College of Cornell University

NewYork-Presbyterian Hospital
Weill Cornell Medical Center
525 East 68th Street
New York, NY 10021

NewYork-Presbyterian Hospital
Columbia University Medical Center
622 West 168th Street
New York, NY 10032

OVERVIEW:

The Digestive Disease Services of NewYork-Presbyterian Hospital provide expert capabilities in research, education and clinical care of patients with gastrointestinal, liver and bile duct, pancreatic and nutritional disorders.

The Hospital offers a wide range of diagnostic tests including,
- Routine procedures, such as endoscopy, capsule endoscopy, colonoscopy and flexible sigmoidoscopy.

- Endoscopic retrograde cholangiopancreatography (ERCP) to evaluate the ducts of the gallbladder, pancreas and liver

- Endoscopic ultrasonography (EUS)to provide detailed images of the upper and lower gastrointestinal tract and for the staging of patients with esophageal, gastric and rectal cancers. The Hospital is one of the few centers using EUS for needle aspiration of pancreatic cysts and tumors.

- Laparoscopy for direct examination of the liver, gallbladder and spleen and in the diagnosis, staging and treatment of pancreatic, gastric, esophageal and colorectal cancer.

The Hospital is a leader in treating gastrointestinal (GI) conditions. For example,
- The Minimal Access Surgery Center (MASC) is at the forefront of developing and applying new technologies, such as robotics, computerized image processing and enhanced optics. It is improving the outcomes of GI surgical patients and speeding their recovery from conditions such as GERD, gallbladder disease, and benign and malignant colon and rectal disease.

- Our surgeons also perform endoscopic sewing (endocinch) and radiofrequency treatment (Stretta procedure) for GERD.

- Our surgeons are internationally renowned in the use of laparoscopic methods for cancer and other colorectal conditions. They are highly experienced with the Whipple procedure to remove a pancreas tumor, which improves the survival rates and life expectancies of patients with pancreatic cancer and other less common pancreas problems.

Additionally, our physicians are involved in numerous clinical trials, (including studies on Cox-2 inhibitors) for preventing colorectal cancer and familial polyposis (a precursor to colorectal cancer), and antiviral therapy for chronic hepatitis C.

Physician Referral: For a physician referral or to learn more about the NewYork-Presbyterian Digestive Disease Services call toll free **1-877-NYP-WELL** (1-877-697-9355) or visit our website at **www.nypdigestive.org**

COMPREHENSIVE CARE

Patients benefit from the collaboration of gastroenterologists, hepatologists, surgeons and diagnostic and pathology experts who develop optimal treatment plans. Areas of expertise include:

- GI Cancer, including esophageal, colorectal, liver, pancreatic and gastric tumors

- Inflammatory Bowel Diseases (Ulcerative Colitis and Crohn's Disease)

- Liver Diseases. The Hospital has a comprehensive Hepatitis C Center and the Center for Liver Disease and Transplantation

- Esophageal Disorders, including gastroesophageal reflux disease (GERD) and Barrett's esophagus

- Pancreatic and Biliary Disorders

- Celiac Disease

- Polyps of the Colon

- Peptic Ulcer Disease/Helicobacter Pylori Infections

- Gallbladder and Bile Duct Disorders

- Restorative surgery to avoid colostomies in diseases like rectal cancer, Crohn's disease, ulcerative colitis, and incontinence

- Anal diseases, such as hemorrhoids, fistulas, vascular tumors, abscesses and others

NYU Langone Medical Center

550 First Avenue (at 31St Stree
New York, NY 1001
Physician Referra
(888)7-NYU-MED (888-769-863
www.nyumc.or

GASTROENTEROLOGY

The mission of the Division of Gastroenterology at NYU Langone Medical Center is excellence in the delivery of patient care, research, and education in diseases of the gastrointestinal tract. Its physicians bring with them a rich body of knowledge in the diagnosis and management of inflammatory bowel disease, peptic ulcer disease, esophageal disorders, gastrointestinal cancer, and liver, biliary, and pancreatic diseases. Their multidisciplinary approach insures the greatest possible patient care at NYU three acclaimed, academically- integrated teaching hospitals Tisch Hospital (New York University Hospital), Bellevue Hospitals Center, and the New York Harbor Health Care System (Manhattan Veterans Hospital).

Members of the Division of Gastroenterology are nationally recognized leaders who are involved in numerous studies in the field of gastroenterology and hepatology, including clinical research in liver diseases (especially hepatitis C), endoscopy, colon cancer screening, acute and chronic 61 bleeding, and Helicobacter pylon.

Always at the forefront of new technologies, NYU's gastroenterologists work side-by-side with radiologists to perform virtual colonoscopies, a new minimally invasive technique for finding early-stage cancers in the colon.

Virtual colonoscopy is a new screening test in which a radiologist uses a CAT (Computer Assisted Tomography) scanner and sophisticated image processing computers to actually recreate and evaluate the inner surface of the colon. The CAT scanner provides the x-ray images; the image-processing computers create the 3-D display for the final interpretation by the referring gastroenterologist. The study gives a complete evaluation of the entire surface of the colon and can be performed quickly, with little discomfort and extremely accurate readings.

Geriatric Medicine

a subspecialty of Internal Medicine
or Family Practice

An internist or family physician with special knowledge of the aging process and special skills in the diagnostic, therapeutic, preventive and rehabilitative aspects of illness in the elderly.   This specialist cares for geriatric patients in the patient's home, the office, long-term care settings such as nursing homes and the hospital.

Family Medicine

A family physician is concerned with the total healthcare of the individual and the family, and is trained to diagnose and treat a wide variety of ailments in patients of all ages. The family physician receives a broad range of training that includes internal medicine, pediatrics, obstetrics and gynecology, psychiatry and geriatrics. Special emphasis is placed on prevention and the primary care of entire families, utilizing consultations and community resources when appropriate.

Training Required: Three years in internal medicine or family practice *plus* additional training and examination for certification in geriatric medicine.

GERIATRIC MEDICINE

New England

Cooney Jr, Leo M MD [Ger] - **Spec Exp:** Rheumatology; **Hospital:** Yale-New Haven Hosp; **Address:** Yale-New Haven Hosp, 20 York St, Tompkins 17, New Haven, CT 06504; **Phone:** 203-688-2204; **Board Cert:** Internal Medicine 1974; Rheumatology 1978; Geriatric Medicine 2000; **Med School:** Yale Univ 1969; **Resid:** Internal Medicine, Boston City Hosp 1971; Internal Medicine, Boston City Hosp 1974; **Fellow:** Rheumatology, Boston Med Ctr 1975; **Fac Appt:** Prof Med, Yale Univ

Lipsitz, Lewis Arnold MD [Ger] - **Spec Exp:** Falls in the Elderly; **Hospital:** Beth Israel Deaconess Med Ctr - Boston; **Address:** Beth Israel Med Ctr, Gerontology, 110 Francis St, LMOB 1B, Boston, MA 02215; **Phone:** 617-632-8696; **Board Cert:** Internal Medicine 1980; Geriatric Medicine 1999; **Med School:** Univ Pennsylvania 1977; **Resid:** Internal Medicine, Beth Israel Hosp 1980; **Fellow:** Geriatric Medicine, Harvard Univ 1983; **Fac Appt:** Prof Med, Harvard Med Sch

Minaker, Kenneth MD [Ger] - **Spec Exp:** Aging; Neuroendocrinology; Cardiovascular Disease; **Hospital:** Mass Genl Hosp, Brigham & Women's Hosp; **Address:** Charles River Plaza, Ste 502, 165 Cambridge St, Boston, MA 02114-2723; **Phone:** 617-726-4600; **Board Cert:** Internal Medicine 1979; Geriatric Medicine 1985; **Med School:** Univ Toronto 1972; **Resid:** Internal Medicine, Univ Toronto 1981; **Fellow:** Geriatric Medicine, Mass Gen Hosp-Harvard 1983; **Fac Appt:** Assoc Prof Med, Harvard Med Sch

Tinetti, Mary E MD [Ger] - **Spec Exp:** Falls in the Elderly; Geriatric Functional Assessment; **Hospital:** Yale-New Haven Hosp; **Address:** Yale-New Haven Hosp, Adler Geriatric Ctr, 20 York St, New Haven, CT 06504; **Phone:** 203-688-6361; **Board Cert:** Internal Medicine 1981; **Med School:** Univ Mich Med Sch 1978; **Resid:** Internal Medicine, Univ Minnesota 1981; **Fellow:** Geriatric Medicine, Univ Rochester 1984; **Fac Appt:** Prof Med, Yale Univ

Mid Atlantic

Bloom, Patricia A MD [Ger] - **Spec Exp:** Dementia; Geriatric Functional Assessment; Osteoporosis; **Hospital:** Mount Sinai Med Ctr (page 64); **Address:** 1440 Madison Ave, New York, NY 10029-6542; **Phone:** 212-659-8552; **Board Cert:** Internal Medicine 1978; Geriatric Medicine 1998; **Med School:** Univ Minn 1975; **Resid:** Internal Medicine, Montefiore Hosp 1978; **Fac Appt:** Assoc Prof Med, Mount Sinai Sch Med

Burton, John R MD [Ger] - **Hospital:** Johns Hopkins Bayview Med Ctr (page 61); **Address:** Division of Geriatric Medicine, 5505 Hopkins Bayview Cir, Baltimore, MD 21224; **Phone:** 410-550-0520; **Board Cert:** Internal Medicine 1980; Geriatric Medicine 1990; Nephrology 1974; **Med School:** McGill Univ 1965; **Resid:** Internal Medicine, Baltimore City Hosp 1971; **Fellow:** Nephrology, Mass Genl Hosp 1972; **Fac Appt:** Prof Med, Johns Hopkins Univ

Finucane, Thomas E MD [Ger] - **Spec Exp:** Pain Management; Swallowing Disorders; Ethics; **Hospital:** Johns Hopkins Bayview Med Ctr (page 61), Johns Hopkins Hosp - Baltimore (page 61); **Address:** 5505 Hopkins Bayview Cir, Level 01, Baltimore, MD 21224; **Phone:** 410-550-0925; **Board Cert:** Internal Medicine 1982; Geriatric Medicine 1998; **Med School:** Emory Univ 1978; **Resid:** Internal Medicine, George Washington Univ Hosp 1982; **Fac Appt:** Prof Med, Johns Hopkins Univ

Freedman, Michael L MD [Ger] - **Spec Exp:** Alzheimer's Disease; Anemia; Nutrition; **Hospital:** NYU Med Ctr (page 68), Bellevue Hosp Ctr; **Address:** 530 First Ave, Ste 4J, New York, NY 10016-6402; **Phone:** 212-263-7043; **Board Cert:** Internal Medicine 1971; Hematology 1974; Geriatric Medicine 1998; **Med School:** Tufts Univ 1963; **Resid:** Internal Medicine, Bellevue Hosp 1965; Internal Medicine, Bellevue Hosp 1969; **Fellow:** Hematology, Natl Inst Hlth-NCI 1968; **Fac Appt:** Prof Med, NYU Sch Med

Gambert, Steven MD [Ger] - **Spec Exp:** Endocrinology; Osteoporosis; Aging; **Hospital:** Sinai Hosp - Baltimore; **Address:** Sinai Hosp Baltimore Hoffberger Bldg, 2401 W Belvedere Ave, Ste 23, Baltimore, MD 21215; **Phone:** 410-601-6340; **Board Cert:** Internal Medicine 1978; **Med School:** Columbia P&S 1975; **Resid:** Internal Medicine, Dartmouth Affl Hosp 1977; **Fellow:** Geriatric Medicine, Beth Israel Hosp-Harvard 1979; Endocrinology, Beth Israel Hosp-Harvard 1979; **Fac Appt:** Prof Med, Johns Hopkins Univ

Lachs, Mark MD [Ger] - **Spec Exp:** Abuse/Neglect; **Hospital:** NY-Presby Hosp/Weill Cornell (page 66); **Address:** Irving Sherwood Wright Center on Aging, 1484 First Ave, New York, NY 10021; **Phone:** 212-746-7000; **Board Cert:** Internal Medicine 1988; Geriatric Medicine 2002; **Med School:** NYU Sch Med 1985; **Resid:** Internal Medicine, Hosp U Penn 1988; **Fellow:** Geriatric Medicine, Yale-New Haven Hosp 1990; **Fac Appt:** Assoc Prof Med, Cornell Univ-Weill Med Coll

Meier, Diane MD [Ger] - **Spec Exp:** Palliative Care; **Hospital:** Mount Sinai Med Ctr (page 64); **Address:** Mt Sinai School Medicine, Box 1070, New York, NY 10029-6501; **Phone:** 212-241-1446; **Board Cert:** Internal Medicine 1981; Geriatric Medicine 1999; Hospice & Palliative Medicine 2006; **Med School:** Northwestern Univ 1977; **Resid:** Internal Medicine, Oregon Hlth Sci Univ 1981; **Fellow:** Geriatric Medicine, VA Med Ctr 1983; **Fac Appt:** Prof Med, Mount Sinai Sch Med

Palmer, Robert M MD [Ger] - **Spec Exp:** Geriatric Functional Assessment; Dementia; **Hospital:** UPMC Presby, Pittsburgh; **Address:** 3471 5th Ave Kaufmann Bldg - Ste 500, Pittsburgh, PA 15213; **Phone:** 412-692-4200; **Board Cert:** Internal Medicine 1975; Geriatric Medicine 1998; **Med School:** Univ Mich Med Sch 1971; **Resid:** Internal Medicine, LA County Med Ctr 1975; **Fellow:** Geriatric Medicine, UCLA Med Ctr 1986; **Fac Appt:** Assoc Clin Prof Med, Case West Res Univ

Resnick, Neil M MD [Ger] - **Spec Exp:** Voiding Dysfunction; Incontinence; **Hospital:** UPMC Presby, Pittsburgh, UPMC Shadyside; **Address:** 3471 5th Ave, Kaufmann Bldg, Ste 500, Pittsburgh, PA 15213-3313; **Phone:** 412-692-2364; **Board Cert:** Internal Medicine 1980; Geriatric Medicine 1998; **Med School:** Stanford Univ 1977; **Resid:** Internal Medicine, Beth Israel Hosp 1980; **Fellow:** Geriatric Medicine, Harvard Univ 1982; Urodynamics, Harvard Univ 1984; **Fac Appt:** Prof Med, Univ Pittsburgh

Studenski, Stephanie A MD [Ger] - **Spec Exp:** Balance Disorders; Mobility Evaluation & Treatment; Falls in the Elderly; **Hospital:** UPMC Presby, Pittsburgh; **Address:** 4 East Montifiore, 200 Lothrop St, Pittsburgh, PA 15213; **Phone:** 412-692-4200; **Board Cert:** Internal Medicine 1982; Rheumatology 1984; Geriatric Medicine 2002; **Med School:** Univ Kans 1979; **Resid:** Internal Medicine, Duke Univ Med Ctr 1982; **Fellow:** Rheumatology, Duke Univ Med Ctr 1984; Geriatric Medicine, Duke Univ Med Ctr 1986; **Fac Appt:** Prof Med, Univ Pittsburgh

Southeast

Ciocon, Jerry O MD [Ger] - **Spec Exp:** Chronic Fatigue-Elderly; Pain-Musculoskeletal; Memory Disorders; **Hospital:** Cleveland Clin - Weston; **Address:** Cleveland Clinic, Div Geriatrics, 2950 Cleveland Clinic Blvd, Weston, FL 33331-3609; **Phone:** 954-659-5867; **Board Cert:** Internal Medicine 1985; Geriatric Medicine 2000; **Med School:** Philippines 1980; **Resid:** Internal Medicine, Mercy Hosp 1985; **Fellow:** Geriatric Medicine, LI Jewish Med Ctr 1987; **Fac Appt:** Asst Clin Prof Med, Ohio State Univ

Geriatric Medicine

Greganti, Mac Andrew MD [Ger] - **Spec Exp:** Diagnostic Problems; Dementia; **Hospital:** Univ NC Hosps; **Address:** Univ North Carolina Hosp, Dept Med, 125 MacNider Bldg, Chapel Hill, NC 27599-7005; **Phone:** 919-966-3063; **Board Cert:** Internal Medicine 1987; **Med School:** Univ Miss 1972; **Resid:** Internal Medicine, Strong Meml Hosp 1975; **Fac Appt:** Prof Med, Univ NC Sch Med

Groene, Linda A MD [Ger] - **Spec Exp:** Osteoporosis; Sleep Disorders/Apnea; Dementia; **Hospital:** Imperial Point Med Ctr, Holy Cross Hosp - Fort Lauderdale; **Address:** 6405 N Federal Hwy, Ste 102, Ft Lauderdale, FL 33308; **Phone:** 954-772-0062; **Board Cert:** Internal Medicine 1986; Geriatric Medicine 2000; **Med School:** Louisiana State U, New Orleans 1981; **Resid:** Pathology, Jackson Meml Hosp 1983; Internal Medicine, Mt Sinai Med Ctr 1986

Hanson, Laura C MD [Ger] - **Spec Exp:** Frailty Syndrome; Palliative Care; **Hospital:** Univ NC Hosps; **Address:** UNC Sch Med, MacNider Bldg - rm 262, CB 7550, Chapel Hill, NC 27599; **Phone:** 919-966-5945 x251; **Board Cert:** Internal Medicine 1989; Geriatric Medicine 2002; **Med School:** Harvard Med Sch 1986; **Resid:** Internal Medicine, Brigham & Womens Hosp 1988; Internal Medicine, Univ North Carolina Hosp 1989; **Fellow:** Geriatric Medicine, Univ North Carolina Hosp 1991; **Fac Appt:** Assoc Prof Med, Univ NC Sch Med

Lyles, Kenneth W MD [Ger] - **Spec Exp:** Bone Disorders-Metabolic; Tumoral Calcinosis; Parathyroid Disease; **Hospital:** Duke Univ Med Ctr, VA Med Ctr - Durham; **Address:** Duke Univ Med Center, Box 3881, Durham, NC 27710; **Phone:** 919-660-7520; **Board Cert:** Internal Medicine 1977; Endocrinology 1979; Geriatric Medicine 2000; **Med School:** Med Coll VA 1974; **Resid:** Internal Medicine, Med Coll VA 1977; **Fellow:** Endocrinology, Diabetes & Metabolism, Duke Univ Med Ctr 1979; Geriatric Medicine, Duke Univ/VA Med Ctr 1981; **Fac Appt:** Prof Med, Duke Univ

Midwest

Carr, David B MD [Ger] - **Spec Exp:** Polypharmacology (Excess Medications); Alzheimer's Disease; **Hospital:** Barnes-Jewish Hosp; **Address:** Wash Univ Sch Med, Div Geriatrics, 660 S Euclid Ave, Box 8303, St Louis, MO 63110; **Phone:** 314-286-2700; **Board Cert:** Internal Medicine 1989; Geriatric Medicine 2000; **Med School:** Univ MO-Columbia Sch Med 1985; **Resid:** Internal Medicine, Mich State Assoc Hosps 1988; **Fellow:** Geriatric Medicine, Duke Univ 1990; **Fac Appt:** Prof Med, Washington Univ, St Louis

Dale, Lowell C MD [Ger] - **Spec Exp:** Tobacco Abuse; Nutrition; **Hospital:** Mayo Med Ctr & Clin - Rochester; **Address:** Mayo Clinic, 200 First St SW, Colonial 3-10, Rochester, MN 55905; **Phone:** 507-266-1093; **Board Cert:** Internal Medicine 1984; **Med School:** Univ Minn 1981; **Resid:** Internal Medicine, Mayo Clinic 1984; **Fellow:** Internal Medicine, Mayo Clinic 1985; **Fac Appt:** Asst Prof Med, Mayo Med Sch

Duthie, Edmund H MD [Ger] - **Spec Exp:** Geriatric Functional Assessment; **Hospital:** Froedtert Meml Lutheran Hosp, Clement J Zablocki VA Med Ctr; **Address:** 9200 W Wisconsin Ave, Milwaukee, WI 53226; **Phone:** 262-253-2455; **Board Cert:** Internal Medicine 1979; Geriatric Medicine 1998; **Med School:** Georgetown Univ 1976; **Resid:** Internal Medicine, Med Coll Wisc Hosps 1979; **Fellow:** Geriatric Medicine, Jewish Inst Geri Care-SUNY 1980; **Fac Appt:** Prof Med, Med Coll Wisc

Gorbien, Martin J MD [Ger] - **Spec Exp:** Dementia; Alzheimer's Disease; Geriatric Functional Assessment; **Hospital:** Rush Univ Med Ctr; **Address:** 1725 W Harrison St, Ste 955, Chicago, IL 60612; **Phone:** 312-942-7030; **Board Cert:** Geriatric Medicine 1998; **Med School:** Mexico 1983; **Resid:** Internal Medicine, Mercy Hosp & Med Ctr 1987; **Fellow:** Geriatric Medicine, UCLA Med Ctr 1989; **Fac Appt:** Assoc Prof Med, Rush Med Coll

America's Top Doctors® 8th Edition

Morley, John MD [Ger] - **Spec Exp:** Endocrinology; Menopause-Male; Alzheimer's Disease; Frailty Syndrome; **Hospital:** St Louis Univ Hosp; **Address:** St Louis Univ Hlth Sci Ctr, Div Ger Med, 3660 Vista, Ste 204, St Louis, MO 63104-1004; **Phone:** 314-977-6055; **Board Cert:** Internal Medicine 1978; Geriatric Medicine 1998; Endocrinology 1981; **Med School:** South Africa 1972; **Resid:** Internal Medicine, Johannesburg Genl Hosp 1974; Internal Medicine, Baragwanath Hosp 1976; **Fellow:** Endocrinology, Diabetes & Metabolism, Wadsworth VA Hosp-UCLA 1979; **Fac Appt:** Prof Med, St Louis Univ

Olson, Jack Conrad MD [Ger] - **Spec Exp:** Dementia; Depression; **Hospital:** Rush Univ Med Ctr; **Address:** Senior Care, Rush Univ Professional Bldg 3, 1725 W Harrison St, Ste 955, Chicago, IL 60612-3836; **Phone:** 312-942-7030; **Board Cert:** Internal Medicine 1987; Geriatric Medicine 2000; **Med School:** Univ Mich Med Sch 1984; **Resid:** Internal Medicine, Univ Wisc Med Sch 1987; **Fellow:** Geriatric Medicine, Univ Wisc Med Sch 1989; **Fac Appt:** Asst Prof Med, Univ Chicago-Pritzker Sch Med

Sachs, Greg A MD [Ger] - **Spec Exp:** Memory Disorders; Alzheimer's Disease; **Hospital:** Indiana Univ Hosp; **Address:** Indiana University Hospital, Dept Medicine & Geriatrics, 1001 W 10th St, rm M200, Indianapolis, IN 46202; **Phone:** 317-630-2564; **Board Cert:** Internal Medicine 1988; Geriatric Medicine 2000; **Med School:** Yale Univ 1985; **Resid:** Internal Medicine, Univ Chicago Hosps 1987; **Fellow:** Geriatric Medicine, Univ Chicago Hosps 1990; **Fac Appt:** Assoc Prof Med, Indiana Univ

Sheehan, Myles MD [Ger] - **Spec Exp:** Dementia; Geriatric Functional Assessment; **Hospital:** Loyola Univ Med Ctr; **Address:** Loyola Univ Med Ctr, 2160 S 1st Ave , Bldg 120 - rm 310, Maywood, IL 60153; **Phone:** 708-216-8887; **Board Cert:** Internal Medicine 1984; Geriatric Medicine 2002; **Med School:** Dartmouth Med Sch 1981; **Resid:** Internal Medicine, Beth Israel Deaconess Med Ctr 1984; **Fellow:** Geriatric Medicine, Beth Israel Deaconess Med Ctr 1991; **Fac Appt:** Assoc Prof Med, Loyola Univ-Stritch Sch Med

Great Plains and Mountains

Schwartz, Robert S MD [Ger] - **Spec Exp:** Diabetes; Exercise Therapy; Hormonal Disorders; **Hospital:** Univ Colorado Hosp, VA Med Ctr; **Address:** Univ Colorado at Denver & Health Sci Ctr, 12631 E 17th Ave Bldg 15 Fl 8111, Box B179, Denver, CO 80262-0001; **Phone:** 303-319-7891; **Board Cert:** Internal Medicine 1977; Endocrinology 1981; Geriatric Medicine 2000; **Med School:** Ohio State Univ 1974; **Resid:** Internal Medicine, Univ Wash Med Ctr 1977; **Fellow:** Endocrinology, Diabetes & Metabolism, Univ Wash Med Ctr 1980; **Fac Appt:** Prof Med, Univ Colorado

Supiano, Mark A MD [Ger] - **Spec Exp:** Hypertension; Geriatric Functional Assessment; **Hospital:** Univ Utah Hosps and Clins; **Address:** Univ Utah, Geriatrics Div, 30 N 1900 E, SOM AB 193, Salt Lake City, UT 84132; **Phone:** 801-587-9103; **Board Cert:** Internal Medicine 1985; Geriatric Medicine 1998; **Med School:** Univ Wisc 1982; **Resid:** Internal Medicine, Univ Mich Med Ctr 1985; **Fellow:** Geriatric Medicine, Univ Mich Med Ctr 1987; **Fac Appt:** Prof Med, Univ Utah

Southwest

Carter, William Jerry MD [Ger] - **Spec Exp:** Geriatric Endocrinology; **Hospital:** John L McClellan VA Med Ctr; **Address:** 2200 Fort Roots Drive, Geriatric Clinic 3B, North Little Rock, AR 72114; **Phone:** 501-257-2061; **Board Cert:** Internal Medicine 1974; Endocrinology, Diabetes & Metabolism 1975; Geriatric Medicine 2005; **Med School:** Univ Ark 1963; **Resid:** Internal Medicine, Univ Ark Med Scis 1967; **Fellow:** Endocrinology, Diabetes & Metabolism, Univ Ark Med Scis 1971; **Fac Appt:** Prof Med, Univ Ark

Geriatric Medicine

Dyer, Carmel B MD [Ger] - **Spec Exp:** Elder Abuse; **Hospital:** Meml Hermann Hosp - Texas Med Ctr, LBJ General Hosp; **Address:** 6431 Fannin St, rm MSB-4.200, Houston, TX 77030; **Phone:** 713-500-6290; **Board Cert:** Internal Medicine 2000; Geriatric Medicine 2000; **Med School:** Baylor Coll Med 1988; **Resid:** Internal Medicine, Baylor Affil Hosps 1991; **Fellow:** Geriatric Medicine, Baylor Affil Hosps 1993; **Fac Appt:** Assoc Prof Med, Baylor Coll Med

Liem, Pham MD [Ger] - **Spec Exp:** Dementia; Alzheimer's Disease; Delirium; **Hospital:** UAMS Med Ctr, Cent Ark Vet Hlthcare Sys; **Address:** Univ Hosp Arkansas Med Sci, 4301 W Markham, Slot #547-13, Little Rock, AR 72205-7101; **Phone:** 501-686-6219; **Board Cert:** Family Medicine 2006; Geriatric Medicine 1998; **Med School:** Vietnam 1973; **Resid:** Family Medicine, Univ Ark Med Sch 1980; **Fellow:** Geriatric Medicine, Univ Ark Med Sch 1982; **Fac Appt:** Prof Med, Univ Ark

Lipschitz, David A MD/PhD [Ger] - **Spec Exp:** Nutrition; Preventive Medicine; **Hospital:** St Vincent Med Ctr; **Address:** Longevity Center-St Vincent Senior Hlth, One St Vincent Circle, Ste 210, Little Rock, AR 72205; **Phone:** 501-552-4777; **Board Cert:** Internal Medicine 1975; Hematology 1976; **Med School:** South Africa 1966; **Resid:** Internal Medicine, Johannesburg Genl Hosp 1972; **Fellow:** Hematology, Univ Washington 1974; Internal Medicine, Montefiore Hosp 1975; **Fac Appt:** Prof Med, Univ Ark

Wei, Jeanne MD/PhD [Ger] - **Spec Exp:** Cardiovascular Disease; **Hospital:** UAMS Med Ctr, John L McClellan VA Med Ctr; **Address:** Donald W Reynolds Ctr on Aging, 4301 W Markham St, Slot 748, Little Rock, AR 72205; **Phone:** 501-296-1000; **Board Cert:** Internal Medicine 1978; Cardiovascular Disease 1979; Geriatric Medicine 2001; **Med School:** Univ IL Coll Med 1975; **Resid:** Internal Medicine, Johns Hopkins Hosp 1977; **Fellow:** Cardiovascular Disease, Johns Hopkins Hosp 1979; Research, Natl Inst Aging 1979; **Fac Appt:** Prof Med, Univ Ark

West Coast and Pacific

Abrass, Itamar B MD [Ger] - **Spec Exp:** Endocrine Disorders; Diabetes; **Hospital:** Harborview Med Ctr, Univ Wash Med Ctr; **Address:** Harborview Medical Ctr, 325 9th Ave, Box 359755, Seattle, WA 98101; **Phone:** 206-744-9100; **Board Cert:** Internal Medicine 1974; Endocrinology, Diabetes & Metabolism 1975; Geriatric Medicine 1988; **Med School:** UCSF 1966; **Resid:** Internal Medicine, Columbia-Pesby Med Ctr 1968; **Fellow:** Endocrinology, Diabetes & Metabolism, UCSD Med Ctr 1971; **Fac Appt:** Prof Med, Univ Wash

Landefeld, C Seth MD [Ger] - **Spec Exp:** Cardiovascular Disease; Incontinence; **Hospital:** UCSF Med Ctr, VA Med Ctr - San Francisco; **Address:** 3333 California St, Ste 380, San Francisco, CA 94118; **Phone:** 415-750-6625; **Board Cert:** Internal Medicine 1982; **Med School:** Yale Univ 1979; **Resid:** Internal Medicine, UCSF Med Ctr 1983; **Fellow:** Geriatric Medicine, Brigham-Womens Hosp 1985; **Fac Appt:** Prof Med, UCSF

McCormick, Wayne MD [Ger] - **Spec Exp:** Dementia; AIDS/HIV; **Hospital:** Univ Wash Med Ctr, Harborview Med Ctr; **Address:** Harborview Medical Ctr, 325 9th Ave Fl 4, Box 359860, Seattle, WA 98104; **Phone:** 206-744-4191; **Board Cert:** Internal Medicine 1986; Geriatric Medicine 1992; Public Health & Genl Preventive Med 1992; **Med School:** Washington Univ, St Louis 1983; **Resid:** Internal Medicine, Michael Reese Hosp 1987; **Fellow:** Geriatric Medicine, Univ Wash Med Ctr 1990; **Fac Appt:** Asst Prof Med, Univ Wash

Reuben, David B MD [Ger] - **Spec Exp:** Geriatric Functional Assessment; **Hospital:** Ronald Reagan UCLA Med Ctr, Santa Monica - UCLA Med Ctr; **Address:** UCLA Sch Med, Div Geriatrics, 10945 Le Conte Ave, Ste 2339, Los Angeles, CA 90095; **Phone:** 310-206-8272; **Board Cert:** Internal Medicine 1980; Geriatric Medicine 2005; **Med School:** Emory Univ 1977; **Resid:** Internal Medicine, Rhode Island Hosp 1980; **Fellow:** Geriatric Medicine, UCLA Med Ctr 1987; **Fac Appt:** Prof Med, UCLA

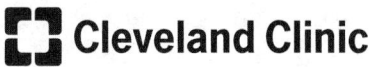 **Cleveland Clinic**

Geriatric Medicine

Cleveland Clinic's Section of Geriatric Medicine specializes in diagnosing and treating frail, elderly patients with complex medical conditions and social problems.

Cleveland Clinic's Section of Geriatric Medicine consists of an interdisciplinary team of health care professionals dedicated to creating comprehensive, coordinated care plans for all patients. The Section of Geriatric Medicine fulfills its "patients first" mission through clinical, educational and research activities with an emphasis on improving the quality of life of older patients. The Section of Geriatric Medicine is an integral part of Cleveland Clinic, a not-for-profit multispecialty academic medical center.

Cleveland Clinic and the Section of Geriatric Medicine offer several specialized programs to help ensure older patients receive the full scope of care necessary for optimal outcomes. These programs include:

Geriatric Evaluation and Management (GEM) Program
Cleveland Clinic's GEM Program is the cornerstone of the comprehensive care offered to older patients and their families. It takes an in-depth look at a patient's physical and psychological health, including the person's medical history, current status, recent changes and special concerns. Older adults appropriate for geriatric assessments include those with cognitive or physical decline; falls; weight loss; depression; social isolation and polypharmacy. Cleveland Clinic specialists from all disciplines are consulted as needed. After the evaluation is complete, the patient and invited family meet with the assessment team to discuss how best to care for the patient, using the most appropriate medications, therapies, community programs and other resources. The Section of Geriatric Medicine also operates a similar comprehensive Geriatric Assessment Program at Euclid Hospital. The Section of Geriatric Medicine also operates a similar comprehensive Geriatric Assessment Program at Euclid Hospital and Cleveland Clinic Independence Family Health Center.

Aging Brain Clinic
Cleveland Clinic's Aging Brain Clinic brings together a medical team that includes physicians who specialize in geriatric medicine, neurology and neurosurgery. Patients appropriate for these clinics are older adults with ventriculomegaly (hydrocephalus) and cognitive, gait and urological problems. Experts in other medical specialties, such as urology and vascular medicine, as well as professionals in social work, nutrition, psychiatry and neuropsychology are involved as needed.

Inpatient Consultations
One of the special features that Cleveland Clinic offers older adults hospitalized for acute medical or surgical problems is an inpatient geriatrics assessment. These assessments can be requested by the attending physician for specific geriatric concerns, including: depression, delirium (acute confusion), dementia, falls, concerns about medications or other geriatric issues.

For more information about Cleveland Clinic Section of Geriatric Medicine, to schedule a second opinion or learn about assistance for out-of-state patients, call 800.890.2467 or visit www.clevelandclinic.org/geriatrictopdocs.

Section of Geriatric Medicine | 9500 Euclid Avenue / AC311 | Cleveland OH 44195

Maimonides Medical Center
MAIMONIDES GERIATRICS PROGRAM

4802 Tenth Avenue • Brooklyn, New York 11219
Phone: (718) 283-7071 • Fax: (718) 635-6417
http://www.maimonidesmed.org

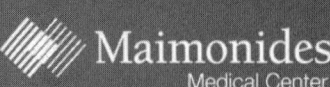

Maimonides
Medical Center

Maimonides serves one of the oldest populations in New York City, with one quarter of our patients over the age of 75. The Geriatrics Program at Maimonides is fully equipped to meet the special needs of this growing segment of the population. Directed by Barbara Paris, MD, the program encompasses inpatient and outpatient services, featuring the Acute Care for Elderly (ACE) Unit. The staff of this unit is focused on the continuity, coordination, quality and dignity of care provided.

Patient Evaluation

ACE Unit services focus on acute medical care and account for the complex needs of hospitalized elderly patients. Special attention is given to the assessment of memory loss and understanding the underlying causes of geriatric syndromes such as incontinence, falls and frailty. Psychosocial issues affecting elderly patients such as loneliness and end-of-life care are also addressed.

Wound Care

Because patients can have wounds that do not heal easily, we provide special attention through our wound care team.

Discharge & Medical Care at Home

Caregiver support groups are initiated while patients are in the hospital and are available after discharge. Once at home, if indicated, patients can receive a home visit from a member of our geriatric team, ensuring the coordination and continuity of their care.

Community & Nursing Home Liaison

The ACE Unit team serves as a bridge between hospital and community health care providers. Discharged patients are given a comprehensive plan that, if needed, includes a one-time home visit by our nurse practitioner, continued follow-up by geriatric specialists and referrals to community services. Maimonides has long established relationships with many nursing and rehabilitation facilities in Brooklyn.

Outpatient Geriatric Services

Our geriatric team offers comprehensive assessment and primary care services throughout Southern Brooklyn.

Physicians at Maimonides are among the ten percent in the US who use computers to enter patient orders, thereby reducing the risk of errors, increasing efficiency, and speeding the healing process.

Maimonides has appeared on the American Hospital Association's "Most Wired" and "Most Wireless" lists more often than any other healthcare institution in the metropolitan area. Advanced technology allows our doctors to focus more attention on caring for their patients.

Maimonides Medical Center – Passionate about medicine, compassionate about people.

www.maimonidesmed.org/geriatrics

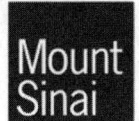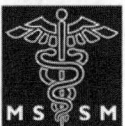

MOUNT SINAI
SCHOOL OF
MEDICINE

**THE MOUNT SINAI MEDICAL CENTER
GERIATRICS AND ADULT DEVELOPMENT**
One Gustave L. Levy Place
Fifth Avenue and 100th Street
New York, NY 10029-6574
Physician Referral: 1-800-MD-SINAI (637-4624)
www.mountsinai.org

THE BEST IN CLINICAL CARE

In recognition of the care offered to older patients, Mount Sinai specialists are cited time and time again as the finest in the nation. In its 2008 *Best Graduate Schools* issue, *U.S. News & World Report* ranked Mount Sinai School of Medicine at number 23 for research. Its *America's Best Hospitals* guide has ranked Mount Sinai's geriatrics specialty at number three for several years running.

We offer a full spectrum of patient care, including a specialized inpatient care team for the elderly (to minimize complications sometimes associated with an older person's hospital stay), a primary care geriatrics practice for older adults living in the community, a hospital-based consultation service for patients throughout Mount Sinai, a number of community-linked programs and partnerships, and a palliative care team dedicated to assuring the highest quality care and support for patients and families facing serious illnesses.

The Martha Stewart Center for Living, a new modern facility designed by renowned architect I.M. Pei, provides clinical care and education for patients and serves as a training ground for physicians.

GROUNDBREAKING RESEARCH

Mount Sinai's researchers continue to advance the understanding, prevention, and treatment of age-related disorders. The extensive research on aging conducted by the Department of Geriatrics and Adult Development includes studies on health services, medical decision making and ethical dilemmas, palliative care, the neurobiology of aging, and clinical interventions to promote independence in old age. The Department's expertise serves as a renowned educational resource for all Mount Sinai affiliates and other institutions in teaching geriatrics and gerontology to medical students, medical residents, geriatrics fellows, established physicians, and health profession trainees in other disciplines.

HISTORY OF EXCELLENCE

The Mount Sinai Medical Center is a pioneer in geriatric medicine. In 1909, a Mount Sinai physician coined the term "geriatrics," and in 1914, he wrote the first textbook on medical care for older adults. Today the Brookdale Department of Geriatrics and Adult Development continues to break new ground, offering comprehensive care, disease prevention, and the promotion of healthy and productive aging. The Department's enhanced expertise in assessing and managing patients with dementia greatly complements its established, interdisciplinary approach to patient care, in which medical staff and social workers address each patient's needs as a team.

THE FIRST FREESTANDING DEPARTMENT OF GERIATRICS AT A U.S. MEDICAL SCHOOL
Mount Sinai's Brookdale Department of Geriatrics and Adult Development was the first freestanding department of geriatrics established by a U.S. medical school, and it continues to be one of the very best. It offers unparalleled inpatient and outpatient care, as well as numerous treatment programs designed to meet the unique needs of older adults. Mount Sinai is also home to world-class researchers dedicated to advancing our understanding of Alzheimer's disease and other common geriatric conditions. At the Department's heart are its patients. The geriatricians of The Mount Sinai Medical Center work hard to improve life and longevity for New York's elderly.

NYU Langone Medical Center

GERIATRIC MEDICINE

Caring for the Elderly

The goal of geriatrics is to keep us all-and for as long as possible- healthy, functional, and vital members of our families and communities.

NYU has a distinguished history in this increasingly important specialty, as a federally designated research center and, since 1973, a leader in the care of older patients. Finding new answers and applying them to patient care are equally important. Among NYU's accomplishments in the care of the elderly are:

The Silberstein Aging and Dementia Research Center, one of the largest in the nation and designated a center of excellence in Alzheimer's treatment by the National Institute on Aging.

The Belfer Geriatrics Center, a multidisciplinary approach to the care of people over 65. Geriatrics, home care, neurology, orthopedics, dentistry, geropsychiatry, and many other disciplines are available to the Center's patients, whether referred from NYU, Bellevue, or the Manhattan Veteran's Administration Hospital.

Inpatient Geriatrics Service at NYU Hospitals Center, a team approach to inpatient care. A senior geriatrician leads the team of nurses, pharmacists, geropsychiatrists, rehabilitation experts, and fellowship trainees in caring for geriatric patients with complex conditions.

The NYU Geriatric Falls Prevention Program, an initiative across the NYU affiliated hospitals to address this major risk to life and independence in the elderly.

The William and Sylvia Silberstein Aging and Dementia Research Center provides:

- Comprehensive diagnostic evaluations to determine if memory loss is "normal" or more serious

- A memory enhancement program for age-related memory decline

- Pharmaceutical clinical trials for mild memory loss and for Alzheimer's treatment

- State-of-the-art brain imaging techniques

- Methods to prevent excess disability in Alzheimer's disease patients

- And comprehensive, on-going counseling and support groups for patients, caregivers and family members. Its longitudinal study of Alzheimer's patients is the most comprehensive ongoing study of its kind in the world.

242

Gynecologic Oncology

a subspecialty of
Obstetrics & Gynecology

An obstetrician/gynecologist who provides consultation and comprehensive management of patients with gynecologic cancer, including those diagnostic and therapeutic procedures necessary
for the total care of the patient with gynecologic cancer and resulting complications.

Training Required: Four years *plus* two years in clinical practice before certification in obstetrics and gynecology is complete *plus* additional training and examination in gynecologic oncology.

GYNECOLOGIC ONCOLOGY

New England

Berkowitz, Ross S MD [GO] - **Spec Exp:** Gynecologic Cancer; **Hospital:** Brigham & Women's Hosp, Dana-Farber Cancer Inst; **Address:** Brigham & Women's Hosp, Dept OB/GYN, 75 Francis St, Boston, MA 02115-6110; **Phone:** 617-732-8843; **Board Cert:** Obstetrics & Gynecology 1981; Gynecologic Oncology 1982; **Med School:** Boston Univ 1973; **Resid:** Surgery, Peter Bent Brigham Hosp 1975; Obstetrics & Gynecology, Boston Hosp for Women 1978; **Fellow:** Gynecologic Oncology, Boston Hosp for Women 1980; **Fac Appt:** Prof ObG, Harvard Med Sch

Brewer, Molly A MD [GO] - **Spec Exp:** Ovarian Cancer; **Hospital:** Univ of Conn Hlth Ctr, John Dempsey Hosp; **Address:** Univ Connecticut Hlth Ctr, Div Gyn Oncology, 263 Farmington Ave, MC2875, Farmington, CT 06032-2875; **Phone:** 860-679-4933; **Board Cert:** Obstetrics & Gynecology 1999; Gynecologic Oncology 2001; **Med School:** SUNY Upstate Med Univ 1991; **Resid:** Obstetrics & Gynecology, Oregon Hlth Scis Univ Hosp 1995; **Fellow:** Gynecologic Oncology, MD Anderson Cancer Ctr 1997

Currie, John L MD [GO] - **Spec Exp:** Gynecologic Cancer; Pelvic Reconstruction; Gynecologic Problems of Obesity; **Hospital:** Hartford Hosp; **Address:** Hartford Hospital, 85 Seymour St Fl 7 - Ste 705, Box 5037, Hartford, CT 06106-5501; **Phone:** 860-545-4341; **Board Cert:** Obstetrics & Gynecology 1991; Gynecologic Oncology 1982; **Med School:** Univ NC Sch Med 1967; **Resid:** Gynecologic Oncology, Hosp Univ Penn 1972; **Fellow:** Gynecologic Oncology, Duke Univ Med Ctr 1980; **Fac Appt:** Prof ObG, Univ Conn

DeMars, Leslie R MD [GO] - **Spec Exp:** Gynecologic Cancer; Colposcopy; Laparoscopic Surgery; **Hospital:** Dartmouth - Hitchcock Med Ctr; **Address:** Dartmouth-Hitchcock Med Ctr, Gyn-Oncology, 1 Medical Center Drive, Lebanon, NH 03756; **Phone:** 603-653-3530; **Board Cert:** Obstetrics & Gynecology 2006; Gynecologic Oncology 2006; **Med School:** Univ VT Coll Med 1987; **Resid:** Obstetrics & Gynecology, Univ N Carolina Hosps 1991; **Fellow:** Gynecologic Oncology, Univ N Carolina Hosps 1994; **Fac Appt:** Asst Prof ObG, Dartmouth Med Sch

Granai, Skip MD [GO] - **Spec Exp:** Complementary Medicine; **Hospital:** Women & Infants Hosp of RI; **Address:** Women's & Infants' Hosp, 101 Dudley St, GYN Oncology Department, Providence, RI 02905; **Phone:** 401-453-7520; **Med School:** Univ VT Coll Med 1977; **Fac Appt:** Assoc Prof ObG, Brown Univ

Muto, Michael G MD [GO] - **Spec Exp:** Ovarian Cancer; Cervical Cancer; Vulvar & Vaginal Cancer; Robotic Surgery; **Hospital:** Dana-Farber Cancer Inst, Brigham & Women's Hosp; **Address:** Dana Farber Cancer Inst, 44 Binney St Fl 9, Boston, MA 02115; **Phone:** 617-582-7931; **Board Cert:** Gynecologic Oncology 2006; Obstetrics & Gynecology 2006; Obstetrics & Gynecology 2006; Obstetrics & Gynecology 2007; **Med School:** Univ Mass Sch Med 1983; **Resid:** Obstetrics & Gynecology, Brigham & Women's Hosp 1987; **Fellow:** Gynecologic Oncology, Brigham & Women's Hosp 1990; **Fac Appt:** Assoc Prof ObG, Harvard Med Sch

Rutherford, Thomas MD [GO] - **Spec Exp:** Ovarian Cancer; Uterine Cancer; Ovarian Cancer-Early Detection; Cervical Cancer; **Hospital:** Yale-New Haven Hosp; **Address:** Yale Univ Sch Med Dept Ob-Gyn, 333 Cedar St, Box 208063, New Haven, CT 06520; **Phone:** 203-785-6301; **Board Cert:** Obstetrics & Gynecology 1997; Gynecologic Oncology 2000; **Med School:** Med Coll OH 1989; **Resid:** Obstetrics & Gynecology, Cooper Hosp 1993; **Fellow:** Gynecologic Oncology, Yale-New Haven Hosp 1995; **Fac Appt:** Assoc Prof ObG, Yale Univ

Schwartz, Peter E MD [GO] - **Spec Exp:** Ovarian Cancer; Uterine Cancer; Gynecologic Surgery-Complex; Cervical Cancer; **Hospital:** Yale-New Haven Hosp, Hosp of St Raphael; **Address:** Yale Univ Sch Med, Dept Ob/Gyn, 333 Cedar St, rm FMB-316, New Haven, CT 06510-3289; **Phone:** 203-785-4014; **Board Cert:** Obstetrics & Gynecology 1973; Gynecologic Oncology 1979; **Med School:** Albert Einstein Coll Med 1966; **Resid:** Obstetrics & Gynecology, Yale-New Haven Hosp 1970; **Fellow:** Gynecologic Oncology, MD Anderson Cancer Ctr 1975; **Fac Appt:** Prof ObG, Yale Univ

Tarraza, Hector M MD [GO] - **Spec Exp:** Gynecologic Cancer; **Hospital:** Maine Med Ctr; **Address:** 102 Campus Drive, rm 116, Scarborough, ME 04074; **Phone:** 207-883-0069; **Board Cert:** Obstetrics & Gynecology 1998; Gynecologic Oncology 1998; **Med School:** Harvard Med Sch 1981; **Resid:** Obstetrics & Gynecology, Mass Genl Hosp 1985; **Fellow:** Gynecologic Oncology, Mass Genl Hosp 1987; **Fac Appt:** Prof ObG, Univ VT Coll Med

Mid Atlantic

Abu-Rustum, Nadeem R MD [GO] - **Spec Exp:** Ovarian Cancer; Uterine Cancer; Cervical Cancer; Vulvar Disease/Cancer; **Hospital:** Meml Sloan-Kettering Cancer Ctr; **Address:** 1275 York Avenue, New York, NY 10065; **Phone:** 800-525-2225; **Board Cert:** Obstetrics & Gynecology 1998; Gynecologic Oncology 2000; **Med School:** Lebanon 1990; **Resid:** Obstetrics & Gynecology, Greater Baltimore Med Ctr 1994; **Fellow:** Gynecologic Oncology, Meml Sloan-Kettering Cancer Ctr 1997; **Fac Appt:** Assoc Prof ObG, Cornell Univ-Weill Med Coll

Barakat, Richard R MD [GO] - **Spec Exp:** Laparoscopic Surgery; Ovarian Cancer; Uterine Cancer; **Hospital:** Meml Sloan-Kettering Cancer Ctr; **Address:** 1275 York Avenue, New York, NY 10065; **Phone:** 800-525-2225; **Board Cert:** Obstetrics & Gynecology 2006; Gynecologic Oncology 2006; **Med School:** SUNY Hlth Sci Ctr 1985; **Resid:** Obstetrics & Gynecology, Bellevue Hosp 1989; **Fellow:** Gynecologic Oncology, Meml Sloan Kettering Cancer Ctr 1991; **Fac Appt:** Assoc Prof ObG, Cornell Univ-Weill Med Coll

Barnes, Willard MD [GO] - **Spec Exp:** Pelvic Tumors; Gynecologic Cancer; **Hospital:** Georgetown Univ Hosp, Virginia Hosp Ctr - Arlington; **Address:** Georgetown Univ Hosp, Lombardi Cancer Ctr, Dept Gyn Oncology, 3800 Reservoir Rd NW, Washington, DC 20007-2194; **Phone:** 202-444-2114; **Board Cert:** Obstetrics & Gynecology 1997; Gynecologic Oncology 1997; **Med School:** Univ Miss 1979; **Resid:** Obstetrics & Gynecology, Univ Miss Med Ctr 1983; **Fellow:** Gynecologic Oncology, Georgetown Univ Med Ctr 1985; **Fac Appt:** Assoc Prof ObG, Georgetown Univ

Barter, James MD [GO] - **Spec Exp:** Laparoscopic Surgery; Ovarian Cancer; Gynecologic Cancer; **Hospital:** Holy Cross Hospital - Silver Spring, Suburban Hosp - Bethesda; **Address:** 6301 Executive Blvd, Rockville, MD 20852; **Phone:** 301-770-4967; **Board Cert:** Obstetrics & Gynecology 1997; Gynecologic Oncology 1997; **Med School:** Univ VA Sch Med 1977; **Resid:** Internal Medicine, Univ Kentucky Med Ctr 1979; Obstetrics & Gynecology, Duke Univ Med Ctr 1983; **Fellow:** Gynecologic Oncology, Univ Alabama 1985; **Fac Appt:** Clin Prof ObG, Georgetown Univ

Bristow, Robert E MD [GO] - **Spec Exp:** Ovarian Cancer; Cervical Cancer; Uterine Cancer; **Hospital:** Johns Hopkins Hosp - Baltimore (page 61); **Address:** Johns Hopkins Hosp, 600 N Wolfe St, Phipps 281, Baltimore, MD 21287; **Phone:** 410-955-6700; **Board Cert:** Obstetrics & Gynecology 1999; Gynecologic Oncology 2003; **Med School:** USC Sch Med 1991; **Resid:** Obstetrics & Gynecology, Johns Hopkins Hosp 1995; **Fellow:** Gynecologic Oncology, UCLA Med Ctr 1998; **Fac Appt:** Assoc Prof ObG, Johns Hopkins Univ

Gynecologic Oncology

Caputo, Thomas A MD [GO] - **Spec Exp:** Cervical Cancer; Ovarian Cancer; Uterine Cancer; Vulvar Disease/Cancer; **Hospital:** NY-Presby Hosp/Weill Cornell (page 66); **Address:** NY Presby Hosp-Weill Cornell, 525 E 68th St, Ste J130, New York, NY 10021; **Phone:** 212-746-3179; **Board Cert:** Obstetrics & Gynecology 1993; Gynecologic Oncology 1977; **Med School:** UMDNJ-NJ Med Sch, Newark 1965; **Resid:** Obstetrics & Gynecology, Martland Hosp 1969; **Fellow:** Gynecologic Oncology, Emory Univ Hosp 1974; **Fac Appt:** Clin Prof ObG, Cornell Univ-Weill Med Coll

Carlson, John A MD [GO] - **Spec Exp:** Gynecologic Cancer; Ovarian Cancer; Gynecologic Surgery-Complex; **Hospital:** St Peter's Univ Hosp; **Address:** St Peter's Univ Hosp, 254 Easton Ave, New Brunswick, NJ 08901; **Phone:** 732-937-6003; **Board Cert:** Obstetrics & Gynecology 1981; Gynecologic Oncology 1982; **Med School:** Georgetown Univ 1974; **Resid:** Obstetrics & Gynecology, Hosp Univ Penn 1978; **Fellow:** Gynecologic Oncology, MD Anderson Hosp 1980; **Fac Appt:** Prof ObG, Drexel Univ Coll Med

Coukos, George MD/PhD [GO] - **Spec Exp:** Ovarian Cancer; Gynecologic Cancer; Vaccine Therapy; Clinical Trials; **Hospital:** Hosp Univ Penn - UPHS (page 60); **Address:** Hosp Univ Penn, 1000 Courtyard Bldg, 3400 Spruce St, Philadelphia, PA 19104; **Phone:** 215-662-3318; **Board Cert:** Obstetrics & Gynecology 2004; Gynecologic Oncology 2004; **Med School:** Italy 1987; **Resid:** Obstetrics & Gynecology, Hosp Univ Penn 1997; **Fellow:** Gynecologic Oncology, Hosp Univ Penn 2000; **Fac Appt:** Assoc Prof ObG, Univ Pennsylvania

Curtin, John P MD [GO] - **Spec Exp:** Uterine Cancer; Ovarian Cancer; Laparoscopic Surgery; **Hospital:** NYU Med Ctr (page 68); **Address:** NYU Clinical Cancer Ctr, 160 E 34th St Fl 4, New York, NY 10016-6402; **Phone:** 212-731-5345; **Board Cert:** Obstetrics & Gynecology 1996; Gynecologic Oncology 1996; **Med School:** Creighton Univ 1979; **Resid:** Obstetrics & Gynecology, Univ Minn Med Ctr 1984; **Fellow:** Gynecologic Oncology, Meml Sloan-Kettering Cancer Ctr 1988; **Fac Appt:** Prof ObG, NYU Sch Med

Dottino, Peter R MD [GO] - **Spec Exp:** Laparoscopic Surgery; Gynecologic Cancer; **Hospital:** Mount Sinai Med Ctr (page 64), Hackensack Univ Med Ctr; **Address:** 800-A 5th Ave, Ste 405, New York, NY 10021-7215; **Phone:** 212-888-8439; **Board Cert:** Obstetrics & Gynecology 1996; Gynecologic Oncology 1996; **Med School:** Georgetown Univ 1979; **Resid:** Obstetrics & Gynecology, SUNY Downstate Med Ctr 1983; **Fellow:** Gynecologic Oncology, Mount Sinai Hosp 1985

Dunton, Charles J MD [GO] - **Spec Exp:** Ovarian Cancer; Uterine Cancer; Cervical Cancer; Pap Smear Abnormalities; **Hospital:** Lankenau Hosp; **Address:** 100 E Lancaster Ave, Med Office Bldg East, Ste 661, Wynnewood, PA 19096; **Phone:** 610-649-8085; **Board Cert:** Obstetrics & Gynecology 1996; Gynecologic Oncology 1996; **Med School:** Jefferson Med Coll 1980; **Resid:** Obstetrics & Gynecology, Lankenau Hosp 1984; **Fellow:** Gynecologic Oncology, Hosp Univ Penn 1989; **Fac Appt:** Prof ObG, Jefferson Med Coll

Edwards, Robert P MD [GO] - **Spec Exp:** Ovarian Cancer; Gynecologic Cancer; Cervical Cancer; Clinical Trials; **Hospital:** Magee-Womens Hosp - UPMC; **Address:** Magee-Womens Hosp, Gynecologic Oncology, 300 Halket St, Pittsburgh, PA 15213; **Phone:** 412-641-5411; **Board Cert:** Obstetrics & Gynecology 2006; Gynecologic Oncology 2006; **Med School:** Univ Pittsburgh 1984; **Resid:** Obstetrics & Gynecology, Magee WomensHosp-UPMC 1989; **Fellow:** Gynecologic Oncology, Univ Alabama Med Ctr 1993; **Fac Appt:** Prof ObG, Univ Pittsburgh

Fishman, David A MD [GO] - **Spec Exp:** Ovarian Cancer; Ovarian Cancer-Early Detection; Gynecologic Cancer; **Hospital:** NYU Med Ctr (page 68); **Address:** NYU Clinical Cancer Ctr, 160 E 34 St Fl 4, New York, NY 10016; **Phone:** 212-731-5345; **Board Cert:** Obstetrics & Gynecology 2005; Gynecologic Oncology 2005; **Med School:** Texas Tech Univ 1988; **Resid:** Obstetrics & Gynecology, Yale-New Haven Hosp 1992; **Fellow:** Gynecologic Oncology, Yale-New Haven Hosp 1994; **Fac Appt:** Prof ObG, NYU Sch Med

Herzog, Thomas J MD [GO] - **Spec Exp:** Cervical Cancer; Gynecologic Cancer; Laparoscopic Surgery; Ovarian Cancer; **Hospital:** NY-Presby Hosp/Columbia (page 66); **Address:** Herbert Irving Pavilion, 161 Fort Washington Ave, 8-837, New York, NY 10032; **Phone:** 212-305-3410; **Board Cert:** Obstetrics & Gynecology 2006; Gynecologic Oncology 2006; **Med School:** Univ Cincinnati 1986; **Resid:** Obstetrics & Gynecology, Good Samaritan Hosp 1990; **Fellow:** Gynecologic Oncology, Barnes Jewish Hosp 1993; **Fac Appt:** Assoc Prof ObG, Columbia P&S

Kelley III, Joseph L MD [GO] - **Spec Exp:** Breast Cancer; Ovarian Cancer; Cervical Cancer; Gynecologic Cancer; **Hospital:** Magee-Womens Hosp - UPMC; **Address:** Magee-Womens Hosp, Gynecologic Oncology, 300 Halket St, Pittsburgh, PA 15213; **Phone:** 412-641-5411; **Board Cert:** Obstetrics & Gynecology 2005; Gynecologic Oncology 2005; **Med School:** St Louis Univ 1985; **Resid:** Obstetrics & Gynecology, Magee-Womens Hosp 1988; **Fellow:** Gynecologic Oncology, MD Anderson Cancer Ctr 1991; **Fac Appt:** Assoc Prof ObG, Univ Pittsburgh

Koulos, John MD [GO] - **Spec Exp:** Cervical Cancer; Uterine Cancer; Ovarian Cancer; **Hospital:** Beth Israel Med Ctr - Petrie Division (page 57); **Address:** Beth Israel Hosp Cancer Ctr, 10 Union Square E, Ste 4C, New York, NY 10003; **Phone:** 212-844-5729; **Board Cert:** Obstetrics & Gynecology 2006; Gynecologic Oncology 2006; **Med School:** Northwestern Univ 1978; **Resid:** Obstetrics & Gynecology, Northwestern Univ Med Sch 1982; **Fellow:** Gynecologic Oncology, Meml Sloan Kettering Cancer Ctr 1984; **Fac Appt:** Assoc Prof ObG, NY Med Coll

Lele, Shashikant B MD [GO] - **Spec Exp:** Gynecologic Cancer; Ovarian Cancer; **Hospital:** Roswell Park Cancer Inst, Buffalo General Hosp; **Address:** Roswell Park Cancer Inst, Dept of Gynecology, Elm & Carlton Sts, Buffalo, NY 14263; **Phone:** 716-845-5776; **Board Cert:** Obstetrics & Gynecology 1976; Gynecologic Oncology 1979; **Med School:** India 1968; **Resid:** Obstetrics & Gynecology, JJ Hosp-Grant Med Ctr 1970; Obstetrics & Gynecology, Mt Sinai Hosp 1973; **Fellow:** Gynecologic Oncology, Roswell Park Cancer Inst 1976; **Fac Appt:** Clin Prof ObG, SUNY Buffalo

Morgan, Mark A MD [GO] - **Spec Exp:** Laparoscopic Surgery; Gynecologic Surgery-Complex; Gynecologic Cancer; Uro-Gynecology; **Hospital:** Fox Chase Cancer Ctr (page 58); **Address:** Fox Chase Cancer Ctr-Gyn Oncology, 333 Cottman Ave, Philadelphia, PA 19111; **Phone:** 215-214-1430; **Board Cert:** Obstetrics & Gynecology 2006; Gynecologic Oncology 2006; **Med School:** SUNY Downstate 1982; **Resid:** Obstetrics & Gynecology, Hosp Univ Penn 1986; **Fellow:** Gynecologic Oncology, Hosp Univ Penn 1988

Odunsi, Adekunle O MD/PhD [GO] - **Spec Exp:** Ovarian Cancer; Immunotherapy; Clinical Trials; **Hospital:** Roswell Park Cancer Inst; **Address:** Roswell Park Cancer Inst, Gyn Oncology, Elm and Carlton Streets, Buffalo, NY 14263; **Phone:** 716-845-3511; **Board Cert:** Obstetrics & Gynecology 2004; Gynecologic Oncology 2004; **Med School:** Nigeria 1984; **Resid:** Obstetrics & Gynecology, Rosie Maternity & Addenbrookes Hosps 1990; Obstetrics & Gynecology, Yale-New Haven Hosp 1999; **Fellow:** Gynecologic Oncology, Roswell Park Cancer Inst 2001; **Fac Appt:** Prof ObG, SUNY Buffalo

Rosenblum, Norman G MD/PhD [GO] - **Spec Exp:** Ovarian Cancer; Uterine Cancer; Vulvar Disease/Cancer; **Hospital:** Thomas Jefferson Univ Hosp; **Address:** 834 Chesnut St, Ste 300, Philadelphia, PA 19107-5127; **Phone:** 215-955-6200; **Board Cert:** Obstetrics & Gynecology 2007; Gynecologic Oncology 2007; **Med School:** Jefferson Med Coll 1978; **Resid:** Obstetrics & Gynecology, Hosp Univ Penn 1982; **Fellow:** Gynecologic Oncology, Hosp Univ Penn 1984; **Fac Appt:** Prof ObG, Jefferson Med Coll

Gynecologic Oncology

Rubin, Stephen C MD [GO] - **Spec Exp:** Gynecologic Cancer; Ovarian Cancer; Cervical Cancer; **Hospital:** Hosp Univ Penn - UPHS (page 60); **Address:** Hosp Univ Penn, Gynecologic Oncology, 3400 Spruce St, 1000 Courtyard Bldg, Philadelphia, PA 19104-4283; **Phone:** 215-662-3318; **Board Cert:** Obstetrics & Gynecology 2006; Gynecologic Oncology 2006; **Med School:** Univ Pennsylvania 1976; **Resid:** Obstetrics & Gynecology, Hosp Univ Penn 1980; **Fellow:** Gynecologic Oncology, Hosp Univ Penn 1982; **Fac Appt:** Prof ObG, Univ Pennsylvania

Southeast

Alleyn, James MD [GO] - **Spec Exp:** Cervical Cancer; Ovarian Cancer; Uterine Cancer; **Hospital:** Mercy Hosp, Baptist Hosp of Miami; **Address:** 3661 S Miami Ave, Ste 308, Miami, FL 33133-4232; **Phone:** 305-854-3603; **Board Cert:** Obstetrics & Gynecology 1978; **Med School:** Indiana Univ 1972; **Resid:** Obstetrics & Gynecology, Miami-Jackson Meml Hosp 1976; **Fellow:** Gynecologic Oncology, Miami-Jackson Meml Hosp 1978; **Fac Appt:** Asst Clin Prof ObG, Univ Miami Sch Med

Alvarez, Ronald D MD [GO] - **Spec Exp:** Gynecologic Cancer; Ovarian Cancer; **Hospital:** Univ of Ala Hosp at Birmingham, Brookwood Med Ctr; **Address:** Univ Alabama, Div Gyn Oncology, 619 19th St S, OHB 538, Birmingham, AL 35249-7333; **Phone:** 205-934-4986; **Board Cert:** Obstetrics & Gynecology 2006; Gynecologic Oncology 2006; **Med School:** Louisiana State U, New Orleans 1983; **Resid:** Obstetrics & Gynecology, Univ Alabama Hosp 1987; **Fellow:** Gynecologic Oncology, Univ Alabama Hosp 1990; **Fac Appt:** Assoc Prof ObG, Univ Ala

Berchuck, Andrew MD [GO] - **Spec Exp:** Ovarian Cancer; Uterine Cancer; **Hospital:** Duke Univ Med Ctr; **Address:** Duke Univ Med Center, DUMC Box 3079, Durham, NC 27710; **Phone:** 919-684-3765; **Board Cert:** Obstetrics & Gynecology 1998; Gynecologic Oncology 1998; **Med School:** Case West Res Univ 1980; **Resid:** Obstetrics & Gynecology, Case Western Resrv 1984; **Fellow:** Gynecology, UT Southwestern 1985; Gynecologic Oncology, Meml Sloan-Kettering 1987; **Fac Appt:** Prof ObG, Duke Univ

Clarke-Pearson, Daniel L MD [GO] - **Spec Exp:** Pelvic Reconstruction; Gynecologic Surgery-Complex; Gynecologic Cancer; **Hospital:** Univ NC Hosps, Wesley Long Comm Hosp; **Address:** Univ of North Carolina, CB #7570, Chapel Hill, NC 27599; **Phone:** 919-966-5280; **Board Cert:** Obstetrics & Gynecology 2006; Gynecologic Oncology 2006; **Med School:** Case West Res Univ 1975; **Resid:** Obstetrics & Gynecology, Duke Univ Med Ctr 1979; **Fellow:** Gynecologic Oncology, Duke Univ Med Ctr 1981; **Fac Appt:** Prof ObG, Univ NC Sch Med

Creasman, William T MD [GO] - **Spec Exp:** Uterine Cancer; Ovarian Cancer; Cervical Cancer; **Hospital:** MUSC Med Ctr; **Address:** Med Univ S Carolina-Dept ObGyn, Charleston, SC 29425; **Phone:** 843-792-4509; **Board Cert:** Obstetrics & Gynecology 1991; Gynecologic Oncology 1974; **Med School:** Baylor Coll Med 1960; **Resid:** Obstetrics & Gynecology, Rochester Med Ctr 1967; **Fellow:** Gynecologic Oncology, Anderson Hosp Tumor Inst 1969; **Fac Appt:** Prof ObG, Med Univ SC

DePriest, Paul D MD [GO] - **Spec Exp:** Ovarian Cancer-Early Detection; Cervical Cancer; Pap Smear Abnormalities; **Hospital:** Univ of Kentucky Chandler Hosp; **Address:** Univ Kentucky Gynecologic Oncology, Whiteney Hendrickson Bldg, 800 Rose St, rm 331E1, Lexington, KY 40536; **Phone:** 859-323-5277; **Board Cert:** Obstetrics & Gynecology 2006; Gynecologic Oncology 2006; **Med School:** Univ KY Coll Med 1985; **Resid:** Obstetrics & Gynecology, Univ Kentucky Med Ctr 1989; **Fellow:** Gynecologic Oncology, Univ Kentucky Med Ctr 1991; **Fac Appt:** Prof ObG, Univ KY Coll Med

Fields, Abbie MD [GO] - **Spec Exp:** Fertility Preservation in Cancer; Robotic Surgery; Cancer Genetics; Pelvic Reconstruction; **Hospital:** Henrico Doctors Hosp; **Address:** 7603 Forest Ave, Ste 207, Richmond, VA 23229; **Phone:** 804-200-7025; **Board Cert:** Obstetrics & Gynecology 2006; Gynecologic Oncology 2006; **Med School:** Ohio State Univ 1987; **Resid:** Obstetrics & Gynecology, Northwestern Univ 1991; **Fellow:** Gynecologic Oncology, Johns Hopkins Hosp 1993

Finan, Michael A MD [GO] - **Spec Exp:** Ovarian Cancer; Cervical Cancer; Uterine Cancer; **Hospital:** Mobile Infirmary Med Ctr, USA Children & Women's Hospital; **Address:** University of S Alabama, Mitchell Cancer Inst, 1 Mobile Infirmary Cir Fl 1, Mobile, AL 36607; **Phone:** 251-665-8000; **Board Cert:** Obstetrics & Gynecology 2005; Gynecologic Oncology 2005; **Med School:** Louisiana State U, New Orleans 1986; **Resid:** Obstetrics & Gynecology, Univ South Fla Affil Hosps 1990; **Fellow:** Gynecologic Oncology, H Lee Moffitt Cancer Ctr 1992; **Fac Appt:** Prof ObG, Univ S Ala Coll Med

Fiorica, James V MD [GO] - **Spec Exp:** Gynecologic Cancer; Breast Cancer; Cervical Cancer; **Hospital:** Sarasota Meml Hosp; **Address:** 1888 Hillview St, Sarasota, FL 34239; **Phone:** 941-917-8383; **Board Cert:** Obstetrics & Gynecology 2006; Gynecologic Oncology 2006; **Med School:** Tufts Univ 1982; **Resid:** Obstetrics & Gynecology, Univ South Fla Affil Hosp 1986; **Fellow:** Gynecologic Oncology, Univ South Fla Affil Hosp 1989; Breast Disease, Tufts Univ 1990; **Fac Appt:** Clin Prof ObG, Univ S Fla Coll Med

Fowler Jr, Wesley C MD [GO] - **Spec Exp:** Vulvar Disease/Cancer; DES-Exposed Females; Cancer Prevention; **Hospital:** Univ NC Hosps; **Address:** U NC Chapel Hill, Div of Ob/Gyn, Campus Box 7570, Chapel Hill, NC 27599-7570; **Phone:** 919-966-1196; **Board Cert:** Obstetrics & Gynecology 1991; Gynecologic Oncology 1979; **Med School:** Univ NC Sch Med 1966; **Resid:** Obstetrics & Gynecology, NC Memorial Hosp 1971; **Fac Appt:** Prof ObG, Univ NC Sch Med

Horowitz, Ira R MD [GO] - **Spec Exp:** Laparoscopic Surgery; Ovarian Cancer; Cervical Cancer; **Hospital:** Emory Univ Hosp, Crawford Long Hosp of Emory Univ; **Address:** Emory Clinic, 1365 Clifton Rd NE A Bldg Fl 4, Atlanta, GA 30322; **Phone:** 404-778-4416; **Board Cert:** Obstetrics & Gynecology 1997; Gynecologic Oncology 1997; **Med School:** Baylor Coll Med 1980; **Resid:** Obstetrics & Gynecology, Baylor Affil Hosp 1984; **Fellow:** Gynecologic Oncology, Johns Hopkins Hosp 1987; **Fac Appt:** Prof ObG, Emory Univ

Kohler, Matthew MD [GO] - **Spec Exp:** Pelvic Reconstruction; **Hospital:** MUSC Med Ctr; **Address:** MUSC Med Ctr- Women's Hlth Ob/Gyn, 86 Jonathan Lucas St, Box 250957, Charleston, SC 29425; **Phone:** 843-792-9300; **Board Cert:** Obstetrics & Gynecology 1995; Gynecologic Oncology 1997; **Med School:** Duke Univ 1987; **Resid:** Obstetrics & Gynecology, Duke University Med Ctr 1991; **Fellow:** Gynecologic Oncology, Duke University Med Ctr 1993; **Fac Appt:** Assoc Prof ObG, Med Univ SC

Lancaster, Johnathan M MD/PhD [GO] - **Spec Exp:** Ovarian Cancer; Cancer Genetics; Gene Therapy; **Hospital:** H Lee Moffitt Cancer Ctr & Research Inst; **Address:** H Lee Moffitt Cancer Ctr - Gyn Oncology, 12902 Magnolia Drive, Tampa, FL 33612; **Phone:** 813-745-7272; **Board Cert:** Obstetrics & Gynecology 2005; **Med School:** Wales 1997; **Resid:** Obstetrics & Gynecology, Duke Univ Med Ctr 2000; **Fellow:** Gynecologic Oncology, Duke Univ Med Ctr 2003; **Fac Appt:** Asst Prof ObG, Univ S Fla Coll Med

Lentz, Samuel S MD [GO] - **Spec Exp:** Gynecologic Cancer; Pelvic Reconstruction; **Hospital:** Wake Forest Univ Baptist Med Ctr (page 73), Forsyth Med Ctr; **Address:** Wake Forest Univ Sch Med, Div Gyn Oncology, Medical Center Blvd, Winston-Salem, NC 27157; **Phone:** 336-716-6673; **Board Cert:** Obstetrics & Gynecology 2006; Gynecologic Oncology 2006; **Med School:** Wake Forest Univ 1978; **Resid:** Obstetrics & Gynecology, NC Baptist Hosp 1982; **Fellow:** Gynecologic Oncology, Mayo Clinic 1989; **Fac Appt:** Prof ObG, Wake Forest Univ

Gynecologic Oncology

Partridge, Edward E MD [GO] - **Spec Exp:** Ovarian Cancer; **Hospital:** Univ of Ala Hosp at Birmingham; **Address:** UAB Cancer Ctr, 1802 6th Ave S, Ste MP2555, Birmingham, AL 35294-3300; **Phone:** 205-934-4986; **Board Cert:** Obstetrics & Gynecology 1993; Gynecologic Oncology 1981; **Med School:** Univ Ala 1973; **Resid:** Obstetrics & Gynecology, Univ Alabama Hosp 1977; **Fellow:** Gynecologic Oncology, Univ Alabama Hosp 1979; **Fac Appt:** Prof ObG, Univ Ala

Penalver, Manuel A MD [GO] - **Spec Exp:** Gynecologic Cancer; Cervical Cancer; Pelvic Tumors; **Hospital:** Doctors' Hosp, Baptist Hosp of Miami; **Address:** South Florida Gyn Oncology, 5000 University Drive, Ste 3300, Coral Gables, FL 33146; **Phone:** 305-663-7001; **Board Cert:** Obstetrics & Gynecology 1997; Gynecologic Oncology 1997; **Med School:** Univ Miami Sch Med 1977; **Resid:** Obstetrics & Gynecology, Univ Miami/Jackson Meml Hosp 1982; **Fellow:** Gynecologic Oncology, Univ Miami/Jackson Meml Hosp 1984

Poliakoff, Steven MD [GO] - **Spec Exp:** Ovarian Cancer; Minimally Invasive Surgery; Cancer Genetics; **Hospital:** Mount Sinai Med Ctr - Miami, South Miami Hosp; **Address:** 6280 Sunset Dr, Ste 502, South Miami, FL 33143-4870; **Phone:** 305-596-0870; **Board Cert:** Obstetrics & Gynecology 1983; **Med School:** Univ NC Sch Med 1975; **Resid:** Obstetrics & Gynecology, Johns Hopkins Hosp 1979; **Fellow:** Gynecologic Oncology, Jackson Meml Hosp/Univ Miami 1981

Sevin, Bernd-Uwe MD [GO] - **Spec Exp:** Ovarian Cancer; Pelvic Reconstruction; Pelvic Tumors; **Hospital:** St Luke's Hosp - Jacksonville; **Address:** Mayo Clinic-Dept Gynecology, 4500 San Pablo Rd, Jacksonville, FL 32224; **Phone:** 904-953-0612; **Board Cert:** Obstetrics & Gynecology 1980; Gynecologic Oncology 1981; **Med School:** Germany 1968; **Resid:** Obstetrics & Gynecology, Stanford U Med Ctr 1977; **Fellow:** Gynecologic Oncology, Jackson Meml Hosp 1979; **Fac Appt:** Prof ObG, Mayo Med Sch

Soper, John T MD [GO] - **Spec Exp:** Gynecologic Cancer; **Hospital:** Univ NC Hosps; **Address:** Univ North Carolina, Dept OB/GYN, 5017 Old Clinic Bldg, Chapel Hill, NC 27599; **Phone:** 919-966-1194; **Board Cert:** Obstetrics & Gynecology 2006; Gynecologic Oncology 2006; **Med School:** Univ Iowa Coll Med 1978; **Resid:** Obstetrics & Gynecology, Univ Utah Med Ctr 1982; **Fellow:** Gynecologic Oncology, Duke Univ Med Ctr 1985; **Fac Appt:** Prof ObG, Univ NC Sch Med

Spann Jr, Cyril O MD [GO] - **Spec Exp:** Gynecologic Cancer; Ovarian Cancer; **Hospital:** Emory Univ Hosp, Crawford Long Hosp of Emory Univ; **Address:** Emory Clinic Crawford Long, 550 Peachtree St, Ste 900, Atlanta, GA 30308; **Phone:** 404-616-3540; **Board Cert:** Obstetrics & Gynecology 2005; Gynecologic Oncology 2005; **Med School:** Meharry Med Coll 1981; **Resid:** Obstetrics & Gynecology, Emory Univ Med Ctr 1985; **Fellow:** Gynecologic Oncology, Univ NC Meml Hosp 1989; **Fac Appt:** Prof ObG, Emory Univ

Taylor Jr, Peyton T MD [GO] - **Spec Exp:** Gynecologic Surgery-Complex; Gynecologic Cancer; **Hospital:** Univ Virginia Med Ctr; **Address:** Univ VA Hlth Sys, Dept Ob/Gyn, PO Box 800712, Charlottesville, VA 22908; **Phone:** 434-924-9933; **Board Cert:** Obstetrics & Gynecology 1994; Gynecologic Oncology 1981; **Med School:** Univ Ala 1968; **Resid:** Obstetrics & Gynecology, Univ VA Hosp 1970; Obstetrics & Gynecology, Univ VA Hosp 1975; **Fellow:** Surgical Oncology, Natl Cancer Inst 1972; Gynecologic Oncology, Univ Va Hosp 1977; **Fac Appt:** Prof ObG, Univ VA Sch Med

Van Nagell Jr, John R MD [GO] - **Spec Exp:** Ovarian Cancer; Cervical Cancer; **Hospital:** Univ of Kentucky Chandler Hosp; **Address:** UKMC, Dept Ob/Gyn, 800 Rose St, Lexington, KY 40536-0001; **Phone:** 859-323-5553; **Board Cert:** Obstetrics & Gynecology 1973; Gynecologic Oncology 1976; **Med School:** Univ Pennsylvania 1967; **Resid:** Obstetrics & Gynecology, Kentucky Med Ctr 1971; **Fac Appt:** Prof ObG, Univ KY Coll Med

Midwest

Belinson, Jerome L MD [GO] - **Spec Exp:** Ovarian Cancer; Cervical Cancer; **Hospital:** Cleveland Clin Fdn (page 56); **Address:** 9500 Euclid Ave, Desk A81, Cleveland, OH 44195; **Phone:** 216-444-7933; **Board Cert:** Obstetrics & Gynecology 1998; Gynecologic Oncology 1980; **Med School:** Univ MO-Columbia Sch Med 1968; **Resid:** Obstetrics & Gynecology, Columbia Presby Med Ctr 1973; **Fellow:** Gynecologic Oncology, Jackson Meml Hosp 1977; **Fac Appt:** Prof ObG, Ohio State Univ

Copeland, Larry J MD [GO] - **Spec Exp:** Ovarian Cancer; Uterine Cancer; Gynecologic Cancer; **Hospital:** Arthur G James Cancer Hosp & Research Inst, Ohio St Univ Med Ctr; **Address:** 1654 Upham Drive, Ste 505, Columbus, OH 43210-1250; **Phone:** 614-293-8697; **Board Cert:** Obstetrics & Gynecology 1991; Gynecologic Oncology 1981; **Med School:** Univ Western Ontario 1973; **Resid:** Obstetrics & Gynecology, McMaster Univ Affil Hosps 1977; **Fellow:** Gynecologic Oncology, MD Anderson Cancer Ctr-Univ Tex 1979; **Fac Appt:** Prof ObG, Ohio State Univ

De Geest, Koen MD [GO] - **Spec Exp:** Ovarian Cancer; Cervical Cancer; Clinical Trials; **Hospital:** Univ Iowa Hosp & Clinics; **Address:** Univ Iowa, Div Gynecological Oncology, 200 Hawkins Drive, rm 4630 JCP, Iowa City, IA 52242; **Phone:** 319-356-2015; **Board Cert:** Obstetrics & Gynecology 1997; Gynecologic Oncology 1997; **Med School:** Belgium 1977; **Resid:** Obstetrics & Gynecology, Univ Ghent 1982; **Fellow:** Gynecologic Oncology, Penn State/Hershey Med Ctr 1990; **Fac Appt:** Prof ObG, Univ Iowa Coll Med

Fowler, Jeffrey M MD [GO] - **Spec Exp:** Laparoscopic Surgery; Gynecologic Cancer; Robotic Surgery; Pelvic Reconstruction; **Hospital:** Ohio St Univ Med Ctr; **Address:** Ohio State Univ, Div Gynecologic Oncology, 320 W Tenth Ave, M-210 SLH, Columbus, OH 43210; **Phone:** 614-293-8737; **Board Cert:** Obstetrics & Gynecology 2005; Gynecologic Oncology 2005; **Med School:** Northwestern Univ 1985; **Resid:** Obstetrics & Gynecology, Ohio State Univ Hosp 1989; **Fellow:** Gynecologic Oncology, UCLA 1991; **Fac Appt:** Prof ObG, Ohio State Univ

Johnston, Carolyn M MD [GO] - **Spec Exp:** Gynecologic Surgery-Complex; Cervical Cancer; **Hospital:** Univ Michigan Hlth Sys; **Address:** Womens Hosp-Div Gyn Oncology, 1500 E Med Ctr Drive, rm L4510, Ann Arbor, MI 48109-0276; **Phone:** 734-647-8906; **Board Cert:** Obstetrics & Gynecology 2000; Gynecologic Oncology 2000; **Med School:** Yale Univ 1984; **Resid:** Obstetrics & Gynecology, Univ Chicago Hosp 1988; **Fellow:** Gynecologic Oncology, Mt Sinai Hosp 1990; **Fac Appt:** Assoc Clin Prof ObG, Univ Mich Med Sch

Look, Katherine Y MD [GO] - **Spec Exp:** Ovarian Cancer; Uterine Cancer; **Hospital:** Indiana Univ Hosp, Methodist Hosp - Indianapolis; **Address:** 535 Barnhill Drive, Ste 434, Indianapolis, IN 46202; **Phone:** 317-274-2130; **Board Cert:** Obstetrics & Gynecology 2005; Gynecologic Oncology 2005; **Med School:** Univ Mich Med Sch 1979; **Resid:** Obstetrics & Gynecology, Univ Illinois Med Ctr 1983; **Fellow:** Gynecologic Oncology, Meml Sloan Kettering Cancer Ctr 1986; **Fac Appt:** Prof ObG, Indiana Univ

Lurain, John R MD [GO] - **Spec Exp:** Gestational Trophoblastic Disease; Uterine Cancer; Ovarian Cancer; **Hospital:** Northwestern Meml Hosp; **Address:** Northwestern Univ Feinberg Sch Med, 250 E Superior St, Chicago, IL 60611-3056; **Phone:** 312-472-4684; **Board Cert:** Obstetrics & Gynecology 1977; Gynecologic Oncology 1981; **Med School:** Univ NC Sch Med 1972; **Resid:** Obstetrics & Gynecology, Univ Pittsburgh Med Ctr 1975; **Fellow:** Gynecologic Oncology, Roswell Park Cancer Inst 1979; **Fac Appt:** Prof ObG, Northwestern Univ

Gynecologic Oncology

Mutch, David G MD [GO] - **Spec Exp:** Gynecologic Cancer; Pelvic Reconstruction; **Hospital:** Barnes-Jewish Hosp; **Address:** 4911 Barnes Jewish Hospital Plaza, St Louis, MO 63110; **Phone:** 314-362-3181; **Board Cert:** Obstetrics & Gynecology 2006; Gynecologic Oncology 2006; **Med School:** Washington Univ, St Louis 1980; **Resid:** Obstetrics & Gynecology, Barnes Hosp-Wash Univ 1984; **Fellow:** Gynecologic Oncology, Duke Univ Med Ctr 1987; **Fac Appt:** Prof ObG, Washington Univ, St Louis

Potkul, Ronald MD [GO] - **Spec Exp:** Ovarian Cancer; Cervical Cancer; **Hospital:** Loyola Univ Med Ctr; **Address:** Loyola Univ Med Ctr, 2160 S 1st Ave Bldg 112 - rm 267, Maywood, IL 60153; **Phone:** 708-327-3500; **Board Cert:** Obstetrics & Gynecology 1997; Gynecologic Oncology 1997; **Med School:** Univ Chicago-Pritzker Sch Med 1981; **Resid:** Obstetrics & Gynecology, Univ Chicago Hosps 1985; **Fellow:** Gynecologic Oncology, Georgetown Univ 1988; **Fac Appt:** Prof ObG, Loyola Univ-Stritch Sch Med

Reynolds, R Kevin MD [GO] - **Hospital:** Univ Michigan Hlth Sys; **Address:** Women's Hosp, Div Gyn Onc, 1500 E Med Ctr Drive, rm L4510, Ann Arbor, MI 48109-0276; **Phone:** 734-764-9106; **Board Cert:** Obstetrics & Gynecology 1998; Gynecologic Oncology 1994; **Med School:** Univ New Mexico 1982; **Resid:** Obstetrics & Gynecology, Univ Vt Hosp 1986; **Fellow:** Gynecologic Oncology, Univ Mich Med Ctr 1991; **Fac Appt:** Asst Prof ObG, Univ Mich Med Sch

Rice, Laurel W MD [GO] - **Spec Exp:** Ovarian Cancer; Uterine Cancer; Cervical Cancer; **Hospital:** Univ WI Hosp & Clins; **Address:** 1 S Park St, Ste 555, Madison, WI 53715; **Phone:** 608-263-3194; **Board Cert:** Obstetrics & Gynecology 2006; Gynecologic Oncology 2006; **Med School:** Univ Colorado 1983; **Resid:** Obstetrics & Gynecology, Brigham-Womens Hosp 1987; **Fellow:** Obstetrics & Gynecology, Brigham-Womens Hosp 1989; **Fac Appt:** Assoc Prof ObG, Univ VA Sch Med

Rose, Peter G MD [GO] - **Spec Exp:** Cervical Cancer; Ovarian Cancer; **Hospital:** Cleveland Clin Fdn (page 56), MetroHealth Med Ctr; **Address:** Cleveland Clinic Fdn, 9500 Euclid Ave A-81, Cleveland, OH 44195; **Phone:** 216-444-1712; **Board Cert:** Obstetrics & Gynecology 2006; Gynecologic Oncology 2006; **Med School:** Boston Univ 1981; **Resid:** Surgery, Vanderbilt Med Ctr 1983; Obstetrics & Gynecology, Ohio State Univ Med Ctr 1986; **Fellow:** Gynecologic Oncology, Roswell Park Med Ctr 1988; **Fac Appt:** Prof ObG, Case West Res Univ

Rotmensch, Jacob MD [GO] - **Spec Exp:** Gynecologic Cancer; Ovarian Cancer; Cervical Cancer; **Hospital:** Rush Univ Med Ctr; **Address:** University Gynecologic Oncology Assocs, 1725 W Harrison St, Ste 842, Chicago, IL 60612; **Phone:** 312-942-6300; **Board Cert:** Obstetrics & Gynecology 2006; Gynecologic Oncology 2006; **Med School:** Meharry Med Coll 1977; **Resid:** Obstetrics & Gynecology, Johns Hopkins Hosp 1981; **Fellow:** Gynecologic Oncology, Johns Hopkins Hosp 1984; **Fac Appt:** Prof ObG, Rush Med Coll

Schink, Julian C MD [GO] - **Spec Exp:** Ovarian Cancer; **Hospital:** Northwestern Meml Hosp; **Address:** 675 N St Clair St, Fl 21 - Ste 100, Chicago, IL 60611; **Phone:** 312-695-0990; **Board Cert:** Obstetrics & Gynecology 2000; Gynecologic Oncology 2000; **Med School:** Univ Tex, San Antonio 1982; **Resid:** Obstetrics & Gynecology, Northwestern Univ Med Sch 1986; **Fellow:** Gynecologic Oncology, UCLA Med Ctr 1988; **Fac Appt:** Prof ObG, Northwestern Univ

Smith, Donna Marie MD [GO] - **Spec Exp:** Cervical Cancer; Ovarian Cancer; **Hospital:** Loyola Univ Med Ctr; **Address:** Cardinal Bernardin Cancer Ctr, Clinic A, 2160 S 1st Ave Bldg 112 - rm 267, Maywood, IL 60153; **Phone:** 708-327-3500; **Board Cert:** Obstetrics & Gynecology 1997; Gynecologic Oncology 1997; **Med School:** Univ MO-Kansas City 1980; **Resid:** Obstetrics & Gynecology, Emory Univ Hosp 1984; **Fellow:** Gynecologic Oncology, Georgetown Univ Med Ctr 1987; **Fac Appt:** Assoc Prof ObG, Loyola Univ-Stritch Sch Med

America's Top Doctors® 8th Edition

Stehman, Frederick B MD [GO] - **Spec Exp:** Clinical Trials; Gynecologic Cancer; **Hospital:** Indiana Univ Hosp, Wishard Hlth Srvs; **Address:** Indiana Univ Hosp, Dept ObGyn, 550 N University Blvd, rm 2440, Indianapolis, IN 46202; **Phone:** 317-274-8609; **Board Cert:** Obstetrics & Gynecology 2005; Gynecologic Oncology 2003; **Med School:** Univ Mich Med Sch 1972; **Resid:** Obstetrics & Gynecology, Univ Kansas Med Ctr 1975; Surgery, Univ Kansas Med Ctr 1977; **Fellow:** Gynecologic Oncology, UCLA Med Ctr 1979; **Fac Appt:** Prof ObG, Indiana Univ

Waggoner, Steven MD [GO] - **Spec Exp:** Ovarian Cancer; Cervical Cancer; Uterine Cancer; **Hospital:** Univ Hosps Case Med Ctr; **Address:** Dept Ob/Gyn, Div Gyn Oncology, 11100 Euclid Ave, MC 5034, Cleveland, OH 44106; **Phone:** 216-844-3954; **Board Cert:** Obstetrics & Gynecology 2006; Gynecologic Oncology 2006; **Med School:** Univ Wash 1984; **Resid:** Obstetrics & Gynecology, Univ Chicago Hosps 1988; **Fellow:** Gynecologic Oncology, Georgetown Univ 1991; **Fac Appt:** Prof ObG, Case West Res Univ

Great Plains and Mountains

Davidson, Susan MD [GO] - **Spec Exp:** Gynecologic Cancer; **Hospital:** Univ Colorado Hosp; **Address:** Univ Colorado Hosp, Dept OB/GYN, 12631 E 17th Ave B198-4 Bldg, Box 6511, Denver, CO 80262; **Phone:** 720-724-2040; **Board Cert:** Obstetrics & Gynecology 2005; Gynecologic Oncology 2005; **Med School:** Univ Tex, San Antonio 1984; **Resid:** Obstetrics & Gynecology, Univ Texas Med Ctr 1988; **Fellow:** Gynecologic Oncology, Meml Sloan Kettering Cancer Ctr 1990; **Fac Appt:** Assoc Prof ObG, Univ Colorado

Remmenga, Steven W MD [GO] - **Spec Exp:** Ovarian Cancer; Cervical Cancer; Gynecologic Cancer; **Hospital:** Nebraska Med Ctr; **Address:** Univ Nebraska Med Ctr, Gyne Oncology, 983255 Nebraska Med Ctr, Omaha, NE 68198-3255; **Phone:** 402-559-5068; **Board Cert:** Obstetrics & Gynecology 1998; Gynecologic Oncology 1998; **Med School:** Univ Nebr Coll Med 1981; **Resid:** Obstetrics & Gynecology, Naval Hospital 1986; **Fellow:** Gynecologic Oncology, Walter Reed Army Med Ctr 1990; **Fac Appt:** Assoc Prof ObG, Univ Nebr Coll Med

Soisson, Andrew MD [GO] - **Spec Exp:** Cervical Cancer; **Hospital:** LDS Hosp, Univ Utah Hosps and Clins; **Address:** Univ Hosp, Div Gyn Oncology, 30 N 1900 E, rm 2B200, Salt Lake City, UT 84132; **Phone:** 801-585-0100; **Board Cert:** Obstetrics & Gynecology 2006; Gynecologic Oncology 2006; **Med School:** Georgetown Univ 1981; **Resid:** Obstetrics & Gynecology, Madigan AMC 1985; **Fellow:** Gynecologic Oncology, Duke Univ Med Ctr 1990; **Fac Appt:** Assoc Prof ObG, Univ Utah

Southwest

Chambers, Setsuko K MD [GO] - **Spec Exp:** Gynecologic Cancer; Breast Cancer; Ovarian Cancer; **Hospital:** Univ Med Ctr - Tucson; **Address:** 1515 N Campbell Ave, Arizona Cancer Center, Tucson, AZ 85724; **Phone:** 520-626-9285; **Board Cert:** Obstetrics & Gynecology 2007; Gynecologic Oncology 2007; **Med School:** Brown Univ 1980; **Resid:** Obstetrics & Gynecology, Yale-New Haven Hosp 1984; **Fellow:** Gynecologic Oncology, Yale-New Haven Hosp 1986; **Fac Appt:** Prof ObG, Univ Ariz Coll Med

Follen, Michele MD/PhD [GO] - **Spec Exp:** Gynecologic Cancer; Clinical Trials; Cervical Cancer; **Hospital:** UT MD Anderson Cancer Ctr; **Address:** MD Anderson Cancer Ctr, 1515 Holcombe Blvd, Unit 1362, Houston, TX 77030; **Phone:** 713-745-2564; **Board Cert:** Obstetrics & Gynecology 1999; Gynecologic Oncology 1999; **Med School:** Univ Mich Med Sch 1980; **Resid:** Obstetrics & Gynecology, Columbia-Presby Med Ctr 1983; **Fellow:** Gynecologic Oncology, MD Anderson Cancer Ctr 1986; **Fac Appt:** Prof ObG, Univ Tex, Houston

Gynecologic Oncology

Gershenson, David M MD [GO] - **Spec Exp:** Ovarian Cancer & Borderline Tumors; Peritoneal Carcinomatosis; Fertility Preservation in Cancer; **Hospital:** UT MD Anderson Cancer Ctr, St Luke's Episcopal Hosp - Houston; **Address:** Univ Tex MD Anderson Cancer Ctr, PO Box 301439, Houston, TX 77030-1439; **Phone:** 713-745-2565; **Board Cert:** Obstetrics & Gynecology 1991; Gynecologic Oncology 1981; **Med School:** Vanderbilt Univ 1971; **Resid:** Obstetrics & Gynecology, Yale-New Haven Hosp 1975; **Fellow:** Gynecologic Oncology, MD Anderson Cancer Ctr 1979; **Fac Appt:** Prof ObG, Univ Tex, Houston

Hatch, Kenneth MD [GO] - **Spec Exp:** Cervical Cancer; Uro-Gynecology; Pelvic Organ Prolapse Repair; **Hospital:** Univ Med Ctr - Tucson, NW Med Ctr; **Address:** Univ Arizona College of Medicine, 1515 N Campbell Ave, rm 1968, Tucson, AZ 85724; **Phone:** 520-626-9285; **Board Cert:** Obstetrics & Gynecology 1993; Gynecologic Oncology 1981; **Med School:** Univ Nebr Coll Med 1971; **Resid:** Obstetrics & Gynecology, Univ AL Med Ctr Birmingham 1976; **Fellow:** Gynecologic Oncology, Univ AL Med Ctr Birmingham 1978; **Fac Appt:** Prof ObG, Univ Ariz Coll Med

Levenback, Charles MD [GO] - **Spec Exp:** Vulvar Disease/Cancer; Cervical Cancer; Gynecologic Cancer; **Hospital:** UT MD Anderson Cancer Ctr; **Address:** PO Box 301439 - Unit 1362, Houston, TX 77230; **Phone:** 713-745-2563; **Board Cert:** Obstetrics & Gynecology 2005; Gynecologic Oncology 2005; **Med School:** Mount Sinai Sch Med 1983; **Resid:** Obstetrics & Gynecology, Albert Einstein Coll Med 1987; **Fellow:** Gynecologic Oncology, Meml Sloan Kettering Cancer Ctr 1989; **Fac Appt:** Prof ObG, Univ Tex, Houston

Magrina, Javier MD [GO] - **Spec Exp:** Gynecologic Cancer; Endometriosis; Hysterectomy Alternatives; Robotic Surgery; **Hospital:** Mayo Clinic - Scottsdale; **Address:** Mayo Clinic, 5779 E Mayo Blvd, Phoenix, AZ 85054; **Phone:** 480-342-2668; **Board Cert:** Obstetrics & Gynecology 1994; Gynecologic Oncology 1982; **Med School:** Spain 1972; **Resid:** Obstetrics & Gynecology, Mayo Clinic 1977; **Fellow:** Gynecologic Oncology, Kansas Med Ctr 1980; **Fac Appt:** Prof ObG, Mayo Med Sch

Walker, Joan L MD [GO] - **Spec Exp:** Ovarian Cancer; Cervical Cancer; Uterine Cancer; **Hospital:** OU Med Ctr; **Address:** OU Health Science Ctr, Dept Ob/Gyn, PO Box 26901, Oklahoma City, OK 73126; **Phone:** 405-271-8707 x4108; **Board Cert:** Obstetrics & Gynecology 2006; Gynecologic Oncology 2006; **Med School:** UCLA 1982; **Resid:** Obstetrics & Gynecology, Hosp Univ Penn 1986; **Fellow:** Gynecologic Oncology, UC-Irvine Med Ctr 1990; **Fac Appt:** Assoc Prof ObG, Univ Okla Coll Med

West Coast and Pacific

Berek, Jonathan S MD [GO] - **Spec Exp:** Ovarian Cancer; Uterine Cancer; Cervical Cancer; **Hospital:** Stanford Univ Med Ctr; **Address:** Stanford Univ School of Medicine, 300 Pasteur Dr, HH333, Stanford, CA 94305-2296; **Phone:** 650-498-5618; **Board Cert:** Obstetrics & Gynecology 2005; Gynecologic Oncology 2005; **Med School:** Johns Hopkins Univ 1975; **Resid:** Obstetrics & Gynecology, Brigham & Womans Hosp 1979; **Fellow:** Gynecologic Oncology, UCLA Sch Med 1981; **Fac Appt:** Prof ObG, Stanford Univ

Berman, Michael L MD [GO] - **Spec Exp:** Gynecologic Cancer; Cervical Cancer; **Hospital:** UC Irvine Med Ctr, Long Beach Meml Med Ctr; **Address:** Cho Family Comprehensive Cancer Ctr, 101 The City Drive Bldg 56 - Ste 260, Orange, CA 92868-3201; **Phone:** 714-456-8020; **Board Cert:** Obstetrics & Gynecology 2005; Gynecologic Oncology 2005; **Med School:** Geo Wash Univ 1967; **Resid:** Obstetrics & Gynecology, GW Univ Hosp 1969; Obstetrics & Gynecology, Los Angeles Co-Harbor 1974; **Fellow:** Gynecologic Oncology, UCLA Med Ctr 1976; **Fac Appt:** Prof ObG, UC Irvine

Cain, Joanna M MD [GO] - **Spec Exp:** Ovarian Cancer; Breast Cancer Risk Assessment; Uterine Cancer; Ovarian Cancer-Early Detection; **Hospital:** OR Hlth & Sci Univ; **Address:** 3181 SW Sam Jackson Park Rd, MC L-466, Portland, OR 97239; **Phone:** 503-494-2999; **Board Cert:** Obstetrics & Gynecology 2006; Gynecologic Oncology 2006; **Med School:** Creighton Univ 1978; **Resid:** Obstetrics & Gynecology, Univ Washington Med Ctr 1981; **Fellow:** Gynecologic Oncology, Meml Sloan Kettering Cancer Ctr 1983; **Fac Appt:** Prof ObG, Oregon Hlth Sci Univ

Di Saia, Philip J MD [GO] - **Spec Exp:** Ovarian Cancer; Gynecologic Cancer; Cervical Cancer; **Hospital:** UC Irvine Med Ctr; **Address:** 101 City Drive Bldg 56 - rm 260, Orange, CA 92668; **Phone:** 714-456-8000; **Board Cert:** Obstetrics & Gynecology 1983; Gynecologic Oncology 1974; **Med School:** Tufts Univ 1963; **Resid:** Obstetrics & Gynecology, Yale-New Haven Hosp 1967; **Fellow:** Gynecologic Oncology, MD Anderson Hosp 1971; **Fac Appt:** Prof ObG, UC Irvine

Goff, Barbara A MD [GO] - **Spec Exp:** Ovarian Cancer; Uterine Cancer; Cervical Cancer; Gynecologic Surgery-Complex; **Hospital:** Univ Wash Med Ctr; **Address:** Univ Washington, Dept ObGyn, Box 356460, Seattle, WA 98195; **Phone:** 206-543-3669; **Board Cert:** Obstetrics & Gynecology 2006; Gynecologic Oncology 2006; **Med School:** Univ Pennsylvania 1986; **Resid:** Obstetrics & Gynecology, Mass Genl Hosp/Brigham & Womens Hosp 1990; **Fellow:** Gynecologic Oncology, Mass Genl Hosp 1993; **Fac Appt:** Prof ObG, Univ Wash

Greer, Benjamin E MD [GO] - **Spec Exp:** Gynecologic Cancer; **Hospital:** Univ Wash Med Ctr; **Address:** Univ Wash, Dept OB/GYN, Box 356460, Seattle, WA 98195; **Phone:** 206-543-3669; **Board Cert:** Obstetrics & Gynecology 2002; Gynecologic Oncology 2002; **Med School:** Univ Pennsylvania 1966; **Resid:** Obstetrics & Gynecology, Univ Colorado Med Ctr 1970; **Fac Appt:** Prof ObG, Univ Wash

Karlan, Beth Y MD [GO] - **Spec Exp:** Ovarian Cancer; Gynecologic Cancer; **Hospital:** Cedars-Sinai Med Ctr, Ronald Reagan UCLA Med Ctr; **Address:** 8700 Beverly Blvd, Ste 290W, Los Angeles, CA 90048; **Phone:** 310-423-3302; **Board Cert:** Obstetrics & Gynecology 1998; Gynecologic Oncology 1998; **Med School:** Harvard Med Sch 1982; **Resid:** Obstetrics & Gynecology, Yale-New Haven Hosp 1986; **Fellow:** Gynecologic Oncology, UCLA Med Sch 1989; **Fac Appt:** Prof ObG, UCLA

Monk, Bradley J MD [GO] - **Spec Exp:** Gynecologic Surgery-Complex; Cervical Cancer; Ovarian Cancer; Gynecologic Cancer; **Hospital:** UC Irvine Med Ctr; **Address:** UC Irvine Comprehensive Cancer Ctr, 101 The City Drive Bldg 56 - rm 260, Irvine, CA 92868; **Phone:** 714-456-6570; **Board Cert:** Obstetrics & Gynecology 2006; Gynecologic Oncology 2006; **Med School:** Univ Ariz Coll Med 1988; **Resid:** Obstetrics & Gynecology, UCLA Med Ctr 1992; **Fellow:** Gynecologic Oncology, UC Irvine Med Ctr 1995; **Fac Appt:** Assoc Prof ObG, UC Irvine

Muntz, Howard G MD [GO] - **Spec Exp:** Gynecologic Cancer; Ovarian Cancer; Clinical Trials; Gynecologic Surgery-Complex; **Hospital:** Northwest Hosp; **Address:** Women's Cancer Care of Seattle, 1560 N 115th St, Ste 101, Seattle, WA 98133; **Phone:** 206-368-6806; **Board Cert:** Obstetrics & Gynecology 2007; Gynecologic Oncology 2007; **Med School:** Harvard Med Sch 1984; **Resid:** Obstetrics & Gynecology, Brigham & Women's Hosp 1988; **Fellow:** Gynecologic Oncology, Mass General Hosp 1991; **Fac Appt:** Assoc Clin Prof ObG, Univ Wash

Powell, Catherine Bethan MD [GO] - **Spec Exp:** Gynecologic Cancer; Cancer Genetics; Complementary Medicine; **Hospital:** UCSF - Mt Zion Med Ctr; **Address:** UCSF Comp Cancer Ctr, 1600 Divisadero St Fl 4, San Francisco, CA 94115; **Phone:** 415-353-9838; **Board Cert:** Obstetrics & Gynecology 2005; Gynecologic Oncology 2005; **Med School:** Univ Pennsylvania 1982; **Resid:** Obstetrics & Gynecology, Pennsylvania Hosp 1987; **Fellow:** Gynecologic Oncology, Wash Univ 1990; **Fac Appt:** Asst Clin Prof ObG, UCSF

Gynecologic Oncology

Smith, Lloyd H MD [GO] - **Spec Exp:** Ovarian Cancer; Uterine Cancer; Vulvar Disease/Cancer; Vaginal Cancer; **Hospital:** UC Davis Med Ctr, Sutter Mem Hospital - Sacramento; **Address:** UC Davis Med Ctr, Dept Ob/Gyn, 4860 Y St, Ste 2500, Sacramento, CA 95817-2307; **Phone:** 916-734-6946; **Board Cert:** Obstetrics & Gynecology 1998; Gynecologic Oncology 1998; **Med School:** UC Davis 1981; **Resid:** Obstetrics & Gynecology, UC Davis Med Ctr 1985; **Fellow:** Gynecologic Oncology, Stanford Univ Hosp 1988; **Fac Appt:** Prof ObG, UC Davis

Spirtos, Nicola Michael MD [GO] - **Spec Exp:** Gynecologic Cancer; Ovarian Cancer; **Hospital:** Univ Med Ctr - Las Vegas; **Address:** 3131 La Canada St, Ste 110, Las Vegas, NV 89169; **Phone:** 702-693-6870; **Board Cert:** Obstetrics & Gynecology 1998; Gynecologic Oncology 1998; **Med School:** Northwestern Univ 1980; **Resid:** Obstetrics & Gynecology, Women's Hosp LAC-USC Med Ctr 1984; **Fellow:** Gynecologic Oncology, Stanford Univ 1987

Stern, Jeffrey L MD [GO] - **Spec Exp:** Laparoscopic Surgery; Vulvar Disease/Cancer; **Hospital:** Alta Bates Summit Med Ctr; **Address:** Womens Cancer Ctr Northern Calif, 2001 Dwight Way, Berkley, CA 94704; **Phone:** 510-204-5770; **Board Cert:** Obstetrics & Gynecology 1983; Gynecologic Oncology 1984; **Med School:** SUNY Upstate Med Univ 1976; **Resid:** Obstetrics & Gynecology, Johns Hopkins Hosp 1980; **Fellow:** Gynecologic Oncology, USC Med Ctr 1982

Teng, Nelson NH MD/PhD [GO] - **Spec Exp:** Ovarian Cancer; Clinical Trials; **Hospital:** Stanford Univ Med Ctr; **Address:** Stanford Univ Sch Med, Dept Gyn Oncology, 300 Pasteur Drive, Ste HH333, Stanford, CA 94305-5317; **Phone:** 650-498-8080; **Board Cert:** Obstetrics & Gynecology 1985; Gynecologic Oncology 1987; **Med School:** Univ Miami Sch Med 1977; **Resid:** Obstetrics & Gynecology, UCLA Med Ctr 1981; **Fellow:** Gynecologic Oncology, Stanford Univ Sch Med 1984; **Fac Appt:** Assoc Prof ObG, Stanford Univ

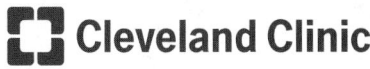 **Cleveland Clinic**

Obstetrics and Gynecology

Reproductive Endocrinology and Infertility: Our Reproductive Endocrinology and Infertility Program involves close collaboration among male and female infertility specialists, andrologists and embryologists, as well as our colleagues in the Minimally Invasive Surgery Center. Cleveland Clinic reproductive surgeons were among the first to routinely remove advanced endometriosis laparoscopically. Many procedures today are performed with robotic assistance.

Urogynecology and Reconstructive Pelvic Surgery: This Center offers cutting-edge and traditional surgery for urinary incontinence and pelvic organ prolapse, along with medical and behavioral therapy.

Center for Female Pelvic Medicine and Reconstructive Surgery: Cleveland Clinic urogynecologists established the Center for Female Pelvic Medicine and Reconstructive Surgery in conjunction with Cleveland Clinic urologists and colorectal surgeons. The sub specialists on this team treat incontinence and prolapse via the abdominal, vaginal and laparoscopic routes.

Maternal-Fetal Medicine/Obstetrics: Cleveland Clinic maternal-fetal medicine specialists provide overall management of complicated pregnancies, beginning with genetic counseling for high-risk patients. Our dedicated Maternal-Fetal Testing Center offers high-risk consults, detailed ultrasound with Doppler wave form analysis, first-trimester nuchal translucency ultrasound screening and other sophisticated diagnostic testing.

The Fetal Care Center: The Fetal Care Center involves a multidisciplinary team of perinatologists, neonatologists, pediatric surgeons and other specialists. Through collaboration and communication, we provide prenatal diagnosis using state-of-the-art techniques such as high-resolution ultrasound, fetal MRI and fetoscopy. We then apply this information as we develop a management plan for pregnancy, delivery and newborn care.

Menstrual Disorders, Fibroids and Hysteroscopic Services: This Center offers unified and streamlined consultations, workups and treatment for menstrual dysfunction and uterine fibroids in the least invasive manner, so as to preserve a woman's reproductive potential.

Gynecologic Oncology: Our gynecologic oncologists have garnered national and international recognition for expertise in complex reproductive cancers, clinical and basic research, and preventive oncology. Cleveland Clinic gynecologists were among the first to treat early cervical and endometrial cancers laparoscopically. In performing less invasive surgical procedures, we always weigh curative potential against preservation of fertility. We offer oocyte, embryo and ovarian tissue cryopreservation for cancer patients.

Women's Health Center: The Cleveland Clinic Women's Health Center offers a full range of specialized women's health services in one location. We manage menopause, hormone therapy, vulvar disorders, and premenstrual dysthymic disorder and hormonally exacerbated mood disorders. We offer evaluation and treatment for women with urinary incontinence, osteoporosis or breast concerns. Breast specialists evaluate and treat breast cancer as well as benign breast disease in our center.

For more information about the Cleveland Clinic Department of Obstetrics and Gynecology, to schedule a second opinion or to learn about assistance for out-of-town patients, call 800.890.2467 or visit www.clevelandclinic.org/obgyntopdocs.

Department of Obstetrics and Gynecology
9500 Euclid Avenue / AC311 | Cleveland OH 44195

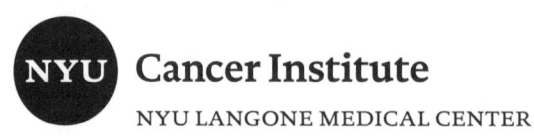

Cancer Institute
NYU LANGONE MEDICAL CENTER

A Collaborative Approach

The NYU Cancer Institute, an NCI designated center, is a "matrix cancer center" without walls operating within the larger NYU Langone Medical Center. With over 175 members and a research funding base of over $81 million, this structure strengthens our capabilities to forge collaborations across medical and scientific disciplines, which translates to comprehensive care for our patients and discoveries that will influence the future of this disease.

Renowned Expertise

Team members' compassion and expertise help patients better manage the symptoms of their disease as well as their special needs. Our highly skilled Magnet™ nursing team not only plays a pivotal role in coordinating direct patient care, but is also a source of invaluable patient education.

A Patient-Focused Setting

The NYU Clinical Cancer Center, with over 70 faculty members from various disciplines at the New York University School of Medicine, is the principal outpatient facility of the Cancer Institute and serves as home for our patients and their caregivers. The center and its multidisciplinary team of experts provide access to the latest treatment options and clinical trials along with a variety of programs in cancer prevention, screening, diagnostics, genetic counseling, and supportive services. When it comes to kids and cancer, the Stephen D. Hassenfeld Children's Center for Cancer and Blood Disorders offers not just innovation but insight. As a leading member of the NCI-sponsored Children's Oncology Group, our physicians are known for developing new ways to treat childhood cancer. Our affiliation with Bellevue Hospital, the oldest public hospital in the country, affords clinically distinctive opportunities to learn and care for patients with cancer by observing its presentation and behavior in a variety of patient groups.

Hand Surgery

a subspecialty of Orthopaedics, Surgery or Plastic Surgery

A specialist trained in the investigation, preservation and restoration by medical, surgical and rehabilitative means of all structures of the upper extremity directly affecting the form and function of the hand and wrist.

For more information about the mentioned specialties or those physicians, see **Orthopaedic Surgery, Surgery** or **Plastic Surgery** section(s).

Training Required: Five years (including general surgery) in orthopaedics *plus* two years in clinical practice before final certification is achieved *plus* additional training and examination in hand surgery OR five to seven years in plastic surgery *plus* additional training and examination in hand surgery.

HAND SURGERY

New England

Akelman, Edward MD [HS] - **Spec Exp:** Carpal Tunnel Syndrome; Arthritis; Wrist/Hand Injuries; **Hospital:** Rhode Island Hosp; **Address:** 2 Dudley St, Ste 200, Providence, RI 02905; **Phone:** 401-457-1510; **Board Cert:** Orthopaedic Surgery 2008; Hand Surgery 2008; **Med School:** Dartmouth Med Sch 1978; **Resid:** Surgery, Peter Bent Brigham Hosp 1980; Orthopaedic Surgery, Yale-New Haven Hosp 1984; **Fellow:** Hand Surgery, Roosevelt Hosp 1985; **Fac Appt:** Prof OrS, Brown Univ

Belsky, Mark R MD [HS] - **Spec Exp:** Arthritis; Nerve Disorders/Surgery; Elbow Surgery; **Hospital:** Newton - Wellesley Hosp; **Address:** 2000 Washington St, Green - Ste 563, Newton, MA 02462-1629; **Phone:** 617-965-4263; **Board Cert:** Orthopaedic Surgery 1982; Hand Surgery 2001; **Med School:** Tufts Univ 1974; **Resid:** Surgery, Peter Bent Brigham Hosp 1976; Orthopaedic Surgery, Tufts-New England Med Ctr 1979; **Fellow:** Hand Surgery, Roosevelt Hosp 1980; **Fac Appt:** Clin Prof OrS, Tufts Univ

Sampson, Christian E MD [HS] - **Spec Exp:** Hand Injuries; Hand & Fingers Vascular Surgery; **Hospital:** Brigham & Women's Hosp; **Address:** Brigham & Women's Hosp, Div Plastic Surg, 75 Francis St, Boston, MA 02115; **Phone:** 617-732-6297; **Board Cert:** Plastic Surgery 2004; Hand Surgery 2003; **Med School:** Boston Univ 1986; **Resid:** Surgery, Boston Univ Med Ctr 1991; Plastic Surgery, Brigham & Women's Hosp 1993; **Fellow:** Hand Surgery, Roosevelt Hosp 1994

Waters, Peter Michael MD [HS] - **Spec Exp:** Brachial Plexus Palsy; Hand-Congenital Anomaly; **Hospital:** Children's Hospital - Boston; **Address:** Chldns Hosp, Dept Ortho Surg, 300 Longwood Ave, Hunnewell - 2, Boston, MA 02115-5724; **Phone:** 617-355-6021; **Board Cert:** Orthopaedic Surgery 2001; Hand Surgery 2004; **Med School:** Tufts Univ 1981; **Resid:** Pediatrics, Mass Genl Hosp 1983; Orthopaedic Surgery, Harvard Combined Prog 1988; **Fellow:** Hand Surgery, Brigham/Chldns Hosp 1989; **Fac Appt:** Assoc Prof OrS, Harvard Med Sch

Weiss, Arnold P MD [HS] - **Spec Exp:** Carpal Tunnel Syndrome; Wrist Surgery; Elbow Replacement; **Hospital:** Rhode Island Hosp; **Address:** Univ Orthopedics, 2 Dudley St, Ste 200, Providence, RI 02905-3248; **Phone:** 401-457-1520; **Board Cert:** Orthopaedic Surgery 2004; Hand Surgery 2004; **Med School:** Johns Hopkins Univ 1985; **Resid:** Orthopaedic Surgery, Johns Hopkins Hosp 1990; **Fellow:** Hand Surgery, Indiana Hand Ctr 1991; **Fac Appt:** Prof OrS, Brown Univ

Mid Atlantic

Athanasian, Edward MD [HS] - **Spec Exp:** Bone & Soft Tissue Tumors; Hand & Upper Extremity Tumors; Hand & Upper Extremity Surgery; **Hospital:** Hosp For Special Surgery (page 59), Meml Sloan-Kettering Cancer Ctr; **Address:** Hospital for Special Surgery, 535 E 70th St, New York, NY 10021; **Phone:** 212-606-1962; **Board Cert:** Orthopaedic Surgery 1997; Hand Surgery 1999; **Med School:** Columbia P&S 1988; **Resid:** Surgery, Beth Israel Hosp 1989; Orthopaedic Surgery, Hosp Special Surgery 1993; **Fellow:** Hand Surgery, Mayo Clinic 1994; Orthopaedic Oncology, Meml Sloan Kettering Cancer Ctr 1995; **Fac Appt:** Asst Prof OrS, Cornell Univ-Weill Med Coll

Baratz, Mark E MD [HS] - **Spec Exp:** Hand Surgery; Upper Extremity Surgery; Elbow Reconstruction; **Hospital:** Allegheny General Hosp; **Address:** 1307 Federal St Fl 2, Pittsburgh, PA 15212; **Phone:** 412-359-4263; **Board Cert:** Orthopaedic Surgery 2004; Hand Surgery 2004; **Med School:** Univ Pittsburgh 1984; **Resid:** Orthopaedic Surgery, Univ Hlth Ctr 1990; **Fellow:** Orthopaedic Surgery, Univ Hlth Ctr 1987; Hand Surgery, Med Coll Penn 1991; **Fac Appt:** Prof OrS, Drexel Univ Coll Med

Culp, Randall MD [HS] - **Spec Exp:** Microsurgery; Hand & Upper Extremity Surgery; Elbow Surgery; **Hospital:** Thomas Jefferson Univ Hosp; **Address:** 700 S Henderson Rd, Ste 200, King of Prussia, PA 19406; **Phone:** 610-768-4474; **Board Cert:** Orthopaedic Surgery 2001; Hand Surgery 2001; **Med School:** Penn State Univ-Hershey Med Ctr 1982; **Resid:** Orthopaedic Surgery, Hosp Univ Penn 1987; **Fellow:** Hand Surgery, Hosp Univ Penn 1988; **Fac Appt:** Assoc Prof OrS, Jefferson Med Coll

Glickel, Steven MD [HS] - **Spec Exp:** Hand & Wrist Surgery; Elbow Surgery; Peripheral Nerve Surgery; **Hospital:** St Luke's - Roosevelt Hosp Ctr - Roosevelt Div (page 57); **Address:** 1000 10th Ave Fl 3, New York, NY 10019-1147; **Phone:** 212-523-7590; **Board Cert:** Orthopaedic Surgery 1985; Hand Surgery 2000; **Med School:** Harvard Med Sch 1976; **Resid:** Surgery, Columbia Presby Hosp 1978; Orthopaedic Surgery, Harvard Comb Ortho 1981; **Fellow:** Hand Surgery, St Luke's-Roosevelt Hosp Ctr 1983; Research, Columbia Presby Hosp 1982; **Fac Appt:** Assoc Clin Prof OrS, Columbia P&S

Graham, Thomas J MD [HS] - **Spec Exp:** Hand & Wrist Surgery; Elbow Surgery; Sports Injuries; Wrist/Hand Injuries; **Hospital:** Union Meml Hosp - Baltimore; **Address:** Curtis National Hand Ctr, 3333 N Calvert St Fl 2, Baltimore, MD 21218; **Phone:** 410-235-3869; **Board Cert:** Orthopaedic Surgery 2007; Hand Surgery 2007; **Med School:** Univ Cincinnati 1988; **Resid:** Orthopaedic Surgery, Univ Michigan Med Ctr 1993; **Fellow:** Hand Surgery, Indiana Hand Ctr 1994; Elbow Surgery, Mayo Clinic 1994; **Fac Appt:** Assoc Clin Prof OrS, Johns Hopkins Univ

Imbriglia, Joseph E MD [HS] - **Spec Exp:** Arthritis; Carpal Tunnel Syndrome; Shoulder Surgery; Rotator Cuff Surgery; **Hospital:** UPMC Passavant-Cranberry, UPMC Passavant; **Address:** 6001 Stonewood Drive, Wexford, PA 15090-7380; **Phone:** 724-933-3850; **Board Cert:** Orthopaedic Surgery 1977; Hand Surgery 2000; **Med School:** Hahnemann Univ 1970; **Resid:** Surgery, Univ Pittsburgh Med Ctr 1972; Orthopaedic Surgery, Columbia Presby Med Ctr 1975; **Fellow:** Hand Surgery, Columbia Presby Med Ctr 1976; **Fac Appt:** Clin Prof OrS, Univ Pittsburgh

Kozin, Scott H MD [HS] - **Spec Exp:** Congenital Hand Deformities; Brachial Plexus Palsy-Pediatric; Spinal Cord Injury-Pediatric; **Hospital:** Philadelphia Shriners Hosp; **Address:** Shriners Hosp for Children, 3551 N Broad St, Philadelphia, PA 19140; **Phone:** 215-430-4074; **Board Cert:** Orthopaedic Surgery 2005; Hand Surgery 2005; **Med School:** Hahnemann Univ 1986; **Resid:** Orthopaedic Surgery, Albert Einstein Med Ctr 1991; **Fellow:** Hand Surgery, Mayo Clinic 1992; **Fac Appt:** Assoc Prof OrS, Temple Univ

Kulick, Roy G MD [HS] - **Spec Exp:** Carpal Tunnel Syndrome; Arthritis; Tendon Surgery; **Hospital:** Montefiore Med Ctr - Weiler-Einstein Div, Westchester Med Ctr; **Address:** The Tower at Montefiore Medical Park, 1695 Eastchester Rd Fl 2, Bronx, NY 10461; **Phone:** 718-920-2060; **Board Cert:** Orthopaedic Surgery 1980; Hand Surgery 2001; **Med School:** Cornell Univ-Weill Med Coll 1973; **Resid:** Surgery, St Lukes-Roosevelt Hosp 1975; Orthopaedic Surgery, Columbia Presbyterian Hosp 1978; **Fellow:** Hand Surgery, Hosp for Special Surgery 1979; **Fac Appt:** Assoc Prof OrS, Albert Einstein Coll Med

Hand Surgery

Lane, Lewis B MD [HS] - **Spec Exp:** Carpal Tunnel Syndrome; Arthritis; Sports Injuries; Hand Reconstruction; **Hospital:** N Shore Univ Hosp, St Francis Hosp - The Heart Ctr (page 72); **Address:** 600 Northern Blvd, Ste 300, Great Neck, NY 11021; **Phone:** 516-627-8717; **Board Cert:** Orthopaedic Surgery 1981; Hand Surgery 2000; **Med School:** Columbia P&S 1974; **Resid:** Surgery, NY Hosp 1975; Orthopaedic Surgery, Hosp for Special Surg 1979; **Fellow:** Research, Hosp for Special Surg 1976; Hand Surgery, St Luke's-Roosevelt Hosp Ctr 1980; **Fac Appt:** Assoc Clin Prof OrS, Albert Einstein Coll Med

Lee, W P Andrew MD [HS] - **Spec Exp:** Reconstructive Surgery; Cartilage Damage; Transplant-Hand; Pediatric Hand Surgery; **Hospital:** UPMC Presby, Pittsburgh, Chldns Hosp of Pittsburgh - UPMC; **Address:** Univ Pittsburgh, Scaife Hall 6B, 3550 Terrace St, Pittsburgh, PA 15261; **Phone:** 412-648-9670; **Board Cert:** Hand Surgery 2005; Plastic Surgery 2005; **Med School:** Johns Hopkins Univ 1983; **Resid:** Surgery, Johns Hopkins Univ Hosp 1989; Plastic Surgery, Mass General Hosp 1991; **Fellow:** Microsurgery, Johns Hopkins Hosp 1987; Hand Surgery, Indiana Hand Ctr 1993; **Fac Appt:** Prof S, Univ Pittsburgh

Lubahn, John D MD [HS] - **Spec Exp:** Microsurgery; **Hospital:** Hamot Med Ctr, St Vincent Hlth Ctr; **Address:** 300 State St, Ste 205, Erie, PA 16507; **Phone:** 814-456-6022; **Board Cert:** Orthopaedic Surgery 2008; Hand Surgery 1998; **Med School:** Case West Res Univ 1975; **Resid:** Surgery, Univ Rochester Med Ctr 1977; Orthopaedic Surgery, Univ Rochester Med Ctr 1980; **Fellow:** Hand Surgery, Univ Louisville Hosp 1981

Melone Jr, Charles P MD [HS] - **Spec Exp:** Arthritis; Wrist Surgery; Fractures; **Hospital:** Beth Israel Med Ctr - Petrie Division (page 57); **Address:** 321 E 34th St, New York, NY 10016; **Phone:** 212-340-0000; **Board Cert:** Orthopaedic Surgery 1976; Hand Surgery 2004; **Med School:** Georgetown Univ 1969; **Resid:** Surgery, Nassau Co Med Ctr 1971; Orthopaedic Surgery, Nassau Co Med Ctr 1974; **Fellow:** Hand Surgery, NYU Med Ctr 1975; **Fac Appt:** Clin Prof OrS, Albert Einstein Coll Med

Osterman Jr, A Lee MD [HS] - **Spec Exp:** Upper Extremity Surgery; Wrist Surgery; Neuromuscular Disorders; **Hospital:** Thomas Jefferson Univ Hosp, Chldns Hosp of Philadelphia, The; **Address:** Philadelphia Hand Ctr, 700 S Henderson Rd, Ste 200, King of Prussia, PA 19406-4207; **Phone:** 610-265-3135; **Board Cert:** Orthopaedic Surgery 1980; Hand Surgery 2001; **Med School:** Univ Pennsylvania 1973; **Resid:** Orthopaedic Surgery, Hosp Univ Penn 1978; **Fellow:** Hand Surgery, Hosp Univ Penn 1979; Microvascular Surgery, Duke Univ Med Ctr 1980; **Fac Appt:** Prof OrS, Jefferson Med Coll

Patel, Mukund MD [HS] - **Spec Exp:** Arthritis; Carpal Tunnel Syndrome; Fractures; **Hospital:** Long Island Coll Hosp (page 57), Richmond Univ Med Ctr; **Address:** Comprehensive Hand Surgery, 4901 Fort Hamilton Pkwy, Brooklyn, NY 11219; **Phone:** 718-435-4944; **Board Cert:** Orthopaedic Surgery 1972; Hand Surgery 2000; **Med School:** India 1967; **Resid:** Orthopaedic Surgery, Maimonides Med Ctr 1970; **Fellow:** Hand Surgery, Mass Genl Hosp 1971; **Fac Appt:** Assoc Clin Prof S, SUNY Hlth Sci Ctr

Raskin, Keith MD [HS] - **Spec Exp:** Wrist/Hand Injuries; Arthritis; Carpal Tunnel Syndrome; **Hospital:** NYU Med Ctr (page 68), Hosp For Joint Diseases (page 70); **Address:** 317 E 34th St, Fl 3, New York, NY 10016; **Phone:** 212-263-4263; **Board Cert:** Orthopaedic Surgery 2002; Hand Surgery 2002; **Med School:** Geo Wash Univ 1983; **Resid:** Orthopaedic Surgery, NYU Med Ctr 1988; **Fellow:** Hand Surgery, Union Mem Hosp 1989; **Fac Appt:** Assoc Clin Prof OrS, NYU Sch Med

       America's Top Doctors® 8th Edition

Rosenwasser, Melvin MD [HS] - **Spec Exp:** Carpal Tunnel Syndrome; Sports Injuries; Elbow Surgery; Trauma; **Hospital:** NY-Presby Hosp/Columbia (page 66); **Address:** 622 W 168th St, PH 11, rm 1119, New York, NY 10032; **Phone:** 212-305-4565; **Board Cert:** Orthopaedic Surgery 1999; Hand Surgery 1999; **Med School:** Columbia P&S 1976; **Resid:** Surgery, Roosevelt Hosp 1979; Orthopaedic Surgery, Columbia Presby Hosp 1982; **Fellow:** Hand Surgery, Columbia Presby Hosp 1983; **Fac Appt:** Prof OrS, Columbia P&S

Strauch, Robert MD [HS] - **Spec Exp:** Hand Reconstruction; Hand & Elbow Nerve Disorders; Hand & Wrist Surgery; Elbow Surgery; **Hospital:** NY-Presby Hosp/Columbia (page 66); **Address:** 622 W 168th St, rm PH-11, New York, NY 10032; **Phone:** 212-305-4272; **Board Cert:** Orthopaedic Surgery 2005; Hand Surgery 2005; **Med School:** Columbia P&S 1986; **Resid:** Orthopaedic Surgery, Columbia-Presby Hosp 1991; **Fellow:** Hand Surgery, Indiana Hand Center 1992; **Fac Appt:** Assoc Prof OrS, Columbia P&S

Weiland, Andrew J MD [HS] - **Spec Exp:** Wrist/Hand Injuries; Hand Reconstruction; **Hospital:** Hosp For Special Surgery (page 59), NY-Presby Hosp/Weill Cornell (page 66); **Address:** Hospital for Special Surgery, 535 E 70th St, New York, NY 10021-4872; **Phone:** 212-606-1575; **Board Cert:** Orthopaedic Surgery 1977; **Med School:** Wake Forest Univ 1968; **Resid:** Surgery, Univ Michigan Med Ctr 1970; Orthopaedic Surgery, Johns Hopkins Hosp 1975; **Fellow:** Hand Surgery, Kleinert Hosp 1975; **Fac Appt:** Prof OrS, Cornell Univ-Weill Med Coll

Wolfe, Scott W MD [HS] - **Spec Exp:** Wrist Surgery; Nerve Disorders/Surgery; Fractures; **Hospital:** Hosp For Special Surgery (page 59), St Vincent's Med Ctr - Bridgeport; **Address:** Hospital for Special Surgery, 535 E 70 St, New York, NY 10021; **Phone:** 212-606-1529; **Board Cert:** Orthopaedic Surgery 2003; Hand Surgery 2003; **Med School:** Cornell Univ-Weill Med Coll 1984; **Resid:** Orthopaedic Surgery, Hosp Special Surg 1989; **Fellow:** Hand & Microvascular Surgery, Columbia Presby Med Ctr 1990; **Fac Appt:** Prof OrS, Cornell Univ-Weill Med Coll

Southeast

Breidenbach, Warren C MD [HS] - **Spec Exp:** Transplant-Hand; **Hospital:** Jewish Hosp HlthCre Svcs Inc; **Address:** 225 Abraham Flexner Way, Ste 700, Louisville, KY 40202; **Phone:** 502-561-4263; **Board Cert:** Plastic Surgery 1988; Hand Surgery 1992; **Med School:** Univ Calgary 1975; **Resid:** Plastic Surgery, McGill Univ 1982; **Fellow:** Microsurgery, Eastern Va Med Sch 1982; Hand Surgery, Univ Med Ctr 1983; **Fac Appt:** Asst Clin Prof PlS, Univ Louisville Sch Med

Carneiro, Ronaldo D S MD [HS] - **Spec Exp:** Carpal Tunnel Syndrome; Wrist Surgery; Arthritis; **Hospital:** Physicians Regl Med Ctr; **Address:** 6101 Pine Ridge Rd, Naples, FL 34119-3900; **Phone:** 239-348-4040; **Board Cert:** Plastic Surgery 1990; Hand Surgery 1994; **Med School:** Brazil 1970; **Resid:** Surgery, Union Meml Hosp 1975; Plastic Surgery, Allentown & Sacred Heart Hosp Ctr 1977; **Fellow:** Hand Surgery, Jackson Meml Hosp-Univ Miami Hosp 1977; Plastic Surgery, Univ Miami Sch Med 1978; **Fac Appt:** Assoc Clin Prof PlS, Univ S Fla Coll Med

Greene, Thomas L MD [HS] - **Spec Exp:** Arthritis; Peripheral Nerve Surgery; Arthroscopic Surgery; Tendon Surgery; **Hospital:** Tampa Genl Hosp, St Joseph's Hosp - Tampa; **Address:** 2727 W Dr Martin Luther King Jr Blvd, Ste 560, Tampa, FL 33607-6009; **Phone:** 813-873-0337; **Board Cert:** Orthopaedic Surgery 1983; Hand Surgery 2000; **Med School:** Ohio State Univ 1975; **Resid:** Surgery, Univ Michigan Med Ctr 1977; Orthopaedic Surgery, Univ Michigan Med Ctr 1980; **Fellow:** Hand Surgery, St Vincent's Hosp 1981

Hand Surgery

Hunt III, Thomas R MD [HS] - **Spec Exp:** Hand & Wrist Surgery; Arthritis; Trauma; Hand Reconstruction; **Hospital:** Univ of Ala Hosp at Birmingham; **Address:** UAB, Div Orthopaedic Surgery, 1313 13th St S, Ste 201, Birmingham, AL 35205-5327; **Phone:** 205-934-9999; **Board Cert:** Orthopaedic Surgery 2006; Hand Surgery 2006; **Med School:** Vanderbilt Univ 1986; **Resid:** Orthopaedic Surgery, Univ Kansas Med Ctr 1992; **Fellow:** Hand Surgery, Hosp Univ Penn 1993; **Fac Appt:** Prof S, Univ Ala

Koman, L Andrew MD [HS] - **Spec Exp:** Pediatric Hand Surgery; Vascular Disorders-Upper Extremity; Pain-Nerve Injury; **Hospital:** Wake Forest Univ Baptist Med Ctr (page 73); **Address:** WFU Hlth Sci, Medical Center Blvd, Dept Orthopaedic Surgery, Winston-Salem, NC 27157-1070; **Phone:** 336-716-8094; **Board Cert:** Orthopaedic Surgery 1981; Hand Surgery 2000; **Med School:** Duke Univ 1974; **Resid:** Surgery, Duke Univ Med Ctr. 1975; Orthopaedic Surgery, Duke Univ Med Ctr. 1979; **Fellow:** Hand Surgery, Duke Univ Med Ctr 1980; **Fac Appt:** Prof OrS, Wake Forest Univ

Midwest

Bishop, Allen T MD [HS] - **Spec Exp:** Microsurgery; Brachial Plexus Palsy; **Hospital:** Mayo Med Ctr & Clin - Rochester; **Address:** Mayo Clinic, Div Hand Surgery, 200 First St SW, Rochester, MN 55905; **Phone:** 507-284-4149; **Board Cert:** Orthopaedic Surgery 2000; Hand Surgery 2000; **Med School:** Mayo Med Sch 1981; **Resid:** Orthopaedic Surgery, Mayo Clinic 1986; **Fellow:** Hand Surgery, St Vincent Hosp 1987; **Fac Appt:** Prof OrS, Mayo Med Sch

Carroll, Charles MD [HS] - **Spec Exp:** Carpal Tunnel Syndrome; Dupuytren's Contracture; Elbow Surgery; Shoulder Surgery; **Hospital:** Northwestern Meml Hosp, NorthShore Univ HlthSys; **Address:** Northwest Orthopaedic Inst, 680 N Lakeshore Drive, Ste 924, Chicago, IL 60611; **Phone:** 312-664-6848; **Board Cert:** Orthopaedic Surgery 2001; Hand Surgery 2001; **Med School:** Univ MD Sch Med 1982; **Resid:** Surgery, Johns Hopkins Hosp 1984; Orthopaedic Surgery, Johns Hopkins Hosp 1987; **Fellow:** Hand Surgery, Indiana Univ Med Ctr 1988; Shoulder Surgery, Univ Western Ontario 1988; **Fac Appt:** Assoc Clin Prof OrS, Northwestern Univ

Chung, Kevin Chi MD [HS] - **Spec Exp:** Reconstructive Surgery; Hand & Microvascular Surgery; Upper Extremity Trauma; Nail Surgery; **Hospital:** Univ Michigan Hlth Sys; **Address:** University of Michigan, 2130 Taubman Health Ctr, 1500 E Medical Ctr Drive, Box 0340, Ann Arbor, MI 48109; **Phone:** 734-936-5885; **Board Cert:** Hand Surgery 2007; Plastic Surgery 2007; **Med School:** Emory Univ 1987; **Resid:** Plastic Surgery, Univ Michigan Hosp & Hlth Ctr 1994; Hand Surgery, Union Meml Hosp 1995; **Fac Appt:** Assoc Prof S, Univ Mich Med Sch

Cohen, Mark S MD [HS] - **Spec Exp:** Hand Surgery; Wrist Surgery; Elbow Surgery; **Hospital:** Rush Univ Med Ctr; **Address:** Midwest Orthopedics at Rush, 1725 W Harrison St, Ste 1042, Chicago, IL 60612-3841; **Phone:** 312-243-4244; **Board Cert:** Orthopaedic Surgery 2006; Hand Surgery 2006; **Med School:** Harvard Med Sch 1986; **Resid:** Orthopaedic Surgery, UCSD Med Ctr 1992; **Fellow:** Hand Surgery, Indiana Hand Ctr 1993; **Fac Appt:** Prof OrS, Rush Med Coll

Derman, Gordon Harris MD [HS] - **Spec Exp:** Carpal Tunnel Syndrome; Tendon Surgery; Repetitive Motion Injuries; Nerve Disorders/Surgery; **Hospital:** Rush Univ Med Ctr, NorthShore Univ HlthSys; **Address:** 1725 W Harrison St, Ste 740, Chicago, IL 60612; **Phone:** 312-432-9200; **Board Cert:** Plastic Surgery 1984; Hand Surgery 1996; **Med School:** Rush Med Coll 1975; **Resid:** Surgery, Loyola Univ Med Ctr 1981; Plastic Surgery, Univ Mich Hosp 1983; **Fellow:** Microsurgery, Rush/Presby St Luke's Med Ctr 1976; **Fac Appt:** Asst Prof S, Rush Med Coll

DeSilva, Stephen P MD [HS] - **Hospital:** Henry Ford Hosp; **Address:** Henry Ford Hospital, 2799 West Grand Blvd Fl 12, Detroit, MI 48202; **Phone:** 313-972-4079; **Board Cert:** Orthopaedic Surgery 2002; Hand Surgery 2002; **Med School:** Johns Hopkins Univ 1983; **Resid:** Orthopaedic Surgery, Mayo Clinic 1988; **Fellow:** Hand Surgery, Union Meml Hosp 1989; **Fac Appt:** Prof OrS, Wayne State Univ

Failla, Joseph M MD [HS] - **Spec Exp:** Hand Surgery; Hand Reconstruction; **Hospital:** Providence Hosp - Southfield, Huron Valley-Sinai Hosp; **Address:** Farmbrook Med Complex One Bldg - Ste 201, 29829 Telegraph Rd, Southfield, MI 48034; **Phone:** 248-352-4263; **Board Cert:** Orthopaedic Surgery 2001; Hand Surgery 2001; **Med School:** SUNY Buffalo 1982; **Resid:** Orthopaedic Surgery, SUNY-Buffalo 1987; **Fellow:** Hand Surgery, Mayo Clinic 1988

Fischer, Thomas J MD [HS] - **Spec Exp:** Microsurgery; Elbow Reconstruction; **Hospital:** St Vincent Hosp & Hlth Svcs - Indianapolis, Methodist Hosp - Indianapolis; **Address:** 8501 Harcourt Rd, Indianapolis, IN 46280-0434; **Phone:** 317-875-9105; **Board Cert:** Orthopaedic Surgery 2000; Hand Surgery 2000; **Med School:** Indiana Univ 1979; **Resid:** Orthopaedic Surgery, Univ Wash Affil Hosp 1984; **Fellow:** Hand Surgery, Hand Surg Assocs 1985; Hand Surgery, Duke Univ Med Ctr; **Fac Appt:** Assoc Clin Prof OrS, Indiana Univ

Gelberman, Richard MD [HS] - **Spec Exp:** Tendon Surgery; Peripheral Nerve Surgery; **Hospital:** Barnes-Jewish Hosp; **Address:** Wash Univ Sch Med, Dept Ortho Surg, 660 S Euclid Ave, Box 8233, St Louis, MO 63110; **Phone:** 314-747-2500; **Board Cert:** Orthopaedic Surgery 2007; Hand Surgery 2007; **Med School:** Univ Tenn Coll Med, Memphis 1969; **Resid:** Surgery, Univ Wisc Med Ctr 1975; **Fellow:** Hand Surgery, Duke Univ Med Ctr 1977; Pediatric Orthopaedic Surgery, Chldns Hosp-Harvard 1986; **Fac Appt:** Prof OrS, Washington Univ, St Louis

Hastings II, Hill MD [HS] - **Spec Exp:** Wrist Surgery; Elbow Reconstruction; Fractures & Tendon Transfers; Arthritis; **Hospital:** St Vincent Hosp & Hlth Svcs - Indianapolis; **Address:** 8501 Harcourt Rd, Indianapolis, IN 46280-0434; **Phone:** 317-875-9105; **Board Cert:** Orthopaedic Surgery 1982; Hand Surgery 2000; **Med School:** USC Sch Med 1974; **Resid:** Surgery, Univ Colorado Med Ctr 1976; Orthopaedic Surgery, Mass Genl Hosp 1980; **Fellow:** Hand Surgery, St Vincent Hosp 1981; **Fac Appt:** Clin Prof OrS, Indiana Univ

Idler, Richard S MD [HS] - **Spec Exp:** Upper Extremity Surgery; **Hospital:** St Vincent Hosp & Hlth Svcs - Indianapolis, Indiana Univ Hosp; **Address:** 8501 Harcourt Rd, Indianapolis, IN 46260; **Phone:** 317-875-9105; **Board Cert:** Orthopaedic Surgery 1985; Hand Surgery 2000; **Med School:** Dartmouth Med Sch 1975; **Resid:** Surgery, UCLA Med Ctr 1977; Plastic Surgery, UCLA Med Ctr 1978; **Fellow:** Orthopaedic Surgery, Mass Genl Hosp-Harvard 1981; Hand Surgery, St Vincent Hosp 1982; **Fac Appt:** Asst Clin Prof OrS, Indiana Univ

Kleinman, William B MD [HS] - **Spec Exp:** Arthritis; Congenital Hand Deformities; **Hospital:** St Vincent Hosp & Hlth Svcs - Indianapolis; **Address:** 8501 Harcourt Rd, Indianapolis, IN 46280; **Phone:** 317-875-9105; **Board Cert:** Orthopaedic Surgery 1979; Hand Surgery 2000; **Med School:** Cornell Univ-Weill Med Coll 1972; **Resid:** Surgery, Univ Colorado 1974; Orthopaedic Surgery, NY Orthopaedic Hosp/Columbia 1977; **Fellow:** Hand Surgery, Columbia-Presby Med Ctr 1978; Microvascular Surgery, Duke Univ; **Fac Appt:** Clin Prof OrS, Indiana Univ

Light, Terry MD [HS] - **Spec Exp:** Hand-Congenital Anomaly; Hand Injuries-Pediatric; Arthritis; **Hospital:** Loyola Univ Med Ctr, Chicago Shriners Hosp; **Address:** Loyola Univ Med Ctr, Dept Ortho, 2160 S First Ave Maguire Bldg - rm 1700, Maywood, IL 60153-5590; **Phone:** 708-216-4570; **Board Cert:** Orthopaedic Surgery 1979; Hand Surgery 2000; **Med School:** Ros Franklin Univ/Chicago Med Sch 1973; **Resid:** Orthopaedic Surgery, Yale-New Haven Hosp 1977; **Fellow:** Hand Surgery, Hartford Combined Prog 1977; **Fac Appt:** Prof OrS, Loyola Univ-Stritch Sch Med

Hand Surgery

Manske, Paul MD [HS] - **Spec Exp:** Congenital Hand Deformities; Pediatric Hand Surgery; **Hospital:** Barnes-Jewish Hosp; **Address:** Wash Univ Sch Med, Dept Ortho Surg, 660 S Euclid Ave, Box 8233, St Louis, MO 63110; **Phone:** 314-747-2500; **Board Cert:** Orthopaedic Surgery 1974; Hand Surgery 2000; **Med School:** Washington Univ, St Louis 1964; **Resid:** Surgery, Univ Wash Med Ctr 1966; Orthopaedic Surgery, Barnes Hosp-Wash Univ 1972; **Fellow:** Hand Surgery, Univ Louisville Hosp 1971; **Fac Appt:** Prof OrS, Washington Univ, St Louis

Mass, Daniel MD [HS] - **Spec Exp:** Tendon Surgery; Shoulder Reconstruction; Elbow Reconstruction; Wrist Surgery; **Hospital:** Univ of Chicago Hosps; **Address:** 5841 S Maryland Ave, MC 3079, Chicago, IL 60637-1448; **Phone:** 773-834-3531; **Board Cert:** Orthopaedic Surgery 1994; Hand Surgery 2000; **Med School:** Univ Chicago-Pritzker Sch Med 1975; **Resid:** Orthopaedic Surgery, Univ Chicago Hosp 1979; **Fellow:** Hand Surgery, St Francis Hosp 1980; **Fac Appt:** Prof S, Univ Chicago-Pritzker Sch Med

Mih, Alexander MD [HS] - **Spec Exp:** Microsurgery; **Hospital:** Indiana Univ Hosp, St Vincent Hosp & Hlth Svcs - Indianapolis; **Address:** Indiana Hand Center, 8501 Harcourt Rd, Indianapolis, IN 46280; **Phone:** 317-274-5648; **Board Cert:** Orthopaedic Surgery 2003; Hand Surgery 2003; **Med School:** Johns Hopkins Univ 1984; **Resid:** Orthopaedic Surgery, Mayo Clinic 1989; **Fellow:** Hand Surgery, Indiana Ctr for Hand Surg 1990; **Fac Appt:** Assoc Prof OrS, Indiana Univ

Nagle, Daniel J MD [HS] - **Spec Exp:** Wrist Surgery; Carpal Tunnel Syndrome; **Hospital:** Northwestern Meml Hosp, Children's Mem Hosp; **Address:** Chicago Hand Surgery, 737 N Michigan Ave, Ste 700, Chicago, IL 60611-7108; **Phone:** 312-337-6960; **Board Cert:** Orthopaedic Surgery 2007; Hand Surgery 2007; **Med School:** Belgium 1978; **Resid:** Orthopaedic Surgery, Northwestern Univ Med Sch 1983; **Fellow:** Hand Surgery, Christine Kleinert 1984; **Fac Appt:** Prof OrS, Northwestern Univ

Putnam, Matthew D MD [HS] - **Spec Exp:** Wrist Surgery; Fracture Deformities/Arm; Arthritis; **Hospital:** Univ Minn Med Ctr, Fairview - Univ Campus, Univ Minn Med Ctr, Fairview - Riverside Campus; **Address:** 2450 Riverside Ave S, Ste R200, Minneapolis, MN 55454; **Phone:** 612-273-9400; **Board Cert:** Hand Surgery 2001; **Med School:** Dartmouth Med Sch 1977; **Resid:** Surgery, Roosevelt Hosp 1979; Orthopaedic Surgery, Univ Pittsburgh 1984; **Fellow:** Hand Surgery, NVOH 1985; **Fac Appt:** Prof OrS, Univ Minn

Seitz, William H MD [HS] - **Spec Exp:** Hand & Upper Extremity Surgery; Shoulder Surgery; **Hospital:** Lutheran Med Ctr - Cleveland (page 56), Cleveland Clin Fdn (page 56); **Address:** 1730 W 25th St, Ste 2C, Beachwood, OH 44113; **Phone:** 216-363-2331; **Board Cert:** Orthopaedic Surgery 1998; Hand Surgery 1998; **Med School:** Columbia P&S 1979; **Resid:** Surgery, St Vincents Med Ctr 1981; Orthopaedic Surgery, Columbia-Presby Med Ctr 1984; **Fellow:** Hand & Microvascular Surgery, Columbia-Presby Med Ctr 1985; **Fac Appt:** Assoc Clin Prof OrS, Case West Res Univ

Steinmann, Scott P MD [HS] - **Spec Exp:** Shoulder Surgery; Elbow Surgery; Brachial Plexus Palsy; Reconstructive Microvascular Surgery; **Hospital:** Mayo Med Ctr & Clin - Rochester; **Address:** Mayo Clinic, Gonda 15, 200 1st St SW, Rochester, MN 55905; **Phone:** 507-284-3399; **Board Cert:** Orthopaedic Surgery 2004; Hand Surgery 2004; **Med School:** Cornell Univ-Weill Med Coll 1988; **Resid:** Orthopaedic Surgery, Hosp for Special Surgery 1992; **Fellow:** Shoulder Surgery, Columbia-Presby Med Ctr 1995; Hand Surgery, Mayo Clinic 1998; **Fac Appt:** Prof OrS, Mayo Med Sch

Stern, Peter J MD [HS] - **Spec Exp:** Hand & Wrist Surgery; Microsurgery; **Hospital:** Good Samaritan Hosp - Cincinnati, Univ Hosp - Cincinnati; **Address:** Hand Surg Specialists, 538 Oak St, Ste 200, Cincinnati, OH 45219; **Phone:** 513-961-4263; **Board Cert:** Orthopaedic Surgery 1993; Hand Surgery 2000; **Med School:** Washington Univ, St Louis 1970; **Resid:** Surgery, Beth Israel Hosp 1972; Orthopaedic Surgery, Harvard Combined Prgm 1977; **Fellow:** Hand Surgery, Univ Louisville Hosps 1979; **Fac Appt:** Prof OrS, Univ Cincinnati

Southwest

Ezaki, Marybeth MD [HS] - **Spec Exp:** Hand-Congenital Anomaly; Hand Reconstruction-Pediatric; **Hospital:** Texas Scottish Rite Hosp for Chldn; **Address:** 2222 Welborn St, Ste 131, Dallas, TX 75219; **Phone:** 214-559-7842; **Board Cert:** Orthopaedic Surgery 1993; Hand Surgery 2000; **Med School:** Yale Univ 1977; **Resid:** Orthopaedic Surgery, Univ Tex SW Med Ctr 1982; **Fellow:** Hand Surgery, Weyham Pk Hosp 1982; **Fac Appt:** Assoc Prof OrS, Univ Tex SW, Dallas

Moneim, Moheb S MD [HS] - **Spec Exp:** Hand Surgery; **Hospital:** Univ NM Hlth & Sci Ctr; **Address:** Univ of New Mexico, Dept Orthopedics, 2211 Lomas Blvd NE, Fl 2nd, Albuquerque, NM 87106; **Phone:** 505-272-4107; **Board Cert:** Orthopaedic Surgery 1998; Hand Surgery 1998; **Med School:** Egypt 1963; **Resid:** Orthopaedic Surgery, Duke Univ Med Ctr 1975; **Fellow:** Hand Surgery, Hosp for Spec Surgery 1976; **Fac Appt:** Prof OrS, Univ New Mexico

Rayan, Ghazi M MD [HS] - **Spec Exp:** Microsurgery; Congenital Limb Deformities; Arthritis; **Hospital:** Integris Baptist Med Ctr - OK, OU Med Ctr; **Address:** 3366 Northwest Expressway, Ste 700, Oklahoma City, OK 73112-4439; **Phone:** 405-945-4888; **Board Cert:** Orthopaedic Surgery 2000; Hand Surgery 2000; **Med School:** Egypt 1973; **Resid:** Surgery, S Baltimore Genl Hosp 1977; Orthopaedic Surgery, Union Meml Hosp 1980; **Fellow:** Hand & Microvascular Surgery, Union Meml Hosp 1980; **Fac Appt:** Clin Prof OrS, Univ Okla Coll Med

West Coast and Pacific

Atkinson, Robert E MD [HS] - **Spec Exp:** Arthritis; Arthroscopic Surgery; Nerve Disorders/Surgery; **Hospital:** Queen's Med Ctr - Honolulu, Kapiolani Med Ctr @ Pali Momi; **Address:** Queen's Physicians' Office Bldg 1, 1380 Lusitana St, Ste 604, Honolulu, HI 96813; **Phone:** 808-521-8128; **Board Cert:** Orthopaedic Surgery 1985; **Med School:** Jefferson Med Coll 1977; **Resid:** Orthopaedic Surgery, Hosp Special Surgery 1982; **Fellow:** Hand Surgery, Mass Genl Hosp 1983; **Fac Appt:** Clin Prof OrS, Univ Hawaii JA Burns Sch Med

Godzik, Cathleen MD [HS] - **Spec Exp:** Congenital Hand Deformities; Sports Injuries; Dupuytren's Contracture; **Hospital:** California Hosp Med Ctr, Good Samaritan Hosp - Los Angeles; **Address:** 1245 Wilshire Blvd, Ste 611, Los Angeles, CA 90017; **Phone:** 213-482-6100; **Board Cert:** Orthopaedic Surgery 2001; Hand Surgery 2001; **Med School:** NY Med Coll 1981; **Resid:** Surgery, Brown Univ Sch Med 1983; Orthopaedic Surgery, Univ Conn Sch Med 1984; **Fellow:** Hand Surgery, Joseph Boyes Hand Fell-USC 1987

Hanel, Douglas P MD [HS] - **Spec Exp:** Reconstructive Microvascular Surgery; Hand-Congenital Anomaly; Elbow Reconstruction; **Hospital:** Harborview Med Ctr, Chldns Hosp and Regl Med Ctr - Seattle; **Address:** Harborview Medical Ctr, 325 9th Ave, Box 359798, Seattle, WA 98104-2420; **Phone:** 206-731-3462; **Board Cert:** Orthopaedic Surgery 2007; Hand Surgery 2007; **Med School:** St Louis Univ 1977; **Resid:** Orthopaedic Surgery, St Louis Univ Hosp 1982; **Fellow:** Hand Surgery, Univ Louisville Hosp 1983; Microsurgery, Univ Louisville Hosp 1983; **Fac Appt:** Prof OrS, Univ Wash

Hentz, Vincent R MD [HS] - **Spec Exp:** Hand Plastic Surgery; **Hospital:** Stanford Univ Med Ctr; **Address:** 1000 Welch Rd, Ste 100, Palto Alto, CA 94304; **Phone:** 650-723-5256; **Board Cert:** Plastic Surgery 1977; **Med School:** Univ Fla Coll Med 1968; **Resid:** Plastic Surgery, Stanford Univ Hosp 1974; **Fellow:** Hand Surgery, Roosevelt Hosp 1975; **Fac Appt:** Prof S, Stanford Univ

Hand Surgery

Jones, Neil MD [HS] - **Spec Exp:** Hand Reconstruction-Pediatric; Nerve Disorders/Surgery; Tendon Surgery; Toe-to-Hand Transfer; **Hospital:** UC Irvine Med Ctr; **Address:** 101 The City Drive S, Route 94, Pavilion 3, Los Angeles, CA 90095; **Phone:** 714-456-7012; **Board Cert:** Plastic Surgery 1985; **Med School:** England 1974; **Resid:** Surgery, Radcliffe Infirmary 1979; Plastic Surgery, Univ Mich Med Ctr 1981; **Fellow:** Plastic Surgery, St Bartholomew's Hosp 1982; Hand & Microvascular Surgery, Mass Gen Hosp/Harvard 1983; **Fac Appt:** Prof PlS, UC Irvine

Meals, Roy Allen MD [HS] - **Hospital:** Ronald Reagan UCLA Med Ctr; **Address:** 100 UCLA Medical Plaza, Ste 305, Los Angeles, CA 90024; **Phone:** 310-206-6337; **Board Cert:** Orthopaedic Surgery 1980; Hand Surgery 2000; **Med School:** Vanderbilt Univ 1971; **Resid:** Surgery, Johns Hopkins Hosp 1973; Orthopaedic Surgery, Johns Hopkins Hosp 1978; **Fellow:** Hand Surgery, Mass Genl Hosp 1979; **Fac Appt:** Clin Prof S, UCLA

Slutsky, David J MD [HS] - **Spec Exp:** Hand Reconstruction; Wrist Surgery; Peripheral Nerve Surgery; **Hospital:** LAC - Harbor - UCLA Med Ctr; **Address:** South Bay Hand Surgery Ctr, 3475 Torrance Blvd, Ste F, Torrance, CA 90503; **Phone:** 310-792-1809; **Board Cert:** Orthopaedic Surgery 2002; Hand Surgery 2002; **Med School:** Univ Manitoba 1981; **Resid:** Orthopaedic Surgery, Univ Manitoba Med Ctr 1987; **Fellow:** Hand & Microvascular Surgery, Loma Linda Univ Med Ctr 1989; **Fac Appt:** Asst Prof OrS, UCLA

Szabo, Robert M MD [HS] - **Spec Exp:** Peripheral Nerve Surgery; Hand Injuries; Hand & Upper Extremity Tumors; **Hospital:** UC Davis Med Ctr, Mercy General Hosp - Sacramento; **Address:** UC Davis, Dept Orthopaedics, 4860 Y St, Ste 3800, Sacramento, CA 95817-2307; **Phone:** 916-734-3678; **Board Cert:** Orthopaedic Surgery 1998; Hand Surgery 1998; **Med School:** SUNY Buffalo 1977; **Resid:** Surgery, Mt Sinai Hosp 1979; Orthopaedic Surgery, Mt Sinai Hosp 1982; **Fellow:** Hand Surgery, UCSD Med Ctr 1983; Epidemiology, UC Berkeley 1995; **Fac Appt:** Prof OrS, UC Davis

Trumble, Thomas MD [HS] - **Spec Exp:** Nerve Disorders/Surgery; Upper Extremity Trauma; Biomechanics-Arms; **Hospital:** Univ Wash Med Ctr, Harborview Med Ctr; **Address:** 4245 Roosevelt Way NE, 325 9th Ave, Box 359798, Seattle, WA 98105; **Phone:** 206-598-4288; **Board Cert:** Orthopaedic Surgery 1999; Hand Surgery 1999; **Med School:** Yale Univ 1979; **Resid:** Orthopaedic Surgery, Yale-New Haven Hosp 1984; **Fellow:** Microvascular Surgery, Duke Univ Med Ctr 1984; Hand Surgery, Mass Genl Hosp 1985; **Fac Appt:** Prof S, Univ Wash

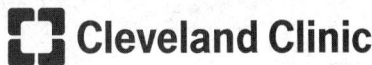 **Cleveland Clinic**

Hand and Upper Extremity Center

Cleveland Clinic Hand and Upper Extremity Center, a division of the Department of Orthopaedic Surgery, provides a centralized, comprehensive and diagnostic treatment center for problems affecting the hand, wrist, elbow and shoulder. If you are among the millions of Americans experiencing hand and upper extremity problems each year, finding expert care is all-important. For the past several years, *U.S.News* & *World Report* has consistently ranked the Department of Orthopaedic Surgery among the nation's top orthopaedic programs.

Our surgeons treat all disorders of the upper extremity. The following is a list of many of the injuries and disorders we treat. We encourage you to ask about our experience with your particular problem.

Shoulder
Fractures and dislocations
Arthritis
Chronic instability
Rotator cuff tears
Brachial plexus injuries

Wrist
Fractures and nonunions
Dislocations
Instability
Carpal tunnel syndrom
Tendinitis
Rheumatoid wrist

Elbow
Fractures and dislocations
Tennis and golfer's elbow
Arthritis
Throwing elbow

Hand
Fractures and dislocations
Trigger finger
Cysts and tumors
Burns

Surgery of the Hand and Upper Extremity
Our surgeons are experts in the operative care of a wide array of upper extremity disorders. For some injuries, this includes the newest surgical techniques, such as microsurgery and minimally invasive surgery.

Work-Related Disorders
Acute injuries and chronic problems of the hand and upper extremity can result from occupational activity. Our surgeons are experts in determining whether a disorder is work-related and at determining a treatment course that will help you meet the physical demands of your job.

For more information about the Cleveland Clinic Hand and Upper Extremity Center, to schedule a second opinion or to learn about assistance for out-of-town patients, call 800.890.2467 or visit www.clevelandclinic.org/orthotopdocs.

Hand and Upper Extremity Center
9500 Euclid Avenue / AC311 | Cleveland OH 44195

NYU Hospital for Joint Diseases
NYU LANGONE MEDICAL CENTER

301 East 17th Street
(at Second Avenue)
New York, NY 10003
212-598-6000 FAX: 212-260-1203
www.nyuhjd.org

HAND SURGERY

NYU Hospital for Joint Diseases provides comprehensive care of patients with hand and wrist disorders, including:
- Fractures
- Congenital anomalies
- Soft tissue and skeletal trauma
- Degenerative and rheumatoid arthritis
- Sports-related injuries of the hand and wrist
- Vascular disorders
- Tumors
- Occupational hand and wrist disorders

Care is provided by 16 specialists encompassing all aspects of diagnosis and treatment of the full spectrum of problems that affect the hand and wrist.

Specific emphases include fractures of the wrist and distal radius and reconstructive aspects of hand surgery, as reflected by the large volume of cases involving post traumatic, arthritis, congenital, neuromuscular, and neoplastic conditions.

The research focus of the NYUHJD Hand Service is on a variety of clinical problems, including wrist fractures, non- unions of the scaphoid, avascular necrosis of the lunate (Kienbock's disease), intercarpal subluxations, and neuropathies of the upper extremity.

After surgery, the Rusk Institute of Rehabilitation Medicine's Hand Therapy Unit helps surgical patients recover full or partial use of their hands, providing comprehensive rehabilitation for a variety of ailments associated with the hand and upper body. The Hand Therapy Unit specializes in fractures, traumatic injuries, tendonitis, sports injuries, work-related injuries, repetitive stress injuries, carpal tunnel syndrome, tendon and nerve repairs, and arthritis. It is staffed by licensed occupational therapists who specialize in the treatment of the hand and upper extremities.

NYU HOSPITAL FOR JOINT DISEASES

Optimal care of hands requires a specialist who has advanced training in the entire spectrum of hand and wrist disorders including rehabilitation techniques.

At NYU Hospital for Joint Diseases, world-class hand surgery and rehabilitation are brought together ensuring patients and their families have a positive outcome.

Physician Referral
NYUHJD offers a free telephone physician referral service, Monday-Friday, 8:30 am to 6:00 pm. The physician referral service can be reached at 1-888-HJD-DOCS (1-888-453-3627)

Hematology &
Medical Oncology
a subspecialty of Internal Medicine

Hematology: An internist with additional training who specializes in diseases of the blood, spleen and lymph glands. This specialist treats conditions such as anemia, clotting disorders, sickle cell disease, hemophilia, leukemia and lymphoma.

Medical Oncology: An internist who specializes in the diagnosis and treatment of all types of cancer and other benign and malignant tumors. This specialist decides on and administers chemotherapy for malignancy, as well as consulting with surgeons and radiotherapists on other treatments for cancer.

Training Required: Three years in internal medicine *plus* additional training and examination for certification in hematology or medical oncology.

HEMATOLOGY

New England

Anderson, Kenneth C MD [Hem] - **Spec Exp:** Multiple Myeloma; Hematologic Malignancies; **Hospital:** Dana-Farber Cancer Inst, Brigham & Women's Hosp; **Address:** 44 Binney St Mayer Bldg - rm 557, Boston, MA 02115; **Phone:** 617-632-2144; **Board Cert:** Internal Medicine 1980; **Med School:** Johns Hopkins Univ 1977; **Resid:** Internal Medicine, Johns Hopkins Hosp 1980; **Fellow:** Hematology & Oncology, Dana Farber Cancer Inst 1983; **Fac Appt:** Prof Med, Harvard Med Sch

Dezube, Bruce J MD [Hem] - **Spec Exp:** AIDS Related Cancers; Clinical Trials; **Hospital:** Beth Israel Deaconess Med Ctr - Boston; **Address:** BIDMC-Division of Hematology/Oncology, 330 Brookline Ave, MASCO 414, Boston, MA 02215; **Phone:** 617-632-9258; **Board Cert:** Internal Medicine 1986; Medical Oncology 1989; Hematology 1988; **Med School:** Tufts Univ 1983; **Resid:** Internal Medicine, New England Med Ctr 1986; **Fellow:** Hematology & Oncology, Beth Israel Deaconess Hosp 1989; **Fac Appt:** Assoc Prof Med, Harvard Med Sch

Duffy, Thomas P MD [Hem] - **Spec Exp:** Mast Cell Diseases; Leukemia; Lymphoma; **Hospital:** Yale-New Haven Hosp; **Address:** Yale Univ, Sect Hematology, 333 Cedar St, rm 403-WWW, Box 208021, New Haven, CT 06520-8021; **Phone:** 203-785-4744; **Board Cert:** Internal Medicine 1972; Hematology 1974; **Med School:** Johns Hopkins Univ 1962; **Resid:** Internal Medicine, Johns Hopkins Hosp 1965; **Fellow:** Hematology, Johns Hopkins Hosp 1970; **Fac Appt:** Prof Med, Yale Univ

Groopman, Jerome E MD [Hem] - **Spec Exp:** AIDS/HIV; AIDS Related Cancers; **Hospital:** Beth Israel Deaconess Med Ctr - Boston; **Address:** Beth Israel Deaconess Medical Ctr, 330 Brookline Ave, Boston, MA 02215; **Phone:** 617-667-0070; **Board Cert:** Internal Medicine 1979; Medical Oncology 1981; Hematology 1984; **Med School:** Columbia P&S 1976; **Resid:** Internal Medicine, Mass Genl Hosp 1978; **Fellow:** Hematology & Oncology, UCLA Med Ctr 1979; Research, Dana Farber Cancer Ctr 1980; **Fac Appt:** Prof Med, Harvard Med Sch

Meehan, Kenneth MD [Hem] - **Spec Exp:** Bone Marrow Transplant; **Hospital:** Dartmouth - Hitchcock Med Ctr; **Address:** Norris Cotton Cancer Ctr, Dartmouth-Hitchcock Med Ctr, 1 Medical Center Drive, Lebanon, NH 03756; **Phone:** 603-650-4628; **Board Cert:** Internal Medicine 1989; Hematology 2003; Medical Oncology 1991; **Med School:** Georgetown Univ 1986; **Resid:** Internal Medicine, Georgetown Univ 1989; **Fellow:** Hematology & Oncology, Dartmouth-Hitchcock Med Ctr 1992; **Fac Appt:** Assoc Prof Med, Dartmouth Med Sch

Miller, Kenneth B MD [Hem] - **Spec Exp:** Bone Marrow Transplant; Leukemia; Myelodysplastic Syndromes; **Hospital:** Tufts Med Ctr; **Address:** Dept Medicine, 750 Washington St, Box 245, Boston, MA 02211; **Phone:** 617-636-2600; **Board Cert:** Internal Medicine 1976; Hematology 1980; **Med School:** NY Med Coll 1972; **Resid:** Internal Medicine, NYU Med Ctr/VA Hosp 1976; Internal Medicine, NYU Med Ctr 1976; **Fellow:** Hematology, New England Med Ctr 1979; **Fac Appt:** Prof Med, Tufts Univ

Spitzer, Thomas R MD [Hem] - **Spec Exp:** Bone Marrow Transplant; Leukemia; **Hospital:** Mass Genl Hosp; **Address:** Mass Genl Hosp-Bone Marrow Tranplant Program, 55 Fruit St, Emerson Pl, Ste 118, Boston, MA 02114; **Phone:** 617-724-1124; **Board Cert:** Internal Medicine 1977; Medical Oncology 1983; Hematology 1984; **Med School:** Univ Rochester 1974; **Resid:** Internal Medicine, NYew York Hosp-Cornell Med Ctr 1977; **Fellow:** Hematology & Oncology, Case West Res Univ 1983; **Fac Appt:** Prof Med, Harvard Med Sch

Stone, Richard M MD [Hem] - **Spec Exp:** Leukemia; **Hospital:** Dana-Farber Cancer Inst, Brigham & Women's Hosp; **Address:** Dana Farber Cancer Inst, Adult Leukemia Prog, 44 Binney St, Ste M1B17, Boston, MA 02115-6084; **Phone:** 617-632-2214; **Board Cert:** Internal Medicine 1984; Medical Oncology 1987; Hematology 1988; **Med School:** Harvard Med Sch 1981; **Resid:** Internal Medicine, Brigham & Womens Hosp 1984; **Fellow:** Medical Oncology, Dana Farber Cancer Inst 1987; **Fac Appt:** Assoc Prof Med, Harvard Med Sch

Mid Atlantic

Abrams, Charles S MD [Hem] - **Spec Exp:** Bleeding/Coagulation Disorders; Thrombotic Disorders; **Hospital:** Hosp Univ Penn - UPHS (page 60); **Address:** Univ Penn, Dept Hem/Onc, 421 Curie Blvd, Bio Medical Research Bldg 2/3, Philadelphia, PA 19104-6160; **Phone:** 215-573-3288; **Board Cert:** Internal Medicine 1987; Medical Oncology 1989; Hematology 1990; **Med School:** Yale Univ 1984; **Resid:** Internal Medicine, Hosp U Penn 1987; **Fellow:** Hematology & Oncology, Hosp U Penn 1988; **Fac Appt:** Assoc Prof Med, Univ Pennsylvania

Baer, Maria R MD [Hem] - **Spec Exp:** Leukemia; Myelodysplastic Syndromes; **Hospital:** Univ of MD Med Sys; **Address:** Univ Maryland, Greenebaum Cancer Ctr, 22 S Greene St, rm S9D04, Baltimore, MD 21201; **Phone:** 410-328-7904; **Board Cert:** Internal Medicine 1983; Hematology 1984; **Med School:** Johns Hopkins Univ 1979; **Resid:** Internal Medicine, Vanderbilt Univ Hosp 1982; **Fellow:** Hematology, Vanderbilt Univ Hosp 1984; **Fac Appt:** Prof Med, Univ MD Sch Med

Cheson, Bruce D MD [Hem] - **Spec Exp:** Leukemia; Hematologic Malignancies; **Hospital:** Georgetown Univ Hosp; **Address:** GUMC - Lombardi Cancer Ctr, 3800 Reservoir Rd NW, Podium B, Washington, DC 20007; **Phone:** 202-444-7932; **Board Cert:** Internal Medicine 1974; Hematology 1976; **Med School:** Tufts Univ 1971; **Resid:** Internal Medicine, Univ Virginia Hosp 1974; **Fellow:** Hematology, New England Med Ctr Hosp 1976

Coller, Barry MD [Hem] - **Spec Exp:** Glanzmann's Thrombasthenia; Bleeding/Coagulation Disorders; **Hospital:** Rockefeller Univ, Mount Sinai Med Ctr (page 64); **Address:** Rockefeller Univ, 1230 York Ave, New York, NY 10065; **Phone:** 212-327-7490; **Board Cert:** Internal Medicine 1973; Hematology 1975; **Med School:** NYU Sch Med 1970; **Resid:** Internal Medicine, Bellevue Hosp 1972; **Fellow:** Hematology, Natl Inst Hlth Clin Ctr 1974; **Fac Appt:** Clin Prof Med, Mount Sinai Sch Med

Diuguid, David L MD [Hem] - **Spec Exp:** Bleeding/Coagulation Disorders; **Hospital:** NY-Presby Hosp/Columbia (page 66); **Address:** 161 Ft Washington Ave, Rm 862, New York, NY 10032; **Phone:** 212-305-0527; **Board Cert:** Internal Medicine 1982; Hematology 1986; Medical Oncology 1985; **Med School:** Cornell Univ-Weill Med Coll 1979; **Resid:** Internal Medicine, Boston Univ Med Ctr 1983; **Fellow:** Hematology & Oncology, New England Med Ctr 1986; **Fac Appt:** Assoc Prof Med, Columbia P&S

Fruchtman, Steven M MD [Hem] - **Spec Exp:** Myeloproliferative Disorders; Polycythemia Rubra Vera; **Address:** 1111 Park Ave, New York, NY 10029; **Phone:** 212-427-7700; **Board Cert:** Internal Medicine 1980; Hematology 1984; **Med School:** NY Med Coll 1977; **Resid:** Internal Medicine, Univ Hosp 1981; **Fellow:** Hematology, Mount Sinai Med Ctr 1984; Hematology, Meml Sloan Kettering Cancer Ctr 1985; **Fac Appt:** Assoc Prof Med, NY Med Coll

Gewirtz, Alan M MD [Hem] - **Spec Exp:** Leukemia; Gene Therapy; **Hospital:** Hosp Univ Penn - UPHS (page 60); **Address:** Univ Penn - Div Hem/Onc, 421 Curie Blvd, 716BRB, Philadelphia, PA 19104; **Phone:** 215-662-3914; **Board Cert:** Internal Medicine 1979; Hematology 1982; Medical Oncology 1981; **Med School:** SUNY Buffalo 1976; **Resid:** Internal Medicine, Mt Sinai Hosp 1979; **Fellow:** Medical Oncology, Yale-New Haven Hosp 1981; Hematology, Yale-New Haven Hosp 1982; **Fac Appt:** Prof Med, Univ Pennsylvania

Hematology

Goldberg, Jack MD [Hem] - **Spec Exp:** Leukemia; Lymphoma; Breast Cancer; Bone Marrow Transplant; **Hospital:** Penn Presby Med Ctr - UPHS (page 60), Virtua West Jersey Hosp - Voorhees; **Address:** 409 Route 70 E, Cherry Hill, NJ 08034; **Phone:** 856-429-1519; **Board Cert:** Internal Medicine 1976; Hematology 1980; Medical Oncology 1989; **Med School:** SUNY Upstate Med Univ 1973; **Resid:** Internal Medicine, Boston Univ Hosp 1975; **Fellow:** Hematology & Oncology, SUNY Syracuse Med Ctr 1977; **Fac Appt:** Clin Prof Med, Univ Pennsylvania

Kempin, Sanford Jay MD [Hem] - **Spec Exp:** Bleeding/Coagulation Disorders; Leukemia; Lymphoma; **Hospital:** St Vincent Cath Med Ctrs - Manhattan; **Address:** St Vincents Cancer Ctr, 325 W 15th St, New York, NY 10011; **Phone:** 212-604-6010; **Board Cert:** Internal Medicine 1976; Medical Oncology 1977; Hematology 1978; **Med School:** Belgium 1971; **Resid:** Internal Medicine, Lemuel Shattuck Hosp 1972; **Fellow:** Hematology, St Jude Chldns Hosp 1975; Medical Oncology, Meml Sloan Kettering Cancer Ctr 1976; **Fac Appt:** Asst Prof Med, NY Med Coll

Kessler, Craig M MD [Hem] - **Spec Exp:** Bleeding/Coagulation Disorders; Hemophilia; Hematologic Malignancies; **Hospital:** Georgetown Univ Hosp; **Address:** GUMC, Lombardi Cancer Ctr, 3800 Reservoir Rd NW, Washington, DC 20007; **Phone:** 202-444-8676; **Board Cert:** Internal Medicine 1976; Hematology 1980; **Med School:** Tulane Univ 1973; **Resid:** Internal Medicine, Ochsner Fdn Hosp 1976; **Fellow:** Hematology, Johns Hopkins Hosp 1978; **Fac Appt:** Prof Med, Georgetown Univ

Marks, Stanley M MD [Hem] - **Spec Exp:** Leukemia; Lymphoma; **Hospital:** UPMC Shadyside; **Address:** 5115 Centre Ave, Fl 3, Pittsburgh, PA 15232; **Phone:** 412-235-1020; **Board Cert:** Internal Medicine 1976; Hematology 1978; **Med School:** Univ Pittsburgh 1973; **Resid:** Internal Medicine, Presby Univ Hosp 1976; **Fellow:** Hematology & Oncology, Peter Bent Brigham Hosp 1978; **Fac Appt:** Assoc Clin Prof Med, Drexel Univ Coll Med

Mears, John G MD [Hem] - **Spec Exp:** Lymphoma; Leukemia; Multiple Myeloma; Breast Cancer; **Hospital:** NY-Presby Hosp/Columbia (page 66); **Address:** 161 Ft Washington Ave, Ste 923, New York, NY 10032; **Phone:** 212-305-3506; **Board Cert:** Internal Medicine 1976; Hematology 1978; **Med School:** Columbia P&S 1973; **Resid:** Internal Medicine, Boston Univ Med Ctr 1975; **Fellow:** Hematology & Oncology, Columbia-Presby Med Ctr 1978; **Fac Appt:** Clin Prof Med, Columbia P&S

Millenson, Michael M MD [Hem] - **Spec Exp:** Leukemia & Lymphoma; Thromboembolic Disorders; Hematologic Malignancies; **Hospital:** Fox Chase Cancer Ctr (page 58); **Address:** Fox Chase Cancer Center, 7701 Burholme Ave, Ste C307, Philadelphia, PA 19111; **Phone:** 215-728-2600; **Board Cert:** Internal Medicine 1987; Medical Oncology 2000; Hematology 2000; **Med School:** Temple Univ 1984; **Resid:** Internal Medicine, Temple Univ Hosp 1987; **Fellow:** Hematology & Oncology, Beth Israel Hosp 1991

Nimer, Stephen D MD [Hem] - **Spec Exp:** Bone Marrow Transplant; Myelodysplastic Syndromes; Leukemia; Stem Cell Transplant; **Hospital:** Meml Sloan-Kettering Cancer Ctr; **Address:** 1275 York Avenue, New York, NY 10065; **Phone:** 800-525-2225; **Board Cert:** Internal Medicine 1982; Hematology 1986; Medical Oncology 1985; **Med School:** Univ Chicago-Pritzker Sch Med 1979; **Resid:** Internal Medicine, UCLA Med Ctr 1982; **Fellow:** Hematology & Oncology, UCLA Med Ctr 1986; **Fac Appt:** Prof Med, Cornell Univ-Weill Med Coll

Porter, David L MD [Hem] - **Spec Exp:** Leukemia; Bone Marrow Transplant; Lymphoma; **Hospital:** Hosp Univ Penn - UPHS (page 60); **Address:** Hosp Univ Penn, Div Hem/Oncology, 3400 Spruce St, 16 Penn Twr, Philadelphia, PA 19104; **Phone:** 215-662-7909; **Board Cert:** Internal Medicine 1990; Medical Oncology 1993; Hematology 1994; **Med School:** Brown Univ 1987; **Resid:** Internal Medicine, Univ Hosp 1990; **Fellow:** Hematology & Oncology, Brigham & Womens Hosp 1992; **Fac Appt:** Assoc Prof Med, Univ Pennsylvania

Rai, Kanti MD [Hem] - **Spec Exp:** Leukemia; Lymphoma; Multiple Myeloma; **Hospital:** Long Island Jewish Med Ctr; **Address:** 410 Lakeville Rd, Ste 212, New Hyde Park, NY 10042; **Phone:** 718-470-4050; **Board Cert:** Pediatrics 1959; **Med School:** India 1955; **Resid:** Pediatrics, Lincoln Hosp 1958; Pediatrics, North Shore Univ Hosp 1959; **Fellow:** Hematology, LI Jewish Med Ctr 1960; **Fac Appt:** Prof Med, Albert Einstein Coll Med

Rand, Jacob H MD [Hem] - **Spec Exp:** Bleeding/Coagulation Disorders; Pregnancy & Hematologic Abnormalities; Thrombotic Disorders; **Hospital:** Montefiore Med Ctr; **Address:** Montefiore Medical Ctr, 111 E 210th St, N8 Silverzone, Bronx, NY 10467-2401; **Phone:** 718-920-5991; **Board Cert:** Internal Medicine 1977; Hematology 1978; **Med School:** Albert Einstein Coll Med 1973; **Resid:** Pathology, Montefiore Med Ctr 1974; Internal Medicine, Mount Sinai Hosp 1976; **Fellow:** Hematology, Montefiore Med Ctr 1978; **Fac Appt:** Prof Med, Albert Einstein Coll Med

Raphael, Bruce MD [Hem] - **Spec Exp:** Lymphoma; Leukemia; Multiple Myeloma; **Hospital:** NYU Med Ctr (page 68), NY Downtown Hosp; **Address:** 160 E 34th Street Ave Fl 7, NYU Clinical Cancer Ctr, New York, NY 10016-6402; **Phone:** 212-731-5185; **Board Cert:** Internal Medicine 1978; Hematology 1980; Medical Oncology 1981; **Med School:** McGill Univ 1975; **Resid:** Internal Medicine, Jewish Genl Hosp 1977; **Fellow:** Medical Oncology, Meml Sloan Kettering Cancer Ctr 1978; Hematology, NYU Med Ctr 1980; **Fac Appt:** Assoc Prof Med, NYU Sch Med

Roodman, G David MD [Hem] - **Spec Exp:** Multiple Myeloma; **Hospital:** UPMC Shadyside, VA Pittsburgh Hlth Care Sys; **Address:** VA Pittsburgh Healthcare System, R&D 151-U, rm 2E113, University Drive C, Pittsburgh, PA 15240; **Phone:** 412-688-6571; **Board Cert:** Internal Medicine 1978; Hematology 1980; **Med School:** Univ KY Coll Med 1973; **Resid:** Internal Medicine, Univ Minnesota Hosp 1978; **Fellow:** Hematology, Univ Minnesota Hosp 1980; **Fac Appt:** Prof Med, Univ Pittsburgh

Savage, David G MD [Hem] - **Spec Exp:** Stem Cell Transplant; Multiple Myeloma; Lymphoma; **Hospital:** NY-Presby Hosp/Columbia (page 66); **Address:** 177 Fort Washington Ave, Millstein Bldg Fl 6 - rm 435, New York, NY 10032; **Phone:** 212-305-9783; **Board Cert:** Internal Medicine 1977; Hematology 1982; Medical Oncology 1985; **Med School:** Columbia P&S 1974; **Resid:** Internal Medicine, Harlem Hosp/Columbia Presby Med Ctr 1977; **Fellow:** Hematology & Oncology, Harlem Hosp/Columbia Presby Med Ctr 1979; **Fac Appt:** Assoc Prof Med, Columbia P&S

Schuster, Michael W MD [Hem] - **Spec Exp:** Bone Marrow Transplant; **Hospital:** NY-Presby Hosp/Weill Cornell (page 66); **Address:** NY Weill Cornell Medical Ctr, 525 E 68th St, Starr 341, New York, NY 10021; **Phone:** 212-746-2119; **Board Cert:** Internal Medicine 1984; Hematology 1986; **Med School:** Dartmouth Med Sch 1980; **Resid:** Internal Medicine, New England Deaconess Hosp 1983; **Fellow:** Hematology & Oncology, Beth Israel Med Ctr 1987; **Fac Appt:** Assoc Prof Med, Cornell Univ-Weill Med Coll

Spivak, Jerry L MD [Hem] - **Spec Exp:** Myeloproliferative Disorders; Polycythemia Rubra Vera; Leukemia; Anemia; **Hospital:** Johns Hopkins Hosp - Baltimore (page 61); **Address:** 720 Rutland Ave Bldg Ross - Ste 1025, Baltimore, MD 21205; **Phone:** 410-614-0167; **Board Cert:** Internal Medicine 1971; Hematology 1974; **Med School:** Cornell Univ-Weill Med Coll 1964; **Resid:** Internal Medicine, Johns Hopkins Hosp 1966; Internal Medicine, Johns Hopkins Hosp 1972; **Fellow:** Hematology, Natl Cancer Inst 1968; Hematology, Johns Hopkins Hosp 1971; **Fac Appt:** Prof Med, Johns Hopkins Univ

Wisch, Nathaniel MD [Hem] - **Spec Exp:** Lymphoma; Breast Cancer; Leukemia; **Hospital:** Lenox Hill Hosp (page 62), Mount Sinai Med Ctr (page 64); **Address:** 12 E 86th St, New York, NY 10028-0506; **Phone:** 212-861-6660; **Board Cert:** Internal Medicine 1965; Hematology 1972; Medical Oncology 1977; **Med School:** Northwestern Univ 1958; **Resid:** Internal Medicine, VA Hosp 1960; Internal Medicine, Montefiore Hosp 1961; **Fellow:** Hematology, Mount Sinai Hosp 1962; **Fac Appt:** Clin Prof Med, Mount Sinai Sch Med

Hematology

Zalusky, Ralph MD [Hem] - **Spec Exp:** Anemia; Leukemia; Lymphoma; **Hospital:** Beth Israel Med Ctr - Petrie Division (page 57); **Address:** Beth Israel Med Ctr, First Ave at 16th St, New York, NY 10003; **Phone:** 212-420-4185; **Board Cert:** Internal Medicine 1964; Hematology 1972; **Med School:** Boston Univ 1957; **Resid:** Internal Medicine, Duke Univ Med Ctr 1962; **Fellow:** Hematology, Boston Med Ctr 1961; **Fac Appt:** Prof Med, Albert Einstein Coll Med

Southeast

Bigelow, Carolyn L MD [Hem] - **Spec Exp:** Bone Marrow Transplant; Sickle Cell Disease; **Hospital:** Univ Hosps & Clins - Jackson; **Address:** Univ Mississippi Med Ctr-Div Hematology, 2500 N State St, Jackson, MS 39216; **Phone:** 601-984-5615; **Board Cert:** Internal Medicine 1982; Hematology 1988; **Med School:** Univ Miss 1979; **Resid:** Internal Medicine, Univ Mississippi Med Ctr 1982; **Fellow:** Hematology & Oncology, Univ Washington Med Ctr 1987; **Fac Appt:** Prof Med, Univ Miss

Djulbegovic, Benjamin MD [Hem] - **Spec Exp:** Multiple Myeloma; Lymphoma; Myeloproliferative Disorders; **Hospital:** H Lee Moffitt Cancer Ctr & Research Inst; **Address:** H Lee Moffitt Cancer Ctr, 12902 Magnolia Drive, MRC Bldg - Ste 2067H, Tampa, FL 33612; **Phone:** 813-745-4605; **Board Cert:** Internal Medicine 2002; Hematology 2004; **Med School:** Bosnia 1976; **Resid:** Internal Medicine, Univ Med Ctr 1983; Internal Medicine, Univ Louisville Med Ctr 1988; **Fellow:** Univ Manchester 1985; Hematology & Oncology, Univ Louisville 1990; **Fac Appt:** Prof Med, Univ S Fla Coll Med

Files, Joe C MD [Hem] - **Spec Exp:** Bone Marrow Transplant; Stem Cell Transplant; Leukemia; **Hospital:** Univ Hosps & Clins - Jackson; **Address:** Univ Miss Med Ctr-Div Hematology, 2500 N State St, Jackson, MS 39216; **Phone:** 601-984-5615; **Board Cert:** Internal Medicine 1976; Hematology 1980; **Med School:** Univ Miss 1972; **Resid:** Internal Medicine, Univ Miss Med Ctr 1976; **Fellow:** Hematology, Univ Wash Sch Med 1979; **Fac Appt:** Prof Med, Univ Miss

Greer, John P MD [Hem] - **Spec Exp:** Leukemia & Lymphoma; Myelodysplastic Syndromes; Stem Cell Transplant; **Hospital:** Vanderbilt Univ Med Ctr; **Address:** 2665 The Vanderbilt Clinic, 1301 22nd Ave S, Nashville, TN 37232-5505; **Phone:** 615-936-1803; **Board Cert:** Pediatrics 1985; Internal Medicine 1979; Hematology 1984; Medical Oncology 1985; **Med School:** Vanderbilt Univ 1976; **Resid:** Internal Medicine, Tulane Univ Med Ctr 1979; Pediatrics, Med Coll Virginia 1981; **Fellow:** Hematology & Oncology, Vanderbilt Univ Med Ctr 1984; **Fac Appt:** Prof Med, Vanderbilt Univ

Lin, Weei-Chin MD/PhD [Hem] - **Spec Exp:** Hematologic Malignancies; Bleeding/Coagulation Disorders; **Hospital:** Univ of Ala Hosp at Birmingham; **Address:** Univ of Alabama, 1530 3rd Ave S, Ste 520A, Birmingham, AL 35294; **Phone:** 205-934-3980; **Board Cert:** Internal Medicine 1996; Hematology 1999; Medical Oncology 1999; **Med School:** Taiwan 1986; **Resid:** Internal Medicine, Duke Univ Med Ctr 1996; **Fellow:** Hematology & Oncology, Duke Univ Med Ctr 1999; **Fac Appt:** Assoc Prof Med, Univ Ala

List, Alan F MD [Hem] - **Spec Exp:** Myelodysplastic Syndromes; Leukemia; **Hospital:** H Lee Moffitt Cancer Ctr & Research Inst; **Address:** 12902 Magnolia Drive, SRB 4, Tampa, FL 33612-9497; **Phone:** 813-745-6086; **Board Cert:** Internal Medicine 1983; Medical Oncology 1985; Hematology 1986; **Med School:** Univ Pennsylvania 1980; **Resid:** Internal Medicine, Good Samaritan Hosp 1983; Oncology, Vanderbilt Univ Med Ctr 1985; **Fellow:** Hematology, Vanderbilt Univ Med Ctr 1986

Ortel, Thomas L MD/PhD [Hem] - **Spec Exp:** Bleeding/Coagulation Disorders; Hemophilia; **Hospital:** Duke Univ Med Ctr; **Address:** Duke Medical Ctr, Box 3422, Durham, NC 27710; **Phone:** 919-668-6688; **Board Cert:** Internal Medicine 1988; Hematology 2002; **Med School:** Indiana Univ 1985; **Resid:** Internal Medicine, Duke Univ Med Ctr 1988; **Fellow:** Hematology & Oncology, Duke Univ Med Ctr 1989; **Fac Appt:** Prof Med, Duke Univ

Powell, Bayard L MD [Hem] - **Spec Exp:** Leukemia; Myelodysplastic Syndromes; **Hospital:** Wake Forest Univ Baptist Med Ctr (page 73); **Address:** Wake Forest Univ Baptist Med Ctr, Med Ctr Blvd-Cancer Center, Winston-Salem, NC 27157; **Phone:** 336-716-7970; **Board Cert:** Internal Medicine 1983; Medical Oncology 1985; **Med School:** Univ NC Sch Med 1980; **Resid:** Internal Medicine, NC Baptist Hospital 1983; **Fellow:** Hematology & Oncology, Wake Forest Univ Sch Med 1986; **Fac Appt:** Prof Med, Wake Forest Univ

Rosenblatt, Joseph D MD [Hem] - **Spec Exp:** Lymphoma; Leukemia; Multiple Myeloma; **Hospital:** Univ of Miami Hosp & Clins/Sylvester Comp Canc Ctr, Jackson Meml Hosp; **Address:** Sylvester Comprehensive Cancer Ctr, 1475 NW 12th Ave, D8-4, Ste 3300, Miami, FL 33136; **Phone:** 305-243-4909; **Board Cert:** Internal Medicine 1983; Medical Oncology 1985; **Med School:** UCLA 1980; **Resid:** Internal Medicine, UCLA Medical Ctr 1983; **Fellow:** Hematology & Oncology, UCLA Medical Ctr 1986; **Fac Appt:** Prof Med, Univ Miami Sch Med

Schwartzberg, Lee S MD [Hem] - **Spec Exp:** Breast Cancer; Lung Cancer; Stem Cell Transplant; **Hospital:** Baptist Memorial Hospital - Memphis; **Address:** The West Clinic, 100 N Humphreys Blvd, Memphis, TN 38120; **Phone:** 901-683-0055; **Board Cert:** Internal Medicine 1983; Hematology 1986; Medical Oncology 1985; **Med School:** NY Med Coll 1980; **Resid:** Internal Medicine, North Shore Univ Hosp 1983; Internal Medicine, Meml Sloan Kettering Cancer Ctr 1985; **Fellow:** Hematology & Oncology, Meml Sloan Kettering Cancer Ctr 1984; Hematology & Oncology, Meml Sloan Kettering Cancer Ctr 1987; **Fac Appt:** Assoc Prof Med, Univ Tenn Coll Med, Memphis

Solberg, Lawrence MD/PhD [Hem] - **Spec Exp:** Bone Marrow Transplant; Myeloproliferative Disorders; Porphyria; **Hospital:** Mayo - Jacksonville, St Luke's Hosp - Jacksonville; **Address:** Mayo Clinic-Dept Hem-Onc, 4500 San Pablo Rd Fl 8, Jacksonville, FL 32224; **Phone:** 904-953-7292; **Board Cert:** Internal Medicine 1978; Hematology 1980; **Med School:** St Louis Univ 1975; **Resid:** Internal Medicine, Mayo Clinic 1978; **Fellow:** Hematology, Mayo Clinic 1980; **Fac Appt:** Prof Med, Mayo Med Sch

Telen, Marilyn J MD [Hem] - **Spec Exp:** Transfusion Medicine; Anemia & Red Cell Disorders; Sickle Cell Disease; **Hospital:** Duke Univ Med Ctr; **Address:** Duke Univ Med Ctr, Box 2615, Durham, NC 27710; **Phone:** 919-684-5426; **Board Cert:** Internal Medicine 1980; Hematology 1984; **Med School:** NYU Sch Med 1977; **Resid:** Internal Medicine, Erie Co Med Cr 1980; **Fellow:** Hematology, Duke Univ Med Ctr 1983; **Fac Appt:** Prof Med, Duke Univ

Zuckerman, Kenneth S MD [Hem] - **Spec Exp:** Myeloproliferative Disorders; Leukemia; Lymphoma; Anemia; **Hospital:** H Lee Moffitt Cancer Ctr & Research Inst, Tampa Genl Hosp; **Address:** H Lee Moffitt Cancer Ctr, 12902 Magnolia Drive, SRB4, Tampa, FL 33612-9416; **Phone:** 813-745-8090; **Board Cert:** Internal Medicine 1975; Hematology 1978; **Med School:** Ohio State Univ 1972; **Resid:** Internal Medicine, Ohio State Univ Hosps 1975; **Fellow:** Hematology, Brigham Hosp/Harvard Univ 1978; **Fac Appt:** Prof Med, Univ S Fla Coll Med

Hematology

Midwest

Baron, Joseph M MD [Hem] - **Spec Exp:** Bleeding/Coagulation Disorders; Lymphoma; Myelo-proliferative Disorders; **Hospital:** Univ of Chicago Hosps; **Address:** 5758 S Maryland Ave, MC 9015, Chicago, IL 60637-1463; **Phone:** 773-702-6149; **Board Cert:** Internal Medicine 1969; Hematology 1972; Medical Oncology 1975; **Med School:** Univ Chicago-Pritzker Sch Med 1962; **Resid:** Internal Medicine, Univ Chicago Hosps 1964; **Fellow:** Hematology, Univ Chicago Hosps 1968; **Fac Appt:** Assoc Prof Med, Univ Chicago-Pritzker Sch Med

Blinder, Morey MD [Hem] - **Spec Exp:** Bleeding/Coagulation Disorders; Anemia; Sickle Cell Disease; **Hospital:** Barnes-Jewish Hosp; **Address:** Barnes Jewish Hospital, Div Hematology, 660 S Euclid Ave, Box 8125, St Louis, MO 63110; **Phone:** 314-362-8808; **Board Cert:** Internal Medicine 1984; Hematology 1988; Medical Oncology 1987; **Med School:** St Louis Univ 1981; **Resid:** Internal Medicine, Univ Illinois Hosp 1984; **Fellow:** Hematology & Oncology, Univ Wash Med Ctr 1986; **Fac Appt:** Assoc Prof Med, Washington Univ, St Louis

Bockenstedt, Paula MD [Hem] - **Spec Exp:** Bleeding/Coagulation Disorders; Leukemia; Von Willebrand's Disease; **Hospital:** Univ Michigan Hlth Sys; **Address:** Div Hematology, 1500 E Med Ctr Dr, MIB, rm C-344, Ann Arbor, MI 48109-8048; **Phone:** 734-647-8921; **Board Cert:** Internal Medicine 1981; Hematology 1984; **Med School:** Harvard Med Sch 1978; **Resid:** Internal Medicine, Brigham-Womens Hosp 1981; **Fellow:** Hematology, Brigham-Womens Hosp 1984; **Fac Appt:** Assoc Clin Prof Med, Univ Mich Med Sch

Di Persio, John MD/PhD [Hem] - **Spec Exp:** Bone Marrow Transplant; Hematologic Malignancies; Leukemia; **Hospital:** Barnes-Jewish Hosp; **Address:** Wash Univ Sch Med, Sect Bone Marrow Transplant & Leukemia, 660 S Euclid Ave, Box 8007, St Louis, MO 63110; **Phone:** 314-454-8306; **Board Cert:** Internal Medicine 1984; Medical Oncology 1987; Hematology 1988; **Med School:** Univ Rochester 1980; **Resid:** Internal Medicine, Parkland Meml Hosp 1984; **Fellow:** Hematology & Oncology, UCLA Sch Med 1987; **Fac Appt:** Prof Med, Washington Univ, St Louis

Erba, Harry P MD/PhD [Hem] - **Spec Exp:** Leukemia; Myelodysplastic Syndromes; Lymphoma; **Hospital:** Univ Michigan Hlth Sys; **Address:** Univ Michigan Medical Ctr, 1500 Medical Center Dr, rm C348 MIB, Ann Arbor, MI 48109-5848; **Phone:** 734-647-8901; **Board Cert:** Internal Medicine 2004; Hematology 2004; Medical Oncology 2005; **Med School:** Stanford Univ 1988; **Resid:** Internal Medicine, Brigham & Womens Hosp 1990; **Fellow:** Hematology & Oncology, Brigham & Womens Hosp 1993; **Fac Appt:** Assoc Prof Med, Univ Mich Med Sch

Farag, Sherif S MD/PhD [Hem] - **Spec Exp:** Multiple Myeloma; Leukemia & Lymphoma; Bone Marrow Transplant; Stem Cell Transplant; **Hospital:** Indiana Univ Hosp; **Address:** 1044 W Walnut St, Ste 202, Indianapolis, IN 46202; **Phone:** 317-274-0843; **Med School:** Australia 1995; **Resid:** Internal Medicine, Univ Melbourne Med Ctr; **Fellow:** Hematology & Oncology, Roswell Park Cancer Inst; **Fac Appt:** Assoc Prof Med, Indiana Univ

Flynn, Patrick MD [Hem] - **Spec Exp:** Hematologic Malignancies; Colon & Rectal Cancer; Clinical Trials; **Hospital:** Abbott - Northwestern Hosp, Fairview Southdale Hosp; **Address:** 800 E 28th St, Piper Bldg, Ste 405, Minneapolis, MN 55407; **Phone:** 612-863-8585; **Board Cert:** Internal Medicine 1978; Medical Oncology 1981; Hematology 1982; **Med School:** Univ Minn 1975; **Resid:** Internal Medicine, Hennepin Co Med Ctr 1978; **Fellow:** Hematology & Oncology, Univ Minnesota Hosp 1981

Gaynor, Ellen MD [Hem] - **Spec Exp:** Lymphoma; Genitourinary Cancer; Breast Cancer; **Hospital:** Loyola Univ Med Ctr; **Address:** Loyola Univ Med Ctr, Dept Hematology, 2160 S First Ave Bldg 112 - rm 108, Maywood, IL 60153-3328; **Phone:** 708-327-3214; **Board Cert:** Internal Medicine 1982; Hematology 1986; Medical Oncology 1985; **Med School:** Univ Wisc 1978; **Resid:** Internal Medicine, Loyola Univ Med Ctr 1982; **Fellow:** Medical Oncology, Loyola Univ Med Ctr 1981; Hematology & Oncology, Univ Chicago Hosp 1984; **Fac Appt:** Prof Med, Loyola Univ-Stritch Sch Med

Gertz, Morris MD [Hem] - **Spec Exp:** Multiple Myeloma; Amyloidosis; Waldenstrom's Macroglobulinemia; Plasma Cell Disorders; **Hospital:** Mayo Med Ctr & Clin - Rochester, Rochester Methodist Hosp; **Address:** 200 SW 1st St Fl W10, Rochester, MN 55905; **Phone:** 507-284-2511; **Board Cert:** Internal Medicine 1979; Hematology 1982; Medical Oncology 1983; **Med School:** Loyola Univ-Stritch Sch Med 1975; **Resid:** Internal Medicine, St Lukes Hosp 1979; **Fellow:** Hematology & Oncology, Mayo Clin 1982; **Fac Appt:** Prof Med, Mayo Med Sch

Godwin, John MD [Hem] - **Spec Exp:** Thrombotic Disorders; Leukemia in Elderly; **Hospital:** St John's Hosp - Springfield, Memorial Med Ctr - Springfield; **Address:** SIU School Medicine, Simmons Cooper Cancer Inst, PO Box 19678, Springfield, IL 62794; **Phone:** 217-545-5817; **Board Cert:** Internal Medicine 1981; Hematology 1986; **Med School:** Univ Ala 1978; **Resid:** Internal Medicine, Baylor Coll Med 1981; Internal Medicine, Baylor Coll Med 1982; **Fellow:** Hematology, Baylor Coll Med 1983; Hematology, North Carolina Meml Hosp 1985; **Fac Appt:** Prof Med, Southern IL Univ

Gordon, Leo I MD [Hem] - **Spec Exp:** Lymphoma, Non-Hodgkin's; Hodgkin's Disease; Bone Marrow Transplant; **Hospital:** Northwestern Meml Hosp; **Address:** 675 N St Clair St, Ste 850, Chicago, IL 60611-3124; **Phone:** 312-695-0990; **Board Cert:** Internal Medicine 1976; Hematology 1978; Medical Oncology 1979; **Med School:** Univ Cincinnati 1973; **Resid:** Internal Medicine, Univ Chicago Hosps 1976; **Fellow:** Hematology, Univ Minnesota Hosps 1978; Hematology & Oncology, Univ Chicago Hosps 1979; **Fac Appt:** Prof Med, Northwestern Univ

Gregory, Stephanie A MD [Hem] - **Spec Exp:** Lymphoma; Leukemia; Plasma Cell Disorders; Multiple Myeloma; **Hospital:** Rush Univ Med Ctr; **Address:** 1725 W Harrison St, Ste 834, Rush Professional Office Bldg, Chicago, IL 60612-3861; **Phone:** 312-942-5982; **Board Cert:** Internal Medicine 1972; Hematology 1972; **Med School:** Med Coll PA Hahnemann 1965; **Resid:** Internal Medicine, Rush/Presby-St Luke's Med Ctr 1969; **Fellow:** Hematology, Rush/Presby-St Luke's Med Ctr 1972; **Fac Appt:** Prof Med, Rush Med Coll

Greipp, Philip R MD [Hem] - **Spec Exp:** Multiple Myeloma; **Hospital:** Mayo Med Ctr & Clin - Rochester; **Address:** Mayo Clinic, Div Hematology, 200 First St SW Mayo Bldg Fl W-10, Rochester, MN 55905-0001; **Phone:** 507-284-3159; **Board Cert:** Internal Medicine 1974; Hematology 1994; **Med School:** Georgetown Univ 1968; **Resid:** Internal Medicine, Mayo Clinic 1973; **Fellow:** Hematology, Mayo Clinic 1975; **Fac Appt:** Prof Med, Mayo Med Sch

Grever, Michael R MD [Hem] - **Spec Exp:** Hematologic Malignancies; Leukemia; Drug Development; Clinical Trials; **Hospital:** Ohio St Univ Med Ctr; **Address:** 215 Means Hall, 1654 Upham Drive, Columbus, OH 43210; **Phone:** 614-293-8724; **Board Cert:** Internal Medicine 1975; Hematology 1988; Medical Oncology 1979; **Med School:** Univ Pittsburgh 1971; **Resid:** Internal Medicine, Presby-Univ Hosp 1974; **Fellow:** Hematology & Oncology, Ohio State Univ 1978; **Fac Appt:** Prof Med, Ohio State Univ

Habermann, Thomas M MD [Hem] - **Spec Exp:** Lymphoma; Hodgkin's Disease; Leukemia; **Hospital:** Mayo Med Ctr & Clin - Rochester; **Address:** Mayo Clinic, 200 1st St SW, Rochester, MN 55905; **Phone:** 507-284-0923; **Board Cert:** Internal Medicine 1982; Hematology 1984; **Med School:** Creighton Univ 1979; **Resid:** Internal Medicine, Mayo Clinic 1982; **Fellow:** Hematology, Mayo Clinic 1985; **Fac Appt:** Prof Med, Mayo Med Sch

Hematology

Kraut, Eric H MD [Hem] - **Spec Exp:** Hematologic Malignancies; Leukemia; Drug Development; Clinical Trials; **Hospital:** Ohio St Univ Med Ctr; **Address:** B405 Starling Loving Hall, 320 W 10th Ave, Columbus, OH 43210; **Phone:** 614-293-2887; **Board Cert:** Internal Medicine 1975; Hematology 1978; Medical Oncology 1977; **Med School:** Temple Univ 1972; **Resid:** Internal Medicine, Univ Pittsburgh 1975; **Fellow:** Hematology & Oncology, Ohio State Univ Hosp 1977; **Fac Appt:** Prof Med, Ohio State Univ

Kuriakose, Philip MD [Hem] - **Spec Exp:** Leukemia; **Hospital:** Henry Ford Hosp; **Address:** Henry Ford Hosp, Hematology/Oncology, 2799 W Grand Blvd, Detroit, MI 48202; **Phone:** 313-916-1841; **Board Cert:** Internal Medicine 1999; Medical Oncology 2002; Hematology 2002; **Med School:** India 1990; **Resid:** Internal Medicine, Christian Med Coll 1992; Internal Medicine, Henry Ford Hosp 1994; **Fellow:** Hematology & Oncology, Mayo Clinic 1995

Kuzel, Timothy M MD [Hem] - **Spec Exp:** Kidney Cancer; Melanoma; Bladder Cancer; Lymphoma; **Hospital:** Northwestern Meml Hosp; **Address:** Northwestern Meml Hosp, 675 N St Clair, Ste 21-100, Chicago, IL 60611; **Phone:** 312-695-0990; **Board Cert:** Internal Medicine 1987; Hematology 2000; Medical Oncology 1989; **Med School:** Univ Mich Med Sch 1984; **Resid:** Internal Medicine, McGraw MC-Northwestern Univ 1987; **Fellow:** Hematology & Oncology, McGraw MC-Northwestern Univ 1990; **Fac Appt:** Prof Med, Northwestern Univ

Larson, Richard A MD [Hem] - **Spec Exp:** Leukemia & Lymphoma; Bone Marrow Transplant; Myelodysplastic Syndromes; **Hospital:** Univ of Chicago Hosps; **Address:** Univ Chicago Hospitals, 5841 S Maryland Ave, MC 2115, Chicago, IL 60637; **Phone:** 773-702-6149; **Board Cert:** Internal Medicine 1980; Hematology 1982; Medical Oncology 1983; **Med School:** Stanford Univ 1977; **Resid:** Internal Medicine, Univ Chicago Hosps 1980; **Fellow:** Hematology & Oncology, Univ Chicago Hosps 1983; **Fac Appt:** Prof Med, Univ Chicago-Pritzker Sch Med

Laughlin, Mary J MD [Hem] - **Spec Exp:** Bone Marrow Transplant; **Hospital:** Univ Hosps Case Med Ctr; **Address:** 2103 Cornell Rd, WRB 2-129, Cleveland, OH 44106; **Phone:** 216-844-5182; **Board Cert:** Internal Medicine 2003; Hematology 2004; **Med School:** SUNY Buffalo 1988; **Resid:** Internal Medicine, Duke Univ Med Ctr 1991; **Fellow:** Hematology & Oncology, Duke Univ Med Ctr 1992; Bone Marrow Transplant, Rosewell Park Cancer Inst 1994; **Fac Appt:** Assoc Prof Med, Case West Res Univ

Lazarus, Hillard M MD [Hem] - **Spec Exp:** Bone Marrow Transplant; Stem Cell Transplant; Leukemia; **Hospital:** Univ Hosps Case Med Ctr; **Address:** 11100 Euclid Ave, Cleveland, OH 44106-5065; **Phone:** 216-844-3629; **Board Cert:** Internal Medicine 1977; Medical Oncology 1979; Hematology 1980; **Med School:** Univ Rochester 1974; **Resid:** Internal Medicine, Univ Hosps 1977; **Fellow:** Hematology & Oncology, Univ Hosps 1979; **Fac Appt:** Prof Med, Case West Res Univ

Litzow, Mark R MD [Hem] - **Spec Exp:** Bone Marrow Transplant; Leukemia; **Hospital:** Mayo Med Ctr & Clin - Rochester; **Address:** Mayo Clinic, Div Hematology, 200 First St SW, Rochester, MN 55905; **Phone:** 507-284-0923; **Board Cert:** Internal Medicine 1983; Hematology 1988; Medical Oncology 1989; **Med School:** Univ Chicago-Pritzker Sch Med 1980; **Resid:** Internal Medicine, Mayo Clinic 1984; **Fellow:** Medical Oncology, Mayo Clinic 1990; **Fac Appt:** Asst Prof Med, Mayo Med Sch

Maciejewski, Jaroslaw P MD/PhD [Hem] - **Spec Exp:** Anemia-Aplastic; Hematologic Malignancies; Stem Cell Transplant; **Hospital:** Cleveland Clin Fdn (page 56); **Address:** Cleveland Clinic, 9500 Euclid Ave, Desk R40, Cleveland, OH 44195; **Phone:** 216-445-5962; **Board Cert:** Internal Medicine 1999; Hematology 2001; **Med School:** Germany 1990; **Resid:** Internal Medicine, Univ Nevada Med Ctr 1997; **Fellow:** Hematology, Natl Inst Hlth 2000

McGlave, Philip B MD [Hem] - **Spec Exp:** Leukemia; Bone Marrow Transplant; **Hospital:** Univ Minn Med Ctr, Fairview - Univ Campus; **Address:** Univ Minn, Dept Med - Div Hem/Onc, Mayo Mail Code 480, 420 Delaware St SE, Minneapolis, MN 55455; **Phone:** 612-626-2446; **Board Cert:** Internal Medicine 1977; Hematology 1980; **Med School:** Univ IL Coll Med 1974; **Resid:** Internal Medicine, Univ Minn 1977; **Fellow:** Hematology & Oncology, Univ Minn 1980; **Fac Appt:** Prof Med, Univ Minn

Mosher, Deane F MD [Hem] - **Hospital:** Univ WI Hosp & Clins; **Address:** Univ Wisc Hosp, Dept Hematology, 600 Highland Ave Fl 5, Madison, WI 53792; **Phone:** 608-263-7022; **Board Cert:** Internal Medicine 1973; Hematology 1980; **Med School:** Harvard Med Sch 1968; **Resid:** Internal Medicine, Beth Israel Hosp 1970; **Fellow:** Hematology, Harvard Med Sch 1972; **Fac Appt:** Prof Med, Univ Wisc

Nand, Sucha MD [Hem] - **Spec Exp:** Myelodysplastic Syndromes; Myeloproliferative Disorders; Leukemia; **Hospital:** Loyola Univ Med Ctr; **Address:** Cardinal Bernardin Cancer Ctr, 2160 S First Ave Bldg 112 - rm 342, Maywood, IL 60153-3304; **Phone:** 708-327-3217; **Board Cert:** Internal Medicine 1979; Medical Oncology 1981; Hematology 1982; **Med School:** India 1971; **Resid:** Physical Medicine & Rehabilitation, Northwestern Meml Hosp 1976; Internal Medicine, North Chicago VA Hosp 1978; **Fellow:** Medical Oncology, Northwestern Meml Hosp 1981; **Fac Appt:** Prof Med, Loyola Univ-Stritch Sch Med

Palascak, Joseph E MD [Hem] - **Spec Exp:** Hemophilia; Bleeding/Coagulation Disorders; Thrombotic Disorders; **Hospital:** Univ Hosp - Cincinnati; **Address:** Univ Cincinnati, Div Hem/Onc, 231 Albert Sabin Way, Box 670562, Cincinnati, OH 45267-0562; **Phone:** 513-584-1937; **Board Cert:** Internal Medicine 1975; Hematology 1978; **Med School:** Jefferson Med Coll 1968; **Resid:** Internal Medicine, Thomas Jefferson Univ Hosp 1971; **Fellow:** Hematology, Thomas Jefferson Univ Hosp 1972; Hematology, Thomas Jefferson Univ Hosp 1976; **Fac Appt:** Prof Med, Univ Cincinnati

Porcu, Pierluigi MD [Hem] - **Spec Exp:** Lymphoma; Lymphoma, Non-Hodgkin's; Immunotherapy; **Hospital:** Ohio St Univ Med Ctr; **Address:** 320 W 10th Ave, B320 Starling Loving Hall, Columbus, OH 43210; **Phone:** 614-293-9273; **Board Cert:** Hematology 1999; Medical Oncology 1999; **Med School:** Italy 1987; **Resid:** Internal Medicine, Indiana Univ Hosp 1996; **Fellow:** Hematology & Oncology, Indiana Univ Hosp 1999; **Fac Appt:** Asst Prof Med, Ohio State Univ

Silverstein, Roy L MD [Hem] - **Spec Exp:** Thrombotic Disorders; Bleeding/Coagulation Disorders; **Hospital:** Cleveland Clin Fdn (page 56); **Address:** Dept Cell Biology, 9500 Euclid Ave, NC10, Cleveland, OH 44195; **Phone:** 216-444-5220; **Board Cert:** Internal Medicine 1982; Hematology 1984; Medical Oncology 1985; **Med School:** Emory Univ 1979; **Resid:** Internal Medicine, New York Hosp-Cornell Med Ctr 1982; Hematology & Oncology, New York Hosp-Cornell Med Ctr 1984; **Fac Appt:** Prof Med, Cleveland Cl Coll Med/Case West Res

Singhal, Seema MD [Hem] - **Spec Exp:** Multiple Myeloma; **Hospital:** Northwestern Meml Hosp; **Address:** 675 N St Claire St, Ste 21-100, Chicago, IL 60611; **Phone:** 312-695-0990; **Board Cert:** Internal Medicine 2005; **Med School:** India 1989; **Resid:** Internal Medicine, King Edward Meml Hosp 1991; Hematology, King Edward Meml Hosp 1991; **Fellow:** Bone Marrow Transplant, Hadassah Univ Hosp 1992; **Fac Appt:** Prof Med, Northwestern Univ

Stiff, Patrick J MD [Hem] - **Spec Exp:** Bone Marrow Transplant; Lymphoma, Non-Hodgkin's; Leukemia; **Hospital:** Loyola Univ Med Ctr; **Address:** Cardinal Bernadin Cancer Ctr, 2160 S First Ave Bldg 112 - rm 255, Maywood, IL 60153; **Phone:** 708-327-3304; **Board Cert:** Internal Medicine 1978; Medical Oncology 1981; Hematology 1982; **Med School:** Loyola Univ-Stritch Sch Med 1975; **Resid:** Internal Medicine, Cleveland Clinic 1978; **Fellow:** Hematology & Oncology, Meml Sloan Kettering Cancer Ctr 1981; **Fac Appt:** Prof Med, Loyola Univ-Stritch Sch Med

Hematology

Tallman, Martin S MD [Hem] - **Spec Exp:** Bone Marrow Transplant; Leukemia; Lymphoma; **Hospital:** Northwestern Meml Hosp; **Address:** 675 N St Clair St, Ste 21-100, Chicago, IL 60611; **Phone:** 312-695-0990; **Board Cert:** Internal Medicine 1983; Medical Oncology 1987; Hematology 1988; **Med School:** Ros Franklin Univ/Chicago Med Sch 1980; **Resid:** Internal Medicine, Evanston Hosp 1983; **Fellow:** Medical Oncology, Fred Hutchinson Cancer Ctr 1987; **Fac Appt:** Prof Med, Northwestern Univ

van Besien, Koen W MD [Hem] - **Spec Exp:** Lymphoma; Stem Cell Transplant; **Hospital:** Univ of Chicago Hosps; **Address:** Stem Cell Transplant Program, 5841 S Maryland Ave, MC 2115, Chicago, IL 60637; **Phone:** 773-702-4400; **Board Cert:** Internal Medicine 2005; Medical Oncology 2005; Hematology 2006; **Med School:** Belgium 1984; **Resid:** Internal Medicine, Univ Leuven Med Ctr 1987; **Fellow:** Hematology & Oncology, Indiana Univ Med Ctr 1990; **Fac Appt:** Prof Med, Univ Chicago-Pritzker Sch Med

Winter, Jane N MD [Hem] - **Spec Exp:** Lymphoma, Non-Hodgkin's; Hodgkin's Disease; Bone Marrow Transplant; **Hospital:** Northwestern Meml Hosp; **Address:** Northwestern Univ - Div Hem/Oncology, 675 N St Clair St, Ste 21-100, Chicago, IL 60611; **Phone:** 312-695-0990; **Board Cert:** Internal Medicine 1980; Hematology 1982; Medical Oncology 1983; **Med School:** Univ Pennsylvania 1977; **Resid:** Internal Medicine, Univ Chicago Hosps 1980; **Fellow:** Hematology & Oncology, Columbia Presby Hosp 1981; Hematology & Oncology, Northwestern Univ 1983; **Fac Appt:** Prof Med, Northwestern Univ

Great Plains and Mountains

Vose, Julie M MD [Hem] - **Spec Exp:** Lymphoma; **Hospital:** Nebraska Med Ctr; **Address:** 987680 Nebraska Med Ctr, Emile @ 42nd St, Omaha, NE 68198-7680; **Phone:** 402-559-5600; **Board Cert:** Internal Medicine 1987; Hematology 2000; Medical Oncology 2000; **Med School:** Univ Nebr Coll Med 1984; **Resid:** Internal Medicine, Univ Nebraska Med Ctr 1987; **Fellow:** Hematology & Oncology, Univ Nebraska Med Ctr 1990; **Fac Appt:** Prof Med, Univ Nebr Coll Med

Southwest

Barlogie, Bart MD/PhD [Hem] - **Spec Exp:** Bone Marrow Transplant; Plasma Cell Disorders; Multiple Myeloma; **Hospital:** UAMS Med Ctr; **Address:** UAMS-Myeloma Inst Rsch & Therapy, 4301 West Markham St, Slot 816, Little Rock, AR 72205; **Phone:** 501-603-1583; **Med School:** Germany 1969; **Resid:** Internal Medicine, Univ Muenster Med Sch; **Fellow:** Medical Oncology, MD Anderson Cancer Ctr-Tumor Inst 1976; **Fac Appt:** Prof Med, Univ Ark

Boldt, David H MD [Hem] - **Spec Exp:** Leukemia; Lymphoma; Multiple Myeloma; **Hospital:** Univ Hlth Sys - Univ Hosp (San Antonio, TX); **Address:** UT Hlth Sci Ctr, Div Hematology, 7703 Floyd Curl Drive, MC 7880, San Antonio, TX 78229; **Phone:** 210-567-4848; **Board Cert:** Internal Medicine 1973; Hematology 1974; Medical Oncology 1975; **Med School:** Tufts Univ 1969; **Resid:** Internal Medicine, Barnes Hosp-Wash Univ 1971; **Fellow:** Hematology & Oncology, Barnes Hosp 1973; **Fac Appt:** Prof Med, Univ Tex, San Antonio

Brenner, Malcolm K MD/PhD [Hem] - **Spec Exp:** Gene Therapy; Bone Marrow Transplant; **Hospital:** Methodist Hosp - Houston, Texas Chldns Hosp - Houston; **Address:** 6621 Fannin St, rm 3-3320, Houston, TX 77030; **Phone:** 832-824-4671; **Med School:** England 1975; **Resid:** Internal Medicine, Cambridge Univ 1979; **Fellow:** Immunology, Clinical Research Ctr 1984; Hematology & Oncology, Royal Free Hospital 1986; **Fac Appt:** Prof Med, Baylor Coll Med

Champlin, Richard E MD [Hem] - **Spec Exp:** Bone Marrow Transplant; Stem Cell Transplant; Leukemia & Lymphoma; **Hospital:** UT MD Anderson Cancer Ctr; **Address:** MD Anderson Cancer Ctr, Stem Cell Transplantation Ctr, 1515 Holcombe Blvd, Box 0423, Houston, TX 77030; **Phone:** 713-792-6100; **Board Cert:** Internal Medicine 1978; Hematology 1980; Medical Oncology 1981; **Med School:** Univ Chicago-Pritzker Sch Med 1975; **Resid:** Internal Medicine, LA Co Harbor/UCLA Med Ctr 1978; **Fellow:** Hematology & Oncology, LA Co Harbor/UCLA Med Ctr 1980; **Fac Appt:** Prof Med, Univ Tex, Houston

Cobos, Everardo MD [Hem] - **Spec Exp:** Bone Marrow Transplant; Bleeding/Coagulation Disorders; **Hospital:** Univ Med Ctr - Lubbock; **Address:** Texas Tech Univ Med Sch, Dept Med, 3601 4th St, MS 9410, Lubbock, TX 79430; **Phone:** 806-743-3155; **Board Cert:** Internal Medicine 1985; Medical Oncology 1987; Hematology 1988; **Med School:** Univ Tex, San Antonio 1981; **Resid:** Internal Medicine, Letterman Army Med Ctr 1985; **Fellow:** Hematology & Oncology, Letterman Army Med Ctr 1988; **Fac Appt:** Prof Med, Texas Tech Univ

Cooper, Barry MD [Hem] - **Spec Exp:** Leukemia; Lymphoma; Bleeding/Coagulation Disorders; **Hospital:** Baylor Univ Medical Ctr; **Address:** 3535 Worth St, Ste 200, Dallas, TX 75246-2096; **Phone:** 214-370-1002; **Board Cert:** Internal Medicine 1974; Medical Oncology 1977; Hematology 1978; **Med School:** Johns Hopkins Univ 1971; **Resid:** Internal Medicine, Johns Hopkins Hosp 1973; **Fellow:** Metabolism, Natl Inst of Health 1975; Hematology, Peter Bent Brigham Hosp 1977; **Fac Appt:** Clin Prof Med, Univ Tex SW, Dallas

Emanuel, Peter D MD [Hem] - **Spec Exp:** Lymphoma; Leukemia; Hodgkin's Disease; Multiple Myeloma; **Hospital:** UAMS Med Ctr; **Address:** 4301 W Markham, Slot 623, Little Rock, AR 72205; **Phone:** 501-526-2272; **Board Cert:** Internal Medicine 1988; **Med School:** Univ Wisc 1985; **Resid:** Internal Medicine, Univ Alabama Hosp 1988; **Fellow:** Hematology & Oncology, Univ Alabama 1991; **Fac Appt:** Prof Med, Univ Ark

Fonseca, Rafael MD [Hem] - **Spec Exp:** Multiple Myeloma; **Hospital:** Mayo Clinic - Scottsdale; **Address:** 13400 E Shea Blvd, MCCRB 3-001, Scottsdale, AZ 85259; **Phone:** 480-301-4280; **Board Cert:** Hematology 1998; Medical Oncology 1997; **Med School:** Mexico 1991; **Resid:** Internal Medicine, Jackson Meml Hosp 1994; **Fellow:** Hematology & Oncology, Mayo Clinic 1998; **Fac Appt:** Assoc Prof Med, Mayo Med Sch

Kantarjian, Hagop M MD [Hem] - **Spec Exp:** Leukemia; **Hospital:** UT MD Anderson Cancer Ctr; **Address:** 1400 Holcombe Blvd, Unit 428, Houston, TX 77030; **Phone:** 713-792-7026; **Board Cert:** Internal Medicine 1983; Medical Oncology 1985; **Med School:** Lebanon 1979; **Resid:** Internal Medicine, Univ Tex MD Anderson Cancer Ctr 1983; **Fellow:** Hematology & Oncology, Univ Tex MD Anderson Cancer Ctr 1983; **Fac Appt:** Prof Med, Univ Tex, Houston

Keating, Michael MD [Hem] - **Spec Exp:** Leukemia; **Hospital:** UT MD Anderson Cancer Ctr; **Address:** MD Anderson Cancer Ctr, 1515 Holcombe Blvd, Box 428, Houston, TX 77030-4000; **Phone:** 713-745-2376; **Med School:** Australia 1966; **Resid:** Internal Medicine, St Vincents Hosp 1973; **Fellow:** Hematology, MD Anderson Cancer Ctr 1975; **Fac Appt:** Prof Med, Univ Tex, Houston

Lyons, Roger M MD [Hem] - **Spec Exp:** Leukemia & Lymphoma; Multiple Myeloma; Bleeding/Coagulation Disorders; Platelet Disorders; **Hospital:** SW TX Meth Hosp, Methodist Spec & Transpl Hosp; **Address:** 4411 Medical Drive, Ste 100, San Antonio, TX 78229-3325; **Phone:** 210-595-5300; **Board Cert:** Internal Medicine 1981; Hematology 1982; **Med School:** Canada 1967; **Resid:** Internal Medicine, Winnipeg Genl Hosp 1969; Internal Medicine, Barnes-Wohl Hosps 1972; **Fellow:** Hematology, Washington Univ Hosps 1975; **Fac Appt:** Clin Prof Med, Univ Tex, San Antonio

Hematology

Maddox, Anne Marie MD [Hem] - **Spec Exp:** Hematologic Malignancies; Lung Cancer; Head & Neck Cancer; Clinical Trials; **Hospital:** UAMS Med Ctr; **Address:** Univ Arkansas Med Ctr, 4301 W Markham St, Slot 74-5, Little Rock, AR 72205; **Phone:** 501-686-8530; **Board Cert:** Internal Medicine 1979; Medical Oncology 1985; Hematology 2004; **Med School:** Dalhousie Univ 1975; **Resid:** Internal Medicine, Univ Toronto 1978; **Fellow:** Medical Oncology, TX MD Anderson Cancer Ctr 1982; **Fac Appt:** Prof, Univ Ark

Miro-Quesada, Miguel MD [Hem] - **Hospital:** Meml Hermann Hosp - Texas Med Ctr, St Luke's Episcopal Hosp - Houston; **Address:** 920 Frostwood, Ste 780, Houston, TX 77030; **Phone:** 713-827-9525; **Board Cert:** Internal Medicine 1972; Hematology 1974; Medical Oncology 1985; **Med School:** Johns Hopkins Univ 1969; **Resid:** Internal Medicine, Northwestern Univ Hosp 1971; Internal Medicine, Rush-Presby-St Luke's Med Ctr 1972; **Fellow:** Hematology, Montefiore Hosp 1974

Strauss, James F MD [Hem] - **Spec Exp:** Bleeding/Coagulation Disorders; Leukemia; Lymphoma; **Hospital:** Presby Hosp of Dallas; **Address:** Texas Oncology at Presbyterian, 8220 Walnut Hill Ln Bldg 2 - Ste 700, Dallas, TX 75231; **Phone:** 214-739-4175; **Board Cert:** Internal Medicine 1976; Hematology 1978; Medical Oncology 1981; **Med School:** NYU Sch Med 1972; **Resid:** Internal Medicine, Baylor Univ Medical Ctr 1976; **Fellow:** Hematology, Univ Texas SW Medical Ctr 1977

Yeager, Andrew M MD [Hem] - **Spec Exp:** Bone Marrow & Stem Cell Transplant; Graft vs Host Disease; Leukemia; **Hospital:** Univ Med Ctr - Tucson; **Address:** Arizona Cancer Ctr, 1515 N Campbell Ave, Ste 2956, Tucson, AZ 85724-0001; **Phone:** 520-626-0662; **Board Cert:** Pediatrics 1979; Pediatric Hematology-Oncology 1980; **Med School:** Johns Hopkins Univ 1975; **Resid:** Pediatrics, Johns Hopkins Hosp 1978; **Fellow:** Pediatric Hematology-Oncology, Johns Hopkins Hosp 1980; **Fac Appt:** Prof Med, Univ Ariz Coll Med

West Coast and Pacific

Damon, Lloyd E MD [Hem] - **Spec Exp:** Leukemia; Lymphoma; Stem Cell Transplant; **Hospital:** UCSF Med Ctr; **Address:** UCSF Comprehensive Cancer Ctr, 400 Parnassus Ave, Ste A502, San Francisco, CA 94143; **Phone:** 415-353-2421; **Board Cert:** Internal Medicine 1985; Hematology 1988; Medical Oncology 1987; **Med School:** Univ Mich Med Sch 1982; **Resid:** Internal Medicine, UCSF Med Ctr 1985; **Fellow:** Hematology & Oncology, UCSF Med Ctr 1988; **Fac Appt:** Prof Med, UCSF

Forman, Stephen J MD [Hem] - **Spec Exp:** Lymphoma; Leukemia; Bone Marrow Transplant; **Hospital:** City of Hope Natl Med Ctr & Beckman Rsch; **Address:** City Hope National Medical Ctr, 1500 E Duarte Rd, rm 3002, Duarte, CA 91010-3012; **Phone:** 626-256-4673 x62403; **Board Cert:** Internal Medicine 1977; **Med School:** USC Sch Med 1974; **Resid:** Internal Medicine, LAC-Harbor-UCLA Med Ctr 1976; **Fellow:** Hematology, LAC-USC Med Ctr 1978; Hematology, City of Hope Med Ctr 1979; **Fac Appt:** Clin Prof Med, USC Sch Med

Heinrich, Michael C MD [Hem] - **Spec Exp:** Hematologic Malignancies; Sarcoma; Gastrointestinal Stromal Tumors; **Hospital:** VA Medical Center - Portland, OR Hlth & Sci Univ; **Address:** 3710 SW US Veteran's Hospital Rd, Portland, OR 97239; **Phone:** 503-220-8262; **Board Cert:** Internal Medicine 1987; Hematology 2000; Medical Oncology 2001; **Med School:** Johns Hopkins Univ 1984; **Resid:** Internal Medicine, Oreg Hlth Scis Univ 1988; **Fellow:** Hematology & Oncology, Oreg Hlth Scis Univ 1991; **Fac Appt:** Prof Med, Oregon Hlth Sci Univ

Leung, Lawrence L MD [Hem] - **Spec Exp:** Thrombotic Disorders; **Hospital:** Stanford Univ Med Ctr, VA Hlth Care Sys - Palo Alto; **Address:** Stanford Univ Med Ctr, Hematology Div, 269 Campus Drive CCSR Bldg - rm 1155, Stanford, CA 94305-5156; **Phone:** 650-723-9729; **Board Cert:** Internal Medicine 1978; Hematology 1980; Medical Oncology 1981; **Med School:** Columbia P&S 1975; **Resid:** Internal Medicine, NY Hosp/Cornell Med Ctr 1978; **Fellow:** Hematology & Oncology, NY Hosp/Cornell Med Ctr 1981; **Fac Appt:** Prof Med, Stanford Univ

Levine, Alexandra M MD [Hem] - **Spec Exp:** Lymphoma; AIDS Related Cancers; AIDS/HIV; **Hospital:** City of Hope Natl Med Ctr & Beckman Rsch; **Address:** 1500 E Duarte Rd, Needleman 213, Duarte, CA 91010; **Phone:** 626-256-4673; **Med School:** USC Sch Med 1971; **Resid:** Internal Medicine, LAC-USC Med Ctr 1974; **Fellow:** Hematology & Oncology, Grady Meml Hosp-Emory Univ 1975; Hematology, LAC-USC Med Ctr 1978; **Fac Appt:** Prof Med, USC Sch Med

Lill, Michael MD [Hem] - **Spec Exp:** Lymphoma; Leukemia; Stem Cell Transplant; Bone Marrow Transplant; **Hospital:** Cedars-Sinai Med Ctr; **Address:** Cedars-Sinai Med Ctr-Outpt Cancer Ctr, 8700 Beverly Blvd, Ste AC 1070, Los Angeles, CA 90048; **Phone:** 310-423-1160; **Med School:** Australia 1982; **Resid:** Internal Medicine, Sir Charles Gairdner Hospital 1985; **Fellow:** Hematology, Royal Perth Hospital 1988; **Fac Appt:** Prof Med, UCLA

Linenberger, Michael MD [Hem] - **Spec Exp:** Bone Marrow Transplant; Leukemia & Lymphoma; Multiple Myeloma; **Hospital:** Univ Wash Med Ctr; **Address:** 825 Eastlake Ave E, MS G6-800, Seattle, WA 98109; **Phone:** 206-288-1260; **Board Cert:** Internal Medicine 1985; Hematology 1988; **Med School:** Univ Kans 1982; **Resid:** Internal Medicine, Rhode Island Hosp 1985; **Fellow:** Hematology, Univ Wash Med Ctr 1989; **Fac Appt:** Assoc Prof Med, Univ Wash

Linker, Charles A MD [Hem] - **Spec Exp:** Leukemia; Bone Marrow Transplant; Multiple Myeloma; **Hospital:** UCSF Med Ctr, St Francis Memorial Hosp; **Address:** 400 Parnassus Ave, Ste A502, San Francisco, CA 94143; **Phone:** 415-353-2421; **Board Cert:** Internal Medicine 1978; Hematology 1980; Medical Oncology 1981; **Med School:** Stanford Univ 1974; **Resid:** Internal Medicine, Stanford Univ Hosp 1978; **Fellow:** Hematology & Oncology, UCSF Med Ctr 1981; **Fac Appt:** Clin Prof Med, UCSF

Maziarz, Richard MD [Hem] - **Spec Exp:** Leukemia; Immunotherapy; Bone Marrow Transplant; Lymphoma; **Hospital:** OR Hlth & Sci Univ; **Address:** OHSU Ctr Hematologic Malignancies, 3181 SW Sam Jackson Park Rd, UHN 73C, Portland, OR 97239; **Phone:** 503-494-4601; **Board Cert:** Internal Medicine 1982; Hematology 1988; Medical Oncology 1989; **Med School:** Harvard Med Sch 1979; **Resid:** Internal Medicine, Univ Hosp 1982; **Fellow:** Hematology & Oncology, Brigham & Womens Hosp 1988; **Fac Appt:** Prof Med, Oregon Hlth Sci Univ

Negrin, Robert S MD [Hem] - **Spec Exp:** Bone Marrow Transplant; **Hospital:** Stanford Univ Med Ctr; **Address:** BMT Program, 300 Pasteur Drive, rm H3249, MC 5623, Stanford, CA 94305; **Phone:** 650-723-0822; **Board Cert:** Internal Medicine 1987; Hematology 1992; **Med School:** Harvard Med Sch 1984; **Resid:** Internal Medicine, Stanford Univ Hosp 1987; **Fellow:** Hematology, Stanford Univ Hosp 1990; **Fac Appt:** Prof Med, Stanford Univ

O'Donnell, Margaret R MD [Hem] - **Spec Exp:** Leukemia; Clinical Trials; **Hospital:** City of Hope Natl Med Ctr & Beckman Rsch; **Address:** City of Hope National Med Ctr, 1500 E Duarte Rd, MOB-rm 3001, Duarte, CA 91010; **Phone:** 626-359-8111 x62405; **Board Cert:** Internal Medicine 1980; Hematology 1980; Medical Oncology 1979; **Med School:** Med Coll PA 1974; **Resid:** Internal Medicine, Montreal Genl Hosp 1976; Hematology, Royal Victoria Hosp-Montreal 1977; **Fellow:** Hematology & Oncology, Fred Hutchinson Cancer Ctr 1979

Hematology

Saven, Alan MD [Hem] - **Spec Exp:** Leukemia; Lymphoma; **Hospital:** Scripps Green Hosp; **Address:** Scripps Green Hosp, 10666 N Torrey Pines Rd, MS 217, La Jolla, CA 92037; **Phone:** 858-554-9489; **Board Cert:** Internal Medicine 1987; Medical Oncology 1989; **Med School:** South Africa 1982; **Resid:** Internal Medicine, Albert Einstein Med Ctr 1986; **Fellow:** Hematology & Oncology, Scripps Clinic 1987

Schiller, Gary J MD [Hem] - **Spec Exp:** Leukemia; **Hospital:** Ronald Reagan UCLA Med Ctr; **Address:** 10833 Le Conte Ave, rm 42-121 CHS, Los Angeles, CA 90095; **Phone:** 310-825-5513; **Board Cert:** Internal Medicine 1987; Hematology 2000; Medical Oncology 1989; **Med School:** USC Sch Med 1984; **Resid:** Internal Medicine, UCLA Med Ctr 1987; **Fellow:** Hematology & Oncology, UCLA Med Ctr 1990; **Fac Appt:** Prof Med, UCLA

Snyder, David S MD [Hem] - **Spec Exp:** Leukemia; Bone Marrow Transplant; **Hospital:** City of Hope Natl Med Ctr & Beckman Rsch; **Address:** 1500 E Duarte Rd, Duarte, CA 91010-3012; **Phone:** 626-256-4673; **Board Cert:** Internal Medicine 1980; Hematology 1984; **Med School:** Harvard Med Sch 1977; **Resid:** Internal Medicine, Beth Israel Hosp 1980; **Fellow:** Immunology, Harvard Med Sch 1982; Hematology & Oncology, New England Med Ctr 1984

MEDICAL ONCOLOGY

New England

Antin, Joseph H MD [Onc] - **Spec Exp:** Bone Marrow Transplant; Stem Cell Transplant; Leukemia; **Hospital:** Brigham & Women's Hosp, Dana-Farber Cancer Inst; **Address:** 44 Binney St, rm D1B20, Boston, MA 02115-6013; **Phone:** 617-632-3667; **Board Cert:** Internal Medicine 1981; Medical Oncology 1983; Hematology 1984; **Med School:** Cornell Univ-Weill Med Coll 1978; **Resid:** Internal Medicine, Peter Bent Brigham Hosp 1981; **Fellow:** Hematology & Oncology, Brigham & Womens Hosp/Dana Farber 1984; **Fac Appt:** Prof Med, Harvard Med Sch

Atkins, Michael B MD [Onc] - **Spec Exp:** Melanoma; Kidney Cancer; Immunotherapy; **Hospital:** Beth Israel Deaconess Med Ctr - Boston; **Address:** Beth Israel Deaconess Med Ctr, Cancer Clinical Trials 375 Longwood Ave, Masco Bldg Fl 4 - Ste 412, Boston, MA 02215; **Phone:** 617-632-9250; **Board Cert:** Internal Medicine 1983; Medical Oncology 1987; **Med School:** Tufts Univ 1980; **Resid:** Internal Medicine, New England Med Ctr 1983; **Fellow:** Hematology & Oncology, New England Med Ctr 1987; **Fac Appt:** Prof Med, Harvard Med Sch

Burstein, Harold J MD [Onc] - **Spec Exp:** Breast Cancer; **Hospital:** Dana-Farber Cancer Inst, Brigham & Women's Hosp; **Address:** Dana Farber Cancer Inst, 44 Binney St, Ste Mayer 2, Boston, MA 02115; **Phone:** 617-632-4587; **Board Cert:** Internal Medicine 1997; Medical Oncology 2000; **Med School:** Harvard Med Sch 1994; **Resid:** Internal Medicine, Mass Genl Hosp 1996; **Fellow:** Medical Oncology, Dana Farber Cancer Inst 1999; **Fac Appt:** Asst Prof Med, Harvard Med Sch

Canellos, George P MD [Onc] - **Spec Exp:** Lymphoma; Leukemia; Breast Cancer; **Hospital:** Dana-Farber Cancer Inst, Brigham & Women's Hosp; **Address:** 44 Binney St, Boston, MA 02115; **Phone:** 617-632-3470; **Board Cert:** Internal Medicine 1967; Hematology 1972; Medical Oncology 1973; **Med School:** Columbia P&S 1960; **Resid:** Internal Medicine, Mass Genl Hosp 1963; Internal Medicine, Mass Genl Hosp 1966; **Fellow:** Medical Oncology, Natl Cancer Inst 1965; Hematology, Hammersmith Hosp 1967; **Fac Appt:** Prof Med, Harvard Med Sch

America's Top Doctors® 8th Edition

Chabner, Bruce A MD [Onc] - **Spec Exp:** Colon & Rectal Cancer; Breast Cancer; **Hospital:** Mass Genl Hosp; **Address:** Mass General Hospital, 55 Fruit St, Lawrence House 214, Boston, MA 02114; **Phone:** 617-724-3200; **Board Cert:** Internal Medicine 1971; Medical Oncology 1973; **Med School:** Harvard Med Sch 1965; **Resid:** Internal Medicine, Peter Bent Brigham Hosp 1967; Internal Medicine, Yale-New Haven Hosp 1970; **Fellow:** Medical Oncology, Natl Inst Hlth 1969; **Fac Appt:** Prof Med, Harvard Med Sch

Chu, Edward MD [Onc] - **Spec Exp:** Colon & Rectal Cancer; Gastrointestinal Cancer; Clinical Trials; **Hospital:** Yale-New Haven Hosp, VA Conn Hlthcre Sys; **Address:** Yale Cancer Ctr, 333 Cedar St, PO Box 208032, rm WWW221, New Haven, CT 06520-8032; **Phone:** 203-785-6879; **Board Cert:** Internal Medicine 1986; Medical Oncology 1989; **Med School:** Brown Univ 1983; **Resid:** Internal Medicine, Roger Williams Hosp 1987; **Fellow:** Hematology & Oncology, Natl Cancer Inst 1990; Internal Medicine, Natl Cancer Inst 1992; **Fac Appt:** Prof Med, Yale Univ

Come, Steven E MD [Onc] - **Spec Exp:** Breast Cancer; Hodgkin's Disease; **Hospital:** Beth Israel Deaconess Med Ctr - Boston, Dana-Farber Cancer Inst; **Address:** Beth Israel Deaconess Hosp, 330 Brookline Ave, Boston, MA 02215-5400; **Phone:** 617-667-4599; **Board Cert:** Internal Medicine 1975; Medical Oncology 1979; **Med School:** Harvard Med Sch 1972; **Resid:** Internal Medicine, Beth Israel Hosp 1977; **Fellow:** Medical Oncology, Natl Cancer Inst 1976; **Fac Appt:** Assoc Prof Med, Harvard Med Sch

Demetri, George D MD [Onc] - **Spec Exp:** Sarcoma; **Hospital:** Dana-Farber Cancer Inst; **Address:** Dana Farber Cancer Inst, 44 Binney St, D1212, Boston, MA 02115; **Phone:** 617-632-3985; **Board Cert:** Internal Medicine 1986; Medical Oncology 1989; **Med School:** Stanford Univ 1983; **Resid:** Internal Medicine, Univ Wash Med Ctr 1986; **Fellow:** Medical Oncology, Dana Farber Cancer Inst 1989; **Fac Appt:** Assoc Prof Med, Harvard Med Sch

DeVita Jr, Vincent T MD [Onc] - **Spec Exp:** Lymphoma Consultation; Hodgkin's Disease Consultation; **Hospital:** Yale-New Haven Hosp; **Address:** Yale Cancer Ctr, 333 Cedar St, rm WWW-211B, New Haven, CT 06520-8028; **Phone:** 203-737-1010; **Board Cert:** Internal Medicine 1974; Hematology 1972; Medical Oncology 1973; **Med School:** Geo Wash Univ 1961; **Resid:** Internal Medicine, Geo Wash Hosp 1963; Internal Medicine, Yale-New Haven Hosp 1966; **Fellow:** Medical Oncology, Natl Cancer Inst 1965; **Fac Appt:** Prof Med, Yale Univ

Earle, Craig C MD [Onc] - **Spec Exp:** Gastrointestinal Cancer; Liver Cancer; Biliary Cancer; **Hospital:** Dana-Farber Cancer Inst; **Address:** Dana Farber Cancer Institute, 44 Binney St, Boston, MA 02115; **Phone:** 617-632-5564; **Board Cert:** Internal Medicine 2004; Medical Oncology 2000; **Med School:** Univ Ottawa 1990; **Resid:** Internal Medicine, Univ Ottawa 1994; **Fellow:** Medical Oncology, Univ Ottawa 1996; **Fac Appt:** Assoc Prof Med, Harvard Med Sch

Erban III, John K MD [Onc] - **Spec Exp:** Breast Cancer; Hematologic Malignancies; Stem Cell Transplant; **Hospital:** Mass Genl Hosp; **Address:** Mass Genl Hosp, Yawkey Center, Ste 9A, 55 Fruit St, Boston, MA 02114; **Phone:** 617-726-6500; **Board Cert:** Internal Medicine 1984; Medical Oncology 1989; Hematology 1999; **Med School:** Tufts Univ 1981; **Resid:** Internal Medicine, Hosp Univ Penn 1984; **Fellow:** Hematology & Oncology, New England Med Ctr 1990; **Fac Appt:** Assoc Prof Med, Harvard Med Sch

Fuchs, Charles S MD [Onc] - **Spec Exp:** Gastrointestinal Cancer; **Hospital:** Dana-Farber Cancer Inst, Brigham & Women's Hosp; **Address:** 44 Binney St, Dana 1220, Boston, MA 02115; **Phone:** 617-632-5840; **Board Cert:** Internal Medicine 1989; Medical Oncology 2002; **Med School:** Harvard Med Sch 1986; **Resid:** Internal Medicine, Brigham & Womens Hosp 1989; **Fellow:** Hematology & Oncology, Dana Farber Cancer Inst 1992; **Fac Appt:** Assoc Prof Med, Harvard Med Sch

Medical Oncology

Garber, Judy E MD [Onc] - **Spec Exp:** Breast Cancer; **Hospital:** Dana-Farber Cancer Inst; **Address:** Dana Farber Cancer Inst, 44 Binney St, Smith 210, Boston, MA 02115; **Phone:** 617-632-5770; **Board Cert:** Internal Medicine 1984; Medical Oncology 1987; Hematology 1988; **Med School:** Yale Univ 1981; **Resid:** Internal Medicine, Brigham & Womens Hosp 1984; **Fellow:** Medical Oncology, Dana Farber Cancer Inst 1988; Epidemiology, Dana Farber Cancer Inst 1990; **Fac Appt:** Assoc Prof Med, Harvard Med Sch

Garnick, Marc B MD [Onc] - **Spec Exp:** Prostate Cancer; Urologic Cancer; **Hospital:** Beth Israel Deaconess Med Ctr - Boston; **Address:** Beth Israel Deaconess Medical Ctr, SCC9, 330 Brookline Ave, Boston, MA 02215; **Phone:** 617-667-9187; **Board Cert:** Internal Medicine 1976; Medical Oncology 1979; **Med School:** Univ Pennsylvania 1972; **Resid:** Internal Medicine, Univ Penn Hosp 1974; **Fellow:** Research, Natl Inst Hlth 1976; Medical Oncology, Dana-Farber Cancer Inst 1978; **Fac Appt:** Clin Prof Med, Harvard Med Sch

Grunberg, Steven M MD [Onc] - **Spec Exp:** Lung Cancer; Head & Neck Cancer; **Hospital:** FAHC - Med Ctr Campus; **Address:** FAHC Division of Hematology/Oncology, 89 Beaumont Ave, Given Bldg, E214, Burlington, VT 05405; **Phone:** 802-847-8400; **Board Cert:** Internal Medicine 1978; Medical Oncology 1983; **Med School:** Cornell Univ-Weill Med Coll 1975; **Resid:** Internal Medicine, Mofitt Hosp-U Calif 1978; **Fellow:** Medical Oncology, Sidney Farber Cancer Ctr 1981; **Fac Appt:** Prof Med, Univ VT Coll Med

Hammond, Denis B MD [Onc] - **Spec Exp:** Breast Cancer; Prostate Cancer; **Hospital:** Elliot Hosp, Catholic Med Ctr; **Address:** NH Oncology-Hematology, 200 Technology Drive, Hooksett, NH 03106; **Phone:** 603-622-6484; **Board Cert:** Internal Medicine 1977; Hematology 1978; **Med School:** Tufts Univ 1973; **Resid:** Internal Medicine, SUNY Buffalo Affil Hosps 1976; **Fellow:** Hematology, Mass Genl Hosp 1977; Medical Oncology, Dartmouth Med Sch 1978

Johnson, Bruce E MD [Onc] - **Spec Exp:** Lung Cancer; Thoracic Cancers; Merkel Cell Carcinoma; **Hospital:** Dana-Farber Cancer Inst, Brigham & Women's Hosp; **Address:** Lowe Ctr Thoracic Oncology, 44 Binney St, Ste D-1234, Boston, MA 02115; **Phone:** 617-632-4790; **Board Cert:** Internal Medicine 1982; Medical Oncology 1985; **Med School:** Univ Minn 1979; **Resid:** Internal Medicine, Univ Chicago Hosps 1982; **Fellow:** Medical Oncology, Natl Cancer Inst 1985; **Fac Appt:** Assoc Prof Med, Harvard Med Sch

Kantoff, Philip W MD [Onc] - **Spec Exp:** Genitourinary Cancer; Prostate Cancer; **Hospital:** Dana-Farber Cancer Inst, Brigham & Women's Hosp; **Address:** 44 Binney St, Ste D-1230, Boston, MA 02115; **Phone:** 617-632-3466; **Board Cert:** Internal Medicine 1982; Medical Oncology 1989; **Med School:** Brown Univ 1979; **Resid:** Internal Medicine, NYU/Bellevue Hosp 1983; **Fellow:** Gene Therapy Research, NIH 1986; **Fac Appt:** Prof Med, Harvard Med Sch

Kaufman, Peter A MD [Onc] - **Spec Exp:** Breast Cancer; Clinical Trials; **Hospital:** Dartmouth - Hitchcock Med Ctr; **Address:** Dept Hematology-Oncology, One Medical Center Drive, Lebanon, NH 03756; **Phone:** 603-653-6181; **Board Cert:** Internal Medicine 1986; Medical Oncology 1989; **Med School:** NYU Sch Med 1983; **Resid:** Internal Medicine, Duke Univ Med Ctr 1986; **Fellow:** Hematology & Oncology, Duke Univ Med Ctr 1989; **Fac Appt:** Assoc Prof Med, Dartmouth Med Sch

Lacy, Jill MD [Onc] - **Spec Exp:** Colon & Rectal Cancer; Brain Tumors; Gastrointestinal Cancer; Lymphoma; **Hospital:** Yale-New Haven Hosp; **Address:** Yale Univ Sch Med-Div Medical Oncology, 333 Cedar St, PO Box 208032, New Haven, CT 06520-8032; **Phone:** 203-785-4191; **Board Cert:** Internal Medicine 1982; Medical Oncology 2005; **Med School:** Yale Univ 1978; **Resid:** Internal Medicine, Yale-New Haven Hosp 1981; **Fellow:** Medical Oncology, Yale-New Haven Hosp 1985; **Fac Appt:** Assoc Prof Med, Yale Univ

Lynch, Thomas MD [Onc] - **Spec Exp:** Lung Cancer; Thoracic Cancers; **Hospital:** Mass Genl Hosp; **Address:** Mass Genl Hosp, Dept Hem/Onc, 55 Fruit St, Yawkey Bldg - Ste 7B, Boston, MA 02114-2617; **Phone:** 617-724-1136; **Board Cert:** Internal Medicine 1989; Medical Oncology 2003; **Med School:** Yale Univ 1986; **Resid:** Internal Medicine, Mass Genl Hosp 1989; **Fellow:** Medical Oncology, Dana-Farber Cancer Inst 1991; **Fac Appt:** Asst Prof Med, Harvard Med Sch

Matulonis, Ursula A MD [Onc] - **Spec Exp:** Gynecologic Cancer; Ovarian Cancer; Breast Cancer; Drug Development; **Hospital:** Dana-Farber Cancer Inst; **Address:** Gynecologic Oncology Program, Dana Farber Cancer Institute, 44 Binney St, Ste Dana 1210, Boston, MA 02115; **Phone:** 617-632-2334; **Board Cert:** Internal Medicine 2000; Medical Oncology 2000; **Med School:** Albany Med Coll 1987; **Resid:** Internal Medicine, Univ Pittsburgh Hosp 1990; **Fellow:** Medical Oncology, Dana Farber Cancer Inst 1993; **Fac Appt:** Asst Prof Med, Harvard Med Sch

Muss, Hyman B MD [Onc] - **Spec Exp:** Breast Cancer; **Hospital:** FAHC - Med Ctr Campus; **Address:** Univ Vermont Div Hematology/Oncology, 89 Beaumont Ave, Burlington, VT 05405; **Phone:** 802-847-8400; **Board Cert:** Internal Medicine 1973; Hematology 1974; Medical Oncology 1975; **Med School:** SUNY Downstate 1968; **Resid:** Internal Medicine, Peter Bent Brigham Hosp 1970; **Fellow:** Hematology & Oncology, Peter Bent Brigham Hosp 1974; **Fac Appt:** Prof Med, Univ VT Coll Med

Nadler, Lee M MD [Onc] - **Spec Exp:** Lymphoma; **Hospital:** Dana-Farber Cancer Inst, Brigham & Women's Hosp; **Address:** Dana Farber Cancer Inst, 44 Binney St, SM 339A, Boston, MA 02115; **Phone:** 617-632-3331; **Board Cert:** Internal Medicine 1976; **Med School:** Harvard Med Sch 1973; **Resid:** Internal Medicine, Columbia-Presby Hosp 1975; **Fellow:** Medical Oncology, Natl Cancer Inst 1977; Medical Oncology, Dana-Farber Cancer Inst 1978; **Fac Appt:** Prof Med, Harvard Med Sch

Posner, Marshall R MD [Onc] - **Spec Exp:** Head & Neck Cancer; Skin Cancer-Head & Neck; **Hospital:** Dana-Farber Cancer Inst, Beth Israel Deaconess Med Ctr - Boston; **Address:** Dana-Farber Cancer Inst, Head & Neck Cancer Ctr, 44 Binney St, rm G430, Boston, MA 02115; **Phone:** 617-632-3090; **Board Cert:** Internal Medicine 1978; Medical Oncology 1981; **Med School:** Tufts Univ 1975; **Resid:** Internal Medicine, Boston City Hosp 1978; **Fellow:** Oncology, Dana-Farber Cancer Inst 1981; **Fac Appt:** Assoc Prof Med, Harvard Med Sch

Schnipper, Lowell E MD [Onc] - **Spec Exp:** Breast Cancer; Lymphoma; **Hospital:** Beth Israel Deaconess Med Ctr - Boston; **Address:** Beth Israel Deaconess Med Ctr, 330 Brookline Ave, Boston, MA 02215; **Phone:** 617-667-1198; **Board Cert:** Internal Medicine 1973; Medical Oncology 1983; **Med School:** SUNY Downstate 1968; **Resid:** Internal Medicine, Yale-New Haven Hosp 1970; Medical Oncology, Natl Cancer Inst 1973; **Fellow:** Hematology & Oncology, Barnes Jewish Hosp 1974; **Fac Appt:** Prof Med, Harvard Med Sch

Shulman, Lawrence N MD [Onc] - **Spec Exp:** Breast Cancer; **Hospital:** Dana-Farber Cancer Inst; **Address:** Dana-Farber Cancer Inst, 44 Binney St, rm Dana-1608, Boston, MA 02115; **Phone:** 617-632-2277; **Board Cert:** Internal Medicine 1978; Medical Oncology 1981; Hematology 1982; **Med School:** Harvard Med Sch 1975; **Resid:** Internal Medicine, Beth Israel Hosp 1977; **Fellow:** Hematology & Oncology, Beth Israel Hosp 1980; **Fac Appt:** Assoc Prof Med, Harvard Med Sch

Strauss, Gary M MD [Onc] - **Spec Exp:** Melanoma; **Hospital:** Tufts Med Ctr; **Address:** Tufts Medical Ctr, 800 Washington St, Box 245, Boston, MA 02111; **Phone:** 617-636-5627; **Board Cert:** Internal Medicine 1975; Medical Oncology 1979; Hematology 1980; **Med School:** Yale Univ 1972; **Resid:** Internal Medicine, Boston City Hosp 1976; **Fellow:** Medical Oncology, Natl Cancer Inst 1976; Hematology & Oncology, Mass General Hosp 1979

Medical Oncology

Taplin, Mary-Ellen MD [Onc] - **Spec Exp:** Prostate Cancer; Genitourinary Cancer; **Hospital:** Dana-Farber Cancer Inst, Brigham & Women's Hosp; **Address:** Dana Farber Cancer Inst, 44 Binney St, rm D1230, Boston, MA 02115; **Phone:** 617-632-3237; **Board Cert:** Internal Medicine 1989; Hematology 1996; Medical Oncology 2003; **Med School:** Univ Mass Sch Med 1986; **Resid:** Internal Medicine, U Mass Med Ctr 1990; **Fellow:** Hematology & Oncology, Beth Israel Deaconess Hosp 1993; **Fac Appt:** Assoc Prof Med

Weisberg, Tracey MD [Onc] - **Spec Exp:** Breast Cancer; **Hospital:** Maine Med Ctr; **Address:** 100 Campus Drive, Unit 108, Scarborough, ME 04074; **Phone:** 207-885-7600; **Board Cert:** Internal Medicine 1987; Medical Oncology 1989; **Med School:** SUNY Stony Brook 1983; **Resid:** Internal Medicine, Mount Sinai Hosp 1985; Internal Medicine, Hartford Hosp 1986; **Fellow:** Medical Oncology, Yale Univ Hosp 1988

Winer, Eric P MD [Onc] - **Spec Exp:** Breast Cancer; **Hospital:** Dana-Farber Cancer Inst, Brigham & Women's Hosp; **Address:** Dana Farber Cancer Inst, 44 Binney St, Mayer 2, Boston, MA 02115; **Phone:** 617-582-7933; **Board Cert:** Internal Medicine 1987; Medical Oncology 1989; **Med School:** Yale Univ 1983; **Resid:** Internal Medicine, Yale-New Haven Hosp 1987; **Fellow:** Hematology & Oncology, Duke Univ 1989; **Fac Appt:** Assoc Prof Med, Harvard Med Sch

Mid Atlantic

Ahlgren, James D MD [Onc] - **Spec Exp:** Gastrointestinal Cancer; **Hospital:** G Washington Univ Hosp; **Address:** Geo Wash Univ Med Ctr, Div Hem/Oncology, 2150 Pennsylvania Ave NW, Ste 3-428, Washington, DC 20037-3201; **Phone:** 202-741-2478; **Board Cert:** Internal Medicine 1980; Medical Oncology 1989; **Med School:** Georgetown Univ 1977; **Resid:** Internal Medicine, Georgetown Univ Hosp 1979; **Fellow:** Medical Oncology, Georgetown Univ Hosp 1981; **Fac Appt:** Prof Med, Geo Wash Univ

Aisner, Joseph MD [Onc] - **Spec Exp:** Lung Cancer; Solid Tumors; **Hospital:** Robert Wood Johnson Univ Hosp - New Brunswick; **Address:** Cancer Inst of New Jersey, 195 Little Albany St, rm 2012, New Brunswick, NJ 08903-2681; **Phone:** 732-235-6777; **Board Cert:** Internal Medicine 1973; Medical Oncology 1975; **Med School:** Wayne State Univ 1970; **Resid:** Internal Medicine, Georgetown Univ Hosp 1972; **Fellow:** Medical Oncology, Natl Cancer Inst 1975

Algazy, Kenneth M MD [Onc] - **Spec Exp:** Lung Cancer; Mesothelioma; Hematologic Malignancies; **Hospital:** Hosp Univ Penn - UPHS (page 60), VA Med Ctr; **Address:** Hosp Univ Pennsylvania, 3400 Spruce St, 12 Penn Tower, Philadelphia, PA 19104; **Phone:** 215-614-1858; **Board Cert:** Internal Medicine 1972; Hematology 1974; Medical Oncology 1979; **Med School:** Temple Univ 1969; **Resid:** Internal Medicine, Univ Rochester-Strong Meml Hosp 1972; **Fellow:** Hematology & Oncology, Johns Hopkins Med Ctr 1974; **Fac Appt:** Clin Prof Med, Univ Pennsylvania

Ambinder, Richard F MD/PhD [Onc] - **Spec Exp:** Lymphoma; Hodgkin's Disease; AIDS Related Cancers; **Hospital:** Johns Hopkins Hosp - Baltimore (page 61); **Address:** Cancer Research Bldg, 1650 Orleans St, rm CRB 389, Baltimore, MD 21231; **Phone:** 410-955-8964; **Board Cert:** Internal Medicine 1982; Medical Oncology 1985; **Med School:** Johns Hopkins Univ 1979; **Resid:** Internal Medicine, Johns Hopkins Hosp 1981; **Fellow:** Internal Medicine, Johns Hopkins Hosp 1982; Medical Oncology, Johns Hopkins Hosp 1985; **Fac Appt:** Prof Med, Johns Hopkins Univ

Argiris, Athanassios MD [Onc] - **Spec Exp:** Lung Cancer; Head & Neck Cancer; Clinical Trials; **Hospital:** UPMC Presby, Pittsburgh; **Address:** UPMC Presbyterian Cancer Ctr, 5115 Centre Ave Fl 2, Pittsburgh, PA 15232; **Phone:** 412-692-4724; **Board Cert:** Internal Medicine 1997; Medical Oncology 2000; **Med School:** Greece 1990; **Resid:** Internal Medicine, Beth Israel Med Ctr 1997; **Fellow:** Medical Oncology, Yale-New Haven Hosp 2000; **Fac Appt:** Assoc Prof Med, Univ Pittsburgh

Arlen, Philip M MD [Onc] - **Spec Exp:** Prostate Cancer-Vaccine Therapy; Vaccine Therapy-Clinical Trials Only; Clinical Trials Only; **Hospital:** Natl Inst of Hlth - Clin Ctr, Natl Naval Med Ctr; **Address:** National Cancer Inst, MSC 1750, 10 Center Drive Bldg 10 - rm 5B52, Bethesda, MD 20892-1750; **Phone:** 301-496-0629; **Board Cert:** Internal Medicine 1997; Medical Oncology 1998; **Med School:** Med Coll GA 1991; **Resid:** Internal Medicine, Georgia Baptist Hlth Care Syst 1994; **Fellow:** Hematology & Oncology, Emory Univ Med Ctr 1994; NCI/NIH 1999

Attas, Lewis MD [Onc] - **Spec Exp:** Breast Cancer; Lymphoma; Bleeding/Coagulation Disorders; **Hospital:** Englewood Hosp & Med Ctr, Holy Name Hosp; **Address:** 25 Rockwood Pl Fl 1, Englewood, NJ 07631-4957; **Phone:** 201-568-5250; **Board Cert:** Internal Medicine 1985; Medical Oncology 1987; Hematology 1988; **Med School:** Mount Sinai Sch Med 1982; **Resid:** Internal Medicine, Montefiore Hosp Med Ctr 1985; **Fellow:** Hematology & Oncology, North Shore Univ Hosp 1988; **Fac Appt:** Assoc Clin Prof Med, Mount Sinai Sch Med

Axelrod, Rita S MD [Onc] - **Spec Exp:** Head & Neck Cancer; Lung Cancer; Complementary Medicine; **Hospital:** Thomas Jefferson Univ Hosp; **Address:** Thomas Jefferson Univ Hosp, 111 S 11th St, Ste 4240, Gibbon Bldg, Philadelphia, PA 19107; **Phone:** 215-955-8874; **Board Cert:** Internal Medicine 1976; Medical Oncology 1977; Hematology 1978; **Med School:** NYU Sch Med 1970; **Resid:** Internal Medicine, Med Coll Georgia Hosps 1973; **Fellow:** Hematology & Oncology, Hosp Univ Penn 1975; **Fac Appt:** Assoc Prof Med, Thomas Jefferson Univ

Belani, Chandra P MD [Onc] - **Spec Exp:** Lung Cancer; Drug Discovery; **Hospital:** Penn State Milton S Hershey Med Ctr; **Address:** Penn State Hershey Cancer Ctr, 500 University Drive, MC H072, Hershey, PA 17033; **Phone:** 717-531-7710; **Board Cert:** Internal Medicine 1986; Medical Oncology 1987; **Med School:** India 1978; **Resid:** Internal Medicine, SMS Med Hosp 1981; Internal Medicine, Good Samaritan/Univ MD Hosps 1984; **Fellow:** Hematology & Oncology, Univ Maryland Hosp 1987; **Fac Appt:** Prof Med, Univ Pittsburgh

Berd, David MD [Onc] - **Spec Exp:** Melanoma; Vaccine Therapy; **Hospital:** Thomas Jefferson Univ Hosp; **Address:** Thomas Jefferson Univ Hosp, Gibbon Bldg - Ste 4240, 111 S 11th St, Philadelphia, PA 19107; **Phone:** 215-955-8874; **Board Cert:** Internal Medicine 1973; Medical Oncology 1975; **Med School:** Thomas Jefferson Univ 1968; **Resid:** Internal Medicine, Hosp U Penn 1972; **Fellow:** Medical Oncology, Yale-New Haven Hosp 1975; **Fac Appt:** Prof Med, Thomas Jefferson Univ

Bookman, Michael A MD [Onc] - **Spec Exp:** Ovarian Cancer; Uterine Cancer; Cervical Cancer; **Hospital:** Fox Chase Cancer Ctr (page 58); **Address:** Fox Chase Cancer Ctr, Dept Medical Oncology, 333 Cottman Ave, Philadelphia, PA 19111; **Phone:** 215-728-2987; **Board Cert:** Internal Medicine 1983; Medical Oncology 1985; **Med School:** Harvard Med Sch 1980; **Resid:** Internal Medicine, Beth Israel Med Ctr 1983; **Fellow:** Medical Oncology, National Cancer Inst 1986

Bosl, George MD [Onc] - **Spec Exp:** Testicular Cancer; Head & Neck Cancer; **Hospital:** Meml Sloan-Kettering Cancer Ctr; **Address:** 1275 York Avenue, New York, NY 10065; **Phone:** 800-525-2225; **Board Cert:** Internal Medicine 1976; Medical Oncology 1979; **Med School:** Creighton Univ 1973; **Resid:** Internal Medicine, New York Hosp 1975; Internal Medicine, Memorial Sloan-Kettering Cancer Ctr 1977; **Fellow:** Medical Oncology, Univ Minn Hosps 1979; **Fac Appt:** Prof Med, Cornell Univ-Weill Med Coll

Brufsky, Adam MD/PhD [Onc] - **Spec Exp:** Breast Cancer; **Hospital:** Magee-Womens Hosp - UPMC, UPMC Presby, Pittsburgh; **Address:** Univ Pitt Cancer Inst/Magee-Women's Hosp, 300 Halket St, Ste 4628, Pittsburgh, PA 15213; **Phone:** 412-641-4530; **Board Cert:** Internal Medicine 2004; Medical Oncology 2005; **Med School:** Univ Conn 1990; **Resid:** Internal Medicine, Brigham & Womens Hosp 1992; **Fellow:** Medical Oncology, Dana Farber Cancer Inst 1995; Medical Microbiology, Brigham & Womens Hosp 1995; **Fac Appt:** Asst Prof Med, Univ Pittsburgh

Medical Oncology

Carabasi, Matthew H MD [Onc] - **Spec Exp:** Bone Marrow Transplant; **Hospital:** Thomas Jefferson Univ Hosp; **Address:** Jefferson Univ Hosp, 111 S 11th St, Gibbon Bldg - Ste 4240, Philadelphia, PA 19107; **Phone:** 215-955-8874; **Board Cert:** Internal Medicine 1983; Medical Oncology 1987; **Med School:** Jefferson Med Coll 1980; **Resid:** Internal Medicine, Hahnemann MC Hosp 1984; **Fellow:** Hematology & Oncology, Meml Sloan-Kettering Cancer Ctr 1988; Research, Meml Sloan-Kettering Cancer Ctr 1989; **Fac Appt:** Assoc Prof Med, Jefferson Med Coll

Carducci, Michael A MD [Onc] - **Spec Exp:** Urologic Cancer; Drug Discovery & Development; Vaccine Therapy; Clinical Trials; **Hospital:** Johns Hopkins Hosp - Baltimore (page 61); **Address:** Sidney Kimmel Cancer Ctr, 1650 Orleans St IM59 BB Bldg, Baltimore, MD 21231; **Phone:** 410-614-3977; **Board Cert:** Internal Medicine 2001; Medical Oncology 2005; **Med School:** Wayne State Univ 1988; **Resid:** Internal Medicine, Univ Colorado Hlth Sci Ctr 1992; **Fellow:** Medical Oncology, Johns Hopkins Hosp 1995; **Fac Appt:** Prof Med, Johns Hopkins Univ

Chanan-Khan, Asher A MD [Onc] - **Spec Exp:** Multiple Myeloma; Leukemia; **Hospital:** Roswell Park Cancer Inst; **Address:** Roswell Park Cancer Inst, Elm & Carlton Sts, Buffalo, NY 14263; **Phone:** 716-845-3221; **Board Cert:** Internal Medicine 1997; Medical Oncology 2001; Hematology 2004; **Med School:** Pakistan 1993; **Resid:** Internal Medicine, Harlem Hosp Ctr 1997; **Fellow:** Hematology & Oncology, NYU Med Ctr 1999; **Fac Appt:** Asst Prof Med, SUNY Buffalo

Chapman, Paul MD [Onc] - **Spec Exp:** Melanoma; Immunotherapy; Vaccine Therapy; **Hospital:** Meml Sloan-Kettering Cancer Ctr; **Address:** 1275 York Avenue, New York, NY 10065; **Phone:** 800-525-2225; **Board Cert:** Internal Medicine 1984; Medical Oncology 1987; **Med School:** Cornell Univ-Weill Med Coll 1981; **Resid:** Internal Medicine, Univ Chicago Hosps 1984; **Fellow:** Medical Oncology, Meml Sloan-Kettering Cancer Ctr 1987; **Fac Appt:** Prof Med, Cornell Univ-Weill Med Coll

Claxton, David F MD [Onc] - **Spec Exp:** Leukemia; Bone Marrow Transplant; Hematologic Malignancies; **Hospital:** Penn State Milton S Hershey Med Ctr; **Address:** MS Hershey Med Ctr, Medical Oncology, 500 University Drive, MC HO46, Hershey, PA 17033; **Phone:** 717-531-8677; **Board Cert:** Internal Medicine 1984; Medical Oncology 2004; **Med School:** McGill Univ 1978; **Resid:** Internal Medicine, Royal Victoria Hosp 1984; **Fellow:** Hematology, Royal Victoria Hosp 1986; Medical Oncology, UTMD Anderson Cancer Ctr 1989; **Fac Appt:** Assoc Prof Med, Penn State Univ-Hershey Med Ctr

Cohen, Philip MD [Onc] - **Spec Exp:** Breast Cancer; **Hospital:** Georgetown Univ Hosp; **Address:** Georgetown Univ Hosp, Lombardi Cancer Ctr, 3800 Reservoir Rd NW, Washington, DC 20007; **Phone:** 202-444-2198; **Board Cert:** Internal Medicine 1973; Medical Oncology 1975; Hematology 1976; **Med School:** Harvard Med Sch 1970; **Resid:** Internal Medicine, Mass Genl Hosp 1972; **Fellow:** Medical Oncology, Natl Cancer Inst 1974; **Fac Appt:** Assoc Prof Med, Geo Wash Univ

Cohen, Roger MD [Onc] - **Spec Exp:** Drug Discovery & Development; Clinical Trials; **Hospital:** Fox Chase Cancer Ctr (page 58); **Address:** Fox Chase Cancer Ctr, 333 Cottman Ave, Ste C307, Philadelphia, PA 19111; **Phone:** 215-728-2570; **Board Cert:** Internal Medicine 1984; Medical Oncology 1993; Hematology 1986; **Med School:** Harvard Med Sch 1980; **Resid:** Internal Medicine, Mt Sinai Hosp 1982; **Fellow:** Research, Sloan Kettering Cancer Inst 1985; Hematology, Mt Sinai Hosp 1986

Cohen, Seymour M MD [Onc] - **Spec Exp:** Melanoma; Breast Cancer; Lung Cancer; Merkel Cell Carcinoma; **Hospital:** Mount Sinai Med Ctr (page 64); **Address:** 1045 5th Ave, New York, NY 10028-0138; **Phone:** 212-249-9141; **Board Cert:** Internal Medicine 1971; Medical Oncology 1973; **Med School:** Univ Pittsburgh 1962; **Resid:** Internal Medicine, Montefiore Med Ctr 1964; Internal Medicine, Mount Sinai Med Ctr 1965; **Fellow:** Hematology, Mount Sinai Med Ctr 1966; Hematology & Oncology, LI Jewish Hosp 1969; **Fac Appt:** Assoc Clin Prof Med, Mount Sinai Sch Med

Coleman, Morton MD [Onc] - **Spec Exp:** Leukemia & Lymphoma; Hodgkin's Disease; Multiple Myeloma; Waldenstrom's Macroglobulinemia; **Hospital:** NY-Presby Hosp/Weill Cornell (page 66); **Address:** 407 E 70th St, FL 3, New York, NY 10021-5302; **Phone:** 212-517-5900; **Board Cert:** Internal Medicine 1971; Hematology 1972; Medical Oncology 1973; **Med School:** Med Coll VA 1963; **Resid:** Internal Medicine, Grady Meml Hosp-Emory 1965; Internal Medicine, New York Hosp-Cornell 1968; **Fellow:** Hematology & Oncology, New York Hosp-Cornell 1970; **Fac Appt:** Clin Prof Med, Cornell Univ-Weill Med Coll

Cullen, Kevin MD [Onc] - **Spec Exp:** Head & Neck Cancer; **Hospital:** Univ of MD Med Sys; **Address:** Univ Md Greenbaum Cancer Ctr, 22 S Greene St, rm N9E22, Baltimore, MD 21201; **Phone:** 410-328-5506; **Board Cert:** Internal Medicine 1986; Medical Oncology 1989; **Med School:** Harvard Med Sch 1983; **Resid:** Internal Medicine, Beth Israel Hosp 1986; Internal Medicine, Hammersmith Hosp 1985; **Fellow:** Medical Oncology, Natl Cancer Inst 1988

Czuczman, Myron S MD [Onc] - **Spec Exp:** Lymphoma; Multiple Myeloma; Leukemia; **Hospital:** Roswell Park Cancer Inst; **Address:** Roswell Park Cancer Inst, Elm & Carlton Sts, Buffalo, NY 14263; **Phone:** 716-845-7695; **Board Cert:** Internal Medicine 1988; **Med School:** Penn State Univ-Hershey Med Ctr 1985; **Resid:** Internal Medicine, North Shore Univ Hosp 1988; **Fellow:** Hematology & Oncology, Meml Sloan-Kettering Cancer Ctr 1992; **Fac Appt:** Assoc Prof Med, SUNY Buffalo

Daly, Mary B MD/PhD [Onc] - **Spec Exp:** Breast Cancer; Breast Cancer Risk Assessment; Cancer Prevention; Ovarian Cancer Risk Assessment; **Hospital:** Fox Chase Cancer Ctr (page 58); **Address:** Fox Chase Cancer Ctr, 333 Cottman Ave, P1054, Philadelphia, PA 19111; **Phone:** 215-728-2791; **Board Cert:** Internal Medicine 1981; Medical Oncology 1983; **Med School:** Univ NC Sch Med 1978; **Resid:** Internal Medicine, Univ Texas Hlth Sci Ctr 1981; **Fellow:** Medical Oncology, Univ Texas Hlth Sci Ctr 1983; **Fac Appt:** Clin Prof Med, Temple Univ

Davidson, Nancy E MD [Onc] - **Spec Exp:** Breast Cancer; **Hospital:** Johns Hopkins Hosp - Baltimore (page 61); **Address:** Johns Hopkins Oncology Center, 1650 Orleans St, Baltimore, MD 21231-1000; **Phone:** 410-955-8964; **Board Cert:** Internal Medicine 1982; Medical Oncology 1985; **Med School:** Harvard Med Sch 1979; **Resid:** Internal Medicine, Johns Hopkins Hosp 1982; **Fellow:** Medical Oncology, Natl Cancer Inst 1986; **Fac Appt:** Prof Med, Johns Hopkins Univ

Dawson, Nancy MD [Onc] - **Spec Exp:** Prostate Cancer; Kidney Cancer; Bladder Cancer; **Hospital:** Georgetown Univ Hosp; **Address:** Lombardi Cancer Ctr, Georgetown Univ Hosp, 3800 Reservoir Rd NW, Washington, DC 20007; **Phone:** 202-444-9094; **Board Cert:** Internal Medicine 1982; Medical Oncology 1985; Hematology 1984; **Med School:** Georgetown Univ 1979; **Resid:** Internal Medicine, Walter Reed AMC 1982; **Fellow:** Hematology & Oncology, Walter Reed AMC 1985; **Fac Appt:** Prof Med, Georgetown Univ

Donehower, Ross Carl MD [Onc] - **Spec Exp:** Pancreatic Cancer; Colon Cancer; Prostate Cancer; **Hospital:** Johns Hopkins Hosp - Baltimore (page 61); **Address:** Hopkins Kimmel Cancer Ctr, 1650 Orleans St, CRB-I, rm 187, Baltimore, MD 21231-1000; **Phone:** 410-955-8838; **Board Cert:** Internal Medicine 1977; Medical Oncology 1979; **Med School:** Univ Minn 1974; **Resid:** Internal Medicine, Johns Hopkins Hosp 1976; **Fellow:** Medical Oncology, Natl Inst Hlth 1980; **Fac Appt:** Prof Med, Johns Hopkins Univ

Medical Oncology

Doroshow, James H MD [Onc] - **Spec Exp:** Drug Discovery & Development; Colon Cancer; Breast Cancer; **Hospital:** Natl Inst of Hlth - Clin Ctr; **Address:** National Cancer Institute, Div Cancer Treatment & Diagnosis, 31 Center, Bldg 31-rm 3A44, Bethesda, MD 20892; **Phone:** 301-496-4291; **Board Cert:** Internal Medicine 1976; Medical Oncology 1977; **Med School:** Harvard Med Sch 1973; **Resid:** Internal Medicine, Mass Genl Hosp 1975; **Fellow:** Medical Oncology, Natl Cancer Inst 1978

Edelman, Martin J MD [Onc] - **Spec Exp:** Thoracic Cancers; Lung Cancer; Mesothelioma; **Hospital:** Univ of MD Med Sys; **Address:** Greenebaum Cancer Ctr-Univ MD, 22 S Greene St, Baltimore, MD 21201; **Phone:** 410-328-2703; **Board Cert:** Internal Medicine 1986; Medical Oncology 1989; **Med School:** Albany Med Coll 1982; **Resid:** Internal Medicine, Naval Hosp 1986; **Fellow:** Hematology & Oncology, Naval Hosp 1990; **Fac Appt:** Prof Med, Univ MD Sch Med

Eisenberger, Mario MD [Onc] - **Spec Exp:** Prostate Cancer; **Hospital:** Johns Hopkins Hosp - Baltimore (page 61); **Address:** 1650 Orleans St, rm 1M51, Baltimore, MD 21231; **Phone:** 410-614-3511; **Board Cert:** Internal Medicine 1976; Medical Oncology 1979; **Med School:** Brazil 1972; **Resid:** Internal Medicine, Michael Reese Hosp 1975; **Fellow:** Hematology, Michael Reese Hosp 1976; Medical Oncology, Jackson Meml Hosp/Univ Miami 1979; **Fac Appt:** Prof Med, Johns Hopkins Univ

Ettinger, David S MD [Onc] - **Spec Exp:** Lung Cancer; Sarcoma; Clinical Trials; **Hospital:** Johns Hopkins Hosp - Baltimore (page 61); **Address:** Bunting Blaustein Cancer Rsrch Bldg, 1650 Orleans St, rm G88, Baltimore, MD 21231-1000; **Phone:** 410-955-8847; **Board Cert:** Internal Medicine 1976; Medical Oncology 1977; **Med School:** Univ Louisville Sch Med 1967; **Resid:** Internal Medicine, Mayo Grad Schl 1971; **Fellow:** Medical Oncology, Johns Hopkins Hosp 1975; **Fac Appt:** Prof Med, Johns Hopkins Univ

Fanucchi, Michael P MD [Onc] - **Spec Exp:** Sarcoma; Aerodigestive Tract Cancer; Lung Cancer; **Hospital:** St Vincent Cath Med Ctrs - Manhattan; **Address:** 325 W 15th St, New York, NY 10011; **Phone:** 212-604-6011; **Board Cert:** Internal Medicine 1980; Medical Oncology 1985; **Med School:** Columbia P&S 1977; **Resid:** Internal Medicine, Bronx Muni Hosp Ctr 1981; **Fellow:** Medical Oncology, Meml Sloan-Kettering Cancer Ctr 1984; **Fac Appt:** Assoc Prof Med, Emory Univ

Fine, Howard Alan MD [Onc] - **Spec Exp:** Brain Tumors; **Hospital:** Natl Inst of Hlth - Clin Ctr; **Address:** NIH/NCI/NOB, Bloch Building 82, Rm 225 MSC 8202, 9030 Old Georgetown Rd, Bethesda, MD 20892-0001; **Phone:** 301-402-6298; **Board Cert:** Internal Medicine 1987; Medical Oncology 1989; **Med School:** Mount Sinai Sch Med 1984; **Resid:** Internal Medicine, Hosp Univ Penn 1987; **Fellow:** Medical Oncology, Dana Farber Cancer Ctr 1990

Fine, Robert MD [Onc] - **Spec Exp:** Pancreatic Cancer; Drug Development; Brain Tumors; Clinical Trials; **Hospital:** NY-Presby Hosp/Columbia (page 66); **Address:** Columbia Univ Comprehensive Cancer Ctr, 650 W 168th St, rm BB 20-05, New York, NY 10032; **Phone:** 212-305-1168; **Board Cert:** Internal Medicine 1983; Medical Oncology 1985; **Med School:** Univ Chicago-Pritzker Sch Med 1979; **Resid:** Internal Medicine, Stanford Univ Med Ctr 1982; **Fellow:** Medical Oncology, National Cancer Inst 1988; **Fac Appt:** Assoc Prof Med, Columbia P&S

Fisher, Richard I MD [Onc] - **Spec Exp:** Lymphoma; Hodgkin's Disease; **Hospital:** Univ of Rochester Strong Meml Hosp; **Address:** James P Wilmot Cancer Ctr, 601 Elmwood Ave, Box 704, Rochester, NY 14642; **Phone:** 585-275-5823; **Board Cert:** Internal Medicine 1973; Medical Oncology 1977; **Med School:** Harvard Med Sch 1970; **Resid:** Internal Medicine, Mass Genl Hosp 1972; **Fac Appt:** Prof Med, Univ Rochester

Flomenberg, Neal MD [Onc] - **Spec Exp:** Bone Marrow Transplant; Stem Cell Transplant; Leukemia & Lymphoma; **Hospital:** Thomas Jefferson Univ Hosp; **Address:** Thomas Jefferson Univ Hosp, 125 S 9th St, Ste 801, Philadelphia, PA 19107; **Phone:** 215-955-0356; **Board Cert:** Internal Medicine 1979; Medical Oncology 1981; Hematology 1982; **Med School:** Jefferson Med Coll 1976; **Resid:** Internal Medicine, Montefiore Med Ctr 1979; **Fellow:** Hematology & Oncology, Meml Sloan Kettering Cancer Ctr 1982; **Fac Appt:** Clin Prof Med, Thomas Jefferson Univ

Flood, William A MD [Onc] - **Spec Exp:** Lung Cancer; Esophageal Cancer; Stomach Cancer; Head & Neck Cancer; **Hospital:** Penn State Milton S Hershey Med Ctr; **Address:** MS Hershey Med Ctr-Hem/Oncology, 500 University Drive, Hershey, PA 17033-0850; **Phone:** 717-531-8677; **Board Cert:** Medical Oncology 1997; **Med School:** Temple Univ 1990; **Resid:** Internal Medicine, Duke Univ Med Ctr 1993; **Fellow:** Medical Oncology, Johns Hopkins Onc Ctr 1996; **Fac Appt:** Assoc Prof Med, Penn State Univ-Hershey Med Ctr

Forastiere, Arlene A MD [Onc] - **Spec Exp:** Esophageal Cancer; Head & Neck Cancer; **Hospital:** Johns Hopkins Hosp - Baltimore (page 61); **Address:** Bunting Blaustein Cancer Research Bldg, 1650 Orleans St, rm G90, Baltimore, MD 21231; **Phone:** 410-955-8964; **Board Cert:** Internal Medicine 1978; Medical Oncology 1981; **Med School:** NY Med Coll 1975; **Resid:** Internal Medicine, Albert Einstein Med Ctr 1977; Internal Medicine, Univ Conn Health Ctr 1978; **Fellow:** Medical Oncology, Meml Sloan Kettering Cancer Ctr 1980; **Fac Appt:** Prof Med, NY Med Coll

Fox, Kevin R MD [Onc] - **Spec Exp:** Breast Cancer; **Hospital:** Hosp Univ Penn - UPHS (page 60); **Address:** 3400 Spruce St, 14 Penn Tower, Philadelphia, PA 19104; **Phone:** 215-662-7469; **Board Cert:** Internal Medicine 1985; Medical Oncology 1987; **Med School:** Johns Hopkins Univ 1981; **Resid:** Internal Medicine, Johns Hopkins Hosp 1984; **Fellow:** Hematology & Oncology, Hosp Univ Penn 1987; **Fac Appt:** Prof Med, Univ Pennsylvania

Friedberg, Jonathan MD [Onc] - **Spec Exp:** Lymphoma; Hodgkin's Disease; **Hospital:** Univ of Rochester Strong Meml Hosp; **Address:** James P Wilmot Cancer Ctr, 601 Elmwood Ave, Box 704, Rochester, NY 14642-8704; **Phone:** 585-273-4150; **Board Cert:** Internal Medicine 1997; Hematology 2000; Medical Oncology 2000; **Med School:** Harvard Med Sch 1994; **Resid:** Internal Medicine, Mass Genl Hosp 1997; Hematology & Oncology, Dana-Farber/Partners Cancer Ctr 1999; **Fac Appt:** Asst Prof Med, Univ Rochester

Gabrilove, Janice MD [Onc] - **Spec Exp:** Myelodysplastic Syndromes; Leukemia; Hematologic Malignancies; Myeloproliferative Disorders; **Hospital:** Mount Sinai Med Ctr (page 64); **Address:** Mount Sinai Med Ctr, One Gustave L Levy Pl, Box 1079, Dept Hem Onc, New York, NY 10029-6574; **Phone:** 212-241-9650; **Board Cert:** Internal Medicine 1980; Medical Oncology 1983; **Med School:** Mount Sinai Sch Med 1977; **Resid:** Internal Medicine, Columbia-Presby Med Ctr 1980; **Fellow:** Hematology & Oncology, Meml Sloan-Kettering Cancer Ctr 1983; **Fac Appt:** Prof Med, Mount Sinai Sch Med

Gelmann, Edward P MD [Onc] - **Spec Exp:** Prostate Cancer; Testicular Cancer; **Hospital:** NY-Presby Hosp/Columbia (page 66); **Address:** Columbia Univ Med Ctr, Milstein Hosp Bldg 6-435, 177 Fort Washington Ave, New York, NY 10032; **Phone:** 212-305-5098; **Board Cert:** Internal Medicine 1979; Medical Oncology 1981; **Med School:** Stanford Univ 1976; **Resid:** Internal Medicine, Univ Chicago Hosps 1978; **Fellow:** Medical Oncology, National Cancer Inst 1981; **Fac Appt:** Prof Med, Columbia P&S

Geyer Jr, Charles E MD [Onc] - **Spec Exp:** Breast Cancer; **Hospital:** Allegheny General Hosp; **Address:** Allegheny Cancer Ctr, 320 E North Ave Fl 5, Pittsburgh, PA 15212; **Phone:** 412-359-6147; **Board Cert:** Internal Medicine 1983; Medical Oncology 1987; **Med School:** Texas Tech Univ 1980; **Resid:** Internal Medicine, Baylor Affil Hosps 1983; **Fellow:** Medical Oncology, Baylor Affil Hosps 1985

Medical Oncology

Glick, John H MD [Onc] - **Spec Exp:** Breast Cancer; Hodgkin's Disease; Lymphoma, Non-Hodgkin's; **Hospital:** Hosp Univ Penn - UPHS (page 60); **Address:** Abramson Cancer Ctr of Univ Penn, 3400 Spruce St, 1218 Penn Tower, Philadelphia, PA 19104; **Phone:** 215-662-6065; **Board Cert:** Internal Medicine 1973; Medical Oncology 1975; **Med School:** Columbia P&S 1969; **Resid:** Internal Medicine, Presbyterian Hosp 1971; **Fellow:** Medical Oncology, Natl Cancer Inst 1973; Medical Oncology, Stanford Univ 1974; **Fac Appt:** Prof Med, Univ Pennsylvania

Goldstein, Lori J MD [Onc] - **Spec Exp:** Breast Cancer; **Hospital:** Fox Chase Cancer Ctr (page 58); **Address:** Fox Chase Cancer Ctr, Dept Med Oncology, 333 Cottman Ave, Philadelphia, PA 19111; **Phone:** 215-728-2689; **Board Cert:** Internal Medicine 1985; Medical Oncology 2002; **Med School:** SUNY Upstate Med Univ 1982; **Resid:** Internal Medicine, Presby Univ Hosp 1985; **Fellow:** Medical Oncology, Natl Cancer Inst/NIH 1990

Goy, Andre MD [Onc] - **Spec Exp:** Lymphoma; Hodgkin's Disease; **Hospital:** Hackensack Univ Med Ctr; **Address:** 20 Prospect Ave, Ste 400, Hackensack, NJ 07601; **Phone:** 201-996-5900; **Med School:** France 1988; **Resid:** Internal Medicine, Grenoble Univ Med Ctr 1992; **Fellow:** Hematology & Oncology, Grenoble Univ Med Ctr 1993; **Fac Appt:** Assoc Clin Prof

Grana, Generosa MD [Onc] - **Spec Exp:** Breast Cancer; Cancer Genetics; Cancer Prevention; **Hospital:** Cooper Univ Hosp, Virtua West Jersey Hosp - Voorhees; **Address:** 900 Centennial Blvd, Ste M, Voorhees, NJ 08043; **Phone:** 856-325-6740; **Board Cert:** Internal Medicine 1988; Medical Oncology 2001; **Med School:** Northwestern Univ 1985; **Resid:** Internal Medicine, Temple Univ Hosp 1988; **Fellow:** Hematology & Oncology, Fox Chase Cancer Ctr 1992; **Fac Appt:** Assoc Prof Med, UMDNJ-RW Johnson Med Sch

Grossbard, Michael L MD [Onc] - **Spec Exp:** Lymphoma; Breast Cancer; Gastrointestinal Cancer; **Hospital:** St Luke's - Roosevelt Hosp Ctr - Roosevelt Div (page 57), Beth Israel Med Ctr - Petrie Division (page 57); **Address:** 1000 10th Ave Fl 11 - Ste C02, New York, NY 10019; **Phone:** 212-523-5419; **Board Cert:** Internal Medicine 1989; Medical Oncology 2001; **Med School:** Yale Univ 1986; **Resid:** Internal Medicine, Mass Genl Hosp 1989; **Fellow:** Medical Oncology, Dana Farber Cancer Inst 1991; **Fac Appt:** Clin Prof Med, Columbia P&S

Grossman, Stuart MD [Onc] - **Spec Exp:** Brain Tumors; Neuro-Oncology; Pain-Cancer; **Hospital:** Johns Hopkins Hosp - Baltimore (page 61); **Address:** Cancer Research Bldg 2, rm 1M16, 1551 Orleans St, Baltimore, MD 21231; **Phone:** 410-955-8837; **Board Cert:** Internal Medicine 1976; Medical Oncology 1983; **Med School:** Univ Rochester 1973; **Resid:** Internal Medicine, Strong Meml Hosp 1976; **Fellow:** Medical Oncology, Johns Hopkins Hosp 1981; **Fac Appt:** Prof Med, Johns Hopkins Univ

Gulley, James L MD/PhD [Onc] - **Spec Exp:** Prostate Cancer-Vaccine Therapy; Vaccine Therapy-Clinical Trials Only; Clinical Trials Only; **Hospital:** Natl Inst of Hlth - Clin Ctr; **Address:** NIH Cancer Research Ctr, MSC 1750, 10 Center Drive Bldg 10 - rm 5B52, Bethesda, MD 20892; **Phone:** 301-435-2956; **Board Cert:** Internal Medicine 1999; Medical Oncology 2000; **Med School:** Loma Linda Univ 1995; **Resid:** Internal Medicine, Emory Univ Med Ctr 1998; **Fellow:** Medical Oncology, Natl Cancer Inst 2000

Haas, Naomi S Balzer MD [Onc] - **Spec Exp:** Melanoma; Genitourinary Cancer; Kidney Cancer; Clinical Trials; **Hospital:** Hosp Univ Penn - UPHS (page 60); **Address:** Abramson Cancer Ctr, 12 Penn Tower, 3400 Spruce St, Philadelphia, PA 19104; **Phone:** 215-615-5121; **Board Cert:** Internal Medicine 1988; Medical Oncology 2005; **Med School:** NE Ohio Univ 1985; **Resid:** Internal Medicine, Abington Meml Hosp 1988; **Fellow:** Hematology & Oncology, Fox Chase Cancer Ctr 1989

Haller, Daniel G MD [Onc] - **Spec Exp:** Gastrointestinal Cancer; Colon & Rectal Cancer; Cancer Prevention; **Hospital:** Hosp Univ Penn - UPHS (page 60); **Address:** Hosp Univ Penn, Div Hematology/Oncology, 3400 Spruce St, 12 Penn Tower, Philadelphia, PA 19104; **Phone:** 215-662-6318; **Board Cert:** Internal Medicine 1976; Medical Oncology 1979; **Med School:** Univ Pittsburgh 1973; **Resid:** Internal Medicine, Georgetown Univ Hosp 1976; **Fellow:** Medical Oncology, Georgetown Univ Hosp 1978; **Fac Appt:** Prof Med, Univ Pennsylvania

Hesdorffer, Charles S MD [Onc] - **Spec Exp:** Stem Cell Transplant; Immunotherapy; Lymphoma; Sarcoma; **Hospital:** Johns Hopkins Hosp - Baltimore (page 61); **Address:** Johns Hopkins Univ Hosp, 720 Rutland Ave, rm 1025, Baltimore, MD 21205; **Phone:** 410-502-7004; **Board Cert:** Medical Oncology 1997; **Med School:** South Africa 1978; **Resid:** Internal Medicine, Univ Wittwatersrand Hosp 1984; **Fellow:** Hematology & Oncology, Columbia-Presby Hosp 1988; **Fac Appt:** Prof Med, Johns Hopkins Univ

Hochster, Howard S MD [Onc] - **Spec Exp:** Gastrointestinal Cancer; Gynecologic Cancer; Colon & Rectal Cancer; **Hospital:** NYU Med Ctr (page 68); **Address:** NYU Cancer Institute, 160 E 34 St Fl 9, New York, NY 10016; **Phone:** 212-731-5100; **Board Cert:** Internal Medicine 1983; Medical Oncology 1985; Hematology 1986; **Med School:** Yale Univ 1980; **Resid:** Internal Medicine, NYU Med Ctr 1983; **Fellow:** Hematology & Oncology, NYU Med Ctr 1985; Medical Oncology, Jules Bordet Inst 1986; **Fac Appt:** Prof Med, NYU Sch Med

Holland, James F MD [Onc] - **Spec Exp:** Breast Cancer; Colon Cancer; Lung Cancer; **Hospital:** Mount Sinai Med Ctr (page 64); **Address:** Ruttenberg Cancer Ctr, Div Med Oncology, 1 Gustave L Levy Pl, Box 1129, New York, NY 10029-6500; **Phone:** 212-241-4495; **Board Cert:** Internal Medicine 1955; **Med School:** Columbia P&S 1947; **Resid:** Internal Medicine, Columbia-Presby Hosp 1949; **Fellow:** Medical Oncology, Francis Delafield Hosp 1953; **Fac Appt:** Prof Med, Mount Sinai Sch Med

Hudes, Gary R MD [Onc] - **Spec Exp:** Prostate Cancer; Genitourinary Cancer; Kidney Cancer; **Hospital:** Fox Chase Cancer Ctr (page 58); **Address:** 333 Cottman Ave, rm C307, Philadelphia, PA 19111; **Phone:** 215-728-3889; **Board Cert:** Internal Medicine 1982; Hematology 1984; Medical Oncology 1985; **Med School:** SUNY Downstate 1979; **Resid:** Internal Medicine, Graduate Hosp 1982; **Fellow:** Hematology & Oncology, Presby-Univ Penn Med Ctr 1985

Hudis, Clifford A MD [Onc] - **Spec Exp:** Breast Cancer; **Hospital:** Meml Sloan-Kettering Cancer Ctr; **Address:** 1275 York Avenue, New York, NY 10065; **Phone:** 800-525-2225; **Board Cert:** Internal Medicine 1986; Medical Oncology 2001; **Med School:** Med Coll PA Hahnemann 1983; **Resid:** Internal Medicine, Hosp Med Coll Penn 1986; **Fellow:** Medical Oncology, Meml Sloan Kettering Cancer Ctr 1991; **Fac Appt:** Prof Med, Cornell Univ-Weill Med Coll

Ilson, David H MD [Onc] - **Spec Exp:** Esophageal Cancer; Colon & Rectal Cancer; Mesothelioma; Unknown Primary Cancer; **Hospital:** Meml Sloan-Kettering Cancer Ctr; **Address:** 1275 York Avenue, New York, NY 10065; **Phone:** 800-525-2225; **Board Cert:** Internal Medicine 1989; Medical Oncology 2002; **Med School:** NYU Sch Med 1986; **Resid:** Internal Medicine, Bellevue-NYU Sch Med 1989; **Fellow:** Medical Oncology, Meml Sloan Kettering Hosp 1992; **Fac Appt:** Assoc Prof Med, Cornell Univ-Weill Med Coll

Isaacs, Claudine J MD [Onc] - **Spec Exp:** Breast Cancer; Breast Cancer Risk Assessment; **Hospital:** Georgetown Univ Hosp; **Address:** Lombardi Cancer Ctr, Podium B, 3800 Reservoir Rd NW, Washington, DC 20007; **Phone:** 202-444-3677; **Board Cert:** Internal Medicine 2002; Medical Oncology 2003; **Med School:** McGill Univ 1987; **Resid:** Internal Medicine, Montreal Genl Hosp 1990; Hematology & Oncology, McGill Univ Hosp 1992; **Fellow:** Medical Oncology, Georgetown Univ Med Ctr 1993; **Fac Appt:** Assoc Prof Med, Georgetown Univ

Medical Oncology

Karp, Judith MD [Onc] - **Spec Exp:** Leukemia; Clinical Trials; Myelodysplastic Syndromes; **Hospital:** Johns Hopkins Hosp - Baltimore (page 61); **Address:** 1650 Orleans St, rm 289, Baltimore, MD 21287; **Phone:** 410-502-7726; **Board Cert:** Internal Medicine 1976; **Med School:** Stanford Univ 1971; **Resid:** Internal Medicine, John Hopkins Hosp 1974; **Fellow:** Medical Oncology, John Hopkins Hosp 1977; **Fac Appt:** Prof Med, Johns Hopkins Univ

Kelsen, David MD [Onc] - **Spec Exp:** Gastrointestinal Cancer; Neuroendocrine Tumors; Unknown Primary Cancer; Merkel Cell Carcinoma; **Hospital:** Meml Sloan-Kettering Cancer Ctr; **Address:** 1275 York Avenue, New York, NY 10065; **Phone:** 800-525-2225; **Board Cert:** Internal Medicine 1976; Medical Oncology 1979; **Med School:** Hahnemann Univ 1972; **Resid:** Internal Medicine, Temple Univ Hosp 1976; **Fellow:** Medical Oncology, Meml Sloan Kettering Cancer Ctr 1978; **Fac Appt:** Prof Med, Cornell Univ-Weill Med Coll

Kemeny, Nancy MD [Onc] - **Spec Exp:** Colon Cancer; Rectal Cancer; Liver Cancer; **Hospital:** Meml Sloan-Kettering Cancer Ctr; **Address:** 1275 York Avenue, New York, NY 10065; **Phone:** 800-525-2225; **Board Cert:** Internal Medicine 1974; Medical Oncology 1981; **Med School:** UMDNJ-NJ Med Sch, Newark 1971; **Resid:** Internal Medicine, St Luke's Hosp 1974; **Fellow:** Medical Oncology, Mem Sloan Kettering Cancer Ctr 1976; **Fac Appt:** Prof Med, Cornell Univ-Weill Med Coll

Kirkwood, John M MD [Onc] - **Spec Exp:** Melanoma; Immunotherapy; **Hospital:** UPMC Presby, Pittsburgh, UPMC Shadyside; **Address:** Hillman Cancer Research Pavilion, 5117 Centre Ave, Ste 1.32, Pittsburgh, PA 15213-1862; **Phone:** 412-623-7707; **Board Cert:** Internal Medicine 1976; Medical Oncology 1981; **Med School:** Yale Univ 1973; **Resid:** Internal Medicine, Yale-New Haven Hosp 1976; **Fellow:** Medical Oncology, Dana Farber Cancer Inst 1979; **Fac Appt:** Prof Med, Univ Pittsburgh

Kris, Mark G MD [Onc] - **Spec Exp:** Lung Cancer; Mediastinal Tumors; Thymoma; Thoracic Cancers; **Hospital:** Meml Sloan-Kettering Cancer Ctr; **Address:** 1275 York Avenue, New York, NY 10065; **Phone:** 800-525-2225; **Board Cert:** Internal Medicine 1980; Medical Oncology 1983; **Med School:** Cornell Univ-Weill Med Coll 1977; **Resid:** Internal Medicine, New York Hosp 1980; **Fellow:** Medical Oncology, Meml Sloan Kettering Cancer Ctr 1983; **Fac Appt:** Prof Med, Cornell Univ-Weill Med Coll

Langer, Corey J MD [Onc] - **Spec Exp:** Lung Cancer; Head & Neck Cancer; Mesothelioma; Thoracic Cancers; **Hospital:** Fox Chase Cancer Ctr (page 58); **Address:** Fox Chase Cancer Ctr, 333 Cottman Ave, Philadelphia, PA 19111-2412; **Phone:** 215-728-2985; **Board Cert:** Internal Medicine 1984; Hematology 1986; Medical Oncology 1987; **Med School:** Boston Univ 1981; **Resid:** Internal Medicine, Graduate Hosp 1984; Hematology & Oncology, Presby Hosp 1986; **Fellow:** Medical Oncology, Fox Chase Cancer Ctr 1987; **Fac Appt:** Assoc Prof Med, Temple Univ

Levine, Ellis G MD [Onc] - **Spec Exp:** Breast Cancer; Testicular Cancer; Kidney Cancer; Urologic Cancer; **Hospital:** Roswell Park Cancer Inst; **Address:** Roswell Park Cancer Inst, Elm & Carlton St, Buffalo, NY 14263-0001; **Phone:** 716-845-8547; **Board Cert:** Internal Medicine 1982; Medical Oncology 1985; **Med School:** Univ Pittsburgh 1979; **Resid:** Internal Medicine, Univ Minn Hosps 1982; **Fellow:** Medical Oncology, Univ Minn Hosps 1984; **Fac Appt:** Assoc Prof Med, SUNY Buffalo

Levy, Michael H MD/PhD [Onc] - **Spec Exp:** Pain Management; Palliative Care; Pain-Cancer; Ethics; **Hospital:** Fox Chase Cancer Ctr (page 58); **Address:** Fox Chase Cancer Ctr, Dept Medical Oncology, 333 Cottman Ave, Ste C307, Philadelphia, PA 19111; **Phone:** 215-728-3637; **Board Cert:** Internal Medicine 1979; Medical Oncology 1981; **Med School:** Jefferson Med Coll 1976; **Resid:** Internal Medicine, Mt Sinai Med Ctr 1978; Internal Medicine, Hosp Univ Penn 1979; **Fellow:** Hematology & Oncology, Hosp Univ Penn 1981

America's Top Doctors® 8th Edition

Livingston, Philip MD [Onc] - **Spec Exp:** Melanoma; Vaccine Therapy; Immunotherapy; **Hospital:** Meml Sloan-Kettering Cancer Ctr; **Address:** 1275 York Avenue, New York, NY 10065; **Phone:** 800-525-2225; **Board Cert:** Internal Medicine 1980; Allergy & Immunology 1974; Rheumatology 1974; Medical Oncology 1981; **Med School:** Harvard Med Sch 1969; **Resid:** Internal Medicine, N Shore Hosp-Cornell Med Ctr 1971; **Fellow:** Immunology, NYU Med Ctr 1973; Medical Oncology, Meml Sloan Kettering Cancer Inst 1977; **Fac Appt:** Prof Med, Cornell Univ-Weill Med Coll

Marshall, John L MD [Onc] - **Spec Exp:** Gastrointestinal Cancer; Drug Development; **Hospital:** Georgetown Univ Hosp; **Address:** Lombardi Cancer Ctr, Podium A, 3800 Reservoir Rd NW, Washington, DC 20007; **Phone:** 202-444-7064; **Board Cert:** Internal Medicine 2001; Medical Oncology 2003; **Med School:** Univ Louisville Sch Med 1988; **Resid:** Internal Medicine, Georgetown Univ Hosp 1991; **Fellow:** Medical Oncology, Georgetown Univ Hosp 1993; **Fac Appt:** Assoc Prof Med, Georgetown Univ

Maslak, Peter G MD [Onc] - **Spec Exp:** Leukemia; Stem Cell Transplant; Myelodysplastic Syndromes; Clinical Trials; **Hospital:** Meml Sloan-Kettering Cancer Ctr; **Address:** 1275 York Avenue, New York, NY 10065; **Phone:** 800-525-2225; **Board Cert:** Internal Medicine 1987; Hematology 2000; Medical Oncology 1989; **Med School:** Mount Sinai Sch Med 1984; **Resid:** Internal Medicine, Univ Michigan Med Ctr 1987; **Fellow:** Hematology & Oncology, Meml Sloan Kettering Cancer Ctr 1990

Masters, Gregory A MD [Onc] - **Spec Exp:** Lung Cancer; Esophageal Cancer; Thoracic Cancers; **Hospital:** Christiana Hospital; **Address:** Med Onc-Hem Consultants, Graham Cancer Ctr, 4701 Ogletown-Stanton Rd, Ste 2200, Newark, DE 19713; **Phone:** 302-366-1200; **Board Cert:** Internal Medicine 2003; Medical Oncology 2005; **Med School:** Northwestern Univ 1990; **Resid:** Internal Medicine, Hosp Univ Penn 1993; **Fellow:** Medical Oncology, Univ Chicago Hosps 1995; **Fac Appt:** Assoc Prof Med, Thomas Jefferson Univ

McGuire III, William P MD [Onc] - **Spec Exp:** Gynecologic Cancer; Ovarian Cancer; Breast Cancer; **Hospital:** Franklin Square Hosp; **Address:** Harry & Jeanette Weinberg Cancer Inst, 9103 Franklin Square Drive, Ste 2200, Baltimore, MD 21287; **Phone:** 443-777-7826; **Board Cert:** Internal Medicine 1974; Medical Oncology 1981; **Med School:** Baylor Coll Med 1971; **Resid:** Internal Medicine, Yale-New Haven Hosp 1973; **Fac Appt:** Clin Prof Med, Univ MD Sch Med

Meropol, Neal J MD [Onc] - **Spec Exp:** Gastrointestinal Cancer; Stomach Cancer; Esophageal Cancer; Colon Cancer; **Hospital:** Fox Chase Cancer Ctr (page 58); **Address:** Fox Chase Cancer Ctr, Medical Oncology, 333 Cottman Ave, Philadelphia, PA 19111; **Phone:** 215-728-2450; **Board Cert:** Internal Medicine 1988; Medical Oncology 2001; **Med School:** Vanderbilt Univ 1985; **Resid:** Internal Medicine, Univ Hosps/Case West Res 1988; **Fellow:** Hematology & Oncology, Hosp Univ Penn 1992; **Fac Appt:** Prof Med, Temple Univ

Mintzer, David M MD [Onc] - **Spec Exp:** Breast Cancer; Gastrointestinal Cancer; Head & Neck Cancer; **Hospital:** Pennsylvania Hosp (page 60); **Address:** 230 W Washington Square Fl 2, Philadelphia, PA 19106; **Phone:** 215-829-6088; **Board Cert:** Internal Medicine 1980; Hematology 1982; Medical Oncology 1983; **Med School:** Jefferson Med Coll 1977; **Resid:** Internal Medicine, Pennsylvania Hosp 1980; **Fellow:** Hematology, Jefferson Med Coll 1982; Medical Oncology, Meml Sloan Kettering Cancer Ctr 1984; **Fac Appt:** Assoc Clin Prof Med, Univ Pennsylvania

Moore, Anne MD [Onc] - **Spec Exp:** Breast Cancer; **Hospital:** NY-Presby Hosp/Weill Cornell (page 66); **Address:** Weill Cornell Breast Ctr, 425 E 61st St Fl 8, New York, NY 10065; **Phone:** 212-821-0654; **Board Cert:** Internal Medicine 1973; Hematology 1976; Medical Oncology 1977; **Med School:** Columbia P&S 1969; **Resid:** Internal Medicine, Cornell Univ Med Ctr 1973; **Fellow:** Medical Oncology, Rockefeller Univ 1973; **Fac Appt:** Prof Med, Cornell Univ-Weill Med Coll

Medical Oncology

Motzer, Robert J MD [Onc] - **Spec Exp:** Kidney Cancer; Testicular Cancer; Prostate Cancer; **Hospital:** Meml Sloan-Kettering Cancer Ctr; **Address:** 1275 York Avenue, New York, NY 10065; **Phone:** 800-525-2225; **Board Cert:** Internal Medicine 1984; Medical Oncology 1987; **Med School:** Univ Mich Med Sch 1981; **Resid:** Internal Medicine, Meml Sloan Kettering Cancer Ctr 1984; **Fellow:** Medical Oncology, Meml Sloan Kettering Cancer Ctr 1987; **Fac Appt:** Assoc Prof Med, Cornell Univ-Weill Med Coll

Muggia, Franco MD [Onc] - **Spec Exp:** Gynecologic Cancer; **Hospital:** NYU Med Ctr (page 68); **Address:** NYU Clinical Cancer Ctr, 160 E 34th St Fl 8, New York, NY 10016; **Phone:** 212-731-5433; **Board Cert:** Internal Medicine 1968; Hematology 1974; Medical Oncology 1973; **Med School:** Cornell Univ-Weill Med Coll 1961; **Resid:** Internal Medicine, Hartford Hosp 1964; Internal Medicine, Francis A Delafield Hosp 1966; **Fac Appt:** Prof Med, NYU Sch Med

Nissenblatt, Michael MD [Onc] - **Spec Exp:** Breast Cancer; Colon Cancer; Hereditary Cancer; Familial Cancer; **Hospital:** Robert Wood Johnson Univ Hosp - New Brunswick, St Peter's Univ Hosp; **Address:** 205 Easton Ave, New Brunswick, NJ 08901-1722; **Phone:** 732-828-9570; **Board Cert:** Internal Medicine 1976; Medical Oncology 1979; **Med School:** Columbia P&S 1973; **Resid:** Internal Medicine, Johns Hopkins Hosp 1976; **Fellow:** Medical Oncology, Johns Hopkins Hosp 1978; **Fac Appt:** Clin Prof Med, Robert W Johnson Med Sch

Norton, Larry MD [Onc] - **Spec Exp:** Breast Cancer; **Hospital:** Meml Sloan-Kettering Cancer Ctr; **Address:** 1275 York Avenue, New York, NY 10065; **Phone:** 800-525-2225; **Board Cert:** Internal Medicine 1975; Medical Oncology 1977; **Med School:** Columbia P&S 1972; **Resid:** Internal Medicine, Bronx Muni Hosp 1974; **Fellow:** Medical Oncology, Natl Cancer Inst 1977; **Fac Appt:** Prof Med, Cornell Univ-Weill Med Coll

O'Reilly, Eileen M MD [Onc] - **Spec Exp:** Pancreatic Cancer; Clinical Trials; Biliary Cancer; Neuroendocrine Tumors; **Hospital:** Meml Sloan-Kettering Cancer Ctr, NY-Presby Hosp/Weill Cornell (page 66); **Address:** 1275 York Avenue, New York, NY 10065; **Phone:** 800-525-2225; **Med School:** Ireland 1990; **Resid:** Internal Medicine, St Vincent's Hosp 1994; **Fellow:** Hematology, St Vincent's Hosp 1995; Medical Oncology, Memorial-Sloan Kettering Cancer Ctr 1997; **Fac Appt:** Asst Prof Med, Cornell Univ-Weill Med Coll

Offit, Kenneth MD [Onc] - **Spec Exp:** Cancer Genetics; Breast Cancer; Lymphoma; **Hospital:** Meml Sloan-Kettering Cancer Ctr; **Address:** 1275 York Avenue, New York, NY 10065; **Phone:** 800-525-2225; **Board Cert:** Internal Medicine 1985; Medical Oncology 1987; **Med School:** Harvard Med Sch 1982; **Resid:** Internal Medicine, Lenox Hill Hosp 1985; **Fellow:** Hematology & Oncology, Meml Sloan Kettering Cancer Ctr 1988; **Fac Appt:** Prof Med, Cornell Univ-Weill Med Coll

Oratz, Ruth MD [Onc] - **Spec Exp:** Breast Cancer; Melanoma; **Hospital:** NYU Med Ctr (page 68); **Address:** 345 E 37th St, Ste 202, New York, NY 10016; **Phone:** 212-400-4904; **Board Cert:** Internal Medicine 1985; Medical Oncology 1989; **Med School:** Albert Einstein Coll Med 1982; **Resid:** Internal Medicine, NYU Med Ctr 1982; **Fellow:** Medical Oncology, NYU Med Ctr 1985; **Fac Appt:** Assoc Clin Prof Med, NYU Sch Med

Oster, Martin W MD [Onc] - **Spec Exp:** Breast Cancer; Gastrointestinal Cancer; Head & Neck Cancer; **Hospital:** NY-Presby Hosp/Columbia (page 66); **Address:** NY Presby Hosp-Columbia Presby Med Ctr, 161 Fort Washington Ave, New York, NY 10032-3713; **Phone:** 212-305-8231; **Board Cert:** Internal Medicine 1974; Medical Oncology 1975; **Med School:** Columbia P&S 1971; **Resid:** Internal Medicine, Mass Genl Hosp 1973; **Fellow:** Medical Oncology, Natl Cancer Inst/NIH 1976; **Fac Appt:** Assoc Clin Prof Med, Columbia P&S

America's Top Doctors® 8th Edition

Pasmantier, Mark MD [Onc] - **Spec Exp:** Lung Cancer; Ovarian Cancer; **Hospital:** NY-Presby Hosp/Weill Cornell (page 66); **Address:** 407 E 70th St Fl 3, New York, NY 10021-5302; **Phone:** 212-517-5900; **Board Cert:** Internal Medicine 1972; Hematology 1974; Medical Oncology 1975; **Med School:** NYU Sch Med 1966; **Resid:** Internal Medicine, Harlem Hosp 1970; **Fellow:** Hematology, Montefiore Hosp Med Ctr 1971; Medical Oncology, New York Hosp 1972; **Fac Appt:** Clin Prof Med, Cornell Univ-Weill Med Coll

Pecora, Andrew L MD [Onc] - **Spec Exp:** Stem Cell Transplant; Myelodysplastic Syndromes; Melanoma; Immunotherapy; **Hospital:** Hackensack Univ Med Ctr; **Address:** The Cancer Ctr-Hackensack Univ Med Ctr, 20 Prospect Ave, Ste 400, Hackensack, NJ 07601; **Phone:** 201-996-5900; **Board Cert:** Internal Medicine 1986; Hematology 1988; Medical Oncology 1989; **Med School:** UMDNJ-NJ Med Sch, Newark 1983; **Resid:** Internal Medicine, NY Hosp-Cornell Med Ctr 1986; **Fellow:** Hematology & Oncology, Meml Sloan Kettering Cancer Ctr 1988; **Fac Appt:** Prof Med, UMDNJ-NJ Med Sch, Newark

Petrylak, Daniel P MD [Onc] - **Spec Exp:** Genitourinary Cancer; Prostate Cancer; Bladder Cancer; Kidney Cancer; **Hospital:** NY-Presby Hosp/Columbia (page 66); **Address:** 161 Fort Washington Ave, New York, NY 10032-3729; **Phone:** 212-305-1731; **Board Cert:** Internal Medicine 2001; Medical Oncology 2003; **Med School:** Case West Res Univ 1985; **Resid:** Internal Medicine, Jacobi Med Ctr 1988; **Fellow:** Oncology, Meml-Sloan Kettering Cancer Ctr 1991; **Fac Appt:** Assoc Prof Med, Columbia P&S

Pfister, David G MD [Onc] - **Spec Exp:** Head & Neck Cancer; Laryngeal Cancer; Thyroid Cancer; **Hospital:** Meml Sloan-Kettering Cancer Ctr; **Address:** 1275 York Avenue, New York, NY 10065; **Phone:** 800-525-2225; **Board Cert:** Internal Medicine 1985; Medical Oncology 1989; **Med School:** Univ Pennsylvania 1982; **Resid:** Internal Medicine, Hosp Univ Penn 1985; **Fellow:** Epidemiology, Yale New Haven Hosp 1987; Hematology & Oncology, Meml Sloan Kettering Cancer Ctr 1989; **Fac Appt:** Prof Med, Cornell Univ-Weill Med Coll

Remick, Scot C MD [Onc] - **Spec Exp:** AIDS Related Cancers; Clinical Trials; Drug Development; **Hospital:** WV Univ Hosp - Ruby Memorial; **Address:** WVU Mary Babb Randolph Cancer Ctr, Box 9300, Morgantown, WV 26506-9300; **Phone:** 304-598-4552; **Board Cert:** Internal Medicine 1985; Medical Oncology 1987; **Med School:** NY Med Coll 1982; **Resid:** Internal Medicine, Johns Hopkins Hosp 1985; **Fellow:** Medical Oncology, Univ Wisconsin Clin Cancer Ctr 1988; **Fac Appt:** Prof Med, Case West Res Univ

Ruggiero, Joseph MD [Onc] - **Spec Exp:** Colon Cancer; Breast Cancer; **Hospital:** NY-Presby Hosp/Weill Cornell (page 66); **Address:** 428 E 72nd St, Ste 300, New York, NY 10021-4635; **Phone:** 212-746-2083; **Board Cert:** Internal Medicine 1980; Hematology 1982; Medical Oncology 1983; **Med School:** NYU Sch Med 1977; **Resid:** Internal Medicine, NY Hosp-Cornell Med Ctr 1980; **Fellow:** Hematology & Oncology, NY Hosp-Cornell Med Ctr 1983; **Fac Appt:** Assoc Clin Prof Med, Cornell Univ-Weill Med Coll

Saltz, Leonard B MD [Onc] - **Spec Exp:** Colon & Rectal Cancer; Gastrointestinal Cancer & Rare Tumors; Liver Cancer; Neuroendocrine Tumors; **Hospital:** Meml Sloan-Kettering Cancer Ctr; **Address:** 1275 York Avenue, New York, NY 10065; **Phone:** 800-525-2225; **Board Cert:** Internal Medicine 1986; Hematology 1988; Medical Oncology 1989; **Med School:** Yale Univ 1983; **Resid:** Internal Medicine, NY Hosp-Cornell Med Ctr 1986; **Fellow:** Hematology & Oncology, NY Hosp-Cornell Med Ctr/Rockefeller Univ 1987; **Fac Appt:** Prof Med, Cornell Univ-Weill Med Coll

Medical Oncology

Scheinberg, David MD/PhD [Onc] - **Spec Exp:** Leukemia; Immunotherapy; Vaccine Therapy; **Hospital:** Meml Sloan-Kettering Cancer Ctr; **Address:** 1275 York Avenue, New York, NY 10065; **Phone:** 800-525-2225; **Board Cert:** Internal Medicine 1986; Medical Oncology 2005; **Med School:** Johns Hopkins Univ 1983; **Resid:** Internal Medicine, NY Hosp-Cornell Med Ctr 1985; **Fellow:** Medical Oncology, Meml Sloan Kettering Cancer Ctr 1987; **Fac Appt:** Prof Med, Cornell Univ-Weill Med Coll

Scher, Howard MD [Onc] - **Spec Exp:** Genitourinary Cancer; Prostate Cancer; Bladder Cancer; **Hospital:** Meml Sloan-Kettering Cancer Ctr; **Address:** 1275 York Avenue, New York, NY 10065; **Phone:** 800-525-2225; **Board Cert:** Internal Medicine 1979; Medical Oncology 1985; **Med School:** NYU Sch Med 1976; **Resid:** Internal Medicine, Bellevue Hosp 1980; **Fellow:** Medical Oncology, Meml Sloan Kettering Cancer Ctr 1983; **Fac Appt:** Prof Med, Cornell Univ-Weill Med Coll

Schilder, Russell J MD [Onc] - **Spec Exp:** Gynecologic Cancer; Hematologic Malignancies; Drug Development; Clinical Trials; **Hospital:** Fox Chase Cancer Ctr (page 58); **Address:** Fox Chase Cancer Center, 333 Cottman Ave, Philadelphia, PA 19111; **Phone:** 215-728-4300; **Board Cert:** Internal Medicine 1986; Hematology 1988; Medical Oncology 1989; **Med School:** Univ Miami Sch Med 1983; **Resid:** Internal Medicine, Temple Univ Hosp 1986; **Fellow:** Hematology & Oncology, Fox Chase Cancer Ctr 1989; **Fac Appt:** Prof Med, Temple Univ

Schuchter, Lynn M MD [Onc] - **Spec Exp:** Melanoma; Breast Cancer; Clinical Trials; **Hospital:** Hosp Univ Penn - UPHS (page 60); **Address:** Univ Penn/Abramson Cancer Ctr, 3400 Spruce St, 16 Penn Tower, Philadelphia, PA 19104-4206; **Phone:** 215-662-7907; **Board Cert:** Internal Medicine 1985; Medical Oncology 1989; **Med School:** Ros Franklin Univ/Chicago Med Sch 1982; **Resid:** Internal Medicine, Michael Reese Hosp 1985; **Fellow:** Medical Oncology, Johns Hopkins Hosp 1989; **Fac Appt:** Prof Med, Univ Pennsylvania

Shields, Peter G MD [Onc] - **Spec Exp:** Hematologic Malignancies; Hematology-Benign; **Hospital:** Georgetown Univ Hosp; **Address:** Lombardi Cancer Ctr, 3800 Reservoir Rd NW, First Floor, Washington, DC 20007; **Phone:** 202-444-9495; **Board Cert:** Internal Medicine 1986; Medical Oncology 1989; **Med School:** Mount Sinai Sch Med 1983; **Resid:** Internal Medicine, George Washington Univ Hosp 1986; **Fellow:** Hematology & Oncology, George Washington Univ Hosp 1990; **Fac Appt:** Prof Med, Georgetown Univ

Sidransky, David MD [Onc] - **Spec Exp:** Head & Neck Cancer; **Hospital:** Johns Hopkins Hosp - Baltimore (page 61); **Address:** 1550 Orleans St, rm 5-N03, Baltimore, MD 21231; **Phone:** 410-502-5153; **Board Cert:** Internal Medicine 1988; **Med School:** Baylor Coll Med 1984; **Resid:** Internal Medicine, Baylor Coll Medicine 1988; **Fellow:** Medical Oncology, Johns Hopkins Hosp 1992; **Fac Appt:** Prof Oto, Johns Hopkins Univ

Smith, Mitchell R MD/PhD [Onc] - **Spec Exp:** Lymphoma; Leukemia; Multiple Myeloma; Hematologic Malignancies; **Hospital:** Fox Chase Cancer Ctr (page 58); **Address:** Fox Chase Cancer Center, 333 Cottman Ave, Ste C307, Philadelphia, PA 19111; **Phone:** 215-728-2570; **Board Cert:** Internal Medicine 1985; Hematology 1988; Medical Oncology 1987; **Med School:** Case West Res Univ 1979; **Resid:** Pathology, Barnes Jewish Hosp 1983; Internal Medicine, Barnes Jewish Hosp 1984; **Fellow:** Medical Oncology, Meml Sloan-Ketter Cancer Ctr 1988

Speyer, James MD [Onc] - **Spec Exp:** Ovarian Cancer; Breast Cancer; Cardiac Toxicity in Cancer Therapy; **Hospital:** NYU Med Ctr (page 68); **Address:** NYU Clinical Cancer Center, 160 E 34th St, New York, NY 10016-4750; **Phone:** 212-731-5432; **Board Cert:** Internal Medicine 1977; Hematology 1978; Medical Oncology 1979; **Med School:** Johns Hopkins Univ 1974; **Resid:** Internal Medicine, Columbia-Presby Med Ctr 1976; Hematology, Columbia-Presby Med Ctr 1977; **Fellow:** Medical Oncology, Natl Cancer Inst 1979; **Fac Appt:** Clin Prof Med, NYU Sch Med

America's Top Doctors® 8th Edition

Spriggs, David MD [Onc] - **Spec Exp:** Ovarian Cancer; Drug Development; Uterine Cancer; **Hospital:** Meml Sloan-Kettering Cancer Ctr; **Address:** 1275 York Avenue, New York, NY 10065; **Phone:** 800-525-2225; **Board Cert:** Internal Medicine 1981; Medical Oncology 2006; **Med School:** Univ Wisc 1977; **Resid:** Internal Medicine, Columbia-Presby Hosp 1981; **Fellow:** Medical Oncology, Dana-Farber Cancer Inst 1985; **Fac Appt:** Prof Med, Cornell Univ-Weill Med Coll

Stadtmauer, Edward A MD [Onc] - **Spec Exp:** Bone Marrow & Stem Cell Transplant; Leukemia; Multiple Myeloma; **Hospital:** Hosp Univ Penn - UPHS (page 60); **Address:** Univ Penn Cancer Ctr, 3400 Spruce St, 16 Penn Tower, Philadelphia, PA 19104; **Phone:** 215-662-3915; **Board Cert:** Internal Medicine 1986; Hematology 1988; Medical Oncology 1989; **Med School:** Univ Pennsylvania 1983; **Resid:** Internal Medicine, Bronx Muni Hosp 1986; **Fellow:** Hematology & Oncology, Hosp Univ Penn 1989; **Fac Appt:** Assoc Prof Med, Univ Pennsylvania

Stoopler, Mark MD [Onc] - **Spec Exp:** Lung Cancer; Esophageal Cancer; Unknown Primary Cancer; **Hospital:** NY-Presby Hosp/Columbia (page 66); **Address:** 161 Fort Washington Ave, Ste 936, New York, NY 10032-3713; **Phone:** 212-305-8230; **Board Cert:** Internal Medicine 1978; Medical Oncology 1981; **Med School:** Cornell Univ-Weill Med Coll 1975; **Resid:** Internal Medicine, North Shore Univ Hosp 1978; Internal Medicine, Memorial Hosp 1978; **Fellow:** Medical Oncology, Meml-Sloan Kettering Cancer Ctr 1980; **Fac Appt:** Assoc Clin Prof Med, Columbia P&S

Straus, David J MD [Onc] - **Spec Exp:** Lymphoma; Multiple Myeloma; **Hospital:** Meml Sloan-Kettering Cancer Ctr; **Address:** 1275 York Avenue, New York, NY 10065; **Phone:** 800-525-2225; **Board Cert:** Internal Medicine 1972; Hematology 1976; Medical Oncology 1977; **Med School:** Marquette Sch Med 1969; **Resid:** Internal Medicine, Montefiore Med Ctr 1972; Medical Oncology, Meml Sloan Kettering Cancer Ctr 1977; **Fellow:** Hematology, Beth Israel Hosp 1973; **Fac Appt:** Prof Med, Cornell Univ-Weill Med Coll

Tkaczuk, Katherine H MD [Onc] - **Spec Exp:** Breast Cancer; **Hospital:** Univ of MD Med Sys; **Address:** Univ MD Cancer Ctr, 22 S Greene St, rm S9D12, Baltimore, MD 21201; **Phone:** 410-328-7904; **Board Cert:** Internal Medicine 1989; Medical Oncology 2001; **Med School:** Poland 1984; **Resid:** Internal Medicine, St Agnes Hosp 1989; **Fellow:** Hematology & Oncology, Univ Maryland Cancer Ctr 1992; **Fac Appt:** Assoc Prof Med, Univ MD Sch Med

Trump, Donald L MD [Onc] - **Spec Exp:** Prostate Cancer; Genitourinary Cancer; Drug Discovery & Development; **Hospital:** Roswell Park Cancer Inst; **Address:** Elm & Carlton St, Buffalo, NY 14263; **Phone:** 716-845-3499; **Board Cert:** Internal Medicine 1973; Medical Oncology 1977; **Med School:** Johns Hopkins Univ 1970; **Resid:** Internal Medicine, Johns Hopkins Hosp 1975; **Fellow:** Medical Oncology, Johns Hopkins Hosp 1974; **Fac Appt:** Prof Med, SUNY Buffalo

Vaughn, David J MD [Onc] - **Spec Exp:** Testicular Cancer; Bladder Cancer; Prostate Cancer; Genitourinary Cancer; **Hospital:** Hosp Univ Penn - UPHS (page 60), Penn Presby Med Ctr - UPHS (page 60); **Address:** Hosp Univ of Pennsylvania-16 Penn Tower, 3400 Spruce St, Philadelphia, PA 19104; **Phone:** 215-349-8140; **Board Cert:** Medical Oncology 2003; **Med School:** Harvard Med Sch 1987; **Resid:** Internal Medicine, NY Hosp-Cornell Med Ctr 1990; **Fellow:** Hematology & Oncology, Hosp U Penn 1993; **Fac Appt:** Assoc Prof Med, Univ Pennsylvania

Vogel, Victor G MD [Onc] - **Spec Exp:** Breast Cancer; Cancer Genetics; Drug Development; Clinical Trials; **Hospital:** Magee-Womens Hosp - UPMC; **Address:** Magee-Womens Hosp, Breast Cancer Prevention, 300 Halket St, rm 3524, Pittsburgh, PA 15213-3180; **Phone:** 412-641-6500; **Board Cert:** Internal Medicine 1984; Medical Oncology 2003; Public Health & Genl Preventive Med 1993; **Med School:** Temple Univ 1978; **Resid:** Internal Medicine, Baltimore City Hosp 1981; **Fellow:** Medical Oncology, Johns Hopkins Hosp 1986; Epidemiology, Johns Hopkins Hosp 1986; **Fac Appt:** Prof Med, Univ Pittsburgh

Medical Oncology

von Mehren, Margaret MD [Onc] - **Spec Exp:** Sarcoma; Melanoma; Immunotherapy; Gastrointestinal Stromal Tumors; **Hospital:** Fox Chase Cancer Ctr (page 58); **Address:** Fox Chase Cancer Ctr, Dept Med Oncology, 333 Cottman Ave, Philadelphia, PA 19111-2434; **Phone:** 215-728-2570; **Board Cert:** Medical Oncology 1997; **Med School:** Albany Med Coll 1989; **Resid:** Internal Medicine, NYU Med Ctr 1993; **Fellow:** Hematology & Oncology, Fox Chase Cancer Ctr 1996; **Fac Appt:** Assoc Prof Med, Temple Univ

Weiner, Louis M MD [Onc] - **Spec Exp:** Gastrointestinal Cancer; Immunotherapy; Liver Cancer; **Hospital:** Georgetown Univ Hosp; **Address:** Lombardi Cancer Ctr, Georgetown Univ, Research Bldg - rm E501, 3970 Reservoir Rd NW, Washington, DC 20057; **Phone:** 202-687-2110; **Board Cert:** Internal Medicine 1980; Medical Oncology 1985; **Med School:** Mount Sinai Sch Med 1977; **Resid:** Internal Medicine, Med Ctr Hosp Vermont 1981; **Fellow:** Hematology & Oncology, New England Med Ctr 1984; **Fac Appt:** Prof Med, Georgetown Univ

Wilson, Wyndham MD [Onc] - **Spec Exp:** Lymphoma; **Hospital:** Natl Inst of Hlth - Clin Ctr; **Address:** National Cancer Inst, Bldg 10 - rm 12N-226, 9000 Rockville Pike, Bethesda, MD 20892; **Phone:** 301-435-2415; **Board Cert:** Internal Medicine 1985; Medical Oncology 1987; **Med School:** Stanford Univ 1981; **Resid:** Internal Medicine, Stanford Univ 1984; **Fellow:** Oncology, NCI-NIH 1987

Wolff, Antonio C MD [Onc] - **Spec Exp:** Breast Cancer; Drug Development; **Hospital:** Johns Hopkins Hosp - Baltimore (page 61); **Address:** 1650 Orleans St, rm 189, Baltimore, MD 21231; **Phone:** 410-614-4192; **Board Cert:** Internal Medicine 2000; Medical Oncology 2000; **Med School:** Brazil 1986; **Resid:** Internal Medicine, Mt Sinai Med Ctr 1991; **Fellow:** Hematology & Oncology, Washington Univ Med Ctr 1992; Medical Oncology, Johns Hopkins Hosp 1995; **Fac Appt:** Assoc Prof Med, Johns Hopkins Univ

Zelenetz, Andrew D MD/PhD [Onc] - **Spec Exp:** Lymphoma; **Hospital:** Meml Sloan-Kettering Cancer Ctr; **Address:** 1275 York Avenue, New York, NY 10065; **Phone:** 800-525-2225; **Med School:** Harvard Med Sch 1984; **Resid:** Internal Medicine, Stanford Univ Med Ctr 1986; **Fellow:** Medical Oncology, Stanford Univ Med Ctr 1991; **Fac Appt:** Asst Prof Med, Cornell Univ-Weill Med Coll

Southeast

Antonia, Scott J MD/PhD [Onc] - **Spec Exp:** Kidney Cancer; Lung Cancer; **Hospital:** H Lee Moffitt Cancer Ctr & Research Inst; **Address:** H Lee Moffitt Cancer Ctr, 12902 Magnolia Drive, Tampa, FL 33612; **Phone:** 813-979-3883; **Board Cert:** Internal Medicine 2002; Medical Oncology 1995; **Med School:** Univ Conn 1989; **Resid:** Internal Medicine, Yale-New Haven Hosp 1991; **Fellow:** Medical Oncology, Yale-New Haven Hosp 1994; **Fac Appt:** Assoc Prof Med, Univ S Fla Coll Med

Arteaga, Carlos L MD [Onc] - **Spec Exp:** Breast Cancer; **Hospital:** Vanderbilt Univ Med Ctr; **Address:** Vanderbilt-Ingram Cancer Ctr, 2220 Pierce Ave, 777-PRB, Nashville, TN 37232-6838; **Phone:** 615-936-3524; **Board Cert:** Internal Medicine 1984; Medical Oncology 1989; **Med School:** Ecuador 1980; **Resid:** Internal Medicine, Grady Meml Hosp 1984; **Fellow:** Hematology & Oncology, Univ Texas Hlth Sci Ctr 1987; **Fac Appt:** Prof Med, Vanderbilt Univ

Balducci, Lodovico MD [Onc] - **Spec Exp:** Genitourinary Cancer; Breast Cancer; **Hospital:** H Lee Moffitt Cancer Ctr & Research Inst, Tampa Genl Hosp; **Address:** H Lee Moffitt Cancer Ctr, 12902 Magnolia Drive, Tampa, FL 33612; **Phone:** 813-745-8658; **Board Cert:** Internal Medicine 1987; Hematology 1978; Medical Oncology 1979; **Med School:** Italy 1968; **Resid:** Internal Medicine, Univ Miss Med Ctr 1976; Hematology & Oncology, Univ Miss Med Ctr 1979; **Fellow:** Internal Medicine, A Gemelli Genl Hosp 1970; **Fac Appt:** Prof Med, Univ S Fla Coll Med

America's Top Doctors® 8th Edition

Benedetto, Pasquale W MD [Onc] - **Spec Exp:** Genitourinary Cancer; Bladder Cancer; Kidney Cancer; Pancreatic Cancer; **Hospital:** Univ of Miami Hosp & Clins/Sylvester Comp Canc Ctr, Jackson Meml Hosp; **Address:** Sylvester Comp Cancer Ctr, Med Oncology, 1475 NW 12th Ave, Ste 3310, Locator D8-4, Miami, FL 33136; **Phone:** 305-243-4909; **Board Cert:** Internal Medicine 1979; Medical Oncology 1981; Hematology 1982; **Med School:** Cornell Univ-Weill Med Coll 1976; **Resid:** Internal Medicine, Johns Hopkins Hosp 1979; **Fellow:** Medical Oncology, Meml Sloan Kettering Cancer Ctr 1981; **Fac Appt:** Prof Med, Univ Miami Sch Med

Berlin, Jordan MD [Onc] - **Spec Exp:** Gastrointestinal Cancer; Pancreatic Cancer; Liver Cancer; **Hospital:** Vanderbilt Univ Med Ctr; **Address:** 777 Preston Research Building, Nashville, TN 37232-0001; **Phone:** 615-322-6053; **Board Cert:** Internal Medicine 2002; Medical Oncology 2005; **Med School:** Univ IL Coll Med 1989; **Resid:** Internal Medicine, Univ Cincinnati 1992; **Fellow:** Medical Oncology, Univ Wisconsin 1995; **Fac Appt:** Assoc Prof Med, Vanderbilt Univ

Bernard, Stephen MD [Onc] - **Spec Exp:** Gastrointestinal Cancer; Palliative Care; Clinical Trials; **Hospital:** Univ NC Hosps; **Address:** Univ North Carolina Sch Med, 3009 Old Clinic, CB 7305, Chapel Hill, NC 27599; **Phone:** 919-966-4431; **Board Cert:** Internal Medicine 1987; Medical Oncology 1979; Hospice & Palliative Medicine 2004; **Med School:** Univ NC Sch Med 1973; **Resid:** Internal Medicine, Columbia-Presby Med Ctr 1976; **Fellow:** Hematology & Oncology, Wash Univ Hosps 1978; **Fac Appt:** Prof Med, Univ NC Sch Med

Bolger, Graeme B MD [Onc] - **Spec Exp:** Prostate Cancer; Testicular Cancer; **Hospital:** Univ of Ala Hosp at Birmingham; **Address:** 1530 3rd Ave S, Ste FOT-1105, Birmingham, AL 35294; **Phone:** 205-975-0088; **Board Cert:** Internal Medicine 1984; Medical Oncology 2000; **Med School:** McGill Univ 1980; **Resid:** Internal Medicine, Johns Hopkins Hosp 1984; **Fellow:** Medical Oncology, Fred Hutchinson Cancer Rsch 1985; Oncology, Meml Sloan-Kettering Cancer Ctr 1992; **Fac Appt:** Assoc Prof Med, Univ Ala

Boston, Barry MD [Onc] - **Spec Exp:** Gastrointestinal Cancer; Genitourinary Cancer; Prostate Cancer; **Hospital:** St Francis Hosp - Memphis, Methodist Univ Hosp - Memphis; **Address:** Univ of Tennessee Cancer Inst, 7945 Wolf River Blvd, Ste 300, Germantown, TN 38138; **Phone:** 901-752-6131; **Board Cert:** Internal Medicine 1974; Medical Oncology 1977; **Med School:** Louisiana State U, New Orleans 1971; **Resid:** Internal Medicine, Univ Tenn Hosp-VA Hosp 1973; Hematology, Univ Tenn Hosp-VA Hosp 1973; **Fellow:** Medical Oncology, Yale-New Haven Hosp 1975; **Fac Appt:** Assoc Prof Med, Univ Tenn Coll Med, Memphis

Brawley, Otis W MD [Onc] - **Spec Exp:** Breast Cancer; Prostate Cancer; **Hospital:** Emory Univ Hosp, Grady Hlth Sys; **Address:** Winship Cancer Inst, 1365 Clifton Rd NE, Atlanta, GA 30322; **Phone:** 404-778-1900; **Board Cert:** Internal Medicine 1988; Medical Oncology 2003; **Med School:** Univ Chicago-Pritzker Sch Med 1985; **Resid:** Internal Medicine, Univ Hosp Cleveland 1988; **Fellow:** Oncology, Natl Cancer Inst 1990; **Fac Appt:** Prof Med, Emory Univ

Brescia, Frank J MD [Onc] - **Spec Exp:** Palliative Care; Breast Cancer; Gastrointestinal Cancer; Ethics; **Hospital:** Roper Hosp, MUSC Med Ctr; **Address:** Low Country Hematology & Oncology, 900 Bowman Drive, Mount Pleasant, SC 29464; **Phone:** 843-881-5844; **Board Cert:** Internal Medicine 1974; Medical Oncology 1975; **Med School:** UMDNJ-NJ Med Sch, Newark 1968; **Resid:** Internal Medicine, North Shore Univ Hosp 1970; **Fellow:** Medical Oncology, Meml Sloan Kettering Cancer Ctr 1974; **Fac Appt:** Prof Med, Med Univ SC

Burris III, Howard A MD [Onc] - **Spec Exp:** Drug Development; Drug Discovery; Breast Cancer; **Hospital:** Centennial Med Ctr, Baptist Hosp - Nashville; **Address:** 250 25th Ave N Atrium Bldg - Ste 100, Nashville, TN 37203; **Phone:** 615-329-7276; **Board Cert:** Internal Medicine 1988; Medical Oncology 2001; **Med School:** Univ S Ala Coll Med 1985; **Resid:** Internal Medicine, Brooke Army Med Ctr 1988; **Fellow:** Medical Oncology, Brooke Army Med Ctr 1991

Medical Oncology

Butler, William M MD [Onc] - **Spec Exp:** Breast Cancer; Prostate Cancer; Lung Cancer; Clinical Trials; **Hospital:** Palmetto Richland Mem Hosp; **Address:** SC Oncology Associates, 166 Stoneridge St, Columbia, SC 29210; **Phone:** 803-461-3000; **Board Cert:** Internal Medicine 1975; Hematology 1980; Medical Oncology 1979; **Med School:** Tulane Univ 1972; **Resid:** Internal Medicine, Charity Hosp 1975; **Fellow:** Hematology & Oncology, Walter Reed AMC 1980; **Fac Appt:** Clin Prof Med, Univ SC Sch Med

Carbone, David MD [Onc] - **Spec Exp:** Lung Cancer; **Hospital:** Vanderbilt Univ Med Ctr; **Address:** Vanderbilt-Ingram Cancer Ctr, 685 Preston Rsch Bldg, 2200 Pierce Ave, Nashville, TN 37232-6838; **Phone:** 615-936-3524; **Board Cert:** Internal Medicine 1988; Medical Oncology 2001; **Med School:** Johns Hopkins Univ 1985; **Resid:** Internal Medicine, Johns Hopkins Hosp 1988; **Fellow:** Oncology, Natl Cancer Inst 1991; **Fac Appt:** Prof Med, Vanderbilt Univ

Carey, Lisa A MD [Onc] - **Spec Exp:** Breast Cancer; **Hospital:** Univ NC Hosps; **Address:** Univ North Carolina-Div Hem/Onc, Campus Box 7305, 3009 Old Clinic Bldg, Chapel Hill, NC 27599; **Phone:** 919-966-4431; **Board Cert:** Internal Medicine 2003; Medical Oncology 1997; **Med School:** Johns Hopkins Univ 1990; **Resid:** Internal Medicine, Johns Hopkins Hosp 1993; **Fellow:** Oncology, Johns Hopkins Hosp 1996; **Fac Appt:** Asst Prof Med, Univ NC Sch Med

Carpenter Jr, John MD [Onc] - **Spec Exp:** Breast Cancer; **Hospital:** Univ of Ala Hosp at Birmingham; **Address:** 1530 3rd Ave S, Birmingham, AL 35294; **Phone:** 205-934-2084; **Board Cert:** Internal Medicine 1972; Hematology 1981; Medical Oncology 1975; **Med School:** Tulane Univ 1968; **Resid:** Internal Medicine, Grady Meml Hosp 1971; **Fellow:** Hematology & Oncology, Emory Univ 1973; **Fac Appt:** Prof Med, Univ Ala

Chao, Nelson Jen An MD [Onc] - **Spec Exp:** Bone Marrow Transplant; Lymphoma; Leukemia; **Hospital:** Duke Univ Med Ctr; **Address:** Duke Univ Med Ctr, Box 3961, Durham, NC 27710; **Phone:** 919-668-1002; **Board Cert:** Internal Medicine 1984; Medical Oncology 1987; **Med School:** Yale Univ 1981; **Resid:** Internal Medicine, Stanford Univ Med Ctr 1984; **Fellow:** Oncology, Stanford Univ Med Ctr 1987; **Fac Appt:** Prof Med, Duke Univ

Colon-Otero, Gerardo MD [Onc] - **Spec Exp:** Ovarian Cancer; Breast Cancer; Hematologic Malignancies; **Hospital:** Mayo - Jacksonville, St Luke's Hosp - Jacksonville; **Address:** Mayo Clinic Jacksonville, 4500 San Pablo Rd S, Jacksonville, FL 32224-1865; **Phone:** 904-953-2000; **Board Cert:** Internal Medicine 1982; Hematology 1984; Medical Oncology 1985; **Med School:** Puerto Rico 1979; **Resid:** Internal Medicine, Mayo Clinic 1982; **Fellow:** Hematology, Mayo Clinic 1984; Medical Oncology, Univ Va Med Ctr 1986; **Fac Appt:** Assoc Prof Med, Mayo Med Sch

Conry, Robert M MD [Onc] - **Spec Exp:** Melanoma; Lung Cancer; Colon & Rectal Cancer; Sarcoma; **Hospital:** Univ of Ala Hosp at Birmingham; **Address:** The Kirklin Clinic At Acton Rd, 2145 Bonner Way, Birmingham, AL 35243; **Phone:** 205-978-0250; **Board Cert:** Medical Oncology 1997; Hematology 2001; **Med School:** Univ Ala 1987; **Resid:** Internal Medicine, Univ Alabama Hosp 1990; **Fellow:** Medical Oncology, Univ Alabama Hosp 1993; **Fac Appt:** Assoc Prof Med, Univ Ala

Crawford, Jeffrey MD [Onc] - **Spec Exp:** Lung Cancer; **Hospital:** Duke Univ Med Ctr; **Address:** Duke Univ Med Ctr, Box 3476, Durham, NC 27710-0001; **Phone:** 919-668-6688; **Board Cert:** Internal Medicine 1977; Hematology 1980; Medical Oncology 1981; **Med School:** Ohio State Univ 1974; **Resid:** Internal Medicine, Duke Univ Med Ctr 1977; **Fellow:** Hematology & Oncology, Duke Univ Med Ctr 1981; **Fac Appt:** Prof Med, Duke Univ

Daud, Adil I MD [Onc] - **Spec Exp:** Melanoma; Skin Cancer; Drug Development; **Hospital:** H Lee Moffitt Cancer Ctr & Research Inst; **Address:** H Lee Moffitt Cancer Ctr & Rsch Inst, 12902 Magnolia Drive, Tampa, FL 33612; **Phone:** 813-745-8581; **Board Cert:** Internal Medicine 1997; Hematology 2000; Medical Oncology 2000; **Med School:** India 1987; **Resid:** Internal Medicine, Indiana Univ; **Fellow:** Hematology & Oncology, Meml Sloan Kettering Cancer Ctr

De Simone, Philip MD [Onc] - **Spec Exp:** Colon Cancer; Pancreatic Cancer; **Hospital:** Univ of Kentucky Chandler Hosp; **Address:** UKMC Markey Cancer Ctr, CC-160, 800 Rose St, Lexington, KY 40536; **Phone:** 859-323-8043; **Board Cert:** Internal Medicine 1972; Hematology 1974; **Med School:** Univ VT Coll Med 1967; **Resid:** Internal Medicine, Univ Kentucky Hosp 1972; **Fellow:** Hematology & Oncology, Univ Kentucky Hosp 1974; **Fac Appt:** Prof Med, Univ KY Coll Med

Dunphy, Frank R MD [Onc] - **Spec Exp:** Lung Cancer; Head & Neck Cancer; **Hospital:** Duke Univ Med Ctr; **Address:** Duke Univ Med Ctr, Box 3198, Durham, NC 27710; **Phone:** 919-668-6688; **Board Cert:** Internal Medicine 1984; Hematology 1986; Medical Oncology 1989; **Med School:** Louisiana State U, New Orleans 1979; **Resid:** Internal Medicine, Lousiana St Univ Hosp 1983; **Fellow:** Hematology & Oncology, Louisiana St Univ Hosp 1985; **Fac Appt:** Assoc Prof Med, Duke Univ

Flinn, Ian W MD/PhD [Onc] - **Spec Exp:** Hematologic Malignancies; Lymphoma; Bone Marrow Transplant; Clinical Trials; **Hospital:** Centennial Med Ctr; **Address:** Tennessee Oncology, 250 25th Ave N, Ste 412, Nashville, TN 37203; **Phone:** 615-986-7600; **Board Cert:** Hematology 2007; Medical Oncology 1997; **Med School:** Johns Hopkins Univ 1990; **Resid:** Internal Medicine, Univ Michigan Med Ctr 1993; **Fellow:** Hematology & Oncology, Johns Hopkins Univ Hosps 1993

Fracasso, Paula M MD/PhD [Onc] - **Spec Exp:** Ovarian Cancer; Gynecologic Cancer; Breast Cancer; **Hospital:** Univ Virginia Med Ctr; **Address:** Dept Medicine, Div Hem/Onc, PO Box 800716, Charlottesville, VA 22908; **Phone:** 434-243-6143; **Board Cert:** Internal Medicine 1987; Medical Oncology 2003; **Med School:** Yale Univ 1984; **Resid:** Internal Medicine, Beth Israel Hosp 1987; **Fellow:** Cancer Research, Mass Inst Tech 1989; Hematology & Oncology, Tufts-New England Med Ctr 1991; **Fac Appt:** Prof Med, Univ VA Sch Med

Garst, Jennifer L MD [Onc] - **Spec Exp:** Lung Cancer; Thoracic Cancers; Cancer Survivors-Late Effects of Therapy; **Hospital:** Duke Univ Med Ctr; **Address:** Duke Univ Med Ctr, 25176 Morris Bldg, Box 3198, Durham, NC 27710-0001; **Phone:** 919-668-6688; **Board Cert:** Medical Oncology 1997; **Med School:** Med Coll GA 1990; **Resid:** Internal Medicine, Univ SW Texas Hosp 1993; **Fellow:** Hematology & Oncology, Duke Univ Med Ctr 1996; **Fac Appt:** Assoc Prof Med, Duke Univ

Gockerman, Jon Paul MD [Onc] - **Spec Exp:** Leukemia; Lymphoma; **Hospital:** Duke Univ Med Ctr; **Address:** Duke Univ Med Ctr, 1 Trent Drive, rm 25153, Box 3872, Morris Bldg, Durham, NC 27710; **Phone:** 919-684-8964; **Board Cert:** Internal Medicine 1972; Hematology 1974; Medical Oncology 1973; **Med School:** Univ Chicago-Pritzker Sch Med 1967; **Resid:** Internal Medicine, Duke Univ Med Ctr 1969; **Fellow:** Hematology & Oncology, Duke Univ Med Ctr 1971

Goldberg, Richard M MD [Onc] - **Spec Exp:** Stomach Cancer; Esophageal Cancer; Colon & Rectal Cancer; Pancreatic Cancer; **Hospital:** Univ NC Hosps; **Address:** Division of Hematology/Oncology, CB 7305, 3009 Old Clinic Bldg SW, Chapel Hill, NC 27599-0001; **Phone:** 919-843-7711; **Board Cert:** Internal Medicine 1982; Medical Oncology 1985; **Med School:** SUNY Upstate Med Univ 1979; **Resid:** Internal Medicine, Emory Univ Med Ctr 1982; **Fellow:** Medical Oncology, Georgetown Univ Med Ctr 1984; **Fac Appt:** Prof Med, Univ NC Sch Med

Medical Oncology

Graham II, Mark L MD [Onc] - **Spec Exp:** Breast Cancer; Breast Cancer Genetics; **Hospital:** WakeMed Cary; **Address:** Waverly Hematology/Oncology, 300 Ashville Ave, Ste 310, Cary, NC 27518; **Phone:** 919-233-8585; **Board Cert:** Internal Medicine 1989; **Med School:** Mayo Med Sch 1982; **Resid:** Internal Medicine, Duke Univ Med Ctr 1985; **Fellow:** Medical Oncology, Univ CO Hlth Sci Ctr 1990; Medical Oncology, Mayo Clinic; **Fac Appt:** Assoc Clin Prof Med, Univ NC Sch Med

Greco, F Anthony MD [Onc] - **Spec Exp:** Lung Cancer; Unknown Primary Cancer; **Hospital:** Centennial Med Ctr; **Address:** Sarah Cannon Research Inst, 250 25th Ave N Atrium Bldg - Ste 100, Nashville, TN 37203; **Phone:** 615-320-5090; **Board Cert:** Internal Medicine 1975; Medical Oncology 1977; **Med School:** W VA Univ 1972; **Resid:** Internal Medicine, Univ West Virginia Hosp 1974; **Fellow:** Medical Oncology, Natl Cancer Inst 1976

Grosh, William W MD [Onc] - **Spec Exp:** Melanoma; Sarcoma; Neuroendocrine Tumors; **Hospital:** Univ Virginia Med Ctr; **Address:** UVA Health System, Div Hem/Oncology, PO Box 800716, Charlottesville, VA 22908; **Phone:** 434-924-1904; **Board Cert:** Internal Medicine 1978; Medical Oncology 1985; **Med School:** Columbia P&S 1974; **Resid:** Internal Medicine, Vanderbilt Univ Med Ctr 1977; **Fellow:** Medical Oncology, Vanderbilt Univ Med Ctr 1983; **Fac Appt:** Assoc Prof Med, Univ VA Sch Med

Hande, Kenneth MD [Onc] - **Spec Exp:** Drug Discovery; Sarcoma; Carcinoid Tumors; **Hospital:** Vanderbilt Univ Med Ctr, VA Med Ctr - Nashville; **Address:** Vanderbilt Univ Med Ctr, 777 Preston Research Building, Nashville, TN 37232-6307; **Phone:** 615-322-4967; **Board Cert:** Internal Medicine 1975; Medical Oncology 1977; **Med School:** Johns Hopkins Univ 1972; **Resid:** Internal Medicine, Barnes Hosp 1974; **Fellow:** Medical Oncology, Natl Cancer Inst 1977; **Fac Appt:** Prof Med, Vanderbilt Univ

Hurd, David MD [Onc] - **Spec Exp:** Lymphoma; Leukemia; Bone Marrow Transplant; **Hospital:** Wake Forest Univ Baptist Med Ctr (page 73); **Address:** Wake Forest Sch Med, Comp Cancer Ctr, Medical Center Boulevard, Winston-Salem, NC 27157-1082; **Phone:** 336-713-5440; **Board Cert:** Internal Medicine 1977; Medical Oncology 1981; **Med School:** Univ IL Coll Med 1974; **Resid:** Internal Medicine, Univ Minn Hosp 1977; **Fellow:** Medical Oncology, Univ Minn Hosp 1979; **Fac Appt:** Prof Med, Wake Forest Univ

Jahanzeb, Mohammad MD [Onc] - **Spec Exp:** Breast Cancer; Lung Cancer; **Hospital:** Methodist Univ Hosp - Memphis, St Francis Hosp - Memphis; **Address:** Univ Tennessee Coll Med, Div Hem/Onc, 1331 Union Ave, Ste 800, Memphis, TN 38104; **Phone:** 901-722-0532; **Board Cert:** Medical Oncology 2003; Hematology 2005; **Med School:** Pakistan 1986; **Resid:** Internal Medicine, New Britain Genl Hosp 1990; **Fellow:** Hematology & Oncology, Washington Univ 1993; **Fac Appt:** Prof Med, Univ Tenn Coll Med, Memphis

Jillella, Anand MD [Onc] - **Spec Exp:** Bone Marrow Transplant; Leukemia; Lymphoma; Multiple Myeloma; **Hospital:** Med Coll of GA Hosp and Clin; **Address:** Med Coll Ga - BMT Program, 1120 15th St, BAA 5407, Augusta, GA 30912-3125; **Phone:** 706-721-2505; **Board Cert:** Medical Oncology 1997; **Med School:** India 1985; **Resid:** Internal Medicine, Med Coll Georgia 1992; **Fellow:** Medical Oncology, Yale-New Haven Hosp 1996; **Fac Appt:** Prof Med, Med Coll GA

Johnson, David H MD [Onc] - **Spec Exp:** Lung Cancer; Breast Cancer; Drug Development; **Hospital:** Vanderbilt Univ Med Ctr; **Address:** Vanderbilt Univ Med Ctr, Div Med Onc, 2220 Pierce Ave, 777 PRB, Nashville, TN 37232-0021; **Phone:** 615-322-6053; **Board Cert:** Internal Medicine 1979; Medical Oncology 1983; **Med School:** Med Coll GA 1976; **Resid:** Internal Medicine, Univ South Alabama Med Ctr 1979; Internal Medicine, Med Coll Georgia Hosps 1980; **Fellow:** Medical Oncology, Vanderbilt Univ Med Ctr 1983; **Fac Appt:** Prof Med, Vanderbilt Univ

Khuri, Fadlo MD [Onc] - **Spec Exp:** Head & Neck Cancer; Lung Cancer; **Hospital:** Emory Univ Hosp; **Address:** Winship Cancer Institute, Emory Univ Hosp, 1365 Clifton Rd NE, Ste 3000, Atlanta, GA 30322; **Phone:** 404-778-4250; **Board Cert:** Medical Oncology 1997; **Med School:** Columbia P&S 1989; **Resid:** Internal Medicine, Boston Univ Sch Med 1992; **Fellow:** Medical Oncology, Tufts Univ Sch Med 1995; **Fac Appt:** Prof Med, Emory Univ

Kraft, Andrew S MD [Onc] - **Spec Exp:** Prostate Cancer; Sarcoma; Drug Development; Clinical Trials; **Hospital:** MUSC Med Ctr; **Address:** 86 Jonathan Lucas St, PO BOX 250955, Charleston, SC 29425; **Phone:** 843-792-8284; **Board Cert:** Internal Medicine 1980; Medical Oncology 1985; **Med School:** Univ Pennsylvania 1975; **Resid:** Internal Medicine, Mt Sinai Hosp 1979; **Fellow:** Medical Oncology, Natl Cancer Inst 1983; **Fac Appt:** Prof Med, Med Univ SC

Kvols, Larry K MD [Onc] - **Spec Exp:** Gastrointestinal Cancer; Carcinoid Tumors; Neuroendocrine Tumors; **Hospital:** H Lee Moffitt Cancer Ctr & Research Inst; **Address:** H Lee Moffitt Cancer Ctr & Research Inst, 12902 Magnolia Drive, WCB-GI Program, Tampa, FL 33612-9497; **Phone:** 813-745-7257; **Board Cert:** Internal Medicine 1976; Medical Oncology 1977; **Med School:** Baylor Coll Med 1970; **Resid:** Internal Medicine, Johns Hopkins Hosp 1972; **Fellow:** Hematology & Oncology, Johns Hopkins Hosp 1973; **Fac Appt:** Prof Med, Mayo Med Sch

Lawson, David H MD [Onc] - **Spec Exp:** Melanoma; **Hospital:** Emory Univ Hosp; **Address:** Winship Cancer Institute, 1365 Clifton Rd NE, Atlanta, GA 30322; **Phone:** 404-778-1900; **Board Cert:** Internal Medicine 1977; Medical Oncology 1979; **Med School:** Emory Univ 1974; **Resid:** Internal Medicine, Emory Univ Hosps 1977; **Fellow:** Medical Oncology, Emory Univ Hosps 1979; **Fac Appt:** Assoc Prof Med, Emory Univ

Lesser, Glenn J MD [Onc] - **Spec Exp:** Neuro-Oncology; Brain Tumors; **Hospital:** Wake Forest Univ Baptist Med Ctr (page 73); **Address:** Wake Forest University-Div of Hem/Onc, Medical Center Blvd, Winston-Salem, NC 27157-1082; **Phone:** 336-716-9527; **Board Cert:** Internal Medicine 1990; Medical Oncology 1993; **Med School:** Penn State Univ-Hershey Med Ctr 1987; **Resid:** Internal Medicine, NC Baptist Hosp/Bowman Gray Sch Med 1991; **Fellow:** Medical Oncology, Johns Hopkins Hosp 1994; **Fac Appt:** Assoc Prof Med, Wake Forest Univ

Lilenbaum, Rogerio MD [Onc] - **Spec Exp:** Lung Cancer; **Hospital:** Mount Sinai Med Ctr - Miami; **Address:** Mount Sinai Cancer Ctr, 4306 Alton Rd, Ste 3, Miami, FL 33140-2840; **Phone:** 305-535-3310; **Board Cert:** Internal Medicine 2005; Hematology 1998; Medical Oncology 1997; **Med School:** Brazil 1986; **Resid:** Internal Medicine, Univ Hosp-Rio de Janeiro 1989; **Fellow:** Hematology & Oncology, Washington Univ Sch Med 1992; Oncology, UCSD 1994; **Fac Appt:** Assoc Clin Prof Med, Univ Miami Sch Med

Limentani, Steven A MD [Onc] - **Spec Exp:** Breast Cancer; Multiple Myeloma; Clinical Trials; **Hospital:** Carolinas Med Ctr; **Address:** 1100 S Tryon St, Ste 400, Charlotte, NC 28203; **Phone:** 704-446-9046; **Board Cert:** Internal Medicine 1989; Hematology 2002; Medical Oncology 2001; **Med School:** Tufts Univ 1986; **Resid:** Internal Medicine, New England Deaconess Hosp 1989; **Fellow:** Hematology & Oncology, New England Med Ctr 1992; **Fac Appt:** Clin Prof Med, Univ NC Sch Med

Lippman, Marc E MD [Onc] - **Spec Exp:** Breast Cancer; **Hospital:** Univ of Miami Hosp & Clins/Sylvester Comp Canc Ctr; **Address:** Leonard M Miller Sch Med, Dept Med, 1430 NW 11th Ave, MTSL, Ste 1001, Miami, FL 33136; **Phone:** 305-243-9120; **Board Cert:** Internal Medicine 1987; Endocrinology 1975; Medical Oncology 1977; **Med School:** Yale Univ 1968; **Resid:** Internal Medicine, Johns Hopkins Hosp 1970; **Fellow:** Medical Oncology, Natl Cancer Inst 1973; Endocrinology, Yale-New Haven Hosp 1974; **Fac Appt:** Prof Med, Univ Mich Med Sch

Medical Oncology

Lossos, Izidore MD [Onc] - **Spec Exp:** Lymphoma; Hodgkin's Disease; Leukemia; **Hospital:** Univ of Miami Hosp & Clins/Sylvester Comp Canc Ctr, Jackson Meml Hosp; **Address:** Univ Miami - Sylvester Comp Cancer Ctr, 1475 NW 12th Ave, D8-4, Miami, FL 33136; **Phone:** 305-243-4785; **Med School:** Israel 1987; **Resid:** Internal Medicine, Hadassah Univ Hosp 1995; **Fellow:** Hematology & Oncology, Hadassah Univ Hosp 1997; Medical Oncology, Stanford Univ 2001; **Fac Appt:** Assoc Prof Med, Univ Miami Sch Med

Lyckholm, Laurel J MD [Onc] - **Spec Exp:** Neuro-Oncology; **Hospital:** Med Coll of VA Hosp; **Address:** Med Coll of VA, Div Hem/Onc, PO Box 980230, Richmond, VA 23298; **Phone:** 804-828-9723; **Board Cert:** Internal Medicine 1989; Medical Oncology 2003; Hematology 2004; **Med School:** Creighton Univ 1985; **Resid:** Internal Medicine, Creighton Univ 1989; **Fellow:** Hematology & Oncology, Univ IA Coll Med 1992; **Fac Appt:** Assoc Prof Med, Med Coll VA

Lyman, Gary H MD [Onc] - **Spec Exp:** Breast Cancer; **Hospital:** Duke Univ Med Ctr; **Address:** Duke Comprehensive Cancer Center, Hock Plaza, 2424 Erwin Rd, Ste 602 - rm 6038, Box 3645, Durham, NC 27710; **Phone:** 919-681-1604; **Board Cert:** Internal Medicine 1987; Medical Oncology 1977; Hematology 1978; **Med School:** SUNY Buffalo 1972; **Resid:** Internal Medicine, Univ North Carolina Hosp 1974; **Fellow:** Medical Oncology, Roswell Park Meml Inst 1976; Biostatistics, Harvard Med Sch 1982

Lynch Jr, James W MD [Onc] - **Spec Exp:** Lymphoma; Immunotherapy; Lung Cancer; **Hospital:** Shands at Univ of FL; **Address:** Shands Hlthcare, Div Hematology/Oncology, PO Box 100278, Gainesville, FL 32610-0277; **Phone:** 352-265-0725; **Board Cert:** Internal Medicine 1987; Medical Oncology 2001; **Med School:** Eastern VA Med Sch 1984; **Resid:** Internal Medicine, Univ Florida 1987; **Fellow:** Medical Oncology, Natl Cancer Inst 1991; **Fac Appt:** Prof Med, Univ Fla Coll Med

Marcom, Paul K MD [Onc] - **Spec Exp:** Breast Cancer; Clinical Trials; Cancer Genetics; **Hospital:** Duke Univ Med Ctr; **Address:** Duke Univ Med Ctr, Box 3147, Ste 3800, Red Zone, Duke South Hosp, Durham, NC 27710; **Phone:** 919-684-3877; **Board Cert:** Internal Medicine 2003; Medical Oncology 2005; **Med School:** Baylor Coll Med 1989; **Resid:** Internal Medicine, Duke Univ Med Ctr 1992; Hematology & Oncology, Duke Univ Med Ctr 1995; **Fac Appt:** Assoc Prof Med, Duke Univ

Miller, Donald M MD/PhD [Onc] - **Spec Exp:** Melanoma; Lung Cancer; **Hospital:** Univ of Louisville Hosp; **Address:** 529 S Jackson St, Louisville, KY 40202; **Phone:** 502-562-4790; **Board Cert:** Internal Medicine 1979; **Med School:** Duke Univ 1973; **Resid:** Internal Medicine, Peter Bent Brigham Hosp 1975; **Fellow:** Internal Medicine, Harvard Univ Hosp 1978; Medical Oncology, Natl Cancer Inst 1979; **Fac Appt:** Prof Med, Univ Louisville Sch Med

Moore, Joseph O MD [Onc] - **Spec Exp:** Leukemia; Hodgkin's Disease; Lymphoma, Non-Hodgkin's; Neuroendocrine Tumors; **Hospital:** Duke Univ Med Ctr; **Address:** Duke Univ Med Ctr, Box 3872, Durham, NC 27710; **Phone:** 919-684-8964; **Board Cert:** Internal Medicine 1975; Medical Oncology 1977; **Med School:** Johns Hopkins Univ 1970; **Resid:** Internal Medicine, Johns Hopkins Hosp 1975; **Fellow:** Hematology & Oncology, Duke Univ 1977; **Fac Appt:** Prof Med, Duke Univ

Nabell, Lisle M MD [Onc] - **Spec Exp:** Breast Cancer; Head & Neck Cancer; **Hospital:** Univ of Ala Hosp at Birmingham; **Address:** Univ of Alabama, 1530 3rd Ave S, Ste WTI237, Birmingham, AL 35294; **Phone:** 205-934-3061; **Board Cert:** Internal Medicine 2000; Medical Oncology 2000; **Med School:** Univ NC Sch Med 1987; **Resid:** Internal Medicine, Univ Alabama Hosp 1990; **Fellow:** Hematology & Oncology, Univ Alabama Hosp 1992; **Fac Appt:** Assoc Prof Med, Univ Ala

O'Regan, Ruth M MD [Onc] - **Spec Exp:** Breast Cancer; Breast Cancer Risk Assessment; Cancer Prevention; Clinical Trials; **Hospital:** Emory Univ Hosp; **Address:** Emory Univ Winship Cancer Inst, 1365 Clifton Rd C Bldg - Ste 4005, Atlanta, GA 30322; **Phone:** 404-778-1900; **Board Cert:** Internal Medicine 1999; Medical Oncology 2000; **Med School:** Ireland 1988; **Resid:** Internal Medicine, Med Coll Wisc 1995; Medical Oncology, Northwestern Univ Hosp 1999; **Fellow:** Medical Oncology, Northwestern Univ Hosp 1998; **Fac Appt:** Assoc Prof Med, Emory Univ

Perez, Edith A MD [Onc] - **Spec Exp:** Breast Cancer; Breast Cancer Risk Assessment; Clinical Trials; **Hospital:** Mayo - Jacksonville; **Address:** Mayo Clinic-Jacksonville, 4500 San Pablo Rd Davis Bldg Fl 8, Jacksonville, FL 32224; **Phone:** 904-953-7283; **Board Cert:** Internal Medicine 1983; Hematology 1986; Medical Oncology 1987; **Med School:** Univ Puerto Rico 1979; **Resid:** Internal Medicine, Loma Linda Univ Med Ctr 1982; **Fellow:** Hematology & Oncology, Martinez VA Hosp/UC Davis 1987; **Fac Appt:** Prof Med, Mayo Med Sch

Posey III, James A MD [Onc] - **Spec Exp:** Gastrointestinal Cancer; Colon Cancer; Liver Cancer; Biliary Cancer; **Hospital:** Univ of Ala Hosp at Birmingham; **Address:** Wallace Tumor Institute, 24 6th Ave S, rm 263A, Birmingham, AL 35294-3300; **Phone:** 205-934-0916; **Board Cert:** Medical Oncology 1997; **Med School:** Howard Univ 1991; **Resid:** Internal Medicine, Georgetown Univ Med Ctr 1994; **Fellow:** Hematology & Oncology, Georgetown Univ Med Ctr 1997; **Fac Appt:** Assoc Prof Med, Univ Ala

Robert, Nicholas J MD [Onc] - **Spec Exp:** Breast Cancer; **Hospital:** Inova Fairfax Hosp; **Address:** 8503 Arlington Blvd, Ste 400, Fairfax, VA 22031; **Phone:** 703-280-5390; **Board Cert:** Internal Medicine 1978; Anatomic Pathology 1979; Medical Oncology 1981; Hematology 1984; **Med School:** McGill Univ 1974; **Resid:** Internal Medicine, Royal Victoria Hosp 1976; Pathology, Mass Genl Hosp 1979; **Fellow:** Hematology, Peter Bent Brigham Hosp 1980; Medical Oncology, Dana Farber Cancer Inst 1981

Robert-Vizcarrondo, Francisco MD [Onc] - **Spec Exp:** Lung Cancer; Mesothelioma; Drug Development; Clinical Trials; **Hospital:** Univ of Ala Hosp at Birmingham; **Address:** 1824 6th Ave S, Room NT-CC-2555D, Birmingham, AL 35294-0001; **Phone:** 205-934-5077; **Board Cert:** Internal Medicine 1973; Hematology 1976; Medical Oncology 1975; **Med School:** Puerto Rico 1969; **Resid:** Internal Medicine, Univ PR Hosp 1972; Hematology, Univ PR Hosp 1974; **Fellow:** Medical Oncology, Univ AL Hosp at Birmingham 1976; **Fac Appt:** Prof Med, Univ Ala

Romond, Edward H MD [Onc] - **Spec Exp:** Breast Cancer; Hemophilia; **Hospital:** Univ of Kentucky Chandler Hosp; **Address:** Univ Kentucky Med Ctr, Div Hematology/Oncology, CC413 Markey Cancer Center, Lexington, KY 40536-0093; **Phone:** 859-323-8043; **Board Cert:** Internal Medicine 1980; Hematology 1984; Medical Oncology 1983; **Med School:** Univ KY Coll Med 1977; **Resid:** Internal Medicine, Michigan State Univ Hosps 1980; **Fellow:** Hematology & Oncology, Michigan State Univ 1983; **Fac Appt:** Prof Med, Univ KY Coll Med

Roth, Bruce J MD [Onc] - **Spec Exp:** Prostate Cancer; Bladder Cancer; Testicular Cancer; **Hospital:** Vanderbilt Univ Med Ctr; **Address:** Vanderbilt Ingram Cancer Center, 777 Preston Research Bldg, Nashville, TN 37232-6307; **Phone:** 615-343-4070; **Board Cert:** Internal Medicine 1983; Medical Oncology 1985; **Med School:** St Louis Univ 1980; **Resid:** Internal Medicine, Indiana Univ Med Ctr 1983; **Fellow:** Hematology & Oncology, Indiana Univ Med Ctr 1986; **Fac Appt:** Prof Med, Vanderbilt Univ

Rothenberg, Mace MD [Onc] - **Spec Exp:** Pancreatic Cancer; Colon & Rectal Cancer; Clinical Trials; **Hospital:** Vanderbilt Univ Med Ctr; **Address:** Vanderbilt Ingram Cancer Center, 777 Preston Research Bldg, Nashville, TN 37232-6307; **Phone:** 615-322-4967; **Board Cert:** Internal Medicine 1985; Medical Oncology 1987; **Med School:** NYU Sch Med 1982; **Resid:** Internal Medicine, Vanderbilt Univ Med Ctr 1985; **Fellow:** Medical Oncology, Natl Cancer Inst 1988; **Fac Appt:** Prof Med, Vanderbilt Univ

Medical Oncology

Sandler, Alan MD [Onc] - **Spec Exp:** Lung Cancer; Sarcoma; **Hospital:** Vanderbilt Univ Med Ctr; **Address:** Vanderbilt Univ Med Ctr-Thoracic Onc, 2220 Pierce Ave, 777 Preston Research Bldg, Nashville, TN 37232-0021; **Phone:** 615-322-6053; **Med School:** Rush Med Coll 1987; **Resid:** Internal Medicine, Yale-New Haven Hosp 1990; **Fellow:** Medical Oncology, Yale Univ 1993; **Fac Appt:** Assoc Prof Med, Vanderbilt Univ

Schwartz, Michael A MD [Onc] - **Spec Exp:** Breast Cancer; Lymphoma; Colon Cancer; **Hospital:** Mount Sinai Med Ctr - Miami, Miami Heart Inst; **Address:** 4306 Alton Rd Fl 3, Miami Beach, FL 33140; **Phone:** 305-535-3310; **Board Cert:** Internal Medicine 1989; Medical Oncology 2004; Hematology 2004; **Med School:** UMDNJ-RW Johnson Med Sch 1986; **Resid:** Internal Medicine, Mt Sinai Medical Ctr 1989; **Fellow:** Hematology & Oncology, Meml Sloan Kettering Cancer Ctr 1992; **Fac Appt:** Asst Clin Prof Med, Univ Miami Sch Med

Serody, Jonathan S MD [Onc] - **Spec Exp:** Breast Cancer Vaccine Therapy; Clinical Trials; Lymphoma; **Hospital:** Univ NC Hosps; **Address:** Lineberger Comprehensive Cancer Ctr, 450 West Drive, CB 7295, Chapel Hill, NC 27599-7295; **Phone:** 919-966-8644; **Board Cert:** Internal Medicine 1989; Hematology 2007; **Med School:** Univ VA Sch Med 1986; **Resid:** Internal Medicine, Univ NC Med Ctr 1989; **Fellow:** Hematology, Univ NC Med Ctr 1992; Bone Marrow Transplant, Fred Hutchinson Transplant Program 1993; **Fac Appt:** Assoc Prof Med, Univ NC Sch Med

Shea, Thomas MD [Onc] - **Spec Exp:** Bone Marrow Transplant; Lymphoma; Leukemia; **Hospital:** Univ NC Hosps; **Address:** Univ N Carolina, Dept Medicine, 3009 Old Clinic Bldg, Box 7305, Chapel Hill, NC 27599; **Phone:** 919-966-7746; **Board Cert:** Internal Medicine 1982; Hematology 1984; Medical Oncology 1985; **Med School:** Univ NC Sch Med 1978; **Resid:** Internal Medicine, Beth Israel Deaconess Med Ctr 1982; **Fellow:** Hematology & Oncology, Beth Israel Deaconess Med Ctr 1985; Bone Marrow Transplant, Dana Farber Cancer Inst 1988; **Fac Appt:** Prof Med, Univ NC Sch Med

Sherman, Carol A MD [Onc] - **Spec Exp:** Lung Cancer; Thoracic Cancers; **Hospital:** MUSC Med Ctr; **Address:** 96 Jonathan Lucas St, Ste CSB-903, Charleston, SC 29425; **Phone:** 843-792-9621; **Board Cert:** Internal Medicine 1987; Medical Oncology 1989; **Med School:** Univ Mass Sch Med 1984; **Resid:** Internal Medicine, Univ Mass Med Ctr 1987; **Fellow:** Hematology & Oncology, Univ Mass Med Ctr 1989; **Fac Appt:** Assoc Prof Med, Med Univ SC

Shin, Dong Moon MD [Onc] - **Spec Exp:** Head & Neck Cancer; Cancer Prevention; Mesothelioma; Thymoma; **Hospital:** Emory Univ Hosp; **Address:** Emory Winship Cancer Inst, 1365 C Clifton Rd NE, Ste 3090, Atlanta, GA 30322; **Phone:** 404-778-5990; **Board Cert:** Internal Medicine 1985; Medical Oncology 1989; **Med School:** South Korea 1975; **Resid:** Internal Medicine, Cook Co Hosp 1985; **Fellow:** Medical Oncology, Univ Texas MD Anderson Cancer Ctr 1986; **Fac Appt:** Prof Med, Emory Univ

Smith, Thomas Joseph MD [Onc] - **Spec Exp:** Breast Cancer; Palliative Care; **Hospital:** Med Coll of VA Hosp; **Address:** Med Coll Va, Div Hem/Onc, PO Box 980230, Richmond, VA 23298-0230; **Phone:** 804-828-9992; **Board Cert:** Internal Medicine 1982; Medical Oncology 1987; Hospice & Palliative Medicine ; **Med School:** Yale Univ 1979; **Resid:** Internal Medicine, Hosp Univ Penn 1982; **Fellow:** Medical Oncology, Med Coll Virginia 1987; **Fac Appt:** Prof Med, Med Coll VA

Socinski, Mark A MD [Onc] - **Spec Exp:** Lung Cancer; **Hospital:** Univ NC Hosps; **Address:** UNC Chapel Hill, Div Hem/Onc, 3009 Old Clinic Bldg, Campus Box 7305, Chapel Hill, NC 27599-7305; **Phone:** 919-966-4431; **Board Cert:** Internal Medicine 1988; Medical Oncology 2002; **Med School:** Univ VT Coll Med 1984; **Resid:** Internal Medicine, Beth Israel Hosp 1986; **Fellow:** Medical Oncology, Dana-Farber Cancer Inst 1989; **Fac Appt:** Assoc Prof Med, Univ NC Sch Med

Sosman, Jeffrey MD [Onc] - **Spec Exp:** Kidney Cancer; Melanoma; Drug Discovery; **Hospital:** Vanderbilt Univ Med Ctr; **Address:** Vanderbilt Ingram Cancer Ctr, 777 Preston Research Bldg, Nashville, TN 37232-6307; **Phone:** 615-322-4967; **Board Cert:** Anatomic Pathology 1985; Internal Medicine 1987; Medical Oncology 1989; **Med School:** Albert Einstein Coll Med 1981; **Resid:** Anatomic Pathology, Univ Chicago Hosps 1985; Internal Medicine, Univ Wisconsin Hosp 1986; **Fellow:** Medical Oncology, Univ Wisconsin 1989; **Fac Appt:** Clin Prof Med, Vanderbilt Univ

Sotomayor, Eduardo M MD [Onc] - **Spec Exp:** Lymphoma; Gene Therapy; Vaccine Therapy; Clinical Trials; **Hospital:** H Lee Moffitt Cancer Ctr & Research Inst; **Address:** H Lee Moffitt Cancer Inst, 12902 Magnolia Drive, MRC 3 East, Ste 3056, Tampa, FL 33612; **Phone:** 813-745-1387; **Board Cert:** Medical Oncology 1997; **Med School:** Peru 1988; **Resid:** Internal Medicine, Univ Miami Sch Med 1995; **Fellow:** Immunology, Univ Mlami Sch Med 1989; Oncology, Johns Hopkins Hosp 1998; **Fac Appt:** Assoc Prof Med, Univ S Fla Coll Med

Stone, Joel MD [Onc] - **Spec Exp:** Lung Cancer; Breast Cancer; **Hospital:** St Vincent's Med Ctr - Jacksonville; **Address:** St Vincent's Med Ctr, 2 Shircliff Way, Ste 800, Jacksonville, FL 32204; **Phone:** 904-388-2619; **Board Cert:** Internal Medicine 1977; Medical Oncology 1979; **Med School:** Univ VA Sch Med 1974; **Resid:** Internal Medicine, Univ KY Med Ctr 1977; **Fellow:** Hematology & Oncology, Emory Univ 1979

Sutton, Linda Marie MD [Onc] - **Spec Exp:** Breast Cancer; Palliative Care; **Hospital:** Duke Univ Med Ctr; **Address:** University Tower, 3100 Tower Blvd, Ste 600, Durham, NC 27707; **Phone:** 919-419-5005; **Board Cert:** Internal Medicine 2002; Medical Oncology 2003; **Med School:** Univ Mass Sch Med 1987; **Resid:** Internal Medicine, Montefiore Med Ctr 1990; **Fellow:** Hematology & Oncology, Duke Univ Med Ctr 1993

Thigpen, James T MD [Onc] - **Spec Exp:** Gynecologic Cancer; Breast Cancer; Lung Cancer; **Hospital:** Univ Hosps & Clins - Jackson; **Address:** Univ Mississippi Med Ctr, Div Med Onc, 2500 N State St, Jackson, MS 39216; **Phone:** 601-984-5590; **Board Cert:** Internal Medicine 1972; Hematology 1974; Medical Oncology 1975; **Med School:** Univ Miss 1973; **Resid:** Internal Medicine, Univ Miss Med Ctr 1971; **Fellow:** Hematology & Oncology, Univ Miss Med Ctr 1973; **Fac Appt:** Prof Med, Univ Miss

Torti, Frank M MD [Onc] - **Spec Exp:** Prostate Cancer; Urologic Cancer; **Hospital:** Wake Forest Univ Baptist Med Ctr (page 73); **Address:** Wake Forest Med Ctr-Comp Cancer Ctr, Medical Center Blvd, Winston-Salem, NC 27157-1082; **Phone:** 336-716-7971; **Board Cert:** Internal Medicine 1976; Medical Oncology 1979; **Med School:** Harvard Med Sch 1974; **Resid:** Internal Medicine, Beth Israel Hosp 1976; **Fellow:** Medical Oncology, Stanford Univ Med Ctr 1979; **Fac Appt:** Prof Med, Wake Forest Univ

Troner, Michael MD [Onc] - **Spec Exp:** Head & Neck Cancer; Urologic Cancer; **Hospital:** Baptist Hosp of Miami; **Address:** 8940 N Kendall Drive, Ste 300, East Tower, Miami, FL 33176-2132; **Phone:** 305-595-2141; **Board Cert:** Internal Medicine 1972; Medical Oncology 1973; **Med School:** SUNY Downstate 1968; **Resid:** Internal Medicine, Univ Maryland Hosp 1971; **Fellow:** Medical Oncology, Univ Miami Med Ctr 1973; **Fac Appt:** Assoc Clin Prof Med, Univ Miami Sch Med

Vance, Ralph MD [Onc] - **Spec Exp:** Lung Cancer; **Hospital:** Univ Hosps & Clins - Jackson; **Address:** Univ Mississippi Med Ctr, Div Med Onc, 2500 N State St, Jackson, MS 39216; **Phone:** 601-984-5590; **Med School:** Univ Miss 1972; **Resid:** Internal Medicine, Univ Hosp; **Fellow:** Hematology & Oncology, Univ Hosp; **Fac Appt:** Prof Med, Univ Miss

Medical Oncology

Vaughan, William P MD [Onc] - **Spec Exp:** Bone Marrow Transplant; Breast Cancer; **Hospital:** Univ of Ala Hosp at Birmingham; **Address:** Univ Ala Birmingham, 1900 Univ Blvd, rm 541, Tinsley Harrison Twr, Birmingham, AL 35294; **Phone:** 205-934-1908; **Board Cert:** Internal Medicine 1975; Medical Oncology 1979; **Med School:** Univ Conn 1972; **Resid:** Internal Medicine, Univ Chicago Hosps 1975; **Fellow:** Oncology, Johns Hopkins Hosp 1977; **Fac Appt:** Prof Med, Univ Ala

Weber, Jeffrey S MD/PhD [Onc] - **Spec Exp:** Kidney Cancer; Melanoma; Breast Cancer; **Hospital:** H Lee Moffitt Cancer Ctr & Research Inst; **Address:** H Lee Moffitt Cancer Ctr, 12902 Magnolia Ave, Tampa, FL 33612; **Phone:** 813-745-2691; **Board Cert:** Internal Medicine 1983; Medical Oncology 1987; **Med School:** NYU Sch Med 1980; **Resid:** Internal Medicine, UCSD Med Ctr 1983; **Fellow:** Medical Oncology, Natl Cancer Inst 1990; **Fac Appt:** Assoc Prof Med, USC Sch Med

Weiss, Geoffrey R MD [Onc] - **Spec Exp:** Gastrointestinal Cancer; Genitourinary Cancer; Melanoma; **Hospital:** Univ Virginia Med Ctr; **Address:** Univ Virginia Hlth System, Div Hem/Onc, PO Box 800716, Charlottesville, VA 22908-0716; **Phone:** 434-243-0066; **Board Cert:** Internal Medicine 1977; Medical Oncology 1981; **Med School:** St Louis Univ 1974; **Resid:** Internal Medicine, Temple Univ Hosp 1978; **Fellow:** Medical Oncology, Dana Farber Cancer Inst 1982; **Fac Appt:** Prof Med, Univ VA Sch Med

Williams, Michael MD [Onc] - **Spec Exp:** Lymphoma; Multiple Myeloma; Leukemia; **Hospital:** Univ Virginia Med Ctr; **Address:** UVA Hlth System, Div Hem/Oncology, PO Box 800716, Charlottesville, VA 22908-0716; **Phone:** 434-924-9637; **Board Cert:** Internal Medicine 1982; Medical Oncology 1987; Hematology 1988; **Med School:** Univ Cincinnati 1979; **Resid:** Internal Medicine, Univ Virginia Med Ctr 1983; **Fellow:** Hematology & Oncology, Univ Virginia Med Ctr 1986; **Fac Appt:** Prof Med, Univ VA Sch Med

Wingard, John R MD [Onc] - **Spec Exp:** Bone Marrow Transplant; Leukemia; Multiple Myeloma; **Hospital:** Shands at Univ of FL; **Address:** 1376 Mowry Rd, Ste 145, Box 103633, Gainesville, FL 32610; **Phone:** 352-273-8010; **Board Cert:** Internal Medicine 1977; Medical Oncology 1981; **Med School:** Johns Hopkins Univ 1973; **Resid:** Internal Medicine, Memphis City Hosps 1976; Internal Medicine, VA Hosp 1977; **Fellow:** Medical Oncology, Johns Hopkins Hosp 1979; **Fac Appt:** Prof Med, Univ Fla Coll Med

Yunus, Furhan MD [Onc] - **Spec Exp:** Multiple Myeloma; Lymphoma; **Hospital:** Methodist Univ Hosp - Memphis, St Jude Children's Research Hosp; **Address:** Univ TN Cancer Inst, 1331 Union Ave, Ste 800, Memphis, TN 38104; **Phone:** 901-722-0561; **Board Cert:** Internal Medicine 1993; Medical Oncology 2008; **Med School:** Pakistan 1986; **Resid:** Internal Medicine, Methodist Hosp 1993; **Fellow:** Hematology & Oncology, Univ Ariz Coll Med 1995; **Fac Appt:** Asst Prof Med, Univ Tenn Coll Med, Memphis

Midwest

Adelstein, David J MD [Onc] - **Spec Exp:** Head & Neck Cancer; Esophageal Cancer; Lung Cancer; **Hospital:** Cleveland Clin Fdn (page 56); **Address:** Cleveland Clinic Fdn, Taussig Cancer Ctr, 9500 Euclid Ave, R35, Cleveland, OH 44195; **Phone:** 216-444-9310; **Board Cert:** Internal Medicine 1197; Medical Oncology 1981; Hematology 1982; **Med School:** NYU Sch Med 1975; **Resid:** Internal Medicine, Univ Hosps Cleveland 1978; **Fellow:** Hematology, Univ Hosps Cleveland 1981; **Fac Appt:** Prof Med, Cleveland Cl Coll Med/Case West Res

Albain, Kathy S MD [Onc] - **Spec Exp:** Breast Cancer; Lung Cancer; Cancer Survivors-Late Effects of Therapy; **Hospital:** Loyola Univ Med Ctr; **Address:** Loyola Univ Med Ctr, 2160 S First Ave, Bldg 112 - Ste 109, Maywood, IL 60153-5590; **Phone:** 708-327-3102; **Board Cert:** Internal Medicine 1981; Medical Oncology 1983; **Med School:** Univ Mich Med Sch 1978; **Resid:** Internal Medicine, Univ Illinois Med Ctr 1981; **Fellow:** Hematology & Oncology, Univ Chicago Hosps 1984; **Fac Appt:** Prof Med, Loyola Univ-Stritch Sch Med

Albertini, Mark R MD [Onc] - **Spec Exp:** Melanoma; Melanoma-Metastatic; **Hospital:** Univ WI Hosp & Clins; **Address:** Univ Wisconsin Medical Oncology, 600 Highland Ave, K4 414 CSC, Madison, WI 53792; **Phone:** 608-265-1700; **Board Cert:** Internal Medicine 1987; Medical Oncology 2002; **Med School:** Univ VT Coll Med 1984; **Resid:** Internal Medicine, Univ Wisc Hosps Clins 1987; **Fellow:** Medical Oncology, Univ Wisconsin 1991; **Fac Appt:** Assoc Prof Med, Univ Wisc

Anderson, Joseph M MD [Onc] - **Spec Exp:** Breast Cancer; Palliative Care; Neuro-Oncology; **Hospital:** Henry Ford Hosp; **Address:** 2799 W Grand Blvd, Ste K13, Detroit, MI 48202; **Phone:** 313-916-1854; **Board Cert:** Internal Medicine 1985; Medical Oncology 1989; **Med School:** Univ Mich Med Sch 1982; **Resid:** Internal Medicine, Henry Ford Hosp 1986; **Fellow:** Medical Oncology, Henry Ford Hosp 1988

Benson III, Al B MD [Onc] - **Spec Exp:** Colon Cancer; Carcinoid Tumors; Pancreatic Cancer; **Hospital:** Northwestern Meml Hosp, Jesse A Brown VA Med Ctr; **Address:** 675 N St Clair, Ste 21-100, Chicago, IL 60611; **Phone:** 312-695-0990; **Board Cert:** Internal Medicine 1979; Medical Oncology 1983; **Med School:** SUNY Buffalo 1976; **Resid:** Internal Medicine, Univ Wisc Hosps 1979; **Fellow:** Medical Oncology, Univ Wisc Hosps 1984; **Fac Appt:** Prof Med, Northwestern Univ

Bitran, Jacob MD [Onc] - **Spec Exp:** Breast Cancer; Bone Marrow Transplant; Lung Cancer; **Hospital:** Adv Luth Genl Hosp, Rush N Shore Med Ctr; **Address:** Lutheran Genl Cancer Care Specialists, 1700 Luther Lane, Park Ridge, IL 60068-1270; **Phone:** 847-268-8200; **Board Cert:** Internal Medicine 1974; Hematology 1986; Medical Oncology 1977; **Med School:** Univ IL Coll Med 1971; **Resid:** Pathology, Rush Presby St Lukes Hosp 1973; Internal Medicine, Michael Reese Hosp 1973; **Fellow:** Hematology & Oncology, Univ Chicago Hosps 1977; **Fac Appt:** Prof Med, Ros Franklin Univ/Chicago Med Sch

Bolwell, Brian J MD [Onc] - **Spec Exp:** Bone Marrow Transplant; Hematologic Malignancies; **Hospital:** Cleveland Clin Fdn (page 56); **Address:** 9500 Euclid Ave, Desk R32, Cleveland, OH 44195; **Phone:** 216-444-6922; **Board Cert:** Internal Medicine 1985; Medical Oncology 1987; **Med School:** Case West Res Univ 1981; **Resid:** Internal Medicine, Univ Hosp 1984; **Fellow:** Hematology & Oncology, Hosp Univ Penn 1987; **Fac Appt:** Prof Med, Cleveland Cl Coll Med/Case West Res

Bonomi, Philip MD [Onc] - **Spec Exp:** Lung Cancer; Thymoma; Mesothelioma; **Hospital:** Rush Univ Med Ctr; **Address:** 1725 W Harrison St, Ste 821, Chicago, IL 60612; **Phone:** 312-942-3312; **Board Cert:** Internal Medicine 1975; Medical Oncology 1977; **Med School:** Univ IL Coll Med 1970; **Resid:** Internal Medicine, Geisinger Med Ctr 1972; Internal Medicine, Geisinger Med Ctr 1975; **Fellow:** Medical Oncology, Rush Presby-St Luke's Med Ctr 1977; **Fac Appt:** Prof Med, Rush Med Coll

Borden, Ernest C MD [Onc] - **Spec Exp:** Melanoma; Immunotherapy; Sarcoma; Vaccine Therapy; **Hospital:** Cleveland Clin Fdn (page 56); **Address:** 9500 Euclid Ave, Desk R40, Cleveland, OH 44195; **Phone:** 216-444-8183; **Board Cert:** Internal Medicine 1973; Medical Oncology 1975; **Med School:** Duke Univ 1966; **Resid:** Internal Medicine, Hosp Univ Penn 1968; **Fellow:** Medical Oncology, Johns Hopkins Hosp 1973; **Fac Appt:** Prof Med, Cleveland Cl Coll Med/Case West Res

Medical Oncology

Bricker, Leslie J MD [Onc] - **Spec Exp:** Palliative Care; **Hospital:** Henry Ford Hosp; **Address:** Henry Ford Hospital, 2799 W Grand Blvd, CFP 5, Detroit, MI 48202; **Phone:** 313-916-1859; **Board Cert:** Internal Medicine 1980; Hematology 1982; Medical Oncology 1983; **Med School:** Wayne State Univ 1977; **Resid:** Internal Medicine, Sinai Hosp 1980; **Fellow:** Hematology & Oncology, Univ Mich Hosp 1983; **Fac Appt:** Assoc Prof Med, Wayne State Univ

Brockstein, Bruce E MD [Onc] - **Spec Exp:** Head & Neck Cancer; Sarcoma; Melanoma; **Hospital:** Evanston Hosp, Highland Park Hosp; **Address:** Evanston Northwestern Healthcare, Div Hematology/Oncology, 2650 Ridge Ave, rm 5134, Evanston, IL 60201; **Phone:** 847-570-2515; **Board Cert:** Internal Medicine 2003; Medical Oncology 2005; **Med School:** Univ Chicago-Pritzker Sch Med 1990; **Resid:** Internal Medicine, Hosp Univ Penn 1993; **Fellow:** Hematology & Oncology, Univ Chicago Hosps 1996; **Fac Appt:** Assoc Prof Med, Northwestern Univ

Buckner, Jan Craig MD [Onc] - **Spec Exp:** Brain Tumors; Neuro-Oncology; **Hospital:** Mayo Med Ctr & Clin - Rochester; **Address:** Mayo Clinic, 200 First St SW, Rochester, MN 55905; **Phone:** 507-284-4320; **Board Cert:** Internal Medicine 1983; Medical Oncology 1985; **Med School:** Univ NC Sch Med 1980; **Resid:** Internal Medicine, Butterworth Hosp 1983; **Fellow:** Medical Oncology, Mayo Clinic 1985; **Fac Appt:** Prof Med, Mayo Med Sch

Budd, George T MD [Onc] - **Spec Exp:** Breast Cancer; **Hospital:** Cleveland Clin Fdn (page 56); **Address:** Cleveland Clinic, Taussig Cancer Ctr, 9500 Euclid Ave, Desk R35, Cleveland, OH 44195; **Phone:** 216-444-6480; **Board Cert:** Internal Medicine 1980; Medical Oncology 1983; **Med School:** Univ Kans 1976; **Resid:** Internal Medicine, Cleveland Clinic 1980; **Fellow:** Hematology & Oncology, Cleveland Clinic 1982

Bukowski, Ronald M MD [Onc] - **Spec Exp:** Kidney Cancer; **Hospital:** Cleveland Clin Fdn (page 56); **Address:** Cleveland Clinic, Taussig Cancer Ctr, 9500 Euclid Ave, Desk R35, Cleveland, OH 44195-0001; **Phone:** 216-444-6825; **Board Cert:** Internal Medicine 1974; Medical Oncology 1975; Hematology 1976; **Med School:** Northwestern Univ 1967; **Resid:** Internal Medicine, Cleveland Clin Fdn 1969; Internal Medicine, Cleveland Clin Fdn 1973; **Fellow:** Hematology, Cleveland Clin Fdn 1975; **Fac Appt:** Prof Med, Cleveland Cl Coll Med/Case West Res

Burt, Richard K MD [Onc] - **Spec Exp:** Stem Cell Transplant in Lupus/Crohn's; Stem Cell Transplant in MS; Autoimmune Disease; **Hospital:** Northwestern Meml Hosp; **Address:** Div Immunotherapy, 750 N Lakeshore Drive, rm 649, Chicago, IL 60611; **Phone:** 312-908-0059; **Board Cert:** Internal Medicine 1989; **Med School:** St Louis Univ 1984; **Resid:** Internal Medicine, Baylor Coll Med 1988; **Fellow:** Medical Oncology, Natl Inst Hlth Clin Ctr 1991; Hematology, Nat Inst Hlth Clin Ctr 1993; **Fac Appt:** Assoc Prof Med, Northwestern Univ

Byrd, John C MD [Onc] - **Spec Exp:** Leukemia-Chronic Lymphocytic; **Hospital:** Arthur G James Cancer Hosp & Research Inst; **Address:** Bl02 Starling-Loving Hall, 320 W 10th Ave, Columbus, OH 43210; **Phone:** 614-293-3196; **Board Cert:** Medical Oncology 1997; **Med School:** Univ Ark 1991; **Resid:** Internal Medicine, Walter Reed AMC 1994; **Fellow:** Hematology & Oncology, Walter Reed AMC 1997; **Fac Appt:** Assoc Prof Med, Ohio State Univ

Chapman, Robert A MD [Onc] - **Spec Exp:** Lung Cancer; **Hospital:** Henry Ford Hosp; **Address:** 2799 W Grand Blvd, Fl K13, Detroit, MI 48202; **Phone:** 313-916-1841; **Board Cert:** Internal Medicine 1985; Medical Oncology 1989; **Med School:** Cornell Univ-Weill Med Coll 1976; **Resid:** Internal Medicine, Henry Ford Hosp 1979; **Fellow:** Medical Oncology, Meml Sloan Kettering Cancer Ctr 1981

Chitambar, Christopher R MD [Onc] - **Spec Exp:** Lymphoma; Leukemia; Breast Cancer; **Hospital:** Froedtert Meml Lutheran Hosp; **Address:** Med Coll Wisconsin, Div Neoplastic Disease, 9200 W Wisconsin Ave, Milwaukee, WI 53226-3522; **Phone:** 414-805-4600; **Board Cert:** Internal Medicine 1980; Hematology 1982; Medical Oncology 1983; **Med School:** India 1977; **Resid:** Internal Medicine, Brackenridge Hosp 1980; **Fellow:** Hematology & Oncology, Univ CO Hlth Sci Ctr 1983; **Fac Appt:** Prof Med, Med Coll Wisc

Clamon, Gerald MD [Onc] - **Spec Exp:** Lung Cancer; Drug Development; **Hospital:** Univ Iowa Hosp & Clinics; **Address:** Univ Iowa Hosps & Clins, Dept Internal Med, 200 Hawkins Drive, rm 5970 JPP, Iowa City, IA 52242; **Phone:** 319-356-1932; **Board Cert:** Internal Medicine 1976; Medical Oncology 1979; **Med School:** Washington Univ, St Louis 1971; **Resid:** Internal Medicine, Barnes Hosp 1976; **Fellow:** Natl Cancer Inst 1974; Medical Oncology, Univ Iowa Hosp & Clinics 1977; **Fac Appt:** Prof Med, Univ Iowa Coll Med

Clark, Joseph I MD [Onc] - **Spec Exp:** Kidney Cancer; Melanoma; Head & Neck Cancer; **Hospital:** Loyola Univ Med Ctr, Hines VA Hosp; **Address:** Cardinal Bernardin Canc Ctr, Loyola Univ Med Ctr, 2160 S 1st Ave, rm 343, Maywood, IL 60153-5500; **Phone:** 708-327-3236; **Board Cert:** Internal Medicine 2002; Medical Oncology 2006; **Med School:** Loyola Univ-Stritch Sch Med 1989; **Resid:** Internal Medicine, Loyola Univ Med Ctr/Hines VA Hosp 1992; **Fellow:** Hematology & Oncology, Fox Chase Cancer Ctr/Temple Univ Hosp 1995; **Fac Appt:** Prof Med, Loyola Univ-Stritch Sch Med

Cleary, James F MD [Onc] - **Spec Exp:** Palliative Care; Head & Neck Cancer; **Hospital:** Univ WI Hosp & Clins; **Address:** K61546 CSC, 600 Highland Ave, Madison, WI 53792; **Phone:** 608-263-8090; **Med School:** Australia 1984; **Resid:** Internal Medicine, Royal Adelaide Hosp 1987; **Fellow:** Medical Oncology, Royal Adelaide Hosp 1990; **Fac Appt:** Assoc Prof Med, Univ Wisc

Clinton, Steven MD/PhD [Onc] - **Spec Exp:** Genitourinary Cancer; Prostate Cancer; Nutrition & Cancer Prevention/Control; **Hospital:** Ohio St Univ Med Ctr; **Address:** A434 Starling Loving Hall, 320 W 10th Ave, Columbus, OH 43210; **Phone:** 614-293-7560; **Board Cert:** Internal Medicine 1987; **Med School:** Univ IL Coll Med 1984; **Resid:** Internal Medicine, Univ Chicago Hosps 1987; **Fellow:** Medical Oncology, Dana Farber Cancer Inst/Harvard 1991; **Fac Appt:** Assoc Prof Med, Ohio State Univ

Cobleigh, Melody A MD [Onc] - **Spec Exp:** Breast Cancer; **Hospital:** Rush Univ Med Ctr; **Address:** Rush Univ Med Ctr, 1725 W Harrison St, Ste 821, Chicago, IL 60612-3828; **Phone:** 312-942-5904; **Board Cert:** Internal Medicine 1979; Medical Oncology 1981; **Med School:** Rush Med Coll 1976; **Resid:** Internal Medicine, Rush Presby-St Lukes Med Ctr 1979; **Fellow:** Medical Oncology, Indiana Univ 1981; **Fac Appt:** Prof Med, Rush Med Coll

Daugherty, Christopher K MD [Onc] - **Spec Exp:** Leukemia & Lymphoma; Stem Cell Transplant; **Hospital:** Univ of Chicago Hosps; **Address:** University of Chicago Hospitals, 5758 S Maryland Ave, MC 2115, Chicago, IL 60637; **Phone:** 773-702-6149; **Board Cert:** Medical Oncology 1997; **Med School:** Indiana Univ 1989; **Resid:** Internal Medicine, Indiana Univ 1993; **Fellow:** Hematology & Oncology, Univ Chicago Hosps 1997; Medical Ethics, Univ Chicago Hosps

Davis, Mellar MD [Onc] - **Spec Exp:** Palliative Care; Lung Cancer (advanced); **Hospital:** Cleveland Clin Fdn (page 56); **Address:** Cleveland Clin Fdn, 9500 Euclid Ave, Desk R35, Cleveland, OH 44195-0002; **Phone:** 216-445-4622; **Board Cert:** Internal Medicine 1980; Hematology 1982; Medical Oncology 1983; Hospice & Palliative Medicine 2002; **Med School:** Ohio State Univ 1977; **Resid:** Internal Medicine, Riverside Methodist Hosp 1979; **Fellow:** Hematology, Mayo Clinic 1981; Medical Oncology, Mayo Clinic 1982

Medical Oncology

Dreicer, Robert MD [Onc] - **Spec Exp:** Breast Cancer; Prostate Cancer; **Hospital:** Cleveland Clin Fdn (page 56); **Address:** Cleveland Clinic, Taussig Cancer Ctr, 9500 Euclid Ave, Desk R35, Cleveland, OH 44195; **Phone:** 216-445-4623; **Board Cert:** Internal Medicine 1986; Medical Oncology 1989; **Med School:** Univ Tex, Houston 1983; **Resid:** Internal Medicine, Ind Univ Med Ctr 1986; **Fellow:** Medical Oncology, Univ Wisconsin Hosp 1989

Einhorn, Lawrence MD [Onc] - **Spec Exp:** Testicular Cancer; Lung Cancer; Urologic Cancer; **Hospital:** Indiana Univ Hosp; **Address:** 535 Barnhill Drive, rm 473, Indianapolis, IN 46202; **Phone:** 317-274-0920; **Board Cert:** Internal Medicine 1972; Medical Oncology 1975; **Med School:** UCLA 1967; **Resid:** Internal Medicine, Indiana Univ Hosp 1969; **Fellow:** Medical Oncology, Indiana Univ Hosp 1972; **Fac Appt:** Prof Med, Indiana Univ

Ellis, Matthew J MD/PhD [Onc] - **Spec Exp:** Breast Cancer; **Hospital:** Barnes-Jewish Hosp; **Address:** Washington University, 660 S Euclid Ave, Box 8056, St Louis, MO 63110; **Phone:** 314-747-1171; **Board Cert:** Internal Medicine 2004; Medical Oncology 2005; **Med School:** England 1984; **Fellow:** Research, Georgetown Univ Med Ctr 1992; Medical Oncology, Georgetwon Univ Med Ctr 1994; **Fac Appt:** Assoc Prof Med, Washington Univ, St Louis

Eng, Charis MD [Onc] - **Spec Exp:** Breast Cancer; Ovarian Cancer; Cancer Genetics; **Hospital:** Cleveland Clin Fdn (page 56); **Address:** Cleveland Clinic Foundation, 9500 Euclid Ave, MC NE50, Cleveland, OH 44195; **Phone:** 216-444-3440; **Board Cert:** Internal Medicine 1991; Medical Oncology 1997; **Med School:** Univ Chicago-Pritzker Sch Med 1988; **Resid:** Internal Medicine, Beth Israel Hosp 1991; **Fellow:** Medical Oncology, Dana-Farber Cancer Inst 1995

Ensminger, William D MD/PhD [Onc] - **Spec Exp:** Gastrointestinal Cancer; Liver Cancer; Clinical Trials; **Hospital:** Univ Michigan Hlth Sys; **Address:** Upjohn Center, rm 3709, 1310 E Catherine, Ann Arbor, MI 48109-5504; **Phone:** 734-764-5468; **Board Cert:** Internal Medicine 1976; Medical Oncology 1979; **Med School:** Harvard Med Sch 1973; **Resid:** Internal Medicine, Beth Israel Hosp 1975; **Fellow:** Medical Oncology, Dana Farber Cancer Inst 1977; **Fac Appt:** Prof Med, Univ Mich Med Sch

Fleming, Gini F MD [Onc] - **Spec Exp:** Breast Cancer; Gynecologic Cancer; **Hospital:** Univ of Chicago Hosps; **Address:** Univ Chicago Hospitals, 5841 S Maryland MC2115, Chicago, IL 60637-1470; **Phone:** 773-839-7924; **Board Cert:** Internal Medicine 1988; Medical Oncology 2001; Hematology 2002; **Med School:** Univ IL Coll Med 1985; **Resid:** Internal Medicine, Univ Chicago Hosps 1988; **Fellow:** Hematology & Oncology, Univ Chicago 1992; **Fac Appt:** Prof Med, Univ Chicago-Pritzker Sch Med

Gerson, Stanton MD [Onc] - **Spec Exp:** Leukemia; Lymphoma, Non-Hodgkin's; Stem Cell Transplant; **Hospital:** Univ Hosps Case Med Ctr; **Address:** Case Comprehensive Cancer Ctr, 11000 Euclid Ave, 1 WEARN 151, Cleveland, OH 44106-5065; **Phone:** 216-844-8562; **Board Cert:** Internal Medicine 1980; Medical Oncology 1983; Hematology 1982; **Med School:** Harvard Med Sch 1977; **Resid:** Internal Medicine, Hosp Univ Penn 1980; **Fellow:** Hematology & Oncology, Hosp Univ Penn 1983; **Fac Appt:** Prof Med, Case West Res Univ

Golomb, Harvey MD [Onc] - **Spec Exp:** Lung Cancer; Leukemia; Lymphoma; **Hospital:** Univ of Chicago Hosps; **Address:** Univ of Chicago Hospital, 5758 S Maryland Ave, MC 9015, Chicago, IL 60637-1463; **Phone:** 773-702-6115; **Board Cert:** Internal Medicine 1975; Medical Oncology 1979; **Med School:** Univ Pittsburgh 1968; **Resid:** Internal Medicine, Johns Hopkins Hosp 1972; Clinical Genetics, Johns Hopkins Hosp 1973; **Fellow:** Hematology & Oncology, Univ Chicago Hosps 1975; **Fac Appt:** Prof Med, Univ Chicago-Pritzker Sch Med

Gradishar, William J MD [Onc] - **Spec Exp:** Breast Cancer; **Hospital:** Northwestern Meml Hosp; **Address:** 676 N St Claire St, Ste 21-100, Chicago, IL 60611; **Phone:** 312-695-0990; **Board Cert:** Internal Medicine 1985; Medical Oncology 1989; **Med School:** Univ IL Coll Med 1982; **Resid:** Internal Medicine, Michael Reese Hosp 1985; **Fellow:** Hematology & Oncology, Univ Chicago Hosps 1990; **Fac Appt:** Prof Med, Northwestern Univ

Gruber, Stephen B MD/PhD [Onc] - **Spec Exp:** Cancer Genetics; Colon & Rectal Cancer; Melanoma; **Hospital:** Univ Michigan Hlth Sys; **Address:** 1524 BSRB, 109 Zina Pitcher Pl, Ann Arbor, MI 48109-2200; **Phone:** 734-647-8906; **Board Cert:** Internal Medicine 1995; Medical Oncology 1998; **Med School:** Univ Pennsylvania 1992; **Resid:** Internal Medicine, Hosp Univ Penn 1994; **Fellow:** Medical Oncology, Johns Hopkins Hosp 1997; Clinical Genetics, Univ Michigan Hlth Sys 1999; **Fac Appt:** Assoc Prof Med, Univ Mich Med Sch

Hartmann, Lynn Carol MD [Onc] - **Spec Exp:** Ovarian Cancer; **Hospital:** Mayo Med Ctr & Clin - Rochester; **Address:** Mayo Clinic Gonda 10 South, 200 First St SW, Rochester, MN 55905; **Phone:** 507-284-3903; **Board Cert:** Internal Medicine 1986; Medical Oncology 1989; **Med School:** Northwestern Univ 1983; **Resid:** Internal Medicine, Univ Ia Hosps/Clinics 1986; **Fellow:** Medical Oncology, Mayo Clinic 1989; **Fac Appt:** Prof Med, Mayo Med Sch

Hayes, Daniel F MD [Onc] - **Spec Exp:** Breast Cancer; **Hospital:** Univ Michigan Hlth Sys; **Address:** Univ Michigan Comprehensive Cancer Ctr, 1500 E Med Ctr Drive, rm 6312, Box 0942, Ann Arbor, MI 48109-5942; **Phone:** 734-615-6725; **Board Cert:** Internal Medicine 1982; Medical Oncology 1985; **Med School:** Indiana Univ 1979; **Resid:** Internal Medicine, Parkland Meml Hosp 1982; **Fellow:** Medical Oncology, Dana Farber Cancer Inst 1985; **Fac Appt:** Prof Med, Univ Mich Med Sch

Hoffman, Philip C MD [Onc] - **Spec Exp:** Lung Cancer; Breast Cancer; Esophageal Cancer; **Hospital:** Univ of Chicago Hosps, Little Company of Mary Hosp & Hlth Care Ctrs; **Address:** 5841 S Maryland Ave, MC 2115, Chicago, IL 60637-1447; **Phone:** 773-834-7424; **Board Cert:** Internal Medicine 1975; Hematology 1980; Medical Oncology 1981; **Med School:** Jefferson Med Coll 1972; **Resid:** Internal Medicine, Hosp Univ Penn 1975; **Fellow:** Hematology & Oncology, Univ Chicago Hosps 1980; **Fac Appt:** Prof Med, Univ Chicago-Pritzker Sch Med

Hussain, Maha H MD [Onc] - **Spec Exp:** Prostate Cancer; Bladder Cancer; Testicular Cancer; Genitourinary Cancer; **Hospital:** Univ Michigan Hlth Sys; **Address:** University of Michigan Cancer Ctr, 1500 E Medical Drive, Ann Arbor, MI 48109; **Phone:** 734-936-8906; **Board Cert:** Internal Medicine 1986; Medical Oncology 1989; **Med School:** Iraq 1980; **Resid:** Internal Medicine, Wayne State Univ Affil Hosps 1986; **Fellow:** Medical Oncology, Wayne State Univ Affil Hosps 1989; **Fac Appt:** Prof Med, Univ Mich Med Sch

Ingle, James N MD [Onc] - **Spec Exp:** Breast Cancer; **Hospital:** Rochester Methodist Hosp; **Address:** Mayo Clinic, 200 First St SW, 12 East, Rochester, MN 55905-0001; **Phone:** 507-284-8432; **Board Cert:** Internal Medicine 1974; Medical Oncology 1975; **Med School:** Johns Hopkins Univ 1971; **Resid:** Internal Medicine, Johns Hopkins Hosp 1976; Medical Oncology, Natl Cancer Inst 1975; **Fac Appt:** Prof Med, Mayo Med Sch

Kalaycio, Matt E MD [Onc] - **Spec Exp:** Leukemia; **Hospital:** Cleveland Clin Fdn (page 56); **Address:** Taussig Cancer Ctr, 9500 Euclid Ave, Desk R35, Cleveland, OH 44195; **Phone:** 216-444-3705; **Board Cert:** Internal Medicine 2002; Hematology 2004; Medical Oncology 2005; **Med School:** W VA Univ 1988; **Resid:** Internal Medicine, Mercy Hosp 1991; **Fellow:** Hematology & Oncology, Cleveland Clinic 1994; **Fac Appt:** Prof Med, Cleveland Cl Coll Med/Case West Res

Medical Oncology

Kalemkerian, Gregory MD [Onc] - **Spec Exp:** Lung Cancer; Mesothelioma; Thymoma; **Hospital:** Univ Michigan Hlth Sys; **Address:** 1500 E Medical Center Dr, C350MIB, Ann Arbor, MI 48109-0848; **Phone:** 734-232-6046; **Board Cert:** Internal Medicine 1988; Medical Oncology 2001; **Med School:** Northwestern Univ 1985; **Resid:** Internal Medicine, Northwestern Meml Hosp 1988; **Fac Appt:** Prof Med, Univ Mich Med Sch

Kaminski, Mark S MD [Onc] - **Spec Exp:** Lymphoma; Bone Marrow Transplant; Drug Development; Clinical Trials; **Hospital:** Univ Michigan Hlth Sys; **Address:** Univ Michigan Cancer Ctr, 1500 E Medical Ctr Drive, rm 4316, Ann Arbor, MI 48109-0936; **Phone:** 734-936-5310; **Board Cert:** Internal Medicine 1981; Medical Oncology 1983; **Med School:** Stanford Univ 1978; **Resid:** Internal Medicine, Barnes Hosp 1981; **Fellow:** Medical Oncology, Stanford Univ Med Ctr 1985; **Fac Appt:** Prof Med, Univ Mich Med Sch

Kindler, Hedy Lee MD [Onc] - **Spec Exp:** Mesothelioma; Pancreatic Cancer; Colon & Rectal Cancer; **Hospital:** Univ of Chicago Hosps; **Address:** Univ of Chicago Hospital, 5841 S Maryland Ave, MC 2115, Chicago, IL 60637-1470; **Phone:** 773-834-7424; **Board Cert:** Internal Medicine 2002; Medical Oncology 2005; **Med School:** SUNY Buffalo 1985; **Resid:** Internal Medicine, UCLA Med Ctr 1992; **Fellow:** Medical Oncology, Meml Sloan Kettering Cancer Ctr 1995; **Fac Appt:** Assoc Prof Med, Univ Chicago-Pritzker Sch Med

Kosova, Leonard MD [Onc] - **Spec Exp:** Breast Cancer; Lymphoma; Lung Cancer; **Hospital:** Adv Luth Genl Hosp; **Address:** 8915 W Golf Rd, Ste 3, Niles, IL 60714-5825; **Phone:** 847-827-9060; **Board Cert:** Internal Medicine 1974; Hematology 1972; Medical Oncology 1975; **Med School:** Univ IL Coll Med 1961; **Resid:** Internal Medicine, Hines VA Hosp 1964; **Fellow:** Hematology & Oncology, Hektoen Inst-Cook Cty Hosp 1965

Locker, Gershon Y MD [Onc] - **Spec Exp:** Gastrointestinal Cancer; Ovarian Cancer; Breast Cancer; Cancer Genetics; **Hospital:** Evanston Hosp; **Address:** Evanston Hospital-Kellog Cancer Ctr, 2650 Ridge Ave, rm 5134, Evanston, IL 60201-1781; **Phone:** 847-570-2515; **Board Cert:** Internal Medicine 1976; Medical Oncology 1977; **Med School:** Harvard Med Sch 1973; **Resid:** Internal Medicine, Univ Chicago Hosps 1976; **Fellow:** Medical Oncology, Natl Cancer Inst 1977; **Fac Appt:** Prof Med, Northwestern Univ

Loehrer, Patrick J MD [Onc] - **Spec Exp:** Gastrointestinal Cancer; Thymoma; Genitourinary Cancer; **Hospital:** Indiana Univ Hosp; **Address:** Indiana Cancer Pavilion, 535 Barnhill Drive, rm 473, Indianapolis, IN 46202-5112; **Phone:** 317-278-7418; **Board Cert:** Internal Medicine 1981; Medical Oncology 2006; **Med School:** Rush Med Coll 1978; **Resid:** Internal Medicine, Rush-Presby-St Lukes Hosp 1981; **Fellow:** Medical Oncology, Indiana Univ 1983; **Fac Appt:** Prof Med, Indiana Univ

Loprinzi, Charles L MD [Onc] - **Spec Exp:** Breast Cancer; **Hospital:** Mayo Med Ctr & Clin - Rochester; **Address:** Mayo Clinic, Dept Med Oncology, 200 First St SW, Rochester, MN 55905-0001; **Phone:** 507-284-4137; **Board Cert:** Internal Medicine 1982; Medical Oncology 1985; **Med School:** Oregon Hlth Sci Univ 1979; **Resid:** Internal Medicine, Maricopa Co Hosp 1982; **Fellow:** Medical Oncology, Univ Wisconsin Med Ctr 1984; **Fac Appt:** Prof Med, Mayo Med Sch

Markowitz, Sanford D MD [Onc] - **Spec Exp:** Colon & Rectal Cancer; Hereditary Cancer; **Hospital:** Univ Hosps Case Med Ctr; **Address:** Ireland Cancer Ctr, 11100 Euclid Ave Fl 6, Cleveland, OH 44106; **Phone:** 216-844-3127; **Board Cert:** Internal Medicine 1984; Medical Oncology 1987; **Med School:** Yale Univ 1980; **Resid:** Internal Medicine, Univ Chicago Hosp 1984; **Fellow:** Medical Oncology, Natl Cancer Inst 1986; **Fac Appt:** Prof Med, Case West Res Univ

Olopade, Olufunmilayo I F MD [Onc] - **Spec Exp:** Breast Cancer; Hereditary Cancer; Cancer Genetics-Breast; **Hospital:** Univ of Chicago Hosps; **Address:** Univ Chicago Hospital, 5841 S Maryland Ave, MC 2115, Section, Hematology-Oncology, Chicago, IL 60637-1470; **Phone:** 773-702-6149; **Board Cert:** Internal Medicine 1986; Hematology 2001; Medical Oncology 1989; **Med School:** Nigeria 1980; **Resid:** Internal Medicine, Cook Co Hosp 1986; **Fellow:** Hematology & Oncology, Univ Chicago Hosps 1991; **Fac Appt:** Prof Med, Univ Chicago-Pritzker Sch Med

Perry, Michael MD [Onc] - **Spec Exp:** Lung Cancer; Breast Cancer; **Hospital:** Univ of Missouri Hosp & Clins; **Address:** Ellis Fischel Cancer Ctr, 115 Business Loop 70 W, DC 116.71, rm 524, Columbia, MO 65203-3299; **Phone:** 573-882-4979; **Board Cert:** Internal Medicine 1987; Hematology 1974; Medical Oncology 1975; **Med School:** Wayne State Univ 1970; **Resid:** Internal Medicine, Mayo Grad Sch 1972; **Fellow:** Hematology, Mayo Grad Sch 1974; Medical Oncology, Mayo Grad Sch 1975; **Fac Appt:** Prof Med, Univ MO-Columbia Sch Med

Peterson, Bruce MD [Onc] - **Spec Exp:** Lymphoma; Leukemia; **Hospital:** Univ Minn Med Ctr, Fairview - Univ Campus; **Address:** Masonics Cancer Center, 424 Harvard St, Ste M100, Minneapolis, MN 55455; **Phone:** 612-624-5631; **Board Cert:** Internal Medicine 1974; Medical Oncology 1977; **Med School:** Univ Minn 1971; **Resid:** Internal Medicine, Fletcher Allen Hlthcare 1973; Internal Medicine, Fairview-Univ Med Ctr 1974; **Fellow:** Medical Oncology, Fairview-Univ Med Ctr 1977; **Fac Appt:** Prof Med, Univ Minn

Picus, Joel MD [Onc] - **Spec Exp:** Pancreatic Cancer; Prostate Cancer; Colon Cancer; **Hospital:** Barnes-Jewish Hosp; **Address:** Washington University School of Medicine, Dept Medicine, 660 S Euclid Ave Campus Box 8056, St Louis, MO 63110; **Phone:** 314-362-5737; **Board Cert:** Internal Medicine 1987; Medical Oncology 1989; **Med School:** Harvard Med Sch 1984; **Resid:** Internal Medicine, Duke Univ Med Ctr 1987; **Fellow:** Hematology & Oncology, UCSF Med Ctr 1991; **Fac Appt:** Assoc Prof Med, Washington Univ, St Louis

Pienta, Kenneth J MD [Onc] - **Spec Exp:** Prostate Cancer; **Hospital:** Univ Michigan Hlth Sys; **Address:** Cancer Center/Geriatrics Center, 1500 E Medical Center Drive, rm 7303 CCGC, Ann Arbor, MI 48109-5946; **Phone:** 734-647-3421; **Board Cert:** Internal Medicine 2001; Medical Oncology 2001; **Med School:** Johns Hopkins Univ 1986; **Resid:** Internal Medicine, Univ Chicago Hosps 1988; **Fellow:** Medical Oncology, Johns Hopkins Hosp 1991; **Fac Appt:** Prof Med, Univ Mich Med Sch

Raghavan, Derek MD/PhD [Onc] - **Spec Exp:** Prostate Cancer; Testicular Cancer; Bladder Cancer; Genitourinary Cancer; **Hospital:** Cleveland Clin Fdn (page 56); **Address:** Cleveland Clinic Taussig Cancer Inst, 9500 Euclid Ave, MC R35, Cleveland, OH 44195; **Phone:** 216-445-6888; **Med School:** Australia 1974; **Resid:** Internal Medicine, Royal Prince Alfred Hosp 1977; **Fellow:** Medical Oncology, Royal Prince Alfred Hosp 1979; Medical Oncology, Royal Marsden Hosp; **Fac Appt:** Prof Med, Cleveland Cl Coll Med/Case West Res

Ratain, Mark J MD [Onc] - **Spec Exp:** Solid Tumors; Drug Discovery & Development; **Hospital:** Univ of Chicago Hosps; **Address:** Univ Chicago Med Ctr, 5841 S Maryland Ave, MC 211, Chicago, IL 60637; **Phone:** 773-702-6149; **Board Cert:** Internal Medicine 1983; Hematology 1986; Medical Oncology 1985; **Med School:** Yale Univ 1980; **Resid:** Internal Medicine, Johns Hopkins Hosp 1983; **Fellow:** Hematology & Oncology, Univ Chicago 1986; **Fac Appt:** Prof Med, Univ Chicago-Pritzker Sch Med

Richards, Jon MD/PhD [Onc] - **Spec Exp:** Testicular Cancer; Prostate Cancer; Melanoma; **Hospital:** Adv Luth Genl Hosp, Rush N Shore Med Ctr; **Address:** Center for Advanced Care, 1700 Luther Ln Fl 2, Park Ridge, IL 60068; **Phone:** 847-268-8200; **Board Cert:** Internal Medicine 1998; **Med School:** Cornell Univ-Weill Med Coll 1983; **Resid:** Internal Medicine, Univ Chicago Hosp 1985; **Fellow:** Hematology & Oncology, Univ Chicago Hosp 1988; **Fac Appt:** Asst Prof Med, Univ IL Coll Med

Medical Oncology

Rosen, Steven T MD [Onc] - **Spec Exp:** Hematologic Malignancies; Breast Cancer; Lymphoma; **Hospital:** Northwestern Meml Hosp; **Address:** Northwestern Univ, 303 E Chicago Ave, Lurie 3-125, Chicago, IL 60611-3013; **Phone:** 312-695-0990; **Board Cert:** Internal Medicine 1979; Medical Oncology 1981; Hematology 1984; **Med School:** Northwestern Univ 1976; **Resid:** Internal Medicine, Northwestern Univ Hosp 1979; **Fellow:** Medical Oncology, Natl Cancer Inst 1981; **Fac Appt:** Prof Med, Northwestern Univ

Ruckdeschel, John C MD [Onc] - **Spec Exp:** Lung Cancer; Mesothelioma; **Hospital:** Karmanos Cancer Inst; **Address:** Karmanos Cancer Inst-Excutive Offices, 4100 John R Fl 2, Detroit, MI 48201-2013; **Phone:** 313-526-8621; **Board Cert:** Internal Medicine 1976; Medical Oncology 1977; **Med School:** Albany Med Coll 1971; **Resid:** Internal Medicine, Johns Hopkins Hosp 1972; Internal Medicine, Beth Israel Hosp 1976; **Fellow:** Medical Oncology, Natl Cancer Inst 1975; **Fac Appt:** Prof Med, Wayne State Univ

Salgia, Ravi MD/PhD [Onc] - **Spec Exp:** Lung Cancer; Mesothelioma; Thoracic Cancers; **Hospital:** Univ of Chicago Hosps; **Address:** University of Chicago Hospitals, 5841 S Maryland Ave, MC 2115, Chicago, IL 60637; **Phone:** 773-702-6149; **Board Cert:** Medical Oncology 2006; **Med School:** Loyola Univ-Stritch Sch Med 1987; **Resid:** Internal Medicine, Johns Hopkins Hospital 1990; **Fellow:** Medical Oncology, Dana-Farber Cancer Inst 1993; **Fac Appt:** Assoc Prof Med, Univ IL Coll Med

Schiffer, Charles A MD [Onc] - **Spec Exp:** Leukemia; Lymphoma; Multiple Myeloma; **Hospital:** Karmanos Cancer Inst, Harper Univ Hosp; **Address:** Karmanos Cancer Inst, Cancer Research Ctr, 4100 John R, 4-Hudson Webber, Detroit, MI 48201; **Phone:** 313-576-8737; **Board Cert:** Internal Medicine 1972; Medical Oncology 1973; **Med School:** NYU Sch Med 1968; **Resid:** Internal Medicine, Bellevue-NY VA Hosp-NYU 1972; **Fellow:** Medical Oncology, Natl Cancer Inst 1974; **Fac Appt:** Prof Med, Wayne State Univ

Schilsky, Richard MD [Onc] - **Spec Exp:** Gastrointestinal Cancer; Pancreatic Cancer; Drug Development; **Hospital:** Univ of Chicago Hosps; **Address:** Univ Chicago- Bio Sciences Div, 5841 S Maryland Ave, MC 2115, Chicago, IL 60637; **Phone:** 773-834-3914; **Board Cert:** Internal Medicine 1978; Medical Oncology 1979; **Med School:** Univ Chicago-Pritzker Sch Med 1975; **Resid:** Internal Medicine, Univ Texas 1977; **Fellow:** Medical Oncology, Natl Cancer Inst 1980; **Fac Appt:** Prof Med, Univ Chicago-Pritzker Sch Med

Schwartz, Burton S MD [Onc] - **Spec Exp:** Lymphoma; Breast Cancer; **Hospital:** Abbott - Northwestern Hosp; **Address:** 800 E 28th St, Piper Bldg, Ste 405, Minneapolis, MN 55407; **Phone:** 612-863-8585; **Board Cert:** Internal Medicine 1980; Hematology 1976; Medical Oncology 1977; **Med School:** Meharry Med Coll 1968; **Resid:** Internal Medicine, Michael Reese Hosp 1971; **Fellow:** Hematology, Univ Minn Hosp 1976; **Fac Appt:** Clin Prof Med, Univ Minn

Shapiro, Charles L MD [Onc] - **Spec Exp:** Breast Cancer; **Hospital:** Arthur G James Cancer Hosp & Research Inst; **Address:** Starling Loving Hall, rm B420, 320 W 10th Ave, Columbus, OH 43210; **Phone:** 614-293-6401; **Board Cert:** Internal Medicine 1987; Medical Oncology 2005; **Med School:** SUNY Buffalo 1984; **Resid:** Internal Medicine, Temple Univ Hosp 1987; **Fellow:** Medical Oncology, Dana Farber Cancer Inst 1991; **Fac Appt:** Assoc Prof Med, Ohio State Univ

Silverman, Paula MD [Onc] - **Spec Exp:** Breast Cancer; **Hospital:** Univ Hosps Case Med Ctr; **Address:** Univ Hosp Cleveland, Ireland Cancer Ctr, 11100 Euclid Ave, Cleveland, OH 44106; **Phone:** 216-844-8510; **Board Cert:** Internal Medicine 1984; Medical Oncology 1989; **Med School:** Case West Res Univ 1981; **Resid:** Internal Medicine, Univ Hosps 1984; **Fellow:** Hematology & Oncology, Case Western Reserve Univ 1987; **Fac Appt:** Assoc Prof Med, Case West Res Univ

America's Top Doctors® 8th Edition

Sledge Jr, George W MD [Onc] - **Spec Exp:** Breast Cancer; **Hospital:** Indiana Univ Hosp; **Address:** 535 Barnhill Drive, rm 473, Indianapolis, IN 46202; **Phone:** 317-274-0920; **Board Cert:** Internal Medicine 1980; Medical Oncology 1983; **Med School:** Tulane Univ 1977; **Resid:** Internal Medicine, St Louis Univ 1980; **Fellow:** Medical Oncology, Univ Texas 1983; **Fac Appt:** Prof Med, Indiana Univ

Stadler, Walter M MD [Onc] - **Spec Exp:** Kidney Cancer; Prostate Cancer; Bladder Cancer; **Hospital:** Univ of Chicago Hosps; **Address:** Univ Chicago Hosps, Div Hem/Onc, 5758 S Maryland Ave, MC 9015, Chicago, IL 60637; **Phone:** 773-834-7424; **Board Cert:** Internal Medicine 2002; Medical Oncology 2003; **Med School:** Yale Univ 1988; **Resid:** Internal Medicine, Michael Reese Hosp 1991; **Fellow:** Medical Oncology, Univ Chicago Hosps 1994; **Fac Appt:** Prof Med, Univ Chicago-Pritzker Sch Med

Todd III, Robert F MD/PhD [Onc] - **Spec Exp:** Gastrointestinal Cancer; Lung Cancer; **Hospital:** Univ Michigan Hlth Sys; **Address:** Univ Michigan Cancer Ctr, 7216CCGC, 1500 E Med Ctr Dr, Box 0948, Ann Arbor, MI 48109; **Phone:** 734-647-8903; **Board Cert:** Internal Medicine 1979; Medical Oncology 1981; **Med School:** Duke Univ 1976; **Resid:** Internal Medicine, Peter Bent Brigham Hosp 1978; **Fellow:** Medical Oncology, Dana Farber Cancer Inst 1981; **Fac Appt:** Prof Med, Univ Mich Med Sch

Urba, Susan G MD [Onc] - **Spec Exp:** Head & Neck Cancer; **Hospital:** Univ Michigan Hlth Sys; **Address:** Comp Cancer Ctr & Geriatrics Ctr, 1500 E Med Ctr Drive, rm 4214, Ann Arbor, MI 48109-0922; **Phone:** 734-647-8902; **Board Cert:** Internal Medicine 1986; Medical Oncology 1991; **Med School:** Univ Mich Med Sch 1983; **Resid:** Internal Medicine, Univ Mich Med Ctr 1986; **Fellow:** Hematology & Oncology, Univ Mich Med Ctr 1988; **Fac Appt:** Assoc Prof Med, Univ Mich Med Sch

Vokes, Everett E MD [Onc] - **Spec Exp:** Lung Cancer; Head & Neck Cancer; Esophageal Cancer; **Hospital:** Univ of Chicago Hosps; **Address:** Univ Chicago Hosps, 5841 S Maryland Ave, MC 2115, Chicago, IL 60637-1470; **Phone:** 773-834-3093; **Board Cert:** Internal Medicine 1983; Medical Oncology 1985; **Med School:** Germany 1980; **Resid:** Internal Medicine, Ravenswood Hosp-Univ Illinois 1982; Internal Medicine, USC Med Ctr 1983; **Fellow:** Medical Oncology, Univ Chicago 1986; **Fac Appt:** Prof Med, Univ Chicago-Pritzker Sch Med

Von Roenn, Jamie H MD [Onc] - **Spec Exp:** Palliative Care; AIDS Related Cancers; Breast Cancer; **Hospital:** Northwestern Meml Hosp; **Address:** 675 N St Clair, Ste 21-100, Chicago, IL 60611; **Phone:** 312-695-0990; **Board Cert:** Internal Medicine 1983; Medical Oncology 1985; **Med School:** Rush Med Coll 1980; **Resid:** Internal Medicine, Rush-Presby-St Lukes Hosp 1983; **Fellow:** Medical Oncology, Rush-Presby-St Lukes Hosp 1985; **Fac Appt:** Prof Med, Northwestern Univ

Wade, James C MD [Onc] - **Spec Exp:** Infections in Cancer Patients; Bone Marrow Transplant; Leukemia; **Hospital:** Froedtert Meml Lutheran Hosp; **Address:** 9200 W Wisconsin Ave, FEC 3963A, Milwaukee, WI 53226-3522; **Phone:** 414-805-4693; **Board Cert:** Internal Medicine 1977; Infectious Disease 1982; Medical Oncology 1981; **Med School:** Univ Utah 1974; **Resid:** Internal Medicine, Johns Hopkins Hosp 1977; **Fellow:** Medical Oncology, Natl Cancer Inst/NIH 1979; Infectious Disease, Univ Wash/Fred Hutchinson Cancer Rsch Ctr 1982; **Fac Appt:** Prof Med, Med Coll Wisc

Weiner, George J MD [Onc] - **Spec Exp:** Lymphoma; Leukemia; Immunotherapy; **Hospital:** Univ Iowa Hosp & Clinics; **Address:** Holden Comprehensive Cancer Center, 200 Hawkins Drive Bldg 5970JPP, Iowa City, IA 52242; **Phone:** 319-356-1932; **Board Cert:** Internal Medicine 1985; Hematology 1988; Medical Oncology 1987; **Med School:** Ohio State Univ 1981; **Resid:** Medical Oncology, Med Coll Ohio 1984; **Fellow:** Hematology & Oncology, Univ Mich Med Ctr 1987; **Fac Appt:** Prof Med, Univ Iowa Coll Med

Medical Oncology

Weissman, David E MD [Onc] - **Spec Exp:** Palliative Care; Pain-Cancer; **Hospital:** Froedtert Meml Lutheran Hosp; **Address:** Med Coll Wisc, Dept Hem/Onc, 9200 W Wisconsin Ave, Milwaukee, WI 53226-3596; **Phone:** 414-805-6800; **Board Cert:** Internal Medicine 1983; Medical Oncology 1985; **Med School:** UCSD 1980; **Resid:** Internal Medicine, UCSD Univ Hosp 1983; **Fellow:** Medical Oncology, Johns Hopkins Hosp 1985; **Fac Appt:** Prof Med, Univ Wisc

Wicha, Max S MD [Onc] - **Spec Exp:** Breast Cancer; Stem Cell Transplant; **Hospital:** Univ Michigan Hlth Sys; **Address:** Comp Cancer Ctr & Geriatrics Ctr, 1500 E Med Ctr Dr, rm 6302 CC, Ann Arbor, MI 48109-5942; **Phone:** 734-936-1831; **Board Cert:** Internal Medicine 1977; Medical Oncology 1983; **Med School:** Stanford Univ 1974; **Resid:** Internal Medicine, Univ Chicago Hosp 1977; **Fellow:** Medical Oncology, Natl Inst Hlth 1980; **Fac Appt:** Prof Med, Univ Mich Med Sch

Wilding, George MD [Onc] - **Spec Exp:** Prostate Cancer; Kidney Cancer; Genitourinary Cancer; Drug Discovery & Development; **Hospital:** Univ WI Hosp & Clins; **Address:** UWCCC, Clinical Science Ctr, K4-614, 600 Highland Ave, MC 6164, Madison, WI 53792; **Phone:** 608-263-8610; **Board Cert:** Internal Medicine 1983; Medical Oncology 1985; **Med School:** Univ Mass Sch Med 1980; **Resid:** Internal Medicine, Univ Mass Med Ctr 1983; **Fellow:** Medical Oncology, Natl Cancer Inst 1985

Williams, Stephen D MD [Onc] - **Spec Exp:** Testicular Cancer; Gynecologic Cancer; Genitourinary Cancer; **Hospital:** Indiana Univ Hosp; **Address:** IU Simon Cancer Center, 535 Barnhill Drive, RT 455, Indianapolis, IN 46202; **Phone:** 317-278-0070; **Board Cert:** Internal Medicine 1976; Medical Oncology 1979; **Med School:** Indiana Univ 1971; **Resid:** Internal Medicine, Indiana Univ Hosp 1975; **Fellow:** Medical Oncology, Indiana Univ Hosp 1978; **Fac Appt:** Prof Med, Indiana Univ

Worden, Francis P MD [Onc] - **Spec Exp:** Head & Neck Cancer; Palliative Care; Clinical Trials; **Hospital:** Univ Michigan Hlth Sys; **Address:** Cancer Center & Geriatric Center, 1500 E Medical Center Drive, rm 4214, Ann Arbor, MI 48109; **Phone:** 734-647-8902; **Board Cert:** Internal Medicine 1997; Medical Oncology 2000; **Med School:** Indiana Univ 1993; **Resid:** Internal Medicine & Pediatrics, Detroit Med Ctr 1997; **Fellow:** Medical Oncology, Detroit Med Ctr 1920; **Fac Appt:** Asst Clin Prof Med, Univ Mich Med Sch

Yee, Douglas MD [Onc] - **Spec Exp:** Breast Cancer; **Hospital:** Univ Minn Med Ctr, Fairview - Univ Campus; **Address:** Univ Minnesota Cancer Ctr, 420 Delaware St SE, MMC 88, Minneapolis, MN 55455; **Phone:** 612-625-5411; **Board Cert:** Internal Medicine 1984; Medical Oncology 1987; **Med School:** Univ Chicago-Pritzker Sch Med 1981; **Resid:** Internal Medicine, Univ NC Med Ctr; **Fellow:** Medical Oncology, NIH-Clin Ctr; **Fac Appt:** Prof Med, Univ Minn

Great Plains and Mountains

Akerley, Wallace MD [Onc] - **Spec Exp:** Lung Cancer; Clinical Trials; **Hospital:** Univ Utah Hosps and Clins; **Address:** Huntsman Cancer Inst, 2000 Circle of Hope, rm 2165, Salt Lake City, UT 84112; **Phone:** 801-585-0100; **Board Cert:** Internal Medicine 1984; Medical Oncology 1987; Hematology 1988; **Med School:** Brown Univ 1981; **Resid:** Internal Medicine, USC Medical Ctr 1985; **Fellow:** Medical Oncology, USC Medical Ctr 1986; Hematology, Norris Cotton Cancer Ctr/Dartmouth 1988; **Fac Appt:** Prof Med, Univ Utah

Armitage, James MD [Onc] - **Spec Exp:** Lymphoma; Bone Marrow Transplant; **Hospital:** Nebraska Med Ctr; **Address:** 987680 Nebraska Medical Center, Omaha, NE 68198-7680; **Phone:** 402-559-7290; **Board Cert:** Internal Medicine 1976; Medical Oncology 1977; Hematology 1984; **Med School:** Univ Nebr Coll Med 1973; **Resid:** Internal Medicine, Univ Nebraska Med Ctr 1975; **Fellow:** Hematology & Oncology, Univ Iowa Hosp 1977; **Fac Appt:** Prof Med, Univ Nebr Coll Med

Beatty, Patrick G MD [Onc] - **Spec Exp:** Hematologic Malignancies; Lymphoma; **Hospital:** St Patrick Hospital - Missoula; **Address:** PO Box 7877, Missoula, MT 59807; **Phone:** 406-728-2539; **Board Cert:** Internal Medicine 1980; Medical Oncology 1985; **Resid:** Internal Medicine, Vanderbilt Univ Med Ctr 1979; **Fellow:** Oncology, Univ Washington Hosps 1982

Bierman, Philip J MD [Onc] - **Spec Exp:** Lymphoma; Bone Marrow Transplant; **Hospital:** Nebraska Med Ctr; **Address:** Nebraska Medical Ctr, Dept Hem/Oncology, 987680 Nebraska Medical Ctr, Omaha, NE 68198-7680; **Phone:** 402-559-5520; **Board Cert:** Internal Medicine 1982; Hematology 1986; Medical Oncology 1985; **Med School:** Univ MO-Kansas City 1979; **Resid:** Internal Medicine, Univ Nebraska Med Ctr 1983; **Fellow:** Medical Oncology, Univ Nebraska Med Ctr 1985; Hematology, City of Hope Natl Med Ctr 1986; **Fac Appt:** Assoc Prof Med, Univ Nebr Coll Med

Bunn Jr, Paul MD [Onc] - **Spec Exp:** Lung Cancer; Lymphoma; **Hospital:** Univ Colorado Hosp; **Address:** Univ Colorado Cancer Ctr, Box 6510, MS F-704, Aurora, CO 80045-0510; **Phone:** 720-848-0300; **Board Cert:** Internal Medicine 1974; Medical Oncology 1975; **Med School:** Cornell Univ-Weill Med Coll 1971; **Resid:** Internal Medicine, Moffitt Hosp/ UCSF Med Ctr 1973; **Fellow:** Medical Oncology, Natl Cancer Inst 1976; **Fac Appt:** Prof Med, Univ Colorado

Buys, Saundra S MD [Onc] - **Spec Exp:** Breast Cancer; Breast Cancer Risk Assessment; Breast Cancer Genetics; **Hospital:** Univ Utah Hosps and Clins; **Address:** Huntsman Cancer Institute, 2000 Circle of Hope, Ste 210, Salt Lake City, UT 84112; **Phone:** 801-585-3525; **Board Cert:** Internal Medicine 1982; Medical Oncology 1985; Hematology 1984; **Med School:** Tufts Univ 1979; **Resid:** Internal Medicine, Univ Utah Hosps 1982; **Fellow:** Hematology & Oncology, Univ Utah Hosps 1985; **Fac Appt:** Prof Med, Univ Utah

Cowan, Kenneth H MD/PhD [Onc] - **Spec Exp:** Breast Cancer; **Hospital:** Nebraska Med Ctr; **Address:** Eppley Cancer Center, 986805 Nebraska Medical Ctr, Omaha, NE 68198-6805; **Phone:** 402-559-4238; **Board Cert:** Internal Medicine 1978; Medical Oncology 1981; **Med School:** Case West Res Univ 1974; **Resid:** Internal Medicine, Parkland Meml Hosp 1977

Dakhil, Shaker MD [Onc] - **Spec Exp:** Leukemia; Mesothelioma; Lymphoma; **Hospital:** Univ of Kansas Hosp; **Address:** Cancer Center Kansas, 818 N Emporia, Ste 403, Wichita, KS 67214; **Phone:** 316-262-4467; **Board Cert:** Internal Medicine 1978; Medical Oncology 1981; **Med School:** Lebanon 1976; **Resid:** Internal Medicine, Wayne State Univ Hosp 1978; **Fellow:** Hematology & Oncology, Univ Michigan Sch Med 1981; **Fac Appt:** Assoc Clin Prof Med, Univ Kans

Eckhardt, S Gail MD [Onc] - **Spec Exp:** Gastrointestinal Cancer; Drug Development; **Hospital:** Univ Colorado Hosp; **Address:** Univ Colorado Hospital, 1665 N Ursula St, Box 6510, MS F-704, Aurora, CO 80045-0510; **Phone:** 720-848-0300; **Board Cert:** Internal Medicine 1988; Medical Oncology 1993; **Med School:** Univ Tex Med Br, Galveston 1985; **Resid:** Internal Medicine, Univ Virginia Med Ctr 1988; **Fellow:** Research, Scripps Clinic 1989; Medical Oncology, UCSD Med Ctr 1992; **Fac Appt:** Prof Med, Univ Colorado

Fabian, Carol J MD [Onc] - **Spec Exp:** Breast Cancer; Breast Cancer Risk Assessment; **Hospital:** Univ of Kansas Hosp; **Address:** Univ Kansas Med Ctr, Div Clinical Onc, 2330 Shawnee Mission Pkwy, Ste 1102, MS 5015, Kansas City, KS 66160-7418; **Phone:** 913-588-7791; **Board Cert:** Internal Medicine 1976; Medical Oncology 1977; **Med School:** Univ Kans 1972; **Resid:** Internal Medicine, Wesley Med Ctr 1975; **Fellow:** Medical Oncology, Univ Kansas Med Ctr 1977; **Fac Appt:** Prof Med, Univ Kans

Medical Oncology

Glode, L Michael MD [Onc] - **Spec Exp:** Prostate Cancer; Genitourinary Cancer; **Hospital:** Univ Colorado Hosp; **Address:** U Colo Hlth Scis Ctr, Div Med Oncology, PO Box 6510, MS F710, Aurora, CO 80045-0510; **Phone:** 720-848-0170; **Board Cert:** Internal Medicine 1975; Medical Oncology 1981; **Med School:** Washington Univ, St Louis 1972; **Resid:** Internal Medicine, Univ Texas SW Med Sch 1973; Immunology, Natl Inst Hlth 1976; **Fellow:** Medical Oncology, Dana Farber Cancer Inst 1978; **Fac Appt:** Prof Med, Univ Colorado

Grem, Jean L MD [Onc] - **Spec Exp:** Colon & Rectal Cancer; Pancreatic Cancer; Stomach Cancer; Esophageal Cancer; **Address:** 987680 Nebraska Medical Ctr, Omaha, NE 68198-7680; **Phone:** 402-559-6210; **Board Cert:** Internal Medicine 1983; Medical Oncology 1985; **Med School:** Jefferson Med Coll 1980; **Resid:** Internal Medicine, Univ Iowa Hosps & Clinics 1983; **Fellow:** Medical Oncology, Univ Wisc Clin Cancer Ctr 1986; **Fac Appt:** Prof Med, Univ Nebr Coll Med

Hauke, Ralph J MD [Onc] - **Spec Exp:** Urologic Cancer; Vaccine Therapy; Clinical Trials; Testicular Cancer; **Hospital:** Methodist Hosp - Omaha, Alegent Hlth - Bergan Mercy Med Ctr; **Address:** 8303 Dodge St, Ste 250, Omaha, NE 68114; **Phone:** 402-354-8124; **Board Cert:** Internal Medicine 1996; Medical Oncology 2001; **Med School:** Panama 1990; **Resid:** Internal Medicine, Univ Nebraska Med Ctr 1996; **Fellow:** Medical Oncology, Univ Nebraska Med Ctr 2001; **Fac Appt:** Assoc Prof Med, Univ Nebr Coll Med

Kane, Madeleine A MD/PhD [Onc] - **Spec Exp:** Head & Neck Cancer; Gastrointestinal Cancer; Neuroendocrine Tumors; **Hospital:** Univ Colorado Hosp, VA Med Ctr; **Address:** Univ Colorado Cancer Ctr, 1665 N Ursula St Cancer Bldg, Box 6510, MS F704, Aurora, CO 80045; **Phone:** 720-848-0300; **Board Cert:** Internal Medicine 1981; Medical Oncology 1983; Hematology 1986; **Med School:** Univ Miami Sch Med 1978; **Resid:** Internal Medicine, Stanford Univ Med Ctr 1981; **Fellow:** Hematology & Oncology, Univ Colo Hlth Sci Ctr 1984; **Fac Appt:** Prof Med, Univ Colorado

Kelly, Karen Lee MD [Onc] - **Spec Exp:** Lung Cancer; **Hospital:** Univ of Kansas Hosp; **Address:** Univ Kansas Cancer Ctr, 4030 Robinson, MS #1027, 3901 Rainbow Blvd, Kansas City, KS 66160; **Phone:** 913-588-4761; **Board Cert:** Internal Medicine 1987; Medical Oncology 2003; **Med School:** Univ Kans 1984; **Resid:** Internal Medicine, Univ Colo Hlth Sci Ctr 1987; **Fellow:** Medical Oncology, Univ Colo Hlth Sci Ctr 1990; **Fac Appt:** Assoc Prof Med, Univ Colorado

Samuels, Brian L MD [Onc] - **Spec Exp:** Sarcoma; **Hospital:** Kootenai Med Ctr; **Address:** North Idaho Cancer Center, 700 W Ironwood Drive, Ste 103, Coeur D'Alene, ID 83814; **Phone:** 208-666-3800; **Board Cert:** Internal Medicine 1984; Medical Oncology 1987; **Med School:** Zimbabwe 1976; **Resid:** Internal Medicine, Albert Einstein Med Ctr 1981; Internal Medicine, Albert Einstein Med Ctr 1984; **Fellow:** Hematology & Oncology, Univ Chicago Hosps 1988

Tschetter, Loren K MD [Onc] - **Spec Exp:** Hematologic Malignancies; Breast Cancer; Colon Cancer; Lung Cancer; **Hospital:** Sanford Health SD; **Address:** Sanford Cancer Ctr, 1020 W 18th St, Sioux Falls, SD 57104; **Phone:** 605-328-8000; **Board Cert:** Internal Medicine 1972; Hematology 1980; **Med School:** Univ Kans 1968; **Resid:** Internal Medicine, Mayo Clinic 1972; **Fellow:** Hematology, Mayo Clinic 1980; **Fac Appt:** Clin Prof Med, Univ SD Sch Med

Ward, John H MD [Onc] - **Spec Exp:** Breast Cancer; Gastrointestinal Cancer; **Hospital:** Univ Utah Hosps and Clins; **Address:** Huntsman Cancer Inst, 2000 Circle of Hope, Ste 2100, Salt Lake City, UT 84112-5550; **Phone:** 801-585-0255; **Board Cert:** Internal Medicine 1979; Medical Oncology 1981; Hematology 1982; **Med School:** Univ Utah 1976; **Resid:** Internal Medicine, Duke Univ Med Ctr 1979; **Fellow:** Hematology & Oncology, Univ Utah 1982; **Fac Appt:** Prof Med, Univ Utah

America's Top Doctors® 8th Edition

Southwest

Abbruzzese, James L MD [Onc] - **Spec Exp:** Gastrointestinal Cancer; Pancreatic Cancer; Clinical Trials; **Hospital:** UT MD Anderson Cancer Ctr; **Address:** Univ Tex MD Anderson Cancer Ctr, 1515 Holcombe Blvd, Unit 426, Houston, TX 77030; **Phone:** 713-792-2828; **Board Cert:** Internal Medicine 1981; Medical Oncology 1983; **Med School:** Univ Chicago-Pritzker Sch Med 1978; **Resid:** Internal Medicine, Johns Hopkins Hosp 1981; **Fellow:** Medical Oncology, Dana-Farber Cancer Inst 1983; **Fac Appt:** Assoc Prof Med, Univ Tex, Houston

Ahmann, Frederick R MD [Onc] - **Spec Exp:** Prostate Cancer; Testicular Cancer; Bladder Cancer; **Hospital:** Univ Med Ctr - Tucson; **Address:** Arizona Cancer Ctr, 1515 N Campbell Ave, Box 245024, Tucson, AZ 85724; **Phone:** 520-694-2873; **Board Cert:** Internal Medicine 1977; Medical Oncology 1981; **Med School:** Univ MO-Columbia Sch Med 1974; **Resid:** Internal Medicine, Georgetown Univ Med Ctr 1977; **Fellow:** Medical Oncology, Univ Med Ctr 1980; **Fac Appt:** Prof Med, Univ Ariz Coll Med

Ajani, Jaffer A MD [Onc] - **Spec Exp:** Gastrointestinal Cancer; Esophageal Cancer; Stomach Cancer; Neuroendocrine Tumors; **Hospital:** UT MD Anderson Cancer Ctr; **Address:** Univ Tex MD Anderson Cancer Ctr, Faculty Ctr Unit 426, Box 301402, Houston, TX 77230; **Phone:** 713-792-2828; **Board Cert:** Internal Medicine 1979; Medical Oncology 1983; **Med School:** India 1971; **Resid:** Family Medicine, Penn Stae Univ-Altoona 1977; Internal Medicine, Tulane Univ Sch Med 1980; **Fellow:** Medical Oncology, MD Anderson Cancer Ctr 1983; **Fac Appt:** Prof Med, Univ Tex, Houston

Alberts, David S MD [Onc] - **Spec Exp:** Cancer Prevention; Ovarian Cancer; **Hospital:** Univ Med Ctr - Tucson; **Address:** Arizona Cancer Center, 1515N Campbell Ave, PO Box 245024, Tucson, AZ 85724; **Phone:** 520-626-7685; **Board Cert:** Internal Medicine 1973; Medical Oncology 1973; **Med School:** Univ VA Sch Med 1966; **Resid:** Medical Oncology, Natl Cancer Inst-NIH 1969; Internal Medicine, Univ Minn Hosps 1971; **Fellow:** Clinical Pharmacology, UC San Francisco 1974; **Fac Appt:** Prof Med, Univ Ariz Coll Med

Anthony, Lowell B MD [Onc] - **Spec Exp:** Gastrointestinal Cancer; Carcinoid Tumors; Neuroendocrine Tumors; **Hospital:** Med Ctr LA @ New Orleans (Univ Hosp); **Address:** 200 W Esplanade, Ste 200, Kenner, LA 70065; **Phone:** 504-464-8500; **Board Cert:** Internal Medicine 1983; Medical Oncology 1989; **Med School:** Vanderbilt Univ 1979; **Resid:** Internal Medicine, Vanderbilt Univ Med Ctr 1982; **Fellow:** Medical Oncology, Vanderbilt Univ Med Ctr 1985; **Fac Appt:** Assoc Prof Med, Louisiana State U, New Orleans

Arun, Banu K MD [Onc] - **Spec Exp:** Breast Cancer; Cancer Prevention; Clinical Trials; **Hospital:** UT MD Anderson Cancer Ctr; **Address:** 1515 Holcombe Blvd, Unit 1354, Houston, TX 77030; **Phone:** 713-792-2817; **Med School:** Turkey 1990; **Resid:** Internal Medicine, Univ Istanbul 1994; **Fellow:** Hematology & Oncology, Lombardi Cancer Ctr-Georgetown Univ 1997; **Fac Appt:** Assoc Prof Med, Univ Tex, Houston

Benjamin, Robert S MD [Onc] - **Spec Exp:** Sarcoma; **Hospital:** UT MD Anderson Cancer Ctr; **Address:** UT MD Anderson Cancer Ctr, 1515 Holcombe Blvd, Unit 450, Houston, TX 77030; **Phone:** 713-792-3626; **Board Cert:** Internal Medicine 1973; Medical Oncology 1973; **Med School:** NYU Sch Med 1968; **Resid:** Internal Medicine, Bellevue Hosp Ctr-NYU 1970; **Fellow:** Medical Oncology, Baltimore Cancer Rsch Ctr 1972; **Fac Appt:** Prof Med, Univ Tex, Houston

Bruera, Eduardo MD [Onc] - **Spec Exp:** Palliative Care; **Hospital:** UT MD Anderson Cancer Ctr; **Address:** 1515 Holcombe Ave, Unit 8, Houston, TX 77030; **Phone:** 713-792-6085; **Med School:** Argentina 1979; **Resid:** Internal Medicine, Hospital Privado; **Fellow:** Medical Oncology, Cross Cancer Inst; **Fac Appt:** Prof Med, Univ Tex, Houston

Medical Oncology

Buzdar, Aman U MD [Onc] - **Spec Exp:** Breast Cancer; **Hospital:** UT MD Anderson Cancer Ctr; **Address:** UT MD Anderson Canc Ctr, 1155 Pressler St, Unit 1354, Houston, TX 77030-4009; **Phone:** 713-792-2817; **Board Cert:** Internal Medicine 1975; Medical Oncology 1979; **Med School:** Pakistan 1967; **Resid:** Internal Medicine, Norwalk Hosp 1973; Internal Medicine, Lakewood Hosp 1971; **Fellow:** Hematology, Norwalk Hosp 1974; Oncology, MD Anderson Cancer Ctr 1975; **Fac Appt:** Prof Med, Univ Tex, Houston

Camoriano, John MD [Onc] - **Spec Exp:** Lymphoma; Breast Cancer; Bone Marrow Transplant; Castleman's Disease; **Hospital:** Mayo Clinic - Scottsdale; **Address:** Mayo Clinic - Scottsdale, 13400 E Shea, Scottsdale, AZ 85259; **Phone:** 480-301-8335; **Board Cert:** Internal Medicine 1985; Medical Oncology 1989; Hematology 1988; **Med School:** Univ Nebr Coll Med 1982; **Resid:** Internal Medicine, Univ OK 1985; **Fellow:** Hematology & Oncology, Mayo Grad Sch Med 1989; **Fac Appt:** Asst Prof Med, Mayo Med Sch

Chang, Jenny C N MD [Onc] - **Spec Exp:** Breast Cancer; Clinical Trials; **Hospital:** Methodist Hosp - Houston; **Address:** One Baylor Plaza, MS BCM600, Houston, TX 77030; **Phone:** 713-798-1609; **Med School:** England 1989; **Resid:** Internal Medicine 1993; **Fellow:** Medical Oncology, Royal Marsden Hosp 1997; **Fac Appt:** Assoc Prof Med, Baylor Coll Med

Fay, Joseph W MD [Onc] - **Spec Exp:** Bone Marrow Transplant; Melanoma; Leukemia & Lymphoma; **Hospital:** Baylor Univ Medical Ctr; **Address:** 3409 Worth St, Sammons Tower, Suite 600, Dallas, TX 75246; **Phone:** 214-370-1500; **Board Cert:** Internal Medicine 1975; Medical Oncology 1977; Hematology 1978; **Med School:** Ohio State Univ 1972; **Resid:** Internal Medicine, Duke Med Ctr 1974; Oncology, Natl Cancer Institute 1976; **Fellow:** Hematology, Duke Med Ctr 1977; **Fac Appt:** Clin Prof Med, Univ Tex SW, Dallas

Fitch, Tom R MD [Onc] - **Spec Exp:** Breast Cancer; Sarcoma; Cancer Prevention; Palliative Care; **Hospital:** Mayo Clinic - Scottsdale; **Address:** Mayo Clinic - Scottsdale, 13400 E Shea Blvd, Scottsdale, AZ 85259; **Phone:** 480-301-8335; **Board Cert:** Internal Medicine 1985; Hematology 1988; Medical Oncology 1987; **Med School:** Univ Kans 1982; **Resid:** Internal Medicine, Univ Michigan Med Ctr 1985; **Fellow:** Hematology & Oncology, Mayo Clinic 1988; **Fac Appt:** Asst Prof Med, Mayo Med Sch

Fossella, Frank V MD [Onc] - **Spec Exp:** Lung Cancer; **Hospital:** UT MD Anderson Cancer Ctr; **Address:** Dept Thoracic Head/Neck Med Oncol, Unit 432, 1400 Holcombe Blvd, Houston, TX 77030; **Phone:** 713-792-6363; **Board Cert:** Internal Medicine 1985; Medical Oncology 1987; **Med School:** Baylor Coll Med 1982; **Resid:** Internal Medicine, Baylor Coll Med 1985; **Fellow:** Medical Oncology, Baylor Coll Med 1987; **Fac Appt:** Prof Med, Univ Tex, Houston

Glisson, Bonnie S MD [Onc] - **Spec Exp:** Head & Neck Cancer; Lung Cancer; **Hospital:** UT MD Anderson Cancer Ctr; **Address:** 1515 Holcombe Blvd, Unit 432, Houston, TX 77030; **Phone:** 713-792-6363; **Board Cert:** Internal Medicine 1982; Medical Oncology 1985; **Med School:** Ohio State Univ 1979; **Resid:** Internal Medicine, Univ Va Med Ctr 1982; **Fellow:** Medical Oncology, Univ Fla Health Sci Ctr 1985; **Fac Appt:** Prof Med, Univ Tex, Houston

Haley, Barbara MD [Onc] - **Spec Exp:** Breast Cancer; **Hospital:** UT Southwestern Med Ctr - Dallas; **Address:** UTSW Med Ctr, 5323 Harry Hines Blvd, Dallas, TX 75390-8852; **Phone:** 214-648-4180; **Board Cert:** Internal Medicine 1979; Hematology 1984; **Med School:** Univ Tex SW, Dallas 1976; **Resid:** Internal Medicine, Parkland Meml Hosp 1979; **Fellow:** Hematology & Oncology, Parkland Meml Hosp 1981; **Fac Appt:** Prof Med, Univ Tex SW, Dallas

Herbst, Roy S MD/PhD [Onc] - **Spec Exp:** Lung Cancer; Head & Neck Cancer; Breast Cancer; Drug Development; **Hospital:** UT MD Anderson Cancer Ctr; **Address:** Thoracic/Head & Neck Med Onc - Unit 432, UT MD Anderson Cancer Ctr, PO Box 301402, Houston, TX 77230-1402; **Phone:** 713-792-6363; **Board Cert:** Medical Oncology 1997; **Med School:** Cornell Univ-Weill Med Coll 1991; **Resid:** Internal Medicine, Brigham & Women's Hosp 1994; **Fellow:** Medical Oncology, Dana Farber Cancer Inst 1996; **Fac Appt:** Assoc Prof Med, Univ Tex, Houston

Hong, Waun Ki MD [Onc] - **Spec Exp:** Lung Cancer; Head & Neck Cancer; Thoracic Cancers; **Hospital:** UT MD Anderson Cancer Ctr; **Address:** 1515 Holcombe Blvd, Unit 421, Houston, TX 77030; **Phone:** 713-745-5353; **Board Cert:** Internal Medicine 1976; Medical Oncology 1979; **Med School:** South Korea 1967; **Resid:** Internal Medicine, Boston VA Hosp 1973; **Fellow:** Medical Oncology, Meml Sloan-Kettering Cancer Ctr 1975; **Fac Appt:** Prof Med, Univ Tex, Houston

Hortobagyi, Gabriel N MD [Onc] - **Spec Exp:** Breast Cancer; Clinical Trials; Gene Therapy; **Hospital:** UT MD Anderson Cancer Ctr; **Address:** UT MD Anderson Cancer Ctr, Dept Breast Oncology, PO Box 301429, Unit 1354, Houston, TX 77030-1439; **Phone:** 713-792-2817; **Board Cert:** Internal Medicine 1975; Medical Oncology 1977; **Med School:** Colombia 1970; **Resid:** Internal Medicine, St Lukes Hosp 1974; **Fellow:** Medical Oncology, MD Anderson Cancer Ctr 1976; **Fac Appt:** Prof Med

Hutchins, Laura MD [Onc] - **Spec Exp:** Breast Cancer; Melanoma; **Hospital:** UAMS Med Ctr; **Address:** Univ Arkansas Med Scis, Dept Hem/Onc, 4301 W Markham St, MS 721-5, Little Rock, AR 72205-7101; **Phone:** 501-686-8511; **Board Cert:** Internal Medicine 1980; Hematology 1984; Medical Oncology 1987; **Med School:** Univ Ark 1977; **Resid:** Internal Medicine, Univ Ark Med Scis 1980; **Fellow:** Hematology & Oncology, Univ Ark Med Scis 1983; **Fac Appt:** Prof Med, Univ Ark

Karp, Daniel D MD [Onc] - **Spec Exp:** Lung Cancer; **Hospital:** UT MD Anderson Cancer Ctr; **Address:** 1515 Holcombe Blvd, Unit 432, Houston, TX 77030-4009; **Phone:** 713-792-6363; **Board Cert:** Internal Medicine 1976; Hematology 1980; Medical Oncology 1981; **Med School:** Duke Univ 1973; **Resid:** Internal Medicine, Dartmouth-Hitchcock Med Ctr 1976; **Fellow:** Hematology, Dartmouth-Hitchcock Med Ctr 1978; Medical Oncology, Dana Farber Cancer Inst 1979; **Fac Appt:** Prof Med, Univ Tex, Houston

Kies, Merrill S MD [Onc] - **Spec Exp:** Head & Neck Cancer; Lung Cancer; **Hospital:** UT MD Anderson Cancer Ctr; **Address:** Dept Thoracic, Head & Neck Oncology, 1515 Holcombe Blvd, Unit 432, Houston, TX 77030; **Phone:** 713-792-6363; **Board Cert:** Internal Medicine 1976; Medical Oncology 1979; **Med School:** Loyola Univ-Stritch Sch Med 1973; **Resid:** Internal Medicine, Walter Reed AMC 1976; **Fellow:** Medical Oncology, Brooke AMC 1978; **Fac Appt:** Prof Med, Univ Tex, Houston

Kwak, Larry W MD/PhD [Onc] - **Spec Exp:** Lymphoma; Multiple Myeloma; Vaccine Therapy; Immunotherapy; **Hospital:** UT MD Anderson Cancer Ctr; **Address:** MD Anderson Cancer Ctr, Dept Lymphoma/Myeloma, 1515 Holcombe Blvd, Unit 429, Houston, TX 77035; **Phone:** 713-745-4244; **Board Cert:** Internal Medicine 1987; Medical Oncology 1989; **Med School:** Northwestern Univ 1982; **Resid:** Internal Medicine, Stanford Univ Hosp 1987; **Fellow:** Oncology, Stanford Univ Hosp 1989

Legha, Sewa Singh MD [Onc] - **Spec Exp:** Melanoma; Breast Cancer; Endocrine Cancers; Sarcoma; **Hospital:** St Luke's Episcopal Hosp - Houston, Methodist Hosp - Houston; **Address:** 6624 Fannin, Ste 1440, Houston, TX 77030; **Phone:** 713-797-9711; **Board Cert:** Internal Medicine 1987; Medical Oncology 1977; **Med School:** India 1970; **Resid:** Internal Medicine, Milwaukee Co Genl Hosp/Med Coll Wisc 1974; Medical Oncology, Natl Cancer Inst 1976; **Fellow:** Medical Oncology, MD Anderson Hosp 1977; **Fac Appt:** Clin Prof Med, Baylor Coll Med

Medical Oncology

Lippman, Scott M MD [Onc] - **Spec Exp:** Cancer Prevention; Lung Cancer; Head & Neck Cancer; **Hospital:** UT MD Anderson Cancer Ctr; **Address:** UT MD Anderson Cancer Ctr, 1515 Holcombe Blvd, Box 432, Houston, TX 77030-1439; **Phone:** 713-745-5439; **Board Cert:** Internal Medicine 1987; Hematology 1988; Medical Oncology 1989; **Med School:** Johns Hopkins Univ 1981; **Resid:** Internal Medicine, Harbor-UCLA Med Ctr 1983; **Fellow:** Hematology, Stanford Univ Med Ctr 1985; Hematology & Oncology, Univ Ariz Hlth Scis Ctr 1987; **Fac Appt:** Prof Med, Univ Tex, Houston

Livingston, Robert B MD [Onc] - **Spec Exp:** Bone Marrow Transplant; Breast Cancer; Lung Cancer; **Hospital:** Univ Med Ctr - Tucson; **Address:** University Medical Center, 3838 N Campbell Ave, Tucson, AZ 85724; **Phone:** 520-694-2873; **Board Cert:** Internal Medicine 1972; Medical Oncology 1973; **Med School:** Univ Okla Coll Med 1965; **Resid:** Internal Medicine, Univ Oklahoma Med Ctr 1971; **Fellow:** Medical Oncology, Univ Texas Cancer Ctr 1973; **Fac Appt:** Prof Med, Univ Wash

Logothetis, Christopher J MD [Onc] - **Spec Exp:** Prostate Cancer; Bladder Cancer; **Hospital:** UT MD Anderson Cancer Ctr; **Address:** UT MD Anderson Cancer Ctr, Dept GU Onc, Unit 1374, Box 301439, Houston, TX 77230-1439; **Phone:** 713-792-2830; **Board Cert:** Internal Medicine 1978; Medical Oncology 1981; **Med School:** Greece 1974; **Resid:** Internal Medicine, Univ Texas 1979; **Fellow:** Hematology & Oncology, Univ Tex-MD Anderson Cancer Ctr 1981; **Fac Appt:** Prof Med, Univ Tex, Houston

Markman, Maurie MD [Onc] - **Spec Exp:** Ovarian Cancer; Gynecologic Cancer; Drug Development; Palliative Care; **Hospital:** UT MD Anderson Cancer Ctr; **Address:** Univ Texas MD Anderson Cancer Ctr, 1515 Holcombe Blvd, Box 121, Houston, TX 77030-4009; **Phone:** 713-745-7140; **Board Cert:** Internal Medicine 1977; Hematology 1982; Medical Oncology 1981; **Med School:** NYU Sch Med 1974; **Resid:** Internal Medicine, Bellevue Hosp Ctr 1978; **Fellow:** Medical Oncology, Johns Hopkins Hosp 1980; **Fac Appt:** Prof Med, Univ Tex, Houston

Miller, Thomas P MD [Onc] - **Spec Exp:** Lymphoma; **Hospital:** Univ Med Ctr - Tucson; **Address:** Arizona Cancer Ctr, 1515 N Campbell Ave, PO Box 245024, Tucson, AZ 85724; **Phone:** 520-626-2667; **Board Cert:** Internal Medicine 1977; Medical Oncology 1981; **Med School:** Univ IL Coll Med 1972; **Resid:** Internal Medicine, Univ Illinois Hosps 1977; **Fellow:** Hematology & Oncology, Univ Med Ctr 1980; **Fac Appt:** Prof Med, Univ Ariz Coll Med

Nemunaitis, John G MD [Onc] - **Spec Exp:** Cancer Genetics; Vaccine Therapy; Lung Cancer; **Hospital:** Baylor Univ Medical Ctr; **Address:** Mary Crowley Med Rsch Ctr, 3535 Worth St, Ste 302, Dallas, TX 75246; **Phone:** 214-370-1870; **Board Cert:** Internal Medicine 1987; **Med School:** Case West Res Univ 1982; **Resid:** Internal Medicine, Boston City Hosp 1985; **Fellow:** Hematology & Oncology, Fred Hutchinson Cancer Rsch Ctr 1989

Northfelt, Donald W MD [Onc] - **Spec Exp:** Breast Cancer; Colon & Rectal Cancer; Lung Cancer; **Hospital:** Mayo Clinic - Scottsdale; **Address:** Mayo Clinic Scottsdale, 13400 E Shea Blvd, Scottsdale, AZ 85259; **Phone:** 480-301-8335; **Board Cert:** Internal Medicine 1988; Medical Oncology 2001; **Med School:** Univ Minn 1985; **Resid:** Internal Medicine, UCLA Med Ctr 1988; **Fellow:** Hematology & Oncology, UCSF Med Ctr 1991; **Fac Appt:** Assoc Prof Med, Mayo Med Sch

O'Brien, Susan M MD [Onc] - **Spec Exp:** Leukemia; Lymphoma; **Hospital:** UT MD Anderson Cancer Ctr; **Address:** Univ Texas MD Anderson Cancer Ctr, Dept Leukemia, Unit 428, Box 301439, Houston, TX 77230; **Phone:** 713-792-7305; **Board Cert:** Internal Medicine 1983; Medical Oncology 1987; **Med School:** UMDNJ-NJ Med Sch, Newark 1980; **Resid:** Internal Medicine, UMDNJ Med Ctr 1983; **Fellow:** Medical Oncology, Univ TX MD Anderson Med Ctr 1987; **Fac Appt:** Prof Med, Univ Tex, Houston

O'Shaughnessy, Joyce A MD [Onc] - **Spec Exp:** Breast Cancer; **Hospital:** Baylor Univ Medical Ctr; **Address:** US Oncology, 3535 Worth St, Ste 600, Dallas, TX 75246; **Phone:** 214-370-1000; **Board Cert:** Internal Medicine 1985; Medical Oncology 1987; **Med School:** Yale Univ 1982; **Resid:** Internal Medicine, Mass Genl Hosp 1985; **Fellow:** Medical Oncology, National Cancer Inst 1988

Orlowski, Robert Z MD/PhD [Onc] - **Spec Exp:** Multiple Myeloma; Lymphoma, Non-Hodgkin's; Leukemia; Clinical Trials; **Hospital:** UT MD Anderson Cancer Ctr; **Address:** MD Anderson Cancer Ctr, Lymphoma & Myeloma Clinic, 1515 Holcombe Blvd, Box 0429, Houston, TX 77030; **Phone:** 713-792-3510; **Board Cert:** Medical Oncology 1997; **Med School:** Yale Univ 1991; **Resid:** Internal Medicine, Barnes Hosp/Wash Univ 1994; **Fellow:** Hematology & Oncology, Johns Hopkins Hosp 1998

Osborne, Charles K MD [Onc] - **Spec Exp:** Breast Cancer; **Hospital:** Methodist Hosp - Houston; **Address:** 1 Baylor Plaza, MS BCM600, Houston, TX 77030; **Phone:** 713-798-1641; **Board Cert:** Internal Medicine 1975; Medical Oncology 1977; **Med School:** Univ MO-Columbia Sch Med 1972; **Resid:** Internal Medicine, Johns Hopkins Hosp 1974; **Fellow:** Medical Oncology, Natl Cancer Inst 1977; **Fac Appt:** Prof Med, Baylor Coll Med

Papadopoulos, Nicholas E MD [Onc] - **Spec Exp:** Melanoma; **Hospital:** UT MD Anderson Cancer Ctr; **Address:** 1515 Holcombe Blvd, Unit 430, Houston, TX 77030; **Phone:** 713-792-2821; **Med School:** Greece 1966; **Resid:** Internal Medicine, Baylor Coll Med 1976; **Fellow:** Medical Oncology, MD Anderson Cancer Ctr 1978; **Fac Appt:** Assoc Prof Med, Univ Tex, Houston

Patt, Yehuda Z MD [Onc] - **Spec Exp:** Liver Cancer; Biliary Cancer; Colon & Rectal Cancer; **Hospital:** Univ NM Hlth & Sci Ctr; **Address:** Univ New Mexico CRTC, Div Hem/Onc, 900 Camino de Salud NE, MSC 084630, Albuquerque, NM 87131-0001; **Phone:** 505-272-5837; **Board Cert:** Internal Medicine 1982; Medical Oncology 1987; **Med School:** Israel 1967; **Resid:** Internal Medicine, Tel Aviv-Sheba Med Ctr 1974; **Fellow:** Medical Oncology, UT MD Anderson Cancer Ctr 1977; **Fac Appt:** Prof Med, Univ New Mexico

Pisters, Katherine M W MD [Onc] - **Spec Exp:** Lung Cancer; **Hospital:** UT MD Anderson Cancer Ctr; **Address:** UT MD Anderson Cancer Ctr, PO Box 301402 Unit 432, Houston, TX 77030-1402; **Phone:** 713-792-6363; **Board Cert:** Internal Medicine 1988; Medical Oncology 2002; **Med School:** Univ Western Ontario 1985; **Resid:** Internal Medicine, N Shore Univ Hosp 1988; **Fellow:** Medical Oncology, Meml Sloan Kettering Cancer Ctr 1991; **Fac Appt:** Prof Med, Univ Tex, Houston

Ross, Helen Jane MD [Onc] - **Spec Exp:** Lung Cancer; Esophageal Cancer; Chest Wall Tumors; Clinical Trials; **Hospital:** Mayo Clinic - Scottsdale; **Address:** Mayo Clinic, 13400 E Shea Blvd, Scottsdale, AZ 85259; **Phone:** 480-301-8335; **Board Cert:** Internal Medicine 1987; Medical Oncology 1989; **Med School:** UCLA 1984; **Resid:** Internal Medicine, Cedars Sinai Med Ctr 1987; **Fellow:** Medical Oncology, UCLA Med Ctr 1989; **Fac Appt:** Assoc Prof Med, Oregon Hlth Sci Univ

Saiki, John H MD [Onc] - **Hospital:** Univ NM Hlth & Sci Ctr; **Address:** Univ of New Mexico Cancer Ctr, 900 Camino de Salud NE, MSC 084630, Albuquerque, NM 87131-0001; **Phone:** 505-272-8740; **Board Cert:** Internal Medicine 1970; Medical Oncology 1973; **Med School:** McGill Univ 1961; **Resid:** Internal Medicine, Univ New Mexico 1968; Hematology, Univ New Mexico 1969; **Fellow:** Medical Oncology, MD Anderson Hosp 1970; **Fac Appt:** Prof Emeritus Med, Univ New Mexico

Medical Oncology

Schiller, Joan H MD [Onc] - **Spec Exp:** Lung Cancer; **Hospital:** UT Southwestern Med Ctr - Dallas; **Address:** Univ Texas SW, 5323 Harry Hines Blvd, Dallas, TX 75390-8852; **Phone:** 214-648-4180; **Board Cert:** Internal Medicine 1983; Medical Oncology 1987; **Med School:** Univ IL Coll Med 1980; **Resid:** Internal Medicine, Northwestern Meml Hosp 1983; **Fellow:** Medical Oncology, Univ Wisconsin Hosp 1986; **Fac Appt:** Prof Med, Univ Wisc

Stopeck, Alison T MD [Onc] - **Spec Exp:** Breast Cancer; Breast Cancer Risk Assessment; **Hospital:** Univ Med Ctr - Tucson; **Address:** 1515 N Campbell Ave, P.O. Box 245024, Tucson, AZ 85724; **Phone:** 520-626-2816; **Board Cert:** Internal Medicine 1988; Medical Oncology 2002; Hematology 2002; **Med School:** Columbia P&S 1985; **Resid:** Internal Medicine, Columbia-Presby Med Ctr 1988; **Fellow:** Hematology & Oncology, New York Hosp 1991; **Fac Appt:** Assoc Prof Med, Univ Ariz Coll Med

Takimoto, Chris Hidemi M MD/PhD [Onc] - **Spec Exp:** Gastrointestinal Cancer; **Hospital:** Metro Methodist Hosp; **Address:** South TX Accelerated Rsch Therapeutics, 4319 Medical Drive, Ste 205, San Antonio, TX 78229; **Phone:** 210-562-1725; **Board Cert:** Internal Medicine 1989; Medical Oncology 2005; **Med School:** Yale Univ 1986; **Resid:** Internal Medicine, UCSF Med Ctr 1989; **Fac Appt:** Assoc Prof Med, Univ Tex, San Antonio

Valero, Vicente MD [Onc] - **Spec Exp:** Breast Cancer; **Hospital:** UT MD Anderson Cancer Ctr, LBJ General Hosp; **Address:** Univ Texas MD Anderson Cancer Ctr, 1515 Holcombe Blvd, Unit 1354, Houston, TX 77030; **Phone:** 713-792-2817; **Board Cert:** Internal Medicine 1985; Hematology 1988; Medical Oncology 1987; **Med School:** Mexico 1980; **Resid:** Internal Medicine, Univ Cincinnati Med Ctr 1985; Hematology & Oncology, Univ Cincinnati Med Ctr 1987; **Fellow:** Hematology & Oncology, Univ Texas Med Br 1988; **Fac Appt:** Prof Med, Univ Tex, Houston

Verschraegen, Claire F MD [Onc] - **Spec Exp:** Ovarian Cancer; Drug Discovery; Mesothelioma; **Hospital:** Univ NM Hlth & Sci Ctr; **Address:** UNM Cancer Research & Treatment Ctr, 900 Camino de Salud NE, rm MS C084630, Albuquerque, NM 87131-0001; **Phone:** 505-272-6760; **Board Cert:** Internal Medicine 2000; Medical Oncology 2000; **Med School:** Belgium 1982; **Resid:** Internal Medicine, Bordet 1985; Internal Medicine, Univ Texas 1991; **Fellow:** Cancer Research, Stehlin Fdn for Cancer Research 1988; Oncology, MD Anderson Cancer Ctr 1994; **Fac Appt:** Prof Med, Univ New Mexico

Von Hoff, Daniel D MD [Onc] - **Spec Exp:** Pancreatic Cancer; Breast Cancer; Drug Discovery; **Hospital:** Scottsdale Hlthcare - Shea; **Address:** Translational Genomics Research Institute, 445 N 5th St, Ste 600, Phoenix, AZ 85004; **Phone:** 602-343-8492; **Board Cert:** Internal Medicine 1976; Medical Oncology 1979; **Med School:** Columbia P&S 1973; **Resid:** Internal Medicine, UCSF Med Ctr 1975; **Fac Appt:** Prof Med, Univ Ariz Coll Med

Willson, James KV MD [Onc] - **Spec Exp:** Gastrointestinal Cancer; Colon Cancer; Pancreatic Cancer; **Hospital:** UT Southwestern Med Ctr - Dallas; **Address:** UTSW Med Ctr, NB2.308, 5323 Harry Hines Blvd, Dallas, TX 75390-8590; **Phone:** 214-645-4673; **Board Cert:** Internal Medicine 1980; Medical Oncology 1981; **Med School:** Univ Ala 1976; **Resid:** Internal Medicine, Johns Hopkins Hosp 1978; **Fellow:** Medical Oncology, Natl Cancer Inst-NIH 1980; **Fac Appt:** Prof Med, Univ Tex SW, Dallas

West Coast and Pacific

Abrams, Donald I MD [Onc] - **Spec Exp:** AIDS Related Cancers; **Hospital:** San Francisco Genl Hosp; **Address:** Positive Hlth Program-SF Genl Hosp, 995 Potrero Ave, Bldg 80, Ward 84, San Francisco, CA 94110; **Phone:** 415-476-4082 x444; **Board Cert:** Internal Medicine 1980; Medical Oncology 1983; **Med School:** Stanford Univ 1977; **Resid:** Internal Medicine, Kaiser Fdn Hosp 1980; **Fellow:** Medical Oncology, UCSF Cancer Rsch 1982; **Fac Appt:** Clin Prof Med, UCSF

Appelbaum, Frederick R MD [Onc] - **Spec Exp:** Bone Marrow Transplant; Leukemia; **Hospital:** Univ Wash Med Ctr; **Address:** 1100 Fairview Ave N, rm D5-310, PO Box 19024, Seattle, WA 98109; **Phone:** 206-288-1024; **Board Cert:** Internal Medicine 1975; Medical Oncology 1977; **Med School:** Tufts Univ 1972; **Resid:** Internal Medicine, Univ Michigan Med Ctr 1974; **Fellow:** Medical Oncology, Natl Cancer Inst 1976; **Fac Appt:** Prof Med, Univ Wash

Ball, Edward D MD [Onc] - **Spec Exp:** Bone Marrow & Stem Cell Transplant; Leukemia & Lymphoma; Multiple Myeloma; **Hospital:** UCSD Med Ctr; **Address:** 3855 Health Sciences Dr, #0960, La Jolla, CA 92093; **Phone:** 858-822-6600; **Board Cert:** Internal Medicine 1979; Medical Oncology 1983; Hematology 2000; **Med School:** Case West Res Univ 1976; **Resid:** Internal Medicine, Hartford Hosp 1979; **Fellow:** Hematology & Oncology, Univ Hosps Cleveland 1981; Hematology & Oncology, Dartmouth-Hitchcock Hosp 1982; **Fac Appt:** Prof Med, UCSD

Beer, Tomasz MD [Onc] - **Spec Exp:** Prostate Cancer; **Hospital:** OR Hlth & Sci Univ; **Address:** 3303 SW Bond Ave, CH7M, Portland, OR 97239; **Phone:** 503-494-6594; **Board Cert:** Internal Medicine 1995; Medical Oncology 2000; **Med School:** Johns Hopkins Univ 1991; **Resid:** Internal Medicine, Oreg Hlth Scis Univ 1994; Internal Medicine, Oreg Hlth Scis Univ 1996; **Fellow:** Hematology & Oncology, Oreg Hlth Scis Univ 1999; **Fac Appt:** Assoc Prof Med, Oregon Hlth Sci Univ

Bensinger, William I MD [Onc] - **Spec Exp:** Multiple Myeloma; Stem Cell Transplant; **Hospital:** Univ Wash Med Ctr; **Address:** Fred Hutchinson Cancer Research Ctr, 825 Eastlake Ave E, MS E5-390, Seattle, WA 98109-1024; **Phone:** 206-288-1024; **Board Cert:** Internal Medicine 1978; Medical Oncology 1979; **Med School:** Northwestern Univ 1973; **Resid:** Internal Medicine, Univ Wash Hosps 1978; **Fellow:** Medical Oncology, Univ Wash Hosps 1979; **Fac Appt:** Assoc Prof Med, Univ Wash

Carlson, Robert Wells MD [Onc] - **Spec Exp:** Breast Cancer; **Hospital:** Stanford Univ Med Ctr; **Address:** Stanford Comprehensive Cancer Ctr, 875 Blake Wilbur Drive, MC 5826, Stanford, CA 94305; **Phone:** 650-723-7621; **Board Cert:** Internal Medicine 1981; Medical Oncology 1983; **Med School:** Stanford Univ 1978; **Resid:** Internal Medicine, Barnes Hosp 1980; Internal Medicine, Stanford Univ Hosp 1981; **Fellow:** Medical Oncology, Stanford Univ Hosp 1983; **Fac Appt:** Prof Med, Stanford Univ

Chap, Linnea MD [Onc] - **Spec Exp:** Breast Cancer; **Hospital:** St John's Hlth Ctr, Santa Monica; **Address:** Premier Oncology, 2020 Santa Monica Blvd, Ste 600, Santa Monica, CA 90404-2023; **Phone:** 310-633-8400; **Board Cert:** Medical Oncology 2005; **Med School:** Univ Chicago-Pritzker Sch Med 1988; **Resid:** Internal Medicine, Northwestern Meml Hosp 1991; **Fellow:** Hematology & Oncology, UCLA Med Ctr 1992

Chlebowski, Rowan T MD/PhD [Onc] - **Spec Exp:** Breast Cancer; Women's Health; **Hospital:** LAC - Harbor - UCLA Med Ctr; **Address:** 1124 W Carson St J3 Bldg, Torrance, CA 90502; **Phone:** 310-222-2218; **Board Cert:** Internal Medicine 1980; Medical Oncology 1981; **Med School:** Case West Res Univ 1974; **Resid:** Internal Medicine, MetroHealth Med Ctr 1976; Medical Oncology, LAC-USC Med Ctr 1979; **Fac Appt:** Prof Med, UCLA

Chow, Warren Allen MD [Onc] - **Spec Exp:** Sarcoma; Bone Cancer; **Hospital:** City of Hope Natl Med Ctr & Beckman Rsch; **Address:** 1500 E Duarte Rd, Duarte, CA 91010; **Phone:** 626-359-8111; **Board Cert:** Hematology 2004; Medical Oncology 2003; **Med School:** Ros Franklin Univ/Chicago Med Sch 1986; **Resid:** Internal Medicine, Cedars-Sinai Med Ctr 1990; **Fellow:** Hematology & Oncology, City of Hope 1992; Molecular Genetics, City of Hope 1994; **Fac Appt:** Assoc Prof Med

Medical Oncology

Deeg, H. Joachim MD [Onc] - **Spec Exp:** Bone Marrow Failure Disorders; Hematologic Malignancies; **Hospital:** Univ Wash Med Ctr; **Address:** Fred Hutchinson Cancer Research Center, 1100 Fairview Avenue N, D1-100, Box 19024, Seattle, WA 98109-1024; **Phone:** 206-667-5985; **Board Cert:** Internal Medicine 1976; Medical Oncology 1979; **Med School:** Germany 1972; **Fac Appt:** Prof Med, Univ Wash

Disis, Mary Lenora MD [Onc] - **Spec Exp:** Breast Cancer; Ovarian Cancer; Clinical Trials; **Hospital:** Univ Wash Med Ctr; **Address:** Univ Washington, Ctr Translational Medicine Women's Hlth, 815 Mercer St Fl 2, Seattle, WA 98109; **Phone:** 206-616-1823; **Board Cert:** Internal Medicine 1989; Medical Oncology 1997; **Med School:** Univ Nebr Coll Med 1986; **Resid:** Internal Medicine, Univ Illinois Med Ctr 1990; **Fellow:** Medical Oncology, Fred Hutchinson Cancer Ctr 1993; **Fac Appt:** Assoc Prof Med, Univ Wash

Druker, Brian MD [Onc] - **Spec Exp:** Leukemia; **Hospital:** OR Hlth & Sci Univ; **Address:** 3181 SW Sam Jackson Park Rd, MC L592, Portland, OR 97239-3098; **Phone:** 503-494-5058; **Board Cert:** Internal Medicine 1984; Medical Oncology 1987; **Med School:** UCSD 1981; **Resid:** Internal Medicine, Barnes Jewish Hosp 1984; **Fellow:** Medical Oncology, Dana-Farber Cancer Inst 1987; **Fac Appt:** Prof Med, Oregon Hlth Sci Univ

Ellis, Georgiana K MD [Onc] - **Spec Exp:** Breast Cancer; Clinical Trials; **Hospital:** Univ Wash Med Ctr; **Address:** Univ Washington Sch Med, Div Oncology, SCCA 825 Eastlake Ave E, Box 358081, MS G3-630, Seattle, WA 98109-1023; **Phone:** 206-288-6989; **Board Cert:** Internal Medicine 1985; Medical Oncology 1987; **Med School:** Univ Wash 1982; **Resid:** Internal Medicine, Univ Washington 1985; **Fellow:** Medical Oncology, Univ Washington 1988; **Fac Appt:** Assoc Prof Med, Univ Wash

Estey, Elihu H MD [Onc] - **Spec Exp:** Leukemia; Myelodysplastic Syndromes; Clinical Trials; **Hospital:** Univ Wash Med Ctr; **Address:** Seattle Cancer Care Alliance, 825 Eastlake Ave E, PO Box 19023, Seattle, WA 98109; **Phone:** 206-288-1024; **Board Cert:** Internal Medicine 1975; Medical Oncology 1981; **Med School:** Johns Hopkins Univ 1972; **Resid:** Internal Medicine, Bellevue Hosp Ctr 1975; **Fellow:** Medical Oncology, MD Anderson Cancer Ctr 1978

Figlin, Robert A MD [Onc] - **Spec Exp:** Urologic Cancer; Kidney Cancer; Immunotherapy; **Hospital:** City of Hope Natl Med Ctr & Beckman Rsch; **Address:** Med Oncology & Therapeutics Research, 1500 E Duarte Rd, Duarte, CA 91010; **Phone:** 626-256-4673; **Board Cert:** Internal Medicine 1979; Medical Oncology 1983; **Med School:** Med Coll PA Hahnemann 1976; **Resid:** Internal Medicine, Cedars Sinai Med Ctr 1980; **Fellow:** Hematology & Oncology, UCLA Ctr Hlth Sci 1982; **Fac Appt:** Prof Med, UCLA

Ford, James M MD [Onc] - **Spec Exp:** Gastrointestinal Cancer; Colon & Rectal Cancer; Cancer Genetics; **Hospital:** Stanford Univ Med Ctr; **Address:** Stanford Comp Cancer Ctr, 875 Blake Wilbur Drive, Ste Clinic B, Stanford, CA 94305-5820; **Phone:** 650-723-7621; **Board Cert:** Internal Medicine 1996; Medical Oncology 2005; **Med School:** Yale Univ 1989; **Resid:** Internal Medicine, Stanford Univ Med Ctr 1991; **Fellow:** Medical Oncology, Stanford Univ Med Ctr 1994; **Fac Appt:** Assoc Prof Med, Stanford Univ

Forscher, Charles A MD [Onc] - **Spec Exp:** Bone Tumors; Sarcoma-Soft Tissue; **Hospital:** Cedars-Sinai Med Ctr, Ronald Reagan UCLA Med Ctr; **Address:** Outpatient Cancer Ctr, Lower Level, 8700 Beverly Blvd, Los Angeles, CA 90048; **Phone:** 310-423-8045; **Board Cert:** Internal Medicine 1981; Hematology 1986; Medical Oncology 1987; **Med School:** Albert Einstein Coll Med 1978; **Resid:** Internal Medicine, Montefiore Med Ctr 1981; **Fellow:** Hematology, Montefiore Med Ctr 1983; Neoplastic Diseases, Mt Sinai Med Ctr 1985; **Fac Appt:** Clin Prof Med, UCLA

Gandara, David R MD [Onc] - **Spec Exp:** Lung Cancer; **Hospital:** UC Davis Med Ctr; **Address:** UC Davis Cancer Ctr, 4501 X St, Sacramento, CA 95817; **Phone:** 916-734-5959; **Board Cert:** Internal Medicine 1976; Medical Oncology 1979; **Med School:** Univ Tex Med Br, Galveston 1973; **Resid:** Internal Medicine, Madigan Med Ctr 1976; **Fellow:** Hematology & Oncology, Letterman AMC 1978; **Fac Appt:** Asst Prof Med, UC Davis

Ganz, Patricia A MD [Onc] - **Spec Exp:** Breast Cancer; Cancer Survivors-Late Effects of Therapy; **Hospital:** Ronald Reagan UCLA Med Ctr; **Address:** UCLA, Cancer Prev/Control Rsch, A2-125 CHS, 650 Charles Young Drive S, Box 956900, Los Angeles, CA 90095-6900; **Phone:** 310-206-1404; **Board Cert:** Internal Medicine 1976; Medical Oncology 1979; **Med School:** UCLA 1973; **Resid:** Internal Medicine, UCLA Med Ctr 1976; **Fellow:** Hematology, UCLA Med Ctr 1978; **Fac Appt:** Prof Med, UCLA

Glaspy, John A MD [Onc] - **Spec Exp:** Breast Cancer; Melanoma; Lymphoma; **Hospital:** Ronald Reagan UCLA Med Ctr; **Address:** 100 UCLA Medical Plaza, Ste 550, Los Angeles, CA 90095; **Phone:** 310-794-4955; **Board Cert:** Internal Medicine 1982; Medical Oncology 1985; Hematology 1986; **Med School:** UCLA 1979; **Resid:** Internal Medicine, UCLA Med Ctr 1982; **Fellow:** Hematology & Oncology, UCLA Med Ctr 1984; **Fac Appt:** Prof Med, UCLA

Gold, Philip J MD [Onc] - **Spec Exp:** Gastrointestinal Cancer; **Hospital:** Swedish Med Ctr - Seattle; **Address:** Swedish Cancer Inst, 1221 Madison St Fl 2, Seattle, WA 98104; **Phone:** 206-386-2121; **Board Cert:** Internal Medicine 2005; Medical Oncology 1997; **Med School:** Univ Miami Sch Med 1991; **Resid:** Internal Medicine, Univ of Washington Med Ctr 1994; **Fellow:** Medical Oncology, Fred Hutchinson Cancer Rsch Ctr 1997

Gralow, Julie MD [Onc] - **Spec Exp:** Breast Cancer; **Hospital:** Univ Wash Med Ctr; **Address:** Seattle Cancer Care Alliance-UW, 825 Eastlake Ave E, Box 358081, MS G4-83, Seattle, WA 98109; **Phone:** 206-288-7222; **Board Cert:** Medical Oncology 2005; **Med School:** USC Sch Med 1988; **Resid:** Internal Medicine, Brigham & Women's Hosp 1991; **Fellow:** Oncology, Univ Wash Med Ctr 1994; **Fac Appt:** Assoc Prof Med, Univ Wash

Higano, Celestia MD [Onc] - **Spec Exp:** Genitourinary Cancer; Prostate Cancer; Bladder Cancer; Testicular Cancer; **Hospital:** Univ Wash Med Ctr; **Address:** Seattle Cancer Care Alliance, 825 Eastlake Ave E, PO Box 19024, Seattle, WA 98109; **Phone:** 206-288-7222; **Board Cert:** Internal Medicine 1982; Medical Oncology 1985; **Med School:** Univ Mass Sch Med 1979; **Resid:** Internal Medicine, Mayo Clinic 1982; **Fellow:** Oncology, Univ Washington 1985; **Fac Appt:** Assoc Prof Med, Univ Wash

Horning, Sandra J MD [Onc] - **Spec Exp:** Hodgkin's Disease; Bone Marrow & Stem Cell Transplant; Lymphoma; **Hospital:** Stanford Univ Med Ctr; **Address:** Stanford Cancer Center, 875 Blake Wilbur Drive, Stanford, CA 94305; **Phone:** 650-723-7621; **Board Cert:** Internal Medicine 1978; Medical Oncology 1981; **Med School:** Univ Iowa Coll Med 1975; **Resid:** Internal Medicine, Strong Meml Hosp 1978; **Fellow:** Medical Oncology, Stanford Univ 1980; **Fac Appt:** Prof Med, Stanford Univ

Jacobs, Charlotte D MD [Onc] - **Spec Exp:** Sarcoma; Unknown Primary Cancer; **Hospital:** Stanford Univ Med Ctr; **Address:** 875 Blake Wilbur Drive, Stanford, CA 94305; **Phone:** 650-723-7621 x2; **Board Cert:** Internal Medicine 1975; Medical Oncology 1977; **Med School:** Washington Univ, St Louis 1972; **Resid:** Internal Medicine, Barnes Hosp 1974; Internal Medicine, UCSF Med Ctr 1975; **Fellow:** Medical Oncology, Stanford Univ 1977; **Fac Appt:** Prof Med, Stanford Univ

Medical Oncology

Jahan, Thierry Marie MD [Onc] - **Spec Exp:** Endocrine Tumors; Lung Cancer; Mesothelioma; Thyroid Cancer; **Hospital:** UCSF Med Ctr; **Address:** UCSF Comprehensive Cancer Center, 1600 Divisadero St, San Francisco, CA 94115; **Phone:** 415-353-9888; **Board Cert:** Hematology 1994; Medical Oncology 1995; Internal Medicine 1990; **Med School:** Geo Wash Univ 1987; **Resid:** Internal Medicine, Cedars-Sinai Med Ctr 1990; **Fac Appt:** Asst Clin Prof Med, UCSF

Kaplan, Lawrence D MD [Onc] - **Spec Exp:** AIDS Related Cancers; Lymphoma; **Hospital:** UCSF Med Ctr; **Address:** UCSF Medical Center, 400 Parnassus Ave, rm A502, San Francisco, CA 94143-0324; **Phone:** 415-353-2737; **Board Cert:** Internal Medicine 1983; Medical Oncology 1985; **Med School:** UCLA 1980; **Resid:** Internal Medicine, Boston City Hosp 1983; **Fellow:** Hematology & Oncology, UCSF Med Ctr 1985; **Fac Appt:** Clin Prof Med, UCSF

Koczywas, Marianna MD [Onc] - **Spec Exp:** Lung Cancer; **Hospital:** City of Hope Natl Med Ctr & Beckman Rsch; **Address:** City of Hope National Medical Center, 1500 E Duarte Rd, Duarte, CA 91010; **Phone:** 626-359-8111; **Board Cert:** Internal Medicine 1997; Hematology 2000; Medical Oncology 2001; **Med School:** Poland 1984; **Resid:** Internal Medicine, Troczewski City Hosp 1988; Internal Medicine, St. Francis Med Ctr 1997; **Fellow:** Hematology & Oncology, City of Hope Natl Med Ctr 2000

Maloney, David G MD/PhD [Onc] - **Spec Exp:** Lymphoma; Bone Marrow & Stem Cell Transplant; Vaccine Therapy; **Hospital:** Univ Wash Med Ctr; **Address:** Fred Hutchinson Cancer, Research Ctr Ave, MS D1-100, 1100 Fairview Ave N, Box 19024, Seattle, WA 98109-1024; **Phone:** 206-667-5616; **Board Cert:** Internal Medicine 1988; Medical Oncology 2005; **Med School:** Stanford Univ 1985; **Resid:** Internal Medicine, Brigham & Women's Hosp 1988; **Fellow:** Medical Oncology, Stanford Univ Med Ctr 1994; **Fac Appt:** Prof Med, Univ Wash

Margolin, Kim Allyson MD [Onc] - **Spec Exp:** Melanoma; Kidney Cancer; Germ Cell Tumors; **Hospital:** City of Hope Natl Med Ctr & Beckman Rsch; **Address:** City of Hope Comprehensive Cancer Ctr, 1500 E Duarte Rd, Duarte, CA 91010-3012; **Phone:** 626-359-8111 x62307; **Board Cert:** Internal Medicine 1982; Hematology 1986; Medical Oncology 2006; **Med School:** Stanford Univ 1979; **Resid:** Internal Medicine, Yale-New Haven Hosp 1982; **Fellow:** Hematology & Oncology, UC San Diego Med Ctr 1983; Hematology & Oncology, City of Hope Med Ctr 1985

Martins, Renato G MD [Onc] - **Spec Exp:** Head & Neck Cancer; Lung Cancer; Mesothelioma; Salivary Gland Tumors; **Hospital:** Univ Wash Med Ctr; **Address:** Seattle Cancer Care Alliance, 825 Eastlake Ave E, MS G4-830, Seattle, WA 98109; **Phone:** 206-288-2048; **Board Cert:** Internal Medicine 1995; Medical Oncology 1998; **Med School:** Brazil 1992; **Resid:** Internal Medicine, Gunderson Clinic 1995; **Fellow:** Medical Oncology, Mass Genl Hosp 1998

Meyskens, Frank MD [Onc] - **Spec Exp:** Cancer Prevention; Melanoma; Sarcoma; **Hospital:** UC Irvine Med Ctr; **Address:** UC Irvine Cancer Ctr, 101 The City Drive Bldg 56 - rm 215, Orange, CA 92868; **Phone:** 714-456-6310; **Board Cert:** Internal Medicine 1975; Medical Oncology 1981; **Med School:** UCSF 1972; **Resid:** Internal Medicine, Moffit-Calif Hosps 1974; **Fellow:** Hematology & Oncology, Natl Cancer Inst 1977; **Fac Appt:** Prof Med, UC Irvine

Mitchell, Beverly MD [Onc] - **Spec Exp:** Hematologic Malignancies; Leukemia; Lymphoma; **Hospital:** Stanford Univ Med Ctr; **Address:** Stanford Cancer Center, 800 Welch Rd, Ste 280, MC 5-5796, Stanford, CA 94305-5402; **Phone:** 650-725-9621; **Board Cert:** Internal Medicine 1973; Hematology 1978; **Med School:** Harvard Med Sch 1969; **Resid:** Internal Medicine, Univ Washington Med Ctr 1972; **Fellow:** Metabolism, Univ Zurich 1975; Hematology & Oncology, Univ Michigan 1977; **Fac Appt:** Prof Med, Stanford Univ

Mortimer, Joanne MD [Onc] - **Spec Exp:** Breast Cancer; Clinical Trials; **Hospital:** City of Hope Natl Med Ctr & Beckman Rsch; **Address:** 1500 E Duarte Rd, Duarte, CA 91010; **Phone:** 626-471-9200; **Board Cert:** Internal Medicine 1980; Medical Oncology 1983; **Med School:** Loyola Univ-Stritch Sch Med 1977; **Resid:** Internal Medicine, Cleveland Clinic 1980; **Fellow:** Medical Oncology, Cleveland Clinic 1982; **Fac Appt:** Prof Med, UCSD

Natale, Ronald B MD [Onc] - **Spec Exp:** Lung Cancer; **Hospital:** Cedars-Sinai Med Ctr; **Address:** Cedars-Sinai Comp Cancer Ctr, 8700 Beverly Blvd, Ste C2000, Los Angeles, CA 90048; **Phone:** 310-423-1101; **Board Cert:** Internal Medicine 1977; Medical Oncology 1979; **Med School:** Wayne State Univ 1974; **Resid:** Internal Medicine, Wayne State Univ 1977; **Fellow:** Hematology & Oncology, Meml Sloan Kettering 1980; **Fac Appt:** Prof Med, Univ Mich Med Sch

Nichols, Craig R MD [Onc] - **Spec Exp:** Testicular Cancer; Hodgkin's Disease; Lymphoma; **Hospital:** Providence Portland Med Ctr; **Address:** Providence Cancer Ctr, Oregon Clinic, 4805 NE Glisan St, Ste 6N40, Portland, OR 97213; **Phone:** 503-215-5696; **Board Cert:** Internal Medicine 1981; Medical Oncology 1985; **Med School:** Oregon Hlth Sci Univ 1978; **Resid:** Internal Medicine, Oschner Foundation Hosp 1981; **Fellow:** Medical Oncology, Indiana Univ 1985; **Fac Appt:** Prof Med, Oregon Hlth Sci Univ

O'Day, Steven J MD [Onc] - **Spec Exp:** Melanoma; Melanoma-Advanced; **Hospital:** St John's Hlth Ctr, Santa Monica; **Address:** 2001 Santa Monica Blvd, Ste 560W, 11818 Wilshire Blvd, Ste 200, Los Angeles, CA 90025; **Phone:** 310-231-2121; **Board Cert:** Internal Medicine 1991; Medical Oncology 1993; **Med School:** Johns Hopkins Univ 1988; **Resid:** Internal Medicine, Johns Hopkins Hosp 1991; **Fellow:** Medical Oncology, Dana Farber Cancer Inst 1992; **Fac Appt:** Assoc Clin Prof Med, USC-Keck School of Medicine

Petersdorf, Stephen MD [Onc] - **Spec Exp:** Lymphoma; Myelodysplastic Syndromes; Leukemia; **Hospital:** Univ Wash Med Ctr; **Address:** Seattle Cancer Care Alliance, 825 Eastlake Ave E, MS G3200, Seattle, WA 98109-1023; **Phone:** 206-288-1024; **Board Cert:** Internal Medicine 1986; Hematology 2001; Medical Oncology 2001; **Med School:** Brown Univ 1983; **Resid:** Internal Medicine, Univ Washington Med Ctr 1986; **Fellow:** Hematology & Oncology, Univ Washington Med Ctr 1989; **Fac Appt:** Assoc Prof Med, Univ Wash

Picozzi Jr, Vincent J MD [Onc] - **Spec Exp:** Pancreatic Cancer; **Hospital:** Virginia Mason Med Ctr; **Address:** Virginia Mason Med Ctr, Div Hem/Onc, MS C2-Hem, Seattle, WA 98111; **Phone:** 206-223-6193; **Board Cert:** Internal Medicine 1981; Hematology 1986; Medical Oncology 1987; **Med School:** Stanford Univ 1978; **Resid:** Internal Medicine, Peter Bent Brigham Med Ctr 1981; **Fellow:** Hematology, Stanford Univ Med Ctr 1983; Medical Oncology, Stanford Univ MEd Ctr 1983; **Fac Appt:** Clin Prof Med, Univ Wash

Pinto, Harlan Andrew MD [Onc] - **Spec Exp:** Head & Neck Cancer; Clinical Trials; **Hospital:** Stanford Univ Med Ctr, VA Hlth Care Sys - Palo Alto; **Address:** Stanford Med Ctr Oncol Div, 875 Blake Wilbur Drive, Stanford, CA 94305; **Phone:** 650-723-7621; **Board Cert:** Internal Medicine 1986; Medical Oncology 2002; **Med School:** Yale Univ 1983; **Resid:** Internal Medicine, Mass Genl Hosp 1986; **Fellow:** Medical Oncology, Stanford Univ Med Sch 1991; **Fac Appt:** Assoc Prof Med, Stanford Univ

Prados, Michael MD [Onc] - **Spec Exp:** Neuro-Oncology; Brain Tumors; **Hospital:** UCSF Med Ctr; **Address:** UCSF Med Ctr, Div Neuro-Oncology, 400 Parnassus Ave, rm A-808, San Francisco, CA 94143; **Phone:** 415-353-2966; **Board Cert:** Internal Medicine 1977; **Med School:** Louisiana State U, New Orleans 1974; **Resid:** Internal Medicine, Earl K Long Hosp 1977; **Fac Appt:** Prof NS, UCSF

Medical Oncology

Press, Oliver W MD/PhD [Onc] - **Spec Exp:** Lymphoma; Bone Marrow Transplant; **Hospital:** Univ Wash Med Ctr; **Address:** 1100 Fairview Ave N, MS D3-19, Seattle, WA 98109; **Phone:** 206-667-1864; **Board Cert:** Internal Medicine 1982; Medical Oncology 1985; **Med School:** Univ Wash 1979; **Resid:** Internal Medicine, Mass Genl Hosp 1982; Internal Medicine, Univ Hosp 1983; **Fellow:** Medical Oncology, Univ Washington 1985; **Fac Appt:** Prof Med, Univ Wash

Quinn, David MD/PhD [Onc] - **Spec Exp:** Testicular Cancer; Prostate Cancer; Kidney Cancer; **Hospital:** USC Norris Comp Cancer Ctr; **Address:** 1441 Eastlake Ave, Ste 3440, Los Angeles, CA 90033; **Phone:** 323-865-3956; **Med School:** Australia 1987; **Resid:** Internal Medicine, St Vincent's Hosp 1992; **Fellow:** Medical Oncology, St Vincent's Hosp 1995; **Fac Appt:** Asst Prof Med, USC Sch Med

Rugo, Hope S MD [Onc] - **Spec Exp:** Breast Cancer; Complementary Medicine; Breast Cancer-Novel Therapies; **Hospital:** UCSF Med Ctr; **Address:** UCSF Comp Cancer Ctr-Breast Care Ctr, 1600 Divisadero St Fl 2, San Francisco, CA 94115; **Phone:** 415-353-7070; **Board Cert:** Internal Medicine 1987; Medical Oncology 1989; **Med School:** Univ Pennsylvania 1984; **Resid:** Internal Medicine, UCSF Med Ctr 1987; **Fellow:** Hematology & Oncology, UCSF Med Ctr 1989; **Fac Appt:** Clin Prof Med, UCSF

Russell, Christy A MD [Onc] - **Spec Exp:** Breast Cancer; **Hospital:** USC Univ Hosp - R K Eamer Med Plz; **Address:** Norris Cancer Ctr, The Breast Ctr, 1441 Eastlake Ave, Los Angeles, CA 90033; **Phone:** 323-865-3371; **Board Cert:** Internal Medicine 1983; Medical Oncology 1985; **Med School:** Med Coll PA Hahnemann 1980; **Fac Appt:** Assoc Prof Med, USC Sch Med

Samlowski, Wolfram E MD [Onc] - **Spec Exp:** Kidney Cancer; Melanoma; Immunotherapy; **Hospital:** Univ Utah Hosps and Clins; **Address:** Nevada Cancer Institute, One Breakthrough Way, Las Vegas, NV 89135; **Phone:** 702-822-5433; **Board Cert:** Internal Medicine 1981; Medical Oncology 1985; **Med School:** Ohio State Univ 1978; **Resid:** Internal Medicine, Wayne State Univ 1981; **Fellow:** Hematology & Oncology, Univ Utah 1984; **Fac Appt:** Prof Med, Univ Utah

Shibata, Stephen I MD [Onc] - **Spec Exp:** Gastrointestinal Cancer; Clinical Trials; **Hospital:** City of Hope Natl Med Ctr & Beckman Rsch; **Address:** City of Hope Cancer Ctr, 1500 E Duarte Rd, Duarte, CA 91010; **Phone:** 626-471-9200 x7; **Board Cert:** Internal Medicine 1988; Medical Oncology 1991; **Med School:** UC Irvine 1985; **Resid:** Internal Medicine, St Mary Med Ctr 1988; **Fellow:** Medical Oncology, City of Hope Cancer Ctr 1990; Bone Marrow Transplant, City of Hope Cancer Ctr 1991; **Fac Appt:** Assoc Prof Med

Sikic, Branimir I MD [Onc] - **Spec Exp:** Unknown Primary Cancer; Clinical Trials; **Hospital:** Stanford Univ Med Ctr; **Address:** Stanford Comp Cancer Ctr, Med Oncology, 875 Blake Wilbur Drive, Stanford, CA 94305; **Phone:** 650-723-7621; **Board Cert:** Internal Medicine 1975; Medical Oncology 1979; **Med School:** Ros Franklin Univ/Chicago Med Sch 1972; **Resid:** Internal Medicine, Georgetown Univ Hosp 1975; **Fellow:** Medical Oncology, Natl Cancer Inst 1978; Medical Oncology, Georgetown Univ Hosp 1979; **Fac Appt:** Prof Med, Stanford Univ

Small, Eric J MD [Onc] - **Spec Exp:** Prostate Cancer; Vaccine Therapy; Genitourinary Cancer; **Hospital:** UCSF Med Ctr; **Address:** UCSF Urologic Oncology Practice, 1600 Divisadero St Fl 3rd, San Francisco, CA 94115-1711; **Phone:** 415-353-7171; **Board Cert:** Internal Medicine 1988; Medical Oncology 2001; **Med School:** Case West Res Univ 1985; **Resid:** Internal Medicine, Beth Israel Hosp 1988; **Fellow:** Hematology & Oncology, Cancer Research Inst/UCSF 1991; **Fac Appt:** Prof Med, UCSF

America's Top Doctors® 8th Edition

Stewart, Forrest M MD [Onc] - **Spec Exp:** Unknown Primary Cancer; Sarcoma; **Hospital:** Univ Wash Med Ctr; **Address:** Seattle Cancer Care Alliance, 825 Eastlake Ave E, Box 19023, Seattle, WA 98109; **Phone:** 206-288-7222; **Board Cert:** Internal Medicine 1980; Hematology 1982; Medical Oncology 1985; **Med School:** Indiana Univ 1977; **Resid:** Internal Medicine, Indiana Univ Med Ctr 1980; Medical Oncology, Indiana Univ Med Ctr 1981; **Fellow:** Hematology, Univ Virginia Med Ctr 1983; **Fac Appt:** Prof Med, Univ Wash

Stockdale, Frank E MD/PhD [Onc] - **Spec Exp:** Breast Cancer; **Hospital:** Stanford Univ Med Ctr; **Address:** Stanford University Medical Ctr, 875 Lake Wilbur Drive, Stanford, CA 94305-5826; **Phone:** 650-723-6449; **Med School:** Univ Pennsylvania 1963; **Resid:** Internal Medicine, Stanford Univ Med Ctr 1967; Hematology & Oncology, Stanford Univ Med Ctr; **Fac Appt:** Prof Emeritus Med, Stanford Univ

Tempero, Margaret MD [Onc] - **Spec Exp:** Pancreatic Cancer; Gastrointestinal Cancer; **Hospital:** UCSF Med Ctr; **Address:** UCSF, Multi-Disciplinary Practice, 1600 Divisadero St, Box 1705, San Francisco, CA 94115; **Phone:** 415-353-9888; **Board Cert:** Internal Medicine 1980; Hematology 1984; Medical Oncology 1983; **Med School:** Univ Nebr Coll Med 1977; **Resid:** Internal Medicine, Univ Nebraska Hosp 1980; **Fellow:** Medical Oncology, Univ Nebraska 1982

Thompson, John A MD [Onc] - **Spec Exp:** Melanoma; **Hospital:** Univ Wash Med Ctr; **Address:** Seattle Cancer Care Alliance, 825 Eastlake Ave E, MS G4-830, Seattle, WA 98109-1023; **Phone:** 206-288-2015; **Board Cert:** Internal Medicine 1982; Medical Oncology 1985; **Med School:** Univ Ala 1979; **Resid:** Internal Medicine, Univ Wash Med Ctr 1982; **Fellow:** Medical Oncology, Univ Washington 1985

Urba, Walter J MD/PhD [Onc] - **Spec Exp:** Breast Cancer; **Hospital:** Providence Portland Med Ctr; **Address:** Oregon Clinic, Div Medical Oncology, 4805 NE Glisan Rd, Ste 6N40, Portland, OR 97213; **Phone:** 503-215-5696; **Board Cert:** Internal Medicine 1985; Medical Oncology 1987; **Med School:** Univ Miami Sch Med 1981; **Resid:** Internal Medicine, Morristown Meml Hosp 1983; **Fellow:** Medical Oncology, Natl Cancer Inst 1986; **Fac Appt:** Assoc Clin Prof Med, Oregon Hlth Sci Univ

Venook, Alan P MD [Onc] - **Spec Exp:** Gastrointestinal Cancer; Colon & Rectal Cancer; Liver Cancer; **Hospital:** UCSF Med Ctr; **Address:** UCSF Comprehensive Cancer Ctr, Multi Disciplinary Practice, 1600 Divisadero St Fl 4, Box 1705, San Francisco, CA 94115; **Phone:** 415-353-9888; **Board Cert:** Internal Medicine 1985; Medical Oncology 1987; Hematology 1988; **Med School:** UCSF 1980; **Resid:** Internal Medicine, UC Davis Med Ctr 1985; **Fellow:** Hematology & Oncology, UCSF Med Ctr 1987; **Fac Appt:** Prof Med

Vescio, Robert A MD [Onc] - **Spec Exp:** Multiple Myeloma; Amyloidosis; **Hospital:** Cedars-Sinai Med Ctr; **Address:** Cedars Sinai Med Ctr, Dept Hem/Oncology, 8700 Beverly Blvd, Los Angeles, CA 90048; **Phone:** 310-423-1825; **Board Cert:** Internal Medicine 1989; Hematology 2004; Medical Oncology 2003; **Med School:** UCSD 1986; **Resid:** Internal Medicine, UCSD Med Ctr 1989; **Fellow:** Hematology & Oncology, UCLA Med Ctr 1993; **Fac Appt:** Assoc Prof Med, UCLA

Vogelzang, Nicholas MD [Onc] - **Spec Exp:** Prostate Cancer; Mesothelioma; Kidney Cancer; **Hospital:** Univ Med Ctr - Las Vegas, Summerlin Hosp Med Ctr; **Address:** Nevada Cancer Institute, One Breakthrough Way, Las Vegas, NV 89135; **Phone:** 702-822-5100; **Board Cert:** Internal Medicine 1978; Medical Oncology 1981; **Med School:** Univ IL Coll Med 1974; **Resid:** Internal Medicine, Rush-Presby St Luke's Med Ctr 1978; **Fellow:** Medical Oncology, Univ Minn Med Ctr 1981; **Fac Appt:** Prof Med, Univ Nevada

Medical Oncology

Volberding, Paul Arthur MD [Onc] - **Spec Exp:** AIDS Related Cancers; **Hospital:** UCSF Med Ctr; **Address:** 4150 Clement St, VAMC 111, San Francisco, CA 94121; **Phone:** 415-750-2203; **Board Cert:** Internal Medicine 1978; Medical Oncology 1981; **Med School:** Univ Minn 1975; **Resid:** Internal Medicine, Univ Utah Med Ctr 1978; **Fellow:** Medical Oncology, UCSF Med Ctr 1981; **Fac Appt:** Prof Med, UCSF

von Gunten, Charles MD/PhD [Onc] - **Spec Exp:** Palliative Care; **Hospital:** San Diego Hospice; **Address:** San Diego Hospice, 4311 Third Ave, San Diego, CA 92103; **Phone:** 619-688-1600; **Board Cert:** Internal Medicine 2002; Medical Oncology 2003; Hospice & Palliative Medicine 2001; **Med School:** Univ Colorado 1988; **Resid:** Internal Medicine, Northwestern Univ 1991; **Fellow:** Medical Oncology, Northwestern Univ 1993; **Fac Appt:** Assoc Clin Prof Med, UCSD

Yen, Yun MD/PhD [Onc] - **Spec Exp:** Liver Cancer; Biliary Cancer; **Hospital:** City of Hope Natl Med Ctr & Beckman Rsch; **Address:** City of Hope Comprehensive Cancer Ctr, 1500 E Duarte Rd, Duarte, CA 91010; **Phone:** 626-359-8111 x62307; **Board Cert:** Medical Oncology 2003; **Med School:** Taiwan 1982; **Resid:** Internal Medicine, St Luke's Hosp 1990; **Fellow:** Hematology & Oncology, Yale-New Haven Hosp 1993; **Fac Appt:** Prof Med, USC Sch Med

Cleveland Clinic

Innovative Research and Outstanding Outcomes

At Cleveland Clinic Taussig Cancer Institute, more than 250 cancer specialists, researchers, nurses and technicians are dedicated to developing and applying the latest and most effective medical techniques to achieve the long-term survival and improve the quality of life for 7,500 new cancer patients every year. Because of our innovative research, 350 clinical trials and state-of-the-art medical technologies, *U.S.News & World Report* has ranked Taussig Cancer Institute one of the top cancer centers in the nation.

The Taussig Cancer Institute has more than 200,000 annual cancer patient visits at its main campus in Cleveland and at 10 locations throughout Northeast Ohio. Our areas of expertise include prostate and other urologic cancers, melanoma, blood and bone marrow cancers, multiple myeloma, colorectal cancer, lung cancer, breast cancer and brain and spinal cord tumors.

Because of Taussig Cancer Institute's extensive cancer care system, the Leukemia & Lymphoma Society forged a groundbreaking partnership with Taussig Cancer Institute to make blood cancer clinical trials available to patients in their communities. This enables patients to stay with their primary doctors and participate in clinical trials near their hometown.

"Patients First"

"Patients First" is the guiding principle of Cleveland Clinic. It declares the primacy of patient care, patient comfort and patient communication in every activity we undertake. It affirms the importance of research and education for their contributions to clinical medicine and the improvement of patient care. At the same time, "Patients First" demands a relentless focus on measurable quality. By setting standards, collecting data and analyzing the results, Cleveland Clinic puts patients first through improved outcomes and better service, providing a healthier future for all.

Outstanding Outcomes: Our Bone Marrow Transplant outcomes are unsurpassed by any program in the world. We have one of the most experienced teams in the nation, having performed more than 2,900 bone marrow transplant procedures since 1977.

Innovative Research: Taussig Cancer Institute is at the forefront of cancer research. Our world-renowned scientists are dedicated to developing novel, effective therapeutic options for cancer patients. Through understanding cellular abnormalities that lead to cancer, our researchers target specific genes with drugs or combinations of drugs to improve outcomes.

Cancer Genetics at the Center for Personalized Genetic Healthcare: Because some families are prone to developing cancer, advances in genetic research help us identify some of the risk factors. Cleveland Clinic's Center for Personalized Genetic Healthcare aims to prevent cancer by identifying high risk individuals and offers personalized medical management to them and their family members.

In our multidisciplinary clinics, medical, radiation and surgical oncologists work closely with pathologists, radiologists, oncology nurses and social workers to optimize the options for individual patients with complex problems.

For more information about the Cleveland Clinic Taussig Cancer Institute, to schedule a second opinion or to learn about assistance for out-of-town patients, call 800.890.2467 or visit www.clevelandclinic.org/cancertopdocs.
Cleveland Clinic Taussig Cancer Institute
9500 Euclid Avenue / AC311 | Cleveland OH 44195

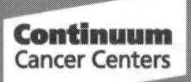

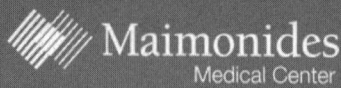

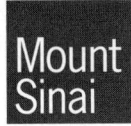
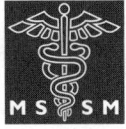

MOUNT SINAI
SCHOOL OF
MEDICINE

THE MOUNT SINAI MEDICAL CENTER
CANCER INSTITUTE
One Gustave L. Levy Place
Fifth Avenue and 100th Street
New York, NY 10029-6574
Physician Referral: 1-800-MD-SINAI (637-4624)
www.mountsinai.org/cancer

OVERVIEW
The Mount Sinai Medical Center Cancer Institute is located on the Upper East Side of Manhattan. The Institute is part of The Mount Sinai Medical Center, which was founded in 1852 and encompasses one of the oldest teaching hospitals in the country. In an atmosphere of learning, cutting-edge basic and clinical research, and superb patient care, the Cancer Institute coordinates a full-service diagnostic and treatment program for cancer patients. As new treatments are developed at the Institute, patients often have access to these therapies before they are available anywhere else in the world.

A HERITAGE OF BREAKTHROUGHS
Teams of physicians and scientists at Mount Sinai work together to rapidly translate laboratory research into new patient treatments. Among the advances pioneered at Mount Sinai are the first successful treatment of tumors of the bladder by transurethral electrocoagulation; the first demonstration of how asbestos can cause cancerous changes in the DNA of cells; and the first development of an ultrasound-guided technique to insert radioactive seeds into the prostate to treat prostate cancer.

THE CANCER INSTITUTE
The Cancer Institute employs a multidisciplinary treatment approach, providing access to clinical breakthroughs, innovative techniques, leading-edge technologies and a wide range of diagnostic, therapeutic, and support services for all types of cancer. These include: head and neck; thoracic (including lung and esophagus); gynecologic; hematological malignancies (including bone marrow transplantation, myelodysplastic syndrome, and myeloproliferative disorders); brain tumors; prostate, bladder, and kidney; and liver. In addition to surgical treatment, radiation and medical oncology therapies are provided.

Our multidisciplinary treatment approach includes collaboration with colleagues across the Medical Center, offering access to a vast network of specialists who are outstanding in their fields. Our experts consist of award-winning physicians and surgeons specializing in cardiac care, neurology, urology, pediatrics, digestive diseases, obstetrics and gynecology, and other therapeutic areas. In addition to our physicians, Mount Sinai's nursing staff is an important part of the Medical Center's focus on delivering exceptional patient care, and has received the prestigious Magnet Award for nursing excellence.

Mount Sinai is renowned for its palliative care program, and provides the highest level of care—focusing on the relief of pain, symptoms, and stress to cancer patients in both an in-patient and out-patient setting.

THE RUTTENBERG TREATMENT CENTER
The mission of the Ruttenberg Treatment Center at The Mount Sinai Medical Center is to reduce the burden of human cancer through its outstanding interdisciplinary programs in patient care and research, including cancer prevention, treatment, early detection, and education. Oncologists, surgeons, and specialists from across the medical spectrum work together to provide the highest quality care to all cancer patients. The members of the Center—scientists and physicians—are developing cancer therapies and prevention strategies to improve cancer care, and patients at the Center are the first to benefit from these treatments.

NewYork-Presbyterian

The University Hospital of Columbia and Cornell

NewYork-Presbyterian Cancer Centers

Affiliated with Columbia University College of Physicians and Surgeons and Weill Medical College of Cornell University

Herbert Irving Comprehensive Cancer Center
At NewYork-Presbyterian Hospital
Columbia University Medical Center
161 Fort Washington Avenue
New York, NY 10032

Weill Cornell Cancer Center
At NewYork-Presbyterian Hospital
Weill Cornell Medical Center
525 East 68th Street
New York, NY 10021

OVERVIEW:

NewYork-Presbyterian Cancer Centers are dedicated to reducing cancer morbidity and mortality by providing

- a full continuum of multidisciplinary, state-of-the-art screening, diagnostic, treatment and support services for all phases of the disease process;
- cutting-edge basic, clinical, and public health research;
- full range of cancer-related educational programs and resources to clinicians, scientists, patients and survivors, families, and the cancer prevention community.

The Cancer Centers, which treat over 6,000 new patients annually, draw on the innovation and excellence of the NCI- designated Herbert Irving Comprehensive Cancer Center at NewYork-Presbyterian Hospital/Columbia University Medical Center and oncology services at NewYork-Presbyterian Hospital/Weill Cornell Medical Center. Programs include:

- AIDS-related Malignancies
- Bone Marrow Transplant
- Breast Cancer
- Dermatologic/Skin Cancer
- Gastrointestinal Cancers
- Genitourinary Cancers
- Gynecologic Cancers
- Head and Neck Cancers
- Hematologic Malignancies, such as lymphoma, myeloma and leukemias
- Lung Cancer
- Neurologic Cancer
- Ophthalmic Cancer
- Pediatric Hematology/Oncology
- Urologic Cancers, including bladder, kidney and prostate cancer
- Sarcomas and Mesotheiliomas

The Centers are frequent recipients of major grants and gifts to support research programs. Recent highlights include:
- Avon Products Foundation $10 million award to NewYork-Presbyterian Hospital/Columbia University Medical Center and Columbia University for establishment of the Avon Products Breast Center to support basic, clinical and public health research in breast cancer;
- The Leukemia and Lymphoma Society five-year $7.5 million grant to NewYork-Presbyterian Hospital/Weill Cornell Medical Center to study fundamental causes of multiple myeloma

Physician Referral: For a physician referral call toll free **1-877-NYP-WELL** (1-877-697-9355) to learn more about our Cancer Centers visit our website at **www.nypcancer.org**

COMPREHENSIVE SERVICES INCLUDE:

- Access to over 400 clinical trials supported by the National Institutes of Health and many prominent pharmaceutical companies.

- Bone marrow and blood stem cell transplant, including New York State approval to perform transplants using unrelated donors for patients with hematologic malignancies

- CT screening for early lung cancer detection

- Sentinel node biopsy to assess spread of breast cancer

- Skin-sparing mastectomy and reconstruction

- Laparoscopic surgery for colon cancer

- Intraoperative brachytherapy for GI, prostate and other cancers

- Stereotactic biopsies for breast cancer and brain cancer

- Stereotactic gamma radiation for brain tumors

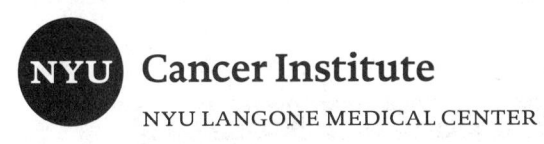

NYU Cancer Institute
NYU LANGONE MEDICAL CENTER

Wake Forest University Baptist
MEDICAL CENTER ®
Comprehensive Cancer Center

Medical Center Boulevard • Winston-Salem, NC 27157
PAL® (Physician-to-physician calls) 1-800-277-7654
Health On-Call® (Patient access) 1-800-446-2255
www.wfubmc.edu/cancer/

TOP RANKINGS

The Comprehensive Cancer Center of Wake Forest University Baptist Medical is among an elite group of only 39 U.S. cancer centers designated by the National Cancer Institute as comprehensive, indicating excellence in research, patient care and education. The comprehensive designation was renewed for an additional five years in late 2006.

RESEARCH ADVANTAGES

Wake Forest Baptist offers more cancer-related clinical trials than any other hospital in western N.C. From gene therapy to vitamin and nutrition studies to new surgical and radiological treatments, patients benefit from the leading edge of cancer knowledge and care. Innovative basic science, public health and clinical research promote new discovery about prevention, detection and treatment of cancers. Wake Forest scientists were first in the world to discover cancer resistant cells in mice.

TECHNOLOGY AND TREATMENT STRENGTHS

Wake Forest University Baptist Medical Center is home to North Carolina's first Gamma Knife, a non-invasive, stereotactic radiosurgical tool used to treat malignant and benign brain tumors once considered inoperable. Operated by one of the nation's most experienced treatment teams, the Gamma Knife painlessly bombards tumors with precisely focused beams of gamma energy – sparing normal tissue -- and is performed on an outpatient basis. Extracranial body stereotactic radiosurgery offers new options for other types of cancers.

Wake Forest Baptist offers an integrated brachytherapy unit (IBU) and highly targeted Intensity Modulated Radiation Therapy (IMRT) for treatment of prostate, brain, lung, head and neck, and gynecological cancers. Other treatment innovations include IPHC (intraperitoneal hyperthermic chemotherapy) for abdominal cavity cancers and radiofrequency ablation for liver malignancies.

MULTIDISCIPLINARY EXPERTISE

Expert, subspecialized oncology teams provide patients a consensus opinion on treatment. Multidisciplinary centers include the Thoracic Oncology Program, the Breast Care Center, the Brain Tumor Clinic and the Head and Neck Cancers Multidisciplinary Clinic.

To make an appointment or find a specialist, call Health On-Call®
at 1-800-446-2255.

HIGHLIGHTS OF EXCELLENCE

- Western North Carolina's only NCI-designated Comprehensive Cancer Center offers the convenience and comfort of a state-of-the-art Outpatient Cancer Center. The nation's first Cancer Patient Support Group was developed here.

- The Cancer Center's Blood and Marrow Transplant Program operates the nation's second-largest collection site.

- The Breast Cancer Risk Assessment Clinic and the Hereditary Cancer Clinic help patients understand their risk profile.

- Minimally invasive treatments include high dose rate (HDR) brachytherapy for prostate cancer. Lymph node mapping increases chance for lymph-sparing breast surgery.

- Clinical trials testing new methods of drug delivery offer patients with brain tumors potentially more effective treatment while minimizing effects on healthy tissue.

KNOWLEDGE MAKES ALL THE DIFFERENCE.

Sponsored Page

Infectious Disease
a subspecialty of Internal Medicine

An internist who deals with infectious diseases of all types and in all organs. Conditions requiring selective use of antibiotics call for this special skill. This physician often diagnoses and treats AIDS patients and patients with fevers which have not been explained. Infectious disease specialists may also have expertise in preventive medicine and conditions associated with travel.

Training Required: Three years in internal medicine *plus* additional training and examination for certification in infectious disease.

INFECTIOUS DISEASE

New England

Craven, Donald Edward MD [Inf] - **Spec Exp:** AIDS/HIV; Hepatitis C; Hospital Acquired Infections; Pneumonia; **Hospital:** Lahey Clin; **Address:** Lahey Clin Med Ctr, Infectious Diseases, 41 Mall Rd, Burlington, MA 01805; **Phone:** 781-744-8608; **Board Cert:** Internal Medicine 1973; Infectious Disease 1982; **Med School:** Albany Med Coll 1970; **Resid:** Internal Medicine, Royal Victoria Hosp-McGill 1973; Internal Medicine, Royal Victoria Hosp 1974; **Fellow:** Infectious Disease, Boston Univ Hosp 1976; NIH/Bureau of Biologics 1979; **Fac Appt:** Prof Med, Tufts Univ

Flanigan, Timothy P MD [Inf] - **Spec Exp:** AIDS/HIV; **Hospital:** Miriam Hosp, Rhode Island Hosp; **Address:** 164 Summit Ave Fain Bldg - Ste E, Providence, RI 02906; **Phone:** 401-793-2928; **Board Cert:** Internal Medicine 1986; Infectious Disease 1988; **Med School:** Cornell Univ-Weill Med Coll 1983; **Resid:** Internal Medicine, Hosp Univ Penn 1986; **Fellow:** Infectious Disease, Case West Res Univ 1987; **Fac Appt:** Prof Med, Brown Univ

Longworth, David L MD [Inf] - **Hospital:** Baystate Med Ctr; **Address:** Baystate Medical Ctr, 759 Chestnut St, Springfield, MA 01199; **Phone:** 413-794-4319; **Board Cert:** Internal Medicine 1981; Infectious Disease 1984; **Med School:** Cornell Univ-Weill Med Coll 1978; **Resid:** Internal Medicine, UCSF-HC Moffitt Hosp 1981; **Fellow:** Infectious Disease, Brigham & Womens Hosp 1983; Research, Harvard Med School 1985; **Fac Appt:** Prof Med, Tufts Univ

Quagliarello, Vincent MD [Inf] - **Spec Exp:** Meningitis; Pneumonia; Endocarditis; **Hospital:** Yale-New Haven Hosp; **Address:** Yale Univ Sch Med, TAC S169A, 300 Cedar St, New Haven, CT 06520-8022; **Phone:** 203-785-7570; **Board Cert:** Internal Medicine 1985; Infectious Disease 1989; **Med School:** Washington Univ, St Louis 1980; **Resid:** Internal Medicine, Yale-New Haven Hosp 1984; **Fellow:** Infectious Disease, Univ VA Hlth Sci Ctr 1987; **Fac Appt:** Prof Med, Yale Univ

Rubin, Robert H MD [Inf] - **Spec Exp:** Infections-Transplant; **Hospital:** Brigham & Women's Hosp; **Address:** Brigham & Women's Hospital, Div Infectious Disease, 15 Francis St, Boston, MA 02115; **Phone:** 617-732-8881; **Board Cert:** Internal Medicine 1972; Infectious Disease 1974; **Med School:** Harvard Med Sch 1966; **Resid:** Internal Medicine, Peter Bent Brigham Hosp 1970; **Fellow:** Infectious Disease, Mass Genl Hosp 1972; **Fac Appt:** Prof Med, Harvard Med Sch

Sax, Paul E MD [Inf] - **Spec Exp:** AIDS/HIV; **Hospital:** Brigham & Women's Hosp; **Address:** Brigham & Women's Hospital, Div Infectious Disease, 15 Francis St, Boston, MA 02115; **Phone:** 617-732-8881; **Board Cert:** Internal Medicine 2000; Infectious Disease 2000; **Med School:** Harvard Med Sch 1987; **Resid:** Internal Medicine, Brigham & Womens Hosp 1990; **Fellow:** Infectious Disease, Mass Genl Hosp 1992

Mid Atlantic

Auwaerter, Paul MD [Inf] - **Spec Exp:** Lyme Disease; Ehrlichiosis; Tick-borne Diseases; Fevers of Unknown Origin; **Hospital:** Johns Hopkins Hosp - Baltimore (page 61); **Address:** 10753 Falls Rd, Ste 325, Lutherville, MD 21093; **Phone:** 410-583-2774; **Board Cert:** Internal Medicine 2002; Infectious Disease 1994; **Med School:** Columbia P&S 1988; **Resid:** Internal Medicine, Johns Hopkins Med Ctr 1992; **Fellow:** Infectious Disease, Johns Hopkins Med Ctr 1996; **Fac Appt:** Assoc Prof Med, Johns Hopkins Univ

Bartlett, John G MD [Inf] - **Spec Exp:** AIDS/HIV; Fevers of Unknown Origin; Pseudomembranous Colitis; **Hospital:** Johns Hopkins Hosp - Baltimore (page 61); **Address:** 1830 E Monument St, Ste 439, Baltimore, MD 21205; **Phone:** 410-955-7634; **Board Cert:** Internal Medicine 1972; **Med School:** SUNY Upstate Med Univ 1963; **Resid:** Internal Medicine, Peter Bent Brigham Hosp 1965; Internal Medicine, Univ Hosp Birmingham 1968; **Fellow:** Infectious Disease, Wadsworth VA Hosp 1970

Berkowitz, Leonard B MD [Inf] - **Spec Exp:** AIDS/HIV; **Hospital:** Brooklyn Hosp Ctr-Downtown; **Address:** 121 DeKalb Ave, rm 5H, Brooklyn, NY 11201-5425; **Phone:** 718-250-6922; **Board Cert:** Internal Medicine 1980; Infectious Disease 1984; **Med School:** SUNY Downstate 1977; **Resid:** Internal Medicine, Kings Co Med Ctr 1981; **Fellow:** Infectious Disease, Kings Co Med Ctr 1983; **Fac Appt:** Asst Clin Prof Med, SUNY Hlth Sci Ctr

Brause, Barry MD [Inf] - **Spec Exp:** Bone/Joint Infections; Skin/Soft Tissue Infection; Infections in Prosthetic Devices; **Hospital:** Hosp For Special Surgery (page 59), NY-Presby Hosp/Weill Cornell (page 66); **Address:** 535 E 70th St, New York, NY 10021-5718; **Phone:** 212-774-7411; **Board Cert:** Internal Medicine 1973; Infectious Disease 1976; **Med School:** Univ Pittsburgh 1970; **Resid:** Internal Medicine, New York Hosp 1973; **Fellow:** Infectious Disease, New York Hosp 1975; **Fac Appt:** Clin Prof Med, Cornell Univ-Weill Med Coll

Chaisson, Richard E MD [Inf] - **Spec Exp:** AIDS/HIV; Tuberculosis; **Hospital:** Johns Hopkins Hosp - Baltimore (page 61); **Address:** 1503 E Jefferson St, Ste 1104, Baltimore, MD 21231; **Phone:** 410-955-1755; **Board Cert:** Internal Medicine 1985; **Med School:** Univ Mass Sch Med 1982; **Resid:** Internal Medicine, UCSF Med Ctr 1985; **Fellow:** Infectious Disease, UCSF Med Ctr 1987; **Fac Appt:** Assoc Prof Med, Johns Hopkins Univ

Cunha, Burke A MD [Inf] - **Spec Exp:** Infections in Immunocompromised Patients; Fevers of Unknown Origin; Pneumonia; Chronic Fatigue Syndrome; **Hospital:** Winthrop - Univ Hosp; **Address:** 222 Station Plz N, Ste 432, Mineola, NY 11501; **Phone:** 516-663-2507; **Board Cert:** Internal Medicine 1977; Infectious Disease 1978; **Med School:** Penn State Univ-Hershey Med Ctr 1972; **Resid:** Internal Medicine, Hartford Hosp 1975; **Fellow:** Infectious Disease, Hartford Hosp 1977; **Fac Appt:** Prof Med, SUNY Stony Brook

Fauci, Anthony S MD [Inf] - **Spec Exp:** AIDS/HIV; Immunotherapy; **Hospital:** Natl Inst of Hlth - Clin Ctr; **Address:** NIAID Bldg 31 - rm 7A03, 31 Center Drive, MSC 2520, Bethesda, MD 20892-2520; **Phone:** 301-496-2263; **Board Cert:** Internal Medicine 1972; Allergy & Immunology 1974; Infectious Disease 1974; **Med School:** Cornell Univ-Weill Med Coll 1966; **Resid:** Internal Medicine, New York Hosp Cornell Med Ctr 1972; **Fellow:** Infectious Disease, Natl Inst Infectious Disease NIH 1971

Frank, Ian MD [Inf] - **Spec Exp:** AIDS/HIV; **Hospital:** Hosp Univ Penn - UPHS (page 60); **Address:** Hosp Univ Penn, Div Infectious Disease, 3400 Spruce St, Sliverstein Bldg, Fl 3 - Ste D, Philadelphia, PA 19104; **Phone:** 215-662-6932; **Board Cert:** Internal Medicine 1983; Infectious Disease 1992; **Med School:** Dartmouth Med Sch 1980; **Resid:** Internal Medicine, Graduate Hosp 1983; **Fellow:** Infectious Disease, Hosp Univ Penn; **Fac Appt:** Assoc Prof Med, Univ Pennsylvania

Gumprecht, Jeffrey Paul MD [Inf] - **Spec Exp:** AIDS/HIV; Travel Medicine; Infections-Surgical; **Hospital:** Mount Sinai Med Ctr (page 64); **Address:** 1100 Park Ave, New York, NY 10128; **Phone:** 212-427-9550; **Board Cert:** Internal Medicine 1987; Infectious Disease 2003; **Med School:** Albany Med Coll 1983; **Resid:** Internal Medicine, Mount Sinai Hosp 1987; **Fellow:** Infectious Disease, Montefiore Med Ctr 1990; **Fac Appt:** Prof Med, Mount Sinai Sch Med

Infectious Disease

Hammer, Glenn MD [Inf] - **Spec Exp:** AIDS/HIV; Hospital Acquired Infections; Infections-Surgical; **Hospital:** Mount Sinai Med Ctr (page 64); **Address:** 1100 Park Ave, New York, NY 10128-1202; **Phone:** 212-427-9550; **Board Cert:** Infectious Disease 1974; Internal Medicine 1973; **Med School:** NYU Sch Med 1969; **Resid:** Internal Medicine, Mount Sinai Hosp 1972; **Fellow:** Infectious Disease, Mount Sinai Hosp 1974; **Fac Appt:** Asst Clin Prof Med, Mount Sinai Sch Med

Hammer, Scott M MD [Inf] - **Spec Exp:** AIDS/HIV; **Hospital:** NY-Presby Hosp/Columbia (page 66); **Address:** 622 W 168th St, PH Bldg - rm 876 West, New York, NY 10032; **Phone:** 212-305-7185; **Board Cert:** Internal Medicine 1975; Infectious Disease 1980; **Med School:** Columbia P&S 1972; **Resid:** Internal Medicine, Columbia-Presby Hosp 1975; Internal Medicine, Stanford Univ Hosp 1976; **Fellow:** Infectious Disease, Mass Genl Hosp 1981; **Fac Appt:** Prof Med, Columbia P&S

Hartman, Barry Jay MD [Inf] - **Spec Exp:** Endocarditis; Infections-Surgical; Parasitic Infections; **Hospital:** NY-Presby Hosp/Weill Cornell (page 66); **Address:** 407 E 70th St, Fl 4, New York, NY 10021-5302; **Phone:** 212-744-4882; **Board Cert:** Internal Medicine 1976; Infectious Disease 1980; **Med School:** Penn State Univ-Hershey Med Ctr 1973; **Resid:** Internal Medicine, New York Hosp /Cornell Med Ctr 1976; **Fellow:** Infectious Disease, New York Hosp/ Cornell Med Ctr 1981; **Fac Appt:** Clin Prof Med, Cornell Univ-Weill Med Coll

Louie, Eddie MD [Inf] - **Spec Exp:** Lyme Disease; AIDS/HIV; Hospital Acquired Infections; **Hospital:** NYU Med Ctr (page 68); **Address:** 345 E 37th St, New York, NY 10016-3256; **Phone:** 212-682-9202; **Board Cert:** Internal Medicine 1982; Infectious Disease 1986; **Med School:** NYU Sch Med 1979; **Resid:** Internal Medicine, Kings County Hosp 1983; **Fellow:** Infectious Disease, NYU Med Ctr 1985; **Fac Appt:** Assoc Clin Prof Med, NYU Sch Med

Masur, Henry MD [Inf] - **Spec Exp:** Critical Care; AIDS/HIV; **Hospital:** Natl Inst of Hlth - Clin Ctr; **Address:** National Institutes of Health, 10 Center Drive, Clinical Ctr 7D43, Bethesda, MD 20892; **Phone:** 301-496-9320; **Board Cert:** Internal Medicine 1975; Infectious Disease 1978; **Med School:** Cornell Univ-Weill Med Coll 1972; **Resid:** Internal Medicine, New York Hosp 1974; Internal Medicine, Johns Hopkins Hosp 1975; **Fellow:** Infectious Disease, New York Hosp-Cornell 1977

Mildvan, Donna MD [Inf] - **Spec Exp:** AIDS/HIV; Clinical Trials; **Hospital:** Beth Israel Med Ctr - Petrie Division (page 57); **Address:** Beth Israel Med Ctr, Div Infectious Dis, 1st Ave at 16th St, 19BH17, New York, NY 10003; **Phone:** 212-420-4005; **Board Cert:** Internal Medicine 1972; Infectious Disease 1972; **Med School:** Johns Hopkins Univ 1967; **Resid:** Internal Medicine, Mount Sinai Hosp 1970; **Fellow:** Infectious Disease, Mount Sinai Hosp 1972; **Fac Appt:** Prof Med, Albert Einstein Coll Med

Nahass, Ronald MD [Inf] - **Spec Exp:** Hepatitis B & C; Wound Healing/Care; Digestive Disorders; Bone Infections; **Hospital:** Robert Wood Johnson Univ Hosp - New Brunswick, Univ Med Ctr - Princeton; **Address:** 105 Raider Rd, Hillsborough, NJ 08844; **Phone:** 908-281-0221; **Board Cert:** Internal Medicine 1985; Infectious Disease 1988; **Med School:** UMDNJ-RW Johnson Med Sch 1982; **Resid:** Internal Medicine, RWJ Univ Hosp 1986; **Fellow:** Infectious Disease, RWJ Univ Hosp 1988; **Fac Appt:** Clin Prof Med, UMDNJ-RW Johnson Med Sch

Perlman, David MD [Inf] - **Spec Exp:** AIDS/HIV; Lyme Disease; Travel Medicine; Tuberculosis; **Hospital:** Beth Israel Med Ctr - Petrie Division (page 57), Lenox Hill Hosp (page 62); **Address:** Beth Israel Med Ctr, 1st Ave at 16th St, New York, NY 10003; **Phone:** 212-420-4470; **Board Cert:** Internal Medicine 1986; Infectious Disease 1988; **Med School:** Albert Einstein Coll Med 1983; **Resid:** Internal Medicine, New York Hosp/Meml Sloan Kettering 1986; **Fellow:** Infectious Disease, Montefiore Hosp 1988; **Fac Appt:** Prof Med, Albert Einstein Coll Med

Polsky, Bruce MD [Inf] - **Spec Exp:** AIDS/HIV; Viral Infections; Infections in Cancer Patients; AIDS Related Cancers; **Hospital:** St Luke's - Roosevelt Hosp Ctr - Roosevelt Div (page 57); **Address:** 1111 Amsterdam Ave, New York, NY 10025; **Phone:** 212-523-2525; **Board Cert:** Internal Medicine 1983; Infectious Disease 1986; **Med School:** Wayne State Univ 1980; **Resid:** Internal Medicine, Montefiore Hosp 1983; **Fellow:** Infectious Disease, Meml Sloan Kettering Cancer Ctr 1986; **Fac Appt:** Prof Med, Columbia P&S

Rahal, James MD [Inf] - **Spec Exp:** West Nile Virus; Antibiotic Resistance; Hospital Acquired Infections; **Hospital:** NY Hosp Queens; **Address:** NY Hosp Queens, Div Infectious Disease, 56-45 Main St, Flushing, NY 11355-5095; **Phone:** 718-670-1525; **Board Cert:** Internal Medicine 1967; Infectious Disease 1972; **Med School:** Tufts Univ 1959; **Resid:** Internal Medicine, Bellevue Hosp Ctr 1961; Internal Medicine, New England Ctr Hosp 1964; **Fellow:** Infectious Disease, New England Ctr Hosp 1965; **Fac Appt:** Prof Med, Cornell Univ-Weill Med Coll

Rao, Nalini G MD [Inf] - **Spec Exp:** Bone/Joint Infections; Tropical Diseases; Travel Medicine; **Hospital:** UPMC Presby, Pittsburgh, UPMC Shadyside; **Address:** Centre Commons, Suite 510, 5750 Centre Ave, Pittsburgh, PA 15206-3721; **Phone:** 412-661-1633; **Board Cert:** Internal Medicine 1975; Infectious Disease 1980; **Med School:** India 1970; **Resid:** Internal Medicine, Geo Wash Univ Hosp 1974; **Fellow:** Infectious Disease, Baylor Coll Med 1975; Infectious Disease, Univ Pittsburgh Sch Med 1977; **Fac Appt:** Clin Prof Med, Univ Pittsburgh

Sepkowitz, Kent MD [Inf] - **Spec Exp:** Tuberculosis; Infections in Cancer Patients; Fungal Infections; **Hospital:** Meml Sloan-Kettering Cancer Ctr; **Address:** 1275 York Avenue, New York, NY 10065; **Phone:** 800-525-2225; **Board Cert:** Internal Medicine 1983; Infectious Disease 2000; **Med School:** Univ Okla Coll Med 1980; **Resid:** Internal Medicine, Roosevelt Hosp 1984; **Fellow:** Infectious Disease, Meml Sloan Kettering Cancer Ctr 1991; **Fac Appt:** Prof Med, Cornell Univ-Weill Med Coll

Welch, Peter MD [Inf] - **Spec Exp:** Lyme Disease; Tick-borne Diseases; **Hospital:** Northern Westchester Hosp; **Address:** 16 Orchard Drive, Armonk, NY 10504; **Phone:** 914-273-3404; **Board Cert:** Internal Medicine 1977; Infectious Disease 1980; **Med School:** SUNY Buffalo 1974; **Resid:** Internal Medicine, New York Hosp 1977; **Fellow:** Infectious Disease, New York Hosp 1979

Wormser, Gary MD [Inf] - **Spec Exp:** Lyme Disease; AIDS/HIV; Diagnostic Problems; **Hospital:** Westchester Med Ctr; **Address:** New York Medical College, Munger Pavilion, rm 245, Valhalla, NY 10595; **Phone:** 914-493-8865; **Board Cert:** Internal Medicine 1978; Infectious Disease 1982; **Med School:** Johns Hopkins Univ 1972; **Resid:** Internal Medicine, Mount Sinai Hosp 1975; **Fellow:** Infectious Disease, Mount Sinai Hosp 1977; **Fac Appt:** Prof Med, NY Med Coll

Yancovitz, Stanley MD [Inf] - **Spec Exp:** Lyme Disease; AIDS/HIV; **Hospital:** Beth Israel Med Ctr - Petrie Division (page 57); **Address:** 1st Ave at 16th St, Ste 17 BH10, New York, NY 10003; **Phone:** 212-420-2600; **Board Cert:** Internal Medicine 1973; Infectious Disease 1976; **Med School:** SUNY Downstate 1967; **Resid:** Internal Medicine, Metropolitan Hosp 1969; Internal Medicine, Beth Israel Med Ctr 1972; **Fellow:** Infectious Disease, Mount Sinai Hosp 1975; **Fac Appt:** Assoc Prof Med, Albert Einstein Coll Med

Yu, Victor L MD [Inf] - **Spec Exp:** Legionnaire's Disease; Pneumonia; Staphylococcal Infections; **Hospital:** UPMC Presby, Pittsburgh; **Address:** University of Pittsburgh, 1401 Forbes Ave, Ste 209, Pittsburgh, PA 15219; **Phone:** 412-434-8484; **Board Cert:** Internal Medicine 1978; Infectious Disease 1982; **Med School:** Univ Minn 1970; **Resid:** Internal Medicine, Univ Colo Med Ctr 1972; Internal Medicine, Stanford Univ Med Ctr 1975; **Fellow:** Infectious Disease, Stanford Univ Med Ctr 1977; **Fac Appt:** Prof Med, Univ Pittsburgh

Infectious Disease

Southeast

Alvarez-Elcoro, Salvador MD [Inf] - **Spec Exp:** Tuberculosis; Travel Medicine; Infections-Transplant; **Hospital:** Mayo - Jacksonville; **Address:** Mayo Clinic, Div Infectious Disease, 4500 San Pablo Rd, Jacksonville, FL 32224; **Phone:** 904-953-2419; **Board Cert:** Internal Medicine 1977; Infectious Disease 1982; **Med School:** Mexico 1972; **Resid:** Internal Medicine, Charity Hosp 1977; **Fellow:** Infectious Disease, Boston City Hosp 1979; **Fac Appt:** Prof Med, Univ Fla Coll Med

Blumberg, Henry MD [Inf] - **Spec Exp:** Tuberculosis; **Hospital:** Grady Hlth Sys, Emory Univ Hosp; **Address:** Emory Univ, Div Infectious Diseases, 49 Jesse Hill Jr Drive, Atlanta, GA 30303; **Phone:** 404-616-6145; **Board Cert:** Internal Medicine 1986; Infectious Disease 2000; **Med School:** Vanderbilt Univ 1983; **Resid:** Internal Medicine, Emory Univ Affil Hosps 1986; Internal Medicine, Crawford-Long Hosp 1988; **Fellow:** Infectious Disease, Emory Univ Affil Hosps 1992; **Fac Appt:** Prof Med, Emory Univ

Cancio, Margarita MD [Inf] - **Spec Exp:** AIDS/HIV; **Hospital:** Tampa Genl Hosp; **Address:** 4 Columbia Dr, Ste 820, Tampa, FL 33606; **Phone:** 813-251-8444; **Board Cert:** Internal Medicine 1985; Infectious Disease 1988; **Med School:** Univ S Fla Coll Med 1982; **Resid:** Internal Medicine, Univ S Florida Affil Hosps 1985; **Fellow:** Infectious Disease, Univ S Florida Affil Hosps 1988; **Fac Appt:** Assoc Prof Med, Univ S Fla Coll Med

Chapman, Stanley W MD [Inf] - **Spec Exp:** Fungal Infections (Systemic Mycoses); **Hospital:** Univ Hosps & Clins - Jackson; **Address:** Univ Mississippi Med Ctr, Div Infectious Disease, 2500 N State St, Jackson, MS 39216; **Phone:** 601-984-5560; **Board Cert:** Internal Medicine 1975; Allergy & Immunology 1977; Infectious Disease 1980; **Med School:** Univ Rochester 1972; **Resid:** Internal Medicine, Emory Affil Hosps 1974; **Fellow:** Allergy & Immunology, NIAID-NIH 1977; Infectious Disease, Univ Rochester Med Ctr 1979; **Fac Appt:** Prof Med, Univ Miss

Cohen, Myron S MD [Inf] - **Spec Exp:** Infections in Immunocompromised Patients; **Hospital:** Univ NC Hosps; **Address:** UNC-Chapel Hill, Div Infectious Disease, 130 Mason Farm Rd, Ste 2115, Box CB 7030, Chapel Hill, NC 27599-7030; **Phone:** 919-843-5719; **Board Cert:** Internal Medicine 1977; Infectious Disease 1982; **Med School:** Rush Med Coll 1974; **Resid:** Internal Medicine, Univ Mich Hlth Ctr 1977; **Fellow:** Infectious Disease, Yale-New Haven Hosp 1979; **Fac Appt:** Prof Med, Univ NC Sch Med

Corey, G Ralph MD [Inf] - **Spec Exp:** Tropical Diseases; Travel Medicine; **Hospital:** Duke Univ Med Ctr; **Address:** 2400 Pratt St, rm 7021, Durham, NC 27710; **Phone:** 919-668-7174; **Board Cert:** Internal Medicine 1977; Infectious Disease 1980; **Med School:** Baylor Coll Med 1973; **Resid:** Internal Medicine, Duke Univ Med Ctr 1978; **Fellow:** Infectious Disease, Duke Univ Med Ctr 1980; **Fac Appt:** Prof Med, Duke Univ

Gorensek, Margaret J MD [Inf] - **Spec Exp:** AIDS/HIV; Infections-Transplant; Chronic Fatigue Syndrome; **Hospital:** Holy Cross Hosp - Fort Lauderdale, Broward General Med Ctr; **Address:** Holy Cross Medical Group, 1930 NE 47th St, Ste 104, Fort Lauderdale, FL 33308; **Phone:** 954-493-9752; **Board Cert:** Internal Medicine 1985; Pediatrics 1986; Infectious Disease 1988; Pediatric Infectious Disease 2002; **Med School:** Case West Res Univ 1981; **Resid:** Internal Medicine & Pediatrics, Cleveland Clinic Fdn 1985; **Fellow:** Infectious Disease, Cleveland Clinic Fdn 1987; Pediatric Infectious Disease, Chldns Med Ctr 1988; **Fac Appt:** Asst Clin Prof Med, Univ Miami Sch Med

Guerrant, Richard MD [Inf] - **Spec Exp:** Tropical Diseases; Infectious Diarrhea; Travel Medicine; **Hospital:** Univ Virginia Med Ctr; **Address:** Ctr Global Hlth, PO Box 801379, Charlottesville, VA 22908-1379; **Phone:** 434-924-5242; **Board Cert:** Infectious Disease 1976; Internal Medicine 1973; **Med School:** Univ VA Sch Med 1968; **Resid:** Internal Medicine, Boston City Hosp 1970; Internal Medicine, Univ Virginia Hosp 1973; **Fellow:** Infectious Disease, Johns Hopkins 1972; Infectious Disease, Univ Virginia Hosp 1974; **Fac Appt:** Prof Med, Univ VA Sch Med

Katner, Harold P MD [Inf] - **Spec Exp:** AIDS/HIV; **Hospital:** Med Ctr of Central GA; **Address:** Mercer Univ Sch Med, Dept Internal Med, 707 Pine St, Macon, GA 31201; **Phone:** 478-301-5809; **Board Cert:** Internal Medicine 1983; Infectious Disease 1986; **Med School:** Louisiana State U, New Orleans 1980; **Resid:** Internal Medicine, Univ Med Ctr 1983; **Fellow:** Infectious Disease, Ochsner Fdn Hosp 1986; **Fac Appt:** Prof Med, Mercer Univ Sch Med

Pearson, Richard D MD [Inf] - **Spec Exp:** Tropical Diseases; Travel Medicine; Infectious Disease; **Hospital:** Univ Virginia Med Ctr; **Address:** Univ VA Sch Med, Dept Internal Med, McKin Hall, Box 800739, Charlottesville, VA 22908-0001; **Phone:** 434-924-5579; **Board Cert:** Internal Medicine 1976; Infectious Disease 1980; **Med School:** Univ Mich Med Sch 1973; **Resid:** Internal Medicine, Strong Meml Hosp 1976; **Fellow:** Infectious Disease, Strong Meml Hosp-Univ Rochester 1979; **Fac Appt:** Prof Med, Univ VA Sch Med

Pegram, Paul S MD [Inf] - **Spec Exp:** AIDS/HIV; **Hospital:** Wake Forest Univ Baptist Med Ctr (page 73); **Address:** Wake Forest Baptist Med Ctr, Medical Ctr Blvd, ID Dept, Winston-Salem, NC 27157-1042; **Phone:** 336-716-2700; **Board Cert:** Infectious Disease 1978; Internal Medicine 1976; **Med School:** Wake Forest Univ 1970; **Resid:** Internal Medicine, NC Baptist Hosp 1975; **Fellow:** Infectious Disease, NC Baptist Hosp 1978; **Fac Appt:** Prof Med, Wake Forest Univ

Ratzan, Kenneth MD [Inf] - **Spec Exp:** AIDS/HIV; **Hospital:** Mount Sinai Med Ctr - Miami, Miami Heart Inst; **Address:** Mount Sinai Medical Ctr, 4300 Alton Rd, Ste 450, Miami Beach, FL 33140-2800; **Phone:** 305-673-5490; **Board Cert:** Internal Medicine 1977; Infectious Disease 1974; **Med School:** Harvard Med Sch 1965; **Resid:** Internal Medicine, Columbia Presby Med Ctr 1967; Infectious Disease, Tufts New England Med Ctr 1972; **Fellow:** Infectious Disease, Tufts New England Med Ctr 1971; **Fac Appt:** Prof Med, Univ Miami Sch Med

Saag, Michael S MD [Inf] - **Spec Exp:** AIDS/HIV; **Hospital:** Univ of Ala Hosp at Birmingham; **Address:** UAB Div Infectious Diseases, 845 19th St S, Birmingham, AL 35294-2170; **Phone:** 205-934-1917; **Board Cert:** Internal Medicine 1985; Infectious Disease 1988; **Med School:** Univ Louisville Sch Med 1981; **Resid:** Internal Medicine, Univ Ala Hosp 1984; **Fellow:** Infectious Disease, Univ Ala Hosp 1987

Scheld, William Michael MD [Inf] - **Spec Exp:** Meningitis; Septic Shock; AIDS/HIV; **Hospital:** Univ Virginia Med Ctr; **Address:** Univ VA Hlth Sci Ctr, PO Box 801342, Charlottesville, VA 22908; **Phone:** 434-924-5991; **Board Cert:** Internal Medicine 1976; Infectious Disease 1978; **Med School:** Cornell Univ-Weill Med Coll 1973; **Resid:** Internal Medicine, Univ VA Med Ctr 1976; **Fellow:** Infectious Disease, Univ VA Med Ctr 1979; **Fac Appt:** Prof Med, Univ VA Sch Med

van der Horst, Charles M MD [Inf] - **Spec Exp:** AIDS/HIV; Fungal Infections; Viral Infections; **Hospital:** Univ NC Hosps; **Address:** Univ NC-Dept Med, Box CB3368, Chapel Hill, NC 27599-0001; **Phone:** 919-843-4375; **Board Cert:** Internal Medicine 1982; Infectious Disease 1986; **Med School:** Harvard Med Sch 1979; **Resid:** Internal Medicine, Montefiore Hosp 1982; **Fellow:** Infectious Disease, NC Meml Hosp 1985; **Fac Appt:** Prof Med, Univ NC Sch Med

Wallace, Mark R MD [Inf] - **Spec Exp:** Fever in Returning Travelers; Travel Medicine; Valley Fever; **Hospital:** Orlando Regl Med Ctr; **Address:** 777 W Underwood, Ste 4B, Orlando, FL 32806; **Phone:** 321-841-7750; **Board Cert:** Internal Medicine 1984; Infectious Disease 2000; **Med School:** St Louis Univ 1981; **Resid:** Internal Medicine, Univ Washington Hosp 1984; **Fellow:** Infectious Disease, Naval Hosp 1989; **Fac Appt:** Prof Med, Uniformed Srvs Univ, Bethesda

Infectious Disease

Midwest

Bakken, Johan S MD/PhD [Inf] - **Spec Exp:** Human Granulocytic Anaplasmosis; Tick-borne Diseases; Antibiotic Resistance; Ehrlichiosis; **Hospital:** St Luke's Hosp - Duluth, St Mary's Med Ctr - Duluth; **Address:** 1001 E Superior St, Ste L201, Duluth, MN 55802; **Phone:** 218-249-7990; **Board Cert:** Internal Medicine 1999; **Med School:** Univ Wash 1972; **Resid:** Internal Medicine, Univ Wash Hosps 1978; Internal Medicine, Lillehammer Fylkessykehus 1981; **Fellow:** Infectious Disease, Ulleval Hosp 1985; Microbiology, Creighton Univ 1987; **Fac Appt:** Assoc Clin Prof FMed, Univ Minn

Campbell, J William MD [Inf] - **Spec Exp:** AIDS/HIV; **Hospital:** St Luke's Hosp - Chesterfield, MO, Barnes-Jewish Hosp; **Address:** 222 S Woods Mill Rd, Ste 750N, Chesterfield, MO 63017; **Phone:** 314-205-6600; **Board Cert:** Internal Medicine 1980; Infectious Disease 1982; **Med School:** Washington Univ, St Louis 1977; **Resid:** Internal Medicine, Barnes Hosp-Wash Univ 1980; **Fellow:** Infectious Disease, Univ Tex Hlth Sci Ctr 1981; Infectious Disease, Wash Univ 1982; **Fac Appt:** Clin Prof Med, Washington Univ, St Louis

Kazanjian Jr, Powel H MD [Inf] - **Spec Exp:** AIDS/HIV; **Hospital:** Univ Michigan Hlth Sys; **Address:** Infectious Disease Clin, TC Level 3, Reception D, 1500 E Med Ctr Drive, Ann Arbor, MI 48109-0999; **Phone:** 734-647-5899; **Board Cert:** Internal Medicine 1982; Infectious Disease 1986; **Med School:** Tufts Univ 1979; **Resid:** Internal Medicine, Univ Chicago Hosp 1982; **Fellow:** Infectious Disease, Brigham & Womens Hosp 1984; **Fac Appt:** Assoc Prof Med, Univ Mich Med Sch

Maki, Dennis G MD [Inf] - **Spec Exp:** Urinary Tract Infections; Critical Care; **Hospital:** Univ WI Hosp & Clins; **Address:** 600 Highland Ave, H4/572, Madison, WI 53792-5158; **Phone:** 608-263-0946; **Board Cert:** Internal Medicine 1972; Infectious Disease 1974; **Med School:** Univ Wisc 1967; **Resid:** Infectious Disease, Mass Genl Hosp 1972; Internal Medicine, Harvard-Boston City Hosp 1973; **Fellow:** Infectious Disease, Mass Genl Hosp 1974; **Fac Appt:** Prof Med, Univ Wisc

Slama, Thomas MD [Inf] - **Spec Exp:** Fungal Infections; Bone Infections; Infective Endocarditis; **Hospital:** St Vincent Hosp & Hlth Svcs - Indianapolis; **Address:** 8240 Naab Rd, Ste 300, Indianapolis, IN 46260; **Phone:** 317-870-1970; **Board Cert:** Internal Medicine 1976; Infectious Disease 1978; **Med School:** India 1973; **Resid:** Internal Medicine, Indianapolis Meth Hosp 1976; **Fellow:** Infectious Disease, Ohio State Univ Hosps 1978; **Fac Appt:** Clin Prof Med, Indiana Univ

Sobel, Jack MD [Inf] - **Spec Exp:** Vaginitis; Fungal Infections; Urinary Tract Infections; **Hospital:** Harper Univ Hosp, Detroit Receiving Hospital; **Address:** 3750 Woodward Ave, Ste 200, Detroit, MI 48201; **Phone:** 313-745-9035; **Board Cert:** Internal Medicine 1978; Infectious Disease 1982; **Med School:** South Africa 1965; **Resid:** Internal Medicine 1970; **Fellow:** Infectious Disease, Univ Penn Hosps 1977; Research, Natl Inst Hlth 1978; **Fac Appt:** Prof Med, Wayne State Univ

Trenholme, Gordon M MD [Inf] - **Spec Exp:** Fevers of Unknown Origin; Malaria; Tropical Diseases; **Hospital:** Rush Univ Med Ctr; **Address:** Rush Univ Med Ctr, Infectious Disease, 600 S Paulina St, Ste 143AAC, Chicago, IL 60612-3809; **Phone:** 312-942-3665; **Board Cert:** Internal Medicine 1972; Infectious Disease 1976; **Med School:** Med Coll Wisc 1970; **Resid:** Internal Medicine, Univ Chicago Hosp 1972; **Fellow:** Infectious Disease, Rush/Presby-St Luke's Med Ctr 1975; **Fac Appt:** Prof Med, Rush Med Coll

Wilson, Walter Ray MD [Inf] - **Spec Exp:** Musculoskeletal Infections; **Hospital:** Mayo Med Ctr & Clin - Rochester; **Address:** Mayo Clinic, Div Infectious Disease, 200 First St SW, Rochester, MN 55905; **Phone:** 507-255-7761; **Board Cert:** Internal Medicine 1973; Infectious Disease 1974; Medical Microbiology 1975; **Med School:** Baylor Coll Med 1967; **Resid:** Internal Medicine, Methodist Hosp 1968; Internal Medicine, Mayo Clinic 1973; **Fellow:** Infectious Disease, Mayo Clinic 1974; Microbiology, Mayo Clinic 1975; **Fac Appt:** Prof Med, Mayo Med Sch

Great Plains and Mountains

Cohn, David L MD [Inf] - **Spec Exp:** Tuberculosis; AIDS/HIV; **Hospital:** Denver Health Med Ctr; **Address:** Denver Public Health, 605 Bannock Street, Denver, CO 80204-4507; **Phone:** 303-602-8763; **Board Cert:** Internal Medicine 1978; Infectious Disease 1982; **Med School:** Univ IL Coll Med 1975; **Resid:** Internal Medicine, Univ Wisconsin Hosp 1978; **Fellow:** Infectious Disease, Univ Colorado Hosp 1981; **Fac Appt:** Prof Med, Univ Colorado

Freifeld, Alison G MD [Inf] - **Spec Exp:** Infectious Disease during Chemotherapy; Infections in Cancer Patients; **Address:** University of Nebraska, 985400 Nebraska Medical Center, Omaha, NE 68198-5400; **Phone:** 402-559-8650; **Board Cert:** Internal Medicine 1985; Infectious Disease 1988; **Med School:** Johns Hopkins Univ 1982; **Resid:** Internal Medicine, Johns Hopkins Univ Med Ctr 1985

Huitt, Gwen A MD [Inf] - **Spec Exp:** Tuberculosis; Cystic Fibrosis-Adult; Mycobacterial Infections; **Hospital:** Natl Jewish Med & Rsch Ctr; **Address:** Natl Jewish Med & Research Ctr, 1400 Jackson St, rm J222, Denver, CO 80206; **Phone:** 303-398-1700; **Board Cert:** Internal Medicine 2003; Infectious Disease 2004; **Med School:** Univ Colorado 1988; **Resid:** Internal Medicine, Univ Colorado Hlth Sci Ctr 1991; **Fellow:** Infectious Disease, Univ Colorado Hlth Sci Ctr 1993; **Fac Appt:** Assoc Prof Med, Univ Colorado

Southwest

DuPont, Herbert L MD [Inf] - **Spec Exp:** Tropical Diseases; Diarrheal Diseases; Travel Medicine; **Hospital:** St Luke's Episcopal Hosp - Houston; **Address:** 6720 Bertner Ave, MC 1-164, Houston, TX 77030-1602; **Phone:** 832-355-4122; **Board Cert:** Internal Medicine 1972; **Med School:** Emory Univ 1965; **Resid:** Internal Medicine, Univ Minn Hosps 1967; **Fellow:** Infectious Disease, Univ Maryland Hosp 1969; **Fac Appt:** Prof Med, Baylor Coll Med

Keiser, Philip MD [Inf] - **Spec Exp:** AIDS/HIV; **Hospital:** UT Southwestern Med Ctr - Dallas; **Address:** 1936 Amelia, Dallas, TX 75235-9173; **Phone:** 214-590-5647; **Board Cert:** Internal Medicine 1989; Infectious Disease 1992; **Med School:** Univ MD Sch Med 1986; **Resid:** Internal Medicine, Francis Scott Key Med Ctr 1989; **Fellow:** Infectious Disease, Univ Maryland 1989; **Fac Appt:** Assoc Prof Med, Univ Tex SW, Dallas

Luby, James P MD [Inf] - **Spec Exp:** Viral Infections; **Hospital:** Parkland Meml Hosp - Dallas, UT Southwestern Med Ctr - Dallas; **Address:** Univ Tex SW Med Ctr, Div Inf Dis, 5323 Harry Hines Blvd, Y7.218A, Dallas, TX 75390-9113; **Phone:** 214-648-3480; **Board Cert:** Internal Medicine 1968; Infectious Disease 1972; **Med School:** Northwestern Univ 1961; **Resid:** Internal Medicine, Northwestern Univ 1964; **Fac Appt:** Prof Med, Univ Tex SW, Dallas

Patterson, Jan E Evans MD [Inf] - **Spec Exp:** Hospital Acquired Infections; Antibiotic Resistance; **Hospital:** Univ Hlth Sys - Univ Hosp (San Antonio, TX); **Address:** Univ Tex Hlth Sci Ctr, Dept Med, 7703 Floyd Curl Drive, San Antonio, TX 78229-3900; **Phone:** 210-592-0340; **Board Cert:** Internal Medicine 1985; Infectious Disease 1988; **Med School:** Univ Tex, Houston 1982; **Resid:** Internal Medicine, Vanderbilt Univ Hosp 1985; **Fellow:** Infectious Disease, Yale-New Haven Hosp 1988; **Fac Appt:** Prof Med, Univ Tex, San Antonio

Patterson, Thomas F MD [Inf] - **Spec Exp:** Fungal Infections; **Hospital:** Univ Hlth Sys - Univ Hosp (San Antonio, TX); **Address:** Univ Texas HSC, Dept Medicine, Div Infectious Dis, 7703 Floyd Curl Drive, MC 7881, San Antonio, TX 78229-3900; **Phone:** 210-567-4823; **Board Cert:** Internal Medicine 1986; Infectious Disease 1988; **Med School:** Univ Tex, Houston 1983; **Resid:** Internal Medicine, Vanderbilt Univ Hosp 1985; Internal Medicine, Yale-New Haven Hosp 1986; **Fellow:** Infectious Disease, Yale-New Haven Hosp 1989; **Fac Appt:** Prof Med, Univ Tex, San Antonio

Infectious Disease

Wallace Jr, Richard James MD [Inf] - **Spec Exp:** Non Tuberculous Mycobacteria; Nocardia Infection; **Hospital:** UT Hlth Ctr at Tyler; **Address:** University of Texas Health Ctr, 11937 US Hwy 271, Tyler, TX 75708; **Phone:** 903-877-5122; **Board Cert:** Internal Medicine 1975; Infectious Disease 1976; **Med School:** Baylor Coll Med 1972; **Resid:** Internal Medicine, Boston City Hosp 1974; **Fellow:** Infectious Disease, Boston City Hosp 1975; Infectious Disease, Baylor Coll Med 1977

West Coast and Pacific

Ballon-Landa, Gonzalo MD [Inf] - **Spec Exp:** Hospital Acquired Infections; AIDS/HIV; Travel Medicine; **Hospital:** Scripps Mercy Hosp & Med Ctr; **Address:** 4136 Bachman Pl, San Diego, CA 92103; **Phone:** 619-298-1443; **Board Cert:** Internal Medicine 1980; Infectious Disease 1984; **Med School:** Northwestern Univ 1977; **Resid:** Internal Medicine, Evanston Hosp 1981; **Fellow:** Infectious Disease, UCSD Med Ctr 1983

Bayer, Arnold MD [Inf] - **Spec Exp:** Infective Endocarditis; Arthritis-Septic; Coccidioidomycosis; **Hospital:** LAC - Harbor - UCLA Med Ctr, Ronald Reagan UCLA Med Ctr; **Address:** 1124 W Carson St, RB2 Fl 2, Torrance, CA 90502; **Phone:** 310-222-3813; **Board Cert:** Internal Medicine 1973; Infectious Disease 1978; **Med School:** Temple Univ 1970; **Resid:** Internal Medicine, Thomas Jefferson Univ Hosp 1972; Internal Medicine, LAC-Harbor UCLA Med Ctr 1974; **Fellow:** Infectious Disease, VA Med Ctr 1976; Infectious Disease, LAC-Harbor UCLA Med Ctr 1977; **Fac Appt:** Prof Med, UCLA

Corey, Lawrence MD [Inf] - **Spec Exp:** Viral Infections; AIDS/HIV; **Hospital:** Univ Wash Med Ctr; **Address:** Fred Hutchinson Cancer Ctr, 1100 Fairview Ave N, Ste LE-500, Seattle, WA 98109; **Phone:** 206-667-6702; **Board Cert:** Internal Medicine 1974; **Med School:** Univ Mich Med Sch 1971; **Resid:** Internal Medicine, Univ Mich Med Ctr 1973; **Fellow:** Infectious Disease, Univ Wash Hosp 1977; **Fac Appt:** Prof Med, Univ Wash

Daar, Eric S MD [Inf] - **Spec Exp:** AIDS/HIV; Infectious Disease; **Hospital:** LAC - Harbor - UCLA Med Ctr; **Address:** 1000 W Carson St, Box 449, Torrance, CA 90502; **Phone:** 310-222-2467; **Board Cert:** Internal Medicine 1988; **Med School:** Georgetown Univ 1985; **Resid:** Internal Medicine, Cedars-Sinai Med Ctr 1988; **Fellow:** Infectious Disease, Cedars-Sinai Med Ctr 1991

Edwards Jr, John Ellis MD [Inf] - **Spec Exp:** Fungal Infections; Infections in Immunocompromised Patients; **Hospital:** LAC - Harbor - UCLA Med Ctr; **Address:** 1124 W Carson St, RB2 Fl 2, Torrance, CA 90502; **Phone:** 310-222-3813; **Board Cert:** Internal Medicine 1980; Infectious Disease 1974; **Med School:** UC Irvine 1968; **Resid:** Internal Medicine, Harbor-UCLA Med Ctr 1971; **Fellow:** Infectious Disease, Harbor-UCLA Med Ctr 1973; **Fac Appt:** Prof Med, UCLA

Holmes, King K MD [Inf] - **Spec Exp:** AIDS/HIV; Sexually Transmitted Diseases; **Hospital:** Harborview Med Ctr; **Address:** Harborview Med Ctr, 325 Ninth Ave, Box 359931, Seattle, WA 98104; **Phone:** 206-744-4239; **Board Cert:** Internal Medicine 1971; Infectious Disease 1974; **Med School:** Cornell Univ-Weill Med Coll 1963; **Resid:** Internal Medicine, Univ Wash Med Ctr 1969; **Fellow:** Infectious Disease, Univ Wash Med Ctr 1970; **Fac Appt:** Prof Med, Univ Wash

Palefsky, Joel M MD [Inf] - **Spec Exp:** AIDS Related Cancers; **Hospital:** UCSF - Mt Zion Med Ctr; **Address:** UCSF Med Ctr, Infectious Disease, 505 Parnassus Ave, rm M1203, San Francisco, CA 94143-0126; **Phone:** 415-476-1574; **Board Cert:** Internal Medicine 1984; Infectious Disease 1988; **Med School:** McGill Univ 1980; **Resid:** Internal Medicine, Royal Victoria Hosp 1984; **Fellow:** Infectious Disease, Stanford Univ 1989

Richman, Douglas MD [Inf] - **Spec Exp:** AIDS/HIV; **Hospital:** VA San Diego Hlthcre Sys, UCSD Med Ctr; **Address:** UCSD-Stein Clin Rsch Bldg, 9500 Gilman, MC 0679, La Jolla, CA 92093-0679; **Phone:** 858-552-7439; **Board Cert:** Internal Medicine 1973; Infectious Disease 1976; **Med School:** Stanford Univ 1970; **Resid:** Internal Medicine, Stanford Univ Hosp 1972; **Fellow:** Infectious Disease, NIAID/NIH 1975; Infectious Disease, Beth Israel/Chldns Hosp-Harvard 1976; **Fac Appt:** Prof Med, UCSD

Schooley, Robert T MD [Inf] - **Spec Exp:** AIDS/HIV; Infectious Disease; **Hospital:** UCSD Med Ctr; **Address:** UCSD - Stein Rsch Bldg, rm 401, MC 071, 9500 Gilman Drive, La Jolla, CA 92023-0665; **Phone:** 858-822-0216; **Board Cert:** Internal Medicine 1977; **Med School:** Johns Hopkins Univ 1974; **Resid:** Internal Medicine, Johns Hopkins Hosp 1976; **Fellow:** Infectious Disease, Natl Inst Hlth 1979; Infectious Disease, Mass Genl Hosp 1981; **Fac Appt:** Prof Med, UCSD

Wiviott, Lory David MD [Inf] - **Spec Exp:** AIDS/HIV; **Hospital:** CA Pacific Med Ctr - Pacific Campus, CA Pacific Med Ctr - Davies Campus; **Address:** 2100 Webster St, Ste 400, San Francisco, CA 94115; **Phone:** 415-923-3883; **Board Cert:** Internal Medicine 1986; Infectious Disease 2000; **Med School:** Albert Einstein Coll Med 1982; **Resid:** Internal Medicine, Columbia Presby Med Ctr 1985; **Fellow:** Infectious Disease, UCSF Med Ctr 1989; **Fac Appt:** Asst Clin Prof Med, UCSF

Yoshikawa, Thomas T MD [Inf] - **Spec Exp:** Infections in the Elderly; **Hospital:** VA Med Ctr - W Los Angeles; **Address:** 11301 Wilshire Blvd, Los Angeles, CA 90073; **Phone:** 310-478-3711; **Board Cert:** Internal Medicine 1971; Infectious Disease 1974; **Med School:** Univ Mich Med Sch 1966; **Resid:** Internal Medicine, Harbor Genl Hosp 1970; **Fellow:** Infectious Disease, Harbor Genl Hosp 1972; **Fac Appt:** Prof Med, Charles Drew Univ Med & Sci

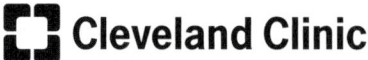
Cleveland Clinic

Infectious Disease

The mission of the Cleveland Clinic Department of Infectious Disease is to provide all patients with the most technologically advanced, compassionate medical care available anywhere. We diagnose and treat patients with a wide range of both opportunistic and acquired infections. The department is an integral part of Cleveland Clinic, a not-for-profit multispecialty academic medical center ranked by *U.S.News* & *World Report* as one of the nation's best hospitals.

We provide around-the-clock inpatient care, including three general infectious disease consultation services as well as dedicated solid organ transplant, bone marrow transplant, cardiothoracic intensive care and medical/surgical intensive infectious disease services. The department also operates several specialty outpatient clinics. Both services are designed to provide patients with optimal care, while supporting research and education initiatives. The department's outpatient subspecialty clinics include:

Granuloma Clinic: Granulomas are tumor-like masses often caused by tissue infections. One of the most common types of infections that cause granulomatous disease in Northeast Ohio is histoplasmosis. Granulomas are non-cancerous, but many types require special care because they can spread from person to person. Tuberculosis is an example of a contagious and potentially fatal granuloma. Other conditions treated by Cleveland Clinic's Granuloma Clinic include coccidoidmycosis, cyptococcosis and mycobacterial avium-intracellulare complex.

Endocarditis Clinic: Endocarditis is an inflammation of the endocardium, or the inner lining of the heart and the heart valves. The disease is most commonly caused by a bacterial pathogen but can be due to fungal pathogens as well. Major symptoms of bacterial endocarditis include fever, fatigue, heart murmur, enlarged spleen and areas of tissue death. In addition to bacterial endocarditis, Cleveland Clinic's Endocarditis Clinic also treats infections of the endocardium caused by cardiac devices, grafts or implants.

HIV/AIDS Clinic: This specialty clinic provides care and support for patients infected with the human immunodeficiency virus, or HIV. This virus attacks the immune system, weakening a person's ability to fight infections and cancer.

International Traveler's Health Clinic: This specialty clinic provides pre-travel health and safety advice to anyone planning to journey abroad. All vaccinations and prescription medications necessary to facilitate safe travel are administered or prescribed. The International Traveler's Health Clinic also provides a comprehensive itinerary review, developing individualized packets of information for every client. Post-travel evaluation is available as needed.

Outpatient Parenteral Antimicrobial Therapy Program: This program works with patients receiving intravenous treatments for serious infections while living at home or outside a hospital setting. We play an integral role in the managing this program, which has one of the highest volumes of any center in the United States.

The Bone and Joint Infection Program: This service at Cleveland Clinic employs a multi-disciplinary team approach in the inpatient and outpatient settings for diagnosis, management, and prevention of infections of the musculoskeletal system. Infectious Disease specialists and orthopaedic surgeons work hand in hand with colleagues in microbiology, pathology, pharmacy, and infection control to treat complex infections such as prosthetic joint infections and osteomyelitis.

For more information about the Cleveland Clinic Department of Infectious Disease, to schedule a second opinion or to learn about assistance for out-of-town patients, call 800.890.2467 or visit www.clevelandclinic.org/infectioustopdocs.

Department of Infectious Disease | 9500 Euclid Avenue / AC311 | Cleveland OH 44195

NYU Langone Medical Center

550 First Avenue (at 31St Street)
New York, NY 10016
Physician Referral:
(888)7-NYU-MED (888-769-8633)
www.nyumc.org

INFECTIOUS DISEASES

Developing effective treatment for infectious diseases is among the miracles of last century's science, but today we are faced with deadly new infections and old ones that were never tamed. These and the rapidly emerging problem of resistance to antibiotics place the study and treatment of infectious diseases (ID) at the forefront of modern medicine.

NYU's ID doctors are actively engaged in research at the laboratory bench and in clinical trials of new antibiotics and other anti-infective strategies.

- A novel program, Population Biology of Infectious Diseases, combines these laboratory and clinical studies with epidemiology and genetics
- The NYU AIDS Clinical Trials Unit is one of the most productive among the 35 such centers nationally. Supported by the National Institutes of Health the NYU unit has played a leading role in drug development and delivering the very latest care to patients with this increasingly controllable infection.
- NYU doctors are deeply involved in local and international research into the early diagnosis, treatment and prevention of such chronic infections as tuberculosis and Helicobacrer (the bacteria associated with stomach ulcers).
- Using lessons learned in their research, NYU ID doctors are actively involved in management of complicated bone and joint infections, prevention of infection in cancer and transplant patients, and developing strategies for managing hepatitis B and C.
- NYU's Department of Medical and Molecular Parasitology, working alongside the Division of Infectious Diseases, is active internationally in bringing malaria and other parasitic diseases under control.

NYU Langone Medical Center

The AIDS Clinical Trial Unit is on of 35 such units designated and supported by the National Institute of Allergy and Infectious Diseases. The NYU Clinical Trials Unit is one of the most productive in the nations and enrolls adult and pediatric patients in clinical trials supported by both the NIH and pharmaceutical companies. The data from the NYU AIDS Clincal Trials Unit have supported the licensing of several drugs and play and essential role in defining optimal therapies, in optimizing, monitoring, and preventing complications.

Internal Medicine

A personal physician who provides long-term, comprehensive care in the office and the hospital, managing both common and complex illness of adolescents, adults and the elderly. Internists are trained in the diagnosis and treatment of cancer, infections and diseases affecting the heart, blood, kidneys, joints and digestive, respiratory and vascular systems. They are also trained in the essentials of primary care internal medicine which incorporates an understanding of disease prevention, wellness, substance abuse, mental health and effective treatment of common problems of the eyes, ears, skin, nervous system and reproductive organs.

Note: *Internal Medicine normally includes many primary care physicians. However, for purposes of this directory, no primary care physicians are included.*

Training Required: Three years

INTERNAL MEDICINE

New England

Barry, Michele MD [IM] - **Spec Exp:** Travel Medicine; Tropical Diseases; **Hospital:** Yale-New Haven Hosp; **Address:** 333 Cedar St, PO Box 208025, New Haven, CT 06520-8025; **Phone:** 203-688-2476; **Board Cert:** Internal Medicine 1980; **Med School:** Albert Einstein Coll Med 1977; **Resid:** Internal Medicine, Yale-New Haven Hosp 1981; **Fellow:** Rheumatology, Yale-New Haven Hosp 1981; Tropical Medicine, Walter Reed AMC 1981; **Fac Appt:** Prof Med, Yale Univ

Mid Atlantic

Braunstein, Seth N MD/PhD [IM] - **Spec Exp:** Diabetes; **Hospital:** Hosp Univ Penn - UPHS (page 60); **Address:** Hosp of Univ Penn, Diabetes Ctr, 3400 Spruce St, 4 Penn Tower, Philadelphia, PA 19104-4219; **Phone:** 215-662-2468; **Board Cert:** Internal Medicine 1975; **Med School:** NYU Sch Med 1972; **Resid:** Internal Medicine, Hosp U Penn 1975; **Fac Appt:** Assoc Prof Med, Univ Pennsylvania

Cirigliano, Michael D MD [IM] - **Spec Exp:** Complementary Medicine; Women's Health; **Hospital:** Hosp Univ Penn - UPHS (page 60); **Address:** Penn Internal Med Practice, UPHS, 3701 Market St, Ste 760, Philadelphia, PA 19104; **Phone:** 215-615-0878; **Board Cert:** Internal Medicine 2005; **Med School:** Univ Pennsylvania 1990; **Resid:** Internal Medicine, Hosp U Penn 1993; **Fac Appt:** Assoc Prof Med, Univ Pennsylvania

Galland, Leo MD [IM] - **Spec Exp:** Nutrition; Chronic Illness; Complementary Medicine; **Address:** 156 5th Ave, Ste 820, New York, NY 10010; **Phone:** 212-989-6733; **Board Cert:** Internal Medicine 1972; **Med School:** NYU Sch Med 1968; **Resid:** Internal Medicine, Bellevue Hosp 1972; **Fellow:** Behavioral Medicine, Univ Conn Hlth Ctr 1981

Legato, Marianne J MD [IM] - **Spec Exp:** Cardiovascular Disease; Women's Health; Gender Specific Medicine; **Hospital:** NY-Presby Hosp/Columbia (page 66), St Luke's - Roosevelt Hosp Ctr - Roosevelt Div (page 57); **Address:** 962 Park Ave, New York, NY 10028-2433; **Phone:** 212-737-5663; **Board Cert:** Internal Medicine 2003; **Med School:** NYU Sch Med 1962; **Resid:** Internal Medicine, Columbia-Presby Med Ctr 1965; **Fellow:** Cardiovascular Disease, Columbia-Presby Med Ctr 1968; **Fac Appt:** Prof Emeritus Med, Columbia P&S

Lewin, Neal MD [IM] - **Spec Exp:** Headache; Preventive Medicine; Toxicology; **Hospital:** NYU Med Ctr (page 68); **Address:** 120 E 36th St, Ste 1B, New York, NY 10016-3426; **Phone:** 212-889-2813; **Board Cert:** Internal Medicine 1977; Emergency Medicine 2002; Medical Toxicology 1983; **Med School:** SUNY Downstate 1974; **Resid:** Internal Medicine, NYU-Bellevue Hosp 1977; **Fac Appt:** Prof Med, NYU Sch Med

Rader, Daniel J MD [IM] - **Spec Exp:** Cholesterol/Lipid Disorders; Preventive Cardiology; Metabolic Disorders; **Hospital:** Hosp Univ Penn - UPHS (page 60), Penn Presby Med Ctr - UPHS (page 60); **Address:** Univ Penn-UPHS, 52 N 39th St, PHI Bldg - Ste 2A, Philadelphia, PA 19104; **Phone:** 215-662-9993; **Board Cert:** Internal Medicine 1987; **Med School:** Med Coll PA Hahnemann 1984; **Resid:** Internal Medicine, Yale-New Haven Hosp 1987; **Fellow:** Research, Natl Inst Hlth 1992; **Fac Appt:** Prof Med, Univ Pennsylvania

Rivlin, Richard S MD [IM] - **Spec Exp:** Nutrition; Nutrition & Cancer Prevention/Control; Endocrinology & Thyroid Disease; **Hospital:** NY-Presby Hosp/Weill Cornell (page 66); **Address:** Director, Anne Fisher Nutrition Ctr, Strang Cancer Research Lab, 428 E 72nd St, Ste 600, New York, NY 10021; **Phone:** 212-794-4900 x152; **Board Cert:** Internal Medicine 1969; **Med School:** Harvard Med Sch 1959; **Resid:** Internal Medicine, Johns Hopkins Hosp 1961; Internal Medicine, Johns Hopkins Hosp 1964; **Fellow:** Endocrinology, Diabetes & Metabolism, Natl Inst Hlth 1963; Biochemistry, Johns Hopkins Hosp 1966; **Fac Appt:** Prof Med, Cornell Univ-Weill Med Coll

Selwyn, Peter MD [IM] - **Spec Exp:** AIDS/HIV; Addiction/Substance Abuse; Palliative Care; **Hospital:** Montefiore Med Ctr; **Address:** Montfiore Med Ctr, 3544 Jerome Ave, Bronx, NY 10467; **Phone:** 718-920-4678; **Board Cert:** Family Medicine 2005; **Med School:** Harvard Med Sch 1981; **Resid:** Family Medicine, Montefiore Med Ctr 1984; **Fac Appt:** Prof Med, Albert Einstein Coll Med

Yaffe, Bruce MD [IM] - **Spec Exp:** Gastroscopy; Colonoscopy; **Hospital:** Lenox Hill Hosp (page 62); **Address:** 201 E 65th St, New York, NY 10021-6701; **Phone:** 212-879-4700; **Board Cert:** Internal Medicine 1979; Gastroenterology 1981; **Med School:** Geo Wash Univ 1976; **Resid:** Internal Medicine, Mount Sinai Hosp 1979; Hepatology, Mount Sinai Hosp 1980; **Fellow:** Gastroenterology, Lenox Hill Hosp 1982

Southeast

Bouldin IV, Marshall J MD [IM] - **Spec Exp:** Diabetes; **Hospital:** Univ Hosps & Clins - Jackson; **Address:** Univ Mississippi Med Ctr, Medicine, 2500 North State St, Annexe 2, rm 155, Jackson, MS 39216; **Phone:** 601-815-1961; **Board Cert:** Internal Medicine 2001; **Med School:** Johns Hopkins Univ 1988; **Resid:** Internal Medicine, Univ Virginia Med Ctr 1991; **Fac Appt:** Assoc Prof Med, Univ Miss

Cushman, William C MD [IM] - **Spec Exp:** Hypertension; Preventive Cardiology; Cholesterol/Lipid Disorders; **Hospital:** VA Med Ctr - Memphis; **Address:** VA Medical Ctr, 1030 Jefferson Ave, MC 111Q, Memphis, TN 38104-2127; **Phone:** 901-523-8990 x6605; **Board Cert:** Internal Medicine 1977; **Med School:** Univ Miss 1974; **Resid:** Internal Medicine, Univ Mississippi Med Ctr 1977; **Fac Appt:** Prof Med, Univ Tenn Coll Med, Memphis

Heimburger, Douglas C MD [IM] - **Spec Exp:** Nutrition & Disease Prevention/Control; Nutrition & Cancer Prevention; **Hospital:** Univ of Ala Hosp at Birmingham, VA Med Ctr; **Address:** Univ Alabama, Dept Nutrition Sci & Med, 1675 University Blvd, Webb 439, Birmingham, AL 35294-3360; **Phone:** 205-996-5400; **Board Cert:** Internal Medicine 1981; **Med School:** Vanderbilt Univ 1978; **Resid:** Internal Medicine, Washington Univ Hosps 1981; **Fellow:** Nutrition, Univ Alabama Med Ctr 1982

Midwest

Weder, Alan B MD [IM] - **Spec Exp:** Hypertension; Renovascular Disease; Peripheral Vascular Disease; Carotid Artery Disease; **Hospital:** Univ Michigan Hlth Sys; **Address:** Univ Mich, Div Cardiovascular Med, 24 Frank Lloyd Wright Drive, Box 322, Ann Arbor, MI 48106-0739; **Phone:** 734-998-7956; **Board Cert:** Internal Medicine 1978; **Med School:** Hahnemann Univ 1975; **Resid:** Internal Medicine, Univ Chicago Hosps 1978; **Fac Appt:** Prof Med, Univ Mich Med Sch

Internal Medicine

Wright Jr, Jackson T MD/PhD [IM] - **Spec Exp:** Hypertension; **Hospital:** Univ Hosps Case Med Ctr; **Address:** CWRU Div Hypertension, 11100 Euclid Ave, Bolwell Bldg - rm 2200, Cleveland, OH 44106; **Phone:** 216-844-5174; **Board Cert:** Internal Medicine 1980; **Med School:** Univ Pittsburgh 1976; **Resid:** Internal Medicine, Univ Michigan Hosps 1987; **Fellow:** Pharmacology, Univ Health Ctr 1980; **Fac Appt:** Prof Med, Case West Res Univ

Great Plains and Mountains

Mehler, Philip S MD [IM] - **Spec Exp:** Eating Disorders; Substance Abuse; Preventive Medicine; **Hospital:** Denver Health Med Ctr; **Address:** Denver Health Med Ctr, 777 Bannock St, MC 0278, Denver, CO 80204; **Phone:** 303-436-3234; **Board Cert:** Internal Medicine 1989; **Med School:** Univ Colorado 1983; **Resid:** Internal Medicine, Univ Colorado Affil Hosp 1987; **Fac Appt:** Prof Med, Univ Colorado

Southwest

Witte, Marlys H MD [IM] - **Spec Exp:** Lymphedema; **Hospital:** Univ Med Ctr - Tucson; **Address:** Univ Arizona Hlth Scis Ctr, 1501 N Campbell Ave, rm 4406, Box 245200, Tucson, AZ 85724-5063; **Phone:** 520-626-6118; **Board Cert:** Internal Medicine 1967; **Med School:** NYU Sch Med 1960; **Resid:** Internal Medicine, Bellevue Hosp 1963; **Fellow:** Internal Medicine, NYU Med Ctr 1966; **Fac Appt:** Prof S, Univ Ariz Coll Med

Wolff, Robert A MD [IM] - **Spec Exp:** Gastrointestinal Cancer; Pancreatic Cancer; Colon & Rectal Cancer; Clinical Trials; **Hospital:** UT MD Anderson Cancer Ctr; **Address:** MD Anderson Cancer Ctr, Faculty Center Unit 421, Box 301402, Houston, TX 77230; **Phone:** 713-745-5476; **Board Cert:** Internal Medicine 1989; **Med School:** Albany Med Coll 1986; **Resid:** Internal Medicine, Duke Univ Med Ctr 1989; **Fellow:** Hematology & Oncology, Duke Univ Med Ctr 1992

West Coast and Pacific

Bissell Jr, Dwight M MD [IM] - **Spec Exp:** Porphyria; **Hospital:** UCSF Med Ctr; **Address:** UCSF Med Ctr, Dept Gastroenterology, 350 Parnassus Ave, Ste 410, San Francisco, CA 94117; **Phone:** 415-353-2318; **Board Cert:** Internal Medicine 1974; **Med School:** Harvard Med Sch 1967; **Resid:** Internal Medicine, Boston City Hosp-Harvard 1970; **Fellow:** Gastroenterology, UCSF Med Ctr 1973; **Fac Appt:** Prof Med, UCSF

INTERNAL MEDICINE

NYU Langone Medical Center

Famous equally for cutting-edge research and for nurturing lifelong physician-patient relationships, the Internal Medicine physicians of NYU are dedicated to treating the whole patient. NYU internists meet the highest standards of the medical profession, addressing physical, social, and psychological aspects of health and disease. Here, experts in very specialized areas of medicine provide state-of-the-art care that brings the latest developments from the laboratory to the care of patients with rare or difficult diseases. In addition, the Division of General Medicine attracts internists whose passion is the care of patients with multiple problems and who specialize in keeping people healthy. The research interests of our doctors span molecular biology, and the social aspects of medicine such as epidemiology and behavioral medicine that guide good clinical decision-making. These and other skills are actively brought to the service of patient care every day.

Below are just a few of the many services offered by the NYU team:

- Primary health care, including physical examinations.
- Specialized care of illnesses involving the heart, lungs gastrointestinal tract, joints, bones, muscles, endocrine organs, and kidneys.
- Comprehensive women's health care, from obstetric and gynecologic needs to osteoporosis prevention and treatment.
- Geriatric care by experts with special interest and training in the particular circumstances of older people
- A wide range of laboratory, imaging, and advanced diagnostic testing from something as simple as a throat culture to complex mapping of the electrical surface of the heart.
- Guidance and treatment for substance abuse, eating disorders and obesity, and high cholesterol.

The physicians of the Division of Internal Medicine at NYU Langone Medical Center treat the full spectrum of conditions, from addiction to rheumatoid arthritis, in an environment that is steeped in NYU's tradition of excellence and a dedication to state-of-the-art patient care and research.
This application of world-class science to bedside medicine is enhanced by interdisciplinary collaboration between departments and physicians, demonstrative of NYU Langone Medical Center's professionalism and dedication to teamwork and collegiality.

Maternal & Fetal Medicine
a subspecialty of Obstetrics & Gynecology

An obstetrician/gynecologist possesses special knowledge, skills and professional capability in the medical and surgical care of the female reproductive system and associated disorders. This physician serves as a consultant to other physicians and as a primary physician for women.

Training Required: Four years *plus* two years in clinical practice before certification in obstetrics and gynecology is complete *plus* additional training and examination in maternal-fetal medicine.

MATERNAL & FETAL MEDICINE

New England

Acker, David B MD [MF] - **Spec Exp:** Multiple Gestation; Pregnancy-High Risk; **Hospital:** Brigham & Women's Hosp; **Address:** Brigham & Womens Hosp, Dept Ob/Gyn, 75 Francis St, ASB1-3, Boston, MA 02115-6110; **Phone:** 617-732-5445; **Board Cert:** Obstetrics & Gynecology 2005; Maternal & Fetal Medicine 2005; **Med School:** NYU Sch Med 1968; **Resid:** Obstetrics & Gynecology, Einstein Affil Hosp 1971; Obstetrics & Gynecology, Vanderbilt Univ Affil Hosp 1974; **Fellow:** Maternal & Fetal Medicine, Boston Lying-In Hosp 1979; **Fac Appt:** Assoc Prof ObG, Harvard Med Sch

Baker, Emily MD [MF] - **Spec Exp:** Ultrasound; **Hospital:** Dartmouth - Hitchcock Med Ctr; **Address:** Dartmouth-Hitchcock Med Ctr, Dept Ob/Gyn, One Medical Center Drive, Desk 5L, Lebanon, NH 03756; **Phone:** 603-653-9306; **Board Cert:** Obstetrics & Gynecology 2003; Maternal & Fetal Medicine 2003; **Med School:** Stanford Univ 1986; **Resid:** Obstetrics & Gynecology, Univ Chicago Hosps 1990; Maternal & Fetal Medicine, Univ Washington Med Ctr 1991; **Fellow:** Maternal & Fetal Medicine, St Margaret's Hosp-Tufts Univ 1992; **Fac Appt:** Assoc Prof ObG, Dartmouth Med Sch

Carr, Stephen R MD [MF] - **Spec Exp:** Twin to Twin Transfusion Syndrome (TTTS); Multiple Gestation; Fetal Surgery; **Hospital:** Women & Infants Hosp of RI; **Address:** Women & Infants Hosp, Div Mat-Fet Med, 101 Dudley St, Providence, RI 02903; **Phone:** 401-274-1122; **Board Cert:** Obstetrics & Gynecology 2000; Maternal & Fetal Medicine 1998; **Med School:** Univ Hawaii JA Burns Sch Med 1982; **Resid:** Obstetrics & Gynecology, Univ Illinois Med Ctr 1986; **Fellow:** Maternal & Fetal Medicine, Brown Univ 1988; **Fac Appt:** Assoc Prof ObG, Brown Univ

Copel, Joshua A MD [MF] - **Spec Exp:** Prenatal Diagnosis; Fetal Echocardiography; Pregnancy-High Risk; Fetal Diagnosis & Therapy; **Hospital:** Yale-New Haven Hosp; **Address:** Yale Univ Sch Med, Dept OB/GYN, 333 Cedar St, Box 208063, New Haven, CT 06520-3206; **Phone:** 203-785-5682; **Board Cert:** Obstetrics & Gynecology 2006; Maternal & Fetal Medicine 2006; **Med School:** Tufts Univ 1979; **Resid:** Obstetrics & Gynecology, Pennsylvania Hosp 1983; **Fellow:** Maternal & Fetal Medicine, Yale-New Haven Hosp 1985; **Fac Appt:** Prof ObG, Yale Univ

Greene, Michael F MD [MF] - **Spec Exp:** Pregnancy-High Risk; Multiple Gestation; Seizure Disorders & Pregnancy; **Hospital:** Mass Genl Hosp; **Address:** Mass Genl Hosp, Dept Ob/Gyn, 32 Fruit St Yawkey Bldg - rm 4F, Boston, MA 02114; **Phone:** 617-724-2229; **Board Cert:** Obstetrics & Gynecology 2007; Maternal & Fetal Medicine 2007; **Med School:** SUNY Downstate 1976; **Resid:** Obstetrics & Gynecology, Boston Hosp Women 1980; **Fellow:** Maternal & Fetal Medicine, Brigham Hosp Women 1982; **Fac Appt:** Prof ObG, Harvard Med Sch

Heffner, Linda MD/PhD [MF] - **Spec Exp:** Pregnancy-Advanced Maternal Age; Pregnancy-High Risk; **Hospital:** Boston Med Ctr; **Address:** 85 E Concord St Fl 6, Boston, MA 02118; **Phone:** 617-414-5175; **Board Cert:** Obstetrics & Gynecology 1998; Maternal & Fetal Medicine 1998; **Med School:** Johns Hopkins Univ 1977; **Resid:** Obstetrics & Gynecology, Hosp Univ Penn 1983; **Fellow:** Maternal & Fetal Medicine, Brigham-Womens Hosp 1987; **Fac Appt:** Prof ObG, Boston Univ

Lockwood, Charles MD [MF] - **Spec Exp:** Prematurity Prevention; Miscarriage-Recurrent; Multiple Gestation; **Hospital:** Yale-New Haven Hosp; **Address:** Yale Univ Sch Med, Dept Ob-Gyn, 333 Cedar St, rm FMB 335, New Haven, CT 06520-8063; **Phone:** 203-737-2970; **Board Cert:** Obstetrics & Gynecology 1997; Maternal & Fetal Medicine 1997; **Med School:** Univ Pennsylvania 1981; **Resid:** Obstetrics & Gynecology, Pennsylvania Hosp 1985; **Fellow:** Maternal & Fetal Medicine, Yale-New Haven Hosp 1987; Thrombosis, Mt Sinai Med Ctr 1991; **Fac Appt:** Prof ObG, Yale Univ

Paidas, Michael J MD [MF] - **Spec Exp:** Pregnancy-High Risk; Clotting Disorders in Pregnancy; Miscarriage-Recurrent; **Hospital:** Yale-New Haven Hosp; **Address:** Dept Ob/Gyn & Reproductive Scis, Yale-New Haven Hosp, 333 Cedar St, FMB 308, New Haven, CT 06520-8063; **Phone:** 203-785-5682; **Board Cert:** Obstetrics & Gynecology 2005; Maternal & Fetal Medicine 2005; **Med School:** Tufts Univ 1987; **Resid:** Obstetrics & Gynecology, Pennsylvania Hosp 1991; **Fellow:** Maternal & Fetal Medicine, Mount Sinai Med Ctr 1993; **Fac Appt:** Assoc Prof ObG, Yale Univ

Riley, Laura E MD [MF] - **Spec Exp:** AIDS/HIV in Pregnancy; Infectious Disease in Pregnancy; Pregnancy-High Risk; **Hospital:** Mass Genl Hosp; **Address:** Mass Genl Hosp, Yawkey Bldg, 32 Fruit St, Ste 4200, Boston, MA 02114; **Phone:** 617-724-2229; **Board Cert:** Obstetrics & Gynecology 2006; Maternal & Fetal Medicine 2006; **Med School:** Univ Pittsburgh 1985; **Resid:** Obstetrics & Gynecology, Univ Pittsburgh Med Ctr 1988; **Fellow:** Maternal & Fetal Medicine, Brigham & Womens Hosp 1990; **Fac Appt:** Assoc Prof ObG, Harvard Med Sch

Mid Atlantic

Berkowitz, Richard MD [MF] - **Spec Exp:** Fetal Therapy; Multiple Gestation; Pregnancy & Hematologic Abnormalities; **Hospital:** NY-Presby Hosp/Columbia (page 66); **Address:** 16 E 60th St Fl 4, New York, NY 10022; **Phone:** 212-326-8952; **Board Cert:** Obstetrics & Gynecology 1974; Maternal & Fetal Medicine 1979; **Med School:** NYU Sch Med 1965; **Resid:** Obstetrics & Gynecology, NY Hosp-Cornell Univ 1972; **Fac Appt:** Prof ObG, Columbia P&S

Caritis, Steve N MD [MF] - **Hospital:** Magee-Womens Hosp - UPMC; **Address:** Magee-Womens Hosp, Maternal/Fetal Med, 300 Halket St, Pittsburgh, PA 15213-3180; **Phone:** 412-641-6361; **Board Cert:** Obstetrics & Gynecology 1999; Maternal & Fetal Medicine 1999; **Med School:** W VA Univ 1969; **Resid:** Obstetrics & Gynecology, Univ Pittsburgh Med Ctr 1973; **Fellow:** Maternal & Fetal Medicine, Columbia-Presby Med Ctr 1975; **Fac Appt:** Prof ObG, Univ Pittsburgh

Chervenak, Francis A MD [MF] - **Spec Exp:** Ultrasound; Pregnancy-High Risk; Ethics; **Hospital:** NY-Presby Hosp/Weill Cornell (page 66); **Address:** 525 E 68th St, Ste J-130, New York, NY 10021-4870; **Phone:** 212-746-3184; **Board Cert:** Obstetrics & Gynecology 1984; Maternal & Fetal Medicine 1985; **Med School:** Jefferson Med Coll 1976; **Resid:** Obstetrics & Gynecology, NY Med Coll-Flower Fifth Ave Hosp 1979; Obstetrics & Gynecology, St Lukes Hosp 1981; **Fellow:** Maternal & Fetal Medicine, Yale-New Haven Hosp 1983; **Fac Appt:** Prof ObG, Cornell Univ-Weill Med Coll

Collea, Joseph Vincent MD [MF] - **Spec Exp:** Multiple Gestation; Obstetric Ultrasound; **Hospital:** Georgetown Univ Hosp, Sibley Mem Hosp; **Address:** GUMC PHC Bldg Fl 3, 3800 Reservoir Rd NW, Washington, DC 20007-2194; **Phone:** 202-444-8531; **Board Cert:** Obstetrics & Gynecology 1974; Maternal & Fetal Medicine 1981; **Med School:** SUNY Upstate Med Univ 1966; **Resid:** Obstetrics & Gynecology, Johns Hopkins Hosp 1972; **Fellow:** Perinatal Medicine, LAC-USC Medical Center 1976; **Fac Appt:** Prof ObG, Georgetown Univ

D'Alton, Mary Elizabeth MD [MF] - **Spec Exp:** Pregnancy-High Risk; Multiple Gestation; Prenatal Diagnosis; **Hospital:** NY-Presby Hosp/Columbia (page 66); **Address:** 16 E 60th St, Ste 480, New York, NY 10032; **Phone:** 212-326-8951; **Board Cert:** Obstetrics & Gynecology 2001; Maternal & Fetal Medicine 2001; **Med School:** Ireland 1976; **Resid:** Obstetrics & Gynecology, Univ Ottawa Med Ctr 1982; **Fellow:** Maternal & Fetal Medicine, New England Med Ctr 1984; **Fac Appt:** Clin Prof ObG, Columbia P&S

Maternal & Fetal Medicine

Edersheim, Terri MD [MF] - **Spec Exp:** Pregnancy-High Risk; Multiple Gestation; Prenatal Diagnosis; **Hospital:** NY-Presby Hosp/Weill Cornell (page 66); **Address:** 523 E 72nd St, FL 9, New York, NY 10021; **Phone:** 212-472-5340; **Board Cert:** Obstetrics & Gynecology 1997; Maternal & Fetal Medicine 1997; **Med School:** Albert Einstein Coll Med 1980; **Resid:** Obstetrics & Gynecology, New York Hosp 1984; **Fellow:** Maternal & Fetal Medicine, New York Hosp 1986; **Fac Appt:** Asst Clin Prof ObG, Cornell Univ-Weill Med Coll

Fox, Harold E MD [MF] - **Spec Exp:** Pregnancy-High Risk; Prematurity Prevention; Multiple Gestation; **Hospital:** Johns Hopkins Hosp - Baltimore (page 61); **Address:** 600 N Wolfe St Phipps Bldg - rm 264, Baltimore, MD 21287; **Phone:** 410-614-0178; **Board Cert:** Obstetrics & Gynecology 2007; Maternal & Fetal Medicine 2007; **Med School:** Univ Rochester 1972; **Resid:** Obstetrics & Gynecology, Strong Meml Hosp 1975; **Fellow:** Maternal & Fetal Medicine, Univ Rochester Hosps 1977; **Fac Appt:** Prof ObG, Johns Hopkins Univ

Landy, Helain J MD [MF] - **Spec Exp:** Pregnancy-High Risk; Miscarriage-Recurrent; Multiple Gestation; Diabetes in Pregnancy; **Hospital:** Georgetown Univ Hosp; **Address:** Georgetown Univ Dept Ob/Gyn, 3800 Reservoir Rd NW, 3PHC, Washington, DC 20007-2113; **Phone:** 202-444-8531; **Board Cert:** Obstetrics & Gynecology 1998; Maternal & Fetal Medicine 1998; **Med School:** Northwestern Univ 1982; **Resid:** Obstetrics & Gynecology, Pennsylvania Hosp 1986; **Fellow:** Maternal & Fetal Medicine, Geo Washington Univ Med Ctr 1988; **Fac Appt:** Prof ObG, Georgetown Univ

Parry, Samuel I MD [MF] - **Hospital:** Hosp Univ Penn - UPHS (page 60); **Address:** Hospital U Penn, Maternal & Fetal Medicine, 3400 Spruce St, Ste 2000 Courtyard St, Philadephia, PA 19104; **Phone:** 215-662-6913; **Board Cert:** Obstetrics & Gynecology 2004; Maternal & Fetal Medicine 2004; **Med School:** Cornell Univ-Weill Med Coll 1990; **Resid:** Obstetrics & Gynecology, SUNY Buffalo Med Ctr 1994; **Fellow:** Maternal & Fetal Medicine, Hosp U Penn 1996; **Fac Appt:** Assoc Prof ObG, Univ Pennsylvania

Pinckert, Thomas L MD [MF] - **Spec Exp:** Pregnancy-High Risk; **Hospital:** Shady Grove Adven Hosp, Holy Cross Hospital - Silver Spring; **Address:** Greater Washington Maternal-Fetal Medicine, 9707 Medical Ctr Drive, Ste 230, Rockville, MD 20850; **Phone:** 301-279-6060; **Board Cert:** Obstetrics & Gynecology 2007; Clinical Genetics 1990; Maternal & Fetal Medicine 2007; **Med School:** Oregon Hlth Sci Univ 1979; **Resid:** Obstetrics & Gynecology, David Grant Med Ctr 1983; **Fellow:** Maternal & Fetal Medicine, UCSF Med Ctr 1989; Clinical Genetics, UCSF Med Ctr 1990

Repke, John T MD [MF] - **Spec Exp:** Pregnancy-High Risk; Hypertension in Pregnancy; Women's Health; **Hospital:** Penn State Milton S Hershey Med Ctr; **Address:** MS Hershey Med Ctr Maternal Fetal Med, 500 University Drive, MC H103, Hershey, PA 17033; **Phone:** 717-531-3503 x4; **Board Cert:** Obstetrics & Gynecology 2006; Maternal & Fetal Medicine 2006; **Med School:** NY Med Coll 1978; **Resid:** Obstetrics & Gynecology, Johns Hopkins Hosp 1982; **Fellow:** Maternal & Fetal Medicine, Johns Hopkins Hosp 1984; **Fac Appt:** Prof ObG, Penn State Univ-Hershey Med Ctr

Wapner, Ronald J MD [MF] - **Spec Exp:** Perinatal Medicine; Genetic Disorders; Multiple Gestation; Vomiting-Cyclic; **Hospital:** NY-Presby Hosp/Columbia (page 66); **Address:** Div Maternal/Fetal Medicine, 16 E 60th St, rm 480, New York, NY 10021; **Phone:** 212-326-8951; **Board Cert:** Obstetrics & Gynecology 2000; Maternal & Fetal Medicine 2000; Clinical Genetics 2006; **Med School:** Jefferson Med Coll 1972; **Resid:** Obstetrics & Gynecology, Jefferson Univ Hosp 1976; **Fellow:** Maternal & Fetal Medicine, Jefferson Med Coll 1978; **Fac Appt:** Prof ObG, Columbia P&S

Watt-Morse, Margaret L MD [MF] - **Hospital:** Magee-Womens Hosp - UPMC; **Address:** Magee-Women's Hosp, Maternal/Fetal Med, Obstetric Outpatient Clinic, 300 Halket St, Pittsburgh, PA 15213; **Phone:** 412-641-4455; **Board Cert:** Obstetrics & Gynecology 2006; Maternal & Fetal Medicine 2006; **Med School:** Univ IL Coll Med 1988; **Resid:** Obstetrics & Gynecology, Univ Illinois Hosps 1992; **Fellow:** Maternal & Fetal Medicine, Univ Pittsburgh Med Ctr 1994; **Fac Appt:** Assoc Prof ObG, Univ Pittsburgh

Southeast

Abuhamad, Alfred Z MD [MF] - **Spec Exp:** Twin to Twin Transfusion Syndrome (TTTS); Prenatal Diagnosis; Prenatal Ultrasound; Multiple Gestation; **Hospital:** Sentara Norfolk Genl Hosp; **Address:** E VA Med Sch, Div Mat Fetal Med, 825 Fairfax Ave, Ste 310, Norfolk, VA 23507; **Phone:** 757-446-7900; **Board Cert:** Obstetrics & Gynecology 2006; Maternal & Fetal Medicine 2006; **Med School:** Amer Univ Beirut 1985; **Resid:** Obstetrics & Gynecology, Jackson Meml Hosp 1989; **Fellow:** Maternal & Fetal Medicine, Jackson Meml Hosp-Univ Miami 1991; Ultrasound, Yale Univ 1991; **Fac Appt:** Prof ObG, Eastern VA Med Sch

Bruner, Joseph P MD [MF] - **Spec Exp:** Fetal Surgery; Spina Bifida; **Hospital:** Fort Sanders Reg Med Ctr; **Address:** Trustees Tower, 501 19th St, Ste 304, Knoxville, TN 37916; **Phone:** 865-541-2020; **Board Cert:** Obstetrics & Gynecology 2007; Maternal & Fetal Medicine 2007; **Med School:** Univ Nebr Coll Med 1979; **Resid:** Obstetrics & Gynecology, Letterman AMC 1983; **Fellow:** Maternal & Fetal Medicine, Hosp U Penn 1988; **Fac Appt:** Assoc Prof ObG, Vanderbilt Univ

Ferguson II, James E MD [MF] - **Spec Exp:** Pregnancy-High Risk; Ultrasound; **Hospital:** Univ of Kentucky Chandler Hosp; **Address:** Univ KY Medical Ctr, Dept Ob/Gyn, 800 Rose St, rm C-375, Lexington, KY 40536-0293; **Phone:** 859-323-6434; **Board Cert:** Obstetrics & Gynecology 2007; Maternal & Fetal Medicine 2007; **Med School:** Wake Forest Univ 1977; **Resid:** Obstetrics & Gynecology, Stanford Univ Med Ctr 1980; **Fellow:** Maternal & Fetal Medicine, Stanford Univ Med Ctr 1984; **Fac Appt:** Prof ObG, Univ KY Coll Med

Malee, Maureen P MD/PhD [MF] - **Spec Exp:** Pregnancy-High Risk; **Hospital:** Vanderbilt Univ Med Ctr; **Address:** Vanderbilt Univ Med Ctr, Dept OB/GYN, 1161 21st Ave S, Ste B1100, Nashville, TN 37232; **Phone:** 615-322-2308; **Board Cert:** Obstetrics & Gynecology 2007; Maternal & Fetal Medicine 2007; **Med School:** Loyola Univ-Stritch Sch Med 1984; **Resid:** Obstetrics & Gynecology, Univ of Illinois; **Fellow:** Maternal & Fetal Medicine, Unive of California; **Fac Appt:** Assoc Prof ObG, Vanderbilt Univ

McLaren, Rodney A MD [MF] - **Spec Exp:** Prenatal Diagnosis; Amniocentesis; Pregnancy-High Risk; **Hospital:** Virginia Hosp Ctr - Arlington, Georgetown Univ Hosp; **Address:** Dept Maternal & Fetal Med, 1635 N George Mason Drive, Ste 190, Arlington, VA 22205-3698; **Phone:** 703-558-6077; **Board Cert:** Obstetrics & Gynecology 2003; Maternal & Fetal Medicine 2003; **Med School:** Tufts Univ 1983; **Resid:** Obstetrics & Gynecology, LI Coll Hosp 1987; **Fellow:** Maternal & Fetal Medicine, Georgetown Univ 1989

Miller, Franklin C MD [MF] - **Spec Exp:** Pregnancy-High Risk; Fetal Assessment; **Hospital:** Univ of Kentucky Chandler Hosp; **Address:** Univ Kentucky Med Ctr, Div High Risk Obstetrics, 800 Rose St, Ste C358, Lexington, KY 40536-0084; **Phone:** 859-257-5158; **Board Cert:** Obstetrics & Gynecology 1999; Maternal & Fetal Medicine 1999; **Med School:** Univ Louisville Sch Med 1962; **Resid:** Obstetrics & Gynecology, Tripler General Hosp 1969; **Fellow:** Maternal & Fetal Medicine, USC Medical Ctr 1974; **Fac Appt:** Prof ObG, Univ KY Coll Med

Maternal & Fetal Medicine

Thorp Jr, John M MD [MF] - **Spec Exp:** Multiple Gestation; Premature Labor; **Hospital:** Univ NC Hosps; **Address:** UNC-Chapel Hill, 101 Manning Drive, Box 7600, Chapel Hill, NC 27599; **Phone:** 919-966-2496; **Board Cert:** Obstetrics & Gynecology 2004; Maternal & Fetal Medicine 2004; **Med School:** E Carolina Univ 1983; **Resid:** Obstetrics & Gynecology, Univ NC Hosp 1987; **Fellow:** Maternal & Fetal Medicine, Univ NC Hosp 1989; **Fac Appt:** Prof ObG, Univ NC Sch Med

Van Dorsten, J Peter MD [MF] - **Spec Exp:** Pregnancy-High Risk; **Hospital:** MUSC Med Ctr; **Address:** MUSC Med Ctr, Dept ObGyn, 96 Jonathan Lucas St, Charleston, SC 29425; **Phone:** 843-792-4509; **Board Cert:** Obstetrics & Gynecology 2007; Maternal & Fetal Medicine 2007; **Med School:** Univ NC Sch Med 1971; **Resid:** Obstetrics & Gynecology, Med Univ SC Hosp 1976; **Fellow:** Maternal & Fetal Medicine, USC-LAC Hosp 1981; **Fac Appt:** Prof ObG, Med Univ SC

Wenstrom, Katharine D MD [MF] - **Spec Exp:** Reproductive Genetics; Pregnancy-High Risk; **Hospital:** Vanderbilt Univ Med Ctr; **Address:** Vanderbilt Med Ctr, Dept OB/GYN, 1161 21st Ave S, Ste B1100, Nashville, TN 37232; **Phone:** 615-322-2308; **Board Cert:** Obstetrics & Gynecology 2006; Maternal & Fetal Medicine 2006; Clinical Genetics 1990; **Med School:** Case West Res Univ 1983; **Resid:** Obstetrics & Gynecology, Univ Illinois Hosp 1987; **Fellow:** Maternal & Fetal Medicine, Univ Illinois Hosp 1989; Clinical Genetics, Univ Iowa Med Ctr 1990; **Fac Appt:** Prof ObG, Vanderbilt Univ

Midwest

Bahado-Singh, Ray O MD [MF] - **Spec Exp:** Pregnancy-High Risk; Genetic Disorders; Obstetric Ultrasound; Twin to Twin Transfusion Syndrome (TTTS); **Hospital:** Hutzel Hosp - Detroit; **Address:** 3990 John R, 4 Webber N, Detroit, MI 48201; **Phone:** 313-745-7066; **Board Cert:** Obstetrics & Gynecology 2007; Maternal & Fetal Medicine 2007; Clinical Genetics 2004; **Med School:** Jamaica 1979; **Resid:** Obstetrics & Gynecology, Metropolitan Hosp 1985; **Fellow:** Perinatal Medicine, UC-Irvine 1987; Clinical Genetics, Yale Univ 1993

Bartelsmeyer, James MD [MF] - **Spec Exp:** Pregnancy-High Risk; Multiple Gestation; **Hospital:** St John's Mercy Med Ctr - St Louis; **Address:** 621 S New Ballas Rd, Ste 2007B, St Louis, MO 63141; **Phone:** 314-991-5000; **Board Cert:** Obstetrics & Gynecology 2007; Maternal & Fetal Medicine 2007; **Med School:** Univ IL Coll Med 1985; **Resid:** Obstetrics & Gynecology, Univ Ill Coll Med Hosps 1989; **Fellow:** Maternal & Fetal Medicine, Barnes Hosp-Univ Wash 1991; **Fac Appt:** Assoc Prof ObG, Washington Univ, St Louis

Besinger, Richard MD [MF] - **Spec Exp:** Prenatal Diagnosis; Premature Labor; Critical Care; **Hospital:** Loyola Univ Med Ctr; **Address:** Loyola Univ Med Ctr, Bldg 103, 2160 S First Ave, Ste 1013, Maywood, IL 60153-5590; **Phone:** 708-216-6444; **Board Cert:** Obstetrics & Gynecology 1998; Maternal & Fetal Medicine 1998; **Med School:** Loyola Univ-Stritch Sch Med 1982; **Resid:** Obstetrics & Gynecology, Univ Mich Med Ctr 1986; **Fellow:** Maternal & Fetal Medicine, Johns Hopkins Hosp 1988; **Fac Appt:** Prof ObG, Loyola Univ-Stritch Sch Med

Dooley, Sharon L MD [MF] - **Spec Exp:** Fetal Abnormalities; Pregnancy-High Risk; Multiple Gestation; **Hospital:** Northwestern Meml Hosp; **Address:** 675 N St Clair Fl 14 - Ste 200, Chicago, IL 60611; **Phone:** 312-695-7542; **Board Cert:** Obstetrics & Gynecology 1989; Maternal & Fetal Medicine 1981; **Med School:** Univ VA Sch Med 1973; **Resid:** Obstetrics & Gynecology, Northwestern Meml Hosp 1977; **Fac Appt:** Prof ObG, Northwestern Univ

Gianopoulos, John MD [MF] - **Spec Exp:** Perinatal Medicine; Premature Labor; Critical Care; **Hospital:** Loyola Univ Med Ctr; **Address:** Loyola Univ Med Ctr, 2160 S 1st Ave, Bldg 103 - Ste 1019, Maywood, IL 60153; **Phone:** 708-216-5423; **Board Cert:** Obstetrics & Gynecology 2004; Maternal & Fetal Medicine 2004; **Med School:** Loyola Univ-Stritch Sch Med 1977; **Resid:** Obstetrics & Gynecology, Loyola Univ Med Ctr 1981; **Fellow:** Maternal & Fetal Medicine, Loyola Univ Med Ctr 1983; **Fac Appt:** Prof ObG, Loyola Univ-Stritch Sch Med

Hibbard, Judith MD [MF] - **Spec Exp:** Pregnancy-High Risk; Heart Disease in Pregnancy; Prenatal Ultrasound; **Hospital:** Univ of IL Med Ctr at Chicago; **Address:** Univ Illinois at Chicago, Dept OB-GYN, 1801 W Taylor St, MS 808, Chicago, IL 60612; **Phone:** 312-413-7500; **Board Cert:** Obstetrics & Gynecology 1999; Maternal & Fetal Medicine 1999; **Med School:** Loyola Univ-Stritch Sch Med 1982; **Resid:** Obstetrics & Gynecology, Univ Chicago Hosps 1986; **Fellow:** Maternal & Fetal Medicine, Univ Chicago Hosps 1988; **Fac Appt:** Prof ObG, Univ IL Coll Med

Hussey, Michael J MD [MF] - **Spec Exp:** Perinatal Medicine; Congenital Anomalies; Multiple Gestation; **Hospital:** Rush Univ Med Ctr; **Address:** 1725 W Harrison St, Ste 408, Chicago, IL 60612; **Phone:** 312-997-2229; **Board Cert:** Obstetrics & Gynecology 2007; Maternal & Fetal Medicine 2007; **Med School:** Univ IL Coll Med 1986; **Resid:** Obstetrics & Gynecology, Loyola Univ Med Ctr 1993; **Fellow:** Maternal & Fetal Medicine, Rush-Presby-St Lukes Hosp 1995; Ultrasound, Univ Col Hlth Sci Ctr 1996; **Fac Appt:** Asst Prof ObG, Rush Med Coll

Ismail, Mahmoud A MD [MF] - **Spec Exp:** Pregnancy-High Risk; Perinatal Medicine; Infections-Neonatal; Infections in Pregnancy; **Hospital:** Univ of Chicago Hosps; **Address:** 5841 S Maryland Ave, MC 2050, Chicago, IL 60637-1463; **Phone:** 773-702-5200; **Board Cert:** Obstetrics & Gynecology 2005; Maternal & Fetal Medicine 2005; **Med School:** Egypt 1970; **Resid:** Obstetrics & Gynecology, Wayne St Univ Affil Hosps 1977; **Fellow:** Maternal & Fetal Medicine, Univ Chicago Hosps 1982; **Fac Appt:** Prof ObG, Univ Chicago-Pritzker Sch Med

Johnson, Timothy R B MD [MF] - **Spec Exp:** Fetal Assessment; Prenatal Diagnosis; **Hospital:** Univ Michigan Hlth Sys; **Address:** Univ Mich, Dept Ob/Gyn, 1500 E Med Ctr, rm L4000, Box 5276, Ann Arbor, MI 48109; **Phone:** 734-764-8123; **Board Cert:** Obstetrics & Gynecology 2001; Maternal & Fetal Medicine 2001; **Med School:** Univ VA Sch Med 1975; **Resid:** Obstetrics & Gynecology, Univ Michigan Med Ctr 1979; **Fellow:** Maternal & Fetal Medicine, Johns Hopkins Hosp 1981; **Fac Appt:** Prof ObG, Univ Mich Med Sch

Landers, Daniel V MD [MF] - **Spec Exp:** Infectious Disease; **Hospital:** Univ Minn Med Ctr, Fairview - Riverside Campus; **Address:** 606 S 24th Ave S, Professional Bldg Fl 4, Minneapolis, MN 55454; **Phone:** 612-273-2223; **Board Cert:** Obstetrics & Gynecology 1998; Maternal & Fetal Medicine 1998; **Med School:** UCSF 1980; **Resid:** Obstetrics & Gynecology, UCSF Med Ctr 1984; **Fellow:** Maternal & Fetal Medicine, UCSF Med Ctr 1986; Infectious Disease, UCSF Med Ctr 1988; **Fac Appt:** Prof ObG, Univ Minn

Macones, George A MD [MF] - **Spec Exp:** Pregnancy-High Risk; Premature Labor; **Hospital:** Barnes-Jewish Hosp, St Louis Chldns Hosp; **Address:** Washington Univ Dept Ob/Gyn, 660 S Euclid Ave, Box 8064, St Louis, MO 63110; **Phone:** 314-996-6096; **Board Cert:** Obstetrics & Gynecology 2006; Maternal & Fetal Medicine 2006; **Med School:** Jefferson Med Coll 1988; **Resid:** Obstetrics & Gynecology, Pennsylvania Hosp 1992; **Fellow:** Maternal & Fetal Medicine, Jefferson Univ Hosp 1994; **Fac Appt:** Prof ObG, Washington Univ, St Louis

Philipson, Elliot MD [MF] - **Spec Exp:** Pregnancy-High Risk; Amniocentesis; **Hospital:** Hillcrest Hosp-Mayfield Hts (page 56), Cleveland Clin Fdn (page 56); **Address:** Hillcrest Hosp, Dept OB/Gyn, 6770 Mayfield Rd, Ste 336, Mayfield Heights, OH 44124; **Phone:** 440-312-7774; **Board Cert:** Obstetrics & Gynecology 2007; Maternal & Fetal Medicine 2007; **Med School:** Italy 1975; **Resid:** Obstetrics & Gynecology, Albany Med Ctr 1980; **Fellow:** Maternal & Fetal Medicine, Metro Genl Hosp 1982; **Fac Appt:** Assoc Prof ObG, Cleveland Cl Coll Med/Case West Res

Maternal & Fetal Medicine

Socol, Michael MD [MF] - **Spec Exp:** Diabetes in Pregnancy; Multiple Gestation; Premature Labor; **Hospital:** Northwestern Meml Hosp; **Address:** Prentice Womens Hosp, 250 E Superior St, Ste 3-2307, Chicago, IL 60611-3056; **Phone:** 312-472-3970; **Board Cert:** Obstetrics & Gynecology 1989; Maternal & Fetal Medicine 1981; **Med School:** Univ IL Coll Med 1974; **Resid:** Obstetrics & Gynecology, Univ Illinois Med Ctr 1977; **Fellow:** Maternal & Fetal Medicine, USC Med Ctr 1979; **Fac Appt:** Prof ObG, Northwestern Univ

Strassner, Howard T MD [MF] - **Spec Exp:** Pregnancy-High Risk; Amniocentesis; Obstetric Ultrasound; **Hospital:** Rush Univ Med Ctr, Resurrection Hlth Care St Joseph Hosp; **Address:** Women's Health Consultants, 1725 W Harrison St, Professional Bldg 1, Ste 408-West, Chicago, IL 60612; **Phone:** 312-997-2229; **Board Cert:** Obstetrics & Gynecology 2005; Maternal & Fetal Medicine 2005; **Med School:** Univ Chicago-Pritzker Sch Med 1974; **Resid:** Obstetrics & Gynecology, Columbia Presby Med Ctr 1978; **Fellow:** Maternal & Fetal Medicine, LA Co-USC Med Ctr 1980; **Fac Appt:** Prof ObG, Rush Med Coll

Treadwell, Marjorie C MD [MF] - **Spec Exp:** Obstetric Ultrasound; Pregnancy-High Risk; Fetal Diagnosis & Therapy; **Hospital:** Univ Michigan Hlth Sys; **Address:** 1500 E Medical Center Drive, F4835 MOTT, Ann Arbor, MI 48109-0264; **Phone:** 734-763-4264; **Board Cert:** Obstetrics & Gynecology 2000; Maternal & Fetal Medicine 2000; **Med School:** Univ Mich Med Sch 1984; **Resid:** Obstetrics & Gynecology, Wayne State Univ 1988; **Fellow:** Maternal & Fetal Medicine, Wayne State Univ 1990; **Fac Appt:** Prof ObG, Wayne State Univ

Wilkins, Isabelle MD [MF] - **Spec Exp:** Multiple Gestation; Congenital Anomalies; Prenatal Ultrasound; **Hospital:** Univ of IL Med Ctr at Chicago; **Address:** Univ Illinois Med Ctr at Chicago, Center for Womens Health, 1801 W Taylor, MS 650, Chicago, IL 60612; **Phone:** 312-413-7500; **Board Cert:** Obstetrics & Gynecology 1996; Maternal & Fetal Medicine 1996; **Med School:** Duke Univ 1980; **Resid:** Obstetrics & Gynecology, Mount Sinai Med Ctr 1984; **Fellow:** Maternal & Fetal Medicine, Mount Sinai Med Ctr 1986; **Fac Appt:** Prof ObG, Univ IL Coll Med

Winn, Hung MD [MF] - **Spec Exp:** Multiple Gestation; Pregnancy-High Risk; **Hospital:** Univ of Missouri Hosp & Clins; **Address:** 500 N Keene St, Ste 405, Columbia, MO 65201; **Phone:** 573-882-6361; **Board Cert:** Obstetrics & Gynecology 2000; Maternal & Fetal Medicine 2000; **Med School:** Univ IL Coll Med 1982; **Resid:** Obstetrics & Gynecology, Univ Ill Hosp 1986; **Fellow:** Maternal & Fetal Medicine, Yale-New Haven Hosp 1988; **Fac Appt:** Prof ObG, Univ MO-Columbia Sch Med

Great Plains and Mountains

Dugoff, Lorraine MD [MF] - **Spec Exp:** Pregnancy-High Risk; Prenatal Diagnosis; Ultrasound; **Hospital:** Univ Colorado Hosp; **Address:** Dept of ObGyn, MS 198-1, 4200 E PO Box 6511 Ave, Aurora, CO 80045; **Phone:** 720-848-1060; **Board Cert:** Maternal & Fetal Medicine 1999; Obstetrics & Gynecology 1997; **Med School:** Georgetown Univ 1989; **Resid:** Obstetrics & Gynecology, Philadelphia Hosp 1990; Obstetrics & Gynecology, U Colorado Hlth Sci Ctr 1993; **Fellow:** Maternal & Fetal Medicine, U Colorado Hlth Sci Ctr 1995; Clinical Genetics, U Colorado Hlth Sci Ctr 1996; **Fac Appt:** Assoc Prof ObG, Univ Colorado

Gibbs, Ronald S MD [MF] - **Spec Exp:** Infectious Disease; **Hospital:** Univ Colorado Hosp; **Address:** Dept of Ob/Gyn, MS B198-1, PO Box 6511, Aurora, CO 80045; **Phone:** 720-848-1060; **Board Cert:** Obstetrics & Gynecology 1989; Maternal & Fetal Medicine 1981; **Med School:** Univ Pennsylvania 1969; **Resid:** Obstetrics & Gynecology, Hosp Univ Penn 1974; **Fellow:** Maternal & Fetal Medicine, Univ Tex Hlth Sci Ctr 1978; **Fac Appt:** Prof ObG, Univ Colorado

Tomich, Paul MD [MF] - **Spec Exp:** Pregnancy-High Risk; Prenatal Ultrasound; **Hospital:** Nebraska Med Ctr; **Address:** 983255 Nebraska Medical Center, Omaha, NE 68198-3255; **Phone:** 402-559-6150; **Board Cert:** Obstetrics & Gynecology 2004; Maternal & Fetal Medicine 2004; **Med School:** Loyola Univ-Stritch Sch Med 1973; **Resid:** Obstetrics & Gynecology, Mayo Clinic 1978; **Fellow:** Maternal & Fetal Medicine, Barnes Hosp-Wash Univ 1980; **Fac Appt:** Prof ObG, Univ Nebr Coll Med

Southwest

Elliott, John P MD [MF] - **Spec Exp:** Twin to Twin Transfusion Syndrome (TTTS); Multiple Gestation; Premature Labor; **Hospital:** Banner Good Samaritan Regl Med Ctr - Phoenix, Banner Desert Med Ctr; **Address:** 6320 W Union Hills Drive, Ste B1400, Glendale, AZ 85308; **Phone:** 623-561-0043; **Board Cert:** Obstetrics & Gynecology 1980; Maternal & Fetal Medicine 1982; **Med School:** Univ Colorado 1972; **Resid:** Obstetrics & Gynecology, Fitzsimmons Army Med Ctr 1976; **Fellow:** Maternal & Fetal Medicine, Long Beach Meml Hosp/UC Irvine 1980; **Fac Appt:** Clin Prof ObG, Univ Ariz Coll Med

Hankins, Gary D V MD [MF] - **Spec Exp:** Pregnancy-High Risk; Hypertension in Pregnancy; **Hospital:** UT Med Br Hosp at Galveston; **Address:** Univ Texas Medical Branch at Galveston, 301 University Blvd, 3.400 JSA, Galveston, TX 77555-0587; **Phone:** 409-772-1957; **Board Cert:** Obstetrics & Gynecology 2000; Maternal & Fetal Medicine 2000; **Med School:** Med Coll VA 1977; **Resid:** Obstetrics & Gynecology, Wilford Hall Med Ctr 1981; **Fellow:** Critical Care Medicine, Wilford Hall Med Ctr 1982; Maternal & Fetal Medicine, Parkland Hosp 1984; **Fac Appt:** Prof ObG, Univ Tex Med Br, Galveston

Horsager, Robyn Boehrer MD [MF] - **Hospital:** UT Southwestern Med Ctr - Dallas; **Address:** UT Southwestern Med Ctr, 5939 Harry Hines Blvd, Ste 300, MC 9102, Dallas, TX 75390-9102; **Phone:** 214-645-3837; **Board Cert:** Obstetrics & Gynecology 2006; Maternal & Fetal Medicine 2006; **Med School:** Univ IL Coll Med 1987; **Resid:** Obstetrics & Gynecology, Parkland Meml Hosp 1991; **Fellow:** Maternal & Fetal Medicine, Univ Texas SW Med Ctr 1993; **Fac Appt:** Assoc Prof ObG, Univ Tex SW, Dallas

Reed, Kathryn L MD [MF] - **Spec Exp:** Prenatal Diagnosis; Ultrasound; Fetal Echocardiography; **Hospital:** Univ Med Ctr - Tucson; **Address:** University Medical Ctr, Womens Resource Ctr, 1501 N Campbell Ave Fl 8, Tucson, AZ 85724; **Phone:** 520-694-6010; **Board Cert:** Obstetrics & Gynecology 1994; Maternal & Fetal Medicine 1987; **Med School:** Univ Ariz Coll Med 1977; **Resid:** Obstetrics & Gynecology, Ariz Hlth Scis Ctr 1981; Maternal & Fetal Medicine, Ariz Hlth Scis Ctr 1983; **Fac Appt:** Prof ObG, Univ Ariz Coll Med

West Coast and Pacific

Benedetti, Thomas J MD [MF] - **Spec Exp:** Prematurity Prevention; Fetal Macrosomia; **Hospital:** Univ Wash Med Ctr, Yakima Valley Mem Hosp; **Address:** 1959 NE Pacific St, Box 356460, Seattle, WA 98195; **Phone:** 206-543-3729; **Board Cert:** Obstetrics & Gynecology 1980; Maternal & Fetal Medicine 1981; **Med School:** Univ Wash 1973; **Resid:** Obstetrics & Gynecology, LAC-USC Med Ctr 1977; **Fellow:** Maternal & Fetal Medicine, LAC-USC Med Ctr 1979; **Fac Appt:** Prof ObG, Univ Wash

Maternal & Fetal Medicine

Druzin, Maurice L MD [MF] - **Spec Exp:** Lupus/SLE in Pregnancy; Fetal Electronic Monitors; Miscarriage-Recurrent; **Hospital:** Lucile Packard Chldns Hosp/Stanford Univ Med Ctr; **Address:** Stanford Univ, Dept Ob/Gyn, 300 Pasteur Drive, rm HH333, MC 5317, Stanford, CA 94305-5317; **Phone:** 650-498-4069; **Board Cert:** Obstetrics & Gynecology 2007; Maternal & Fetal Medicine 2007; **Med School:** South Africa 1970; **Resid:** Obstetrics & Gynecology, Rose Med Ctr-Univ Colo 1977; **Fellow:** Maternal & Fetal Medicine, LAC-USC Med Ctr 1979; **Fac Appt:** Prof ObG, Stanford Univ

Goldberg, James D MD [MF] - **Spec Exp:** Prenatal Diagnosis; Fetal Diagnosis & Therapy; **Hospital:** CA Pacific Med Ctr - Pacific Campus; **Address:** San Francisco Perinatal Assoc, One Daniel Burnham Ct, Ste 230C, San Francisco, CA 94109; **Phone:** 415-202-1200; **Board Cert:** Obstetrics & Gynecology 1994; Clinical Genetics 1987; **Med School:** Univ Minn 1979; **Resid:** Obstetrics & Gynecology, UCSF Med Ctr 1983; **Fellow:** Maternal & Fetal Medicine, Mt Sinai Hosp 1985; Clinical Genetics, Mt Sinai Hosp 1985

Gravett, Michael Glen MD [MF] - **Spec Exp:** Infectious Disease-Perinatal; **Hospital:** Univ Wash Med Ctr; **Address:** Univ Washington, Dept OB/GYN, Box 356460, Seattle, WA 98195-6460; **Phone:** 206-598-4070; **Board Cert:** Obstetrics & Gynecology 1985; Maternal & Fetal Medicine 1987; **Med School:** UCLA 1977; **Resid:** Obstetrics & Gynecology, Univ Wash Med Ctr 1981; **Fellow:** Maternal & Fetal Medicine, Univ Wash Med Ctr 1983; **Fac Appt:** Prof ObG, Univ Wash

Hobel, Calvin MD [MF] - **Spec Exp:** Prematurity Prevention; Fetal Diagnosis & Therapy; **Hospital:** Cedars-Sinai Med Ctr; **Address:** 8635 W Third St, #160W, Los Angeles, CA 90048; **Phone:** 310-423-3365; **Board Cert:** Obstetrics & Gynecology 1971; Maternal & Fetal Medicine 1975; **Med School:** Univ Nebr Coll Med 1963; **Resid:** Obstetrics & Gynecology, Harbor Genl Hosp 1968; **Fellow:** Maternal & Fetal Medicine, Natl Womens Hosp 1967; **Fac Appt:** Prof ObG, UCLA

Koos, Brian J MD [MF] - **Spec Exp:** Pregnancy-High Risk; Fetal Diagnosis & Therapy; Heart Disease in Pregnancy; **Hospital:** Ronald Reagan UCLA Med Ctr; **Address:** UCLA Medical Ctr, 10833 Le Conte Ave, MC 3075, Los Angeles, CA 90095-3075; **Phone:** 310-794-7852; **Board Cert:** Obstetrics & Gynecology 1999; Maternal & Fetal Medicine 1999; **Med School:** Loma Linda Univ 1974; **Resid:** Obstetrics & Gynecology, Brigham & Womens Hosp 1979; **Fellow:** Maternal & Fetal Medicine, Womens Hosp 1983; **Fac Appt:** Prof ObG, UCLA

Moore, Thomas R MD [MF] - **Spec Exp:** Diabetes in Pregnancy; Fetal Diagnosis & Therapy; **Hospital:** UCSD Med Ctr; **Address:** 200 W Arbor Drive, MC 8433, San Diego, CA 92103; **Phone:** 619-543-7900; **Board Cert:** Obstetrics & Gynecology 2006; Maternal & Fetal Medicine 2006; **Med School:** Yale Univ 1979; **Resid:** Obstetrics & Gynecology, Naval Hosp 1983; **Fellow:** Maternal & Fetal Medicine, UCSD 1985; **Fac Appt:** Prof ObG, UCSD

Platt, Lawrence D MD [MF] - **Spec Exp:** Maternal & Fetal Medicine; Ultrasound; Prenatal Diagnosis; **Hospital:** Cedars-Sinai Med Ctr, St John's Hlth Ctr, Santa Monica; **Address:** 6310 W San Vincente Blvd, Ste 520, Los Angeles, CA 90048; **Phone:** 323-857-1952; **Board Cert:** Obstetrics & Gynecology 1979; Maternal & Fetal Medicine 1981; **Med School:** Wayne State Univ 1972; **Resid:** Obstetrics & Gynecology, Sinai Hosp 1976; **Fellow:** Maternal & Fetal Medicine, USC Med Ctr 1978; **Fac Appt:** Prof ObG, UCLA

Tabsh, Khalil M A MD [MF] - **Spec Exp:** Pregnancy-High Risk; **Hospital:** Ronald Reagan UCLA Med Ctr, Santa Monica - UCLA Med Ctr; **Address:** 200 Medical Plaza, Ste 430, Los Angeles, CA 90095; **Phone:** 310-208-4492; **Board Cert:** Obstetrics & Gynecology 1981; Maternal & Fetal Medicine 1982; **Med School:** Lebanon 1974; **Resid:** Obstetrics & Gynecology, American Univ Beirut Med Ctr 1976; Obstetrics & Gynecology, Yale-New Haven Hosp 1978; **Fellow:** Maternal & Fetal Medicine, UCLA Med Ctr 1979; **Fac Appt:** Clin Prof ObG, UCLA-David Geffen Sch Med

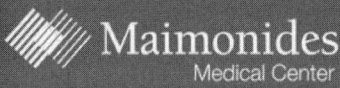

Maimonides
Medical Center

The Birthing Center at Maimonides is ranked among the best hospitals in the nation for maternity care by HealthGrades, the nation's leading source for independent healthcare quality information. More babies are delivered at Maimonides Medical Center than at any other hospital in New York State.

The Maimonides Birthing Center features private suites with hardwood floors and a homelike environment. At the same time, physician coverage is provided 24/7 in our advanced Neonatal Intensive Care Unit. Our 36 obstetricians and 26 midwives have found that most families appreciate having the best of both worlds available to them.

Maimonides provides other unique services to its maternity patients. The largest doula program in the metropolitan area can be found at Maimonides. These fully-trained childbirth assistants are available to patients before, during and after delivery at no cost to families. And the maternity units utilize an electronic patient record that sets industry standards for patient safety and hospital efficiency.

This combination of family-centered services and advanced technology continues to have enormous appeal to the women we serve – over 6,700 of them last year alone. Our highly trained staff includes the finest nurses, physicians, midwives and specialists to ensure the safety and comfort of our patients. Several physicians specialize in high-risk pregnancy, including the Chairman of Obstetrics & Gynecology, Howard Minkoff, MD.

In recognition of its excellence in obstetrics and pediatrics, Maimonides was designated a Regional Perinatal Center by the New York State Department of Health. Women who give birth at Maimonides also have a variety of other services available to them, including:

- A Perinatal Testing Center, directed by Shoshana Haberman, MD, offering amniocentesis, 3-D ultrasound, fetal echocardiograms and other diagnostic exams.

- Neonatologists onsite around-the-clock. The Norma Sutton Center for Neonatology adjoins the Payson Birthing Center and provides the most sophisticated care in a family-friendly environment.

Physicians at Maimonides are among the ten percent in the US who use computers to enter patient orders, thereby reducing the risk of errors, increasing efficiency, and speeding the healing process. Maimonides has appeared on the American Hospital Association's "Most Wired" and "Most Wireless" lists more often than any other healthcare institution in the metropolitan area. Advanced technology allows our doctors to focus more attention on caring for their patients.

Maimonides Medical Center – Passionate about medicine, compassionate about people.

www.maimonidesmed.org/obgyn

NYU **Langone Medical Center**

550 First Avenue (at 31St Street)
New York, NY 10016
Physician Referral:
(888)7-NYU-MED (888-769-8633)
www.nyumc.org

MATERNAL-FETAL MEDICINE

The NYU Langone Medical Center Program for Maternal Fetal Medicine offers prenatal care for high-risk pregnancies as well as detailed consultations before, during, and after pregnancy. Special attention is given to multifetal pregnancies and to women who have other medical conditions that complicate their pregnancy, like diabetes, heart problems, high blood pressure, and lupus, among others.

The Program's primary concern is making sure each patient delivers a healthy baby. Many of the patients referred to the specialists at NYU are able to conceive but have difficulty carrying babies to term. In response to their particular needs, NYU Medical has conducted extensive research into the causes of recurrent miscarriage and pre-term delivery, with impressive results.

Of course, the ideal time to correct fetal problems is when infants are still in the womb. Using minimally invasive techniques, doctors at NYU Langone Medical Center are able to repair a number of life-threatening conditions in a child before it is even born. These techniques reduce the risks of pre-term labor and the need for cesarean births.

The program's high success rates are testimony to the immediate impact research has on treatment at NYU Medical Center This program has generated numerous new treatment
modalities for high-risk obstetrics around the nation and around the world.

The Program for Maternal Fetal Medicine enjoys a close, synergistic relationship with the Prenatal Diagnostic Unit. Several of the perinatologists from the Maternal Fetal Medicine Practice provide coverage at the ultrasound unit, and refer patients for sonography and other procedures. From this partnership, our physicians use state-of-the-art techniques for in-utero diagnosis and treatment, and our experienced physicians gain immediate access to the latest findings.

Neonatal-Perinatal Medicine
a subspecialty of Pediatrics

A subspecialist in neonatal-perinatal medicine is a pediatrician who is the principal care provider for sick newborn infants. Clinical expertise is used for direct patient care and for consulting with obstetrical colleagues to plan for the care of mothers who have high-risk pregnancies.

Training Required: Three years in pediatrics *plus* additional training and examination.

NEONATAL-PERINATAL MEDICINE

New England

Cloherty, John MD [NP] - **Spec Exp:** Neonatology; **Hospital:** Children's Hospital - Boston, Brigham & Women's Hosp; **Address:** 319 Longwood Ave, Fl 4, Boston, MA 02115; **Phone:** 617-277-7320; **Board Cert:** Pediatrics 1986; Neonatal-Perinatal Medicine 1986; **Med School:** Boston Univ 1962; **Resid:** Pediatrics, Mass Genl Hosp 1969; **Fellow:** Neonatal-Perinatal Medicine, Chldns Hosp; **Fac Appt:** Assoc Clin Prof Ped, Harvard Med Sch

Ehrenkranz, Richard MD [NP] - **Spec Exp:** Neonatal Critical Care; Nutrition; **Hospital:** Yale-New Haven Hosp; **Address:** Yale Univ-Dept Ped, PO Box 208064, New Haven, CT 06520-8064; **Phone:** 203-688-2320; **Board Cert:** Neonatal-Perinatal Medicine 1979; Pediatrics 1977; **Med School:** SUNY Downstate 1972; **Resid:** Pediatrics, Yale-New Haven Hosp 1974; **Fellow:** Neonatal-Perinatal Medicine, Yale-New Haven Hosp 1978; **Fac Appt:** Prof Ped, Yale Univ

Gross, Ian MD [NP] - **Spec Exp:** Breathing Disorders; Critical Care; **Hospital:** Yale-New Haven Hosp; **Address:** Yale Sch Med, Dept Peds, 333 Cedar St, PO Box 208064, New Haven, CT 06520-8064; **Phone:** 203-688-2320; **Board Cert:** Pediatrics 1974; Neonatal-Perinatal Medicine 1977; **Med School:** South Africa 1967; **Resid:** Pediatrics, Univ Witwatersrand Affil Hosps 1971; Pediatrics, Chldns Hosp Med Ctr 1972; **Fellow:** Pediatrics, Mass Genl Hosp 1973; Neonatal-Perinatal Medicine, Yale-New Haven Hosp 1974; **Fac Appt:** Prof Ped, Yale Univ

Horbar, Jeffrey D MD [NP] - **Hospital:** FAHC - Med Ctr Campus; **Address:** Vermont Oxford Mutual, 33 Kilburn St, Burlington, VT 05401; **Phone:** 802-865-4814; **Board Cert:** Pediatrics 1982; Neonatal-Perinatal Medicine 1983; **Med School:** SUNY Downstate 1977; **Resid:** Pediatrics, Med Ctr Hosp Vermont 1979; **Fellow:** Obstetrics & Gynecology, Med Ctr Hosp Vermont 1981; **Fac Appt:** Assoc Prof Ped, Univ VT Coll Med

Van Marter, Linda J MD [NP] - **Spec Exp:** Neonatal Chronic Lung Disease (CLD); Lung Disease in Newborns; Pulmonary Hypertension of Newborn (PPHN); **Hospital:** Brigham & Women's Hosp, Children's Hospital - Boston; **Address:** 300 Longwood Ave, Hunnewell 430 - Newborn Med, Boston, MA 02115; **Phone:** 617-355-6027; **Board Cert:** Pediatrics 1985; Neonatal-Perinatal Medicine 1985; **Med School:** Univ Pittsburgh 1980; **Resid:** Pediatrics, Childrens Hosp Med Ctr 1983; **Fellow:** Neonatology, Harvard Med Sch 1986; **Fac Appt:** Assoc Prof Ped, Harvard Med Sch

Mid Atlantic

Davidson, Dennis MD [NP] - **Spec Exp:** Lung Disease in Newborns; **Hospital:** Schneider Chldn's Hosp; **Address:** Schneider Chldns Hosp, Neonatal Div, 269-01 76th Ave, Ste 344, New Hyde Park, NY 11040; **Phone:** 718-470-3440; **Board Cert:** Pediatrics 1980; Neonatal-Perinatal Medicine 1981; **Med School:** Loyola Univ-Stritch Sch Med 1974; **Resid:** Pediatrics, Babies Hosp-Columbia Univ 1978; **Fellow:** Neonatal-Perinatal Medicine, Babies Hosp-Columbia Univ 1981; **Fac Appt:** Assoc Prof Ped, Albert Einstein Coll Med

Delivoria-Papadopoulos, Maria MD [NP] - **Spec Exp:** Neonatology; **Hospital:** St Christopher's Hosp for Chldn, Hahnemann Univ Hosp; **Address:** St Christopher's Hosp for Children, Erie Ave at Front St, Ste 2212, Neonatology, Philadelphia, PA 19134; **Phone:** 215-427-5202; **Board Cert:** Pediatrics 1971; Neonatal-Perinatal Medicine 1975; **Med School:** Greece 1957; **Resid:** Pediatrics, Chldns Hosp 1959; Psychiatry, Colo State Hosp 1962; **Fellow:** Neonatology, Hosp Sick Chldn 1964; **Fac Appt:** Prof Ped

Hendricks-Munoz, Karen MD [NP] - **Spec Exp:** Breathing Disorders; Neonatal Neurology; Retinopathy of Prematurity; **Hospital:** NYU Med Ctr (page 68), Bellevue Hosp Ctr; **Address:** NYU Med Ctr, Dept Neonatology, 530 1st Ave, Ste HCC-7A, New York, NY 10016-6402; **Phone:** 212-263-7477; **Board Cert:** Pediatrics 1985; Neonatal-Perinatal Medicine 1987; **Med School:** Yale Univ 1978; **Resid:** Pediatrics, Yale-New Haven Hosp 1981; **Fellow:** Neonatology, Strong Meml Hosp 1984; **Fac Appt:** Assoc Prof Ped, NYU Sch Med

Holzman, Ian R MD [NP] - **Spec Exp:** Neonatal Nutrition; Necrotizing Enterocolitis; Prematurity/Low Birth Weight Infants; **Hospital:** Mount Sinai Med Ctr (page 64); **Address:** Newborn Assocs, 1 Gustave L Levy Pl, Box 1508, New York, NY 10029-6500; **Phone:** 212-241-5446; **Board Cert:** Pediatrics 1975; Neonatal-Perinatal Medicine 1977; **Med School:** Univ Pittsburgh 1971; **Resid:** Pediatrics, Chldns Hosp 1975; **Fellow:** Neonatal-Perinatal Medicine, Univ Colorado Hosp 1977; **Fac Appt:** Prof Ped, Mount Sinai Sch Med

Hurt, Hallam MD [NP] - **Spec Exp:** Neonatology; **Hospital:** Chldns Hosp of Philadelphia, The, Hosp Univ Penn - UPHS (page 60); **Address:** Chldns Hosp of Philadelphia, 3535 Market St, rm 1509, Philadelphia, PA 19104; **Phone:** 215-590-0560; **Board Cert:** Pediatrics 1976; Neonatal-Perinatal Medicine 2002; **Med School:** Univ VA Sch Med 1971; **Resid:** Pediatrics, Univ Virginia Hosp 1974; **Fellow:** Neonatal-Perinatal Medicine, Univ Virginia Hosp 1976; **Fac Appt:** Prof Ped, Temple Univ

La Gamma, Edmund F MD [NP] - **Spec Exp:** Neonatal Infections; Prematurity/Low Birth Weight Infants; Necrotizing Enterocolitis; **Hospital:** Westchester Med Ctr; **Address:** Maria Fareri Chldns Hosp, Grasslands Rd Fl 2, Valhalla, NY 10595-0001; **Phone:** 914-493-8558; **Board Cert:** Pediatrics 1981; Neonatal-Perinatal Medicine 1981; **Med School:** NY Med Coll 1976; **Resid:** Pediatrics, NY Hosp-Cornell Med Ctr 1978; **Fellow:** Neonatal-Perinatal Medicine, NY Hosp-Cornell Med Ctr 1980; Cardiovascular Disease, UCSF Med Ctr 1981; **Fac Appt:** Prof Ped, NY Med Coll

Lawson, Edward E MD [NP] - **Spec Exp:** Neonatal Critical Care; Breathing Disorders; Prematurity/Low Birth Weight Infants; **Hospital:** Johns Hopkins Hosp - Baltimore (page 61), Johns Hopkins Bayview Med Ctr (page 61); **Address:** Johns Hopkins Chldns Ctr, 600 N Wolfe St, Nelson 2-133, Baltimore, MD 21287; **Phone:** 410-955-5259; **Board Cert:** Pediatrics 1990; Neonatal-Perinatal Medicine 1997; **Med School:** Northwestern Univ 1972; **Resid:** Pediatrics, Chldns Hosp Med Ctr 1975; **Fellow:** Neonatal-Perinatal Medicine, Harvard Med Sch 1977; **Fac Appt:** Prof Ped, Johns Hopkins Univ

Nogee, Lawrence M MD [NP] - **Spec Exp:** Lung Disease in Newborns-Genetic; **Hospital:** Johns Hopkins Hosp - Baltimore (page 61); **Address:** Johns Hopkins Hosp, Div Neonatolgy, 600 N Wolfe St, Nelson 2-133, Baltimore, MD 21287-3200; **Phone:** 410-955-5259; **Board Cert:** Pediatrics 1986; Neonatal-Perinatal Medicine 1987; **Med School:** Johns Hopkins Univ 1981; **Resid:** Pediatrics, Johns Hopkins Hosp 1984; **Fellow:** Neonatal-Perinatal Medicine, Chldns Hosp Med Ctr 1986; **Fac Appt:** Assoc Prof Ped, Johns Hopkins Univ

Perlman, Jeffrey M MD [NP] - **Spec Exp:** Neonatal Critical Care; Prematurity/Low Birth Weight Infants; Neonatal Neurology; Lung Disease in Newborns; **Hospital:** NY-Presby Hosp/Weill Cornell (page 66); **Address:** 525 E 68th St, Ste N 506, New York, NY 10021; **Phone:** 212-746-3530; **Board Cert:** Pediatrics 1983; Neonatal-Perinatal Medicine 1983; **Med School:** South Africa 1974; **Resid:** Pediatrics, Johannesburg Chlds Hosp 1979; Pediatrics, St Louis Chldns Hosp 1981; **Fellow:** Neonatology, St Louis Chldns Hosp 1983; **Fac Appt:** Prof Ped, Cornell Univ-Weill Med Coll

Neonatal-Perinatal Medicine

Polin, Richard MD [NP] - **Spec Exp:** Neonatal Infections; **Hospital:** NYPresby-Morgan Stanley Children's Hosp (page 66); **Address:** Morgan Stanley Chlds Hosp of NY-Presby, 3959 Broadway, CHC 115, New York, NY 10032; **Phone:** 212-305-5827; **Board Cert:** Pediatrics 1975; Neonatal-Perinatal Medicine 1977; **Med School:** Temple Univ 1970; **Resid:** Pediatrics, Chldns Meml Hosp 1972; Pediatrics, Babies Hosp-Columbia Presby 1975; **Fellow:** Neonatal-Perinatal Medicine, Babies Hosp-Columbia Presby 1974; **Fac Appt:** Prof Ped, Columbia P&S

Short, Billie Lou MD [NP] - **Hospital:** Chldns Natl Med Ctr; **Address:** Div Neonatology, 111 Michigan Ave NW, Washington, DC 20010; **Phone:** 202-476-3314; **Board Cert:** Pediatrics 1979; Neonatal-Perinatal Medicine 1979; **Med School:** Univ Okla Coll Med 1974; **Resid:** Pediatrics, Chldn's Hosp-Oklahoma 1977; **Fellow:** Neonatal-Perinatal Medicine, Chldn's Hosp Med Ctr 1979; **Fac Appt:** Prof Ped, Geo Wash Univ

Sison, Joseph MD [NP] - **Spec Exp:** Neonatology; **Hospital:** Englewood Hosp & Med Ctr, Mount Sinai Med Ctr (page 64); **Address:** 350 Engle St, Englewood, NJ 07631-1808; **Phone:** 201-894-3321; **Board Cert:** Pediatrics 2007; Neonatal-Perinatal Medicine 2005; **Med School:** Philippines 1984; **Resid:** Pediatrics, Jersey Shore Med Ctr 1992; Neonatal-Perinatal Medicine, Vanderbilt Univ Hosp 1993; **Fellow:** Neonatal-Perinatal Medicine, New York Hosp 1995; **Fac Appt:** Clin Prof Ped, Mount Sinai Sch Med

Sola, Augusto MD [NP] - **Spec Exp:** Brain Injury; Breathing Disorders; **Hospital:** Morristown Mem Hosp; **Address:** Mid-Atlantic Neonatology Assocs, 100 Madison Ave, Box 85, Morristown, NJ 07962; **Phone:** 973-971-5488; **Board Cert:** Pediatrics 1979; Neonatal-Perinatal Medicine 1979; **Med School:** Argentina 1973; **Resid:** Pediatrics, St Vincents Hosp 1976; Pediatrics, Univ Mass Meml Med Ctr 1977; **Fellow:** Neonatal-Perinatal Medicine, Univ Mass Meml Med Ctr 1978

Zubrow, Alan B MD [NP] - **Spec Exp:** Neonatology; **Hospital:** St Christopher's Hosp for Chldn, Hahnemann Univ Hosp; **Address:** St Christopher's Hosp for Chldn, Erie Ave at Front St, Ste 2212, Philadelphia, PA 19134; **Phone:** 215-427-5202; **Board Cert:** Pediatrics 1980; Neonatal-Perinatal Medicine 1981; **Med School:** Univ Pennsylvania 1976; **Resid:** Pediatrics, Chldns Hosp 1979; **Fellow:** Neonatology, Columbia-Presby Med Ctr 1981; **Fac Appt:** Prof Ped, Drexel Univ Coll Med

Southeast

Bancalari, Eduardo MD [NP] - **Spec Exp:** Neonatology; **Hospital:** Jackson Meml Hosp; **Address:** Dept Pediatrics (R-131), PO Box 016960, Miami, FL 33101; **Phone:** 305-585-2328; **Board Cert:** Neonatal-Perinatal Medicine 1993; Pediatrics 1993; **Med School:** Chile 1966; **Resid:** Pediatrics, Hosp Luis Calvo Mackenna 1969; **Fellow:** Pediatric Cardiology, Univ Miami Med Ctr; **Fac Appt:** Prof Ped, Univ Miami Sch Med

Boyle, Robert J MD [NP] - **Spec Exp:** Neonatology; Ethics; **Hospital:** Univ Virginia Med Ctr; **Address:** UVA Hlth Sci Ctr, Dept Peds, PO Box 800386, Charlottesville, VA 22908; **Phone:** 434-924-5429; **Board Cert:** Pediatrics 1978; Neonatal-Perinatal Medicine 1979; **Med School:** Johns Hopkins Univ 1973; **Resid:** Pediatrics, Rainbow Babies Chldns Hosp 1976; **Fellow:** Neonatal-Perinatal Medicine, Women & Infants Hosp 1978; **Fac Appt:** Prof Ped, Univ VA Sch Med

Bucciarelli, Richard L MD [NP] - **Spec Exp:** Neonatal Cardiology; **Hospital:** Shands at Univ of FL; **Address:** Shands Healthcare, 1600 SW Archer Rd, rm M105, Gainesville, FL 32610; **Phone:** 352-392-3337; **Board Cert:** Pediatrics 1977; Neonatal-Perinatal Medicine 1977; Pediatric Cardiology 1977; **Med School:** Univ Mich Med Sch 1972; **Resid:** Pediatrics, Shands Hosp-Univ Fla 1975; **Fellow:** Neonatal-Perinatal Medicine, Shands Hosp-Univ Fla 1977; **Fac Appt:** Prof Ped, Univ Fla Coll Med

America's Top Doctors® 8th Edition

Holtzman, Ronald B MD [NP] - **Spec Exp:** Neonatology; Lung Disease in Newborns; **Hospital:** Gaston Meml Hosp; **Address:** Gaston Meml Hosp, NICU Office, 2525 Court Drive, Gastonia, NC 28054-2140; **Phone:** 704-834-3390; **Board Cert:** Pediatrics 1987; Neonatal-Perinatal Medicine 2004; **Med School:** Rush Med Coll 1983; **Resid:** Pediatrics, Chldns Meml/Northwestern Univ 1986; **Fellow:** Neonatal-Perinatal Medicine, Chldns Meml/Northwestern Univ 1986

Kattwinkel, John MD [NP] - **Spec Exp:** Lung Disease in Newborns; Sudden Infant Death Syndrome (SIDS); **Hospital:** Univ Virginia Med Ctr; **Address:** Univ Va Hosp, Div Neonatology, Dept Peds, PO Box 800386, Charlottesville, VA 22908-0386; **Phone:** 434-924-5428; **Board Cert:** Pediatrics 1986; Neonatal-Perinatal Medicine 1986; **Med School:** Harvard Med Sch 1968; **Resid:** Pediatrics, Duke Univ Med Ctr 1970; **Fellow:** Neonatology, Case-West Res Univ 1974; **Fac Appt:** Prof Ped, Univ VA Sch Med

Neu, Josef MD [NP] - **Spec Exp:** Neonatal Nutrition; Neonatal Gastroenterology; **Hospital:** Shands at Univ of FL; **Address:** Shands Healthcare-Univ Fla, 1600 SW Archer Rd, rm HD513, Gainesville, FL 32610; **Phone:** 352-392-3020; **Board Cert:** Pediatrics 1980; Neonatal-Perinatal Medicine 1981; **Med School:** Univ Wisc 1975; **Resid:** Pediatrics, Johns Hopkins Hosp 1978; **Fellow:** Neonatal-Perinatal Medicine, Stanford Univ 1980; **Fac Appt:** Prof Ped, Univ Fla Coll Med

Stiles, Alan MD [NP] - **Spec Exp:** Neonatology; **Hospital:** Univ NC Hosps; **Address:** 130 Mason Farm Rd, CB7220, Chapel Hill, NC 27599-7220; **Phone:** 919-966-4427; **Board Cert:** Pediatrics 1984; Neonatal-Perinatal Medicine 1985; **Med School:** Univ NC Sch Med 1977; **Resid:** Pediatrics, North Carolina Meml Hosp 1982; **Fellow:** Neonatal-Perinatal Medicine, Chldns Hosp/Brigham Hosp 1985; **Fac Appt:** Prof Ped, Univ NC Sch Med

Midwest

Bell, Edward F MD [NP] - **Spec Exp:** Neonatal Critical Care; Prematurity/Low Birth Weight Infants; **Hospital:** Univ Iowa Hosp & Clinics, Genesis Med Ctr; **Address:** Univ Iowa Hosps, Dept Pediatrics, 200 Hawkins Drive, rm 8811 JPP, Iowa City, IA 52242; **Phone:** 319-356-4006; **Board Cert:** Pediatrics 1978; Neonatal-Perinatal Medicine 1995; **Med School:** Columbia P&S 1973; **Resid:** Pediatrics, Babies Hosp-Columbia Presby 1976; **Fellow:** Neonatology, McMaster Univ Med Ctr 1977; Neonatology, Women & Infants Hosp-Brown Univ 1979; **Fac Appt:** Prof Ped, Univ Iowa Coll Med

Cole, Francis Sessions MD [NP] - **Spec Exp:** Neonatal Chronic Lung Disease (CLD); Respiratory Distress Syndrome (RDS); Surfactant Biology; Prematurity/Low Birth Weight Infants; **Hospital:** St Louis Chldns Hosp, Barnes-Jewish Hosp; **Address:** St Louis Chldns Hosp, 1 Children's Pl, Box 8116/NWT, St Louis, MO 63110; **Phone:** 314-454-6148; **Board Cert:** Pediatrics 1980; Neonatal-Perinatal Medicine 1983; **Med School:** Yale Univ 1973; **Resid:** Pediatrics, Chldns Hosp Med Ctr 1978; **Fellow:** Neonatology, Brigham & Womens Hosp 1981; **Fac Appt:** Prof Ped, Washington Univ, St Louis

Donn, Steven M MD [NP] - **Spec Exp:** Breathing Disorders; Respiratory Distress Syndrome (RDS); Pulmonary Hypertension of Newborn (PPHN); Surfactant Biology; **Hospital:** Mott Chldns Hosp; **Address:** F5790 Mott Hosp/ 0254, 1500 E Med Ctr Drive, Ann Arbor, MI 48109-0999; **Phone:** 734-763-4109; **Board Cert:** Pediatrics 1981; Neonatal-Perinatal Medicine 1981; **Med School:** Tulane Univ 1974; **Resid:** Pediatrics, Univ Vermont Med Ctr 1978; **Fellow:** Neonatology, Univ Michigan 1980; **Fac Appt:** Prof Ped, Univ Mich Med Sch

Gewolb, Ira MD [NP] - **Spec Exp:** Breathing Disorders; **Hospital:** Mich State Univ-Sparrow Hos; **Address:** Sparrow Hosp, Div Neonatology, 1215 E Michigan Ave, Lansing, MI 48912; **Phone:** 517-364-2670; **Board Cert:** Pediatrics 1980; Neonatal-Perinatal Medicine 1981; **Med School:** Yale Univ 1976; **Resid:** Pediatrics, Childrens Hosp Med Ctr 1979; **Fellow:** Neonatology, Yale Univ 1981; **Fac Appt:** Prof Ped, Mich State Univ

Neonatal-Perinatal Medicine

Hamvas, Aaron MD [NP] - **Spec Exp:** Lung Disease in Newborns-Genetic; **Hospital:** St Louis Chldns Hosp, Barnes-Jewish Hosp; **Address:** St Louis Chldns Hosp, One Childrens Place, NICU-5th Fl, St Louis, MO 63110; **Phone:** 314-454-6148; **Board Cert:** Pediatrics 1989; Neonatal-Perinatal Medicine 2006; **Med School:** Washington Univ, St Louis 1981; **Resid:** Pediatrics, St Louis Chldns Hosp 1984; **Fellow:** Neonatology, St Louis Chldns Hosp 1990; **Fac Appt:** Prof Ped, Washington Univ, St Louis

Lemons, James A MD [NP] - **Spec Exp:** Nutrition; Ethics; **Hospital:** Riley Hosp for Children, Indiana Univ Hosp; **Address:** 699 West Drive, RR-208, Indianapolis, IN 46202-5119; **Phone:** 317-274-4716; **Board Cert:** Pediatrics 1993; Neonatal-Perinatal Medicine 1993; **Med School:** North-western Univ 1969; **Resid:** Pediatrics, Univ Mich Med Sch 1972; **Fellow:** Neonatal-Perinatal Medicine, Univ Colo Med Ctr 1975; **Fac Appt:** Prof Ped, Indiana Univ

Martin, Richard J MD [NP] - **Spec Exp:** Breathing Disorders; **Hospital:** Rainbow Babies & Chldns Hosp; **Address:** 11100 Euclid Ave, Cleveland, OH 44106-6010; **Phone:** 216-844-3387; **Board Cert:** Pediatrics 1976; Neonatal-Perinatal Medicine 2005; **Med School:** Australia 1970; **Resid:** Pediatrics, Univ Missouri 1973; **Fellow:** Neonatal-Perinatal Medicine, Case West Res Univ 1975; **Fac Appt:** Prof Ped, Case West Res Univ

Meadow, William MD/PhD [NP] - **Spec Exp:** Infections-Neonatal; Ethics; **Hospital:** Univ of Chicago Hosps; **Address:** 5841 S Maryland Ave, MC-6060, Chicago, IL 60637; **Phone:** 773-702-6210; **Board Cert:** Pediatrics 1979; Neonatal-Perinatal Medicine 1981; **Med School:** Univ Pennsyl-vania 1974; **Resid:** Pediatrics, Chldns Meml Hosp 1978; **Fellow:** Neonatology, Wyler Chldns Hosp 1981; Infectious Disease, Wyler Chldns Hosp 1981; **Fac Appt:** Prof Ped, Univ Chicago-Pritzker Sch Med

Muraskas, Jonathan MD [NP] - **Spec Exp:** Prematurity/Low Birth Weight Infants; Multiple Gestation; Conjoined Twins; Ethics; **Hospital:** Loyola Univ Med Ctr; **Address:** Loyola University Med-ical Ctr, Bldg 107, 2160 S First Ave Fl 5 - rm 5810, Maywood, IL 60153-5500; **Phone:** 708-216-1067; **Board Cert:** Pediatrics 1987; Neonatal-Perinatal Medicine 1987; **Med School:** Loyola Univ-Stritch Sch Med 1982; **Resid:** Pediatrics, Loyola Univ Med Ctr 1985; **Fellow:** Neonatal-Perinatal Medicine, Loyola Univ Med Ctr 1987; **Fac Appt:** Prof Ped, Loyola Univ-Stritch Sch Med

Steinhorn, Robin H MD [NP] - **Spec Exp:** Pulmonary Hypertension; **Hospital:** Children's Mem Hosp, Northwestern Meml Hosp; **Address:** 2300 Children's Plaza, Box 45, Chicago, IL 60614; **Phone:** 773-880-4142; **Board Cert:** Pediatrics 2000; Neonatal-Perinatal Medicine 2002; **Med School:** Washington Univ, St Louis 1980; **Resid:** Obstetrics & Gynecology, Barnes Hosp 1983; Pedi-atrics, Univ Minn 1986; **Fellow:** Neonatal-Perinatal Medicine, Univ Minn 1988; **Fac Appt:** Prof Ped, Northwestern Univ

Whitsett, Jeffrey A MD [NP] - **Spec Exp:** Lung Disease in Newborns-Genetic; **Hospital:** Cincinnati Chldns Hosp Med Ctr, Good Samaritan Hosp - Cincinnati; **Address:** Cincinnati Chldns Hosp, Div Neonatalogy, 3333 Burnet Ave, Cincinnati, OH 45229-3039; **Phone:** 513-636-4830; **Board Cert:** Pediatrics 1979; Neonatal-Perinatal Medicine 1979; **Med School:** Columbia P&S 1973; **Resid:** Pediatrics, Mt Sinai Hosp 1976; **Fellow:** Neonatology, Chldns Hosp Med Ctr 1977; **Fac Appt:** Prof Ped, Univ Cincinnati

America's Top Doctors® 8th Edition

Great Plains and Mountains

Milley, J Ross MD/PhD [NP] - **Spec Exp:** Nutrition; **Hospital:** Primary Children's Med Ctr, Univ Utah Hosps and Clins; **Address:** Univ Utah - Dept Pediatrics/Neonatology, Williams Bldg, PO Box 581289, Salt Lake City, UT 84158; **Phone:** 801-581-7085; **Board Cert:** Pediatrics 1980; Neonatal-Perinatal Medicine 1981; **Med School:** Univ Chicago-Pritzker Sch Med 1975; **Resid:** Pediatrics, Johns Hopkins Hosp 1978; **Fellow:** Neonatology, Johns Hopkins Hosp 1980; **Fac Appt:** Prof Ped, Univ Utah

Zach, Terence MD [NP] - **Spec Exp:** Neonatal Critical Care; **Hospital:** Creighton Univ Med Ctr; **Address:** 600 S 42nd St, Omaha, NE 68198; **Phone:** 402-559-6750; **Board Cert:** Pediatrics 1987; Neonatal-Perinatal Medicine 2004; **Med School:** Univ Nebr Coll Med 1983; **Resid:** Pediatrics, Univ Nebr Med Ctr 1986; **Fellow:** Neonatology, Univ Minnesota 1986; **Fac Appt:** Prof Ped, Creighton Univ

Southwest

Adams, James M MD [NP] - **Spec Exp:** Lung Disease in Newborns; **Hospital:** Texas Chldns Hosp - Houston; **Address:** 6621 Fannin St, MC WT-6104, Houston, TX 77030; **Phone:** 832-826-1380; **Board Cert:** Pediatrics 1975; Neonatal-Perinatal Medicine 1975; **Med School:** Baylor Coll Med 1970; **Resid:** Pediatrics, Baylor Affil Hosps 1973; **Fellow:** Neonatal-Perinatal Medicine, Baylor Affil Hosps 1975; **Fac Appt:** Prof Ped, Baylor Coll Med

Denson, Susan E MD [NP] - **Spec Exp:** Neonatology; **Hospital:** Meml Hermann Hosp - Texas Med Ctr, LBJ General Hosp; **Address:** Univ Tex Houston Med Sch, Dept Peds, 6431 Fannin, Ste 3.256, Houston, TX 77030; **Phone:** 713-500-5727; **Board Cert:** Pediatrics 1978; Neonatal-Perinatal Medicine 1979; **Med School:** Univ Tex SW, Dallas 1972; **Resid:** Pediatrics, Univ Ariz 1974; **Fellow:** Neonatal-Perinatal Medicine, Univ Ariz 1975; Neonatal-Perinatal Medicine, Univ Tex Med Sch 1976; **Fac Appt:** Prof Ped, Univ Tex, Houston

Escobedo, Marilyn B MD [NP] - **Spec Exp:** Neonatology; Nutrition; **Hospital:** Chldns Hosp OU Med Ctr; **Address:** 1200 Everett Dr, 7th Fl, North Pavilion, Oklahoma City, OK 73104; **Phone:** 405-271-5215; **Board Cert:** Pediatrics 1986; Neonatal-Perinatal Medicine 2004; **Med School:** Washington Univ, St Louis 1970; **Resid:** Pediatrics, Chldns Hosp 1972; Neonatal-Perinatal Medicine, Chldns Hosp 1973; **Fellow:** Neonatal-Perinatal Medicine, Vanderbilt Univ 1976; **Fac Appt:** Prof Ped, Univ Okla Coll Med

Garcia-Prats, Joseph MD [NP] - **Spec Exp:** Lung Disease in Newborns; Neonatology; **Hospital:** Texas Chldns Hosp - Houston, Ben Taub Genl Hosp; **Address:** 6621 Fannin St, MC WT-6104, Houston, TX 77030-1608; **Phone:** 832-826-1380; **Board Cert:** Pediatrics 1977; Neonatal-Perinatal Medicine 1977; **Med School:** Tulane Univ 1972; **Resid:** Pediatrics, Baylor Affil Hosp 1975; **Fellow:** Neonatal-Perinatal Medicine, Baylor Affil Hosp 1977; **Fac Appt:** Prof Ped, Baylor Coll Med

Odom, Michael W MD [NP] - **Spec Exp:** Neonatology; **Hospital:** Univ Hlth Sys - Univ Hosp (San Antonio, TX); **Address:** Dept Peds, 7703 Floyd Curl Drive, MC 7812, San Antonio, TX 78229-3900; **Phone:** 210-567-5225; **Board Cert:** Pediatrics 1987; Neonatal-Perinatal Medicine 2004; **Med School:** Univ Tex SW, Dallas 1983; **Resid:** Pediatrics, Vanderbilt Univ Affil Hosps 1986; **Fellow:** Neonatal-Perinatal Medicine, Mt Zion Med Ctr-UCSF 1989; **Fac Appt:** Assoc Prof Ped, Univ Tex, San Antonio

Neonatal-Perinatal Medicine

Seidner, Steven R MD [NP] - **Spec Exp:** Neonatal Chronic Lung Disease (CLD); Respiratory Distress Syndrome (RDS); Pulmonary Hypertension of Newborn (PPHN); **Hospital:** Univ Hlth Sys - Univ Hosp (San Antonio, TX); **Address:** Univ Texas Hlth Sci Ctr, Dept Peds, 7703 Floyd Curl Drive, MC 7812, San Antonio, TX 78229-3901; **Phone:** 210-567-5229; **Board Cert:** Pediatrics 1987; Neonatal-Perinatal Medicine 1987; **Med School:** Univ Ariz Coll Med 1982; **Resid:** Pediatrics, Harbor-UCLA Med Ctr 1985; **Fellow:** Neonatal-Perinatal Medicine, Harbor-UCLA Med Ctr 1988; **Fac Appt:** Prof Ped, Univ Tex, San Antonio

Tyson, Jon E MD [NP] - **Spec Exp:** Neonatology; Epidemiology; **Hospital:** Meml Hermann Hosp - Texas Med Ctr; **Address:** Univ Tex, Ctr Clin Rsch, 6431 Fannin St, Ste 2.106, Houston, TX 77030; **Phone:** 713-500-5651; **Board Cert:** Pediatrics 1973; Neonatal-Perinatal Medicine 1975; **Med School:** Tulane Univ 1968; **Resid:** Pediatrics, Univ Tenn/Memphis Hosp 1971; **Fellow:** Neonatology, McMaster Univ 1975; **Fac Appt:** Prof Ped, Univ Tex, Houston

West Coast and Pacific

Ariagno, Ronald L MD [NP] - **Spec Exp:** Sudden Infant Death Syndrome (SIDS); Breathing Disorders; **Hospital:** Stanford Univ Med Ctr; **Address:** Stanford Univ, Div Neonatology, 750 Welch Rd, Ste 315, Palo Alto, CA 94304; **Phone:** 650-723-5711; **Board Cert:** Pediatrics 1973; Neonatal-Perinatal Medicine 1975; **Med School:** Univ IL Coll Med 1968; **Resid:** Pediatrics, Presby-St Lukes Hosp 1971; **Fellow:** Neonatology, Chldns Hosp, UCSF 1975; **Fac Appt:** Prof Ped, Stanford Univ

Stevenson, David K MD [NP] - **Spec Exp:** Neonatology; **Hospital:** Lucile Packard Chldns Hosp/Stanford Univ Med Ctr; **Address:** 750 Welch Rd, Ste 315, Palo Alto, CA 94304-1510; **Phone:** 650-723-5711; **Board Cert:** Pediatrics 1979; Neonatal-Perinatal Medicine 2004; **Med School:** Univ Wash 1975; **Resid:** Pediatrics, Univ Washington 1977; **Fellow:** Neonatal-Perinatal Medicine, Stanford Univ 1979; **Fac Appt:** Prof Ped, Stanford Univ

NYU Langone Medical Center

550 First Avenue (at 31St Street)
New York, NY 10016
Physician Referral:
(888)7-NYU-MED (888-769-8633)
www.nyumc.org

NEONATAL PERINATAL MEDICINE

The typical NICU is full of bright lights, loud noises and round-the-clock activity. So much sensory input at such an early age can give newborn babies a lot of stress, which may have a negative impact on their development.

Recently, NYU Langone Medical Center redesigned its NICU surroundings to provide positive early experiences — and simultaneously enhance the quality of medical care. Visitors to the NICU at Tisch Hospital will see covered incubators, drawn shades, and parents holding pre-term infants skin-to-skin in a quiet, relaxed setting. NYU School of Medicine's studies have shown dramatic decreases in length of hospitalization and in the number and severity of complications. This approach has also decreased the need for ventilator support and the risk of chronic lung disease. It has also been shown to enhance weight gain and improve overall neurological development.

Because many premature babies may be at increased risk for problems in growth and development, our Continuing Care Program is designed to follow these infants from birth through pre-school, providing evaluation and assessment of any problems as soon as they arise.

Of course, the ideal time to correct fetal problems is when infants are still in the womb. Using minimally invasive techniques, doctors at NYU Langone Medical Center are able to repair a number of life-threatening conditions in a child before it is even born. These techniques reduce the risks of pre-term labor and the need for cesarean births.

Nephrology
a subspecialty of Internal Medicine

An internist who treats disorders of the kidney, high blood pressure, fluid and mineral balance and dialysis of body wastes when the kidneys do not function. This specialist consults with surgeons about kidney transplantation.

Training Required: Three years in internal medicine *plus* additional training and examination for certification in nephrology.

NEPHROLOGY

New England

Aronson, Peter S MD [Nep] - **Spec Exp:** Electrolyte Disorders; Kidney Stones; **Hospital:** Yale-New Haven Hosp, VA Conn Hlthcre Sys; **Address:** Yale Sch Med, Dept Medicine, PO Box 208029, New Haven, CT 06520-8029; **Phone:** 203-785-4186; **Board Cert:** Internal Medicine 1973; Nephrology 1976; **Med School:** NYU Sch Med 1970; **Resid:** Internal Medicine, NC Meml Hosp 1972; **Fellow:** Nephrology, Yale-New Haven Hosp 1977; **Fac Appt:** Prof Med, Yale Univ

Bazari, Hasan MD [Nep] - **Spec Exp:** Kidney Failure-Acute; Nephrotic Syndrome; Hypertension; **Hospital:** Mass Genl Hosp; **Address:** Renal Assocs, Mass Genl Hospital, 55 Fruit St Gray Bldg - Ste 1003, Boston, MA 02114; **Phone:** 617-726-5050; **Board Cert:** Internal Medicine 1986; Nephrology 1988; **Med School:** Albert Einstein Coll Med 1983; **Resid:** Internal Medicine, Mass Genl Hosp 1986; **Fellow:** Nephrology, Mass Genl Hosp 1988

Brenner, Barry M MD [Nep] - **Spec Exp:** Hypertension; Diabetic Kidney Disease; Kidney Failure-Acute; Kidney Failure-Chronic; **Hospital:** Brigham & Women's Hosp; **Address:** Brigham & Women's Hosp, Renal Div, 75 Francis St, Boston, MA 02115; **Phone:** 617-732-5850; **Med School:** Univ Pittsburgh 1962; **Resid:** Internal Medicine, Albert Einstein Coll Med 1966; **Fellow:** Nephrology, Nat Inst Health 1969; **Fac Appt:** Prof Med, Harvard Med Sch

Coggins, Cecil MD [Nep] - **Spec Exp:** Kidney Disease; Hypertension; **Hospital:** Mass Genl Hosp; **Address:** 185 Cambridge St, Ste 501, Boston, MA 02114-2712; **Phone:** 617-726-4900; **Board Cert:** Internal Medicine 1965; Nephrology 1974; **Med School:** Harvard Med Sch 1958; **Resid:** Internal Medicine, Stanford Univ Med Ctr 1965; Internal Medicine; **Fellow:** Nephrology, Stanford Univ Med Ctr 1963; Nephrology, Mass Genl Hosp 1967; **Fac Appt:** Assoc Prof Med, Harvard Med Sch

Kliger, Alan MD [Nep] - **Spec Exp:** Kidney Disease; Kidney Disease-Metabolic; **Hospital:** Hosp of St Raphael; **Address:** 136 Sherman Ave, New Haven, CT 06511-5238; **Phone:** 203-787-0117 x307; **Board Cert:** Internal Medicine 1973; Nephrology 1976; **Med School:** SUNY Upstate Med Univ 1970; **Resid:** Internal Medicine, SUNY Upstate Med Ctr 1973; **Fellow:** Nephrology, Georgetown Univ Hosp 1975; **Fac Appt:** Clin Prof Med, Yale Univ

Perrone, Ronald MD [Nep] - **Spec Exp:** Kidney Disease-Chronic; Kidney Failure-Acute; Polycystic Kidney Disease; **Hospital:** Tufts Med Ctr; **Address:** Tufts-New Eng Med Ctr, Div Nephrology, 750 Washington St, Box 391, Boston, MA 02111; **Phone:** 617-636-5866; **Board Cert:** Internal Medicine 1979; Nephrology 1982; **Med School:** Hahnemann Univ 1975; **Resid:** Internal Medicine, Grady Meml Hosp 1978; **Fellow:** Nephrology, Boston Med Ctr 1982; **Fac Appt:** Prof Med, Tufts Univ

Salant, David MD [Nep] - **Spec Exp:** Kidney Disease-Glomerular; Kidney Disease-Autoimmune; Lupus Nephritis; **Hospital:** Boston Med Ctr; **Address:** 720 Harrison Ave, Boston, MA 02118-2371; **Phone:** 617-638-7480; **Board Cert:** Internal Medicine 1978; Nephrology 1980; **Med School:** South Africa 1969; **Resid:** Internal Medicine, Johannesburg Genl Hosp 1973; **Fellow:** Nephrology, Boston Univ Med Ctr 1978; **Fac Appt:** Prof Med, Boston Univ

Seifter, Julian L MD [Nep] - **Spec Exp:** Diabetic Kidney Disease; Kidney Failure-Chronic; Kidney Stones; **Hospital:** Brigham & Women's Hosp; **Address:** Brigham & Women's Hosp, Div Renal Med, 75 Francis St, MRB-4, Boston, MA 02115; **Phone:** 617-732-6383; **Board Cert:** Internal Medicine 1978; Nephrology 1980; **Med School:** Albert Einstein Coll Med 1975; **Resid:** Internal Medicine, Bronx Muni Hosp Ctr 1981; **Fellow:** Nephrology, Yale-New Haven Hosp 1982; **Fac Appt:** Assoc Prof Med, Harvard Med Sch

Tolkoff-Rubin, Nina MD [Nep] - **Spec Exp:** Transplant Medicine-Kidney; Hypertension; Kidney Failure-Acute; **Hospital:** Mass Genl Hosp; **Address:** 55 Fruit St, GRB 103J, Boston, MA 02114; **Phone:** 617-726-3706; **Board Cert:** Nephrology 1974; Internal Medicine 1972; **Med School:** Harvard Med Sch 1968; **Resid:** Internal Medicine, Mass Genl Hosp 1970; Internal Medicine, Mass Genl Hosp 1972; **Fellow:** Nephrology, Mass Genl Hosp 1971; **Fac Appt:** Assoc Prof Med, Harvard Med Sch

Mid Atlantic

Appel, Gerald MD [Nep] - **Spec Exp:** Glomerulonephritis; Lupus Nephritis; Nephrotic Syndrome; **Hospital:** NY-Presby Hosp/Columbia (page 66); **Address:** 622 W 168th St, Ste PH4-124, New York, NY 10032-3720; **Phone:** 212-305-3273; **Board Cert:** Internal Medicine 1975; Nephrology 1978; **Med School:** Albert Einstein Coll Med 1972; **Resid:** Internal Medicine, Columbia Presby Hosp 1975; **Fellow:** Nephrology, Columbia Presby Hosp 1976; Nephrology, Yale-New Haven Hosp 1978; **Fac Appt:** Clin Prof Med, Columbia P&S

August, Phyllis MD [Nep] - **Spec Exp:** Hypertension; Hypertension in Pregnancy; **Hospital:** NY-Presby Hosp/Weill Cornell (page 66); **Address:** 525 E 68th St, Ste L-1, Hypertension Center, New York, NY 10021-4870; **Phone:** 212-746-2210; **Board Cert:** Internal Medicine 1980; Nephrology 1982; **Med School:** Yale Univ 1977; **Resid:** Internal Medicine, NY Hosp-Cornell Med Ctr 1980; **Fellow:** Nephrology, NY Hosp-Cornell Med Ctr 1983; **Fac Appt:** Prof Med, Cornell Univ-Weill Med Coll

Black, Henry R MD [Nep] - **Spec Exp:** Hypertension; Cholesterol/Lipid Disorders; Preventive Cardiology; **Hospital:** NYU Med Ctr (page 68); **Address:** NYU Medical Ctr, 530 First Ave, Skirvul 9U, New York, NY 10016; **Phone:** 212-263-5571; **Board Cert:** Internal Medicine 1972; Nephrology 1974; **Med School:** NYU Sch Med 1967; **Resid:** Internal Medicine, Johns Hopkins Hosp 1971; Internal Medicine, Yale-New Haven Hosp 1972; **Fellow:** Nephrology, Yale-New Haven Hosp 1974; **Fac Appt:** Prof Med, NYU Sch Med

Blumenfeld, Jon D MD [Nep] - **Spec Exp:** Hypertension; Polycystic Kidney Disease; Adrenal Disorders; **Hospital:** NY-Presby Hosp/Weill Cornell (page 66), Rockefeller Univ; **Address:** The Rogosin Institute, 505 E 70th St, rm HT230, New York, NY 10021; **Phone:** 212-746-1495; **Board Cert:** Internal Medicine 1984; Nephrology 1986; **Med School:** Yale Univ 1981; **Resid:** Internal Medicine, NY Hosp-Cornell Med Ctr 1984; **Fellow:** Nephrology, Brigham & Womens Hosp 1988; **Fac Appt:** Prof Med, Cornell Univ-Weill Med Coll

Cohen, David J MD [Nep] - **Spec Exp:** Transplant Medicine-Kidney; Glomerulonephritis; **Hospital:** NY-Presby Hosp/Columbia (page 66); **Address:** Columbia Univ Med Ctr, 622 W 168th St, rm PH 4-124, New York, NY 10032-3720; **Phone:** 212-305-3273; **Board Cert:** Internal Medicine 1980; Nephrology 1984; **Med School:** Albert Einstein Coll Med 1977; **Resid:** Internal Medicine, Mount Sinai Hosp 1980; **Fellow:** Nephrology, Columbia Presby Med Ctr 1981; Transplant Immunobiology, Brigham & Women's Hosp 1983; **Fac Appt:** Assoc Prof Med, Columbia P&S

Nephrology

Johnston, James R MD [Nep] - **Spec Exp:** Diabetic Kidney Disease; Hypertension; **Hospital:** UPMC Presby, Pittsburgh; **Address:** Univ Pittsburgh Physicians, Renal Div, 3550 Terrace St, Scaife Hall, rm A915, Pittsburgh, PA 15261; **Phone:** 412-802-3043; **Board Cert:** Internal Medicine 1982; Nephrology 1984; **Med School:** Univ Pittsburgh 1979; **Resid:** Internal Medicine, Montefiore Hosp 1982; **Fellow:** Nephrology, Univ Pittsburgh Med Ctr 1983; Nephrology, Brigham & Women's Hosp 1986; **Fac Appt:** Prof Med, Univ Pittsburgh

Kelepouris, Ellie MD [Nep] - **Spec Exp:** Kidney Stones; Hypertension; **Hospital:** Temple Univ Hosp; **Address:** 3322 N Broad St, Medical Office Bldg, Ste 201, Philadelphia, PA 19140; **Phone:** 215-707-7944; **Board Cert:** Nephrology 1997; **Med School:** Greece 1976; **Resid:** Internal Medicine, Mercy Cath Med Ctr 1979; **Fellow:** Nephrology, Hosp U Penn 1982; **Fac Appt:** Prof Med, Temple Univ

Kobrin, Sidney M MD [Nep] - **Spec Exp:** Diabetic Kidney Disease; Kidney Failure; Hypertension; **Hospital:** Hosp Univ Penn - UPHS (page 60); **Address:** Hosp Univ Penn, Div Nephrology, 3400 Spruce St 210 White Bldg, Philadelphia, PA 19104; **Phone:** 215-662-2638; **Board Cert:** Nephrology 2002; **Med School:** South Africa 1978; **Resid:** Internal Medicine, Johannesburg Tchg Hosp 1984; **Fellow:** Nephrology, Einstein Med Ctr 1988; **Fac Appt:** Assoc Prof Med, Univ Pennsylvania

Piraino, Beth Marie MD [Nep] - **Spec Exp:** Kidney Failure; Hypertension; **Hospital:** UPMC Presby, Pittsburgh; **Address:** 3504 Fifth Ave, Ste 200, Pittsburgh, PA 15213; **Phone:** 412-383-4899; **Board Cert:** Internal Medicine 1980; Nephrology 1982; **Med School:** Med Coll PA Hahnemann 1977; **Resid:** Internal Medicine, Presby Univ Hosp 1980; **Fellow:** Nephrology, Presby Univ Hosp 1982; **Fac Appt:** Prof Med, Univ Pittsburgh

Rudnick, Michael R MD [Nep] - **Spec Exp:** Hypertension; Kidney Disease; **Hospital:** Penn Presby Med Ctr - UPHS (page 60); **Address:** Presbyterian Medical Ctr, Medical Office Bldg, 39th and Market Sts, Ste 240, Philadelphia, PA 19104; **Phone:** 215-662-8730; **Board Cert:** Internal Medicine 1975; Nephrology 1976; **Med School:** Hahnemann Univ 1972; **Resid:** Internal Medicine, Hahnemann U Med Ctr 1974; **Fellow:** Nephrology, Hosp U Penn 1976; **Fac Appt:** Assoc Prof Med, Univ Pennsylvania

Scheinman, Steven J MD [Nep] - **Spec Exp:** Kidney Stones; Bartter's Syndrome; Gitelman's Syndrome; **Hospital:** Univ. Hosp.- SUNY Upstate, Crouse Hosp; **Address:** SUNY Upstate Med Univ, Office of the Dean, 750 E Adams St, Syracuse, NY 13210; **Phone:** 315-464-9720; **Board Cert:** Internal Medicine 1980; Nephrology 1984; **Med School:** Yale Univ 1977; **Resid:** Internal Medicine, Yale New Haven Hosp 1990; Internal Medicine, Upstate Med Ctr 1981; **Fellow:** Nephrology, Upstate Med Ctr 1983; Nephrology, Yale New Haven Hosp 1984; **Fac Appt:** Prof Med, SUNY Upstate Med Univ

Townsend, Raymond R MD [Nep] - **Spec Exp:** Hypertension-Complex; Renal Artery Stenosis; **Hospital:** Hosp Univ Penn - UPHS (page 60); **Address:** Hosp Univ Pennsylvania, Renal Electrolyte/Hypertension Div, 3400 Spruce St, 210 White Bldg, Philadelphia, PA 19104; **Phone:** 215-662-2638; **Board Cert:** Internal Medicine 1982; Nephrology 1984; **Med School:** Hahnemann Univ 1979; **Resid:** Internal Medicine, Allegheny Genl Hosp 1982; **Fellow:** Nephrology, Temple Univ Hosp 1984; **Fac Appt:** Assoc Prof Med, Univ Pennsylvania

Umans, Jason MD/PhD [Nep] - **Spec Exp:** Hypertension/Kidney Disease in Pregnancy; Kidney Disease; Hypertension; **Hospital:** Georgetown Univ Hosp, Washington Hosp Ctr; **Address:** 3800 Reservoir Rd NW, PHC Bldg- Fl 6, Washington, DC 20007; **Phone:** 202-444-9183; **Board Cert:** Internal Medicine 1988; Nephrology 2000; **Med School:** Cornell Univ-Weill Med Coll 1984; **Resid:** Internal Medicine, Univ Chicago Hosps 1987; **Fellow:** Nephrology, Univ Chicago Hosps 1988; **Fac Appt:** Assoc Prof Med, Georgetown Univ

Wilcox, Christopher S MD [Nep] - **Spec Exp:** Hypertension-Renovascular; Hypertension-Drug Resistent; **Hospital:** Georgetown Univ Hosp; **Address:** Georgetown Univ Med Ctr, 3800 Reservoir Rd NW, PHC Fl 6th, Washington, DC 20007-2113; **Phone:** 202-444-9183; **Board Cert:** Internal Medicine 1983; Nephrology 1986; **Med School:** England 1968; **Resid:** Internal Medicine, Middlesex Hosp 1971; Nephrology, Middlesex Hosp 1972; **Fellow:** Nephrology, Middlesex Hosp 1975; **Fac Appt:** Prof Med, Georgetown Univ

Southeast

Allon, Michael MD [Nep] - **Spec Exp:** Dialysis Care; **Hospital:** Univ of Ala Hosp at Birmingham; **Address:** 1530 3rd Ave S, PB226, Birmingham, AL 35294; **Phone:** 205-975-9676; **Board Cert:** Internal Medicine 1985; Nephrology 1988; **Med School:** Univ Mich Med Sch 1982; **Resid:** Internal Medicine, Emory Univ Hosp 1985; **Fellow:** Nephrology, Emory Univ 1987; **Fac Appt:** Prof Med, Univ Ala

Bolton, W Kline MD [Nep] - **Spec Exp:** Kidney Disease-Glomerular; Kidney Disease-Chronic; **Hospital:** Univ Virginia Med Ctr; **Address:** Univ VA Hlth Scis Ctr, Box 800 133, Charlottesville, VA 22908-0001; **Phone:** 434-924-5125; **Board Cert:** Internal Medicine 1972; Nephrology 1974; **Med School:** Univ VA Sch Med 1969; **Resid:** Internal Medicine, Boston City Hosp 1971; **Fellow:** Nephrology, Univ Chicago 1973; **Fac Appt:** Prof Med, Univ VA Sch Med

Coffman, Thomas M MD [Nep] - **Spec Exp:** Transplant Medicine-Kidney; Hypertension; **Hospital:** VA Med Ctr - Durham, Duke Univ Med Ctr; **Address:** Duke Univ Med Center, Box 103015, Durham, NC 27710; **Phone:** 919-684-9788; **Board Cert:** Internal Medicine 1983; Nephrology 1988; **Med School:** Ohio State Univ 1980; **Resid:** Internal Medicine, Duke Univ Med Ctr 1983; **Fellow:** Nephrology, Duke Univ Med Ctr 1985; **Fac Appt:** Prof Med, Duke Univ

Falk, Ronald J MD [Nep] - **Spec Exp:** Glomerulonephritis; Lupus Nephritis; Wegener's Granulomatosis; Vasculitis; **Hospital:** Univ NC Hosps; **Address:** Univ North Carolina Kidney Ctr, 7024 Burnett Womack Bldg CB #7155, Chapel Hill, NC 27599-7155; **Phone:** 919-966-2561; **Board Cert:** Internal Medicine 1980; Nephrology 1982; **Med School:** Univ NC Sch Med 1977; **Resid:** Internal Medicine, Univ North Carolina Hosps 1980; Nephrology, Univ NC 1981; **Fellow:** Research, Univ Minn 1983; **Fac Appt:** Prof Med, Univ NC Sch Med

Helderman, J Harold MD [Nep] - **Spec Exp:** Transplant Medicine-Kidney; Kidney Disease; **Hospital:** Vanderbilt Univ Med Ctr; **Address:** Vanderbilt-Div Nephrology & Hypertension, 1161 21st Ave S, S-3223 MCN, Nashville, TN 37232-2372; **Phone:** 615-343-7592; **Board Cert:** Internal Medicine 1974; **Med School:** SUNY Downstate 1971; **Resid:** Internal Medicine, Johns Hopkins Hosp 1973; **Fellow:** Nephrology, Brigham & Womens Hosp-Harvard 1976; **Fac Appt:** Prof Med, Vanderbilt Univ

Okusa, Mark D MD [Nep] - **Spec Exp:** Kidney Failure-Chronic; Nephrotic Syndrome; Kidney Failure-Acute; **Hospital:** Univ Virginia Med Ctr; **Address:** Univ VA Hlth Sci Ctr, Div Nephrology, Lee St, Box 800-133, Charlottesville, VA 22908-0001; **Phone:** 434-924-5125; **Board Cert:** Internal Medicine 1985; Nephrology 1988; **Med School:** Med Coll VA 1982; **Resid:** Internal Medicine, Med Coll Virginia 1985; **Fellow:** Nephrology, Yale Univ Sch Med 1988; **Fac Appt:** Prof Med, Univ VA Sch Med

Rakowski, Thomas A MD [Nep] - **Spec Exp:** Polycystic Kidney Disease; Kidney Disease-Glomerular; **Hospital:** Virginia Hosp Ctr - Arlington, Inova Fairfax Hosp; **Address:** Virginia Nephrology Group, 1635 N George Mason Drive, Ste 215, Arlington, VA 22205; **Phone:** 703-841-0707; **Board Cert:** Internal Medicine 1972; Nephrology 1974; **Med School:** Hahnemann Univ 1969; **Resid:** Internal Medicine, Georgetown Univ 1971; **Fellow:** Nephrology, Georgetown Univ 1972; **Fac Appt:** Assoc Prof Med, Georgetown Univ

Nephrology

Roth, David MD [Nep] - **Spec Exp:** Transplant Medicine-Kidney; Kidney Failure-Chronic; **Hospital:** Jackson Meml Hosp, Univ of Miami Hosp & Clins/Sylvester Comp Canc Ctr; **Address:** Nephrology & Hypertension, PO Box 016960 (R-126), Miami, FL 33101; **Phone:** 305-243-6251; **Board Cert:** Internal Medicine 1980; Nephrology 1982; **Med School:** SUNY Downstate 1977; **Resid:** Internal Medicine, Jackson Meml Hosp 1980; **Fellow:** Nephrology, Jackson Meml Hosp 1982; **Fac Appt:** Prof Med, Univ Miami Sch Med

Warnock, David G MD [Nep] - **Spec Exp:** Liddle's Syndrome; Kidney Stones; Nephrotic Syndrome; **Hospital:** Univ of Ala Hosp at Birmingham; **Address:** UAB Dept Medicine, 1530 3rd Ave S, ZRB 614, Birmingham, AL 35294-0006; **Phone:** 205-996-5374 x2; **Board Cert:** Internal Medicine 1973; Nephrology 2000; **Med School:** UCSF 1970; **Resid:** Internal Medicine, UCSF Med Ctr 1973; **Fellow:** Nephrology, Natl Inst Hlth 1975; **Fac Appt:** Prof Med, Univ Ala

Weiner, I David MD [Nep] - **Spec Exp:** Kidney Disease; Fluid/Electrolyte Balance; Kidney Stones; Hypertension; **Hospital:** Shands at Univ of FL; **Address:** Shands at Univ Florida, Dept Nephrology, PO Box 100224, Gainesville, FL 32610-0224; **Phone:** 352-392-4008; **Board Cert:** Internal Medicine 1987; Nephrology 2000; **Med School:** Vanderbilt Univ 1984; **Resid:** Internal Medicine, Univ Texas Hlth Sci Ctr 1987; **Fellow:** Nephrology, Wash Univ 1990; **Fac Appt:** Assoc Prof Med, Univ Fla Coll Med

Midwest

Brennan, Daniel C MD [Nep] - **Spec Exp:** Transplant Medicine-Kidney; **Hospital:** Barnes-Jewish Hosp; **Address:** Wash Univ School Med, Div Renal Diseases, 660 S Euclid Ave, Box 8126, St Louis, MO 63110; **Phone:** 314-362-7603; **Board Cert:** Internal Medicine 1988; Nephrology 2002; **Med School:** Univ Iowa Coll Med 1985; **Resid:** Internal Medicine, U Iowa Hosps 1988; **Fellow:** Nephrology, Brigham & Womens Hosp 1992; **Fac Appt:** Assoc Prof Med, Washington Univ, St Louis

Coe, Fredric MD [Nep] - **Spec Exp:** Kidney Stones; Fluid/Electrolyte Balance; **Hospital:** Univ of Chicago Hosps; **Address:** 5841 S Maryland Ave, MC 5100, Chicago, IL 60637-1463; **Phone:** 773-702-1475; **Board Cert:** Internal Medicine 1968; **Med School:** Univ Chicago-Pritzker Sch Med 1961; **Resid:** Internal Medicine, Michael Reese Hosp 1965; **Fellow:** Renal Disease, Univ Texas SW 1969; **Fac Appt:** Prof Med, Univ Chicago-Pritzker Sch Med

Delmez, James MD [Nep] - **Spec Exp:** Kidney Disease; **Hospital:** Barnes-Jewish Hosp, Washington Univ Med Ctr; **Address:** Wash Univ Sch Med, Div Renal Disease, 4921 Parkview Pl, St Louis, MO 63110; **Phone:** 314-362-7603; **Board Cert:** Internal Medicine 1976; Nephrology 1982; **Med School:** Univ Rochester 1973; **Resid:** Internal Medicine, Barnes Hosp 1976; **Fellow:** Nephrology, Barnes Hosp 1978; **Fac Appt:** Prof Med, Washington Univ, St Louis

Hruska, Keith MD [Nep] - **Spec Exp:** Kidney Disease-Pediatric & Adult; Kidney Stones; Bone Disorders; **Hospital:** St Louis Chldns Hosp, Barnes-Jewish Hosp; **Address:** St Louis Chldn's Hospital, Dept Peds, 660 S Euclid Ave Fl 5MPRB, Box 8208, St Louis, MO 63110-1010; **Phone:** 314-286-2772; **Board Cert:** Internal Medicine 1972; Nephrology 1976; **Med School:** Creighton Univ 1969; **Resid:** Internal Medicine, New York Hosp-Cornell 1971; Internal Medicine, Barnes Hosp-Wash Univ 1972; **Fellow:** Nephrology, Barnes Hosp-Wash Univ 1974; **Fac Appt:** Prof Ped, Washington Univ, St Louis

Josephson, Michelle A MD [Nep] - **Spec Exp:** Transplant Medicine-Kidney; Hypertension; **Hospital:** Univ of Chicago Hosps; **Address:** Univ Chicago, Div Nephrology, 5841 S Maryland Ave, MC 5100, Chicago, IL 60637; **Phone:** 773-702-6134; **Board Cert:** Internal Medicine 1986; Nephrology 2000; **Med School:** Univ Pennsylvania 1983; **Resid:** Internal Medicine, Univ Chicago Hosps 1986; **Fellow:** Nephrology, Univ Chicago Hosps 1991; **Fac Appt:** Assoc Clin Prof Med, Univ Chicago-Pritzker Sch Med

Kasiske, Bertram MD [Nep] - **Spec Exp:** Transplant Medicine-Kidney; Kidney Disease-Geriatric; **Hospital:** Hennepin Cnty Med Ctr; **Address:** Div Nephrology, Hennepin Co Med Ctr, 701 Park Ave, Minneapolis, MN 55415; **Phone:** 612-347-6088; **Board Cert:** Internal Medicine 1980; Nephrology 1982; **Med School:** Univ Iowa Coll Med 1976; **Resid:** Internal Medicine, Hennepin Co Med Ctr 1980; **Fellow:** Nephrology, Hennepin Co Med Ctr 1983; **Fac Appt:** Prof Med, Univ Minn

Kraus, Michael A MD [Nep] - **Spec Exp:** Dialysis; Kidney Failure-Acute; **Hospital:** Indiana Univ Hosp, Wishard Hlth Srvs; **Address:** Indiana University Hosp, 550 N University Blvd, Ste 1115, Indianapolis, IN 46202; **Phone:** 317-274-5292; **Board Cert:** Internal Medicine 1988; Nephrology 2002; **Med School:** Indiana Univ 1985; **Resid:** Internal Medicine, Indiana Univ Med Ctr 1988; **Fellow:** Nephrology, Univ Iowa Hosps/Clinics 1991; **Fac Appt:** Clin Prof Med, Indiana Univ

Lewis, Edmund J MD [Nep] - **Spec Exp:** Lupus Nephritis; Diabetic Kidney Disease; Glomerulonephritis; **Hospital:** Rush Univ Med Ctr; **Address:** 1426 W Washington Blvd, Chicago, IL 60607; **Phone:** 312-850-8434; **Board Cert:** Internal Medicine 1969; **Med School:** Univ British Columbia Fac Med 1962; **Resid:** Internal Medicine, Johns Hopkins Hosp 1965; **Fellow:** Nephrology, Peter Bent Brigham Hosp 1966; Research, Peter Bent Brigham Hosp 1970; **Fac Appt:** Prof Med, Rush Med Coll

Pohl, Marc MD [Nep] - **Spec Exp:** Hypertension; Kidney Disease; Diabetes; **Hospital:** Cleveland Clin Fdn (page 56); **Address:** Div Nephrology & Hypertension, 9500 Euclid Ave, Desk A51, Cleveland, OH 44195; **Phone:** 216-444-6776; **Board Cert:** Internal Medicine 1972; Nephrology 1978; **Med School:** Case West Res Univ 1966; **Resid:** Internal Medicine, Univ Hosps 1968; Internal Medicine, Mass Genl Hosp 1971; **Fellow:** Nephrology, Boston City Hosp-Boston Univ 1972; Nephrology, Mass Genl Hosp 1973

Schwartz, Gary Lee MD [Nep] - **Spec Exp:** Hypertension; Hypotension; Diabetic Kidney Disease; **Hospital:** St Mary's Hosp - Rochester, Mayo Med Ctr & Clin - Rochester; **Address:** Mayo Clinic, 200 1st St SW, Rochester, MN 55905-0002; **Phone:** 507-284-4083; **Board Cert:** Internal Medicine 1980; Nephrology 1982; **Med School:** Univ Wisc 1977; **Resid:** Internal Medicine, Mayo Clinic 1980; **Fellow:** Nephrology, Mayo Clinic 1982; **Fac Appt:** Assoc Clin Prof Med, Mayo Med Sch

Somerville, James MD [Nep] - **Hospital:** Fairview Southdale Hosp, Fairview Ridges Hosp; **Address:** 6363 France Ave S, Ste 400, Edina, MN 55435; **Phone:** 952-920-2070; **Board Cert:** Internal Medicine 1978; Nephrology 1982; **Med School:** Univ MD Sch Med 1975; **Resid:** Internal Medicine, Hennepin Co Med Ctr 1978; **Fellow:** Nephrology, Hennepin Co Med Ctr 1980

Swartz, Richard D MD [Nep] - **Spec Exp:** Kidney Failure; Dialysis Care; **Hospital:** Univ Michigan Hlth Sys; **Address:** Univ Mich, Div Nephrology, 1500 E Med Ctr Drive, 3914 Taubman Ctr, Ann Arbor, MI 48109-0364; **Phone:** 734-647-9342; **Board Cert:** Internal Medicine 1975; Nephrology 1978; **Med School:** Univ Mich Med Sch 1970; **Resid:** Internal Medicine, Boston City Hosp 1975; Nephrology, Beth Israel Hosp-Harvard 1977; **Fac Appt:** Prof Med, Univ Mich Med Sch

Nephrology

Textor, Stephen C MD [Nep] - **Spec Exp:** Transplant Medicine-Kidney; Hypertension; Renal Artery Stenosis; **Hospital:** Mayo Med Ctr & Clin - Rochester; **Address:** Mayo Clinic, Div Nephrology/Hypertension Fl W19A, 200 First St SW, Rochester, MN 55905; **Phone:** 507-284-4083; **Board Cert:** Internal Medicine 1977; Nephrology 1980; **Med School:** UCLA 1973; **Resid:** Internal Medicine, Boston City Hosp 1977; **Fellow:** Nephrology, Boston Univ 1978; Hypertension, Fogarty Inst 1980; **Fac Appt:** Prof Med, Mayo Med Sch

Torres, Vicente Esbarranch MD [Nep] - **Spec Exp:** Polycystic Kidney Disease; **Hospital:** Mayo Med Ctr & Clin - Rochester; **Address:** Mayo Clinic, Eisenberg Bldg-Rm SL 24, 200 First St SW, Rochester, MN 55905; **Phone:** 507-266-7093; **Board Cert:** Internal Medicine 1977; Nephrology 1980; **Med School:** Spain 1969; **Resid:** Internal Medicine, Mayo Grad Sch Med 1977; **Fellow:** Nephrology, Mayo Grad Sch Med 1979; **Fac Appt:** Prof Med, Mayo Med Sch

Venkat, K K MD [Nep] - **Spec Exp:** Transplant Medicine-Kidney; Kidney Disease; **Hospital:** Henry Ford Hosp; **Address:** Henry Ford Hosp, Div Nephrology, 2799 W Grand Blvd, rm CFP5, Detroit, MI 48202-2689; **Phone:** 313-916-2702; **Board Cert:** Internal Medicine 1977; Nephrology 1978; **Med School:** India 1970; **Resid:** Internal Medicine, Henry Ford Hosp 1976; **Fellow:** Nephrology, Henry Ford Hosp 1978

Great Plains and Mountains

Berl, Tomas MD [Nep] - **Spec Exp:** Fluid/Electrolyte Balance; Kidney Failure-Chronic; **Hospital:** Univ Colorado Hosp; **Address:** Univ Colorado-Denver, Div of Renal Dis & Hypertention, 12700 E 19th Ave, rm C281, Aurora, CO 80045; **Phone:** 303-372-8069; **Board Cert:** Internal Medicine 1972; Nephrology 1976; **Med School:** NYU Sch Med 1968; **Resid:** Internal Medicine, Bronx Municipal Hosp 1970; **Fellow:** Renal Disease, Moffit Hosp-UCSF 1971

Schrier, Robert W MD [Nep] - **Spec Exp:** Hypertension; Polycystic Kidney Disease; **Hospital:** Univ Colorado Hosp; **Address:** Univ Colorado Denver, 12700 E 19th Ave, Box 6511, Box C281, Aurora, CO 80045; **Phone:** 303-315-7297; **Board Cert:** Internal Medicine 1969; **Med School:** Indiana Univ 1962; **Resid:** Internal Medicine, Univ Wash Hosp 1965; **Fellow:** Research, PB Brigham Hosp/Harvard 1966; **Fac Appt:** Prof Med, Univ Colorado

Southwest

Brennan, Stephen T MD [Nep] - **Spec Exp:** Transplant Medicine-Kidney; Kidney Stones; Kidney Failure-Chronic; **Hospital:** Methodist Hosp - Houston, St Luke's Episcopal Hosp - Houston; **Address:** 1415 La Concha Ln, Houston, TX 77054; **Phone:** 713-790-9080; **Board Cert:** Internal Medicine 1983; Nephrology 1988; **Med School:** Loyola Univ-Stritch Sch Med 1979; **Resid:** Internal Medicine, Loyola Univ Med Ctr 1983; **Fellow:** Nephrology, Univ Wash-Barnes Hosp 1986; **Fac Appt:** Assoc Clin Prof Med, Baylor Coll Med

Hura, Claudia E MD [Nep] - **Spec Exp:** Transplant Medicine-Kidney; Glomerulonephritis; Lupus Nephritis; **Hospital:** Methodist Spec & Transpl Hosp, SW TX Meth Hosp; **Address:** 8042 Wurzbach St, Physician Plaza 2, Ste 500, San Antonio, TX 78229; **Phone:** 210-692-7228; **Board Cert:** Internal Medicine 1982; Nephrology 1986; **Med School:** Ohio State Univ 1979; **Resid:** Internal Medicine, Indiana Univ Med Ctr 1983; **Fellow:** Nephrology, Univ Tex Hlth Sci Ctr 1986; **Fac Appt:** Assoc Clin Prof Med, Univ Tex, San Antonio

Kasinath, Balakuntalam S MD [Nep] - **Spec Exp:** Glomerulonephritis; Diabetic Kidney Disease; **Hospital:** Univ Hlth Sys - Univ Hosp (San Antonio, TX), Audie L Murphy Meml Vets Hosp; **Address:** Univ Tex Hlth Sci Ctr, Dept Med/Div Neph, 7703 Floyd Curl Drive, MC 7882, San Antonio, TX 78229-3901; **Phone:** 210-567-4707; **Board Cert:** Internal Medicine 1980; Nephrology 1982; **Med School:** India 1975; **Resid:** Internal Medicine, Ill Masonic Med Ctr 1980; **Fellow:** Nephrology, Univ Chicago Hosp 1983; **Fac Appt:** Prof Med, Univ Tex, San Antonio

Mitch, William MD [Nep] - **Spec Exp:** Nutrition; Hypertension; Kidney Failure; **Hospital:** Baylor Univ Medical Ctr, Ben Taub Genl Hosp; **Address:** Baylor College of Medicine, Nephrology Div, MIS:BCM 285, One Baylor Plaza, Ste N-620, Houston, TX 77030; **Phone:** 713-798-2500; **Board Cert:** Internal Medicine 1972; Nephrology 1978; **Med School:** Harvard Med Sch 1967; **Resid:** Internal Medicine, Brigham & Women's Hosp 1974; Nat Cancer Inst-NIH 1972; **Fellow:** Nephrology, Johns Hopkins Hosp 1973; **Fac Appt:** Prof Med, Baylor Coll Med

Olivero, Juan J MD [Nep] - **Spec Exp:** Kidney Failure; Fluid/Electrolyte Balance; **Hospital:** Methodist Hosp - Houston; **Address:** 6560 Fannin St, Scurlock Twr, Ste 2206, Houston, TX 77030; **Phone:** 713-790-4615; **Board Cert:** Internal Medicine 1974; Nephrology 1976; **Med School:** Guatemala 1970; **Resid:** Internal Medicine, Baylor Affil Hosps 1973; Internal Medicine, Ben Taub Genl Hosp 1974; **Fellow:** Nephrology, Baylor Affil Hosps 1975; **Fac Appt:** Clin Prof Med, Baylor Coll Med

Suki, Wadi N MD [Nep] - **Spec Exp:** Transplant Medicine-Kidney; Hypertension; Lupus Nephritis; **Hospital:** Methodist Hosp - Houston, St Luke's Episcopal Hosp - Houston; **Address:** 1415 La Concha Ln, Houston, TX 77054; **Phone:** 713-790-9080; **Board Cert:** Internal Medicine 1967; Nephrology 1972; **Med School:** Sudan 1959; **Resid:** Internal Medicine, Parkland Meml Hosp 1963; **Fellow:** Nephrology, Univ Tex SW Med Ctr 1961; Nephrology, Univ Tex SW Med Ctr 1965; **Fac Appt:** Clin Prof Med, Baylor Coll Med

Toto, Robert D MD [Nep] - **Spec Exp:** Hypertension/Kidney Disease; Dialysis Care; Diabetic Kidney Disease; Kidney Failure-Acute; **Hospital:** UT Southwestern Med Ctr - Dallas; **Address:** UT Southwestern Medical Ctr, 5323 Harry Hines Blvd, MC 8856, Dallas, TX 75390-8856; **Phone:** 214-648-3442; **Board Cert:** Internal Medicine 1980; Nephrology 1982; **Med School:** Univ IL Coll Med 1977; **Resid:** Internal Medicine, Univ Michigan Med Ctr 1979; Internal Medicine, Baylor Univ Med Ctr 1980; **Fellow:** Nephrology, US Public Health Service Hosp 1981; Nephrology, UTSW Med Ctr 1983; **Fac Appt:** Prof Med, Univ Tex SW, Dallas

West Coast and Pacific

Ahmad, Suhail MD [Nep] - **Spec Exp:** Hypertension; Kidney Failure-Chronic; Kidney Stones; **Hospital:** Univ Wash Med Ctr; **Address:** 2150 N 107th St, Ste 160, Seattle, WA 98133; **Phone:** 206-363-5090; **Med School:** India 1968; **Resid:** Internal Medicine, Univ Allahabad 1971; **Fellow:** Nephrology, Univ Washington 1978; **Fac Appt:** Assoc Prof Med, Univ Wash

Bennett, William M MD [Nep] - **Spec Exp:** Polycystic Kidney Disease; Transplant Medicine-Kidney; Drug Toxicity-Kidneys; **Hospital:** Legacy Good Samaritan Hosp and Med Ctr, Legacy Emanuel Hospitals; **Address:** Legacy Good Samaritan Hosp, Transplant Svcs, 1040 NW 22nd, Ste 480, Portland, OR 97210; **Phone:** 503-413-6555; **Board Cert:** Internal Medicine 2003; Nephrology 2003; **Med School:** Northwestern Univ 1963; **Resid:** Internal Medicine, Northwestern Univ 1965; Internal Medicine, Ore Hlth Sci Univ 1966; **Fellow:** Nephrology, Mass Genl Hosp 1970

Nephrology

Ellison, David H MD [Nep] - **Spec Exp:** Bartter's Syndrome; Gitelman's Syndrome; Hypertension; **Hospital:** OR Hlth & Sci Univ, VA Medical Center - Portland; **Address:** Oregon Hlth Scis Univ - Div Nephrology, 3314 SW US Veteran's Hospital Rd, MC PP262, Portland, OR 97239-3098; **Phone:** 503-494-8490; **Board Cert:** Internal Medicine 1981; Nephrology 1986; **Med School:** Rush Med Coll 1978; **Resid:** Internal Medicine, Oregon Hlth Scis Univ 1981; **Fellow:** Research, Oregon Hlth Scis Univ 1982; Nephrology, Yale Univ 1985; **Fac Appt:** Prof Med, Oregon Hlth Sci Univ

Gluck, Stephen L MD [Nep] - **Spec Exp:** Kidney Disease; Fluid/Electrolyte Balance; Hypertension; Kidney Stones; **Hospital:** UCSF Med Ctr; **Address:** UCSF, Div Nephrology, C442, 526 Parnassus Ave, Box 0532, San Francisco, CA 94143-0532; **Phone:** 415-476-2173; **Board Cert:** Internal Medicine 1980; Nephrology 1984; **Med School:** UCLA 1977; **Resid:** Internal Medicine, Columbia Presby Med Ctr 1980; **Fellow:** Nephrology, Columbia Presby Med Ctr 1983; **Fac Appt:** Prof Med, UCSF

Kaysen, George Alan MD/PhD [Nep] - **Spec Exp:** Kidney Disease-Metabolic; Kidney Failure-Chronic; **Hospital:** UC Davis Med Ctr; **Address:** UC Davis Med Ctr, Div Nephr, 451 Hlth Sciences Drive, GBSF Bldg - rm 6310, Davis, CA 95616; **Phone:** 530-752-4010; **Board Cert:** Internal Medicine 1975; Nephrology 1980; **Med School:** Albert Einstein Coll Med 1972; **Resid:** Internal Medicine, Bronx Muni Hosp 1975; **Fellow:** Renal Disease, Bronx Muni Hosp 1977; **Fac Appt:** Prof Med, UC Davis

King, Andrew J MD [Nep] - **Spec Exp:** Kidney Disease-Chronic; Hypertension; Dialysis Care; **Hospital:** Scripps Green Hosp; **Address:** Scripps Green Hospital, 10666 N Torrey Pines Rd, MC N239, La Jolla, CA 92037-1027; **Phone:** 858-554-9765; **Board Cert:** Internal Medicine 1986; Nephrology 1988; **Med School:** Northwestern Univ 1983; **Resid:** Internal Medicine, Northwestern Meml Hosp 1986; **Fellow:** Nephrology, Brigham & Women's Hosp 1990; **Fac Appt:** Clin Prof Med, UCSD

Ott, Susan M MD [Nep] - **Spec Exp:** Metabolic Bone Disease; Osteoporosis; **Hospital:** Univ Wash Med Ctr; **Address:** Bone & Joint Center, UWMC- Roosevelt, 4245 Roosevelt Way NE, Box 354740, Seattle, WA 98105-6920; **Phone:** 206-598-4288; **Board Cert:** Internal Medicine 1978; Nephrology 1982; **Med School:** Univ Wash 1974; **Resid:** Family Medicine, UC Davis Med Ctr 1978; **Fellow:** Nephrology, Univ Wash Med Ctr 1982; **Fac Appt:** Assoc Prof Med, Univ Wash

Riordan, John W MD [Nep] - **Hospital:** CA Pacific Med Ctr - Pacific Campus; **Address:** 2100 Webster St, Ste 412, San Francisco, CA 94115; **Phone:** 415-923-3815; **Board Cert:** Nephrology 2005; **Med School:** Univ Tex Med Br, Galveston 1987; **Resid:** Internal Medicine, Univ Texas Hlth Sci Ctr 1990; **Fellow:** Nephrology, UCSF Med Ctr 1995

Scandling Jr, John David MD [Nep] - **Spec Exp:** Transplant Medicine-Kidney; **Hospital:** Stanford Univ Med Ctr; **Address:** 750 Welch Rd, Ste 200, Palo Alto, CA 94304-1509; **Phone:** 650-725-9891; **Board Cert:** Internal Medicine 1981; Nephrology 1984; **Med School:** Med Coll VA 1978; **Resid:** Internal Medicine, West Virginia Univ Hosp 1981; **Fellow:** Nephrology, Univ Rochester 1983; **Fac Appt:** Prof Med, Stanford Univ

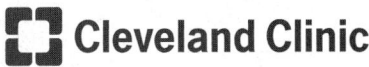 **Cleveland Clinic**

Glickman Urological and Kidney Institute

The Glickman Urological and Kidney Institute's Department of Nephrology and Hypertension provides comprehensive diagnostic and therapeutic services for patients with kidney disease and hypertension. The department participates in an active kidney transplant program, all modalities of dialysis care, and clinical research studies of diabetic and other glomerular disease. In addition to unique diagnostic capabilities, the department is renowned for its expertise in the areas of renovascular hypertension, primary aldosteronism and pheochromocytoma.

Intensive Care Nephrology Services

The Department of Nephrology and Hypertension is a major participant in the intensive care setting. Institute nephrologists are leaders in research into the risk factors for acute renal failure after surgeries and in evaluations of different techniques for treatment of acute renal failure such as slow continuous ultrafiltration, continuous arteriovenous hemofiltration and venovenous hemofiltration.

Research and Clinical Trials

The Department of Nephrology and Hypertension is actively involved in clinical and basic research. Its legacy of excellence in hypertension research began in 1945.

For more than 30 years, the Clinic has received support from the National Institutes of Health (NIH) for its research into the causes of hypertension.

Kidney/Kidney-Pancreas Transplant

Cleveland Clinic's kidney transplant program dates to January 1963. Since then, more than 3,000 kidney transplants have been performed here. Each year, between 75 and 100 kidney transplants are performed.

For more information about Glickman Urological and Kidney Institute's Department of Nephrology and Hypertension, to schedule a second opinion or learn about assistance for out-of-state patients, call 800.890.2467 or visit www.clevelandclinic.org/nephrologytopdocs.

Glickman Urological & Kidney Institute
Department of Nephrology and Hypertension
Cleveland Clinic | 9500 Euclid Avenue / AC311 | Cleveland OH 44195

Neurological Surgery

A neurological surgeon provides the operative and non-operative management (i.e., prevention, diagnosis, evaluation, treatment, critical care and rehabilitation) of disorders of the central, peripheral and autonomic nervous systems, including their supporting structures and vascular supply; the evaluation and treatment of pathological processes which modify function or activity of the nervous system; and the operative and non-operative management of pain. A neurological surgeon treats patients with disorders of the nervous system; disorders of the brain, meninges, skull and their blood supply, including the extracranial carotid and vertebral arteries; disorders of the pituitary gland; disorders of the spinal cord, meninges and vertebral column, including those which may require treatment by spinal fusion or instrumentation; and disorders of the cranial and spinal nerves throughout their distribution.

Training Required: Seven years (including general surgery)

The American Board of Pediatric Neurological Surgery (ABPNS) is not a recognized ABMS subspecialty. However, this designation has been included because the certification process is meaningful and rigorous. It is awarded to those doctors who hold a current ABMS certification in Neurological Surgery, have completed a fully accredited one year, post-graduate fellowship in pediatric neurological surgery, and have submitted surgical logs indicating a practice of pediatric neurological surgery for one year, followed by a written examination.

NEUROLOGICAL SURGERY

New England

Black, Peter MD/PhD [NS] - **Spec Exp:** Brain Tumors; Pituitary Tumors; Seizure Disorders; **Hospital:** Brigham & Women's Hosp, Children's Hospital - Boston; **Address:** Brigham & Women's Hosp, Dept Neurosurg, 75 Francis St, Boston, MA 02115-6106; **Phone:** 617-732-6600; **Board Cert:** Neurological Surgery 1984; **Med School:** McGill Univ 1970; **Resid:** Surgery, Mass Genl Hosp 1972; Neurological Surgery, Mass Genl Hosp 1980; **Fellow:** Neurosurgical Oncology, Mass Genl Hosp 1976; **Fac Appt:** Prof NS, Harvard Med Sch

Borges, Lawrence F MD [NS] - **Spec Exp:** Spinal Surgery; Spinal Tumors; **Hospital:** Mass Genl Hosp; **Address:** Mass Genl Hosp, Div Neurosurg Svcs, 55 Fruit St, Ste 1205, Boston, MA 02114-2696; **Phone:** 617-726-6156; **Board Cert:** Neurological Surgery 1986; **Med School:** Johns Hopkins Univ 1977; **Resid:** Neurological Surgery, Mass Genl Hosp 1983; **Fac Appt:** Assoc Prof S, Harvard Med Sch

Cosgrove, G Rees MD [NS] - **Spec Exp:** Epilepsy/Seizure Disorders; Brain Tumors; **Hospital:** Lahey Clin, Emerson Hosp; **Address:** Lahey Clinic, 41 Mall Rd, Burlington, MA 01805; **Phone:** 781-744-1990; **Board Cert:** Neurological Surgery 1989; **Med School:** Queens Univ 1980; **Resid:** Neurological Surgery, Montreal Neur Inst 1986; **Fac Appt:** Prof NS, Tufts Univ

David, Carlos MD [NS] - **Spec Exp:** Cerebrovascular Surgery; Skull Base Tumors & Surgery; **Hospital:** Lahey Clin, Emerson Hosp; **Address:** Lahey Clinic, Dept Neurosurgery, 41 Mall Rd, Burlington, MA 01805; **Phone:** 781-744-8643; **Board Cert:** Neurological Surgery 2001; **Med School:** Univ Miami Sch Med 1990; **Resid:** Neurological Surgery, Jackson Memorial Hosp 1995; **Fellow:** Cerebrovascular & Skull Base Surgery, Barrow Neuro Inst 1997; **Fac Appt:** Assoc Clin Prof NS, Tufts Univ

Day, Arthur L MD [NS] - **Spec Exp:** Cerebrovascular Surgery; Orbital Tumors/Cancer; Carotid Artery Surgery; Skull Base Tumors; **Hospital:** Brigham & Women's Hosp, Children's Hospital - Boston; **Address:** Brigham & Womens Hosp, Dept Neurosurgery, 75 Francis St, Boston, MA 02115; **Phone:** 617-732-6600; **Board Cert:** Neurological Surgery 1980; **Med School:** Louisiana State U, New Orleans 1972; **Resid:** Neurological Surgery, Shands-Univ Florida Hosp 1977; **Fellow:** Neurological Pathology, Shands-Univ Florida Hosp 1978; **Fac Appt:** Prof NS, Harvard Med Sch

Duhaime, Ann Christine MD [NS] - **Spec Exp:** Pediatric Neurosurgery; Brain Tumors; Epilepsy; Craniofacial Surgery; **Hospital:** Dartmouth - Hitchcock Med Ctr; **Address:** Chldns Hosp at Dartmouth-Hitchcock Med Ctr, One Medical Center Drive, Lebanon, NH 03756; **Phone:** 603-653-9880; **Board Cert:** Neurological Surgery 1990; Pediatric Neurological Surgery 2005; **Med School:** Univ Pennsylvania 1981; **Resid:** Neurological Surgery, Hosp Univ Penn 1987; **Fellow:** Pediatric Neurological Surgery, Chldns Hosp 1987; **Fac Appt:** Prof S, Dartmouth Med Sch

Heilman, Carl B MD [NS] - **Spec Exp:** Skull Base Surgery; Pediatric Neurosurgery; **Hospital:** Tufts Med Ctr; **Address:** Tufts-NE Med Ctr, Dept Neurosurgery, 800 Washington St, Box 178, Bsoton, MA 02111; **Phone:** 617-636-5858; **Board Cert:** Neurological Surgery 1996; **Med School:** Univ Pennsylvania 1986; **Resid:** Neurological Surgery, Tufts New England Med Ctr 1993; **Fellow:** Skull Base Surgery, Baptist Meml Hosp 1993; **Fac Appt:** Assoc Prof NS, Tufts Univ

Madsen, Joseph MD [NS] - **Spec Exp:** Pediatric Neurosurgery; Epilepsy/Seizure Disorders; **Hospital:** Children's Hospital - Boston; **Address:** 300 Longwood Ave, Bader 3, Boston, MA 02115; **Phone:** 617-355-6005; **Board Cert:** Neurological Surgery 1994; Pediatric Neurological Surgery 1997; **Med School:** Harvard Med Sch 1981; **Resid:** Neurological Surgery, Mass Genl Hosp 1989; **Fellow:** Research, Beth Israel Hosp 1983; **Fac Appt:** Assoc Prof NS, Harvard Med Sch

Martuza, Robert L MD [NS] - **Spec Exp:** Brain Tumors; Acoustic Neuroma; Skull Base Surgery; **Hospital:** Mass Genl Hosp; **Address:** Mass General Hosp, 55 Fruit St, MGH-White 502, Boston, MA 02114; **Phone:** 617-726-8581; **Board Cert:** Neurological Surgery 1983; **Med School:** Harvard Med Sch 1973; **Resid:** Neurological Surgery, Mass Genl Hosp 1980; **Fac Appt:** Prof NS, Harvard Med Sch

Penar, Paul L MD [NS] - **Spec Exp:** Brain & Spinal Tumors; Epilepsy/Seizure Disorders; Movement Disorders; Stereotactic Radiosurgery; **Hospital:** FAHC - Med Ctr Campus; **Address:** Fletcher Allen Health Care, 111 Colchester Ave, Fletcher 5-247FL5, Burlington, VT 05401; **Phone:** 802-847-4590; **Board Cert:** Neurological Surgery 1989; **Med School:** Univ Mich Med Sch 1981; **Resid:** Neurological Surgery, Yale-New Haven Hosp 1987

Piepmeier, Joseph MD [NS] - **Spec Exp:** Neuro-Oncology; Brain & Spinal Cord Tumors; **Hospital:** Yale-New Haven Hosp; **Address:** Yale Sch Med, Dept Neurosurgery, 333 Cedar St Fl TMP-410, New Haven, CT 06520; **Phone:** 203-785-2791; **Board Cert:** Neurological Surgery 1984; **Med School:** Univ Tenn Coll Med, Memphis 1975; **Resid:** Neurological Surgery, Yale-New Haven Hosp 1982; **Fac Appt:** Prof NS, Yale Univ

Spencer, Dennis D MD [NS] - **Spec Exp:** Epilepsy/Seizure Disorders; Brain Tumors; **Hospital:** Yale-New Haven Hosp, Hosp of St Raphael; **Address:** Yale Univ Sch Med, Dept Neurosurgery, 333 Cedar St, TMP-4, New Haven, CT 06520; **Phone:** 203-785-4891; **Board Cert:** Neurological Surgery 1980; **Med School:** Washington Univ, St Louis 1971; **Resid:** Surgery, Barnes Hosp 1972; Neurological Surgery, Yale-New Haven Hosp 1976; **Fac Appt:** Prof NS, Yale Univ

Mid Atlantic

Adelson, P David MD [NS] - **Spec Exp:** Pediatric Neurosurgery; Brain Injury; Epilepsy/Seizure Disorders; Spinal Cord Injury; **Hospital:** Chldns Hosp of Pittsburgh - UPMC, UPMC Presby, Pittsburgh; **Address:** Children's Hosp Pittsburgh, Neurosurgery, 3705 Fifth Ave, Ste 3705, Pittsburgh, PA 15213-2583; **Phone:** 412-692-5090; **Board Cert:** Neurological Surgery 1997; Pediatric Neurological Surgery 1998; **Med School:** Columbia P&S 1986; **Resid:** Neurological Surgery, UCLA Med Ctr 1992; **Fellow:** Pediatric Neurological Surgery, Children's Hosp 1994; **Fac Appt:** Prof NS, Univ Pittsburgh

Andrews, David MD [NS] - **Spec Exp:** Brain Tumors; Stereotactic Radiosurgery; **Hospital:** Thomas Jefferson Univ Hosp; **Address:** Thom Jefferson Univ Hosp, Dept Neurosurg, 909 Walnut St Fl 2, Philadelphia, PA 19107-5109; **Phone:** 215-503-7005; **Board Cert:** Neurological Surgery 1992; **Med School:** Univ Colorado 1983; **Resid:** Neurological Surgery, NY Presby Hos-Cornell Med Ctr 1989; **Fellow:** Neuro-Oncology, Meml Sloan Kettering Cancer Ctr 1987; **Fac Appt:** Prof NS, Thomas Jefferson Univ

Baltuch, Gordon MD/PhD [NS] - **Spec Exp:** Movement Disorders; Parkinson's Disease; Epilepsy/Seizure Disorders; **Hospital:** Hosp Univ Penn - UPHS (page 60), Pennsylvania Hosp (page 60); **Address:** Penn Neurological Institute, 3400 Spruce St, Silverstein Bldg Fl 3, Philadelphia, PA 19104; **Phone:** 215-662-7788; **Board Cert:** Neurological Surgery 1998; **Med School:** McGill Univ 1986; **Resid:** Surgery, Montreal Genl Hosp 1988; Neurological Surgery, Montreal Neuro Inst 1994; **Fellow:** Neurological Surgery, Centre Hospitalier Univ Vaudois 1995; **Fac Appt:** Assoc Prof NS, Univ Pennsylvania

Neurological Surgery

Bederson, Joshua MD [NS] - **Spec Exp:** Aneurysm-Cerebral; Brain & Spinal Cord Tumors; Trigeminal Neuralgia; Skull Base Tumors; **Hospital:** Mount Sinai Med Ctr (page 64); **Address:** Mount Sinai Med Ctr, 1 Gustave Levy Pl Box 1136, New York, NY 10029; **Phone:** 212-241-2377; **Board Cert:** Neurological Surgery 1993; **Med School:** UCSF 1984; **Resid:** Neurological Surgery, UCSF Med Ctr 1990; **Fellow:** Neurological Vascular Surgery, Barrow Neur Inst 1990; Neurological Vascular Surgery, Univ Hosp Zurich 1990; **Fac Appt:** Prof NS, Mount Sinai Sch Med

Bilsky, Mark H MD [NS] - **Spec Exp:** Spinal Tumors; Skull Base Tumors; Brain Tumors; Spinal Reconstructive Surgery; **Hospital:** Meml Sloan-Kettering Cancer Ctr, NY-Presby Hosp/Weill Cornell (page 66); **Address:** 1275 York Avenue, New York, NY 10065; **Phone:** 800-525-2225; **Board Cert:** Neurological Surgery 1999; **Med School:** Emory Univ 1988; **Resid:** Neurological Surgery, NY Hosp-Cornell Med Ctr 1994; **Fellow:** Neuro-Oncology, Louisville Univ Med Ctr 1995; **Fac Appt:** Assoc Prof NS, Cornell Univ-Weill Med Coll

Brem, Henry MD [NS] - **Spec Exp:** Brain & Spinal Cord Tumors; Skull Base Tumors; Pituitary Tumors; **Hospital:** Johns Hopkins Hosp - Baltimore (page 61), Johns Hopkins Bayview Med Ctr (page 61); **Address:** Johns Hopkins Med Ctr-Dept Neuro Surgery, 600 N Wolfe St Bldg Meyer 7-113, Baltimore, MD 21287; **Phone:** 410-955-2248; **Board Cert:** Neurological Surgery 1986; **Med School:** Harvard Med Sch 1978; **Resid:** Neurological Surgery, Columbia-Presby Med Ctr 1984; **Fellow:** Neurological Surgery, Johns Hopkins Hosp 1980; **Fac Appt:** Prof NS, Johns Hopkins Univ

Bruce, Jeffrey MD [NS] - **Spec Exp:** Brain Tumors; Pituitary Tumors; Skull Base Surgery; **Hospital:** NY-Presby Hosp/Columbia (page 66); **Address:** NY Presby Hosp, Dept Neurosurgery, 710 W 168th St N1 Bldg Fl 4 - rm 434, New York, NY 10032-3726; **Phone:** 212-305-7346; **Board Cert:** Neurological Surgery 1993; **Med School:** UMDNJ-RW Johnson Med Sch 1983; **Resid:** Neurological Surgery, Columbia-Presby Med Ctr 1990; **Fellow:** Neurological Surgery, Nat Inst Health 1985; **Fac Appt:** Prof NS, Columbia P&S

Campbell, James N MD [NS] - **Spec Exp:** Spinal Tumors; Pain-Chronic; Nerve Disorders/Surgery; Spinal Disorders; **Hospital:** Johns Hopkins Hosp - Baltimore (page 61); **Address:** Johns Hopkins Hospital, 600 N Wolfe St Meyer Bldg - Ste 5-109, Baltimore, MD 21287-7509; **Phone:** 410-955-3046; **Board Cert:** Neurological Surgery 1982; **Med School:** Yale Univ 1973; **Resid:** Neurological Surgery, Johns Hopkins Hosp 1979; **Fellow:** Neurological Surgery, Johns Hopkins 1977; **Fac Appt:** Prof NS, Johns Hopkins Univ

Caputy, Anthony J MD [NS] - **Spec Exp:** Epilepsy/Seizure Disorders; Spinal Surgery; **Hospital:** G Washington Univ Hosp, Inova Fairfax Hosp; **Address:** Geo Wash Univ, Dept Neurosurgery, 2150 Pennsylvania Ave NW, Ste 7-420, Washington, DC 20037; **Phone:** 202-741-2735; **Board Cert:** Neurological Surgery 1989; **Med School:** Univ VA Sch Med 1980; **Resid:** Neurological Surgery, Georgetown Univ Hosp 1986; **Fac Appt:** Prof NS, Geo Wash Univ

Carson, Benjamin S MD [NS] - **Spec Exp:** Brain Injury; Brain & Spinal Cord Tumors; Pediatric Neurosurgery; Rasmussen's Syndrome; **Hospital:** Johns Hopkins Hosp - Baltimore (page 61); **Address:** 600 N Wolfe St, Harvey 811, Baltimore, MD 21287-8811; **Phone:** 410-955-7888; **Board Cert:** Neurological Surgery 1988; Pediatric Neurological Surgery 1997; **Med School:** Univ Mich Med Sch 1977; **Resid:** Neurological Surgery, Johns Hopkins Hosp 1983; **Fellow:** Pediatric Neurological Surgery, Queen Elizabeth II Med Ctr 1984; **Fac Appt:** Assoc Prof NS, Johns Hopkins Univ

Chen, Chun Siang MD [NS] - **Spec Exp:** Skull Base Tumors; Skull Base Surgery; Microsurgery; **Hospital:** Mount Sinai Med Ctr (page 64); **Address:** Mount Sinai Med Ctr, Annenberg Bldg, One Gustave L Levy Pl Fl 8 - rm 10, New York, NY 10029; **Phone:** 212-241-8480; **Med School:** Brazil 1978; **Resid:** Neurological Surgery, Santa Casa de Misericordia of Sao Paulo Med Sch 1983; Neurological Surgery, Mount Sinai Med Ctr 2005; **Fellow:** Skull Base Surgery, St Lukes Roosevelt Hosp 2006; **Fac Appt:** Asst Prof NS, Mount Sinai Sch Med

Di Giacinto, George V MD [NS] - **Spec Exp:** Spinal Surgery; Pain Management; **Hospital:** St Luke's - Roosevelt Hosp Ctr - Roosevelt Div (page 57); **Address:** 425 W 59th St, Ste 4E, New York, NY 10019; **Phone:** 212-523-8500; **Board Cert:** Neurological Surgery 1981; **Med School:** Harvard Med Sch 1970; **Resid:** Neurological Surgery, Columbia-Presby Hosp 1978

Dias, Mark S MD [NS] - **Spec Exp:** Pediatric Neurosurgery; Spinal Bifida; Hydrocephalus; Trauma; **Hospital:** Penn State Milton S Hershey Med Ctr; **Address:** Penn State-Hersey Med Ctr, Dept Neurosurg, 500 Univ Dr, C3830-Biomed Rsch Bldg, Hersey, PA 17033-0850; **Phone:** 717-531-8807; **Board Cert:** Neurological Surgery 1995; Pediatric Neurological Surgery 2006; **Med School:** Johns Hopkins Univ 1982; **Resid:** Neurological Surgery, Univ Pittsburgh Med Ctr 1989; **Fellow:** Pediatric Neurological Surgery, Univ Utah-Primary Chldns Hosp 1991

Eisenberg, Howard M MD [NS] - **Spec Exp:** Acoustic Neuroma; Parkinson's Disease/Movement Disorders; Epilepsy/Seizure Disorders; **Hospital:** Univ of MD Med Sys, Greater Baltimore Med Ctr; **Address:** Univ MD Sch Med, Dept Neurosurg, 22 S Greene St, Ste S-12-D, Baltimore, MD 21201-1544; **Phone:** 410-328-3514; **Board Cert:** Neurological Surgery 1973; **Med School:** SUNY Downstate 1964; **Resid:** Surgery, New York Hosp 1966; Neurological Surgery, Peter Bent Brigham Hosp/Chldns Hosp 1970; **Fellow:** Harvard Univ 1970; **Fac Appt:** Prof NS, Univ MD Sch Med

Feldstein, Neil A MD [NS] - **Spec Exp:** Pediatric Neurosurgery; Chiari's Deformity; Brain Tumors-Pediatric; Spinal Cord Surgery-Pediatric; **Hospital:** NY-Presby Hosp/Columbia (page 66); **Address:** Neurological Inst, 710 W 168th St Fl 2 - rm 213, New York, NY 10032; **Phone:** 212-305-1396; **Board Cert:** Neurological Surgery 1995; Pediatric Neurological Surgery 1995; **Med School:** NYU Sch Med 1984; **Resid:** Neurological Surgery, Baylor Coll Med 1989; **Fellow:** Pediatric Neurological Surgery, NYU Med Ctr 1991; **Fac Appt:** Assoc Prof NS, Columbia P&S

Flamm, Eugene S MD [NS] - **Spec Exp:** Aneurysm-Cerebral; Brain Tumors; Cerebrovascular Surgery; **Hospital:** Montefiore Med Ctr; **Address:** Montefiore Med Ctr, 111 E 210th St, Bronx, NY 10467-2841; **Phone:** 718-920-2339; **Board Cert:** Neurological Surgery 1973; **Med School:** SUNY Buffalo 1962; **Resid:** Surgery, New York Hosp 1964; Neurological Surgery, NYU Med Ctr 1970; **Fellow:** Neurological Surgery, Univ Zurich 1971; **Fac Appt:** Prof NS, Albert Einstein Coll Med

Gokaslan, Ziya L MD [NS] - **Spec Exp:** Spinal Tumors; Spinal Surgery-Complex; Spinal Reconstructive Surgery; **Hospital:** Johns Hopkins Hosp - Baltimore (page 61); **Address:** Johns Hopkins Hosp, Dept Neurosurg, 600 N Wolfe St, Meyer 7-109, Baltimore, MD 21287; **Phone:** 410-955-4424; **Board Cert:** Neurological Surgery 1997; **Med School:** Turkey 1983; **Resid:** Neurological Surgery, Baylor Coll Med 1993; **Fellow:** Neurological Trauma, Baylor Coll Med 1988; Spinal Surgery, NYU Med Ctr 1994; **Fac Appt:** Prof NS, Johns Hopkins Univ

Golfinos, John G MD [NS] - **Spec Exp:** Brain Tumors; Acoustic Neuroma; Stereotactic Radiosurgery; Skull Base Surgery; **Hospital:** NYU Med Ctr (page 68), Lenox Hill Hosp (page 62); **Address:** NYU Med Ctr, Dept Neurosurgery, 530 1st Ave, Ste 8R, New York, NY 10016-6402; **Phone:** 212-263-2950; **Board Cert:** Neurological Surgery 1998; **Med School:** Columbia P&S 1988; **Resid:** Neurological Surgery, Barrow Neuro Inst 1995; **Fac Appt:** Assoc Prof NS, NYU Sch Med

Goodman, Robert R MD/PhD [NS] - **Spec Exp:** Parkinson's Disease; Epilepsy; Trigeminal Neuralgia; **Hospital:** NY-Presby Hosp/Columbia (page 66); **Address:** 710 W 168th St, rm 426, New York, NY 10032-2603; **Phone:** 212-305-3774; **Board Cert:** Neurological Surgery 1993; **Med School:** Johns Hopkins Univ 1982; **Resid:** Neurological Surgery, Columbia-Presby Med Ctr 1989; **Fac Appt:** Assoc Prof NS, Columbia P&S

Neurological Surgery

Goodrich, James T MD [NS] - **Spec Exp:** Craniofacial Surgery/Reconstruction; Spina Bifida; Brain Tumors-Pediatric; Pediatric Neurosurgery; **Hospital:** Montefiore Med Ctr, Jacobi Med Ctr; **Address:** Montefiore Med Ctr, Dept Ped Neurosurgery, 111 E 210th St, Bronx, NY 10467-2401; **Phone:** 718-920-4197; **Board Cert:** Neurological Surgery 1989; Pediatric Neurological Surgery 1996; **Med School:** Columbia P&S 1980; **Resid:** Neurological Surgery, NY Neurological Inst 1986; **Fac Appt:** Prof NS, Albert Einstein Coll Med

Grady, M Sean MD [NS] - **Spec Exp:** Cerebrovascular Surgery; Aneurysm-Cerebral; Arteriovenous Malformations; **Hospital:** Hosp Univ Penn - UPHS (page 60), Pennsylvania Hosp (page 60); **Address:** Hosp Univ Penn, Dept Neurosurgery, 3400 Spruce St, Silverstein Bldg Fl 3, Philadelphia, PA 19104; **Phone:** 215-662-3483; **Board Cert:** Neurological Surgery 1990; **Med School:** Georgetown Univ 1981; **Resid:** Neurological Surgery, Univ Virginia Hosp 1987; **Fac Appt:** Prof NS, Univ Pennsylvania

Gutin, Philip MD [NS] - **Spec Exp:** Brain Tumors; Meningioma; Acoustic Neuroma; **Hospital:** Meml Sloan-Kettering Cancer Ctr, NY-Presby Hosp/Weill Cornell (page 66); **Address:** 1275 York Avenue, New York, NY 10065; **Phone:** 800-525-2225; **Board Cert:** Neurological Surgery 1981; **Med School:** Univ Pennsylvania 1971; **Resid:** Neurological Surgery, UCSF Med Ctr 1979; **Fellow:** Natl Cancer Inst 1976; **Fac Appt:** Prof NS, Cornell Univ-Weill Med Coll

Harbaugh, Robert E MD [NS] - **Spec Exp:** Carotid Artery Surgery; Aneurysm-Cerebral; Arteriovenous Malformations; **Hospital:** Penn State Milton S Hershey Med Ctr; **Address:** Penn State-Hershey Med Ctr, H110 Neurosurg, C3830-Biomed Rsch Bldg, 500 University Drive, Hershey, PA 17033-0850; **Phone:** 717-531-8807; **Board Cert:** Neurological Surgery 1989; **Med School:** Penn State Univ-Hershey Med Ctr 1978; **Resid:** Surgery, Dartmouth-Hitchcock Med Ctr 1980; Neurological Surgery, Dartmouth-Hitchcock Med Ctr 1985; **Fac Appt:** Prof NS, Penn State Univ-Hershey Med Ctr

Hopkins, L Nelson MD [NS] - **Spec Exp:** Cerebrovascular Disease; Endovascular Surgery; **Hospital:** Millard Fillmore Gates Cir Hosp; **Address:** Millard Fillmore Hosp, Dept Neurosurgery, 3 Gates Cir, Buffalo, NY 14209; **Phone:** 716-887-5210; **Board Cert:** Neurological Surgery 1977; **Med School:** Albany Med Coll 1969; **Resid:** Neurological Surgery, SUNY Buffalo Med Ctr 1975; **Fac Appt:** Prof NS, SUNY Buffalo

Jallo, George I MD [NS] - **Spec Exp:** Pediatric Neurosurgery; Spinal Cord Tumors; Brain & Spinal Cord Tumors; **Hospital:** Johns Hopkins Hosp - Baltimore (page 61); **Address:** Johns Hopkins Hosp, Dept of Neurosurgery, 600 N Wolfe St, Ste Harvey 811, Baltimore, MD 21287; **Phone:** 410-955-7851; **Board Cert:** Neurological Surgery 2002; **Med School:** Univ VA Sch Med 1991; **Resid:** Neurological Surgery, NY Univ Med Ctr; **Fellow:** Pediatric Surgery, Beth Israel Med Ctr; **Fac Appt:** Asst Prof NS, Johns Hopkins Univ

Jho, Hae-Dong MD/PhD [NS] - **Spec Exp:** Minimally Invasive Neurosurgery; **Hospital:** Allegheny General Hosp; **Address:** Inst for Minimally Invasive Neurosurgery, 320 E North Ave, Snyder Pavilion, Fl 7, Pittsburgh, PA 15212-4746; **Phone:** 412-359-6110; **Board Cert:** Neurological Surgery 1991; **Med School:** Korea 1971; **Resid:** Neurological Surgery, Hanyang Univ Hosp 1979; Neurological Surgery, Univ Pittsburgh 1989; **Fellow:** Microsurgery, Univ Pittsburgh 1983; **Fac Appt:** Prof NS, Drexel Univ Coll Med

Judy, Kevin MD [NS] - **Spec Exp:** Brain Tumors; **Hospital:** Hosp Univ Penn - UPHS (page 60), Pennsylvania Hosp (page 60); **Address:** Hosp Univ Penn-Dept Neurosurg, 3400 Spruce St, 3 Silverstein, Philadelphia, PA 19104; **Phone:** 215-662-7854; **Board Cert:** Neurological Surgery 1997; **Med School:** Univ Pittsburgh 1984; **Resid:** Surgery, Mercy Hosp 1986; Neurological Surgery, Johns Hopkins Hosp 1992; **Fellow:** Neurological Surgery, Johns Hopkins Hosp 1991; **Fac Appt:** Assoc Prof NS, Univ Pennsylvania

America's Top Doctors® 8th Edition

Kassam, Amin MD [NS] - **Spec Exp:** Skull Base Tumors & Surgery; Cranial Nerve Disorders; Cerebrovascular Surgery; Endoscopic Surgery; **Hospital:** UPMC Presby, Pittsburgh; **Address:** Univ Pittsburgh Med Ctr, Dept Neurosurgery, 200 Lothrop St, Ste B400, Pittburgh, PA 15213; **Phone:** 412-647-3685; **Med School:** Univ Toronto 1991; **Resid:** Neurological Surgery, Univ Ottawa Med Ctr 1997; **Fac Appt:** Assoc Prof NS, Univ Pittsburgh

Khan, Agha S MD [NS] - **Spec Exp:** Skull Base Surgery; Spinal Surgery; **Hospital:** Sinai Hosp - Baltimore; **Address:** 2411 W Belvedere Ave, Ste 402, Baltimore, MD 21215; **Phone:** 410-601-8314; **Board Cert:** Neurological Surgery 1995; **Med School:** Pakistan 1979; **Resid:** Neurological Surgery, Univ Wisconsin Hosp 1990; **Fellow:** Surgical Oncology, Roswell Park Meml Inst 1982; Neurological Surgery, Allegheny Genl Hosp 1991

Kobrine, Arthur MD/PhD [NS] - **Spec Exp:** Spinal Cord Surgery; Brain & Spinal Cord Tumors; **Hospital:** Sibley Mem Hosp, Georgetown Univ Hosp; **Address:** 2440 M St NW, Ste 315, Washington, DC 20037-1404; **Phone:** 202-293-7136; **Board Cert:** Neurological Surgery 1976; **Med School:** Northwestern Univ 1968; **Resid:** Neurological Surgery, Northwestern Univ Hosp 1970; Neurological Surgery, Walter Reed Army Hosp 1973; **Fellow:** Physiology, Geo Wash Univ 1979; **Fac Appt:** Clin Prof NS, Georgetown Univ

Kondziolka, Douglas MD [NS] - **Spec Exp:** Brain Tumors-Adult & Pediatric; Brain Tumors-Metastatic; Stereotactic Radiosurgery; Movement Disorders; **Hospital:** UPMC Presby, Pittsburgh, Chldns Hosp of Pittsburgh - UPMC; **Address:** Univ Pittsburgh Med Ctr, Dept Neurological Surgery, 200 Lothrop St, Ste B400, Pittsburgh, PA 15213; **Phone:** 412-647-9990; **Board Cert:** Neurological Surgery 1994; **Med School:** Univ Toronto 1985; **Resid:** Neurological Surgery, Univ Toronto 1991; **Fellow:** Stereo Neurological Surgery, UPMC Presby Med Ctr 1991; **Fac Appt:** Prof NS, Univ Pittsburgh

Lavyne, Michael H MD [NS] - **Spec Exp:** Spinal Surgery; Spinal Tumors; Spinal Disorders; **Hospital:** NY-Presby Hosp/Weill Cornell (page 66), Hosp For Special Surgery (page 59); **Address:** 110 E 55th St Fl 9, New York, NY 10022; **Phone:** 212-486-9100; **Board Cert:** Neurological Surgery 1982; **Med School:** Cornell Univ-Weill Med Coll 1972; **Resid:** Neurological Surgery, Mass Genl Hosp 1979; **Fellow:** Neurology, Beth Israel Hosp 1974; **Fac Appt:** Clin Prof NS, Cornell Univ-Weill Med Coll

Loftus, Christopher M MD [NS] - **Spec Exp:** Carotid Artery Surgery; Aneurysm-Cerebral; Arteriovenous Malformations; Cerebrovascular Surgery; **Hospital:** Temple Univ Hosp; **Address:** Temple Univ School Med, 3401 N Broad St, Parkinson Pavilion 540, Philadelphia, PA 19140; **Phone:** 215-707-4109; **Board Cert:** Neurological Surgery 1987; **Med School:** SUNY Downstate 1979; **Resid:** Neurological Surgery, Columbia-Presby Med Ctr 1985; **Fac Appt:** Prof NS, Temple Univ

Lunsford, L Dade MD [NS] - **Spec Exp:** Brain Tumors; Stereotactic Radiosurgery; Movement Disorders; Vascular Malformations; **Hospital:** UPMC Presby, Pittsburgh, Chldns Hosp of Pittsburgh - UPMC; **Address:** UPMC Presbyterian Hosp, 200 Lothrop St, Ste B400, Pittsburgh, PA 15213-2536; **Phone:** 412-647-9990; **Board Cert:** Neurological Surgery 1983; **Med School:** Columbia P&S 1974; **Resid:** Neurological Surgery, Univ Pittsburgh Med Ctr 1980; **Fellow:** Stereo Neurological Surgery, Karolinska Hospital 1981; **Fac Appt:** Prof NS, Univ Pittsburgh

Maroon, Joseph C MD [NS] - **Spec Exp:** Minimally Invasive Surgery; Microdiscectomy; Brain Injury-Traumatic; **Hospital:** UPMC Presby, Pittsburgh; **Address:** UPMC Presbyterian, Dept Neuro Surg, 200 Lothrop St, Ste 5-C, Pittsburgh, PA 15213; **Phone:** 412-647-3604; **Board Cert:** Neurological Surgery 1973; **Med School:** Indiana Univ 1965; **Resid:** Surgery, Georgetown Univ Hosp 1967; Neurological Surgery, Indiana Univ Med Ctr 1971; **Fellow:** Neurological Surgery, Radcliffe Infirmary 1969; Microsurgery, Univ Vermont 1972; **Fac Appt:** Clin Prof NS, Univ Pittsburgh

Neurological Surgery

McCormick, Paul C MD [NS] - **Spec Exp:** Spinal Surgery; Spinal Tumors; **Hospital:** NY-Presby Hosp/Columbia (page 66), Valley Hosp; **Address:** 710 W 168th St, Ste 406, New York, NY 10032-2603; **Phone:** 212-305-7976; **Board Cert:** Neurological Surgery 1993; **Med School:** Columbia P&S 1982; **Resid:** Neurological Surgery, Columbia Presby Med Ctr 1989; **Fellow:** Neurological Surgery, Natl Inst Hlth 1984; Spinal Surgery, Med Coll Wisconsin 1990; **Fac Appt:** Prof NS, Columbia P&S

Murali, Raj MD [NS] - **Spec Exp:** Trigeminal Neuralgia; Skull Base Surgery; Aneurysm-Cerebral; Pituitary Tumors; **Hospital:** Westchester Med Ctr, St Vincent Cath Med Ctrs - Manhattan; **Address:** Westchester Med Ctr, Dept Neurosurgery, Munger Pavilion, Ste 329, Valhalla, NY 10595; **Phone:** 914-493-8392; **Board Cert:** Neurological Surgery 1982; **Med School:** India 1968; **Resid:** Neurological Surgery, Royal Infirm-Univ Edinburgh 1974; Neurological Surgery, NYU Med Ctr 1979; **Fac Appt:** Prof NS, NY Med Coll

O'Rourke, Donald MD [NS] - **Spec Exp:** Neuro-Oncology; Brain Tumors; Spinal Surgery-Cervical; **Hospital:** Hosp Univ Penn - UPHS (page 60); **Address:** Hosp Univ Penn - Dept Neurosurg, 3400 Spruce St, 3 Silverstein, Philadelphia, PA 19104; **Phone:** 215-662-3490; **Board Cert:** Neurological Surgery 1998; **Med School:** Univ Pennsylvania 1987; **Resid:** Neurological Surgery, Hosp Univ Penn 1994; **Fac Appt:** Assoc Prof NS, Univ Pennsylvania

Piatt, Joseph H MD [NS] - **Spec Exp:** Brachial Plexus Palsy-Pediatric; Spasticity & Movement Disorders; Chiari's Deformity; Syringomyelia & Spinal Cord Diseases; **Hospital:** St Christopher's Hosp for Chldn; **Address:** St Christopher's Hosp-Div Neurosurg, Erie Ave & Front St, Ste 2202, Philadelphia, PA 19134; **Phone:** 215-427-5196; **Board Cert:** Neurological Surgery 1989; Pediatric Neurological Surgery 2006; **Med School:** Univ Pennsylvania 1979; **Resid:** Neurological Surgery, Duke Univ Med Ctr 1986; **Fellow:** Pediatric Neurological Surgery, Hosp Sick Chldn 1987; **Fac Appt:** Prof NS, Drexel Univ Coll Med

Pollack, Ian MD [NS] - **Spec Exp:** Pediatric Neurosurgery; Brain Tumors; Craniofacial Surgery; Neuro-Oncology; **Hospital:** Chldns Hosp of Pittsburgh - UPMC, UPMC Presby, Pittsburgh; **Address:** Chldns Hosp Pittsburgh, Div Neurosurgery, 3705 Fifth Ave, Ste 3670A, Pittsburgh, PA 15213-2524; **Phone:** 412-692-5881; **Board Cert:** Neurological Surgery 1996; Pediatric Neurological Surgery 1997; **Med School:** Johns Hopkins Univ 1984; **Resid:** Neurological Surgery, Univ Pittsburgh Med Ctr 1991; **Fellow:** Pediatric Neurological Surgery, Hosp Sick Chldn 1992; **Fac Appt:** Prof NS, Univ Pittsburgh

Rigamonti, Daniele MD [NS] - **Spec Exp:** Hydrocephalus-Adult; Brain Tumors; Spinal Disorders; Vascular Neurosurgery; **Hospital:** Johns Hopkins Hosp - Baltimore (page 61); **Address:** Johns Hopkins Hosp, Dept Neurosurgery, 600 N Wolfe St, Phipps 100, Baltimore, MD 21287; **Phone:** 410-955-2259; **Board Cert:** Neurological Surgery 1988; **Med School:** Italy 1976; **Resid:** Neurological Surgery, Mt Sinai Hosp Med Ctr 1984; **Fellow:** Neurological Vascular Surgery, Barrow Neuro Inst 1987; **Fac Appt:** Prof NS, Johns Hopkins Univ

Rosenwasser, Robert H MD [NS] - **Spec Exp:** Aneurysm-Cerebral; Cerebrovascular Surgery; Arteriovenous Malformations; **Hospital:** Thomas Jefferson Univ Hosp; **Address:** Thomas Jefferson University Hospital, 909 Walnut St Fl 2, Philadelphia, PA 19107; **Phone:** 215-955-7000; **Board Cert:** Neurological Surgery 1987; **Med School:** Louisiana State U, New Orleans 1979; **Resid:** Neurological Surgery, Temple Univ Hosp 1984; **Fellow:** Neurological Vascular Surgery, Univ West Ontarion 1985; Interventional Neuroradiology, NYU Med Ctr 1993; **Fac Appt:** Prof NS, Thomas Jefferson Univ

Sen, Chandranath MD [NS] - **Spec Exp:** Brain Tumors; Skull Base Tumors; Skull Base Surgery; **Hospital:** St Luke's - Roosevelt Hosp Ctr - Roosevelt Div (page 57); **Address:** St Lukes Roosevelt Hosp Ctr, Dept Neurosurgery, 1000 10th Ave, Ste 5G-80, New York, NY 10019; **Phone:** 212-523-6720; **Board Cert:** Neurological Surgery 1989; **Med School:** India 1976; **Resid:** Surgery, Univ Wisconsin Hosps 1980; Neurological Surgery, Univ Wisconsin Hosps 1985; **Fellow:** Microsurgery, Univ Pittsburgh Med Ctr 1986

Solomon, Robert A MD [NS] - **Spec Exp:** Aneurysm-Cerebral; Arteriovenous Malformations; **Hospital:** NY-Presby Hosp/Columbia (page 66); **Address:** 710 W 168th St, Ste 439, New York, NY 10032; **Phone:** 212-305-4118; **Board Cert:** Neurological Surgery 1988; **Med School:** Johns Hopkins Univ 1980; **Resid:** Neurological Surgery, Neuro Inst-Columbia Univ 1986; **Fac Appt:** Prof NS, Columbia P&S

Stieg, Philip E MD/PhD [NS] - **Spec Exp:** Cerebrovascular Surgery; Acoustic Neuroma; Skull Base Surgery; Meningioma; **Hospital:** NY-Presby Hosp/Weill Cornell (page 66); **Address:** 525 E 68th St, STARR 651, New York, NY 10021-9800; **Phone:** 212-746-4684; **Board Cert:** Neurological Surgery 1992; **Med School:** Med Coll Wisc 1983; **Resid:** Neurological Surgery, Dallas Chldns Hosp/Parkland Meml Hosp 1988; **Fellow:** Neurological Biology, Karolinska Inst 1988; **Fac Appt:** Prof NS, Cornell Univ-Weill Med Coll

Sutton, Leslie N MD [NS] - **Spec Exp:** Brain Tumors-Pediatric; Fetal Neurosurgery; Hydrocephalus; **Hospital:** Chldns Hosp of Philadelphia, The; **Address:** Childrens Hosp of Phila -Div Neurosurgery, 34th St & Civic Ctr Blvd Wood 6 Bldg, Philadelphia, PA 19104; **Phone:** 215-590-2780; **Board Cert:** Neurological Surgery 1984; Pediatric Neurological Surgery 1996; **Med School:** Univ Pennsylvania 1975; **Resid:** Neurological Surgery, Hosp Univ Penn 1981; **Fac Appt:** Prof NS, Univ Pennsylvania

Tamargo, Rafael J MD [NS] - **Spec Exp:** Vascular Neurosurgery; Skull Base Surgery; **Hospital:** Johns Hopkins Hosp - Baltimore (page 61); **Address:** Johns Hopkins Hosp, Dept Neurosurgery, 600 N Wolfe St, Meyer 8-181, Baltimore, MD 21287; **Phone:** 410-614-1533; **Board Cert:** Neurological Surgery 1995; **Med School:** Columbia P&S 1984; **Resid:** Neurological Surgery, Johns Hopkins Hosps 1992; **Fac Appt:** Prof NS, Johns Hopkins Univ

Turtz, Alan R MD [NS] - **Spec Exp:** Brain Tumors; Pituitary Tumors; Spinal Surgery; **Hospital:** Cooper Univ Hosp; **Address:** 3 Cooper Plaza, Ste 403, Camden, NJ 08103; **Phone:** 856-968-7898; **Board Cert:** Neurological Surgery 1995; **Med School:** Med Coll PA 1986; **Resid:** Neurological Surgery, Med Coll Penn 1992; **Fac Appt:** Asst Prof NS, Jefferson Med Coll

Weiner, Howard L MD [NS] - **Spec Exp:** Pediatric Neurosurgery; Epilepsy; Brain Tumors; Tuberous Sclerosis; **Hospital:** NYU Med Ctr (page 68); **Address:** NYU Med Ctr, Div Pediatric Neurosurgery, 317 E 34th St, Ste 1002, New York, NY 10016; **Phone:** 212-263-6419; **Board Cert:** Neurological Surgery 2001; **Med School:** Cornell Univ 1989; **Resid:** Neurological Surgery, NYU Med Ctr 1996; **Fellow:** Pediatric Neurological Surgery, NYU Med Ctr 1997; **Fac Appt:** Assoc Prof NS, NYU Sch Med

Welch, William C MD [NS] - **Spec Exp:** Spinal Surgery; **Hospital:** Pennsylvania Hosp (page 60); **Address:** Pennsylvania Hospital, Garfield-Duncan Bldg, 301 S 8th St, Ste 4B, Philadelphia, PA 19106; **Phone:** 215-829-6700; **Board Cert:** Neurological Surgery 1995; **Med School:** SUNY Downstate 1985; **Resid:** Neurological Surgery, Univ Rochester/Strong Meml Hosp 1991; **Fellow:** Neuro-Oncology, Montefiore Med Ctr 1992; Spinal Surgery, Montefiore Med Ctr/Albert Einstein 1993; **Fac Appt:** Prof NS, Univ Pennsylvania

Neurological Surgery

Whiting, Donald M MD [NS] - **Spec Exp:** Movement Disorders; Pain & Spasticity; Spinal Disorders; **Hospital:** Allegheny General Hosp, Washington Hosp, The; **Address:** 380 West Chestnut St, Washington, PA 15301-4657; **Phone:** 724-228-1414; **Board Cert:** Neurological Surgery 1995; **Med School:** Jefferson Med Coll 1985; **Resid:** Surgery, Geisinger Med Ctr 1986; Neurological Surgery, Cleveland Clinic 1991; **Fellow:** Neurological Trauma, Allegheny Genl Hosp 1990; **Fac Appt:** Assoc Prof NS, Drexel Univ Coll Med

Wisoff, Jeffrey H MD [NS] - **Spec Exp:** Pediatric Neurosurgery; Brain Tumors-Pediatric; Hydrocephalus; **Hospital:** NYU Med Ctr (page 68), Maimonides Med Ctr (page 63); **Address:** 317 E 34th St, Ste 1002, New York, NY 10016-4974; **Phone:** 212-263-6419; **Board Cert:** Neurological Surgery 1990; Pediatric Neurological Surgery 1996; **Med School:** Geo Wash Univ 1978; **Resid:** Neurological Surgery, NYU/Bellevue Hosp 1984; **Fellow:** Pediatric Neurological Surgery, NYU Med Ctr 1985; **Fac Appt:** Assoc Prof NS, NYU Sch Med

Southeast

Asher, Anthony MD [NS] - **Spec Exp:** Brain Tumors; Stereotactic Radiosurgery; Epilepsy; **Hospital:** Carolinas Med Ctr, Presby Hosp - Charlotte; **Address:** 225 Baldwin Ave, Charlotte, NC 28204; **Phone:** 704-376-1605; **Board Cert:** Neurological Surgery 1998; **Med School:** Wayne State Univ 1987; **Resid:** Neurological Surgery, Univ Mich Med Ctr 1995; **Fellow:** Surgical Oncology, Natl Cancer Inst 1991

Boop, Frederick A MD [NS] - **Spec Exp:** Pediatric Neurosurgery; Epilepsy; Brain Tumors; **Hospital:** Le Bonheur Chldns Med Ctr, Methodist Univ Hosp - Memphis; **Address:** Semmes Murphy Clinic, 1211 Union Ave, Ste 200, Memphis, TN 38104; **Phone:** 901-259-5340; **Board Cert:** Neurological Surgery 1993; Pediatric Neurological Surgery 2005; **Med School:** Univ Ark 1983; **Resid:** Neurological Surgery, Univ Tex Hlth Sci Ctr 1989; Neurological Surgery, Inst Neur/Hosp Sick Chldn 1987; **Fellow:** Epilepsy, Univ Minn 1989; Pediatric Neurological Surgery, Ark Chldns Hosp 1990; **Fac Appt:** Assoc Prof NS, Univ Tenn Coll Med, Memphis

Branch Jr, Charles L MD [NS] - **Spec Exp:** Spinal Reconstructive Surgery; Minimally Invasive Spinal Surgery; Stereotactic Radiosurgery; **Hospital:** Wake Forest Univ Baptist Med Ctr (page 73), Forsyth Med Ctr; **Address:** WFU Baptist Med Ctr, Medical Center Blvd, Winston-Salem, NC 27157-1029; **Phone:** 336-716-4083; **Board Cert:** Neurological Surgery 1991; **Med School:** Univ Tex SW, Dallas 1981; **Resid:** Neurological Surgery, NC Baptist Hosp 1987; **Fac Appt:** Prof NS, Wake Forest Univ

Brem, Steven MD [NS] - **Spec Exp:** Brain Tumors; Pituitary Tumors; Clinical Trials; **Hospital:** H Lee Moffitt Cancer Ctr & Research Inst; **Address:** H. Lee Moffitt Cancer Ctr/ Neurosurgery, 12902 Magnolia Drive, Tampa, FL 33612-9497; **Phone:** 813-745-3063; **Board Cert:** Neurological Surgery 1983; **Med School:** Harvard Med Sch 1972; **Resid:** Neurological Surgery, Massachusetts Genl Hosp 1981; **Fellow:** Oncology, Natl Cancer Inst 1976; **Fac Appt:** Prof NS, Univ S Fla Coll Med

Ewend, Matthew MD [NS] - **Spec Exp:** Brain Tumors; Pituitary Tumors; Pediatric Neurosurgery; Epilepsy; **Hospital:** Univ NC Hosps; **Address:** Univ North Carolina Neurosurgery, 3015 Burnett Womack Bldg, CB# 7060, Chapel Hill, NC 27599; **Phone:** 919-966-1374; **Board Cert:** Neurological Surgery 2001; **Med School:** Johns Hopkins Univ 1990; **Resid:** Neurological Surgery, Johns Hopkins Hospital 1994; **Fellow:** Neuro-Oncology, National Institutes of Health 1996; **Fac Appt:** Asst Prof NS, Univ NC Sch Med

Foley, Kevin MD [NS] - **Spec Exp:** Spinal Surgery; Minimally Invasive Spinal Surgery; **Hospital:** Methodist Univ Hosp - Memphis, Baptist Memorial Hospital - Memphis; **Address:** Semmes-Murphy Clinic, 1211 Union Ave, Ste 200, Memphis, TN 38104; **Phone:** 901-259-5340; **Board Cert:** Neurological Surgery 1987; **Med School:** UCLA 1979; **Resid:** Neurological Surgery, UCLA Med Ctr 1985; **Fac Appt:** Prof NS, Univ Tenn Coll Med, Memphis

Freeman, Thomas B MD [NS] - **Spec Exp:** Parkinson's Disease; Nerve Surgery & Transplantation; Spinal Surgery; **Hospital:** Tampa Genl Hosp; **Address:** 2 A Columbia Drive USF Bldg, Tampa, FL 33606; **Phone:** 813-259-0889; **Board Cert:** Neurological Surgery 1993; **Med School:** Johns Hopkins Univ 1981; **Resid:** Neurological Surgery, NYU Med Ctr 1988; **Fac Appt:** Prof NS, Univ S Fla Coll Med

Friedman, Allan H MD [NS] - **Spec Exp:** Brain Tumors; Skull Base Tumors; Cerebrovascular Surgery; **Hospital:** Duke Univ Med Ctr; **Address:** Duke Univ Med Ctr, DUMC 3807, Durham, NC 27710; **Phone:** 919-681-6421; **Board Cert:** Neurological Surgery 1983; **Med School:** Univ IL Coll Med 1974; **Resid:** Neurological Surgery, Duke Univ Med Ctr 1980; **Fellow:** Vascular Surgery, Univ Western Ontario 1981; **Fac Appt:** Prof S, Duke Univ

Green, Barth MD [NS] - **Spec Exp:** Spinal Surgery; **Hospital:** Jackson Meml Hosp, Univ of Miami Hosp & Clins/Sylvester Comp Canc Ctr; **Address:** 1095 NW 14th Terr Fl 2, Miami, FL 33136; **Phone:** 305-243-6946; **Board Cert:** Neurological Surgery 1978; **Med School:** Indiana Univ 1969; **Resid:** Neurological Surgery, Northwestern Univ Sch Med 1975; **Fac Appt:** Prof NS, Univ Miami Sch Med

Guthrie, Barton L MD [NS] - **Spec Exp:** Brain Tumors; Stereotactic Radiosurgery; Parkinson's Disease/Movement Disorders; **Hospital:** Univ of Ala Hosp at Birmingham; **Address:** Univ Alabama, Div Neurosurg, 510 20th St S, FOT 1038, Birmingham, AL 35294-3410; **Phone:** 205-934-8136; **Board Cert:** Neurological Surgery 1992; **Med School:** Univ Ala 1980; **Resid:** Neurological Surgery, Mayo Clinic 1988; **Fellow:** Neurological Surgery, Stanford Univ Med Ctr 1988; **Fac Appt:** Assoc Prof NS, Univ Ala

Hadley, Mark N MD [NS] - **Spec Exp:** Spinal Surgery-Complex; Spinal Disorders-Degenerative; **Hospital:** Univ of Ala Hosp at Birmingham; **Address:** UAB Sch Med, Div Neurosurgery, 510 20th St S, Ste FOT 1030, Birmingham, AL 35294-3410; **Phone:** 205-934-1439; **Board Cert:** Neurological Surgery 1992; **Med School:** Albany Med Coll 1982; **Resid:** Neurological Surgery, St Josephs Hosp Med Ctr 1988; **Fac Appt:** Prof NS, Univ Ala

Haid Jr, Regis W MD [NS] - **Spec Exp:** Spinal Surgery; Minimally Invasive Spinal Surgery; Spinal Disc Replacement; Microdiscectomy; **Hospital:** Piedmont Hosp; **Address:** Atlanta Brain & Spine Care, 2001 Peachtree Rd NE, Ste 645, Atlanta, GA 30309; **Phone:** 404-350-0106; **Board Cert:** Neurological Surgery 2000; **Med School:** W VA Univ 1982; **Resid:** Surgery, W Va Univ Hosps 1983; Neurological Surgery, W Va Univ Hosps 1988; **Fellow:** Spinal Surgery, Univ Fl Affil Hosps 1989; **Fac Appt:** Assoc Prof NS, Emory Univ

Heros, Roberto MD [NS] - **Spec Exp:** Cerebrovascular Surgery; Skull Base Surgery; Brain Tumors; **Hospital:** Jackson Meml Hosp; **Address:** Univ Miami, Dept Neurosurgery, 1095 NW 14th Terrace, Miami, FL 33136; **Phone:** 305-243-4572; **Board Cert:** Neurological Surgery 1979; **Med School:** Univ Tenn Coll Med, Memphis 1968; **Resid:** Surgery, Mass Genl Hosp 1970; Neurological Surgery, Mass Genl Hosp 1976; **Fac Appt:** Prof NS, Univ Miami Sch Med

Landy, Howard J MD [NS] - **Spec Exp:** Epilepsy/Seizure Disorders; Spinal Cord Injury; Brain Injury; Stereotactic Radiosurgery; **Hospital:** Jackson Meml Hosp; **Address:** University of Miami, Neurosurgery, 1095 NW 14th Terrace Fl 2, Miami, FL 33136; **Phone:** 305-243-4675; **Board Cert:** Neurological Surgery 1991; **Med School:** Univ Miami Sch Med 1980; **Resid:** Neurological Surgery, Jackson Meml Hosp 1987; **Fac Appt:** Prof NS, Univ Miami Sch Med

Neurological Surgery

Markert Jr, James M MD [NS] - **Spec Exp:** Brain Tumors; Stereotactic Radiosurgery; Clinical Trials; **Hospital:** Univ of Ala Hosp at Birmingham; **Address:** Univ Alabama, Div Neurosurgery, 510 20th St S, FOT 1060, Birmingham, AL 35294; **Phone:** 205-975-6985; **Board Cert:** Neurological Surgery 1999; **Med School:** Columbia P&S 1988; **Resid:** Neurological Surgery, Univ Mich Med Ctr 1995; **Fellow:** Neuro-Oncology, Mass Genl Hosp; **Fac Appt:** Prof NS, Univ Ala

Morrison, Glenn MD [NS] - **Spec Exp:** Pediatric Neurosurgery; Epilepsy; Craniofacial Surgery; Spinal Cord Tumors; **Hospital:** Miami Children's Hosp, Jackson Meml Hosp; **Address:** Ambulatory Care Bldg, 3215 SW 62nd Ave, Ste 3109, Miami, FL 33155; **Phone:** 305-662-8386; **Board Cert:** Neurological Surgery 1976; Pediatric Neurological Surgery 1996; **Med School:** Case West Res Univ 1967; **Resid:** Neurological Surgery, Case Western Univ Hosp 1974; **Fac Appt:** Prof NS, Univ Miami Sch Med

Myseros, John S MD [NS] - **Spec Exp:** Pediatric Neurosurgery; Brain Tumors; Congenital Nervous System Malformations; **Hospital:** Inova Fairfax Hosp for Chldn; **Address:** 8501 Arlington Blvd, Fairfax, VA 22031; **Phone:** 571-226-8330; **Board Cert:** Neurological Surgery 2000; **Med School:** Johns Hopkins Univ 1990; **Resid:** Neurological Surgery, Med Coll Virginia 1996; **Fellow:** Pediatric Neurological Surgery, Hosp for Sick Children 1997; **Fac Appt:** Assoc Prof NS, Geo Wash Univ

Oakes, W Jerry MD [NS] - **Spec Exp:** Pediatric Neurosurgery; Chiari's Deformity; Occult Spinal Dysraphism (OSD); **Hospital:** Children's Hospital - Birmingham; **Address:** Children's Hosp Alabama, 1600 7th Ave S ACC 400 Bldg, Birmingham, AL 35233; **Phone:** 205-939-9653; **Board Cert:** Neurological Surgery 1981; Pediatric Neurological Surgery 1996; **Med School:** Duke Univ 1972; **Resid:** Neurological Surgery, Duke Univ Hosp 1978; **Fellow:** Neurological Surgery, Hosp for Sick Chldn 1975; Neurological Surgery, Great Ormond St Hosp 1979; **Fac Appt:** Prof NS, Univ Ala

Olson, Jeffrey J MD [NS] - **Spec Exp:** Neuro-Oncology; Brain Tumors; Stereotactic Radiosurgery; **Hospital:** Emory Univ Hosp, Crawford Long Hosp of Emory Univ; **Address:** Emory Univ, Dept Neurosurgery, 1365B Clifton Rd NE, Ste 2200, Atlanta, GA 30322; **Phone:** 404-778-5770; **Board Cert:** Neurological Surgery 1989; **Med School:** Univ Minn 1981; **Resid:** Neurological Surgery, Univ Iowa Hosps & Clinics 1987; **Fellow:** Neurological Surgery, Natl Inst Hlth 1990; **Fac Appt:** Prof NS, Emory Univ

Parent, Andrew D MD [NS] - **Spec Exp:** Pediatric Neurosurgery; Neuroendocrine Tumors; Pituitary Tumors; **Hospital:** Univ Hosps & Clins - Jackson; **Address:** Univ Miss Med Ctr- Dept Neurosurgery, 2500 N State St, Jackson, MS 39216-4500; **Phone:** 601-984-5702; **Board Cert:** Neurological Surgery 1981; **Med School:** Univ VT Coll Med 1970; **Resid:** Neurological Surgery, Emory Univ 1978; **Fellow:** Neurological Surgery, Univ Tex Med Br 1974; **Fac Appt:** Prof NS, Univ Miss

Patel, Sunil J MD [NS] - **Spec Exp:** Brain Tumors; Skull Base Surgery; Pain-Facial; Trigeminal Neuralgia; **Hospital:** MUSC Med Ctr; **Address:** MUSC - Department of Neurosciences, Division of Neurosurgery, CSB, Ste 428, Charleston, SC 29425; **Phone:** 843-792-7700; **Board Cert:** Neurological Surgery 1996; **Med School:** Med Univ SC 1985; **Resid:** Neurology, Univ South Carolina 1991; **Fellow:** Neurology, Nagoya Univ Med School 1991; Skull Base Surgery, Univ Pittsburgh 1993; **Fac Appt:** Assoc Prof NS, Med Univ SC

Reid, William S MD [NS] - **Spec Exp:** Spinal Surgery; Spinal Cord Surgery; Brain & Spinal Cord Tumors; **Hospital:** Univ of Tennessee Mem Hosp, Fort Sanders Reg Med Ctr; **Address:** 1932 Alcoa Hwy, Bldg C, Ste 280, Knoxville, TN 37920; **Phone:** 865-329-4003; **Board Cert:** Neurological Surgery 1980; **Med School:** Univ Ariz Coll Med 1971; **Resid:** Neurological Surgery, Univ Texas Hlth Sci Ctr 1975; **Fac Appt:** Assoc Clin Prof NS, Univ Tex SW, Dallas

America's Top Doctors® 8th Edition

Rodts Jr, Gerald E MD [NS] - **Spec Exp:** Spinal Surgery; **Hospital:** Crawford Long Hosp of Emory Univ, Emory Univ Hosp; **Address:** Emory Spine Center, 59 Executive Park South, Ste 3000, Atlanta, GA 30329; **Phone:** 404-778-6227; **Board Cert:** Neurological Surgery 1998; **Med School:** Columbia P&S 1987; **Resid:** Neurological Surgery, UCLA Med Ctr 1994; **Fellow:** Spinal Surgery, Emory Univ Hosp 1995; **Fac Appt:** Prof NS, Emory Univ

Sampson, John H MD/PhD [NS] - **Spec Exp:** Brain Tumors; Clinical Trials; **Hospital:** Duke Univ Med Ctr; **Address:** Duke Univ Med Ctr, Box 3050, Durham, NC 27710; **Phone:** 919-684-9041; **Board Cert:** Neurological Surgery 2002; **Med School:** Univ Manitoba 1990; **Resid:** Neurological Surgery, Duke Univ Med Ctr 1998; **Fellow:** Neurological Intensive Care, Duke Univ Med Ctr 1999; **Fac Appt:** Assoc Prof S, Duke Univ

Sanford, Robert A MD [NS] - **Spec Exp:** Pediatric Neurosurgery; Brain Tumors-Pediatric; **Hospital:** Le Bonheur Chldns Med Ctr, St Jude Children's Research Hosp; **Address:** 6325 Humphreys Blvd, Memphis, TN 38120; **Phone:** 901-522-7762; **Board Cert:** Neurological Surgery 1976; Pediatric Neurological Surgery 2005; **Med School:** Univ Ark 1967; **Resid:** Neurological Surgery, Univ Minneapolis Med Ctr 1973; **Fac Appt:** Prof NS, Univ Tenn Coll Med, Memphis

Shaffrey, Christopher I MD [NS] - **Spec Exp:** Spinal Surgery; Spinal Surgery-Pediatric; **Hospital:** Univ Virginia Med Ctr; **Address:** Univ Virg, Dept Neurosurg, Hosp Drive, Private Clinic 3rd Fl, Rm 3508, Charlottesville, VA 22908; **Phone:** 434-243-7026; **Board Cert:** Neurological Surgery 1997; Orthopaedic Surgery 1997; **Med School:** Univ VA Sch Med 1986; **Resid:** Neurological Surgery, Univ Virginia Med Ctr 1992; Orthopaedic Surgery, Univ Virginia Med Ctr 1995; **Fellow:** Spinal Surgery, Univ Virginia Med Ctr 1996; **Fac Appt:** Prof NS, Univ VA Sch Med

Shaffrey, Mark E MD [NS] - **Spec Exp:** Brain Tumors; Clinical Trials; Spinal Cord Tumors; Spinal Tumors; **Hospital:** Univ Virginia Med Ctr; **Address:** UVA Health System, Dept Neurosurgery, PO Box 800212, Charlottesville, VA 22908; **Phone:** 434-924-1843; **Board Cert:** Neurological Surgery 2000; **Med School:** Univ VA Sch Med 1987; **Resid:** Neurological Surgery, Univ Virginia Med Ctr 1991; **Fellow:** Microvascular Physiology, NIH 1992; Neurological Pathology, Univ Virginia Med Ctr 1993; **Fac Appt:** Prof NS, Univ VA Sch Med

Sills Jr, Allen MD [NS] - **Spec Exp:** Brain & Spinal Tumors; Stereotactic Radiosurgery; Cerebrovascular Disease; **Hospital:** Methodist Univ Hosp - Memphis; **Address:** Semmes-Murphey Clinic, 1211 Union Ave, Ste 200, Memphis, TN 38104; **Phone:** 901-259-5340; **Board Cert:** Neurological Surgery 2002; **Med School:** Johns Hopkins Univ 1990; **Resid:** Neurological Surgery, Johns Hopkins Hosp 1994; **Fellow:** Neuro-Oncology, Hunterian Neurosurg Lab/Johns Hopkins 1996; **Fac Appt:** Prof NS, Univ Tenn Coll Med, Memphis

Swaid, Swaid N MD [NS] - **Spec Exp:** Stereotactic Radiosurgery; **Hospital:** UAB Highlands Hosp; **Address:** 513 Brookwood Blvd, Ste 372, Birmingham, AL 35209; **Phone:** 205-802-6844; **Board Cert:** Neurological Surgery 1983; **Med School:** Univ Ala 1976; **Resid:** Neurological Surgery, Univ Alabama 1981; **Fac Appt:** Assoc Prof NS, Univ Ala

Tatter, Stephen MD/PhD [NS] - **Spec Exp:** Brain Tumors; Pituitary Tumors; Stereotactic Radiosurgery; **Hospital:** Wake Forest Univ Baptist Med Ctr (page 73); **Address:** Wake Forest Univ Sch Med, Dept Neurosurg, Medical Center Blvd, Winston-Salem, NC 27157-1029; **Phone:** 336-716-4047; **Board Cert:** Neurological Surgery 2004; **Med School:** Cornell Univ-Weill Med Coll 1990; **Resid:** Neurological Surgery, Mass Genl Hosp 1996; **Fellow:** Neurological Surgery, Mass Genl Hosp 1997; **Fac Appt:** Assoc Prof NS, Wake Forest Univ

Neurological Surgery

Thompson, Reid C MD [NS] - **Spec Exp:** Neuro-Oncology; Brain & Spinal Cord Tumors; Neurovascular Surgery; Skull Base Tumors; **Hospital:** Vanderbilt Univ Med Ctr; **Address:** Vanderbilt Univ Med Ctr, Dept Neurosurg, 1500 21st Ave S, Ste 1506, Nashville, TN 37212; **Phone:** 615-322-7417; **Board Cert:** Neurological Surgery 2001; **Med School:** Johns Hopkins Univ 1989; **Resid:** Neurological Surgery, Johns Hopkins Hosp 1995; **Fellow:** Neuro-Oncology, Rsch-Johns Hopkins Hosp 1996; Cerebrovascular Neurosurgery, Stanford Univ Med Ctr 1997; **Fac Appt:** Assoc Prof NS, Vanderbilt Univ

Tiel, Robert L MD [NS] - **Hospital:** Univ Hosps & Clins - Jackson; **Address:** Univ Mississippi Med Ctr, 2500 N State St, Jackson, MS 39216-4505; **Phone:** 601-984-6445; **Board Cert:** Neurological Surgery 1991; **Med School:** Univ Minn 1980; **Resid:** Neurological Surgery, Henry Ford Hosp 1986; **Fac Appt:** Prof NS, Univ Miss

Van Loveren, Harry R MD [NS] - **Spec Exp:** Trigeminal Neuralgia; Skull Base Surgery; **Hospital:** Tampa Genl Hosp; **Address:** Harbourside Medical Tower, 4 Columbia Drive, Ste 650, Tampa, FL 33606; **Phone:** 813-259-0929; **Board Cert:** Neurological Surgery 1988; **Med School:** Univ Cincinnati 1979; **Resid:** Neurological Surgery, Good Samaritan Hosp 1984; **Fellow:** Neurological Surgery, Universitatspital 1985; **Fac Appt:** Prof NS, Univ S Fla Coll Med

Wharen Jr, Robert E MD [NS] - **Spec Exp:** Parkinson's Disease; Brain Tumors; Epilepsy; **Hospital:** Mayo - Jacksonville; **Address:** Mayo Clinic, Dept Neurosurgery, 4500 San Pablo Rd, Jacksonville, FL 32224-1865; **Phone:** 904-953-2103; **Board Cert:** Neurological Surgery 1988; **Med School:** Penn State Univ-Hershey Med Ctr 1979; **Resid:** Neurological Surgery, Mayo Clinic 1985; **Fac Appt:** Prof NS, Mayo Med Sch

Wilson, John A MD [NS] - **Spec Exp:** Cerebrovascular Surgery; Skull Base Surgery; Spinal Surgery; **Hospital:** Wake Forest Univ Baptist Med Ctr (page 73); **Address:** Wake Forest Univ Medical Ctr, Medical Center Blvd, Box 1029, Winston-Salem, NC 27157-1029; **Phone:** 336-716-4020; **Board Cert:** Neurological Surgery 1996; **Med School:** Jefferson Med Coll 1982; **Resid:** Surgery, Allegheny Gen Hosp 1985; Neurological Surgery, NYU Med Ctr 1986; **Fellow:** Neurological Surgery, New England Med Ctr 1990; **Fac Appt:** Assoc Prof NS, Wake Forest Univ

Young, A Byron MD [NS] - **Spec Exp:** Brain Tumors; Stereotactic Radiosurgery; Parkinson's Disease; **Hospital:** Univ of Kentucky Chandler Hosp; **Address:** Div Neurosurgery, MS 101, 800 Rose St, Lexington, KY 40536-0298; **Phone:** 859-323-5861; **Board Cert:** Neurological Surgery 1974; **Med School:** Univ KY Coll Med 1965; **Resid:** Surgery, Vanderbilt Hosp 1967; Neurological Surgery, Vanderbilt Hosp 1971; **Fac Appt:** Prof S, Univ KY Coll Med

Midwest

Albright, A Leland MD [NS] - **Spec Exp:** Pediatric Neurosurgery; Spasticity & Movement Disorders; Brain Tumors; **Hospital:** Univ WI Hosp & Clins; **Address:** UW Hosp & Clinics, 600 Highland Ave, rm K4/836, Madison, WI 53792; **Phone:** 608-263-9651; **Board Cert:** Neurological Surgery 1981; Pediatric Neurological Surgery 1996; **Med School:** Louisiana State U, New Orleans 1969; **Resid:** Surgery, Wash Hosps 1971; Neurological Surgery, Univ Pittsburgh Med Ctr 1978; **Fellow:** Neurological Surgery, Natl Inst Hlth 1974; Immunopathology, Univ Pittsburgh Med Ctr 1978; **Fac Appt:** Prof NS, Univ Wisc

Atkinson, John MD [NS] - **Spec Exp:** Pituitary Surgery; Stroke; Cerebrovascular Disease; **Hospital:** Mayo Med Ctr & Clin - Rochester; **Address:** Mayo Clinic, Dept Neurosurgery, 200 First St SW, Rochester, MN 55905; **Phone:** 507-284-2376; **Board Cert:** Neurological Surgery 1992; **Med School:** Univ Ala 1984; **Resid:** Neurological Surgery, Mayo Clinic 1990; **Fac Appt:** Assoc Prof NS, Mayo Med Sch

Bakay, Roy MD [NS] - **Spec Exp:** Parkinson's Disease/Movement Disorders; Epilepsy; Brain Tumors; **Hospital:** Rush Univ Med Ctr; **Address:** Rush Univ Med Ctr, 1725 W Harrison St, Ste 970, Chicago, IL 60612; **Phone:** 312-942-6644; **Board Cert:** Neurological Surgery 1985; **Med School:** Northwestern Univ 1975; **Resid:** Neurological Surgery, Univ Washington Sch Med 1981; **Fellow:** Neuronal Plasticity, Natl Inst Hlth 1982; **Fac Appt:** Prof NS, Rush Med Coll

Barnett, Gene H MD [NS] - **Spec Exp:** Brain Tumors; Stereotactic Radiosurgery; **Hospital:** Cleveland Clin Fdn (page 56); **Address:** Cleveland Clinic Brain Tumor Inst, 9500 Euclid Ave, Desk R20, Cleveland, OH 44195; **Phone:** 216-444-5381; **Board Cert:** Neurological Surgery 1990; **Med School:** Case West Res Univ 1980; **Resid:** Neurological Surgery, Cleveland Clinic 1986; **Fellow:** Neurology, Cleveland Clinic 1982; Research, Mass Genl Hosp-Harvard 1987; **Fac Appt:** Prof NS, Cleveland Cl Coll Med/Case West Res

Batjer, Hunt Henry MD [NS] - **Spec Exp:** Aneurysm-Cerebral; Arteriovenous Malformations; Stroke; **Hospital:** Northwestern Meml Hosp, Evanston Hosp; **Address:** 675 N St Clair, Galter Bldg Fl 20 - Ste 250, Chicago, IL 60611; **Phone:** 312-695-8143; **Board Cert:** Neurological Surgery 1986; **Med School:** Univ Tex SW, Dallas 1977; **Resid:** Neurological Surgery, Parkland Meml Hosp 1981; **Fellow:** Neurological Surgery, Univ W Ontario Med Ctr 1982; **Fac Appt:** Prof NS, Northwestern Univ

Bauer, Jerry MD [NS] - **Spec Exp:** Pain-Back & Neck; Brain Tumors; Spinal Surgery; Minimally Invasive Spinal Surgery; **Hospital:** Adv Luth Genl Hosp; **Address:** Ctr Brain & Spine Surg-Parkside Ctr, 1875 Dempster St, Ste 605, Park Ridge, IL 60068-1168; **Phone:** 847-698-1088; **Board Cert:** Neurological Surgery 1982; **Med School:** Univ IL Coll Med 1974; **Resid:** Neurological Surgery, Univ Illinios Med Ctr 1979; **Fac Appt:** Asst Clin Prof NS, Univ IL Coll Med

Benzel, Edward C MD [NS] - **Spec Exp:** Spinal Surgery; **Hospital:** Cleveland Clin Fdn (page 56); **Address:** 9500 Euclid Ave, Ste S80, Cleveland, OH 44195; **Phone:** 216-445-5514; **Board Cert:** Neurological Surgery 1986; **Med School:** Univ Wisc 1974; **Resid:** Neurological Surgery, Med Coll Wisc Clins 1980; **Fellow:** Spinal Cord Injury Medicine, Wood VA Med Ctr 1981; **Fac Appt:** Prof NS, Case West Res Univ

Bierbrauer, Karin S MD [NS] - **Spec Exp:** Pediatric Neurosurgery; Spina Bifida; Craniosynostosis; Hydrocephalus; **Hospital:** Cincinnati Chldns Hosp Med Ctr; **Address:** Cincinnati Children's Hospital, 3333 Burnet Ave, MC 2016, Cincinnati, OH 45229; **Phone:** 513-636-7124; **Board Cert:** Neurological Surgery 1994; Pediatric Neurological Surgery 1995; **Med School:** Med Univ SC 1984; **Resid:** Neurological Surgery, Emory Univ Hosp 1990; **Fellow:** Pediatric Neurological Surgery, Chldns Meml Hosp 1991; **Fac Appt:** Assoc Clin Prof NS, Ohio State Univ

Brown, Frederick D MD [NS] - **Spec Exp:** Minimally Invasive Spinal Surgery; Spinal Surgery; Pain-Chronic; **Hospital:** Univ of Chicago Hosps; **Address:** Univ Chicago Hosp, Dept Neurosurgery, 5841 S Maryland Ave, MC 3026, Chicago, IL 60617; **Phone:** 773-702-2123; **Board Cert:** Neurological Surgery 1982; **Med School:** Ohio State Univ 1972; **Resid:** Neurological Surgery, Univ Chicago Hosps 1978; **Fac Appt:** Assoc Prof NS, Univ Chicago-Pritzker Sch Med

Chandler, William F MD [NS] - **Spec Exp:** Pituitary Surgery; Brain Tumors; **Hospital:** Univ Michigan Hlth Sys; **Address:** 1500 E Med Center Drive, Ste 3470, Tauban Center, Ann Arbor, MI 48109; **Phone:** 734-936-5020; **Board Cert:** Neurological Surgery 1980; **Med School:** Univ Mich Med Sch 1971; **Resid:** Neurological Surgery, Michigan Hosp 1977; **Fac Appt:** Prof NS, Univ Mich Med Sch

Neurological Surgery

Chiocca, E Antonio MD [NS] - **Spec Exp:** Brain Tumors; Spinal Cord Tumors; **Hospital:** Arthur G James Cancer Hosp & Research Inst, Ohio St Univ Med Ctr; **Address:** OSU Med Ctr, Dept Neurosurgery, 410 W 10th Ave, 1021-N Doan Hall, Columbus, OH 43210; **Phone:** 614-293-9312; **Board Cert:** Neurological Surgery 2000; **Med School:** Univ Tex, Houston 1988; **Resid:** Neurological Surgery, Mass Genl Hosp 1995; **Fac Appt:** Prof NS, Ohio State Univ

Cohen, Alan R MD [NS] - **Spec Exp:** Pediatric Neurosurgery; Brain & Spinal Tumors-Pediatric; Minimally Invasive Neurosurgery; **Hospital:** Rainbow Babies & Chldns Hosp, Univ Hosps Case Med Ctr; **Address:** 11100 Euclid Ave, Ste B501, Cleveland, OH 44106; **Phone:** 216-844-5741; **Board Cert:** Neurological Surgery 1991; Pediatric Neurological Surgery 2007; **Med School:** Cornell Univ-Weill Med Coll 1978; **Resid:** Surgery, NYU Medical Ctr 1980; Neurological Surgery, NYU Medical Ctr 1987; **Fellow:** Neurology, Natl Hosp Queen's Square 1982; **Fac Appt:** Prof NS, Case West Res Univ

Dacey Jr, Ralph G MD [NS] - **Spec Exp:** Cerebrovascular Surgery; Aneurysm-Cerebral; Brain Tumors; **Hospital:** Barnes-Jewish Hosp, Barnes-Jewish West County Hosp; **Address:** Wash Univ Dept Neurosurgery, 660 S Euclid Ave, Box 8057, St Louis, MO 63110; **Phone:** 314-362-3577; **Board Cert:** Internal Medicine 1978; Neurological Surgery 1985; **Med School:** Univ VA Sch Med 1974; **Resid:** Internal Medicine, Strong Meml Hosp 1977; Neurological Surgery, Univ Virginia Med Ctr 1983; **Fac Appt:** Prof NS, Washington Univ, St Louis

Dempsey, Robert J MD [NS] - **Spec Exp:** Vascular Neurosurgery; Aneurysm-Cerebral; Stroke; **Hospital:** Univ WI Hosp & Clins; **Address:** Univ Wisc Hosp, Dept Neurosurgery, 600 Highland Ave, rm K4-822, Madison, WI 53792; **Phone:** 608-265-5967; **Board Cert:** Neurological Surgery 1985; **Med School:** Univ Chicago-Pritzker Sch Med 1977; **Resid:** Neurological Surgery, Univ Mich Hosps 1983; **Fac Appt:** Prof NS, Univ Wisc

Diaz, Fernando G MD/PhD [NS] - **Spec Exp:** Arteriovenous Malformations; Spinal Surgery; **Hospital:** Providence Hosp - Southfield, Harper Univ Hosp; **Address:** Michigan Head & Spine Institute, 29275 Northwestern Hwy, Ste 100, Southfield, MI 48034; **Phone:** 248-784-3667; **Board Cert:** Neurological Surgery 1980; **Med School:** Mexico 1968; **Resid:** Surgery, Univ Kansas Med Ctr 1973; Neurological Surgery, Univ Minn Med Ctr 1978; **Fellow:** Cerebrovascular Disease, Univ Minn Med Ctr 1979; **Fac Appt:** Prof NS, Wayne State Univ

Fessler, Richard G MD/PhD [NS] - **Spec Exp:** Skull Base Surgery; Spinal Surgery; Minimally Invasive Spinal Surgery; **Hospital:** Northwestern Meml Hosp; **Address:** 676 N St Clair, Ste 2210, Chicago, IL 60611; **Phone:** 312-695-8143; **Board Cert:** Neurological Surgery 1992; **Med School:** Univ Chicago-Pritzker Sch Med 1983; **Resid:** Neurological Surgery, Univ Chicago Hosp 1989; **Fac Appt:** Prof NS, Northwestern Univ

Frim, David M MD/PhD [NS] - **Spec Exp:** Pediatric Neurosurgery; Hydrocephalus; Brain & Spinal Tumors; Brain & Spinal Malformations; **Hospital:** Univ of Chicago Hosps; **Address:** Univ of Chicago Hosps, Pediatric Neurosurgery, 5841 S Maryland Ave, MC 3026, Chicago, IL 60637-1463; **Phone:** 773-702-2475; **Board Cert:** Neurological Surgery 1998; Pediatric Neurological Surgery 1998; **Med School:** Harvard Med Sch 1988; **Resid:** Neurological Surgery, Mass Genl Hosp 1995; **Fellow:** Pediatric Neurological Surgery, Children's Hosp 1996; **Fac Appt:** Assoc Prof S, Univ Chicago-Pritzker Sch Med

Greene Jr, Clarence S MD [NS] - **Spec Exp:** Pediatric Neurosurgery; Congenital Nervous System Malformations; Brain Tumors; **Hospital:** Chldns Mercy Hosps & Clinics; **Address:** 2401 Gillham Rd, Kansas City, MO 64108; **Phone:** 816-234-3000; **Board Cert:** Neurological Surgery 1984; Pediatric Neurological Surgery 2007; **Med School:** Howard Univ 1974; **Resid:** Neurological Surgery, Chldns Hosp 1981; Neurological Surgery, Peter Bent Brigham Hosp 1981; **Fellow:** Pediatric Neurological Surgery, Chldns Hosp 1985; **Fac Appt:** Assoc Clin Prof NS, UC Irvine

Grubb Jr, Robert L MD [NS] - **Spec Exp:** Brain Tumors; Acoustic Neuroma; Trigeminal Neuralgia; Skull Base Tumors; **Hospital:** Barnes-Jewish Hosp, St Louis Chldns Hosp; **Address:** Wash Univ Sch Med, Dept Neurosurgery, 660 S Euclid Ave, Box 8057, St Louis, MO 63110; **Phone:** 314-362-3577; **Board Cert:** Neurological Surgery 1976; **Med School:** Univ NC Sch Med 1965; **Resid:** Surgery, Barnes Jewish Hosp 1967; Neurological Surgery, Barnes Jewish Hosp 1973; **Fellow:** Neurological Surgery, National Inst Health 1969; **Fac Appt:** Prof NS, Washington Univ, St Louis

Guthikonda, Murali MD [NS] - **Spec Exp:** Skull Base Tumors; Pituitary Tumors; Aneurysm-Cerebral; Spinal Tumors; **Hospital:** Detroit Med Ctr, Harper Univ Hosp; **Address:** Univ Neurologic Surgeons, 4160 John R, Ste 930, Detroit, MI 48201; **Phone:** 313-831-0777; **Board Cert:** Neurological Surgery 1982; **Med School:** India 1971; **Resid:** Surgery, St Elizabeth Hosp 1976; Neurological Surgery, Med Ctr Hosp VT 1980; **Fellow:** Skull Base Surgery, Univ Cincinnati 1993; **Fac Appt:** Assoc Prof NS, Wayne State Univ

Gutierrez, Francisco A MD [NS] - **Spec Exp:** Brain Tumors; Cerebrovascular Surgery; Spinal Surgery; **Hospital:** Northwestern Meml Hosp, Resurrection Med Ctr; **Address:** 201 E Huron St, Ste 9-160, Galter Pavilion, Chicago, IL 60611; **Phone:** 312-926-3490; **Board Cert:** Neurological Surgery 1976; **Med School:** Colombia 1965; **Resid:** Neurological Surgery, San Juan de Dios Hosp 1967; Neurological Surgery, Northwestern Meml Hosp 1973; **Fac Appt:** Assoc Prof NS, Northwestern Univ

Kaufman, Bruce A MD [NS] - **Spec Exp:** Pediatric Neurosurgery; Brain & Spinal Cord Tumors; Spasticity & Movement Disorders; **Hospital:** Chldns Hosp - Wisconsin; **Address:** Chldns Hosp, Dept Neurosurg, 999 N 92nd St, Ste 310, Milwaukee, WI 53226; **Phone:** 414-266-6435; **Board Cert:** Neurological Surgery 1992; Pediatric Neurological Surgery 2006; **Med School:** Case West Res Univ 1982; **Resid:** Neurological Surgery, Univ Hosp Cleveland/Case West Res 1988; **Fellow:** Pediatric Neurological Surgery, Chldns Meml Hosp/Northwestern Univ 1989; **Fac Appt:** Prof NS, Med Coll Wisc

Levy, Robert M MD/PhD [NS] - **Spec Exp:** Stereotactic Radiosurgery; Brain Tumors; Pain-Chronic; **Hospital:** Northwestern Meml Hosp, Evanston Hosp; **Address:** 675 N Saint Clair St, Ste 2210, Gaulter Pavilion, Chicago, IL 60611-2922; **Phone:** 312-695-8143; **Board Cert:** Neurological Surgery 1991; **Med School:** Stanford Univ 1981; **Resid:** Neurological Surgery, UCSF Med Ctr 1987; **Fellow:** Neurological Surgery, UCSF Med Ctr 1986; **Fac Appt:** Prof NS, Northwestern Univ

Link, Michael J MD [NS] - **Spec Exp:** Skull Base Tumors; Brain Tumors; Cerebrovascular Surgery; **Hospital:** Mayo Med Ctr & Clin - Rochester; **Address:** Mayo Clinic, Dept Neurosurgery, 200 First St SW, Rochester, MN 55905; **Phone:** 507-284-8008; **Board Cert:** Neurological Surgery 2000; **Med School:** Mayo Med Sch 1990; **Resid:** Neurological Surgery, Mayo Clinic 1996; **Fellow:** Cerebrovascular & Skull Base Surgery, Univ Cincinnati/Mayfield Clinic 1998; **Fac Appt:** Assoc Prof NS, Mayo Med Sch

Luken, Martin MD [NS] - **Spec Exp:** Brain Tumors; Spinal Surgery; Chiari's Deformity; **Hospital:** Ingalls Meml Hosp, Northern Illinois Med Ctr; **Address:** 71 W 156th St, Ste 208, Harvey, IL 60426; **Phone:** 708-331-6669; **Board Cert:** Neurological Surgery 1983; **Med School:** Columbia P&S 1973; **Resid:** Surgery, Univ Illinois Med Ctr 1976; Neurological Surgery, Neurological Inst-Columbia Presby 1980; **Fac Appt:** Asst Prof NS, Rush Med Coll

Malik, Ghaus MD [NS] - **Spec Exp:** Trigeminal Neuralgia; Cerebrovascular Surgery; Brain & Spinal Cord Tumors; **Hospital:** Henry Ford Hosp, William Beaumont Hosp; **Address:** Henry Ford Hosp, Dept Neurosurg, 2799 W Grand Blvd, Detroit, MI 48202; **Phone:** 313-916-1093; **Board Cert:** Neurological Surgery 1978; **Med School:** Pakistan 1968; **Resid:** Surgery, Henry Ford Hosp 1971; Neurological Surgery, Henry Ford Hosp 1975

Menezes, Arnold MD [NS] - **Spec Exp:** Pediatric Neurosurgery; Craniocervical Disorders; Spinal Surgery-Pediatric; **Hospital:** Univ Iowa Hosp & Clinics; **Address:** Univ Iowa Hosp, Dept Neurosurgery, 200 Hawkins Drive, rm 1824JPP, Iowa City, IA 52242; **Phone:** 319-356-2768; **Board Cert:** Neurological Surgery 1976; Pediatric Neurological Surgery 1997; **Med School:** India 1967; **Resid:** Surgery, Univ Iowa Hosps 1970; Neurological Surgery, Univ Iowa Hosps 1974; **Fellow:** Child Neurology, Univ Iowa Hosps; **Fac Appt:** Prof NS, Univ Iowa Coll Med

Nagib, Mahmoud MD [NS] - **Spec Exp:** Pediatric Neurosurgery; Skull Base Surgery; **Hospital:** Chldns Hosp and Clinics - Minneapolis, Abbott - Northwestern Hosp; **Address:** 800 E 28th St Piper Bldg - Ste 305, Minneapolis, MN 55407-3723; **Phone:** 612-871-7278; **Board Cert:** Neurological Surgery 1985; **Med School:** Egypt 1973; **Resid:** Neurological Surgery, Univ Minn Hosps 1982; **Fellow:** Neurological Physiology, Univ Oslo 1976; **Fac Appt:** Asst Clin Prof NS, Univ Minn

Ondra, Stephen MD [NS] - **Spec Exp:** Spinal Surgery; **Hospital:** Northwestern Meml Hosp; **Address:** Neurological Surgery, 676 N St. Clair St, Ste 2210, Chicago, IL 60611; **Phone:** 312-695-6282; **Board Cert:** Neurological Surgery 1994; **Med School:** Rush Med Coll 1984; **Resid:** Neurological Surgery, Walter Reed Army Med Ctr 1990; **Fac Appt:** Assoc Prof NS, Northwestern Univ

Origitano, Thomas MD/PhD [NS] - **Spec Exp:** Skull Base Tumors & Surgery; Cerebrovascular Surgery; Brain Tumors; **Hospital:** Loyola Univ Med Ctr; **Address:** Loyola Univ Medical Ctr, Dept Neurosurgery, 2160 S First Ave Bldg 105 - rm 1900, Maywood, IL 60153-3304; **Phone:** 708-216-8920; **Board Cert:** Neurological Surgery 1995; **Med School:** Loyola Univ-Stritch Sch Med 1984; **Resid:** Neurological Surgery, Loyola Univ Med Ctr 1990; **Fac Appt:** Prof NS, Loyola Univ-Stritch Sch Med

Park, Tae Sung MD [NS] - **Spec Exp:** Pediatric Neurosurgery; Cerebral Palsy-Select Dorsal Rhizotomy; Chiari's Deformity; Neuro-Oncology; **Hospital:** St Louis Chldns Hosp; **Address:** St Louis Children's Hospital, 1 Children's Place, Ste 4-S20, St Louis, MO 63110; **Phone:** 314-454-4629; **Board Cert:** Neurological Surgery 1985; Pediatric Neurological Surgery 2006; **Med School:** Korea 1971; **Resid:** Neurological Surgery, Univ Virginia Hosp 1981; **Fellow:** Neuropathology, Mass General; Pediatric Neurological Surgery, Hospital for Sick Children; **Fac Appt:** Prof NS, St Louis Univ

Piepgras, David MD [NS] - **Spec Exp:** Vascular Neurosurgery; Minimally Invasive Spinal Surgery; Pain-Facial; **Hospital:** Mayo Med Ctr & Clin - Rochester, St Mary's Hosp - Rochester; **Address:** Mayo Clinic, Dept Neuro Surg, 200 First St SW, Rochester, MN 55905; **Phone:** 507-284-3331; **Board Cert:** Neurological Surgery 1977; **Med School:** Univ Minn 1965; **Resid:** Surgery, Hennipin Co Genl Hosp 1970; Neurological Surgery, Mayo Clinic 1974; **Fac Appt:** Prof NS, Mayo Med Sch

Raffel, Corey MD/PhD [NS] - **Spec Exp:** Pediatric Neurosurgery; Brain Tumors; Medulloblastoma; **Hospital:** Nationwide Chldn's Hosp; **Address:** Nationwide Chldn's Hosp, Dept Neurosurgery, 700 Children's Drive, Columbus, OH 43205; **Phone:** 614-722-2014; **Board Cert:** Neurological Surgery 1990; Pediatric Neurological Surgery 1996; **Med School:** UCSD 1980; **Resid:** Neurological Surgery, UCSF Med Ctr 1986; **Fellow:** Pediatric Neurological Surgery, Hosp Sick Chldn 1988

Rezai, Ali R MD [NS] - **Spec Exp:** Parkinson's Disease; Pain-Chronic; Deep Brain Stimulation; **Hospital:** Cleveland Clin Fdn (page 56); **Address:** 9500 Euclid Ave, Desk S31, Cleveland, OH 44195; **Phone:** 216-444-2210; **Board Cert:** Neurological Surgery 2003; **Med School:** USC Sch Med 1990; **Resid:** Neurological Surgery, NYU Med Ctr 1997; **Fellow:** Stereo Neurological Surgery, Univ Toronto Med Ctr 1998; Neurological Surgery, Karolinska Inst; **Fac Appt:** Assoc Prof NS, Cleveland Cl Coll Med/Case West Res

Rich, Keith M MD [NS] - **Spec Exp:** Brain Tumors; Neurovascular Surgery; Stereotactic Radiosurgery; **Hospital:** Barnes-Jewish Hosp; **Address:** Wash Univ Dept Neurosurgery, 660 S Euclid Ave, Box 8057, St Louis, MO 63110; **Phone:** 314-362-3577; **Board Cert:** Neurological Surgery 1987; **Med School:** Indiana Univ 1977; **Resid:** Neurological Surgery, Barnes Jewish Hosp 1982; **Fellow:** Neurological Pharmacology, Barnes Jewish Hosp 1984; **Fac Appt:** Assoc Prof NS, Washington Univ, St Louis

Rock, Jack P MD [NS] - **Spec Exp:** Neuro-Oncology; Pituitary Surgery; Skull Base Surgery; Brain Tumors; **Hospital:** Henry Ford Hosp; **Address:** Henry Ford Hosp, Dept Neurosurg, 2799 W Grand Blvd, Detroit, MI 48202; **Phone:** 313-916-2241; **Board Cert:** Neurological Surgery 1989; **Med School:** Univ Miami Sch Med 1979; **Resid:** Neurological Surgery, NY Hosp-Cornell Med Ctr 1985; **Fellow:** Univ Maryland 1986

Rosenblum, Mark L MD [NS] - **Spec Exp:** Brain Tumors; Spinal Surgery; Infections-Neurologic; Neuro-Oncology; **Hospital:** Henry Ford Hosp; **Address:** Henry Ford Hospital, K11, 2799 W Grand Blvd, Detroit, MI 48202; **Phone:** 313-916-1340; **Board Cert:** Neurological Surgery 1982; **Med School:** NY Med Coll 1969; **Resid:** Surgery, UCLA Med Ctr 1973; Neurological Surgery, UCSF Med Ctr 1979; **Fellow:** Neuro-Oncology, Natl Cancer Inst 1972; **Fac Appt:** Prof NS, Case West Res Univ

Ruge, John MD [NS] - **Spec Exp:** Pediatric Neurosurgery; Brain Tumors; Hydrocephalus; **Hospital:** Adv Luth Genl Hosp; **Address:** Ctr Brain & Spine Surg-Parkside Ctr, 1875 Dempster St, Ste 605, Park Ridge, IL 60068; **Phone:** 847-698-1088; **Board Cert:** Neurological Surgery 1993; **Med School:** Northwestern Univ 1983; **Resid:** Neurological Surgery, Northwestern Meml Hosp 1989; **Fellow:** Pediatric Neurological Surgery, Childrens Hosp 1990; **Fac Appt:** Asst Prof S, Rush Med Coll

Ryken, Timothy MD [NS] - **Spec Exp:** Brain Tumors; Spinal Surgery; **Hospital:** Univ Iowa Hosp & Clinics; **Address:** Univ Iowa Hosps & Clinics, Div Neurosurg, 200 Hawkins Drive, rm 1844 JPP, Iowa City, IA 52242; **Phone:** 319-356-2237; **Board Cert:** Neurological Surgery 1998; **Med School:** Univ Iowa Coll Med 1988; **Resid:** Neurological Surgery, Univ Iowa 1995; **Fellow:** Cambridge Univ 1996; **Fac Appt:** Assoc Prof NS, Univ Iowa Coll Med

Selman, Warren R MD [NS] - **Spec Exp:** Stroke; Pituitary Surgery; Aneurysm-Cerebral; Microsurgery; **Hospital:** Univ Hosps Case Med Ctr; **Address:** Dept Neurosurgery, 11100 Euclid Ave, 5th Fl Hanna House, Cleveland, OH 44106; **Phone:** 216-844-5745; **Board Cert:** Neurological Surgery 1986; **Med School:** Case West Res Univ 1977; **Resid:** Neurological Surgery, Univ Hosps 1984; **Fellow:** Research, Univ Hosps 1980; Neurological Surgery, Mayo Clinic 1984; **Fac Appt:** Prof NS, Case West Res Univ

Shapiro, Scott A MD [NS] - **Spec Exp:** Brain Tumors; Aneurysm-Cerebral; Spinal Cord Injury; Pituitary Tumors; **Hospital:** Indiana Univ Hosp; **Address:** Inidiana Univ, Wishard Memorial Hosp, 1001 W 10th St, Ste EOP323, Indianapolis, IN 46202; **Phone:** 317-630-7625; **Board Cert:** Neurological Surgery 1990; **Med School:** Indiana Univ 1981; **Resid:** Neurological Surgery, Indiana Univ Med Ctr 1987; **Fac Appt:** Prof NS, Indiana Univ

Thompson, B Gregory MD [NS] - **Spec Exp:** Acoustic Neuroma; Neurovascular Surgery; Skull Base Tumors & Surgery; Aneurysm-Cerebral; **Hospital:** Univ Michigan Hlth Sys; **Address:** Dept Neurosurgery, 3552 Taubman, 1500 E Medical Center Drive, Ann Arbor, MI 48109; **Phone:** 734-936-7493; **Board Cert:** Neurological Surgery 1998; **Med School:** Univ Kans 1986; **Resid:** Neurological Surgery, Univ Pittsburgh 1993; Research, Natl Inst Hlth 1992; **Fellow:** Neurological Surgery, Barrow Neuro Inst 1994; Interventional Radiology, Thomas Jefferson Univ 2005

Neurological Surgery

Tomita, Tadanori MD [NS] - **Spec Exp:** Pediatric Neurosurgery; Brain Tumors-Pediatric; Hydrocephalus; **Hospital:** Children's Mem Hosp, Northwestern Meml Hosp; **Address:** Chldns Meml Hosp, Div Ped Neurosurg, 2300 Children's Plaza, Box 28, Chicago, IL 60614-3363; **Phone:** 773-880-4373; **Board Cert:** Neurological Surgery 1984; Pediatric Neurological Surgery 1996; **Med School:** Japan 1970; **Resid:** Neurological Surgery, Kobe Univ 1974; Neurological Surgery, Northwestern Meml Hosp 1980; **Fellow:** Surgery, Meml Sloan Kettering Canc Ctr 1981; **Fac Appt:** Prof NS, Northwestern Univ

Traynelis, Vincent C MD [NS] - **Spec Exp:** Spinal Surgery; **Hospital:** Univ Iowa Hosp & Clinics; **Address:** Univ Iowa Hosp, Dept Neurosurgery, 200 Hawkins Drive, rm 3005BT, Iowa City, IA 52242; **Phone:** 319-356-2774; **Board Cert:** Neurological Surgery 1992; **Med School:** W VA Univ 1983; **Resid:** Neurological Surgery, Univ West Virginia Med Ctr 1989; **Fac Appt:** Prof NS, Univ Iowa Coll Med

Warnick, Ronald E MD [NS] - **Spec Exp:** Neuro-Oncology; Brain Tumors; **Hospital:** Univ Hosp - Cincinnati, Good Samaritan Hosp - Cincinnati; **Address:** 222 Piedmont Ave, Ste 3100, Cincinnati, OH 45219; **Phone:** 513-475-8629; **Board Cert:** Neurological Surgery 1995; **Med School:** Univ Rochester 1982; **Resid:** Neurological Surgery, NYU Med Ctr 1989; **Fellow:** Neuro-Oncology, UCSF Med Ctr 1991; **Fac Appt:** Prof NS, Univ Cincinnati

Great Plains and Mountains

Apfelbaum, Ronald I MD [NS] - **Spec Exp:** Spinal Surgery; **Hospital:** Univ Utah Hosps and Clins; **Address:** Univ Utah Hosp, Dept Neurosurgery, 175 N Medical Drive E Bldg 550 Fl 5th, Salt Lake City, UT 84132-2303; **Phone:** 801-585-6040; **Board Cert:** Neurological Surgery 1976; **Med School:** Hahnemann Univ 1965; **Resid:** Surgery, Montefiore Med Ctr 1969; Neurological Surgery, Montefiore Med Ctr 1974; **Fac Appt:** Prof NS, Univ Utah

Cherny, W Bruce MD [NS] - **Spec Exp:** Pediatric Neurosurgery; Brain Tumors; Spina Bifida; **Hospital:** St. Luke's Reg Med Ctr - Boise; **Address:** 100 E Idaho St, Ste 202, Boise, ID 83712; **Phone:** 208-381-7360; **Board Cert:** Neurological Surgery 2000; **Med School:** Univ Ariz Coll Med 1987; **Resid:** Neurological Surgery, Barrow Neuro Inst/St Joseph's Med Ctr 1994; **Fellow:** Pediatric Neurological Surgery, Primary Chldns Hosp 1995

Couldwell, William MD/PhD [NS] - **Spec Exp:** Brain Tumors; Epilepsy/Movement Disorders; Parkinson's Disease; Pituitary Tumors; **Hospital:** Univ Utah Hosps and Clins; **Address:** Univ Utah, Dept Neurological Surgery, 175 N Medical Drive E, Salt Lake City, UT 84132-2303; **Phone:** 801-581-6908; **Board Cert:** Neurological Surgery 1994; **Med School:** McGill Univ 1984; **Resid:** Neurological Surgery, LAC/USC Med Ctr 1989; **Fellow:** Neurological Immunology, Montreal Neur Inst/McGill Univ 1991; Neurological Surgery, CHUV; **Fac Appt:** Prof NS, Univ Utah

Johnson, Stephen D MD [NS] - **Spec Exp:** Skull Base Tumors & Surgery; **Hospital:** Presby - St Luke's Med Ctr; **Address:** Western Neurological Group, 1601 E 19th Ave, Ste 4400, Denver, CO 80218; **Phone:** 303-861-2266; **Board Cert:** Neurological Surgery 1988; **Med School:** Univ Tenn Coll Med, Memphis 1974; **Resid:** Neurological Surgery, Virginia Mason Med Ctr; Neurological Surgery, New York Hosp; **Fellow:** Neurological Surgery, Univ Tennessee; **Fac Appt:** Assoc Prof NS, Univ Colorado

Kestle, John RW MD [NS] - **Spec Exp:** Pediatric Neurosurgery; Epilepsy/Seizure Disorders; **Hospital:** Primary Children's Med Ctr; **Address:** 100 N Medical Drive, Ste 2400, Salt Lake City, UT 84113; **Phone:** 801-662-5340; **Board Cert:** Neurological Surgery 2002; **Med School:** Canada 1984; **Resid:** Neurology, Univ Toronto 1990; **Fellow:** Pediatric Neurological Surgery, Hosp Sick Chldn/Univ Toronto 1992; **Fac Appt:** Assoc Prof NS, Univ Utah

Lillehei, Kevin O MD [NS] - **Spec Exp:** Neuro-Oncology; Pituitary Tumors; Peripheral Nerve Surgery; **Hospital:** Univ Colorado Hosp, Exempla Lutheran Med Ctr; **Address:** Univ Colorado Hosp, 12631 E 17th Ave, Aurora, CO 80045; **Phone:** 303-724-2280; **Board Cert:** Neurological Surgery 1989; **Med School:** Univ Minn 1979; **Resid:** Neurological Surgery, Univ Mich Med Ctr 1985; **Fac Appt:** Prof NS, Univ Colorado

Nazzaro, Jules M MD [NS] - **Spec Exp:** Parkinson's Disease; Movement Disorders; Stereotactic Radiosurgery; **Hospital:** Univ of Kansas Hosp; **Address:** Kansas University Medical Ctr, 3901 Rainbow Blvd, MS 3021, Kansas City, KS 66160; **Phone:** 913-588-5129; **Board Cert:** Neurological Surgery 1996; **Med School:** Albert Einstein Coll Med 1984; **Resid:** Neurological Surgery, NYU Med Ctr 1991; **Fellow:** Neurosurgical Oncology, Meml Sloan-Kettering Cancer Ctr 1992; **Fac Appt:** Assoc Prof NS, Univ Kans

Taylon, Charles MD [NS] - **Spec Exp:** Spinal Surgery-Cervical; Spinal Surgery-Low Back; Carpal Tunnel Syndrome; Trauma; **Hospital:** Creighton Univ Med Ctr; **Address:** Creighton Univ, Dept Surg, 601 N 30th St, Ste 3700, Omaha, NE 68131; **Phone:** 402-280-4497; **Board Cert:** Neurological Surgery 1984; **Med School:** Creighton Univ 1975; **Resid:** Neurological Surgery, Univ Wisc Hosps 1981; **Fac Appt:** Assoc Prof NS, Creighton Univ

Walker, Marion L MD [NS] - **Spec Exp:** Pediatric Neurosurgery; Spasticity & Movement Disorders; Hydrocephalus; Brain Tumors; **Hospital:** Primary Children's Med Ctr, Univ Utah Hosps and Clins; **Address:** Primary Children's Med Ctr, Div Ped Neurosurgery, 100 N Mario Capecchi Drive, Ste 1475, Salt Lake City, UT 84113-1103; **Phone:** 801-662-5340; **Board Cert:** Neurological Surgery 1979; Pediatric Neurological Surgery 1996; **Med School:** Univ Tenn Coll Med, Memphis 1969; **Resid:** Surgery, St Joseph's Hosp 1971; Neurological Surgery, St Joseph's Hosp-Barrow Neuro Inst 1976; **Fellow:** Pediatric Neurological Surgery, Hosp for Sick Chldn 1973; **Fac Appt:** Prof NS, Univ Utah

Winston, Ken R MD [NS] - **Spec Exp:** Pediatric Neurosurgery; Craniosynostosis; Epilepsy/Seizure Disorders; **Hospital:** Chldn's Hosp - Aurora, The, Univ Colorado Hosp; **Address:** 12631 E 17th Ave, Box C307, Aurora, CO 80045; **Phone:** 303-724-2305; **Board Cert:** Neurological Surgery 1973; **Med School:** Univ Tenn Coll Med, Memphis 1963; **Resid:** Surgery, Colorado Genl Hosp 1967; Neurological Surgery, Colorado Genl Hosp 1971; **Fac Appt:** Prof NS, Univ Colorado

Southwest

Al-Mefty, Ossama MD [NS] - **Spec Exp:** Skull Base Surgery; Brain Tumors; Cerebrovascular Surgery; **Hospital:** UAMS Med Ctr, Arkansas Chldns Hosp; **Address:** Univ Hosp of Arkansas for Med Scis, 4301 W Markham Slot 507, Little Rock, AR 72205; **Phone:** 501-686-8757; **Board Cert:** Neurological Surgery 1980; **Med School:** Syria 1972; **Resid:** Surgery, Med Coll Ohio 1974; Neurological Surgery, West Va Med Ctr 1978; **Fac Appt:** Prof NS, Univ Ark

De Monte, Franco MD [NS] - **Spec Exp:** Skull Base Tumors & Surgery; Neuro-Oncology; **Hospital:** UT MD Anderson Cancer Ctr; **Address:** UT MD Anderson Cancer Ctr, Dept Neurosurgery, 1515 Holcombe Blvd, Ste 442, Houston, TX 77030; **Phone:** 713-792-2400; **Board Cert:** Neurological Surgery 1995; **Med School:** Canada 1985; **Resid:** Neurological Surgery, Univ Western Ontario 1991; **Fellow:** Skull Base Surgery, Loyola Univ-Stritch Sch Med 1992

Hankinson, Hal L MD [NS] - **Spec Exp:** Brain Tumors; **Hospital:** St Vincent Hosp - Santa Fe; **Address:** 465 St Michael's Drive, Ste 107, Sante Fe, NM 87102; **Phone:** 505-988-3233; **Board Cert:** Neurological Surgery 1977; **Med School:** Tulane Univ 1967; **Resid:** Neurological Surgery, UCSF Med Ctr 1975; **Fac Appt:** Clin Prof NS, Univ New Mexico

Neurological Surgery

Harper, Richard L MD [NS] - **Spec Exp:** Spinal Surgery; Brain Tumors & Hemifacial Spasms; **Hospital:** Methodist Hosp - Houston; **Address:** 6560 Fannin St, Ste 1200, Houston, TX 77030; **Phone:** 713-790-1211; **Board Cert:** Neurological Surgery 1983; **Med School:** Baylor Coll Med 1971; **Resid:** Neurological Surgery, Baylor Hosps 1978; **Fac Appt:** Asst Clin Prof NS, Baylor Coll Med

Jimenez, David MD [NS] - **Spec Exp:** Pediatric Neurosurgery; Craniosynostosis; Endoscopic Strip Craniectomy; Spinal Surgery; **Hospital:** Univ Hlth Sys - Univ Hosp (San Antonio, TX), St Luke's Baptist Hosp; **Address:** Dept of Neurosurgery, 7703 Floyd Curl Drive, MC 7843, San Antonio, TX 78229-3900; **Phone:** 210-567-5625; **Board Cert:** Neurological Surgery 1995; **Med School:** Temple Univ 1985; **Resid:** Neurological Surgery, Temple Univ Hosp 1991; **Fellow:** Pediatric Neurological Surgery, Montefiore Hosp/Einstein Coll Med 1992; **Fac Appt:** Prof NS, Univ Tex, San Antonio

Lang Jr, Frederick F MD [NS] - **Spec Exp:** Brain & Spinal Tumors; Neuro-Oncology; **Hospital:** UT MD Anderson Cancer Ctr; **Address:** Univ Texas MD Anderson Cancer Ctr, 1515 Holcombe Blvd, Unit 442, Houston, TX 77030; **Phone:** 713-792-6660; **Board Cert:** Neurological Surgery 2000; **Med School:** Yale Univ 1988; **Resid:** Neurological Surgery, NYU Med Ctr 1995; **Fellow:** Neurosurgical Oncology, MD Anderson Cancer Ctr 1996; **Fac Appt:** Prof NS, Univ Tex, Houston

Luerssen, Thomas G MD [NS] - **Spec Exp:** Pediatric Neurosurgery; Brain Injury-Traumatic; **Hospital:** Texas Chldns Hosp - Houston; **Address:** Texas Children's Hosp, Ped Neurosurgery, Clinical Care Center, Ste 1230, 6621 Fannin St, MC CC 1230.01, Houston, TX 77030-2399; **Phone:** 832-822-3950; **Board Cert:** Neurological Surgery 1985; Pediatric Neurological Surgery 2005; **Med School:** Indiana Univ 1976; **Resid:** Neurological Surgery, Indiana Univ Hosp 1981; **Fellow:** Pediatric Neurological Surgery, Chldns Hosp 1984; **Fac Appt:** Prof NS, Baylor Coll Med

Mapstone, Timothy B MD [NS] - **Spec Exp:** Brain Tumors-Adult & Pediatric; Pediatric Neurosurgery; Congenital Anomalies; **Hospital:** OU Med Ctr, Chldns Hosp OU Med Ctr; **Address:** Univ OK Hlth Sci Ctr, Dept Neurosurgery, 1000 N Lincoln Blvd, Ste 400, Oklahoma City, OK 73104; **Phone:** 405-271-4912; **Board Cert:** Neurological Surgery 1985; Pediatric Neurological Surgery 2005; **Med School:** Case West Res Univ 1977; **Resid:** Neurological Surgery, Univ Hosps 1983; **Fellow:** Research, Case West Reserve Univ; **Fac Appt:** Prof NS, Univ Okla Coll Med

Mickey, Bruce E MD [NS] - **Spec Exp:** Brain Tumors; Skull Base Surgery; **Hospital:** UT Southwestern Med Ctr - Dallas; **Address:** UTSW Med Ctr, Dept Neurosurgery, 5323 Harry Hines Blvd, Dallas, TX 75390-8855; **Phone:** 214-645-2300; **Board Cert:** Neurological Surgery 1987; **Med School:** Univ Tex SW, Dallas 1978; **Resid:** Neurological Surgery, Parkland Meml Hosp 1984; **Fellow:** Research, Righospitalet 1983; **Fac Appt:** Prof NS, Univ Tex SW, Dallas

Papadopoulos, Stephen M MD [NS] - **Spec Exp:** Spinal Surgery; Stereotactic Radiosurgery; **Hospital:** St Joseph's Hosp & Med Ctr - Phoenix; **Address:** Barrow Neurosurg Assocs, 2910 N 3rd Ave, Phoenix, AZ 85013; **Phone:** 602-406-3159; **Board Cert:** Neurological Surgery 1991; **Med School:** Univ Tex, Houston 1978; **Resid:** Neurological Surgery, Univ Mich Med Ctr 1988; **Fellow:** Spinal Surgery, Barrow Neuro Inst 1989

Samson, Duke S MD [NS] - **Spec Exp:** Vascular Neurosurgery; Cerebrovascular Disease; Arteriovenous Malformations; **Hospital:** UT Southwestern Med Ctr - Dallas, Parkland Meml Hosp - Dallas; **Address:** Univ Tex SW Med Ctr, Dept Neuro Surg, 5323 Harry Hines Blvd, Dallas, TX 75390-8855; **Phone:** 214-648-3529; **Board Cert:** Neurological Surgery 1978; **Med School:** Washington Univ, St Louis 1969; **Resid:** Neurological Surgery, Univ Texas SW Med Ctr 1975; **Fellow:** Neurological Surgery, Ctr Medico-Chirurgical Fech 1973; Neurological Surgery, Univ Zurich 1973; **Fac Appt:** Prof NS, Univ Tex SW, Dallas

Sawaya, Raymond MD [NS] - **Spec Exp:** Brain Tumors; **Hospital:** UT MD Anderson Cancer Ctr, Baylor Univ Medical Ctr; **Address:** MD Anderson Cancer Ctr, 1515 Holcombe Blvd, Unit 442, Houston, TX 77030; **Phone:** 713-563-8749; **Board Cert:** Neurological Surgery 1985; **Med School:** Lebanon 1974; **Resid:** Neurological Surgery, Univ Cincinnati Med Ctr 1980; Neurological Surgery, Johns Hopkins Med Ctr 1981; **Fellow:** Neuro-Oncology, Natl Inst Hlth 1982; **Fac Appt:** Prof NS, Univ Tex, Houston

Sklar, Frederick H MD [NS] - **Spec Exp:** Pediatric Neurosurgery; Craniofacial Surgery; Hydro-cephalus; **Hospital:** Chldns Med Ctr of Dallas, Texas Scottish Rite Hosp for Chldn; **Address:** Center for Pediatric Neurosurgery, 1935 Medical District Drive, Dallas, TX 75235; **Phone:** 214-456-6660; **Board Cert:** Neurological Surgery 1978; Pediatric Neurological Surgery ; **Med School:** Johns Hopkins Univ 1970; **Resid:** Neurological Surgery, Johns Hopkins Hosp 1976; **Fac Appt:** Assoc Clin Prof NS, Univ Tex SW, Dallas

Sonntag, Volker MD [NS] - **Spec Exp:** Spinal Surgery; **Hospital:** St Joseph's Hosp & Med Ctr - Phoenix; **Address:** Barrow Neurosurgery Associates, 2910 N Third Ave, Phoenix, AZ 85013; **Phone:** 602-406-3458; **Board Cert:** Neurological Surgery 1980; **Med School:** Univ Ariz Coll Med 1971; **Resid:** Neurological Surgery, New England Med Ctr 1977; **Fac Appt:** Clin Prof NS, Univ Ariz Coll Med

Spetzler, Robert F MD [NS] - **Spec Exp:** Skull Base Tumors & Surgery; Cerebrovascular Surgery; **Hospital:** St Joseph's Hosp & Med Ctr - Phoenix; **Address:** Barrow Neurosurgical Assocs, 2910 N Third Ave, Phoenix, AZ 85013; **Phone:** 602-406-3489; **Board Cert:** Neurological Surgery 1979; **Med School:** Northwestern Univ 1971; **Resid:** Neurological Surgery, UCSF Med Ctr 1976; **Fac Appt:** Prof S, Univ Ariz Coll Med

Walsh, John W MD/PhD [NS] - **Spec Exp:** Pediatric Neurosurgery; Epilepsy; **Hospital:** Tulane Univ Hosp & Clin; **Address:** 4720 S I-10 Service Rd, New Orleans, LA 70001; **Phone:** 504-988-8000; **Board Cert:** Neurological Surgery 1997; Pediatric Neurological Surgery 1996; **Med School:** UCLA 1966; **Resid:** Neurological Surgery, Peter Bent Brigham Hosp 1974; **Fellow:** Neurological Surgery, Lahey Clin Fdn 1975; **Fac Appt:** Prof NS, Tulane Univ

Yonas, Howard MD [NS] - **Spec Exp:** Vascular Neurosurgery; Stroke; Skull Base Surgery; Trigeminal Neuralgia; **Hospital:** Univ Hosp of Albquerque; **Address:** 1 University of New Mexico, MSC10 5615, Albuquerque, NM 87131-0001; **Phone:** 505-272-9494; **Board Cert:** Neurological Surgery 1981; **Med School:** Ohio State Univ 1970; **Resid:** Neurological Surgery, Case West Res 1976; **Fellow:** Univ Pittsburgh 1978; **Fac Appt:** Prof NS, Univ New Mexico

West Coast and Pacific

Adler Jr, John R MD [NS] - **Spec Exp:** Stereotactic Radiosurgery; Brain Tumors; Acoustic Neuroma; **Hospital:** Stanford Univ Med Ctr; **Address:** Stanford Univ Med Ctr, Dept Neurosurg, 300 Pasteur Drive, rm R 205, Stanford, CA 94305-5327; **Phone:** 650-723-5573; **Board Cert:** Neurological Surgery 1990; **Med School:** Harvard Med Sch 1980; **Resid:** Neurological Surgery, Chldns Hosp 1987; Neurological Surgery, Mass Genl Hosp 1985; **Fellow:** Cerebrovascular Disease, Karolinska Inst 1986; **Fac Appt:** Prof NS, Stanford Univ

Apuzzo, Michael L J MD [NS] - **Spec Exp:** Brain Tumors; Epilepsy/Seizure Disorders; Stereotactic Radiosurgery; **Hospital:** LAC & USC Med Ctr, USC Norris Comp Cancer Ctr; **Address:** 1420 N San Pablo Street, PMBA106, Los Angeles, CA 90033-1029; **Phone:** 323-226-7421; **Board Cert:** Neurological Surgery 1975; **Med School:** Boston Univ 1965; **Resid:** Neurological Surgery, Hartford Hosp 1970; Neurological Surgery, Hartford Hosp 1973; **Fellow:** Neurological Physiology, Yale Univ Hosp 1972; **Fac Appt:** Prof NS, USC Sch Med

Neurological Surgery

Badie, Behnam MD [NS] - **Spec Exp:** Brain Tumors; **Hospital:** City of Hope Natl Med Ctr & Beckman Rsch; **Address:** 1500 E Duarte Rd, City Of Hope Natl Mem Ctr, Duarte, CA 91010; **Phone:** 626-471-7100; **Board Cert:** Neurological Surgery 1998; **Med School:** UCLA 1989; **Resid:** Neurological Surgery, UCLA Med Ctr 1996; **Fac Appt:** Assoc Prof NS, UCLA

Berger, Mitchel S MD [NS] - **Spec Exp:** Brain & Spinal Cord Tumors; Pituitary Tumors; Neuro-Oncology; Pain Management; **Hospital:** UCSF Med Ctr; **Address:** UCSF Med Ctr, Dept Neuro-surgery, 505 Parnassus Avenue, M-786, San Francisco, CA 94143-0112; **Phone:** 415-353-3933; **Board Cert:** Neurological Surgery 1991; **Med School:** Univ Miami Sch Med 1979; **Resid:** Neurological Surgery, UCSF Med Ctr 1984; **Fellow:** Neuro-Oncology, UCSF Med Ctr 1985; Pediatric Neurological Surgery, Hosp Sick Chldn 1986; **Fac Appt:** Prof NS, UCSF

Black, Keith L MD [NS] - **Spec Exp:** Brain Tumors; Pituitary Surgery; Trigeminal Neuralgia; **Hospital:** Cedars-Sinai Med Ctr; **Address:** Maxine Dunitz Neurosurgical Inst, 8631 W 3rd St, Ste 800E, Los Angeles, CA 90048; **Phone:** 310-423-7900; **Board Cert:** Neurological Surgery 1990; **Med School:** Univ Mich Med Sch 1981; **Resid:** Neurological Surgery, Univ Michigan Med Ctr 1987; **Fac Appt:** Prof NS, UCLA

Boggan, James E MD [NS] - **Spec Exp:** Skull Base Tumors & Surgery; Pediatric Neurosurgery; **Hospital:** UC Davis Med Ctr; **Address:** Dept Neurological Surgery, 4860 Y St, Ste 3740, Sacramento, CA 95817-2307; **Phone:** 916-734-2371; **Board Cert:** Neurological Surgery 1985; **Med School:** Univ Chicago-Pritzker Sch Med 1976; **Resid:** Neurological Surgery, UCSF Med Ctr 1982; **Fac Appt:** Prof NS, UC Davis

Burchiel, Kim J MD [NS] - **Spec Exp:** Pain Management; Stereotactic Radiosurgery; Epilepsy/Movement Disorders; **Hospital:** OR Hlth & Sci Univ; **Address:** Oregon Hlth & Sci Univ, Dept Neurosurgery, 3303 SW Bond Ave, MC CH8N, Portland, OR 97239; **Phone:** 503-494-4314; **Board Cert:** Neurological Surgery 1984; **Med School:** UCSD 1976; **Resid:** Neurological Surgery, Univ Wash Med Ctr 1982; **Fac Appt:** Prof NS, Oregon Hlth Sci Univ

Edwards, Michael S MD [NS] - **Spec Exp:** Brain Tumors-Pediatric; Pediatric Neurosurgery; Stereotactic Radiosurgery; **Hospital:** Lucile Packard Chldns Hosp/Stanford Univ Med Ctr; **Address:** Pediatric Neurosurgery, 300 Pasteur Drive, Ste R211, MC 5327, Stanford, CA 94305-5327; **Phone:** 650-497-8775; **Board Cert:** Neurological Surgery 1980; Pediatric Neurological Surgery 2006; **Med School:** Tulane Univ 1970; **Resid:** Neurological Surgery, Oschner Fdn Hosp/Charity Hosp 1977; **Fellow:** Pediatric Neuro-Oncology, UCSF Med Ctr 1978; **Fac Appt:** Prof NS, Stanford Univ

Ellenbogen, Richard MD [NS] - **Spec Exp:** Pediatric Neurosurgery; Chiari's Deformity; Brain Tumors; **Hospital:** Chldns Hosp and Regl Med Ctr - Seattle, Univ Wash Med Ctr; **Address:** 4800 Sand Point Way NE, MS W-7729, Seattle, WA 98105; **Phone:** 206-987-2544; **Board Cert:** Neurological Surgery 1992; Pediatric Neurological Surgery 1998; **Med School:** Brown Univ 1983; **Resid:** Neurological Surgery, Brigham Womens Hosp/Childrens Hosp 1989; **Fac Appt:** Prof NS, Univ Wash

Frazee, John G MD [NS] - **Spec Exp:** Vascular Neurosurgery; Spinal Surgery; Neuro-Endoscopy; **Hospital:** Ronald Reagan UCLA Med Ctr, VA Med Ctr - W Los Angeles; **Address:** UCLA Med Ctr, Div Neurosurgery, 760 Westwood Ave, Los Angeles, CA 90095-7039; **Phone:** 310-206-1231; **Board Cert:** Neurological Surgery 1984; **Med School:** Univ Rochester 1975; **Resid:** Neurological Surgery, UCLA Med Ctr 1982; **Fac Appt:** Clin Prof NS, UCLA

Giannotta, Steven L MD [NS] - **Spec Exp:** Aneurysm-Cerebral; Skull Base Tumors; Acoustic Neuroma; **Hospital:** USC Univ Hosp - R K Eamer Med Plz, LAC & USC Med Ctr; **Address:** 1520 San Pablo St, Ste 3800, Los Angeles, CA 90033; **Phone:** 323-442-5720; **Board Cert:** Neurological Surgery 1980; **Med School:** Univ Mich Med Sch 1972; **Resid:** Neurological Surgery, Univ Michigan Med Ctr 1978; **Fac Appt:** Prof NS, USC Sch Med

America's Top Doctors® 8th Edition

Harsh IV, Griffith MD [NS] - **Spec Exp:** Brain & Spinal Cord Tumors; Skull Base Tumors; Pituitary Tumors; Acoustic Neuroma; **Hospital:** Stanford Univ Med Ctr; **Address:** Stanford Center for Advanced Medicine, 875 Blake Wilbur Drive, MC 5826, Stanford, CA 94305; **Phone:** 650-736-9976; **Board Cert:** Neurological Surgery 1989; **Med School:** Harvard Med Sch 1980; **Resid:** Neurological Surgery, UCSF Med Ctr 1986; **Fellow:** Neuro-Oncology, UCSF Med Ctr 1987; **Fac Appt:** Prof NS, Stanford Univ

Levy, Michael L MD/PhD [NS] - **Spec Exp:** Pediatric Neurosurgery; **Hospital:** Rady Children's Hosp - San Diego; **Address:** 8010 Frost St, Ste 502, San Diego, CA 92123; **Phone:** 858-966-8574; **Board Cert:** Neurological Surgery 1997; Pediatric Neurological Surgery 1998; **Med School:** UCSF 1986; **Resid:** Neurological Surgery, USC 1993; **Fellow:** Pediatric Neurological Surgery, Chldns Hosp 1995; **Fac Appt:** Asst Prof NS, USC Sch Med

Liau, Linda MD/PhD [NS] - **Spec Exp:** Brain Tumors; Neuro-Oncology; **Hospital:** Ronald Reagan UCLA Med Ctr; **Address:** CHS 74-145, Box 956901, 10833 Le Conte Ave, Los Angeles, CA 90095-6901; **Phone:** 310-267-2621; **Board Cert:** Neurological Surgery 2002; **Med School:** Stanford Univ 1991; **Resid:** Neurological Surgery, UCLA Med Ctr 1998; **Fellow:** Neuro-Oncology, UCLA Med Ctr 1998; **Fac Appt:** Prof NS, UCLA

Linskey, Mark E MD [NS] - **Spec Exp:** Brain Tumors; Stereotactic Radiosurgery; Skull Base Surgery; **Hospital:** UC Irvine Med Ctr, Chldns Hosp Orange Co - CHOC; **Address:** UCI Med Ctr, Dept Neurosurgery-Route 81, 101 The City Drive S Bldg 56 - Ste 400, Orange, CA 92868-3298; **Phone:** 714-456-6392; **Board Cert:** Neurological Surgery 1996; **Med School:** Columbia P&S 1986; **Resid:** Neurological Surgery, Univ Pittsburgh Hlth Ctrs 1993; **Fellow:** Neuro-Oncology, Ludwig Inst Cancer Rsch/Univ Coll London 1994; Neuro-Oncology, Pittsburgh Cancer Inst/Univ Pittsburgh 1992; **Fac Appt:** Assoc Prof NS, UC Irvine

Mamelak, Adam N MD [NS] - **Spec Exp:** Brain Tumors; Epilepsy; Spinal Tumors; **Hospital:** Cedars-Sinai Med Ctr, Huntington Memorial Hosp; **Address:** Maxine Dunitz Neurosurgical Institute, 8631 W Third St, Ste 800-East, Los Angeles, CA 90048; **Phone:** 310-423-7900; **Board Cert:** Neurological Surgery 2000; **Med School:** Harvard Med Sch 1990; **Resid:** Neurological Surgery, UCSF Med Ctr 1994; **Fellow:** Epilepsy, UCSF Epilepsy Research Lab 1996

Marshall, Lawrence F MD [NS] - **Spec Exp:** Spinal Surgery; Spinal Cord Surgery; Brain Tumors; Head Injury; **Hospital:** UCSD Med Ctr; **Address:** UCSD Medical Ctr, Dept Neurosurgery, 200 W Arbor Drive, rm 8893, San Diego, CA 92103; **Phone:** 619-543-5540; **Board Cert:** Neurological Surgery 1977; **Med School:** Univ Mich Med Sch 1969; **Resid:** Neurological Surgery, Hosp U Penn 1975; **Fellow:** Neurological Pathology, Glasgow Univ Med Research 1976; **Fac Appt:** Prof NS, UCSD

Martin, Neil A MD [NS] - **Spec Exp:** Vascular Neurosurgery; **Hospital:** Ronald Reagan UCLA Med Ctr; **Address:** UCLA Med Ctr, Div Neuro Surgery, 10833 LeConte Ave, Box 95-7039, Los Angeles, CA 90095-7039; **Phone:** 310-825-5482; **Board Cert:** Neurological Surgery 1989; **Med School:** Med Coll VA 1978; **Resid:** Neurological Surgery, UCSF Med Ctr 1984; **Fellow:** Neurological Vascular Surgery, Barrow Neuro Inst 1985; **Fac Appt:** Prof NS, UCLA

Mayberg, Marc R MD [NS] - **Spec Exp:** Pituitary Surgery; Stroke/Cerebrovascular Disease; Skull Base Tumors; Acoustic Neuroma; **Hospital:** Swedish Med Ctr - Seattle; **Address:** Seattle Neuroscience Inst, 550 17th Ave, Ste 500, Seattle, WA 98122; **Phone:** 206-320-2800; **Board Cert:** Neurological Surgery 1988; **Med School:** Mayo Med Sch 1978; **Resid:** Neurological Surgery, Mass Genl Hosp 1984; **Fellow:** Neurological Surgery, Natl Hosp for Nervous Dis 1985

Neurological Surgery

McDermott, Michael W MD [NS] - **Spec Exp:** Brain Tumors; Meningioma; Stereotactic Radiosurgery; Skull Base Tumors; **Hospital:** UCSF Med Ctr; **Address:** UCSF Dept Neurosurgery, 400 Parnassus Ave, rm A808, San Francisco, CA 94143; **Phone:** 415-353-7500; **Board Cert:** Neurological Surgery 2003; **Med School:** Univ Toronto 1982; **Resid:** Neurological Surgery, Univ British Columbia 1988; **Fellow:** Neuro-Oncology, UCSF Med Ctr 1990; **Fac Appt:** Prof NS, UCSF

Neuwelt, Edward A MD [NS] - **Spec Exp:** Neuro-Oncology; Brain Tumors; **Hospital:** OR Hlth & Sci Univ; **Address:** Oregon Hlth Sci Univ, Dept NS, 3181 SW Sam Jackson Pk Rd, MC-L603, Portland, OR 97239; **Phone:** 503-494-5626; **Board Cert:** Neurological Surgery 1980; **Med School:** Univ Colorado 1972; **Resid:** Neurological Surgery, Univ Tex SW Med Sch 1978; **Fellow:** Neuro-Oncology, Natl Canc Inst, NIH 1976; **Fac Appt:** Prof NS, Oregon Hlth Sci Univ

Ott, Kenneth H MD [NS] - **Spec Exp:** Brain Tumors; Stereotactic Radiosurgery; **Hospital:** Scripps Meml Hosp - La Jolla; **Address:** Neurosurgical Medical Clinic, 501 Washington St, Ste 700, San Diego, CA 92103-2231; **Phone:** 619-297-4481; **Board Cert:** Neurological Surgery 1980; **Med School:** UCSF 1970; **Resid:** Surgery, Mass Genl Hosp 1972; Neurological Surgery, Mass Genl Hosp 1976; **Fac Appt:** Assoc Clin Prof S, UCSD

Pitts, Lawrence H MD [NS] - **Spec Exp:** Acoustic Neuroma; Skull Base Surgery; Spinal Surgery; **Hospital:** UCSF Med Ctr; **Address:** UCSF Dept of Neurosurgery, 400 Parnassus Ave, rm A808, San Francisco, CA 94143; **Phone:** 415-353-7500; **Board Cert:** Neurological Surgery 1978; **Med School:** Case West Res Univ 1969; **Resid:** Neurological Surgery, UCSF Med Ctr 1975; **Fac Appt:** Prof NS, UCSF

Sekhar, Laligam N MD [NS] - **Spec Exp:** Aneurysm-Cerebral; Arteriovenous Malformations; Brain Tumors; Skull Base Tumors; **Hospital:** Harborview Med Ctr, Univ Wash Med Ctr; **Address:** Harborview Med Ctr, UW Dept Neurosurgery, 325 Ninth Ave, Box 359766, Seattle, WA 98104-2420; **Phone:** 206-744-9300; **Board Cert:** Neurological Surgery 1986; **Med School:** India 1973; **Resid:** Neurology, Univ Cincinnati Med Ctr 1977; Neurology, Univ Pittsburgh Med Ctr 1982; **Fellow:** Skull Base Surgery, Norstadt Krankenhaus 1983; Cerebrovascular Neurosurgery, Univ Zurich Hospital; **Fac Appt:** Prof NS, Univ Wash

Selden, Nathan R MD/PhD [NS] - **Spec Exp:** Pediatric Neurosurgery; Epilepsy; Spasticity & Movement Disorders; Chiari's Deformity; **Hospital:** OR Hlth & Sci Univ; **Address:** 3303 SW Bond Ave, MC CH8N, Portland, OR 97239; **Phone:** 503-494-4314; **Board Cert:** Neurological Surgery 2004; **Med School:** Harvard Med Sch 1993; **Resid:** Neurological Surgery, Univ Michigan Med Ctr 1999; **Fac Appt:** Assoc Prof NS, Oregon Hlth Sci Univ

Shuer, Lawrence M MD [NS] - **Spec Exp:** Pediatric Neurosurgery; Craniosynostosis; Epilepsy; Chiari's Deformity; **Hospital:** Stanford Univ Med Ctr; **Address:** Stanford Univ Med Ctr, Dept Neurosurgery, 300 Pasteur Drive, rm R229, Stanford, CA 94305; **Phone:** 650-723-5574; **Board Cert:** Neurological Surgery 1986; **Med School:** Univ Mich Med Sch 1978; **Resid:** Neurological Surgery, Stanford Univ 1984; **Fac Appt:** Prof NS, Stanford Univ

Silbergeld, Daniel MD [NS] - **Spec Exp:** Brain Tumors; Brain Tumors-Metastatic; Brain Mapping; **Hospital:** Univ Wash Med Ctr; **Address:** Univ Wash Med Ctr, Dept Neurosurg, 1959 NE Pacific, Box 356470, Seattle, WA 98195; **Phone:** 206-598-5637; **Board Cert:** Neurological Surgery 1995; **Med School:** Univ Cincinnati 1984; **Resid:** Neurological Surgery, Univ Wash Med Ctr 1990; Research, Univ Wash Med Ctr 1988; **Fellow:** Neuro-Oncology, Univ Wash Med Ctr 1991; Epilepsy, Univ Wash Med Ctr 1991; **Fac Appt:** Assoc Prof NS, Univ Wash

Steinberg, Gary K MD/PhD [NS] - **Spec Exp:** Aneurysm-Cerebral; Moya Moya; Arteriovenous Malformations; **Hospital:** Stanford Univ Med Ctr; **Address:** Stanford Univ Hosp, Dept Neurosurg, 300 Pasteur Drive, rm R281, Stanford, CA 94305-5327; **Phone:** 650-723-5575; **Board Cert:** Neurological Surgery 1989; **Med School:** Stanford Univ 1980; **Resid:** Neuropathology, Stanford Univ Med Ctr 1982; Neurological Surgery, Stanford Univ Med Ctr 1987; **Fellow:** Cerebrovascular Neurosurgery, Univ West Ontario 1985; **Fac Appt:** Assoc Prof NS, Stanford Univ

Yu, John S MD [NS] - **Spec Exp:** Brain Tumors; Spinal Tumors; Clinical Trials; Spinal Surgery; **Hospital:** Cedars-Sinai Med Ctr; **Address:** 8631 W 3rd St, Ste 800E, Los Angeles, CA 90048; **Phone:** 310-423-7900; **Board Cert:** Neurological Surgery 2002; **Med School:** Harvard Med Sch 1990; **Resid:** Neurological Surgery, Mass General Hosp 1997

Cleveland Clinic

Neurological Institute

The Cleveland Clinic Neurological Institute is a fully integrated entity with a disease-specific focus, combining all physicians and other healthcare providers in neurology, neurosurgery, neuroradiology, the behavioral sciences and nursing who treat children and adults with neurological and neurobehavioral disorders. Our staff of more than 220 specialists sees one of the largest and most diverse patient populations in the country. Because of our clinical expertise, academic achievement and innovative research, the Cleveland Clinic Neurological Institute has earned an international reputation for excellence.

U.S.News & World Report's "America's Best Hospitals" survey has consistently ranked our Neurology and Neurosurgery programs among the Top 10 in the nation and best in Ohio.

Our unique clinical structure allows us to deliver coordinated, comprehensive, multidisciplinary care to our patients through more efficient treatment decision making and consultation for complex cases. Fully integrating specialties along disease lines creates an exciting synergy among Institute physicians who share similar clinical, research and educational interests, to the benefit of patients and physicians alike.

Major advances in the treatment of brain tumors, epilepsy, mood disorders, stroke, movement disorders, pain and spinal disorders are improving quality of life and survival for thousands of patients. For those diseases resistant to available treatments, we believe the innovative model of medicine created within the Neurological Institute will speed research and advances in treatment, resulting in better clinical care and more rapid breakthroughs in the full range of neurological and behavioral disorders.

Centers in the Neurological Institute include: Brain Tumor & Neuro-Oncology Center, Center for Headache & Pain, Center for Neuroimaging, Center for Neurological Restoration, Center for Pediatric Neurology & Neurosurgery, Center for Spine Health, Cerebrovascular Center, Epilepsy Center, Mellen Center for Multiple Sclerosis Treatment & Research, Neuromuscular Center, Psychiatry and Psychology and Sleep Disorders Center

For more information about the Cleveland Clinic Neurological Institute, to schedule a second opinion or to learn about assistance for out-of-town patients, call 800.890.2467 or visit www.clevelandclinic.org/neurotopdocs.

Cleveland Clinic Neurological Institute
9500 Euclid Avenue / AC311 | Cleveland OH 44195

Comprehensive Neurological Care

Cleveland Clinic offers expert diagnostic and treatment options for all neurologic conditions affecting children and adults, including:

- Alzheimer's disease
- ALS (Amyotrophic Lateral Sclerosis)
- Aneurysms
- Arteriovenous Malformations (AVMs)
- Back and Neck Disorders
- Brain and Spine Tumors
- Cerebral Palsy
- Chronic Pain Rehabilitation
- Congenital Disorders
- Craniofacial Disorders
- Epilepsy
- Headache
- Hydrocephalus
- Metastatic Tumors
- Movement Disorders
- Neonatal Disorders
- Neurofibromatosis
- Parkinson's Disease
- Peripheral Neuropathies
- Pituitary Disorders
- Psychiatric Disorders
- Skull Base Disorders
- Sleep Disorders
- Stroke

PENN NEUROSURGERY

The Department of Neurosurgery at the University of Pennsylvania provides comprehensive medical and surgical care for people with disorders of the brain, spinal cord and peripheral nervous system. One of the hallmarks of Penn's neurosurgery program is its integration of research and clinical practice, embracing new technologies and seeking the highest quality and best outcomes possible.

More Penn neurosurgeons are listed in *The Best Doctors in America®* than are found at any other hospital or medical center in the Philadelphia region.

The department of Neurosurgery is a component of the Penn Comprehensive Neuroscience Center, which facilitates and strengthens the integration of Penn's world-class neuroscience programs within the areas of clinical care, research and education.

Penn's neurosurgical specialists, backed by the most extensive neurodiagnostic and imaging facilities in the region, perform more than 4,500 operations each year. The neurosurgical faculty all have a particular subspecialty focus, covering the entire spectrum of surgically treated disorders of the nervous system.

Excellence and Expertise

The Penn Gamma Knife® Center at Pennsylvania Hospital offers power, precision and hope to patients suffering from brain tumors and other serious brain disorders. Gamma Knife radiosurgery is noninvasive, effective, and safe for treating conditions including benign or malignant brain tumors, blood vessel malformations and trigeminal neuralgia.

The Center for Functional and Restorative Neurosurgery at Pennsylvania Hospital performed more deep brain stimulation procedures for the treatment of Parkinson's disease and epilepsy in the past year than any other hospital or health system in the U.S.

The Center for Cranial Base Surgery offers expert evaluation and treatment of tumors of the head, neck, face and other complex skull-base disorders. With the development of innovative and endoscopic surgical procedures and state-of-the-art imaging, many of these tumors, previously inaccessible, can now be successfully treated.

The Neuro-Oncology Program provides evaluation, diagnosis and treatment to patients with brain and spinal tumors and other cancer-related neurological central nervous system and peripheral nervous system problems. The program utilizes a patient-oriented team approach bringing together some of the nation's leading experts in the field.

The Neurosurgical Spine Center provides medical and surgical care for the most complex disorders of the spinal cord. Penn is a regional and national leader in providing quality spine care utilizing a multidisciplinary team approach, implementing the latest advances in techniques and technology.

The Neurovascular Center offers minimally invasive (endovascular) coiling and stent treatments of brain aneurysms, vascular malformations and atherosclerotic narrowing of the blood vessels of the brain, combining the skill sets of neurosurgeons and interventional neuroradiologists to obtain the best possible outcomes.

Programs

- The Center for Brain Injury and Repair
- The Center for Cranial Base Surgery
- The Center for Functional and Restorative Neurosurgery
- Penn Gamma Knife® Center
- Neuro Intensive Care
- The Neuro-Oncology Program
- The Neurovascular Center
- The Neurosurgical Spine Center

Gamma Knife and Leksell Gamma Knife are U.S. federally registered trademarks of Elekta Instrument S.A., Geneva, Switzerland.

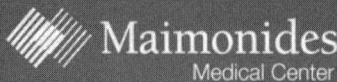

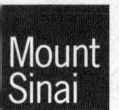
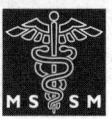

MOUNT SINAI
SCHOOL OF
MEDICINE

THE MOUNT SINAI MEDICAL CENTER
NEUROSURGERY
One Gustave L. Levy Place
Fifth Avenue and 100th Street
New York, NY 10029-6574
Physician Referral: 1-800-MD-SINAI (637-4624)
www.mountsinai.org

The Department of Neurosurgery at The Mount Sinai Medical Center was established in 1920 and has gained a distinguished international reputation. Areas of expertise include the skull base, cerebrovascular, pituitary, acoustic, spinal reconstruction, epilepsy, radiosurgery, stereotactic, primary brain tumor surgery, functional, minimally invasive, and neuroendoscopy. Neurosurgery research at Mount Sinai includes clinical programs, case presentations, and laboratories in the following areas: cerebrovascular, skull-base dissection, spinal cord injury, pituitary endocrinology, cerebral blood flow regulation, gene therapy and brain tumors, and movement disorders.

The Mount Sinai Brain Tumor Program provides comprehensive care to patients with peripheral and central nervous system tumors and with neurological complications of systemic cancer. Our physicians utilize the latest techniques, including computer-assisted image-guided tumor resections and biopsies, advanced skull-base approaches, and minimally invasive, endoscopic procedures. The most advanced stereotactic radiosurgery program gives patients a treatment option that does not require open surgery, and gene therapy is an option for selected patients. An interdisciplinary approach includes members of the Departments of Neurology, Radiation Oncology, and Rehabilitation Medicine. Mount Sinai physicians focus not only on survival but also on the quality of the patient's life during and after treatment.

The Mount Sinai Clinical Center for Cranial Base Surgery provides a comprehensive, highly advanced treatment program for lesions of nerve, blood vessel, and brain in the complex structures and remote recesses at the base of the skull. The multidisciplinary Center unites the expertise of surgical specialists in neurosurgery, otolaryngology/head and neck cancer, craniofacial surgery, oral and maxillofacial surgery, and microvascular and reconstructive procedures. Together they have pioneered the development of minimally invasive techniques, including purely endoscopic tumor resection and stereotactic radiosurgery to treat complex skull-base lesions. The Center also offers patients the benefit of a wide range of experts in the related fields of neurology, electrophysiology, pathology, radiation oncology, rehabilitation medicine, and medical oncology. Our program is world-renowned for the treatment of pituitary adenomas, acoustic neuromas, meningiomas, and skull-base lesions.

The Clinical Program for Cerebrovascular Disorders and Stroke at Mount Sinai provides expertise in the evaluation, treatment, and rehabilitation of patients with cerebrovascular diseases. The team evaluates each patient to determine whether vascular lesions can be treated with minimally invasive endovascular techniques from the inside of the blood vessel. Pathologies treated include intracranial aneurysms, arteriovenous malformations of the brain, dura, and spinal cord, carotid artery stenosis, intracerebral cerebral hemorrhage, stroke/cerebral infarction, lesions of the skull base, and trigeminal neuralgia.

The Division of Functional and Restorative Neurosurgery utilizes the latest technology to precisely target locations and abnormalities in the brain and spinal cord. Our physicians are focused on the development of minimally invasive neurosurgical techniques that either modulate neural function, replace lost neuronal populations, or halt the neurodegenerative process altogether. Currently, deep brain stimulation (DBS) dominates this field, but many technologies with great potential are on the horizon. Our physicians have been honored by the Dystonia Medical Research Foundation for their pioneering work treating dystonia with DBS. They also use cutting-edge techniques in the treatment of patients with Parkinson's disease, essential tremor, facial nerve disorders, epilepsy, and pain.

The Mount Sinai Clinical Program for Stereotactic Neurosurgery has extended the scope of operative tumors by using techniques such as frame-based or frameless stereotaxy, awake and asleep brain mapping, microneurosurgery, and endoscopic surgery. Our physicians have been pioneers in computer-assisted techniques since 1993. The development of a precision navigation system and the addition of the Novalis Shaped Beam Surgery system at Mount Sinai have resulted in substantial reductions of wound and neurosurgical morbidity, length of surgery, length of stay, and hospital costs.

The Mount Sinai Center for Spinal Disorders offers comprehensive treatment for all disorders of the spinal column and spinal cord, including degenerative disorders (disc herniations, spinal stenosis, spinal instability), trauma, infections, congenital disorders (including scoliosis), and tumors. The Center's neurosurgeons have pioneered endoscopic, minimally invasive surgical approaches to treat disorders of the spine. These approaches have the potential to reduce postoperative pain, speed recovery, shorten hospital stays, reduce disability, and facilitate an early return to work, while providing the same or improved decompression or stabilization.

NYU Langone Medical Center

550 First Avenue (at 31St Street
New York, NY 10016
Physician Referra
(888)7-NYU-MED (888-769-8633)
www.nyumc.org

NEUROSURGERY

The Department of Neurosurgery at NYU Langone Medical Center offers the most advanced surgical procedures available anywhere in the world, along with compassionate care and supportive services for patients and their families. In an environment of leading-edge research and medical education, the department's interdisciplinary team of physicians, nurses, and allied health professionals are world-renowned for their highly specialized training and their down-to-earth approach to clinical care. The department also is home to some of the most sophisticated equipment in the region.

Because neurosurgery encompasses the surgical treatment of disorders of the entire nervous system and its coverings — the brain, spinal cord, skull, scalp, and vertebral column — many physicians subspecialize in a particular aspect of the field. At NYU Langone Medical Center, neurosurgeons treat a broad range of conditions, including tumors, vascular disorders, Parkinson's disease, and epilepsy, among others.

THE CENTER FOR THE STUDY AND TREATMENT OF MOVEMENT DISORDERS

The Center for Study and Treatment of Movement Disorders provides surgical care for patients with Parkinson's disease and other movement disorders. Its highly focused surgeons perform pallidotomy surgery when a patient suffers from severe stiffness, rigidity, and movement difficulties; and thalamotomy for those with disabling tremor. One of the center's most innovative treatments is deep brain stimulation, used to relieve the disabling symptoms of Parkinson's disease. NYU's neurosurgeons perform these procedures using the latest computer technology in conjunction with electrophysiologic monitoring.

THE GAMMA KNIFE

In the recent past, patients with brain abnormalities considered too deep or too delicate to reach with a scalpel had little reason for hope. But with the Gamma Knife, neurosurgeons at NYU Langone Medical Center can now remove deep-seated tumors, vascular malformations, and other sites of dysfunction with outstanding results. The Leksell Ganima Knife® — a revolutionary tool developed in Sweden for performing stereotactic radiosurgery — is the latest such technology in the New York and New England regions. Aided by three-dimensional MRI technology that pinpoints the problem area, the neurosurgeon uses the Gamma Knife to bombard its target with precise doses of radiation.

Neurology

A neurologist specializes in the diagnosis and treatment of all types of disease or impaired function of the brain, spinal cord, peripheral nerves, muscles and autonomic nervous system, as well as the blood vessels that relate to these structures. A child neurologist has special skills in the diagnosis and management of neurologic disorders of the neonatal period, infancy, early childhood and adolescence.

Training Required: Four years

NEUROLOGY

New England

Amato, Anthony A MD [N] - **Spec Exp:** Peripheral Neuropathy; Neuromuscular Disorders; Muscular Dystrophy; **Hospital:** Brigham & Women's Hosp; **Address:** Brigham & Women's Hosp, Dept Neurology, 75 Francis St, Boston, MA 02115; **Phone:** 617-732-8046; **Board Cert:** Neurology 1991; **Med School:** Univ Cincinnati 1986; **Resid:** Neurology, Wilford Hall USAF Med Ctr 1990; **Fellow:** Neuromuscular Medicine, Ohio State Med Ctr 1992; **Fac Appt:** Assoc Prof N, Harvard Med Sch

Armon, Carmel MD [N] - **Spec Exp:** Epilepsy/Seizure Disorders; Amyotrophic Lateral Sclerosis (ALS); **Hospital:** Baystate Med Ctr; **Address:** Baystate Neurology, 759 Chestnut St, Springfield, MA 01199; **Phone:** 413-794-7033; **Board Cert:** Neurology 1990; Clinical Neurophysiology 2002; Vascular Neurology 2005; Sleep Medicine 2007; **Med School:** Israel 1980; **Resid:** Neurology, Mayo Clinic 1988; **Fellow:** Neurology, Mayo Clinic 1989; Clinical Neurophysiology, Duke Univ Med Ctr 1991

Blumenfeld, Hal MD/PhD [N] - **Spec Exp:** Epilepsy/Seizure Disorders; **Hospital:** Yale-New Haven Hosp; **Address:** Yale Dept of Neurology, PO Box 208018, New Haven, CT 06520-8018; **Phone:** 203-785-3865; **Board Cert:** Neurology 1998; **Med School:** Columbia P&S 1992; **Resid:** Neurology, Mass Genl Hosp 1996; **Fellow:** Epilepsy, Yale-New Haven Hosp 1998; **Fac Appt:** Assoc Prof N, Yale Univ

Bromfield, Edward B MD [N] - **Spec Exp:** Epilepsy/Seizure Disorders; Sleep Disorders/Apnea; **Hospital:** Brigham & Women's Hosp, Mass Genl Hosp; **Address:** Brigham & Women's Hosp, Dept Neurology, Division of Epilepsy and EEG, 75 Francis St, Boston, MA 02115; **Phone:** 617-732-7547; **Board Cert:** Neurology 1989; **Med School:** Harvard Med Sch 1983; **Resid:** Neurology, New York Hosp 1987; **Fellow:** Epilepsy, Natl Inst Hlth/NINDS 1989; **Fac Appt:** Assoc Prof N, Harvard Med Sch

Caplan, Louis Robert MD [N] - **Spec Exp:** Stroke; **Hospital:** Beth Israel Deaconess Med Ctr - Boston; **Address:** Palmer 127 West Campus BIDMC, 330 Brookline Ave, Boston, MA 02215; **Phone:** 617-632-8911; **Board Cert:** Internal Medicine 1969; Neurology 1972; **Med School:** Univ MD Sch Med 1962; **Resid:** Neurology, Boston City Hosp 1969; **Fellow:** Neurology, Harvard 1970; **Fac Appt:** Prof N, Harvard Med Sch

Cole, Andrew J MD [N] - **Spec Exp:** Epilepsy/Seizure Disorders; Rasmussen's Syndrome; **Hospital:** Mass Genl Hosp; **Address:** Mass Genl Hosp-Epilepsy Svc, 55 Fruit St, rm Wang 735, Boston, MA 02114; **Phone:** 617-726-3311; **Board Cert:** Neurology 1987; **Med School:** Dartmouth Med Sch 1982; **Resid:** Neurology, Neuro Inst-McGill 1986; **Fellow:** Electroencephalography, Neuro Inst-McGill 1987; Neurological Surgery, Johns Hopkins Hosp 1988; **Fac Appt:** Asst Prof N, Harvard Med Sch

Feldmann, Edward MD [N] - **Spec Exp:** Cerebrovascular Disease; Stroke; **Hospital:** Rhode Island Hosp; **Address:** 110 Lockwood St, Ste 324, Providence, RI 02903; **Phone:** 401-444-8806; **Board Cert:** Neurology 1988; Vascular Neurology 2005; **Med School:** Harvard Med Sch 1983; **Resid:** Neurology, New York Hosp 1987; **Fellow:** Cerebrovascular Disease, Tufts New Eng Med Ctr 1988; **Fac Appt:** Prof N, Brown Univ

Hafler, David A MD [N] - **Spec Exp:** Multiple Sclerosis; **Hospital:** Brigham & Women's Hosp; **Address:** Harvard Med Sch, 77 Ave Louis Pasteur, NRB 641-D, Boston, MA 02115; **Phone:** 617-525-5330; **Board Cert:** Neurology 1987; **Med School:** Univ Miami Sch Med 1978; **Resid:** Neurology, NY Hosp-Cornell Med Ctr 1982; **Fellow:** Neurological Immunology, Harvard Med Sch 1984; **Fac Appt:** Prof N, Harvard Med Sch

Jobst, Barbara Christine MD [N] - **Spec Exp:** Epilepsy in Pregnancy; Women's Health; **Hospital:** Dartmouth - Hitchcock Med Ctr; **Address:** One Medical Center Drive, Lebanon, NH 03756-1000; **Phone:** 603-650-8309; **Board Cert:** Neurology 2002; **Med School:** Germany 1993; **Resid:** Neurology, Krankenhaus Barmherzigen Bruder 1996; Neurology, Dartmouth-Hitchcock Med Ctr 2000; **Fellow:** Epilepsy, Dartmouth-Hitchcock Med Ctr 2001; **Fac Appt:** Asst Prof N, Dartmouth Med Sch

Kase, Carlos S MD [N] - **Spec Exp:** Stroke; Seizure Disorders; **Hospital:** Boston Med Ctr; **Address:** Boston Univ Sch of Med, 715 Albany St, Neurology C-329, Boston, MA 02118; **Phone:** 617-638-5102; **Board Cert:** Neurology 1980; **Med School:** Chile 1967; **Resid:** Neurology, Mass Genl Hosp 1973; Neurology, Mass Genl Hosp 1978; **Fac Appt:** Prof N, Boston Univ

Ropper, Allan MD [N] - **Spec Exp:** Trauma Neurology; Guillain-Barre Syndrome; **Hospital:** Brigham & Women's Hosp; **Address:** 75 Francis St, Box BB204, Boston, MA 02115; **Phone:** 617-732-8047; **Board Cert:** Internal Medicine 1977; Neurology 1980; **Med School:** Cornell Univ-Weill Med Coll 1974; **Resid:** Internal Medicine, UCSF Med Ctr 1976; Neurology, Mass Genl Hosp 1979; **Fac Appt:** Prof N, Tufts Univ

Samuels, Martin Allen MD [N] - **Spec Exp:** Neurologic Aspects of Systemic Disease; **Hospital:** Brigham & Women's Hosp, Mass Genl Hosp; **Address:** Brigham & Women's Hosp, Dept Neurology, 75 Francis St, Neurology ASB-1, rm 158, Boston, MA 02115; **Phone:** 617-732-7432; **Board Cert:** Internal Medicine 1974; Neurology 1978; **Med School:** Univ Cincinnati 1971; **Resid:** Internal Medicine, Boston City Hosp 1975; Neurology, Mass Genl Hosp 1977; **Fellow:** Neurological Pathology, Mass Genl Hosp 1976; **Fac Appt:** Prof N, Harvard Med Sch

Selkoe, Dennis MD [N] - **Spec Exp:** Alzheimer's Disease; **Hospital:** Brigham & Women's Hosp; **Address:** 77 Ave Louis Pasteur HIM 730 Bldg, Boston, MA 02115-5716; **Phone:** 617-525-5200; **Board Cert:** Neurology 1977; **Med School:** Univ VA Sch Med 1969; **Resid:** Neurology, Peter Bent Brigham 1975; **Fellow:** Neurological Biology, Chldns Hosp Med Ctr 1978; **Fac Appt:** Prof N, Harvard Med Sch

Spencer, Susan S MD [N] - **Spec Exp:** Epilepsy/Seizure Disorders; **Hospital:** Yale-New Haven Hosp; **Address:** Yale Univ Sch Med, Dept Neurology, 333 Cedar St, Box 208018, New Haven, CT 06520-8018; **Phone:** 203-785-3865; **Board Cert:** Neurology 1980; Clinical Neurophysiology 1988; **Med School:** Univ Rochester 1974; **Resid:** Neurology, Yale-New Haven Hosp 1978; **Fellow:** Epilepsy, Yale New Haven Hosp 1980; **Fac Appt:** Prof N, Yale Univ

Weiner, Howard L MD [N] - **Spec Exp:** Multiple Sclerosis; Autoimmune Disease; **Hospital:** Brigham & Women's Hosp; **Address:** Harvard Inst Med-Ctr Neuro Disease, 77 Ave Louis Pasteur, Bldg HIM 730, Boston, MA 02115; **Phone:** 617-525-5300; **Board Cert:** Neurology 1978; **Med School:** Univ Colorado 1969; **Resid:** Internal Medicine, Beth Israel 1971; Neurology, Longwood Prog 1974; **Fellow:** Immunology, Univ Colo 1976; **Fac Appt:** Prof N, Harvard Med Sch

Young, Anne MD [N] - **Spec Exp:** Huntington's Disease; Parkinson's Disease; Movement Disorders; **Hospital:** Mass Genl Hosp; **Address:** Mass Genl Hosp, Dept Neurology, 55 Fruit Street, WAC 915, Boston, MA 02114; **Phone:** 617-726-2385; **Board Cert:** Neurology 1981; **Med School:** Johns Hopkins Univ 1973; **Resid:** Neurology, UCSF Med Ctr 1978; **Fac Appt:** Prof N, Harvard Med Sch

Neurology

Mid Atlantic

Apatoff, Brian R MD/PhD [N] - **Spec Exp:** Multiple Sclerosis; Neuro-Immunology; **Hospital:** NY-Presby Hosp/Weill Cornell (page 66); **Address:** 1305 York Ave, Ste Y217, New York, NY 10021; **Phone:** 646-808-5454; **Board Cert:** Neurology 1991; **Med School:** Univ Chicago-Pritzker Sch Med 1984; **Resid:** Neurology, Columbia Presby Med Ctr 1990; **Fellow:** Multiple Sclerosis, Neuro Inst-Columbia Univ 1992; **Fac Appt:** Assoc Prof N, Cornell Univ-Weill Med Coll

Baser, Susan M MD [N] - **Spec Exp:** Parkinson's Disease; Huntington's Disease; Dystonia; Movement Disorders; **Hospital:** Allegheny General Hosp; **Address:** Allegheny Neurology Assocs, 490 E North Ave Prof Bldg - Ste 500, Pittsburgh, PA 15212; **Phone:** 412-359-8860; **Board Cert:** Neurology 1990; **Med School:** Loyola Univ-Stritch Sch Med 1983; **Resid:** Neurology, Univ Pittsburgh 1987; **Fellow:** Neuropharmacology, Natl Inst Hlth 1990; **Fac Appt:** Assoc Prof N, Thomas Jefferson Univ

Bell, Rodney D MD [N] - **Spec Exp:** Stroke; **Hospital:** Thomas Jefferson Univ Hosp; **Address:** Thomas Jefferson Univ Dept Neurology, 900 Walnut St, Ste 200, Philadelphia, PA 19107; **Phone:** 215-955-6488; **Board Cert:** Internal Medicine 1975; Neurotology 1981; Vascular Neurology 2005; **Med School:** Oregon Hlth Sci Univ 1971; **Resid:** Internal Medicine, Parkland Meml Hosp 1975; Neurology, Parkland Meml Hosp 1978; **Fac Appt:** Prof N, Thomas Jefferson Univ

Bergey, Gregory K MD [N] - **Spec Exp:** Epilepsy/Seizure Disorders; Epilepsy in Women; Epilepsy in Pregnancy; **Hospital:** Johns Hopkins Hosp - Baltimore (page 61); **Address:** Johns Hopkins Epilepsy Ctr, 600 N Wolfe St, Meyer 2-147, Baltimore, MD 21287; **Phone:** 410-955-7338; **Board Cert:** Internal Medicine 1978; Neurology 1984; **Med School:** Univ Pennsylvania 1975; **Resid:** Internal Medicine, Yale-New Haven Hosp 1977; Neurology, Johns Hopkins Hosp 1981; **Fellow:** Neurological Physiology, Natl Inst Health 1983; **Fac Appt:** Prof N, Johns Hopkins Univ

Bressman, Susan MD [N] - **Spec Exp:** Parkinson's Disease; Movement Disorders; Dystonia; **Hospital:** Beth Israel Med Ctr - Petrie Division (page 57); **Address:** 10 Union Square East, Ste 2-Q, New York, NY 10003-3314; **Phone:** 212-844-8379; **Board Cert:** Neurology 1983; **Med School:** Columbia P&S 1977; **Resid:** Internal Medicine, New York Hosp 1978; Neurology, Columbia-Presby Med Ctr 1981; **Fellow:** Movement Disorders, Columbia-Presby Med Ctr 1983; **Fac Appt:** Prof N, Albert Einstein Coll Med

Brust, John C M MD [N] - **Spec Exp:** Stroke; Substance Abuse; **Hospital:** Harlem Hosp Ctr, NY-Presby Hosp/Columbia (page 66); **Address:** 506 Lenox Ave, rm 16-101, New York, NY 10037-1802; **Phone:** 212-939-4244; **Board Cert:** Neurology 1971; **Med School:** Columbia P&S 1962; **Resid:** Internal Medicine, Columbia Presby 1966; Neurology, Columbia Presby 1969; **Fac Appt:** Clin Prof N, Columbia P&S

Buchholz, David W MD [N] - **Spec Exp:** Migraine; Restless Legs Syndrome; Headache; **Hospital:** Johns Hopkins Hosp - Baltimore (page 61); **Address:** Johns Hopkins at Green Spring Station, 10753 Falls Rd, Ste 315, Lutherville, MD 21093; **Phone:** 410-583-2830; **Board Cert:** Neurology 1984; **Med School:** Univ Pennsylvania 1979; **Resid:** Neurology, Johns Hopkins Hosp 1983; **Fac Appt:** Assoc Prof N, Johns Hopkins Univ

Caronna, John J MD [N] - **Spec Exp:** Cerebrovascular Disease; Stroke; **Hospital:** NY-Presby Hosp/Weill Cornell (page 66); **Address:** Dept Neurology, Cornell Univ-Weill Med College, 520 E 70th St, Ste 607, New York, NY 10021; **Phone:** 212-746-2304; **Board Cert:** Neurology 1974; **Med School:** Cornell Univ-Weill Med Coll 1965; **Resid:** Internal Medicine, NY Hosp 1967; Neurology, NY Hosp 1971; **Fellow:** Neurology, NY Hosp 1973; **Fac Appt:** Prof N, Cornell Univ-Weill Med Coll

Charney, Jonathan MD [N] - **Spec Exp:** Headache; Stroke; **Hospital:** Mount Sinai Med Ctr (page 64); **Address:** 1111 Park Ave, Ste 1H, New York, NY 10128-1234; **Phone:** 212-831-2886; **Board Cert:** Neurology 1977; **Med School:** NY Med Coll 1969; **Resid:** Neurology, Methodist Hosp-Baylor 1971; Neurology, Columbia-Presby Med Ctr 1973; **Fac Appt:** Asst Prof N, Mount Sinai Sch Med

Cook, Stuart D MD [N] - **Spec Exp:** Multiple Sclerosis; Infectious & Demyelinating Diseases; **Hospital:** UMDNJ-Univ Hosp-Newark; **Address:** 65 Bergen St, rm 1435, Newark, NJ 07101-1709; **Phone:** 973-972-9181; **Board Cert:** Neurology 1970; **Med School:** Univ VT Coll Med 1962; **Resid:** Neurology, Albert Einstein Coll Med 1968; **Fac Appt:** Prof N, UMDNJ-NJ Med Sch, Newark

Cornblath, David R MD [N] - **Spec Exp:** Peripheral Neuropathy; **Hospital:** Johns Hopkins Hosp - Baltimore (page 61); **Address:** 600 N Wolfe St Meyer 6-181A, Baltimore, MD 21287-6965; **Phone:** 410-955-2229; **Board Cert:** Neurology 1982; Clinical Neurophysiology 1994; **Med School:** Case West Res Univ 1977; **Resid:** Neurology, Hosp Univ Penn 1981; **Fellow:** Neurology, Hosp Univ Penn 1982; **Fac Appt:** Prof N, Johns Hopkins Univ

Coyle, Patricia K MD [N] - **Spec Exp:** Multiple Sclerosis; Neuro-Immunology; Lyme Disease; Infectious-Neurologic; **Hospital:** Stony Brook Univ Med Ctr; **Address:** Dept Neurology, HSC T-12, rm 020, Stonybrook Univ Med Ctr, East Setauket, NY 11794; **Phone:** 631-444-2599; **Board Cert:** Neurology 2004; **Med School:** Johns Hopkins Univ 1974; **Resid:** Neurology, Johns Hopkins Hosp 1978; **Fellow:** Neurological Immunology, Johns Hopkins Hosp 1980; **Fac Appt:** Prof N, SUNY Stony Brook

Dalakas, Marinos C MD [N] - **Spec Exp:** Neuromuscular Disorders; **Hospital:** Thomas Jefferson Univ Hosp; **Address:** 900 Walnut St, Ste 200, JHN Bldg, Philadelphia, PA 19107; **Phone:** 215-955-7952; **Board Cert:** Neurology 1980; **Med School:** Greece 1972; **Resid:** Neurology, UMDNJ-Univ Hosp 1977; **Fellow:** Neuromuscular Medicine, Natl Inst Hlth 1980

De Angelis, Lisa MD [N] - **Spec Exp:** Neuro-Oncology; **Hospital:** Meml Sloan-Kettering Cancer Ctr; **Address:** 1275 York Avenue, New York, NY 10065; **Phone:** 800-525-2225; **Board Cert:** Neurology 1986; **Med School:** Columbia P&S 1980; **Resid:** Neurology, Neuro Inst-Presby Hosp 1984; **Fellow:** Neuro-Oncology, Neuro Inst-Presby Hosp 1985; Neuro-Oncology, Meml Sloan-Kettering Cancer Ctr 1986; **Fac Appt:** Prof N, Cornell Univ-Weill Med Coll

DeKosky, Steven T MD [N] - **Spec Exp:** Alzheimer's Disease; **Hospital:** UPMC Presby, Pittsburgh; **Address:** Univ Pittsburgh Physicians, Dept Neurology, 3471 Fifth Ave, Ste 811, Pittsburgh, PA 15213-2593; **Phone:** 412-692-2700; **Board Cert:** Neurology 2004; **Med School:** Univ Fla Coll Med 1974; **Resid:** Internal Medicine, Johns Hopkins Hosp 1975; Neurology, Univ Florida 1978; **Fellow:** Neurological Chemistry, Univ Virginia Hosp 1979; **Fac Appt:** Prof N, Univ Pittsburgh

Devinsky, Orrin MD [N] - **Spec Exp:** Epilepsy; Tuberous Sclerosis; Behavioral Neurology; **Hospital:** NYU Med Ctr (page 68), St Barnabas Med Ctr; **Address:** 403 E 34th St Fl 4, New York, NY 10016-4972; **Phone:** 212-263-8871; **Board Cert:** Neurology 1987; Clinical Neurophysiology 1990; **Med School:** Harvard Med Sch 1982; **Resid:** Neurology, New York Hosp-Cornell Med Ctr 1986; **Fellow:** Epilepsy, Natl Inst Health 1988; **Fac Appt:** Prof N, NYU Sch Med

Dewberry, Robert G MD [N] - **Hospital:** Maryland Genl Hosp; **Address:** Maryland Genl Hosp, Div Neurology, 827 Linden Ave Fl Basement, Baltimore, MD 21201; **Phone:** 410-225-8290; **Board Cert:** Neurology 1992; **Med School:** Univ MD Sch Med 1987; **Resid:** Neurology, Barnes Hospital 1991; **Fellow:** Neurological Muscular Disease, Univ Virginia Hosp 1993

Neurology

Dichter, Marc A MD [N] - **Spec Exp:** Epilepsy/Seizure Disorders; **Hospital:** Hosp Univ Penn - UPHS (page 60); **Address:** Hosp Univ Pennsylvania, Dept Neurology, 3400 Spruce St 3W Gates Bldg, Philadelphia, PA 19104; **Phone:** 215-349-5166; **Board Cert:** Neurology 1978; **Med School:** NYU Sch Med 1969; **Resid:** Neurology, Beth Israel Hosp/Chldns Hosp/ Brigham Hosp 1975; **Fac Appt:** Prof N, Univ Pennsylvania

Drachman, Daniel B MD [N] - **Spec Exp:** Muscular Dystrophy; Neuromuscular Disorders; Myasthenia Gravis; Amyotrophic Lateral Sclerosis (ALS); **Hospital:** Johns Hopkins Hosp - Baltimore (page 61); **Address:** Johns Hopkins Med Ctr, 600 N Wolfe St, Meyer 5-119, Baltimore, MD 21287-7519; **Phone:** 410-955-5406; **Board Cert:** Neurology 1963; **Med School:** NYU Sch Med 1956; **Resid:** Neurology, Boston City Hosp 1959; Neuropathology, Mallory Inst Path/Boston City Hosp 1960; **Fellow:** Neurology, Harvard Med Sch 1960; **Fac Appt:** Prof N, Johns Hopkins Univ

Dromerick, Alexander MD [N] - **Spec Exp:** Stroke Rehabilitation; **Hospital:** Natl Rehab Hosp, Washington Hosp Ctr; **Address:** NRH-Neuroscience Rsch Ctr, 102 Irving St NW, Washington, DC 20010; **Phone:** 202-877-1000; **Board Cert:** Neurology 1992; **Med School:** Univ MD Sch Med 1986; **Resid:** Neurology, Hosp Univ Penn 1991; **Fellow:** Neurological Rehabilitation, Univ Penn 1992; Neurological Rehabilitation, Cornell-Burke Rehab Ctr 1993

Fahn, Stanley MD [N] - **Spec Exp:** Movement Disorders; Parkinson's Disease; **Hospital:** NY-Presby Hosp/Columbia (page 66); **Address:** 710 W 168th St, Fl 3rd - rm 350, Neurological Institute Bldg, New York, NY 10032; **Phone:** 212-305-5277; **Board Cert:** Neurology 1968; **Med School:** UCSF 1958; **Resid:** Neurology, Neuro Inst-Columbia Presby Hosp 1962; **Fac Appt:** Prof N, Columbia P&S

Feinberg, Todd E MD [N] - **Spec Exp:** Alzheimer's Disease; Stroke Rehabilitation; Brain Injury; **Hospital:** Beth Israel Med Ctr - Petrie Division (page 57); **Address:** Beth Israel Med Ctr, Yarmon Neurobehavioral Ctr, First Ave at 16th St, New York, NY 10003; **Phone:** 212-420-4111; **Board Cert:** Psychiatry 1984; Neurology 1987; **Med School:** Mount Sinai Sch Med 1978; **Resid:** Psychiatry, Mount Sinai 1982; Neurology, Mount Sinai 1984; **Fellow:** Behavioral Neurology, Univ Florida 1986; **Fac Appt:** Clin Prof N, Albert Einstein Coll Med

Fink, Matthew E MD [N] - **Spec Exp:** Cerebrovascular Disease; Stroke; **Hospital:** NY-Presby Hosp/Weill Cornell (page 66); **Address:** NY Cornell Med Ctr Dept Neurology, 525 E 68th St, rm 607, New York, NY 10021-4870; **Phone:** 212-746-4564; **Board Cert:** Internal Medicine 1980; Vascular Neurology 2005; **Med School:** Univ Pittsburgh 1976; **Resid:** Internal Medicine, Boston Med Ctr 1980; Neurology, Columbia-Presby Hosp 1982; **Fac Appt:** Prof N, Cornell Univ

Foo, Sun-Hoo MD [N] - **Spec Exp:** Stroke; Headache; Parkinson's Disease; Dementia; **Hospital:** NYU Med Ctr (page 68), NY Downtown Hosp; **Address:** 650 1st Ave, FL 4, New York, NY 10016-3240; **Phone:** 212-213-0270; **Board Cert:** Internal Medicine 1976; Neurology 1980; **Med School:** Taiwan 1972; **Resid:** Internal Medicine, St Vincent's Hosp 1976; Neurology, NYU Med Ctr 1979; **Fac Appt:** Prof N, NYU Sch Med

French, Jacqueline MD [N] - **Spec Exp:** Epilepsy/Seizure Disorders; **Hospital:** NYU Med Ctr (page 68); **Address:** 403 E 34th St Fl 4, New York, NY 10016; **Phone:** 212-263-8327; **Board Cert:** Neurology 1987; **Med School:** Brown Univ 1982; **Resid:** Neurological Surgery, Mount Sinai Hosp 1986; **Fellow:** Epilepsy, Mount Sinai Hosp 1988; Epilepsy, Yale-New Haven Hosp 1989; **Fac Appt:** Prof N, NYU Sch Med

Galetta, Steven MD [N] - **Spec Exp:** Neuro-Ophthalmology; Optic Nerve Disorders; Multiple Sclerosis; **Hospital:** Hosp Univ Penn - UPHS (page 60); **Address:** Hosp Univ Penn, Dept Neurology, 3W Gates Bldg, 3400 Spruce St, Philadelphia, PA 19104; **Phone:** 215-662-3381; **Board Cert:** Neurology 1988; **Med School:** Cornell Univ-Weill Med Coll 1983; **Resid:** Neurology, Hosp Univ Penn 1987; **Fellow:** Neurological Ophthalmology, Bascom Palmer Eye Inst 1988; **Fac Appt:** Prof N, Univ Pennsylvania

Gendelman, Seymour MD [N] - **Spec Exp:** Parkinson's Disease; Dementia; Headache; **Hospital:** Mount Sinai Med Ctr (page 64); **Address:** 5 E 98th St Fl 7, Box 1139, New York, NY 10029-6501; **Phone:** 212-241-8172; **Board Cert:** Neurology 1971; **Med School:** Geo Wash Univ 1964; **Resid:** Neurology, Mount Sinai Hosp 1968; **Fac Appt:** Clin Prof N, Mount Sinai Sch Med

Gizzi, Martin S MD/PhD [N] - **Spec Exp:** Neuro-Ophthalmology; Balance Disorders; Progressive Supranuclear Palsy (PSP); **Hospital:** JFK Med Ctr - Edison; **Address:** NJ Neuroscience Insitute, 65 James St, Edison, NJ 08820-3947; **Phone:** 732-321-7010; **Board Cert:** Neurology 1990; **Med School:** Univ Miami Sch Med 1985; **Resid:** Neurology, Mount Sinai Hosp 1989; **Fellow:** Neurological Ophthalmology, Mount Sinai Hosp 1991; **Fac Appt:** Prof N, Seton Hall Univ Sch Grad Med Ed

Glass, Jon MD [N] - **Spec Exp:** Neuro-Oncology; Brain Tumors; Spinal Tumors; **Hospital:** Thomas Jefferson Univ Hosp; **Address:** 909 Walnut St Fl 2, Philadelphia, PA 19107; **Phone:** 215-503-7005; **Board Cert:** Neurology 1993; **Med School:** SUNY Downstate 1986; **Resid:** Neurology, Boston Univ 1989; **Fellow:** Neuro-Oncology, Mass Genl Hosp 1991; **Fac Appt:** Asst Prof N, NYU Sch Med

Golbe, Lawrence MD [N] - **Spec Exp:** Parkinson's Disease; Progressive Supranuclear Palsy (PSP); Movement Disorders; **Hospital:** Robert Wood Johnson Univ Hosp - New Brunswick; **Address:** 97 Paterson St Fl 2 - rm 204, New Brunswick, NJ 08901-2160; **Phone:** 732-235-7733; **Board Cert:** Neurology 1984; **Med School:** NYU Sch Med 1978; **Resid:** Internal Medicine, Hahnemann Univ Hosp 1980; Neurology, Bellevue Hosp 1983; **Fac Appt:** Prof N, UMDNJ-RW Johnson Med Sch

Goodgold, Albert MD [N] - **Spec Exp:** Parkinson's Disease; Spinal Cord Disorders; Multiple Sclerosis; Movement Disorders; **Hospital:** NYU Med Ctr (page 68); **Address:** 530 First Ave Fl 5 - Ste 5A, New York, NY 10016; **Phone:** 212-263-7205; **Med School:** Switzerland 1955; **Resid:** Neurology, Bellevue Hosp 1960; **Fac Appt:** Prof N, NYU Sch Med

Griffin, John W MD [N] - **Spec Exp:** Peripheral Neuropathy; Guillain-Barre Syndrome; Diabetic Polyneuropathy; **Hospital:** Johns Hopkins Hosp - Baltimore (page 61); **Address:** 600 N Wolfe St, Meyer 6-113, Baltimore, MD 21287; **Phone:** 410-955-2227; **Board Cert:** Internal Medicine 1974; Neurology 1976; **Med School:** Stanford Univ 1968; **Resid:** Internal Medicine, Johns Hopkins Hosp 1970; Neurology, Johns Hopkins Hosp 1973; **Fac Appt:** Prof N, Johns Hopkins Univ

Hiesiger, Emile MD [N] - **Spec Exp:** Pain Management; Neuro-Oncology; **Hospital:** NYU Med Ctr (page 68), VA Med Ctr - Manhattan; **Address:** 530 1st Ave, Ste 5A, New York, NY 10016-6402; **Phone:** 212-263-6123; **Board Cert:** Neurology 1983; **Med School:** NY Med Coll 1978; **Resid:** Neurology, NYU Med Ctr 1982; **Fellow:** Neurology, Meml Sloan-Kettering Cancer Ctr 1984; **Fac Appt:** Assoc Clin Prof N, NYU Sch Med

Hurtig, Howard MD [N] - **Spec Exp:** Parkinson's Disease; Movement Disorders; **Hospital:** Pennsylvania Hosp (page 60); **Address:** Pennsylvania Hosp Neurological Inst, 330 S 9th St Fl 3, Philadelphia, PA 19107; **Phone:** 215-829-6500; **Board Cert:** Neurology 1976; **Med School:** Tulane Univ 1966; **Resid:** Internal Medicine, New York Hosp 1968; Neurology, Hosp Univ Penn 1973; **Fac Appt:** Prof N, Univ Pennsylvania

Neurology

Jordan, Barry D MD [N] - **Spec Exp:** Brain Injury-Traumatic; Sports Neurology; Alzheimer's Disease; Memory Disorders; **Hospital:** Burke Rehab Hosp; **Address:** Burke Rehabilitation Hosp, 785 Mamaroneck Ave, White Plains, NY 10605; **Phone:** 914-597-2332; **Board Cert:** Neurology 1989; **Med School:** Harvard Med Sch 1981; **Resid:** Neurology, New York Hosp 1986; **Fellow:** Hosp Spec Surgery 1987; UCLA Med Ctr 1998; **Fac Appt:** Assoc Prof N, Cornell Univ-Weill Med Coll

Kolodny, Edwin H MD [N] - **Spec Exp:** Pediatric Neurology; Inherited Disorders of Nervous System; Gaucher Disease; Fabry's Disease; **Hospital:** NYU Med Ctr (page 68), Bellevue Hosp Ctr; **Address:** 403 E 34 St Fl 2, New York, NY 10016-6402; **Phone:** 212-263-8344; **Board Cert:** Neurology 1971; Clinical Genetics 1984; Clinical Biochemical Genetics 1987; **Med School:** NYU Sch Med 1962; **Resid:** Internal Medicine, Bellevue Hosp 1964; Neurology, Mass Genl Hosp 1967; **Fellow:** Neurological Pathology, Mass Genl Hosp 1966; Neurology, Nat Inst Neurol Dis & Stroke 1970; **Fac Appt:** Prof N, NYU Sch Med

Krauss, Gregory L MD [N] - **Spec Exp:** Epilepsy/Seizure Disorders; **Hospital:** Johns Hopkins Hosp - Baltimore (page 61); **Address:** Johns Hopkins Hosp, Dept Neurology, 600 N Wolfe St, Meyer 2-147, Baltimore, MD 21287; **Phone:** 410-955-2822; **Board Cert:** Neurology 1990; **Med School:** Oregon Hlth Sci Univ 1985; **Resid:** Neurology, Johns Hopkins Hosp 1989; **Fellow:** Epilepsy, Johns Hopkins Hosp 1991; **Fac Appt:** Assoc Prof N, Johns Hopkins Univ

Krumholz, Allan MD [N] - **Spec Exp:** Epilepsy/Seizure Disorders; **Hospital:** Univ of MD Med Sys; **Address:** Univ Maryland Med System, Dept Neurology, 22 S Greene St, rm N4W46, Baltimore, MD 21201-1544; **Phone:** 410-328-6267; **Board Cert:** Neurology 1977; Clinical Neurophysiology 2006; **Med School:** Ros Franklin Univ/Chicago Med Sch 1970; **Resid:** Internal Medicine, Baltimore City Hosp 1972; Neurology, Johns Hopkins Hosp 1975; **Fellow:** Electroencephalography, Johns Hopkins Hosp 1980; **Fac Appt:** Prof N, Univ MD Sch Med

Kula, Roger W MD [N] - **Spec Exp:** Neuromuscular Disorders; Myasthenia Gravis; Syringomyelia & Spinal Cord Diseases; **Hospital:** N Shore Univ Hosp, Long Island Jewish Med Ctr; **Address:** 865 Northern Blvd, Ste 302, Great Neck, NY 11021; **Phone:** 516-570-4400; **Board Cert:** Internal Medicine 1975; Neurology 1977; **Med School:** Johns Hopkins Univ 1970; **Resid:** Internal Medicine, New York Hosp 1972; Neurology, UCSF Med Ctr 1974; **Fellow:** Neuromuscular Medicine, Natl Inst Hlth 1977; **Fac Appt:** Assoc Prof N, SUNY Hlth Sci Ctr

Kunschner, Lara MD [N] - **Spec Exp:** Neuro-Oncology; Brain Tumors; **Hospital:** Allegheny General Hosp; **Address:** 420 E North Ave, Ste 206, Pittsburgh, PA 15212; **Phone:** 412-359-8850; **Board Cert:** Neurology 1999; **Med School:** Univ Pittsburgh 1994; **Resid:** Neurology, Univ Michigan Hosps 1999; **Fellow:** Neurology, MD Anderson Cancer Ctr 2000

Kuzniecky, Ruben MD [N] - **Spec Exp:** Epilepsy/Seizure Disorders; MRI; Developmental Neurologic Disorders; **Hospital:** NYU Med Ctr (page 68); **Address:** 403 E 34th St Fl 4, New York, NY 10016; **Phone:** 212-263-8870; **Board Cert:** Neurology 1990; **Med School:** Argentina 1980; **Resid:** Neurology, McGill Univ 1986; **Fellow:** Epilepsy, McGill Univ 1988; **Fac Appt:** Prof N, NYU Sch Med

Lacomis, David MD [N] - **Spec Exp:** Amyotrophic Lateral Sclerosis (ALS); Muscle Disorders; Myasthenia Gravis; Neuromuscular Disorders; **Hospital:** UPMC Presby, Pittsburgh; **Address:** Dept Neurology -Kaufmann Med Bldg, 3471 Fifth Ave, Ste 810, Pittsburgh, PA 15213; **Phone:** 412-692-4917; **Board Cert:** Neurology 1992; Clinical Neurophysiology 2004; **Med School:** Penn State Univ-Hershey Med Ctr 1987; **Resid:** Neurology, Harvard Affil Hosp 1991; **Fellow:** Neurological Muscular Disease, U Mass Med Ctr 1993; **Fac Appt:** Prof N, Univ Pittsburgh

Laterra, John J MD/PhD [N] - **Spec Exp:** Neuro-Oncology; Brain Tumors; **Hospital:** Johns Hopkins Hosp - Baltimore (page 61); **Address:** Phipps 115, 600 N Wolfe St, Baltimore, MD 21287; **Phone:** 410-614-3853; **Board Cert:** Neurology 1990; **Med School:** Case West Res Univ 1984; **Resid:** Neurology, Univ Mich Hosps 1988; **Fellow:** Research, Johns Hopkins Hosp 1989; **Fac Appt:** Prof N, Johns Hopkins Univ

Levine, David N MD [N] - **Spec Exp:** Dementia; Stroke; Spinal Cord Disorders; **Hospital:** NYU Med Ctr (page 68); **Address:** 400 E 34th St, Ste RIRM-311, New York, NY 10016-4901; **Phone:** 212-263-7744; **Board Cert:** Neurology 1976; **Med School:** Harvard Med Sch 1968; **Resid:** Neurology, Mass Genl Hosp 1974; **Fellow:** Neurology, Mass Genl Hosp 1976; **Fac Appt:** Prof N, NYU Sch Med

Levine, Steven R MD [N] - **Spec Exp:** Stroke; Cerebrovascular Disease; **Hospital:** Mount Sinai Med Ctr (page 64); **Address:** Mt Sinai Sch Med, Neurology, Stroke Center, 1 Gustave L Levy Pl, Box 1137, New York, NY 10029-6500; **Phone:** 212-241-1970; **Board Cert:** Neurology 1986; Vascular Neurology 2005; **Med School:** Med Coll Wisc 1981; **Resid:** Neurology, Univ Mich Hosps 1985; **Fellow:** Cerebrovascular Disease, Henry Ford Hosp 1987; **Fac Appt:** Prof N, Mount Sinai Sch Med

Liporace, Joyce D MD [N] - **Spec Exp:** Epilepsy in Women; Women's Health; Epilepsy in Pregnancy; **Hospital:** Riddle Meml Hosp; **Address:** Riddle Healthcare 2, 1088 Baltimore Pike, Ste 2205, Media, PA 19063; **Phone:** 610-744-2960; **Board Cert:** Neurological Surgery 1993; Clinical Neurophysiology 1999; **Med School:** Johns Hopkins Univ 1988; **Resid:** Neurology, Hosp U Penn 1992; **Fellow:** Clinical Neurophysiology, Hosp U Penn 1994; **Fac Appt:** Assoc Prof Med, Thomas Jefferson Univ

Lipton, Richard MD [N] - **Spec Exp:** Headache; Migraine; Clinical Trials; **Hospital:** Montefiore Med Ctr - Weiler-Einstein Div; **Address:** Montefiore Headache Center, 1575 Blondell Ave, Ste 225, Bronx, NY 10461-2662; **Phone:** 718-405-8360; **Board Cert:** Neurology 1985; **Med School:** Univ Chicago-Pritzker Sch Med 1980; **Resid:** Neurology, Montefiore Med Ctr 1984; **Fellow:** Neurological Physiology, Montefiore Med Ctr 1985; NeuroEpidemiology, Columbia Univ 1990; **Fac Appt:** Prof N, Albert Einstein Coll Med

Liu, Grant T MD [N] - **Spec Exp:** Pediatric Neuro-Ophthalmology; Neuro-Ophthalmology; **Hospital:** Hosp Univ Penn - UPHS (page 60), Chldns Hosp of Philadelphia, The; **Address:** Hosp Univ Penn, Dept Neurology, 3W Gates Bldg, 3400 Spruce St, Philadelphia, PA 19104; **Phone:** 215-349-8460; **Board Cert:** Neurology 1993; **Med School:** Columbia P&S 1988; **Resid:** Neurology, Harvard-Nolgwood Neurology Program 1992; **Fellow:** Neurological Ophthalmology, Bascom Palmer Eye Inst 1993; **Fac Appt:** Assoc Prof N, Univ Pennsylvania

Logigian, Eric L MD [N] - **Spec Exp:** Neuromuscular Disorders; Electromyography; Lyme Disease; **Hospital:** Univ of Rochester Strong Meml Hosp; **Address:** Univ Rochester, Dept of Neurology, 601 Elmwood Ave, Box 673, Rochester, NY 14642; **Phone:** 585-275-4568; **Board Cert:** Internal Medicine 1981; Neurology 1985; Clinical Neurophysiology 1999; **Med School:** Boston Univ 1978; **Resid:** Internal Medicine, Beth Israel Hosp 1981; Neurology, Mass Genl Hosp 1984; **Fellow:** Clinical Neurophysiology, Mass General Hosp 1985; **Fac Appt:** Prof N, Univ Rochester

Lublin, Fred MD [N] - **Spec Exp:** Multiple Sclerosis; **Hospital:** Mount Sinai Med Ctr (page 64); **Address:** Dickinson Ctr for Multiple Sclerosis, 5 E 98th St, Box 1138, New York, NY 10029-6574; **Phone:** 212-241-6854; **Board Cert:** Neurology 1977; **Med School:** Jefferson Med Coll 1972; **Resid:** Neurology, NY Hosp/Cornell Med Ctr 1976; **Fac Appt:** Prof N, Mount Sinai Sch Med

Neurology

McArthur, Justin C MD [N] - **Spec Exp:** AIDS/HIV; Multiple Sclerosis; **Hospital:** Johns Hopkins Hosp - Baltimore (page 61); **Address:** Johns Hopkins Hosp, Dept Neurology, 600 N Wolfe St, Meyer 6-109, Baltimore, MD 21287; **Phone:** 410-955-3730; **Board Cert:** Neurology 1986; Internal Medicine 1984; **Med School:** England 1979; **Resid:** Internal Medicine, Johns Hopkins Hosp 1982; Neurology, Johns Hopkins Hosp 1985; **Fac Appt:** Prof N, Johns Hopkins Univ

McCluskey, Leo MD [N] - **Spec Exp:** Amyotrophic Lateral Sclerosis (ALS); **Hospital:** Hosp Univ Penn - UPHS (page 60); **Address:** 330 S 9th St, Philadelphia, PA 19107; **Phone:** 215-829-3053; **Board Cert:** Neurology 1986; **Med School:** Columbia P&S 1980; **Resid:** Internal Medicine, Univ Mich 1982; Neurology, Hosp Univ Penn 1985; **Fellow:** Neurological Muscular Disease, Hosp Univ Penn 1986; **Fac Appt:** Assoc Prof N, Univ Pennsylvania

McDonald, John W MD/PhD [N] - **Spec Exp:** Spinal Cord Injury; Stroke Rehabilitation; **Hospital:** Kennedy Krieger Inst; **Address:** Kennedy Krieger Inst, 707 N Broadway, Ste 518, Baltimore, MD 21205; **Phone:** 443-923-9210; **Med School:** Univ Mich Med Sch 1991; **Resid:** Neurology, Barnes-Jewish Hosp 1995; **Fac Appt:** Assoc Prof N, Johns Hopkins Univ

Miller, Aaron MD [N] - **Spec Exp:** Multiple Sclerosis; Alzheimer's Disease; Autoimmune Disease; **Hospital:** Mount Sinai Med Ctr (page 64), Maimonides Med Ctr (page 63); **Address:** Corinne Goldsmith Dickinson Ctr for MS, 5 E 98th St, Box 1138, New York, NY 10029; **Phone:** 212-241-6854; **Board Cert:** Internal Medicine 1972; Neurology 1977; **Med School:** NYU Sch Med 1968; **Resid:** Internal Medicine, Jacobi Med Ctr 1970; Neurology, Montefiore Med Ctr 1975; **Fellow:** Neurovirology, Johns Hopkins Hosp 1977; **Fac Appt:** Prof N, Mount Sinai Sch Med

Mitsumoto, Hiroshi MD [N] - **Spec Exp:** Amyotrophic Lateral Sclerosis (ALS); Neuromuscular Disorders; Clinical Trials; **Hospital:** NY-Presby Hosp/Columbia (page 66); **Address:** Neurological Inst, 710 W 168th St Fl 9 - rm 9001, New York, NY 10032; **Phone:** 212-305-1319; **Board Cert:** Neurology 1978; **Med School:** Japan 1968; **Resid:** Internal Medicine, Toho Univ Hosps 1972; Neurology, Univ Hosps 1976; **Fellow:** Neurological Pathology, Cleveland Clinic 1978; Neuromuscular Medicine, Tufts Univ 1981; **Fac Appt:** Prof N, Columbia P&S

Mohr, Jay P MD [N] - **Spec Exp:** Aphasia; Stroke; Aneurysm-Cerebral; Brain Arteriovenous Malformation; **Hospital:** NY-Presby Hosp/Columbia (page 66); **Address:** Neurological Inst-Dept Neurology, 710 W 168 St, Ste 615, New York, NY 10032-2603; **Phone:** 212-305-8033; **Board Cert:** Neurology 1971; Vascular Neurology 2005; **Med School:** Univ VA Sch Med 1963; **Resid:** Neurology, Columbia Presby Med Ctr 1966; Neurology, Mass Genl Hosp 1968; **Fellow:** Neurology, Mass Genl Hosp 1969; **Fac Appt:** Clin Prof N, Columbia P&S

Newman, Lawrence C MD [N] - **Spec Exp:** Headache; Pain-Facial; **Hospital:** St Luke's - Roosevelt Hosp Ctr - Roosevelt Div (page 57); **Address:** St Luke's-Roosevelt Hosp-Headache Inst, 1000 Tenth Ave Fl 1 - Ste 1C10, New York, NY 10019-1192; **Phone:** 212-523-5869; **Board Cert:** Neurology 2005; Headache Medicine 2006; **Med School:** Mexico 1983; **Resid:** Internal Medicine, Elmhurst Hosp 1986; Neurology, Montefiore Med Ctr 1989; **Fac Appt:** Assoc Prof N, Albert Einstein Coll Med

Olanow, C Warren MD [N] - **Spec Exp:** Parkinson's Disease; Movement Disorders; **Hospital:** Mount Sinai Med Ctr (page 64); **Address:** 5 E 98th St, New York, NY 10029; **Phone:** 212-241-8435; **Med School:** Univ Toronto 1965; **Resid:** Neurology, Toronto Genl Hosp 1968; Neurology, Columbia Presby Hosp 1970; **Fellow:** Neurological Anatomy, Columbia Presby Hosp 1971; **Fac Appt:** Prof N, Mount Sinai Sch Med

Pedley, Timothy A MD [N] - **Spec Exp:** Epilepsy/Seizure Disorders; **Hospital:** NY-Presby Hosp/Columbia (page 66); **Address:** The Neurological Inst, 710 W 168th St, rm 1406, New York, NY 10032; **Phone:** 212-305-6489; **Board Cert:** Neurology 1975; **Med School:** Yale Univ 1969; **Resid:** Neurology, Stanford Univ Hosp 1973; **Fellow:** Clinical Neurophysiology, Stanford Univ Hosp 1975; **Fac Appt:** Prof N, Columbia P&S

Petito, Frank MD [N] - **Spec Exp:** Multiple Sclerosis; Headache; Lyme Disease; **Hospital:** NY-Presby Hosp/Weill Cornell (page 66); **Address:** 525 E 68th St, Ste 607, New York, NY 10021-4870; **Phone:** 212-746-2309; **Board Cert:** Neurology 1972; **Med School:** Columbia P&S 1967; **Resid:** Neurology, New York Hosp 1971; **Fac Appt:** Prof N, Cornell Univ-Weill Med Coll

Posner, Jerome MD [N] - **Spec Exp:** Neuro-Oncology; Brain Tumors; **Hospital:** Meml Sloan-Kettering Cancer Ctr; **Address:** 1275 York Avenue, New York, NY 10065; **Phone:** 800-525-2225; **Board Cert:** Neurology 1962; **Med School:** Univ Wash 1955; **Resid:** Neurology, Univ WA Affil Hosp 1959; **Fellow:** Biochemistry, Univ WA Affil Hosp 1963; **Fac Appt:** Prof N, Cornell Univ-Weill Med Coll

Pula, Thaddeus MD [N] - **Spec Exp:** Neurophysiology; Electromyography; **Hospital:** Maryland Genl Hosp; **Address:** Maryland Genl Hosp, Div Neurology, 827 Linden Ave Fl Basement, Baltimore, MD 21201-4606; **Phone:** 410-225-8290; **Board Cert:** Neurology 1981; **Med School:** Univ MD Sch Med 1976; **Resid:** Internal Medicine, Mercy Hosp Med Ctr; **Fellow:** Neurology, Univ Maryland

Reich, Stephen G MD [N] - **Spec Exp:** Movement Disorders; Parkinson's Disease; Ataxia; Dystonia-Botox Therapy; **Hospital:** Univ of MD Med Sys; **Address:** Univ Maryland Med System, Frenkil Bldg, 16 S Eutaw St Fl 3, Baltimore, MD 21201; **Phone:** 410-328-5858; **Board Cert:** Neurology 1989; **Med School:** Tulane Univ 1983; **Resid:** Neurology, Case West Res Univ Hosp 1987; **Fellow:** Movement Disorders, Johns Hopkins Hosp 1988; **Fac Appt:** Assoc Prof N, Univ MD Sch Med

Relkin, Norman MD/PhD [N] - **Spec Exp:** Alzheimer's Disease; Dementia; Memory Disorders; **Hospital:** NY-Presby Hosp/Columbia (page 66); **Address:** Weill Cornell Memory Disorders Program, 428 E 72nd St, Ste 500, New York, NY 10021; **Phone:** 212-746-2441; **Board Cert:** Neurology 1992; **Med School:** Albert Einstein Coll Med 1987; **Resid:** Neurology, New York Hosp 1991; **Fellow:** Behavioral Neurology, New York Hosp-Cornell 1992; **Fac Appt:** Asst Prof N, Cornell Univ-Weill Med Coll

Rosenfeld, Myrna MD/PhD [N] - **Spec Exp:** Neuro-Oncology; Brain Tumors; **Hospital:** Hosp Univ Penn - UPHS (page 60); **Address:** Hosp Univ Penn, Dept Neurology, 3400 Spruce St, 3W Gates, Philadelphia, PA 19104; **Phone:** 215-746-4707; **Board Cert:** Neurology 1990; **Med School:** Northwestern Univ 1985; **Resid:** Neurology, Northwestern Univ Hosp 1987; Neurology, Univ Hosp Cleveland 1989; **Fellow:** Neuro-Oncology, Meml Sloan Kettering Cancer Ctr; **Fac Appt:** Assoc Prof N, Univ Pennsylvania

Rosenfeld, Steven S MD [N] - **Spec Exp:** Brain Tumors; Gliomas; Neuro-Oncology; **Hospital:** NY-Presby Hosp/Columbia (page 66); **Address:** Neurological Inst of NY-Brain Tumor Ctr, 710 W 168th St, rm 204, New York, NY 10032; **Phone:** 212-305-1718; **Board Cert:** Neurology 1994; **Med School:** Northwestern Univ 1985; **Resid:** Neurology, Duke Univ Med Ctr 1989; **Fellow:** Neuro-Oncology, Duke Univ Med Ctr 1990; **Fac Appt:** Prof N, Columbia P&S

Sage, Jacob MD [N] - **Spec Exp:** Parkinson's Disease; **Hospital:** Robert Wood Johnson Univ Hosp - New Brunswick; **Address:** UMDNJ, Dept Neurology, 97 Paterson St, New Brunswick, NJ 08901-2160; **Phone:** 732-235-7733; **Board Cert:** Neurology 1979; **Med School:** Univ Pittsburgh 1972; **Resid:** Neurology, Univ Pittsburgh Hosps 1978; **Fellow:** Neurological Chemistry, NY Hosp-Cornell 1980; **Fac Appt:** Prof N, UMDNJ-RW Johnson Med Sch

Neurology

Schwartzman, Robert J MD [N] - **Spec Exp:** Reflex Sympathetic Dystrophy (RSD); Pain Management; **Hospital:** Hahnemann Univ Hosp; **Address:** Drexel Neurological Assocs, 219 N Broad St Fl 7, Philadelphia, PA 19107; **Phone:** 215-762-6915; **Board Cert:** Internal Medicine 1971; Neurology 1974; **Med School:** Univ Pennsylvania 1965; **Resid:** Internal Medicine, Duke Univ Hosp 1967; Neurology, Hosp Univ Penn 1969; **Fellow:** Neurology, NIH-Med Neur Br 1971; **Fac Appt:** Prof N, Drexel Univ Coll Med

Shefner, Jeremy MD/PhD [N] - **Spec Exp:** Amyotrophic Lateral Sclerosis (ALS); Neuromuscular Disorders; **Hospital:** Univ. Hosp.- SUNY Upstate; **Address:** 750 E Adams Rd, Syracuse, NY 13210-1834; **Phone:** 315-464-4243; **Board Cert:** Neurology 1989; Clinical Neurophysiology 2004; **Med School:** Northwestern Univ 1983; **Resid:** Neurology, Harvard-Longwood Neur Trng 1988; **Fellow:** Neurological Muscular Disease, Brigham & Womens Hosp 1990; **Fac Appt:** Prof N, SUNY Upstate Med Univ

Shoulson, Ira MD [N] - **Spec Exp:** Parkinson's Disease; Movement Disorders; Huntington's Disease; **Hospital:** Univ of Rochester Strong Meml Hosp; **Address:** 1351 Mount Hope Ave, Ste 218, Rochester, NY 14620; **Phone:** 585-275-2585; **Board Cert:** Internal Medicine 1974; Neurology 1980; **Med School:** Univ Rochester 1971; **Resid:** Internal Medicine, Strong Meml Hosp 1973; Neurology, Strong Meml Hosp 1977; **Fellow:** Neurology, Natl Inst Hlth 1975; **Fac Appt:** Prof N, Univ Rochester

Shulman, Lisa M MD [N] - **Spec Exp:** Movement Disorders; Movement Disorders-Botox Therapy; Parkinson's Disease; **Hospital:** Univ of MD Med Sys; **Address:** Univ Maryland Med System, Frenkil Bldg, 16 S Eutaw St Fl 3, Baltimore, MD 21201; **Phone:** 410-328-2164; **Board Cert:** Neurology 1994; **Med School:** Univ Miami Sch Med 1988; **Resid:** Neurology, Jackson Meml Hosp 1992; **Fellow:** Movement Disorders, Jackson Meml Hosp 1994; **Fac Appt:** Assoc Prof N, Univ MD Sch Med

Silberstein, Stephen D MD [N] - **Spec Exp:** Headache; Migraine; Pain-Facial; **Hospital:** Thomas Jefferson Univ Hosp; **Address:** Jefferson Headache Center, 111 S 11th St, Gibbon Bldg, Philadelphia, PA 19107; **Phone:** 215-955-2243; **Board Cert:** Neurology 1975; Headache Medicine 2006; **Med School:** Univ Pennsylvania 1967; **Resid:** Internal Medicine, Hosp Univ Penn 1969; Neurology, Hosp Univ Penn 1975; **Fac Appt:** Clin Prof N, Temple Univ

Sirdofsky, Michael D MD [N] - **Spec Exp:** Neuromuscular Disorders; Electrodiagnosis; **Hospital:** Georgetown Univ Hosp; **Address:** Pasquerilla Health Care Bldg, Entrance 1 Fl 7, 3800 Resevoir Rd NW, Washington, DC 20007; **Phone:** 202-444-8525; **Board Cert:** Neurology 1981; **Med School:** Georgetown Univ 1976; **Resid:** Neurology, Georgetown Univ Hosp 1980; **Fac Appt:** Assoc Prof N, Georgetown Univ

Sperling, Michael R MD [N] - **Spec Exp:** Epilepsy/Seizure Disorders; **Hospital:** Thomas Jefferson Univ Hosp; **Address:** Thos Jefferson Univ Hosp, Dept Neurology, 900 Walnut St, Ste 200, Philadelphia, PA 19107; **Phone:** 215-955-1222; **Board Cert:** Neurology 1984; Clinical Neurophysiology 1999; **Med School:** Temple Univ 1978; **Resid:** Neurology, Mt Sinai Hosp 1982; **Fellow:** Epilepsy, UCLA Med Ctr 1984; **Fac Appt:** Prof N, Thomas Jefferson Univ

Stern, Matthew MD [N] - **Spec Exp:** Parkinson's Disease; Movement Disorders; Botox Therapy; **Hospital:** Pennsylvania Hosp (page 60); **Address:** Pennsylvania Hosp, Dept Neurology, 330 S 9th St Fl 3, Philadelphia, PA 19107; **Phone:** 215-829-6500; **Board Cert:** Neurology 1983; **Med School:** Duke Univ 1978; **Resid:** Neurology, Hosp Univ Penn 1982; **Fac Appt:** Prof Med, Univ Pennsylvania

Swerdlow, Michael MD [N] - **Spec Exp:** Myasthenia Gravis; Spinal Disorders; Multiple Sclerosis; **Hospital:** Montefiore Med Ctr; **Address:** 3400 Bainbridge Ave, Bronx, NY 10467-2401; **Phone:** 718-920-4178; **Board Cert:** Neurology 1975; **Med School:** Univ Pennsylvania 1967; **Resid:** Internal Medicine, Mount Sinai Hosp 1969; Neurology, Albert Einstein Coll 1972; **Fellow:** Neurology, Natl Inst Hlth 1974; **Fac Appt:** Prof N, Albert Einstein Coll Med

Vas, George A MD [N] - **Spec Exp:** Stroke; Multiple Sclerosis; **Hospital:** SUNY Downstate Med Ctr, Kings County Hosp Ctr; **Address:** 450 Clarkson Ave, Ste A, Brooklyn, NY 11203-2056; **Phone:** 718-270-2502; **Board Cert:** Internal Medicine 1973; Neurology 1977; Clinical Neurophysiology 2002; **Med School:** Univ Pittsburgh 1970; **Resid:** Internal Medicine, New York Hosp 1972; Neurology, New York Hosp 1975; **Fac Appt:** Prof N, SUNY Downstate

Wechsler, Lawrence R MD [N] - **Spec Exp:** Cerebrovascular Disease; Stroke; **Hospital:** UPMC Presby, Pittsburgh, UPMC Shadyside; **Address:** UPMC Stroke Institute, 3471 Fifth Ave, Ste 810, Pittsburgh, PA 15213; **Phone:** 412-692-4920; **Board Cert:** Internal Medicine 1983; Neurology 1984; Clinical Neurophysiology 1994; Vascular Neurology 2005; **Med School:** Univ Pennsylvania 1978; **Resid:** Internal Medicine, Presby-Univ Hosp 1980; Neurology, Mass Genl Hosp 1983; **Fellow:** Clinical Neurophysiology, Mass Genl Hosp 1984; Cerebrovascular Disease, Mass Genl Hosp 1985; **Fac Appt:** Prof N, Univ Pittsburgh

Weinberg, Harold MD [N] - **Spec Exp:** Headache; Spinal Disorders; Neuromuscular Disorders; **Hospital:** NYU Med Ctr (page 68); **Address:** 650 1st Ave Fl 4, New York, NY 10016-3240; **Phone:** 212-213-9339; **Board Cert:** Neurology 1983; **Med School:** Albert Einstein Coll Med 1978; **Resid:** Neurology, Columbia-Presby Med Ctr 1982; **Fellow:** Neuromuscular Medicine, Columbia-Presby Med Ctr 1982; **Fac Appt:** Clin Prof N, NYU Sch Med

Weiner, William J MD [N] - **Spec Exp:** Movement Disorders; Parkinson's Disease; Huntington's Disease; Progressive Supranuclear Palsy (PSP); **Hospital:** Univ of MD Med Sys; **Address:** Univ Maryland Med System, Dept Neurology, 22 S Greene St, rm N4W46, Baltimore, MD 21201; **Phone:** 410-328-2172; **Board Cert:** Neurology 1975; **Med School:** Univ IL Coll Med 1969; **Resid:** Neurology, Univ Minn 1971; Neurology, Rush-Presby Med Ctr 1973; **Fac Appt:** Prof N, Univ MD Sch Med

Wityk, Robert J MD [N] - **Spec Exp:** Stroke; Cerebrovascular Disease; **Hospital:** Johns Hopkins Hosp - Baltimore (page 61); **Address:** 601 N Caroline St, Ste 5073A, Baltimore, MD 21287; **Phone:** 410-955-2228; **Board Cert:** Internal Medicine 1988; Neurology 1992; **Med School:** Case West Res Univ 1985; **Resid:** Internal Medicine, UCSD Med Ctr 1988; Neurology, Mass Genl Hosp 1991; **Fellow:** Cardiovascular Disease, Tufts U-New Eng MC 1992; **Fac Appt:** Assoc Prof N, Johns Hopkins Univ

Zimmerman, Earl A MD [N] - **Spec Exp:** Memory Disorders; Alzheimer's Disease; Dementia; **Hospital:** Albany Med Ctr; **Address:** Albany Med Ctr-Neurology, 47 New Scotland Ave, MC 70, Albany, NY 12208; **Phone:** 518-262-5226; **Board Cert:** Neurology 1970; Internal Medicine 1970; **Med School:** Univ Pennsylvania 1963; **Resid:** Internal Medicine, Presbyterian Hosp 1965; Neurology, Neurological Inst 1968; **Fellow:** Endocrinology, Presbyterian Hosp 1972; **Fac Appt:** Prof N, Albany Med Coll

Southeast

Abou-Khalil, Bassel MD [N] - **Spec Exp:** Epilepsy; **Hospital:** Vanderbilt Univ Med Ctr; **Address:** Vanderbilt Univ-Dept Neurology, 1161 21st Ave, rm A-0118 MCN, Nashville, TN 37232-2551; **Phone:** 615-936-0060; **Board Cert:** Neurology 1986; Clinical Neurophysiology 2002; **Med School:** Amer Univ Beirut 1978; **Resid:** Neurology, Strong Meml Hosp 1980; Neurology, Univ Mich Hosps 1982; **Fellow:** Epilepsy, Univ Mich Hosps 1985; Electroencephalography, Univ Mich Hosps 1985; **Fac Appt:** Prof N, Vanderbilt Univ

Neurology

Adams, Robert J MD [N] - **Spec Exp:** Stroke; **Hospital:** MUSC Med Ctr; **Address:** MUSC Stroke Center, 96 Jonathan Lucas St, Ste 307, Charleston, SC 29425; **Phone:** 843-792-7058; **Board Cert:** Neurology 1987; **Med School:** Univ Ark 1980; **Resid:** Neurology, Med Coll Georgia 1985; **Fac Appt:** Assoc Prof N, Med Coll GA

Berger, Joseph MD [N] - **Spec Exp:** Multiple Sclerosis; AIDS/HIV; Infectious & Demyelinating Diseases; **Hospital:** Univ of Kentucky Chandler Hosp; **Address:** Univ Kentucky, Dept Neurology, Kentucky Clinic, Rm L-445, 740 S Limestone, Lexington, KY 40536; **Phone:** 859-323-5661; **Board Cert:** Neurology 1983; Internal Medicine 1977; **Med School:** Jefferson Med Coll 1974; **Resid:** Internal Medicine, Georgetown Univ Hosp 1977; Neurology, Jackson Meml Hosp 1981; **Fac Appt:** Prof N, Univ KY Coll Med

Bernad, Peter MD [N] - **Spec Exp:** Stroke; Headache; Migraine; Head Injury; **Hospital:** Inova Fairfax Hosp, G Washington Univ Hosp; **Address:** 2296 Opitz Blvd, Ste 360, Woodbridge, VA 22191; **Phone:** 703-878-0600; **Board Cert:** Internal Medicine 1979; Neurology 1981; **Med School:** McGill Univ 1974; **Resid:** Internal Medicine, USC Univ Hosp 1976; Neurology, Mass Genl Hosp-Harvard 1979; **Fellow:** Neurological Muscular Disease, Natl Inst Hlth 1981; **Fac Appt:** Assoc Clin Prof N, Geo Wash Univ

Brooks, Benjamin R MD [N] - **Spec Exp:** Neuromuscular Disorders; Multiple Sclerosis; Neurotoxicology; **Hospital:** Carolinas Med Ctr; **Address:** Carolinas Neuromuscular/ALS-MDA Ctr, Neuroscience & Spine Inst, PO Box 32861, Charlotte, NC 28207; **Phone:** 704-446-4360; **Board Cert:** Internal Medicine 1974; Neurology 1978; **Med School:** Harvard Med Sch 1970; **Resid:** Neurology, Mass Genl Hosp 1974; Neurology, Natl Inst Neuro Disorders & Stroke-NIH 1976; **Fellow:** Neurovirology, Johns Hopkins Hosp 1978

Corbett, James MD [N] - **Spec Exp:** Neuro-Ophthalmology; Pseudotumor Cerebri; Neurosarcoidosis; **Hospital:** Univ Hosps & Clins - Jackson; **Address:** Univ Mississippi Med Ctr, Dept Neurology, 2500 N State St, Jackson, MS 39216-4505; **Phone:** 601-984-5501; **Board Cert:** Neurology 2004; **Med School:** Ros Franklin Univ/Chicago Med Sch 1966; **Resid:** Internal Medicine, Rhode Island Hosp 1968; Neurology, Univ Hosp-Case Western Reserve 1971; **Fac Appt:** Prof N, Univ Miss

De Long, Mahlon R MD [N] - **Spec Exp:** Parkinson's Disease; Movement Disorders; **Hospital:** Emory Univ Hosp; **Address:** Emory Clinic, Dept Neurology, 101 Woodruff Cir, Ste 6000, Atlanta, GA 30322; **Phone:** 404-727-9107; **Board Cert:** Neurology 1980; **Med School:** Harvard Med Sch 1966; **Resid:** Internal Medicine, Boston City Hosp 1968; Neurology, Johns Hopkins Hosp 1976; **Fellow:** Neurology, NIMH 1973; **Fac Appt:** Prof N, Emory Univ

Dure IV, Leon S MD [N] - **Spec Exp:** Huntington's Disease; Tourette's Syndrome; Movement Disorders; **Hospital:** Univ of Ala Hosp at Birmingham; **Address:** 1600 7th Ave S CHB Bldg - Ste 314, Birmingham, AL 35233-0011; **Phone:** 205-996-7865; **Board Cert:** Child Neurology 1991; **Med School:** Baylor Coll Med 1984; **Resid:** Pediatrics, Columbia Presby Hosp 1986; Child Neurology, Texas Chldns Hosp 1989; **Fellow:** Child Neurology, Univ Michigan 1990; **Fac Appt:** Assoc Prof N, Univ Ala

Finkel, Alan G MD [N] - **Spec Exp:** Headache; Pain-Facial; Migraine; **Hospital:** Univ NC Hosps; **Address:** Univ North Carolina Dept Neurology, 3114 Bioinformatics Bldg, CB# 7025, Chapel Hill, NC 27599-7025; **Phone:** 919-966-2527; **Board Cert:** Neurology 1991; Pain Medicine 2003; Headache Medicine 2006; **Med School:** SUNY Buffalo 1985; **Resid:** Neurology, NC Meml HOsp 1989; **Fellow:** Pain & Headache Medicine, Univ NC; **Fac Appt:** Prof N, Univ NC Sch Med

Finkel, Michael F MD [N] - **Spec Exp:** Movement Disorders-Lower Limb; ADD/ADHD; Headache in Women; Trauma Neurology; **Hospital:** Physicians Regl Med Ctr; **Address:** Medical Surgical Specialists, 6101 Pine Ridge Rd, Naples, FL 34119; **Phone:** 239-348-4397; **Board Cert:** Neurology 1979; **Med School:** Washington Univ, St Louis 1973; **Resid:** Neurology, Strong Meml Hosp 1977

Glass, Jonathan D MD [N] - **Spec Exp:** Neuro-Pathology; Amyotrophic Lateral Sclerosis (ALS); Peripheral Neuropathy; **Hospital:** Emory Univ Hosp, Grady Hlth Sys; **Address:** 1365 Clifton Rd NE, Ste A3100, Atlanta, GA 30322; **Phone:** 404-778-3444; **Board Cert:** Neurology 1990; Neuropathology 1997; **Med School:** Univ VT Coll Med 1985; **Resid:** Neurology, Johns Hopkins Univ 1989; **Fellow:** Neuropathology, Johns Hopkins Univ 1991; **Fac Appt:** Prof N, Emory Univ

Goldstein, Larry B MD [N] - **Spec Exp:** Stroke; Carotid Artery Disease; **Hospital:** Duke Univ Med Ctr, VA Med Ctr - Durham; **Address:** Duke Univ Med Ctr, Box 3651, Durham, NC 27710-0001; **Phone:** 919-684-3801; **Board Cert:** Neurology 1987; Vascular Neurology 2005; **Med School:** Mount Sinai Sch Med 1981; **Resid:** Neurology, Mt Sinai Hosp 1985; **Fellow:** Cerebrovascular Disease, Duke Univ Med Ctr 1986; **Fac Appt:** Prof N, Duke Univ

Gress, Daryl Ray MD [N] - **Spec Exp:** Critical Care; Stroke; **Hospital:** Univ Virginia Med Ctr; **Address:** Box 800394, Charlottesville, VA 22908; **Phone:** 434-924-8371; **Board Cert:** Neurology 1989; **Med School:** Washington Univ, St Louis 1982; **Resid:** Internal Medicine, Johns Hopkins Hosp 1984; Neurology, Mass Genl Hosp 1987; **Fellow:** Stroke, Mass Genl Hosp 1988

Haley Jr, Elliott C MD [N] - **Spec Exp:** Stroke; **Hospital:** Univ Virginia Med Ctr; **Address:** Univ VA Hlth Sys, Dept Neurology, PO Box 800394, Charlottesville, VA 22908; **Phone:** 434-924-8041; **Board Cert:** Internal Medicine 1978; Neurology 1985; **Med School:** Tulane Univ 1974; **Resid:** Internal Medicine, Univ Va Hosp 1978; Neurology, Univ Va Hosp 1982; **Fellow:** Cerebrovascular Disease, Mass Genl Hosp 1984; **Fac Appt:** Prof N, Univ VA Sch Med

Heilman, Kenneth M MD [N] - **Spec Exp:** Behavioral Neurology; Memory Disorders; **Hospital:** Shands at Univ of FL, Malcolm Randall VA Med Ctr; **Address:** Hlth Ctr Univ Fla Coll Med, Dept Neur, P.O. Box 100236, Gainesville, FL 32610-0236; **Phone:** 352-273-5550; **Board Cert:** Neurology 1973; **Med School:** Univ VA Sch Med 1963; **Resid:** Internal Medicine, Bellevue Hosp Ctr 1965; Neurology, Boston City Hosp 1970; **Fac Appt:** Prof N, Univ Fla Coll Med

Hess, David C MD [N] - **Spec Exp:** Stroke; Antiphospholipid Syndrome (APS); Autoimmune Cerebrovascular Disease; **Hospital:** Med Coll of GA Hosp and Clin; **Address:** Med Coll Ga Dept Neurology, 1120 15th St, rm BI-3080, Augusta, GA 30912; **Phone:** 706-721-1691; **Board Cert:** Internal Medicine 1986; Neurology 1990; **Med School:** Univ MD Sch Med 1983; **Resid:** Internal Medicine, Allegheny Genl Hosp 1985; Neurology, Med Coll Ga 1989; **Fellow:** Cerebrovascular Disease, Med Coll Ga 1990; **Fac Appt:** Prof N, Med Coll GA

Hurwitz, Barrie J MD [N] - **Spec Exp:** Multiple Sclerosis; Parkinson's Disease; Stroke/Cerebrovascular Disease; **Hospital:** Duke Univ Med Ctr; **Address:** Duke Univ Med Ctr, 122 Baker House, Box 3184, Durham, NC 27710; **Phone:** 919-684-4126; **Board Cert:** Neurology 1979; **Med School:** South Africa 1968; **Resid:** Internal Medicine, Johannesburg Genl Hosp 1973; Neurology, New York Hosp/Sloan Kettering Hosp 1977; **Fellow:** Neurology, New York Hosp-Cornell 1976; **Fac Appt:** Assoc Prof Med, Duke Univ

Janss, Anna J MD/PhD [N] - **Spec Exp:** Brain Tumors-Pediatric; Clinical Trials; Cancer Survivors-Late Effects of Therapy; **Hospital:** Chldns Hlthcare Atlanta - Egleston; **Address:** Aflac Cancer & Blood Disorders Ctr, Outpatient Clin, Tower 1 Fl 4, 1405 Clifton Rd NE, Atlanta, GA 30322; **Phone:** 404-785-1200; **Board Cert:** Neurology 1993; **Med School:** Univ Iowa Coll Med 1988; **Resid:** Neurology, Hosp Univ Penn 1992; **Fellow:** Pediatric Neuro-Oncology, Chldns Hosp 1996; **Fac Appt:** Assoc Prof N, Emory Univ

Neurology

Kirshner, Howard S MD [N] - **Spec Exp:** Stroke; Aphasia; Neurorehabilitation; Dementia; **Hospital:** Vanderbilt Univ Med Ctr, Vanderbilt Stallworth Rehab Hosp Lp; **Address:** Vanderbilt Univ Med Ctr, Dept Neurology, 2311 Pierce Ave, SGOB-Ste 2306, Nashville, TN 37232-3375; **Phone:** 615-936-1354; **Board Cert:** Neurology 1980; Vascular Neurology 2005; **Med School:** Harvard Med Sch 1972; **Resid:** Neurology, Mass Genl Hosp 1978; **Fellow:** Neurological Science, Natl Inst Hlth 1975; **Fac Appt:** Prof N, Vanderbilt Univ

Kurtzke, Robert N MD [N] - **Spec Exp:** Electromyography; Nerve/Muscle Disorders; **Hospital:** Inova Fairfax Hosp, Reston Hosp Ctr; **Address:** Neurology Ctr of Fairfax, 3020 Hamaker Ct, Ste 400, Fairfax, VA 22031-2220; **Phone:** 703-876-0800; **Board Cert:** Neurology 1990; Clinical Neurophysiology 2004; **Med School:** Georgetown Univ 1985; **Resid:** Neurology, Neurology Inst-Columbia Presby 1989; **Fellow:** Neurological Muscular Disease, Duke Univ Med Ctr 1990

Lavin, Patrick J MD [N] - **Spec Exp:** Neuro-Ophthalmology; Eye Movement Disorders; Headache; Neuro-Otology; **Hospital:** Vanderbilt Univ Med Ctr; **Address:** Vanderbilt Dept Neurology, 1161 21st Ave S, A-0118 MCN, Nashville, TN 37232-2551; **Phone:** 615-936-0060; **Board Cert:** Neurology 1985; **Med School:** Ireland 1970; **Resid:** Internal Medicine, St Vincent Hosp Elm Pk 1973; Internal Medicine, Genl Hosp-Royal Infirm 1976; **Fellow:** Neurology, Case Western Reserve Univ 1981; Neurological Ophthalmology, Case Western Reserve Univ 1983; **Fac Appt:** Prof N, Vanderbilt Univ

Morgenlander, Joel Charles MD [N] - **Spec Exp:** Nerve/Muscle Disorders; **Hospital:** Duke Univ Med Ctr; **Address:** Duke Univ Med Ctr, Box 3394, Durham, NC 27710; **Phone:** 919-684-6887; **Board Cert:** Neurology 1992; **Med School:** Univ Pittsburgh 1986; **Resid:** Neurology, Duke Univ Med Ctr 1990; **Fellow:** Neurological Muscular Disease, Duke Univ Med Ctr 1991; **Fac Appt:** Assoc Prof N, Duke Univ

Nabors III, Louis Burt MD [N] - **Spec Exp:** Neuro-Oncology; Brain Tumors; **Hospital:** Univ of Ala Hosp at Birmingham; **Address:** UAB, FOT 1020, 510 20th St S, Birmingham, AL 35294-0001; **Phone:** 205-934-1432; **Board Cert:** Neurology 1999; **Med School:** Univ Tenn Coll Med, Memphis 1991; **Resid:** Neurology, Univ Alabama; **Fellow:** Neuro-Oncology, Univ Alabama; **Fac Appt:** Assoc Prof N, Univ Ala

Newman, Nancy Jean MD [N] - **Spec Exp:** Neuro-Ophthalmology; **Hospital:** Emory Univ Hosp; **Address:** Emory Eye Center, 1365B Clifton Rd NE, Ste 3500, Atlanta, GA 30322; **Phone:** 404-778-5360; **Board Cert:** Neurology 1989; **Med School:** Harvard Med Sch 1984; **Resid:** Neurology, Mass Genl Hosp 1988; **Fellow:** Neurological Ophthalmology, Mass EE Infirmary 1989; **Fac Appt:** Prof N, Emory Univ

Nolan, Bruce A MD [N] - **Spec Exp:** Sleep Disorders/Apnea; **Hospital:** Jackson Meml Hosp; **Address:** Univ Miami, Dept Neurology, U Health Sleep Program, 1501 NW 9th Ave, Miami, FL 33136; **Phone:** 305-243-5195; **Board Cert:** Neurology 1974; **Med School:** Wayne State Univ 1966; **Resid:** Neurology, Univ Miami Med Ctr 1970; **Fac Appt:** Assoc Prof N, Univ Miami Sch Med

Oh, Shin Joong MD [N] - **Spec Exp:** Neuromuscular Disorders; Electromyography; **Hospital:** Univ of Ala Hosp at Birmingham; **Address:** Dept of Neurology, 1530 3rd Ave S SC Bldg - rm 200, Birmingham, AL 35294; **Phone:** 205-934-2121; **Board Cert:** Neurology 1973; Clinical Neurophysiology 2001; **Med School:** Korea 1960; **Resid:** Internal Medicine, Seoul National Univ Hosp 1964; Neurology, Georgetown Univ Hosp 1967; **Fellow:** NeuroEpidemiology, Univ Minnesota Hosps 1968; **Fac Appt:** Prof N, Univ Ala

Patchell, Roy MD [N] - **Spec Exp:** Neuro-Oncology; Brain Tumors; Spinal Tumors; **Hospital:** Univ of Kentucky Chandler Hosp; **Address:** Univ Kentucky Neurosurgery, Chandler Med Ctr, 800 Rose St, MS 105, Lexington, KY 40536; **Phone:** 859-257-1532; **Board Cert:** Neurology 1984; **Med School:** Univ KY Coll Med 1979; **Resid:** Neurology, Johns Hopkins Hosp 1983; **Fellow:** Neuro-Oncology, Meml Sloan-Kettering Canc Ctr 1985; **Fac Appt:** Prof N, Univ KY Coll Med

Rothrock, John F MD [N] - **Spec Exp:** Headache; Stroke; **Hospital:** Univ of Ala Hosp at Birmingham; **Address:** UAB, Dept Neurology, 1720 7th Ave S, SC350, Birmingham, AL 35249; **Phone:** 205-801-8986; **Board Cert:** Neurology 1984; **Med School:** Univ VA Sch Med 1977; **Resid:** Neurology, Univ Ariz Med Ctr 1981; **Fac Appt:** Prof N, Univ S Ala Coll Med

Sacco, Ralph L MD [N] - **Spec Exp:** Stroke; Stroke Prevention; **Hospital:** Univ of Miami Hosp & Clins/Sylvester Comp Canc Ctr; **Address:** Univ of Miami, Chairman of Neurology, 1120 NW 14th St Fl 13 - Ste 52, Miami, FL 33136; **Phone:** 305-243-7519; **Board Cert:** Neurology 1989; **Med School:** Boston Univ 1983; **Resid:** Neurology, Columbia-Presby Med Ctr 1987; **Fellow:** Cerebrovascular Disease, Columbia-Presby Med Ctr 1989; **Fac Appt:** Prof N, Univ Miami Sch Med

Sadowsky, Carl H MD [N] - **Spec Exp:** Memory Disorders; Alzheimer's Disease; Dementia; **Hospital:** Good Sam Med Ctr - W Palm Beach, Columbia Hosp - W Palm Beach; **Address:** 4631 N Congress Ave, Ste 200, West Palm Beach, FL 33407-2234; **Phone:** 561-845-0500 x129; **Board Cert:** Neurology 1977; **Med School:** Cornell Univ 1971; **Resid:** Internal Medicine, Dartmouth-Hitchcock Med Ctr 1973; Neurology, Dartmouth-Hitchcock Med Ctr 1976; **Fac Appt:** Assoc Clin Prof N, Nova SE Univ, Coll Osteo Med

Schatz, Norman J MD [N] - **Spec Exp:** Neuro-Ophthalmology; Multiple Sclerosis & Visual Loss; Vision-Unexplained Loss; **Hospital:** Mount Sinai Med Ctr - Miami, Cleveland Clin - Weston; **Address:** 4701 N Meridian Ave, Adams Bldg - Ste 500A, Miami Beach, FL 33140; **Phone:** 305-532-2885; **Board Cert:** Neurology 1969; **Med School:** Hahnemann Univ 1961; **Resid:** Neurology, Jefferson Hosp 1965; **Fellow:** Neurological Ophthalmology, Bascom Palmer Eye Inst 1966; **Fac Appt:** Clin Prof N, Univ Pennsylvania

Schiff, David MD [N] - **Spec Exp:** Brain Tumors; Spinal Cord Tumors; Neurological Complications of Cancer; Neuro-Oncology; **Hospital:** Univ Virginia Med Ctr; **Address:** Univ VA, Div of Neuro-Oncology, PO Box 800432, Charlottesville, VA 22908; **Phone:** 434-982-4415; **Board Cert:** Neurology 1994; **Med School:** Harvard Med Sch 1988; **Resid:** Neurology, Harvard Longwood 1992; **Fellow:** Neuro-Oncology, Meml Sloan Kettering Cancer Ctr 1993; Mayo Clinic 1994; **Fac Appt:** Assoc Prof NS, Univ VA Sch Med

Schold Jr, S Clifford MD [N] - **Spec Exp:** Brain Tumors; Neuro-Oncology; **Hospital:** H Lee Moffitt Cancer Ctr & Research Inst; **Address:** H Lee Moffitt Cancer Ctr, 12902 Magnolia Dr, MCC VP Admin, Tampa, FL 33612; **Phone:** 813-745-7426; **Board Cert:** Neurology 1980; **Med School:** Univ Ariz Coll Med 1973; **Resid:** Neurology, Colorado Med Ctr 1977; **Fellow:** Neuro-Oncology, Sloan-Kettering Cancer Ctr 1978; **Fac Appt:** Prof N, Univ S Fla Coll Med

Sethi, Kapil D MD [N] - **Spec Exp:** Parkinson's Disease; Restless Legs Syndrome; Movement Disorders; Botox Therapy; **Hospital:** Med Coll of GA Hosp and Clin; **Address:** Med College Georgia, Dept Neurology, 1429 Harper St, Augusta, GA 30912-0004; **Phone:** 706-721-2798; **Board Cert:** Neurology 1987; **Med School:** India 1976; **Resid:** Neurology, Pgimer 1981; Neurology, Med Coll Georgia 1985; **Fac Appt:** Prof N, Med Coll GA

Neurology

Singer, Carlos MD [N] - **Spec Exp:** Parkinson's Disease; Movement Disorders; Botox Therapy; **Hospital:** Jackson Meml Hosp; **Address:** Univ Miami Dept Neurology, 1501 NW 9th Ave, Miami, FL 33136; **Phone:** 305-243-3876; **Board Cert:** Neurology 1981; Internal Medicine 1976; **Med School:** Venezuela 1972; **Resid:** Internal Medicine, Montefiore Hosp 1976; Neurology, Albert Einstein Affil Hosp 1979; **Fellow:** Electromyography, Jackson Meml Hosp 1981; Movement Disorders, Univ Miami 1989; **Fac Appt:** Prof N, Univ Miami Sch Med

Valenstein, Edward MD [N] - **Spec Exp:** Neuromuscular Disorders; Multiple Sclerosis; Amyotrophic Lateral Sclerosis (ALS); **Hospital:** Shands at Univ of FL; **Address:** 100 S Newell Drive, Box 100263, Gainesville, FL 32610; **Phone:** 352-265-8408; **Board Cert:** Neurology 1976; Clinical Neurophysiology 2006; **Med School:** Albert Einstein Coll Med 1967; **Resid:** Neurology, Boston City Hosp 1971; **Fac Appt:** Prof N, Univ Fla Coll Med

Watts, Ray L MD [N] - **Spec Exp:** Parkinson's Disease; Movement Disorders; **Hospital:** Univ of Ala Hosp at Birmingham; **Address:** Kirkland Clinic, 2000 6th Ave S Fl 5, Birmingham, AL 35233; **Phone:** 205-934-0683; **Board Cert:** Neurology 1985; **Med School:** Washington Univ, St Louis 1980; **Resid:** Neurology, Mass Genl Hosp 1984; **Fellow:** Electromyography, Mass Genl Hosp 1983; **Fac Appt:** Prof N, Univ Ala

Wooten Jr, George F MD [N] - **Spec Exp:** Movement Disorders; Parkinson's Disease; Tremor & Dystonia; **Hospital:** Univ Virginia Med Ctr; **Address:** Univ VA Hlth Sys, Dept Neuro-McKim Hall, PO Box 800394, Charlottesville, VA 22908; **Phone:** 434-924-8369; **Board Cert:** Neurology 1977; **Med School:** Cornell Univ-Weill Med Coll 1970; **Resid:** Neurology, New York Hosp-Cornell 1977; **Fellow:** Pharmacology, Natl Inst Hlth-NIMH 1974; **Fac Appt:** Prof N, Univ VA Sch Med

Midwest

Adams Jr, Harold P MD [N] - **Spec Exp:** Stroke; Cerebrovascular Disease; **Hospital:** Univ Iowa Hosp & Clinics; **Address:** Univ Iowa Hosp, Dept Neurology, 200 Hawkins Drive, rm 2148-RCP, Iowa City, IA 52242; **Phone:** 319-356-4110; **Board Cert:** Neurology 2004; Vascular & Interventional Radiology 2005; **Med School:** Northwestern Univ 1970; **Resid:** Neurology, Univ Iowa Hosp 1974; **Fac Appt:** Prof N, Univ Iowa Coll Med

Ahlskog, J Eric MD/PhD [N] - **Spec Exp:** Parkinson's Disease; Movement Disorders; **Hospital:** Mayo Med Ctr & Clin - Rochester, St Mary's Hosp - Rochester; **Address:** Mayo Clinic, Dept Neurology, 200 First St SW, Rochester, MN 55905; **Phone:** 507-538-1038; **Board Cert:** Neurology 1984; **Med School:** Dartmouth Med Sch 1976; **Resid:** Internal Medicine, Univ Chicago Hosps Clins 1978; Neurology, Mayo Grad Sch Med 1981; **Fac Appt:** Prof N, Mayo Med Sch

Alberts, Mark J MD [N] - **Spec Exp:** Stroke/Cerebrovascular Disease; **Hospital:** Northwestern Meml Hosp; **Address:** 675 N St Clair, Galter Bldg Fl 20 - Ste 100, Chicago, IL 60611; **Phone:** 312-695-7950; **Board Cert:** Neurology 1987; **Med School:** Tufts Univ 1982; **Resid:** Neurology, Duke Univ Med Ctr 1986; **Fellow:** Cerebrovascular Disease, Duke Univ Med Ctr 1987; **Fac Appt:** Prof N, Northwestern Univ

Arnason, Barry G W MD [N] - **Spec Exp:** Multiple Sclerosis; Guillain-Barre Syndrome; Myasthenia Gravis; **Hospital:** Univ of Chicago Hosps; **Address:** 5841 S Maryland Ave, MC 2030, Chicago, IL 60637; **Phone:** 773-702-6222; **Board Cert:** Neurology 1971; **Med School:** Univ Manitoba 1957; **Resid:** Neurology, Mass Genl Hosp 1959; Neurology, Mass Genl Hosp 1962; **Fac Appt:** Prof N, Univ Chicago-Pritzker Sch Med

Barger, Geoffrey R MD [N] - **Spec Exp:** Neuro-Oncology; Brain Tumors; **Hospital:** Harper Univ Hosp; **Address:** Wayne State Univ Hlth Ctr, 4201 St Antoine, Ste 8D-UHC, Detroit, MI 48201; **Phone:** 313-745-4275; **Board Cert:** Neurology 1981; **Med School:** Jefferson Med Coll 1975; **Resid:** Neurology, Penn Hosp 1979; **Fellow:** Neuro-Oncology, Moffitt Hosp & Brain Tumor Ctr/UCSF 1982; **Fac Appt:** Assoc Prof N, Wayne State Univ

Broderick, Joseph P MD [N] - **Spec Exp:** Stroke; **Hospital:** Univ Hosp - Cincinnati; **Address:** Univ Cincinnati, Dept Neurology, 222 Piedmont Ave, Ste 3200, Cincinnati, OH 45267-0525; **Phone:** 513-475-8730; **Board Cert:** Neurotology 1988; Vascular Neurology 2005; **Med School:** Univ Cincinnati 1982; **Resid:** Neurology, Mayo Clinic 1986; **Fac Appt:** Clin Prof N, Univ Cincinnati

Brown, Robert D MD [N] - **Spec Exp:** Stroke; **Hospital:** Mayo Med Ctr & Clin - Rochester; **Address:** Mayo Clinic, Dept Neurology, 200 First St SW, Rochester, MN 55905; **Phone:** 507-266-4143; **Board Cert:** Neurology 1994; **Med School:** Mayo Med Sch 1989; **Resid:** Neurology, Mayo Clinic 1994; **Fellow:** Mayo Clinic 1995; **Fac Appt:** Prof N, Mayo Med Sch

Burke, Allan M MD [N] - **Spec Exp:** Cerebrovascular Disease; Neurologic Imaging; **Hospital:** Northwestern Meml Hosp; **Address:** 233 E Eerie St, Ste 500, Chicago, IL 60611-2912; **Phone:** 312-944-0063; **Board Cert:** Neurology 1982; Neuroimaging 2002; **Med School:** Columbia P&S 1976; **Resid:** Internal Medicine, NY Hosp 1978; Neurology, Columbia-Presby Med Ctr 1981; **Fellow:** Cerebrovascular Disease, Hosp Univ Penn 1983; **Fac Appt:** Assoc Clin Prof N, Northwestern Univ

Cascino, Terrence L MD [N] - **Spec Exp:** Neuro-Oncology; **Hospital:** Mayo Med Ctr & Clin - Rochester; **Address:** Mayo Clinic, Dept Neurology, 200 1st St SW, Rochester, MN 55905-0001; **Phone:** 507-284-2576; **Board Cert:** Neurology 1984; **Med School:** Loyola Univ-Stritch Sch Med 1972; **Resid:** Neurology, Mayo Clinic 1980; **Fellow:** Neuro-Oncology, Meml Sloan Kettering Cancer Ctr; **Fac Appt:** Assoc Prof N, Mayo Med Sch

Cohen, Jeffrey Alan MD [N] - **Spec Exp:** Multiple Sclerosis; Neuro-Immunology; **Hospital:** Cleveland Clin Fdn (page 56); **Address:** Cleveland Clin - Mellen Ctr, 9500 Euclid Ave, Desk U10, Cleveland, OH 44195; **Phone:** 216-445-8110; **Board Cert:** Neurology 1985; **Med School:** Univ Chicago-Pritzker Sch Med 1980; **Resid:** Neurology, Hosp Univ Penn 1984; **Fellow:** Neurological Immunology, Hosp Univ Penn 1987

Cutrer, F Michael MD [N] - **Spec Exp:** Headache; Pain-Facial; Migraine; **Hospital:** Mayo Med Ctr & Clin - Rochester, Rochester Methodist Hosp; **Address:** Mayo Clinic, Dept Neurology, 200 First St NW, Rochester, MN 55905-0001; **Phone:** 507-284-4409; **Board Cert:** Neurology 1993; **Med School:** Univ Miss 1988; **Resid:** Neurology, UCLA Med Ctr 1992; **Fellow:** Neurology, Mass Genl Hosp-Harvard 1994; **Fac Appt:** Asst Prof N, Mayo Med Sch

Elias, Stanton B MD [N] - **Spec Exp:** Multiple Sclerosis; Myasthenia Gravis; **Hospital:** Henry Ford Hosp; **Address:** Henry Ford Hosp, Dept Neurology, 2799 W Grand Blvd, Fl K-11, Detroit, MI 48202-2689; **Phone:** 313-916-7207; **Board Cert:** Neurology 1979; **Med School:** Univ Pittsburgh 1972; **Resid:** Neurology, Duke Univ Med Ctr 1976; **Fellow:** Neurology, Duke Univ Med Ctr 1977

Farlow, Martin MD [N] - **Spec Exp:** Alzheimer's Disease; Neurodegenerative Disorders; Multiple Sclerosis; **Hospital:** Indiana Univ Hosp, Wishard Hlth Srvs; **Address:** Indiana Univ Sch Med, Dept Neurology, 541 Clinical Drive, rm 291, Indianapolis, IN 46202; **Phone:** 317-274-2291; **Board Cert:** Neurology 1988; **Med School:** Indiana Univ 1979; **Resid:** Neurology, Indiana Univ Hosp 1983; **Fac Appt:** Prof N, Indiana Univ

Neurology

Feldman, Eva L MD/PhD [N] - **Spec Exp:** Neuromuscular Disorders; Amyotrophic Lateral Sclerosis (ALS); Peripheral Neuropathy; **Hospital:** Univ Michigan Hlth Sys; **Address:** Univ Mich, Dept Neurology, 1500 E Med Ctr Drive, SPC 5322, rm 1324 Taubman, Ann Arbor, MI 48109-0322; **Phone:** 734-936-9020; **Board Cert:** Neurology 1988; **Med School:** Univ Mich Med Sch 1983; **Resid:** Neurology, Johns Hopkins Hosp 1987; **Fellow:** Neuromuscular Medicine, Univ Mich Hosps 1988; **Fac Appt:** Prof N, Univ Mich Med Sch

Furlan, Anthony J MD [N] - **Spec Exp:** Stroke; Thrombolytic Therapy; **Hospital:** Univ Hosps Case Med Ctr; **Address:** Dept Neurology, 11100 Euclid Ave, Fl 5, Hanna House, Cleveland, OH 44106; **Phone:** 216-844-3192; **Board Cert:** Neurology 1979; Vascular Neurology 2005; **Med School:** Loyola Univ-Stritch Sch Med 1973; **Resid:** Neurology, Cleveland Clinic 1977; **Fellow:** Cerebrovascular Disease, Mayo Clinic 1978; **Fac Appt:** Assoc Prof N, Ohio State Univ

Gilman, Sid MD [N] - **Spec Exp:** Parkinson's Disease/Movement Disorders; Alzheimer's Disease; Multiple Sclerosis; Epilepsy; **Hospital:** Univ Michigan Hlth Sys; **Address:** Univ Mich, Dept Neurology, 300 N Ingalls 3D15, Ann Arbor, MI 48109-0489; **Phone:** 734-936-1808; **Board Cert:** Neurology 1966; **Med School:** UCLA 1957; **Resid:** Neurology, Boston City Hosp-Harvard 1963; **Fellow:** Neurological Physiology, Boston City Hosp-Harvard 1965; **Fac Appt:** Prof N, Univ Mich Med Sch

Goetz, Christopher G MD [N] - **Spec Exp:** Movement Disorders; Parkinson's Disease; Dyskinesias; **Hospital:** Rush Univ Med Ctr; **Address:** 1725 W Harrison St, Ste 755, Chicago, IL 60612-3835; **Phone:** 312-563-2030; **Board Cert:** Neurology 1982; **Med School:** Rush Med Coll 1975; **Resid:** Neurology, Rush-Presby-St Luke's Med Ctr 1976; Neurology, Michael Reese Med Ctr 1977; **Fellow:** Neurology, Rush-Presby-St Luke's Med Ctr 1979; **Fac Appt:** Prof N, Rush Med Coll

Greenberg, Harry S MD [N] - **Spec Exp:** Neuro-Oncology; Brain Tumors; **Hospital:** Univ Michigan Hlth Sys, Vail Valley Med Ctr; **Address:** Taubman Ctr 1914, 1500 E Med Ctr Dr, Ann Arbor, MI 48109-5316; **Phone:** 734-936-9055; **Board Cert:** Neurology 1980; **Med School:** SUNY Upstate Med Univ 1973; **Resid:** Neurology, Stanford Univ Hosp 1977; **Fellow:** Neuro-Oncology, Sloan Kettering Cancer Ctr 1979; **Fac Appt:** Prof N, Univ Mich Med Sch

Hain, Timothy C MD [N] - **Spec Exp:** Neuro-Otology; Balance Disorders; Motion Sickness; **Hospital:** Northwestern Meml Hosp; **Address:** 645 N Michigan Ave, Ste 410, Chicago, IL 60611; **Phone:** 312-274-0197; **Board Cert:** Neurology 1983; **Med School:** Univ IL Coll Med 1978; **Resid:** Neurology, Univ IL 1982; **Fellow:** Neurology, Johns Hopkins Hosp 1984; Psychiatry, Johns Hopkins Hosp 1984; **Fac Appt:** Prof N, Northwestern Univ

Hecox, Kurt E MD [N] - **Spec Exp:** Pediatric Neurology; Epilepsy/Seizure Disorders; Hearing Loss; **Hospital:** Chldns Hosp - Wisconsin; **Address:** Med College Wisconsin, Dept of Neurology, 9000 W Wisconsin Ave, MS CCC540, PO Box 1997, Milwaukee, WI 53226; **Phone:** 414-266-3464; **Board Cert:** Clinical Neurophysiology 1977; **Med School:** UCSD 1971; **Resid:** Neurology, Univ Texas Southwestern Med Ctr 1975; **Fellow:** Pediatric Neurology, Children's Med Ctr/Parkland Hosp 1978; **Fac Appt:** Prof N, Med Coll Wisc

Josephson, David A MD [N] - **Spec Exp:** Electromyography; Epilepsy; Stroke; **Hospital:** St Vincent Hosp & Hlth Svcs - Indianapolis, Comm Hosp N - Indianapolis; **Address:** 8402 Harcourt Rd, Ste 615, Indianapolis, IN 46260; **Phone:** 317-355-1555; **Board Cert:** Neurology 1976; **Med School:** Indiana Univ 1971; **Resid:** Neurology, Univ Mich Med Ctr 1973; Neurology, Indiana Univ Med Ctr 1975; **Fac Appt:** Assoc Clin Prof N, Indiana Univ

Kincaid, John C MD [N] - **Spec Exp:** Neuromuscular Disorders; Electromyography; Pain-Facial; **Hospital:** Indiana Univ Hosp; **Address:** Indiana Univ Hosp, 550 N University Blvd, Ste 1711, Indianapolis, IN 46202; **Phone:** 317-274-0311; **Board Cert:** Neurology 1982; Clinical Neurophysiology 1997; **Med School:** Indiana Univ 1975; **Resid:** Neurology, Indiana Univ 1979; **Fellow:** Electromyography, Mayo Clinic 1980; **Fac Appt:** Prof N, Indiana Univ

Lisak, Robert P MD [N] - **Spec Exp:** Multiple Sclerosis; Myasthenia Gravis; Vasculitis; **Hospital:** Harper Univ Hosp, Detroit Receiving Hospital; **Address:** Wayne State Univ Sch Med, 4201 St Antoine, Hlth Ctr 8D, Detroit, MI 48201; **Phone:** 313-745-4240; **Board Cert:** Neurology 1975; **Med School:** Columbia P&S 1965; **Resid:** Internal Medicine, Bronx Municipal Hosp-Einstein 1969; Neurology, Hosp Univ Penn 1972; **Fac Appt:** Prof N, Wayne State Univ

Logan, William R MD [N] - **Hospital:** St John's Mercy Med Ctr - St Louis; **Address:** St Johns Mercy Med Ctr, Tower B, 621 New Ballas Rd, Ste 5003, St Louis, MO 63141; **Phone:** 314-251-5910; **Board Cert:** Internal Medicine 1981; Neurology 1986; **Med School:** Univ Okla Coll Med 1978; **Resid:** Internal Medicine, Univ MO Hosps 1982; Neurology, Unix Texas Hlth Sci Ctr 1984

Luders, Hans MD/PhD [N] - **Spec Exp:** Epilepsy; **Hospital:** Univ Hosps Case Med Ctr; **Address:** University Hosps-Case Med Ctr, 11100 Euclid Ave, Dept Neurology, Lakeside Bldg - Ste 3200, Cleveland, OH 44195-0001; **Phone:** 216-844-3650; **Board Cert:** Neurology 1985; **Med School:** Chile 1965; **Resid:** Neurology, Neur Inst-Kyushu Univ 1971; **Fellow:** Neurological Physiology, Mayo Grad Sch Med 1975; **Fac Appt:** Prof N, Ohio State Univ

Mahowald, Mark W MD [N] - **Spec Exp:** Sleep Disorders/Apnea; **Hospital:** Hennepin Cnty Med Ctr; **Address:** Minn Regional Sleep Disorders Ctr, 701 Park Ave S, Minneapolis, MN 55415; **Phone:** 612-873-6201; **Board Cert:** Neurology 1976; **Med School:** Univ Minn 1968; **Resid:** Neurology, Fairview Univ Med Ctr 1974; **Fac Appt:** Prof N, Univ Minn

Mesulam, Marel MD [N] - **Spec Exp:** Alzheimer's Disease; Tourette's Syndrome; Dementia; **Hospital:** Northwestern Meml Hosp; **Address:** 320 E Superior St, Chicago, IL 60611; **Phone:** 312-908-9339; **Board Cert:** Neurology 1977; **Med School:** Harvard Med Sch 1972; **Resid:** Neurology, Boston City Hosp 1976; **Fac Appt:** Prof N, Northwestern Univ

Mikkelsen, Tommy MD [N] - **Spec Exp:** Brain Tumors; Gliomas; **Hospital:** Henry Ford Hosp, William Beaumont Hosp; **Address:** Henry Ford Hospital, ER 3096, 2799 W Grand Blvd, Detroit, MI 48202; **Phone:** 313-916-8641; **Board Cert:** Neurology 1998; **Med School:** Univ Calgary 1983; **Resid:** Internal Medicine, Calgary General Hosp 1985; Neurology, Montreal Neurological Inst 1988; **Fellow:** Neuro-Oncology, Royal Victoria Hosp 1990; Neuro-Oncology, Ludwig Inst for Cancer Rsch 1992; **Fac Appt:** Assoc Prof N, Case West Res Univ

Montgomery Jr, Erwin B MD [N] - **Spec Exp:** Parkinson's Disease; **Hospital:** Univ WI Hosp & Clins; **Address:** 600 Highland Ave, MS 2425, Madison, WI 53792; **Phone:** 608-263-5442; **Board Cert:** Neurology 1982; **Med School:** SUNY Buffalo 1976; **Resid:** Neurology, Wahington Univ Med Ctr 1980; **Fellow:** Neurological Physiology, Washington Univ Med Ctr 1981; **Fac Appt:** Prof N, Univ Wisc

Morris, John MD [N] - **Spec Exp:** Alzheimer's Disease; **Hospital:** Barnes-Jewish Hosp; **Address:** Memory Diagnostic Ctr, 4488 Forest Park, Ste 160, St Louis, MO 63108-2215; **Phone:** 314-286-1967; **Board Cert:** Internal Medicine 1979; Neurology 1985; **Med School:** Univ Rochester 1974; **Resid:** Internal Medicine, Akron Genl Med Ctr 1979; Neurology, Cleveland Metro Genl Hosp 1982; **Fellow:** Neuropharmacology, Washington Univ 1985; **Fac Appt:** Prof N, Washington Univ, St Louis

Neurology

Newton, Herbert B MD [N] - **Spec Exp:** Neuro-Oncology; Brain & Spinal Tumors; **Hospital:** Ohio St Univ Med Ctr, Arthur G James Cancer Hosp & Research Inst; **Address:** 465 Means Hall, 1654 Upham Dr Fl 4, Columbus, OH 43210; **Phone:** 614-293-8930; **Board Cert:** Neurology 1989; **Med School:** SUNY Buffalo 1984; **Resid:** Neurology, Univ Michigan Med Ctr 1988; **Fellow:** Neuro-Oncology, Meml Sloan-Kettering Cancer Ctr 1990; **Fac Appt:** Prof N, Ohio State Univ

Pascuzzi, Robert M MD [N] - **Spec Exp:** Neuromuscular Disorders; Amyotrophic Lateral Sclerosis (ALS); Myasthenia Gravis; **Hospital:** Indiana Univ Hosp, Wishard Hlth Srvs; **Address:** Clarian Hlth-Indiana Univ Sch Med, 545 Barnhill Drive, EH 125, Indianapolis, IN 46202; **Phone:** 317-274-4455; **Board Cert:** Neurology 2004; **Med School:** Indiana Univ 1979; **Resid:** Neurology, Univ Va Med Ctr 1983; **Fellow:** Neuromuscular Medicine, Univ Va Med Ctr 1985; **Fac Appt:** Prof N, Indiana Univ

Perlmutter, Joel S MD [N] - **Spec Exp:** Parkinson's Disease; Movement Disorders; Huntington's Disease; **Hospital:** Barnes-Jewish Hosp; **Address:** Wash Univ Sch Med, Dept Neurology, 660 S Euclid Ave, Box 8111, St Louis, MO 63110; **Phone:** 314-362-6908; **Board Cert:** Neurology 1985; **Med School:** Univ MO-Columbia Sch Med 1979; **Resid:** Neurology, Barnes Hosp-Wash Univ 1983; **Fellow:** Movement Disorders, Barnes Hosp-Wash Univ 1984; **Fac Appt:** Prof N, Washington Univ, St Louis

Pestronk, Alan MD [N] - **Spec Exp:** Neuromuscular Disorders; Peripheral Neuropathy; **Hospital:** Barnes-Jewish Hosp; **Address:** Washington Univ Sch Med, Dept Neurology, 660 S Euclid Ave, Box 8111, St Louis, MO 63110; **Phone:** 314-362-6981; **Board Cert:** Neurology 1978; **Med School:** Johns Hopkins Univ 1970; **Resid:** Neurology, Johns Hopkins Hosp 1974; **Fellow:** Neuromuscular Medicine, Johns Hopkins Hosp 1977; **Fac Appt:** Prof NPath, Washington Univ, St Louis

Petersen, Ronald C MD/PhD [N] - **Spec Exp:** Alzheimer's Disease; **Hospital:** Mayo Med Ctr & Clin - Rochester; **Address:** Mayo Clinic, Dept Neurology, 200 1st St SW, Rochester, MN 55905; **Phone:** 507-538-1038; **Board Cert:** Neurology 1986; **Med School:** Mayo Med Sch 1980; **Resid:** Neurology, Mayo Clinic 1984; **Fellow:** Behavioral Neurology, Beth Israel Med Ctr 1986; **Fac Appt:** Prof N, Mayo Med Sch

Reder, Anthony T MD [N] - **Spec Exp:** Multiple Sclerosis; Tetanus; Myasthenia Gravis; Reflex Sympathetic Dystrophy (RSD); **Hospital:** Univ of Chicago Hosps; **Address:** Ctr Advanced Medicine, 5758 S Maryland Ave, rm 4D, Chicago, IL 60637-1426; **Phone:** 773-702-6222; **Board Cert:** Neurology 1984; **Med School:** Univ Mich Med Sch 1978; **Resid:** Neurology, Univ Minn Hosps 1982; **Fellow:** Neurological Immunology, Univ Chicago 1984; **Fac Appt:** Assoc Prof N, Univ Chicago-Pritzker Sch Med

Reed, Robert L MD [N] - **Spec Exp:** Multiple Sclerosis; Stroke; **Hospital:** Good Samaritan Hosp - Cincinnati; **Address:** 111 Wellington Pl, Cincinnati, OH 45219; **Phone:** 513-241-2370; **Board Cert:** Neurology 1975; **Med School:** Univ Cincinnati 1966; **Resid:** Internal Medicine, Mayo Grad Sch Med 1970; Neurology, Mayo Grad Sch Med 1973

Rogers, Lisa R DO [N] - **Spec Exp:** Neuro-Oncology; Brain Tumors; Brain Radiation Toxicity; **Hospital:** Univ Michigan Hlth Sys; **Address:** Univ Michigan, Dept Neurology, 1914 Taubman Center, Ann Arbor, MI 48109-5316; **Phone:** 734-615-2994; **Board Cert:** Neurology 1982; **Med School:** Kirksville Coll Osteo Med 1976; **Resid:** Neurology, Cleveland Clinic Fdn 1980; **Fellow:** Neuro-Oncology, Meml-Sloan Kettering Cancer Ctr 1982; **Fac Appt:** Prof N, Univ Mich Med Sch

Roos, Karen MD [N] - **Spec Exp:** Infections-Neurologic; Encephalitis; **Hospital:** Indiana Univ Hosp, Wishard Hlth Srvs; **Address:** Indiana Univ Med Ctr, 550 N University Blvd, rm 1711, Indianapolis, IN 46202-5149; **Phone:** 317-278-6785; **Board Cert:** Neurology 1986; **Med School:** Hahnemann Univ 1981; **Resid:** Neurology, Univ Virginia Med Ctr 1985; **Fac Appt:** Prof N, Indiana Univ

Roos, Raymond MD [N] - **Spec Exp:** Amyotrophic Lateral Sclerosis (ALS); Multiple Sclerosis; Neuromuscular Disorders; **Hospital:** Univ of Chicago Hosps; **Address:** Univ Chicago, Dept Neurology, 5841 S Maryland Ave, MC-2030, Chicago, IL 60637; **Phone:** 773-702-5659; **Board Cert:** Neurology 1976; **Med School:** SUNY Downstate 1968; **Resid:** Neurology, Johns Hopkins Hosp 1974; **Fellow:** Neurology, Natl Inst Neur Dis & Stroke 1971; Neurological Viral Immunology, Johns Hopkins Hosp 1976; **Fac Appt:** Prof N, Univ Chicago-Pritzker Sch Med

Rubin, Susan M MD [N] - **Spec Exp:** Multiple Sclerosis in Women; Epilepsy in Pregnancy; Headache in Women; Migraine in Women; **Hospital:** Glenbrook Hosp, Evanston Hosp; **Address:** Glenbrook Hosp, Dept Neurology, 2100 Pfingsten Rd, Glenview, IL 60026; **Phone:** 847-657-5875; **Board Cert:** Neurology 2006; **Med School:** Univ IL Coll Med 1988; **Resid:** Neurology, Northwestern Meml Hosp 1993; **Fellow:** Neurology, Northwestern Meml Hosp 1994

Ruff, Robert L MD/PhD [N] - **Spec Exp:** Spinal Cord Injury; Neuro-Rehabilitation; Muscle Disorders; **Hospital:** VA Med Ctr - Cleveland; **Address:** Department of Neurology, 10701 East Blvd, Cleveland, OH 44106; **Phone:** 216-791-3800; **Board Cert:** Neurology 1982; Spinal Cord Injury Medicine 2002; **Med School:** Univ Wash 1976; **Resid:** Neurology, NY-Cornell Hosp 1980; **Fac Appt:** Prof N, Case West Res Univ

Saper, Joel R MD [N] - **Spec Exp:** Headache; Pain-Chronic after Head Injury; **Hospital:** Chelsea Comm Hosp; **Address:** Michigan Head Pain & Neurological Inst, 3120 Professional Drive, Ann Arbor, MI 48104; **Phone:** 734-677-6000; **Board Cert:** Neurology 1975; Pain Medicine 1996; Headache Medicine 2006; **Med School:** Univ IL Coll Med 1969; **Resid:** Neurology, Univ Mich Med Ctr 1973; **Fac Appt:** Clin Prof N, Mich State Univ

Schapiro, Randall T MD [N] - **Spec Exp:** Multiple Sclerosis; **Hospital:** Univ Minn Med Ctr, Fairview - Univ Campus; **Address:** Schapiro Center for MS, 4225 Golden Valley Rd, Golden Valley, MN 55422; **Phone:** 763-302-4199; **Board Cert:** Neurology 1976; **Med School:** Univ Minn 1970; **Resid:** Internal Medicine, Wadsworth VA Hosp 1972; Neurology, Univ Minn 1975; **Fac Appt:** Clin Prof N, Univ Minn

Siddique, Teepu MD [N] - **Spec Exp:** Amyotrophic Lateral Sclerosis (ALS); Muscular Dystrophy; Neurogenetics; **Hospital:** Northwestern Meml Hosp; **Address:** Northwestern Univ-Feinberg, Dept Neuro, 303 E Chicago Ave, Tarry Bldg, rm 13-715, Chicago, IL 60611-5935; **Phone:** 312-695-5886; **Board Cert:** Neurology 1980; **Med School:** Pakistan 1973; **Resid:** Neurology, UMDNJ-RW Johnson Med Sch 1979; **Fellow:** Electromyography, Hosp Special Surg-Cornell 1980; Neurological Muscular Disease, Natl Inst Hlth 1981; **Fac Appt:** Prof N, Northwestern Univ

Swanson, Jerry W MD [N] - **Spec Exp:** Headache; Migraine; **Hospital:** Mayo Med Ctr & Clin - Rochester; **Address:** Mayo Clinic, Dept Neurology, 200 First St SW, Rochester, MN 55905-0001; **Phone:** 507-538-1036; **Board Cert:** Neurology 1984; Headache Medicine 2006; **Med School:** Northwestern Univ 1977; **Resid:** Neurology, Mayo Clinic 1982; **Fellow:** Electroencephalography, Mayo Clinic 1983; **Fac Appt:** Prof N, Mayo Med Sch

Taylor, Frederick R MD [N] - **Spec Exp:** Headache; Pain-Facial; **Hospital:** Methodist Hosp - Minnesota; **Address:** Park Nicollet Headache Clinic, 6490 Excelsior Blvd, Meadowbrook Bldg, Ste E-500, Minneapolis, MN 55426; **Phone:** 952-993-3432; **Board Cert:** Pediatrics 1982; Neurology 1985; Headache Medicine 2006; **Med School:** Univ New Mexico 1977; **Resid:** Pediatrics, Univ Wisc Hlth Sci Ctr 1980; Neurology, Univ Wisc Hlth Sci Ctr 1983; **Fellow:** Neurological Physiology, Univ Wisc Hlth Sci Ctr 1984; **Fac Appt:** Assoc Prof N, Univ Minn

Neurology

Vick, Nicholas A MD [N] - **Spec Exp:** Brain Tumors; Neuro-Oncology; **Hospital:** Evanston Hosp; **Address:** Evanston Hosp, Dept Neurology, 2650 Ridge Ave, Evanston, IL 60201; **Phone:** 847-570-2570; **Board Cert:** Neurology 1971; **Med School:** Univ Chicago-Pritzker Sch Med 1965; **Resid:** Neurology, Univ Chicago Hosps 1968; **Fellow:** Neurology, Natl Inst Hlth 1970; **Fac Appt:** Prof N, Northwestern Univ

Vitek, Jerrold Lee MD/PhD [N] - **Spec Exp:** Parkinson's Disease/Movement Disorders; Tremor & Dystonia; **Hospital:** Cleveland Clin Fdn (page 56); **Address:** 9500 Euclid Ave, MC NC30, Cleveland, OH 44195; **Phone:** 216-445-9897; **Board Cert:** Neurology 1992; **Med School:** Univ Minn 1984; **Resid:** Neurology, Johns Hopkins Hosp 1988; **Fac Appt:** Prof N, Cleveland Cl Coll Med/Case West Res

Windebank, Anthony J MD [N] - **Spec Exp:** Peripheral Neuropathy; Amyotrophic Lateral Sclerosis (ALS); Multiple Sclerosis; **Hospital:** Mayo Med Ctr & Clin - Rochester; **Address:** Mayo Clinic, Dept Neurology, 200 First St SW, Rochester, MN 55905; **Phone:** 507-284-2798; **Board Cert:** Neurology 1982; **Med School:** England 1974; **Resid:** Internal Medicine, Radcliffe Infirm 1977; Neurology, Mayo Clinic 1981; **Fellow:** Neurology, Mayo Clinic 1982; **Fac Appt:** Prof N, Mayo Med Sch

Wright, Robert B MD [N] - **Spec Exp:** Myasthenia Gravis; Migraine; **Hospital:** Rush Univ Med Ctr; **Address:** 1725 W Harrison St, Ste 1118, Chicago, IL 60612-3841; **Phone:** 312-942-5936; **Board Cert:** Neurology 1988; **Med School:** Univ IL Coll Med 1982; **Resid:** Neurology, Rush Presby-St Luke's Med Ctr 1986; **Fellow:** Neuromuscular Medicine, Rush Presby-St Luke's Med Ctr 1987; **Fac Appt:** Asst Prof N, Rush Med Coll

Great Plains and Mountains

Barohn, Richard J MD [N] - **Spec Exp:** Peripheral Neuropathy; Myasthenia Gravis; Amyotrophic Lateral Sclerosis (ALS); **Hospital:** Univ of Kansas Hosp; **Address:** Univ Kansas Medical Ctr, Dept Neurology, 3599 Rainbow Blvd, MS 2012, Kansas City, KS 66160; **Phone:** 913-588-6970; **Board Cert:** Neurology 1987; Clinical Neurophysiology 2004; **Med School:** Univ MO-Kansas City 1980; **Resid:** Neurology, Lackland AFB 1985

Bromberg, Mark B MD/PhD [N] - **Spec Exp:** Peripheral Neuropathy; Neuromuscular Disorders; **Hospital:** Univ Utah Hosps and Clins; **Address:** 175 N Medical Drive Fl 6th, Salt Lake City, UT 84132; **Phone:** 801-585-6837; **Board Cert:** Neurology 1988; Clinical Neurophysiology 2002; **Med School:** Univ Mich Med Sch 1982; **Resid:** Neurology, Univ Mich Med Ctr 1986; **Fellow:** Electromyography, Univ Mich Med Ctr 1987; **Fac Appt:** Prof N, Univ Utah

Cilo, Mark P MD [N] - **Spec Exp:** Brain Injury; Spinal Cord Injury; **Hospital:** Craig Hosp, Swedish Med Ctr - Englewood; **Address:** 3425 S Clarkson St, Englewood, CO 80113; **Phone:** 303-789-8220; **Board Cert:** Neurology 1979; Spinal Cord Injury Medicine 2003; **Med School:** Mount Sinai Sch Med 1972; **Resid:** Neurology, Mount Sinai Hosp 1976; **Fellow:** Spinal Cord & Brain Injury Rehab, Craig Hosp 1978; **Fac Appt:** Asst Clin Prof Med, Univ Colorado

Filley, Christopher M MD [N] - **Spec Exp:** Leukoencephalopathy; Alzheimer's Disease; Brain Injury-Traumatic; Multiple Sclerosis; **Hospital:** Univ Colorado Hosp, VA Med Ctr; **Address:** Univ CO, Neurology Dept, Behavioral Neurology Section, 12631 E 17th Ave, Ste B183, Aurora, CO 80045; **Phone:** 303-724-2187; **Board Cert:** Neurology 1984; **Med School:** Johns Hopkins Univ 1979; **Resid:** Neurology, Univ Colorado Hosp 1983; **Fellow:** Behavioral Neurology, Boston VA Hosp 1984; **Fac Appt:** Prof N, Univ Colorado

Kelly, James P MD [N] - **Spec Exp:** Brain Injury; Memory Disorders; Neurologic Rehabilitation; **Hospital:** Univ Colorado Hosp; **Address:** PO Box 6510, Campus Box F727, Aurora, CO 80045; **Phone:** 720-848-2086; **Board Cert:** Neurology 1991; **Med School:** Northwestern Univ 1983; **Resid:** Neurology, Univ Colorado Med Ctr 1988; **Fellow:** Behavioral Neurology, Univ Colorado Med Ctr 1989; **Fac Appt:** Prof N, Univ Colorado

Kelts, K Alan MD/PhD [N] - **Spec Exp:** Pediatric Neurology; Sleep Disorders/Apnea; Neuromuscular Disorders; **Hospital:** Rapid City Reg Hosp; **Address:** Black Hills Neurology, 2929 5th St, Ste 240, Rapid City, SD 57701; **Phone:** 605-341-3770; **Board Cert:** Pediatrics 1977; Child Neurology 1978; **Med School:** Univ Rochester 1971; **Resid:** Pediatrics, Chldns & Univ Hosps 1973; Child Neurology, Colorado Med Ctr 1976; **Fellow:** Neurological Muscular Disease, Muscular Dystrophy Assn 1975; **Fac Appt:** Clin Prof N, Univ SD Sch Med

Ringel, Steven MD [N] - **Spec Exp:** Neuromuscular Disorders; **Hospital:** Univ Colorado Hosp; **Address:** Neuromuscular Dept, 12631 E 17th Ave, Box B185, Denver, CO 80045; **Phone:** 303-714-2188; **Board Cert:** Neurology 1974; **Med School:** Univ Mich Med Sch 1968; **Resid:** Neurology, Rush-Presby-St Lukes Med Ctr 1972; **Fellow:** Neurology, Natl Inst Neuro Dis-NIH 1976; **Fac Appt:** Prof N, Univ Colorado

Southwest

Ahern, Geoffry L MD/PhD [N] - **Spec Exp:** Behavioral Neurology; Dementia; Alzheimer's Disease; **Hospital:** Univ Med Ctr - Tucson; **Address:** Univ Arizona, Dept Neurology, 1501 N Campbell Ave, Box 245094, Tucson, AZ 85724-5094; **Phone:** 520-694-8888; **Board Cert:** Neurology 1992; **Med School:** Yale Univ 1984; **Resid:** Neurology, Boston Univ Affil Hosps 1988; **Fellow:** Behavioral Neurology, Beth Israel Hosp 1990; **Fac Appt:** Prof N, Univ Ariz Coll Med

Burns, Richard S MD [N] - **Spec Exp:** Movement Disorders; Ataxia; Neurodegenerative Disorders; **Hospital:** St Joseph's Hosp & Med Ctr - Phoenix; **Address:** Barrow Neurological Institute, 500 W Thomas Rd, Ste 720, Phoenix, AZ 85013; **Phone:** 602-406-4931; **Board Cert:** Neurology 1985; **Med School:** Univ Minn 1969; **Resid:** Internal Medicine, Huntington Meml Hosp 1971; Neurology, UC Irvine Med Ctr 1978; **Fellow:** Clinical Pharmacology, Natl Inst Genl Med Sci 1980

Carter, John E MD [N] - **Spec Exp:** Neuro-Ophthalmology; **Hospital:** Univ Hlth Sys - Univ Hosp (San Antonio, TX); **Address:** Univ Tex Hlth Sci Ctr, Div Neurology, 7703 Floyd Curl, rm 5.318T, MC 7883, San Antonio, TX 78229-3900; **Phone:** 210-567-5088; **Board Cert:** Neurology 1978; **Med School:** Univ Ark 1969; **Resid:** Neurology, Boston Univ Med Ctr 1978; Neurological Ophthalmology, Tufts Univ 1979; **Fac Appt:** Assoc Prof N, Univ Tex, San Antonio

Couch Jr, James R MD/PhD [N] - **Spec Exp:** Headache; Stroke; **Hospital:** OU Med Ctr, VA Med Ctr - Oklahoma City; **Address:** 711 S L Young Blvd, Ste 210, Oklahoma City, OK 73104-5021; **Phone:** 405-271-3635; **Board Cert:** Neurology 1974; Clinical Neurophysiology 2002; Headache Medicine 2006; **Med School:** Baylor Coll Med 1965; **Resid:** Neurology, Washington Univ Med Ctr 1972; **Fellow:** Neuropharmacology, Natl Inst Hlth 1969; **Fac Appt:** Prof N, Univ Okla Coll Med

Coull, Bruce M MD [N] - **Spec Exp:** Stroke; Cerebrovascular Disease; **Hospital:** Univ Med Ctr - Tucson; **Address:** 2800 E Ajo Way, Tucson, AZ 85713; **Phone:** 520-874-2700; **Board Cert:** Neurology 1979; Vascular Neurology 2005; **Med School:** Univ Pittsburgh 1972; **Resid:** Neurology, Stanford Univ Med Ctr 1976; **Fac Appt:** Prof N, Univ Ariz Coll Med

Dodick, David W MD [N] - **Spec Exp:** Headache; Migraine; **Hospital:** Mayo Clinic - Scottsdale; **Address:** Mayo Clinic, Dept of Neurology, 13400 E Shea Blvd, Scottsdale, AZ 85259; **Phone:** 480-301-8100; **Board Cert:** Neurology 2006; Vascular Neurology 2005; Headache Medicine 2006; **Med School:** Dalhousie Univ 1990; **Resid:** Neurology, Mayo Clinic 1994; **Fellow:** Headache, Sunnybrook Hlth Sci Ctr 1996; **Fac Appt:** Assoc Prof N, Mayo Med Sch

Ferrendelli, James A MD [N] - **Spec Exp:** Epilepsy/Seizure Disorders; Geriatric Neurology; **Hospital:** Meml Hermann Hosp - Texas Med Ctr; **Address:** UT Houston Sch Med, Dept Neurology, 6431 Fannin St, Ste 7.044, Houston, TX 77030-1501; **Phone:** 713-500-7070; **Board Cert:** Neurology 1973; **Med School:** Univ Colorado 1962; **Resid:** Neurology, Cleveland Metro Genl Hosp 1968; **Fellow:** Neuropharmacology, Washington Univ Med Sch 1971; **Fac Appt:** Prof N, Univ Tex, Houston

Fox, Peter Thornton MD [N] - **Spec Exp:** PET Imaging; **Hospital:** Univ Hlth Sys - Univ Hosp (San Antonio, TX); **Address:** UT Hlth Sci Ctr San Antonio, Rsch Imaging Ctr, 7703 Floyd Curl Drive, MS 6240, San Antonio, TX 78229-3900; **Phone:** 210-567-8150; **Board Cert:** Neurology 1985; **Med School:** Georgetown Univ 1979; **Resid:** Neurology, Washington Univ 1983; **Fellow:** Radiotracer Imaging, Washington Univ 1984; **Fac Appt:** Prof N, Univ Tex, San Antonio

Gilbert, Mark R MD [N] - **Spec Exp:** Brain Tumors; Neuro-Oncology; **Hospital:** UT MD Anderson Cancer Ctr; **Address:** Univ Tex MD Anderson Cancer Ctr, 1515 Holcombe Blvd, Unit 431, Houston, TX 77030; **Phone:** 713-792-4008; **Board Cert:** Internal Medicine 1985; Neurology 1990; **Med School:** Johns Hopkins Univ 1982; **Resid:** Internal Medicine, Johns Hopkins Hosp 1985; Neurology, Johns Hopkins Hosp 1988; **Fellow:** Neuro-Oncology, Johns Hopkins Hosp 1988; **Fac Appt:** Assoc Prof N, Univ Tex, Houston

Grotta, James C MD [N] - **Spec Exp:** Stroke; **Hospital:** Meml Hermann Hosp - Texas Med Ctr; **Address:** UT Houston Med Sch, Dept Neur, 6410 Fannin St, Ste 1014, Houston, TX 77030; **Phone:** 832-325-7080; **Board Cert:** Neurology 1978; Vascular Neurology 2005; **Med School:** Univ VA Sch Med 1971; **Resid:** Neurology, Univ Colorado Hlth Sci Ctr 1977; **Fellow:** Diagnostic Radiology, Mass Genl Hosp 1979; **Fac Appt:** Prof N, Univ Tex, Houston

Hart, Robert G MD [N] - **Spec Exp:** Stroke; **Hospital:** Univ Hlth Sys - Univ Hosp (San Antonio, TX); **Address:** Univ Tex Hlth & Sci Ctr, Dept Neurology, 7703 Floyd Curl, MC 7883, San Antonio, TX 78229-3901; **Phone:** 210-592-0404; **Board Cert:** Neurology 1985; Vascular Neurology 2005; **Med School:** Univ MO-Columbia Sch Med 1977; **Resid:** Neurology, Univ Hosp & Clinic 1981; **Fellow:** Stroke, Oregon Hlth Sci Ctr 1982; **Fac Appt:** Prof N, Univ Tex, San Antonio

Infante, Ernesto MD [N] - **Spec Exp:** Neuromuscular Disorders; Movement Disorders; Headache; **Hospital:** Meml Hermann Hosp - Texas Med Ctr; **Address:** 6410 Fannin St, Ste 1014, UT Professional Building Fl 10, Houston, TX 77030; **Phone:** 832-325-7080; **Board Cert:** Neurology 1973; **Med School:** Spain 1964; **Resid:** Neurology, Univ Minn Hosps 1969; **Fellow:** Electromyography, Mayo Clinic 1970; **Fac Appt:** Assoc Clin Prof N, Univ Tex, Houston

Jankovic, Joseph MD [N] - **Spec Exp:** Movement Disorders; Parkinson's Disease; Tourette's Syndrome; **Hospital:** Methodist Hosp - Houston, St Luke's Episcopal Hosp - Houston; **Address:** Parkinson's Dis Ctr & Movement Disorders Clin, 6550 Fannin St, Smith Twr, Ste 1801, Houston, TX 77030; **Phone:** 713-798-5998; **Board Cert:** Neurology 1979; **Med School:** Univ Ariz Coll Med 1973; **Resid:** Neurology, Columbia-Presby Med Ctr 1977; **Fac Appt:** Prof N, Baylor Coll Med

Knoefel, Janice E MD [N] - **Spec Exp:** Geriatric Neurology; Neuro-Rehabilitation; **Hospital:** VA Med Ctr, Univ NM Hlth & Sci Ctr; **Address:** New Mexico VA Hlth Care System, 1501 San Pedro SE, MC 111K, Albuquerque, NM 87108-5153; **Phone:** 505-256-2795; **Board Cert:** Neurology 1983; **Med School:** Ohio State Univ 1977; **Resid:** Internal Medicine, Univ Cincinnati Med Ctr 1979; Neurology, Boston Univ Med Ctr 1982; **Fellow:** Geriatric Medicine, Boston Univ Med Ctr 1983; **Fac Appt:** Prof N, Univ New Mexico

Labiner, David M MD [N] - **Spec Exp:** Epilepsy; Seizure Disorders; **Hospital:** Univ Med Ctr - Tucson; **Address:** Univ Arizona HSC, Dept Neurology, 1501 N Campbell Ave, PO Box 245023, Tucson, AZ 85724-5023; **Phone:** 520-626-2006; **Board Cert:** Neurology 1992; **Med School:** Med Coll GA 1984; **Resid:** Neurology, Neuro Inst/Columbia 1988; **Fellow:** Epilepsy, Duke Univ Med Ctr 1989; **Fac Appt:** Prof N, Univ Ariz Coll Med

Levin, Victor A MD [N] - **Spec Exp:** Brain Tumors; Neuro-Oncology; Clinical Trials; **Hospital:** UT MD Anderson Cancer Ctr; **Address:** 1515 Holcombe Blvd, Unit #431, Houston, TX 77030-4009; **Phone:** 713-792-8297; **Board Cert:** Neurology 1976; **Med School:** Univ Wisc 1966; **Resid:** Neurology, Mass Genl Hosp 1972; **Fac Appt:** Prof Med, Univ Tex, Houston

Nicholl, Jeffrey S MD [N] - **Spec Exp:** Seizure Disorders; Epilepsy; **Hospital:** Tulane Univ Hosp & Clin; **Address:** Tulane Univ Sch Med Dept Neuro TB-52, 1440 Canal St, New Orleans, LA 70112; **Phone:** 504-988-2241; **Board Cert:** Neurology 1999; Psychiatry 1981; Clinical Neurophysiology 2001; Emergency Medicine 2004; **Med School:** Georgetown Univ 1974; **Resid:** Psychiatry, UCLA Neuro Psyc Inst 1979; Neurology, Tulane Univ 1997; **Fellow:** Clinical Neurophysiology, Tulane Univ 1998; Epilepsy, UCLA 2000; **Fac Appt:** Asst Prof N, Tulane Univ

Oommen, Kalarickal MD [N] - **Spec Exp:** Epilepsy; **Hospital:** OU Med Ctr; **Address:** 711 Stanton L Young Blvd, Ste 210, Oklahoma City, OK 73104; **Phone:** 405-271-3635; **Board Cert:** Neurology 1983; **Med School:** India 1973; **Resid:** Psychiatry, Arizona Hlth Sci Ctr 1979; Neurology, Arizona Hlth Sci Ctr 1982; **Fellow:** Electroencephalography, Med Coll Georgia 1983; **Fac Appt:** Assoc Prof N, Univ Okla Coll Med

Shapiro, William R MD [N] - **Spec Exp:** Neuro-Oncology; **Hospital:** St Joseph's Hosp & Med Ctr - Phoenix; **Address:** Barrow Neurology Clinics, 500 W Thomas Rd, Ste 300, Phoenix, AZ 85013; **Phone:** 602-406-6262; **Board Cert:** Neurology 1969; **Med School:** UCSF 1961; **Resid:** Internal Medicine, Univ Wash Hosp 1963; Neurology, NY Hosp-Cornell Med Ctr 1966; **Fellow:** Neuro-Oncology, Natl Inst Hlth 1969; **Fac Appt:** Prof N, Univ Ariz Coll Med

Wolinsky, Jerry S MD [N] - **Spec Exp:** Multiple Sclerosis; Clinical Trials; MRI; **Hospital:** Meml Hermann Hosp - Texas Med Ctr; **Address:** Univ Texas Med Sch, 6431 Fannin St, MSMB 7.044, Houston, TX 77030-1503; **Phone:** 713-500-7135; **Board Cert:** Neurology 1975; **Med School:** Univ IL Coll Med 1969; **Resid:** Neurology, UCSF Med Ctr 1973; **Fellow:** Neuropathology, VA Hosp 1975; **Fac Appt:** Prof N, Univ Tex, Houston

Yung, Wai-Kwan Alfred MD [N] - **Spec Exp:** Neuro-Oncology; Brain Tumors; **Hospital:** UT MD Anderson Cancer Ctr; **Address:** 1515 Holcombe Blvd, Unit 0431, Houston, TX 77030-4017; **Phone:** 713-794-1285; **Board Cert:** Neurology 1980; **Med School:** Univ Chicago-Pritzker Sch Med 1975; **Resid:** Neurology, UCSD Med Ctr 1978; **Fellow:** Neuro-Oncology, Meml Sloan Kettering Cancer Ctr 1981; **Fac Appt:** Prof N, Univ Tex, Houston

Neurology

West Coast and Pacific

Adornato, Bruce T MD [N] - **Spec Exp:** Stroke; Neuropathy; Sleep Disorders/Apnea; **Hospital:** Stanford Univ Med Ctr; **Address:** 1101 Welch Rd, Ste C5, Palo Alto, CA 94304-1926; **Phone:** 650-324-4300; **Board Cert:** Internal Medicine 1975; Neurology 1978; **Med School:** UCSD 1972; **Resid:** Internal Medicine, UCSF-Moffitt Hosp 1974; Neurology, UCSF-Moffitt Hosp 1976; **Fellow:** Neurology, Natl Inst Hlth 1978; **Fac Appt:** Clin Prof N, Stanford Univ

Albers, Gregory W MD [N] - **Spec Exp:** Cerebrovascular Disease; Stroke; **Hospital:** Stanford Univ Med Ctr; **Address:** Stanford Univ Med Ctr, Dept Neurology, 300 Pasteur Drive, rm A301, Stanford, CA 94305; **Phone:** 650-723-4448; **Board Cert:** Neurology 1990; **Med School:** UCSD 1984; **Resid:** Neurology, Standford Univ Med Ctr 1988; **Fellow:** Stroke, Standford Univ Med Ctr 1989; **Fac Appt:** Assoc Prof N, Stanford Univ

Aminoff, Michael J MD [N] - **Spec Exp:** Movement Disorders; Parkinson's Disease; **Hospital:** UCSF Med Ctr; **Address:** 505 Parnassus Ave, Fl 3 - rm M348, San Francisco, CA 94143-0216; **Phone:** 415-353-2904; **Board Cert:** Neurology 2004; Clinical Neurophysiology 2000; **Med School:** England 1965; **Resid:** Internal Medicine, Univ London Hosps 1970; Neurology, Middlesex Hosp/Natl Hosp Queen Sq 1972; **Fac Appt:** Prof N, UCSF

Aurora, Sheena K MD [N] - **Spec Exp:** Headache; Migraine; Electromyography; Movement Disorders; **Hospital:** Swedish Med Ctr - Seattle; **Address:** Swedish Headache Center, 1101 Madison Med Tower, Ste 200, Seattle, WA 98104-1306; **Phone:** 206-215-2243; **Board Cert:** Neurology 2006; Electrodiagnostic Medicine 1998; Clinical Neurophysiology 1999; Headache Medicine 2006; **Med School:** India 1990; **Resid:** Neurology, Henry Ford Hosp 1997

Becker, Kyra J MD [N] - **Spec Exp:** Stroke/Cerebrovascular Disease; Neuro-Immunology; Stroke-Young Adults; **Hospital:** Harborview Med Ctr, Univ Wash Med Ctr; **Address:** Harborview Medical Ctr, Dept Neurology, 325 9th Ave, Box 359775, Seattle, WA 98104; **Phone:** 206-744-6285; **Board Cert:** Neurology 1995; **Med School:** Duke Univ 1989; **Resid:** Neurology, Johns Hopkins Hosp 1993; **Fellow:** Critical Care Neurology, Johns Hopkins Hosp 1995; Research, NIH-NINDS 1996; **Fac Appt:** Assoc Prof N, Univ Wash

Bourdette, Dennis MD [N] - **Spec Exp:** Multiple Sclerosis; Guillain-Barre Syndrome; Myasthenia Gravis; **Hospital:** OR Hlth & Sci Univ; **Address:** Oregon Hlth & Sci Univ, Dept Neurology, 3181 SW Sam Jackson Park Rd, MS L226, Portland, OR 97239; **Phone:** 503-494-5759; **Board Cert:** Neurology 1985; **Med School:** UC Davis 1978; **Resid:** Neurology, Oregon Hlth Sci Univ Hosp 1982; **Fellow:** Neurological Immunology, VA Med Ctr 1985; **Fac Appt:** Prof N, Oregon Hlth Sci Univ

Bowen, James MD [N] - **Spec Exp:** Multiple Sclerosis; **Hospital:** Evergreen Hosp Med Ctr; **Address:** Evergreen Multiple Sclerosis Ctr, 12333 NE 130th Ln, Ste 225, Kirkland, WA 98034; **Phone:** 425-899-5350; **Board Cert:** Neurology 1990; **Med School:** Johns Hopkins Univ 1982; **Resid:** Internal Medicine, Univ Washington Med Ctr 1984; Neurology, Univ Washington Med Ctr 1987; **Fac Appt:** Asst Clin Prof N, Univ Wash

Charles, Andrew C MD [N] - **Spec Exp:** Headache; **Hospital:** Ronald Reagan UCLA Med Ctr; **Address:** UCLA Neurological Services, 300 Medical Plaza, Ste B200, Los Angeles, CA 90024; **Phone:** 310-794-1195; **Board Cert:** Neurology 1992; **Med School:** UCLA 1986; **Resid:** Neurology, UCLA Med Ctr 1990; **Fellow:** Neurology, UCLA Med Ctr 1992; **Fac Appt:** Prof N, UCLA

Chui, Helena Chang MD [N] - **Spec Exp:** Stroke; Dementia; Alzheimer's Disease; **Hospital:** USC Univ Hosp - R K Eamer Med Plz, Rancho Los Amigos Natl Rehab Ctr; **Address:** Health Care Consultation Center II, 1510 San Pablo St, Ste 618, Los Angeles, CA 90033; **Phone:** 323-442-7591; **Board Cert:** Neurology 1984; **Med School:** Johns Hopkins Univ 1977; **Resid:** Neurology, Univ Iowa Med Ctr 1981; **Fellow:** Behavioral Neurology, Univ Iowa Med Ctr 1979; **Fac Appt:** Prof N, USC Sch Med

Cloughesy, Timothy F MD [N] - **Spec Exp:** Neuro-Oncology; Seizure Disorders; Brain Tumors; **Hospital:** Ronald Reagan UCLA Med Ctr; **Address:** UCLA Neurological Services, 710 Westwood Plaza, Ste 1-230, Los Angeles, CA 90095; **Phone:** 310-825-5321; **Board Cert:** Neurology 1993; **Med School:** Tulane Univ 1987; **Resid:** Neurology, UCLA Med Ctr 1991; **Fellow:** Neuro-Oncology, Meml Sloan-Kettering Canc Ctr; **Fac Appt:** Clin Prof N, UCLA

Cummings, Jeffrey Lee MD [N] - **Spec Exp:** Neuro-Psychiatry; Alzheimer's Disease; Parkinson's Disease; **Hospital:** Ronald Reagan UCLA Med Ctr; **Address:** UCLA Med Ctr, Alzheimer's Disease Ctr, 10911 Weyburn Ave, Ste 200, Los Angeles, CA 90095-7226; **Phone:** 310-794-3665; **Board Cert:** Neurology 1979; **Med School:** Univ Wash 1974; **Resid:** Neurology, Boston Univ Sch Med 1978; **Fellow:** Behavioral Neurology and Psychiatry, Boston Univ Sch Med 1979; Neurological Pathology, The Natl Hosp 1980; **Fac Appt:** Assoc Prof N, UCLA

DeGiorgio, Christopher M MD [N] - **Spec Exp:** Epilepsy; Seizure Disorders; Neurocysticercosis; Parasitic Infections; **Hospital:** Ronald Reagan UCLA Med Ctr; **Address:** UCLA Med Ctr, Dept Neurology, 710 Westwood Plaza, Los Angeles, CA 90095; **Phone:** 310-825-5521; **Board Cert:** Neurology 1987; **Med School:** Loyola Univ-Stritch Sch Med 1981; **Resid:** Neurology, West Los Angeles VA Hosp 1985; **Fellow:** Epilepsy, UCLA Med Ctr 1987; **Fac Appt:** Assoc Prof N, UCLA

Engel, William King MD [N] - **Spec Exp:** Neuromuscular Disorders; **Hospital:** Good Samaritan Hosp - Los Angeles, USC Univ Hosp - R K Eamer Med Plz; **Address:** 637 S Lucas Ave Fl 3, Los Angeles, CA 90017; **Phone:** 213-975-9950; **Board Cert:** Neurology 1962; **Med School:** McGill Univ 1955; **Resid:** Neurology, Natl Inst Hlth 1959; Neurology, Natl Hosp 1960; **Fellow:** Neuromuscular Medicine, Natl Inst Hlth 1961; **Fac Appt:** Prof N, USC Sch Med

Engstrom, John W MD [N] - **Spec Exp:** Peripheral Neuropathy; Neuromuscular Disorders; Spinal Cord Disorders; **Hospital:** UCSF Med Ctr; **Address:** UCSF Med Ctr, Dept Neurology, 400 Parnassus Ave Fl 8, Box 0348, San Francisco, CA 94143; **Phone:** 415-353-2273; **Board Cert:** Internal Medicine 1984; Neurology 1991; Clinical Neurophysiology 2002; **Med School:** Stanford Univ 1981; **Resid:** Internal Medicine, Johns Hopkins Hosp 1984; Neurology, UCSF Med Ctr 1988; **Fellow:** Neurology, UCSF Med Ctr 1989; **Fac Appt:** Prof N, UCSF

Fisher, Mark MD [N] - **Spec Exp:** Stroke; Cerebrovascular Disease; **Hospital:** UC Irvine Med Ctr; **Address:** UC Irvine Med Ctr, Dept Neurology, 101 The City Drive S Bldg 55 - rm 121, Orange, CA 92868; **Phone:** 714-456-6856; **Board Cert:** Neurology 1981; Vascular Neurology 2005; **Med School:** Univ Cincinnati 1975; **Resid:** Neurology, UCLA-Wadsworth VA Hosp 1980; **Fac Appt:** Prof N, UC Irvine

Fisher, Robert S MD [N] - **Spec Exp:** Epilepsy/Seizure Disorders; **Hospital:** Stanford Univ Med Ctr; **Address:** 300 Pasteur Drive, rm A-343, Dept of Neurology, Stanford, CA 94305-5235; **Phone:** 650-498-3056; **Board Cert:** Neurology 1983; Clinical Neurophysiology 2002; **Med School:** Stanford Univ 1977; **Resid:** Internal Medicine, Stanford Univ 1979; Neurology, Johns Hopkins Hosp 1982

Goodin, Douglas MD [N] - **Spec Exp:** Multiple Sclerosis; **Hospital:** UCSF Med Ctr, VA Med Ctr - San Francisco; **Address:** UCSF MS Ctr, 400 Parnassus Ave Fl 8, San Francisco, CA 94117; **Phone:** 415-353-2069; **Board Cert:** Neurology 1985; **Med School:** UC Irvine 1978; **Resid:** Neurology, UCSF Med Ctr 1981; **Fac Appt:** Assoc Prof N, UCSF

Neurology

Graves, Michael C MD [N] - **Spec Exp:** Amyotrophic Lateral Sclerosis (ALS); **Hospital:** Ronald Reagan UCLA Med Ctr; **Address:** UCLA Neurological Svcs, 300 Medical Plaza, Ste B200, Box 956975, Los Angeles, CA 90095-6975; **Phone:** 310-825-7266; **Board Cert:** Neurology 1977; **Med School:** Stanford Univ 1970; **Resid:** Internal Medicine, UCSD Med Ctr 1972; Neurology, Johns Hopkins Hosp 1975; **Fellow:** Rockefeller Univ Hosp; **Fac Appt:** Assoc Prof N, UCLA

Hauser, Stephen Lawrence MD [N] - **Spec Exp:** Multiple Sclerosis; Epilepsy; **Hospital:** UCSF Med Ctr; **Address:** UCSF MS Ctr, 400 Parnassus Ave Fl 8th, Box 0114, San Francisco, CA 94143-0164; **Phone:** 415-353-2069; **Board Cert:** Internal Medicine 1978; Neurology 1981; **Med School:** Harvard Med Sch 1975; **Resid:** Internal Medicine, NY Presby-Cornell 1977; Neurology, Mass Genl Hosp 1980; **Fellow:** Neurology, Harvard Univ 1980; **Fac Appt:** Prof N, UCSF

Henderson, Victor W MD [N] - **Spec Exp:** Alzheimer's Disease; Dementia; Memory Disorders; **Hospital:** Stanford Univ Med Ctr; **Address:** Stanford Univ Hosp, Dept Neurology, 300 Pasteur Drive, rm A343, Stanford, CA 94305-5235; **Phone:** 650-723-5184; **Board Cert:** Neurology 1981; **Med School:** Johns Hopkins Univ 1976; **Resid:** Internal Medicine, Duke Univ Med Ctr 1977; Neurology, Barnes Hosp- Wash Univ 1980; **Fellow:** Behavioral Neurology, Aphasia Rsch Ctr-Boston Univ 1981; **Fac Appt:** Prof N, Stanford Univ

Langston, J William MD [N] - **Spec Exp:** Parkinson's Disease; Movement Disorders; Tremor; **Hospital:** Parkinson's Inst/Movement Disorders Trmt Ctr, The; **Address:** The Parkinsons Institute, 675 Almanor Ave, Sunnyvale, CA 94085; **Phone:** 408-542-5633; **Board Cert:** Neurology 1986; **Med School:** Univ MO-Columbia Sch Med 1967; **Resid:** Neurology, Stanford Univ 1974; **Fellow:** Electroencephalography, Stanford Univ

Lutsep, Helmi L MD [N] - **Spec Exp:** Stroke/Cerebrovascular Disease; **Hospital:** OR Hlth & Sci Univ; **Address:** Oregon Stroke Ctr, Oregon HSU, 3181 SW Sam Jackson Park Rd, CR-131, Portland, OR 97239; **Phone:** 503-494-7225; **Board Cert:** Neurology 1994; Vascular Neurology 2005; **Med School:** Mayo Med Sch 1988; **Resid:** Neurology, Mayo Clinic 1992; **Fellow:** Behavioral Neurology, UC Davis Med Ctr 1995; Stroke, Stanford Univ Med Ctr 1996; **Fac Appt:** Assoc Prof N, Oregon Hlth Sci Univ

Morrell, Martha J MD [N] - **Spec Exp:** Epilepsy; Epilepsy in Women; **Hospital:** Stanford Univ Med Ctr; **Address:** 300 Pasteur Drive, rm A-343, MC 5235, Stanford, CA 94305; **Phone:** 650-498-6648; **Board Cert:** Neurology 1989; Clinical Neurophysiology 2003; **Med School:** Stanford Univ 1984; **Resid:** Neurology, Hosp Univ Penn 1988; **Fellow:** Epilepsy, Graduate Hosp-Univ Penn 1990; **Fac Appt:** Prof N, Stanford Univ

Nutt Jr, John G MD [N] - **Spec Exp:** Movement Disorders; Parkinson's Disease; **Hospital:** OR Hlth & Sci Univ; **Address:** Oregon Health Science Univ, MC OP-32, 3181 SW Sam Jackson Park Rd, Portland, OR 97239; **Phone:** 503-494-7230; **Board Cert:** Neurology 1978; **Med School:** Baylor Coll Med 1970; **Resid:** Neurology, Univ Wash Med Ctr 1976; **Fellow:** Pharmacology, Natl Inst Neuro Disorders /Stroke 1978; **Fac Appt:** Prof N, Oregon Hlth Sci Univ

Phuphanich, Surasak MD [N] - **Spec Exp:** Neuro-Oncology; Brain Tumors; Spinal Tumors; **Hospital:** Cedars-Sinai Med Ctr; **Address:** 8631 W 3rd St, Ste 410E, Los Angeles, CA 90048; **Phone:** 310-423-8100; **Board Cert:** Neurology 1983; **Med School:** Thailand 1975; **Resid:** Neurology, Univ Illinois Med Ctr 1981; **Fellow:** Neuro-Oncology, UCSF Med Ctr 1984; **Fac Appt:** Prof, Emory Univ

Raskin, Neil H MD [N] - **Spec Exp:** Headache; Migraine; **Hospital:** UCSF Med Ctr; **Address:** UCSF Neurology Faculty Practice, 400 Parnassus Ave Fl 8, Box 0348, San Francisco, CA 94143; **Phone:** 415-353-2273; **Board Cert:** Neurology 1969; **Med School:** Harvard Med Sch 1959; **Resid:** Internal Medicine, Bellevue Hosp Ctr 1961; Neurology, Neuro Inst/Columbia 1964; **Fellow:** Neurology, Neuro Inst/Columbia 1965; **Fac Appt:** Prof N, UCSF

Rosenbaum, Richard B MD [N] - **Spec Exp:** Neuromuscular Disorders; **Hospital:** OR Hlth & Sci Univ; **Address:** Oregon Clinic Neurology Department, 5050 NE Hoyt St, Ste 315, Portland, OR 97213-2975; **Phone:** 503-963-3100; **Board Cert:** Neurology 1979; Internal Medicine 1975; **Med School:** Harvard Med Sch 1971; **Resid:** Internal Medicine, Stanford Med Ctr 1974; Neurology, UCSF Med Ctr 1977; **Fac Appt:** Clin Prof N, Oregon Hlth Sci Univ

Smith, Wade S MD/PhD [N] - **Spec Exp:** Stroke; Pain-Back & Shoulder; **Hospital:** UCSF Med Ctr; **Address:** UCSF, Dept Neurology, 505 Parnassus Ave, Ste M830, Box 0114, San Francisco, CA 94143; **Phone:** 415-353-1489; **Board Cert:** Neurology 2006; **Med School:** Univ Wash 1989; **Resid:** Neurology, UCSF-Moffitt Hosp 1993; **Fellow:** Critical Care Medicine, UCSF-Moffitt Hosp 1994; **Fac Appt:** Asst Clin Prof N, UCSF

Starr, Arnold MD [N] - **Spec Exp:** Hearing Disorders; Neurophysiology-Aging; Neurophysiology-Dementia; Hearing Disorders; **Hospital:** UC Irvine Med Ctr; **Address:** Dept Neurology, 1 Medical Plaza Drive, Irvine, CA 92697; **Phone:** 714-456-7239; **Board Cert:** Neurology 1970; **Med School:** NYU Sch Med 1957; **Resid:** Neurology, Boston City Hosp 1959; **Fellow:** Neurology, Natl Inst Hlth 1962; Clinical Neurophysiology, Inst Neurophysiology 1963; **Fac Appt:** Prof N, UC Irvine

Tanner, Caroline M MD/PhD [N] - **Spec Exp:** Parkinson's Disease; Movement Disorders; Dystonia; **Hospital:** Parkinson's Inst/Movement Disorders Trmt Ctr, The; **Address:** The Parkinson's Institute, 675 Almanor Ave, Sunnyvale, CA 94085; **Phone:** 408-734-2800; **Board Cert:** Neurology 1982; **Med School:** Loyola Univ-Stritch Sch Med 1976; **Resid:** Neurology, Rush-Presby-St Luke's Med Ctr 1980; **Fellow:** Neurological Pharmacology, Rush-Presby-St Luke's Med Ctr 1982

Tetrud, James W MD [N] - **Spec Exp:** Movement Disorders; Parkinson's Disease; Tremor; **Hospital:** Parkinson's Inst/Movement Disorders Trmt Ctr, The; **Address:** The Parkinson's Institute, 675 Almanor Ave, Sunnyvale, CA 94085; **Phone:** 408-734-2800; **Board Cert:** Neurology 1981; **Med School:** NYU Sch Med 1973; **Resid:** Internal Medicine, VetVA Med Ctr-West Los Angeles 1974; Neurology, VA Med Ctr-West Los Angeles 1978

Weiner, Leslie P MD [N] - **Spec Exp:** Multiple Sclerosis; Amyotrophic Lateral Sclerosis (ALS); **Hospital:** USC Univ Hosp - R K Eamer Med Plz, LAC & USC Med Ctr; **Address:** Keck Sch Med, Dept Neurology, 2025 Zonal Ave, RMR - 506, Los Angeles, CA 90089; **Phone:** 323-442-3020; **Board Cert:** Neurology 1969; **Med School:** Univ Cincinnati 1961; **Resid:** Neurology, Baltimore City Hosp 1963; Neurology, Johns Hopkins Hosp 1965; **Fellow:** Neurology, Johns Hopkins Hosp 1969; **Fac Appt:** Prof N, USC Sch Med

:: Cleveland Clinic

Neurological Institute

The Cleveland Clinic Neurological Institute is a fully integrated entity with a disease-specific focus, combining all physicians and other healthcare providers in neurology, neurosurgery, neuroradiology, the behavioral sciences and nursing who treat children and adults with neurological and neurobehavioral disorders. Our staff of more than 220 specialists sees one of the largest and most diverse patient populations in the country. Because of our clinical expertise, academic achievement and innovative research, the Cleveland Clinic Neurological Institute has earned an international reputation for excellence.

U.S.News & World Report's "America's Best Hospitals" survey has consistently ranked our Neurology and Neurosurgery programs among the Top 10 in the nation and best in Ohio.

Our unique clinical structure allows us to deliver coordinated, comprehensive, multidisciplinary care to our patients through more efficient treatment decision making and consultation for complex cases. Fully integrating specialties along disease lines creates an exciting synergy among Institute physicians who share similar clinical, research and educational interests, to the benefit of patients and physicians alike.

Major advances in the treatment of brain tumors, epilepsy, mood disorders, stroke, movement disorders, pain and spinal disorders are improving quality of life and survival for thousands of patients. For those diseases resistant to available treatments, we believe the innovative model of medicine created within the Neurological Institute will speed research and advances in treatment, resulting in better clinical care and more rapid breakthroughs in the full range of neurological and behavioral disorders.

Centers in the Neurological Institute include: Brain Tumor & Neuro-Oncology Center, Center for Headache & Pain, Center for Neuroimaging, Center for Neurological Restoration, Center for Pediatric Neurology & Neurosurgery, Center for Spine Health, Cerebrovascular Center, Epilepsy Center, Mellen Center for Multiple Sclerosis Treatment & Research, Neuromuscular Center, Psychiatry and Psychology and Sleep Disorders Center

For more information about the Cleveland Clinic Neurological Institute, to schedule a second opinion or to learn about assistance for out-of-town patients, call 800.890.2467 or visit www.clevelandclinic.org/neurotopdocs.

Cleveland Clinic Neurological Institute
9500 Euclid Avenue / AC311 | Cleveland OH 44195

Comprehensive Neurological Care

Cleveland Clinic offers expert diagnostic and treatment options for all neurologic conditions affecting children and adults, including:

- Alzheimer's disease
- ALS (Amyotrophic Lateral Sclerosis)
- Aneurysms
- Arteriovenous Malformations (AVMs)
- Back and Neck Disorders
- Brain and Spine Tumors
- Cerebral Palsy
- Chronic Pain Rehabilitation
- Congenital Disorders
- Craniofacial Disorders
- Epilepsy
- Headache
- Hydrocephalus
- Metastatic Tumors
- Movement Disorders
- Neonatal Disorders
- Neurofibromatosis
- Parkinson's Disease
- Peripheral Neuropathies
- Pituitary Disorders
- Psychiatric Disorders
- Skull Base Disorders
- Sleep Disorders
- Stroke

PENN NEUROLOGY

The University of Pennsylvania's history of excellence in the treatment of neurological diseases dates back to the establishment of the Department of Neurology in 1874. *The Best Doctors in America*® lists more neurologists and neurosurgeons from the Hospital of the University of Pennsylvania than from any other hospital or medical center in the Philadelphia region.

The Department of Neurology is a component of the new Penn Comprehensive Neuroscience Center, which is dedicated to the advancement of the understanding of the brain, spine and peripheral nervous system and will facilitate and strengthen the integration of Penn's world-class neuroscience programs within the areas of clinical care, research and education.

Excellence and Expertise

Recognized by the National Parkinson Foundation as one of its worldwide Centers of Excellence, **the Parkinson's Disease and Movement Disorders Center** is committed to providing exceptional patient care, education, social support services and ongoing research into the causes of Parkinson's disease. Research is an important and ongoing mission of the Parkinson's Disease and Movement Disorders Center, which actively pursues the investigation of the disease as well as exploration of new medications.

The Multiple Sclerosis Center (MS) program provides comprehensive evaluation, diagnosis and treatment for patients with MS and other demyelinating disorders of the central nervous system. The Center specializes in quality, state-of-the-art care with a personal approach. The comprehensive multidisciplinary team includes neurologists, nurse practitioners and specialists from other disciplines who are available for consultation in the management of genitourinary complications, spasticity and pain. In addition to maintaining high standards for clinical service, the Penn MS program is a leader in MS training and in clinical and laboratory-based research.

The Neuro-Oncology Program has set the standard for the region and provides comprehensive evaluation, diagnosis and treatment to patients with brain and spinal tumors and other cancer-related neurological central nervous system and peripheral nervous system problems. The program utilizes a patient-oriented team approach and brings together some of the nation's leading experts in the field. Each patient's case is reviewed by a multidisciplinary team to ensure that the patient is offered the most up-to-date therapy that is appropriate for them. The goal is to provide the best chance for a cure while preserving quality of life for each patient.

The Penn Epilepsy Center provides the highest standard of care to patients with epilepsy and related problems. The Center offers a comprehensive, full continuum of care including state-of-the-art diagnostic techniques, cutting-edge research, medical treatments, surgery, and support services to patients with epilepsy. Both outpatient evaluation and inpatient care are available via this multi-disciplinary, full-service facility.

Programs

- The Cognitive Neurology Program
- The Center for Brain Injury and Repair
- The Interventional Neuro Center
- The Memory Disorders Clinic
- Multiple Sclerosis Center
- Neuro Intensive Care
- The Neurogenetics Center
- Neuromuscular Disorders Program
- Neuro-Oncology Program
- The Neuro-Ophthalmology Service
- The Neuropsychology Service
- The Neurovascular Center
- The Parkinson's Disease and Movement Disorders Center
- The Penn Epilepsy Center
- Penn Center for Sleep Disorders
- Penn Memory Center
- The Stroke Center

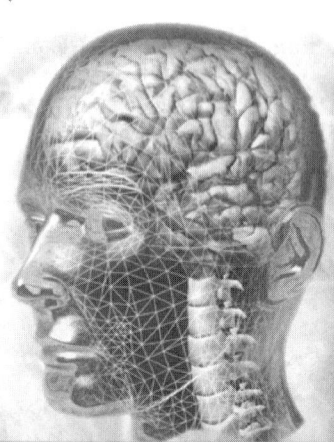

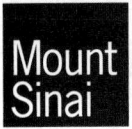
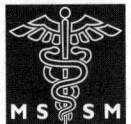

MOUNT SINAI
SCHOOL OF
MEDICINE

THE MOUNT SINAI MEDICAL CENTER
NEUROLOGY
One Gustave L. Levy Place
Fifth Avenue and 100th Street
New York, NY 10029-6574
Physician Referral: 1-800-MD-SINAI (637-4624)
www.mountsinai.org/cancer

The Robert and John M. Bendheim Parkinson's Disease Center is one of the world's first multidisciplinary centers for the study of Parkinson's disease and related disorders and serves as a forum for collaboration among world-renowned neuroscientists. The Center offers state-of-the-art clinical care, translational research, and basic science programs aimed at discovering the cause of and cure for Parkinson's disease. The Center incorporates a renowned deep brain stimulation (DBS) and functional neurosurgery program and has played a major role in evaluating cell-based and gene therapies for the treatment of movement disorders.

The Corinne Goldsmith Dickinson Center for Multiple Sclerosis is one of the most comprehensive centers of its kind, uniting the efforts of leading physicians and scientists from many disciplines to understand the causes and overcome the consequences of multiple sclerosis (MS). The Center provides services in all aspects of diagnosis, disease management, rehabilitation, and patient support, as well as the opportunity for patients to participate in potentially groundbreaking experimental trials.

The Clinical Program for Cerebrovascular Disorders provides a highly qualified team of medical experts who specialize in the most advanced approaches in the evaluation, treatment, and rehabilitation of patients with cerebrovascular diseases. Services include the early diagnosis of stroke, a specialized Neurointensive Care Unit, and a new inpatient stroke unit. As part of our commitment to excellence in patient care, the Program's physicians are available at all times for emergency consultation with referring physicians.

The NeuroAIDS Program is designed to diagnose and treat disorders associated with HIV disease. The program at Mount Sinai is one of the few in the world to treat the various central and peripheral nervous systems complications of the disease that affect as many as 70 percent of patients.

The MDA/ALS Program has been established in conjunction with the Muscular Dystrophy Association and provides state-of-the-art diagnosis and treatment of muscular dystrophy and amyotrophic lateral sclerosis (ALS). Our clinical care team specializes in improving the quality of life for those afflicted with these disorders, and the research team engages in both clinical and laboratory research projects aimed at finding enhanced treatments for these conditions.

The Division of Neuromuscular Diseases provides unparalleled diagnosis, treatment, and compassionate care of patients with disorders in neuromuscular transmission, diseases of the muscles, and peripheral nerve problems.

THE ESTELLE AND DANIEL MAGGIN DEPARTMENT OF NEUROLOGY at The Mount Sinai Medical Center is the oldest neurology department in the nation. The Department is renowned for its strong basic science laboratories, which study the causes and mechanisms underlying Parkinson's disease, ALS, MS, and other neurological disorders. One of the nation's top programs in the field for research and patient care, the Department is led by some of the most prominent figures in American neurology and receives annual grants of more than $15 million.

Mount Sinai's Neurological Tumor Program is world-acclaimed for the treatment of pituitary adenomas, acoustic neuromas, meningiomas, skull-base lesions, and cancerous brain tumors. The Program's multispecialty group of physicians works together to provide individualized therapy for each patient and delivers outstanding care through state-of-the-art surgical procedures, radiation therapy, cancer-related chemotherapy, and supportive therapy. Our physicians have pioneered the treatment of tumors with stereotactic radiosurgery and have developed and participated in a number of experimental treatment protocols to improve the lives of patients with tumors of the nervous system.

The Eye Movement and Vestibular Disorder Program at Mount Sinai is one of the finest in the world. Our physicians participate in NASA programs, employing state-of-the-art equipment that has been used to assess these disorders in space. Scientists who participate in this Program have helped to define the physiologic basis of these disorders and are performing groundbreaking research toward understanding such problems as gait dysfunction and motion sickness.

NEUROLOGY

Dedicated to exceptional patient care, advanced scientific research, and high-quality graduate education, the Department of Neurology at NYU Langone Medical Center evaluates and treats children and adults with a broad spectrum of neurological diseases. Specialty groups within the department deliver integrated care to patients with stroke, cerebrovascular behavioral disorders and dementia, brain tumors, genetic and degenerative diseases, headache and pain syndromes, movement disorders including Parkinson's disease, multiple sclerosis, neuromuscular diseases, and enologic diseases of children. NYU Langone Medical Center is home to the largest multiple sclerosis program in New York.

The clinical mission especially benefits from a 30-bed neurorehabilitation unit, a state-of-the-art neurophysiology laboratory, and a neurogenetics testing facility, each conducted under departmental auspices.

472

Sponsored Page

Nuclear Medicine

A nuclear medicine specialist employs the properties of radioactive atoms and molecules in the diagnosis and treatment of disease, and in research. Radiation detection and imaging instrument systems are used to detect disease as it changes the function and metabolism of normal cells, tissues and organs. A wide variety of diseases can be found in this way, usually before the structure of the organ involved by the disease can be seen to be abnormal by any other techniques. Early detection of coronary artery disease (including acute heart attack); early cancer detection and evaluation of the effect of tumor treatment; diagnosis of infection and inflammation anywhere in the body; and early detection of blood clot in the lungs, are all possible with these techniques. Unique forms of radioactive molecules can attack and kill cancer cells (e.g., lymphoma, thyroid cancer) or can relieve the severe pain of cancer that has spread to bone.

The nuclear medicine specialist has special knowledge in the biologic effects of radiation exposure, the fundamentals of the physical sciences and the principles and operation of radiation detection and imaging instrumentation systems.

Training required: Three years

NUCLEAR MEDICINE

Mid Atlantic

Alavi, Abass MD [NuM] - **Spec Exp:** Brain Tumors; Neurologic Imaging; PET Imaging-Brain; Brain Infections; **Hospital:** Hosp Univ Penn - UPHS (page 60), Chldns Hosp of Philadelphia, The; **Address:** Hosp Univ Penn, Div Nuclear Med, 3400 Spruce St, Donner Bldg rm 110, Philadelphia, PA 19104; **Phone:** 215-662-3014; **Board Cert:** Nuclear Medicine 1973; Internal Medicine 1972; **Med School:** Iran 1964; **Resid:** Internal Medicine, Albert Einstein Med Ctr/Phila VA Hosp 1969; Hematology, Hosp Univ Penn 1970; **Fellow:** Nuclear Medicine, Hosp Univ Penn 1973; **Fac Appt:** Prof Rad, Univ Pennsylvania

Carrasquillo, Jorge A MD [NuM] - **Spec Exp:** Radioimmunotherapy of Cancer; PET Imaging; **Hospital:** Meml Sloan-Kettering Cancer Ctr; **Address:** 1275 York Avenue, New York, NY 10065; **Phone:** 800-525-2225; **Board Cert:** Internal Medicine 1977; Nuclear Medicine 1982; **Med School:** Univ Puerto Rico 1974; **Resid:** Internal Medicine, Univ Dist Hosp 1977; Nuclear Medicine, Univ Wash Hosp 1982

Freeman, Leonard M MD [NuM] - **Spec Exp:** Nuclear Oncology; Gastrointestinal Disorders; PET Imaging; CT Scan; **Hospital:** Montefiore Med Ctr; **Address:** 111 E 210th St, Bronx, NY 10467-2401; **Phone:** 718-920-6060; **Board Cert:** Diagnostic Radiology 1966; Nuclear Medicine 1972; Nuclear Radiology 1974; **Med School:** Ros Franklin Univ/Chicago Med Sch 1961; **Resid:** Diagnostic Radiology, Bronx Municipal Hosp 1965; **Fac Appt:** Prof NuM, Albert Einstein Coll Med

Goldsmith, Stanley J MD [NuM] - **Spec Exp:** Thyroid Cancer; Neuroendocrine Tumors; PET Imaging; Lymphoma; **Hospital:** NY-Presby Hosp/Weill Cornell (page 66); **Address:** 525 E 68th St Starr Bldg - rm 2-21, New York, NY 10021-9800; **Phone:** 212-746-4588; **Board Cert:** Internal Medicine 1969; Nuclear Medicine 1972; Endocrinology 1972; **Med School:** SUNY Downstate 1962; **Resid:** Internal Medicine, Kings Co Hosp 1967; **Fellow:** Endocrinology, Diabetes & Metabolism, Mt Sinai Hosp 1968; Nuclear Medicine, Bronx VA Hosp 1969; **Fac Appt:** Prof Rad, Cornell Univ-Weill Med Coll

Lamonica, Dominick M MD [NuM] - **Spec Exp:** Thyroid Cancer; **Hospital:** Roswell Park Cancer Inst; **Address:** Roswell Park Cancer Inst, Elm & Carlton St, Dept of Nuclear Medicine, Buffalo, NY 14263; **Phone:** 716-845-3282; **Board Cert:** Internal Medicine 2005; Nuclear Medicine 2006; **Med School:** Mount Sinai Sch Med 1987; **Resid:** Internal Medicine, Univ Hosp-SUNY Stony Brook 1991; Diagnostic Radiology, Nassau City Med Ctr 1992; **Fellow:** Nuclear Medicine, DVAMC North Port-SUNY Stony Brook 1994; Nuclear Medicine, SUNY Buffalo-RPCI 1995; **Fac Appt:** Asst Prof, SUNY Buffalo

Larson, Steven M MD [NuM] - **Spec Exp:** Thyroid Cancer; PET Imaging; **Hospital:** Meml Sloan-Kettering Cancer Ctr; **Address:** 1275 York Avenue, New York, NY 10065; **Phone:** 800-525-2225; **Board Cert:** Nuclear Medicine 1972; Internal Medicine 1973; **Med School:** Univ Wash 1965; **Resid:** Internal Medicine, Virginia Mason Hosp 1970; Nuclear Medicine, Natl Inst Hlth 1972; **Fac Appt:** Prof NuM, Cornell Univ-Weill Med Coll

Majd, Massoud MD [NuM] - **Spec Exp:** Pediatric Nuclear Medicine; **Hospital:** Chldns Natl Med Ctr; **Address:** 111 Michigan Ave NW, Washington, DC 20010-2978; **Phone:** 202-476-3698; **Board Cert:** Diagnostic Radiology 1972; Nuclear Medicine 1973; **Med School:** Iran 1960; **Resid:** Diagnostic Radiology, Georgetown Univ Hosp 1965; **Fac Appt:** Prof NuM, Geo Wash Univ

Mountz, James M MD/PhD [NuM] - **Spec Exp:** Neurologic Imaging; Brain Imaging; **Hospital:** UPMC Presby, Pittsburgh, Agnews Dev Ctr; **Address:** UPMC Hlth Sys, Presby Univ Hosp, 200 Lothrop St, PET Facility, rm B 932, Pittsburgh, PA 15213; **Phone:** 412-647-0104; **Board Cert:** Diagnostic Radiology 1985; Nuclear Medicine 1986; **Med School:** Case West Res Univ 1981; **Resid:** Diagnostic Radiology, Univ Michigan Hosps 1985; **Fellow:** Nuclear Medicine, Univ Michigan Hosps 1986; **Fac Appt:** Prof Rad, Univ Pittsburgh

Neumann, Ronald D MD [NuM] - **Hospital:** Natl Inst of Hlth - Clin Ctr; **Address:** NIH Bldg 10, Box 1C-401, 10 Center Dr, MSC 1180, Bethesda, MD 20892-1180; **Phone:** 301-496-6455; **Board Cert:** Nuclear Medicine 1979; **Med School:** Yale Univ 1974; **Resid:** Pathology, Yale-New Haven Hosp 1977; Nuclear Medicine, Yale-New Haven Hosp 1979

Sanger, Joseph J MD [NuM] - **Spec Exp:** Nuclear Cardiology; **Hospital:** NYU Med Ctr (page 68); **Address:** NYU Medical Ctr, 545 1st Ave, rm SC2-184, New York, NY 10016-6402; **Phone:** 212-263-3434; **Board Cert:** Nuclear Medicine 1981; **Med School:** NYU Sch Med 1977; **Resid:** Diagnostic Radiology, NYU Med Ctr 1979; **Fellow:** Nuclear Medicine, NYU Med Ctr 1981; **Fac Appt:** Assoc Clin Prof, NYU Sch Med

Strashun, Arnold M MD [NuM] - **Spec Exp:** Neurologic Imaging; Nuclear Cardiology; Thyroid Disorders; PET Imaging-Brain; **Hospital:** SUNY Downstate Med Ctr, Kings County Hosp Ctr; **Address:** SUNY Hlth Sci Ctr, Dept Radiology, 450 Clarkson Ave, Box 1198, Brooklyn, NY 11203; **Phone:** 718-270-1603; **Board Cert:** Internal Medicine 1977; Nuclear Medicine 1979; **Med School:** Baylor Coll Med 1974; **Resid:** Internal Medicine, Baylor Med Ctr 1975; Internal Medicine, Texas Med Ctr 1977; **Fellow:** Nuclear Medicine, VA Med Ctr 1978; Nuclear Medicine, Mount Sinai Hosp 1979; **Fac Appt:** Prof NuM, SUNY Downstate

Strauss, H William MD [NuM] - **Spec Exp:** Cardiac Imaging in Cancer Therapy; Thyroid Disorders; Cardiac Imaging; **Hospital:** Meml Sloan-Kettering Cancer Ctr; **Address:** 1275 York Avenue, New York, NY 10065; **Phone:** 800-525-2225; **Board Cert:** Nuclear Medicine 1988; **Med School:** SUNY Downstate 1965; **Resid:** Internal Medicine, Downstate Med Ctr 1967; Internal Medicine, Bellevue Hosp 1968; **Fellow:** Nuclear Medicine, Johns Hopkins Hosp 1970; **Fac Appt:** Prof NuM, Cornell Univ-Weill Med Coll

Van Heertum, Ronald L MD [NuM] - **Spec Exp:** PET Imaging; PET Imaging in Alzheimer's Disease; **Hospital:** NY-Presby Hosp/Columbia (page 66); **Address:** NY Presby Hosp, Dept Radiology, 622 W 168th St, Ste HP 3-320, New York, NY 10032; **Phone:** 212-305-7132; **Board Cert:** Diagnostic Radiology 1971; Nuclear Medicine 1973; **Med School:** UMDNJ-NJ Med Sch, Newark 1966; **Resid:** Diagnostic Radiology, St Vincents Hosp 1970; **Fellow:** Diagnostic Radiology, St Vincents Hosp Med Ctr 1971; Nuclear Medicine, SUNY-Upstate Med Ctr 1975; **Fac Appt:** Prof Rad, Columbia P&S

Wahl, Richard L MD [NuM] - **Spec Exp:** Radioimmunotherapy of Cancer; PET Imaging; PET Imaging-Breast; **Hospital:** Johns Hopkins Hosp - Baltimore (page 61); **Address:** Johns Hopkins Hosp, Radiology Dept, Nuclear Medicine Fl 3, 601 N Caroline St, JHOC-3223, Baltimore, MD 21287; **Phone:** 410-955-7226; **Board Cert:** Diagnostic Radiology 1982; Nuclear Radiology 1983; Nuclear Medicine 1985; **Med School:** Washington Univ, St Louis 1978; **Resid:** Diagnostic Radiology, Mallinckrodt Inst 1982; **Fellow:** Nuclear Radiology, Mallinckrodt Inst 1983; **Fac Appt:** Prof Rad, Johns Hopkins Univ

Nuclear Medicine

Southeast

Alazraki, Naomi P MD [NuM] - **Spec Exp:** Nuclear Oncology; **Hospital:** VA Med Ctr - Atlanta, Emory Univ Hosp; **Address:** VA Medical Ctr - Atlanta, 1670 Clairmont Rd, MC 115, Decatur, GA 30033; **Phone:** 404-728-7629; **Board Cert:** Nuclear Medicine 1972; Diagnostic Radiology 1972; **Med School:** Albert Einstein Coll Med 1966; **Resid:** Diagnostic Radiology, Univ Hospital 1971; **Fac Appt:** Prof, Emory Univ

Coleman, Ralph E MD [NuM] - **Spec Exp:** PET Imaging; SPECT Imaging; Tumor Imaging; **Hospital:** Duke Univ Med Ctr; **Address:** Duke Univ Med Ctr, Erwin Rd, Box 3949, Durham, NC 27710-0001; **Phone:** 919-684-7244; **Board Cert:** Nuclear Medicine 1974; Internal Medicine 1973; **Med School:** Washington Univ, St Louis 1968; **Resid:** Internal Medicine, Royal Victoria Hosp 1970; **Fellow:** Nuclear Medicine, Mallinckrodt Inst Radiology 1974; **Fac Appt:** Prof Rad, Duke Univ

Sandler, Martin P MD [NuM] - **Spec Exp:** Nuclear Endocrinology; Cardiac Imaging; PET Imaging; **Hospital:** Vanderbilt Univ Med Ctr; **Address:** Vanderbilt Univ Med Ctr, O-3300 MCN, 1161 21st Ave S, Nashville, TN 37232-2104; **Phone:** 615-322-0860; **Board Cert:** Nuclear Medicine 1983; **Med School:** South Africa 1972; **Resid:** Internal Medicine, Groote Schur Hosp; **Fellow:** Endocrinology, Diabetes & Metabolism, Vanderbilt Univ Med Ctr 1980; Nuclear Medicine, Vanderbilt Univ Med Ctr 1982; **Fac Appt:** Prof Rad, Vanderbilt Univ

Midwest

Dillehay, Gary MD [NuM] - **Spec Exp:** Lymphoma; Bone Densitometry; PET Imaging; **Hospital:** Northwestern Meml Hosp; **Address:** Northwestern Meml Hosp, Dept Nuclear Medicine, 675 N St Clair St, Galter 8-110, Chicago, IL 60611; **Phone:** 312-926-5119; **Board Cert:** Nuclear Medicine 1985; Nuclear Radiology 1987; **Med School:** Mayo Med Sch 1979; **Resid:** Diagnostic Radiology, Northwestern Meml Hosp 1983; Nuclear Medicine, Northwestern Meml Hosp 1984

Neumann, Donald R MD [NuM] - **Spec Exp:** Nuclear Oncology; Nuclear Cardiology; Parathyroid Disease; Pheochromocytoma; **Hospital:** Cleveland Clin Fdn (page 56); **Address:** Cleveland Clinic, MFI Dept, 9500 Euclid Ave, MS Gb3, Cleveland, OH 44195; **Phone:** 216-444-2193; **Board Cert:** Diagnostic Radiology 1987; Nuclear Radiology 1990; **Med School:** Wright State Univ 1980; **Resid:** Diagnostic Radiology, Mount Sinai Med Ctr 1987; **Fellow:** Magnetic Resonance Imaging, Mount Sinai Med Ctr 1987

Siegel, Barry A MD [NuM] - **Spec Exp:** Cancer Detection & Staging; PET Imaging; **Hospital:** Barnes-Jewish Hosp, St Louis Chldns Hosp; **Address:** Mallinckrodt Inst of Radiology, 510 S Kingshighway Blvd, St Louis, MO 63110-1016; **Phone:** 314-362-2809; **Board Cert:** Diagnostic Radiology 1977; Nuclear Medicine 1973; Nuclear Radiology 1981; **Med School:** Washington Univ, St Louis 1969; **Resid:** Diagnostic Radiology, Mallinckrodt Inst Radiology 1973; **Fellow:** Nuclear Medicine, Mallinckrodt Inst Radiology 1973; **Fac Appt:** Prof, Washington Univ, St Louis

Wiseman, Gregory MD [NuM] - **Spec Exp:** Lymphoma, Non-Hodgkin's; Multiple Myeloma; Radioimmunotherapy of Cancer; **Hospital:** Mayo Med Ctr & Clin - Rochester; **Address:** Mayo Clinic, Dept Nuc Med, 200 First St SW, Charlton Bldg, Rochester, MN 55905; **Phone:** 507-284-9599; **Board Cert:** Internal Medicine 1986; Hematology 1988; Nuclear Medicine 2002; **Med School:** Univ Utah 1983; **Resid:** Internal Medicine, Mayo Clinic 1986; Nuclear Medicine, Univ Washington Med Ctr 1992; **Fellow:** Hematology, Mayo Clinic 1989; Medical Oncology, Univ Washington 1991; **Fac Appt:** Asst Prof, Mayo Med Sch

Southwest

Podoloff, Donald MD [NuM] - **Spec Exp:** Prostate Cancer; Breast Cancer; Lymphoma; **Hospital:** UT MD Anderson Cancer Ctr; **Address:** UT MD Anderson Cancer Ctr, 1515 Holcombe Blvd, Box 57, Houston, TX 77030; **Phone:** 713-745-1160; **Board Cert:** Diagnostic Radiology 1973; Nuclear Medicine 1975; Nuclear Radiology 1975; **Med School:** SUNY Downstate 1964; **Resid:** Internal Medicine, Beth Israel Med Ctr 1968; Diagnostic Radiology, Wilford Hall USAF Med Ctr 1973; **Fac Appt:** Prof Rad, Univ Tex, Houston

West Coast and Pacific

Dae, Michael W MD [NuM] - **Spec Exp:** Nuclear Cardiology; Pediatric Nuclear Medicine; **Hospital:** UCSF Med Ctr; **Address:** UCSF, Dept Nuclear Medicine, 505 Parnassus Ave, Box 0252, San Francisco, CA 94143-0252; **Phone:** 415-353-1521; **Board Cert:** Pediatrics 1983; Nuclear Medicine 1984; **Med School:** Duke Univ 1976; **Resid:** Pediatrics, Chldns Hosp 1978; **Fellow:** Pediatric Cardiology, UCSF Med Ctr 1982; Nuclear Cardiology, UCSF Med Ctr 1983; **Fac Appt:** Prof, UCSF

Scheff, Alice M MD [NuM] - **Spec Exp:** PET Imaging; Thyroid Disorders; Neurologic Imaging; Cardiac Imaging; **Hospital:** Santa Clara Vly Med Ctr; **Address:** 751 S Bascom Ave, San Jose, CA 95128; **Phone:** 408-885-6970; **Board Cert:** Nuclear Medicine 1982; Nuclear Radiology 1983; **Med School:** Penn State Univ-Hershey Med Ctr 1978; **Resid:** Diagnostic Radiology, Penn State-Hershey Med Ctr 1982; Nuclear Medicine, Penn State-Hershey Med Ctr 1982; **Fellow:** Magnetic Resonance Imaging, Long Beach Meml Med Ctr 1993

Schelbert, Heinrich R MD/PhD [NuM] - **Spec Exp:** Nuclear Cardiology; Coronary Artery Disease; **Hospital:** Ronald Reagan UCLA Med Ctr; **Address:** B2-085J CHS, Box 95648, Los Angeles, CA 90095-6948; **Phone:** 310-825-3076; **Board Cert:** Nuclear Medicine 1976; **Med School:** Germany 1964; **Resid:** Internal Medicine, Mercy Med Ctr 1968; Cardiovascular Disease, Univ Duesseldorf Sch Med 1972; **Fellow:** Nuclear Medicine, UCSD 1973; Cardiovascular Disease, UCSD 1969

Waxman, Alan D MD [NuM] - **Spec Exp:** PET Imaging-Brain; Thyroid Cancer; Cancer Detection & Staging; **Hospital:** Cedars-Sinai Med Ctr, USC Univ Hosp - R K Eamer Med Plz; **Address:** Cedars-Sinai Med Ctr, Taper Imaging, 8700 Beverly Blvd, rm 1251, Los Angeles, CA 90048-1804; **Phone:** 310-423-4216; **Board Cert:** Nuclear Medicine 1972; **Med School:** USC Sch Med 1963; **Resid:** Nuclear Medicine, Wadsworth VA Hosp 1965; **Fellow:** Internal Medicine, Natl Inst Hlth 1967; **Fac Appt:** Clin Prof, USC Sch Med

NUCLEAR MEDICINE

Nuclear Medicine is an integral part of patient care, offering safe and cost-effective techniques to image the body physiology in order to provide diagnosis, management, treatment, and prevention of disease.

The Division of Nuclear Medicine in the Department of Radiology at NYU Medical Center is an integral component of its world-renowned multidisciplinary care. Offering the latest in technological expertise to medical specialties from pediatrics to cardiology to oncology to psychiatry, nuclear medicine truly cuts across all fields to deliver life-saving diagnoses. There are nearly one hundred different nuclear medicine imaging procedures available, with every major organ system imaged by Positron Emission Tomography (PET) scans.

PET scans are simple imaging studies that allow physicians to view the metabolic function of various organs and tissues in the body. Patients receive a simple injection in the arm of radiolabeled sugar. One hour later patients lie on the imaging table of the scanner while images are taken.

NYU Medical Center houses some of the most advanced radiology equipment in the world, including remote- controlled digital fluoroscopy and advanced digital subtraction angiography with three-dimensional capabilities. There are six high-field, large bore Magnetic Resonance Imaging (Mm) units, an open MRI unit, 10 Computed Tomography (CT) units (seven of which are the latest spiral units) and one of the largest concentration of Single-Photon Emission Computed Tomography (SPECT) gamma cameras in the United States. Over 90% of the reports at Tisch Hospital are dictated directly into the radiology information system using computerized voice recognition technology.

The NYU Department of Radiology has a large and distinguished faculty. In a recent year, department members wrote 146 peer-reviewed scientific papers as well as 11 complete texts and 55 chapters for other academic texts. Among the faculty are officers of national and regional scientific and professional societies, members of selective societies, and frequent peer reviewers and editors of professional journals.

Obstetrics & Gynecology

An obstetrician/gynecologist possesses special knowledge, skills and professional capability in the medical and surgical care of the female reproductive system and associated disorders. This physician serves as a consultant to other physicians and as a primary physician for women.

Training Required: Four years *plus* two years in clinical practice before certification is complete.

OBSTETRICS & GYNECOLOGY

New England

Cramer, Daniel W MD [ObG] - **Spec Exp:** Ovarian Cancer; Ovarian Cancer-High Risk; **Hospital:** Brigham & Women's Hosp, Dana-Farber Cancer Inst; **Address:** Brigham & Women's Hosp, Ob/Gyn Epidemiology Ctr, 221 Longwood Ave, RFB 336, Boston, MA 02115; **Phone:** 617-732-4895; **Board Cert:** Obstetrics & Gynecology 1979; **Med School:** Univ Colorado 1970; **Resid:** Obstetrics & Gynecology, Boston Womens Hosp 1976; **Fellow:** Public Health, Harvard Med Sch 1982; **Fac Appt:** Prof ObG, Harvard Med Sch

Laufer, Marc MD [ObG] - **Spec Exp:** Adolescent Gynecology; Endometriosis; Congenital Anomalies-Gynecologic; Pediatric Gynecology; **Hospital:** Children's Hospital - Boston, Brigham & Women's Hosp; **Address:** Chldns Hosp, Dept of Ped Gynecology, 300 Longwood Ave, Boston, MA 02115; **Phone:** 617-355-5785; **Board Cert:** Obstetrics & Gynecology 2007; **Med School:** Univ Pennsylvania 1986; **Resid:** Obstetrics & Gynecology, Brigham & Womens Hosp/Mass Genl Hosp 1990; **Fellow:** Reproductive Endocrinology, Brigham & Womens Hosp/Chldns Hosp 1992; Gynecology, Chldns Hosp 1992; **Fac Appt:** Assoc Prof ObG, Harvard Med Sch

Noller, Kenneth L MD [ObG] - **Spec Exp:** DES-Exposed Females; Gynecology Only; Cervical Cancer; **Hospital:** Tufts Med Ctr; **Address:** Tufts New England Med Ctr, Box 324, 750 Washington St, Boston, MA 02111; **Phone:** 617-636-2382; **Board Cert:** Obstetrics & Gynecology 1991; **Med School:** Creighton Univ 1970; **Resid:** Obstetrics & Gynecology, Mayo Clinic 1974; **Fac Appt:** Prof ObG, Tufts Univ

Nour, Nawal M MD [ObG] - **Spec Exp:** Female Genital Cutting (FGC) Education; **Hospital:** Brigham & Women's Hosp; **Address:** Brigham & Women's Hosp, Dept Ob/Gyn, 75 Francis St, Connors Ctr, 3rd Fl, Boston, MA 02115; **Phone:** 617-732-4740; **Board Cert:** Obstetrics & Gynecology 2002; **Med School:** Harvard Med Sch 1994; **Resid:** Obstetrics & Gynecology, Brgham & Women's Hosp 1998

Reilly, Raymond J MD [ObG] - **Spec Exp:** Gynecologic Surgery; **Hospital:** Brigham & Women's Hosp; **Address:** 1 Brookline Pl, Ste 522, Brookline, MA 02445; **Phone:** 617-731-3400; **Board Cert:** Obstetrics & Gynecology 1969; **Med School:** Ireland 1958; **Resid:** Obstetrics & Gynecology, Johns Hopkins Hosp 1964; **Fac Appt:** Assoc Prof ObG, Harvard Med Sch

Mid Atlantic

Brodman, Michael MD [ObG] - **Spec Exp:** Incontinence-Female; Laparoscopic Surgery; Pelvic Organ Prolapse Repair; Uro-Gynecology; **Hospital:** Mount Sinai Med Ctr (page 64); **Address:** Div of Obstetrics & Gynecology, 5 E 98th St Fl 2, Box 1170, New York, NY 10029; **Phone:** 212-241-7952; **Board Cert:** Obstetrics & Gynecology 2006; **Med School:** Mount Sinai Sch Med 1982; **Resid:** Obstetrics & Gynecology, Mount Sinai Hosp 1986; **Fellow:** Pelvic Surgery, Mount Sinai Hosp 1987; **Fac Appt:** Assoc Prof ObG, Mount Sinai Sch Med

Carson, Donald G MD [ObG] - **Hospital:** Magee-Womens Hosp - UPMC; **Address:** Ob/Gyn Assocs of Pittsburgh, 3380 Boulevard of the Allies, Ste 1, Pittsburgh, PA 15213; **Phone:** 412-621-7575; **Board Cert:** Obstetrics & Gynecology 2006; **Med School:** Univ Pittsburgh 1977; **Resid:** Obstetrics & Gynecology, Magee-Women's Hosp 1981; **Fac Appt:** Clin Prof ObG, Univ Pittsburgh

De Cherney, Alan Hersh MD [ObG] - **Spec Exp:** Infertility-Female; Reproductive Endocrinology; **Hospital:** Natl Inst of Hlth - Clin Ctr; **Address:** NICHD, NIH, Bldg 10, CRC, 1 East, 10 Center Drive, rm 1-3140, MS 1109, Bethesda, MD 20892-5800; **Phone:** 301-770-9667; **Board Cert:** Obstetrics & Gynecology 1989; Reproductive Endocrinology 1979; **Med School:** Temple Univ 1967; **Resid:** Obstetrics & Gynecology, Hosp Univ Penn 1972; **Fac Appt:** Prof ObG, UCLA

Evans, Mark I MD [ObG] - **Spec Exp:** Prenatal Diagnosis; Multiple Gestation; Fetal Therapy; Reproductive Genetics; **Hospital:** Mount Sinai Med Ctr (page 64); **Address:** Comprehensive Genetics, 131 E 65th St, New York, NY 10021; **Phone:** 212-744-2590; **Board Cert:** Obstetrics & Gynecology 2006; Clinical Genetics 1984; **Med School:** SUNY Downstate 1978; **Resid:** Obstetrics & Gynecology, Lying-In Hosp 1982; **Fellow:** Clinical Genetics, Natl Inst Hlth 1984; **Fac Appt:** Prof ObG, Mount Sinai Sch Med

Goldstein, Martin S MD [ObG] - **Spec Exp:** Incontinence; Laparoscopic Surgery; Uterine Fibroids; Pelvic Organ Prolapse Repair; **Hospital:** Mount Sinai Med Ctr (page 64); **Address:** 40 E 84th St, New York, NY 10028-1314; **Phone:** 212-472-6500; **Board Cert:** Obstetrics & Gynecology 1980; **Med School:** SUNY Hlth Sci Ctr 1966; **Resid:** Obstetrics & Gynecology, Mount Sinai Hosp 1971; **Fac Appt:** Assoc Clin Prof ObG, Mount Sinai Sch Med

Lucente, Vincent R MD [ObG] - **Spec Exp:** Uro-Gynecology; Pelvic Floor Reconstruction; Incontinence-Female; **Hospital:** St Luke's Hosp - Bethlehem, Abington Mem Hosp; **Address:** Park Professional Bldg, 2200 W Hamilton St, Ste 111, Allentown, PA 18104; **Phone:** 610-435-9575; **Board Cert:** Obstetrics & Gynecology 2006; **Med School:** SUNY Stony Brook 1985; **Resid:** Obstetrics & Gynecology, N Shore Univ Hosp 1989; **Fellow:** Uro-Gynecology, Methodist Hosp 1990; **Fac Appt:** Clin Prof ObG, Temple Univ

Minkoff, Howard L MD [ObG] - **Spec Exp:** AIDS/HIV in Pregnancy-Consultation; Pregnancy-High Risk, Consultation; **Hospital:** Maimonides Med Ctr (page 63); **Address:** Maimonides Med Ctr, Dept Ob-Gyn, 4802 Tenth Ave, Brooklyn, NY 11219; **Phone:** 718-283-7973; **Board Cert:** Obstetrics & Gynecology 1995; Maternal & Fetal Medicine 1995; **Med School:** Penn State Univ-Hershey Med Ctr 1975; **Resid:** Obstetrics & Gynecology, Kings Co Hosp Ctr 1979; Obstetrics & Gynecology, SUNY Hlth Sci Ctr 1981; **Fellow:** Maternal & Fetal Medicine, Kings Co Hosp Ctr 1981; **Fac Appt:** Prof ObG, SUNY Hlth Sci Ctr

Plante, Lauren A MD [ObG] - **Spec Exp:** Pregnancy-High Risk; **Hospital:** Thomas Jefferson Univ Hosp; **Address:** 834 Chestnut St, Ste 400, Philadelphia, PA 19107-5113; **Phone:** 215-955-5000; **Board Cert:** Anesthesiology 2004; Obstetrics & Gynecology 2006; Maternal & Fetal Medicine 2006; Critical Care Medicine 1993; **Med School:** Albert Einstein Coll Med 1984; **Resid:** Anesthesiology, Montefiore Med Ctr 1989; Obstetrics & Gynecology, Hahnemann Univ Hosp 1994; **Fellow:** Critical Care Medicine, Montefiore Med Ctr 1990; Maternal & Fetal Medicine, Temple Univ Med Ctr 1998

Scher, Jonathan MD [ObG] - **Spec Exp:** Miscarriage-Recurrent; Pregnancy-High Risk; **Hospital:** Mount Sinai Med Ctr (page 64); **Address:** 1126 Park Ave, New York, NY 10128-1203; **Phone:** 212-427-7400; **Board Cert:** Obstetrics & Gynecology 1981; **Med School:** South Africa 1964; **Resid:** Obstetrics & Gynecology, Groote Schuur Hosp 1970; Obstetrics & Gynecology, Kings College Hosp 1972; **Fac Appt:** Asst Clin Prof ObG, Mount Sinai Sch Med

Wiesenfeld, Harold C MD [ObG] - **Spec Exp:** Infectious Diseases-Gynecologic; Sexually Transmitted Diseases; **Hospital:** Magee-Womens Hosp - UPMC; **Address:** Magee-Women's Hosp, Dept Ob/Gyn, 300 Halket St, Pittsburgh, PA 15213; **Phone:** 412-641-6412; **Board Cert:** Obstetrics & Gynecology 2006; **Med School:** McGill Univ 1987; **Resid:** Obstetrics & Gynecology, McGill Univ 1990; **Fac Appt:** Assoc Prof ObG, Univ Pittsburgh

Obstetrics & Gynecology

Witter, Frank R MD [ObG] - **Spec Exp:** Pregnancy-High Risk; Multiple Gestation; Lupus/SLE in Pregnancy; **Hospital:** Johns Hopkins Hosp - Baltimore (page 61); **Address:** 600 N Wolfe St, Nelson 2170, Baltimore, MD 21287; **Phone:** 410-955-1421; **Board Cert:** Obstetrics & Gynecology 1997; Maternal & Fetal Medicine 1997; **Med School:** Univ Chicago-Pritzker Sch Med 1976; **Resid:** Obstetrics & Gynecology, Johns Hopkins Hosp 1980; **Fellow:** Maternal & Fetal Medicine, Johns Hopkins Hosp 1982; Clinical Pharmacology, Johns Hopkins Hosp 1984; **Fac Appt:** Prof ObG, Johns Hopkins Univ

Young, Bruce MD [ObG] - **Spec Exp:** Infertility; Minimally Invasive Surgery; Twin to Twin Transfusion Syndrome (TTTS); Miscarriage-Recurrent; **Hospital:** NYU Med Ctr (page 68); **Address:** 530 1st Ave, HCC-5th Fl, Ste 5G, New York, NY 10016; **Phone:** 212-263-6359; **Board Cert:** Obstetrics & Gynecology 1970; Maternal & Fetal Medicine 1975; **Med School:** NYU Sch Med 1963; **Resid:** Obstetrics & Gynecology, New York Univ Med Ctr 1968; **Fellow:** Reproductive Endocrinology, New York Univ Med Ctr 1968; **Fac Appt:** Prof ObG, NYU Sch Med

Southeast

Duff, W Patrick MD [ObG] - **Spec Exp:** Pregnancy-High Risk; Infectious Disease; Maternal & Fetal Medicine; **Hospital:** Shands at Univ of FL; **Address:** Magnolia Park Women's Health, 3951 NW 48th Terr, Ste 101, Gainesville, FL 32606; **Phone:** 352-265-6200; **Board Cert:** Obstetrics & Gynecology 2003; Maternal & Fetal Medicine 2003; **Med School:** Georgetown Univ 1974; **Resid:** Obstetrics & Gynecology, Walter Reed Med Ctr 1978; **Fellow:** Maternal & Fetal Medicine, UT - San Antonio 1983; **Fac Appt:** Prof ObG, Univ S Fla Coll Med

Filip, Stanley J MD [ObG] - **Spec Exp:** Uterine Fibroids; Menopause Problems; Hysterectomy Alternatives; Endometriosis; **Hospital:** Duke Univ Med Ctr, Durham Regional Hosp; **Address:** 3116 N Duke St, Durham, NC 27704; **Phone:** 919-684-2471; **Board Cert:** Obstetrics & Gynecology 1985; **Med School:** Mount Sinai Sch Med 1979; **Resid:** Obstetrics & Gynecology, Univ Colo Hlth Scis Ctr 1983

Hager, W David MD [ObG] - **Spec Exp:** Infectious Diseases-Gynecologic; Sexually Transmitted Diseases; **Hospital:** Central Baptist Hosp; **Address:** 1720 Nicholasville Rd, Lexington, KY 40503; **Phone:** 859-278-0363; **Board Cert:** Obstetrics & Gynecology 1993; **Med School:** Univ KY Coll Med 1972; **Resid:** Obstetrics & Gynecology, Univ Kentucky Med Ctr 1976; **Fac Appt:** Prof ObG, Univ KY Coll Med

Kovac, S Robert MD [ObG] - **Spec Exp:** Pelvic Reconstruction; **Hospital:** Emory Univ Hosp, Grady Hlth Sys; **Address:** Emory Clinic A, Dept Ob/Gyn, 1365 Clifton Rd NE Fl 4, Atlanta, GA 30322; **Phone:** 404-778-3401; **Board Cert:** Obstetrics & Gynecology 1979; **Med School:** Univ MO-Columbia Sch Med 1964; **Resid:** Obstetrics & Gynecology, Barnes JewishHosp 1970; **Fellow:** Reconstructive Pelvic Surgery, Barnes Hosp 1969; **Fac Appt:** Prof ObG, Emory Univ

Morgan, Linda S MD [ObG] - **Spec Exp:** Gynecologic Cancer; Women's Health; **Hospital:** Shands at Univ of FL; **Address:** Univ of Florida, PO Box 100294, Dept Ob/Gyn, Gainesville, FL 32610; **Phone:** 352-392-4161; **Board Cert:** Obstetrics & Gynecology 2006; Gynecologic Oncology 2006; **Med School:** Med Coll PA Hahnemann 1975; **Resid:** Obstetrics & Gynecology, Shands Hosp 1979; **Fellow:** Gynecologic Oncology, Mass Genl Hosp 1981; **Fac Appt:** Prof ObG, Univ Fla Coll Med

Sanz, Luis E MD [ObG] - **Spec Exp:** Uro-Gynecology; Hysteroscopic Surgery; Vaginal Reconstructive Surgery; Pelvic Reconstruction; **Hospital:** Virginia Hosp Ctr - Arlington; **Address:** 1625 N George Mason Drive, Ste 475, Arlington, VA 22205; **Phone:** 703-717-4000; **Board Cert:** Obstetrics & Gynecology 1982; **Med School:** Georgetown Univ 1976; **Resid:** Obstetrics & Gynecology, Georgetown Univ Hosp 1980; **Fellow:** Advanced Pelvic Surgery, Georgetown Univ 1982; **Fac Appt:** Prof ObG, Georgetown Univ

Simpson, Joe Leigh MD [ObG] - **Spec Exp:** Prenatal Diagnosis; Ovarian Failure; Infertility/Genetics; **Hospital:** Mount Sinai Med Ctr - Miami; **Address:** Florida International University, University Park HLS 693, 11200 SW H St, Miami, FL 33199; **Phone:** 305-348-0613; **Board Cert:** Obstetrics & Gynecology 2004; Clinical Genetics 1982; **Med School:** Duke Univ 1968; **Resid:** Obstetrics & Gynecology, NY Hosp-Cornell Med Ctr 1973; **Fac Appt:** Prof ObG, Baylor Coll Med

Steege, John F MD [ObG] - **Spec Exp:** Laparoscopic Surgery; Endometriosis; Pain-Pelvic & Perineal; Gynecologic Surgery; **Hospital:** Univ NC Hosps; **Address:** Univ NC-Dept OB/GYN, CB 7570, Chapel Hill, NC 27599-7570; **Phone:** 919-966-7764; **Board Cert:** Obstetrics & Gynecology 1978; **Med School:** Yale Univ 1972; **Resid:** Obstetrics & Gynecology, Yale - New Haven Hosp 1976; **Fac Appt:** Prof ObG, Univ NC Sch Med

Underwood, Paul B MD [ObG] - **Spec Exp:** Pelvic Reconstruction; Women's Health over age 40; **Hospital:** MUSC Med Ctr; **Address:** 1280 Johnnie Dodds Blvd, Ste 200, Mt Pleasant, SC 29464; **Phone:** 843-881-1312; **Board Cert:** Obstetrics & Gynecology 1989; Gynecologic Oncology 1974; **Med School:** Med Univ SC 1959; **Resid:** Obstetrics & Gynecology, Med University SC 1964; **Fellow:** Gynecologic Oncology, MD Anderson Hosp 1967; **Fac Appt:** Prof ObG, Med Univ SC

Midwest

De Lia, Julian E MD [ObG] - **Spec Exp:** Fetal Surgery; Twin to Twin Transfusion Syndrome (TTTS); **Hospital:** Wheaton Franciscan Hlthcare-St Joseph-Milwaukee; **Address:** TTTS Inst, WFHC-St Joseph, 5000 W Chambers St, Milwaukee, WI 53210-1688; **Phone:** 414-447-3535; **Board Cert:** Obstetrics & Gynecology 1993; **Med School:** UMDNJ-NJ Med Sch, Newark 1972; **Resid:** Obstetrics & Gynecology, St Barnabas Med Ctar 1976; **Fac Appt:** Assoc Prof ObG, Med Coll Wisc

DeLancey, John O MD [ObG] - **Spec Exp:** Uro-Gynecology; Incontinence; Pelvic Organ Prolapse Repair; **Hospital:** Univ Michigan Hlth Sys; **Address:** Univ Mich Med Ctr, Dept ObGyn, 1500 E Med Ctr Drive, rm L4100-WH, Ann Arbor, MI 48109-0276; **Phone:** 734-763-6295; **Board Cert:** Obstetrics & Gynecology 1997; **Med School:** Univ Mich Med Sch 1977; **Resid:** Obstetrics & Gynecology, Univ Mich Med Ctr 1981; **Fac Appt:** Prof ObG, Univ Mich Med Sch

Gonik, Bernard MD [ObG] - **Spec Exp:** Maternal & Fetal Medicine; Infectious Disease; Prenatal Diagnosis; Vaccinations in Pregnancy; **Hospital:** Sinai-Grace Hosp - Detroit; **Address:** Womens Diagnostic Unit, 6071 W Outer Drive, Detroit, MI 48235-2624; **Phone:** 313-966-1880; **Board Cert:** Obstetrics & Gynecology 2006; Maternal & Fetal Medicine 2006; **Med School:** Mich State Univ 1978; **Resid:** Obstetrics & Gynecology, Univ Texas Med Sch 1982; **Fellow:** Maternal & Fetal Medicine, Univ Texas Med Sch 1985; **Fac Appt:** Prof ObG, Wayne State Univ

Hale, Douglass S MD [ObG] - **Spec Exp:** Uro-Gynecology; Pelvic Floor Reconstruction; Reconstructive Surgery; Robotic Surgery; **Hospital:** Methodist Hosp - Indianapolis; **Address:** Urogynecology Assocs, 1633 N Capital Ave, Ste 436, Indianapolis, IN 46202; **Phone:** 317-962-6600; **Board Cert:** Obstetrics & Gynecology 2006; **Med School:** Med Coll OH 1989; **Resid:** Obstetrics & Gynecology, T Jefferson Univ Hosp 1993; **Fellow:** Uro-Gynecology, Methodist Hosp 1995; Reconstructive Surgery, Methodist Hosp 1995; **Fac Appt:** Assoc Clin Prof ObG, Indiana Univ

Obstetrics & Gynecology

Karram, Mickey M MD [ObG] - **Spec Exp:** Uro-Gynecology; Pelvic Floor Reconstruction; Incontinence-Female; **Hospital:** Good Samaritan Hosp - Cincinnati; **Address:** Good Samaritan Hosp, 7759 University Drive, Ste D, Westchester, OH 45069; **Phone:** 513-463-2500; **Board Cert:** Obstetrics & Gynecology 1998; **Med School:** Egypt 1982; **Resid:** Obstetrics & Gynecology, Good Samaritan Hosp 1985; **Fellow:** Gynecologic Urology, Harbor Hosp-UCLA 1986; **Fac Appt:** Prof ObG, Univ Cincinnati

Levine, Elliot MD [ObG] - **Spec Exp:** Sexually Transmitted Diseases; Sexual Dysfunction; Vulvar & Vaginal Disorders; **Hospital:** Adv Illinois Masonic Med Ctr, Weiss Meml Hosp; **Address:** 4646 N Marine Drive, Ste 8A, Chicago, IL 60640; **Phone:** 773-564-5355; **Board Cert:** Obstetrics & Gynecology 1984; **Med School:** Ros Franklin Univ/Chicago Med Sch 1978; **Resid:** Obstetrics & Gynecology, Illinois Masonic Med Ctr 1982; **Fac Appt:** Asst Prof ObG, Rush Med Coll

Lipscomb, Gary H MD [ObG] - **Spec Exp:** Pregnancy-High Risk; Cervical Cancer; Uro-Gynecology; **Hospital:** Northwestern Meml Hosp; **Address:** 675 N St Clair Fl 14 - rm 200, Galter Pavilion, Chicago, IL 60611; **Phone:** 312-695-7382; **Board Cert:** Obstetrics & Gynecology 1997; **Med School:** Univ Tenn Coll Med, Memphis 1981; **Resid:** Obstetrics & Gynecology, Univ Tenn Affil Hosps 1985; **Fac Appt:** Prof ObG, Northwestern Univ

Merritt, Diane F MD [ObG] - **Spec Exp:** Adolescent Gynecology; Pediatric Gynecology; Endometriosis; **Hospital:** Barnes-Jewish Hosp, St Louis Chldns Hosp; **Address:** Washington Univ Sch Medicine, 660 S Euclid Ave, St Louis, MO 63110; **Phone:** 314-362-4211; **Board Cert:** Obstetrics & Gynecology 1984; **Med School:** NYU Sch Med 1975; **Resid:** Surgery, Barnes Hosp-Wash Univ 1977; Obstetrics & Gynecology, Barnes Hosp-Wash Univ 1980; **Fac Appt:** Prof ObG, Washington Univ, St Louis

Shulman, Lee MD [ObG] - **Spec Exp:** Prenatal Diagnosis; Breast Cancer Genetics; Ovarian Cancer Genetics; **Hospital:** Northwestern Meml Hosp, Rush Univ Med Ctr; **Address:** Northwestern Univ, Dept Ob/Gyn, 333 E Superior St, Ste 484, Chicago, IL 60611; **Phone:** 312-926-6622; **Board Cert:** Obstetrics & Gynecology 1999; Clinical Genetics 1990; **Med School:** Cornell Univ-Weill Med Coll 1983; **Resid:** Obstetrics & Gynecology, North Shore Univ Hosp 1987; **Fellow:** Reproductive Genetics, Univ Tenn Med Ctr 1989; **Fac Appt:** Prof ObG, Northwestern Univ

Great Plains and Mountains

Bury, Robert J MD [ObG] - **Spec Exp:** Infertility; Laser Surgery; Microsurgery; **Hospital:** St. Alexius Med Ctr - Bismarck; **Address:** Mid Dakota Clinic-Center for Women, PO Box 5538, Bismarck, ND 58506; **Phone:** 701-530-6000; **Board Cert:** Obstetrics & Gynecology 1981; **Med School:** Baylor Coll Med 1975; **Resid:** Obstetrics & Gynecology, Baylor Affil Hosp 1979; **Fac Appt:** Clin Prof ObG, Univ ND Sch Med

Byrne, Janice LB MD [ObG] - **Hospital:** Univ Utah Hosps and Clins; **Address:** 50 N Medical Drive, Salt Lake City, UT 84132; **Phone:** 801-581-2719; **Board Cert:** Obstetrics & Gynecology 2005; Clinical Genetics 2006; Maternal & Fetal Medicine 2005; **Med School:** Univ Tex SW, Dallas 1987; **Resid:** Obstetrics & Gynecology, Univ Utah Hosps & Clins 1991; **Fellow:** Clinical Genetics, Univ Utah Hosps & Clins 1993; Maternal & Fetal Medicine, Univ Utah Hosps & Clins 1994; **Fac Appt:** Assoc Clin Prof ObG, Univ Utah

Southwest

Carr, Bruce MD [ObG] - **Spec Exp:** Infertility-Female; **Hospital:** UT Southwestern Med Ctr - Dallas, Parkland Meml Hosp - Dallas; **Address:** 5323 Harry Hines Blvd, Outpatient Bldg Fl 6, Dallas, TX 75390-8865; **Phone:** 214-648-8846; **Board Cert:** Obstetrics & Gynecology 2000; Reproductive Endocrinology 2000; **Med School:** Univ Mich Med Sch 1971; **Resid:** Obstetrics & Gynecology, Parkland Meml Hosp 1975; **Fellow:** Reproductive Endocrinology, Univ Texas SW Med Ctr 1980; **Fac Appt:** Prof ObG, Univ Tex SW, Dallas

Cornella, Jeffrey L MD [ObG] - **Spec Exp:** Pelvic Reconstructive Surgery; Robotic Surgery; Laparoscopic Surgery; Vaginal Reconstruction; **Hospital:** Mayo Clinic - Scottsdale; **Address:** Mayo Clinic Scottsdale, 13400 E Shea Blvd, Scottsdale, AZ 85259; **Phone:** 480-342-2867; **Board Cert:** Obstetrics & Gynecology 1998; **Med School:** Washington Univ, St Louis 1981; **Resid:** Obstetrics & Gynecology, Mayo Clinic 1986; **Fellow:** Uro-Gynecology, UC Irvine 1987; **Fac Appt:** Prof ObG, Mayo Med Sch

Faro, Sebastian MD/PhD [ObG] - **Spec Exp:** Infections in Pregnancy; Infectious Diseases-Gynecologic; Sexually Transmitted Diseases; **Hospital:** Woman's Hosp TX, The, St Luke's Episcopal Hosp - Houston; **Address:** 7400 Fannin, Ste 840, Houston, TX 77054; **Phone:** 713-799-9091; **Board Cert:** Obstetrics & Gynecology 2006; **Med School:** Creighton Univ 1975; **Resid:** Obstetrics & Gynecology, Creighton Univ 1978; **Fac Appt:** Clin Prof ObG, Univ Tex, Houston

Young, Amy E MD [ObG] - **Hospital:** Baylor Univ Medical Ctr; **Address:** 6620 Main St, Ste 1450, Houston, TX 77030-2717; **Phone:** 713-798-7500; **Board Cert:** Obstetrics & Gynecology 2005; **Med School:** Univ Miss 1994; **Resid:** Obstetrics & Gynecology, Baylor Coll Med 1999

West Coast and Pacific

Eschenbach, David A MD [ObG] - **Spec Exp:** Gynecologic Surgery-Complex; Infectious Disease; Vulvar & Vaginal Disorders; **Hospital:** Univ Wash Med Ctr; **Address:** Univ Washington Women's Health Care, 4245 Roosevelt Way NE, Box 354765, Seattle, WA 98105-6920; **Phone:** 206-598-5500; **Board Cert:** Obstetrics & Gynecology 1975; **Med School:** Univ Wisc 1968; **Resid:** Obstetrics & Gynecology, Univ Wash Hosp 1973; **Fellow:** Infectious Disease, Univ Wash Hosp 1974; **Fac Appt:** Prof ObG, Univ Wash

Sweet, Richard L MD [ObG] - **Spec Exp:** Sexually Transmitted Diseases; Infectious Diseases-Gynecologic; Women's Health; Infections in Pregnancy; **Hospital:** UC Davis Med Ctr; **Address:** UC Davis Women's Center for Health, 4860 Y St, Ste 2500, Sacramento, CA 95817; **Phone:** 916-734-6670; **Board Cert:** Obstetrics & Gynecology 1975; **Med School:** Univ Mich Med Sch 1966; **Resid:** Obstetrics & Gynecology, Univ Mich Med Ctr 1973; **Fac Appt:** Prof ObG, UC Davis

Cleveland Clinic

Obstetrics and Gynecology

Reproductive Endocrinology and Infertility: Our Reproductive Endocrinology and Infertility Program involves close collaboration among male and female infertility specialists, andrologists and embryologists, as well as our colleagues in the Minimally Invasive Surgery Center. Cleveland Clinic reproductive surgeons were among the first to routinely remove advanced endometriosis laparoscopically. Many procedures today are performed with robotic assistance.

Urogynecology and Reconstructive Pelvic Surgery: This Center offers cutting-edge and traditional surgery for urinary incontinence and pelvic organ prolapse, along with medical and behavioral therapy.

Center for Female Pelvic Medicine and Reconstructive Surgery: Cleveland Clinic urogynecologists established the Center for Female Pelvic Medicine and Reconstructive Surgery in conjunction with Cleveland Clinic urologists and colorectal surgeons. The sub specialists on this team treat incontinence and prolapse via the abdominal, vaginal and laparoscopic routes.

Maternal-Fetal Medicine/Obstetrics: Cleveland Clinic maternal-fetal medicine specialists provide overall management of complicated pregnancies, beginning with genetic counseling for high-risk patients. Our dedicated Maternal-Fetal Testing Center offers high-risk consults, detailed ultrasound with Doppler wave form analysis, first-trimester nuchal translucency ultrasound screening and other sophisticated diagnostic testing.

The Fetal Care Center: The Fetal Care Center involves a multidisciplinary team of perinatologists, neonatologists, pediatric surgeons and other specialists. Through collaboration and communication, we provide prenatal diagnosis using state-of-the-art techniques such as high-resolution ultrasound, fetal MRI and fetoscopy. We then apply this information as we develop a management plan for pregnancy, delivery and newborn care.

Menstrual Disorders, Fibroids and Hysteroscopic Services: This Center offers unified and streamlined consultations, workups and treatment for menstrual dysfunction and uterine fibroids in the least invasive manner, so as to preserve a woman's reproductive potential.

Gynecologic Oncology: Our gynecologic oncologists have garnered national and international recognition for expertise in complex reproductive cancers, clinical and basic research, and preventive oncology. Cleveland Clinic gynecologists were among the first to treat early cervical and endometrial cancers laparoscopically. In performing less invasive surgical procedures, we always weigh curative potential against preservation of fertility. We offer oocyte, embryo and ovarian tissue cryopreservation for cancer patients.

Women's Health Center: The Cleveland Clinic Women's Health Center offers a full range of specialized women's health services in one location. We manage menopause, hormone therapy, vulvar disorders, and premenstrual dysthymic disorder and hormonally exacerbated mood disorders. We offer evaluation and treatment for women with urinary incontinence, osteoporosis or breast concerns. Breast specialists evaluate and treat breast cancer as well as benign breast disease in our center.

For more information about the Cleveland Clinic Department of Obstetrics and Gynecology, to schedule a second opinion or to learn about assistance for out-of-town patients, call 800.890.2467 or visit www.clevelandclinic.org/obgyntopdocs.

Department of Obstetrics and Gynecology
9500 Euclid Avenue / AC311 | Cleveland OH 44195

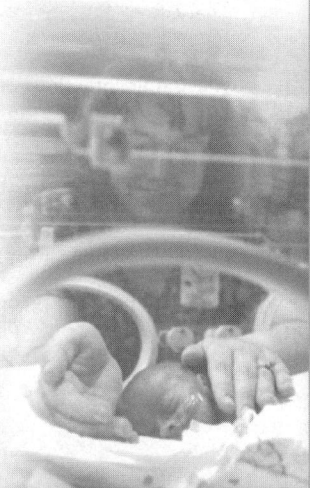

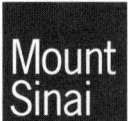
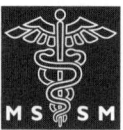

MOUNT SINAI
SCHOOL OF
MEDICINE

Building on more than a century of leadership in providing healthcare to women, the Department of Obstetrics, Gynecology, and Reproductive Science at The Mount Sinai Medical Center offers special expertise in:

- **General obstetrics,** including genetic counseling, prenatal care, labor and delivery management, and postpartum care. In addition to our talented physicians, other healthcare professionals are integrated into our practice, including genetic counselors, nutritionists, social workers, nurse midwives, childbirth educators, and lactation/breastfeeding specialists.

- **High-risk obstetrics,** including advanced techniques in prenatal diagnosis and consultations in the management of complicated pregnancies. Our ultrasound unit is recognized for its expertise in fetal anatomy ultrasound assessments. The latest technology, including 4D imaging, is employed. Antepartum testing, including amniocentesis, chorionic villus sampling, and fetal blood sampling are all routinely performed at Mount Sinai.

- **Reproductive endocrinology and infertility,** including diagnosis and treatment of both female and male factor infertility. Treatment options for women include fertility medications, intrauterine insemination, in vitro fertilization, intracytoplasmic sperm injections, and ovum donation.

- **General gynecology,** including cancer screening, management of abnormal Pap smears, family planning, and surgical management of fibroids, endometriosis, and other benign gynecologic conditions.

- **Gynecologic infectious diseases,** including the treatment and prevention of sexually transmitted infections and consultations on obstetrical and gynecological infections.

- **Gynecologic oncology,** including care for women with cancers of the ovary, uterus, cervix, vulva, and vagina.

- **Minimally invasive surgery** for many conditions.

- **Urogynecology and reconstructive pelvic surgery,** including lower urinary tract disorders.

INNOVATIVE APPROACHES TO PRENATAL CARE AND THE TREATMENT OF GYNECOLOGIC CANCERS
Known worldwide for excellence and innovative approaches to prenatal diagnosis and fetal therapy, Mount Sinai's Department of Obstetrics, Gynecology, and Reproductive Science has a long tradition of advancing clinical practice through patient-oriented research. Faculty members are pioneering work in diverse areas, including first- and second-trimester screening for fetal chromosomal abnormalities, vaccines for the prevention of sexually transmitted infections, minimally invasive surgical techniques, and new approaches to the diagnosis and treatment of gender-specific cancers.

NYU Langone Medical Center

550 First Avenue (at 31St Street)
New York, NY 10016
Physician Referral:
(888)7-NYU-MED (888-769-8633)
www.nyumc.org

WOMEN'S HEALTH

NYU Langone Medical Center supports a comprehensive group of programs and services designed specifically for women's medical needs. Services range from primary care to the most specialized clinical care programs available in the nation. Supported by the most sophisticated research and advanced training at NYU School of Medicine, the Department of Obstetrics and Gynecology at NYU Langone Medical Center offers a unique, abundant blend of high quality therapies and regimens, as well as leading-edge research technologies and methods.

Along with routine gynecological care, many other services are offered including: pelvic ultrasound; aspiration of breast cysts; evaluation of infertility, including the special needs of same-sex couples; colposcopy (a diagnostic evaluation of abnormal pap smears); LEEP (a loop electrosurgical procedure used to diagnose and treat cervical cancer); cryotherapy for vaginal wafts; and bone density testing for osteoporosis prevention and treatment.

The Obstetrics program also offers a broad range of services. Among these are prenatal care that gives equal emphasis to the well-being of the mother and of the fetus; fetal monitoring through ultrasound and other techniques; childbirth preparedness and breastfeeding classes; and consultation for high-risk pregnancies, including treatment for women who experience recurrent pregnancy loss.

At NYU Langone Medical Center, the backbone of patient care is the continued research into gynecologic diseases. With world-class faculty leading clinical investigations into disorders that can occur at any stage of a woman's life, doctors at NYU Langone Medical Center are equipped with the latest findings to treat women throughout their lives.

Ophthalmology

An ophthalmologist has the knowledge and professional skills needed to provide comprehensive eye and vision care. Ophthalmologists are medically trained to diagnose, monitor and medically or surgically treat all ocular and visual disorders. This includes problems affecting the eye and its component structures, the eyelids, the orbit and the visual pathways. In so doing, an ophthalmologist prescribes vision services, including glasses and contact lenses.

Training Required: Four years

OPHTHALMOLOGY

New England

Aiello, Lloyd M MD [Oph] - **Spec Exp:** Diabetic Eye Disease/Retinopathy; **Hospital:** Beth Israel Deaconess Med Ctr - Boston; **Address:** Beetham Eye Inst-Joslin Diabetes Ctr, 1 Joslin Pl, Boston, MA 02215-5397; **Phone:** 617-732-2520; **Board Cert:** Ophthalmology 1966; **Med School:** Boston Univ 1960; **Resid:** Ophthalmology, Mass Eye & Ear Infirm 1964; **Fac Appt:** Assoc Clin Prof Oph, Harvard Med Sch

Dana, Reza MD [Oph] - **Spec Exp:** Corneal Disease & Transplant; Dry Eye Syndrome; **Hospital:** Mass Eye & Ear Infirmary, Mass Eye & Ear Infirmary; **Address:** Mass Eye & Ear Infirmary, 243 Charles St, Boston, MA 02114; **Phone:** 617-573-4331; **Board Cert:** Ophthalmology 2006; **Med School:** Johns Hopkins Univ 1989; **Resid:** Ophthalmology, Illinois Eye & Ear Infirmary 1993; **Fellow:** Cornea & Ext Eye Disease, Wills Eye Hosp 1994; Uveitis, Mass Eye & Ear Infirmary 1995; **Fac Appt:** Assoc Prof Oph, Harvard Med Sch

Duker, Jay S MD [Oph] - **Spec Exp:** Retinal Disorders; Retinal Disorders-Pediatric; Diabetic Eye Disease/Retinopathy; **Hospital:** Tufts Med Ctr; **Address:** New England Eye Ctr, 750 Washington St, Box 450, Boston, MA 02111; **Phone:** 617-636-4600; **Board Cert:** Ophthalmology 1989; **Med School:** Jefferson Med Coll 1984; **Resid:** Ophthalmology, Wills Eye Hosp 1988; **Fellow:** Vitreoretinal Surgery & Disease, Wills Eye Hosp 1990; **Fac Appt:** Assoc Prof Oph, Tufts Univ

Foster, Charles Stephen MD [Oph] - **Spec Exp:** Uveitis; Corneal Disease; Cataract Surgery; **Hospital:** Mass Eye & Ear Infirmary; **Address:** 5 Cambridge Ctr Fl 8, Cambridge, MA 02142; **Phone:** 866-353-6377; **Board Cert:** Ophthalmology 1976; **Med School:** Duke Univ 1969; **Resid:** Ophthalmology, Barnes Hosp 1975; **Fellow:** Cornea, Mass EE Infirm-Harvard 1976; Ocular Immunology, Mass EE Infirm-Harvard 1977; **Fac Appt:** Prof Oph, Harvard Med Sch

Hedges, Thomas R MD [Oph] - **Spec Exp:** Neuro-Ophthalmology; **Hospital:** Tufts Med Ctr; **Address:** New England Med Ctr, 750 Washington St, Box 450, Boston, MA 02111; **Phone:** 617-636-5488; **Board Cert:** Ophthalmology 1980; **Med School:** Tufts Univ 1975; **Resid:** Ophthalmology, Mass EE Infirm 1980; **Fellow:** Neurological Ophthalmology, UCSF Med Ctr 1981; **Fac Appt:** Prof Oph, Tufts Univ

Hunter, David G MD/PhD [Oph] - **Spec Exp:** Pediatric Ophthalmology; Eye Muscle Disorders; Strabismus; Cataract-Pediatric; **Hospital:** Children's Hospital - Boston; **Address:** Chlds Hosp Boston, Dept Ophthalmology, 300 Longwood Ave, Fegan 4, Boston, MA 02115; **Phone:** 617-355-6401; **Board Cert:** Ophthalmology 2003; **Med School:** Baylor Coll Med 1987; **Resid:** Ophthalmology, Mass EE Infirm 1991; **Fellow:** Pediatric Ophthalmology, Wilmer Ophthalmic Inst 1992; **Fac Appt:** Assoc Prof Oph, Harvard Med Sch

Kornmehl, Ernest W MD [Oph] - **Spec Exp:** Laser Vision Surgery; Cornea & External Eye Disease; Dry Eye Syndrome; **Hospital:** Mass Eye & Ear Infirmary, Brigham & Women's Hosp; **Address:** Kornmehl Laser Eye Assoc, 54 Washington St, Wellesley, MA 02481; **Phone:** 617-232-2090; **Board Cert:** Ophthalmology 1989; **Med School:** SUNY Downstate 1984; **Resid:** Ophthalmology, Yale-New Haven Hosp 1988; **Fellow:** Cornea & Ext Eye Disease, Mass E&E Infirmary 1990; **Fac Appt:** Assoc Clin Prof Oph, Tufts Univ

Miller, Joan W MD [Oph] - **Spec Exp:** Macular Degeneration; Retinal Disorders; **Hospital:** Mass Eye & Ear Infirmary; **Address:** Mass Eye & Ear Infirmary - Ophthalmology, 243 Charles St, Boston, MA 02114; **Phone:** 617-573-3915; **Board Cert:** Ophthalmology 1991; **Med School:** Harvard Med Sch 1985; **Resid:** Ophthalmology, Mass Eye & Ear Infirm 1989; **Fellow:** Retina, Mass Eye & Ear Infirm 1991; **Fac Appt:** Assoc Prof Oph, Harvard Med Sch

Mitchell, Paul Ralph MD [Oph] - **Spec Exp:** Pediatric Ophthalmology; **Hospital:** CT Chldns Med Ctr, Hartford Hosp; **Address:** 366 Colt Hwy, Route 6, Farmington, CT 06032-2547; **Phone:** 860-409-0449; **Board Cert:** Ophthalmology 1977; **Med School:** Geo Wash Univ 1970; **Resid:** Ophthalmology, Wills Eye Hosp 1976; **Fellow:** Pediatric Ophthalmology, Chldns Hosp MC/Geo Wash 1977; **Fac Appt:** Asst Clin Prof Oph, Univ Conn

Rizzo III, Joseph F MD [Oph] - **Spec Exp:** Neuro-Ophthalmology; Retinal Disorders; **Hospital:** Mass Eye & Ear Infirmary; **Address:** Mass Eye and Ear Infirmary, 243 Charles St, Boston, MA 02114; **Phone:** 617-573-3412; **Board Cert:** Neurology 1984; Ophthalmology 1987; **Med School:** Louisiana State U, New Orleans 1978; **Resid:** Neurology, Tufts-New Engl Med Ctr 1982; Ophthalmology, Boston Univ 1985; **Fellow:** Neurological Ophthalmology, Harvard Univ 1986; **Fac Appt:** Assoc Prof Oph, Harvard Med Sch

Rubin, Peter A D MD [Oph] - **Spec Exp:** Oculoplastic Surgery; Orbital & Eyelid Tumors/Cancer; Eyelid Cancer & Reconstruction; Eyelid Cosmetic & Reconstructive Surgery; **Hospital:** Beth Israel Deaconess Med Ctr - Boston; **Address:** Boston Eye Physicians, 44 Washington St, Brookline, MA 02445; **Phone:** 617-232-9600; **Board Cert:** Ophthalmology 1991; **Med School:** Yale Univ 1985; **Resid:** Ophthalmology, Manhattan EET Hosp 1989; **Fellow:** Oculoplastic Surgery, Mass EE Infirm 1990; **Fac Appt:** Assoc Prof Oph, Harvard Med Sch

Tsai, James C MD [Oph] - **Spec Exp:** Glaucoma; **Hospital:** Yale-New Haven Hosp; **Address:** Yale Eye Center, 40 Temple St, New Haven, CT 06520-8061; **Phone:** 203-785-2020; **Board Cert:** Ophthalmology 2006; **Med School:** Stanford Univ 1989; **Resid:** Ophthalmology, Doheny Eye Inst/USC 1993; **Fellow:** Glaucoma, Bascom Palmer Eye Inst 1994; Glaucoma, Moorfields Eye Hosp 1995; **Fac Appt:** Prof Oph, Yale Univ

Walton, David S MD [Oph] - **Spec Exp:** Glaucoma-Pediatric; Cataract-Pediatric; Neuro-Ophthalmology; **Hospital:** Mass Eye & Ear Infirmary, Mass Genl Hosp; **Address:** 2 Longfellow Pl, Ste 201, Boston, MA 02114; **Phone:** 617-227-3011; **Board Cert:** Ophthalmology 1969; Pediatrics 1983; **Med School:** Duke Univ 1961; **Resid:** Ophthalmology, Mass EE Infirm 1967; **Fellow:** Glaucoma, Mass EE Infirm 1968; **Fac Appt:** Prof Oph, Harvard Med Sch

Mid Atlantic

Abramson, David H MD [Oph] - **Spec Exp:** Eye Tumors/Cancer; Orbital Tumors/Cancer; Retinoblastoma; Melanoma-Choroidal (eye); **Hospital:** Meml Sloan-Kettering Cancer Ctr; **Address:** 1275 York Avenue, New York, NY 10065; **Phone:** 800-525-2225; **Board Cert:** Ophthalmology 1975; **Med School:** Albert Einstein Coll Med 1969; **Resid:** Ophthalmology, Harkness Eye Inst 1974; **Fellow:** Ocular Oncology, Columbia-Presby Med Ctr 1975; **Fac Appt:** Clin Prof Oph, Cornell Univ-Weill Med Coll

Behrens, Myles MD [Oph] - **Spec Exp:** Neuro-Ophthalmology; **Hospital:** NY-Presby Hosp/Columbia (page 66); **Address:** 635 W 165th St, New York, NY 10032-3701; **Phone:** 212-305-5415; **Board Cert:** Ophthalmology 1971; **Med School:** Columbia P&S 1962; **Resid:** Internal Medicine, Columbia Presby Hosp 1964; Ophthalmology, Columbia Presby Hosp 1970; **Fellow:** Neurological Ophthalmology, UCSF Med Ctr 1971; **Fac Appt:** Clin Prof Oph, Columbia P&S

Ophthalmology

Bressler, Neil M MD [Oph] - **Spec Exp:** Retinal Disorders; **Hospital:** Johns Hopkins Hosp - Baltimore (page 61); **Address:** Wilmer Eye Institute, 550 N Broadway, Ste 115, Baltimore, MD 21205; **Phone:** 410-955-8342; **Board Cert:** Ophthalmology 1987; **Med School:** Johns Hopkins Univ 1982; **Resid:** Internal Medicine, Johns Hopkins Hosp 1983; Ophthalmology, Mass Eye & Ear Infirm 1986; **Fellow:** Retina, Wilmer Inst/Johns Hopkins Hosp 1987; **Fac Appt:** Assoc Prof Oph, Johns Hopkins Univ

Brown, Gary C MD [Oph] - **Spec Exp:** Retinal Disorders; Retinal Vascular Diseases; **Hospital:** Wills Eye Hosp; **Address:** 910 E Willow Grove Ave, Wyndmoor, PA 19038; **Phone:** 215-233-4300; **Board Cert:** Ophthalmology 2003; **Med School:** SUNY Upstate Med Univ 1975; **Resid:** Ophthalmology, Wills Eye Hosp 1979; **Fellow:** Vitreoretinal Disease, Wills Eye Hosp 1981; **Fac Appt:** Prof Oph, Jefferson Med Coll

Brucker, Alexander J MD [Oph] - **Spec Exp:** Retinal Disorders; Retina/Vitreous Surgery; Macular Degeneration; **Hospital:** Penn Presby Med Ctr - UPHS (page 60); **Address:** Univ Penn, Scheie Eye Inst, 51 N 39th St, rm 517, Philadelphia, PA 19104; **Phone:** 215-662-8100; **Board Cert:** Ophthalmology 1977; **Med School:** NY Med Coll 1972; **Resid:** Ophthalmology, Friedenwald Inst 1976; **Fellow:** Retina/Vitreous, Johns Hopkins Hosp 1977; **Fac Appt:** Prof Oph, Univ Pennsylvania

Campochiaro, Peter MD [Oph] - **Spec Exp:** Retina/Vitreous Surgery; **Hospital:** Johns Hopkins Hosp - Baltimore (page 61); **Address:** Wilmer Ophthalmological Inst, 600 N Wolfe St, 719 Maumenee, Baltimore, MD 21287-9277; **Phone:** 410-955-5106; **Board Cert:** Ophthalmology 1983; **Med School:** Johns Hopkins Univ 1978; **Resid:** Ophthalmology, Univ Virginia 1982; **Fellow:** Retina/Vitreous, John Hopkins Univ 1984; **Fac Appt:** Prof Oph, Johns Hopkins Univ

Caputo, Anthony R MD [Oph] - **Spec Exp:** Pediatric Ophthalmology; Strabismus; **Hospital:** Columbus Hosp; **Address:** 556 Eagle Rock Ave, Ste 203, Roseland, NJ 07068-1500; **Phone:** 973-228-3111; **Board Cert:** Ophthalmology 1976; **Med School:** Italy 1969; **Resid:** Ophthalmology, UMDNJ-Univ Hosp 1974; **Fellow:** Ophthalmology, Wills Eye Hosp 1975; **Fac Appt:** Prof Oph, UMDNJ-NJ Med Sch, Newark

Chang, Stanley MD [Oph] - **Spec Exp:** Diabetic Eye Disease/Retinopathy; Macular Disease/Degeneration; Retina/Vitreous Surgery; Retinal Disorders; **Hospital:** NY-Presby Hosp/Columbia (page 66); **Address:** 635 W 165th St, Box 20, New York, NY 10032; **Phone:** 212-305-9535; **Board Cert:** Ophthalmology 1979; **Med School:** Columbia P&S 1974; **Resid:** Ophthalmology, Mass Eye & Ear Infirmary 1978; **Fellow:** Vitreoretinal Surgery, Bascom Palmer Eye Inst 1979; **Fac Appt:** Prof Oph, Columbia P&S

D'Amico, Donald MD [Oph] - **Spec Exp:** Diabetic Eye Disease/Retinopathy; Retinal Detachment; Retinal Disorders; **Hospital:** NY-Presby Hosp/Weill Cornell (page 66); **Address:** Weill Cornell Medical College, Dept of Ophthalmology, 1305 York Ave Fl 11th, New York, NY 10021; **Phone:** 212-746-2860; **Board Cert:** Ophthalmology 1982; **Med School:** Univ IL Coll Med 1977; **Resid:** Ophthalmology, Mass Eye & Ear Infirm 1981; **Fellow:** Vitreoretinal Surgery, Bascom Palmer Eye Inst 1982; **Fac Appt:** Prof Oph, Cornell Univ-Weill Med Coll

Del Priore, Lucian MD/PhD [Oph] - **Spec Exp:** Diabetic Eye Disease/Retinopathy; Macular Degeneration; Retinal Detachment; **Hospital:** NY-Presby Hosp/Columbia (page 66), Manhattan Eye, Ear & Throat Hosp; **Address:** Harkness Eye Inst, 635 W 165th St, New York, NY 10032; **Phone:** 212-305-9535; **Board Cert:** Ophthalmology 1989; **Med School:** Univ Rochester 1982; **Resid:** Ophthalmology, Wilmer Eye Inst/Johns HopkinsHosp 1987; **Fellow:** Glaucoma, Wilmer Eye Inst/Johns Hopkins Hosp 1988; Vitreoretinal Surgery, Wilmer Eye Inst/Johns Hopkins Hosp 1989; **Fac Appt:** Prof Oph, Columbia P&S

Della Rocca, Robert MD [Oph] - **Spec Exp:** Orbital Tumors/Cancer; Eyelid Tumors/Cancer; Thyroid Eye Disease; Oculoplastic Surgery; **Hospital:** New York Eye & Ear Infirm (page 65), Sound Shore Med Ctr - Westchester; **Address:** 310 E 14th St, South Bldg, rm 319, New York, NY 10003; **Phone:** 212-979-4575; **Board Cert:** Ophthalmology 1975; **Med School:** Creighton Univ 1967; **Resid:** Ophthalmology, NY Eye & Ear Infirm 1973; **Fellow:** Oculoplastic Surgery, Albany Med Ctr

Dodick, Jack M MD [Oph] - **Spec Exp:** Cataract Surgery-Lens Implant; Laser Vision Surgery; **Hospital:** Manhattan Eye, Ear & Throat Hosp, NYU Med Ctr (page 68); **Address:** 535 Park Ave, New York, NY 10021-8167; **Phone:** 212-288-7638; **Board Cert:** Ophthalmology 1969; **Med School:** Univ Toronto 1963; **Resid:** Ophthalmology, Manhattan EE&T Hosp 1967; **Fellow:** Anterior Segment - External Disease, Westchester Co Med Ctr 1968; **Fac Appt:** Prof Oph, NYU Sch Med

Eagle, Ralph C MD [Oph] - **Spec Exp:** Ophthalmic Pathology; **Hospital:** Wills Eye Hosp; **Address:** Wills Eye Hosp, Dept Pathology, 840 Walnut St, Ste 1410, Philadelphia, PA 19107; **Phone:** 215-928-3280; **Board Cert:** Ophthalmology 1976; **Med School:** Univ Pennsylvania 1970; **Resid:** Ophthalmology, Scheie Eye Inst 1975; **Fellow:** Ophthalmic Pathology, Armed Forces Inst Path 1978; **Fac Appt:** Prof Oph, Jefferson Med Coll

Eggers, Howard M MD [Oph] - **Spec Exp:** Pediatric Ophthalmology; Strabismus-Adult & Pediatric; **Hospital:** NY-Presby Hosp/Columbia (page 66); **Address:** 635 W 165th St, Box 21, New York, NY 10032-3724; **Phone:** 212-305-5409; **Board Cert:** Ophthalmology 1978; **Med School:** Columbia P&S 1971; **Resid:** Ophthalmology, Harkness Inst - Presby Hosp 1975; **Fac Appt:** Prof Oph, Columbia P&S

Feldon, Steven E MD [Oph] - **Spec Exp:** Neuro-Ophthalmology; Orbital Surgery; Strabismus; **Hospital:** Univ of Rochester Strong Meml Hosp, Rochester Genl Hosp; **Address:** 601 Elmwood Ave, Box 659, Rochester, NY 14642; **Phone:** 585-275-1126; **Board Cert:** Ophthalmology 1979; **Med School:** Albert Einstein Coll Med 1973; **Resid:** Ophthalmology, Mass Eye & Ear Infirmary 1978; **Fellow:** Ophthalmology, UCSF Med Ctr 1979; **Fac Appt:** Prof Oph, Univ Rochester

Finger, Paul T MD [Oph] - **Spec Exp:** Eye Tumors/Cancer; Orbital Diseases; **Hospital:** New York Eye & Ear Infirm (page 65), NYU Med Ctr (page 68); **Address:** The New York Eye Cancer Ctr, 115 E 61st St, New York, NY 10021-8183; **Phone:** 212-832-8170; **Board Cert:** Ophthalmology 1990; **Med School:** Tulane Univ 1982; **Resid:** Ophthalmology, Manhattan EET Hosp 1986; **Fellow:** Ocular Oncology, N Shore Univ Hosp 1987; **Fac Appt:** Clin Prof Oph, NYU Sch Med

Flynn, John T MD [Oph] - **Spec Exp:** Pediatric Ophthalmology; Strabismus; Retinopathy of Prematurity; **Hospital:** NY-Presby Hosp/Columbia (page 66); **Address:** Harkness Eye Inst, 635 W 165th St, Flanzer Ste, New York, NY 10032; **Phone:** 212-305-3908; **Board Cert:** Ophthalmology 1967; **Med School:** Northwestern Univ 1956; **Resid:** Ophthalmology, New York Hosp 1964; **Fellow:** Strabismus, Natl Inst Hlth 1965; **Fac Appt:** Prof Oph, Columbia P&S

Friberg, Thomas R MD [Oph] - **Spec Exp:** Retinal Disorders; Diabetic Eye Disease; Macular Degeneration; **Hospital:** UPMC Presby, Pittsburgh; **Address:** UPMC Eye Center, 203 Lothrop St, rm 825, Pittsburgh, PA 15213-2548; **Phone:** 412-647-2200; **Board Cert:** Ophthalmology 1979; **Med School:** Univ Minn 1973; **Resid:** Ophthalmology, Stanford Univ Med Ctr 1977; **Fellow:** Retina, Mass EE Infirmary 1978; Vitreoretinal Surgery, Duke Univ Med Ctr 1979; **Fac Appt:** Prof Oph, Univ Pittsburgh

Fuchs, Wayne MD [Oph] - **Spec Exp:** Diabetic Eye Disease/Retinopathy; Macular Disease/Degeneration; Retina/Vitreous Surgery; Retinal Disorders; **Hospital:** Mount Sinai Med Ctr (page 64), Manhattan Eye, Ear & Throat Hosp; **Address:** 121 E 60th St, Ste 5B, New York, NY 10022-1186; **Phone:** 212-319-8205; **Board Cert:** Ophthalmology 1985; **Med School:** Mount Sinai Sch Med 1979; **Resid:** Ophthalmology, Mount Sinai Hosp 1983; **Fellow:** Vitreoretinal Surgery & Disease, New York Hosp/Cornell 1984; **Fac Appt:** Clin Prof Oph, Mount Sinai Sch Med

Ophthalmology

Gaasterland, Douglas E MD [Oph] - **Spec Exp:** Glaucoma; Laser Surgery; Anterior Segment Surgery; **Hospital:** Georgetown Univ Hosp, G Washington Univ Hosp; **Address:** 2 Wisconsin Cir, Ste 200, Chevy Chase, MD 20815; **Phone:** 301-215-7100; **Board Cert:** Ophthalmology 1971; **Med School:** Johns Hopkins Univ 1965; **Resid:** Ophthalmology, Yale-New Haven Hosp 1970; **Fellow:** Glaucoma, National Eye Inst-NIH 1971; **Fac Appt:** Clin Prof Oph, Geo Wash Univ

Gallin, Pamela F MD [Oph] - **Spec Exp:** Pediatric Ophthalmology; Amblyopia; Strabismus; Tear Duct Problems; **Hospital:** NY-Presby Hosp/Columbia (page 66), Manhattan Eye, Ear & Throat Hosp; **Address:** Columbia Presby Med Ctr, 635 W 165th St, Ste 224, New York, NY 10032-3701; **Phone:** 212-305-5407; **Board Cert:** Ophthalmology 1983; **Med School:** Washington Univ, St Louis 1978; **Resid:** Ophthalmology, Mount Sinai Med Ctr 1982; **Fellow:** Pediatric Ophthalmology, Chldns Natl Med Ctr 1983; Strabismus, Columbia-Presby Med Ctr 1983; **Fac Appt:** Clin Prof Oph, Columbia P&S

Gentile, Ronald MD [Oph] - **Spec Exp:** Retina/Vitreous Surgery; Diabetic Eye Disease; Macular Degeneration; Retinal Disorders; **Hospital:** New York Eye & Ear Infirm (page 65); **Address:** 2nd Ave at 14th St, South Bldg - Ste 319, New York, NY 10003-4201; **Phone:** 212-979-4120; **Board Cert:** Ophthalmology 1997; **Med School:** SUNY Downstate 1991; **Resid:** Ophthalmology, New York Eye & Ear Infirm 1995; **Fellow:** Vitreoretinal Surgery & Disease, Kresge Eye Inst 1998; **Fac Appt:** Assoc Prof Oph, NY Med Coll

Gibralter, Richard P MD [Oph] - **Spec Exp:** Cataract Surgery; Laser Vision Surgery; Cornea Transplant; Corneal Disease & Surgery; **Hospital:** Manhattan Eye, Ear & Throat Hosp, New York Eye & Ear Infirm (page 65); **Address:** 154 E 71st St, New York, NY 10021-5123; **Phone:** 212-628-2202; **Board Cert:** Ophthalmology 1981; **Med School:** Mount Sinai Sch Med 1976; **Resid:** Ophthalmology, Manhattan EE&T Hosp 1980; **Fellow:** Cornea, Manhattan EE&T Hosp 1981; **Fac Appt:** Asst Prof Oph, NYU Sch Med

Goldberg, Morton MD [Oph] - **Spec Exp:** Macular Disease/Degeneration; Diabetic Eye Disease; Retinal Disorders; **Hospital:** Johns Hopkins Hosp - Baltimore (page 61); **Address:** Johns Hopkins Hosp, 600 N Wolfe St, Maumenee 713, Baltimore, MD 21287-9128; **Phone:** 410-955-6846; **Board Cert:** Ophthalmology 1968; **Med School:** Harvard Med Sch 1962; **Resid:** Ophthalmology, Wilmer Ophth Inst 1966; **Fellow:** Ophthalmology, Wilmer Ophth Inst 1967; Research, Johns Hopkins Hosp 1967; **Fac Appt:** Prof Oph, Johns Hopkins Univ

Guyton, David MD [Oph] - **Spec Exp:** Strabismus; Pediatric Ophthalmology; **Hospital:** Johns Hopkins Hosp - Baltimore (page 61); **Address:** Johns Hopkins Hosp, 600 N Wolfe, Wilmer 233, Baltimore, MD 21287; **Phone:** 410-955-8314; **Board Cert:** Ophthalmology 1977; **Med School:** Harvard Med Sch 1969; **Resid:** Ophthalmology, Johns Hopkins Hosp 1976; **Fellow:** Pediatric Ophthalmology, Baylor Coll Med 1977; **Fac Appt:** Prof Oph, Johns Hopkins Univ

Hall, Lisabeth MD [Oph] - **Spec Exp:** Pediatric Ophthalmology; Strabismus; Eye Muscle Disorders; Cataract-Pediatric; **Hospital:** New York Eye & Ear Infirm (page 65), Lenox Hill Hosp (page 62); **Address:** 40 W 72nd St, New York, NY 10023; **Phone:** 212-979-4614; **Board Cert:** Ophthalmology 1998; **Med School:** SUNY Stony Brook 1992; **Resid:** Ophthalmology, Manhattan Eye & Ear Infirm 1996; **Fellow:** Pediatric Ophthalmology, Jules Stein Eye Inst 1997; **Fac Appt:** Asst Prof Oph, NY Med Coll

Handa, James T MD [Oph] - **Spec Exp:** Macular Degeneration; Melanoma-Choroidal (eye); Retinoblastoma; **Hospital:** Johns Hopkins Hosp - Baltimore (page 61); **Address:** Johns Hopkins-Wilmer Eye Inst, 1550 Orleans St, rm CRB-144, Baltimore, MD 21287; **Phone:** 410-614-4211; **Board Cert:** Ophthalmology 1991; **Med School:** Univ Pennsylvania 1986; **Resid:** Ophthalmology, Wills Eye Hosp 1990; **Fellow:** Retina/Vitreous, Duke Eye Ctr 1992; Ophthalmic Oncololgy, USC Sch Med 1993; **Fac Appt:** Assoc Prof Oph, Johns Hopkins Univ

Hersh, Peter MD [Oph] - **Spec Exp:** LASIK-Refractive Surgery; Cornea Transplant; Keratoconus; **Hospital:** Holy Name Hosp, Hackensack Univ Med Ctr; **Address:** 300 Frank W Burr Blvd, Ste 71, Teaneck, NJ 07666-6704; **Phone:** 201-883-0505; **Board Cert:** Ophthalmology 1987; **Med School:** Johns Hopkins Univ 1982; **Resid:** Internal Medicine, Lenox Hill Hosp 1983; Ophthalmology, Mass Eye & Ear Infirm 1986; **Fellow:** Cornea & Ext Eye Disease, Mass Eye & Ear Infirm 1987; **Fac Appt:** Prof Oph, UMDNJ-NJ Med Sch, Newark

Ho, Allen C MD [Oph] - **Spec Exp:** Retina/Vitreous Surgery; Macular Degeneration; Diabetic Eye Disease/Retinopathy; **Hospital:** Wills Eye Hosp; **Address:** 910 E Willow Grove Ave, Wyndmoor, PA 19038; **Phone:** 215-233-4300; **Board Cert:** Ophthalmology 2004; **Med School:** Columbia P&S 1988; **Resid:** Ophthalmology, Wills Eye Hosp 1992; **Fellow:** Retina/Vitreous, Manhattan E&E Hosp 1994; **Fac Appt:** Prof Oph, Jefferson Med Coll

Iliff, Nicholas T MD [Oph] - **Spec Exp:** Oculoplastic Surgery; Orbital & Eyelid Tumors/Cancer; **Hospital:** Johns Hopkins Hosp - Baltimore (page 61); **Address:** Wilmer at Bayview Med Ctr, 4940 Eastern Ave, Baltimore, MD 21224; **Phone:** 410-550-2360; **Board Cert:** Ophthalmology 1978; **Med School:** Johns Hopkins Univ 1972; **Resid:** Ophthalmology, Johns Hopkins-Wilmer Inst 1977; **Fellow:** Retinal Surgery, Johns Hopkins-Wilmer Inst 1978; Oculoplastic & Reconstructive Surgery, Johns Hopkins-Wilmer Inst 1980; **Fac Appt:** Prof Oph, Johns Hopkins Univ

Jaafar, Mohamad S MD [Oph] - **Spec Exp:** Pediatric Ophthalmology; Strabismus-Adult & Pediatric; Glaucoma-Pediatric; **Hospital:** Chldns Natl Med Ctr, G Washington Univ Hosp; **Address:** Dept Ophthalmology, 111 Michigan Ave NW, Washington, DC 20010-2970; **Phone:** 202-476-3110; **Board Cert:** Ophthalmology 1997; **Med School:** Amer Univ Beirut 1978; **Resid:** Ophthalmology, Am Univ Beirut Med Ctr 1981; Ophthalmology, Washington Hosp Ctr 1994; **Fellow:** Pediatric Ophthalmology, Chldns Hosp 1982; Pediatric Ophthalmology, Baylor Coll Med 1983; **Fac Appt:** Prof Oph, Geo Wash Univ

Jabs, Douglas MD [Oph] - **Spec Exp:** Uveitis; **Hospital:** Mount Sinai Med Ctr (page 64); **Address:** 17 E 102 St Fl 8, New York, NY 10029; **Phone:** 212-241-6752; **Board Cert:** Ophthalmology 1982; Internal Medicine 1983; **Med School:** Johns Hopkins Univ 1977; **Resid:** Ophthalmology, Wilmer Eye Institute 1981; Internal Medicine, Johns Hopkins Hosp 1983; **Fellow:** Rheumatology, Johns Hoskins Hosp 1984; **Fac Appt:** Prof Oph, Mount Sinai Sch Med

Katowitz, James A MD [Oph] - **Spec Exp:** Oculoplastic & Orbital Surgery; Pediatric Ophthalmology; Corneal Disease & Surgery; **Hospital:** Chldns Hosp of Philadelphia, The, Hosp Univ Penn - UPHS (page 60); **Address:** Childrens Hosp, Div Ophthalmology, 34th St & Civic Center Blvd, Wood Bldg Fl 1, Philadelphia, PA 19104; **Phone:** 215-590-2791; **Board Cert:** Ophthalmology 1969; **Med School:** Univ Pennsylvania 1963; **Resid:** Ophthalmology, Hosp Univ Penn 1967; **Fellow:** Oculoplastic Surgery, Queen Victoria Hosp 1968; Oculoplastic Surgery, Moorfield Eye Hosp 1968; **Fac Appt:** Prof Oph, Univ Pennsylvania

Kidwell, Earl MD [Oph] - **Spec Exp:** Oculoplastic Surgery; **Hospital:** Howard Univ Hosp; **Address:** Ophthalmology Associates, 2041 Georgia Ave NW, Ste 2000, Washington, DC 20060; **Phone:** 202-865-1257; **Board Cert:** Ophthalmology 1978; **Med School:** Johns Hopkins Univ 1973; **Resid:** Ophthalmology, Johns Hopkins Hosp 1977; **Fellow:** Oculoplastic Surgery, Univ Miami Hosps 1978

Koller, Harold Paul MD [Oph] - **Spec Exp:** Pediatric Ophthalmology; Eye Muscle Surgery; Visual Perception & Learning Disorders; **Hospital:** Wills Eye Hosp, St Christopher's Hosp for Chldn; **Address:** 1650 Huntington Pike, Ste 150, Meadowbrook, PA 19046-8001; **Phone:** 215-947-6660; **Board Cert:** Ophthalmology 1971; **Med School:** Tulane Univ 1964; **Resid:** Ophthalmology, Tulane Hosp Med Ctr 1968; **Fellow:** Pediatric Ophthalmology, Washington Chldn's Hosp 1970; **Fac Appt:** Clin Prof Oph, Thomas Jefferson Univ

Ophthalmology

Kupersmith, Mark MD [Oph] - **Spec Exp:** Neuro-Ophthalmology; **Hospital:** St Luke's - Roosevelt Hosp Ctr - Roosevelt Div (page 57); **Address:** 1000 10th Ave, New York, NY 10009; **Phone:** 212-870-9418; **Board Cert:** Ophthalmology 1981; Neurology 1981; **Med School:** Northwestern Univ 1974; **Resid:** Neurology, NYU Med Ctr 1978; Ophthalmology, NYU Med Ctr 1980; **Fac Appt:** Prof Oph, NYU Sch Med

Lewis, Hilel MD [Oph] - **Spec Exp:** Macular Degeneration; Diabetic Eye Disease/Retinopathy; Retinal Disorders; **Hospital:** NY-Presby Hosp/Columbia (page 66); **Address:** Edward Harkness Eye Inst, 635 W 165th St, rm 516, New York, NY 10032; **Phone:** 212-305-4606; **Board Cert:** Ophthalmology 1990; **Med School:** Mexico 1980; **Resid:** Ophthalmology, Jules Stein Eye Inst-UCLA 1986; **Fellow:** Ocular Pathology, Jules Stein Eye Inst-UCLA 1983; Vitreoretinal Surgery, Med Coll Wisconsin 1987; **Fac Appt:** Prof Oph, Cleveland Cl Coll Med/Case West Res

Liebmann, Jeffrey MD [Oph] - **Spec Exp:** Glaucoma; Cataract Surgery; **Hospital:** New York Eye & Ear Infirm (page 65), Manhattan Eye, Ear & Throat Hosp; **Address:** 121 E 60th St, New York, NY 10022; **Phone:** 212-477-7540 x330; **Board Cert:** Ophthalmology 1989; **Med School:** Boston Univ 1983; **Resid:** Ophthalmology, SUNY Downstate Med Ctr 1987; **Fellow:** Glaucoma, New York EE Infirmary 1988; **Fac Appt:** Clin Prof Oph, NYU Sch Med

Lisman, Richard D MD [Oph] - **Spec Exp:** Oculoplastic Surgery; Eyelid/Tear Duct Reconstruction; Eyelid Cosmetic & Reconstructive Surgery; **Hospital:** NYU Med Ctr (page 68), Manhattan Eye, Ear & Throat Hosp; **Address:** 635 Park Ave, New York, NY 10021-6546; **Phone:** 212-585-1405; **Board Cert:** Ophthalmology 1981; **Med School:** NYU Sch Med 1976; **Resid:** Ophthalmology, Manhattan EE Hosp 1980; **Fellow:** Ophthalmic Plastic Surgery, NY Eye & Ear Infirmary 1981; Plastic Surgery, Manhattan EE&T Hosp 1982; **Fac Appt:** Clin Prof Oph, NYU Sch Med

Mackool, Richard J MD [Oph] - **Spec Exp:** Cataract Surgery; LASIK-Refractive Surgery; Lens Implants-Multifocal (Restor); Corneal Disease & Surgery; **Hospital:** New York Eye & Ear Infirm (page 65); **Address:** 31-27 41st St, Astoria, NY 11103; **Phone:** 718-728-3400; **Board Cert:** Ophthalmology 1975; **Med School:** Boston Univ 1968; **Resid:** Ophthalmology, New York EE Infirm 1973; **Fac Appt:** Clin Prof Oph, NYU Sch Med

Magramm, Irene MD [Oph] - **Spec Exp:** Pediatric Ophthalmology; Strabismus; Cataract Surgery; **Hospital:** Manhattan Eye, Ear & Throat Hosp, New York Eye & Ear Infirm (page 65); **Address:** 225 E 64th St, New York, NY 10021; **Phone:** 212-644-5100; **Board Cert:** Ophthalmology 1987; **Med School:** Cornell Univ-Weill Med Coll 1981; **Resid:** Ophthalmology, North Shore Univ Hosp 1985; **Fellow:** Pediatric Ophthalmology, Manhattan EE&T Hosp 1986; **Fac Appt:** Asst Clin Prof Oph, Cornell Univ-Weill Med Coll

Mandel, Eric R MD [Oph] - **Spec Exp:** LASIK-Refractive Surgery; Corneal Disease; PRK-Refractive Surgery; **Hospital:** New York Eye & Ear Infirm (page 65), Lenox Hill Hosp (page 62); **Address:** 211 E 70th St, New York, NY 10021-5106; **Phone:** 212-734-0111; **Board Cert:** Ophthalmology 1988; **Med School:** SUNY Stony Brook 1982; **Resid:** Ophthalmology, Lenox Hill Hosp 1986; **Fellow:** Cornea & Ext Eye Disease, Mass EE Infirm 1987

Medow, Norman MD [Oph] - **Spec Exp:** Cataract-Pediatric; Glaucoma-Pediatric; Corneal Disease-Pediatric; **Hospital:** Manhattan Eye, Ear & Throat Hosp, NY-Presby Hosp/Weill Cornell (page 66); **Address:** 225 E 64th St, Ste 6, New York, NY 10021-6690; **Phone:** 212-644-5100; **Board Cert:** Ophthalmology 1975; **Med School:** SUNY Hlth Sci Ctr 1966; **Resid:** Ophthalmology, Manhattan EE&T Hosp 1972; **Fellow:** Cataract/Lens Implant Surgery, Charles Kelman, MD 1973; **Fac Appt:** Assoc Clin Prof Oph, Cornell Univ-Weill Med Coll

Miller, Neil MD [Oph] - **Spec Exp:** Neuro-Ophthalmology; Orbital Diseases; Thyroid Eye Disease; **Hospital:** Johns Hopkins Hosp - Baltimore (page 61); **Address:** Johns Hopkins - Wilmer Eye Inst, 600 N Wolfe St, rm 233, Baltimore, MD 21287-0001; **Phone:** 410-955-8679; **Board Cert:** Ophthalmology 1976; **Med School:** Johns Hopkins Univ 1971; **Resid:** Ophthalmology, Johns Hopkins Hosp 1975; **Fellow:** Neurological Ophthalmology, UCSF Med Ctr 1975; **Fac Appt:** Prof Oph, Johns Hopkins Univ

Mills, Monte D MD [Oph] - **Spec Exp:** Pediatric Ophthalmology; Eye Muscle Disorders; Strabismus; **Hospital:** Chldns Hosp of Philadelphia, The; **Address:** Chldns Hosp, Richard D Wood Bldg, 34th St and Civic Center Blvd, Wood Bldg Fl 1, Philadelphia, PA 19104; **Phone:** 215-590-2791; **Board Cert:** Ophthalmology 1993; **Med School:** Baylor Coll Med 1988; **Resid:** Ophthalmology, Mass E&E Infirm 1992; **Fellow:** Pediatric Ophthalmology, Chldns Hosp 1993; **Fac Appt:** Prof Oph, Univ Pennsylvania

Muldoon, Thomas O MD [Oph] - **Spec Exp:** Retina/Vitreous Surgery; Macular Disease/Degeneration; Diabetic Eye Disease/Retinopathy; **Hospital:** New York Eye & Ear Infirm (page 65); **Address:** 310 E 14th St, Ste 402, New York, NY 10003-4201; **Phone:** 212-979-4595; **Board Cert:** Ophthalmology 1971; **Med School:** Univ Rochester 1962; **Resid:** Surgery, St Lukes Hosp 1966; Ophthalmology, New York EE Infirm 1969; **Fellow:** Retinal Surgery, New York EE Infirm 1970; **Fac Appt:** Assoc Clin Prof Oph, NY Med Coll

Nelson, Leonard B MD [Oph] - **Spec Exp:** Pediatric Ophthalmology; Strabismus; Eye Muscle Disorders; **Hospital:** Wills Eye Hosp; **Address:** Wills Eye Hospital, 840 Walnut St, Ste 1210, Philadelphia, PA 19107; **Phone:** 215-928-3244; **Board Cert:** Ophthalmology 1981; **Med School:** Harvard Med Sch 1976; **Resid:** Ophthalmology, Bellevue Hosp Ctr-NYU 1980; **Fellow:** Pediatric Ophthalmology, Chldns Hosp Med Ctr 1981; **Fac Appt:** Assoc Prof Oph, Jefferson Med Coll

Odel, Jeffrey G MD [Oph] - **Spec Exp:** Neuro-Ophthalmology; Retinal Disorders; Optic Nerve Disorders; **Hospital:** NY-Presby Hosp/Columbia (page 66); **Address:** 635 W 165th St, rm 316, New York, NY 10032-3701; **Phone:** 212-305-5415; **Board Cert:** Ophthalmology 1981; **Med School:** Univ Rochester 1975; **Resid:** Ophthalmology, Mt Sinai Hosp 1981; **Fellow:** Ophthalmology, Bascom-Palmer Eye Inst 1977; Ophthalmology, Columbia Presby Med Ctr 1982; **Fac Appt:** Assoc Clin Prof Oph, Columbia P&S

Podos, Steven M MD [Oph] - **Spec Exp:** Glaucoma-Consultation; **Hospital:** Mount Sinai Med Ctr (page 64); **Address:** 1465 Madison Ave, New York, NY 10029; **Phone:** 212-241-6752; **Board Cert:** Ophthalmology 1968; **Med School:** Harvard Med Sch 1962; **Resid:** Ophthalmology, Washington Univ-Barnes Hosp 1967; **Fac Appt:** Prof Oph, Mount Sinai Sch Med

Quigley, Harry A MD [Oph] - **Spec Exp:** Glaucoma; **Hospital:** Johns Hopkins Hosp - Baltimore (page 61); **Address:** 600 N Wolfe St, Maumenee B-110, Baltimore, MD 21287-9205; **Phone:** 410-955-6052; **Board Cert:** Ophthalmology 1976; **Med School:** Johns Hopkins Univ 1971; **Resid:** Ophthalmology, Wilmer Inst-Johns Hopkins Hosp 1975; **Fellow:** Ophthalmology, Bascom Palmer Eye Inst 1977; **Fac Appt:** Prof Oph, Johns Hopkins Univ

Quinn, Graham E MD [Oph] - **Spec Exp:** Pediatric Ophthalmology; Eye Growth/Development; **Hospital:** Chldns Hosp of Philadelphia, The; **Address:** Chldns Hosp of Philadelphia, Div Ophthalmology, 34th St & Civic Center Blvd, Wood Bldg Fl 1, Philadelphia, PA 19104-4399; **Phone:** 215-590-2791; **Board Cert:** Ophthalmology 1979; **Med School:** Duke Univ 1973; **Resid:** Pathology, Metro Genl Hosp 1975; Ophthalmology, Hosp Univ Penn 1978; **Fellow:** Pediatric Ophthalmology, Childrens Hosp 1979; **Fac Appt:** Prof Oph, Univ Pennsylvania

Ophthalmology

Regillo, Carl D MD [Oph] - **Spec Exp:** Retinal Disorders; **Hospital:** Wills Eye Hosp; **Address:** 910 E Willow Grove Ave, Wyndmoor, PA 19038; **Phone:** 215-233-4300; **Board Cert:** Ophthalmology 2004; **Med School:** Harvard Med Sch 1988; **Resid:** Ophthalmology, Wills Eye Hosp 1992; **Fellow:** Retinal Surgery, Wills Eye Hosp 1994; **Fac Appt:** Prof Oph, Jefferson Med Coll

Reynolds, James D MD [Oph] - **Spec Exp:** Pediatric Ophthalmology; Strabismus; Retinopathy of Prematurity; **Hospital:** Women's & Chldn's Hosp of Buffalo, The; **Address:** 3580 Sheridan Drive, Ste 150, Amherst, NY 14226; **Phone:** 716-834-0113; **Board Cert:** Ophthalmology 1982; **Med School:** SUNY Buffalo 1978; **Resid:** Ophthalmology, Erie Co Med Ctr 1981; **Fellow:** Pediatric Ophthalmology, Pittsburgh EE Hospital 1982; **Fac Appt:** Prof Oph, SUNY Buffalo

Ritch, Robert MD [Oph] - **Spec Exp:** Glaucoma; **Hospital:** New York Eye & Ear Infirm (page 65); **Address:** 310 E 14th St, rm 304S, New York, NY 10003-4201; **Phone:** 212-477-7540; **Board Cert:** Ophthalmology 1977; **Med School:** Albert Einstein Coll Med 1972; **Resid:** Ophthalmology, Mount Sinai Hosp 1976; **Fellow:** Glaucoma, Mount Sinai Hosp 1978; **Fac Appt:** Clin Prof Oph, NY Med Coll

Savino, Peter J MD [Oph] - **Spec Exp:** Neuro-Ophthalmology; **Hospital:** Thomas Jefferson Univ Hosp; **Address:** Wills Eye Hosp, Dept Neuro-Ophthalmology, 840 Walnut St Fl 9 - Ste 930, Philadelphia, PA 19107; **Phone:** 215-928-3130; **Board Cert:** Ophthalmology 1975; **Med School:** Italy 1968; **Resid:** Ophthalmology, Georgetown Med Ctr 1973; **Fellow:** Neurological Ophthalmology, Bascom Palmer Eye Inst 1974; **Fac Appt:** Prof Oph, Thomas Jefferson Univ

Schein, Oliver D MD [Oph] - **Spec Exp:** Cataract Surgery; Corneal Disease & Surgery; **Hospital:** Johns Hopkins Hosp - Baltimore (page 61); **Address:** Johns Hopkins Hosp, 600 N Wolfe St, Maumenee 317, Baltimore, MD 21287; **Phone:** 410-955-7677; **Board Cert:** Internal Medicine 1984; Ophthalmology 1990; **Med School:** Johns Hopkins Univ 1981; **Resid:** Internal Medicine, Johns Hopkins Hosp 1984; Ophthalmology, Mass Eye & Ear Infirm 1987; **Fellow:** Cornea & Ext Eye Disease, Mass Eye & Ear Infirm 1988; **Fac Appt:** Prof Oph, Johns Hopkins Univ

Schiff, William M MD [Oph] - **Spec Exp:** Macular Disease/Degeneration; Diabetic Eye Disease/Retinopathy; Retinal Detachment; **Hospital:** NY-Presby Hosp/Columbia (page 66), St Luke's - Roosevelt Hosp Ctr - Roosevelt Div (page 57); **Address:** Columbia Ophthalmic Consultants, 635 W 165th St, New York, NY 10032; **Phone:** 212-305-9535; **Board Cert:** Ophthalmology 2006; **Med School:** NYU Sch Med 1988; **Resid:** Ophthalmology, New York Eye & Ear Infirm 1994; **Fellow:** Retina/Vitreous, NY Hosp-Harkness Eye Inst 1996; **Fac Appt:** Assoc Prof Oph, Columbia P&S

Schuman, Joel S MD [Oph] - **Spec Exp:** Glaucoma; Cataract Surgery; **Hospital:** UPMC Presby, Pittsburgh, UPMC Shadyside; **Address:** Eye & Ear Institute, Ste 816, 203 Lothrop St, Pittsburgh, PA 15213; **Phone:** 412-647-2200; **Board Cert:** Ophthalmology 1990; **Med School:** Mount Sinai Sch Med 1984; **Resid:** Ophthalmology, Med Coll Virginia Hosps 1988; **Fellow:** Glaucoma, Mass EE Infirmary 1990; **Fac Appt:** Prof Oph, Univ Pittsburgh

Sergott, Robert C MD [Oph] - **Spec Exp:** Neuro-Ophthalmology; Optic Nerve Disorders; Glaucoma; Thyroid Eye Disease; **Hospital:** Thomas Jefferson Univ Hosp, Wills Eye Hosp; **Address:** Wills Eye Hosp, Dept Neuro-Opthalmology, 840 Walnut St Fl 9 - Ste 930, Philadelphia, PA 19107; **Phone:** 215-928-3130; **Board Cert:** Ophthalmology 1982; **Med School:** Johns Hopkins Univ 1975; **Resid:** Internal Medicine, Mary Imogene Bassett Hosp 1976; Ophthalmology, Jackson Meml Hosp 1980; **Fellow:** Ophthalmology, Jackson Meml Hosp 1980

Shabto, Uri MD [Oph] - **Spec Exp:** Retinopathy of Prematurity; Macular Disease/Degeneration; Diabetic Eye Disease/Retinopathy; **Hospital:** New York Eye & Ear Infirm (page 65), Beth Israel Med Ctr - Petrie Division (page 57); **Address:** 310 E 14th St South Bldg - Ste 419, New York, NY 10003-4201; **Phone:** 212-677-2000; **Board Cert:** Ophthalmology 1991; **Med School:** Harvard Med Sch 1986; **Resid:** Ophthalmology, NY Eye & Ear Infirm 1990; **Fellow:** Vitreoretinal Surgery, Montefiore Hosp 1991; **Fac Appt:** Asst Prof Oph, NYU Sch Med

Shields, Carol L MD [Oph] - **Spec Exp:** Orbital Tumors/Cancer; Melanoma; Retinoblastoma; Pediatric Ophthalmology; **Hospital:** Wills Eye Hosp, Jefferson Hosp - Pittsburgh; **Address:** Wills Eye Hosp, Ocular Oncology Service, 840 Walnut St, Ste 1440, Phildelphia, PA 19107; **Phone:** 215-928-3105; **Board Cert:** Ophthalmology 1989; **Med School:** Univ Pittsburgh 1983; **Resid:** Ophthalmology, Willis Eye Hosp 1988; **Fellow:** Ophthalmic Pathology, Willis Eye Hosp 1988; Ophthalmic Oncololgy, Willis Eye Hosp 1989; **Fac Appt:** Prof Oph, Jefferson Med Coll

Shields, Jerry MD [Oph] - **Spec Exp:** Eye Tumors/Cancer; Pediatric Ophthalmology; Retinoblastoma; **Hospital:** Wills Eye Hosp; **Address:** Wills Eye Hosp, Ocular Oncology Service, 840 Walnut St, Ste 1440, Philadelphia, PA 19107; **Phone:** 215-928-3105; **Board Cert:** Ophthalmology 1972; **Med School:** Univ Mich Med Sch 1964; **Resid:** Ophthalmology, Wills Eye Hosp 1970; **Fellow:** Ophthalmology, Wills Eye Hosp 1972; **Fac Appt:** Prof Oph, Thomas Jefferson Univ

Simon, John W MD [Oph] - **Spec Exp:** Pediatric Ophthalmology; Strabismus; **Hospital:** Albany Med Ctr, St Peter's Hosp - Albany; **Address:** 1220 New Scotland Rd, Ste 202, Slingerlands, NY 12159; **Phone:** 518-533-6502; **Board Cert:** Ophthalmology 1981; **Med School:** Mount Sinai Sch Med 1976; **Resid:** Ophthalmology, Mt Sinai Hosp 1980; **Fellow:** Pediatric Ophthalmology, Wills Eye Hosp 1981; **Fac Appt:** Prof Oph, Albany Med Coll

Stark, Walter J MD [Oph] - **Spec Exp:** Corneal Disease & Transplant; Cataract Surgery; Refractive Surgery; **Hospital:** Johns Hopkins Hosp - Baltimore (page 61); **Address:** Wilmer Eye Institute, 600 N Wolfe St Maumenee Bldg - rm 327, Baltimore, MD 21287-9238; **Phone:** 410-955-5490; **Board Cert:** Ophthalmology 1973; **Med School:** Univ Okla Coll Med 1967; **Resid:** Ophthalmology, Wilmer Inst-Johns Hopkins 1971; **Fac Appt:** Prof Oph, Johns Hopkins Univ

Sterns, Gwen MD [Oph] - **Spec Exp:** Geriatric Ophthalmology; Low Vision; **Hospital:** Rochester Genl Hosp, Univ of Rochester Strong Meml Hosp; **Address:** 1425 Portland Ave, Box 224, Ophthalmology Dept, Rochester, NY 14621; **Phone:** 585-922-4794; **Board Cert:** Ophthalmology 1976; **Med School:** Med Coll PA 1970; **Resid:** Ophthalmology, Nassau Co Med Ctr 1974; **Fellow:** Ophthalmology, Colum-Presby Eye Inst 1975

Vander, James F MD [Oph] - **Spec Exp:** Diabetic Eye Disease; Retinal Disorders; Macular Degeneration; **Hospital:** Wills Eye Hosp; **Address:** 910 E Willow Grove Ave, Wyndmoor, PA 19038-7910; **Phone:** 215-233-4300; **Board Cert:** Ophthalmology 1989; **Med School:** Univ Mich Med Sch 1984; **Resid:** Ophthalmology, Univ Michigan Med Ctr 1988; **Fellow:** Retina/Vitreous, Wills Eye Hosp 1990; **Fac Appt:** Prof Oph, Thomas Jefferson Univ

Walsh, Joseph MD [Oph] - **Spec Exp:** Diabetic Eye Disease; Macular Degeneration; Retinal Disorders; **Hospital:** New York Eye & Ear Infirm (page 65), Beth Israel Med Ctr - Petrie Division (page 57); **Address:** 310 E 14th St Bldg S Fl 3, New York, NY 10003-4201; **Phone:** 212-979-4500; **Board Cert:** Ophthalmology 2005; **Med School:** Georgetown Univ 1966; **Resid:** Ophthalmology, NY Eye & Ear Infirm 1973; **Fellow:** Retina, Montefiore Hosp Med Ctr 1974; **Fac Appt:** Prof Oph, NY Med Coll

Ophthalmology

Wang, Frederick MD [Oph] - **Spec Exp:** Pediatric Ophthalmology; Strabismus; Eye Muscle Disorders; **Hospital:** New York Eye & Ear Infirm (page 65), Montefiore Med Ctr; **Address:** 30 E 40th St, Ste 405, New York, NY 10016-1201; **Phone:** 212-684-3980; **Board Cert:** Pediatrics 1978; Ophthalmology 1980; **Med School:** Albert Einstein Coll Med 1972; **Resid:** Pediatrics, Jacobi Med Ctr 1974; Ophthalmology, Albert Einstein 1979; **Fellow:** Pediatric Ophthalmology, Children's Hosp Natl Med Ctr 1980; **Fac Appt:** Clin Prof Oph, Albert Einstein Coll Med

Yannuzzi, Lawrence MD [Oph] - **Spec Exp:** Retina/Vitreous Surgery; Macular Disease/De-generation; Diabetic Eye Disease; **Hospital:** Manhattan Eye, Ear & Throat Hosp; **Address:** 460 Park Ave Fl 5, New York, NY 10021-4028; **Phone:** 212-861-9797; **Board Cert:** Ophthalmology 1970; **Med School:** Boston Univ 1964; **Resid:** Ophthalmology, Manhattan EE&T Hosp 1968; **Fellow:** Ophthalmology, Manhattan EE&T Hosp 1971; **Fac Appt:** Clin Prof Oph, Columbia P&S

Zaidman, Gerald MD [Oph] - **Spec Exp:** Laser Vision Surgery; Cornea Transplant; Cataract Surgery; **Hospital:** Westchester Med Ctr, Our Lady of Mercy Med Ctr; **Address:** Westchester Med Ctr, Macy Pavilion, Dept Opth, rm 1100, Valhalla, NY 10595; **Phone:** 914-493-1599; **Board Cert:** Ophthalmology 1981; **Med School:** Albert Einstein Coll Med 1975; **Resid:** Ophthalmology, Beth Abraham Hosp 1977; Ophthalmology, Lenox Hill Hosp 1980; **Fellow:** Cornea & Ext Eye Disease, Univ Pittsburgh 1982; **Fac Appt:** Prof Oph, NY Med Coll

Southeast

Alfonso, Eduardo MD [Oph] - **Spec Exp:** Corneal Disease & Surgery; LASIK-Refractive Sur-gery; Cataract Surgery; **Hospital:** Bascom Palmer Eye Inst (page 55), Jackson Meml Hosp; **Address:** Bascom Palmer Eye Institute, 900 NW 17th St, Miami, FL 33136-1119; **Phone:** 305-326-6366; **Board Cert:** Ophthalmology 1985; **Med School:** Yale Univ 1980; **Resid:** Ophthalmology, Bascom Palmer Eye Inst-Univ Miami 1984; **Fellow:** Cornea, Mass Eye & Ear Hosp 1986; Ophthalmological Pathology, Mass Eye & Ear Hosp 1986; **Fac Appt:** Prof Oph, Univ Miami Sch Med

Buckley, Edward G MD [Oph] - **Spec Exp:** Pediatric Ophthalmology; Strabismus; Cataract-Pediatric; **Hospital:** Duke Univ Med Ctr; **Address:** 2351 Erwin Rd, Durham, NC 27705; **Phone:** 919-684-6084; **Board Cert:** Ophthalmology 1982; **Med School:** Duke Univ 1977; **Resid:** Oph-thalmology, Duke Univ Eye Ctr 1981; **Fellow:** Ophthalmology, Bascom Palmer Eye Inst 1983; **Fac Appt:** Prof Oph, Duke Univ

Budenz, Donald L MD [Oph] - **Spec Exp:** Glaucoma; **Hospital:** Bascom Palmer Eye Inst (page 55); **Address:** Bascom Palmer Eye Inst, 900 NW 17th St, Ste 341, Miami, FL 33136; **Phone:** 305-326-6384; **Board Cert:** Ophthalmology 2003; **Med School:** Harvard Med Sch 1987; **Resid:** Ophthalmology, Scheie Eye Inst 1991; **Fellow:** Glaucoma, Bascom Palmer Eye Inst 1992; **Fac Appt:** Assoc Prof Oph, Univ Miami Sch Med

Capo, Hilda MD [Oph] - **Spec Exp:** Pediatric Ophthalmology; Strabismus; Neuro-Ophthalmol-ogy; **Hospital:** Bascom Palmer Eye Inst (page 55); **Address:** Bascom Palmer Eye Institute, 900 NW 17th St, Miami, FL 33136; **Phone:** 305-326-6555; **Board Cert:** Ophthalmology 1989; **Med School:** Puerto Rico 1982; **Resid:** Ophthalmology, Univ PR Med Sch 1987; **Fellow:** Neurological Ophthalmology, NYU Med Ctr 1989; Pediatric Ophthalmology, Johns Hopkins Hosp 1988; **Fac Appt:** Prof Oph, Univ Miami Sch Med

Culbertson, William MD [Oph] - **Spec Exp:** LASIK-Refractive Surgery; Corneal Disease & Sur-gery; Cataract Surgery; **Hospital:** Bascom Palmer Eye Inst (page 55); **Address:** Bascom Palmer Eye Institute, 900 NW 17th St, Miami, FL 33136-1119; **Phone:** 305-326-6364; **Board Cert:** Ophthal-mology 1976; **Med School:** Emory Univ 1970; **Resid:** Ophthalmology, Vanderbilt Univ Hosp 1974; **Fellow:** Ophthalmology, Bascom Palmer Eye Inst 1979; **Fac Appt:** Prof Oph, Univ Miami Sch Med

Dutton, Jonathan J MD/PhD [Oph] - **Spec Exp:** Oculoplastic Surgery; Eye Tumors/Cancer; Melanoma-Choroidal (eye); **Hospital:** Univ NC Hosps; **Address:** Univ North Carolina - Dept Ophthalmology, 130 Mason Farm Rd, 5156 Bioinformatics, CB 7040, Chapel Hill, NC 27599; **Phone:** 919-966-5296; **Board Cert:** Ophthalmology 1983; **Med School:** Washington Univ, St Louis 1977; **Resid:** Ophthalmology, Washington Univ Med Ctr 1982; **Fellow:** Oculoplastic Surgery, Univ Iowa Med Ctr 1983; **Fac Appt:** Prof Oph, Univ NC Sch Med

Flynn Jr, Harry W MD [Oph] - **Spec Exp:** Retina/Vitreous Surgery; Diabetic Eye Disease/Retinopathy; **Hospital:** Bascom Palmer Eye Inst (page 55), Univ of Miami Hosp & Clins/Sylvester Comp Canc Ctr; **Address:** Bascom Palmer Eye Institute, 900 NW 17th St, Miami, FL 33136-1119; **Phone:** 305-326-6118; **Board Cert:** Ophthalmology 1976; **Med School:** Univ VA Sch Med 1971; **Resid:** Ophthalmology, Univ VA Hosp 1975; **Fellow:** Retina, Pacific Med Ctr 1976; **Fac Appt:** Prof Oph, Univ Miami Sch Med

Forster, Richard K MD [Oph] - **Spec Exp:** Cornea Transplant; Cataract Surgery; **Hospital:** Bascom Palmer Eye Inst (page 55); **Address:** Bascom Palmer Eye Institute, 900 NW 17th St, Miami, FL 33136; **Phone:** 305-243-2020; **Board Cert:** Ophthalmology 1971; **Med School:** Boston Univ 1963; **Resid:** Ophthalmology, Bascom Palmer Eye Inst 1969; **Fellow:** Ophthalmology, Fl Proctor Fdn/UCSF 1970; **Fac Appt:** Prof Oph, Univ Miami Sch Med

Freedman, Sharon F MD [Oph] - **Spec Exp:** Pediatric Ophthalmology; Glaucoma-Pediatric; Strabismus-Pediatric; Retinopathy of Prematurity; **Hospital:** Duke Univ Med Ctr; **Address:** Duke Eye Center, DUMC 3082, Durham, NC 27710-0001; **Phone:** 919-684-4584; **Board Cert:** Ophthalmology 1991; **Med School:** Harvard Med Sch 1985; **Resid:** Ophthalmology, Mass Eye & Ear Infirm 1989; **Fellow:** Pediatric Ophthalmology, Childns Hosp 1990; Glaucoma, Duke Eye Ctr 1992; **Fac Appt:** Assoc Prof Oph, Duke Univ

Glaser, Joel MD [Oph] - **Spec Exp:** Neuro-Ophthalmology; Orbital Diseases; **Hospital:** Bascom Palmer Eye Inst (page 55); **Address:** 4701 N Meridian Ave, Adams Bldg - Ste 500 A, Miami Beach, FL 33140; **Phone:** 305-532-2885; **Board Cert:** Ophthalmology 1968; **Med School:** Duke Univ 1963; **Resid:** Ophthalmology, Univ Miami Med Coll 1965; **Fellow:** Neurological Ophthalmology, UCSF Med Ctr 1970; **Fac Appt:** Prof Oph, Univ Miami Sch Med

Gorovoy, Mark S MD [Oph] - **Spec Exp:** LASIK-Refractive Surgery; Corneal Disease & Transplant; Glaucoma; Cataract Surgery; **Hospital:** Southwest Florida Regional Medical Center, Lee Memorial Hlth Systems; **Address:** 12381 S Cleveland Ave, Ste 300, Fort Myers, FL 33907; **Phone:** 239-939-1444; **Board Cert:** Ophthalmology 1982; **Med School:** Geo Wash Univ 1973; **Resid:** Ophthalmology, George Washington Univ Hosp 1980; **Fellow:** Cornea & Ext Eye Disease, Univ Florida 1982

Grossniklaus, Hans E MD [Oph] - **Spec Exp:** Ophthalmic Pathology; Melanoma-Choroidal (eye); Macular Disease/Degeneration; Retinal Disorders; **Hospital:** Emory Univ Hosp; **Address:** Emory Clinic - LF Montgomery Lab, 1365-B Clifton Rd NE, rm BT428, Atlanta, GA 30322; **Phone:** 404-778-4611; **Board Cert:** Ophthalmology 1985; Anatomic Pathology 1987; **Med School:** Ohio State Univ 1980; **Resid:** Ophthalmology, Case West Res Univ Hosp 1984; Pathology, Case West Res Univ Hosp 1987; **Fellow:** Ophthalmological Pathology, Johns Hopkins Hosp 1985; **Fac Appt:** Prof Oph, Emory Univ

Haik, Barrett MD [Oph] - **Spec Exp:** Eye Tumors/Cancer; **Hospital:** St Jude Children's Research Hosp; **Address:** Univ Tenn Med Group, Ophthamology, 930 Madison Ave, Ste 200, Memphis, TN 38103-3452; **Phone:** 901-448-6650; **Board Cert:** Ophthalmology 1981; **Med School:** Louisiana State U, New Orleans 1976; **Resid:** Ophthalmology, Columbia-Presby/Harkness Eye Inst 1980; **Fac Appt:** Prof Oph, Univ Tenn Coll Med, Memphis

Ophthalmology

Hess, J Bruce MD [Oph] - **Spec Exp:** Pediatric Ophthalmology; Strabismus; **Hospital:** All Children's Hosp, Bayfront Med Ctr; **Address:** 880 6th St S, Ste 350, St Petersburg, FL 33701; **Phone:** 727-767-4393; **Board Cert:** Ophthalmology 1978; **Med School:** Baylor Coll Med 1971; **Resid:** Ophthalmology, Geisinger Med Ctr 1977; **Fellow:** Ophthalmology, Wills Eye Hosp 1978; **Fac Appt:** Assoc Prof Oph, Univ S Fla Coll Med

Holliday, James N MD/PhD [Oph] - **Spec Exp:** Cataract Surgery; Glaucoma; Diabetic Eye Disease; **Hospital:** St Francis Hosp - Memphis, Baptist Memorial Hospital - Memphis; **Address:** 4571 Summer Ave, Memphis, TN 38122; **Phone:** 901-680-0043; **Board Cert:** Ophthalmology 2005; **Med School:** Duke Univ 1987; **Resid:** Ophthalmology, UC Irvine Med Ctr 1992; **Fellow:** Anterior Segment - External Disease, Mayo Clinic 1993

Lambert, Scott R MD [Oph] - **Spec Exp:** Pediatric Ophthalmology; Strabismus; Cataract-Pediatric; **Hospital:** Chldns Hlthcare Atlanta - Egleston, Chldns Hlthcare Atlanta - Scottish Rite; **Address:** Emory Eye Ctr, Dept Ped Opth, 1365 Clifton Rd B Bldg - Ste 4513, Atlanta, GA 30322; **Phone:** 404-778-3431; **Board Cert:** Ophthalmology 1989; **Med School:** Yale Univ 1983; **Resid:** Ophthalmology, UCSF Med Ctr 1987; **Fellow:** Pediatric Ophthalmology, Hosp for Sick Chldn 1988; **Fac Appt:** Prof Oph, Emory Univ

Lee, Paul P MD [Oph] - **Spec Exp:** Glaucoma; **Hospital:** Duke Univ Med Ctr; **Address:** Duke Univ Eye Ctr, DUMC, Erwin Rd, Box 3802, Durham, NC 27710; **Phone:** 919-681-2793; **Board Cert:** Ophthalmology 1991; **Med School:** Univ Mich Med Sch 1986; **Resid:** Ophthalmology, Wilmer Eye Inst/Johns Hopkins 1990; **Fellow:** Glaucoma, Mass EE Infirm 1991; **Fac Appt:** Prof Oph, Duke Univ

McKeown, Craig A MD [Oph] - **Spec Exp:** Pediatric Ophthalmology; Strabismus-Adult & Pediatric; Eye Muscle Disorders; **Hospital:** Bascom Palmer Eye Inst (page 55); **Address:** Bascolm Palmer Eye Institute, 900 NW 14th St, Miami, FL 33136; **Phone:** 305-243-2020; **Board Cert:** Ophthalmology 1982; **Med School:** Northwestern Univ 1971; **Resid:** Ophthalmology, Walter Reed Med Ctr 1980; **Fellow:** Pediatric Ophthalmology, Chldns Hosp Natl Med Ctr 1984; Pediatric Ophthalmology, Wilmer Inst-Johns Hospkins 1985; **Fac Appt:** Assoc Prof Oph, Univ Miami Sch Med

Meredith, Travis A MD [Oph] - **Spec Exp:** Retina/Vitreous Surgery; Macular Degeneration; Diabetic Eye Disease/Retinopathy; **Hospital:** Univ NC Hosps; **Address:** 5113 Bio Informatics, Box CB#7040, Chapel Hill, NC 27599-7040; **Phone:** 919-966-5509; **Board Cert:** Ophthalmology 1976; **Med School:** Johns Hopkins Univ 1969; **Resid:** Ophthalmology, Wilmer Inst-Johns Hopkins 1971; Ophthalmology, Wilmer Inst-Johns Hopkins 1975; **Fellow:** Vitreoretinal Surgery, Med Coll Wisconsin 1976; **Fac Appt:** Prof Oph, Univ NC Sch Med

Murray, Timothy MD [Oph] - **Spec Exp:** Retinal Disorders; Eye Tumors/Cancer; **Hospital:** Bascom Palmer Eye Inst (page 55); **Address:** Bascom Palmer Eye Inst, 900 NW 17th St, rm 254, Miami, FL 33136-1119; **Phone:** 305-326-6166; **Board Cert:** Ophthalmology 1990; **Med School:** Johns Hopkins Univ 1985; **Resid:** Ophthalmology, UCSF Med Ctr 1989; **Fellow:** Ophthalmology, UCSF 1999; Ophthalmology, Med Coll Wisconsin 1991; **Fac Appt:** Prof Oph, Univ Miami Sch Med

Nunery, William R MD [Oph] - **Spec Exp:** Orbital Surgery; Oculoplastic Surgery; Thyroid Eye Disease; **Hospital:** Univ of Louisville Hosp; **Address:** Eye Specialists of Louisville, PSC, 301 E Muhammad Ali Blvd, Louisville, KY 40202; **Phone:** 502-852-7665; **Board Cert:** Ophthalmology 1980; **Med School:** Case West Res Univ 1975; **Resid:** Ophthalmology, Indiana Univ Hosp 1979; **Fellow:** Ophthalmic Plastic Surgery, Emory Univ 1980

Nussbaum, Julian MD [Oph] - **Spec Exp:** Diabetic Eye Disease/Retinopathy; Macular Degeneration; Retinopathy of Prematurity; **Hospital:** Med Coll of GA Hosp and Clin; **Address:** Med Coll Georgia, 1120 15th St BA Bldg - rm 2701, Augusta, GA 30912; **Phone:** 706-721-1148; **Board Cert:** Ophthalmology 1981; **Med School:** Univ Miami Sch Med 1976; **Resid:** Internal Medicine, Jackson Memorial Hosp 1977; Ophthalmology, Med Coll Georgia 1980; **Fellow:** Vitreoretinal Surgery, Mass Eye & Ear Infirmary 1982; **Fac Appt:** Prof Oph, Med Coll GA

Palmberg, Paul MD/PhD [Oph] - **Spec Exp:** Glaucoma; **Hospital:** Bascom Palmer Eye Inst (page 55); **Address:** 900 NW 17th St, Miami, FL 33136; **Phone:** 305-243-2020; **Board Cert:** Ophthalmology 1976; **Med School:** Northwestern Univ 1970; **Resid:** Ophthalmology, Washington Univ 1974; Ophthalmology, Barnes Hosp 1977; **Fellow:** Glaucoma, Washington Univ 1976; **Fac Appt:** Prof Oph, Univ Miami Sch Med

Parrish, Richard K MD [Oph] - **Spec Exp:** Glaucoma; Cataract Surgery; Anterior Segment Surgery; **Hospital:** Bascom Palmer Eye Inst (page 55), Jackson Meml Hosp; **Address:** Bascom Palmer Eye Institute, 900 NW 17th St, Miami, FL 33136; **Phone:** 305-243-2020; **Board Cert:** Ophthalmology 1981; **Med School:** Indiana Univ 1976; **Resid:** Ophthalmology, Wills Eye Hosp 1980; **Fellow:** Glaucoma, Bascom Palmer Eye Inst 1982; **Fac Appt:** Prof Oph, Univ Miami Sch Med

Pollard, Zane F MD [Oph] - **Spec Exp:** Pediatric Ophthalmology; Strabismus; Tear Duct Problems; **Hospital:** Chldns Hlthcare Atlanta - Scottish Rite, Piedmont Hosp; **Address:** 5445 Meridian Mark Rd, Ste 220, Atlanta, GA 30342-4722; **Phone:** 404-255-2419; **Board Cert:** Ophthalmology 1975; **Med School:** Tulane Univ 1966; **Resid:** Surgery, UCSF Med Ctr 1968; Ophthalmology, USC Med Ctr 1973; **Fellow:** Pediatric Ophthalmology, Wills Eye Hosp 1975

Rosenfeld, Philip MD [Oph] - **Spec Exp:** Macular Disease/Degeneration; Diabetic Eye Disease/Retinopathy; Retinal Detachment; Retina/Vitreous Surgery; **Hospital:** Bascom Palmer Eye Inst (page 55); **Address:** Bascom Palmer Eye Institute, 900 NW 17th St, Miami, FL 33136; **Phone:** 305-243-2020; **Board Cert:** Ophthalmology 1997; **Med School:** Johns Hopkins Univ 1988; **Resid:** Ophthalmology, Mass Eye & Ear Infirm 1995; **Fellow:** Retina, Bascom Palmer Eye Inst 1996; **Fac Appt:** Assoc Prof Oph, Univ Fla Coll Med

Sherwood, Mark MD [Oph] - **Spec Exp:** Glaucoma; **Hospital:** Shands at Univ of FL; **Address:** Shands at University of Florida, Dept of Ophthalmology, 1600 SW Archer Rd, Box 100284, Gainesville, FL 32610-0393; **Phone:** 352-392-3451; **Board Cert:** Ophthalmology 1983; **Med School:** England 1976; **Resid:** Ophthalmology, Moorefield's Eye Hosp 1980; **Fellow:** Glaucoma, Wills Eye Hosp 1982; Glaucoma, Moorefield's Eye Hosp 1983; **Fac Appt:** Prof Oph, Univ Fla Coll Med

Sternberg Jr, Paul MD [Oph] - **Spec Exp:** Retina/Vitreous Surgery; Macular Degeneration; Eye Tumors/Cancer; **Hospital:** Vanderbilt Univ Med Ctr, Vanderbilt Children's Hosp; **Address:** Vanderbilt Eye Institute, 8000 Medical Center E, Nashville, TN 37232-8808; **Phone:** 615-936-1453; **Board Cert:** Ophthalmology 1985; **Med School:** Univ Chicago-Pritzker Sch Med 1979; **Resid:** Ophthalmology, Johns Hopkins Hosp 1983; **Fellow:** Vitreoretinal Surgery, Duke Univ Med Ctr 1984; **Fac Appt:** Prof Oph, Vanderbilt Univ

Stulting, R Doyle MD [Oph] - **Spec Exp:** Corneal Disease & Transplant; Laser Vision Surgery; Cataract Surgery; **Hospital:** Emory Univ Hosp; **Address:** The Emory Clinic, Dept Ophthalmology, 1365B Clifton Rd NE, Ste 4500, Atlanta, GA 30322; **Phone:** 404-778-5818; **Board Cert:** Ophthalmology 1982; **Med School:** Duke Univ 1976; **Resid:** Internal Medicine, Barnes Hosp 1978; Ophthalmology, Bascom Palmer Eye Inst 1981; **Fellow:** Cornea, Emory Univ Clinic 1982; **Fac Appt:** Prof Oph, Emory Univ

Ophthalmology

Tse, David MD [Oph] - **Spec Exp:** Oculoplastic Surgery; Orbital Tumors/Cancer; Lacrimal Gland Disorders; Eyelid Tumors/Cancer; **Hospital:** Bascom Palmer Eye Inst (page 55), Jackson Meml Hosp; **Address:** Bascom Palmer Eye Inst, 900 NW 17th St, Miami, FL 33136-1119; **Phone:** 305-326-6086; **Board Cert:** Ophthalmology 2002; **Med School:** Univ Miami Sch Med 1976; **Resid:** Ophthalmology, LAC/USC Med Ctr 1981; **Fellow:** Oculoplastic Surgery, Univ Iowa Hosps 1982; **Fac Appt:** Prof Oph, Univ Miami Sch Med

Wang, Ming X MD/PhD [Oph] - **Spec Exp:** Laser Vision Surgery; Anterior Segment Surgery; Corneal Disease; **Hospital:** Saint Thomas Hosp - Nashville; **Address:** 1801 West End Ave, Palmer Plaza, Ste 1150, Nashville, TN 37203; **Phone:** 615-321-8881; **Board Cert:** Ophthalmology 1998; **Med School:** Harvard Med Sch 1991; **Resid:** Ophthalmology, Wills Eye Hosp 1996; **Fellow:** Refractive Surgery, Bascom Palmer Eye Inst 1997; **Fac Appt:** , UC Davis

Waring III, George O MD [Oph] - **Spec Exp:** LASIK-Refractive Surgery; Cataract Surgery; Lens Implants; **Hospital:** Northside Hosp; **Address:** 301 Perimeter Center N, Ste 600, Atlanta, GA 30346; **Phone:** 678-222-5102; **Board Cert:** Ophthalmology 1975; **Med School:** Baylor Coll Med 1967; **Resid:** Ophthalmology, Wills Eye Hosp 1973; **Fellow:** Cornea & Ext Eye Disease, Wills Eye Hosp 1974

Wilson Jr, M Edward MD [Oph] - **Spec Exp:** Cataract-Pediatric; Strabismus-Pediatric; Lens Implants-Pediatric; Pediatric Ophthalmology; **Hospital:** MUSC Chldns Hosp; **Address:** MUSC Storm Eye Inst, 167 Ashley Ave, PO Box 250676, Charleston, SC 29425; **Phone:** 843-792-7622; **Board Cert:** Ophthalmology 1987; **Med School:** Med Univ SC 1980; **Resid:** Ophthalmology, Natl Naval Med Ctr 1986; **Fellow:** Pediatric Ophthalmology, Chldns Hosp - Naval Med Ctr 1987; **Fac Appt:** Prof Oph, Med Univ SC

Wilson, Matthew W MD [Oph] - **Spec Exp:** Eye Tumors/Cancer; Retinoblastoma; Melanoma-Choroidal (eye); **Hospital:** St Jude Children's Research Hosp, Methodist Univ Hosp - Memphis; **Address:** Univ Tenn Med Grp, Ophthalmology, 930 Madison Ave, Ste 200, Memphis, TN 38103; **Phone:** 901-448-6650; **Board Cert:** Ophthalmology 2007; **Med School:** Emory Univ 1990; **Resid:** Ophthalmology, Emory Univ Med Ctr 1994; Ophthalmic Pathology, Emory Univ 1995; **Fellow:** Ocular Oncology, Moorfields Eye Hosp 1996; Ophthalmic Plastic & Reconstructive Surgery, Casey Eye Inst 1998; **Fac Appt:** Assoc Prof Oph, Univ Tenn Coll Med, Memphis

Midwest

Abrams, Gary W MD [Oph] - **Spec Exp:** Retina/Vitreous Surgery; **Hospital:** Hutzel Hosp - Detroit; **Address:** Kresge Eye Institute, 4717 St Antoine St, Detroit, MI 48201; **Phone:** 313-577-8900; **Board Cert:** Ophthalmology 1977; **Med School:** Univ Okla Coll Med 1968; **Resid:** Ophthalmology, Med Coll Wisc Affil Hosps 1976; **Fellow:** Vitreoretinal Surgery, Bascom Palmer Eye Inst 1978; **Fac Appt:** Prof Oph, Wayne State Univ

Albert, Daniel M MD [Oph] - **Spec Exp:** Eye Tumors/Cancer; Ophthalmic Pathology; **Hospital:** Univ WI Hosp & Clins; **Address:** 2880 University Ave, Madison, WI 53705; **Phone:** 608-263-7171; **Board Cert:** Ophthalmology 1969; **Med School:** Univ Pennsylvania 1962; **Resid:** Ophthalmology, Hosp Univ Penn 1966; Neurological Ophthalmology, Natl Inst Hlth 1968; **Fellow:** Pathology, Armed Forces Inst Path 1969; **Fac Appt:** Prof Oph, Univ Wisc

Alward, Wallace MD [Oph] - **Spec Exp:** Glaucoma; **Hospital:** Univ Iowa Hosp & Clinics, VA Med Ctr - Iowa City; **Address:** 200 Hawkins Drive, Iowa City, IA 52242-1009; **Phone:** 319-356-3938; **Board Cert:** Ophthalmology 1987; **Med School:** Ohio State Univ 1976; **Resid:** Ophthalmology, Univ Louisville 1986; **Fellow:** Glaucoma, Univ Miami-Bascom Palmer Eye Inst 1987; **Fac Appt:** Prof Oph, Univ Iowa Coll Med

Archer, Steven M MD [Oph] - **Spec Exp:** Pediatric Ophthalmology; **Hospital:** Univ Michigan Hlth Sys; **Address:** Kellogg Eye Center, 1000 Wall St, Ann Arbor, MI 48105-1912; **Phone:** 734-764-7558; **Board Cert:** Ophthalmology 1986; **Med School:** Univ Chicago-Pritzker Sch Med 1978; **Resid:** Ophthalmology, Univ Chicago 1984; **Fellow:** Pediatric Ophthalmology, Indiana Univ 1986; **Fac Appt:** Asst Prof Oph, Univ Mich Med Sch

Augsburger, James MD [Oph] - **Spec Exp:** Eye Tumors/Cancer; Melanoma-Choroidal (eye); Retinoblastoma; **Hospital:** Univ Hosp - Cincinnati, Cincinnati Chldns Hosp Med Ctr; **Address:** Medical Arts Bldg, Ste 1500, 222 Piedmont Ave, rm ML 665-E, Cincinnati, OH 45267-0665; **Phone:** 513-475-7300; **Board Cert:** Ophthalmology 1979; **Med School:** Univ Cincinnati 1974; **Resid:** Ophthalmology, Univ Hosp-Cincinnati 1978; **Fellow:** Ocular Oncology, Wills Eye Hosp 1980; **Fac Appt:** Prof Oph, Univ Cincinnati

Azar, Dimitri T MD [Oph] - **Spec Exp:** Cornea Transplant; Cornea & External Eye Disease; Refractive Surgery; **Hospital:** Univ of IL at Chicago Eye & Ear Infirm; **Address:** Univ of Illinois, 30 N Michigan, Ste 410, Chicago, IL 60602; **Phone:** 312-996-2020; **Board Cert:** Ophthalmology 1991; **Med School:** Lebanon 1983; **Resid:** Ophthalmology, American Univ Medical Ctr 1986; Ophthalmology, Mass E&E Infirm 1991; **Fellow:** Cornea & Ext Eye Disease, Mass E&E Infirm 1988; Cornea Research, Harvard Med Sch 1991

Baker, John D MD [Oph] - **Spec Exp:** Pediatric Ophthalmology; **Hospital:** Chldns Hosp of Michigan; **Address:** 2355 Monroe Blvd, Dearborn, MI 48124-3009; **Phone:** 313-561-1777; **Board Cert:** Ophthalmology 1974; **Med School:** Wayne State Univ 1967; **Resid:** Ophthalmology, Detroit Genl Hosp 1971; **Fellow:** Pediatric Ophthalmology, Chldns Natl Med Ctr 1972; **Fac Appt:** Clin Prof Oph, Wayne State Univ

Burke, Miles J MD [Oph] - **Spec Exp:** Pediatric Ophthalmology; Eye Muscle Surgery; Amblyopia & Vision Development; **Hospital:** Cincinnati Chldns Hosp Med Ctr, Jewish Hosp - Kenwood - Cincinnati; **Address:** 10475 Montgomery Rd, Ste 4F, Cincinnati, OH 45242-5200; **Phone:** 513-984-4949; **Board Cert:** Ophthalmology 1979; **Med School:** Univ Ariz Coll Med 1974; **Resid:** Ophthalmology, Univ Michigan Med Ctr 1978; **Fellow:** Pediatric Ophthalmology, Wills Eye Hosp 1979

Carter, Keith D MD [Oph] - **Spec Exp:** Oculoplastic & Orbital Surgery; Eyelid Surgery / Blepharoplasty; Botox Therapy; **Hospital:** Univ Iowa Hosp & Clinics; **Address:** Univ Iowa, Dept Ophthalmology, 200 Hawkins Dr, PFP 11136-F, Iowa City, IA 52242; **Phone:** 319-356-2852; **Board Cert:** Ophthalmology 1988; **Med School:** Indiana Univ 1983; **Resid:** Ophthalmology, Univ Michigan Med Ctr 1987; **Fellow:** Oculoplastic Surgery, Univ Iowa 1988; **Fac Appt:** Prof Oph, Univ Iowa Coll Med

Cionni, Robert J MD [Oph] - **Spec Exp:** Cataract Surgery-Lens Implant; **Hospital:** Bethesda North Hosp; **Address:** 1945 CEI Drive, Cincinnati, OH 45242; **Phone:** 513-984-5133; **Board Cert:** Ophthalmology 1991; **Med School:** Univ Cincinnati 1985; **Resid:** Ophthalmology, Univ Louisville Hosp 1987; **Fellow:** Cataract/Lens Implant Surgery, Cincinnati Eye Inst

Del Monte, Monte A MD [Oph] - **Spec Exp:** Pediatric Ophthalmology; Strabismus; Glaucoma-Pediatric; Cataract-Pediatric; **Hospital:** Univ Michigan Hlth Sys; **Address:** Kellogg Eye Center, 1000 Wall St, Ann Arbor, MI 48105-1912; **Phone:** 734-764-3111; **Board Cert:** Ophthalmology 1982; **Med School:** Johns Hopkins Univ 1974; **Resid:** Pediatrics, Chldns Hosp Med Ctr 1977; Ophthalmology, Wilmer Eye Inst 1981; **Fellow:** Ophthalmology, Wilmer Eye Inst 1978; Pediatric Ophthalmology, Chldns Hosp 1981; **Fac Appt:** Prof Oph, Univ Mich Med Sch

Ophthalmology

Feder, Robert S MD [Oph] - **Spec Exp:** Corneal Disease; LASIK-Refractive Surgery; Cataract Surgery; **Hospital:** Northwestern Meml Hosp; **Address:** 675 N St Clair St, Fl 15, Chicago, IL 60611-5975; **Phone:** 312-695-8150; **Board Cert:** Ophthalmology 1983; **Med School:** Northwestern Univ 1978; **Resid:** Ophthalmology, Barnes Jewish Hosp 1982; **Fellow:** Cornea & Ext Eye Disease, Univ Iowa Med Ctr 1983; **Fac Appt:** Assoc Prof Oph, Northwestern Univ

France, Thomas D MD [Oph] - **Spec Exp:** Pediatric Ophthalmology; Strabismus-Adult & Pediatric; Amblyopia & Vision Development; **Hospital:** Univ WI Hosp & Clins; **Address:** Univ Station Clinics, Dept Pediatric Ophthalmology, 2880 University Ave, Madison, WI 53705; **Phone:** 608-263-6414; **Board Cert:** Ophthalmology 1971; **Med School:** Northwestern Univ 1962; **Resid:** Ophthalmology, UCSF Med Ctr 1969; **Fellow:** Pediatric Ophthalmology, Chldns Hosp Natl Med Ctr 1970; Pediatric Ophthalmology, Hosp Sick Chldn 1970; **Fac Appt:** Prof Oph, Univ Wisc

Greenwald, Mark MD [Oph] - **Spec Exp:** Pediatric Ophthalmology; **Hospital:** Univ of Chicago Hosps; **Address:** Univ of Chicago, Dept Ophthalmology, 5841 S Maryland Ave, MC 2114, Chicago, IL 60637; **Phone:** 773-834-5685; **Board Cert:** Ophthalmology 1981; **Med School:** Harvard Med Sch 1976; **Resid:** Ophthalmology, Univ Illinois Hosp 1980; **Fellow:** Pediatric Ophthalmology, Children's Hosp 1981; **Fac Appt:** Assoc Prof Oph, Univ Wash

Harbour, J William MD [Oph] - **Spec Exp:** Eye Tumors/Cancer; Melanoma-Choroidal (eye); Retinoblastoma; **Hospital:** Barnes-Jewish Hosp, St Louis Chldns Hosp; **Address:** Washington Univ Sch Med, Dept Ophthalmology, 660 S Euclid Ave, Box 8096, St Louis, MO 63110-1010; **Phone:** 314-362-3315; **Board Cert:** Ophthalmology 2007; **Med School:** Johns Hopkins Univ 1990; **Resid:** Ophthalmology, Wills Eye Hosp 1994; **Fellow:** Retina/Vitreous, Bascom Palmer Eye Inst 1995; Ocular Oncology, UCSF Med Ctr 1996; **Fac Appt:** Prof Oph, Washington Univ, St Louis

Heuer, Dale K MD [Oph] - **Spec Exp:** Glaucoma; **Hospital:** Froedtert Meml Lutheran Hosp; **Address:** The Eye Institute, 925 N 87th St, Milwaukee, WI 53226; **Phone:** 414-456-2020; **Board Cert:** Ophthalmology 1983; **Med School:** Northwestern Univ 1978; **Resid:** Ophthalmology, Med Coll Wisc Affil Hosp 1982; **Fellow:** Glaucoma, Bascom Palmer Eye Inst 1984; **Fac Appt:** Prof Oph, Med Coll Wisc

Holland, Edward J MD [Oph] - **Spec Exp:** Corneal Disease; Refractive Surgery; Cataract Surgery; **Hospital:** St Elizabeth Med Ctr (South Unit), Bethesda North Hosp; **Address:** 1945 CEI Drive, Cincinnati, OH 45242; **Phone:** 513-984-5133; **Board Cert:** Ophthalmology 1986; **Med School:** Loyola Univ-Stritch Sch Med 1981; **Resid:** Ophthalmology, Univ Minn Med Ctr 1985; **Fellow:** Ophthalmology, Univ Iowa 1986; Ocular Immunology, Natl Eye Inst 1987; **Fac Appt:** Clin Prof Oph, Univ Cincinnati

John, Thomas MD [Oph] - **Spec Exp:** Cornea Transplant & Artificial Cornea; Amniotic Membrane Transplant; Cataract Surgery; Refractive Surgery; **Hospital:** Loyola Univ Med Ctr, Adv S Suburban Hosp; **Address:** 16532 S Oak Park Ave, Ste 201, Tinley Park, IL 60477; **Phone:** 708-429-2223; **Board Cert:** Ophthalmology 1987; **Med School:** India 1977; **Resid:** Ophthalmology, Hosp U Penn 1984; **Fellow:** Cornea & Ext Eye Disease, Univ Rochester Sch Med & Dentistry 1985; Cornea & Ext Eye Disease, Mass Eye & Ear Infirmary 1987; **Fac Appt:** Assoc Clin Prof Oph, Loyola Univ-Stritch Sch Med

Kaufman, Paul L MD [Oph] - **Spec Exp:** Glaucoma; **Hospital:** Univ WI Hosp & Clins; **Address:** Univ Wisconsin Hosp, Dept Ophthalmology, 3310 University Ave, Ste 206, Madison, WI 53705-2135; **Phone:** 608-263-7171; **Board Cert:** Ophthalmology 1976; **Med School:** NYU Sch Med 1967; **Resid:** Ophthalmology, Barnes Hospital 1973; **Fellow:** Ocular Pharmacology, Univ Uppsala 1975; **Fac Appt:** Prof Oph, Univ Wisc

Krachmer, Jay H MD [Oph] - **Spec Exp:** Corneal Disease; **Hospital:** Univ Minn Med Ctr, Fairview - Univ Campus; **Address:** Dept Ophthalmology, 420 Delaware St SE, MMC 88, Minneapolis, MN 55455; **Phone:** 612-625-4400; **Board Cert:** Ophthalmology 1972; **Med School:** Tulane Univ 1966; **Resid:** Ophthalmology, Univ Hosp 1970; **Fellow:** Cornea, Wills Eye Hosp 1974; **Fac Appt:** Prof Oph, Univ Minn

Krueger, Ronald MD [Oph] - **Spec Exp:** Corneal Disease; Refractive Surgery; **Hospital:** Cleveland Clin Fdn (page 56); **Address:** Cleveland Clinic Fdn - Cole Eye Inst, 9500 Euclid Ave, Desk i32, Cleveland, OH 44195; **Phone:** 216-444-8158; **Board Cert:** Ophthalmology 2003; **Med School:** UMDNJ-NJ Med Sch, Newark 1987; **Resid:** Ophthalmology, Columbia Presby Med Ctr 1991; **Fellow:** Refractive Surgery, Univ Okla Hlth Sci Ctr-McGee Eye Inst; Cornea, USC-Doheny Eye Inst 1993

Kushner, Burton J MD [Oph] - **Spec Exp:** Pediatric Ophthalmology; Strabismus-Adult & Pediatric; **Hospital:** Univ WI Hosp & Clins; **Address:** Dept Ophth-UNW Hosp, 2870 University Ave, Ste 102, Madison, WI 53705; **Phone:** 608-263-7171; **Board Cert:** Ophthalmology 1975; **Med School:** Northwestern Univ 1969; **Resid:** Ophthalmology, Univ Wisc Hosp 1973; **Fellow:** Pediatric Ophthalmology, Bascom Palmer Eye Inst 1974; **Fac Appt:** Prof Oph, Univ Wisc

Lane, Stephen S MD [Oph] - **Spec Exp:** Laser Vision Surgery; Cataract Surgery; **Hospital:** United Hosp; **Address:** Associated Eye Care, 2950 Curve Crest Blvd, Stillwater, MN 55082; **Phone:** 651-275-3000; **Board Cert:** Ophthalmology 1986; **Med School:** Univ Minn 1980; **Resid:** Ophthalmology, MS Hershey Med Ctr 1984; **Fellow:** Cornea & Ext Eye Disease, Univ Minn 1984; **Fac Appt:** Clin Prof Oph, Univ Minn

Lee, Andrew G MD [Oph] - **Spec Exp:** Neuro-Ophthalmology; Optic Nerve Disorders; Optic Nerve Tumors; **Hospital:** Univ Iowa Hosp & Clinics; **Address:** Univ Iowa, Dept Ophthalmology, 200 Hawkins Dr, PFP 11290-E, Iowa City, IA 52242; **Phone:** 319-356-2548; **Board Cert:** Ophthalmology 1995; **Med School:** Univ VA Sch Med 1989; **Resid:** Ophthalmology, Cullen Eye Inst-Baylor 1993; **Fellow:** Neurological Ophthalmology, Wilmer Eye Inst-Johns Hopkins 1994; **Fac Appt:** Prof Oph, Univ Iowa Coll Med

Lichter, Paul R MD [Oph] - **Spec Exp:** Cataract Surgery; Glaucoma; **Hospital:** Univ Michigan Hlth Sys; **Address:** 1000 Wall St, Ann Arbor, MI 48105; **Phone:** 734-763-5874; **Board Cert:** Ophthalmology 1970; **Med School:** Univ Mich Med Sch 1964; **Resid:** Ophthalmology, Univ Mich Med Ctr 1968; **Fellow:** Ophthalmology, UCSF Med Ctr 1969; **Fac Appt:** Prof Oph, Univ Mich Med Sch

Lindstrom, Richard L MD [Oph] - **Spec Exp:** Corneal Disease; Cataract Surgery; Refractive Surgery; **Hospital:** Abbott - Northwestern Hosp, Phillips Eye Inst; **Address:** 9801 DuPont Ave, Bloomington, MN 55443; **Phone:** 612-813-3600; **Board Cert:** Ophthalmology 1978; **Med School:** Univ Minn 1972; **Resid:** Ophthalmology, Univ Minn 1979; Ophthalmology, Univ Minn 1980; **Fellow:** Anterior Segment - External Disease, Mary Shields Eye Hosp; Glaucoma, Univ Hosps; **Fac Appt:** Prof Oph, Univ Minn

Lueder, Gregg T MD [Oph] - **Spec Exp:** Retinoblastoma; Eye Tumors-Pediatric; Pediatric Ophthalmology; **Hospital:** St Louis Chldns Hosp; **Address:** St Louis Children's Hospital, One Children's Pl, Ste 2S89, St Louis, MO 63110; **Phone:** 314-454-6026; **Board Cert:** Ophthalmology 2003; **Med School:** Univ Iowa Coll Med 1985; **Resid:** Pediatrics, St Louis Children's Hosp 1988; Ophthalmology, Univ Iowa Med Ctr 1991; **Fellow:** Pediatric Ophthalmology, Hosp for Sick Children 1993; **Fac Appt:** Assoc Prof Oph, Washington Univ, St Louis

Ophthalmology

Maguire, Leo J MD [Oph] - **Spec Exp:** Cornea Transplant; Refractive Surgery; Boston Scleral Lens Prosthesis; **Hospital:** Mayo Med Ctr & Clin - Rochester; **Address:** Mayo Clinic, Dept Ophthalmology, 200 First St SW, Rochester, MN 55905; **Phone:** 507-284-4152; **Board Cert:** Ophthalmology 1986; **Med School:** Jefferson Med Coll 1980; **Resid:** Ophthalmology, Univ Michigan Med Ctr 1984; **Fellow:** Cornea & Ext Eye Disease, LSU Eye Ctr 1986; **Fac Appt:** Assoc Prof Oph, Mayo Med Sch

Mets, Marilyn MD [Oph] - **Spec Exp:** Pediatric Ophthalmology; Ophthalmic Genetics; Strabismus; Retinal Disorders; **Hospital:** Children's Mem Hosp; **Address:** 2300 Children's Plaza, Box 70, Chicago, IL 60614; **Phone:** 773-880-4346; **Board Cert:** Ophthalmology 2005; **Med School:** Geo Wash Univ 1976; **Resid:** Ophthalmology, Cleveland Clinic Fdn 1980; **Fellow:** Ophthalmology, Natl Chldns Hosp 1981; **Fac Appt:** Prof Oph, Northwestern Univ

Mieler, William F MD [Oph] - **Spec Exp:** Retina/Vitreous Surgery; Eye Tumors/Cancer; **Hospital:** Univ of Chicago Hosps, Weiss Meml Hosp; **Address:** Univ Chicago, Dept Opth & Vis Sci, 5841 S Maryland, rm S-209, MC 211, Chicago, IL 60637; **Phone:** 773-702-3838; **Board Cert:** Ophthalmology 1984; **Med School:** Univ Wisc 1979; **Resid:** Ophthalmology, Bascom-Palmer Eye Inst 1983; **Fellow:** Vitreoretinal Surgery & Disease, Med Ctr Wisconsin Eye Inst 1984; Oculoplastic Surgery, Wills Eye Hosp 1986; **Fac Appt:** Prof Oph, Univ Chicago-Pritzker Sch Med

Nerad, Jeffrey MD [Oph] - **Spec Exp:** Orbital Tumors/Cancer; Eyelid Cancer & Reconstruction; Oculoplastic Surgery; **Hospital:** Univ Iowa Hosp & Clinics; **Address:** Univ Iowa, Dept Ophthalmology, 200 Hawkins Drive, Iowa City, IA 52242; **Phone:** 319-356-2864; **Board Cert:** Ophthalmology 1984; **Med School:** St Louis Univ 1979; **Resid:** Ophthalmology, St Louis Univ Med Ctr 1983; **Fellow:** Oculoplastic & Reconstructive Surgery, Univ Iowa 1984; **Fac Appt:** Prof Oph, Univ Iowa Coll Med

Olitsky, Scott E MD [Oph] - **Spec Exp:** Pediatric Ophthalmology; Strabismus; **Hospital:** Chldns Mercy Hosps & Clinics; **Address:** Chldns Mercy Hosp, Dept Oph, 2401 Gillham Rd, Kansas City, MO 64108; **Phone:** 816-234-3046; **Board Cert:** Ophthalmology 2004; **Med School:** Jefferson Med Coll 1988; **Resid:** Ophthalmology, SUNY Buffalo Med Ctr 1992; **Fellow:** Pediatric Ophthalmology, Wills Eye Hosp 1993; **Fac Appt:** Prof Oph, Univ MO-Kansas City

Osher, Robert H MD [Oph] - **Spec Exp:** Cataract Surgery-Lens Implant; **Address:** 1945 CEI Drive, Cincinnati, OH 45242; **Phone:** 513-984-5133; **Board Cert:** Ophthalmology 1981; **Med School:** Univ Rochester 1976; **Resid:** Ophthalmology, Bascom Palmer Eye Inst 1980; **Fellow:** Ophthalmology, Wills Eye Hosp 1977; Ophthalmology, Bascom Palmer Eye Inst 1981; **Fac Appt:** Prof Oph, Univ Cincinnati

Pepose, Jay MD [Oph] - **Spec Exp:** LASIK-Refractive Surgery; Cataract Surgery; Corneal & External Eye Disease; **Hospital:** Barnes-Jewish Hosp, St John's Mercy Med Ctr - St Louis; **Address:** 1815 Clarkson Rd, Chesterfield, MO 63017; **Phone:** 636-728-0111; **Board Cert:** Ophthalmology 1989; **Med School:** UCLA 1982; **Resid:** Ophthalmology, Johns Hopkins Hosp 1987; **Fellow:** Cornea & Ext Eye Disease, Georgetown Univ Med Ctr 1988; **Fac Appt:** Prof Oph, Washington Univ, St Louis

Putterman, Allen M MD [Oph] - **Spec Exp:** Oculoplastic & Orbital Surgery; Cosmetic Surgery-Face & Eyes; Thyroid Eye Disease; **Hospital:** Michael Reese Hosp & Med Ctr, Univ of IL Med Ctr at Chicago; **Address:** 111 N Wabash Ave, Ste 1722, Chicago, IL 60602-2002; **Phone:** 312-372-2256; **Board Cert:** Ophthalmology 1971; **Med School:** Univ Wisc 1963; **Resid:** Ophthalmology, Michael Reese Hosp 1969; **Fellow:** Oculoplastic Surgery, Manhattan Eye/Ear Infirm 1970; **Fac Appt:** Prof Oph, Univ IL Coll Med

Rogers, Gary L MD [Oph] - **Spec Exp:** Strabismus-Adult & Pediatric; **Hospital:** Nationwide Chldn's Hosp; **Address:** 555 S 18th St, Ste 4C, Columbus, OH 43205; **Phone:** 614-224-6222; **Board Cert:** Ophthalmology 1974; **Med School:** Ohio State Univ 1968; **Resid:** Ophthalmology, Mt Sinai Hosp 1972; **Fellow:** Pediatric Ophthalmology, Chldns Hosp Natl Med Ctr 1974; **Fac Appt:** Clin Prof Oph, Ohio State Univ

Rosenberg, Michael A MD [Oph] - **Spec Exp:** Refractive Surgery; Cataract Surgery; Eye Muscle Surgery; **Hospital:** Northwestern Meml Hosp, Evanston Hosp; **Address:** Northwestern Med Fac Fdn, 675 N St Clair, Ste 15-150, Chicago, IL 60611-5967; **Phone:** 312-695-8150; **Board Cert:** Ophthalmology 1975; **Med School:** Northwestern Univ 1967; **Resid:** Ophthalmology, Bascom Palmer Eye Inst 1973; **Fellow:** Neurological Ophthalmology, UCSF Med Ctr 1974; Refractive Surgery, Univ Monterrey 1998; **Fac Appt:** Assoc Clin Prof Oph, Northwestern Univ

Samuelson, Thomas MD [Oph] - **Spec Exp:** Glaucoma; Cataract Surgery; Anterior Segment Surgery; Refractive Surgery; **Hospital:** Phillips Eye Inst, Regions Hosp - St Paul; **Address:** Minnesota Eye Consultants, 710 E 24th St, Ste 100, Minneapolis, MN 55404-3810; **Phone:** 612-813-3600; **Board Cert:** Ophthalmology 1991; **Med School:** Univ Minn 1985; **Resid:** Ophthalmology, Univ S Fla 1990; **Fellow:** Glaucoma, Wills Eye Hosp 1991; **Fac Appt:** Assoc Clin Prof Oph, Univ Minn

Schachat, Andrew P MD [Oph] - **Spec Exp:** Retina/Vitreous Surgery; Diabetic Eye Disease/Retinopathy; Melanoma-Choroidal (eye); **Hospital:** Cleveland Clin Fdn (page 56); **Address:** The Cleveland Clinic Fdn, Cole Eye Inst, 9500 Euclid Ave, Desk i30, Cleveland, OH 44195; **Phone:** 216-444-0430; **Board Cert:** Ophthalmology 1983; **Med School:** Johns Hopkins Univ 1979; **Resid:** Ophthalmology, Wilmer Inst-John Hopkins Hosp 1982; **Fellow:** Vitreoretinal Surgery & Disease, Wilmer Eye Inst-Johns Hopkins Hosp 1983; **Fac Appt:** Prof Oph

Stone, Edwin MD [Oph] - **Spec Exp:** Retinal Disorders; Eye Diseases-Hereditary; **Hospital:** Univ Iowa Hosp & Clinics; **Address:** Dept Ophthalmology, 200 Hawkins Dr, Pomerantz Bldg, Iowa City, IA 52242; **Phone:** 319-356-2864; **Board Cert:** Ophthalmology 1990; **Med School:** Baylor Coll Med 1985; **Resid:** Ophthalmology, Univ Iowa Hosps 1989; **Fellow:** Retina, Univ Iowa Hosps 1992; **Fac Appt:** Prof Oph, Univ Iowa Coll Med

Summers, C Gail MD [Oph] - **Hospital:** Univ Minn Med Ctr, Fairview - Univ Campus; **Address:** Dept Ophthalmology, 420 Delaware St SE, MMC 88, Minneapolis, MN 55455-0356; **Phone:** 612-625-4400; **Board Cert:** Ophthalmology 1984; **Med School:** Univ Minn 1979; **Resid:** Ophthalmology, Univ Minnesota Med Ctr 1983; **Fellow:** Pediatric Ophthalmology, Unin Minnesota Med Ctr 1984; **Fac Appt:** Prof Oph, Univ Minn

Traboulsi, Elias Iskan MD [Oph] - **Spec Exp:** Pediatric Ophthalmology; Glaucoma-Pediatric; **Hospital:** Cleveland Clin Fdn (page 56); **Address:** Cleveland Clinic Fdn, Cole Eye Inst, 9500 Euclid Ave, Desk i32, Cleveland, OH 44195; **Phone:** 216-444-0430; **Board Cert:** Clinical Genetics 1987; Ophthalmology 1991; **Med School:** Amer Univ Beirut 1982; **Resid:** Ophthalmology, American Univ Beirut Hosp 1985; Ophthalmology, Georgetown Hosp 1989; **Fellow:** Ophthalmology, Johns Hopkins Hosp 1986; Pediatric Ophthalmology, Chldns Hosp Natl Med Ctr 1990; **Fac Appt:** Prof Oph, Ohio State Univ

Trese, Michael T MD [Oph] - **Spec Exp:** Retina/Vitreous Surgery; Retinal Disorders-Pediatric; **Hospital:** William Beaumont Hosp, Chldns Hosp of Michigan; **Address:** 3535 W 13 Mile Rd, Ste 344, Royal Oak, MI 48073-6710; **Phone:** 248-288-2280; **Board Cert:** Ophthalmology 1981; **Med School:** Georgetown Univ 1976; **Resid:** Ophthalmology, Jules Stein Eye Inst-UCLA 1980; **Fellow:** Retina, Duke Univ Med Ctr 1981; **Fac Appt:** Assoc Clin Prof Oph, Wayne State Univ

Ophthalmology

Trobe, Jonathan Daniel MD [Oph] - **Spec Exp:** Neuro-Ophthalmology; Optic Nerve Disorders; **Hospital:** Univ Michigan Hlth Sys; **Address:** WK Kellogg Eye Ctr, 1000 Wall St, Ann Arbor, MI 48105-1912; **Phone:** 734-763-5114; **Board Cert:** Ophthalmology 1974; Neurology 1988; **Med School:** Harvard Med Sch 1968; **Resid:** Ophthalmology, Wills Eye Hosp 1972; Neurology, Jackson Meml Hosp/U Miami 1986; **Fellow:** Neurological Ophthalmology, Bascom Palmer Eye Inst 1977; **Fac Appt:** Prof Oph, Univ Mich Med Sch

Tychsen, Lawrence MD [Oph] - **Spec Exp:** Pediatric Ophthalmology; Strabismus; Amblyopia; **Hospital:** St Louis Chldns Hosp, Barnes-Jewish Hosp; **Address:** Chldns Eye Care Ctr, 1 Children's Pl, Ste 2S89, St Louis, MO 63110; **Phone:** 314-454-6026; **Board Cert:** Ophthalmology 1984; **Med School:** Georgetown Univ 1979; **Resid:** Ophthalmology, Univ Iowa Hosp 1983; **Fellow:** Pediatric Ophthalmology, UCSF Med Ctr 1985; **Fac Appt:** Assoc Prof Oph, Washington Univ, St Louis

Vine, Andrew K MD [Oph] - **Spec Exp:** Melanoma-Choroidal (eye); Retinal Disorders; Macular Degeneration; **Hospital:** Univ Michigan Hlth Sys; **Address:** Univ Michigan-Kellogg Eye Ctr, 1000 Wall St, Ann Arbor, MI 48105; **Phone:** 734-763-5906; **Board Cert:** Ophthalmology 1979; **Med School:** McGill Univ 1972; **Resid:** Ophthalmology, Royal Victoria Hosp 1978; **Fellow:** Pathology, McGill Univ 1975; Retina, UCSF Med Ctr 1980; **Fac Appt:** Prof Oph, Univ Mich Med Sch

Weingeist, Thomas A MD/PhD [Oph] - **Spec Exp:** Retinal Disorders; Eye Tumors/Cancer; **Hospital:** Univ Iowa Hosp & Clinics; **Address:** Univ Iowa, Dept Ophthalmology, 200 Hawkins Drive, Iowa City, IA 52242; **Phone:** 319-356-2864; **Board Cert:** Ophthalmology 1976; **Med School:** Univ Iowa Coll Med 1972; **Resid:** Ophthalmology, Univ Iowa Hosp 1975; **Fellow:** Vitreoretinal Surgery, Univ Iowa 1976; **Fac Appt:** Prof Oph, Univ Iowa Coll Med

Williams, George A MD [Oph] - **Spec Exp:** Retinal Disorders; Macular Degeneration; **Hospital:** William Beaumont Hosp; **Address:** Associated Retinal Consultants, 3535 W 13 Mile Rd MOB Bldg - Ste 344, Royal Oak, MI 48073; **Phone:** 248-288-2280; **Board Cert:** Ophthalmology 2005; **Med School:** Northwestern Univ 1978; **Resid:** Ophthalmology, Med Coll Wisconsin 1982; **Fellow:** Retina/Vitreous, Med Coll Wisconsin 1984; **Fac Appt:** Clin Prof Oph, Univ Mich Med Sch

Wilson, Steven E MD [Oph] - **Spec Exp:** PRK-Refractive Surgery; Corneal Disease; **Hospital:** Cleveland Clin Fdn (page 56); **Address:** Cleveland Clinic Fdn - Cole Eye Inst, 9500 Euclid Ave, Ste I32, Cleveland, OH 44195; **Phone:** 216-444-5887; **Board Cert:** Ophthalmology 1990; **Med School:** UCSD 1984; **Resid:** Ophthalmology, Mayo Clinic 1988; **Fellow:** Refractive Surgery, Med Ctr Louisiana-LSU 1990; **Fac Appt:** Prof Oph, Case West Res Univ

Younge, Brian R MD [Oph] - **Spec Exp:** Neuro-Ophthalmology; Temporal Arteritis; Ocular Palsies; **Hospital:** Mayo Med Ctr & Clin - Rochester; **Address:** Mayo Clinic, Dept Ophthalmology, 200 First St SW, Rochester, MN 55905-0001; **Phone:** 507-284-4567; **Board Cert:** Ophthalmology 1974; **Med School:** Univ Alberta 1965; **Resid:** Ophthalmology, Montreal Genl Hosp 1972; **Fellow:** Neurological Ophthalmology, Mayo Clinic 1974; **Fac Appt:** Prof Oph, Mayo Med Sch

Great Plains and Mountains

Anderson, Richard L MD [Oph] - **Spec Exp:** Orbital & Eyelid Tumors/Cancer; Eyelid Problems/Ptosis/Blepharospasm; Cosmetic Surgery-Face & Eyes; **Hospital:** Salt Lake Regional Med Ctr, Intermountain Shriners Hosp; **Address:** 1002 E South Temple, Ste 308, Salt Lake City, UT 84102-1525; **Phone:** 801-363-3355; **Board Cert:** Ophthalmology 1976; **Med School:** Univ Iowa Coll Med 1971; **Resid:** Ophthalmology, Univ Iowa Hosps-Clins 1975; **Fellow:** Oculoplastic & Reconstructive Surgery, Albany Med Ctr 1975; Oculoplastic & Reconstructive Surgery, UCSF Med Ctr 1976; **Fac Appt:** Prof Pls, Univ Utah

Crandall, Alan S MD [Oph] - **Spec Exp:** Glaucoma; Cataract Surgery; **Hospital:** Univ Utah Hosps and Clins; **Address:** Moran Eye Ctr- Univ Utah Hosp, 65 N Mario Cappecchi Drive, Salt Lake City, UT 84132; **Phone:** 801-581-2352; **Board Cert:** Ophthalmology 1977; **Med School:** Univ Utah 1973; **Resid:** Ophthalmology, Hosp Univ Penn 1976; **Fellow:** Glaucoma, Scheie Eye Inst; **Fac Appt:** Clin Prof Oph, Univ Utah

Durrie, Daniel MD [Oph] - **Spec Exp:** LASIK-Refractive Surgery; Corneal Disease; **Hospital:** Univ of Kansas Hosp; **Address:** 5520 College Blvd, Ste 201, Leawood, KS 66211; **Phone:** 913-491-3330; **Board Cert:** Ophthalmology 1979; **Med School:** Univ Nebr Coll Med 1975; **Resid:** Ophthalmology, Univ Nebr Med Coll 1979; **Fellow:** Cornea, Filkins Eye Inst 1980; **Fac Appt:** Asst Clin Prof Oph, Univ Kans

Gigantelli, James W MD [Oph] - **Spec Exp:** Orbital Tumors/Cancer; Eyelid Cancer & Reconstruction; Lymphoma-Ocular (eye); **Hospital:** Nebraska Med Ctr; **Address:** Univ Nebraska Med Ctr, Ophthalmology, 985540 Nebraska Medical Ctr, Omaha, NE 68198-5540; **Phone:** 402-559-4276; **Board Cert:** Ophthalmology 1991; **Med School:** Vanderbilt Univ 1985; **Resid:** Ophthalmology, Baylor Coll Med 1989; **Fellow:** Oculoplastic Surgery, Duke Unv Med Ctr 1990; **Fac Appt:** Assoc Prof Oph, Univ Nebr Coll Med

Southwest

Ellis Jr, George S MD [Oph] - **Spec Exp:** Pediatric Ophthalmology; Eye Muscle Disorders; **Hospital:** Children's Hospital - New Orleans, E Jefferson Genl Hosp; **Address:** Children's Hospital, 200 Henry Clay Ave, Ste 3106, New Orleans, LA 70118; **Phone:** 504-896-9426; **Board Cert:** Ophthalmology 1982; **Med School:** Tulane Univ 1977; **Resid:** Ophthalmology, Duke Univ-Eye Ctr 1982; Pediatric Ophthalmology, Hall Eye Clinic 1982; **Fellow:** Pediatric Ophthalmology, Chldns Hosp 1983; **Fac Appt:** Assoc Clin Prof Oph, Tulane Univ

Eustis, Horatio S MD [Oph] - **Spec Exp:** Pediatric Ophthalmology; **Hospital:** Ochsner Fdn Hosp; **Address:** Ochsner Clinic, Dept Oph, 1514 Jefferson Hwy, Fl 10, New Orleans, LA 70121; **Phone:** 504-842-3995; **Board Cert:** Ophthalmology 1985; **Med School:** Louisiana State U, New Orleans 1980; **Resid:** Ophthalmology, LSU Eye Ctr 1984; **Fellow:** Pediatric Ophthalmology, Hosp Sick Chldn 1985; Pediatric Ophthalmology, Chldns Hosp; **Fac Appt:** Clin Prof Oph, Louisiana State U, New Orleans

Holladay, Jack T MD [Oph] - **Spec Exp:** LASIK-Refractive Surgery; PRK-Refractive Surgery; **Hospital:** Park Plaza Hosp; **Address:** Holladay LASIK Institute, 6802 Mapleridge, Ste 200, Houston, TX 77401; **Phone:** 713-668-7337; **Board Cert:** Ophthalmology 1979; **Med School:** Univ Tex, Houston 1974; **Resid:** Ophthalmology, Univ Texas Hlth Sci Ctr 1978; **Fellow:** Ophthalmology, Univ Texas Hlth Sci Ctr 1975; **Fac Appt:** Clin Prof Oph, Baylor Coll Med

Koch, Douglas D MD [Oph] - **Spec Exp:** Cataract Surgery; Refractive Surgery; **Hospital:** Methodist Hosp - Houston; **Address:** 7200 Cambridge St, Houston, TX 77030-2704; **Phone:** 713-798-6100; **Board Cert:** Ophthalmology 1982; **Med School:** Harvard Med Sch 1977; **Resid:** Ophthalmology, Baylor Coll Med 1981; **Fellow:** Cornea, Moorfields Eye Hosp 1982; Ophthalmology, Baylor Coll Med 1982; **Fac Appt:** Prof Oph, Baylor Coll Med

Lambert, H Michael MD [Oph] - **Spec Exp:** Retina/Vitreous Surgery; Macular Disease/Degeneration; Diabetic Eye Disease/Retinopathy; **Hospital:** Methodist Hosp - Houston, St Luke's Episcopal Hosp - Houston; **Address:** 2727 Gramercy, Ste 200, Houston, TX 77025-1633; **Phone:** 713-799-9975; **Board Cert:** Ophthalmology 1983; **Med School:** Baylor Coll Med 1977; **Resid:** Ophthalmology, Wilford Hall USAF Med Ctr 1982; **Fellow:** Vitreoretinal Surgery, Duke Univ Eye Ctr 1983; **Fac Appt:** Assoc Clin Prof Oph, Baylor Coll Med

Ophthalmology

Lewis, Richard Alan MD [Oph] - **Spec Exp:** Eye Diseases-Hereditary; Ophthalmic Genetics; Retinal Disorders; **Hospital:** St Luke's Episcopal Hosp - Houston, Texas Chldns Hosp - Houston; **Address:** Cullen Eye Institute NC-206, Baylor College of Medicine, One Baylor Plaza, Houston, TX 77030; **Phone:** 713-798-6100; **Board Cert:** Ophthalmology 1976; **Med School:** Univ Mich Med Sch 1969; **Resid:** Ophthalmology, Univ Michigan Hospital 1973; **Fellow:** Retina, Univ Michigan Hospital 1974; Macular Disease, Bascom Palmer Eye Inst 1975; **Fac Appt:** Prof Oph, Baylor Coll Med

Mazow, Malcolm L MD [Oph] - **Spec Exp:** Strabismus-Adult; Pediatric Ophthalmology; **Hospital:** Meml Hermann Hosp - Texas Med Ctr; **Address:** 2855 Gramercy St, Houston, TX 77025; **Phone:** 713-668-6828; **Board Cert:** Ophthalmology 1967; **Med School:** Univ Tex Med Br, Galveston 1961; **Resid:** Ophthalmology, Univ Iowa Hosp 1965; **Fellow:** Strabismus, Univ Iowa Hosp 1966; **Fac Appt:** Clin Prof Oph, Univ Tex, Houston

McCulley, James P MD [Oph] - **Spec Exp:** Corneal & External Eye Disease; Laser Vision Surgery; Cataract Surgery; **Hospital:** UT Southwestern Med Ctr - Dallas, Univ Med Ctr - Lubbock; **Address:** Univ Tex SW Med Ctr, Dept Oph, 5323 Harry Hines Blvd, Dallas, TX 75390-9057; **Phone:** 214-645-2020; **Board Cert:** Ophthalmology 1974; **Med School:** Washington Univ, St Louis 1968; **Resid:** Ophthalmology, Mass EE Infirm 1973; **Fellow:** Cornea, Cornea Rsch-Retina Fdn 1974; Cornea, Mass EE Infirm 1974; **Fac Appt:** Prof Oph, Univ Tex SW, Dallas

Miller, Joseph M MD [Oph] - **Spec Exp:** Pediatric Ophthalmology; Strabismus; Amblyopia; **Hospital:** Univ Med Ctr - Tucson; **Address:** Univ Ariz, Dept Ophthalmology, 655 N Alvernon Way, Ste 108, Tucson, AZ 85711; **Phone:** 520-694-1460; **Board Cert:** Ophthalmology 1991; **Med School:** NE Ohio Univ 1985; **Resid:** Ophthalmology, Yale New Haven Hosp 1990; **Fellow:** Pediatric Ophthalmology, Johns Hopkins Hosp 1991; Refractive Surgery, Univ Arizona Hosp 2001; **Fac Appt:** Prof Oph, Univ Ariz Coll Med

Mims III, James Luther MD [Oph] - **Spec Exp:** Pediatric Ophthalmology; Strabismus-Adult & Pediatric; **Hospital:** Baptist Med Ctr - San Antonio, Methodist Chldns Hosp of South Texas; **Address:** 311 Camden St, Ste 511, San Antonio, TX 78215-2015; **Phone:** 210-225-0084; **Board Cert:** Ophthalmology 1977; **Med School:** Tulane Univ 1968; **Resid:** Ophthalmology, Wills Eye Hosp 1976; **Fellow:** Pediatric Ophthalmology, Wills Eye Hosp 1977; **Fac Appt:** Clin Prof Oph, Univ Tex, San Antonio

Pflugfelder, Stephen C MD [Oph] - **Spec Exp:** Corneal & External Eye Disease; Refractive Surgery; Cataract Surgery; Lens Implants; **Hospital:** Baylor Univ Medical Ctr; **Address:** Cullen Eye Inst-Baylor College of Medicine, 6501 Fannin, Ste NC307, Houston, TX 77030; **Phone:** 713-798-4730; **Board Cert:** Ophthalmology 1987; **Med School:** SUNY Upstate Med Univ 1981; **Resid:** Ophthalmology, Baylor Univ Med Ctr 1985; **Fellow:** Cornea & Ext Eye Disease, Bascom Palmer Eye Inst 1986; **Fac Appt:** Prof Oph, Baylor Coll Med

Richard, James M MD [Oph] - **Spec Exp:** Pediatric Ophthalmology; Eye Muscle Surgery; **Hospital:** Integris Baptist Med Ctr - OK, Deaconess Hosp - Oklahoma; **Address:** 11013 Hefner Pointe Drive, Oklahoma City, OK 73120-5050; **Phone:** 405-751-2020; **Board Cert:** Ophthalmology 1979; **Med School:** Univ Okla Coll Med 1974; **Resid:** Ophthalmology, Baylor Coll Med 1978; **Fellow:** Pediatric Ophthalmology, Chldns Hosp 1979; Ophthalmology, Johns Hopkins Hosp 1980; **Fac Appt:** Clin Prof Oph, Univ Okla Coll Med

Siatkowski, R Michael MD [Oph] - **Spec Exp:** Pediatric Ophthalmology; Neuro-Ophthalmology; Retinopathy of Prematurity; **Hospital:** OU Med Ctr; **Address:** Dean A Mcgee Eye Institute, 608 Stanton L Young Blvd, Oklahoma City, OK 73104; **Phone:** 405-271-1094; **Board Cert:** Ophthalmology 2003; **Med School:** Jefferson Med Coll 1987; **Resid:** Ophthalmology, St Francis Med Ctr 1991; **Fellow:** Neurological Ophthalmology, Bascom Palmer Eye Inst 1992; Pediatric Ophthalmology, Bascom Palmer Eye Inst 1993; **Fac Appt:** Prof Oph, Univ Okla Coll Med

Soparkar, Charles MD [Oph] - **Spec Exp:** Eye Tumors/Cancer; Orbital & Eyelid Tumors/Cancer; Oculoplastic Surgery; **Hospital:** Methodist Hosp - Houston, Texas Chldns Hosp - Houston; **Address:** Plastic Eye Surg Assocs, 3730 Kirby Drive, Ste 900, Houston, TX 77098; **Phone:** 713-795-0705; **Board Cert:** Ophthalmology 1996; **Med School:** Univ Mass Sch Med 1990; **Resid:** Ophthalmology, Baylor Affil Hosps 1994; **Fellow:** Ophthalmic Oncololgy, Texas Med Ctr 1995

Wallace, R Bruce MD [Oph] - **Spec Exp:** Refractive Surgery; Cataract Surgery; **Hospital:** St Francis Med Ctr; **Address:** 4110 Parliament Drive, Alexandria, LA 71303; **Phone:** 318-448-4488; **Board Cert:** Ophthalmology 1979; **Med School:** Tulane Univ 1974; **Resid:** Ophthalmology, Tulane Univ 1979; **Fac Appt:** Clin Prof Oph, Louisiana State U, New Orleans

Wilhelmus, Kirk R MD/PhD [Oph] - **Spec Exp:** Corneal & External Eye Disease; **Hospital:** Methodist Hosp - Houston; **Address:** Cullen Eye Inst, 7200 Cambridge St, Houston, TX 77030; **Phone:** 713-798-6100; **Board Cert:** Ophthalmology 1981; **Med School:** Vanderbilt Univ 1975; **Resid:** Ophthalmology, Baylor Coll Med 1979; **Fellow:** Cornea & Ext Eye Disease, Moorfields Eye Hosp 1981; **Fac Appt:** Prof Oph, Baylor Coll Med

West Coast and Pacific

Abbott, Richard L MD [Oph] - **Spec Exp:** Cornea & External Eye Disease; **Hospital:** UCSF Med Ctr; **Address:** UCSF, Dept Ophthalmology, 8 Koret Way, K301, San Francisco, CA 94143-0730; **Phone:** 415-476-3705; **Board Cert:** Ophthalmology 1978; **Med School:** Geo Wash Univ 1971; **Resid:** Ophthalmology, Presby-Pacific Med Ctr 1977; **Fellow:** Cornea & Ext Eye Disease, Bascom Palmer Eye Inst 1978; **Fac Appt:** Clin Prof Oph, UCSF

Arnold, Anthony C MD [Oph] - **Spec Exp:** Neuro-Ophthalmology; **Hospital:** Ronald Reagan UCLA Med Ctr; **Address:** 100 Stein Plaza, Box 957000, Los Angeles, CA 90095-7005; **Phone:** 310-825-4344; **Board Cert:** Ophthalmology 2008; **Med School:** UCLA 1975; **Resid:** Ophthalmology, Jules Stein Eye Inst-UCLA 1979; **Fellow:** Neurological Ophthalmology, Jules Stein Eye Inst-UCLA 1983; **Fac Appt:** Clin Prof Oph, UCLA

Baerveldt, George MD [Oph] - **Spec Exp:** Glaucoma; **Hospital:** UC Irvine Med Ctr; **Address:** UC Irvine Med Ctr, Dept Ophthalmology, 118 Med-Surg I, Irvine, CA 92697-4375; **Phone:** 949-824-2020; **Med School:** South Africa 1967; **Resid:** Ophthalmology, Univ of Witwatersrand 1975; **Fellow:** Neurological Ophthalmology, SUNY Downstate Med Ctr 1975; **Fac Appt:** Prof Oph, UC Irvine

Baylis, Henry I MD [Oph] - **Spec Exp:** Oculoplastic Surgery; Eyelid Surgery; **Hospital:** Ronald Reagan UCLA Med Ctr, Hoag Meml Hosp Presby; **Address:** 1260 15 St, Ste 600, Santa Monica, CA 90404; **Phone:** 310-207-0300; **Board Cert:** Ophthalmology 1969; **Med School:** Univ Mich Med Sch 1960; **Resid:** Ophthalmology, UCLA Med Ctr 1966; **Fellow:** Oculoplastic Surgery, Manhattan EET Hosp 1967; **Fac Appt:** Clin Prof Oph, UCLA

Binder, Perry S MD [Oph] - **Spec Exp:** Refractive Surgery; **Hospital:** Sharp Meml Hosp; **Address:** 2500 6th Ave, Ste 307, San Diego, CA 92103; **Phone:** 619-702-7938; **Board Cert:** Ophthalmology 1975; **Med School:** Northwestern Univ 1969; **Resid:** Ophthalmology, USC Med Ctr 1973; **Fellow:** Cornea, Univ Fla Hosps 1974

Blumenkranz, Mark S MD [Oph] - **Spec Exp:** Retinal Disorders; Macular Degeneration; **Hospital:** Stanford Univ Med Ctr; **Address:** 1225 Crane St, Ste 202, Menlo Park, CA 94025; **Phone:** 650-323-0231; **Board Cert:** Ophthalmology 1980; **Med School:** Brown Univ 1975; **Resid:** Ophthalmology, Stanford Univ Hosp 1979; **Fellow:** Vitreoretinal Surgery, Bascom Palmer Eye Inst 1980; **Fac Appt:** Prof Oph, Stanford Univ

Ophthalmology

Borchert, Mark S MD [Oph] - **Spec Exp:** Pediatric Ophthalmology; Vision-Unexplained Loss; Optic Nerve Disorders; **Hospital:** Chldns Hosp - Los Angeles; **Address:** Chldns Hosp, Div Ophthalmology, MS 88, 4650 Sunset Blvd, Los Angeles, CA 90027-6062; **Phone:** 323-361-4510; **Board Cert:** Ophthalmology 1989; **Med School:** Baylor Coll Med 1983; **Resid:** Ophthalmology, LAC-USC Med Ctr 1987; **Fellow:** Neurological Ophthalmology, Mass EE Infirm-Harvard 1988; **Fac Appt:** Assoc Prof Oph, USC Sch Med

Boxer Wachler, Brian S MD [Oph] - **Spec Exp:** LASIK-Refractive Surgery; Keratoconus; Corneal Disease & Surgery; **Address:** Boxer Wachler Vision Inst, 465 N Roxbury Drive, Ste 902, Los Angeles, CA 90210; **Phone:** 310-860-1900; **Board Cert:** Ophthalmology 1999; **Med School:** Dartmouth Med Sch 1993; **Resid:** Ophthalmology, St Louis Univ Eye Inst 1997; **Fellow:** Refractive Surgery, Univ Kansas Med Ctr 1998

Boxrud, Cynthia Ann MD [Oph] - **Spec Exp:** Oculoplastic Surgery; Eye Tumors/Cancer; Orbital Diseases; **Hospital:** Ronald Reagan UCLA Med Ctr, St John's Hlth Ctr, Santa Monica; **Address:** 2021 Santa Monica Blvd, Ste 700E, Santa Monica, CA 90404-2208; **Phone:** 310-829-9060; **Board Cert:** Ophthalmology 1997; **Med School:** Case West Res Univ 1986; **Resid:** Ophthalmology, NYU-Bellevue Hosp Ctr 1990; **Fellow:** Ophthalmic Oncololgy, New York Hosp-Cornell Med Ctr 1992; Ophthalmic Plastic Surgery, UCLA-Jules Stein Eye Inst 1993; **Fac Appt:** Asst Prof Oph, UCLA

Caprioli, Joseph MD [Oph] - **Spec Exp:** Glaucoma; Cataract Surgery; **Hospital:** Ronald Reagan UCLA Med Ctr; **Address:** UCLA-Jules Stein Eye Institute, 100 Stein Plaza Fl 2 - Ste 2-273, Los Angeles, CA 90095-7006; **Phone:** 310-794-9442; **Board Cert:** Ophthalmology 1985; **Med School:** SUNY Buffalo 1979; **Resid:** Ophthalmology, Yale-New Haven Hosp. 1983; **Fellow:** Glaucoma, Wills Eye Hosp 1984; **Fac Appt:** Prof Oph, UCLA

Caster, Andrew I MD [Oph] - **Spec Exp:** LASIK-Refractive Surgery; Laser Vision Surgery; Pediatric Ophthalmology; Strabismus; **Hospital:** Cedars-Sinai Med Ctr; **Address:** 9100 Wilshire Blvd, Ste 265E, Beverly Hills, CA 90212; **Phone:** 310-274-1221; **Board Cert:** Ophthalmology 1986; **Med School:** Harvard Med Sch 1980; **Resid:** Ophthalmology, UCLA Jules Stein Eye Inst 1984

Char, Devron H MD [Oph] - **Spec Exp:** Eye Tumors/Cancer; Thyroid Eye Disease; Oculoplastic Surgery; **Hospital:** CA Pacific Med Ctr - Pacific Campus, UCSF Med Ctr; **Address:** 45 Castro St, Ste 309, San Francisco, CA 94114; **Phone:** 415-522-0700; **Board Cert:** Ophthalmology 1978; **Med School:** Univ Minn 1970; **Resid:** Internal Medicine, Mass Genl Hosp 1972; Ophthalmology, UCSF Med Ctr 1977; **Fellow:** Medical Oncology, Natl Cancer Inst 1974; Ophthalmology, UCSF Med Ctr 1978; **Fac Appt:** Prof Oph, Stanford Univ

Choy, Andrew MD [Oph] - **Spec Exp:** Eye Muscle Disorders; Oculoplastic & Orbital Surgery; **Hospital:** Long Beach Meml Med Ctr, Los Alamitos Med Ctr; **Address:** 4100 Long Beach Blvd, Ste 108, Long Beach, CA 90807-2619; **Phone:** 562-426-3925; **Board Cert:** Ophthalmology 1976; **Med School:** USC Sch Med 1969; **Resid:** Neurology, LAC-USC Med Ctr 1971; Ophthalmology, Bellevue Hosp Ctr-NYU 1974; **Fellow:** Strabismus, Columbia-Presby Med Ctr 1975; **Fac Appt:** Assoc Clin Prof Oph, UCLA

Cockerham, Kimberly P MD [Oph] - **Spec Exp:** Meningioma-Orbital (eye); Orbital Tumors/Cancer; Eyelid Cancer & Reconstruction; Neuro-Ophthalmology; **Address:** 762 Altos Oaks Drive, Ste 2, Los Altos, CA 94024; **Phone:** 650-559-9150; **Board Cert:** Ophthalmology 2004; **Med School:** Geo Wash Univ 1987; **Resid:** Ophthalmology, Walter Reed Army Med Ctr 1992; **Fellow:** Neurological Ophthalmology, Walter Reed Army Med Ctr 1993; Neurological Ophthalmology, Allegheny General Hosp 1995

Day, Susan H MD [Oph] - **Spec Exp:** Pediatric Ophthalmology; Strabismus; **Hospital:** CA Pacific Med Ctr - Pacific Campus; **Address:** 2340 Clay St, Ste 100, San Francisco, CA 94115; **Phone:** 415-202-1500; **Board Cert:** Ophthalmology 1980; **Med School:** Louisiana State U, New Orleans 1975; **Resid:** Ophthalmology, California Pacific Med Ctr 1979; **Fellow:** Pediatric Ophthalmology, Hosp Sick Chldn 1980

De Juan Jr, Eugene MD [Oph] - **Spec Exp:** Retina/Vitreous Surgery; **Hospital:** UCSF Med Ctr; **Address:** 400 Parnassus Ave, Box 0344, San Francisco, CA 94143; **Phone:** 415-353-2800; **Board Cert:** Ophthalmology 1985; **Med School:** Univ S Ala Coll Med 1979; **Resid:** Ophthalmology, Johns Hopkins Hosp 1983; **Fellow:** Vitreoretinal Surgery, Duke Univ Eye Ctr 1984; **Fac Appt:** Prof Oph, UCSF

Demer, Joseph L MD/PhD [Oph] - **Spec Exp:** Pediatric Ophthalmology; Strabismus; Nystagmus; **Hospital:** Ronald Reagan UCLA Med Ctr; **Address:** Jules Stein Eye Institute, 100 Stein Plaza, MC 700219, Los Angeles, CA 90095-7065; **Phone:** 310-825-5931; **Board Cert:** Ophthalmology 1988; **Med School:** Johns Hopkins Univ 1983; **Resid:** Ophthalmology, Baylor Coll Med 1987; **Fellow:** Pediatric Ophthalmology, Texas Chldns Hosp 1988; **Fac Appt:** Prof Oph, UCLA

Gorin, Michael B MD/PhD [Oph] - **Spec Exp:** Retinal Disorders; Macular Disease/Degeneration; Eye Diseases-Hereditary; **Hospital:** Ronald Reagan UCLA Med Ctr; **Address:** Dept Ophthalmology, Jules Stein Eye Inst, 100 Stein Plaza, DSERC 3-310-B, Los Angeles, CA 90095-7000; **Phone:** 310-794-5400; **Board Cert:** Ophthalmology 1987; **Med School:** Univ Pennsylvania 1980; **Resid:** Ophthalmology, Jules Stein Eye Inst/UCLA 1986; **Fellow:** Medical Retina, Moorfields Eye Hosp 1987; **Fac Appt:** Prof Oph, UCLA-David Geffen Sch Med

Granet, David Bruce MD [Oph] - **Spec Exp:** Pediatric Ophthalmology; Eye Muscle Disorders; Strabismus; **Hospital:** UCSD Med Ctr, Rady Children's Hosp - San Diego; **Address:** UCSD-Shiley Eye Ctr, 9415 Campus Point Drive, La Jolla, CA 92093; **Phone:** 858-534-2020; **Board Cert:** Ophthalmology 1994; **Med School:** Yale Univ 1987; **Resid:** Ophthalmology, Bellevue Hosp-NYU 1991; **Fellow:** Pediatric Ophthalmology, Chldns Hosp 1993; **Fac Appt:** Assoc Prof Oph, UCSD

Irvine, John A MD [Oph] - **Spec Exp:** Corneal & External Eye Disease; **Hospital:** USC Univ Hosp - R K Eamer Med Plz; **Address:** USC-Doheny Eye Institute, 1450 San Pablo St, Ste 5703, Los Angeles, CA 90033; **Phone:** 323-442-6335; **Board Cert:** Ophthalmology 1989; **Med School:** USC Sch Med 1982; **Resid:** Ophthalmology, Mass EE Infirm/Harvard 1986; **Fellow:** Cornea & Ext Eye Disease, Mass EE Infirm 1987; **Fac Appt:** Prof Oph, USC Sch Med

Isenberg, Sherwin Jay MD [Oph] - **Spec Exp:** Strabismus; Pediatric Ophthalmology; **Hospital:** LAC - Harbor - UCLA Med Ctr, Ronald Reagan UCLA Med Ctr; **Address:** Jules Stein Eye Institute, 100 Stein Plaza, Los Angeles, CA 90095-7000; **Phone:** 310-825-8840; **Board Cert:** Ophthalmology 1978; **Med School:** UCLA 1973; **Resid:** Ophthalmology, Illinois Ear & Eye Infirm 1977; **Fellow:** Pediatric Ophthalmology, Chldns Hosp Natl Med Ctr 1978; **Fac Appt:** Prof Oph, UCLA

Iwach, Andrew G MD [Oph] - **Spec Exp:** Glaucoma; **Hospital:** UCSF Med Ctr, CA Pacific Med Ctr; **Address:** Glaucoma Ctr of San Francisco, 55 Stevenson St, San Francisco, CA 94105; **Phone:** 415-981-2020; **Board Cert:** Ophthalmology 1991; **Med School:** UCLA 1984; **Resid:** Ophthalmology, Stanford Univ Med Ctr 1988; **Fellow:** Glaucoma, UCSF Med Ctr 1989; **Fac Appt:** Assoc Prof Oph, UCSF

Ophthalmology

Mahon, Kathleen M K MD [Oph] - **Spec Exp:** Pediatric Ophthalmology; Retinopathy of Prematurity; Eye Muscle Disorders; Glaucoma; **Hospital:** Sunrise Hosp & Med Ctr/Sunrise Chldn's Hosp, Univ Med Ctr - Las Vegas; **Address:** Nevada Eye & Ear, 2598 Windmill Pkwy, Henderson, NV 89074; **Phone:** 702-896-6043; **Board Cert:** Ophthalmology 1980; **Med School:** Univ New Mexico 1975; **Resid:** Ophthalmology, Univ Florida Med Ctr 1979; **Fellow:** Pediatric Ophthalmology, Univ Tex Hlth Sci Ctr 1980; **Fac Appt:** Clin Prof Oph, Univ Nevada

Maloney, Robert K MD [Oph] - **Spec Exp:** Refractive Surgery; LASIK-Refractive Surgery; **Hospital:** Ronald Reagan UCLA Med Ctr; **Address:** Maloney Vision Inst, 10921 Wilshire Blvd, Ste 900, Los Angeles, CA 90024-4002; **Phone:** 310-208-3937; **Board Cert:** Ophthalmology 1991; **Med School:** UCSF 1985; **Resid:** Ophthalmology, Johns Hopkins Hosp 1989; **Fellow:** Refractive Surgery, Emory Univ Hosp 1991; **Fac Appt:** Clin Prof Oph, UCLA

Manche, Edward E MD [Oph] - **Spec Exp:** LASIK-Refractive Surgery; Corneal Disease & Transplant; PRK-Refractive Surgery; **Hospital:** Stanford Univ Med Ctr; **Address:** 900 Blake Wilbur Dr, rm W3002, Palo Alto, CA 94304-2201; **Phone:** 650-498-7020; **Board Cert:** Ophthalmology 2007; **Med School:** Albert Einstein Coll Med 1990; **Resid:** Ophthalmology, UMDNJ-NJ Med Sch 1994; **Fellow:** Cornea & Ext Eye Disease, Jules Stein Eye Inst-UCLA 1996; **Fac Appt:** Assoc Prof Oph, Stanford Univ

Mannis, Mark J MD [Oph] - **Spec Exp:** Cornea Transplant; Refractive Surgery; **Hospital:** UC Davis Med Ctr; **Address:** UC Davis Med Ctr, Dept Ophthalmology, 4860 Y St, Ste 2400, Sacramento, CA 95817; **Phone:** 916-734-6602; **Board Cert:** Ophthalmology 1980; **Med School:** Univ Fla Coll Med 1975; **Resid:** Ophthalmology, Univ Washington 1979; **Fellow:** Cornea & Ext Eye Disease, Univ IA Hosps & Clins 1980; **Fac Appt:** Prof Oph, UC Davis

Marmor, Michael F MD [Oph] - **Spec Exp:** Retinal Disorders; Retinal Dystrophies; Electroretinograms (ERG); Macular Degeneration; **Hospital:** Stanford Univ Med Ctr; **Address:** California Vitreoretinal Ctr, 1225 Crane St, Ste 202, Menlo Park, CA 94025; **Phone:** 650-323-0231; **Board Cert:** Ophthalmology 1974; **Med School:** Harvard Med Sch 1966; **Resid:** Ophthalmology, Mass EE Infirm 1973; **Fellow:** Neurological Physiology, Natl Inst Mntl Hlth 1970; **Fac Appt:** Prof Oph, Stanford Univ

Masket, Samuel MD [Oph] - **Spec Exp:** Cataract Surgery; Cataract Surgery Revision; **Address:** 2080 Century Park E, Ste 911, Los Angeles, CA 90067; **Phone:** 310-229-1220; **Board Cert:** Ophthalmology 1974; **Med School:** NY Med Coll 1968; **Resid:** Ophthalmology, Metropolitan Hosp Ctr 1972; **Fellow:** Ophthalmology, Columbia Presby Med Ctr 1973; **Fac Appt:** Clin Prof Oph, UCLA

Minckler, Donald S MD [Oph] - **Spec Exp:** Glaucoma; **Hospital:** UC Irvine Med Ctr; **Address:** UC Irvine Medical Center, 118 Med Surge 1 Bldg 810, Irvine, CA 92697; **Phone:** 949-824-2020; **Board Cert:** Ophthalmology 2007; Pathology 1978; **Med School:** Oregon Hlth Sci Univ 1964; **Resid:** Anatomic Pathology, Univ Wash Med Ctr 1970; Ophthalmology, Univ Wash Med Ctr 1973; **Fellow:** Pathology, Armed Forces Inst Path 1975; Glaucoma, Shaffer Assocs-UCSF 1982; **Fac Appt:** Prof Oph, USC Sch Med

Mondino, Bartly MD [Oph] - **Spec Exp:** Cornea & External Eye Disease; **Hospital:** Ronald Reagan UCLA Med Ctr; **Address:** 100 Stein Plaza, MC 700019, Los Angeles, CA 90095-7065; **Phone:** 310-825-5053; **Board Cert:** Ophthalmology 1976; **Med School:** Stanford Univ 1971; **Resid:** Ophthalmology, NY Hosp/Cornell Univ 1975; **Fellow:** Cornea & Ext Eye Disease, Univ Pittsburgh Eye & Ear Hosp 1976; **Fac Appt:** Prof Oph, UCLA

America's Top Doctors® 8th Edition

Murphree, A Linn MD [Oph] - **Spec Exp:** Pediatric Ophthalmology; Eye Diseases-Hereditary; Retinoblastoma; Orbital Tumors/Cancer; **Hospital:** Chldns Hosp - Los Angeles, USC Univ Hosp - R K Eamer Med Plz; **Address:** Chldns Hosp, Div Oph, 4650 Sunset Blvd, MS 88, Los Angeles, CA 90027-6016; **Phone:** 323-669-2299; **Board Cert:** Ophthalmology 1978; **Med School:** Baylor Coll Med 1972; **Resid:** Clinical Genetics, Baylor Heed 1973; Ophthalmology, Baylor Coll Med 1976; **Fellow:** Ophthalmology, Wilmer Inst/Johns Hopkins 1977; **Fac Appt:** Prof Oph, USC Sch Med

O'Brien, Joan M MD [Oph] - **Spec Exp:** Eye Tumors/Cancer; Retinoblastoma; **Hospital:** UCSF Med Ctr; **Address:** UCSF, Dept Ophthalmology, 533 Parnassus Ave Fl 5 - Ste 525, San Francisco, CA 94143; **Phone:** 415-476-3705; **Board Cert:** Ophthalmology 1996; **Med School:** Dartmouth Med Sch 1986; **Resid:** Ophthalmology, Mass Eye & Ear Infirm 1992; **Fellow:** Ophthalmic Pathology, Mass Eye & Ear Infirm 1989; UCSF Med Ctr 1993; **Fac Appt:** Prof Oph, UCSF

Palmer, Earl A MD [Oph] - **Spec Exp:** Strabismus; Retinopathy of Prematurity; **Hospital:** OR Hlth & Sci Univ; **Address:** Casey Eye Institute, 3375 SW Terwilliger Blvd, Portland, OR 97239-4197; **Phone:** 503-494-7675; **Board Cert:** Pediatrics 1975; Ophthalmology 1976; **Med School:** Duke Univ 1966; **Resid:** Pediatrics, Univ Colo Med Ctr 1968; Ophthalmology, Oregon Hlth & Sciences Univ 1974; **Fellow:** Pediatric Ophthalmology, Texas Chldns Hosp 1975; **Fac Appt:** Prof Oph, Oregon Hlth Sci Univ

Paul, T Otis MD [Oph] - **Spec Exp:** Pediatric Ophthalmology; Strabismus; **Hospital:** CA Pacific Med Ctr - Pacific Campus, Chldns Hosp - Oakland; **Address:** 2100 Webster St, Ste 214, San Francisco, CA 94115; **Phone:** 415-923-3007; **Board Cert:** Ophthalmology 1974; **Med School:** UCLA 1967; **Resid:** Ophthalmology, Naval Hosp 1972; **Fellow:** Pediatric Ophthalmology, Ca Pacific Med Ctr 1974

Puliafito, Carmen A MD [Oph] - **Spec Exp:** Retinal Disorders; Macular Degeneration; **Address:** Doheny Eye Inst, 1537 Norfolk St, Los Angeles, CA 90033; **Phone:** 323-442-1900; **Board Cert:** Ophthalmology 1983; **Med School:** Harvard Med Sch 1978; **Resid:** Ophthalmology, Mass Eye & Ear Infirm 1982; **Fellow:** Vitreoretinal Surgery, Mass Eye & Ear Infirm 1983; **Fac Appt:** Prof Oph, USC-Keck School of Medicine

Rao, Narsing A MD [Oph] - **Spec Exp:** Uveitis/AIDS; Eye Pathology; **Hospital:** USC Univ Hosp - R K Eamer Med Plz; **Address:** USC Doheny Eye Inst, 1450 San Pablo St, rm DVRZ 211, Los Angeles, CA 90033-4697; **Phone:** 323-442-6645; **Board Cert:** Pathology 1974; Ophthalmology 1977; **Med School:** India 1967; **Resid:** Pathology, Georgetown Hosp 1972; Ophthalmology, Georgetown Hosp 1975; **Fac Appt:** Prof Oph, USC Sch Med

Salz, James J MD [Oph] - **Spec Exp:** LASIK-Refractive Surgery; PRK-Refractive Surgery; Cataract Surgery; **Hospital:** Cedars-Sinai Med Ctr; **Address:** 240 S La Cienega Blvd, Ste 250, Beverly Hills, CA 90211; **Phone:** 323-653-3800; **Board Cert:** Ophthalmology 1971; **Med School:** Duke Univ 1965; **Resid:** Ophthalmology, LAC-USC Med Ctr 1969; **Fac Appt:** Clin Prof Oph, USC Sch Med

Seibel, Barry S MD [Oph] - **Spec Exp:** Cataract Surgery; **Hospital:** Ronald Reagan UCLA Med Ctr; **Address:** 11620 Wilshire Blvd, Ste 711, Los Angeles, CA 90025; **Phone:** 310-273-0323; **Board Cert:** Ophthalmology 1991; **Med School:** Univ Tex, Houston 1985; **Resid:** Ophthalmology, Hollywood Presby Med Ctr 1987; Ophthalmology, USC-Doheny Eye Clin 1989; **Fac Appt:** Asst Clin Prof Oph, UCLA

Ophthalmology

Seiff, Stuart R MD [Oph] - **Spec Exp:** Oculoplastic Surgery; Orbital Tumors/Cancer; **Hospital:** UCSF Med Ctr, CA Pacific Med Ctr; **Address:** 2100 Webster St, Ste 214, San Francisco, CA 94115; **Phone:** 415-923-3007; **Board Cert:** Ophthalmology 1986; **Med School:** UCSF 1980; **Resid:** Ophthalmology, UCSF Med Ctr 1984; **Fellow:** Ophthalmic Plastic & Reconstructive Surgery, UCLA Med Ctr 1985; Oculoplastic Surgery, Moorfield's Eye Hosp 1986; **Fac Appt:** Prof Oph, UCSF

Serafano, Donald N MD [Oph] - **Spec Exp:** LASIK-Refractive Surgery; Cataract Surgery; Lens Implants; **Hospital:** Los Alamitos Med Ctr, Long Beach Meml Med Ctr; **Address:** 10861 Cherry St, Ste 204, Box 250, Los Alamitos, CA 90720-5403; **Phone:** 562-598-3160; **Board Cert:** Ophthalmology 1978; **Med School:** Wayne State Univ 1971; **Resid:** Ophthalmology, Mayo Clinic 1978; **Fac Appt:** Assoc Clin Prof Oph, USC Sch Med

Smith, Ronald E MD [Oph] - **Spec Exp:** Corneal Disease; Uveitis; **Hospital:** USC Univ Hosp - R K Eamer Med Plz; **Address:** USC-Doheny Eye Institute, 1450 San Pablo Rd, Ste 5703, Los Angeles, CA 90033; **Phone:** 323-442-6335; **Board Cert:** Ophthalmology 1974; **Med School:** Johns Hopkins Univ 1967; **Resid:** Ophthalmology, Wilmer Oph Inst/Johns Hopkins 1973; **Fellow:** Research, Proctor Fdn/Univ California 1972; **Fac Appt:** Prof Oph, USC Sch Med

Steinert, Roger F MD [Oph] - **Spec Exp:** Refractive Surgery; Cataract Surgery; Cornea Transplant; **Hospital:** UC Irvine Med Ctr; **Address:** Gottschalk Med Plaza, 1 Medical Plaza Drive Fl 2, Irvine, CA 92697; **Phone:** 949-824-2020; **Board Cert:** Ophthalmology 1982; **Med School:** Harvard Med Sch 1977; **Resid:** Ophthalmology, Mass EE Infirm 1981; **Fac Appt:** Prof Oph, UC Irvine

Stout, John Timothy MD/PhD [Oph] - **Spec Exp:** Retinal Disorders-Pediatric; Retinoblastoma; Retinopathy of Prematurity; **Hospital:** OR Hlth & Sci Univ, Providence St Vincent Med Ctr; **Address:** 3375 SW Terwilliger Blvd, Portland, OR 97239; **Phone:** 503-494-2435; **Board Cert:** Ophthalmology 1999; **Med School:** Baylor Coll Med 1989; **Resid:** Ophthalmology, Doheny Eye Inst 1993; **Fellow:** Ophthalmology, Moorfields Eye Hosp 1994; Retinal Surgery, Doheny Eye Inst 1995; **Fac Appt:** Assoc Prof Oph, Oregon Hlth Sci Univ

Weiss, Avery H MD [Oph] - **Spec Exp:** Pediatric Ophthalmology; Strabismus; Amblyopia; **Hospital:** Chldns Hosp and Regl Med Ctr - Seattle; **Address:** 4800 Sand Point Way NE, MS W-4753, Seattle, WA 98105; **Phone:** 206-987-2177; **Board Cert:** Ophthalmology 1981; **Med School:** Univ Miami Sch Med 1974; **Resid:** Internal Medicine, Barnes Hosp 1976; Ophthalmology, Barnes Hosp 1980; **Fellow:** Research, Barnes Hosp 1977; Pediatric Ophthalmology, Chldns Hosp Natl Med Ctr 1981; **Fac Appt:** Assoc Prof Oph, Univ Wash

Wilson, David Jean MD [Oph] - **Spec Exp:** Eye Tumors/Cancer; Ophthalmic Pathology; **Hospital:** OR Hlth & Sci Univ; **Address:** 3375 SW Terwilliger Blvd, Portland, OR 97239; **Phone:** 503-494-7891; **Board Cert:** Ophthalmology 1986; **Med School:** Baylor Coll Med 1981; **Resid:** Ophthalmology, Univ Oregon 1985; **Fellow:** Ophthalmic Pathology, John Hopkins Hosp 1987; Retina/Vitreous, Mass Eye & Ear Infirm 1988; **Fac Appt:** Prof Oph, Oregon Hlth Sci Univ

Wright, Kenneth W MD [Oph] - **Spec Exp:** Cataract Surgery-Lens Implant; Strabismus-Adult & Pediatric; Pediatric Eye Surgery-Ptosis; Pediatric Ophthalmology; **Hospital:** Cedars-Sinai Med Ctr; **Address:** 520 S San Vincente Blvd, Los Angeles, CA 90048; **Phone:** 310-652-6420; **Board Cert:** Ophthalmology 1983; **Med School:** Boston Univ 1977; **Resid:** Ophthalmology, LAC-USC Med Ctr 1981; **Fellow:** Pediatric Ophthalmology, Johns Hopkins Hosp 1981; Pediatric Ophthalmology, Children's Hosp Natl Med Ctr 1982; **Fac Appt:** Clin Prof Oph, USC Sch Med

Cleveland Clinic

Cole Eye Institute

Cleveland Clinic Cole Eye Institute is one of the few dedicated, comprehensive eye institutes in the world. We are here to serve the needs of patients and referring physicians for early, accurate diagnosis and excellent, effective patient care. Here, the lines between research and patient care blur. The belief that the two are interdependent and synergistic is the foundation for everything we do. We believe that this approach enhances diagnosis and advances treatment, to the benefit of our patients today and tomorrow.

Our Specialized, Experienced Staff

All of our ophthalmologists have advanced expertise in treating disorders and diseases of a specific part or parts of the eye. This specialized approach offers patients a higher level of care and the assurance that their physicians are experienced in treating even the most unusual eye problems.

Why choose Cole Eye Institute?

- Internationally recognized, all subspecialty medical staff.

- Among the world's most advanced eye institutes, dedicated to comprehensive and highly specialized ophthalmologic care.

- One of the highest patient volumes in the United States.

- Aggressive research program that bridges the gap between laboratory and patient care and offers access to the latest clinical trials.

- State-of-the-art diagnostic technology and outpatient surgical center.

- Retina and Vitreous Surgery: Age-related macular degeneration, diabetic retinopathy, inherited retinal diseases and infectious retinopathies.
- Cornea and External Diseases: Diseases of the eye's external surface and cornea, such as inflammatory, infectious and degenerative diseases of the cornea, conjunctiva and lens; corneal tumors; and contact lens-related problems.
- Glaucoma: All forms of this silent thief of sight.
- Neuro-Ophthalmology: Vision problems related to neurologic disorders such as stroke, multiple sclerosis and tumors.
- Oculoplastics and Orbital Surgery: Problems of the orbit and eyelids.
- Ocular Oncology: Primary and metastatic tumors of the eye and eyelids.
- Pediatric Ophthalmology: Strabismus, amblyopia and congenital cataracts.
- Refractive Surgery: Correction of nearsightedness, farsightedness and astigmatism.
- Uveitis: Internal ocular inflammation and infection-related immune system disturbances.

Emergency Services

A Cole Eye Institute ophthalmologist is on-call 24 hours a day for immediate consultation on or treatment of eye emergencies. When necessary, a complete surgical team can be assembled in less than an hour to provide emergency treatment for the most serious cases.

For more information about the Cleveland Clinic Cole Eye Institute, to schedule a second opinion or to learn about assistance for out-of-town patients, call 800.890.2467 or visit www.clevelandclinic.org/eyetopdocs.

Cole Eye Institute | 9500 Euclid Avenue / AC311 | Cleveland OH 44195

PENN EYE CARE

Penn Eye Care and the Scheie Eye Institute are dedicated to excellence in patient care, education of future clinical ophthalmologists and vision scientists, community eye care needs through outreach and advancing the frontier of research to prevent blindness and vision loss. Penn Eye Care serves as the department of ophthalmology of Penn Medicine and its physicians are members of the faculty of the University of Pennsylvania School of Medicine. A world leader in research on retinal degeneration, especially age-related macular degeneration (AMD), Penn was ranked number one in the nation in funding by the National Eye Institute in 2007.

Penn Eye Care is one of the few programs in the country that provides complete eye care by a team of ophthalmologists who are on-site full-time. The highly qualified physicians provide the most up-to-date methods of treatment for the full-range of eye disorders. Complete diagnostic and treatment services in comprehensive ophthalmology are offered as well as in all subspecialty areas. Services range from routine eye examinations for glasses to the most advanced refractive surgery and oculoplastics.

Penn Eye Care specialists have experience and expertise in:

- Adult Strabismus
- Cataracts and Cataract Surgery
- Contact Lenses
- Cornea and External Diseases
- Cosmetic Eye Surgery
- Diabetic Retinopathy
- Glaucoma
- Low Vision Rehabilitation
- Macular Degeneration
- Neuro-Ophthalmology
- Ocular Genetics
- Oculoplastics/Orbital Surgery
- Pediatric Ophthalmology
- Refractive Surgery/LASIK
- Retina and Vitreous Diseases/Surgery

At Scheie's F.M. Kirby Center for Molecular Ophthalmology, scientists investigate the causes of important eye conditions including macular degeneration, diabetic retinopathy, hereditary retinal degenerations, cataract and severe myopia that may be treatable with molecular therapies.

Penn Eye Care Locations

Scheie Eye Institute
Penn Presbyterian
Medical Center
38th and Market Streets
Philadelphia, PA 19104

Hospital of the University
of Pennsylvania
3400 Spruce Street
Philadelphia, PA 19104

Penn Medicine at Radnor
250 King of Prussia Road
Radnor, PA 19087

Penn Center for Low Vision
at Ralston House
3615 Chestnut Street, 1st floor
Philadelphia, PA 19104

Penn Eye Care at Mercy
Fitzgerald Hospital
1501 Lansdowne Avenue,
Suite 208
Darby, PA 19023

Penn Eye Care at Media
601 West State Street
Media, PA 19063

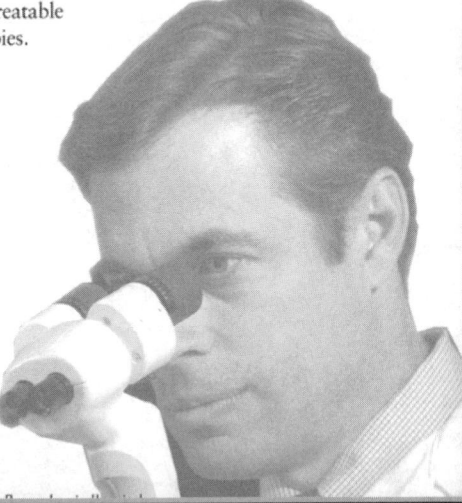

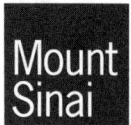 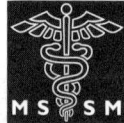

MOUNT SINAI
SCHOOL OF
MEDICINE

THE MOUNT SINAI MEDICAL CENTER
OPHTHALMOLOGY

One Gustave L. Levy Place
Fifth Avenue and 100th Street
New York, NY 10029-6574
Physician Referral: 1-800-MD-SINAI (637-4624)
www.mountsinai.org

Specializing in the prevention, diagnosis, and treatment of eye disorders, The Department of Ophthalmology at Mount Sinai features faculty with wide experience in special eye problems. The Department provides comprehensive eye care for the full range of eye disorders and needs, including refractive errors, glaucoma, eye infections, corneal and external diseases of the eye, retinal disorders (diabetic retinopathy, macular degeneration, and inherited retinal diseases), dry eyes (Sjogren's syndrome), contact lenses, neuro-ophthalmic disorders (double vision and optic nerve problems), trauma, orbital tumors and thyroid-related eye problems, pediatric eye care and strabismus, and uveitis (inflammation inside the eye).

The Department offers the full range of sophisticated diagnostic tests for evaluating patient conditions, including optical coherence tomography (OCT), fundus photography, fluorescein angiography, diagnostic ultrasound, electroretinography, visually evoked potentials, electro-oculography, computerized tomography (CT scanning), magnetic resonance imaging (MRI), corneal topography, and confocal microscopy, as well as state-of-the-art techniques for assessing glaucoma. These techniques include perimetry HRT II imaging, and ultrasound biomicroscopy (UBM), a noninvasive method to achieve high-resolution imaging of the inside of the eye. In certain cases of glaucoma, it is the only noninvasive way to identify the exact cause of the condition and ascertain optimal treatment. These methods allow for faster, more accurate diagnosis and help determine the best treatment plan for each individual patient.

Our highly skilled eye surgeons perform cataract surgery, corneal transplants, refractive surgery, glaucoma surgery, strabismus surgery, ophthalmic plastic and reconstructive surgery, laser surgery, and vitreoretinal surgery for complicated retinal problems. We also offer minimally invasive procedures to treat eye disease, including non-laser refractive surgeries, small-incision cataract surgery, bladeless laser procedures, and Intacs for keratoconus.

A PIONEERING METHOD OF CORRECTING FARSIGHTEDNESS

Mount Sinai ophthalmologists helped pioneer a new radiofrequency method of correcting farsightedness. Known as Conductive Keratoplasty (CK), the brief procedure is performed in the doctor's office with only topical anesthesia (eye drops). For most farsighted patients—especially those over age 40 whose eyes are naturally aging—the CK procedure eliminates the need for glasses.

Orthopaedic Surgery

An orthopaedic surgeon is trained in the preservation, investigation and restoration of the form and function of the extremities, spine and associated structures by medical, surgical and physical means.

An orthopaedic surgeon is involved with the care of patients whose musculoskeletal problems include congenital deformities, trauma, infections, tumors, metabolic disturbances of the musculoskeletal system, deformities, injuries and degenerative diseases of the spine, hands, feet, knee, hip, shoulder and elbow in children and adults. An orthopaedic surgeon is also concerned with primary and secondary muscular problems and the effects of central or peripheral nervous system lesions of the musculoskeletal system.

Note: *There are many Orthopaedic Surgeons who are trained in Sports Medicine and prefer to be listed under that heading; some trained in Sports Medicine prefer to be listed under Orthopaedics.*

Training Required: Five years (including general surgery training) *plus* two years in clinical practice before final certification is achieved.

ORTHOPAEDIC SURGERY

New England

Browner, Bruce D MD [OrS] - **Spec Exp:** Fractures-Complex; Osteomyelitis; Bone Infections; Trauma; **Hospital:** Univ of Conn Hlth Ctr, John Dempsey Hosp, Hartford Hosp; **Address:** Med Arts & Rsch Bldg, 263 Farmington Ave Fl 3 - Ste 2, Farmington, CT 06034-4037; **Phone:** 860-679-6650; **Board Cert:** Orthopaedic Surgery 1997; **Med School:** SUNY Downstate 1973; **Resid:** Orthopaedic Surgery, Albany Med Ctr 1978; **Fellow:** Trauma, Albany Med Ctr 1975; **Fac Appt:** Prof OrS, Univ Conn

Einhorn, Thomas A MD [OrS] - **Spec Exp:** Metabolic Bone Disease; Fractures-Complex; Hip & Knee Replacement; Hip & Knee Reconstruction; **Hospital:** Boston Med Ctr; **Address:** Boston Medical Ctr, Doctors Office Bldg, 720 Harrison Ave, Ste 808, Boston, MA 02118-2393; **Phone:** 617-638-5633; **Board Cert:** Orthopaedic Surgery 1998; **Med School:** Cornell Univ-Weill Med Coll 1976; **Resid:** Orthopaedic Surgery, St Lukes-Roosevelt Hosp 1981; Pediatric Orthopaedic Surgery, Alfred DuPont Inst 1981; **Fellow:** Orthopaedic Surgery, Hosp Special Surgery 1982; **Fac Appt:** Prof OrS, Boston Univ

Friedlaender, Gary E MD [OrS] - **Spec Exp:** Bone & Soft Tissue Tumors; Limb Surgery/Reconstruction; Fractures-Non Union; Bone Tumors-Metastatic; **Hospital:** Yale-New Haven Hosp; **Address:** Yale Univ Sch Med, Dept Orthopedic Surg, 800 Howard Ave YPB Bldg - rm 133, Box 208071, New Haven, CT 06520-8071; **Phone:** 203-737-5656; **Board Cert:** Orthopaedic Surgery 1975; **Med School:** Univ Mich Med Sch 1969; **Resid:** Surgery, Michigan Med Ctr 1971; Orthopaedic Surgery, Yale-New Haven Hosp 1974; **Fellow:** Musculoskeletal Oncology, Mass Genl Hosp 1983; **Fac Appt:** Prof OrS, Yale Univ

Gebhardt, Mark MD [OrS] - **Spec Exp:** Musculoskeletal Tumors; Bone Tumors; **Hospital:** Beth Israel Deaconess Med Ctr - Boston, Children's Hospital - Boston; **Address:** 330 Brookline Ave, Shapiro 2, Boston, MA 02215; **Phone:** 617-667-3940; **Board Cert:** Orthopaedic Surgery 2007; **Med School:** Univ Cincinnati 1975; **Resid:** Surgery, Univ Pittsburg Med Ctr 1977; Orthopaedic Surgery, Harvard 1982; **Fellow:** Pediatric Orthopaedic Surgery, Boston Chldns Hosp 1983; Orthopaedic Oncology, Mass Genl Hosp 1983; **Fac Appt:** Prof OrS, Harvard Med Sch

Jokl, Peter MD [OrS] - **Spec Exp:** Knee Surgery; Sports Medicine; Shoulder Surgery; **Hospital:** Yale-New Haven Hosp; **Address:** Yale Sports Med, Dept Orthopaedics, 800 Howard Ave, New Haven, CT 06519-1369; **Phone:** 203-785-2579; **Board Cert:** Orthopaedic Surgery 1974; **Med School:** Yale Univ 1968; **Resid:** Orthopaedic Surgery, Yale-New Haven Hosp 1972; **Fac Appt:** Prof OrS, Yale Univ

Jupiter, Jesse B MD [OrS] - **Spec Exp:** Upper Extremity Trauma; Hand Surgery; **Hospital:** Mass Genl Hosp, Newton - Wellesley Hosp; **Address:** Yawkey Center, Ste 2100, 55 Fruit St, Boston, MA 02114-2621; **Phone:** 617-726-8530; **Board Cert:** Orthopaedic Surgery 1982; **Med School:** Yale Univ 1972; **Resid:** Surgery, Mass Genl Hosp 1976; Orthopaedic Surgery, Mass Genl Hosp 1979; **Fellow:** Hand Surgery, Univ Louisville 1981; Trauma, AO/ASIF 1980; **Fac Appt:** Prof OrS, Harvard Med Sch

Kasser, James MD [OrS] - **Spec Exp:** Pediatric Orthopaedic Surgery; **Hospital:** Children's Hospital - Boston; **Address:** Chldns Hosp, Dept Ortho Surgery, 300 Longwood Ave, Boston, MA 02115; **Phone:** 617-355-6617; **Board Cert:** Orthopaedic Surgery 1984; **Med School:** Tufts Univ 1976; **Resid:** Orthopaedic Surgery, Tufts Univ 1981; **Fellow:** Pediatric Orthopaedic Surgery, Dupont Inst; **Fac Appt:** Prof OrS, Harvard Med Sch

Kocher, Mininder S MD [OrS] - **Spec Exp:** Pediatric Orthopaedic Surgery; Bone Infections in Children; Limb Lengthening; Pediatric Sports Medicine; **Hospital:** Children's Hospital - Boston, Children's Hospital - Boston; **Address:** Children's Hosp, Dept Orthopaedic Surg, 300 Longwood Ave, Boston, MA 02115; **Phone:** 617-355-6021; **Board Cert:** Orthopaedic Surgery 2002; **Med School:** Duke Univ 1993; **Resid:** Orthopaedic Surgery, Beth Israel Hosp 1999; **Fellow:** Pediatric Orthopaedic Surgery, Chldns Hosp 1999; Sports Medicine, Steadman Hawkins Clin 2000; **Fac Appt:** Asst Prof OrS, Harvard Med Sch

Laurencin, Cato T MD/PhD [OrS] - **Spec Exp:** Shoulder & Knee Surgery; Sports Medicine; **Hospital:** Univ of Conn Hlth Ctr, John Dempsey Hosp; **Address:** U Conn Hlth Ctr, 263 Farmington Ave, Farmington, CT 06030-3800; **Phone:** 860-679-2594; **Board Cert:** Orthopaedic Surgery 2004; **Med School:** Harvard Med Sch 1987; **Resid:** Orthopaedic Surgery, Harvard Combined Program 1993; **Fellow:** Sports Medicine & Shoulder Surgery, New York Hosp-Cornell Med Ctr 1994; **Fac Appt:** Clin Prof OrS, Univ VA Sch Med

Marsh, James S MD [OrS] - **Spec Exp:** Pediatric Orthopaedic Surgery; **Hospital:** Yale-New Haven Hosp; **Address:** 1200 Boston Post Rd, Ste 201B, Gullford, CT 06437; **Phone:** 203-453-1088; **Board Cert:** Orthopaedic Surgery 2000; **Med School:** Harvard Med Sch 1981; **Resid:** Orthopaedic Surgery, Stanford Univ 1986; **Fellow:** Pediatric Orthopaedic Surgery, Mass Genl Hosp 1987; **Fac Appt:** Assoc Prof OrS, Yale Univ

Ready, John E MD [OrS] - **Spec Exp:** Bone Cancer; Sarcoma-Soft Tissue; Hip & Knee Replacement in Bone Tumors; Hip & Knee Replacement; **Hospital:** Brigham & Women's Hosp, Dana-Farber Cancer Inst; **Address:** Brigham & Women's Hospital, Dept Orthopaedics, 75 Francis St, Boston, MA 02115; **Phone:** 617-732-5368; **Board Cert:** Orthopaedic Surgery 2002; **Med School:** Dalhousie Univ 1982; **Resid:** Orthopaedic Surgery, Dalhousie Univ Hosp 1987; **Fellow:** Orthopaedic Oncology, St Michael's Hosp 1988; Orthopaedic Oncology, Mass Genl Hosp/Childns Hosp 1989

Reilly, Donald T MD [OrS] - **Spec Exp:** Hip & Knee Replacement; **Hospital:** New England Bapt Hosp; **Address:** 125 Parker Hill Ave, Ste 550, Boston, MA 02120; **Phone:** 617-232-6025; **Board Cert:** Orthopaedic Surgery 1984; **Med School:** Case West Res Univ 1975; **Resid:** Orthopaedic Surgery, Harvard Combined Ortho 1981

Scott, Richard David MD [OrS] - **Spec Exp:** Hip Replacement; Knee Replacement; **Hospital:** Brigham & Women's Hosp, New England Bapt Hosp; **Address:** 125 Parker Hill Ave, Boston, MA 02120; **Phone:** 617-738-9151; **Board Cert:** Orthopaedic Surgery 1975; **Med School:** Temple Univ 1968; **Resid:** Orthopaedic Surgery, Mass Genl Hosp 1974; **Fellow:** Orthopaedic Surgery, Mass Genl Hosp 1974; **Fac Appt:** Prof OrS, Harvard Med Sch

Springfield, Dempsey MD [OrS] - **Spec Exp:** Bone Tumors; Soft Tissue Tumors; **Hospital:** Mass Genl Hosp; **Address:** 55 Fruit St, Ste YAW 3700, Boston, MA 02114-2621; **Phone:** 617-724-3700; **Board Cert:** Orthopaedic Surgery 2007; **Med School:** Univ Fla Coll Med 1971; **Resid:** Orthopaedic Surgery, Univ Florida/Shands 1978; **Fellow:** Orthopaedic Surgery, Univ Florida/Shands 1979

Thornhill, Thomas S MD [OrS] - **Spec Exp:** Hip & Knee Replacement; Arthritis; **Hospital:** Brigham & Women's Hosp; **Address:** Brigham & Women's Hosp, Dept Orth Surg, 75 Francis St, Boston, MA 02115; **Phone:** 617-732-5322; **Board Cert:** Internal Medicine 1973; Orthopaedic Surgery 1979; **Med School:** Cornell Univ-Weill Med Coll 1970; **Resid:** Internal Medicine, Peter Brent Brigham Hosp 1972; Orthopaedic Surgery, Harvard Combined Prgm 1978; **Fellow:** Joint Replacement Surgery, Robert Breck Brigham Hosp; **Fac Appt:** Prof OrS, Harvard Med Sch

Orthopaedic Surgery

Weinstein, James DO [OrS] - **Spec Exp:** Pain-Back; Spinal Tumors; **Hospital:** Dartmouth - Hitchcock Med Ctr; **Address:** DHMC, Dept Orthopaedic Surgery, One Medical Ctr Drive, Lebanon, NH 03756; **Phone:** 603-650-2225; **Board Cert:** Orthopaedic Surgery 2002; **Med School:** Chicago Coll Osteo Med 1973; **Resid:** Orthopaedic Surgery, Rush Presby-St Lukes Med Ctr 1983; **Fac Appt:** Prof OrS, Dartmouth Med Sch

Zarins, Bertram MD [OrS] - **Spec Exp:** Knee Injuries/ACL; Arthroscopic Surgery; Shoulder Injuries; **Hospital:** Mass Genl Hosp; **Address:** MGH Sports Medicine, 175 Cambridge St Fl 4, Boston, MA 02114; **Phone:** 617-726-3421; **Board Cert:** Orthopaedic Surgery 1975; **Med School:** SUNY Upstate Med Univ 1967; **Resid:** Surgery, Johns Hopkins Hosp 1969; Orthopaedic Surgery, Harvard Ortho Prog 1973; **Fellow:** Sports Medicine, Mass Genl Hosp 1976; **Fac Appt:** Assoc Clin Prof OrS, Harvard Med Sch

Mid Atlantic

Albert, Todd J MD [OrS] - **Spec Exp:** Spinal Surgery; Scoliosis; Spinal Deformity; **Hospital:** Thomas Jefferson Univ Hosp; **Address:** Rothman Institute, 925 Chesnut St Fl 5, Philadelphia, PA 19107; **Phone:** 267-339-3500; **Board Cert:** Orthopaedic Surgery 2006; **Med School:** Univ VA Sch Med 1987; **Resid:** Orthopaedic Surgery, Thomas Jefferson Univ Hosp 1992; **Fellow:** Spinal Surgery, Minnesota Spine Ctr 1993; **Fac Appt:** Prof OrS, Thomas Jefferson Univ

Balderston, Richard MD [OrS] - **Spec Exp:** Scoliosis; Spinal Surgery; Spinal Disc Replacement; **Hospital:** Pennsylvania Hosp (page 60); **Address:** 800 Spruce St, 3B Orthopaedics, Philadelphia, PA 19107; **Phone:** 215-829-2222; **Board Cert:** Orthopaedic Surgery 1985; **Med School:** Univ Pennsylvania 1977; **Resid:** Orthopaedic Surgery, Hosp Univ Penn 1982; **Fellow:** Spinal Surgery, Univ Minn Affil Hosp 1983; **Fac Appt:** Clin Prof OrS, Univ Pennsylvania

Bartolozzi, Arthur R MD [OrS] - **Spec Exp:** Sports Medicine; Arthroscopic Surgery-Knee; Knee Ligament Reconstruction; **Hospital:** Pennsylvania Hosp (page 60); **Address:** 800 Spruce St Fl 1, Philadelphia, PA 19107; **Phone:** 215-829-2222; **Board Cert:** Orthopaedic Surgery 2000; **Med School:** UCSD 1981; **Resid:** Orthopaedic Surgery, Hosp Univ Penn 1986; **Fellow:** Sports Medicine, UCLA Med Ctr 1987; **Fac Appt:** Assoc Clin Prof OrS, Univ Pennsylvania

Bauman, Phillip MD [OrS] - **Spec Exp:** Foot & Ankle Surgery; Knee Surgery; Dance/Sports Medicine; **Hospital:** St Luke's - Roosevelt Hosp Ctr - Roosevelt Div (page 57), NY-Presby Hosp/Columbia (page 66); **Address:** Orthopaedic Assocs of NY, 343 W 58th St, rm 1, New York, NY 10019; **Phone:** 212-765-2260; **Board Cert:** Orthopaedic Surgery 2001; **Med School:** Columbia P&S 1981; **Resid:** Surgery, St Luke's-Roosevelt Hosp Ctr 1983; Orthopaedic Surgery, Columbia-Presby Med Ctr 1987; **Fac Appt:** Asst Prof OrS, Columbia P&S

Benevenia, Joseph MD [OrS] - **Spec Exp:** Limb Sparing Surgery; Bone Cancer; Sarcoma-Soft Tissue; **Hospital:** UMDNJ-Univ Hosp-Newark; **Address:** 90 Bergen St, Ste 1200, Newark, NJ 07103; **Phone:** 973-972-2153; **Board Cert:** Orthopaedic Surgery 2003; **Med School:** UMDNJ-NJ Med Sch, Newark 1984; **Resid:** Orthopaedic Surgery, UMDNJ-NJ Med Sch Hosp 1988; **Fellow:** Orthopaedic Oncology, Case Western Reserve Univ 1991; **Fac Appt:** Prof OrS, UMDNJ-NJ Med Sch, Newark

Betz, Randal R MD [OrS] - **Spec Exp:** Spinal Cord Injury-Pediatric; Praxis Functional Electrical Stim (FES); Scoliosis; Spinal Deformity-Pediatric; **Hospital:** Philadelphia Shriners Hosp; **Address:** Shriners Hospital for Children, 3351 N Broad St, Philadelphia, PA 19140; **Phone:** 215-430-4026; **Board Cert:** Orthopaedic Surgery 1998; Spinal Cord Injury Medicine 1998; **Med School:** Temple Univ 1977; **Resid:** Orthopaedic Surgery, Shriners Hospital 1980; Orthopaedic Surgery, Temple Univ Hospital 1982; **Fellow:** Pediatric Orthopaedic Surgery, DuPont Inst 1983; **Fac Appt:** Prof OrS, Temple Univ

Bigliani, Louis MD [OrS] - **Spec Exp:** Shoulder Surgery; Sports Medicine; Arthroscopic Surgery; **Hospital:** NY-Presby Hosp/Columbia (page 66); **Address:** 622 W 168th St, rm 1130, New York, NY 10032-3720; **Phone:** 212-305-5564; **Board Cert:** Orthopaedic Surgery 1979; **Med School:** Loyola Univ-Stritch Sch Med 1973; **Resid:** Surgery, Roosevelt Hosp 1974; Orthopaedic Surgery, Columbia Presby Med Ctr 1977; **Fac Appt:** Prof OrS, Columbia P&S

Bitan, Fabien D MD [OrS] - **Spec Exp:** Spinal Surgery-Pediatric & Adult; Spinal Disc Replacement; Spinal Deformity; Spinal Disorders-Degenerative; **Hospital:** Lenox Hill Hosp (page 62); **Address:** Lenox Hill Hosp, Spine Surgery, 130 E 77th St Fl 7, New York, NY 10021; **Phone:** 212-744-8114; **Med School:** France 1981; **Resid:** Orthopaedic Surgery, Hospital Beaujon 1987; Pediatric Orthopaedic Surgery, Hosp des Enfants Malades 1990; **Fellow:** Pediatric Orthopaedic Surgery, Hosp Special Surgery 1997; Spinal Surgery, Beth Israel Med Ctr 1998

Boachie-Adjei, Oheneba MD [OrS] - **Spec Exp:** Spinal Surgery; Scoliosis; **Hospital:** Hosp For Special Surgery (page 59); **Address:** Hospital for Special Surgery, 535 E 70th St, New York, NY 10021; **Phone:** 212-606-1948; **Board Cert:** Orthopaedic Surgery 2000; **Med School:** Columbia P&S 1980; **Resid:** Surgery, St Vincents Hosp 1982; Orthopaedic Surgery, Hosp Spec Surg 1986; **Fellow:** Orthopaedic Pathology, Hosp Spec Surg 1983; Spinal Surgery, Twin Cities Scoliosis Ctr/Minn Spine Ctr 1987; **Fac Appt:** Assoc Clin Prof S, Cornell Univ-Weill Med Coll

Booth Jr, Robert E MD [OrS] - **Spec Exp:** Knee Replacement; **Hospital:** Pennsylvania Hosp (page 60); **Address:** 800 Spruce St Fl 1, Philadelphia, PA 19107; **Phone:** 215-829-2222; **Board Cert:** Orthopaedic Surgery 1978; **Med School:** Univ Pennsylvania 1971; **Resid:** Surgery, Penn Hosp 1973; Orthopaedic Surgery, Hosp Univ Penn 1977; **Fac Appt:** Clin Prof OrS, Jefferson Med Coll

Brushart, Thomas M MD [OrS] - **Spec Exp:** Hand Surgery; Peripheral Nerve Surgery; **Hospital:** Johns Hopkins Hosp - Baltimore (page 61); **Address:** 601 N Caroline St, rm 5221, Baltimore, MD 21287-0882; **Phone:** 410-955-9663; **Board Cert:** Orthopaedic Surgery 1985; Hand Surgery 1989; **Med School:** Harvard Med Sch 1978; **Resid:** Orthopaedic Surgery, Harvard Affil Hosps 1981; **Fellow:** Hand Surgery, Curtis Hand Ctr 1983; **Fac Appt:** Prof OrS, Johns Hopkins Univ

Buly, Robert L MD [OrS] - **Spec Exp:** Hip Replacement; Minimally Invasive Surgery; Arthritis; **Hospital:** Hosp For Special Surgery (page 59), NY-Presby Hosp/Weill Cornell (page 66); **Address:** Hospital for Special Surgery, 535 E 70th St, New York, NY 10021; **Phone:** 212-606-1971; **Board Cert:** Orthopaedic Surgery 2004; **Med School:** Cornell Univ-Weill Med Coll 1985; **Resid:** Orthopaedic Surgery, Hosp for Special Surg 1990; **Fellow:** Hip Surgery, Mueller Fdn 1991; Joint Reconstruction, Case Western Res/ Univ Hosp 1992; **Fac Appt:** Asst Prof OrS, Cornell Univ-Weill Med Coll

Cammisa Jr, Frank P MD [OrS] - **Spec Exp:** Spinal Surgery; Spinal Disc Replacement; Scoliosis; **Hospital:** Hosp For Special Surgery (page 59), NY-Presby Hosp/Weill Cornell (page 66); **Address:** 523 E 72nd St, Fl 3, New York, NY 10021; **Phone:** 212-606-1946; **Board Cert:** Orthopaedic Surgery 2001; **Med School:** Columbia P&S 1982; **Resid:** Surgery, Columbia-Presby Hosp 1983; Orthopaedic Surgery, Hosp for Special Surgery 1987; **Fellow:** Spinal Surgery, Jackson Meml Hosp 1988; **Fac Appt:** Assoc Prof OrS, Cornell Univ-Weill Med Coll

Cappuccino, Andrew MD [OrS] - **Spec Exp:** Spinal Surgery; Spinal Disc Replacement; **Hospital:** Millard Fillmore Gates Cir Hosp; **Address:** Buffalo Spine Surgery, 46 Davison Ct, Lockport, NY 14094; **Phone:** 716-438-2976; **Board Cert:** Orthopaedic Surgery 2007; **Med School:** SUNY Buffalo 1988; **Resid:** Orthopaedic Surgery, Monmouth Med Ctr 1993; Pediatric Orthopaedic Surgery, Childrens Hosp 1992; **Fellow:** Orthopaedic Surgery, Johns Hopkins/Paul McAfee, MD 1994

Orthopaedic Surgery

Craig, Edward V MD [OrS] - **Spec Exp:** Shoulder Arthroscopic Surgery; Shoulder Replacement; Sports Medicine; Elbow Surgery; **Hospital:** Hosp For Special Surgery (page 59); **Address:** 535 E 70th St, New York, NY 10021-4892; **Phone:** 212-606-1966; **Board Cert:** Orthopaedic Surgery 1984; **Med School:** Columbia P&S 1973; **Resid:** Internal Medicine, Columbia-Presby Hosp 1976; Orthopaedic Surgery, Columbia-Presby Hosp 1980; **Fellow:** Shoulder Surgery, Columbia-Presby Hosp 1981; Hand Surgery, Columbia-Presby Hosp 1982; **Fac Appt:** Clin Prof OrS, Cornell Univ-Weill Med Coll

Crossett, Lawrence MD [OrS] - **Spec Exp:** Hip Surgery; Knee Surgery; **Hospital:** UPMC Presby, Pittsburgh, UPMC Shadyside; **Address:** Univ Pittsburgh Physicians, Orthopaedics, 5200 Centre Ave, Ste 415, Pittsburgh, PA 15232; **Phone:** 412-802-4100; **Board Cert:** Orthopaedic Surgery 2000; **Med School:** Temple Univ 1981; **Resid:** Orthopaedic Surgery, Temple Univ Hosp 1986; Orthopaedic Surgery, Shriners Children's Hosp 1984; **Fac Appt:** Assoc Prof OrS, Univ Pittsburgh

Davidson, Richard S MD [OrS] - **Spec Exp:** Limb Lengthening (Ilizarov Procedure); Limb Deformities; Foot Deformities; Clubfoot; **Hospital:** Chldns Hosp of Philadelphia, The; **Address:** Children's Hospital, Dept Orthopaedics, 34th St & Civic Ctr Blvd, Wood Center Fl 2, Philadelphia, PA 19104; **Phone:** 215-590-1527; **Board Cert:** Orthopaedic Surgery 1997; **Med School:** NYU Sch Med 1976; **Resid:** Orthopaedic Surgery, Hosp Special Surgery 1981; **Fellow:** Pediatric Orthopaedic Surgery, Hosp for Sick Children 1982; **Fac Appt:** Assoc Clin Prof OrS, Univ Pennsylvania

Delahay, John N MD [OrS] - **Spec Exp:** Pediatric Orthopaedic Surgery; Trauma; **Hospital:** Georgetown Univ Hosp; **Address:** 3800 Reservoir Rd NW, PHC Bldg, Ground FL, Washington, DC 20007; **Phone:** 202-444-1438; **Board Cert:** Orthopaedic Surgery 1975; **Med School:** Georgetown Univ 1969; **Resid:** Orthopaedic Surgery, Georgetown Univ Hosp 1974; **Fac Appt:** Prof OrS, Georgetown Univ

Deland, Jonathan T MD [OrS] - **Spec Exp:** Foot & Ankle Surgery; Sports Medicine; Arthritis; **Hospital:** Hosp For Special Surgery (page 59); **Address:** Hosp Spec Surg, Foot & Ankle Service, 535 E 70th St, New York, NY 10021-4099; **Phone:** 212-606-1665; **Board Cert:** Orthopaedic Surgery 2003; **Med School:** Columbia P&S 1980; **Resid:** Orthopaedic Surgery, St Luke's-Roosevelt Hosp Ctr 1982; Orthopaedic Surgery, Mass Genl Hosp 1987; **Fac Appt:** Asst Prof S, Cornell Univ-Weill Med Coll

Dines, David M MD [OrS] - **Spec Exp:** Shoulder Surgery; Sports Medicine; Shoulder Replacement; **Hospital:** Long Island Jewish Med Ctr, Hosp For Special Surgery (page 59); **Address:** 935 Northern Blvd, Ste 303, Great Neck, NY 11021-5309; **Phone:** 516-482-1037; **Board Cert:** Orthopaedic Surgery 1980; **Med School:** UMDNJ-NJ Med Sch, Newark 1974; **Resid:** Surgery, NY Hosp-Cornell Med Ctr 1976; Orthopaedic Surgery, Hosp Special Surg 1979; **Fac Appt:** Clin Prof OrS, Albert Einstein Coll Med

Donaldson III, William F MD [OrS] - **Spec Exp:** Spinal Surgery; **Hospital:** UPMC Presby, Pittsburgh; **Address:** Univ Pittsburgh Physicians, Orthopaedics, 3471 5th Ave, Ste 1010, Pittsburgh, PA 15213; **Phone:** 412-605-3218; **Board Cert:** Orthopaedic Surgery 1999; **Med School:** Rush Med Coll 1980; **Resid:** Surgery, Rush Presby-St Luke's Med Ctr 1981; Orthopaedic Surgery, Hosp Special Surg 1985; **Fellow:** Spinal Surgery, Hosp Special Surg 1986; **Fac Appt:** Assoc Prof OrS, Univ Pittsburgh

Dormans, John P MD [OrS] - **Spec Exp:** Tumor Surgery-Pediatric; Spinal Surgery-Pediatric; Pediatric Orthopaedic Surgery; **Hospital:** Chldns Hosp of Philadelphia, The; **Address:** Childrens Hosp Philadelphia, 34 St & Civic Center Blvd, Wood Bldg Fl 2 - rm 2315, Philadelphia, PA 19104; **Phone:** 215-590-1534; **Board Cert:** Orthopaedic Surgery 2002; **Med School:** Indiana Univ 1983; **Resid:** Orthopaedic Surgery, Michigan State Univ Hosps 1988; **Fellow:** Pediatric Orthopaedic Surgery, Hosp for Sick Children 1989; **Fac Appt:** Prof OrS, Univ Pennsylvania

Errico, Thomas MD [OrS] - **Spec Exp:** Spinal Surgery; Spinal Disc Replacement; Scoliosis; **Hospital:** NYU Med Ctr (page 68), Hosp For Joint Diseases (page 70); **Address:** 530 1st Ave, Ste 8U, New York, NY 10016-6402; **Phone:** 212-263-7182; **Board Cert:** Orthopaedic Surgery 1986; **Med School:** UMDNJ-NJ Med Sch, Newark 1978; **Resid:** Orthopaedic Surgery, NYU Med Ctr 1983; **Fellow:** Spinal Surgery, Toronto Genl Hosp 1984; **Fac Appt:** Assoc Prof OrS, NYU Sch Med

Feldman, David S MD [OrS] - **Spec Exp:** Limb Deformities; Spinal Surgery; Pediatric Orthopaedic Surgery; **Hospital:** Hosp For Joint Diseases (page 70), NYU Med Ctr (page 68); **Address:** 67 Irving Pl Fl 8, New York, NY 10003; **Phone:** 212-533-5310; **Board Cert:** Orthopaedic Surgery 2007; **Med School:** Albert Einstein Coll Med 1988; **Resid:** Orthopaedic Surgery, Hosp for Joint Diseases 1993; **Fellow:** Pediatric Surgery, Hosp For Sick Chldn 1994; **Fac Appt:** Asst Prof OrS, NYU Sch Med

Flatow, Evan MD [OrS] - **Spec Exp:** Rotator Cuff Surgery; Shoulder Injuries; Shoulder Replacement; Shoulder Arthroscopic Surgery; **Hospital:** Mount Sinai Med Ctr (page 64); **Address:** 5 E 98th St Fl 9, Box 1188, New York, NY 10029; **Phone:** 212-241-1663; **Board Cert:** Orthopaedic Surgery 2000; **Med School:** Columbia P&S 1981; **Resid:** Surgery, Roosevelt Hosp 1983; Orthopaedic Surgery, Columbia-Presby Med Ctr 1985; **Fellow:** Shoulder Surgery, Columbia-Presby Med Ctr 1987; **Fac Appt:** Prof OrS, Mount Sinai Sch Med

Frassica, Frank J MD [OrS] - **Spec Exp:** Bone Cancer; **Hospital:** Johns Hopkins Hosp - Baltimore (page 61); **Address:** 601 N Caroline St, Ste 5215, Baltimore, MD 21287-0882; **Phone:** 410-955-9300; **Board Cert:** Orthopaedic Surgery 2001; **Med School:** Univ SC Sch Med 1982; **Resid:** Orthopaedic Surgery, Mayo Clinic 1987; **Fellow:** Orthopaedic Oncology, Mayo Clinic 1988; **Fac Appt:** Prof OrS, Johns Hopkins Univ

Fu, Freddie H MD [OrS] - **Spec Exp:** Sports Medicine; Knee Injuries/ACL; Shoulder Injuries; **Hospital:** UPMC Presby, Pittsburgh; **Address:** Presbyterian Univ Hospital, Kaufmann Bldg, 3471 5th Ave, Ste 1011, Pittsburgh, PA 15213; **Phone:** 412-432-3611; **Board Cert:** Orthopaedic Surgery 1994; **Med School:** Univ Pittsburgh 1977; **Resid:** Orthopaedic Surgery, Univ Pittsburgh Med Ctr 1982; **Fellow:** Orthopaedic Research, Univ Pittsburgh Med Ctr 1979; **Fac Appt:** Prof OrS, Univ Pittsburgh

Glashow, Jonathan L MD [OrS] - **Spec Exp:** Sports Medicine; Shoulder Surgery; Knee Surgery; Arthroscopic Surgery; **Hospital:** Mount Sinai Med Ctr (page 64), Lenox Hill Hosp (page 62); **Address:** 159 E 74th St Fl 1, New York, NY 10021; **Phone:** 212-794-5096; **Board Cert:** Orthopaedic Surgery 2004; **Med School:** Cornell Univ-Weill Med Coll 1984; **Resid:** Orthopaedic Surgery, Lenox Hill Hosp 1989; **Fellow:** Arthroscopic Surgery, S Calif Ortho Inst 1990; Shoulder Surgery, Univ Texas Med Ctr 1990; **Fac Appt:** Assoc Clin Prof OrS, Mount Sinai Sch Med

Grelsamer, Ronald P MD [OrS] - **Spec Exp:** Knee-Patella Problems; Sports Medicine; Knee Reconstruction; Arthritis-Hip & Knee; **Hospital:** Mount Sinai Med Ctr (page 64); **Address:** Mount Sinai Medical Ctr, Dept Orthopaedics, 5 E 98th St, Box 1188, New York, NY 10029-6574; **Phone:** 212-241-2914; **Board Cert:** Orthopaedic Surgery 2007; **Med School:** Columbia P&S 1979; **Resid:** Orthopaedic Surgery, Columbia Presby Med Ctr 1984; **Fellow:** Hip & Knee Surgery, Columbia Presby Med Ctr 1985; **Fac Appt:** Assoc Prof OrS, Mount Sinai Sch Med

Haas, Steven B MD [OrS] - **Spec Exp:** Knee Surgery; Knee Replacement; Minimally Invasive Surgery; **Hospital:** Hosp For Special Surgery (page 59); **Address:** Hospital for Special Surgery, 535 E 70th St, New York, NY 10021; **Phone:** 212-606-1852; **Board Cert:** Orthopaedic Surgery 2004; **Med School:** Univ Rochester 1985; **Resid:** Orthopaedic Surgery, Hosp Special Surgery 1990; **Fellow:** Knee Surgery, Hosp Special Surgery 1991; **Fac Appt:** Assoc Prof OrS, Cornell Univ-Weill Med Coll

Orthopaedic Surgery

Hannafin, Jo A MD/PhD [OrS] - **Spec Exp:** Sports Medicine-Women; Shoulder Arthroscopic Surgery; Knee Injuries/Ligament Surgery; Ligament Reconstruction; **Hospital:** Hosp For Special Surgery (page 59), NY-Presby Hosp/Weill Cornell (page 66); **Address:** 535 E 70th St, New York, NY 10021-4872; **Phone:** 212-606-1469; **Board Cert:** Orthopaedic Surgery 2005; **Med School:** Albert Einstein Coll Med 1985; **Resid:** Orthopaedic Surgery, Montefiore Hosp Med Ctr 1990; **Fellow:** Sports Medicine, Hosp Special Surg-Cornell 1992; **Fac Appt:** Assoc Prof OrS, Cornell Univ-Weill Med Coll

Hausman, Michael R MD [OrS] - **Spec Exp:** Hand Reconstruction; Elbow Reconstruction; Arthroscopic Surgery; **Hospital:** Mount Sinai Med Ctr (page 64); **Address:** 5 E 98th St, Box 1188, New York, NY 10029-6501; **Phone:** 212-241-1658; **Board Cert:** Orthopaedic Surgery 2000; Hand Surgery 2000; **Med School:** Yale Univ 1979; **Resid:** Surgery, Yale-New Haven Hosp 1981; Orthopaedic Surgery, Yale-New Haven Hosp 1985; **Fellow:** Hand Surgery, Roosevelt Hosp 1987; **Fac Appt:** Assoc Clin Prof OrS, Mount Sinai Sch Med

Healey, John H MD [OrS] - **Spec Exp:** Bone Tumors; Hip & Knee Replacement in Bone Tumors; Sarcoma; Sarcoma-Soft Tissue; **Hospital:** Meml Sloan-Kettering Cancer Ctr, Hosp For Special Surgery (page 59); **Address:** 1275 York Avenue, New York, NY 10065; **Phone:** 800-525-2225; **Board Cert:** Orthopaedic Surgery 2007; **Med School:** Univ VT Coll Med 1978; **Resid:** Orthopaedic Surgery, Hosp Special Surg 1983; **Fellow:** Orthopaedic Oncology, Meml Sloan Kettering Cancer Ctr 1984; Orthopaedic Surgery, Hosp Special Surgery 1984; **Fac Appt:** Prof OrS, Cornell Univ-Weill Med Coll

Helfet, David L MD [OrS] - **Spec Exp:** Fractures-Complex; Fractures-Non Union; Trauma; **Hospital:** Hosp For Special Surgery (page 59), NY-Presby Hosp/Weill Cornell (page 66); **Address:** 535 E 70th St, New York, NY 10021; **Phone:** 212-606-1888; **Board Cert:** Orthopaedic Surgery 1984; **Med School:** South Africa 1975; **Resid:** Surgery, Edendale Hosp 1977; Orthopaedic Surgery, Johns Hopkins 1981; **Fellow:** Orthopaedic Surgery, Inselspita Hosp 1981; Orthopaedic Surgery, UCLA Med Ctr 1982; **Fac Appt:** Prof OrS, Cornell Univ-Weill Med Coll

Herzenberg, John E MD [OrS] - **Spec Exp:** Limb Lengthening (Ilizarov Procedure); Limb Deformities; Pediatric Orthopaedic Surgery; Clubfoot; **Hospital:** Sinai Hosp - Baltimore; **Address:** Rubin Inst for Advanced Orthopaedics, 2401 W Belvedere Ave, Baltimore, MD 21215; **Phone:** 410-601-8700; **Board Cert:** Orthopaedic Surgery 1999; **Med School:** Boston Univ 1979; **Resid:** Orthopaedic Surgery, Duke Univ Med Ctr 1985; **Fellow:** Pediatric Orthopaedic Surgery, Hosp for Sick Children 1986; **Fac Appt:** Prof S, Univ MD Sch Med

Hilibrand, Alan S MD [OrS] - **Spec Exp:** Spinal Surgery; Spinal Trauma; Scoliosis; Spinal Deformity; **Hospital:** Thomas Jefferson Univ Hosp; **Address:** Rothman Institute, 925 Chestnut St Fl 5, Philadelphia, PA 19107; **Phone:** 267-339-3500; **Board Cert:** Orthopaedic Surgery 2008; **Med School:** Yale Univ 1990; **Resid:** Orthopaedic Surgery, Univ Michigan Hlth System 1995; **Fellow:** Spinal Surgery, Cleveland Spine Inst 1996; **Fac Appt:** Prof OrS, Jefferson Med Coll

Hotchkiss, Robert MD [OrS] - **Spec Exp:** Hand Surgery; Wrist Surgery; Elbow Reconstruction; **Hospital:** Hosp For Special Surgery (page 59), NY-Presby Hosp/Weill Cornell (page 66); **Address:** 523 E 72nd St Fl 4, New York, NY 10021; **Phone:** 212-606-1964; **Board Cert:** Orthopaedic Surgery 2000; Hand Surgery 2000; **Med School:** Johns Hopkins Univ 1980; **Resid:** Surgery, Johns Hopkins Hosp 1982; Orthopaedic Surgery, Johns Hopkins Hosp 1985; **Fellow:** Hand Surgery, Union Meml Hosp 1987; **Fac Appt:** Assoc Prof OrS, Cornell Univ-Weill Med Coll

Hozack, William J MD [OrS] - **Spec Exp:** Hip Surgery; Knee Surgery; Joint Replacement; **Hospital:** Thomas Jefferson Univ Hosp; **Address:** Rothman Institute, 925 Chestnut St Fl 5, Philadelphia, PA 19107; **Phone:** 215-955-3458; **Board Cert:** Orthopaedic Surgery 2000; **Med School:** McGill Univ 1981; **Resid:** Orthopaedic Surgery, Hosp Univ Penn 1986; **Fellow:** Joint Reconstruction, Penn Hosp/Thomas Jefferson Univ 1987; **Fac Appt:** Prof OrS, Jefferson Med Coll

Johanson, Norman A MD [OrS] - **Spec Exp:** Hip & Knee Replacement; Joint Replacement; Juvenile Arthritis; Joint Replacement Revision; **Hospital:** Hahnemann Univ Hosp; **Address:** Drexel Orthopaedic Assocs, 216-220 N Broad St, Feinstein Bldg, Fl 2, Philadelphia, PA 19102; **Phone:** 215-762-2663; **Board Cert:** Orthopaedic Surgery 2007; **Med School:** Cornell Univ ; **Resid:** Orthopaedic Surgery, Hosp Special Surg; **Fellow:** Hosp Special Surg; **Fac Appt:** Prof OrS, Drexel Univ Coll Med

Johnson, Carl A MD [OrS] - **Spec Exp:** Knee Surgery; **Hospital:** Johns Hopkins Bayview Med Ctr (page 61), Johns Hopkins Hosp - Baltimore (page 61); **Address:** Johns Hopkins at Whitemarsh, 4924 Campbell Blvd, Ste 130, Nottingham, MD 21236; **Phone:** 443-442-2086; **Board Cert:** Orthopaedic Surgery 1983; **Med School:** Johns Hopkins Univ 1976; **Resid:** Surgery, Johns Hopkins Hosp 1978; Orthopaedic Surgery, Johns Hopkins Hosp 1981; **Fac Appt:** Assoc Prof OrS, Johns Hopkins Univ

Kaplan, Frederick S MD [OrS] - **Spec Exp:** Metabolic Bone Disease; Fibrodysplasia Ossificans Progressiv FOP; Progressive Osseous Heteroplasia POH; **Hospital:** Hosp Univ Penn - UPHS (page 60), Thomas Jefferson Univ Hosp; **Address:** U Penn Medical Ctr, Orthopaedic Inst, 3400 Spruce St, 2 Silverstein, MC 4283, Philadelphia, PA 19104; **Phone:** 215-349-8727; **Med School:** Johns Hopkins Univ 1976; **Resid:** Orthopaedic Surgery, Hosp U Penn 1981; **Fellow:** Orthopaedic Research, Hosp U Penn 1982; Musculoskeletal Disorders, Dr Michael Zasloff/U Penn 1991; **Fac Appt:** Prof OrS, Univ Pennsylvania

Keenan, Mary Ann MD [OrS] - **Spec Exp:** Neuro-Orthopaedic Surgery; Arthritis; Deformity Reconstruction; **Hospital:** Hosp Univ Penn - UPHS (page 60), Pennsylvania Hosp (page 60); **Address:** Hosp Univ Penn, Dept Orthopaedic Surg, 3400 Spruce St, 2 Fl- Silverstein, Philadelphia, PA 19104; **Phone:** 215-662-3340; **Board Cert:** Orthopaedic Surgery 1997; **Med School:** Med Coll PA 1976; **Resid:** Orthopaedic Surgery, Albert Einstein Med Ctr 1981; **Fellow:** Arthritis Surgery, Rancho Los Amigos Med Ctr 1981; Neurological Orthopaedic Surgery, Rancho Los Amigos Med Ctr 1982; **Fac Appt:** Prof OrS, Univ Pennsylvania

Kenan, Samuel MD [OrS] - **Spec Exp:** Bone Tumors; Hip Replacement; Knee Replacement; **Hospital:** Hosp For Joint Diseases (page 70), NYU Med Ctr (page 68); **Address:** 317 E 34th St Fl 9 - Ste 903, New York, NY 10016; **Phone:** 212-684-5511; **Med School:** Israel 1976; **Resid:** Orthopaedic Surgery, Hadassah Univ Hosp 1984; **Fellow:** Orthopaedic Pathology, Hosp for Joint Diseases 1987; **Fac Appt:** Prof OrS, NYU Sch Med

Krackow, Kenneth A MD [OrS] - **Spec Exp:** Knee Replacement; Knee Reconstruction; Hip Replacement & Revision; **Hospital:** Buffalo General Hosp; **Address:** Bufffalo Genl Hosp, Dept Orthopaedic Surgery, 100 High St, Ste B276, Buffalo, NY 14203; **Phone:** 716-859-1256; **Board Cert:** Orthopaedic Surgery 1993; **Med School:** Duke Univ 1971; **Resid:** Surgery, Johns Hopkins Hosp 1973; **Fellow:** Orthopaedic Surgery, Johns Hopkins Hosp 1976; **Fac Appt:** Prof OrS, SUNY Buffalo

Lackman, Richard D MD [OrS] - **Spec Exp:** Bone Cancer; Sarcoma; Limb Sparing Surgery; **Hospital:** Hosp Univ Penn - UPHS (page 60), Pennsylvania Hosp (page 60); **Address:** Hosp Univ Penn-Dept Orthopaedic Surg, 301 S 8th St, Garfield Duncan Bldg, Ste 2C, Philadelphia, PA 19104; **Phone:** 215-829-5022; **Board Cert:** Orthopaedic Surgery 1985; **Med School:** Univ Pennsylvania 1977; **Resid:** Orthopaedic Surgery, Hosp Univ Penn 1982; **Fellow:** Orthopaedic Oncology, Mayo Clinic 1983; **Fac Appt:** Assoc Prof OrS, Univ Pennsylvania

Orthopaedic Surgery

Lane, Joseph MD [OrS] - **Spec Exp:** Bone Disorders-Metabolic; Osteoporosis Spinal Fracture; Osteoporosis Spine-Kyphoplasty; Bone Cancer; **Hospital:** Hosp For Special Surgery (page 59), NY-Presby Hosp/Weill Cornell (page 66); **Address:** Hosp for Special Surgery, 535 E 70th St, New York, NY 10021; **Phone:** 212-606-1172; **Board Cert:** Orthopaedic Surgery 1998; **Med School:** Harvard Med Sch 1965; **Resid:** Surgery, Hosp Univ Penn 1967; Orthopaedic Surgery, Hosp Univ Penn 1973; **Fac Appt:** Prof OrS, Cornell Univ-Weill Med Coll

Lauerman, William MD [OrS] - **Spec Exp:** Spinal Deformity-Pediatric & Adult; Spinal Surgery; Pain-Back; Scoliosis; **Hospital:** Georgetown Univ Hosp; **Address:** 3800 Reservoir Rd NW, Spine Surgery Clinic-1 Gorman, Washington, DC 20007; **Phone:** 202-444-8766 x2; **Board Cert:** Orthopaedic Surgery 2001; **Med School:** Georgetown Univ 1982; **Resid:** Orthopaedic Surgery, Georgetown Univ Med Ctr 1987; **Fellow:** Orthopaedic Surgery, Univ Minn-Twin Cities Scoliosis Ctr 1988; **Fac Appt:** Prof OrS, Georgetown Univ

Lee, Francis Y MD/PhD [OrS] - **Spec Exp:** Bone Tumors; Pediatric Orthopaedic Cancers; Pediatric Orthopaedic Surgery; **Hospital:** NY-Presby Hosp/Columbia (page 66); **Address:** 16 E 16th St, New York, NY 10022; **Phone:** 212-305-4565; **Board Cert:** Orthopaedic Surgery 2001; **Med School:** South Korea 1986; **Resid:** Orthopaedic Surgery, NJ Med Ctr 1997; **Fellow:** Orthopaedic Oncology, Harvard Med Sch 1998; Pediatric Orthopaedic Surgery, Hosp for Sick Chldn/Univ Toronto 1999; **Fac Appt:** Asst Prof OrS, Columbia P&S

Lehman, Wallace B MD [OrS] - **Spec Exp:** Clubfoot/Foot Deformities in Children; Hip Disorders-Pediatric; Limb Deformities; Blount's Disease; **Hospital:** Hosp For Joint Diseases (page 70), NYU Med Ctr (page 68); **Address:** NYU Hosp Joint Diseases, Dept Ped Orth Surg, 301 E 17th St, Ste 413, New York, NY 10003-3804; **Phone:** 212-598-6403; **Board Cert:** Orthopaedic Surgery 1966; **Med School:** SUNY Hlth Sci Ctr 1958; **Resid:** Orthopaedic Surgery, Hosp Joint Diseases 1963; **Fac Appt:** Prof OrS, NYU Sch Med

Malawer, Martin M MD [OrS] - **Spec Exp:** Bone Tumors; Limb Sparing Surgery; Pediatric Orthopaedic Surgery; Sarcoma; **Hospital:** Washington Hosp Ctr; **Address:** Washington Cancer Institute, 110 Irving St NW, Ste C2173, Washington, DC 20010; **Phone:** 202-877-3970; **Board Cert:** Orthopaedic Surgery 1993; **Med School:** NYU Sch Med 1969; **Resid:** Surgery, Bronx Muni Hosp 1972; Orthopaedic Surgery, Bellevue Hosp Ctr 1975; **Fellow:** Orthopaedic Oncology, Shands Hosp-Univ Florida 1978; **Fac Appt:** Prof OrS, Geo Wash Univ

McAfee, Paul C MD [OrS] - **Spec Exp:** Spinal Reconstructive Surgery; Spinal Disc Replacement; Scoliosis; **Hospital:** St Joseph Med Ctr; **Address:** Scoliosis & Spine Ctr, 7505 Osler Drive, Ste 104, Towson, MD 21204; **Phone:** 410-337-8888; **Board Cert:** Orthopaedic Surgery 2007; **Med School:** SUNY Upstate Med Univ 1979; **Resid:** Orthopaedic Surgery, SUNY Upstate Med Ctr 1984; **Fellow:** Spinal Surgery, Case West Res Univ Hosps 1986; **Fac Appt:** Assoc Prof OrS, Johns Hopkins Univ

McCann, Peter D MD [OrS] - **Spec Exp:** Shoulder Surgery; Elbow Surgery; **Hospital:** Beth Israel Med Ctr - Petrie Division (page 57); **Address:** 10 Union Square E, Ste 3M, New York, NY 10003; **Phone:** 212-844-6735; **Board Cert:** Orthopaedic Surgery 1999; **Med School:** Columbia P&S 1980; **Resid:** Surgery, St Vincent's Hosp 1982; Orthopaedic Surgery, Columbia-Presby Med Ctr 1985; **Fellow:** Shoulder Surgery, Columbia-Presby Med Ctr 1986; **Fac Appt:** Assoc Prof OrS, Albert Einstein Coll Med

McFarland, Edward G MD [OrS] - **Spec Exp:** Sports Medicine; **Hospital:** Johns Hopkins Hosp - Baltimore (page 61); **Address:** 10753 Falls Rd, Ste 215, Lutherville, MD 21093; **Phone:** 410-583-2850; **Board Cert:** Orthopaedic Surgery 2001; **Med School:** Univ Louisville Sch Med 1982; **Resid:** Orthopaedic Surgery, Mayo Clinic 1987; **Fellow:** Sports Medicine, Kerlan-Jobe Orthopaedic Group 1989; **Fac Appt:** Assoc Prof OrS, Johns Hopkins Univ

Myerson, Mark MD [OrS] - **Spec Exp:** Foot & Ankle Surgery; **Hospital:** Mercy Medical Center Inc; **Address:** 301 St Paul Pl, Baltimore, MD 21202; **Phone:** 410-659-2800; **Board Cert:** Orthopaedic Surgery 1999; **Med School:** South Africa 1979; **Resid:** Surgery, Sinai Hospital 1981; Orthopaedic Surgery, Johns Hopkins Hosp 1985; **Fellow:** Foot & Ankle Surgery, Hospital Joint Disease

Neuwirth, Michael MD [OrS] - **Spec Exp:** Scoliosis; Spinal Surgery; **Hospital:** Beth Israel Med Ctr - Petrie Division (page 57), Palisades Med Ctr; **Address:** Beth Israel Med Ctr - Spine Institute, 10 Union Square E, Ste 5P, New York, NY 10003-3314; **Phone:** 212-844-8692; **Board Cert:** Orthopaedic Surgery 1980; **Med School:** SUNY Hlth Sci Ctr 1974; **Resid:** Orthopaedic Surgery, Hosp for Joint Diseases 1978; **Fellow:** Spinal Surgery, Rush-Presby Med Ctr 1979; **Fac Appt:** Assoc Clin Prof OrS, NYU Sch Med

Nicholas, Stephen J MD [OrS] - **Spec Exp:** Sports Medicine; Shoulder & Knee Surgery; Arthroscopic Surgery; **Hospital:** Lenox Hill Hosp (page 62); **Address:** 159 E 74 St, New York, NY 10021-1803; **Phone:** 212-737-3301; **Board Cert:** Orthopaedic Surgery 2005; **Med School:** NY Med Coll 1986; **Resid:** Orthopaedic Surgery, Hosp for Special Surgery 1991; **Fellow:** Sports Medicine, Lenox Hill Hosp 1992

O'Keefe, Regis J MD/PhD [OrS] - **Spec Exp:** Bone & Soft Tissue Tumors; Reconstructive Surgery; Metabolic Bone Disease; **Hospital:** Univ of Rochester Strong Meml Hosp, Highland Hosp - Rochester; **Address:** Univ Rochester, Dept Orthopaedic Surgery, 601 Elmwood Ave, Box 665, Rochester, NY 14642; **Phone:** 585-275-3100; **Board Cert:** Orthopaedic Surgery 1996; **Med School:** Harvard Med Sch 1985; **Resid:** Surgery, New Eng Deaconess Hosp/Harvard 1986; Orthopaedic Surgery, Univ Rochester 1992; **Fellow:** Orthopaedic Oncology, Mass Genl Hosp 1993; **Fac Appt:** Prof S, Univ Rochester

O'Leary, Patrick MD [OrS] - **Spec Exp:** Spinal Surgery; **Hospital:** Hosp For Special Surgery (page 59); **Address:** 1015 Madison Ave Fl 4, New York, NY 10021; **Phone:** 212-249-8100; **Board Cert:** Orthopaedic Surgery 1983; **Med School:** Ireland 1968; **Resid:** Surgery, Roosevelt Hosp. 1972; Orthopaedic Surgery, Hosp Spec Surg-Cornell 1975; **Fellow:** Spinal Surgery, Univ Toronto Genl Ortho Hosp 1976; **Fac Appt:** Assoc Clin Prof OrS, Cornell Univ-Weill Med Coll

Okereke, Enyi MD [OrS] - **Spec Exp:** Foot & Ankle Surgery; **Hospital:** Hosp Univ Penn - UPHS (page 60); **Address:** Univ Penn Orthopaedic Surgery, 3400 Spruce St, 2 Silverstein, Philadelphia, PA 19104; **Phone:** 215-662-3340; **Board Cert:** Orthopaedic Surgery 1996; **Med School:** Howard Univ 1987; **Resid:** Orthopaedic Surgery, Hosp Univ Penn 1992; **Fellow:** Foot & Ankle Surgery, Hosp Joint Disease 1993; **Fac Appt:** Assoc Prof OrS, Univ Pennsylvania

Padgett, Douglas E MD [OrS] - **Spec Exp:** Hip & Knee Replacement; Arthroscopic Surgery-Hip; Arthroscopic Surgery-Knee; Dance Medicine; **Hospital:** Hosp For Special Surgery (page 59); **Address:** Hosp for Special Surgery, 535 E 70 St, New York, NY 10021; **Phone:** 212-606-1642; **Board Cert:** Orthopaedic Surgery 2002; **Med School:** NY Med Coll 1982; **Resid:** Orthopaedic Surgery, Hosp Spec Surg 1989; **Fellow:** Orthopaedic Surgery, Rush Presby Med Cr 1990; **Fac Appt:** Assoc Prof OrS, Cornell Univ-Weill Med Coll

Paley, Dror MD [OrS] - **Spec Exp:** Limb Lengthening (Ilizarov Procedure); Limb Deformities; Pediatric Orthopaedic Surgery; **Hospital:** Sinai Hosp - Baltimore, Univ of MD Med Sys; **Address:** Rubin Inst for Advanced Orthopaedics, 2401 W Belvedere Ave, Baltimore, MD 21215; **Phone:** 410-601-4200; **Board Cert:** Orthopaedic Surgery 2000; **Med School:** Univ Toronto 1979; **Resid:** Orthopaedic Surgery, Univ Toronto Hosp 1985; **Fellow:** Hand Surgery, SunnyBrook Hosp 1986; Pediatric Orthopaedic Surgery, Hosp for Sick Children 1987; **Fac Appt:** Assoc Prof S, Univ MD Sch Med

Orthopaedic Surgery

Pellicci, Paul MD [OrS] - **Spec Exp:** Hip Replacement-Young Adults; Hip Resurfacing; Knee Replacement; Joint Replacement; **Hospital:** Hosp For Special Surgery (page 59), NY-Presby Hosp/Weill Cornell (page 66); **Address:** 535 E 70th St, New York, NY 10021-4872; **Phone:** 212-606-1010; **Board Cert:** Orthopaedic Surgery 1982; **Med School:** Cornell Univ-Weill Med Coll 1975; **Resid:** Surgery, New York Hosp 1976; Orthopaedic Surgery, Hosp for Special Surgery 1980; **Fellow:** Joint Replacement Surgery, Brigham & Womens Hosp 1981; **Fac Appt:** Prof OrS, Cornell Univ-Weill Med Coll

Ramsey, Matthew L MD [OrS] - **Spec Exp:** Shoulder Surgery; Elbow Surgery; Sports Medicine; **Hospital:** Thomas Jefferson Univ Hosp; **Address:** Rothman Institute, 925 Chestnut St Fl 5, Philadelphia, PA 19107; **Phone:** 267-339-3500; **Board Cert:** Orthopaedic Surgery 1998; **Med School:** SUNY Hlth Sci Ctr 1990; **Resid:** Orthopaedic Surgery, Thomas Jefferson Univ Hosp 1996; **Fellow:** Shoulder Surgery, Hosp Univ Penn 1996; **Fac Appt:** Assoc Prof OrS, Univ Pennsylvania

Ranawat, Chitranjan MD [OrS] - **Spec Exp:** Hip Replacement; Knee Replacement; **Hospital:** Hosp For Special Surgery (page 59); **Address:** Hospital for Special Surgery, 535 E 70th St, New York, NY 10021; **Phone:** 646-797-8700; **Board Cert:** Orthopaedic Surgery 1969; **Med School:** India 1958; **Resid:** Surgery, MY Hosp 1963; Orthopaedic Surgery, Albany Med Ctr 1965; **Fellow:** Orthopaedic Surgery, Hosp Special Surg 1969; **Fac Appt:** Prof OrS, Cornell Univ-Weill Med Coll

Rechtine, Glenn MD [OrS] - **Spec Exp:** Spinal Surgery; **Hospital:** Univ of Rochester Strong Meml Hosp; **Address:** Strong Meml Hosp, Dept Orthopaedics, 601 Elmwood Ave, Box 665, Rochester, NY 14618; **Phone:** 585-275-2225; **Board Cert:** Orthopaedic Surgery 1982; **Med School:** Univ S Fla Coll Med 1975; **Resid:** Orthopaedic Surgery, Naval Regional Med Ctr 1980; **Fellow:** Spinal Surgery, Case West Res Univ 1981; **Fac Appt:** Prof OrS, Univ Rochester

Rodosky, Mark W MD [OrS] - **Spec Exp:** Sports Medicine; Shoulder Surgery; Rotator Cuff Surgery; **Hospital:** UPMC South Side; **Address:** UPMC Center for Sports Medicine, 3200 S Water St, Pittsburgh, PA 15203; **Phone:** 412-432-3621; **Board Cert:** Orthopaedic Surgery 1997; **Med School:** Mount Sinai Sch Med 1987; **Resid:** Surgery, Univ Pittsburgh Med Ctr 1993; **Fellow:** Orthopaedic Surgery, NY Presby-Columbia Presby Med Ctr 1994; **Fac Appt:** Asst Prof OrS, Univ Pittsburgh

Rosier, Randy MD/PhD [OrS] - **Spec Exp:** Bone Disorders-Metabolic; **Hospital:** Univ of Rochester Strong Meml Hosp; **Address:** Univ Rochester, Dept Orthopaedic Surgery, 601 Elmwood Ave, Box 665, Rochester, NY 14642; **Phone:** 585-275-3100; **Board Cert:** Orthopaedic Surgery 1998; **Med School:** Univ Rochester 1978; **Resid:** Orthopaedic Surgery, Univ Iowa Hosp 1984; **Fellow:** Univ Iowa Hosp 1983; **Fac Appt:** Prof OrS, Univ Rochester

Rothman, Richard H MD/PhD [OrS] - **Spec Exp:** Hip Replacement; Knee Replacement; Joint Replacement; **Hospital:** Thomas Jefferson Univ Hosp; **Address:** Rothman Institute, 925 Chestnut St Fl 5, Philadelphia, PA 19107; **Phone:** 267-339-3500; **Board Cert:** Orthopaedic Surgery 1970; **Med School:** Univ Pennsylvania 1962; **Resid:** Orthopaedic Surgery, Jefferson Hosp 1968; **Fac Appt:** Prof OrS, Jefferson Med Coll

Roye, David MD [OrS] - **Spec Exp:** Pediatric Orthopaedic Surgery; Scoliosis; Hip Disorders-Pediatric; **Hospital:** NY-Presby Hosp/Columbia (page 66), Greenwich Hosp; **Address:** Morgan Stanley Chlds Hosp NewYork-Presby, 3959 Broadway, 8 North, New York, NY 10032-1559; **Phone:** 212-305-5475; **Board Cert:** Orthopaedic Surgery 1981; **Med School:** Columbia P&S 1975; **Resid:** Orthopaedic Surgery, Columbia-Presby Med Ctr 1979; **Fellow:** Orthopaedic Surgery, Hosp for Sick Chldn 1980; **Fac Appt:** Prof OrS, Columbia P&S

Rozbruch, S Robert MD [OrS] - **Spec Exp:** Limb Lengthening; Limb Deformities; Limb Surgery/Reconstruction; Fractures-Complex; **Hospital:** Hosp For Special Surgery (page 59), NY-Presby Hosp/Weill Cornell (page 66); **Address:** 535 E 70th St, New York, NY 10021; **Phone:** 212-606-1415; **Board Cert:** Orthopaedic Surgery 1998; **Med School:** Cornell Univ-Weill Med Coll 1990; **Resid:** Orthopaedic Surgery, Hosp Special Surgery 1995; **Fellow:** Trauma, Univ Bern Hosp 1997; Limb Lengthening, Intl Ctr Limb Length/Univ MD 1999; **Fac Appt:** Asst Prof OrS, Cornell Univ-Weill Med Coll

Salvati, Eduardo A MD [OrS] - **Spec Exp:** Hip Surgery; Hip & Knee Replacement; **Hospital:** Hosp For Special Surgery (page 59); **Address:** Hosp for Spec Surg, 535 E 70th Street, New York, NY 10021; **Phone:** 212-606-1472; **Board Cert:** Orthopaedic Surgery 1972; **Med School:** Argentina 1963; **Resid:** Orthopaedic Surgery, Univ Florence Ortho Clinic 1965; Orthopaedic Surgery, Hosp Buenos Aires 1969; **Fellow:** Hip Surgery, Hosp For Spec Surg 1972; **Fac Appt:** Clin Prof OrS, Cornell Univ-Weill Med Coll

Sandhu, Harvinder S MD [OrS] - **Spec Exp:** Minimally Invasive Surgery; Spinal Disc Replacement; Spinal Surgery; **Hospital:** Hosp For Special Surgery (page 59), NY-Presby Hosp/Weill Cornell (page 66); **Address:** 535 E 70th St, New York, NY 10021; **Phone:** 212-606-1798; **Board Cert:** Orthopaedic Surgery 2007; **Med School:** Northwestern Univ 1987; **Resid:** Orthopaedic Surgery, Univ Hosp-SUNY Hlth Sci Ctr 1992; **Fellow:** Spinal Surgery, UCLA Med Ctr 1993; **Fac Appt:** Assoc Prof OrS, Cornell Univ-Weill Med Coll

Schmidt, Richard G MD [OrS] - **Spec Exp:** Bone Tumors; Sarcoma-Soft Tissue; Limb Sparing Surgery; Metastatic Bone Disease; **Hospital:** Lankenau Hosp, Fox Chase Cancer Ctr (page 58); **Address:** Musculoskeletal Tumor Ctr, 15 N Presidential Blvd, Ste 300, Bala Cynwyd, PA 19004; **Phone:** 610-667-2663; **Board Cert:** Orthopaedic Surgery 1999; **Med School:** Penn State Univ-Hershey Med Ctr 1980; **Resid:** Orthopaedic Surgery, Hosp Univ Penn 1985; **Fellow:** Orthopaedic Oncology, Shands Hosp 1986

Scott, W Norman MD [OrS] - **Spec Exp:** Knee Injuries; Knee Replacement; Sports Medicine; **Hospital:** Lenox Hill Hosp (page 62), Franklin Hosp; **Address:** 210 E 64th St Fl 4, New York, NY 10021-7471; **Phone:** 212-434-4301; **Board Cert:** Orthopaedic Surgery 1978; **Med School:** Cornell Univ-Weill Med Coll 1972; **Resid:** Surgery, St Luke's-Roosevelt Hosp Ctr 1974; Orthopaedic Surgery, Hosp Special Surg 1977; **Fac Appt:** Clin Prof OrS, Cornell Univ-Weill Med Coll

Sculco, Thomas P MD [OrS] - **Spec Exp:** Hip Replacement; Knee Replacement; Minimally Invasive Surgery; Joint Replacement; **Hospital:** Hosp For Special Surgery (page 59); **Address:** 535 E 70th St, Ste 238, New York, NY 10021-4872; **Phone:** 212-606-1475; **Board Cert:** Orthopaedic Surgery 1976; **Med School:** Columbia P&S 1969; **Resid:** Surgery, Roosevelt Hosp 1971; Orthopaedic Surgery, Hosp For Special Surgery 1974; **Fellow:** Orthopaedic Surgery, The London Hosp 1975; **Fac Appt:** Prof OrS, Cornell Univ-Weill Med Coll

Spivak, Jeffrey M MD [OrS] - **Spec Exp:** Spinal Surgery; Scoliosis; Sports Medicine Back Injuries; **Hospital:** Hosp For Joint Diseases (page 70), NYU Med Ctr (page 68); **Address:** Hospital for Joint Diseases, Spine Ctr, 301 E 17th St, Ste 400, New York, NY 10003-3804; **Phone:** 212-598-6696; **Board Cert:** Orthopaedic Surgery 2006; **Med School:** Cornell Univ-Weill Med Coll 1986; **Resid:** Orthopaedic Surgery, Hosp for Joint Diseases 1992; **Fellow:** Spinal Surgery, Thomas Jefferson Univ Hosp 1993; **Fac Appt:** Asst Prof OrS, NYU Sch Med

Sponseller, Paul D MD [OrS] - **Spec Exp:** Cerebral Palsy; Scoliosis; Pediatric Orthopaedic Surgery; **Hospital:** Johns Hopkins Hosp - Baltimore (page 61); **Address:** 601 N Caroline St, Ste 5212, Baltimore, MD 21287-0882; **Phone:** 410-955-3136; **Board Cert:** Orthopaedic Surgery 2000; **Med School:** Univ Mich Med Sch 1980; **Resid:** Orthopaedic Surgery, Univ Wisc Hosp 1985; **Fellow:** Pediatric Orthopaedic Surgery, Chldns Hosp-Harvard 1986; **Fac Appt:** Prof OrS, Johns Hopkins Univ

Orthopaedic Surgery

Strongwater, Allan MD [OrS] - **Spec Exp:** Pediatric Orthopaedic Surgery; Cerebral Palsy; Deformity Reconstruction; **Hospital:** Hosp For Joint Diseases (page 70), NYU Med Ctr (page 68); **Address:** 301 E 17th St, New York, NY 10003; **Phone:** 212-598-6190; **Board Cert:** Orthopaedic Surgery 1997; **Med School:** Rush Med Coll 1978; **Resid:** Orthopaedic Surgery, Yale-New Haven Hosp 1983; Pediatric Orthopaedic Surgery, Hosp Joint Diseases 1984; **Fac Appt:** Clin Prof OrS, NYU Sch Med

Stuchin, Steven MD [OrS] - **Spec Exp:** Hand Surgery; Arthritis; Hip & Knee Replacement; Hip Resurfacing; **Hospital:** Hosp For Joint Diseases (page 70), Lenox Hill Hosp (page 62); **Address:** 301 E 17th St, Ste 1402, New York, NY 10003-3804; **Phone:** 212-598-6708; **Board Cert:** Orthopaedic Surgery 1984; **Med School:** Columbia P&S 1976; **Resid:** Surgery, Roosevelt Hosp 1978; Orthopaedic Surgery, Hosp For Special Surg 1981; **Fellow:** Hand Surgery, Thomas Jefferson Univ Hosp 1982; **Fac Appt:** Assoc Prof OrS, NYU Sch Med

Tischler, Henry MD [OrS] - **Spec Exp:** Hip Replacement; Knee Replacement; **Hospital:** New York Methodist Hosp, St Vincent Cath Med Ctrs - Manhattan; **Address:** Brooklyn Spine & Arthritis Ctr, 263 7th Ave, Ste 2B, Brooklyn, NY 11215; **Phone:** 718-246-8700; **Board Cert:** Orthopaedic Surgery 2006; **Med School:** SUNY Downstate 1985; **Resid:** Orthopaedic Surgery, SUNY Downstate Med Ctr 1990; **Fellow:** Orthopaedic Surgery, Tampa Gen Hosp/Fla Osteo Inst 1991; **Fac Appt:** Asst Prof OrS, SUNY Hlth Sci Ctr

Vaccaro, Alexander R MD/PhD [OrS] - **Spec Exp:** Spinal Surgery; Spinal Trauma; Spinal Cord Injury; **Hospital:** Thomas Jefferson Univ Hosp; **Address:** Rothman Institute, 925 Chestnut St Fl 5, Philadelphia, PA 19107; **Phone:** 267-339-3500; **Board Cert:** Orthopaedic Surgery 2006; **Med School:** Georgetown Univ 1987; **Resid:** Orthopaedic Surgery, Thos Jefferson Univ Hosp 1992; **Fellow:** Spinal Surgery, UCSD Med Ctr 1993; **Fac Appt:** Prof OrS, Thomas Jefferson Univ

Wapner, Keith L MD [OrS] - **Spec Exp:** Foot & Ankle Surgery; Tendon Surgery; Arthritis; **Hospital:** Pennsylvania Hosp (page 60); **Address:** The Farm Journal Bldg Fl 5, 230 W Washington Square, Philadelphia, PA 19106-3500; **Phone:** 215-829-3668; **Board Cert:** Orthopaedic Surgery 1999; **Med School:** Temple Univ 1980; **Resid:** Surgery, Hosp Univ Penn 1981; Orthopaedic Surgery, Hosp Univ Penn 1985; **Fellow:** Joint Reconstruction, Ohio St Univ Med Ctr 1986; Foot & Ankle Surgery, UCSF Med Ctr 1987; **Fac Appt:** Clin Prof OrS, Univ Pennsylvania

Warren, Russell MD [OrS] - **Spec Exp:** Knee Injuries/Ligament Surgery; Shoulder Reconstruction; Shoulder Replacement; Sports Medicine; **Hospital:** Hosp For Special Surgery (page 59), NY-Presby Hosp/Weill Cornell (page 66); **Address:** 535 E 70th St, New York, NY 10021-4892; **Phone:** 212-606-1178; **Board Cert:** Orthopaedic Surgery 1974; **Med School:** SUNY Upstate Med Univ 1966; **Resid:** Surgery, St Lukes Hosp 1968; Orthopaedic Surgery, Hosp For Special Surgery 1973; **Fellow:** Shoulder Surgery, Columbia-Presby Med Ctr 1977; **Fac Appt:** Prof OrS, Cornell Univ-Weill Med Coll

Weinfeld, Steven B MD [OrS] - **Spec Exp:** Foot & Ankle Surgery; Diabetic Leg/Foot; **Hospital:** Mount Sinai Med Ctr (page 64); **Address:** 5 E 98th St Fl 9, Box 1188, New York, NY 10029; **Phone:** 212-241-1634; **Board Cert:** Orthopaedic Surgery 1998; **Med School:** Albany Med Coll 1990; **Resid:** Orthopaedic Surgery, Albany Med Ctr 1995; **Fellow:** Ankle and Foot Surgery, Union Meml Hosp 1996; **Fac Appt:** Assoc Prof OrS, Mount Sinai Sch Med

Wickiewicz, Thomas L MD [OrS] - **Spec Exp:** Shoulder Surgery; Sports Medicine; Knee Surgery; **Hospital:** Hosp For Special Surgery (page 59), NY-Presby Hosp/Weill Cornell (page 66); **Address:** 535 E 70th St, New York, NY 10021; **Phone:** 212-606-1450; **Board Cert:** Orthopaedic Surgery 1984; **Med School:** UMDNJ-NJ Med Sch, Newark 1976; **Resid:** Orthopaedic Surgery, Hosp for Special Surg 1981; **Fellow:** Sports Medicine, UCLA Med Ctr 1982; **Fac Appt:** Clin Prof OrS, Cornell Univ-Weill Med Coll

Wiesel, Sam W MD [OrS] - **Spec Exp:** Spinal Surgery; **Hospital:** Georgetown Univ Hosp; **Address:** 3800 Reservoir Rd NW, PHC Bldg Fl Ground, Washington, DC 20007-2113; **Phone:** 202-444-8766 x2; **Board Cert:** Orthopaedic Surgery 1977; **Med School:** Univ Pennsylvania 1971; **Resid:** Orthopaedic Surgery, Hosp Univ Penn 1976; **Fellow:** Orthopaedic Surgery, Hosp Univ Penn 1973; **Fac Appt:** Prof OrS, Georgetown Univ

Williams, Gerald MD [OrS] - **Spec Exp:** Shoulder Arthroscopic Surgery; Shoulder Reconstruction; Shoulder Cartilage Implant; Shoulder Replacement; **Hospital:** Methodist Hosp, Thomas Jefferson Univ Hosp; **Address:** Rothman Institute, 925 Chestnut St Fl 5, Philadelphia, PA 19107; **Phone:** 267-339-3500; **Board Cert:** Orthopaedic Surgery 2003; **Med School:** Temple Univ 1984; **Resid:** Orthopaedic Surgery, Univ Texas San Antonio Afill Hosp 1989; **Fellow:** Shoulder Surgery, Univ Texas San Antonio 1990; **Fac Appt:** Prof OrS, Thomas Jefferson Univ

Zuckerman, Joseph MD [OrS] - **Spec Exp:** Shoulder Surgery; Hip Replacement; Knee Replacement; Joint Replacement; **Hospital:** Hosp For Joint Diseases (page 70), NYU Med Ctr (page 68); **Address:** NYU Hosp for Joint Diseases, Dept Ortho Surg, 301 E 17th St Fl 14 - Ste 1402, New York, NY 10003; **Phone:** 212-598-6674; **Board Cert:** Orthopaedic Surgery 2006; **Med School:** Med Coll Wisc 1978; **Resid:** Orthopaedic Surgery, Univ WA Med Ctr 1983; **Fellow:** Arthritis Surgery, Brigham & Womans Hosp 1984; Shoulder Surgery, Mayo Clinic 1984; **Fac Appt:** Prof OrS, NYU Sch Med

Southeast

Beaty, James H MD [OrS] - **Spec Exp:** Pediatric Orthopaedic Surgery; Clubfoot; Fractures-Pediatric; **Hospital:** Le Bonheur Chldns Med Ctr, Baptist Memorial Hospital - Memphis; **Address:** Campbell Clinic, 1211 Union Ave, Ste 500, Memphis, TN 38104; **Phone:** 901-759-3125; **Board Cert:** Orthopaedic Surgery 2007; **Med School:** Univ Tenn Coll Med, Memphis 1976; **Resid:** Surgery, Baptist Meml Hosp 1979; Orthopaedic Surgery, Campbell Clin Fdn 1981; **Fellow:** Pediatric Orthopaedic Surgery, Alfred I Dupont Inst 1982; **Fac Appt:** Prof OrS, Univ Tenn Coll Med, Memphis

Berrey, B Hudson MD [OrS] - **Spec Exp:** Musculoskeletal Tumors; Bone Cancer; Soft Tissue Tumors; Sarcoma; **Hospital:** Shands Jacksonville, Wolfson Chldns Hosp; **Address:** Univ Florida Coll Med, Dept Orth Surg, 655 W Eighth St, Jacksonville, FL 32209; **Phone:** 904-244-5942; **Board Cert:** Orthopaedic Surgery 1982; **Med School:** Univ Tex Med Br, Galveston 1977; **Resid:** Orthopaedic Surgery, Tripler Army Med Ctr 1981; **Fellow:** Medical Oncology, Mass Genl Hosp Harvard 1985; **Fac Appt:** Prof OrS, Univ Fla Coll Med

Boden, Scott D MD [OrS] - **Spec Exp:** Spinal Disorders; Spinal Surgery; Spinal Disc Replacement; Microdiscectomy; **Hospital:** Emory Univ Hosp; **Address:** 59 Executive Park S, Ste 3000, Atlanta, GA 30329; **Phone:** 404-778-7143; **Board Cert:** Orthopaedic Surgery 2005; **Med School:** Univ Pennsylvania 1986; **Resid:** Orthopaedic Surgery, George Washington Univ Hosp 1991; **Fellow:** Spinal Surgery, Case Western Res Univ Hosp 1992; **Fac Appt:** Prof OrS, Emory Univ

Cuckler, John MD [OrS] - **Spec Exp:** Hip Replacement & Revision; Knee Replacement & Revision; Knee Cartilage Transplant; Minimally Invasive Surgery; **Hospital:** Brookwood Med Ctr; **Address:** Alabama Spine & Joint Center, 513 Brookwood Blvd, Ste 375, Birmingham, AL 35209; **Phone:** 205-802-4577; **Board Cert:** Orthopaedic Surgery 1999; **Med School:** NYU Sch Med 1975; **Resid:** Orthopaedic Surgery, Hosp Univ Penn 1980; **Fellow:** Orthopaedic Surgery, Hosp Univ Penn; **Fac Appt:** Prof OrS, Univ Ala

Orthopaedic Surgery

Curl, Walton W MD [OrS] - **Spec Exp:** Sports Medicine; **Hospital:** Wake Forest Univ Baptist Med Ctr (page 73); **Address:** Wake Forest Med Ctr, Comp Rehab, 131 Miller St, Winston-Salem, NC 27103; **Phone:** 336-716-8091; **Board Cert:** Orthopaedic Surgery 1980; **Med School:** Duke Univ 1974; **Resid:** Orthopaedic Surgery, Letterman Army Med Ctr 1978; **Fellow:** Sports Medicine, Keller Army Hosp 1979; **Fac Appt:** Prof OrS, Wake Forest Univ

DeOrio, James K MD [OrS] - **Spec Exp:** Ankle Replacement & Revision; Foot & Ankle Surgery; Foot Deformities; **Hospital:** Duke Univ Med Ctr; **Address:** Duke Univ Medical Ctr, Box 3332, Durham, NC 27710; **Phone:** 919-684-6166; **Board Cert:** Orthopaedic Surgery 1983; **Med School:** Geo Wash Univ 1977; **Resid:** Orthopaedic Surgery, Mayo Clinic 1982; **Fellow:** Orthopaedic Surgery, Chur Hosp 1983

Eismont, Frank MD [OrS] - **Spec Exp:** Spinal Surgery; **Hospital:** Jackson Meml Hosp; **Address:** Univ Miami Sch Med, Dept Orth Surg, PO Box 016960, D-27, Miami, FL 33101; **Phone:** 305-243-3000; **Board Cert:** Orthopaedic Surgery 1994; **Med School:** Univ Rochester 1973; **Resid:** Orthopaedic Surgery, Case Western Res Univ Hosp 1978; **Fellow:** Spinal Surgery, Case Western Res Univ Hosp 1979; Spinal Surgery, PA Hosp 1980; **Fac Appt:** Prof OrS, Univ Miami Sch Med

Garrett, William MD [OrS] - **Spec Exp:** Sports Medicine; Shoulder & Knee Surgery; Shoulder & Knee Reconstruction; **Hospital:** Duke Univ Med Ctr; **Address:** Duke Univ Med Ctr, Box 3338, Durham, NC 27710; **Phone:** 919-684-5678; **Board Cert:** Orthopaedic Surgery 1985; **Med School:** Duke Univ 1976; **Resid:** Orthopaedic Surgery, Duke Univ Med Ctr 1982; **Fac Appt:** Prof OrS, Duke Univ

Goldner, Richard MD [OrS] - **Spec Exp:** Upper Extremity Surgery; Hand Surgery; **Hospital:** Duke Univ Med Ctr; **Address:** DUMC, Box 3480, Durham, NC 27710; **Phone:** 919-613-7797; **Board Cert:** Orthopaedic Surgery 1982; Hand Surgery 2000; **Med School:** Duke Univ 1974; **Resid:** Orthopaedic Surgery, Univ Virginia 1980; Surgery, Duke Univ Med Ctr 1976; **Fellow:** Hand Surgery, Duke Univ Med Ctr 1981; **Fac Appt:** Assoc Prof OrS, Duke Univ

Johnson, Darren L MD [OrS] - **Spec Exp:** Knee Injuries; Sports Medicine; Knee Ligament Reconstruction; Arthroscopic Surgery; **Hospital:** Univ of Kentucky Chandler Hosp; **Address:** Univ Kentucky, Dept Orthopaedic Surgery, 740 S Limestone, Ste K-401, Lexington, KY 40536-0284; **Phone:** 859-257-4969; **Board Cert:** Orthopaedic Surgery 2006; **Med School:** UCLA 1987; **Resid:** Orthopaedic Surgery, LAC-USC Med Ctr 1992; **Fellow:** Sports Medicine, Univ Pittsburgh 1993; **Fac Appt:** Assoc Prof OrS, Univ KY Coll Med

Karas, Spero G MD [OrS] - **Spec Exp:** Sports Medicine; Shoulder Reconstruction; Elbow Reconstruction; Knee Reconstruction; **Hospital:** Emory Univ Hosp; **Address:** Emory Healthcare Sports Medicine, 59 Executive Park S, Ste 1000, Atlanta, GA 30329; **Phone:** 404-778-3350; **Board Cert:** Orthopaedic Surgery 2002; **Med School:** Indiana Univ 1993; **Resid:** Orthopaedic Surgery, Duke Univ Med Ctr 1999; **Fellow:** Orthopaedic Surgery, Steadman Hawkins Clinic 2000; **Fac Appt:** Assoc Prof OrS, Emory Univ

Kneisl, Jeffrey S MD [OrS] - **Spec Exp:** Bone Cancer; Musculoskeletal Tumors; **Hospital:** Carolinas Med Ctr; **Address:** Carolinas Med Ctr, 1001 Blythe Blvd, Ste 602, Charlotte, NC 28203; **Phone:** 704-355-5982; **Board Cert:** Orthopaedic Surgery 2000; **Med School:** Northwestern Univ 1980; **Resid:** Orthopaedic Surgery, Northwestern Univ 1987; **Fellow:** Orthopaedic Oncology, Univ Chicago 1990

Nunley, James MD [OrS] - **Spec Exp:** Arthritis; Ankle Replacement & Revision; Foot & Ankle Surgery; Hand & Wrist Surgery; **Hospital:** Duke Univ Med Ctr; **Address:** Duke Hospital S, Box 3670, Durham, NC 27710-0001; **Phone:** 919-613-7797; **Board Cert:** Orthopaedic Surgery 1981; **Med School:** Tulane Univ 1973; **Resid:** Orthopaedic Surgery, Duke Univ Med Ctr 1979; **Fellow:** Hand Surgery, Duke Univ Med Ctr 1980; **Fac Appt:** Prof OrS, Duke Univ

Paulos, Leon MD [OrS] - **Spec Exp:** Sports Medicine; Shoulder & Knee Surgery; **Hospital:** Gulf Breeze Hosp, Baptist Hosp - Pensacola; **Address:** 1040 Gulf Breeze Pkwy, Ste 203, Gulf Breeze, FL 32561; **Phone:** 850-817-8761; **Board Cert:** Orthopaedic Surgery 1980; **Med School:** Univ Utah 1973; **Resid:** Orthopaedic Surgery, Univ Utah Sch Med 1978; **Fellow:** Sports Medicine, Atlanta Sports Med Fdn 1978; Sports Medicine, Univ Hosp 1979

Pettrone, Frank A MD [OrS] - **Spec Exp:** Sports Medicine; Shoulder & Knee Surgery; **Hospital:** Virginia Hosp Ctr - Arlington; **Address:** Commonwealth Ortho & Rehabilitation, 1635 N George Mason Drive, Ste 310, Arlington, VA 22205-3616; **Phone:** 703-525-6100; **Board Cert:** Orthopaedic Surgery 1975; **Med School:** Georgetown Univ 1969; **Resid:** Orthopaedic Surgery, Georgetown Hosp 1974; **Fac Appt:** Clin Prof OrS, Georgetown Univ

Poehling, Gary G MD [OrS] - **Spec Exp:** Hand Surgery; Arthroscopic Surgery; Sports Medicine; **Hospital:** Wake Forest Univ Baptist Med Ctr (page 73); **Address:** 131 Miller St, Winston-Salem, NC 27103; **Phone:** 336-716-8091; **Board Cert:** Orthopaedic Surgery 1977; **Med School:** Marquette Sch Med 1968; **Resid:** Surgery, Duke Univ Med Ctr 1970; Orthopaedic Surgery, Duke Univ Med Ctr 1976; **Fac Appt:** Prof OrS, Wake Forest Univ

Richardson, William J MD [OrS] - **Spec Exp:** Spinal Surgery; Spinal Deformity; Spinal Disc Replacement; Spinal Trauma; **Hospital:** Duke Univ Med Ctr; **Address:** DUMC, PO Box 3077, Durham, NC 27710; **Phone:** 919-613-7797; **Board Cert:** Orthopaedic Surgery 2000; **Med School:** Eastern VA Med Sch 1979; **Resid:** Orthopaedic Surgery, Duke Univ Med Ctr 1986; **Fellow:** Spinal Surgery, Totonto General Hosp 1987

Scarborough, Mark MD [OrS] - **Spec Exp:** Bone Tumors; Sarcoma; **Hospital:** Shands at Univ of FL; **Address:** Shands Healthcare Univ FL, 3450 Hull Rd, Gainesville, FL 32607; **Phone:** 352-273-7000; **Board Cert:** Orthopaedic Surgery 2003; **Med School:** Univ Fla Coll Med 1985; **Resid:** Orthopaedic Surgery, Univ Texas Med Ctr 1990; **Fellow:** Orthopaedic Surgery, Mass Genl Hosp 1991; **Fac Appt:** Prof OrS, Univ Fla Coll Med

Schwartz, Herbert S MD [OrS] - **Spec Exp:** Bone Tumors-Metastatic; Bone Tumors; Pelvic Surgery-Complex; **Hospital:** Vanderbilt Univ Med Ctr, Baptist Hosp - Nashville; **Address:** Vanderbilt Med Ctr Ortho Institute, South Tower, rm 4200, Medical Ctr East, Nashville, TN 37232-8774; **Phone:** 615-343-8612; **Board Cert:** Orthopaedic Surgery 2007; **Med School:** Univ Chicago-Pritzker Sch Med 1981; **Resid:** Orthopaedic Surgery, Univ Chicago Hosps 1986; **Fellow:** Orthopaedic Oncology, Mayo Clinic 1987; **Fac Appt:** Prof OrS, Vanderbilt Univ

Scully, Sean P MD [OrS] - **Spec Exp:** Bone Cancer; Sarcoma; Musculoskeletal Tumors; Knee Replacement & Revision; **Hospital:** Univ of Miami Hosp & Clins/Sylvester Comp Canc Ctr, Jackson Meml Hosp; **Address:** Univ Miami Hospital, 1400 NW 12th Ave, Ste 4035, Miami, FL 33136; **Phone:** 305-325-4683; **Board Cert:** Orthopaedic Surgery 2006; **Med School:** Univ Rochester 1980; **Resid:** Orthopaedic Surgery, Duke Univ Med Ctr 1985; **Fellow:** Orthopaedic Oncology, Mass General Hosp 1987; Research, Natl Inst Health 1988; **Fac Appt:** Prof OrS, Univ Miami Sch Med

Siegel, Herrick J MD [OrS] - **Spec Exp:** Bone Cancer; Sarcoma; Bone Tumors-Benign; Soft Tissue Tumors-Benign; **Hospital:** Univ of Ala Hosp at Birmingham, UAB Highlands Hosp; **Address:** UAB Kirklin Clinic, 2000 6th Ave S, Birmingham, AL 35294; **Phone:** 205-975-0415; **Board Cert:** Orthopaedic Surgery 2005; **Med School:** NYU Sch Med 1995; **Resid:** Orthopaedic Surgery, USC 2000; **Fellow:** Orthopaedic Oncology, Mayo Clinic 2002; **Fac Appt:** Assoc Prof OrS, Univ Ala

Spengler, Dan M MD [OrS] - **Spec Exp:** Spinal Surgery; **Hospital:** Vanderbilt Univ Med Ctr, Saint Thomas Hosp - Nashville; **Address:** Vanderbilt Orthopedic Inst, Medical Ctr E, S Tower Rm#4200, Nashville, TN 37232-8774; **Phone:** 615-343-6364; **Board Cert:** Orthopaedic Surgery 1988; **Med School:** Univ Mich Med Sch 1966; **Resid:** Orthopaedic Surgery, Univ Mich Med Ctr 1968; Orthopaedic Surgery, Univ Mich Med Ctr 1973; **Fellow:** Orthopaedic Surgery, Case West Res Hosps 1974; **Fac Appt:** Prof OrS, Vanderbilt Univ

Spindler, Kurt P MD [OrS] - **Spec Exp:** Sports Medicine; Arthroscopic Surgery; **Hospital:** Vanderbilt Univ Med Ctr; **Address:** Vanderbilt Orthopaedic Inst, 1215 21st Ave S, Ste 3200, Med Ctr East, Nashville, TN 37232-8828; **Phone:** 615-322-7878; **Board Cert:** Orthopaedic Surgery 2004; **Med School:** Univ Pennsylvania 1985; **Resid:** Orthopaedic Surgery, Hosp Univ Penn 1990; **Fellow:** Sports Medicine, Cleveland Clinic Fdn 1991; **Fac Appt:** Prof OrS, Vanderbilt Univ

Taft, Timothy N MD [OrS] - **Spec Exp:** Sports Medicine; Knee Injuries/ACL; Shoulder Surgery; **Hospital:** Univ NC Hosps; **Address:** UNC Orthopaedics, CB # 7055, Bioinformatics Bldg, Chapel Hill, NC 27599-7055; **Phone:** 919-962-6637; **Board Cert:** Orthopaedic Surgery 1976; **Med School:** Univ MO-Columbia Sch Med 1969; **Resid:** Orthopaedic Surgery, UNC Hosps 1974; Orthopaedic Surgery, N Carolina Ortho Hosp 1972; **Fac Appt:** Prof OrS, Univ NC Sch Med

Uribe, John MD [OrS] - **Spec Exp:** Shoulder & Elbow Surgery; Arthroscopic Surgery; Sports Medicine; **Hospital:** Doctors' Hosp, Jackson Meml Hosp; **Address:** 1150 Campo Sano Ave, Ste 200, Coral Gables, FL 33146-6960; **Phone:** 305-669-3320; **Board Cert:** Orthopaedic Surgery 1982; **Med School:** Univ NC Sch Med 1976; **Resid:** Orthopaedic Surgery, Jackson Memorial Hosp 1981; **Fellow:** Sports Medicine, Hughston Sports Med Hosp 1985; **Fac Appt:** Assoc Prof OrS, Univ Miami Sch Med

Walling, Arthur K MD [OrS] - **Spec Exp:** Bone Tumors; Soft Tissue Tumors; Foot & Ankle Surgery; **Hospital:** Tampa Genl Hosp; **Address:** Florida Orthopaedic Inst, 13020 Telecom Pkwy N, Tampa, FL 33637; **Phone:** 813-978-9700; **Board Cert:** Orthopaedic Surgery 1982; **Med School:** Creighton Univ 1976; **Resid:** Orthopaedic Surgery, Univ South Florida Affil Hosps 1980; **Fellow:** Surgical Oncology, Univ Florida 1981; **Fac Appt:** Assoc Clin Prof OrS, Univ S Fla Coll Med

Ward, William G MD [OrS] - **Spec Exp:** Bone Tumors; Soft Tissue Tumors; Reconstructive Surgery; **Hospital:** Wake Forest Univ Baptist Med Ctr (page 73), Forsyth Med Ctr; **Address:** Wake Forest Med Ctr, Comprehensive Rehab, Medical Center Blvd, Winston-Salem, NC 27157; **Phone:** 336-716-8200; **Board Cert:** Orthopaedic Surgery 2004; **Med School:** Duke Univ 1975; **Resid:** Surgery, Duke Univ Med Ctr 1985; Orthopaedic Surgery, Duke Univ Med Ctr 1989; **Fellow:** Sports Medicine, Cleveland Clinic 1990; Orthopaedic Oncology, UCLA Med Ctr 1991; **Fac Appt:** Prof OrS, Wake Forest Univ

Webb, Lawrence MD [OrS] - **Spec Exp:** Trauma; Pelvic & Acetabular Fractures; Fractures-Complex & Non Union; **Hospital:** Wake Forest Univ Baptist Med Ctr (page 73); **Address:** Wake Forest Med Ctr, Dept of Orth Surgery, 1 Med Ctr Blvd, Winston-Salem, NC 27157-1070; **Phone:** 336-716-3606; **Board Cert:** Orthopaedic Surgery 2005; **Med School:** Temple Univ 1978; **Resid:** Orthopaedic Surgery, Bowman Gray Affil Hosp 1983; **Fellow:** Trauma, Harborview Med Ctr 1984; **Fac Appt:** Prof OrS, Wake Forest Univ

Weiner, Richard L MD [OrS] - **Spec Exp:** Knee Surgery; Shoulder Surgery; Hip Surgery; **Hospital:** St Mary's Med Ctr - W Palm Bch, Palm Beach Gardens Med Ctr; **Address:** 733 US Highway 1, North Palm Beach, FL 33408-4508; **Phone:** 561-840-1090; **Board Cert:** Orthopaedic Surgery 2004; **Med School:** Univ Pennsylvania 1986; **Resid:** Orthopaedic Surgery, UMDNJ-Univ Hosp 1991

Midwest

An, Howard MD [OrS] - **Spec Exp:** Spinal Surgery; Scoliosis; Spinal Microdiscectomy; **Hospital:** Rush Univ Med Ctr; **Address:** 1725 W Harrison, Ste 1063, Chicago, IL 60612; **Phone:** 312-243-4244; **Board Cert:** Orthopaedic Surgery 2002; **Med School:** Med Coll OH 1982; **Resid:** Orthopaedic Surgery, Med College Ohio Hosps 1988; **Fellow:** Spinal Surgery, Jefferson Med College 1989; **Fac Appt:** Prof OrS, Rush Med Coll

Bach Jr, Bernard R MD [OrS] - **Spec Exp:** Sports Medicine; Knee Surgery; Knee Injuries/ACL; **Hospital:** Rush Univ Med Ctr; **Address:** Midwest Orthopaedics at Rush, 1725 W Harrison St, Ste 1063, Chicago, IL 60612; **Phone:** 312-243-4244; **Board Cert:** Orthopaedic Surgery 2000; **Med School:** Univ Cincinnati 1979; **Resid:** Surgery, New Eng Deaconess Hosp 1981; Orthopaedic Surgery, Mass Genl Hosp 1985; **Fellow:** Sports Medicine, Hosp Special Surgery 1986; **Fac Appt:** Prof OrS, Rush Med Coll

Bergfeld, John A MD [OrS] - **Spec Exp:** Sports Medicine; Knee Ligament Reconstruction; Cartilage Damage; Musculoskeletal Disorders; **Hospital:** Cleveland Clin Fdn (page 56); **Address:** The Cleveland Clinic, 9500 Euclid Ave, E21, Cleveland, OH 44195-5027; **Phone:** 216-444-2618; **Board Cert:** Orthopaedic Surgery 1972; **Med School:** Temple Univ 1964; **Resid:** Surgery, Cleveland Clinic 1966; Orthopaedic Surgery, Cleveland Clinic 1970

Biermann, J Sybil MD [OrS] - **Spec Exp:** Sarcoma; Bone Cancer; Multiple Myeloma; Limb Sparing Surgery; **Hospital:** Univ Michigan Hlth Sys; **Address:** Univ Michigan Cancer Ctr, 1500 E Medical Ctr Drive, 7304 CCGC, Ann Arbor, MI 48109-5946; **Phone:** 734-647-8902; **Board Cert:** Orthopaedic Surgery 2006; **Med School:** Stanford Univ 1987; **Resid:** Orthopaedic Surgery, Univ Iowa Hosp 1992; **Fellow:** Orthopaedic Oncology, Univ Chicago Hosps 1993; **Fac Appt:** Assoc Prof OrS, Univ Mich Med Sch

Blaha, John D MD [OrS] - **Spec Exp:** Hip & Knee Replacement; **Hospital:** Univ Michigan Hlth Sys; **Address:** Univ Michigan, Dept Orthopaedic Surg, 1500 E Medical Ctr Dr, 2912 Taubman, Ann Arbor, MI 48109; **Phone:** 734-647-9961; **Board Cert:** Orthopaedic Surgery 1979; **Med School:** Univ Mich Med Sch 1973; **Resid:** Surgery, Univ Mich Hosp 1975; Orthopaedic Surgery, Univ Mich Hosp 1978; **Fellow:** Joint Replacement Surgery, Univ London 1980; **Fac Appt:** Prof OrS, Univ Mich Med Sch

Bohlman, Henry H MD [OrS] - **Spec Exp:** Spinal Surgery-Cervical; **Hospital:** Univ Hosps Case Med Ctr; **Address:** Univ Hosps of Cleveland, Dept Ortho Surg, 11100 Euclid Ave, Cleveland, OH 44106-1736; **Phone:** 216-844-1025; **Board Cert:** Orthopaedic Surgery 1972; **Med School:** Univ MD Sch Med 1964; **Resid:** Surgery, Univ Hosp 1966; Orthopaedic Surgery, Johns Hopkins Hosp 1970; **Fellow:** Spinal Surgery, Johns Hopkins Hosp 1968; **Fac Appt:** Prof OrS, Case West Res Univ

Bridwell, Keith MD [OrS] - **Spec Exp:** Spinal Deformity; Scoliosis; Spinal Surgery; **Hospital:** Barnes-Jewish Hosp, St Louis Chldns Hosp; **Address:** 1 Barnes Jewish Hosp Plaza, Ste 11300, West Pav, Dept Ortho Surg, Campus Box 8233, St Louis, MO 63110; **Phone:** 314-747-2500; **Board Cert:** Orthopaedic Surgery 1985; **Med School:** Washington Univ, St Louis 1977; **Resid:** Orthopaedic Surgery, Barnes Hosp-Wash Univ 1981; **Fellow:** Spinal Surgery, Rush Presby-St Lukes Med Ctr 1982; **Fac Appt:** Prof OrS, Washington Univ, St Louis

Buckwalter, Joseph MD [OrS] - **Spec Exp:** Bone Cancer; Bone Tumors-Metastatic; Fractures-Complex; **Hospital:** Univ Iowa Hosp & Clinics; **Address:** Univ Iowa Hosps, Dept Orthopaedics, 200 Hawkins Drive, Iowa City, IA 52242; **Phone:** 319-356-2595; **Board Cert:** Orthopaedic Surgery 1980; **Med School:** Univ Iowa Coll Med 1974; **Resid:** Orthopaedic Surgery, Iowa Hosp 1979; **Fac Appt:** Prof OrS, Univ Iowa Coll Med

Orthopaedic Surgery

Callaghan, John J MD [OrS] - **Spec Exp:** Hip & Knee Replacement; Sports Medicine; **Hospital:** Univ Iowa Hosp & Clinics; **Address:** Univ Iowa, Dept Orthopaedics, 200 Hawkins Drive, Iowa City, IA 52242; **Phone:** 319-356-3110; **Board Cert:** Orthopaedic Surgery 2000; **Med School:** Loyola Univ-Stritch Sch Med 1978; **Resid:** Orthopaedic Surgery, Univ Iowa Hosp 1983; **Fellow:** Orthopaedic Surgery, Hosp Special Surg 1984; **Fac Appt:** Prof OrS, Univ Iowa Coll Med

Cheng, Edward MD [OrS] - **Spec Exp:** Bone & Soft Tissue Tumors; **Hospital:** Univ Minn Med Ctr, Fairview - Univ Campus; **Address:** Dept Orthopedic Surgery, Univ Minnesota, 2450 Riverside Ave S, Ste R-200, Minneapolis, MN 55455; **Phone:** 612-273-1177; **Board Cert:** Orthopaedic Surgery 2003; **Med School:** Northwestern Univ 1983; **Resid:** Surgery, Northwestern Univ 1985; Orthopaedic Surgery, Beth Israel Hosp 1989; **Fellow:** Surgical Oncology, Mass Genl Hosp 1990; **Fac Appt:** Prof OrS, Univ Minn

Clohisy, Denis MD [OrS] - **Spec Exp:** Bone Cancer; **Hospital:** Univ Minn Med Ctr, Fairview - Univ Campus; **Address:** Dept Orthopaedic Surgery, 2450 Riverside Ave S, Ste R200, Minneapolis, MN 55454; **Phone:** 612-273-1177; **Board Cert:** Orthopaedic Surgery 2004; **Med School:** Northwestern Univ 1983; **Resid:** Orthopaedic Surgery, Univ Minn 1990; **Fellow:** Pathology, Wash Univ Med Ctr 1987; Musculoskeletal Oncology, Mass Genl Hosp/Harvard 1991; **Fac Appt:** Prof OrS, Univ Minn

Ebraheim, Nabil A MD [OrS] - **Spec Exp:** Trauma; Fractures-Complex; **Hospital:** Univ of Toledo Med Ctr; **Address:** Univ of Toledo Med Ctr, Orthopaedics, 3065 Arlington Ave, MS 1094, Toledo, OH 43614; **Phone:** 419-383-4020; **Board Cert:** Orthopaedic Surgery 2008; **Med School:** Egypt 1975; **Resid:** Surgery, St Clare's Hosp 1980; Orthopaedic Surgery, SUNY-Downstate Med Ctr 1983; **Fellow:** Trauma, Univ Maryland Hosps 1984; Orthopaedic Surgery, Hanover Trauma Ctr 1985; **Fac Appt:** Prof OrS, Univ Toledo, Med Univ OH

Gitelis, Steven MD [OrS] - **Spec Exp:** Bone Cancer; Soft Tissue Tumors; Limb Sparing Surgery; Hip Replacement; **Hospital:** Rush Univ Med Ctr; **Address:** 1725 W Harrison St, Ste 440, Chicago, IL 60612-3828; **Phone:** 312-563-2600; **Board Cert:** Orthopaedic Surgery 1982; **Med School:** Rush Med Coll 1975; **Resid:** Orthopaedic Surgery, Rush Presby-St Lukes Med Ctr 1980; **Fellow:** Orthopaedic Oncology, Mayo Clinic; **Fac Appt:** Prof OrS, Rush Med Coll

Goitz, Henry MD [OrS] - **Spec Exp:** Sports Medicine; Arthroscopic Surgery; **Hospital:** Henry Ford Hosp; **Address:** Henry Ford Lakeside Med Ctr, 14500 Hall Rd, Sterling Heights, MI 48313; **Phone:** 313-972-4066; **Board Cert:** Orthopaedic Surgery 2006; **Med School:** UMDNJ-Rutgers Med Sch 1985; **Resid:** Surgery, Univ Virginia 1987; Orthopaedic Surgery, Univ Virginia 1991; **Fellow:** Sports Medicine & Hand Surgery, Univ Virginia 1992; Sports Medicine, American Sports Med Inst 1993

Goldberg, Victor M MD [OrS] - **Spec Exp:** Hip & Knee Replacement; Arthritis; **Hospital:** Univ Hosps Case Med Ctr; **Address:** Univ Hosps of Cleveland, Dept Ortho Surg, 11100 Euclid Ave, Cleveland, OH 44106; **Phone:** 216-844-3044; **Board Cert:** Orthopaedic Surgery 1992; **Med School:** SUNY Downstate 1964; **Resid:** Surgery, Univ Hosp 1966; Orthopaedic Surgery, Hosp Special Surg 1971; **Fac Appt:** Prof OrS, Case West Res Univ

Goldstein, Wayne MD [OrS] - **Spec Exp:** Hip Replacement; Knee Replacement; **Hospital:** Adv Luth Genl Hosp; **Address:** 9000 Waukegan Rd, Ste 200, Morton Grove, IL 60053; **Phone:** 847-375-3000; **Board Cert:** Orthopaedic Surgery 1997; **Med School:** Univ IL Coll Med 1978; **Resid:** Orthopaedic Surgery, Univ Ilinois Med Ctr 1983; **Fellow:** Arthritis Surgery, Brigham & Women's Hosp 1984; **Fac Appt:** Assoc Clin Prof OrS, Univ Chicago-Pritzker Sch Med

Graf, Ben K MD [OrS] - **Spec Exp:** Sports Medicine; **Hospital:** Univ WI Hosp & Clins; **Address:** 600 Highland Ave, rm K4-735, Madison, WI 53792-3228; **Phone:** 608-263-8850; **Board Cert:** Orthopaedic Surgery 1998; **Med School:** Univ Wisc 1979; **Resid:** Orthopaedic Surgery, Univ Wisc Hosps 1984; **Fellow:** Sports Medicine, Long Beach Meml Hosp 1985; **Fac Appt:** Assoc Prof S, Univ Wisc

Grant, Richard E MD [OrS] - **Spec Exp:** Hip & Knee Replacement; Spinal Surgery-Low Back; Sickle Cell Disease-Hip Surgery; **Hospital:** Univ Hosps Case Med Ctr; **Address:** Univ Hosps Cleveland, Dept Ortho Surgery, 11100 Euclid Ave, Cleveland, OH 44106; **Phone:** 216-844-1118; **Board Cert:** Orthopaedic Surgery 2007; **Med School:** Howard Univ 1976; **Resid:** Orthopaedic Surgery, Wilford Hall Med Ctr-Lackland 1984; **Fellow:** Joint Arthroplasty, Ohio State Univ Hosp; Spinal Cord Injury Medicine, St Lukes/Baylor Univ; **Fac Appt:** Prof OrS, Howard Univ

Hensinger, Robert MD [OrS] - **Spec Exp:** Pediatric Orthopaedic Surgery; Spinal Surgery-Pediatric; **Hospital:** Univ Michigan Hlth Sys; **Address:** Univ Michigan Med Ctr, Dept Ortho Surg, 2912 Taubman Ctr, 1500 E Medical Ctr Dr, Ann Arbor, MI 48109-0328; **Phone:** 734-936-5780; **Board Cert:** Orthopaedic Surgery 2007; **Med School:** Univ Mich Med Sch 1964; **Resid:** Orthopaedic Surgery, Univ Michigan 1966; Orthopaedic Surgery, Univ Michigan 1971; **Fellow:** Pediatric Orthopaedic Surgery, Al DuPont Inst 1972; **Fac Appt:** Prof OrS, Univ Mich Med Sch

Iannotti, Joseph MD/PhD [OrS] - **Spec Exp:** Shoulder Surgery; **Hospital:** Cleveland Clin Fdn (page 56); **Address:** Cleveland Clinic, Dept Orthopaedic Surg, 9500 Euclid Ave, Cleveland, OH 44195-5027; **Phone:** 216-445-5151; **Board Cert:** Orthopaedic Surgery 2007; **Med School:** Northwestern Univ 1979; **Resid:** Orthopaedic Surgery, Hosp Univ Penn 1984; **Fellow:** Orthopaedic Research, Hosp Univ Penn 1985; **Fac Appt:** Prof OrS, Cleveland Cl Coll Med/Case West Res

Joyce, Michael J MD [OrS] - **Spec Exp:** Bone & Soft Tissue Tumors; Fractures-Complex & Non Union; Musculoskeletal Tissue Banking; Pelvic & Acetabular Fractures; **Hospital:** Cleveland Clin Fdn (page 56); **Address:** Cleveland Clinic, Dept Orthopaedic Surgery, 9500 Euclid Ave, Desk A41, Cleveland, OH 44195-0001; **Phone:** 216-444-4282; **Board Cert:** Orthopaedic Surgery 1985; **Med School:** Univ Louisville Sch Med 1976; **Resid:** Surgery, Johns Hopkins Hosp 1978; Orthopaedic Surgery, Harvard Combined Program 1981; **Fellow:** Orthopaedic Oncology, Mass General Hosp 1982; Trauma, Univ Toronto-Sunnybrook Hosp 1983; **Fac Appt:** Assoc Clin Prof OrS, Case West Res Univ

Lenke, Lawrence G MD [OrS] - **Spec Exp:** Spinal Surgery; Spinal Deformity; Scoliosis; **Hospital:** Barnes-Jewish Hosp, St Louis Chldns Hosp; **Address:** Washington Univ Sch Med, 660 S Euclid Ave, Campus Box 8233, St Louis, MO 63110; **Phone:** 314-747-2500; **Board Cert:** Orthopaedic Surgery 2005; **Med School:** Northwestern Univ 1986; **Resid:** Orthopaedic Surgery, Barnes-Jewish Hosp 1990; **Fellow:** Spinal Surgery, Barnes-Jewish Hosp 1992; **Fac Appt:** Prof OrS, Washington Univ, St Louis

Lock, Terrence Ralph MD [OrS] - **Spec Exp:** Sports Medicine; Arthroscopic Surgery; Shoulder & Knee Reconstruction; **Hospital:** Henry Ford Hosp, Bon Secours Cottage Hosp; **Address:** Henry Ford Hosp, Ctr for Athletic Med, 625 2nd St, Detroit, MI 48202; **Phone:** 313-972-4085; **Board Cert:** Orthopaedic Surgery 2002; **Med School:** Wayne State Univ 1983; **Resid:** Orthopaedic Surgery, Wayne St Univ Sch Med 1988; **Fellow:** Sports Medicine, Mass Genl Hosp 1989

Manoli II, Arthur MD [OrS] - **Spec Exp:** Foot & Ankle Surgery; Reconstructive Surgery; **Hospital:** St Joseph Mercy Oakland Hosp; **Address:** 44555 Woodward Ave, Ste 503, Pontiac, MI 48341; **Phone:** 248-858-6773; **Board Cert:** Orthopaedic Surgery 2007; **Med School:** Univ Mich Med Sch 1970; **Resid:** Surgery, Oakwood Hosp 1972; Orthopaedic Surgery, Wayne St Univ Affil Hosps 1975; **Fellow:** Ankle and Foot Surgery, Univ Wash/Vanderbilt Univ 1990

Orthopaedic Surgery

McDonald, Douglas J MD [OrS] - **Spec Exp:** Bone & Soft Tissue Tumors; Ewing's Sarcoma; Bone Cancer; Hip & Knee Reconstruction; **Hospital:** Barnes-Jewish Hosp; **Address:** Ctr Advanced Med, Orthopaedic Surg Ctr, 4921 Parkview Pl Fl 6 - Ste A, Box 8605, St Louis, MO 63110; **Phone:** 314-747-2500; **Board Cert:** Orthopaedic Surgery 2001; **Med School:** Univ Minn 1982; **Resid:** Orthopaedic Surgery, Mayo Clinic 1987; **Fellow:** Orthopaedic Oncology, Mayo Clinic 1988; **Fac Appt:** Prof OrS, Washington Univ, St Louis

Mott, Michael P MD [OrS] - **Spec Exp:** Bone Tumors; Musculoskeletal Tumors; Pediatric Orthopaedic Surgery; **Hospital:** Henry Ford Hosp; **Address:** Henry Ford Hosp, Ctr for Athletc Med, 6525 2nd St Fl 2, Detroit, MI 48202; **Phone:** 313-972-4079; **Board Cert:** Orthopaedic Surgery 2007; **Med School:** Univ Mich Med Sch 1989; **Resid:** Orthopaedic Surgery, Wayne State Univ Sch Med 1994; **Fellow:** Musculoskeletal Oncology, Mass Genl Hosp 1995; Orthopaedic Oncology, Wayne State Univ Sch Med 1996; **Fac Appt:** Assoc Prof OrS, Wayne State Univ

Muschler, George F MD [OrS] - **Spec Exp:** Hip Replacement; Knee Replacement; Fractures-Non Union; Fractures-Complex; **Hospital:** Cleveland Clin Fdn (page 56); **Address:** Cleveland Clinic, Dept Orthopaedic Surg, 9500 Euclid Ave, Desk A41, Cleveland, OH 44195-0001; **Phone:** 216-444-5338; **Board Cert:** Orthopaedic Surgery 2001; **Med School:** Northwestern Univ 1981; **Resid:** Orthopaedic Surgery, Univ Texas SW Med Ctr 1986; **Fellow:** Metabolic Bone Research, Hosp Special Surgery 1988; Musculoskeletal Oncology, Meml Sloan Kettering Cancer Ctr 1988; **Fac Appt:** Prof OrS, Cleveland Cl Coll Med/Case West Res

Nuber, Gordon MD [OrS] - **Spec Exp:** Shoulder Reconstruction; Cartilage Damage; Elbow Surgery; **Hospital:** Northwestern Meml Hosp; **Address:** Northwestern Orthopaedic Institute, 680 N Lakeshore Dr, Ste 1028, Chicago, IL 60611-4451; **Phone:** 312-664-6848; **Board Cert:** Orthopaedic Surgery 2004; **Med School:** Wayne State Univ 1978; **Resid:** Orthopaedic Surgery, Northwestern Meml Hosp 1983; **Fellow:** Sports Medicine, Natl Hlth Inst 1984; **Fac Appt:** Clin Prof OrS, Northwestern Univ

O'Driscoll, Shawn MD/PhD [OrS] - **Spec Exp:** Sports Medicine; Shoulder Surgery; Elbow Surgery; Cartilage Damage; **Hospital:** Mayo Med Ctr & Clin - Rochester; **Address:** Mayo Clinic, Gonda 14, 200 1st St SW, Rochester, MN 55905; **Phone:** 507-538-1284; **Board Cert:** Orthopaedic Surgery 2003; Orthopaedic Sports Medicine 2007; **Med School:** Univ Toronto 1980; **Resid:** Orthopaedic Surgery, Univ Toronto; **Fellow:** Arthroscopic Surgery, Toronto Western Hosp; Elbow & Shoulder Surgery, Mayo Clinic; **Fac Appt:** Prof OrS, Mayo Med Sch

Parsons III, Theodore W MD [OrS] - **Spec Exp:** Bone & Soft Tissue Tumors; Pediatric Orthopaedic Surgery; **Hospital:** Henry Ford Hosp; **Address:** Henry Ford Hosp, Dept Orthopaedics, 2799 West Grand, Detroit, MI 48202; **Phone:** 313-972-4079; **Board Cert:** Orthopaedic Surgery 2005; **Med School:** Uniformed Srvs Univ, Bethesda 1986; **Resid:** Orthopaedic Surgery, Wilford Hall USAF Med Ctr 1991; **Fellow:** Pediatric Orthopaedic Surgery, Boston Chldn's Hosp 1992; Orthopaedic Oncology, Mass Genl Hosp 1992; **Fac Appt:** Prof OrS, Wayne State Univ

Peabody, Terrance MD [OrS] - **Spec Exp:** Soft Tissue Tumors; Bone Tumors; Pediatric Orthopaedic Cancers; **Hospital:** Univ of Chicago Hosps; **Address:** Univ Chicago Hospital, 5841 S Maryland Ave, MC 3079, Chicago, IL 60637-1463; **Phone:** 773-702-3442; **Board Cert:** Orthopaedic Surgery 2004; **Med School:** UC Irvine 1985; **Resid:** Orthopaedic Surgery, UC Irvine Med Ctr 1990; **Fellow:** Orthopaedic Oncology, Univ Chicago Hosps 1991; **Fac Appt:** Prof S, Univ Chicago-Pritzker Sch Med

Pinzur, Michael S MD [OrS] - **Spec Exp:** Diabetes-Amputation; Foot & Ankle Surgery; Amputation Surgery; **Hospital:** Loyola Univ Med Ctr; **Address:** Loyola Univ Med Ctr, Dept Orth Surg, 2160 S 1st Ave, Maywood, IL 60153-3304; **Phone:** 708-216-4993; **Board Cert:** Orthopaedic Surgery 1980; **Med School:** Rush Med Coll 1974; **Resid:** Orthopaedic Surgery, Northwestern Meml Hosp 1979; **Fac Appt:** Prof OrS, Loyola Univ-Stritch Sch Med

Polly, David W MD [OrS] - **Spec Exp:** Spinal Surgery; Amputation Surgery; Scoliosis; **Hospital:** Univ Minn Med Ctr, Fairview - Univ Campus; **Address:** Univ Minnesota, Orthopaedic Dept, 2450 Riverside Ave S, rm 200, Minneapolis, MN 55454; **Phone:** 612-273-9400; **Board Cert:** Orthopaedic Surgery 2005; **Med School:** Uniformed Srvs Univ, Bethesda 1985; **Resid:** Orthopaedic Surgery, Walter Reed Army Med Ctr 1991; **Fellow:** Spinal Surgery, Univ Minn 1992

Riew, K Daniel MD [OrS] - **Spec Exp:** Spinal Surgery-Cervical; Minimally Invasive Spinal Surgery; Spinal Microdiscectomy; **Hospital:** Barnes-Jewish Hosp; **Address:** Ctr for Advanced Med-Spine Ctr, 4921 Parkview Pl, CAM Bldg Fl 12 - Ste A, St Louis, MO 63110; **Phone:** 314-747-2500; **Board Cert:** Internal Medicine 1987; Orthopaedic Surgery 2008; **Med School:** Case West Res Univ 1984; **Resid:** Internal Medicine, NY Hosp-Cornell Med Ctr 1987; Orthopaedic Surgery, George Wash Univ Med Ctr 1994; **Fellow:** Spinal Surgery, Case West Res Univ 1995; **Fac Appt:** Prof OrS, Washington Univ, St Louis

Rosenberg, Aaron G MD [OrS] - **Spec Exp:** Hip & Knee Replacement; Hip & Knee Reconstruction; **Hospital:** Rush Univ Med Ctr; **Address:** 1725 W Harrison St, Ste 1063, Chicago, IL 60612-3828; **Phone:** 312-432-2340; **Board Cert:** Orthopaedic Surgery 1997; **Med School:** Albany Med Coll 1978; **Resid:** Orthopaedic Surgery, Rush Presby-St Lukes Med Ctr 1983; **Fellow:** Arthritis Surgery, Mass Genl Hosp 1984; **Fac Appt:** Prof OrS, Rush Med Coll

Schafer, Michael F MD [OrS] - **Spec Exp:** Sports Medicine; Spinal Surgery; Scoliosis; **Hospital:** Northwestern Meml Hosp, Children's Mem Hosp; **Address:** 675 N St Clair Fl 17 - Ste 100, Galter Pavillion, Chicago, IL 60611-5968; **Phone:** 312-695-6800; **Board Cert:** Orthopaedic Surgery 1983; **Med School:** Univ Iowa Coll Med 1967; **Resid:** Orthopaedic Surgery, Northwestern Univ Hosp 1972; **Fellow:** Spinal Surgery, Natl Fdn Traveling Fellowship 1973; **Fac Appt:** Prof OrS, Northwestern Univ

Shelbourne, K Donald MD [OrS] - **Spec Exp:** Knee Surgery; Arthroscopic Surgery; Knee Rehabilitation (Non-Surgical); Knee Ligament Reconstruction; **Hospital:** Methodist Hosp - Indianapolis; **Address:** 1815 N Capitol Ave, Ste 600, Indianapolis, IN 46202-1288; **Phone:** 317-924-8636; **Board Cert:** Orthopaedic Surgery 1984; **Med School:** Indiana Univ 1976; **Resid:** Orthopaedic Surgery, Indiana Univ Hosp 1981; **Fellow:** Sports Medicine, Univ Wisconsin 1982; **Fac Appt:** Assoc Clin Prof OrS, Indiana Univ

Simon, Michael MD [OrS] - **Spec Exp:** Bone Tumors; Soft Tissue Tumors; Pediatric Orthopaedic Cancers; **Hospital:** Univ of Chicago Hosps; **Address:** 5841 S Maryland Ave, MC 3079, Univ Chicago, Chicago, IL 60637; **Phone:** 773-702-6144; **Board Cert:** Orthopaedic Surgery 1992; **Med School:** Univ Mich Med Sch 1967; **Resid:** Surgery, Univ Mich Med Ctr 1969; Orthopaedic Surgery, Univ Mich Med Ctr 1974; **Fellow:** Orthopaedic Oncology, Shands/Univ Fla 1975; **Fac Appt:** Prof S, Univ Chicago-Pritzker Sch Med

Stulberg, S David MD [OrS] - **Spec Exp:** Hip & Knee Replacement; **Hospital:** Northwestern Meml Hosp; **Address:** 680 N Lake Shore Drive, Ste 1028, Chicago, IL 60611; **Phone:** 312-664-6848; **Board Cert:** Orthopaedic Surgery 1977; **Med School:** Univ Mich Med Sch 1969; **Resid:** Orthopaedic Surgery, Mass General Hosp 1974; **Fellow:** Research, Toronto Hosp Sick Chldn 1976; **Fac Appt:** Prof OrS, Northwestern Univ

Swiontkowski, Marc F MD [OrS] - **Spec Exp:** Osteomyelitis; Fractures-Non Union; Trauma; Bone Infections; **Hospital:** Univ Minn Med Ctr, Fairview - Univ Campus; **Address:** Univ Minnesota, Orthopaedic Dept, 2450 Riverside Ave S, rm 102, Minneapolis, MN 55454; **Phone:** 612-273-9400; **Board Cert:** Orthopaedic Surgery 2008; **Med School:** USC Sch Med 1979; **Resid:** Orthopaedic Surgery, Univ Washington Med Ctr 1984; **Fac Appt:** Prof OrS, Univ Minn

Orthopaedic Surgery

Weinstein, Stuart L MD [OrS] - **Spec Exp:** Scoliosis; Hip Disorders & Dysplasia; Hip Disorders-Pediatric; Spinal Deformity; **Hospital:** Univ Iowa Hosp & Clinics; **Address:** Univ Iowa, Dept Orthopaedics, 200 Hawkins Drive, Iowa City, IA 52242-1009; **Phone:** 319-356-1872; **Board Cert:** Orthopaedic Surgery 2007; **Med School:** Univ Iowa Coll Med 1972; **Resid:** Orthopaedic Surgery, Univ Iowa Hosps 1976; **Fac Appt:** Prof OrS, Univ Iowa Coll Med

Wixson, Richard L MD [OrS] - **Spec Exp:** Hip & Knee Replacement; **Hospital:** Northwestern Meml Hosp; **Address:** 680 N Lake Shore Drive Fl 10 - rm 1028, Chicago, IL 60611; **Phone:** 312-664-6848; **Board Cert:** Orthopaedic Surgery 1979; **Med School:** Univ Wisc 1972; **Resid:** Orthopaedic Surgery, Henry Ford Hosp 1977; Orthopaedic Surgery, New Eng Baptist Hosp 1979; **Fellow:** Orthopaedic Surgery, Mass Genl Hosp 1978; **Fac Appt:** Clin Prof OrS, Northwestern Univ

Yamaguchi, Ken MD [OrS] - **Spec Exp:** Shoulder Surgery; Elbow Surgery; Rotator Cuff Surgery; **Hospital:** Barnes-Jewish Hosp; **Address:** One Barnes Hosp Plaza, Dept Orthopaedic Surg, 11300 West Pavilion, St Louis, MO 63110-1036; **Phone:** 314-747-2534; **Board Cert:** Orthopaedic Surgery 1997; **Med School:** Geo Wash Univ 1989; **Resid:** Orthopaedic Surgery, George Wash Univ Med Ctr 1994; **Fellow:** Shoulder Surgery, Columbia Presby Med Ctr 1995; **Fac Appt:** Prof OrS, Washington Univ, St Louis

Yasko, Alan MD [OrS] - **Spec Exp:** Pediatric Orthopaedic Surgery; Pediatric Orthopaedic Cancers; Sarcoma; **Hospital:** Northwestern Meml Hosp, Children's Mem Hosp; **Address:** Dept Orthopaedics, 676 N St Clair St, Ste 1350, Chicago, IL 60611; **Phone:** 312-926-4444; **Board Cert:** Orthopaedic Surgery 2004; **Med School:** Northwestern Univ 1984; **Resid:** Orthopaedic Surgery, Case Western 1989; **Fellow:** Orthopaedic Oncology, Meml Sloan Kettering 1991; Metabolic Diseases, Hosp for Special Surgery 1991; **Fac Appt:** Prof S, Northwestern Univ-Feinberg Sch Med

Zdeblick, Thomas MD [OrS] - **Spec Exp:** Spinal Surgery; **Hospital:** Univ WI Hosp & Clins; **Address:** 600 Highland Ave, rm K4-739 CSC, Madison, WI 53792-7375; **Phone:** 608-265-3207; **Board Cert:** Orthopaedic Surgery 2002; **Med School:** Tufts Univ 1982; **Resid:** Orthopaedic Surgery, Case West Res Univ 1988; **Fellow:** Spinal Surgery, Johns Hopkins Univ 1989; **Fac Appt:** Prof OrS, Univ Wisc

Great Plains and Mountains

Coughlin, Michael J MD [OrS] - **Spec Exp:** Foot & Ankle Surgery; **Hospital:** St Alphonsus Regl Med Ctr; **Address:** 901 N Curtis Rd, Ste 503, Boise, ID 83706; **Phone:** 208-377-1000; **Board Cert:** Orthopaedic Surgery 1980; **Med School:** Oregon Hlth Sci Univ 1974; **Resid:** Orthopaedic Surgery, UCSF Med Ctr 1978; **Fellow:** Foot & Ankle Surgery, Samuel Merrit Hosp 1979; **Fac Appt:** Clin Prof OrS, Oregon Hlth Sci Univ

Garvin, Kevin L MD [OrS] - **Spec Exp:** Hip Surgery; Knee Surgery; Joint Replacement; **Hospital:** Nebraska Med Ctr; **Address:** Orthopaedic Clinic, 989265 Nebraska Medical Ctr Fl 2, Omaha, NE 68198-9265; **Phone:** 402-559-8000; **Board Cert:** Orthopaedic Surgery 2001; **Med School:** Med Coll Wisc 1982; **Resid:** Orthopaedic Surgery, Univ Arizona Hosp 1987; **Fellow:** Hip Surgery, Hosp for Special Surgery 1988; **Fac Appt:** Prof OrS, Univ Nebr Coll Med

Millett, Peter J MD [OrS] - **Spec Exp:** Shoulder Surgery; Sports Medicine; Arthroscopic Surgery; **Hospital:** Vail Valley Med Ctr; **Address:** Steadman-Hawkins Clinic, 181 W Meadow Drive, Ste 400, Vail, CO 81657; **Phone:** 970-476-1100; **Board Cert:** Orthopaedic Surgery 2003; **Med School:** Dartmouth Med Sch 1995; **Resid:** Orthopaedic Surgery, Hosp Special Surgery 2000; **Fellow:** Sports Medicine, Steadman Hawkins Clinic 2001

Randall, R Lor MD [OrS] - **Spec Exp:** Bone Tumors; Sarcoma-Soft Tissue; Pediatric Orthopaedic Surgery; **Hospital:** Univ Utah Hosps and Clins, Primary Children's Med Ctr; **Address:** Ped Ortho Surg, Primary Chlds Med Ctr, 100 N Medical Drive, Ste 4550, SLC, UT 84113, Salt Lake City, UT 84113; **Phone:** 801-662-5600; **Board Cert:** Orthopaedic Surgery 2001; **Med School:** Yale Univ 1992; **Resid:** Orthopaedic Surgery, UCSF Med Ctr 1997; **Fellow:** Musculoskeletal Oncology, Univ WA Med Ctr 1998; **Fac Appt:** Assoc Prof OrS, Univ Utah

Rosenberg, Thomas D MD [OrS] - **Spec Exp:** Knee Surgery; Sports Medicine; **Hospital:** Ortho Spec Hosp, The (TOSH); **Address:** 1820 Sidewinder Drive, Park City, UT 84060; **Phone:** 435-655-6600; **Board Cert:** Orthopaedic Surgery 1979; **Med School:** Univ Utah 1973; **Resid:** Orthopaedic Surgery, Univ Utah Affil Hosps 1977; **Fellow:** Sports Medicine, Univ Wisconsin Hosp 1978

Saltzman, Charles L MD [OrS] - **Spec Exp:** Foot & Ankle Surgery; **Hospital:** Univ Utah Hosps and Clins; **Address:** Univ Utah, Dept Orthopaedic Surgery, 590 Wakara Way, Salt Lake City, UT 84108; **Phone:** 801-587-5404; **Board Cert:** Orthopaedic Surgery 2004; **Med School:** Univ NC Sch Med 1985; **Resid:** Orthopaedic Surgery, Univ Michigan Med Ctr; **Fellow:** Orthopaedic Surgery, Mayo Clinic; **Fac Appt:** Prof OrS, Univ Utah

Steadman, J Richard MD [OrS] - **Spec Exp:** Knee-Microfracture Surgery; Sports Medicine; **Hospital:** Vail Valley Med Ctr; **Address:** Steadman-Hawkins Sports Medicine Clinic, 181 W Meadow Drive, Ste 400, Vail, CO 81657; **Phone:** 970-476-1100; **Board Cert:** Orthopaedic Surgery 1972; **Med School:** Univ Tex SW, Dallas 1963; **Resid:** Orthopaedic Surgery, Charity Hosp 1966; Orthopaedic Surgery, Louisiana St Univ Hosp 1967

Wiedel, Jerome D MD [OrS] - **Spec Exp:** Hip/Knee Replacement; Reconstructive Surgery; **Hospital:** Univ Colorado Hosp; **Address:** 1635 N Ursula St, Ste 4100, PO Box 6510, MS F722, Aurora, CO 80045; **Phone:** 720-848-1900; **Board Cert:** Orthopaedic Surgery 1993; **Med School:** Univ Nebr Coll Med 1964; **Resid:** Orthopaedic Surgery, Univ Colorado Med Ctr 1971; **Fellow:** Reconstructive Surgery, Robert Jones-A Hunt Ortho Hosp 1972; **Fac Appt:** Prof OrS, Univ Colorado

Wilkins, Ross M MD [OrS] - **Spec Exp:** Bone Cancer; **Hospital:** Presby - St Luke's Med Ctr, Porter Adventist Hosp; **Address:** 1601 E 19th Ave, Ste 3300, Denver, CO 80218; **Phone:** 303-837-0072; **Board Cert:** Orthopaedic Surgery 2006; **Med School:** Wayne State Univ 1978; **Resid:** Orthopaedic Surgery, Univ Colorado Med Ctr 1983; **Fellow:** Orthopaedic Oncology, Mayo Clinic 1984

Southwest

Aronson, James MD [OrS] - **Spec Exp:** Limb Lengthening (Ilizarov Procedure); Hip Disorders & Dysplasia; Clubfoot; Limb Deformities; **Hospital:** Arkansas Chldns Hosp; **Address:** Arkansas Chldns Hosp, Dept Orthopaedics, 800 Marshall St, Slot 839, Little Rock, AR 72202; **Phone:** 501-364-1468; **Board Cert:** Orthopaedic Surgery 1997; **Med School:** Univ Pittsburgh 1975; **Resid:** Surgery, Maine Med Ctr 1977; Orthopaedic Surgery, Duke Univ Med Ctr 1982; **Fellow:** Pediatric Orthopaedic Surgery, Alfred I DuPont Inst 1983; **Fac Appt:** Prof OrS, Univ Ark

Brodsky, James W MD [OrS] - **Spec Exp:** Foot & Ankle Surgery; **Hospital:** Baylor Univ Medical Ctr; **Address:** 411 N Washington Ave, Ste 7000, Dallas, TX 75246-1777; **Phone:** 214-823-7090; **Board Cert:** Orthopaedic Surgery 2008; **Med School:** Case West Res Univ 1979; **Resid:** Orthopaedic Surgery, Bellevue Hosp Ctr/NYU 1981; Orthopaedic Surgery, Baylor Coll Med 1984; **Fellow:** Foot & Ankle Surgery, Rancho Los Amigos/USC/LAC Hosp 1985; **Fac Appt:** Clin Prof OrS, Univ Tex SW, Dallas

Orthopaedic Surgery

Bucholz, Robert W MD [OrS] - **Spec Exp:** Trauma; **Hospital:** UT Southwestern Med Ctr - Dallas, Parkland Meml Hosp - Dallas; **Address:** Univ Tex SW Med Sch, Dept Ortho Surg, 1801 Inwood Rd, Dallas, TX 75390-8882; **Phone:** 214-648-3068; **Board Cert:** Orthopaedic Surgery 2005; **Med School:** Yale Univ 1973; **Resid:** Orthopaedic Surgery, Yale-New Haven Hosp 1977; **Fac Appt:** Prof OrS, Univ Tex SW, Dallas

Cooper, Daniel E MD [OrS] - **Spec Exp:** Sports Medicine; Knee Injuries/ACL; Arthroscopic Surgery; Reconstructive Surgery; **Hospital:** Baylor Univ Medical Ctr, Mary Shiels Hosp; **Address:** The Carrell Clinic, 9301 N Central Expwy, Ste 400, Dallas, TX 75231; **Phone:** 214-220-2468; **Board Cert:** Orthopaedic Surgery 2003; **Med School:** Univ Tex SW, Dallas 1984; **Resid:** Orthopaedic Surgery, Univ Texas Health Scis Ctr 1989; **Fellow:** Sports Medicine, Hospital for Special Surgery 1990

Gugenheim Jr, Joseph J MD [OrS] - **Spec Exp:** Limb Lengthening (Ilizarov Procedure); Limb Deformities; **Hospital:** Texas Ortho Hosp; **Address:** Foundren Orthopaedic Group, 7401 S Main St, Houston, TX 77030; **Phone:** 713-799-2300; **Board Cert:** Orthopaedic Surgery 1978; **Med School:** Northwestern Univ 1972; **Resid:** Orthopaedic Surgery, Baylor Univ Hosp 1976; **Fellow:** Pediatric Orthopaedic Surgery, Boston Chldns Hosp 1977; **Fac Appt:** Assoc Prof S, Baylor Coll Med

Hochschuler, Stephen H MD [OrS] - **Spec Exp:** Spinal Surgery; **Hospital:** Presby Hosp - Plano; **Address:** Texas Back Institute, 6020 W Parker Rd, Ste 200, Plano, TX 75093-7916; **Phone:** 972-608-5000; **Board Cert:** Orthopaedic Surgery 1978; **Med School:** Harvard Med Sch 1968; **Resid:** Surgery, Boston City Hosp 1971; Orthopaedic Surgery, Univ Texas SW Med Ctr 1976

Mabrey, Jay D MD [OrS] - **Spec Exp:** Knee Replacement & Revision; Hip Replacement & Revision; Arthroscopic Surgery-Hip; **Hospital:** Baylor Univ Medical Ctr; **Address:** Baylor Univ Med Ctr, Dept Orthopaedics, 3500 Gaston Ave Bldg Hob Fl 6, Dallas, TX 75246-9990; **Phone:** 214-820-3434; **Board Cert:** Orthopaedic Surgery 2000; **Med School:** Cornell Univ-Weill Med Coll 1981; **Resid:** Orthopaedic Surgery, Duke Univ MC 1987; Surgery, Duke Univ MC 1983; **Fellow:** Joint Replacement Surgery, Hosp Special Surg 1991; **Fac Appt:** Clin Prof OrS, Univ Tex SW, Dallas

Simmons Jr, James W MD [OrS] - **Spec Exp:** Spinal Surgery; **Hospital:** Methodist Spec & Transpl Hosp; **Address:** 12770 Cimarron Path, Ste 132, San Antonio, TX 78249; **Phone:** 210-614-3900; **Board Cert:** Orthopaedic Surgery 1969; **Med School:** Univ Miss 1962; **Resid:** Orthopaedic Surgery, Martin AMC 1964; Orthopaedic Surgery, Brooke Genl Hosp 1967; **Fac Appt:** Clin Prof OrS, Univ Tex Med Br, Galveston

Souryal, Tarek O MD [OrS] - **Spec Exp:** Sports Medicine; Knee Injuries/ACL; **Hospital:** Presby Hosp of Dallas; **Address:** 6901 Snider Plaza, Ste 200, Dallas, TX 75205; **Phone:** 214-369-7733; **Board Cert:** Orthopaedic Surgery 2001; **Med School:** Univ Tex, San Antonio 1982; **Resid:** Orthopaedic Surgery, UTSW Med Ctr 1987; **Fellow:** Sports Medicine, Sports Med Clin N Tex 1987; Sports Medicine, Hughston Ortho Clinic 1988; **Fac Appt:** Clin Prof OrS, Univ Tex SW, Dallas

Trick, Lorence W MD [OrS] - **Spec Exp:** Hip Replacement; Knee Replacement; **Hospital:** SW TX Meth Hosp, Univ Hlth Sys - Univ Hosp (San Antonio, TX); **Address:** 4647 Medical Drive, San Antonio, TX 78229; **Phone:** 210-567-0924; **Board Cert:** Orthopaedic Surgery 1973; **Med School:** Geo Wash Univ 1967; **Resid:** Orthopaedic Surgery, Wilford Hall USAF Med Ctr 1972; **Fellow:** Orthopaedic Surgery, New Eng Baptist Med Ctr; **Fac Appt:** Clin Prof OrS, Univ Tex, San Antonio

Williams, Ronald Paul MD [OrS] - **Spec Exp:** Bone Tumors; **Hospital:** Univ Hlth Sys - Univ Hosp (San Antonio, TX); **Address:** Dept of Orthopaedics, 7703 Floyd Curl Drive, MC 7774, San Antonio, TX 78229-3900; **Phone:** 210-567-5125; **Board Cert:** Orthopaedic Surgery 2003; **Med School:** Univ Tex, San Antonio 1984; **Resid:** Orthopaedic Surgery, U Kans Sch Med. 1989; **Fellow:** Orthopaedic Surgery, Case West Res. U. 1990; **Fac Appt:** Prof OrS, Univ Tex, San Antonio

America's Top Doctors® 8th Edition

Wirth, Michael A MD [OrS] - **Spec Exp:** Shoulder Surgery; Shoulder Replacement; **Hospital:** Univ Hlth Sys - Univ Hosp (San Antonio, TX); **Address:** Univ Tex Hlth Sci Ctr, Dept Orth, 7703 Floyd Curl Drive, MC 7774, San Antonio, TX 78229-3900; **Phone:** 210-567-5135; **Board Cert:** Orthopaedic Surgery 2004; **Med School:** Oregon Hlth Sci Univ 1985; **Resid:** Orthopaedic Surgery, Univ Texas Hlth Sci Ctr 1990; **Fellow:** Shoulder Surgery, Charles Rockwood Jr MD 1991; **Fac Appt:** Prof OrS, Univ Tex, San Antonio

West Coast and Pacific

Anderson, Lesley J MD [OrS] - **Spec Exp:** Knee Injuries/ACL; Knee Cartilage/Meniscus Transplants; Cartilage Damage; Shoulder Surgery; **Hospital:** CA Pacific Med Ctr; **Address:** 2100 Webster St, Ste 309, San Francisco, CA 94115; **Phone:** 415-923-3029; **Board Cert:** Orthopaedic Surgery 2007; **Med School:** Penn State Univ-Hershey Med Ctr 1976; **Resid:** Orthopaedic Surgery, UCLA Med Ctr 1983; **Fellow:** Sports Medicine/Knee Surgery, Blazina Ortho Clinic 1984; **Fac Appt:** Asst Clin Prof OrS, UCSF

Bos, Gary D MD [OrS] - **Spec Exp:** Musculoskeletal Tumors; Sarcoma; Reconstructive Surgery; **Hospital:** Yakima Valley Mem Hosp; **Address:** 16th Avenue Station, 1470 16th Ave, Yakima, WA 98902; **Phone:** 509-574-3300; **Board Cert:** Orthopaedic Surgery 2008; **Med School:** Univ Chicago-Pritzker Sch Med 1978; **Resid:** Orthopaedic Surgery, Case West Reserve 1984; **Fellow:** Orthopaedic Surgery, Case West Reserve 1980; Orthopaedic Oncology, Mayo Clinic 1985

Cannon Jr, W Dilworth MD [OrS] - **Spec Exp:** Sports Medicine; Knee Surgery; **Hospital:** UCSF Med Ctr; **Address:** 1701 Divisadero St, Ste 240, San Francisco, CA 94115-1351; **Phone:** 415-353-7566; **Board Cert:** Orthopaedic Surgery 1972; **Med School:** Columbia P&S 1963; **Resid:** Surgery, St Vincents Hosp 1965; Orthopaedic Surgery, NY Ortho Hosp 1970; **Fellow:** Orthopaedic Surgery, Royal Natl Ortho Hosp 1971; **Fac Appt:** Clin Prof OrS, UCSF

Carragee, Eugene J MD [OrS] - **Spec Exp:** Spinal Surgery; Spinal Disc Replacement; **Hospital:** Stanford Univ Med Ctr; **Address:** Stanford Univ, Orthopaedics/Spine Ctr, 300 Pasteur Drive, rm R171, Stanford, CA 94304; **Phone:** 650-725-5905; **Board Cert:** Orthopaedic Surgery 2005; **Med School:** Stanford Univ 1982; **Resid:** Internal Medicine, Stanford Univ Hosp 1984; Orthopaedic Surgery, Stanford Univ Hosp 1988; **Fac Appt:** Prof OrS, Stanford Univ

Chambers, Richard Byron MD [OrS] - **Spec Exp:** Diabetes-Amputation; **Hospital:** Rancho Los Amigos Natl Rehab Ctr; **Address:** 7601 E Imperial Hwy, rm HB-145, Downey, CA 90242; **Phone:** 562-401-7166; **Board Cert:** Orthopaedic Surgery 1977; **Med School:** Columbia P&S 1971; **Resid:** Surgery, NY Hosp; Orthopaedic Surgery, Hosp Special Surg

Conrad, Ernest U MD [OrS] - **Spec Exp:** Pediatric Orthopaedic Surgery; Bone Tumors; Sarcoma; **Hospital:** Chldns Hosp and Regl Med Ctr - Seattle, Univ Wash Med Ctr; **Address:** Children's Hosp & Regional Med Ctr, W-7706, Box 359300, Seattle, WA 98105; **Phone:** 206-543-3690; **Board Cert:** Orthopaedic Surgery 1999; **Med School:** Univ VA Sch Med 1979; **Resid:** Orthopaedic Surgery, Hosp for Special Surgery 1984; **Fellow:** Orthopaedic Oncology, Univ Fla Coll Med 1985; Pediatric Orthopaedic Surgery, Hosp for Sick Chldn 1986; **Fac Appt:** Prof OrS, Univ Wash

Copp, Steven N MD [OrS] - **Spec Exp:** Foot & Ankle Surgery; Hip & Knee Replacement; **Hospital:** Scripps Green Hosp; **Address:** Scripps Clinic, Dept Orthopedic Surgery, 10666 N Torrey Pines Rd, La Jolla, CA 92037; **Phone:** 858-554-8519; **Board Cert:** Orthopaedic Surgery 2002; **Med School:** UCSD 1983; **Resid:** Orthopaedic Surgery, UCSD Med Ctr 1988

Orthopaedic Surgery

Delamarter, Rick B MD [OrS] - **Spec Exp:** Spinal Surgery; Minimally Invasive Spinal Surgery; Spinal Disc Replacement; Spinal Reconstructive Surgery; **Hospital:** St John's Hlth Ctr, Santa Monica; **Address:** Spine Institute of Santa Monica, 1301 20th St, Ste 400, Santa Monica, CA 90404; **Phone:** 310-828-7757; **Board Cert:** Orthopaedic Surgery 2000; **Med School:** Oregon Hlth Sci Univ 1981; **Resid:** Orthopaedic Surgery, UCLA Med Ctr 1986; **Fac Appt:** Assoc Prof S, UCLA

Dillingham, Michael F MD [OrS] - **Spec Exp:** Sports Medicine; **Hospital:** Stanford Univ Med Ctr, CA Pacific Med Ctr; **Address:** 500 Arguello St, Ste 100, Redwood City, CA 94063; **Phone:** 650-851-4900; **Board Cert:** Orthopaedic Surgery 1977; Physical Medicine & Rehabilitation 1979; **Med School:** Stanford Univ 1971; **Resid:** Orthopaedic Surgery, Standford Univ Med Ctr 1975; Physical Medicine & Rehabilitation, Santa Clara Valley Med Ctr 1977; **Fellow:** Spinal Surgery, Santa Clara Valley Med Ctr 1976; **Fac Appt:** Clin Prof OrS, Stanford Univ

Dorr, Lawrence Douglas MD [OrS] - **Spec Exp:** Hip & Knee Replacement; **Hospital:** Good Samaritan Hosp - Los Angeles; **Address:** Dorr Arthritis Institute, 637 S Lucas Ave, Ste 500, Los Angeles, CA 90017; **Phone:** 213-977-2280; **Board Cert:** Orthopaedic Surgery 1978; **Med School:** Univ Iowa Coll Med 1967; **Resid:** Orthopaedic Surgery, LAC-USC Med Ctr 1976; **Fellow:** Joint Replacement Surgery, Hosp Special Surg 1977

Eckardt, Jeffrey J MD [OrS] - **Spec Exp:** Bone Tumors; Soft Tissue Tumors; Limb Sparing Surgery; **Hospital:** Santa Monica - UCLA Med Ctr, Ronald Reagan UCLA Med Ctr; **Address:** UCLA Med Ctr, Dept Ortho Surg/Oncology, 1250 16th St Tower # 745, Santa Monica, CA 90404; **Phone:** 310-319-3816; **Board Cert:** Orthopaedic Surgery 1981; **Med School:** Cornell Univ-Weill Med Coll 1971; **Resid:** Orthopaedic Surgery, UCLA Med Ctr 1979; **Fellow:** Orthopaedic Oncology, Mayo Clinic 1980; **Fac Appt:** Prof OrS, UCLA

Eckardt, Jeffrey J MD [OrS] - **Spec Exp:** Limb Sparing Surgery; Bone Cancer; Sarcoma; Soft Tissue Tumors; **Hospital:** Ronald Reagan UCLA Med Ctr; **Address:** UCLA Hosp Dept of Orth Surg, 1250 16 St, Ste 745 tower7, Santa Monica, CA 90404; **Phone:** 310-319-3816; **Board Cert:** Orthopaedic Surgery 1981; **Med School:** Cornell Univ-Weill Med Coll 1971; **Resid:** Orthopaedic Surgery, UCLA Hosp 1979; **Fellow:** Orthopaedic Oncology, Mayo Clinic 1980; **Fac Appt:** Prof OrS, UCLA

Finerman, Gerald MD [OrS] - **Spec Exp:** Sports Medicine; Hip & Knee Replacement; **Hospital:** Ronald Reagan UCLA Med Ctr, Santa Monica - UCLA Med Ctr; **Address:** 1245 16 St, Santa Monica, CA 90404; **Phone:** 310-825-6019; **Board Cert:** Orthopaedic Surgery 1971; **Med School:** Johns Hopkins Univ 1962; **Resid:** Surgery, Johns Hopkins Hosp 1964; Orthopaedic Surgery, Johns Hopkins Hosp 1969; **Fac Appt:** Prof OrS, UCLA

Garfin, Steven R MD [OrS] - **Spec Exp:** Spinal Surgery; **Hospital:** UCSD Med Ctr; **Address:** UCSD, Dept Orthopedic Surgery, 4150 Regents Park Row, La Jolla, CA 92037; **Phone:** 858-657-8200; **Board Cert:** Orthopaedic Surgery 1982; **Med School:** Univ Minn 1972; **Resid:** Orthopaedic Surgery, UCSD Med Ctr 1979; **Fellow:** Spinal Surgery, Pennsylvania Hosp 1981; **Fac Appt:** Prof OrS, UCSD

Goodman, Stuart B MD/PhD [OrS] - **Spec Exp:** Arthritis; Joint Replacement; Reconstructive Surgery; **Hospital:** Stanford Univ Med Ctr, Lucile Packard Chldns Hosp/Stanford Univ Med Ctr; **Address:** Stanford Univ, Div Ortho Surgery, 300 Pasteur, rm R-I05, Stanford, CA 94305-2200; **Phone:** 650-723-7072; **Board Cert:** Orthopaedic Surgery 1998; **Med School:** Univ Toronto 1978; **Resid:** Orthopaedic Surgery, Univ Toronto 1984; **Fellow:** Orthopaedic Surgery, Univ Toronto 1985; **Fac Appt:** Prof OrS, Stanford Univ

Hansen, Sigvard MD [OrS] - **Spec Exp:** Ankle Replacement & Revision; Deformity Reconstruction; Neuromuscular Disorders; **Hospital:** Harborview Med Ctr, Univ Wash Med Ctr; **Address:** Foot & Ankle Institute, 325 9th Ave, Box 359799, Seattle, WA 98104; **Phone:** 206-744-4830; **Board Cert:** Orthopaedic Surgery 1993; **Med School:** Univ Wash 1961; **Resid:** Orthopaedic Surgery, Univ Washington Affil Hosps 1969; **Fellow:** Orthopaedic Surgery, Sheffield Chldrns Hosp 1970; **Fac Appt:** Prof OrS, Univ Wash

Lowenberg, David W MD [OrS] - **Spec Exp:** Osteomyelitis; Limb Lengthening (Ilizarov Procedure); Fractures-Complex & Non Union; Bone Infections; **Hospital:** CA Pacific Med Ctr; **Address:** Dept of Orthopaedic Surgery, 2100 Webster St, Ste 117, San Francisco, CA 94115; **Phone:** 415-600-3835; **Board Cert:** Orthopaedic Surgery 2003; **Med School:** UCLA 1985; **Resid:** Orthopaedic Surgery, UCSF Med Ctr 1990; **Fac Appt:** Assoc Prof OrS, UCSF

Luck Jr, James V MD [OrS] - **Spec Exp:** Hemophilia Related Disease; Hip & Knee Replacement; Musculoskeletal Tumors; **Hospital:** Santa Monica - UCLA Med Ctr; **Address:** 2400 S Flower St, Fl 3, Los Angeles, CA 90007-2660; **Phone:** 213-749-8255; **Board Cert:** Orthopaedic Surgery 2000; **Med School:** USC Sch Med 1967; **Resid:** Orthopaedic Surgery, Orthopaedic Hosp 1973; **Fellow:** Orthopaedic Oncology, Orthopaedic Hosp 1974; Reconstructive Surgery, Rancho Los Amigos 1974; **Fac Appt:** Prof OrS, UCLA

Matsen, Frederick MD [OrS] - **Spec Exp:** Shoulder Replacement; Elbow Replacement; Rotator Cuff Surgery; **Hospital:** Univ Wash Med Ctr; **Address:** Bone & Joint Ctr, UWMC-Roosevelt, 4245 Roosevelt Way NE, Box 354740, Seattle, WA 98105; **Phone:** 206-598-4288; **Board Cert:** Orthopaedic Surgery 1978; **Med School:** Baylor Coll Med 1968; **Resid:** Orthopaedic Surgery, Univ Washington Med Ctr 1974; **Fac Appt:** Prof OrS, Univ Wash

O'Donnell, Richard John MD [OrS] - **Spec Exp:** Bone Cancer; Sarcoma-Soft Tissue; Pediatric Orthopaedic Cancers; **Hospital:** UCSF Med Ctr; **Address:** 1600 Divisadero St Fl 4th, San Francisco, CA 94115; **Phone:** 415-885-3800; **Board Cert:** Orthopaedic Surgery 1999; **Med School:** Harvard Med Sch 1989; **Resid:** Orthopaedic Surgery, Mass Genl Hosp 1995; **Fellow:** Musculoskeletal Oncology, Univ WA Med Ctr 1996; **Fac Appt:** Assoc Prof OrS, UCSF

Oppenheim, William L MD [OrS] - **Spec Exp:** Limb Lengthening; Scoliosis; Clubfoot/Foot Deformities in Children; Pediatric Orthopaedic Surgery; **Hospital:** Ronald Reagan UCLA Med Ctr; **Address:** 10833 Le Conte Ave, UCLA Med Ctr-Div Orth—Rm 76-134CHS, Los Angeles, CA 90024-1300; **Phone:** 310-206-6345; **Board Cert:** Orthopaedic Surgery 1992; **Med School:** Georgetown Univ 1970; **Resid:** Orthopaedic Surgery, Univ Washington Hosp 1978; **Fellow:** Pediatric Orthopaedic Surgery, Orthopaedic Hosp UCLA 1979; **Fac Appt:** Prof OrS, UCLA

Patzakis, Michael J MD [OrS] - **Spec Exp:** Osteomyelitis; Fractures-Non Union; Joint Infections; **Hospital:** USC Univ Hosp - R K Eamer Med Plz; **Address:** 1200 N State St GNH3900, Los Angeles, CA 90033-1029; **Phone:** 323-226-7201; **Board Cert:** Orthopaedic Surgery 1983; **Med School:** Ohio State Univ 1963; **Resid:** Orthopaedic Surgery, LAC-USC Med Ctr 1968; **Fellow:** Rheumatology, Univ CO Med Ctr 1969; **Fac Appt:** Prof OrS, USC Sch Med

Peterson, Davis C MD [OrS] - **Spec Exp:** Spinal Surgery; Scoliosis; Trauma; **Hospital:** Providence Alaska Med Ctr, Alaska Regl Hosp; **Address:** 3260 Providence Drive, Ste 200, Anchorage, AK 99508-4603; **Phone:** 907-563-3145; **Board Cert:** Orthopaedic Surgery 1999; **Med School:** Baylor Coll Med 1980; **Resid:** Orthopaedic Surgery, Madigan Army Med Ctr 1986; **Fellow:** Spinal Surgery, St Luke's Med Ctr 1990

Orthopaedic Surgery

Sangeorzan, Bruce J MD [OrS] - **Spec Exp:** Foot & Ankle Surgery; Trauma; Ankle Replacement & Revision; **Hospital:** Harborview Med Ctr, Univ Wash Med Ctr; **Address:** 325 9th Ave, Box 359799, Seattle, WA 98104-2499; **Phone:** 206-744-4830; **Board Cert:** Orthopaedic Surgery 2000; **Med School:** Wayne State Univ 1981; **Resid:** Orthopaedic Surgery, Wayne State Univ 1986; **Fellow:** Trauma, Univ Wash 1986; Foot & Ankle Reconstruction, Univ Wash 1987; **Fac Appt:** Prof OrS, Univ Wash

Schmalzried, Thomas P MD [OrS] - **Spec Exp:** Hip Replacement; **Hospital:** St Vincent's Med Ctr - Los Angeles; **Address:** The Joint Replacement Institute, St Vincent Med Ctr, 2200 W 3rd St, Ste 400, Los Angeles, CA 90057; **Phone:** 213-484-7600; **Board Cert:** Orthopaedic Surgery 2004; **Med School:** UCLA 1984; **Resid:** Orthopaedic Surgery, UCLA Med Ctr 1990; **Fellow:** Orthopaedic Surgery, UCLA Med Ctr 1987; Hip Surgery, Mass Genl Hosp/Harvard 1991; **Fac Appt:** Asst Prof OrS, UCLA

Schurman, David J MD [OrS] - **Spec Exp:** Hip & Knee Replacement; Sports Medicine; Bone Infections; **Hospital:** Stanford Univ Med Ctr; **Address:** 300 Pasteur Drive, Ste R144, Stanford, CA 94305-5341; **Phone:** 650-723-7608; **Board Cert:** Orthopaedic Surgery 1994; **Med School:** Columbia P&S 1965; **Resid:** Surgery, Mount Sinai Hosp 1967; Orthopaedic Surgery, UCLA Med Ctr 1972; **Fellow:** Arthritis Surgery, UCLA Med Ctr 1973; **Fac Appt:** Prof OrS, Stanford Univ

Singer, Daniel I MD [OrS] - **Spec Exp:** Hand Surgery; Bone Cancer; Hand & Upper Extremity Tumors; **Hospital:** Queen's Med Ctr - Honolulu, Kapiolani Med Ctr @ Pali Momi; **Address:** Queen's Physicians' Office Blg 1, 1380 Lusitana St, Ste 615, Honolulu, HI 96813-2442; **Phone:** 808-521-8109; **Board Cert:** Orthopaedic Surgery 2000; Hand Surgery 2000; **Med School:** Boston Univ 1979; **Resid:** Surgery, Univ Conn Hlth Ctr 1981; Orthopaedic Surgery, Univ Hawaii 1984; **Fellow:** Hand Surgery, Thomas Jefferson Univ Med Ctr 1985; Microvascular Surgery, St Vincent's Hosp 1985; **Fac Appt:** Assoc Prof OrS, Univ Hawaii JA Burns Sch Med

Teitz, Carol C MD [OrS] - **Spec Exp:** Sports Injuries; Arthroscopic Surgery-Knee; Musculoskeletal Injuries in Dancers; Pain-Back; **Hospital:** Univ Wash Med Ctr; **Address:** UW Sports Medicine Clinic, Bank of America Edmundson Pavilion, 3950 Montlake Blvd NE, rm 148, Seattle, WA 98195; **Phone:** 206-543-1552; **Board Cert:** Orthopaedic Surgery 1981; **Med School:** Yale Univ 1974; **Resid:** Orthopaedic Surgery, Univ Wash Affil Hosps 1980; **Fellow:** Arthroscopic Surgery, J McGinty MD,Newton-Wellesley Hosp 1993; **Fac Appt:** Prof OrS, Univ Wash

Tolo, Vernon T MD [OrS] - **Spec Exp:** Pediatric Orthopaedic Surgery; Spinal Deformity-Pediatric; Skeletal Dysplasia; **Hospital:** Chldns Hosp - Los Angeles, USC Univ Hosp - R K Eamer Med Plz; **Address:** Chldns Hosp LA, Orthopaedic Surgery, 4650 W Sunset Blvd, MS 69, Los Angeles, CA 90027-6062; **Phone:** 323-361-4658; **Board Cert:** Orthopaedic Surgery 1977; **Med School:** Johns Hopkins Univ 1968; **Resid:** Orthopaedic Surgery, Johns Hopkins Hosp 1975; **Fellow:** Pediatric Orthopaedic Surgery, Hosp Sick Chldn 1976; **Fac Appt:** Prof OrS, USC Sch Med

Vail, Thomas Parker MD [OrS] - **Spec Exp:** Hip & Knee Replacement; Hip Resurfacing; Arthritis; Osteonecrosis; **Hospital:** UCSF Med Ctr; **Address:** UCSF Med Center, Box 0728, MU326W, 500 Parnassus Ave, San Francisco, CA 94143; **Phone:** 415-502-7335; **Board Cert:** Orthopaedic Surgery 1994; **Med School:** Loyola Univ-Stritch Sch Med 1985; **Resid:** Thoracic Surgery, Duke Univ Med Ctr 1987; Orthopaedic Surgery, Duke Univ Med Ctr 1991; **Fellow:** Reconstructive Surgery, North Amer/Euro Trav Prgm 1992; **Fac Appt:** Prof OrS, UCSF

Wang, Jeffrey MD [OrS] - **Spec Exp:** Spinal Surgery; **Hospital:** Ronald Reagan UCLA Med Ctr; **Address:** Westwood Clinic, 200 UCLA Medical Plaza, Ste 140, Los Angeles, CA 90095; **Phone:** 310-319-3475; **Board Cert:** Orthopaedic Surgery 1999; **Med School:** Univ Pittsburgh 1991; **Resid:** Orthopaedic Surgery, Orthopaedic Hosp UCLA 1996; **Fellow:** Spinal Cord Injury Medicine, Case Western Reserve Univ 1997; **Fac Appt:** Prof OrS, UCLA

Watkins III, Robert G MD [OrS] - **Spec Exp:** Spinal Surgery; Spinal Disc Replacement; **Address:** 13160 Mindanao Way, Ste 325, Marina Del Rey, CA 90292; **Phone:** 310-448-7890; **Board Cert:** Orthopaedic Surgery 1982; **Med School:** Univ Tenn Coll Med, Memphis 1969; **Resid:** Orthopaedic Surgery, LAC-USC Med Ctr 1978; **Fellow:** Spinal Surgery, Jones-Hunt Orth Hosp 1979; **Fac Appt:** Assoc Prof OrS, USC Sch Med

Yoo, Jung MD [OrS] - **Spec Exp:** Spinal Surgery; **Hospital:** OR Hlth & Sci Univ; **Address:** 3181 SW Sam Jackson Park Rd, MC OP-31, Portland, OR 97239; **Phone:** 503-494-6406; **Board Cert:** Orthopaedic Surgery 2004; **Med School:** Univ Chicago-Pritzker Sch Med 1984; **Resid:** Orthopaedic Surgery, Case Western Reserve Univ 1990; **Fellow:** Orthopaedic Surgery, SUNY Hlth Sci Ctr 1991; **Fac Appt:** Prof OrS, Oregon Hlth Sci Univ

Cleveland Clinic

Orthopaedic Surgery

The Cleveland Clinic Department of Orthopaedic Surgery has a long history of excellence and innovation in treating musculoskeletal injuries and diseases. For the past several years, *U.S.News & World Report* has consistently ranked the Department of Orthopaedic Surgery among the nation's top five orthopaedic programs.

Foot & Ankle Center: All specialists and surgeons in the Cleveland Clinic Foot and Ankle Center have extensive training in the diagnosis and care of foot and ankle disorders. Our staff of orthopaedic surgeons, podiatrists, nurse clinicians, certified pedorthists and technicians deliver state-of-the-art care exclusively for the foot and ankle.

Joint Replacement: Cleveland Clinic Section of Adult Reconstruction treats osteoarthritis and rheumatoid arthritis of the hip and knee joints, fractures of these joints, and performs joint replacement and revision surgery. At the frontier of surgical developments, our experienced surgeons offer the most advanced implants and minimally invasive techniques to restore patient mobility.

Pediatrics: The Section of Pediatric Orthopaedic Surgery handles more than 11,000 outpatient visits each year. Our physicians offer expertise in the management of all musculoskeletal conditions, including treatment of spinal deformity, hip dysplasia, clubfoot, leg lengthening and limb deformity correction, fractures and growth plate injuries, neuromuscular disorders and sports injuries.

Research and Education

Established in 2001, the Cleveland Clinic Orthopaedic Research Center (ORC) is a unique collaboration that taps into the synergy between Orthopaedic Surgery and Biomedical Engineering. The Center's mission is to advance the health and treatment of people with disorders of the musculoskeletal system through basic and applied scientific investigation, and to train future leaders in musculoskeletal care, research and education. Recent developments, such as harvesting bone marrow cells to generate new bone tissue, help to advance patient care.

Spine Institute: Cleveland Clinic Spine Institute (CCSI) diagnoses and treats more than 13,000 patients annually. The institute brings together the expertise of specialists in neurosurgery, orthopaedic surgery and non-surgical spine care. CCSI integrates the functions of research, clinical practice and education.

Trauma: Cleveland Clinic has been a leader in the treatment of fracture non-union and in the development of methods to improve outcomes through advanced bone-grafting techniques. Innovative procedures offered are the Ilizarov/Taylor Spatial Frame techniques and the use of fresh frozen osteochondral allografts for traumatic defects in and around the knee.

Tumor: One of the largest multi-disciplinary musculoskeletal tumor centers, we have expertise in treating bone and soft tissue sarcomas and performing limb salvage.

For more information about the Cleveland Clinic Department of Orthopaedic Surgery, to schedule a second opinion or to learn about assistance for out-of-town patients, call 800.890.2467 or visit www.clevelandclinic.org/orthotopdocs.

Department of Orthopaedic Surgery
9500 Euclid Avenue / AC311 | Cleveland OH 44195

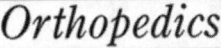

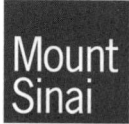
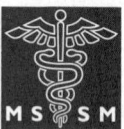

THE MOUNT SINAI MEDICAL CENTER
ORTHOPAEDICS
One Gustave L. Levy Place
Fifth Avenue and 100th Street
New York, NY 10029-6574
Physician Referral: 1-800-MD-SINAI 637-4624)
www.mountsinai.org

Beyond its reputation for depth and breadth of expertise, **The Leni and Peter W. May Department of Orthopaedics** is known for personalized care. The faculty and staff invest the time to get to know their patients as individuals, ensuring that they receive direct care from subspecialty-trained orthopedists. The faculty share expertise in surgery of the foot and ankle, knee, hip, hand, elbow, shoulder, and spine; total joint replacement (knee, hip, foot and ankle, and shoulder); microvascular surgery; cancer surgery; and minimally invasive surgery. Taking a whole-patient approach to care, they work in close collaboration with specialists in geriatrics, neurology, oncology, pathology, and rehabilitation medicine.

INVESTIGATION AND INNOVATION
Recent years have seen successive refinements in the techniques of orthopedic surgery at Mount Sinai, including the design and composition of the prostheses used in joint replacements that have led to improved postoperative function. Faculty members have also been instrumental in the design and perfection of hip and shoulder prostheses. Additionally, Mount Sinai has broadened the applications of arthroscopic surgery—the fiberoptic technology that first heralded the arrival of minimally invasive surgery.

Mount Sinai orthopedic scientists are known for their studies of "wear and tear" diseases of the skeletal system. Researchers are currently investigating bone wear at the microscopic level, rotator cuff degeneration, the effects of microgravity on aging of bones and tissue, how joints of the foot degenerate, methods of determining bone strength, and how genetic alterations change the skeleton's function.

USE OF CUTTING-EDGE TECHNIQUES
Mount Sinai uses innovative, minimally invasive approaches for joint replacement and fracture repair. The Department's oncology service is renowned for saving limbs with both bone and joint malignancies.

GROUNDBREAKING PROCEDURES ENHANCE QUALITY OF LIFE
Today at Mount Sinai, arthroscopy is used to repair not only the knee but virtually every joint. Converting what used to be major open surgery to outpatient procedures has dramatically shortened rehabilitation and return-to-work times. More significantly, it has allowed many more patients to get help for painful, function-limiting conditions. That is the case for many elderly or frail patients who are physically unable to undergo major surgery. The fact that such procedures are now more widely accessible is enhancing the quality of life for many patients and allowing them to lead more active lives.

NYU Hospital for Joint Diseases
NYU LANGONE MEDICAL CENTER

301 East 17th Street
(at Second Avenue)
New York, NY 10003
212-598-6000 FAX: 212-260-1203
www.nyuhjd.org

ORTHOPAEDIC SERVICES
Leaders in the treatment of bone and joint disorders.

NYUHJD Orthopaedic Programs and Services
More than 12,000 surgical procedures are performed at NYU Hospital for Joint Diseases annually. Among our programs and services, we offer the following:

The Joint Replacement Center of NYC: Patients have access to physicians and surgeons highly specialized in treating degenerative joint conditions. Utilizing state-of--the--art techniques, the Center's surgeons are for their expertise in knee, hip and shoulder replacements, complex joint revisions, as well as minimally invasive surgeries. Our center is one of the most active in the world, performing over 2,500 joint replacements annually minimally invasive techniques including anterior approach hip replacement are utilized.

The Spine Center: Provides comprehensive treatment of adult and pediatric spine disorders including lower back pain, neck pain, scoliosis, osteoporosis and the most complex spine problems. We perform minimally invasive spinal fusions that reduce incision size and lead to a speedier recovery. Our Spine Center is distinguished as one of the first in the country to successfully perform artificial disc implantation. We perform over 1,400 spinal procedures each year.

Pediatric Orthopaedic Service: Our skilled specialists provide orthopaedic care for children of all ages with the full spectrum of clinical conditions including neuromuscular diseases such as cerebral palsy, spina bifida and muscular dystrophies and congenital conditions such a clubfoot, hip dysplasia, and limb deformities. Our interdisciplinary approach teams orthopaedic surgeons with pediatric specialists to provide the most up-to-date continuity of care.

Diabetes Foot and Ankle Center: Our main goal is the prevention of foot problems and their recurrence. Dedicated medical professionals provide the most advanced treatment for those complications.

The NYU Hospital for Joint Diseases Department of Orthopaedic Surgery offers the following services and treatments:

- The Spine Center
- Pediatric Orthopaedics
- Foot and Ankle Surgery
- Limb Lengthening and Bone Growth
- Sports Medicine
- Center for Neuromuscular and Developmental Disorders
- General Orthopaedics
Orthopaedic Urgent Care Center
- Arthritis and Joint Replacement Center
- Arthroscopic Surgery
- Bone Tumors/Orthopaedic Oncology
- Hand Surgery
- Shoulder and Elbow Service
- The Harkness Center for Dance Injuries
- Occupational and Industrial Orthopaedic Care

NYU Hospital for Joint Diseases provides care at NYU Tisch Hospital, NYU Hospital for Joint Diseases, Manhattan VA, Jamaica Hospital, and Bellevue Hospital Center, where more than 18,000 surgical procedures are performed each year. The orthopaedic faculty maintains offices in all five boroughs as well as in Rockland County and New Jersey.

Wake Forest University Baptist
MEDICAL CENTER ®
Orthopaedics

Medical Center Boulevard • Winston-Salem, NC 27157 • 336-716-2011
Health On-Call® (Patient access) 1-800-446-2255
PAL® (Physician-to-physician calls) 1-800-277-7654
www.wfubmc.edu

Wake Forest University Baptist Medical Center offers comprehensive programs in all facets of adult and pediatric bone and joint care including joint preservation and replacement, sports medicine, world-class pediatric care, spine care, hand and upper extremity services and innovative therapies that are setting the standards for orthopaedics.

PROGRAM HIGHLIGHTS

The **Comprehensive Joint Replacement Program** employs the most advanced technologies and surgical techniques for hip and knee replacements and specialized after-surgery care. The program is one of only a few in North Carolina to offer hip resurfacing and hip preservation, alternatives to hip replacement. Following surgery, patients recover in a dedicated Joint Replacement Unit where the staff is specialty trained in joint replacement.

The **Hand and Upper Extremity Program** offers nationally and internationally recognized experts with experience in a broad range of disorders... from the shoulder to the finger, from pediatrics to geriatrics, and from congenital to traumatic. Multiple specialists provide replacements of all joints in the arm. Others specialize in the treatment of complex nerve disorders, micro-vascular reconstruction, peripheral neurotization and the treatment of brachial plexus injuries. The Hand Therapy Program, the first in North Carolina, offers integrated physician and therapy teams specially trained in upper extremity disorders.

The **Sports Medicine Program** is comprised of the region's most qualified physicians and therapists working collaboratively to provide a comprehensive, evidence-based approach to treatment of sports-related injuries. The team utilizes an individualized approach to treating athletes and people of all ages whose physical abilities have been limited by injury, degenerative disease or aging. The Sports Medicine Program is the only program in the state to use Motion Monitor technology in a clinical setting. This sophisticated system allows therapists to analyze motion – such as running, pitching or a golf swing – on a computer. Therapists are able to look at the body as an interconnected system and to develop more comprehensive treatment and performance enhancement programs.

Pediatric Orthopaedic Services employs experts with specialty training in acquired and congenital disorders of children and draws patients nationwide and worldwide. The program offers multidisciplinary treatment for cerebral palsy. Surgeons here are pioneers in the use of Botox® injections for treating spasticity disorders. We are also leaders in treating spinal deformities and hip disorders in children. The Pediatric Physical and Occupational Therapy Program boasts a specialty-trained dedicated staff.

The **Orthopaedic Oncology Program** offers a comprehensive team of specialists who provide the most advanced diagnostic technologies and treatment modalities available for patients with benign or malignant bone and soft tissue tumors. The program utilizes limb-sparing techniques and offers expertise in limb salvage and reconstruction.

A TEAM APPROACH

Inpatient and outpatient physical therapy programs supporting the orthopaedic team include acute inpatient therapy services, an outpatient sports medicine therapy program, an outpatient musculoskeletal therapy program, an outpatient spine therapy program, an outpatient hand and upper extremity therapy program, and an outpatient pediatric therapy program offering both single and multidisciplinary therapy services and therapeutic massage.

The Wake Forest Institute for Regenerative Medicine is leading the way in the use of patients' own cells to develop tissues and organs in the laboratory. Multiple projects underway that will benefit patients with orthopaedic injuries include the development of ligament and meniscus replacements, technologies to improve nerve regeneration and methods of bone regeneration.

Wake Forest Baptist has 13 digital operating rooms for orthopaedic surgeries – more than any other center in the United States. This technology enables physicians to capture procedures on video and still images so the patient can be followed appropriately.

KNOWLEDGE MAKES ALL THE DIFFERENCE.

Sponsored Page

Otolaryngology

An otolaryngologist-head and neck surgeon provides comprehensive medical and surgical care for patients with diseases and disorders that affect the ears, nose, throat, the respiratory and upper alimentary systems and related structures of the head and neck.

An otolaryngologist diagnoses and provides medical and/or surgical therapy or prevention of diseases, allergies, neoplasms, deformities, disorders and/or injuries of the ears, nose, sinuses, throat, respiratory and upper alimentary systems, face, jaws and the other head and neck systems. Head and neck oncology, facial plastic and reconstructive surgery and the treatment of disorders of hearing and voice are fundamental areas of expertise.

Training Required: Five years

Certification in the following subspecialty requires additional training and examination.

Plastic Surgery within the Head and Neck: An otolaryngologist with additional training in plastic and reconstructive procedures within the head, face, neck and associated structures, including cutaneous head and neck oncology and reconstruction, management of maxillofacial trauma, soft tissue repair and neural surgery.

Facial Plastic and Reconstructive Surgery is not a recognized ABMS subspecialty. However this designation has been included because the certification process is meaningful and rigorous. It is awarded to those doctors who hold a current ABMS certification in Otolaryngology, but those board certified in Plastic Surgery, Ophthalmology, or Dermatology are also eligible. Certification requires a post-graduate fellowship in Facial Plastic and Reconstructive Surgery followed by a written examination.

This field is diverse and involves a wide age range of patients, from the newborn to the aged. While both cosmetic and reconstructive surgeries are practiced, there are many additional procedures which interface with them.

OTOLARYNGOLOGY

New England

Deschler, Daniel G MD [Oto] - **Spec Exp:** Head & Neck Cancer; Head & Neck Reconstruction; Salivary Gland Tumors & Surgery; **Hospital:** Mass Eye & Ear Infirmary; **Address:** Mass Eye & Ear Infirmary, Head & Neck Surgery, 243 Charles St, Boston, MA 02114; **Phone:** 617-573-4100; **Board Cert:** Otolaryngology 1996; **Med School:** Harvard Med Sch 1990; **Resid:** Otolaryngology, UCSF Med Ctr 1995; **Fellow:** Facial Plastic & Reconstructive Surgery, Hahneman U Med Ctr 1996; **Fac Appt:** Assoc Prof Oto, Harvard Med Sch

Gliklich, Richard E MD [Oto] - **Spec Exp:** Cosmetic Surgery-Face & Neck; Rhinoplasty; Skin Laser Surgery-Resurfacing; **Hospital:** Mass Eye & Ear Infirmary; **Address:** Mass Eye & Ear Infirmary, 243 Charles St Fl 9, Boston, MA 02114; **Phone:** 617-573-4105; **Board Cert:** Otolaryngology 1994; Facial Plastic & Reconstructive Surgery 1996; **Med School:** Harvard Med Sch 1988; **Resid:** Otolaryngology, Mass E&E Infirmary 1993; **Fellow:** Otolaryngology, Mass E&E Infirmary 1994; **Fac Appt:** Assoc Prof Oto, Harvard Med Sch

Grillone, Gregory A MD [Oto] - **Spec Exp:** Laryngeal Disorders; Voice Disorders; Laryngeal Cancer; Head & Neck Cancer & Surgery; **Hospital:** Boston Med Ctr; **Address:** Boston Univ Med Ctr, Dept Otolaryngology, 88 E Newton St, Boston, MA 02118; **Phone:** 617-638-8124; **Board Cert:** Otolaryngology 1988; **Med School:** Mount Sinai Sch Med 1983; **Resid:** Oncology, Boston Univ Med Ctr 1988; **Fac Appt:** Asst Prof Oto, Boston Univ

Grundfast, Kenneth MD [Oto] - **Spec Exp:** Hearing Loss; Pediatric Otolaryngology; **Hospital:** Boston Med Ctr; **Address:** Boston Medical Center, 830 Harrison Ave, Ste 1400, Boston, MA 02119; **Phone:** 617-638-8124; **Board Cert:** Otolaryngology 1977; **Med School:** SUNY Upstate Med Univ 1969; **Resid:** Surgery, Sibley Meml Hosp 1974; Otolaryngology, Boston-Affil Hosps 1977; **Fellow:** Pediatric Otolaryngology, Chldns Hosp 1978; **Fac Appt:** Prof Oto, Boston Univ

Kveton, John MD [Oto] - **Spec Exp:** Ear Disorders; Cochlear Implants; Acoustic Neuroma; **Hospital:** Yale-New Haven Hosp, Hosp of St Raphael; **Address:** 46 Prince St, Ste 601, New Haven, CT 06519-1634; **Phone:** 203-752-1726; **Board Cert:** Otolaryngology 1982; Neurotology 2004; **Med School:** St Louis Univ 1978; **Resid:** Otolaryngology, Yale-New Haven Hosp 1982; **Fellow:** Neurotology, The Otology Group 1983; **Fac Appt:** Clin Prof Oto, Yale Univ

McKenna, Michael J MD [Oto] - **Spec Exp:** Skull Base Surgery; Otology; Neuro-Otology; **Hospital:** Mass Eye & Ear Infirmary; **Address:** Massachusetts Eye & Ear Infirmary, 243 Charles St, Boston, MA 02114-3002; **Phone:** 617-573-3672; **Board Cert:** Otolaryngology 1988; Neurotology 2004; **Med School:** USC Sch Med 1982; **Resid:** Otolaryngology, Mass Eye & Ear Infirm 1988; **Fellow:** Neurotology, Otologic Med Group 1989; **Fac Appt:** Prof Oto, Harvard Med Sch

Metson, Ralph MD [Oto] - **Spec Exp:** Sinus Disorders/Surgery; Facial Plastic Surgery; **Hospital:** Mass Eye & Ear Infirmary; **Address:** Zero Emerson Pl, Ste 2D, Boston, MA 02114; **Phone:** 617-227-4366; **Board Cert:** Otolaryngology 1985; **Med School:** UCSD 1979; **Resid:** Otolaryngology, UCLA Med Ctr 1985; **Fac Appt:** Assoc Clin Prof Oto, Harvard Med Sch

Nadol, Joseph B MD [Oto] - **Spec Exp:** Ear Disorders/Surgery; Hearing Disorders; Cochlear Implants; **Hospital:** Mass Eye & Ear Infirmary; **Address:** Mass Eye & Ear Infirmary, 243 Charles St, Boston, MA 02114-3096; **Phone:** 617-573-3632; **Board Cert:** Otolaryngology 1975; Neurotology 2005; **Med School:** Johns Hopkins Univ 1970; **Resid:** Surgery, Beth Israel Hosp 1972; Otolaryngology, Mass Eye & Ear Infirmary 1975; **Fac Appt:** Prof Oto, Harvard Med Sch

Otolaryngology

Randolph, Gregory W MD [Oto] - **Spec Exp:** Thyroid Disorders; Thyroid Cancer; Parathyroid Disease; **Hospital:** Mass Eye & Ear Infirmary; **Address:** Mass Eye & Ear Infirmary, 243 Charles St Fl 2, Boston, MA 02114; **Phone:** 617-573-4115; **Board Cert:** Otolaryngology 1993; **Med School:** Cornell Univ-Weill Med Coll 1987; **Resid:** Otolaryngology, Mass E&E Infirmary 1992; **Fellow:** Thyroid Oncology, Mass E&E Infirmary 1993; **Fac Appt:** Asst Prof Oto, Harvard Med Sch

Rauch, Steven D MD [Oto] - **Spec Exp:** Hearing & Balance Disorders; Meniere's Disease; Neuro-Otology; **Hospital:** Mass Eye & Ear Infirmary; **Address:** Mass Eye & Ear Infirmary, Dept Otolary, 243 Charles St, Boston, MA 02114; **Phone:** 617-573-3644; **Board Cert:** Otolaryngology 1984; **Med School:** Univ Cincinnati 1979; **Resid:** Surgery, U Mass Med Ctr 1981; Otolaryngology, Mass E&E Infirmary 1984; **Fac Appt:** Assoc Prof Oto, Harvard Med Sch

Sasaki, Clarence T MD [Oto] - **Spec Exp:** Head & Neck Cancer; Skull Base Surgery; Voice Disorders; Swallowing Disorders; **Hospital:** Yale-New Haven Hosp, Hosp of St Raphael; **Address:** Yale Sch Med, Dept Otolaryngology, 333 Cedar St, Box 208041, New Haven, CT 06520-8041; **Phone:** 203-785-2592; **Board Cert:** Otolaryngology 1973; **Med School:** Yale Univ 1966; **Resid:** Surgery, Mary Hitchcock Hosp 1968; Otolaryngology, Yale-New Haven Hosp 1973; **Fellow:** Head and Neck Surgery, Univ of Milan 1978; Skull Base Surgery, Univ Zurich 1982; **Fac Appt:** Prof Oto, Yale Univ

Vining, Eugenia MD [Oto] - **Spec Exp:** Sinus Disorders/Surgery; Skull Base Tumors; Sinus Tumors; **Hospital:** Yale-New Haven Hosp, Hosp of St Raphael; **Address:** 46 Prince St, Ste 601, New Haven, CT 06519; **Phone:** 203-752-1726; **Board Cert:** Otolaryngology 1993; **Med School:** Yale Univ 1987; **Resid:** Otolaryngology, Yale-New Haven Hosp 1991; Otolaryngology, Yale-New Haven Hosp 1992; **Fellow:** Sinus Surgery, Univ Penn Med Ctr 1993

Zeitels, Steven MD [Oto] - **Spec Exp:** Laryngeal Disorders; Voice Disorders; Laryngeal Cancer; Head & Neck Cancer & Surgery; **Hospital:** Mass Genl Hosp; **Address:** Mass Genl Hospital, 1 Bowdoin Square Fl 11, Boston, MA 02114; **Phone:** 617-726-1444; **Board Cert:** Otolaryngology 1988; **Med School:** Boston Univ 1982; **Resid:** Surgery, Univ Hosp-Boston City Hosp 1983; Otolaryngology, Boston Univ-Tufts Univ 1987; **Fellow:** Head and Neck Surgery, Boston VA Med Ctr-Boston Univ 1988; **Fac Appt:** Assoc Prof Oto, Harvard Med Sch

Mid Atlantic

Arriaga, Moises A MD [Oto] - **Spec Exp:** Hearing Loss; Acoustic Neuroma; Balance Disorders; Otology & Neuro-Otology; **Hospital:** Allegheny General Hosp, UPMC Mercy, Pittsburgh; **Address:** 420 E North Ave, Ste 402, Pittsburgh, PA 15212; **Phone:** 412-359-6690; **Board Cert:** Otolaryngology 1990; Neurotology 2004; **Med School:** Brown Univ 1985; **Resid:** Otolaryngology, Univ Pittsburgh Med Ctr 1990; **Fellow:** Neurotology, House Ear Clinic 1991; **Fac Appt:** Assoc Clin Prof Oto, Univ Pittsburgh

Aviv, Jonathan MD [Oto] - **Spec Exp:** Voice Disorders; Swallowing Disorders; Vocal Cord Disorders; Endoscopy; **Hospital:** NY-Presby Hosp/Columbia (page 66); **Address:** 16 E 60th St, Ste 470, New York, NY 10022-1002; **Phone:** 212-326-8475; **Board Cert:** Otolaryngology 1990; **Med School:** Columbia P&S 1985; **Resid:** Surgery, Mount Sinai Med Ctr 1987; Otolaryngology, Mount Sinai Med Ctr 1990; **Fellow:** Otolaryngology, Mount Sinai Med Ctr 1991; **Fac Appt:** Prof Oto, Columbia P&S

Blitzer, Andrew MD/DDS [Oto] - **Spec Exp:** Voice Disorders; Swallowing Disorders; Nasal & Sinus Surgery; Botox Therapy; **Hospital:** NY-Presby Hosp/Columbia (page 66), St Luke's - Roosevelt Hosp Ctr - Roosevelt Div (page 57); **Address:** 425 W 59th St Fl 10, New York, NY 10019-1104; **Phone:** 212-262-9500; **Board Cert:** Otolaryngology 1977; **Med School:** Mount Sinai Sch Med 1973; **Resid:** Surgery, Beth Israel Med Ctr 1974; Otolaryngology, Mount Sinai Hosp 1977; **Fac Appt:** Clin Prof Oto, Columbia P&S

Bolger, William E MD [Oto] - **Spec Exp:** Nasal & Sinus Surgery; Encephalocele; **Hospital:** Suburban Hosp - Bethesda; **Address:** Suburban ENT Associates, 6420 Rockledge Drive, Ste 4200, Bethesda, MD 20817; **Phone:** 301-896-6840; **Board Cert:** Otolaryngology 1992, **Med School:** Uniformed Srvs Univ, Bethesda 1986; **Resid:** Otolaryngology, Willford Hall USAF Med Ctr 1991; **Fellow:** Rhinoplasty, Hosp U Penn 1992; **Fac Appt:** Prof Oto, Uniformed Srvs Univ, Bethesda

Carrau, Ricardo L MD [Oto] - **Spec Exp:** Skull Base Tumors & Surgery; Nasal & Sinus Cancer & Surgery; Swallowing Disorders; **Hospital:** UPMC Presby, Pittsburgh; **Address:** Eye & Ear Institute, 200 Lothrop St, Ste 500, Pittsburgh, PA 15213; **Phone:** 412-647-2100; **Board Cert:** Otolaryngology 1987; **Med School:** Univ Puerto Rico 1981; **Resid:** Surgery, University Hosp 1984; Head and Neck Surgery, University Hosp 1987; **Fellow:** Head and Neck Oncology, Univ Pittsburgh Med Ctr 1990; **Fac Appt:** Assoc Prof Oto, Univ Pittsburgh

Chalian, Ara A MD [Oto] - **Spec Exp:** Head & Neck Cancer; Head & Neck Reconstruction; Thyroid Cancer; Reconstructive Plastic Surgery; **Hospital:** Hosp Univ Penn - UPHS (page 60); **Address:** Hosp Univ Penn, Dept Otolaryngology, 3400 Spruce St, Silverstein Bldg, Philadelphia, PA 19104; **Phone:** 215-349-5559; **Board Cert:** Otolaryngology 1994; **Med School:** Indiana Univ 1988; **Resid:** Surgery, Indiana Univ Hosp 1990; Otolaryngology, Indiana Univ Hosp 1993; **Fellow:** Molecular Biology, Hosp U Penn 1994; Head and Neck Surgery, Hosp U Penn 1995; **Fac Appt:** Assoc Prof Oto, Univ Pennsylvania

Close, Lanny G MD [Oto] - **Spec Exp:** Skull Base Surgery; Head & Neck Cancer; Sinus Disorders/Surgery; Endoscopic Sinus Surgery; **Hospital:** NY-Presby Hosp/Columbia (page 66); **Address:** 16 E 60th St, Ste 470, New York, NY 10022; **Phone:** 212-326-8475; **Board Cert:** Otolaryngology 1977; **Med School:** Baylor Coll Med 1972; **Resid:** Surgery, Johns Hopkins Hosp 1974; Otolaryngology, Baylor Affil Hosps 1977; **Fellow:** Head and Neck Surgery, MD Anderson Cancer Ctr 1979; **Fac Appt:** Prof Oto, Columbia P&S

Costantino, Peter D MD [Oto] - **Spec Exp:** Skull Base Tumors; Head & Neck Cancer; Craniofacial Surgery/Reconstruction; **Hospital:** St Luke's - Roosevelt Hosp Ctr - Roosevelt Div (page 57), NY-Presby Hosp/Columbia (page 66); **Address:** 1000 W 10th Ave, Ste 5G-80, New York, NY 10019-1104; **Phone:** 212-523-6756; **Board Cert:** Otolaryngology 1990; Facial Plastic & Reconstructive Surgery 2000; **Med School:** Northwestern Univ 1984; **Resid:** Surgery, Northwestern Meml Hosp 1986; Otolaryngology, Northwestern Meml Hosp 1989; **Fellow:** Head and Neck Surgery, Northwestern Meml Hosp 1990; Skull Base Surgery, Univ Pittsburgh 1991; **Fac Appt:** Prof Oto, Columbia P&S

Cummings, Charles W MD [Oto] - **Spec Exp:** Head & Neck Cancer & Surgery; Laryngeal Disorders; Laryngeal Cancer; **Hospital:** Johns Hopkins Hosp - Baltimore (page 61); **Address:** Johns Hopkins Outpt Ctr, Otolaryngology, 601 N Caroline St Fl 6, Baltimore, MD 21287; **Phone:** 410-955-7400; **Board Cert:** Otolaryngology 1968; **Med School:** Univ VA Sch Med 1961; **Resid:** Surgery, Univ Virginia Hosp 1965; Otolaryngology, Mass Genl Hosp 1968; **Fac Appt:** Prof Oto, Johns Hopkins Univ

Otolaryngology

Davidson, Bruce J MD [Oto] - **Spec Exp:** Head & Neck Cancer; Thyroid Disorders; **Hospital:** Georgetown Univ Hosp; **Address:** Georgetown Univ Med Ctr, Dept Otolaryngology-Head & Neck Surgery, 3800 Reservoir Rd NW Gorman Bldg Fl 1, Washington, DC 20007; **Phone:** 202-444-8186; **Board Cert:** Otolaryngology 1993; **Med School:** W VA Univ 1987; **Resid:** Otolaryngology, Georgetown Univ Med Ctr 1992; **Fellow:** Otolaryngology, Memorial Sloan-Kettering Cancer Ctr 1994; **Fac Appt:** Asst Prof Oto, Georgetown Univ

Edelstein, David R MD [Oto] - **Spec Exp:** Nasal & Sinus Disorders; Endoscopic Sinus Surgery; Sleep Disorders/Apnea; **Hospital:** Manhattan Eye, Ear & Throat Hosp, Lenox Hill Hosp (page 62); **Address:** 1421 3rd Ave Fl 4, New York, NY 10028; **Phone:** 212-452-1500; **Board Cert:** Otolaryngology 1985; **Med School:** Boston Univ 1980; **Resid:** Otolaryngology, Mount Sinai Hosp 1984; **Fac Appt:** Clin Prof Oto, Cornell Univ-Weill Med Coll

Feghali, Joseph G MD [Oto] - **Spec Exp:** Ear Disorders/Surgery; Acoustic Neuroma; Hearing Disorders; Neuro-Otology; **Hospital:** Montefiore Med Ctr; **Address:** 182 E 210th St, Bronx, NY 10467; **Phone:** 718-881-3277; **Board Cert:** Otolaryngology 1990; **Med School:** Lebanon 1978; **Resid:** Otolaryngology, American Univ Beirut 1982; Otolaryngology, Montefiore Med Ctr 1990; **Fellow:** Otology & Neurotology, House Ear Inst 1983; Neurological Surgery, Meml Sloan Kettering Cancer Ctr 1984; **Fac Appt:** Clin Prof Oto, Albert Einstein Coll Med

Fried, Marvin P MD [Oto] - **Spec Exp:** Endoscopic Sinus Surgery; Head & Neck Tumors; Laryngeal & Voice Disorders; Sinus Disorders/Surgery; **Hospital:** Montefiore Med Ctr, Montefiore Med Ctr - Weiler-Einstein Div; **Address:** 3400 Bainbridge Ave Fl 3, Bronx, NY 10467; **Phone:** 718-920-4646; **Board Cert:** Otolaryngology 1975; **Med School:** Tufts Univ 1969; **Resid:** Surgery, Jewish Hosp 1971; Otolaryngology, Barnes Hosp 1975; **Fellow:** Stroke, Washington Univ 1976; **Fac Appt:** Prof Oto, Albert Einstein Coll Med

Genden, Eric M MD [Oto] - **Spec Exp:** Head & Neck Cancer & Surgery; Head & Neck Cancer Reconstruction; Airway Reconstruction; Thyroid & Parathyroid Cancer & Surgery; **Hospital:** Mount Sinai Med Ctr (page 64); **Address:** Mt Sinai Sch Med Dept Otolar, 1 Gustave L. Levy Pl, Box 1191, New York, NY 10029; **Phone:** 212-241-9410; **Board Cert:** Otolaryngology 1999; Facial Plastic & Reconstructive Surgery 2000; **Med School:** Mount Sinai Sch Med 1992; **Resid:** Otolaryngology, Barnes Jewish Hosp 1998; **Fellow:** Head and Neck Surgery, Mount Sinai Med Ctr 1999; **Fac Appt:** Assoc Prof Oto, Mount Sinai Sch Med

Gold, Scott D MD [Oto] - **Spec Exp:** Endoscopic Sinus Surgery; Sinus Disorders/Surgery; **Hospital:** Beth Israel Med Ctr - Petrie Division (page 57), Mount Sinai Med Ctr (page 64); **Address:** 36A E 36th St, Ste 200, New York, NY 10016-3401; **Phone:** 212-889-8575; **Board Cert:** Otolaryngology 1983; **Med School:** Mount Sinai Sch Med 1979; **Resid:** Otolaryngology, Mount Sinai Med Ctr 1983; **Fac Appt:** Asst Clin Prof Oto, Mount Sinai Sch Med

Grandis, Jennifer R MD [Oto] - **Spec Exp:** Head & Neck Cancer; **Hospital:** UPMC Presby, Pittsburgh, Magee-Womens Hosp - UPMC; **Address:** Univ Pittsburgh Med Ctr EELB, 200 Lothrop St, Ste 500, Pittsburgh, PA 15213; **Phone:** 412-647-5280; **Board Cert:** Otolaryngology 1994; **Med School:** Univ Pittsburgh 1987; **Resid:** Otolaryngology, Univ Pittsburgh Med Ctr 1993; **Fac Appt:** Prof Oto, Univ Pittsburgh

Har-El, Gady MD [Oto] - **Spec Exp:** Head & Neck Cancer; Thyroid & Parathyroid Surgery; Skull Base Surgery; **Hospital:** Lenox Hill Hosp (page 62), Manhattan Eye, Ear & Throat Hosp; **Address:** 186 E 76th St Fl 2, New York, NY 10021; **Phone:** 212-434-2323; **Board Cert:** Otolaryngology 1992; **Med School:** Israel 1982; **Resid:** Otolaryngology, SUNY Downstate Med Ctr 1991; **Fac Appt:** Prof Oto, SUNY Hlth Sci Ctr

Hicks Jr, Wesley L MD/DDS [Oto] - **Spec Exp:** Head & Neck Cancer & Surgery; Reconstructive Surgery; **Hospital:** Roswell Park Cancer Inst; **Address:** Roswell Park Cancer Inst, Head & Neck Surg, Elm & Carlton Sts, Buffalo, NY 14263; **Phone:** 716-845-3158; **Board Cert:** Otolaryngology 1993; **Med School:** SUNY Buffalo 1984; **Resid:** Otolaryngology, Manhattan Eye Ear & Throat Hosp 1988; Otolaryngology, New York Hosp/Meml Sloan Kettering Cancer Ctr 1989; **Fellow:** Head and Neck Surgery, Stanford Univ Med Ctr 1990; **Fac Appt:** Assoc Prof Oto, SUNY Buffalo

Hirsch, Barry MD [Oto] - **Spec Exp:** Hearing Loss; Ear Infections; Ear Tumors; Skull Base Tumors; **Hospital:** UPMC Presby, Pittsburgh; **Address:** 200 Lothrop St, Ste 500, Ear Nose Throat Inst, Dept Otolaryngology, Pittsburgh, PA 15213; **Phone:** 412-647-2100; **Board Cert:** Otolaryngology 1982; Neurotology 2005; **Med School:** Univ Pennsylvania 1977; **Resid:** Otolaryngology, Univ Pittsburgh Med Ctr 1982; **Fellow:** Neurotology, Univ Pittsburgh 1985; Neurotology, Univ Zurich 1986; **Fac Appt:** Prof Oto, Univ Pittsburgh

Holliday, Michael J MD [Oto] - **Spec Exp:** Neuro-Otology; Skull Base Surgery; Otology; **Hospital:** Johns Hopkins Hosp - Baltimore (page 61), Johns Hopkins Bayview Med Ctr (page 61); **Address:** Johns Hopkins Hosp-Otology Division, 601 N Caroline St Fl 6, Baltimore, MD 21287; **Phone:** 410-955-3492; **Board Cert:** Otolaryngology 1976; **Med School:** Marquette Sch Med 1969; **Resid:** Otolaryngology, Johns Hopkins Hosp 1976; **Fellow:** Neurotology, Univ Zurich 1979; **Fac Appt:** Assoc Prof Oto, Johns Hopkins Univ

Hopping, Steven B MD [Oto] - **Spec Exp:** Cosmetic Surgery-Face; Hair Restoration/Transplant; **Hospital:** G Washington Univ Hosp; **Address:** The Center for Cosmetic Surgery, 2440 M St NW, Ste 205, Washington, DC 20037-1449; **Phone:** 202-785-3175; **Board Cert:** Otolaryngology 1980; Facial Plastic & Reconstructive Surgery 1986; Hair Restoration Surgery 1990; **Med School:** Univ Cincinnati 1975; **Resid:** Surgery, George Washington Hosp 1977; Otolaryngology, Maa E&E Infirmary 1980; **Fellow:** Plastic Surgery, Mass E&E Infirmary 1981; **Fac Appt:** Clin Prof S, Geo Wash Univ

Hurst, Michael K MD/DDS [Oto] - **Spec Exp:** Nasal Allergy; Sleep Disorders/Apnea; Thyroid Surgery; **Hospital:** WV Univ Hosp - Ruby Memorial, Monongalia Genl Hosp; **Address:** 1188 Pineview Drive, Morgantown, WV 26505; **Phone:** 304-599-3959; **Board Cert:** Otolaryngology 1994; **Med School:** Marshall Univ 1988; **Resid:** Otolaryngology, Univ West Virginia Hosps 1993; **Fac Appt:** Assoc Prof Oto, W VA Univ

Jacobs, Joseph B MD [Oto] - **Spec Exp:** Endoscopic Sinus Surgery; Sinus Disorders/Surgery; Sinus Surgery-Revision; **Hospital:** NYU Med Ctr (page 68); **Address:** NYU Med Ctr, 530 1st Ave, Ste 3C, New York, NY 10016-6402; **Phone:** 212-263-7398; **Board Cert:** Otolaryngology 1978; **Med School:** Albert Einstein Coll Med 1974; **Resid:** Otolaryngology, NYU Med Ctr 1978; **Fellow:** Plastic Reconstructive Surgery, UCLA Med Ctr 1979; **Fac Appt:** Prof Oto, NYU Sch Med

Johnson, Jonas T MD [Oto] - **Spec Exp:** Head & Neck Surgery; Head & Neck Cancer; Sleep Disorders/Apnea/Snoring; Parotid Gland Tumors; **Hospital:** UPMC Montefiore, UPMC South Side; **Address:** Univ Physicians UPMC, Eye & Ear Inst, 200 Lothrop St, Ste 300, Pittsburgh, PA 15213; **Phone:** 412-647-2100; **Board Cert:** Otolaryngology 1977; **Med School:** SUNY Upstate Med Univ 1972; **Resid:** Surgery, Med Coll Virginia Hosps 1974; Otolaryngology, SUNY-Univ Hosp 1977; **Fac Appt:** Prof Oto, Univ Pittsburgh

Josephson, Jordan S MD [Oto] - **Spec Exp:** Endoscopic Sinus Surgery; Nasal & Sinus Disorders; Sleep Apnea; **Hospital:** Manhattan Eye, Ear & Throat Hosp, Lenox Hill Hosp (page 62); **Address:** 111 E 77th St, New York, NY 10021-1802; **Phone:** 212-717-1773; **Board Cert:** Otolaryngology 1988; **Med School:** SUNY Downstate 1983; **Resid:** Otolaryngology, LI Jewish Med Ctr 1988; **Fellow:** Sinus Surgery, Johns Hopkins Hosp 1989

Otolaryngology

Keane, William M MD [Oto] - **Spec Exp:** Head & Neck Cancer & Surgery; Thyroid Cancer; **Hospital:** Thomas Jefferson Univ Hosp; **Address:** Thomas Jefferson Hosp, 925 Chestnut St Fl 6, Philadelphia, PA 19107; **Phone:** 215-955-6760; **Board Cert:** Otolaryngology 1978; **Med School:** Harvard Med Sch 1970; **Resid:** Surgery, Strong Meml Hosp 1972; Otolaryngology, Univ Penn Hosp 1977; **Fac Appt:** Prof Oto, Thomas Jefferson Univ

Kennedy, David W MD [Oto] - **Spec Exp:** Sinus Disorders/Surgery; Skull Base Tumors & Surgery; Endoscopic Sinus Surgery; Minimally Invasive Transnasal Surgery; **Hospital:** Hosp Univ Penn - UPHS (page 60), Pennsylvania Hosp (page 60); **Address:** Hosp Univ Penn, Dept Oto/Head & Neck Surg, 3400 Spruce St Ravdin Bldg Fl 5, Philadelphia, PA 19104-4229; **Phone:** 215-662-6971; **Board Cert:** Otolaryngology 1978; **Med School:** Ireland 1972; **Resid:** Surgery, Johns Hopkins Hosp 1974; Otolaryngology, Johns Hopkins Hosp 1978; **Fac Appt:** Prof Oto, Univ Pennsylvania

Koch, Wayne Martin MD [Oto] - **Spec Exp:** Head & Neck Cancer; Sinus Tumors; **Hospital:** Johns Hopkins Hosp - Baltimore (page 61); **Address:** Johns Hopkins Hosp, Dept Otolaryngology, 601 N Caroline St, rm 6221, Baltimore, MD 21287; **Phone:** 410-955-4906; **Board Cert:** Otolaryngology 1987; **Med School:** Univ Pittsburgh 1982; **Resid:** Otolaryngology, Tufts-Boston Univ Hosps 1987; **Fellow:** Surgical Oncology, Johns Hopkins Hosp 1989; **Fac Appt:** Assoc Prof Oto, Johns Hopkins Univ

Koufman, Jamie A MD [Oto] - **Spec Exp:** Voice Disorders; Laryngeal Disorders; **Hospital:** New York Eye & Ear Infirm (page 65); **Address:** 200 W 57th St, Ste 1203, New York, NY 10019; **Phone:** 212-463-8014; **Board Cert:** Otolaryngology 1978; **Med School:** Boston Univ 1973; **Resid:** Surgery, Hartford Hosp 1975; Otolaryngology, Boston Univ Med Ctr 1978

Kraus, Dennis H MD [Oto] - **Spec Exp:** Head & Neck Cancer; Skull Base Tumors; Thyroid & Parathyroid Surgery; **Hospital:** Meml Sloan-Kettering Cancer Ctr; **Address:** 1275 York Avenue, New York, NY 10065; **Phone:** 800-525-2225; **Board Cert:** Otolaryngology 1990; **Med School:** Univ Rochester 1985; **Resid:** Surgery, Cleveland Clinic 1987; Otolaryngology, Cleveland Clinic 1990; **Fellow:** Head and Neck Surgery, Meml Sloan Kettering Cancer Ctr 1991; **Fac Appt:** Prof Oto, Cornell Univ-Weill Med Coll

Krespi, Yosef MD [Oto] - **Spec Exp:** Nasal & Sinus Cancer & Surgery; Sleep Disorders/Apnea; Head & Neck Cancer & Surgery; Snoring/Sleep Apnea; **Hospital:** St Luke's - Roosevelt Hosp Ctr - Roosevelt Div (page 57); **Address:** 425 W 59th St Fl 10, New York, NY 10019-1128; **Phone:** 212-262-4444; **Board Cert:** Otolaryngology 1981; **Med School:** Israel 1973; **Resid:** Surgery, Mount Sinai Hosp 1976; Otolaryngology, Mount Sinai Hosp 1980; **Fellow:** Surgery, Northwestern Meml Hosp 1981; **Fac Appt:** Clin Prof Oto, Columbia P&S

Kuhel, William MD [Oto] - **Spec Exp:** Head & Neck Surgery; Thyroid Surgery; Parathyroid Surgery; **Hospital:** NY-Presby Hosp/Weill Cornell (page 66), Hosp For Special Surgery (page 59); **Address:** 1305 York Ave Fl 5, New York, NY 10021; **Phone:** 646-962-6325; **Board Cert:** Otolaryngology 1988; **Med School:** Univ Mich Med Sch 1983; **Resid:** Surgery, St Vincent's Hosp & Med Ctr 1985; Otolaryngology, Indiana Univ 1988; **Fellow:** Head and Neck Surgery, MD Anderson Hosp 1989; **Fac Appt:** Assoc Clin Prof Oto, Cornell Univ-Weill Med Coll

Lalwani, Anil Kumar MD [Oto] - **Spec Exp:** Ear Disorders/Surgery; Facial Nerve Disorders; Pediatric Otolaryngology; Skull Base Surgery; **Hospital:** NYU Med Ctr (page 68); **Address:** 540 1st Ave, Ste 8S, New York, NY 10016; **Phone:** 212-263-7167; **Board Cert:** Otolaryngology 1992; **Med School:** Univ Mich Med Sch 1985; **Resid:** Surgery, Duke Univ Med Ctr 1987; Otolaryngology, UCSF Med Ctr 1991; **Fellow:** Skull Base Surgery, UCSF Med Ctr 1992; **Fac Appt:** Prof Oto, NYU Sch Med

Lawson, William MD [Oto] - **Spec Exp:** Sinus Disorders/Surgery; Cosmetic Surgery-Face; Head & Neck Cancer; Skull Base Surgery; **Hospital:** Mount Sinai Med Ctr (page 64); **Address:** 5 E 98th St Fl 8, Box 1191, New York, NY 10029-6501; **Phone:** 212-241-9410; **Board Cert:** Otolaryngology 1974; **Med School:** NYU Sch Med 1965; **Resid:** Surgery, Bronx VA Hosp 1967; Otolaryngology, Mount Sinai Hosp 1973; **Fellow:** Otolaryngology, Mount Sinai Hosp 1970; **Fac Appt:** Prof Oto, Mount Sinai Sch Med

Linstrom, Christopher MD [Oto] - **Spec Exp:** Cochlear Implants; Acoustic Neuroma; Encephalocele; Cholesteatoma; **Hospital:** New York Eye & Ear Infirm (page 65), St Vincent Cath Med Ctrs - Manhattan; **Address:** NY Eye & Ear Infirmary, Dept Otolaryngology, 310 E 14th St Fl 6, New York, NY 10003-4201; **Phone:** 212-979-4200; **Board Cert:** Otolaryngology 1987; **Med School:** McGill Univ 1982; **Resid:** Surgery, Geo Wash Med Ctr 1984; Otolaryngology, New York Hosp 1987; **Fellow:** Otology & Neurotology, Michigan Ear Inst 1989; **Fac Appt:** Assoc Prof Oto, NY Med Coll

Minor, Lloyd B MD [Oto] - **Spec Exp:** Balance Disorders; Neuro-Otology; Meniere's Disease; **Hospital:** Johns Hopkins Hosp - Baltimore (page 61); **Address:** 601 N Caroline St, rm 6210, Baltimore, MD 21287; **Phone:** 410-955-3403; **Board Cert:** Otolaryngology 1993; Neurotology 2004; **Med School:** Brown Univ 1982; **Resid:** Otolaryngology, Univ Chicago Hosps 1992; **Fellow:** Otolaryngology, Ear Foundation/Baptist Hosp 1993; **Fac Appt:** Prof Oto, Johns Hopkins Univ

Moscatello, Augustine L MD [Oto] - **Spec Exp:** Nasal & Sinus Disorders; Head & Neck Surgery; **Hospital:** Westchester Med Ctr; **Address:** 1055 Sawmill River Rd, Ste 101, Ardsley, NY 10502; **Phone:** 914-693-7636; **Board Cert:** Otolaryngology 1987; **Med School:** Mount Sinai Sch Med 1982; **Resid:** Surgery, Mount Sinai Hosp 1987; Otolaryngology, Mount Sinai Hosp 1987; **Fac Appt:** Assoc Prof Oto, NY Med Coll

Niparko, John MD [Oto] - **Spec Exp:** Ear Disorders/Surgery; Neuro-Otology; **Hospital:** Johns Hopkins Hosp - Baltimore (page 61); **Address:** Johns Hopkins Hosp, Dept Otolaryngology, 601 N Caroline St, rm 6223, Baltimore, MD 21287-0910; **Phone:** 410-955-2689; **Board Cert:** Otolaryngology 1986; Neurotology 2004; **Med School:** Univ Mich Med Sch 1980; **Resid:** Surgery, William Beaumont Hosp 1982; Otolaryngology, Univ Michigan Hosp 1986; **Fellow:** Otolaryngology, Univ Michigan Hosp; **Fac Appt:** Prof Oto, Johns Hopkins Univ

O'Malley Jr, Bert W MD [Oto] - **Spec Exp:** Head & Neck Cancer; Sinus Tumors; Skull Base Tumors; **Hospital:** Hosp Univ Penn - UPHS (page 60); **Address:** Hosp Univ Penn, Dept Otolaryngology, 3400 Spruce St, 5 Ravdin, Philadelphia, PA 19104; **Phone:** 215-615-4325; **Board Cert:** Otolaryngology 1995; **Med School:** Univ Tex SW, Dallas 1988; **Resid:** Surgery, UTSW Med Ctr/Parkland Meml Hosp 1989; Otolaryngology, Baylor Coll Med 1993; **Fellow:** Head and Neck Oncology, Univ Pittsburgh 1994; Skull Base Surgery, Univ Pittsburgh 1995; **Fac Appt:** Prof Oto, Univ Pennsylvania

Papel, Ira D MD [Oto] - **Spec Exp:** Rhinoplasty; Cosmetic Surgery-Face; Reconstructive Surgery-Face; Skin Cancer/Facial Reconstruction; **Hospital:** Greater Baltimore Med Ctr, Johns Hopkins Hosp - Baltimore (page 61); **Address:** 1838 Greene Tree Rd, Ste 370, Baltimore, MD 21208; **Phone:** 410-486-3400; **Board Cert:** Otolaryngology 1986; Facial Plastic & Reconstructive Surgery 1991; **Med School:** Boston Univ 1981; **Resid:** Otolaryngology, Johns Hopkins Hosp 1986; **Fellow:** Facial Plastic Surgery, UCSF Med Ctr 1987; **Fac Appt:** Assoc Prof Oto, Johns Hopkins Univ

Parisier, Simon C MD [Oto] - **Spec Exp:** Cochlear Implants; Hearing Loss; Ear Disorders/Surgery; Cholesteatoma; **Hospital:** New York Eye & Ear Infirm (page 65), Beth Israel Med Ctr - Petrie Division (page 57); **Address:** NY Eye & Ear Infirmary - Otolaryngology, 310 E 14th St, 6th Fl - Window 5, New York, NY 10003-4297; **Phone:** 212-979-4542; **Board Cert:** Otolaryngology 1967; **Med School:** Boston Univ 1961; **Resid:** Otolaryngology, Mount Sinai Hosp 1966; **Fac Appt:** Prof Oto, NY Med Coll

Otolaryngology

Persky, Mark S MD [Oto] - **Spec Exp:** Head & Neck Cancer; Skull Base Tumors; Thyroid Cancer; **Hospital:** Beth Israel Med Ctr - Petrie Division (page 57); **Address:** 10 Union Square East, Ste 4J, New York, NY 10003; **Phone:** 212-844-8648; **Board Cert:** Otolaryngology 1976; **Med School:** SUNY Upstate Med Univ 1972; **Resid:** Otolaryngology, Bellevue Hosp 1976; **Fellow:** Head and Neck Surgery, Beth Israel Med Ctr 1977; **Fac Appt:** Clin Prof Oto, Albert Einstein Coll Med

Picken, Catherine A MD [Oto] - **Spec Exp:** Head & Neck Reconstruction; Thyroid Disorders; Sinus Disorders/Surgery; **Hospital:** Georgetown Univ Hosp; **Address:** 2021 K St, Ste 206, Washington, DC 20006; **Phone:** 202-785-5000; **Board Cert:** Otolaryngology 1989; **Med School:** Northwestern Univ 1979; **Resid:** Surgery, Natl Heart Lung Blood Inst 1983; Otolaryngology, Georgetown Univ Hosp 1989; **Fac Appt:** Assoc Prof Oto, Georgetown Univ

Quatela, Vito C MD [Oto] - **Spec Exp:** Facial Plastic Surgery; Rhinoplasty; **Hospital:** Univ of Rochester Strong Meml Hosp, Rochester Genl Hosp; **Address:** 973 East Ave, Ste 100, Rochester, NY 14607; **Phone:** 585-244-1000; **Board Cert:** Otolaryngology 1985; Facial Plastic & Reconstructive Surgery 1991; **Med School:** Northwestern Univ 1979; **Resid:** Surgery, Med Ctr Hosp Vermont 1981; Otolaryngology, Northwestern Univ Hosp 1985; **Fellow:** Facial Plastic Surgery, Tulane Univ 1986; Facial Plastic Surgery, Oregon Hlth Science Univ 1987; **Fac Appt:** Assoc Clin Prof Oto, Univ Rochester

Rassekh, Christopher MD [Oto] - **Spec Exp:** Laryngeal Cancer-Organ Preservation; Skull Base Tumors; Salivary Gland Tumors & Surgery; **Hospital:** WV Univ Hosp - Ruby Memorial, Monongalia Genl Hosp; **Address:** West Virginia Univ, Dept Otolaryngology, Robin C Byrd Hlth Scis Ctr, Head & Neck Surgery, PO Box 9200, Morgantown, WV 26506-9200; **Phone:** 304-293-3233; **Board Cert:** Otolaryngology 1993; **Med School:** Univ Iowa Coll Med 1986; **Resid:** Otolaryngology, U Iowa Med Ctr 1992; **Fellow:** Head and Neck Surgery, U Pittsburgh Med Ctr 1993; **Fac Appt:** Assoc Prof Oto, W VA Univ

Rosen, Clark A MD [Oto] - **Spec Exp:** Voice Disorders; **Hospital:** UPMC Presby, Pittsburgh; **Address:** UPMC The Voice Ctr, 200 Lothrop St, Ste 214, Pittsburgh, PA 15213; **Phone:** 412-647-7464; **Board Cert:** Otolaryngology 1995; **Med School:** Rush Med Coll 1989; **Resid:** Otolaryngology, Oregon Hlth Sci Univ 1994; **Fellow:** Otolaryngology, Univ Tenn Med Ctr 1995; **Fac Appt:** Assoc Prof Oto, Univ Pittsburgh

Sataloff, Robert T MD [Oto] - **Spec Exp:** Neuro-Otology; Voice Disorders; Laryngeal Disorders; Throat Disorders; **Hospital:** Hahnemann Univ Hosp, Thomas Jefferson Univ Hosp; **Address:** 1721 Pine Street, Philadelphia, PA 19103-6701; **Phone:** 215-545-3322; **Board Cert:** Otolaryngology 1980; **Med School:** Jefferson Med Coll 1975; **Resid:** Otolaryngology, Univ Mich Hosp 1980; **Fellow:** Neurotology, Univ Mich Hosp 1981; **Fac Appt:** Prof Oto, Drexel Univ Coll Med

Schaefer, Steven D MD [Oto] - **Spec Exp:** Sinus Disorders/Surgery; Head & Neck Surgery; Endoscopic Sinus Surgery; **Hospital:** New York Eye & Ear Infirm (page 65), Beth Israel Med Ctr - Petrie Division (page 57); **Address:** NY Eye & Ear Infirm, Dept Otolaryngology, 310 E 14th St, New York, NY 10003-4201; **Phone:** 212-979-4200; **Board Cert:** Otolaryngology 1978; **Med School:** UC Irvine 1972; **Resid:** Surgery, UCLA Med Ctr 1974; Otolaryngology, Stanford Med Ctr 1977; **Fac Appt:** Prof Oto, NY Med Coll

Schantz, Stimson P MD [Oto] - **Spec Exp:** Head & Neck Surgery; Head & Neck Cancer; Thyroid Cancer; **Hospital:** New York Eye & Ear Infirm (page 65), Beth Israel Med Ctr - Petrie Division (page 57); **Address:** 310 E 14th St Fl 6N, New York, NY 10003; **Phone:** 212-979-4535; **Board Cert:** Surgery 2005; **Med School:** Univ Cincinnati 1975; **Resid:** Surgery, Georgetown Univ Med Ctr 1982; Otolaryngology, Univ Illinois Eye & Ear Infirm 1980; **Fellow:** Surgical Oncology, MD Anderson Cancer Ctr 1984; **Fac Appt:** Prof Oto, NY Med Coll

Schley, W Shain MD [Oto] - **Spec Exp:** Nasal & Sinus Disorders; Throat Disorders; Voice Disorders; Ear Disorders; **Hospital:** NY-Presby Hosp/Weill Cornell (page 66); **Address:** 449 E 68th St Fl 2 - Ste DS 10, New York, NY 10021-6310; **Phone:** 212-746-2223; **Board Cert:** Otolaryngology 1973; **Med School:** Emory Univ 1966; **Resid:** Surgery, St Luke's-Roosevelt Hosp Ctr 1968; Otolaryngology, New York Hosp 1973; **Fac Appt:** Assoc Clin Prof Oto, Cornell Univ-Weill Med Coll

Setzen, Michael MD [Oto] - **Spec Exp:** Nasal & Sinus Surgery; Rhinoplasty; Sleep Disorders/Apnea; Snoring/Sleep Apnea; **Hospital:** N Shore Univ Hosp, St Francis Hosp - The Heart Ctr (page 72); **Address:** 333 E Shore Rd, Ste 102, Manhasset, NY 11030-2900; **Phone:** 516-482-8778; **Board Cert:** Otolaryngology 1982; **Med School:** South Africa 1974; **Resid:** Surgery, Cleveland Clinic Fdn 1978; Otolaryngology, Barnes Jewish Hosp 1982; **Fac Appt:** Assoc Clin Prof Oto, NYU Sch Med

Shapshay, Stanley M MD [Oto] - **Spec Exp:** Laryngeal Cancer; Vocal Cord Disorders; **Hospital:** Albany Med Ctr; **Address:** University Ear, Nose & Throat Ctr, 35 Hackett Blvd, Albany, NY 12208-3420; **Phone:** 518-262-5575; **Board Cert:** Otolaryngology 1975; **Med School:** Med Coll VA 1968; **Resid:** Surgery, New England Med Ctr 1971; Otolaryngology, Boston Med Ctr 1975; **Fellow:** Surgery, Serafimer Hosp/Karolinska Med Sch 1972; **Fac Appt:** Prof Oto, Albany Med Coll

Shindo, Maisie L MD [Oto] - **Spec Exp:** Head & Neck Cancer & Surgery; Thyroid Cancer; Laryngeal Cancer; Parathyroid Cancer; **Hospital:** Stony Brook Univ Med Ctr; **Address:** Stony Brook Univ Hosp, HSC T19-064, Stony Brook, NY 11794-8191; **Phone:** 631-444-8410; **Board Cert:** Otolaryngology 1989; **Med School:** Univ Saskatchewan 1984; **Resid:** Otolaryngology, LAC-USC Med Ctr 1989; **Fellow:** Head and Neck Surgery, Northwestern Univ 1991; **Fac Appt:** Assoc Prof Oto, SUNY Stony Brook

Snyderman, Carl H MD [Oto] - **Spec Exp:** Skull Base Tumors & Surgery; Sinus Tumors; Head & Neck Cancer; Endoscopic Surgery; **Hospital:** UPMC Presby, Pittsburgh; **Address:** Eye Ear Inst, Dept of Otolaryngology, 200 Lothrop St, Ste 500, Pittsburgh, PA 15213; **Phone:** 412-647-2100; **Board Cert:** Otolaryngology 1987; **Med School:** Univ Chicago-Pritzker Sch Med 1982; **Resid:** Otolaryngology, Eye-Ear Hosp/Univ Pittsburgh 1987; **Fellow:** Skull Base Surgery, Eye-Ear Hosp/Univ Pittsburgh 1988; **Fac Appt:** Prof Oto, Univ Pittsburgh

Stewart, Michael G MD [Oto] - **Spec Exp:** Nasal & Sinus Disorders; Sleep Disorders/Apnea; Head & Neck Surgery; **Hospital:** NY-Presby Hosp/Weill Cornell (page 66); **Address:** Weill Cornell Physicians, 1305 York Ave Fl 5th, New York, NY 10011; **Phone:** 646-962-6673; **Board Cert:** Otolaryngology 1995; **Med School:** Johns Hopkins Univ 1988; **Resid:** Otolaryngology, Baylor Coll Med 1993; **Fac Appt:** Prof Oto, Cornell Univ-Weill Med Coll

Strome, Marshall MD [Oto] - **Spec Exp:** Sleep Disorders/Apnea; Voice Disorders; Head & Neck Cancer; Swallowing Disorders; **Hospital:** St Luke's - Roosevelt Hosp Ctr - St Luke's Hosp (page 57); **Address:** 110 E 59th St, Ste 10A, New York, NY 10022; **Phone:** 212-223-1333; **Board Cert:** Otolaryngology 1970; **Med School:** Univ Mich Med Sch 1964; **Resid:** Surgery, Harper Hosp 1966; Otolaryngology, Univ Michigan Hosp 1970; **Fac Appt:** Prof Oto

Strome, Scott MD [Oto] - **Spec Exp:** Microvascular Surgery; Head & Neck Cancer; Head & Neck Reconstruction; **Hospital:** Univ of MD Med Sys; **Address:** 16 S Eutaw St, Ste 500, Baltimore, MD 21201; **Phone:** 410-328-6467; **Board Cert:** Otolaryngology 1998; **Med School:** Harvard Med Sch 1991; **Resid:** Otolaryngology, Univ Michigan 1997; **Fellow:** Head and Neck Surgery, Allegheny Genl Hosp 1998; Microvascular Surgery, Allegheny Genl Hosp 1998; **Fac Appt:** Prof Oto, Univ MD Sch Med

Otolaryngology

Sulica, Radu Lucian MD [Oto] - **Spec Exp:** Laryngeal & Vocal Cord Surgery; Voice Disorders; Vocal Cord Disorders; Botox Therapy; **Hospital:** NY-Presby Hosp/Weill Cornell (page 66); **Address:** Weill Cornell Otorhinolaryngology, 1305 York Ave Fl 5, New York, NY 10021; **Phone:** 646-962-4734; **Board Cert:** Otolaryngology 2000; **Med School:** Georgetown Univ 1993; **Resid:** Surgery, Georgetown Univ Hosp 1995; Otolaryngology, Georgetown Univ Hosp 1999; **Fellow:** Laryngology, Roosevelt-St. Lukes 2000; **Fac Appt:** Assoc Prof Oto, Cornell Univ-Weill Med Coll

Urken, Mark MD [Oto] - **Spec Exp:** Head & Neck Cancer & Surgery; Head & Neck Cancer Reconstruction; Thyroid & Parathyroid Cancer & Surgery; Salivary Gland Tumors & Surgery; **Hospital:** Beth Israel Med Ctr - Petrie Division (page 57); **Address:** Inst for Head, Neck & Thyroid Cancer, 10 Union Square E, Ste 5B, New York, NY 10003-3314; **Phone:** 212-844-8775; **Board Cert:** Otolaryngology 1986; **Med School:** Univ VA Sch Med 1981; **Resid:** Otolaryngology, Mount Sinai Hosp 1986; **Fellow:** Microvascular Surgery, Mercy Hosp 1987; **Fac Appt:** Prof Oto, Albert Einstein Coll Med

Waner, Milton MD [Oto] - **Spec Exp:** Pediatric Facial Plastic Surgery; Hemangiomas/Birthmarks; Vascular Malformations; **Hospital:** St Luke's - Roosevelt Hosp Ctr - St Luke's Hosp (page 57), Beth Israel Med Ctr - Petrie Division (page 57); **Address:** Vascular Birthmark Institute, 126 W 60th St, New York, NY 10023; **Phone:** 212-636-3970; **Med School:** South Africa 1977; **Resid:** Surgery, Univ of Witwatersrand 1980; Otolaryngology, Univ of Witwatersrand 1984; **Fellow:** Otolaryngology, Univ Cincinnatti Med Ctr 1985

Weinstein, Gregory MD [Oto] - **Spec Exp:** Head & Neck Cancer; Laryngeal Cancer; **Hospital:** Hosp Univ Penn - UPHS (page 60); **Address:** Hosp Univ Penn, Dept Otolaryngology, 3400 Spruce St, 5 Ravdin, Philadelphia, PA 19104; **Phone:** 215-349-5390; **Board Cert:** Otolaryngology 1990; **Med School:** NY Med Coll 1985; **Resid:** Otolaryngology, Univ Iowa Hosp 1990; **Fellow:** Head and Neck Oncology, UC Davis Med Ctr 1991; **Fac Appt:** Assoc Prof Oto, Univ Pennsylvania

Woo, Peak MD [Oto] - **Spec Exp:** Voice Disorders; Laryngeal Disorders; Laryngeal Cancer; **Hospital:** Mount Sinai Med Ctr (page 64); **Address:** 5 E 98th St Fl 1, Box 1653, New York, NY 10029-6501; **Phone:** 212-241-9425; **Board Cert:** Otolaryngology 1983; **Med School:** Boston Univ 1978; **Resid:** Otolaryngology, Boston Univ Med Ctr 1983; **Fac Appt:** Prof Oto, Mount Sinai Sch Med

Zalzal, George MD [Oto] - **Spec Exp:** Airway Disorders; Laryngeal & Tracheal Disorders; Ear Disorders/Surgery; **Hospital:** Chldns Natl Med Ctr; **Address:** Childrens Natl Med Ctr, Dept Otolaryngology, 111 Michigan Ave NW Fl 1 - rm 1000, Washington, DC 20010; **Phone:** 202-476-2159; **Board Cert:** Otolaryngology 1996; **Med School:** Lebanon 1979; **Resid:** Otolaryngology, American Univ Hosp 1983; **Fellow:** Pediatric Otolaryngology, Univ Cincinnati 1985; **Fac Appt:** Prof Ped, Geo Wash Univ

Southeast

Balkany, Thomas Jay MD [Oto] - **Spec Exp:** Ear Disorders/Surgery; Neuro-Otology; Cochlear Implants; Hearing Loss; **Hospital:** Bascom Palmer Eye Inst (page 55), Jackson Meml Hosp; **Address:** PO Box 016960, Miami, FL 33101; **Phone:** 305-585-7129; **Board Cert:** Otolaryngology 1977; **Med School:** Univ Miami Sch Med 1972; **Resid:** Surgery, St Joseph Hosp 1974; Otolaryngology, Colo Med Ctr 1977; **Fellow:** Otology & Neurotology, House Ear Inst; **Fac Appt:** Clin Prof Oto, Univ Miami Sch Med

Becker, Ferdinand F MD [Oto] - **Spec Exp:** Cosmetic Surgery-Face; **Hospital:** Indian River Mem Hosp; **Address:** 5070 N A1A, Ste A, Vero Beach, FL 32963-1229; **Phone:** 772-234-3700; **Board Cert:** Otolaryngology 1972; **Med School:** Tulane Univ 1965; **Resid:** Surgery, Charity Hosp 1969; Otolaryngology, Charity Hosp 1972; **Fac Appt:** Asst Clin Prof Oto, Univ Fla Coll Med

Bumpous, Jeffrey MD [Oto] - **Spec Exp:** Head & Neck Cancer; Head & Neck Reconstruction; Thyroid & Parathyroid Cancer & Surgery; **Hospital:** Univ of Louisville Hosp, Norton Hosp; **Address:** 601 S Floyd St, Ste 700, Louisville, KY 40202-1845; **Phone:** 502-583-8303; **Board Cert:** Otolaryngology 1994; **Med School:** Univ Louisville Sch Med 1988; **Resid:** Otolaryngology, Univ Louisville Hosp 1993; **Fellow:** Head and Neck Surgery, Univ Pittsburgh 1994; **Fac Appt:** Prof Oto, Univ Louisville Sch Med

Burkey, Brian MD [Oto] - **Spec Exp:** Parotid Gland Tumors; Head & Neck Cancer; Reconstructive Microvascular Surgery; **Hospital:** Vanderbilt Univ Med Ctr, Saint Thomas Hosp - Nashville; **Address:** Vanderbilt Univ, Dept Otolaryngology, 1215 21st Ave South, 7209 MCE-South Tower, Nashville, TN 37232-0014; **Phone:** 615-322-6180; **Board Cert:** Otolaryngology 1992; **Med School:** Univ VA Sch Med 1986; **Resid:** Otolaryngology, Univ Mich Med Ctr 1991; **Fellow:** Microsurgery, Ohio State Univ 1991; **Fac Appt:** Assoc Prof Oto, Vanderbilt Univ

Cassisi, Nicholas J MD [Oto] - **Spec Exp:** Head & Neck Cancer; Voice Disorders; **Hospital:** Shands at Univ of FL; **Address:** Shands Healthcare at Univ FL, 1600 SW Archer Rd, Box 100383, Gainesville, FL 32610; **Phone:** 352-265-8989; **Board Cert:** Otolaryngology 1971; **Med School:** Univ Miami Sch Med 1965; **Resid:** Surgery, Jackson Memorial Hosp 1967; Otolaryngology, Barnes Hosp - Washington U 1971; **Fac Appt:** Prof Oto, Univ Fla Coll Med

Civantos, Francisco J MD [Oto] - **Spec Exp:** Head & Neck Cancer; **Hospital:** Univ of Miami Hosp & Clins/Sylvester Comp Canc Ctr; **Address:** Sylvester CAncer Ctr, Otolaryngology, 1475 NW 12th Ave, Ste 4027, Miami, FL 33136; **Phone:** 205-243-5276; **Board Cert:** Otolaryngology 1992; **Med School:** Columbia P&S 1986; **Resid:** Otolaryngology, Univ Illinois Coll Med 1991; **Fellow:** Head and Neck Oncology, Vanderbilt Univ 1992; **Fac Appt:** Assoc Prof Oto, Univ Miami Sch Med

Couch, Marion E MD [Oto] - **Spec Exp:** Head & Neck Cancer; Thyroid Cancer; **Hospital:** Univ NC Hosps; **Address:** Univ N Carolina Sch Med, Dept Otolaryngology, CB 7070, Chapel Hill, NC 27599-7070; **Phone:** 919-966-3342; **Board Cert:** Otolaryngology 1997; **Med School:** Rush Med Coll 1990; **Resid:** Surgery, Johns Hopkins Hosp 1991; Otolaryngology, Johns Hopkins Hosp 1995; **Fac Appt:** Asst Prof Oto, Univ NC Sch Med

Day, Terrence A MD [Oto] - **Spec Exp:** Head & Neck Cancer; Reconstructive Microvascular Surgery; Skull Base Surgery; Facial Plastic & Reconstructive Surgery; **Hospital:** MUSC Med Ctr; **Address:** MUSC, Dept Otolaryngology, 135 Rutledge Ave, Ste 1130, Box MSC550, Charleston, SC 29425; **Phone:** 843-792-0719; **Board Cert:** Otolaryngology 1996; **Med School:** Univ Okla Coll Med 1989; **Resid:** Otolaryngology, LSU Med Ctr 1995; **Fellow:** Head & Neck Surgical Oncology, UC Davis Med Ctr 1996; Maxillofacial Surgery, Univ Hosp 1994; **Fac Appt:** Assoc Prof Oto, Med Univ SC

Farrior, Edward MD [Oto] - **Spec Exp:** Rhinoplasty; Ear Reshaping (Otoplasty); Facial Plastic Surgery; **Hospital:** Tampa Genl Hosp; **Address:** 2908 W Azeele St, Tampa, FL 33609-3109; **Phone:** 813-875-3223; **Board Cert:** Otolaryngology 1987; Facial Plastic & Reconstructive Surgery 1992; **Med School:** Univ VA Sch Med 1982; **Resid:** Otolaryngology, Univ Mich Hosps 1987; **Fellow:** Facial Plastic & Reconstructive Surgery, Tampa Genl Hosp 1988; **Fac Appt:** Assoc Clin Prof S, Univ S Fla Coll Med

Farrior, Joseph Brown MD [Oto] - **Spec Exp:** Otosclerosis/Stapedectomy; Hearing Loss; Meniere's Disease; Otology; **Hospital:** St Joseph's Hosp - Tampa, Tampa Genl Hosp; **Address:** Farrior Ear Clinic, 2727 Martin Luther King Jr Blvd, Ste 520, Tampa, FL 33607; **Phone:** 800-342-3277; **Board Cert:** Otolaryngology 1981; **Med School:** Emory Univ 1975; **Resid:** Surgery, Johns Hopkins Hosp 1977; Otolaryngology, Johns Hopkins Hosp 1981; **Fellow:** Otolaryngology, Farrior Clin/St Josephs Hosp 1980; **Fac Appt:** Assoc Clin Prof Oto, Univ S Fla Coll Med

Otolaryngology

Goodwin, W Jarrard MD [Oto] - **Spec Exp:** Head & Neck Cancer; **Hospital:** Univ of Miami Hosp & Clins/Sylvester Comp Canc Ctr, Jackson Meml Hosp; **Address:** Dept Otolaryngology, 1475 NW 12th Ave, Ste 4037, Miami, FL 33136-1015; **Phone:** 305-243-4387; **Board Cert:** Otolaryngology 1978; **Med School:** Albany Med Coll 1972; **Resid:** Surgery, Univ Miami/Jackson Hosp Meml Hosp 1973; Otolaryngology, Univ Miami/Jackson Hosp 1977; **Fellow:** Head & Neck Surgical Oncology, MD Anderson Hosp 1980; **Fac Appt:** Prof Oto, Univ Miami Sch Med

Kesser, Bradley W MD [Oto] - **Spec Exp:** Aural Atresia Repair; Neurotology; **Hospital:** Univ Virginia Med Ctr; **Address:** Univ VA Dept Otolaryngology, PO Box 800713, Charlottesville, VA 22908; **Phone:** 434-924-2040; **Board Cert:** Otolaryngology 1999; **Med School:** Univ VA Sch Med 1993; **Resid:** Otolaryngology, Univ Va Med Ctr 1998; **Fellow:** Otology & Neurotology, House Ear Clinic 2000; **Fac Appt:** Asst Prof Oto, Univ VA Sch Med

Kuhn, Frederick MD [Oto] - **Spec Exp:** Endoscopic Sinus Surgery; Allergic Fungal Sinusitis; Rhinoplasty Revision; **Hospital:** Meml Hlth Univ Med Ctr - Savannah, St Joseph's-Candler Hosp; **Address:** Georgia Nasal & Sinus Inst, 4750 Waters Ave, Ste 112, Savannah, GA 31404; **Phone:** 912-355-1070; **Board Cert:** Otolaryngology 1972; **Med School:** Univ Okla Coll Med 1966; **Resid:** Surgery, Univ Oklahoma Hosp 1967; Surgery, St Lukes Hosp 1968; **Fellow:** Otolaryngology, Barnes Hosp/Wash Univ 1972

Lambert, Paul R MD [Oto] - **Spec Exp:** Neuro-Otology; Acoustic Neuroma; **Hospital:** MUSC Med Ctr; **Address:** MUSC, Dept Otolaryngology, 135 Rutledge Ave, Box 250550, Charleston, SC 29425; **Phone:** 843-792-3531; **Board Cert:** Otolaryngology 1981; Neurotology 2004; **Med School:** Duke Univ 1976; **Resid:** Surgery, UCLA Med Ctr 1978; Otolaryngology, UCLA Med Ctr 1981; **Fellow:** Neurotology, Otologic Med Group 1982; **Fac Appt:** Prof Oto, Med Univ SC

Lanza, Donald C MD [Oto] - **Spec Exp:** Skull Base Tumors; Sinus Disorders/Surgery; Rhinitis; Graves' Disease-Eye; **Hospital:** St Anthony's Hosp - St Petersburg, All Children's Hosp; **Address:** 900 Carillon Pkwy, Ste 200, St. Petersburg, FL 33716-1108; **Phone:** 727-573-0074; **Board Cert:** Otolaryngology 1990; **Med School:** SUNY Hlth Sci Ctr 1985; **Resid:** Surgery, Albany Med Ctr 1987; Otolaryngology, Albany Med Ctr 1990; **Fellow:** Rhinology, Johns Hopkins Univ 1990; Rhinology, Univ Penn 1991

Levine, Paul A MD [Oto] - **Spec Exp:** Head & Neck Cancer; Head & Neck Reconstruction; Skull Base Tumors; **Hospital:** Univ Virginia Med Ctr; **Address:** Dept Otolaryngology, PO Box 800713, Charlottesville, VA 22908; **Phone:** 434-924-5593; **Board Cert:** Otolaryngology 1978; **Med School:** Albany Med Coll 1973; **Resid:** Otolaryngology, Yale-New Haven Hosp 1977; **Fellow:** Head and Neck Surgery, Stanford Med Ctr 1978; **Fac Appt:** Prof Oto, Univ VA Sch Med

Mangat, Devinder S MD [Oto] - **Spec Exp:** Cosmetic & Reconstructive Surgery-Face; **Hospital:** St Elizabeth Med Ctr (South Unit); **Address:** 133 Barnwood Drive, Edgewood, KY 41017; **Phone:** 859-331-9600; **Board Cert:** Otolaryngology 1978; Facial Plastic & Reconstructive Surgery 1991; **Med School:** Univ KY Coll Med 1973; **Resid:** Surgery, Univ Ky Med Ctr 1975; Otolaryngology, Univ Okla Hlth Scis Ctr 1978; **Fellow:** Facial Plastic Surgery, McCullough Clinic 1979; **Fac Appt:** Assoc Prof Oto, Univ Cincinnati

Mattox, Douglas MD [Oto] - **Spec Exp:** Neuro-Otology; Ear Tumors; Skull Base Surgery; **Hospital:** Emory Univ Hosp, Chldns Hlthcare Atlanta - Scottish Rite; **Address:** Emory Univ Hospital, Dept Otolaryngology, 1365 Clifton Rd NE A Bldg - Ste 2100, Atlanta, GA 30322; **Phone:** 404-778-3381; **Board Cert:** Otolaryngology 1977; Neurotology 2004; **Med School:** Yale Univ 1973; **Resid:** Otolaryngology, Stanford Univ Hosp 1977; **Fellow:** Neurotology, Ugo Fisch, MD 1985; **Fac Appt:** Prof Oto, Emory Univ

McCaffrey, Thomas MD [Oto] - **Spec Exp:** Head & Neck Cancer; Thyroid Cancer; Tracheal Surgery; **Hospital:** H Lee Moffitt Cancer Ctr & Research Inst, Tampa Genl Hosp; **Address:** H Lee Moffitt Cancer Ctr, Dept Otolaryngology-HNS, 12902 Magnolia Drive, Tampa, FL 33612; **Phone:** 813-745-8463; **Board Cert:** Otolaryngology 1980; **Med School:** Loyola Univ-Stritch Sch Med 1974; **Resid:** Surgery, Mayo Grad Sch Med 1976; Otolaryngology, Mayo Grad Med 1980; **Fac Appt:** Prof Oto, Univ S Fla Coll Med

Netterville, James L MD [Oto] - **Spec Exp:** Head & Neck Surgery; Head & Neck Cancer; Vocal Cord Disorders; Skull Base Tumors; **Hospital:** Vanderbilt Univ Med Ctr, Vanderbilt Children's Hosp; **Address:** Vanderbilt Univ Med Ctr, Dept Oto, 7209 Med Ctr East, South Twr, 1215 21st Ave S, Nashville, TN 37232-8605; **Phone:** 615-343-8840; **Board Cert:** Otolaryngology 1985; **Med School:** Univ Tenn Coll Med, Memphis 1980; **Resid:** Surgery, Methodist Hosp 1982; Otolaryngology, Univ Tenn Med Ctr 1985; **Fellow:** Surgical Oncology, Univ Iowa 1986; **Fac Appt:** Prof Oto, Vanderbilt Univ

Osguthorpe, John D MD [Oto] - **Spec Exp:** Head & Neck Cancer; Thyroid & Parathyroid Cancer & Surgery; Nasal & Sinus Disorders; Salivary Gland Tumors & Surgery; **Hospital:** MUSC Med Ctr; **Address:** MUSC Med Ctr-Dept Otolaryngology, 135 Rutledge Ave, Ste 1130, Box 250550, Charleston, SC 29425; **Phone:** 843-792-3533; **Board Cert:** Otolaryngology 1978; **Med School:** Univ Utah 1973; **Resid:** Surgery, UCLA Med Ctr 1975; Otolaryngology, UCLA Med Ctr 1978; **Fellow:** Skull Base Surgery, Univ Zurich 1989; **Fac Appt:** Prof Oto, Med Univ SC

Peters, Glenn E MD [Oto] - **Spec Exp:** Head & Neck Cancer & Surgery; Skull Base Surgery; Thyroid & Parathyroid Cancer & Surgery; **Hospital:** Univ of Ala Hosp at Birmingham; **Address:** UAB Med Ctr, Div of Head & Neck Surgery, 1530 3rd Ave S, BDB 563 Ave S, Birmingham, AL 35294-0012; **Phone:** 205-934-9777; **Board Cert:** Otolaryngology 1985; **Med School:** Louisiana State U, New Orleans 1980; **Resid:** Surgery, Baptist Med Ctr 1982; Otolaryngology, Univ Alabama Hosp 1984; **Fellow:** Head & Neck Surgical Oncology, Johns Hopkins Hosp 1987; **Fac Appt:** Prof S, Univ Ala

Pillsbury, Harold C MD [Oto] - **Spec Exp:** Cochlear Implants; Neuro-Otology; Ear Disorders/Surgery; **Hospital:** Univ NC Hosps; **Address:** 170 Manning Drive, Physicians Bldg, Box CB 7070, Chapel Hill, NC 27599-7070; **Phone:** 919-966-8926; **Board Cert:** Otolaryngology 1978; Neurotology 2004; **Med School:** Geo Wash Univ 1972; **Resid:** Surgery, Univ NC Hosp 1973; Otolaryngology, NC Meml Hosp 1976; **Fac Appt:** Prof Oto, Univ NC Sch Med

Pitman, Karen MD [Oto] - **Spec Exp:** Head & Neck Cancer & Surgery; Thyroid & Parathyroid Cancer & Surgery; Sentinel Node Surgery; **Hospital:** Univ Hosps & Clins - Jackson; **Address:** Univ Mississippi Med Ctr, 2500 N State St, Jackson, MS 39216; **Phone:** 601-984-5160; **Board Cert:** Otolaryngology 1995; **Med School:** Uniformed Srvs Univ, Bethesda 1987; **Resid:** Otolaryngology, Naval Med Ctr 1994; **Fellow:** Head and Neck Oncology, Univ Pittsburgh 1996; **Fac Appt:** Prof Oto, Univ Miss

Poole, Michael D MD/PhD [Oto] - **Spec Exp:** Pediatric Otolaryngology; Ear Infections; Sleep Disorders/Apnea; Sinus Disorders; **Hospital:** Meml Hlth Univ Med Ctr - Savannah, St Joseph's-Candler Hosp; **Address:** Georgia Ear Institute, 4700 Waters Ave, Savannah, GA 31404; **Phone:** 912-356-1515; **Board Cert:** Otolaryngology 1986; **Med School:** Univ NC Sch Med 1981; **Resid:** Otolaryngology, NC Meml Hosp 1986; **Fac Appt:** Prof Oto, Mercer Univ Sch Med

Postma, Gregory N MD [Oto] - **Spec Exp:** Voice Disorders; **Hospital:** Med Coll of GA Hosp and Clin; **Address:** Med Coll Georgia, Voice & Swallowing Center, 1120 15th St, BP-4109, Augusta, GA 30912; **Phone:** 706-721-6100; **Board Cert:** Otolaryngology 1994; **Med School:** Hahnemann Univ 1984; **Resid:** Otolaryngology, Oakland Naval Hosp 1992; Otolaryngology, Univ N Carolina Hosps 1993; **Fellow:** Otolaryngology, Vanderbilt Univ 1996; **Fac Appt:** Prof Oto, Med Coll GA

Otolaryngology

Senior, Brent A MD [Oto] - **Spec Exp:** Sinus Disorders/Surgery; Nasal Allergy; Sleep Disorders; **Hospital:** Univ NC Hosps; **Address:** UNC-Chapel Hill, Dept Oto-H&N Surg, 610 Burnett-Womack, CB 7070, Chapel Hill, NC 27599-0001; **Phone:** 919-966-6483; **Board Cert:** Otolaryngology 1996; **Med School:** Univ Mich Med Sch 1990; **Resid:** Otolaryngology, Boston Univ/Tufts Univ 1995; **Fellow:** Sinus Surgery, Univ Penn 1996; **Fac Appt:** Prof Oto, Univ NC Sch Med

Sillers, Michael J MD [Oto] - **Spec Exp:** Nasal & Sinus Disorders; Sinus Disorders/Surgery; **Hospital:** St Vincent's Hosp - Birmingham, Brookwood Med Ctr; **Address:** Alabama Nasal & Sinus Ctr, 7191 Cahaba Valley Rd, Ste 301, Birmingham, AL 35242; **Phone:** 205-408-6600; **Board Cert:** Otolaryngology 1994; **Med School:** Univ Ala 1988; **Resid:** Otolaryngology, Univ Alabama Hosp 1993; **Fellow:** Sinus Surgery, Med Coll Georgia 1994; **Fac Appt:** Asst Prof S, Univ Ala

Silverstein, Herbert MD [Oto] - **Spec Exp:** Ear Disorders/Surgery; Meniere's Disease; **Hospital:** Sarasota Meml Hosp; **Address:** Silverstein Institute, 1901 Floyd St, Sarasota, FL 34239; **Phone:** 941-366-9222; **Board Cert:** Otolaryngology 1967; **Med School:** Temple Univ 1961; **Resid:** Surgery, Hosp Univ Penn 1963; Otolaryngology, Mass EE Infirm 1966; **Fac Appt:** Clin Prof S, Univ S Fla Coll Med

Stringer, Scott P MD [Oto] - **Spec Exp:** Nasal & Sinus Disorders; Head & Neck Cancer; Thyroid & Parathyroid Cancer & Surgery; **Hospital:** Univ Hosps & Clins - Jackson; **Address:** Dept Otolaryngology, 2500 N State St, Jackson, MS 39216-4505; **Phone:** 601-984-5160; **Board Cert:** Otolaryngology 1987; **Med School:** Univ Tex SW, Dallas 1982; **Resid:** Surgery, Univ Tex SW Med Ctr 1984; Otolaryngology, Univ Tex SW Med Ctr 1987; **Fac Appt:** Prof Oto, Univ Miss

Terris, David J MD [Oto] - **Spec Exp:** Head & Neck Cancer; Thyroid Cancer; Parathyroid Disease; Sleep Disorders/Apnea; **Hospital:** Med Coll of GA Hosp and Clin; **Address:** MCG Health System-Dept of Otolaryngology, 1120 15th St, rm BP4101, Augusta, GA 30912; **Phone:** 706-721-4400; **Board Cert:** Otolaryngology 1994; **Med School:** Duke Univ 1988; **Resid:** Surgery, Stanford Univ Med Ctr 1989; Otolaryngology, Stanford Univ Med Ctr 1993; **Fellow:** Head and Neck Surgery, Stanford Univ Med Ctr 1994; **Fac Appt:** Prof Oto, Med Coll GA

Tucci, Debara Lyn MD [Oto] - **Spec Exp:** Skull Base Surgery; Middle Ear Disorders; Otology; Hearing Disorders; **Hospital:** Duke Univ Med Ctr; **Address:** 1559 Stead-Blue Zone, South Hospital, Durham, NC 27710; **Phone:** 919-684-6968; **Board Cert:** Otolaryngology 1990; **Med School:** Univ VA Sch Med 1985; **Resid:** Otolaryngology, Univ Va Hlth Sci Ctr 1990; **Fellow:** Otology & Neurotology, Univ Mich Med Ctr 1992; **Fac Appt:** Assoc Prof S, Duke Univ

Valentino, Joseph MD [Oto] - **Spec Exp:** Head & Neck Cancer; Reconstructive Microvascular Surgery; Thyroid Cancer; **Hospital:** Univ of Kentucky Chandler Hosp; **Address:** 740 S Limestone St, rm B-317, Lexington, KY 40536-0284; **Phone:** 859-257-5405; **Board Cert:** Otolaryngology 1993; **Med School:** UMDNJ-RW Johnson Med Sch 1987; **Resid:** Otolaryngology, Univ Minn 1992; **Fellow:** Otolaryngology, Univ Iowa Coll Med 1993; **Fac Appt:** Assoc Prof Oto, Univ KY Coll Med

Wazen, Jack J MD [Oto] - **Spec Exp:** Skull Base Surgery; Meniere's Disease; Acoustic Neuroma; Hearing & Balance Disorders; **Hospital:** Sarasota Meml Hosp; **Address:** Silverstein Institute, 1901 Floyd St, Sarasota, FL 34239; **Phone:** 941-366-9222; **Board Cert:** Otolaryngology 1983; **Med School:** Lebanon 1978; **Resid:** Surgery, St Lukes Hosp 1980; Otolaryngology, Columbia Presby Hosp 1983; **Fellow:** Neurotology, Ear Rsch Fdn 1984; **Fac Appt:** Assoc Clin Prof Oto, Columbia P&S

Weissler, Mark Christian MD [Oto] - **Spec Exp:** Head & Neck Cancer; Laryngeal & Tracheal Disorders; Voice Disorders; **Hospital:** Univ NC Hosps; **Address:** G0412 Neurosciences Hosp UNC, CB 7070, Chapel Hill, NC 27599-7070; **Phone:** 919-843-3796; **Board Cert:** Otolaryngology 1985; **Med School:** Boston Univ 1980; **Resid:** Surgery, Mass Genl Hosp 1982; Otolaryngology, Mass Eye & Ear Infirm 1985; **Fellow:** Head and Neck Oncology, Univ Cincinnati 1986; **Fac Appt:** Prof Oto, Univ NC Sch Med

Yarbrough, Wendell G MD [Oto] - **Spec Exp:** Head & Neck Cancer; **Hospital:** Vanderbilt Univ Med Ctr; **Address:** Vanderbilt Otolaryngology, 1215 21st Ave S, Ste 7209, Nashville, TN 37232-8605; **Phone:** 615-322-6180; **Board Cert:** Otolaryngology 1995; **Med School:** Univ NC Sch Med 1989; **Resid:** Otolaryngology, Univ NC Hosps 1994; **Fellow:** Surgical Oncology, Univ NC Hosps 1996; **Fac Appt:** Assoc Prof Oto, Vanderbilt Univ

Midwest

Arts, H Alexander MD [Oto] - **Spec Exp:** Skull Base Tumors & Surgery; Neuro-Otology; Hearing Loss; Cochlear Implants; **Hospital:** Univ Michigan Hlth Sys; **Address:** Univ Michigan Health Systems, Dept Otolaryngology, 1500 E Medical Ctr Dr, 1904 Taubman Ctr, Ann Arbor, MI 48109; **Phone:** 734-936-8006; **Board Cert:** Otolaryngology 1992; Neurotology 2004; **Med School:** Baylor Coll Med 1983; **Resid:** Surgery, Univ Washington Med Ctr 1985; Otolaryngology, Univ Washington Med Ctr 1990; **Fellow:** Neurotology, Univ Virginia 1991; **Fac Appt:** Prof Oto, Univ Mich Med Sch

Baim, Howard M MD [Oto] - **Spec Exp:** Head & Neck Surgery; Sleep Disorders/Apnea; Sinus Disorders; **Hospital:** Adv Illinois Masonic Med Ctr, Highland Park Hosp; **Address:** 2532 N Lincoln Ave, Chicago, IL 60614-2468; **Phone:** 773-883-1177; **Board Cert:** Otolaryngology 1978; **Med School:** Univ IL Coll Med 1973; **Resid:** Surgery, Illinois Met Grp Hosps 1975; Otolaryngology, Illinois EE Infirmary 1978; **Fac Appt:** Asst Clin Prof Oto, Univ IL Coll Med

Baker, Shan Ray MD [Oto] - **Spec Exp:** Cosmetic Surgery-Face & Neck; Reconstructive Surgery; **Hospital:** Univ Michigan Hlth Sys; **Address:** Ctr Facial & Cosmetic Surgery, 19900 Haggerty Rd, Ste 103, Livonia, MI 48152-1054; **Phone:** 734-432-7634; **Board Cert:** Otolaryngology 1977; Facial Plastic & Reconstructive Surgery 1990; **Med School:** Univ Iowa Coll Med 1971; **Resid:** Surgery, UCSD Med Ctr 1973; Otolaryngology, Univ Iowa Hosps 1977; **Fac Appt:** Prof Oto, Univ Mich Med Sch

Bastian, Robert W MD [Oto] - **Spec Exp:** Voice Disorders; Swallowing Disorders; Laryngeal Disorders; **Hospital:** Adv Good Samaritan Hosp; **Address:** Bastian Voice Inst, 3010 Highland Parkway, Ste 550, Downers Grove, IL 60515-5500; **Phone:** 630-724-1100; **Board Cert:** Otolaryngology 1983; **Med School:** Washington Univ, St Louis 1978; **Resid:** Surgery, Barnes Hosp 1979; Otolaryngology, Barnes Hosp 1983; **Fellow:** Otolaryngology, Hosp Foch 1983

Beatty, Charles W MD [Oto] - **Spec Exp:** Otology & Neuro-Otology; Acoustic Neuroma; Meniere's Disease; **Hospital:** Mayo Med Ctr & Clin - Rochester; **Address:** Mayo Clinic, Dept Otolaryngology, 200 First St SW Fl W5, Rochester, MN 55905; **Phone:** 507-284-8532; **Board Cert:** Otolaryngology 1982; **Med School:** Univ Iowa Coll Med 1977; **Resid:** Otolaryngology, Mayo Clinic 1982; **Fac Appt:** Prof Oto, Mayo Med Sch

Benninger, Michael S MD [Oto] - **Spec Exp:** Voice Disorders; Nasal & Sinus Disorders; Sinus Disorders/Surgery; **Hospital:** Cleveland Clin Fdn (page 56); **Address:** Cleveland Clinic Main Campus, MC A71, 9500 Euclid Ave, Cleveland, OH 44195; **Phone:** 216-444-6686; **Board Cert:** Otolaryngology 1988; **Med School:** Case West Res Univ 1983; **Resid:** Surgery, Cleveland Clin Fdn 1985; Otolaryngology, Cleveland Clin Fdn 1988

Otolaryngology

Bojrab, Dennis I MD [Oto] - **Spec Exp:** Otology & Neuro-Otology; Facial Nerve Disorders; Skull Base Tumors; **Hospital:** Providence Hosp - Southfield, William Beaumont Hosp; **Address:** Michigan Ear Inst, 30055 Northwestern Hwy, Ste 101, Farmington Hills, MI 48334; **Phone:** 248-865-4444; **Board Cert:** Otolaryngology 1985; **Med School:** Indiana Univ 1979; **Resid:** Surgery, Butterworth Hosp 1981; Otolaryngology, Univ Indiana Sch Med 1984; **Fellow:** Skull Base Surgery, Vanderbilt Univ Med Ctr 1985; **Fac Appt:** Prof Oto, Wayne State Univ

Bradford, Carol MD [Oto] - **Spec Exp:** Head & Neck Cancer; Melanoma-Head & Neck; Skin Cancer-Head & Neck; **Hospital:** Univ Michigan Hlth Sys; **Address:** University of Michigan Health System, 1500 E Medical Center Drive, rm 1904-TC, Ann Arbor, MI 48109-0312; **Phone:** 734-936-8050; **Board Cert:** Otolaryngology 1993; **Med School:** Univ Mich Med Sch 1986; **Resid:** Otolaryngology, Univ Michigan Med Ctr 1992; **Fellow:** Head and Neck Surgery, Univ Michigan Med Ctr 1988; **Fac Appt:** Prof Oto, Univ Mich Med Sch

Branham, Gregory H MD [Oto] - **Spec Exp:** Cosmetic & Reconstructive Surgery-Face; Nasal Surgery; Botox Therapy; Skin Laser Surgery-Resurfacing; **Hospital:** Washington Univ Med Ctr, Barnes-Jewish Hosp; **Address:** 605 Old Ballas Rd, Ste 100, St Louis, MO 63141; **Phone:** 314-432-7760; **Board Cert:** Otolaryngology 1989; Facial Plastic & Reconstructive Surgery 1993; **Med School:** Washington Univ, St Louis 1983; **Resid:** Otolaryngology, St Louis Univ Hosp 1989; **Fellow:** Facial Plastic & Reconstructive Surgery, Washington Univ 1990; **Fac Appt:** Assoc Prof Oto, St Louis Univ

Caldarelli, David D MD [Oto] - **Spec Exp:** Laryngeal & Vocal Cord Surgery; Sinus Disorders/Surgery; Ear Disorders/Surgery; Meniere's Disease; **Hospital:** Rush Univ Med Ctr; **Address:** 1725 W Harrison St, rm 308, Chicago, IL 60612; **Phone:** 312-733-4341; **Board Cert:** Otolaryngology 1970; **Med School:** Univ IL Coll Med 1965; **Resid:** Surgery, Presby-St Lukes Hosp 1967; Otolaryngology, Univ Illinois Eye/Ear Infirm 1970; **Fac Appt:** Prof Oto, Rush Med Coll

Campbell, Bruce H MD [Oto] - **Spec Exp:** Head & Neck Surgery; Head & Neck Cancer; **Hospital:** Froedtert Meml Lutheran Hosp, Chldns Hosp - Wisconsin; **Address:** Med Coll Wisc-Dept Oto, 9200 W Wisconsin Ave, Milwaukee, WI 53226; **Phone:** 414-805-5583; **Board Cert:** Otolaryngology 1986; **Med School:** Rush Med Coll 1980; **Resid:** Otolaryngology, Med Coll Wisconsin 1985; **Fellow:** Head and Neck Surgery, MD Anderson Cancer Ctr 1987; **Fac Appt:** Prof Oto, Med Coll Wisc

Corey, Jacquelynne P MD [Oto] - **Spec Exp:** Nasal & Sinus Disorders; Allergy; Voice Disorders; **Hospital:** Univ of Chicago Hosps; **Address:** Univ Chicago Hosps-Otolaryngology, 5758 S Maryland Ave, Chicago, IL 60637; **Phone:** 773-702-1865; **Board Cert:** Otolaryngology 1985; **Med School:** Univ IL Coll Med 1979; **Resid:** Otolaryngology, Rush Presby-St Lukes Med Ctr 1984; **Fac Appt:** Assoc Prof Oto, Univ Chicago-Pritzker Sch Med

Driscoll, Colin L W MD [Oto] - **Spec Exp:** Acoustic Neuroma; Cochlear Implants; Meniere's Disease; Cholesteatoma; **Hospital:** Mayo Med Ctr & Clin - Rochester; **Address:** Mayo Clinic, Dept Otolaryngology, 200 First St SW, W5, Rochester, MN 55905-0001; **Phone:** 507-284-4065; **Board Cert:** Otolaryngology 1998; **Med School:** Univ New Mexico 1992; **Resid:** Otolaryngology, Mayo Clinic 1997; **Fellow:** Neurotology, UCSF Med Ctr 1998; Skull Base Surgery, UCSF Med Ctr 1999; **Fac Appt:** Assoc Prof Oto, Mayo Med Sch

Ford, Charles N MD [Oto] - **Spec Exp:** Voice Disorders; Laryngeal Disorders; **Hospital:** Univ WI Hosp & Clins; **Address:** Univ of WI Hosp & Clinics, 600 Highland Avenue-K4-714, Madison, WI 53792-3284; **Phone:** 608-263-0192; **Board Cert:** Otolaryngology 1971; **Med School:** Univ Louisville Sch Med 1965; **Resid:** Otolaryngology, Henry Ford Hosp 1970; **Fac Appt:** Prof Oto, Univ Wisc

      America's Top Doctors® 8th Edition

Friedman, Michael MD [Oto] - **Spec Exp:** Sleep Disorders/Apnea/Snoring; Thyroid & Parathyroid Surgery; Sinus Disorders/Surgery; **Hospital:** Adv Illinois Masonic Med Ctr, Rush Univ Med Ctr; **Address:** 30 N Michigan St, Ste 1107, Chicago, IL 60602-3747; **Phone:** 312-236-3642; **Board Cert:** Otolaryngology 1977; **Med School:** Univ IL Coll Med 1972; **Resid:** Surgery, Illinois Masonic Hosp 1974; Otolaryngology, Univ Illinois Med Ctr 1977; **Fac Appt:** Prof Oto, Rush Med Coll

Funk, Gerry F MD [Oto] - **Spec Exp:** Head & Neck Cancer; Head & Neck Reconstruction; Head & Neck Trauma; **Hospital:** Univ Iowa Hosp & Clinics; **Address:** UIHC, Dept Otolaryngology, 200 Hawkins Drive, Iowa City, IA 52242-1009; **Phone:** 319-356-2165; **Board Cert:** Otolaryngology 1992; **Med School:** Univ Chicago-Pritzker Sch Med 1986; **Resid:** Surgery, LAC-USC Med Ctr 1987; Otolaryngology, LAC-USC Med Ctr 1991; **Fellow:** Head and Neck Surgery, Univ Iowa Hosp 1992; **Fac Appt:** Prof Oto, Univ Iowa Coll Med

Gantz, Bruce MD [Oto] - **Spec Exp:** Cochlear Implants; Neuro-Otology; Skull Base Surgery; **Hospital:** Univ Iowa Hosp & Clinics; **Address:** Univ Hosp & Clins, Dept Otolaryngology, 200 Hawkins Drive, rm 21201PFP, Iowa City, IA 52242-1078; **Phone:** 319-356-2173; **Board Cert:** Otolaryngology 1980; Neurotology 2004; **Med School:** Univ Iowa Coll Med 1974; **Resid:** Otolaryngology, Univ Iowa Hosps 1980; **Fellow:** Neurotology, Univ Zurich 1982; **Fac Appt:** Prof Oto, Univ Iowa Coll Med

Gluckman, Jack L MD [Oto] - **Spec Exp:** Head & Neck Cancer; Head & Neck Surgery; **Hospital:** Univ Hosp - Cincinnati, Good Samaritan Hosp - Cincinnati; **Address:** Univ Cincinnati Medical Center, Head & Neck Surgery MSB 6505, 231 Albert B Sabin Way, Box 670528, Cincinnati, OH 45267-0528; **Phone:** 513-558-0017; **Board Cert:** Otolaryngology 1990; **Med School:** South Africa 1967; **Resid:** Surgery, St James Hosp 1971; Otolaryngology, Groote Schuur Hosp 1974; **Fellow:** Otolaryngology, Univ Cincinnati Med Ctr 1979; **Fac Appt:** Prof Oto, Univ Cincinnati

Goebel, Joel Alan MD [Oto] - **Spec Exp:** Dizziness; Hearing Disorders; Otology & Neuro-Otology; **Hospital:** Barnes-Jewish Hosp, St Louis Chldns Hosp; **Address:** Barnes Jewish Hosp South, 660 S Euclid, Box 8115, St Louis, MO 63110; **Phone:** 314-362-7509; **Board Cert:** Otolaryngology 1985; **Med School:** Washington Univ, St Louis 1980; **Resid:** Otolaryngology, Barnes Hosp/Wash Univ 1985; **Fac Appt:** Prof Oto, Washington Univ, St Louis

Haughey, Bruce MD [Oto] - **Spec Exp:** Reconstructive Surgery-Face; Head & Neck Cancer; Head & Neck Reconstruction; **Hospital:** Barnes-Jewish Hosp; **Address:** Barnes Jewish Hosp South, 660 S Euclid Ave, Box 8115, St Louis, MO 63110; **Phone:** 314-362-7509; **Board Cert:** Otolaryngology 1984; **Med School:** New Zealand 1976; **Resid:** Surgery, Univ Auckland 1981; Otolaryngology, Univ Iowa Med Ctr 1984; **Fellow:** Otolaryngology, Univ Iowa Med Ctr 1985; **Fac Appt:** Prof Oto, Washington Univ, St Louis

Hilger, Peter A MD [Oto] - **Spec Exp:** Head & Neck Surgery; Facial Plastic Surgery; **Hospital:** Regions Hosp - St Paul, Fairview Southdale Hosp; **Address:** Centennial Lakes Med Bldg, 7373 France Ave S, Ste 410, Edina, MN 55435; **Phone:** 952-844-0404; **Board Cert:** Otolaryngology 1979; **Med School:** Univ Minn 1974; **Resid:** Surgery, Univ Minn Hosp 1975; Otolaryngology, Univ Minn Hosp 1979; **Fellow:** Plastic Surgery, Mass Eye & Ear Infirm 1980; **Fac Appt:** Asst Prof Oto, Univ Minn

Hoffman, Henry T MD [Oto] - **Spec Exp:** Head & Neck Cancer; Head & Neck Surgery; Voice Disorders; **Hospital:** Univ Iowa Hosp & Clinics; **Address:** Univ Iowa Hosp & Clins-Dept Oto, 200 Hawkins Drive, Iowa City, IA 52242; **Phone:** 319-356-2166; **Board Cert:** Otolaryngology 1985; **Med School:** UCSD 1980; **Resid:** Otolaryngology, Univ Iowa Hosp & Clinics 1985; **Fellow:** Head and Neck Oncology, Univ Michigan Hosp 1989; **Fac Appt:** Clin Prof Oto, Univ Iowa Coll Med

Otolaryngology

Hogikyan, Norman D MD [Oto] - **Spec Exp:** Voice Disorders; Vocal Cord Disorders; Swallowing Disorders; Airway Disorders; **Hospital:** Univ Michigan Hlth Sys; **Address:** University og Michigan Health System, Taubman Ctr, rm 1904, 1500 E Medical Ctr Drive, Ann Arbor, MI 48109; **Phone:** 734-936-9598; **Board Cert:** Otolaryngology 1995; **Med School:** Univ Mich Med Sch 1988; **Resid:** Otolaryngology, Barnes Jewish Med Ctr 1994; **Fellow:** Loyola Univ Med Ctr 1995; **Fac Appt:** Assoc Prof Oto, Univ Mich Med Sch

Hotaling, Andrew J MD [Oto] - **Spec Exp:** Pediatric Otolaryngology; Sleep Disorders/Apnea; Neck Masses; **Hospital:** Loyola Univ Med Ctr, Children's Mem Hosp; **Address:** Loyola Univ Med Ctr, 2160 S 1st Ave Bldg 105 - rm 1870, Maywood, IL 60153-5590; **Phone:** 708-216-9183; **Board Cert:** Otolaryngology 1985; **Med School:** Case West Res Univ 1979; **Resid:** Surgery, Case Western 1981; Otolaryngology, Northwestern Meml Hosp 1984; **Fellow:** Pediatric Otolaryngology, Univ Pittsburgh Med Ctr 1985; **Fac Appt:** Prof Oto, Loyola Univ-Stritch Sch Med

Jones, Paul J MD [Oto] - **Spec Exp:** Pediatric Otolaryngology; **Hospital:** Rush Univ Med Ctr; **Address:** 1725 W Harrison St, Ste 938, Chicago, IL 60612; **Phone:** 312-942-2175; **Board Cert:** Otolaryngology 1989; **Med School:** Rush Med Coll 1983; **Resid:** Otolaryngology, Rush Presby-St Lukes Med Ctr 1988; **Fac Appt:** Asst Prof Oto, Rush Med Coll

Kartush, Jack MD [Oto] - **Spec Exp:** Ear Disorders/Surgery; Balance Disorders; **Hospital:** Providence Hosp - Southfield; **Address:** Michigan Ear Inst, 30055 Northwestern Hwy, Ste 101, Farmington Hills, MI 48334; **Phone:** 248-865-4444; **Board Cert:** Otolaryngology 1984; **Med School:** Univ Mich Med Sch 1978; **Resid:** Otolaryngology, Univ Mich Med Ctr 1984; **Fellow:** Neurotology, Univ Mich Med Ctr 1985; **Fac Appt:** Assoc Clin Prof Oto, Wayne State Univ

Kern, Robert MD [Oto] - **Spec Exp:** Head & Neck Cancer; Sinus Disorders/Surgery; Rhinoplasty; **Hospital:** Northwestern Meml Hosp, Stroger Hosp of Cook Co; **Address:** Northwestern Medical Faculty Fdn, 675 N St Clair St, Ste 15-200, Chicago, IL 60611; **Phone:** 312-695-8182; **Board Cert:** Otolaryngology 1990; **Med School:** Jefferson Med Coll 1985; **Resid:** Otolaryngology, Wayne State Affil Hosp 1990; **Fellow:** Research, Natl Inst Hlth 1991; **Fac Appt:** Prof Oto, Northwestern Univ

Lavertu, Pierre MD [Oto] - **Spec Exp:** Thyroid Cancer; Head & Neck Cancer; Skull Base Tumors; **Hospital:** Univ Hosps Case Med Ctr; **Address:** Univ Hosps, Dept Oto-Head & Neck Surg, 11100 Euclid Ave, Cleveland, OH 44106-5045; **Phone:** 216-844-4773; **Board Cert:** Otolaryngology 1981; **Med School:** Univ Montreal 1976; **Resid:** Otolaryngology, Univ Montreal Med Ctr 1981; **Fellow:** Head and Neck Surgery, Univ Montreal Med Ctr 1982; Head and Neck Surgery, Cleveland Clinic 1983; **Fac Appt:** Prof Oto, Case West Res Univ

Leonetti, John P MD [Oto] - **Spec Exp:** Skull Base Tumors & Surgery; Acoustic Neuroma; Neuro-Otology; **Hospital:** Loyola Univ Med Ctr; **Address:** Loyola University Medical Ctr, Dept Otolaryngology, 2160 S First Ave Bldg 105 - rm 1870, Maywood, IL 60153; **Phone:** 708-216-4804; **Board Cert:** Otolaryngology 1987; **Med School:** Loyola Univ-Stritch Sch Med 1982; **Resid:** Otolaryngology, Loyola Univ Med Ctr 1987; Research, House Ear Inst 1987; **Fellow:** Neurotology, Barnes Jewish Hosp 1988; **Fac Appt:** Prof Oto, Loyola Univ-Stritch Sch Med

Marentette, Lawrence MD [Oto] - **Spec Exp:** Skull Base Tumors & Surgery; Facial Plastic & Reconstructive Surgery; **Hospital:** Univ Michigan Hlth Sys; **Address:** Univ Michigan Health Systems, Dept Oto, 1500 E Med Ctr Drive, 1904 Taubman Ctr, Ann Arbor, MI 48109; **Phone:** 734-936-8051; **Board Cert:** Otolaryngology 1981; Facial Plastic & Reconstructive Surgery 1995; **Med School:** Wayne State Univ 1976; **Resid:** Otolaryngology, Wayne State Univ 1980; **Fellow:** Maxillofacial Surgery, Univ of Zurich 1985; **Fac Appt:** Prof Oto, Univ Mich Med Sch

Miyamoto, Richard T MD [Oto] - **Spec Exp:** Neuro-Otology; Acoustic Neuroma; Middle Ear Disorders; Cochlear Implants; **Hospital:** St Vincent Hosp & Hlth Svcs - Indianapolis, Riley Hosp for Children; **Address:** 8402 Harcourt Rd, Ste 732, Indianapolis, IN 46260; **Phone:** 317-338-6815; **Board Cert:** Otolaryngology 1975; Neurotology 2004; **Med School:** Univ Mich Med Sch 1970; **Resid:** Surgery, Butterworth Hosp 1972; Otolaryngology, Indiana Univ Hosps 1975; **Fellow:** Otology & Neurotology, Otologic Med Grp 1978; **Fac Appt:** Prof Oto, Indiana Univ

Naclerio, Robert M MD [Oto] - **Spec Exp:** Head & Neck Surgery; Pediatric Otolaryngology; Sinus Disorders/Surgery; **Hospital:** Univ of Chicago Hosps; **Address:** Univ Chicago Hosps, 5801 S Maryland Ave, MC 1035, AMB E102E, Chicago, IL 60637; **Phone:** 773-702-0080; **Board Cert:** Otolaryngology 1983; **Med School:** Baylor Coll Med 1976; **Resid:** Surgery, Johns Hopkins Hosp 1978; Otolaryngology, Baylor Coll Med 1980; **Fellow:** Clinical Immunology, Johns Hopkins Hosp 1982; **Fac Appt:** Prof Oto, Univ Chicago-Pritzker Sch Med

Olsen, Kerry D MD [Oto] - **Spec Exp:** Head & Neck Cancer & Surgery; Esthesioneuroblastoma; Salivary Gland Tumors & Surgery; Skull Base Tumors; **Hospital:** Mayo Med Ctr & Clin - Rochester; **Address:** Mayo Clinic, Dept Otolaryngology, 200 1st St SW, Rochester, MN 55905-0001; **Phone:** 507-284-3542; **Board Cert:** Otolaryngology 1981; **Med School:** Mayo Med Sch 1976; **Resid:** Otolaryngology, Mayo Clinic 1981; **Fac Appt:** Prof Oto, Mayo Med Sch

Paparella, Michael M MD [Oto] - **Spec Exp:** Hearing Disorders; Neuro-Otology; Meniere's Disease; **Hospital:** Univ Minn Med Ctr, Fairview - Riverside Campus; **Address:** 701 25th Ave S, Ste 200, Minneapolis, MN 55454-1443; **Phone:** 612-339-2836; **Board Cert:** Otolaryngology 1963; **Med School:** Univ Mich Med Sch 1957; **Resid:** Otolaryngology, Henry Ford Hosp 1961; **Fac Appt:** Clin Prof Oto, Univ Minn

Pelzer, Harold J MD/DDS [Oto] - **Spec Exp:** Head & Neck Cancer; Swallowing Disorders; **Hospital:** Northwestern Meml Hosp; **Address:** Northwestern Medical Faculty Fdn, 675 N St Clair St, Ste 15-200, Chicago, IL 60611; **Phone:** 312-695-8182; **Board Cert:** Otolaryngology 1985; **Med School:** Northwestern Univ 1979; **Resid:** Surgery, Northwestern Meml Hosp 1983; **Fellow:** Head and Neck Surgery, Northwestern Meml Hosp 1985; **Fac Appt:** Assoc Prof Oto, Northwestern Univ

Pensak, Myles MD [Oto] - **Spec Exp:** Skull Base Tumors; Facial Paralysis; Hearing & Balance Disorders; **Hospital:** Univ Hosp - Cincinnati, Good Samaritan Hosp - Cincinnati; **Address:** Univ Medical Arts Building, 222 Piedmont Ave, Ste 5200, Cincinnati, OH 45219; **Phone:** 513-475-8400; **Board Cert:** Otolaryngology 1983; Neurotology 2004; **Med School:** NY Med Coll 1978; **Resid:** Surgery, Upstate Med Ctr 1980; Otolaryngology, Yale Univ 1983; **Fellow:** Otology & Neurotology, The Otology Group 1984; **Fac Appt:** Prof Oto, Univ Cincinnati

Petruzzelli, Guy MD/PhD [Oto] - **Spec Exp:** Head & Neck Cancer & Surgery; Skull Base Tumors; Thyroid Cancer; **Hospital:** Rush Univ Med Ctr; **Address:** Rush Univ Med Ctr, 1725 W Harrison St, Ste 218, Chicago, IL 60612; **Phone:** 312-942-6100; **Board Cert:** Otolaryngology 1993; **Med School:** Rush Med Coll 1987; **Resid:** Otolaryngology, Univ Pittsburgh Med Ctr 1992; **Fellow:** Head and Neck Oncology, Univ Pittsburgh Med Ctr 1993; Skull Base Surgery, Univ Pittsburgh Ctr Cranial Base Surg; **Fac Appt:** Prof Oto, Rush Med Coll

Piccirillo, Jay MD [Oto] - **Spec Exp:** Sleep Disorders/Apnea; Sinus Disorders/Surgery; **Hospital:** Barnes-Jewish Hosp; **Address:** Barnes Jewish Hosp South, 660 S Euclid, Box 8115, St Louis, MO 63110; **Phone:** 314-362-7509; **Board Cert:** Otolaryngology 1990; **Med School:** Univ VT Coll Med 1985; **Resid:** Otolaryngology, Albany Med Ctr 1990; **Fellow:** Yale Univ 1992; **Fac Appt:** Asst Prof Oto, Washington Univ, St Louis

Otolaryngology

Schuller, David MD [Oto] - **Spec Exp:** Head & Neck Cancer; Head & Neck Surgery; **Hospital:** Arthur G James Cancer Hosp & Research Inst, Ohio St Univ Med Ctr; **Address:** 300 W 10th Ave, rm 518, Columbus, OH 43210; **Phone:** 614-293-8074; **Board Cert:** Otolaryngology 1975; **Med School:** Ohio State Univ 1970; **Resid:** Otolaryngology, Ohio State Univ Affil Hosps 1975; Surgery, Univ Hosps 1973; **Fellow:** Head and Neck Surgery, Pack Med Fdn 1973; Head and Neck Oncology, Univ Iowa 1976; **Fac Appt:** Prof Oto, Ohio State Univ

Siegel, Gordon J MD [Oto] - **Spec Exp:** Head & Neck Cancer; Nasal & Sinus Disorders; **Hospital:** Northwestern Meml Hosp; **Address:** 3 E Huron St Fl 1, Chicago, IL 60611-2705; **Phone:** 312-988-7777; **Board Cert:** Otolaryngology 1984; **Med School:** Ros Franklin Univ/Chicago Med Sch 1978; **Resid:** Otolaryngology, Northwestern Univ 1982; **Fac Appt:** Asst Clin Prof Oto, Northwestern Univ

Stankiewicz, James MD [Oto] - **Spec Exp:** Endoscopic Sinus Surgery; Rhinosinusitis; Nasal & Sinus Disorders; **Hospital:** Loyola Univ Med Ctr; **Address:** Loyola Univ Med Ctr, Dept Oto, 2160 S First Ave, Maywood, IL 60153-5590; **Phone:** 708-216-8563; **Board Cert:** Otolaryngology 1978; **Med School:** Univ Chicago-Pritzker Sch Med 1974; **Resid:** Otolaryngology, Univ Chicago Hosp 1978; **Fac Appt:** Prof Oto, Loyola Univ-Stritch Sch Med

Szachowicz II, Edward H MD [Oto] - **Spec Exp:** Cosmetic Surgery-Face; Rhinoplasty; **Hospital:** Abbott - Northwestern Hosp; **Address:** Centennial Lakes Med Bldg, 7373 France Ave S, Ste 508, Edina, MN 55435-4538; **Phone:** 952-835-5665; **Board Cert:** Otolaryngology 1984; **Med School:** Univ IL Coll Med 1979; **Resid:** Surgery, Fairview Univ Med Ctr 1980; Otolaryngology, Fairview Univ Med Ctr 1984; **Fellow:** Facial Plastic Surgery, Fairview Univ Med Ctr 1986; **Fac Appt:** Asst Clin Prof Oto, Univ Minn

Teknos, Theodoros N MD [Oto] - **Spec Exp:** Head & Neck Cancer; Thyroid Cancer; Facial Plastic & Reconstructive Surgery; Reconstructive Microvascular Surgery; **Hospital:** Univ Michigan Hlth Sys; **Address:** Univ Mich Med Ctr, TC 1904, 1500 E Med Ctr Drive, Ann Arbor, MI 48109; **Phone:** 734-936-3172; **Board Cert:** Otolaryngology 1997; **Med School:** Harvard Med Sch 1991; **Resid:** Otolaryngology, Mass Eye & Ear Hosp 1996; **Fellow:** Head and Neck Surgery, Vanderbilt Univ Med Ctr 1997; **Fac Appt:** Assoc Prof Oto, Univ Mich Med Sch

Telian, Steven A MD [Oto] - **Spec Exp:** Cochlear Implants; Ear Disorders/Surgery; Acoustic Neuroma; **Hospital:** Univ Michigan Hlth Sys; **Address:** Univ Mich Med Ctr, Dept Otolaryngology-Head & Neck Surgery, 1500 E Med Ctr Drive, 1904 Taubman Ctr, Ann Arbor, MI 48109-0312; **Phone:** 734-936-8006; **Board Cert:** Otolaryngology 1985; **Med School:** Univ Pennsylvania 1980; **Resid:** Otolaryngology, Hosp Univ Penn 1985; **Fellow:** Neurotology, Univ Mich Med Ctr 1986; **Fac Appt:** Prof Oto, Univ Mich Med Sch

Toriumi, Dean MD [Oto] - **Spec Exp:** Rhinoplasty; Cosmetic Surgery-Face; Reconstructive Plastic Surgery; **Hospital:** Univ of IL Med Ctr at Chicago; **Address:** 900 N Michigan Surgery Ctr, 60 E Delaware Pl Fl 14 - Ste 1460, Chicago, IL 60611; **Phone:** 312-255-8812; **Board Cert:** Otolaryngology 1988; **Med School:** Rush Med Coll 1981; **Resid:** Surgery, Univ Illinois Med Ctr 1985; Otolaryngology, Northwestern Univ Med Sch 1987; **Fellow:** Facial Plastic Surgery, Tulane Med Sch 1988; Facial Plastic Surgery, Virginia Mason Med Ctr 1989; **Fac Appt:** Assoc Prof Oto, Univ IL Coll Med

Wackym, P Ashley MD [Oto] - **Spec Exp:** Cochlear Implants; Acoustic Neuroma; Head & Neck Surgery; **Hospital:** Froedtert Meml Lutheran Hosp, Chldns Hosp - Wisconsin; **Address:** Med Coll Wisconsin, Dept Otolaryngology, 9200 W Wisconsin Ave, Milwaukee, WI 53226; **Phone:** 414-805-5625; **Board Cert:** Otolaryngology 1992; Neurotology 2004; **Med School:** Vanderbilt Univ 1985; **Resid:** Neurological Surgery, UCLA Med Ctr 1987; Head and Neck Surgery, UCLA Med Ctr 1991; **Fellow:** Otology & Neurotology, Univ Iowa 1992; Neurological Science, UCLA Med Ctr 1995; **Fac Appt:** Prof Oto, Med Coll Wisc

Wiet, Richard J MD [Oto] - **Spec Exp:** Acoustic Neuroma; Hearing Loss; Otosclerosis/Stapedectomy; **Hospital:** Hinsdale Hosp, Northwestern Meml Hosp; **Address:** 11 Salt Creek Rd, Ste 101, Hinsdale, IL 60521; **Phone:** 630-789-3110; **Board Cert:** Otolaryngology 1976; Neurotology 2004; **Med School:** Loyola Univ-Stritch Sch Med 1971; **Resid:** Otolaryngology, Cincinnati Med Ctr 1976; **Fellow:** Neurotology, Univ Zurich/Ear Fdn 1979; **Fac Appt:** Clin Prof Oto, Northwestern Univ

Wilson, Keith M MD [Oto] - **Spec Exp:** Head & Neck Cancer & Surgery; Voice Disorders; **Hospital:** Univ Hosp - Cincinnati; **Address:** Univ Cincinnati Medical Ctr, 222 Piedmont Ave, Ste 5200, Cincinnati, OH 45219-4222; **Phone:** 513-475-8351; **Board Cert:** Otolaryngology 1992; **Med School:** Cornell Univ-Weill Med Coll 1986; **Resid:** Otolaryngology, St Louis Univ Med Ctr 1991; **Fellow:** Head & Neck Surgical Oncology, Ohio State Med Ctr 1992; **Fac Appt:** Assoc Prof Oto, Univ Cincinnati

Wolf, Gregory T MD [Oto] - **Spec Exp:** Head & Neck Cancer; Laryngeal Cancer; **Hospital:** Univ Michigan Hlth Sys; **Address:** Univ Mich Med Ctr, Dept Oto-HNS, 1500 E Med Ctr, Taubman Ctr, rm 1904, Ann Arbor, MI 48109-0312; **Phone:** 734-936-8029; **Board Cert:** Otolaryngology 1978; **Med School:** Univ Mich Med Sch 1973; **Resid:** Surgery, Georgetown Univ Hosp 1975; Otolaryngology, SUNY Upstate Med Ctr 1978; **Fac Appt:** Prof Oto, Univ Mich Med Sch

Woodson, B Tucker MD [Oto] - **Spec Exp:** Sleep Disorders/Apnea; **Hospital:** Froedtert Meml Lutheran Hosp, Chldns Hosp - Wisconsin; **Address:** 9200 W Wisconsin Ave, Froedtert West ENT Clinic, Milwaukee, WI 53226-3522; **Phone:** 414-805-7667; **Board Cert:** Otolaryngology 1988; **Med School:** Univ MO-Columbia Sch Med 1983; **Resid:** Surgery, Henry Ford Hosp 1984; Otolaryngology, Henry Ford Hosp 1988; **Fac Appt:** Assoc Prof Oto, Med Coll Wisc

Woodson, Gayle Ellen MD [Oto] - **Spec Exp:** Voice Disorders; Swallowing Disorders; **Hospital:** St John's Hosp - Springfield, Memorial Med Ctr - Springfield; **Address:** SIU Sch Med, Div Oto - Head & Neck Surg, 301 N 8 St, PO Box 19662, Springfield, IL 62701; **Phone:** 217-545-6099; **Board Cert:** Otolaryngology 1981; **Med School:** Baylor Coll Med 1976; **Resid:** Surgery, Johns Hopkins Hosp 1978; Otolaryngology, Baylor Coll Med 1981; **Fellow:** Laryngology, Inst Laryngology and Otology 1982; **Fac Appt:** Prof Oto, Southern IL Univ

Young, Nancy MD [Oto] - **Spec Exp:** Cochlear Implants; Cholesteatoma; Hearing Loss; Baha Implant; **Hospital:** Children's Mem Hosp, Glenbrook Hosp; **Address:** Children's Memorial, Div Oto-laryngology, 2300 Children's Plaza, Box 265, Chicago, IL 60614; **Phone:** 773-880-3020; **Board Cert:** Otolaryngology 1987; **Med School:** NYU Sch Med 1982; **Resid:** Surgery, Montefiore Med Ctr 1984; Otolaryngology, Northwestern Univ Hosp 1987; **Fellow:** Neurotology, Hinsdale Hosp 1988; **Fac Appt:** Assoc Prof Oto, Northwestern Univ

Yueh, Bevan MD [Oto] - **Spec Exp:** Head & Neck Cancer; Hearing Loss; **Hospital:** Univ Minn Med Ctr, Fairview - Univ Campus; **Address:** Dept Otolaryngology/Head & Neck Surgery, MMC 396, 420 Delaware St, Minneapolis, MN 55455-0932; **Phone:** 612-625-2410; **Board Cert:** Otolaryngology 1995; **Med School:** Stanford Univ 1989; **Resid:** Otolaryngology, Johns Hopkins Hosp 1994; **Fellow:** Otolaryngology, Johns Hopkins Hosp 1995; **Fac Appt:** Assoc Prof Oto, Univ Minn

Otolaryngology

Great Plains and Mountains

Chowdhury, Khalid MD [Oto] - **Spec Exp:** Skull Base Tumors & Surgery; Craniofacial Surgery; Cosmetic Surgery-Face; **Hospital:** Presby - St Luke's Med Ctr, Chldn's Hosp - Aurora, The; **Address:** Center for Craniofacial Surgery, 1601 E 19th Ave, Ste 3000, Denver, CO 80218; **Phone:** 303-839-5155; **Board Cert:** Otolaryngology 1990; Facial Plastic & Reconstructive Surgery 1995; **Med School:** Univ Saskatchewan 1982; **Resid:** Surgery, Univ Saskatchewan Hosp 1985; Otolaryngology, McGill Univ Hosps 1989; **Fellow:** Craniofacial Surgery, Univ Bern Hosp 1990; Facial Plastic & Reconstructive Surgery, Univ Bern Hosp 1990; **Fac Appt:** Assoc Prof Oto, Univ Colorado

Denenberg, Steven M MD [Oto] - **Spec Exp:** Cosmetic Surgery-Face; Rhinoplasty; **Hospital:** Nebraska Meth Hosp; **Address:** 7640 Pacific St, Omaha, NE 68114-5421; **Phone:** 402-391-7640; **Board Cert:** Otolaryngology 1984; Facial Plastic & Reconstructive Surgery 1992; **Med School:** Univ Nebr Coll Med 1980; **Resid:** Otolaryngology, Stanford Univ Med Ctr 1984; **Fellow:** Facial Plastic Surgery, McCollough Ctr 1985; **Fac Appt:** Asst Clin Prof Oto, Univ Nebr Coll Med

Jenkins, Herman A MD [Oto] - **Spec Exp:** Ear Disorders/Surgery; Neuro-Otology; Acoustic Neuroma; **Hospital:** Univ Colorado Hosp, Chldn's Hosp - Aurora, The; **Address:** Univ Colorado Hosp, Dept Otolaryngology, PO Box 6510, MS F737, Aurora, CO 80045; **Phone:** 720-848-2820; **Board Cert:** Otolaryngology 1977; Neurotology 2004; **Med School:** Vanderbilt Univ 1970; **Resid:** Surgery, UCLA Med Ctr 1972; Otolaryngology, UCLA Med Ctr 1977; **Fellow:** Neurotology, Univ Hosp 1980; **Fac Appt:** Prof Oto, Univ Colorado

Leopold, Donald Arthur MD [Oto] - **Spec Exp:** Olfactory Disorders; Sinus Disorders/Surgery; **Hospital:** Nebraska Med Ctr; **Address:** Univ Nebr, Dept Oto-Head & Neck Surg, 981225 Nebraska Med Ctr, Omaha, NE 68198-1225; **Phone:** 402-559-5208; **Board Cert:** Otolaryngology 1978; Facial Plastic & Reconstructive Surgery 1991; **Med School:** Ohio State Univ 1973; **Resid:** Surgery, St Luke's Med Ctr 1974; Otolaryngology, Univ Iowa 1978; **Fac Appt:** Prof Oto, Univ Nebr Coll Med

Lydiatt, Daniel D MD/DDS [Oto] - **Spec Exp:** Head & Neck Cancer; **Address:** 981225 Nebraska Medical Ctr, Omaha, NE 68198-1225; **Phone:** 402-559-5268; **Board Cert:** Otolaryngology 1992; **Med School:** Univ Nebr Coll Med 1983; **Resid:** Otolaryngology, Univ Nebraska Med Ctr 1990; **Fellow:** Head and Neck Surgery, MD Anderson Med Ctr 1991; **Fac Appt:** Assoc Prof Oto, Univ Nebr Coll Med

Lydiatt, William M MD [Oto] - **Spec Exp:** Head & Neck Cancer; Thyroid Cancer; Salivary Gland Tumors & Surgery; **Hospital:** Nebraska Meth Hosp; **Address:** 981225 Nebraska Medical Ctr, Omaha, NE 68198-1225; **Phone:** 402-559-6500; **Board Cert:** Otolaryngology 1994; **Med School:** Univ Nebr Coll Med 1988; **Resid:** Otolaryngology, Univ Nebraska Med Ctr 1993; **Fellow:** Head and Neck Surgery, Meml Sloan Kettering Cancer Ctr 1995; **Fac Appt:** Prof Oto, Univ Nebr Coll Med

Shelton, Clough MD [Oto] - **Spec Exp:** Facial Nerve Disorders; Acoustic Neuroma; Hearing & Balance Disorders; Cochlear Implants; **Hospital:** Univ Utah Hosps and Clins; **Address:** Univi Utah Sch Med, 50 N Medical Drive, 1-900 East, Ste 3C120, Salt Lake City, UT 84132; **Phone:** 801-585-5450; **Board Cert:** Otolaryngology 1981; Neurotology 2004; **Med School:** Univ Tex SW, Dallas 1981; **Resid:** Otolaryngology, Stanford Univ Med Ctr 1986; **Fellow:** Neurotology, Otologic Med Group 1987; **Fac Appt:** Prof Oto, Univ Utah

Southwest

Clayman, Gary Lee MD/DMD [Oto] - **Spec Exp:** Thyroid Cancer & Surgery; Salivary Gland Tumors & Surgery; Head & Neck Cancer; **Hospital:** UT MD Anderson Cancer Ctr; **Address:** Univ TX/MD Anderson Cancer Center, 1515 Holcombe Blvd, Box 441, Houston, TX 77030-4009; **Phone:** 713-792-8837; **Board Cert:** Otolaryngology 1992; **Med School:** NE Ohio Univ 1986; **Resid:** Surgery, Hennepin Co Med Ctr 1987; Otolaryngology, Univ Minn Med Ctr 1991; **Fellow:** Head and Neck Surgery, MD Anderson Cancer Ctr 1993; **Fac Appt:** Prof Oto, Univ Tex, Houston

Daspit, C Phillip MD [Oto] - **Spec Exp:** Hearing & Balance Disorders; Cochlear Implants; Chronic Ear Disease; **Hospital:** St Joseph's Hosp & Med Ctr - Phoenix; **Address:** 222 W Thomas Rd, Ste 114, Phoenix, AZ 85013; **Phone:** 602-279-5444; **Board Cert:** Otolaryngology 1977; **Med School:** Louisiana State U, New Orleans 1968; **Resid:** Surgery, UCSF Med Ctr 1973; Otolaryngology, Ft Miley VA Hosp 1977; **Fellow:** Otology & Neurotology, House Ear Inst 1978; Skull Base Surgery, House Ear Inst 1978; **Fac Appt:** Clin Prof S, Univ Ariz Coll Med

Donovan, Donald T MD [Oto] - **Spec Exp:** Head & Neck Cancer; Voice Disorders; Vocal Cord Disorders; Thyroid Disorders; **Hospital:** Methodist Hosp - Houston, St Luke's Episcopal Hosp - Houston; **Address:** 6550 Fannin St, Ste 1727, Houston, TX 77030; **Phone:** 713-798-3380; **Board Cert:** Otolaryngology 1981; **Med School:** Baylor Coll Med 1976; **Resid:** Surgery, Baylor Affil Hosps 1978; Otolaryngology, Baylor Affil Hosps 1981; **Fellow:** Head and Neck Surgery, Columbia-Presby Med Ctr 1982; **Fac Appt:** Prof Oto, Baylor Coll Med

Gianoli, Gerard MD [Oto] - **Spec Exp:** Dizziness; Hearing Loss; Ear Disorders; **Hospital:** North Oaks Med Ctr; **Address:** 17050 Medical Center Drive, Ste 315, The Ear & Balance Institute, Baton Rouge, LA 70816-3249; **Phone:** 225-293-6973; **Board Cert:** Otolaryngology 1993; Neurotology 2004; **Med School:** Tulane Univ 1986; **Resid:** Pediatrics, Tulane Univ 1988; Otolaryngology, Tulane Univ 1992; **Fellow:** Otology & Neurotology, Michigan Ear Inst; **Fac Appt:** Assoc Clin Prof Oto, Tulane Univ

Hanna, Ehab YN MD [Oto] - **Spec Exp:** Skull Base Tumors & Surgery; Head & Neck Cancer & Surgery; **Hospital:** UT MD Anderson Cancer Ctr; **Address:** Univ Tex MD Anderson Cancer Ctr, 1515 Holcolmbe Blvd, Unit 441, Houston, TX 77030; **Phone:** 713-745-1815; **Board Cert:** Otolaryngology 1994; **Med School:** Egypt 1982; **Resid:** Otolaryngology, Cleveland Clinic 1989; Otolaryngology, Cleveland Clinic 1993; **Fellow:** Otolaryngology, Univ Pittsburgh Med Ctr 1994; **Fac Appt:** Asst Prof Oto, Univ Tex, Houston

Hayden, Richard E MD [Oto] - **Spec Exp:** Head & Neck Surgery; Facial Plastic & Reconstructive Surgery; Microvascular Surgery; **Hospital:** Mayo Clinic - Phoenix; **Address:** Mayo Clinic, Dept Otolaryngology, 5777 E Mayo Blvd, Phoenix, AZ 85054; **Phone:** 480-342-2912; **Board Cert:** Otolaryngology 1978; **Med School:** McGill Univ 1974; **Resid:** Otolaryngology, Univ Toronto 1978; **Fellow:** Head and Neck Oncology, MD Anderson Hosp 1979; Radiation Oncology, Princess Margaret Hosp 1980; **Fac Appt:** Prof Oto, Mayo Med Sch

Johnson Jr, Calvin M MD [Oto] - **Spec Exp:** Ear Disorders/Surgery; Nasal Surgery; Cosmetic Surgery-Face; **Address:** Hedgewood Surgical Ctr, 2427 St Charles Ave, New Orleans, LA 70130; **Phone:** 504-895-7642; **Board Cert:** Otolaryngology 1974; **Med School:** Tulane Univ 1967; **Resid:** Surgery, Tulane Univ Sch Med 1971; Otolaryngology, Tulane Univ Sch Med 1974; **Fellow:** Facial Plastic Surgery, Amer Academy Facial Plastic & Recon Surg 1975

Macias, John D MD [Oto] - **Spec Exp:** Otology; Neuro-Otology; Cochlear Implants; **Hospital:** Banner Good Samaritan Regl Med Ctr - Phoenix, Phoenix Children's Hosp; **Address:** 1515 N 9th St, Ste B, Phoenix, AZ 85006-2523; **Phone:** 602-257-4228; **Board Cert:** Otolaryngology 1994; Neurotology 2005; **Med School:** Stanford Univ 1988; **Resid:** Otolaryngology, Univ Iowa Hosps & Clins 1993; **Fellow:** Otology, Ear Fdn/Otology Grp 1994

Otolaryngology

Medina, Jesus E MD [Oto] - **Spec Exp:** Head & Neck Cancer; **Hospital:** OU Med Ctr; **Address:** Univ Okla Hlth Sci Ctr, Dept Oto-WP 1290, PO Box 26901, Oklahoma City, OK 73126; **Phone:** 405-271-8047; **Board Cert:** Otolaryngology 1980; **Med School:** Peru 1974; **Resid:** Surgery, Wayne St Univ Affil Hosp 1977; Otolaryngology, Wayne St Univ Affil Hosp 1980; **Fellow:** Head and Neck Surgery, Univ Tex Sys Cancer Ctrs 1981; **Fac Appt:** Prof Oto, Univ Okla Coll Med

Myers, Jeffrey N MD/PhD [Oto] - **Spec Exp:** Head & Neck Cancer; Melanoma-Head & Neck; Tongue Cancer; **Hospital:** UT MD Anderson Cancer Ctr; **Address:** Univ Texas MD Anderson Cancer Ctr, 1515 Holcombe Blvd, Box 441, Houston, TX 77030; **Phone:** 713-745-2667; **Board Cert:** Otolaryngology 1997; **Med School:** Univ Pennsylvania 1991; **Resid:** Otolaryngology, Univ Pittsburgh Med Ctr 1996; **Fellow:** Head & Neck Surgical Oncology, MD Anderson Cancer Ctr 1997; **Fac Appt:** Assoc Prof Oto, Univ Tex, Houston

Nuss, Daniel W MD [Oto] - **Spec Exp:** Head & Neck Cancer; Skull Base Tumors & Surgery; **Hospital:** Our Lady of the Lake Regl Med Ctr; **Address:** Our Lady of the Lake Regl Med Ctr, 7777 Hennessy Blvd, Ste 409, Baton Rouge, LA 70808; **Phone:** 225-765-1765; **Board Cert:** Otolaryngology 1987; **Med School:** Louisiana State U, New Orleans 1981; **Resid:** Surgery, Charity Hosp 1983; Otolaryngology, LSU Med Ctr 1987; **Fellow:** Surgical Oncology, MD Anderson Hosp & Tumor Inst 1984; Head and Neck Surgery, Ctr Cranial Base Surg-Univ Pittsburgh 1991; **Fac Appt:** Prof Oto, Louisiana State U, New Orleans

Otto, Randal A MD [Oto] - **Spec Exp:** Head & Neck Cancer; Thyroid & Parathyroid Cancer & Surgery; Sinus Disorders/Surgery; **Hospital:** Univ Hlth Sys - Univ Hosp (San Antonio, TX), Audie L Murphy Meml Vets Hosp; **Address:** 7703 Floyd Curl Drive, MS 7777, San Antonio, TX 78229-3900; **Phone:** 210-358-0490; **Board Cert:** Otolaryngology 1987; **Med School:** Univ MO-Columbia Sch Med 1981; **Resid:** Pathology, Queens Med Ctr 1982; Otolaryngology, Univ of Missouri 1987; **Fac Appt:** Prof Oto, Univ Tex, San Antonio

Stasney, C Richard MD [Oto] - **Spec Exp:** Voice Disorders; Vocal Cord Disorders; Laryngeal Disorders; **Hospital:** Methodist Hosp - Houston; **Address:** Texas ENT Consultants, 6550 Fannin St, Ste 2025, Houston, TX 77030; **Phone:** 713-796-2001; **Board Cert:** Otolaryngology 1974; **Med School:** Baylor Coll Med 1969; **Resid:** Surgery, Baylor Affil Hosps 1971; Otolaryngology, Baylor Affil Hosps 1974; **Fac Appt:** Assoc Clin Prof Oto, Univ Tex, Houston

Suen, James Y MD [Oto] - **Spec Exp:** Head & Neck Cancer; Vascular Lesions-Head & Neck; Laryngeal Disorders; Thyroid Cancer; **Hospital:** UAMS Med Ctr, Arkansas Chldns Hosp; **Address:** Univ Hosp Arkansas Med Scis, 4301 W Markham St, Slot 543, Little Rock, AR 72205; **Phone:** 501-686-8224; **Board Cert:** Otolaryngology 1973; **Med School:** Univ Ark 1966; **Resid:** Surgery, Univ Arkansas Med Ctr 1970; Otolaryngology, Univ Arkansas Med Ctr 1973; **Fellow:** Head and Neck Surgery, MD Anderson Cancer Ctr-Tumor Inst 1974; **Fac Appt:** Prof Oto, Univ Ark

Weber, Randal S MD [Oto] - **Spec Exp:** Skin Cancer; Thyroid & Parathyroid Cancer & Surgery; Salivary Gland Tumors & Surgery; Head & Neck Cancer; **Hospital:** UT MD Anderson Cancer Ctr; **Address:** 1515 Holcombe Blvd, Unit 441, Houston, TX 77030-4009; **Phone:** 713-745-0497; **Board Cert:** Otolaryngology 1985; **Med School:** Univ Tenn Coll Med, Memphis 1976; **Resid:** Surgery, Baylor Coll Med 1982; Otolaryngology, Baylor Coll Med 1985; **Fellow:** Head and Neck Surgery, MD Anderson Cancer Ctr 1986; **Fac Appt:** Prof Oto, Univ Tex, Houston

Weber, Samuel C MD [Oto] - **Spec Exp:** Thyroid Cancer; Parathyroid Cancer; Nasal & Sinus Cancer & Surgery; Head & Neck Surgery; **Hospital:** St Luke's Episcopal Hosp - Houston, Texas Chldns Hosp - Houston; **Address:** 6624 Fannin St, Ste 1480, Houston, TX 77030-2385; **Phone:** 713-795-5343; **Board Cert:** Otolaryngology 1972; **Med School:** Univ Tenn Coll Med, Memphis 1965; **Resid:** Surgery, Baylor Coll Med 1971; Otolaryngology, Baylor Coll Med 1972; **Fac Appt:** Clin Prof Oto, Baylor Coll Med

West Coast and Pacific

Berke, Gerald S MD [Oto] - **Spec Exp:** Head & Neck Surgery; Head & Neck Cancer; Voice Disorders; Laryngeal Disorders; **Hospital:** Ronald Reagan UCLA Med Ctr; **Address:** 200 UCLA Med Plaza, Ste 550, Los Angeles, CA 90095; **Phone:** 310-825-5179; **Board Cert:** Otolaryngology 1984; **Med School:** USC Sch Med 1978; **Resid:** Otolaryngology, LAC-USC Med Ctr 1979; **Fellow:** Head and Neck Surgery, UCLA Med Ctr 1984; **Fac Appt:** Prof Oto, UCLA

Brackmann, Derald E MD [Oto] - **Spec Exp:** Ear Disorders/Surgery; Facial Nerve Disorders; Acoustic Neuroma; **Hospital:** St Vincent's Med Ctr - Los Angeles, USC Univ Hosp - R K Eamer Med Plz; **Address:** House Clinic, 2100 W 3rd St, Fl 1st, Los Angeles, CA 90057-1902; **Phone:** 213-483-9930; **Board Cert:** Otolaryngology 1971; Neurotology 2005; **Med School:** Univ IL Coll Med 1962; **Resid:** Otolaryngology, LAC/USC Med Ctr 1970; **Fellow:** Otology & Neurotology, House Ear Clinic 1971; **Fac Appt:** Clin Prof Oto, USC-Keck School of Medicine

Cohen, James I MD [Oto] - **Spec Exp:** Thyroid & Parathyroid Cancer & Surgery; **Hospital:** OR Hlth & Sci Univ, Providence St Vincent Med Ctr; **Address:** Oregon Hlth Scis U-PV-01, 3181 SW Sam Jackson Park Rd, Portland, OR 97239; **Phone:** 503-494-5355; **Board Cert:** Otolaryngology 1984; **Med School:** Canada 1978; **Resid:** Surgery, Univ Minn Med Ctr 1980; Otolaryngology, Univ Minn Med Ctr 1984; **Fellow:** Head & Neck Surgical Oncology, MD Anderson Cancer Ctr 1985; **Fac Appt:** Prof Oto, Oregon Hlth Sci Univ

Courey, Mark S MD [Oto] - **Spec Exp:** Laryngeal Disorders; Swallowing Disorders; Laryngeal Cancer; **Hospital:** UCSF - Mt Zion Med Ctr, UCSF Med Ctr; **Address:** UCSF Voice & Swallowing Ctr, 2330 Post St Fl 5, San Francisco, CA 94115; **Phone:** 415-885-7700; **Board Cert:** Otolaryngology 1993; **Med School:** SUNY Buffalo 1987; **Resid:** Otolaryngology, SUNY-Buffalo Med Ctr 1992; **Fellow:** Laryngology, Vanderbilt Univ 1993; **Fac Appt:** Prof Oto, UCSF

De la Cruz, Antonio MD [Oto] - **Spec Exp:** Otosclerosis/Stapedectomy; Skull Base Surgery; Otology; **Hospital:** St Vincent's Med Ctr - Los Angeles, Torrance Memorial Med Ctr; **Address:** 2100 W 3rd St Fl 1, Los Angeles, CA 90057; **Phone:** 213-483-9930; **Board Cert:** Otolaryngology 1973; **Med School:** Costa Rica 1967; **Resid:** Surgery, Univ Miami Med Ctr 1970; Otolaryngology, Univ Miami Med Ctr 1973; **Fellow:** Otology & Neurotology, House Ear Clinic 1974; **Fac Appt:** Clin Prof Oto, USC Sch Med

Donald, Paul MD [Oto] - **Spec Exp:** Skull Base Tumors & Surgery; Head & Neck Cancer; **Hospital:** UC Davis Med Ctr; **Address:** 2521 Stockton Blvd, rm 7200, Sacramento, CA 95817; **Phone:** 916-734-2832; **Board Cert:** Otolaryngology 1973; **Med School:** Univ British Columbia Fac Med 1964; **Resid:** Surgery, St Pauls Hosp 1969; Otolaryngology, Univ Iowa Hosp 1973; **Fac Appt:** Prof Oto, UC Davis

Eisele, David W MD [Oto] - **Spec Exp:** Salivary Gland Tumors & Surgery; Head & Neck Cancer; Thyroid Cancer; **Hospital:** UCSF Med Ctr; **Address:** UCSF, Dept Head & Neck Surgery, 400 Parnassus Ave, Ste A 730, San Francisco, CA 94143-2202; **Phone:** 415-885-7528; **Board Cert:** Otolaryngology 1988; **Med School:** Cornell Univ-Weill Med Coll 1982; **Resid:** Surgery, Univ Wash Med Ctr 1984; Otolaryngology, Univ Wash Med Ctr 1988; **Fac Appt:** Prof Oto, UCSF

Fee Jr, Willard E MD [Oto] - **Spec Exp:** Head & Neck Cancer; Parotid Gland Tumors; Thyroid Cancer; **Hospital:** Stanford Univ Med Ctr; **Address:** Stanford Cancer Ctr, 875 Lake Wilbur Dr, CC-2227, Stanford, CA 94305-5826; **Phone:** 650-723-6500; **Board Cert:** Otolaryngology 1974; **Med School:** Univ Colorado 1969; **Resid:** Surgery, Wadsworth VA Hosp 1971; Otolaryngology, UCLA Med Ctr 1974; **Fac Appt:** Prof Oto, Stanford Univ

Otolaryngology

Futran, Neal D MD/DMD [Oto] - **Spec Exp:** Head & Neck Cancer & Surgery; Head & Neck Cancer Reconstruction; Skull Base Tumors & Surgery; **Hospital:** Univ Wash Med Ctr, Harborview Med Ctr; **Address:** U Wash Med Ctr, Oto Office, 1959 NE Pacific St, Box 356515, Seattle, WA 98195-6515; **Phone:** 206-543-3060; **Board Cert:** Otolaryngology 1993; **Med School:** SUNY Downstate 1987; **Resid:** Surgery, Kings Co-SUNY Downstate 1985; Otolaryngology, Univ Rochester Med Ctr 1992; **Fellow:** Microvascular Surgery, Mt Sinai Hosp 1993; **Fac Appt:** Prof Oto, Univ Wash

Harris, Jeffrey P MD/PhD [Oto] - **Spec Exp:** Neuro-Otology; Hearing & Balance Disorders; Skull Base Surgery; **Hospital:** UCSD Med Ctr, VA San Diego Hlthcre Sys; **Address:** UCSD Med Ctr, 200 W Arbor Drive, MC 8895, San Diego, CA 92103-8895; **Phone:** 619-543-7896; **Board Cert:** Otolaryngology 1974; Neurotology 2004; **Med School:** Univ Pennsylvania 1974; **Resid:** Otolaryngology, Mass EE Infirmary 1979; **Fellow:** Neurological Surgery, Univ Zurich Med Ctr 1983; **Fac Appt:** Prof S, UCSD

Jackler, Robert K MD [Oto] - **Spec Exp:** Neuro-Otology; Skull Base Surgery; Ear Tumors; **Hospital:** Stanford Univ Med Ctr; **Address:** Stanford Univ Med Ctr, Dept Head & Neck Surg, 801 Welch Rd, Stanford, CA 94305-5739; **Phone:** 650-725-6500; **Board Cert:** Otolaryngology 1984; Neurotology 2004; **Med School:** Boston Univ 1979; **Resid:** Otolaryngology, UCSF Med Ctr 1984; **Fellow:** Otolaryngology, Oto Med Grp 1985; **Fac Appt:** Prof Oto, Stanford Univ

Kaplan, Michael J MD [Oto] - **Spec Exp:** Head & Neck Surgery; Skull Base Surgery; Head & Neck Cancer; **Hospital:** Stanford Univ Med Ctr; **Address:** Stanford Cancer Ctr, Dept Otolaryngology, 801 Welch Rd, Stanford, CA 94305-5739; **Phone:** 650-723-5416; **Board Cert:** Otolaryngology 1982; **Med School:** Harvard Med Sch 1977; **Resid:** Surgery, Beth Israel-Chldns Hosps 1979; Otolaryngology, Mass EE Infirm 1982; **Fellow:** Head and Neck Surgery, Univ Virginia 1984; **Fac Appt:** Prof Oto, Stanford Univ

Keller, Gregory S MD [Oto] - **Spec Exp:** Cosmetic Surgery-Face; **Hospital:** Santa Barbara Cottage Hosp, Ronald Reagan UCLA Med Ctr; **Address:** 221 E Pueblo St, Ste A, Santa Barbara, CA 93105; **Phone:** 805-687-6408; **Board Cert:** Otolaryngology 1976; **Med School:** Univ IL Coll Med 1971; **Resid:** Surgery, Cottage Hosp 1973; Otolaryngology, Univ Illinois 1976; **Fac Appt:** Assoc Clin Prof S, UCLA

Larrabee Jr, Wayne F MD [Oto] - **Spec Exp:** Cosmetic Surgery-Face; Eyelid Surgery; Rhinoplasty; Nasal Surgery; **Hospital:** Swedish Med Ctr - Seattle, Univ Wash Med Ctr; **Address:** Facial Plastic Surgery Ctr, 600 Broadway Ste 280, Seattle, WA 98122-5371; **Phone:** 206-386-3550; **Board Cert:** Otolaryngology 1979; Facial Plastic & Reconstructive Surgery 1999; **Med School:** Tulane Univ 1971; **Resid:** Surgery, Charity Hosp 1976; Otolaryngology, Tulane Univ Med Ctr 1979; **Fac Appt:** Clin Prof Oto, Univ Wash

McMenomey, Sean O MD [Oto] - **Spec Exp:** Otology & Neuro-Otology; Skull Base Tumors & Surgery; Head & Neck Surgery; Stereotactic Radiosurgery; **Hospital:** OR Hlth & Sci Univ, Providence St Vincent Med Ctr; **Address:** Oregon Hlth & Sci Univ, Dept Otolaryngology, 3181 SW Sam Jackson Park Rd, MC PV-01, Portland, OR 97239; **Phone:** 503-494-8135; **Board Cert:** Otolaryngology 1993; Neurotology 2004; **Med School:** St Louis Univ 1987; **Resid:** Otolaryngology, Oregon Health Sci Ctr 1992; **Fellow:** Otology & Neurotology, Baptist Hosp 1993; **Fac Appt:** Assoc Prof Oto, Oregon Hlth Sci Univ

Powell, Nelson B MD/DDS [Oto] - **Spec Exp:** Sleep Disorders/Apnea; Maxillofacial Surgery; **Hospital:** Stanford Univ Med Ctr; **Address:** 750 Welch Rd, Ste 317, Palo Alto, CA 94304; **Phone:** 650-328-0511; **Board Cert:** Otolaryngology 1984; **Med School:** Univ Wash 1979; **Resid:** Surgery, Stanford Univ Hosp & Clinics 1980; Otolaryngology, Stanford Univ Hosp 1983; **Fac Appt:** Clin Prof S, Stanford Univ

Rice, Dale MD [Oto] - **Spec Exp:** Head & Neck Cancer; Sinus Disorders/Surgery; **Hospital:** USC Univ Hosp - R K Eamer Med Plz; **Address:** USC Keck Sch Med, 1200 N State St, rm 4316, Los Angeles, CA 90033-1029; **Phone:** 323-442-5790; **Board Cert:** Otolaryngology 1976; **Med School:** Univ Mich Med Sch 1968; **Resid:** Surgery, Univ Mich Med Ctr 1976; Otolaryngology, Univ Mich Med Ctr 1976; **Fac Appt:** Prof Oto, USC Sch Med

Senders, Craig W MD [Oto] - **Spec Exp:** Pediatric Otolaryngology; Cleft Palate/Lip; Endoscopic Sinus Surgery; Sleep Disorders/Apnea; **Hospital:** UC Davis Med Ctr; **Address:** UC Davis, Dept Oto-Head & Neck Surg, 2521 Stockton Blvd, Ste 7200, Sacramento, CA 95817; **Phone:** 916-734-5400; **Board Cert:** Otolaryngology 1984; **Med School:** Oregon Hlth Sci Univ 1979; **Resid:** Otolaryngology, Univ Iowa Hosps & Clins 1983; **Fellow:** Maxillofacial Surgery, Univ Iowa Hosps & Clins 1984; **Fac Appt:** Prof Oto, UC Davis

Singer, Mark I MD [Oto] - **Spec Exp:** Head & Neck Surgery; Head & Neck Cancer; Melanoma; **Hospital:** CA Pacific Med Ctr; **Address:** 3801 Sacramento St, Ste 230, San Francisco, CA 94118; **Phone:** 415-600-2450; **Board Cert:** Otolaryngology 1976; **Med School:** Columbia P&S 1970; **Resid:** Surgery, Northwestern Meml Hosp 1973; Otolaryngology, Northwestern Meml Hosp 1976; **Fellow:** Oncology, Northwestern Meml Hosp 1976

Sinha, Uttam K MD [Oto] - **Spec Exp:** Head & Neck Cancer; Voice Disorders; **Hospital:** USC Univ Hosp - R K Eamer Med Plz, House Ear Inst; **Address:** 1200 N State St, rm 4136, Los Angeles, CA 90033; **Phone:** 323-226-7315; **Board Cert:** Otolaryngology 1998; **Med School:** India 1985; **Resid:** Otolaryngology, LAC-USC Med Ctr 1995; **Fellow:** Mount Sinai Med Sch 1988; LAC-USC Med Ctr 1990; **Fac Appt:** Asst Prof Oto, USC Sch Med

Wax, Mark K MD [Oto] - **Spec Exp:** Facial Nerve Disorders; Skull Base Tumors & Surgery; Facial Plastic & Reconstructive Surgery; **Hospital:** OR Hlth & Sci Univ; **Address:** Oregon Hlth Scis Univ, Dept Ototlaryngology, 3181 SW Sam Jackson Park Rd, Ste PV-01, Portland, OR 97201; **Phone:** 503-494-5355; **Board Cert:** Otolaryngology 1985; Facial Plastic & Reconstructive Surgery 1987; **Med School:** Univ Toronto 1980; **Resid:** Otolaryngology, Univ Toronto 1985; Surgery, Cedars-Sinai Med Ctr 1983; **Fellow:** Head and Neck Surgery, St Michaels Hosp 1991; **Fac Appt:** Prof Oto, Oregon Hlth Sci Univ

Weisman, Robert A MD [Oto] - **Spec Exp:** Head & Neck Cancer; Clinical Trials; Thyroid & Parathyroid Cancer & Surgery; Head & Neck Cancer Reconstruction; **Hospital:** UCSD Med Ctr; **Address:** Moores-UCSD Cancer Center, 3855 Health Sciences Drive, MC 0987, La Jolla, CA 92093-0987; **Phone:** 858-822-6197; **Board Cert:** Otolaryngology 1978; **Med School:** Washington Univ, St Louis 1973; **Resid:** Head and Neck Surgery, UCLA Med Ctr 1978; **Fac Appt:** Prof S, UCSD

Weymuller, Ernest MD [Oto] - **Spec Exp:** Head & Neck Cancer; Sinus Disorders/Surgery; **Hospital:** Univ Wash Med Ctr; **Address:** 1959 NE Pacific St, Box 356161, Seattle, WA 98195-6161; **Phone:** 206-598-4022; **Board Cert:** Otolaryngology 1973; **Med School:** Harvard Med Sch 1966; **Resid:** Surgery, Vanderbilt Univ Hosp 1968; Otolaryngology, Mass Eye and Ear Infirm 1973; **Fac Appt:** Prof Oto, Univ Wash

Cleveland Clinic

Head and Neck Institute

The specialists at the Cleveland Clinic Head and Neck Institute have been recognized nationally and internationally as leaders in this multidisciplinary field. The Institute is composed of specialists with extensive training in all areas, including:

Audiology: Audiologists provide the non-medical management of hearing disorders including comprehensive audiologic evaluation and treatment through the use of assistive listening devices, hearing aids, Baha Hearing Systems, and cochlear implants.

Facial Aesthetic and Reconstructive Surgery: Surgeons perform a broad range of procedures, from office-based treatments including Botox and Restylane injections to operative procedures ranging from rhinoplasty and facelifts to major facial reconstructive surgery.

> The Cleveland Clinic Head and Neck Institute has been routinely recognized among the best programs in the United States by *U.S.News & World Report* magazine.
>
> With more than 25 full-time faculty members caring for adult and pediatric patients with routine or complex ear, nose and throat disorders, the Institute is one of the largest otolaryngology programs in the United States.

Head and Neck Surgery: Evaluation and treatment of both benign and malignant head and neck tumors. Patients are seen in a team fashion by surgeons, radiation therapists and oncologists to facilitate optimal treatment.

Laryngotracheal Reconstruction: Laryngeal airway obstruction, esophageal reflux, tracheal aspiration, and voice preservation and rehabilitation and removal of upper and lower respiratory foreign bodies.

Nasal and Sinus Disorders: Treatment of a wide variety of sinonasal conditions, including rhinosinusitis, nasal polyps, fungal sinusitis, septal deviation, nasal obstruction and inhalant allergies. Minimally invasive, computer-aided, endoscopic techniques for revision sinus surgery, CSF leaks and neoplasms of the nose, sinuses and skull base.

Otology-Neurotology: Care of all forms of otologic disorders, including middle and posterior cranial fossa surgery for cerebellopontine and skull base tumors. Immune-mediated inner ear disease (deafness), Meniere's disease and cochlear implantation are also handled here.

Pediatric Otolaryngology: Treatment of all forms of pediatric otolaryngologic disorders, with support from Cleveland Clinic Children's Hospital, a pediatric intensive care unit and numerous other pediatric specialists on staff.

Speech-Language Pathology: Comprehensive evaluation and treatment for all speech, language, voice, cognitive and swallowing disorders. Services are provided to pediatric through geriatric patient populations via an interdisciplinary medical care model.

Vestibular and Balance Disorders: Diagnosis and vestibular rehabilitation from dizziness, disequilibrium.

For more information about the Cleveland Clinic Head and Neck Institute, to schedule a second opinion or to learn about assistance for out-of-town patients, call 800.890.2467 or visit www.clevelandclinic.org/headandnecktopdocs.

Head and Neck Institute | 9500 Euclid Avenue / AC311 | Cleveland OH 44195

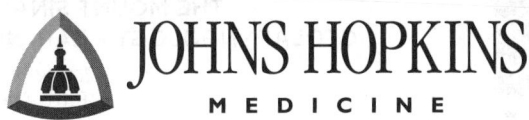

JOHNS HOPKINS
M E D I C I N E

Otolaryngology–Head and Neck Surgery
601 North Caroline Street, Suite 6210, Baltimore, Maryland 21287

For patient appointments: 443-735-4872
www.hopkinsmedicine.org/otolaryngology

Johns Hopkins Otolaryngology–Head and Neck Surgery is consistently recognized by peers around the country for our research, advanced treatments, effective use of technology and focus on patient care.

Named the best Ear, Nose and Throat program in the nation for 11 consecutive years by *U.S. News & World Report*, our faculty and staff devote themselves to patient safety and care every day. Our physicians are clinical scientists who, in addition to taking care of patients, are engaged in research to better understand the diseases and conditions they treat in an effort to develop new and more effective therapies.

Our team includes head and neck surgeons, facial plastic reconstructive surgeons, speech-language pathologists, audiologists, otologists, neurotologists, laryngologists, pediatric otolaryngologists, swallowing therapists, dentists and oral surgeons who collaborate to provide comprehensive services to each of our patients.

Johns Hopkins' expertise ranges from common problems like tonsillitis, snoring and ear infections to such complex conditions as sinusitis, Ménière's disease, speech disorders, skull base tumors and oral and throat cancers.

Innovation and Discovery

■ As the nation's leading cochlear implant program, the Johns Hopkins Listening Center specializes in treating children and adults with profound hearing loss. Our physicians implanted nearly 200 devices last year, more than any other cochlear implant program in North America.

■ Our head and neck surgeons are investigating causes of head and neck cancer and searching for new methods of early cancer detection and prevention as part of a multidisciplinary center.

■ In addition to diagnosing and treating a range of nasal and sinus problems, our sinus and rhinology physicians are also engaged in unparalleled basic science and clinical research to explore the causes of nasal and sinus disorders.

■ Hopkins otologists specialize in treating disorders of the ear, including Ménière's disease, and are researching ways to identify genes associated with the disease that could lead to a diagnostic test and ultimately, effective treatments.

Centers of Excellence include:

■ *Center for Facial Plastic and Reconstructive Surgery*

■ *Head and Neck Cancer Center*

■ *Hopkins Hearing*

■ *Center for Laryngeal and Voice Disorders*

■ *The Listening Center*

■ *Pediatric Otolaryngology*

■ *Sinus Center*

■ *Skull Base Surgery Center*

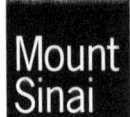 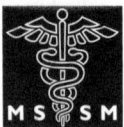

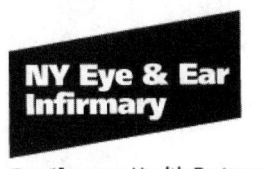

NY Eye & Ear Infirmary

Continuum Health Partners, Inc.

THE NEW YORK EYE AND EAR INFIRMARY

310 East 14th Street
New York, New York 10003
Tel. 212.979.4000   Fax. 212.228.0664
http://www.nyee.edu

PROVIDING EXCEPTIONAL CARE OF THE EAR, NOSE, THROAT, AND HEAD & NECK

Established in 1820 the Department of Otolaryngology/Head & Neck Surgery is the first training program in this specialty in the Western Hemisphere. Over nearly two centuries the department has evolved to be an international referral center for the medical and surgical treatment of diseases of the ear, nose, and throat.

OUTSTANDING SERVICES:

Ear Institute (Otology – Neuro-otology): Specializing in the care of chronic ear disease including hearing loss, cochlear implantation, dizziness, tinnitus, intra cranial tumors and facial nerve disorders. Our advanced otologic and vestibular diagnostic labs assist physicians in treatment.

Facial Plastic Surgery: In-office or ambulatory procedures utilizing computer imaging, new techniques and materials produce outstanding results with minimal incisions, rapid recovery and a natural, youthful appearance.

Facial Paralysis: Comprehensive center treating all causes and offering reconstruction of the paralyzed face.

Head & Neck Oncology: A multi-disciplinary team including board-certified surgeons, medical & radiation oncologists, nutritionists and rehabilitation specialists insure rapid recovery from complex, life-saving surgical procedures and return to daily activities.

Pediatric Otolaryngology: Treating children has long been a priority at the Infirmary. Pediatric care ranges from middle ear infection, tonsil and adenoid disease, and neck masses to complex sinus and airway diseases.

Rhinology and Sinus Surgery: Internationally known specialists utilize minimally invasive techniques to treat disorders from sinusitis to intra cranial tumors.

Thyroid Center: A comprehensive program to streamline the diagnosis and treatment of thyroid diseases and cancers. A highly skilled team of surgeons, endocrinologists and radiologists manage the patient's care.

Voice & Swallowing Institute: Combining the expertise of physicians, speech pathologists and a voice physiologist to diagnose and treat voice problems – not only for performing artists but also for teachers, stockbrokers, receptionists, salespeople – anyone for whom voice is an important part of life.

Otolaryngology Clinical Services

General Otolaryngology *plus*
Facial Plastic & Reconstructive Surgery
Cochlear Implantation
Voice & Vocal Dynamics
Head & Neck Oncology
Laryngology
Otology & Neuro-otology
Pediatric Otolaryngology
Rhinology & Sinus Surgery
Swallowing Disorders
Thyroid Center

Facilities

Ambulatory Care Services
Faculty Practice
Teaching Practice
Hearing Aid Dispensary
Vestibular Rehabilitation

About The New York Eye and Ear Infirmary

The Infirmary is the nation's oldest, continuously operating specialty hospital and one of the most experienced in terms of the number of patients it treats and complexity of its cases. Each year the otolaryngology department performs more than 6,000 surgeries and sees more than 70,000 visits from outpatients

Physician Referral
1.800.449.HOPE (4673)

OTOLARYNGOLOGY

(Ear, Nose, and Throat)

Treating the full spectrum of ear, nose, throat, head and neck disorders, the Department of Otolaryngology at NYU Medical Center (www.med.nyu/ent) provides state-of-the-art patient care and research through the following programs:

Cochlear Implants— the first center in the U.S. to use a multichannel cochlear implant in a profoundly deaf adult, in 1984. Since then we have implanted more than 1700 adults and children from the age of 6 months to 85 years.

Sinus and Nasal Disorders — comprehensive diagnosis and minimally invasive treatment of sinus and nasal disorders

Facial Plastic Surgery — plastic and reconstructive surgery for a variety of problems, including nasal obstruction, facial trauma, defects left after removing skin and other facial cancers, facial paralysis and spasm, congenital malformations.

Head and Neck Surgery — state of the art treatment for benign and cancerous diseases of the nasopharynx, larynx, tongue, mouth, mandible, neck and face.

Sleep Apnea — repairing the collapse of soft tissue that leads to snoring and sleep apnea (a dangerous condition in which snorers stop breathing repeatedly during the night, taxing the heart and leaving the snorer unrested)

Skull Base Surgery — minimally invasive and advanced surgical approaches to the tumors of the anterior and posterior skull base such as acoustic neuroma, esthesioneuroblastoma, NF2, chordoma, chondrosarcoma, encephalocele.

Swallowing Disorders — the only center of its kind in New York City, providing comprehensive diagnosis, treatment and therapy for swallowing disorders.

Voice Center — state-of-the-art biofeedback and therapy to rectify problems in speech

Advanced Otologic Medicine & Surgery — treating patients with disorders of the ear and conditions that affect hearing, balance and facial nerve function

The cochlear implant program at NYU Cochlear Implant Center is one of the nation's finest. Since it set the standard in 1984 by implanting a profoundly deaf adult, the Center has been the site of numerous studies and research trials that will continue to improve the technologies available. www.med.nyu.edu/cochlear

Adults and children travel from all over the world to get their cochlear implant at NYU Langone Medical Center.

Pain Medicine

subspecialty of Anesthesiology, Neurology,
and in Physical Medicine and Rehabilitation
or Psychiatry

Some physicians who have their primary board certification in anesthesiology, neurology, physical medicine and rehabilitation, or psychiatry have completed additional training and passed an examination in the subspecialty called pain management. These doctors provide a high level of care, either as a primary physician or consultant, for patients experiencing problems with acute, chronic and/or cancer pain in both hospital and ambulatory settings.

For more information about the main specialties of these physicians, see **Anesthesiology, Neurology, Physical Medicine** and **Rehabilitation** or **Psychiatry** section(s).

Training Required: Number of years required for primary specialty *plus* additional training and examination

PAIN MEDICINE

New England

Abrahm, Janet L MD [PM] - **Spec Exp:** Palliative Care; Pain-Cancer; **Hospital:** Dana-Farber Cancer Inst, Brigham & Women's Hosp; **Address:** Dana-Farber Cancer Institute, 44 Binney St, Shields-Warren 420, Boston, MA 02115; **Phone:** 617-632-6464; **Board Cert:** Internal Medicine 1976; Medical Oncology 1981; Hematology 1978; **Med School:** UCSF 1973; **Resid:** Internal Medicine, Mass Genl Hosp 1975; Internal Medicine, Moffitt Hosp-UCSF 1977; **Fellow:** Hematology, Mass Genl Hosp 1976; Hematology & Oncology, Hosp Univ Penn 1980; **Fac Appt:** Assoc Prof Med, Harvard Med Sch

Berde, Charles Benjamin MD/PhD [PM] - **Spec Exp:** Pain Management-Pediatric; Critical Care; Reflex Sympathetic Dystrophy (RSD); **Hospital:** Children's Hospital - Boston, Spaulding Rehab Hosp; **Address:** Chldns Hosp, Dept Anes, 300 Longwood Ave, Bader 3, Boston, MA 02115; **Phone:** 617-355-6995; **Board Cert:** Pediatrics 1988; Anesthesiology 1988; Pain Medicine 2004; **Med School:** Stanford Univ 1980; **Resid:** Pediatrics, Chldns Hosp 1983; Anesthesiology, Mass Genl Hosp 1985; **Fellow:** Pediatric Anesthesiology, Chldns Hosp 1985; **Fac Appt:** Prof Ped, Harvard Med Sch

Billings, J Andrew MD [PM] - **Spec Exp:** Palliative Care; Pain Management; **Hospital:** Mass Genl Hosp; **Address:** 55 Fruit St, FND 600, Boston, MA 02114; **Phone:** 617-724-9197; **Board Cert:** Internal Medicine 1975; Hospice & Palliative Medicine ; **Med School:** Harvard Med Sch 1972; **Resid:** Internal Medicine, Univ California Hosps 1975; **Fellow:** Internal Medicine, Mass Genl Hosp 1977; **Fac Appt:** Assoc Prof Med, Harvard Med Sch

Hurwitz, Craig A MD [PM] - **Spec Exp:** Pain-Cancer; Palliative Care; **Hospital:** Maine Med Ctr; **Address:** Center for Pain & Palliative Care, 22 Bramhall St, rm 4670, Portland, ME 04102; **Phone:** 207-662-3500; **Board Cert:** Pediatrics 1986; Pediatric Hematology-Oncology 2007; Hospice & Palliative Medicine 2005; **Med School:** Univ Tex SW, Dallas 1982; **Resid:** Pediatrics, Duke Univ Med Ctr 1985; **Fellow:** Pediatric Hematology-Oncology, Duke Univ Med Ctr 1988; **Fac Appt:** Assoc Clin Prof Ped, Univ VT Coll Med

Loder, Elizabeth W MD [PM] - **Spec Exp:** Headache; Migraine; **Hospital:** Brigham & Women's Hosp, Faulkner Hosp; **Address:** 1153 Centre St, Ste 4970, Boston, MA 02130; **Phone:** 617-983-7580; **Board Cert:** Internal Medicine 2000; **Med School:** Univ ND Sch Med 1985; **Resid:** Internal Medicine, Faulkner Hosp 1989; **Fellow:** Pain Medicine, Graham Headache Ctr 1990; **Fac Appt:** Asst Prof Med, Harvard Med Sch

Mid Atlantic

De Leon-Casasola, Oscar A MD [PM] - **Spec Exp:** Pain-Acute; Pain-Chronic; Pain-Cancer; **Hospital:** Roswell Park Cancer Inst; **Address:** Roswell Park Cancer Inst, Anesthesia/Pain Med, Elm & Carlton Sts, Buffalo, NY 14263; **Phone:** 716-845-4595; **Board Cert:** Anesthesiology 1991; Critical Care Medicine 1993; Pain Medicine 2005; **Med School:** Guatemala 1982; **Resid:** Surgery, SUNY-Downstate Med Ctr 1986; Anesthesiology, Univ Buffalo 1989; **Fac Appt:** Prof Anes, SUNY Buffalo

Diwan, Sudhir MD [PM] - **Spec Exp:** Pain-after Spinal Intervention; Pain-Musculoskeletal; Pain-Neuropathic; Pain-Cancer; **Hospital:** NY-Presby Hosp/Weill Cornell (page 66); **Address:** 1305 York Ave Fl 10, Box 120, New York, NY 10021; **Phone:** 646-962-7246; **Board Cert:** Anesthesiology 2001; Pain Medicine 2002; **Med School:** India 1983; **Resid:** Surgery, St Luke's-Roosevelt Hosp Ctr 1994; Anesthesiology, St Luke's-Roosevelt Hosp Ctr 1997

Dubois, Michel MD [PM] - **Spec Exp:** Pain-Back & Neck; Pain-Neuropathic; **Hospital:** NYU Med Ctr (page 68), Bellevue Hosp Ctr; **Address:** 317 E 34th St, Ste 902, New York, NY 10016-4974; **Phone:** 212-201-1004; **Board Cert:** Anesthesiology 1985; Pain Medicine 2004; **Med School:** France 1974; **Resid:** Anesthesiology, Georgetown Univ Hosp 1980; London Hosp 1976; **Fellow:** Pain Medicine, Georgetown Univ Hosp 1983; **Fac Appt:** Prof Anes, NYU Sch Med

Foley, Kathleen M MD [PM] - **Spec Exp:** Palliative Care; Pain-Cancer; **Hospital:** Meml Sloan-Kettering Cancer Ctr; **Address:** 1275 York Avenue, New York, NY 10065; **Phone:** 800-525-2225; **Board Cert:** Neurology 1977; **Med School:** Cornell Univ-Weill Med Coll 1969; **Resid:** Neurology, New York Hosp 1974; **Fellow:** Clinical Genetics, New York Hosp 1971; **Fac Appt:** Prof N, Cornell Univ-Weill Med Coll

Jain, Subhash MD [PM] - **Spec Exp:** Pain-Cancer; Pain-Pelvic; Reflex Sympathetic Dystrophy (RSD); Pain-Neuropathic; **Hospital:** Beth Israel Med Ctr - Petrie Division (page 57); **Address:** 360 S 72nd St, Ste C, New York, NY 10021; **Phone:** 212-439-6100; **Board Cert:** Anesthesiology 1994; Pain Medicine 1998; **Med School:** India 1968; **Resid:** Surgery, St Vincent Med Ctr 1977; Anesthesiology, New York Hosp 1979; **Fellow:** Pain Medicine, New York Hosp/Meml Sloan Kettering Cancer Ctr 1980; **Fac Appt:** Assoc Prof Anes, Cornell Univ-Weill Med Coll

Kreitzer, Joel MD [PM] - **Spec Exp:** Pain-Back; Pain-Cancer; Pain-Neuropathic; **Hospital:** Mount Sinai Med Ctr (page 64), Mount Sinai Hosp of Queens (page 64); **Address:** Upper East Side Pain Medicine, 1540 York Ave, New York, NY 10028; **Phone:** 212-288-2180; **Board Cert:** Anesthesiology 1990; Pain Medicine 2004; **Med School:** Albert Einstein Coll Med 1985; **Resid:** Anesthesiology, Mount Sinai Hosp 1989; **Fellow:** Pain Medicine, Mount Sinai Hosp 1989; **Fac Appt:** Assoc Clin Prof Anes, Mount Sinai Sch Med

Ngeow, Jeffrey MD [PM] - **Spec Exp:** Pain-Musculoskeletal-Spine & Neck; Acupuncture; Reflex Sympathetic Dystrophy (RSD); Pain-Neuropathic; **Hospital:** Hosp For Special Surgery (page 59); **Address:** 535 E 70th St, New York, NY 10021-4872; **Phone:** 212-606-1059; **Board Cert:** Anesthesiology 1980; Pain Medicine 2005; **Med School:** England 1971; **Resid:** Anesthesiology, Peter Bent Brigham Hosp 1977; **Fellow:** Pain Medicine, Tufts New England Med Ctr 1978; **Fac Appt:** Assoc Clin Prof Anes, Cornell Univ-Weill Med Coll

Portenoy, Russell MD [PM] - **Spec Exp:** Pain-Cancer; Palliative Care; **Hospital:** Beth Israel Med Ctr - Petrie Division (page 57); **Address:** Beth Israel Med Ctr, Dept Pain Medicine/Palliative Care, First Ave at 16th St, New York, NY 10003; **Phone:** 212-844-1403; **Board Cert:** Neurology 1985; **Med School:** Univ MD Sch Med 1980; **Resid:** Neurology, Albert Einstein 1984; **Fellow:** Pain Medicine, Meml Sloan-Kettering Cancer Ctr 1985; **Fac Appt:** Prof N, Albert Einstein Coll Med

Raja, Srinivasa MD [PM] - **Spec Exp:** Pain-Neuropathic; Herpetic Neuralgia (Shingles); Reflex Sympathetic Dystrophy (RSD); **Hospital:** Johns Hopkins Hosp - Baltimore (page 61); **Address:** 600 N Wolfe St Bldg Osler Fl 2 - rm 292, Baltimore, MD 21287; **Phone:** 410-955-7246; **Board Cert:** Anesthesiology 1982; Pain Medicine 1993; **Med School:** India 1974; **Resid:** Anesthesiology, Univ Washington Med Ctr 1979; **Fellow:** Pain Medicine, Univ Virginia Hosp 1981; **Fac Appt:** Prof Anes, Johns Hopkins Univ

Staats, Peter MD [PM] - **Spec Exp:** Pain-Cancer; Pain-Back; **Hospital:** Riverview Med Ctr, CentraState Med Ctr; **Address:** Metzger Staats Pain Mgmt, 160 Avenue at the Commons, Ste 1, Shrewsbury, NJ 07702; **Phone:** 732-380-0200; **Board Cert:** Anesthesiology 1994; Pain Medicine 2005; **Med School:** Univ Mich Med Sch 1989; **Resid:** Anesthesiology, Johns Hopkins Hosp 1993; **Fellow:** Pain Medicine, Johns Hopkins Hosp 1994

Pain Medicine

Weinberger, Michael L MD [PM] - **Spec Exp:** Pain-Cancer; Pain-Back; **Hospital:** NY-Presby Hosp/Columbia (page 66); **Address:** 630 W 168th St, PH5, rm 500, New York, NY 10032-3720; **Phone:** 212-305-7114; **Board Cert:** Internal Medicine 1986; Anesthesiology 1990; Pain Medicine 2004; Hospice & Palliative Medicine 2006; **Med School:** Columbia P&S 1983; **Resid:** Internal Medicine, St Vincent's Hosp 1986; Anesthesiology, Columbia-Presby Med Ctr 1989; **Fellow:** Pain Medicine, Meml Sloan Kettering Cancer Ctr 1990; **Fac Appt:** Assoc Prof Anes, Columbia P&S

Southeast

Anghelescu, Doralina L MD [PM] - **Spec Exp:** Pain Management-Pediatric; Pain-Cancer; **Hospital:** St Jude Children's Research Hosp; **Address:** St Jude Chldn's Rsch Hosp, Anesthesiology, 332 N Lauderdale, rm B3035, MS 130, Memphis, TN 38105; **Phone:** 901-495-4034; **Board Cert:** Anesthesiology 1998; Pain Medicine 2001; **Med School:** Romania 1985; **Resid:** Anesthesiology, Univ NMex Hosp 1997; **Fellow:** Pain Medicine, Chldns Natl Med Ctr 1998; Pain Medicine, Univ NMex Hosp 1999

Baumann, Patricia L MD [PM] - **Hospital:** Crawford Long Hosp of Emory Univ, Emory Univ Hosp; **Address:** 550 Peachtree St Fl 7 - Ste 7085, Atlanta, GA 30308; **Phone:** 404-686-2410; **Board Cert:** Anesthesiology 1993; Pain Medicine 2005; **Med School:** Emory Univ 1988; **Resid:** Anesthesiology, Emory Univ Med Ctr 1992; **Fac Appt:** Asst Prof Anes, Emory Univ

Rauck, Richard L MD [PM] - **Spec Exp:** Pain-Cancer; Spinal Cord Stimulation; Complex Regional Pain Syndrome-CRPS; **Hospital:** Forsyth Med Ctr, Wake Forest Univ Baptist Med Ctr (page 73); **Address:** Carolinas Pain Institute, 145 Kimel Park Drive, Ste 330, Winston-Salem, NC 27103; **Phone:** 336-765-6181; **Board Cert:** Anesthesiology 1987; Pain Medicine 2005; **Med School:** Bowman Gray 1982; **Resid:** Anesthesiology, Univ Cincinnati Hosp 1985; **Fellow:** Pain Medicine, Univ Cincinnati Hosp 1986; **Fac Appt:** Assoc Prof Anes, Wake Forest Univ

Midwest

Abram, Stephen E MD [PM] - **Hospital:** Froedtert Meml Lutheran Hosp; **Address:** Med Coll Wisconsin-Pain Mgmt Ctr, Tosa Ctr Fl 1st, 1155 N Mayfair Rd, Wauwatosa, WI 53226; **Phone:** 414-456-7600; **Board Cert:** Anesthesiology 2001; Pain Medicine 2004; **Med School:** Jefferson Med Coll 1970; **Resid:** Anesthesiology, Mary Hitchcock Meml Hosp 1973; **Fac Appt:** Prof Anes, Med Coll Wisc

Amin, Sandeep D MD [PM] - **Spec Exp:** Headache-Supraorbital stimulation; Complex Regional Pain Syndrome-CRPS; Pain-Cancer; Pain-after Spinal Intervention; **Hospital:** Rush Univ Med Ctr; **Address:** Rush Pain Ctr, 1725 W Harrison St, Ste 550, Chicago, IL 60612; **Phone:** 312-942-6631; **Board Cert:** Anesthesiology 1998; Pain Medicine 2000; **Med School:** India 1991; **Resid:** Anesthesiology, Univ of Illinois Hosps 1997; **Fellow:** Pain Medicine, Univ of Illinois Hosps 1998; Pain Medicine, Johns Hopkins Hosp 1999; **Fac Appt:** Prof Anes, Rush Med Coll

Benedetti, Costantino MD [PM] - **Spec Exp:** Pain-Cancer; Palliative Care; Pain-Acute; Pain-Chronic; **Hospital:** Ohio St Univ Med Ctr, Arthur G James Cancer Hosp & Research Inst; **Address:** Ohio State Univ Med Ctr, 300 W 10th Ave, Ste 519, Columbus, OH 43210; **Phone:** 614-293-6599; **Board Cert:** Hospice & Palliative Medicine 1997; **Med School:** Italy 1972; **Resid:** Anesthesiology, Univ Colorado Hosp 1976; Anesthesiology, Univ Wash Med Ctr 1976; **Fellow:** Pain Medicine, Univ Wash Med Ctr 1978; **Fac Appt:** Clin Prof Anes, Ohio State Univ

Benzon, Honorio T MD [PM] - **Spec Exp:** Pain-Back; Complex Regional Pain Syndrome-CRPS; Pain-Neuropathic; Pain-Cancer; **Hospital:** Northwestern Meml Hosp; **Address:** 675 N Saint Clair St Fl 20, Ste 20-100, Chicago, IL 60611-3015; **Phone:** 312-695-2500; **Board Cert:** Anesthesiology 1995; Pain Medicine 2004; **Med School:** Philippines 1971; **Resid:** Anesthesiology, Univ Cincinnati Med Ctr 1975; Anesthesiology, Northwestern Meml Hosp 1976; **Fellow:** Research, Brigham & Womens Hosp 1986; **Fac Appt:** Prof Anes, Northwestern Univ

Covington, Edward C MD [PM] - **Spec Exp:** Pain-Chronic; **Hospital:** Cleveland Clin Fdn (page 56); **Address:** 9500 Euclid Ave, Desk C21, Cleveland, OH 44195; **Phone:** 216-444-5964; **Board Cert:** Psychiatry 1978; Addiction Psychiatry 1998; Pain Medicine 2001; **Med School:** Univ Tenn Coll Med, Memphis 1970; **Resid:** Psychiatry, Mayo Clinic 1975

Green, Carmen R MD [PM] - **Spec Exp:** Racial/Ethnic Disparities in Pain Care; **Hospital:** Univ Michigan Hlth Sys; **Address:** Univ Mich Hlth Sys, Dept Anesthesiology, rm 1H247 Univ Hosp, 1500 E Med Ctr Drive, SPC5048, Ann Arbor, MI 48109-5048; **Phone:** 734-936-4240; **Board Cert:** Anesthesiology 1996; Pain Medicine 1998; **Med School:** Mich State Univ 1987; **Resid:** Anesthesiology, Univ Mich Med Ctr 1989; **Fellow:** Pain Medicine, Univ Mich Med Ctr 1992; **Fac Appt:** Asst Prof Anes, Univ Mich Med Sch

Harden, R Norman MD [PM] - **Spec Exp:** Pain-Back; Reflex Sympathetic Dystrophy (RSD); Fibromyalgia; Headache; **Hospital:** Rehab Inst - Chicago; **Address:** 980 N Michigan Ave, Ste 800, Chicago, IL 60611; **Phone:** 312-238-7800; **Med School:** Med Coll GA 1984; **Resid:** Neurology, Univ South Carolina Med Ctr 1985; **Fellow:** Pain Medicine, Rehab Inst - Georgia 1989; **Fac Appt:** Asst Prof PMR, Northwestern Univ

Huntoon, Marc MD [PM] - **Spec Exp:** Pain-Cancer; Pain-after Spinal Intervention; Palliative Care; **Hospital:** Mayo Med Ctr & Clin - Rochester; **Address:** Mayo Clinic - Pain Medicine, 200 First St SW, Rochester, MN 55905; **Phone:** 507-266-9240; **Board Cert:** Anesthesiology 2003; Pain Medicine 2004; **Med School:** Wayne State Univ 1985; **Resid:** Anesthesiology, Naval Hosp Med Ctr 1991; **Fellow:** Pain Medicine, Naval Hosp Med Ctr 1992

Robbins, Lawrence D MD [PM] - **Spec Exp:** Headache; Migraine; Psychopharmacology; **Address:** 1535 Lake Cook Rd, Ste 506, Northbrook, IL 60062-1451; **Phone:** 847-480-9399; **Board Cert:** Pain Medicine 1995; **Med School:** Univ IL Coll Med 1981; **Resid:** Neurology, Univ Illinois 1985; **Fellow:** Pain Medicine, Diamond Headache Clinic 1986; **Fac Appt:** Asst Prof N, Rush Med Coll

Rosenquist, Richard W MD [PM] - **Spec Exp:** Complex Regional Pain Syndrome-CRPS; Pain-Back; Pain-Facial; Headache; **Hospital:** Univ Iowa Hosp & Clinics, VA Med Ctr - Iowa City; **Address:** Center Pain Medicine-Dept Anesthesia, 200 Hawkins Drive, Iowa City, IA 52242; **Phone:** 319-356-2320; **Board Cert:** Anesthesiology 1988; Pain Medicine 2004; **Med School:** Northwestern Univ 1984; **Resid:** Anesthesiology, Northwestern Univ Med Ctr 1987; **Fellow:** Anesthesiology & Pain Management, Emory Univ 1988; **Fac Appt:** Prof Anes, Univ Iowa Coll Med

Swarm, Robert A MD [PM] - **Spec Exp:** Pain-Acute; Pain-Chronic; Pain-Cancer; **Hospital:** Barnes-Jewish Hosp; **Address:** Ctr for Advanced Med-Pain Mngmt Ctr, 4921 Parkview Pl, Ste 10A, MS 90-35-706, St Louis, MO 63110; **Phone:** 314-362-8820; **Board Cert:** Anesthesiology 1990; Pain Medicine 2004; **Med School:** Washington Univ, St Louis 1983; **Resid:** Surgery, Barnes Hosp 1986; Anesthesiology, Barnes Hosp 1989; **Fellow:** Pain Medicine, Univ Sydney; **Fac Appt:** Assoc Prof Anes, Washington Univ, St Louis

Pain Medicine

Weisman, Steven Jay MD [PM] - **Spec Exp:** Pain Management-Pediatric; Palliative Care-Pediatric; Reflex Sympathetic Dystrophy (RSD); **Hospital:** Chldns Hosp - Wisconsin; **Address:** Chldns Hosp Wisconsin, 9000 W Wisconsin Ave, MS 792, Milwaukee, WI 53226-3518; **Phone:** 414-266-2775; **Board Cert:** Pediatrics 1982; Pediatric Hematology-Oncology 1984; Anesthesiology 1996; **Med School:** Albert Einstein Coll Med 1978; **Resid:** Pediatrics, Chldns Hosp 1981; Anesthesiology, Univ Conn Hlth Ctr 1994; **Fellow:** Pediatric Hematology-Oncology, Indiana Univ Sch Med 1984; **Fac Appt:** Prof Anes, Med Coll Wisc

Great Plains and Mountains

Fine, Perry G MD [PM] - **Spec Exp:** Pain-Cancer; Palliative Care; Pain-Chronic; **Hospital:** Univ Utah Hosps and Clins; **Address:** 546 S Chipeta Way, Ste 200, Salt Lake City, UT 84108; **Phone:** 801-581-7246; **Board Cert:** Anesthesiology 1985; Pain Medicine 2004; **Med School:** Med Coll VA 1981; **Resid:** Anesthesiology, Univ Utah Hlth Sci Ctr 1984; **Fellow:** Pain Medicine, Univ Toronto 1985; **Fac Appt:** Prof Anes, Univ Utah

Waldman, Steven D MD [PM] - **Spec Exp:** Pain-Neuropathic; **Hospital:** Doctors Hosp; **Address:** The Headache & Pain Ctr, 4801 College Blvd, Leawood, KS 66211; **Phone:** 913-491-6451; **Board Cert:** Anesthesiology 1983; Pain Medicine 2004; **Med School:** Univ MO-Kansas City 1977; **Resid:** Anesthesiology, Mayo Clinic 1980; **Fac Appt:** Clin Prof Anes, Univ MO-Kansas City

Weinstein, Sharon M MD [PM] - **Spec Exp:** Pain-Cancer; Palliative Care; **Hospital:** Univ Utah Hosps and Clins; **Address:** Huntsman Cancer Institute, 2000 Circle of Hope, Salt Lake City, UT 84112; **Phone:** 801-585-0112; **Board Cert:** Neurology 1993; Pain Medicine 2000; **Med School:** Albert Einstein Coll Med 1986; **Resid:** Neurology, Montefiore Med Ctr 1990; **Fellow:** Pain Medicine, Meml Sloan Kettering Cancer Ctr 1991; **Fac Appt:** Assoc Prof Anes, Univ Utah

Southwest

Burton, Allen W MD [PM] - **Spec Exp:** Pain-Cancer; Palliative Care; **Hospital:** UT MD Anderson Cancer Ctr; **Address:** MD Anderson Cancer Ctr, Dept Anesth, 1400 Holcombe Blvd, Unit 409, Houston, TX 77030; **Phone:** 713-745-7246; **Board Cert:** Anesthesiology 1996; Pain Medicine 1998; **Med School:** Baylor Coll Med 1991; **Resid:** Anesthesiology, Brigham & Women's Hosp 1995; **Fellow:** Pain Medicine, U Texas Med Branch Hosp 1998; **Fac Appt:** Assoc Prof Anes, Univ Tex Med Br, Galveston

Driver, Larry C MD [PM] - **Spec Exp:** Pain-Cancer; Palliative Care; **Hospital:** UT MD Anderson Cancer Ctr; **Address:** UT MD Anderson Cancer Ctr, Dept Pain Medicine, 1400 Holcombe Blvd, Unit 409, Houston, TX 77030; **Phone:** 713-745-7246; **Board Cert:** Anesthesiology 1992; Pain Medicine 2002; **Med School:** Univ Tex, San Antonio 1980; **Resid:** Anesthesiology, Univ Colorado Hlth Sci Ctr 1984; **Fellow:** Pain Medicine, MD Anderson Cancer Ctr 1999; **Fac Appt:** Assoc Prof Anes, Univ Tex, Houston

Racz, Gabor MD [PM] - **Spec Exp:** Pain-after Spinal Intervention; Reflex Sympathetic Dystrophy (RSD); Pain-Back, Head & Neck; Headache/Facial Pain; **Hospital:** Univ Med Ctr - Lubbock; **Address:** 3601 4th St, rm 1C282, Lubbock, TX 79430-0002; **Phone:** 806-743-3112; **Board Cert:** Anesthesiology 1993; Pain Medicine 1993; **Med School:** England 1962; **Resid:** Anesthesiology, SUNY Upstate Med Ctr 1969; **Fac Appt:** Prof Anes, Texas Tech Univ

Ramamurthy, Somayaji MD [PM] - **Spec Exp:** Pain-Back; Pain-Chronic; **Hospital:** Univ Hlth Sys - Univ Hosp (San Antonio, TX); **Address:** Univ Tex Hlth Sci Ctr, Dept Anes, 7703 Floyd Curl Drive, MC 7838, San Antonio, TX 78229-3900; **Phone:** 210-567-4543; **Board Cert:** Anesthesiology 1972; Pain Medicine 2003; **Med School:** India 1965; **Resid:** Anesthesiology, Cook Co Hosp 1970; **Fac Appt:** Prof Anes, Univ Tex, San Antonio

Walsh, Nicolas MD [PM] - **Spec Exp:** Pain-Back; Trauma Rehabilitation; Post Polio Syndrome (PPS); **Hospital:** Univ Hlth Sys - Univ Hosp (San Antonio, TX), Audie L Murphy Meml Vets Hosp; **Address:** Univ Tex Hlth Sci Ctr, Rehab Med (7798), 7703 Floyd Curl Drive, San Antonio, TX 78229-3901; **Phone:** 210-567-5350; **Board Cert:** Physical Medicine & Rehabilitation 1983; Pain Medicine 2000; **Med School:** Univ Colorado 1979; **Resid:** Physical Medicine & Rehabilitation, Univ Tex Hlth Sci Ctr 1982; **Fac Appt:** Prof PMR, Univ Tex, San Antonio

West Coast and Pacific

Anderson, Corrie MD [PM] - **Spec Exp:** Pain Management-Pediatric; **Hospital:** Chldns Hosp and Regl Med Ctr - Seattle, Univ Wash Med Ctr; **Address:** Chldns Hosp & Regl Med Ctr, Dept Anesth, 4800 Sands Point Way NE, rm W9825, Seattle, WA 98105; **Phone:** 206-987-2704; **Board Cert:** Anesthesiology 1994; **Med School:** Stanford Univ 1982; **Resid:** Pediatrics, Childrens Hosp 1985; Anesthesiology, Brigham & Womens Hosp 1987; **Fellow:** Pediatric Anesthesiology, Childrens Hosp 1988; **Fac Appt:** Prof Anes, Univ Wash

Audell, Laura G MD [PM] - **Spec Exp:** Complex Regional Pain Syndrome-CRPS; Reflex Sympathetic Dystrophy (RSD); Herpetic Neuralgia (Shingles); Pain-Cancer; **Hospital:** Cedars-Sinai Med Ctr; **Address:** 444 S San Vincente, Ste 1101, Los Angeles, CA 90048; **Phone:** 310-423-9600; **Board Cert:** Internal Medicine 1988; Anesthesiology 1988; Pain Medicine 1996; **Med School:** Univ Wash 1982; **Resid:** Internal Medicine, UCLA-Hosps 1985; Anesthesiology, UCLA-Hosps 1987; **Fellow:** Pain Medicine, UCLA-Hosps 1988

Ferrante, F Michael MD [PM] - **Spec Exp:** Pain-Back & Neck; Reflex Sympathetic Dystrophy (RSD); Botox for Pain; Pain-Neuropathic; **Hospital:** Santa Monica - UCLA Med Ctr, Ronald Reagan UCLA Med Ctr; **Address:** UCLA Pain Program, 1245 16th St, Ste 225, Santa Monica, CA 90404; **Phone:** 310-319-2241; **Board Cert:** Internal Medicine 1985; Anesthesiology 1987; Pain Medicine 2004; **Med School:** NY Med Coll 1980; **Resid:** Internal Medicine, Emroy Univ Affil Hosp 1983; Anesthesiology, Emroy Univ Affil Hosp 1986; **Fellow:** Infectious Disease, Barnes Hosp-Wash Univ 1984; Pain Medicine, Brigham & Women's Hosp 1987; **Fac Appt:** Prof Anes, UCLA

Fishman, Scott M MD [PM] - **Spec Exp:** Pain-Cancer; Pain-Chronic; **Hospital:** UC Davis Med Ctr; **Address:** UC Davis Med Ctr, Pain Management Clinic, 4860 Y St, Ste 2700, Sacramento, CA 95817; **Phone:** 916-734-6824; **Board Cert:** Psychiatry 1998; Pain Medicine 1995; **Med School:** Univ Mass Sch Med 1990; **Resid:** Internal Medicine, Greenwich Hosp 1993; Psychiatry, Mass Genl Hosp 1996; **Fellow:** Pain Medicine, Mass Genl Hosp 1995; **Fac Appt:** Prof Anes, UC Davis

Fitzgibbon, Dermot R MD [PM] - **Spec Exp:** Pain-Cancer; **Hospital:** Univ Wash Med Ctr; **Address:** Univ Wash Med Ctr, Dept Anesthiology, 1959 NE Pacific St, Box 356540, Seattle, WA 98195; **Phone:** 206-598-4260; **Board Cert:** Anesthesiology 1996; Pain Medicine 1998; **Med School:** Ireland 1983; **Resid:** Anesthesiology, St Vincent's Hosp 1992; Anesthesiology, Univ Washington Med Ctr 1995; **Fellow:** Pain Medicine, Univ Wash-Pain Mngmt Clinic 1994; **Fac Appt:** Assoc Prof Anes, Univ Wash

Pain Medicine

Prager, Joshua Philip MD [PM] - **Spec Exp:** Complex Regional Pain Syndrome-CRPS; **Hospital:** Ronald Reagan UCLA Med Ctr; **Address:** 100 UCLA Med Plaza, Ste 760, Los Angeles, CA 90095; **Phone:** 310-264-7246 x100; **Board Cert:** Internal Medicine 1984; Anesthesiology 1987; Pain Medicine 2004; **Med School:** Stanford Univ 1981; **Resid:** Internal Medicine, UCLA Med Ctr 1984; Anesthesiology, Mass Genl Hosp 1986; **Fac Appt:** Asst Clin Prof Anes, UCLA

Ready, L Brian MD [PM] - **Spec Exp:** Pain-Cancer; **Hospital:** Allenmore Hosp; **Address:** 1901 S Union Ave, Ste A244, Tacoma, WA 98405; **Phone:** 253-459-6509; **Med School:** Canada 1967; **Resid:** Anesthesiology, Univ Washington Med Ctr 1975

Rosner, Howard L MD [PM] - **Spec Exp:** Pain-after Spinal Intervention; Pain-Cancer; Pain-Back; **Hospital:** Cedars-Sinai Med Ctr; **Address:** 444 S San Vincente Blvd, Ste 1101, Cedars-Sinai Med Ctr,Mark Goodson Bldg, Los Angeles, CA 90048; **Phone:** 310-423-9612; **Board Cert:** Anesthesiology 1989; Pain Medicine 2004; **Med School:** Univ Miami Sch Med 1980; **Resid:** Anesthesiology, Mass Genl Hosp 1983; **Fellow:** Pain Medicine, Columbia-Presby Med Ctr

Rowbotham, Michael C MD [PM] - **Spec Exp:** Reflex Sympathetic Dystrophy (RSD); Pain-Nerve Injury; Herpetic Neuralgia (Shingles); **Hospital:** UCSF - Mt Zion Med Ctr; **Address:** 1701 Divisadero St, Ste 480, San Francisco, CA 94115; **Phone:** 415-885-7246; **Board Cert:** Neurology 1989; **Med School:** UCSF 1979; **Resid:** Neurology, Boston Univ 1986; Neurology, UCSF Med Ctr 1987; **Fellow:** Neurological Pharmacology, UCSF Med Ctr 1980; Pain Medicine, UCSF Med Ctr 1989; **Fac Appt:** Assoc Prof N, UCSF

Slatkin, Neal E MD [PM] - **Spec Exp:** Pain-Cancer; Palliative Care; **Hospital:** City of Hope Natl Med Ctr & Beckman Rsch; **Address:** City of Hope Supportive Care NW Bldg, 1500 E Duarte Rd, rm 1218, Duarte, CA 91010; **Phone:** 626-256-4673 x63991; **Board Cert:** Neurology 1982; Pain Medicine 2000; **Med School:** SUNY Stony Brook 1976; **Resid:** Neurology, Bellevue Hosp Ctr-NYU 1978; Neurology, Med Coll Va 1981; **Fellow:** Neurology, Med Coll Va 1982; Neuro-Oncology, Meml Sloan-Kettering Cancer Ctr 1984; **Fac Appt:** Asst Clin Prof Med, USC-Keck School of Medicine

Wallace, Mark S MD [PM] - **Spec Exp:** Pain-Chronic; Pain-Cancer; Palliative Care; **Hospital:** UCSD Med Ctr; **Address:** 9300 Campus Point Drive, MC 7651, La Jolla, CA 92037; **Phone:** 858-657-6035; **Board Cert:** Anesthesiology 1992; Pain Medicine 2005; **Med School:** Creighton Univ 1987; **Resid:** Anesthesiology, Univ Maryland Hosp 1991; **Fellow:** Pain Medicine, UCSD Med Ctr 1994; **Fac Appt:** Assoc Prof Anes, UCSD

Pathology

A pathologist deals with the causes and nature of disease and contributes to diagnosis, prognosis and treatment through knowledge gained by the laboratory application of the biologic, chemical and physical sciences.

A pathologist uses information gathered from the microscopic examination of tissue specimens, cells and body fluids, and from clinical laboratory tests on body fluids and secretions for the diagnosis, exclusion and monitoring of disease.

Training Required: Five to seven years

Certification in the following subspecialty requires additional training and examination.

Dermatopathology: A dermatopathologist has the expertise to diagnose and monitor diseases of the skin including infectious, immunologic, degenerative and neoplastic diseases. This entails the examination and interpretation of specially prepared tissue sections, cellular scrapings and smears of skin lesions by means of routine and special (electron and flourescent) microscopes.

PATHOLOGY

New England

Bhan, Atul Kumar MD [Path] - **Spec Exp:** Immunopathology; Liver Pathology; Liver Cancer; **Hospital:** Mass Genl Hosp; **Address:** Mass Genl Hosp, Dept Path, 55 Fruit St, Warren 501, Boston, MA 02114-2620; **Phone:** 617-726-2588; **Board Cert:** Anatomic Pathology 1976; Immunopathology 1985; **Med School:** India 1965; **Resid:** Pathology, Boston Univ Hosp 1971; Pathology, Chldns Univ Hosp 1974; **Fac Appt:** Prof Path, Harvard Med Sch

Connolly, James Leo MD [Path] - **Spec Exp:** Breast Pathology; Breast Cancer; **Hospital:** Beth Israel Deaconess Med Ctr - Boston; **Address:** Beth Israel Deaconess Med Ctr, Dept Path, 330 Brookline Ave, rm ES 112, Boston, MA 02215-5400; **Phone:** 617-667-4344; **Board Cert:** Anatomic Pathology 1980; **Med School:** Vanderbilt Univ 1974; **Resid:** Anatomic Pathology, Beth Israel Hosp 1978; **Fac Appt:** Prof Path, Harvard Med Sch

DeLellis, Ronald A MD [Path] - **Spec Exp:** Thyroid Cancer; Endocrine Pathology; **Hospital:** Rhode Island Hosp, Miriam Hosp; **Address:** Rhode Island Hospital, Dept Pathology, 593 Eddy St, Providence, RI 02903-4923; **Phone:** 401-444-5154; **Board Cert:** Anatomic Pathology 1997; **Med School:** Tufts Univ 1966; **Resid:** Anatomic Pathology, Natl Inst Hlth 1971; **Fellow:** Pathology, Univ Hosp 1973; **Fac Appt:** Prof Path, Brown Univ

Fletcher, Christopher MD [Path] - **Spec Exp:** Soft Tissue Tumors; Sarcoma; Surgical Pathology; **Hospital:** Brigham & Women's Hosp, Dana-Farber Cancer Inst; **Address:** Brigham & Women's Hospital, Dept Pathology, 75 Francis St, Boston, MA 02115-6110; **Phone:** 617-732-8558; **Med School:** England 1981; **Resid:** Pathology, St Thomas Hosp 1985; **Fellow:** Pathology, St Thomas Hosp 1986; **Fac Appt:** Prof Path, Harvard Med Sch

Harris, Nancy L MD [Path] - **Spec Exp:** Lymphoma; Hematopathology; **Hospital:** Mass Genl Hosp; **Address:** Mass Genl Hosp, Dept Path, 55 Fruit St, Warren 211, Boston, MA 02114; **Phone:** 617-726-5155; **Board Cert:** Anatomic Pathology 1978; Clinical Pathology 1978; **Med School:** Stanford Univ 1970; **Resid:** Pathology, Beth Israel Hosp 1978; **Fellow:** Immunopathology, Mass Genl Hosp 1980; **Fac Appt:** Prof Path, Harvard Med Sch

Mark, Eugene J MD [Path] - **Spec Exp:** Lung Pathology; Cardiac Pathology; Forensic Pathology; **Hospital:** Mass Genl Hosp; **Address:** Mass Genl Hosp, Dept Path, 55 Fruit St, Warren 246, Boston, MA 02114; **Phone:** 617-726-8891; **Board Cert:** Anatomic & Clinical Pathology 1973; Dermatopathology 1975; **Med School:** Harvard Med Sch 1967; **Resid:** Pathology, Mass Genl Hosp 1972; **Fellow:** Pathology, Kantons Hospital 1966; **Fac Appt:** Prof Path, Harvard Med Sch

Odze, Robert D MD [Path] - **Spec Exp:** Gastrointestinal Pathology; Liver Pathology; Esophageal Cancer; **Hospital:** Brigham & Women's Hosp; **Address:** Brigham & Women's Hosp, Dept Pathology, 75 Francis St, Boston, MA 02115; **Phone:** 617-732-7549; **Board Cert:** Anatomic Pathology 1990; **Med School:** McGill Univ 1984; **Resid:** Surgery, McGill Univ 1987; Pathology, McGill Univ 1990; **Fellow:** Gastrointestinal Pathology, New England Deaconess Med Ctr 1991; **Fac Appt:** Assoc Prof Path, Harvard Med Sch

Rennke, Helmut G MD [Path] - **Spec Exp:** Kidney Pathology; **Hospital:** Brigham & Women's Hosp; **Address:** Brigham & Womens Hosp, Dept Pathology, 75 Francis St Emory Bldg, Boston, MA 02115; **Phone:** 617-732-6518; **Board Cert:** Anatomic Pathology 1980; **Med School:** Chile 1971; **Resid:** Pathology, Boston City Hosp 1974; Pathology, Peter Bent Brigham Hosp 1977; **Fac Appt:** Prof Path, Harvard Med Sch

America's Top Doctors® 8th Edition

Schnitt, Stuart J MD [Path] - **Spec Exp:** Breast Pathology; Breast Cancer; **Hospital:** Beth Israel Deaconess Med Ctr - Boston; **Address:** Beth Israel Deaconess Med Ctr, Dept Pathology, 330 Brookline Ave, rm ES 112, Boston, MA 02215-5400; **Phone:** 617-667-4344; **Board Cert:** Anatomic & Clinical Pathology 1983; **Med School:** Albany Med Coll 1979; **Resid:** Anatomic Pathology, Beth Israel Deaconess Med Ctr 1983; **Fellow:** Surgical Pathology, Beth Israel Deaconess Med Ctr 1984; **Fac Appt:** Assoc Prof Path, Harvard Med Sch

Smith, Thomas W MD [Path] - **Spec Exp:** Neuropathology; **Hospital:** UMass Meml - Univ Campus; **Address:** U Mass Hospital, 55 Lake Ave N, Worcester, MA 01655; **Phone:** 508-856-2331; **Board Cert:** Neuropathology 1999; **Med School:** Cornell Univ 1972; **Resid:** Neuropathology, Peter Bent Brigham Hosp 1976; Radiology, Mass General Hosp 1977; **Fellow:** Anatomic Pathology, Peter Bent Brigham Hosp 1978; **Fac Appt:** Prof Path, Univ Mass Sch Med

Young, Robert H MD [Path] - **Spec Exp:** Ovarian Cancer; Gynecologic Cancer; **Hospital:** Mass Genl Hosp; **Address:** Mass Genl Hosp, Dept Pathology, 55 Fruit St, Warren 215, Boston, MA 02114; **Phone:** 617-726-8892; **Board Cert:** Anatomic Pathology 1980; **Med School:** Ireland 1974; **Resid:** Pathology, Mass Genl Hosp 1979; Pathology, Dublin Univ 1977; **Fac Appt:** Prof Path, Harvard Med Sch

Mid Atlantic

Brooks, John S MD [Path] - **Spec Exp:** Tumor Diagnosis; Sarcoma; Bone & Soft Tissue Pathology; **Hospital:** Pennsylvania Hosp (page 60), Hosp Univ Penn - UPHS (page 60); **Address:** Pennsylvania Hospital, Preston 6 FL, 800 Spruce St, Philadelphia, PA 19107; **Phone:** 215-829-3541; **Board Cert:** Anatomic Pathology 1978; Immunopathology 1983; **Med School:** Thomas Jefferson Univ 1974; **Resid:** Pathology, Hosp U Penn 1978; **Fellow:** Immunopathology, Hosp U Penn 1978; **Fac Appt:** Prof Path, Univ Pennsylvania

Burger, Peter MD [Path] - **Spec Exp:** Brain Tumors; Neuro-Pathology; **Hospital:** Johns Hopkins Hosp - Baltimore (page 61); **Address:** Johns Hopkins Hosp-Dept Pathology, 600 N Wolfe St, rm 710, Baltimore, MD 21287; **Phone:** 410-955-8378; **Board Cert:** Anatomic Pathology 1976; Neuropathology 1976; **Med School:** Northwestern Univ 1966; **Resid:** Anatomic Pathology, Duke Univ Med Ctr 1973; **Fellow:** Neuropathology, Duke Univ Med Ctr 1973

Demetris, Anthony J MD [Path] - **Spec Exp:** Transplant Pathology; Liver Pathology; **Hospital:** UPMC Montefiore; **Address:** UPMC - Montefiore, 3459 5th Ave, rm E741, Pittsburgh, PA 15213; **Phone:** 412-647-2067; **Board Cert:** Anatomic & Clinical Pathology 1987; **Med School:** Univ Pittsburgh 1982; **Resid:** Anatomic & Clinical Pathology, Univ Pittsburgh Med Ctr 1986; **Fac Appt:** Prof Path, Univ Pittsburgh

Ehya, Hormoz MD [Path] - **Spec Exp:** Cytopathology; Breast Pathology; Lung Pathology; **Hospital:** Fox Chase Cancer Ctr (page 58); **Address:** Fox Chase Cancer Center, 333 Cottman Ave, rm C427, Philadelphia, PA 19111-2497; **Phone:** 215-728-5389; **Board Cert:** Anatomic Pathology 1979; Cytopathology 1989; **Med School:** Iran 1974; **Resid:** Pathology, Univ Miss Med Ctr 1979; **Fellow:** Cytopathology, Meml Sloan-Kettering Cancer Ctr 1980

Epstein, Jonathan MD [Path] - **Spec Exp:** Bladder Cancer; Prostate Cancer; Urologic Pathology; **Hospital:** Johns Hopkins Hosp - Baltimore (page 61); **Address:** 401 N Broadway, Weinberg 2242, Baltimore, MD 21231; **Phone:** 410-955-5043; **Board Cert:** Anatomic Pathology 1986; **Med School:** Boston Univ 1981; **Resid:** Pathology, Johns Hopkins Hosp 1985; **Fellow:** Pathology, Meml Sloan Kettering Cancer Ctr 1984; **Fac Appt:** Prof Path, Johns Hopkins Univ

Pathology

Fogt, Franz MD/PhD [Path] - **Spec Exp:** Gastrointestinal Pathology; **Hospital:** Penn Presby Med Ctr - UPHS (page 60); **Address:** Presbyterian Medical Ctr, Dept Pathology, 551 Wright Saunders Bldg, Philadelphia, PA 19104; **Phone:** 215-662-8077; **Board Cert:** Anatomic & Clinical Pathology 1995; **Med School:** Germany 1988; **Resid:** Anatomic & Clinical Pathology, New England Deaconess Hosp 1995; **Fellow:** Gastrointestinal Pathology, New England Deaconess Hosp 1996; **Fac Appt:** Assoc Prof Path, Univ Pennsylvania

Gottlieb, Geoffrey MD [Path] - **Spec Exp:** Dermatopathology; Melanoma; **Address:** Ackerman Academy Dermatopathology, 145 E 32nd St Fl 10, New York, NY 10016; **Phone:** 212-889-6225; **Board Cert:** Anatomic Pathology 1979; Dermatology 1982; **Med School:** Cornell Univ-Weill Med Coll 1976; **Resid:** Pathology, NY Hosp-Cornell Med Ctr 1979; **Fellow:** Dermatopathology, NYU Med Ctr 1982

Gupta, Prabodh K MD [Path] - **Spec Exp:** Lung Pathology; Cervical Cancer; Fine Needle Aspiration Biopsy; **Hospital:** Hosp Univ Penn - UPHS (page 60); **Address:** Hosp Univ Penn - Cytopathology, 3400 Spruce St, 6 Founders, Philadelphia, PA 19104; **Phone:** 215-662-3238; **Board Cert:** Anatomic Pathology 1975; Cytopathology 1989; **Med School:** India 1965; **Resid:** Pathology, All India Inst Med Scis 1967; **Fellow:** Pathology, Mass Genl Hosp 1968; Johns Hopkins Hosp 1969; **Fac Appt:** Prof Path, Univ Pennsylvania

Heller, Debra S MD [Path] - **Spec Exp:** Gynecologic Pathology; Pediatric Pathology; **Hospital:** UMDNJ-Univ Hosp-Newark; **Address:** UMDNJ-NJ Med Sch Dept Pathology, 185 S Orange Ave, Newark, NJ 07101; **Phone:** 973-972-0751; **Board Cert:** Anatomic Pathology 1988; Obstetrics & Gynecology 2006; Pediatric Pathology 1999; **Med School:** NY Med Coll 1977; **Resid:** Obstetrics & Gynecology, Beth Israel Med Ctr 1981; Anatomic Pathology, Mt Sinai Med Ctr 1988; **Fellow:** Pediatric Pathology, Mt Sinai Med Ctr 1987; Gynecologic Pathology, Mt Sinai Med Ctr 1989; **Fac Appt:** Prof Path, UMDNJ-NJ Med Sch, Newark

Hoda, Syed A MD [Path] - **Spec Exp:** Breast Cancer; Surgical Pathology; **Hospital:** NY-Presby Hosp/Weill Cornell (page 66); **Address:** 525 E 68th St, 1028 Starr, New York, NY 10021-4870; **Phone:** 212-746-2700; **Board Cert:** Anatomic & Clinical Pathology 1990; Cytopathology 1991; Pathology 2001; **Med School:** Pakistan 1984; **Resid:** Anatomic & Clinical Pathology, Tulane Univ Affil Hosps 1990; **Fellow:** Cytopathology, Meml Sloan Kettering Cancer Ctr 1991; Pathology, Meml Sloan Kettering Cancer Ctr 1992; **Fac Appt:** Clin Prof Path, Cornell Univ-Weill Med Coll

Hruban, Ralph H MD [Path] - **Spec Exp:** Gastrointestinal Pathology; Pancreatic Cancer; **Hospital:** Johns Hopkins Hosp - Baltimore (page 61); **Address:** Johns Hopkins Hosp, Dept Pathology, 401 N Broadway Bldg Weinberg - rm 2242, Baltimore, MD 21231; **Phone:** 410-955-9132; **Board Cert:** Anatomic Pathology 1990; **Med School:** Johns Hopkins Univ 1985; **Resid:** Pathology, Johns Hopkins Hosp 1990; **Fellow:** Meml Sloan Kettering Cancer Ctr 1989; **Fac Appt:** Prof Path, Johns Hopkins Univ

Jaffe, Elaine S MD [Path] - **Spec Exp:** Lymphoma; Hematopathology; **Hospital:** Natl Inst of Hlth - Clin Ctr; **Address:** NIH/NCI - Lab Pathology, 10 Center Drive Bldg 10 - rm 2N202, Bethesda, MD 20892; **Phone:** 301-496-0183; **Board Cert:** Anatomic Pathology 1974; **Med School:** Univ Pennsylvania 1969; **Resid:** Pathology, Clinical Ctr/NIH 1972; **Fellow:** Hematopathology, Natl Cancer Inst 1974; **Fac Appt:** Clin Prof Path, Geo Wash Univ

Jones, Robert V MD [Path] - **Spec Exp:** Neuro-Pathology; Brain Tumors; **Hospital:** Georgetown Univ Hosp; **Address:** GWUMC, Dept Path, 2300 Eye St NW, Ross Hall, Ste 502, Washington, DC 20037; **Phone:** 202-994-3391; **Board Cert:** Anatomic & Clinical Pathology 1981; Neuropathology 1994; **Med School:** Univ VA Sch Med 1977; **Resid:** Anatomic & Clinical Pathology, Walter Reed AMC 1981; **Fellow:** Neurological Pathology, ARmed Forces Inst Path 1990; **Fac Appt:** Assoc Prof Path, Geo Wash Univ

America's Top Doctors® 8th Edition

Kahn, Leonard B MD [Path] - **Spec Exp:** Bone Pathology; Head & Neck Pathology; Soft Tissue Tumors; **Hospital:** Long Island Jewish Med Ctr, N Shore Univ Hosp; **Address:** 270-05 76th Ave, rm B67, New Hyde Park, NY 11040-1433; **Phone:** 718-470-7491; **Board Cert:** Anatomic Pathology 1980; **Med School:** South Africa 1960; **Resid:** Pathology, Univ Cape Town 1966; **Fellow:** Pathology, Washington Univ Sch Med 1969; **Fac Appt:** Prof Path, Albert Einstein Coll Med

Katzenstein, Anna-Luise A MD [Path] - **Spec Exp:** Lung Cancer; Pulmonary Pathology; Interstitial Lung Disease; **Hospital:** Univ. Hosp.- SUNY Upstate, Crouse Hosp; **Address:** SUNY Upstate Medical Univ, 766 Irving Ave, Weiskotten, rm 2106, Syracuse, NY 13210; **Phone:** 315-464-7125; **Board Cert:** Anatomic Pathology 1976; **Med School:** Johns Hopkins Univ 1971; **Resid:** Pathology, Univ Hospital 1975; **Fellow:** Surgical Pathology, Barnes Hosp-Wash Univ 1976; **Fac Appt:** Prof Path, SUNY Upstate Med Univ

Knowles, Daniel M MD [Path] - **Spec Exp:** Lymph Node Pathology; Bone Marrow Pathology; Lymphoma; **Hospital:** NY-Presby Hosp/Weill Cornell (page 66); **Address:** Cornell-Weill Med Coll-Dept Pathology, 1300 York Ave, rm C302, New York, NY 10021; **Phone:** 212-746-6464; **Board Cert:** Anatomic Pathology 1978; Immunopathology 1984; **Med School:** Univ Chicago-Pritzker Sch Med 1973; **Resid:** Anatomic Pathology, Columbia-Presby Med Ctr 1975; **Fellow:** Immunopathology, Rockefeller Univ 1977; **Fac Appt:** Prof Path, Cornell Univ-Weill Med Coll

Kurman, Robert J MD [Path] - **Spec Exp:** Gynecologic Pathology; Ovarian Cancer; Uterine Cancer; **Hospital:** Johns Hopkins Hosp - Baltimore (page 61); **Address:** Johns Hopkins Hosp, Dept Pathology, 401 N Broadway, Weinberg-2242, Baltimore, MD 21231; **Phone:** 410-955-0471; **Board Cert:** Anatomic Pathology 1972; Obstetrics & Gynecology 1980; **Med School:** SUNY Upstate Med Univ 1968; **Resid:** Pathology, Peter Bent Brigham Hosp/Mass Genl Hosp 1977; Obstetrics & Gynecology, LAC Hosp/USC 1978; **Fellow:** Obstetrics & Gynecology, Harvard Univ 1973; **Fac Appt:** Prof Path, Johns Hopkins Univ

Li Volsi, Virginia A MD [Path] - **Spec Exp:** Endocrine Cancers; Thyroid Cancer; Gynecologic Cancer; **Hospital:** Hosp Univ Penn - UPHS (page 60); **Address:** Hosp Univ Penn - Pathology, 3400 Spruce St 6 Founders Bldg - Ste 6030, Philadelphia, PA 19104; **Phone:** 215-662-6545; **Board Cert:** Anatomic Pathology 1974; **Med School:** Columbia P&S 1969; **Resid:** Anatomic Pathology, Presbyterian Hosp 1974; **Fac Appt:** Prof Path, Univ Pennsylvania

McNutt, N Scott MD [Path] - **Spec Exp:** Dermatopathology; **Hospital:** Rockefeller Univ; **Address:** Rockefeller Univ, Krueger Laboratory, 1230 York Ave, New York, NY 10021; **Phone:** 212-327-8000; **Board Cert:** Anatomic Pathology 1973; Dermatopathology 1979; **Med School:** Harvard Med Sch 1966; **Resid:** Pathology, Mass Genl Hosp 1970; **Fellow:** Pathology, Mass Genl Hosp 1972

Melamed, Jonathan MD [Path] - **Spec Exp:** Prostate Cancer; Tumor Banking; **Hospital:** NYU Med Ctr (page 68); **Address:** NYU Medical Ctr, Dept Pathology, TH-461, 560 First Ave, New York, NY 10016; **Phone:** 212-263-8927; **Board Cert:** Anatomic & Clinical Pathology 1992; **Med School:** South Africa 1985; **Resid:** Pathology, Lenox Hill Hosp 1991; **Fellow:** Pathology, Meml Sloan Kettering Cancer Ctr 1992; Urologic Pathology, Meml Sloan Kettering Cancer Ctr 1993; **Fac Appt:** Assoc Prof Path, NYU Sch Med

Mies, Carolyn MD [Path] - **Spec Exp:** Breast Cancer; **Hospital:** Hosp Univ Penn - UPHS (page 60); **Address:** Hosp Univ Penn-Surgical Pathology, 3400 Spruce St, Founders 6, Philadelphia, PA 19104; **Phone:** 215-662-6503; **Board Cert:** Anatomic Pathology 1984; **Med School:** Rush Med Coll 1980; **Resid:** Pathology, Tufts-New England Med Ctr 1982; Pathology, New England Deaconess Hosp 1984; **Fellow:** Surgical Pathology, Meml Sloan Kettering Cancer Ctr 1986; **Fac Appt:** Assoc Prof Path, Univ Pennsylvania

Pathology

Montgomery, Elizabeth A MD [Path] - **Spec Exp:** Barrett's Esophagus; Esophageal Cancer; Gastrointestinal Pathology; **Hospital:** Johns Hopkins Hosp - Baltimore (page 61); **Address:** Johns Hopkins Univ, Dept Pathology, 401 N Broadway Weinberg Bldg - rm 2242, Baltimore, MD 21231; **Phone:** 410-614-2308; **Board Cert:** Anatomic Pathology 1988; Cytopathology 1994; **Med School:** Geo Wash Univ 1984; **Resid:** Pathology, Walter Reed AMC 1988; **Fac Appt:** Assoc Prof Path, Johns Hopkins Univ

Orenstein, Jan M MD/PhD [Path] - **Spec Exp:** Prostate Cancer; Tumor Banking; AIDS/HIV; **Hospital:** G Washington Univ Hosp; **Address:** Ross Hall 502, Geo Wash Univ Med Ctr Dept Path, 2300 Eye St NW, Washington, DC 20037; **Phone:** 202-994-2943; **Board Cert:** Anatomic Pathology 1977; **Med School:** SUNY Downstate 1971; **Resid:** Pathology, Presby Hosp 1973; Pathology, Natl Cancer Inst 1977; **Fac Appt:** Prof Path, Geo Wash Univ

Patchefsky, Arthur S MD [Path] - **Spec Exp:** Breast Cancer; Pulmonary Pathology; Sarcoma; **Hospital:** Fox Chase Cancer Ctr (page 58); **Address:** Fox Chase Cancer Center, 333 Cottman Ave, rm C4333, Philadelphia, PA 19111; **Phone:** 215-728-5390; **Board Cert:** Anatomic Pathology 1969; **Med School:** Hahnemann Univ 1963; **Resid:** Pathology, John Hopkins Hosp 1966; Pathology, Hosp U Penn 1967; **Fellow:** Pathology, Meml Sloan Kettering Cancer Ctr 1968; **Fac Appt:** Prof Path, Thomas Jefferson Univ

Reuter, Victor E MD [Path] - **Spec Exp:** Prostate Cancer; Genitourinary Pathology; Bladder Cancer; Urologic Pathology; **Hospital:** Meml Sloan-Kettering Cancer Ctr; **Address:** Memorial Sloan Kettering Cancer Ctr, Dept Pathology, 1275 York Ave, New York, NY 10021; **Phone:** 212-639-8225; **Board Cert:** Anatomic & Clinical Pathology 1983; **Med School:** Dominican Republic 1978; **Resid:** Anatomic Pathology, Thos Jefferson Univ Hosp 1981; Clinical Pathology, Thos Jefferson Univ Hosp 1983; **Fellow:** Surgical Pathology, Meml Sloan Kettering Cancer Ctr 1985; **Fac Appt:** Prof Path, Cornell Univ-Weill Med Coll

Rosen, Paul P MD [Path] - **Spec Exp:** Breast Pathology; Breast Cancer; **Hospital:** NY-Presby Hosp/Weill Cornell (page 66); **Address:** New York Presbyterian, Dept Pathology, 525 E 68th St, Starr 1031, New York, NY 10065; **Phone:** 212-746-6482; **Board Cert:** Anatomic & Clinical Pathology 1969; Pathology 1998; **Med School:** Columbia P&S 1964; **Resid:** Pathology, Presby Hosp 1966; Pathology, VA Hosp 1968; **Fellow:** Pathology, Meml Hosp Cancer Ctr 1970; **Fac Appt:** Prof Path, Cornell Univ-Weill Med Coll

Rosenblum, Marc MD [Path] - **Spec Exp:** Neuropathology; Brain Tumors; **Hospital:** Meml Sloan-Kettering Cancer Ctr; **Address:** 1275 York Avenue, New York, NY 10065; **Phone:** 800-525-2225; **Board Cert:** Anatomic Pathology 1984; Pathology 1998; Neuropathology 1988; **Med School:** Univ Miami Sch Med 1979; **Resid:** Anatomic Pathology, Mount Sinai Med Ctr 1984; **Fellow:** Pathology, Meml Sloan-Kettering Cancer Ctr 1985; Neurological Pathology, Bellevue-NYU Med Ctr 1987; **Fac Appt:** Prof Path, Cornell Univ

Ross, Jeffrey S MD [Path] - **Spec Exp:** Urologic Cancer; Prostate Cancer; Breast Cancer; **Hospital:** Albany Med Ctr; **Address:** Albany Med Coll, Dept Path, 47 New Scotland Ave, MC 81, Albany, NY 12208; **Phone:** 518-262-5471; **Board Cert:** Anatomic & Clinical Pathology 1974; **Med School:** SUNY Buffalo 1970; **Resid:** Pathology, Mass Genl Hosp 1974; **Fellow:** Pathology, Harvard Med Sch 1974; **Fac Appt:** Prof Path, Albany Med Coll

Sanchez, Miguel A MD [Path] - **Spec Exp:** Breast Cancer; Thyroid Cancer; **Hospital:** Englewood Hosp & Med Ctr; **Address:** Englewood Hosp & Med Ctr, Dept Pathology, 350 Engle St, Englewood, NJ 07631-1898; **Phone:** 201-894-3423; **Board Cert:** Anatomic Pathology 1975; Clinical Pathology 1979; Cytopathology 1991; **Med School:** Spain 1969; **Resid:** Pathology, Englewood Hosp 1972; Pathology, Temple Univ 1973; **Fellow:** Pathology, Meml Sloan Kettering Cancer Ctr 1974; Clinical Pathology, St Vincent's Hosp 1975; **Fac Appt:** Assoc Prof Path, Mount Sinai Sch Med

Schiller, Alan L MD [Path] - **Spec Exp:** Bone & Joint Pathology; Soft Tissue Pathology; Bone Tumors; **Hospital:** Mount Sinai Med Ctr (page 64); **Address:** Mt Sinai Sch Med, Dept Pathology, 1 Gustave Levy Pl, Box 1194, New York, NY 10029-6500; **Phone:** 212-241-8014; **Board Cert:** Anatomic Pathology 1973; **Med School:** Ros Franklin Univ/Chicago Med Sch 1967; **Resid:** Pathology, Mass Genl Hosp 1972; **Fac Appt:** Prof Path, Mount Sinai Sch Med

Silverberg, Steven G MD [Path] - **Spec Exp:** Gynecologic Pathology; Breast Pathology; Urologic Pathology; Endocrine Pathology; **Hospital:** Univ of MD Med Sys; **Address:** Univ Maryland Med Ctr, Dept Pathology, 22 S Greene St, Baltimore, MD 21201; **Phone:** 410-328-5072; **Board Cert:** Anatomic Pathology 1969; **Med School:** Johns Hopkins Univ 1962; **Resid:** Pathology, Yale-New Haven Hosp 1965; **Fellow:** Surgical Pathology, Meml Sloan Kettering Cancer Ctr 1966; **Fac Appt:** Prof Path, Univ MD Sch Med

Silverman, Jan F MD [Path] - **Spec Exp:** Breast Cancer; Lung Cancer; Gastrointestinal Pathology; Fine Needle Aspiration Biopsy; **Hospital:** Allegheny General Hosp; **Address:** Allegheny Gen Hosp-Dept Lab Medicine, 320 E North Ave, Pittsburgh, PA 15212; **Phone:** 412-359-6886; **Board Cert:** Anatomic & Clinical Pathology 1975; Cytopathology 1989; **Med School:** Med Coll VA 1970; **Resid:** Pathology, Med Coll Virginia 1975; **Fellow:** Surgical Pathology, Med Coll Virginia 1975; **Fac Appt:** Prof Path, Drexel Univ Coll Med

Swerdlow, Steven H MD [Path] - **Spec Exp:** Lymphoma; Hematopathology; Transplant Pathology; **Hospital:** UPMC Presby, Pittsburgh; **Address:** Div Hematopathology, 200 Lothrop St, rm C606, Pittsburgh, PA 15213-2536; **Phone:** 412-647-5191; **Board Cert:** Anatomic Pathology 2005; Clinical Pathology 2005; **Med School:** Harvard Med Sch 1975; **Resid:** Pathology, Beth Israel Hosp 1979; **Fellow:** Hematopathology, Vanderbilt Univ 1981; Hematopathology, St Bartholmew's Hosp 1983; **Fac Appt:** Prof Path, Univ Pittsburgh

Tomaszewski, John E MD [Path] - **Spec Exp:** Kidney Pathology; Immunopathology; Kidney Pathology; Uterine Cancer; **Hospital:** Hosp Univ Penn - UPHS (page 60); **Address:** Hosp Univ Penn, Dept Pathology & Lab Med, 3400 Spruce St, 6 Founders Bldg, Ste 6042, Philadelphia, PA 19104; **Phone:** 215-662-6852; **Board Cert:** Anatomic Pathology 1982; Immunopathology 1983; **Med School:** Univ Pennsylvania 1977; **Resid:** Pathology, Hosp Univ Penn 1982; **Fellow:** Surgical Pathology, Hosp Univ Penn 1983; **Fac Appt:** Prof Path, Univ Pennsylvania

Travis, William MD [Path] - **Spec Exp:** Pulmonary Pathology; Lung Cancer; Interstitial Lung Disease; **Hospital:** Meml Sloan-Kettering Cancer Ctr; **Address:** 1275 York Avenue, New York, NY 10065; **Phone:** 800-525-2225; **Board Cert:** Anatomic & Clinical Pathology 1985; **Med School:** Univ Fla Coll Med 1981; **Resid:** Anatomic Pathology, New England Deaconess Hosp 1983; Clinical Pathology, Mayo Clinic 1985; **Fellow:** Surgical Pathology, Mayo Clinic 1986

Yousem, Samuel A MD [Path] - **Spec Exp:** Pulmonary Pathology; Transplant-Lung (Pathology); Lung Cancer; **Hospital:** UPMC Presby, Pittsburgh; **Address:** Dept Pathology, A-610, Presbyterian Campus, 200 Lothrop St, Pittsburgh, PA 15213; **Phone:** 412-647-6193; **Board Cert:** Anatomic Pathology 1985; Cytopathology 1997; **Med School:** Univ MD Sch Med 1981; **Resid:** Pathology, Stanford Univ Med Ctr 1983; **Fellow:** Surgical Pathology, Stanford Univ Med Ctr 1984; **Fac Appt:** Prof Path, Univ Pittsburgh

Southeast

Banks, Peter MD [Path] - **Spec Exp:** Hematopathology; Lymphoma; **Hospital:** Carolinas Med Ctr; **Address:** Dept Pathology, 1000 Blythe Blvd, 4th Fl Pathology Lab, Charlotte, NC 28203; **Phone:** 704-355-2251; **Board Cert:** Anatomic Pathology 1976; **Med School:** Harvard Med Sch 1971; **Resid:** Pathology, National Cancer Inst 1974; Pathology, Duke Univ Med Ctr 1975; **Fellow:** Surgical Pathology, Univ Minn Med Ctr 1976; **Fac Appt:** Prof Path, Univ NC Sch Med

Pathology

Bostwick, David MD [Path] - **Spec Exp:** Urologic Pathology; Prostate Cancer; Bladder Cancer; **Address:** 4355 Innslake Drive, Glen Allen, VA 23060; **Phone:** 804-967-9225; **Board Cert:** Anatomic Pathology 1985; **Med School:** Univ MD Sch Med 1979; **Resid:** Pathology, Stanford Univ Med Ctr 1981; **Fellow:** Surgical Pathology, Stanford Univ Med Ctr 1984

Braylan, Raul MD [Path] - **Spec Exp:** Hematopathology; Leukemia; Lymphoma; **Hospital:** Shands at Univ of FL; **Address:** Univ Florida, Dept Hematopathology, PO Box 100275, Gainesville, FL 32610; **Phone:** 352-265-9900; **Board Cert:** Anatomic Pathology 1972; **Med School:** Argentina 1960; **Resid:** Anatomic Pathology, Mt Sinai Hosp 1965; Anatomic Pathology, Einstein Affil Hosps 1967; **Fellow:** Anatomic Pathology, Meml Sloan Kettering Cancer Hosp 1968; Hematopathology, Univ Chicago Hosps 1973; **Fac Appt:** Prof Path, Univ Fla Coll Med

Chesney, Carolyn M MD [Path] - **Spec Exp:** Hematopathology; Bleeding/Coagulation Disorders; **Hospital:** Univ of Tennessee Mem Hosp; **Address:** Dept of Pathology-Coag Lab, 6019 Walnut Grove, Memphis, TN 38120; **Phone:** 901-226-5650; **Board Cert:** Internal Medicine 1972; Hematology 1999; **Med School:** Vanderbilt Univ 1968; **Resid:** Internal Medicine, Vanderbilt Univ Hosp 1970; **Fellow:** Internal Medicine, Mass Genl Hosp 1972; **Fac Appt:** Prof Med, Univ Tenn Coll Med, Memphis

Crawford, James M MD/PhD [Path] - **Spec Exp:** Liver Pathology; Gastrointestinal Pathology; Gastrointestinal Cancer; **Hospital:** Shands at Univ of FL; **Address:** Univ Florida, Dept Pathology, 1600 SW Archer Rd, rm M649, Box 100275, Gainesville, FL 32610-0275; **Phone:** 352-273-7839; **Board Cert:** Anatomic Pathology 1987; **Med School:** Duke Univ 1982; **Resid:** Pathology, Brigham & Women's Hosp 1984; **Fellow:** Gastrointestinal Pathology, Brigham & Women's Hosp 1987; **Fac Appt:** Prof Path, Univ Fla Coll Med

Faye-Petersen, Ona MD [Path] - **Spec Exp:** Perinatal Pathology; Fetal Pathology; Neonatal Pathology; Pediatric Pathology; **Hospital:** Univ of Ala Hosp at Birmingham, UAB Highlands Hosp; **Address:** UAB Hospital, 1802 6th Ave S, Birmingham, AL 35249; **Phone:** 205-975-8880; **Board Cert:** Anatomic & Clinical Pathology 1987; Pediatric Pathology 1991; **Med School:** Univ Colorado 1980; **Resid:** Pathology, Presby-Denver Hosp 1985; **Fellow:** Surgical Pathology, Meml Sloan Ketter Cancer Ctr 1986; Pediatric Pathology, Mt Sinai Hosp 1987; **Fac Appt:** Assoc Prof Path, Univ Ala

Lage, Janice MD [Path] - **Spec Exp:** Obstetric Pathology; Gynecologic Pathology; Breast Pathology; **Hospital:** MUSC Med Ctr; **Address:** MUSC Med Ctr, Dept Path, 165 Ashley Ave, Ste 309, Box 250908, Charleston, SC 29425; **Phone:** 843-792-3121; **Board Cert:** Anatomic Pathology 2001; **Med School:** Washington Univ, St Louis 1980; **Resid:** Pathology, Barnes Hosp/Wash Univ 1982; Obstetrics & Gynecology, Barnes Hosp/Wash Univ 1983; **Fellow:** Surgical Pathology, Barnes Hosp/Wash Univ 1984; **Fac Appt:** Prof Path, Med Univ SC

Masood, Shahla MD [Path] - **Spec Exp:** Breast Cancer; Breast Pathology; **Hospital:** Shands Jacksonville; **Address:** Univ of Florida, Dept Pathology, 655 W 8th St, Jacksonville, FL 32209-6511; **Phone:** 904-244-4387; **Board Cert:** Anatomic & Clinical Pathology 1998; Cytopathology 1990; **Med School:** Iran 1973; **Resid:** Anatomic Pathology, University Hosp 1977; **Fac Appt:** Prof Path, Univ Fla Coll Med

McCurley, Thomas L MD [Path] - **Spec Exp:** Hematopathology; Immunopathology; **Hospital:** Vanderbilt Univ Med Ctr, VA Med Ctr - Nashville; **Address:** Vanderbilt Univ Hosp, Dept Pathology, 21st & Garland Ave, Nashville, TN 37232-0001; **Phone:** 615-343-9167; **Board Cert:** Anatomic & Clinical Pathology 1981; Immunopathology 1986; Hematology 1999; **Med School:** Vanderbilt Univ 1974; **Resid:** Internal Medicine, UCSF Med Ctr 1976; Pathology, Vanderbilt Univ Med Ctr 1981; **Fellow:** Hematopathology, Vanderbilt Univ Med Ctr 1984; **Fac Appt:** Assoc Prof Path, Vanderbilt Univ

Mills, Stacey E MD [Path] - **Spec Exp:** Breast Pathology; Ear, Nose & Throat Cancer; Surgical Pathology; **Hospital:** Univ Virginia Med Ctr; **Address:** Univ VA Hlth System, Dept Pathology, PO Box 800214, Charlottesville, VA 22908-0214; **Phone:** 434-982-4406; **Board Cert:** Anatomic Pathology 1999; **Med School:** Univ VA Sch Med 1977; **Resid:** Pathology, Univ Virginia Med Ctr 1980; **Fellow:** Pathology, Univ Virginia 1981; **Fac Appt:** Prof Path, Univ VA Sch Med

Nicosia, Santo MD [Path] - **Spec Exp:** Ovarian Cancer; **Hospital:** H Lee Moffitt Cancer Ctr & Research Inst; **Address:** 12901 Bruce B Downs Blvd, MDC Box 11, Tampa, FL 33612-4742; **Phone:** 813-974-3133; **Board Cert:** Anatomic Pathology 1978; Cytopathology 1990; **Med School:** Italy 1967; **Resid:** Anatomic Pathology, Michael Reese Hosp 1972; **Fellow:** Hosp Univ Penn 1973; **Fac Appt:** Prof Path, Univ S Fla Coll Med

Norenberg, Michael D MD [Path] - **Spec Exp:** Liver Pathology; Parkinson's Disease; **Hospital:** Jackson Meml Hosp; **Address:** Jackson Meml Hosp, Dept Pathology, 1611 NW 12th Ave Holtz Ctr, rm 2142, Miami, FL 33136; **Phone:** 305-585-7017; **Board Cert:** Anatomic Pathology 1972; Neuropathology 1974; **Med School:** Univ Rochester 1965; **Resid:** Pathology, Strong Meml Hosp 1970; **Fellow:** Neuropathology, Strong Meml Hosp 1972; **Fac Appt:** Prof Path, Univ Miami Sch Med

Page, David L MD [Path] - **Spec Exp:** Breast Cancer; **Hospital:** Vanderbilt Univ Med Ctr; **Address:** Vanderbilt Univ, 1161 21st Ave S, rm C 3309, Nashville, TN 37232-2561; **Phone:** 615-322-3759; **Board Cert:** Anatomic Pathology 1972; Dermatopathology 1974; **Med School:** Johns Hopkins Univ 1966; **Resid:** Pathology, Mass Genl Hosp 1969; Pathology, Johns Hopkins Hosp 1972; **Fac Appt:** Prof Path, Vanderbilt Univ

Petito, Carol MD [Path] - **Spec Exp:** Neuro-Pathology; **Hospital:** Jackson Meml Hosp; **Address:** Univ Miami Sch Med, Dept Pathology (R-5), 1550 NW 10th Ave, PAP Bldg - Fl 4, rm 417, Miami, FL 33136; **Phone:** 305-243-3584; **Board Cert:** Anatomic Pathology 1973; Neuropathology 1973; **Med School:** Columbia P&S 1967; **Resid:** Pathology, NY Hosp-Cornell Med Ctr 1970; Neuropathology, Armed Forces Inst; **Fac Appt:** Prof Path, Univ Miami Sch Med

Sewell, C Whitaker MD [Path] - **Spec Exp:** Breast Pathology; Surgical Pathology; **Hospital:** Emory Univ Hosp; **Address:** Emory Univ Hosp, Dept Pathology, 1364 Clifton Rd NE, rm H185, Atlanta, GA 30322; **Phone:** 404-712-7003; **Board Cert:** Anatomic Pathology 1974; Clinical Pathology 1974; **Med School:** Emory Univ 1969; **Resid:** Pathology, Emory Univ Hosp 1974; **Fac Appt:** Prof Path, Emory Univ

Weiss, Sharon MD [Path] - **Spec Exp:** Soft Tissue Pathology; Surgical Pathology; Sarcoma; **Hospital:** Emory Univ Hosp; **Address:** Emory Univ Hosp, Dept Path, 1364 Clifton Rd NE, rm H180, Atlanta, GA 30322; **Phone:** 404-712-0708; **Board Cert:** Anatomic Pathology 1974; **Med School:** Johns Hopkins Univ 1971; **Resid:** Pathology, Johns Hopkins Hosp 1975; **Fac Appt:** Prof Path, Emory Univ

Midwest

Allred, D Craig MD [Path] - **Spec Exp:** Breast Cancer; Breast Pathology; Breast Cancer Risk Assessment; **Hospital:** Barnes-Jewish Hosp; **Address:** Washington Univ Sch Med, Path & Immunology, 660 S Euclid Ave, Box 8118, St Louis, MO 63110; **Phone:** 314-362-6313; **Board Cert:** Anatomic Pathology 1984; **Med School:** Univ Utah 1979; **Resid:** Anatomic Pathology, Univ Conn Hlth Ctr 1983; **Fellow:** Immunopathology, Univ Conn Hlth Ctr 1982; **Fac Appt:** Prof Path, Baylor Coll Med

Pathology

Appelman, Henry MD [Path] - **Spec Exp:** Gastrointestinal Pathology; Liver Pathology; **Hospital:** Univ Michigan Hlth Sys; **Address:** Univ Michigan, Dept of Pathology, 1500 E Medical Center Drive, Ann Arbor, MI 48109-0054; **Phone:** 734-936-6770; **Board Cert:** Anatomic & Clinical Pathology 1966; **Med School:** Univ Mich Med Sch 1961; **Resid:** Pathology, Univ Mich Med Ctr 1966; **Fac Appt:** Prof Path, Univ Mich Med Sch

Balla, Andre K MD/PhD [Path] - **Spec Exp:** Prostate Cancer; Gynecologic Pathology; Tumor Banking; **Hospital:** Univ of IL Med Ctr at Chicago; **Address:** Univ IL at Chicago, Dept Path, 840 S Wood St, rm 130, MC 847, Chicago, IL 60612; **Phone:** 312-996-3879; **Board Cert:** Anatomic & Clinical Pathology 1988; **Med School:** Brazil 1972; **Resid:** Pathology, Hahnemann Univ Hosp 1988; **Fellow:** Clinical Immunology, Scripps Clin Rsch Fdn 1981; **Fac Appt:** Prof Path, Univ IL Coll Med

Behm, Frederick G MD [Path] - **Spec Exp:** Hematopathology; **Hospital:** Univ of IL Med Ctr at Chicago; **Address:** Univ Illinois Chicago, Dept Pathology, 130 CSN, MC 847, 840 S Wood St, Chicago, IL 60612-7335; **Phone:** 312-996-3150; **Board Cert:** Anatomic & Clinical Pathology 1980; Hematology 1983; **Med School:** Med Coll Wisc 1974; **Resid:** Pathology, Med Coll Va Hosps 1979; **Fac Appt:** Prof Path, Univ IL Coll Med

Bell, Debra A MD [Path] - **Spec Exp:** Gynecologic Pathology; Ovarian Cancer; **Hospital:** Mayo Med Ctr & Clin - Rochester; **Address:** 200 First St SW, Rochester, MN 55905; **Phone:** 507-284-1800; **Board Cert:** Anatomic Pathology 1980; Cytopathology 1989; **Med School:** Albany Med Coll 1976; **Resid:** Pathology, NYU Med Ctr 1981; **Fellow:** Cytopathology, Meml Sloan Kettering Cancer Ctr 1982; **Fac Appt:** Assoc Prof Path, Mayo Med Sch

Cho, Kathleen R MD [Path] - **Spec Exp:** Gynecologic Pathology; Ovarian Cancer; Cervical Cancer; **Hospital:** Univ Michigan Hlth Sys; **Address:** Univ Michigan Med Sch, 109 Zina Pitcher Pl, rm 1506, Ann Arbor, MI 48109-2200; **Phone:** 734-764-1549; **Board Cert:** Anatomic Pathology 1990; **Med School:** Vanderbilt Univ 1984; **Resid:** Pathology, Johns Hopkins Hosp 1988; **Fellow:** Gynecologic Pathology, Johns Hopkins Hosp 1990; **Fac Appt:** Prof Path, Univ Mich Med Sch

Cohen, Michael B MD [Path] - **Spec Exp:** Urologic Cancer; Cytopathology; **Hospital:** Univ Iowa Hosp & Clinics, VA Med Ctr - Iowa City; **Address:** Univ Iowa - Dept Pathology, 200 Hawkins Drive, C670GH, Iowa City, IA 52242; **Phone:** 319-384-9609; **Board Cert:** Anatomic Pathology 2007; Cytopathology 1996; **Med School:** Albany Med Coll 1982; **Resid:** Pathology, UCSF Hosps & Clinics 1986; **Fellow:** Cytopathology, UCSF Hosps & Clinics 1987; **Fac Appt:** Prof Path, Univ Iowa Coll Med

Gambetti, Pierluigi MD [Path] - **Spec Exp:** Neuro-Pathology; Neurodegenerative Disorders; Creutzfeldt-Jakob Disease (CJD); **Hospital:** Univ Hosps Case Med Ctr; **Address:** Case Western Reserve Univ, Inst Path, 2085 Adelbert Rd, rm 419, Cleveland, OH 44106; **Phone:** 216-368-0587; **Board Cert:** Neuropathology 1981; **Med School:** Italy 1960; **Resid:** Neurology, Univ Bologna Med Ctr 1963; **Fellow:** Neurological Pathology, Institut Bunge 1965; Neurological Pathology, Hosp Univ Penn 1968; **Fac Appt:** Prof Path, Case West Res Univ

Goldblum, John R MD [Path] - **Spec Exp:** Soft Tissue Pathology; Esophageal Cancer; Gastrointestinal Pathology; Sarcoma; **Hospital:** Cleveland Clin Fdn (page 56); **Address:** Cleveland Clinic, Anatomic Pathology L25, 9500 Euclid Ave, Cleveland, OH 44195; **Phone:** 216-444-8238; **Board Cert:** Anatomic Pathology 1993; **Med School:** Univ Mich Med Sch 1989; **Resid:** Anatomic Pathology, Univ Michigan Hosps 1993; **Fac Appt:** Prof Path, Cleveland Cl Coll Med/Case West Res

America's Top Doctors® 8th Edition

Greenson, Joel K MD [Path] - **Spec Exp:** Liver Cancer; Gastrointestinal Pathology; Liver Pathology; **Hospital:** Univ Michigan Hlth Sys; **Address:** Univ Michigan Hospitals, Dept Pathology, 1500 E Medical Center Drive, rm 2G332, Ann Arbor, MI 48109-0054; **Phone:** 734-936-6776; **Board Cert:** Anatomic & Clinical Pathology 1988; **Med School:** Univ Mich Med Sch 1984; **Resid:** Pathology, Cedars-Sinai Med Ctr 1988; **Fellow:** Gastrointestinal Pathology, Johns Hopkins Hosp 1990; **Fac Appt:** Prof Path, Univ Mich Med Sch

Kurtin, Paul J MD [Path] - **Spec Exp:** Lymph Node Pathology; Bone Marrow Pathology; Lymphoma; **Hospital:** Mayo Med Ctr & Clin - Rochester; **Address:** Mayo Clinic - Dept Pathology, 200 First St SW, Hilton 1156A, Rochester, MN 55905; **Phone:** 507-284-4939; **Board Cert:** Anatomic & Clinical Pathology 1983; Hematology 1988; **Med School:** Med Coll Wisc 1979; **Resid:** Anatomic & Clinical Pathology, Vanderbilt Univ mED cTR 1983; **Fellow:** Hematopathology, Brigham & Women's Hosp 1984; Surgical Pathology, Brigham & Women's Hosp 1986; **Fac Appt:** Prof Path, Mayo Med Sch

Mitros, Frank A MD [Path] - **Spec Exp:** Liver Pathology; Gastrointestinal Pathology; Surgical Pathology; **Hospital:** Univ Iowa Hosp & Clinics; **Address:** Univ Iowa Hosp & Clins, Dept Pathology, 200 Hawkins Dr, 5244B RCP, Iowa City, IA 52242; **Phone:** 319-356-1760; **Board Cert:** Anatomic Pathology 1979; **Med School:** UMDNJ-NJ Med Sch, Newark 1969; **Resid:** Pathology, Univ Chicago Hosps 1976; **Fac Appt:** Prof Path, Univ Iowa Coll Med

Myers, Jeffrey L MD [Path] - **Spec Exp:** Lung Cancer; Lung Pathology; **Hospital:** Univ Michigan Hlth Sys; **Address:** Univ Michigan, 2G332 UH, 1500 E Medical Ctr Drive, Ann Arbor, MI 48109; **Phone:** 734-936-1888; **Board Cert:** Anatomic Pathology 1986; **Med School:** Washington Univ, St Louis 1981; **Resid:** Anatomic Pathology, Barnes Jewish Hosp 1984; **Fellow:** Surgical Pathology, U Alabama Med Ctr 1985; **Fac Appt:** Prof Path, Univ Mich Med Sch

Nascimento, Antonio G MD [Path] - **Spec Exp:** Bone & Soft Tissue Pathology; Head & Neck Pathology; **Hospital:** Mayo Med Ctr & Clin - Rochester; **Address:** Mayo Clinic - Dept Pathology, 200 First St SW, Hilton 1160A, Rochester, MN 55905; **Phone:** 507-284-1187; **Board Cert:** Anatomic Pathology 1979; **Med School:** Brazil ; **Resid:** Pathology, Univ Mississippi Med Ctr; **Fellow:** Anatomic Pathology, Meml Sloan-Kettering Cancer Ctr; Surgical Pathology, Mayo Clinic

Perry, Arie MD [Path] - **Spec Exp:** Neuro-Pathology; Brain Tumors; **Hospital:** Washington Univ Med Ctr; **Address:** Washington Univ Sch Med, Dept Path-Div Neuropath, 660 S Euclid Ave, St Louis, MO 63110; **Phone:** 314-362-7765; **Board Cert:** Anatomic & Clinical Pathology 1995; Neuropathology 1997; **Med School:** Univ Tex SW, Dallas 1990; **Resid:** Pathology, Univ Tex SW 1994; **Fellow:** Surgical Pathology, Mayo Clinic 1995; Neurological Pathology, Mayo Clinic 1998; **Fac Appt:** Assoc Prof Path, Washington Univ, St Louis

Petras, Robert E MD [Path] - **Spec Exp:** Gastrointestinal Pathology; **Address:** Ameripath GI Institute, 7730 First Pl, Ste A, Oakwood Village, OH 44146; **Phone:** 440-703-2100; **Board Cert:** Anatomic & Clinical Pathology 2004; **Med School:** Ohio State Univ 1978; **Resid:** Anatomic & Clinical Pathology, Cleveland Clinic 1982; **Fellow:** Gastrointestinal Pathology, St Marks Hosp; **Fac Appt:** Assoc Prof Path, NE Ohio Univ

Rubin, Brian P MD [Path] - **Spec Exp:** Bone & Soft Tissue Tumors; Sarcoma; **Hospital:** Cleveland Clin Fdn (page 56); **Address:** Cleveland Clinic, Dept Anatomic Pathology, L25, 9500 Euclid Ave, Cleveland, OH 44195; **Phone:** 216-445-5551; **Board Cert:** Anatomic Pathology 1999; **Med School:** Cornell Univ-Weill Med Coll 1995; **Resid:** Pathology, Brigham & Women's Hosp 2000; **Fac Appt:** Asst Prof Path, Univ Wash

Pathology

Scheithauer, Bernd MD [Path] - **Spec Exp:** Brain Tumors; Pituitary Tumors; Neuro-Pathology; Pituitary Disorders; **Hospital:** Mayo Med Ctr & Clin - Rochester; **Address:** Dept Pathology, 200 First St SW, Rochester, MN 55905; **Phone:** 507-284-8350; **Board Cert:** Anatomic Pathology 1979; Neuropathology 1979; **Med School:** Loma Linda Univ 1973; **Resid:** Anatomic Pathology, Stanford Univ Med Ctr 1976; Neuropathology, Stanford Univ Med Ctr 1978; **Fellow:** Surgical Pathology, Stanford Univ Med Ctr 1979; **Fac Appt:** Prof Path, Mayo Med Sch

Suster, Saul M MD [Path] - **Spec Exp:** Lung Cancer; Mediastinal Tumors; Surgical Pathology; **Hospital:** Froedtert Meml Lutheran Hosp; **Address:** Med College of Wisconsin, Dept Pathology, Dynacare Lab Bldg, rm 226, 9200 W Wisconsin Ave, Milwaukee, WI 53226; **Phone:** 414-805-6968; **Board Cert:** Anatomic & Clinical Pathology 1988; **Med School:** Ecuador 1976; **Resid:** Anatomic Pathology, Tel Aviv Univ Med Ctr 1984; Anatomic & Clinical Pathology, Mt Sinai Med Ctr 1988; **Fellow:** Surgical Pathology, Yale-New Haven Hosp 1990; **Fac Appt:** Prof Path, Univ Wisc

Ulbright, Thomas M MD [Path] - **Spec Exp:** Testicular Cancer; Gynecologic Pathology; **Hospital:** Indiana Univ Hosp; **Address:** Clarion Pathology Laboratory, 350 W 11th St, rm 4014, Indianapolis, IN 46202; **Phone:** 317-491-6498; **Board Cert:** Anatomic Pathology 1980; **Med School:** Washington Univ, St Louis 1975; **Resid:** Pathology, Barnes Jewish Hosp 1978; Surgical Pathology, Barnes Jewish Hosp 1979; **Fellow:** Gynecologic Pathology, St Johns Mercy Med Ctr 1980; **Fac Appt:** Prof Path, Indiana Univ

Great Plains and Mountains

De Masters, Bette K MD [Path] - **Spec Exp:** Neuro-Pathology; Brain Tumors; **Hospital:** Univ Colorado Hosp, Chldn's Hosp - Aurora, The; **Address:** Univ Colo Hlth Sci Ctr, Dept Path, Box 6511, MS 8104, Aurora, CO 80045-0508; **Phone:** 303-724-3704; **Board Cert:** Anatomic & Clinical Pathology 1982; Neuropathology 1985; **Med School:** Univ Wisc 1977; **Resid:** Internal Medicine, Presby Hosp 1979; Pathology, Univ Colo Med Sch 1982; **Fellow:** Neurological Pathology, Univ Colo/Univ Kansas 1984; **Fac Appt:** Prof Path, Univ Colorado

Rodgers III, George M MD/PhD [Path] - **Spec Exp:** Hematopathology; Anemia-Cancer Related; **Hospital:** Univ Utah Hosps and Clins; **Address:** Univ Utah Med Ctr - Div Hematology, 30 N 1900 E, rm 5C402, Salt Lake City, UT 84132; **Phone:** 801-585-3229; **Board Cert:** Internal Medicine 1979; Hematology 1984; **Med School:** Tulane Univ 1976; **Resid:** Internal Medicine, Baylor Affil Hosps 1979; **Fellow:** Hematology, UCSF Med Ctr 1982; **Fac Appt:** Prof Med, Univ Utah

Thor, Ann D MD [Path] - **Spec Exp:** Breast Cancer; Gynecologic Cancer; **Hospital:** Univ Colorado Hosp; **Address:** Univ Colorado Hlth Sci Ctr, Dept Pathology, Box 6511, MS 8104, Aurora, CO 80045-0508; **Phone:** 303-724-3704; **Board Cert:** Anatomic Pathology 1987; Cytopathology 1989; **Med School:** Vanderbilt Univ 1981; **Resid:** Pathology, Vanderbilt Univ 1983; **Fellow:** Immunopathology, Natl Cancer Inst 1986; Gynecologic Pathology, Mass Genl Hosp 1990; **Fac Appt:** Prof Path, Univ Colorado

Weisenburger, Dennis MD [Path] - **Spec Exp:** Hematopathology; Lymphoma; **Hospital:** Nebraska Med Ctr; **Address:** Univ Nebraska Med Ctr, Dept Pathology, 983135 Nebraska Medical Center, Omaha, NE 68198-3135; **Phone:** 402-559-7688; **Board Cert:** Anatomic & Clinical Pathology 1979; **Med School:** Univ Minn 1974; **Resid:** Anatomic Pathology, Univ Iowa Hosps 1978; **Fellow:** Hematopathology, City of Hope Natl Med Ctr 1980; **Fac Appt:** Prof Path, Univ Nebr Coll Med

Southwest

Bruner, Janet M MD [Path] - **Spec Exp:** Brain Tumors; Neuro-Pathology; **Hospital:** UT MD Anderson Cancer Ctr; **Address:** MD Anderson Cancer Ctr, 1515 Holcombe Blvd, Ste 85, Houston, TX 77030; **Phone:** 713-792-6127; **Board Cert:** Anatomic Pathology 1997; Neuropathology 1984; **Med School:** Med Coll OH 1979; **Resid:** Anatomic & Clinical Pathology, Med Coll Ohio Hosp 1982; **Fellow:** Neurological Pathology, Baylor Coll Med 1984

Cagle, Philip MD [Path] - **Spec Exp:** Pulmonary Pathology; Lung Cancer; Mesothelioma; **Hospital:** Methodist Hosp - Houston; **Address:** Methodist Hospital, Dept Pathology, 6565 Fannin St, Ste 227, Houston, TX 77030; **Phone:** 713-441-6478; **Board Cert:** Anatomic & Clinical Pathology 1985; **Med School:** Univ Tenn Coll Med, Memphis 1981; **Fac Appt:** Prof Path, Baylor Coll Med

Foucar, M Kathryn MD [Path] - **Spec Exp:** Leukemia; Lymph Node Pathology; Bone Marrow Pathology; **Hospital:** Univ NM Hlth & Sci Ctr; **Address:** TriCore Reference Lab, Hematopathology, 1001 Woodward Pl NE, Albuquerque, NM 87102; **Phone:** 505-938-8456; **Board Cert:** Anatomic & Clinical Pathology 1978; **Med School:** Ohio State Univ 1974; **Resid:** Anatomic Pathology, Univ NM Health & Sci Ctr 1976; Anatomic Pathology, Univ Minn Med Ctr 1978; **Fellow:** Surgical Pathology, Univ Minn Med Ctr 1979; **Fac Appt:** Prof Path, Univ New Mexico

Grogan, Thomas M MD [Path] - **Spec Exp:** Immunopathology; Lymphoma; **Hospital:** Univ Med Ctr - Tucson; **Address:** Univ Med Ctr, Dept Pathology, 1501 N Campbell Ave, rm 5212, Tucson, AZ 85724; **Phone:** 520-626-7477; **Board Cert:** Anatomic Pathology 1976; **Med School:** Geo Wash Univ 1971; **Resid:** Pathology, Letterman Army Med Ctr 1976; **Fellow:** Immunopathology, Stanford Univ Sch Med 1979; **Fac Appt:** Prof Path, Univ Ariz Coll Med

Hamilton, Stanley R MD [Path] - **Spec Exp:** Surgical Pathology; Gastrointestinal Pathology; Liver Pathology; **Hospital:** UT MD Anderson Cancer Ctr; **Address:** Univ Texas MD Anderson Cancer Ctr, 1515 Holcombe Blvd, Unit 85, Houston, TX 77030-4009; **Phone:** 713-792-2040; **Board Cert:** Anatomic & Clinical Pathology 1978; **Med School:** Indiana Univ 1973; **Resid:** Pathology, Johns Hopkins Hosp 1978; **Fellow:** St Marks Hosp 1979; **Fac Appt:** Prof Path, Univ Tex, Houston

Kinney, Marsha C MD [Path] - **Spec Exp:** Hematopathology; Lymphoma; Leukemia; **Hospital:** Univ Hlth Sys - Univ Hosp (San Antonio, TX); **Address:** Univ Tex Hlth & Sci Ctr, Dept Path, 7703 Floyd Curl Drive, MC 775, San Antonio, TX 78229-3900; **Phone:** 210-567-4098; **Board Cert:** Anatomic & Clinical Pathology 1985; Hematology 1998; **Med School:** Univ Tex SW, Dallas 1981; **Resid:** Pathology, Vanderbilt Univ Med Ctr 1985; **Fellow:** Hematopathology, Vanderbilt Univ Med Ctr 1988; **Fac Appt:** Prof Path, Univ Tex, San Antonio

Leslie, Kevin O MD [Path] - **Spec Exp:** Pulmonary Pathology; Lung Cancer; Surgical Pathology; **Hospital:** Mayo Clinic - Scottsdale; **Address:** Mayo Clinic, Scottsdale, 13400 E Shea Blvd, Scottsdale, AZ 85259; **Phone:** 480-301-8021; **Board Cert:** Anatomic & Clinical Pathology 1982; **Med School:** Albert Einstein Coll Med 1976; **Resid:** Anatomic & Clinical Pathology, Univ Colorado Health Sci Ctr 1982; **Fellow:** Surgical Pathology, Stanford Univ Med Ctr 1983; **Fac Appt:** Prof Path, Mayo Med Sch

Moran, Cesar A MD [Path] - **Spec Exp:** Lung Cancer; Mediastinal Tumors; Mesothelioma; **Hospital:** UT MD Anderson Cancer Ctr; **Address:** MD Anderson Cancer Ctr, Dept Pathology, 1515 Holcombe Blvd, rm G1-3738, Houston, TX 77030; **Phone:** 713-792-8134; **Board Cert:** Anatomic Pathology 1992; **Med School:** Guatemala 1981; **Resid:** Anatomic Pathology, Mt Sinai Med Ctr 1988; **Fellow:** Surgical Pathology, Yale- New Haven Med Ctr 1989; **Fac Appt:** Prof Path, Univ Tex, Houston

Pathology

Prieto, Victor G MD/PhD [Path] - **Spec Exp:** Dermatopathology; Melanoma; Skin Cancer; **Hospital:** UT MD Anderson Cancer Ctr; **Address:** MD Anderson Cancer Ctr, Dept Pathology, 1515 Holcombe Blvd, Box 85, Houston, TX 77030-4000; **Phone:** 713-792-0918; **Board Cert:** Anatomic Pathology 1995; Dermatopathology 1997; **Med School:** Spain 1986; **Resid:** Pathology, New York Hosp-Cornell Med Ctr 1993; **Fellow:** Pathology, Meml Sloan Kettering Cancer Ctr 1995; Dermatopathology, New York Hosp-Cornell Med Ctr 1996; **Fac Appt:** Prof Path, Univ Tex, Houston

Rashid, Asif MD/PhD [Path] - **Spec Exp:** Gastrointestinal Pathology; Liver Pathology; **Hospital:** UT MD Anderson Cancer Ctr; **Address:** MD Anderson Cancer Ctr, Dept Pathology, 1515 Holcombe Blvd, Box 85, Houston, TX 77030; **Phone:** 713-745-1101; **Board Cert:** Anatomic Pathology 1994; **Med School:** Pakistan 1984; **Resid:** Anatomic Pathology, Mass Genl Hosp 1993; **Fellow:** Anatomic Pathology, Mass Genl Hosp 1994; Anatomic Pathology, Johns Hopkins Med Inst 1996

Roberts, William C MD [Path] - **Spec Exp:** Cardiac Pathology; **Hospital:** Baylor Univ Medical Ctr; **Address:** Baylor Univ Med Ctr, Heart & Vascular Inst, 3500 Gaston Ave, Dallas, TX 75246-2017; **Phone:** 214-820-7911; **Board Cert:** Anatomic Pathology 1965; **Med School:** Emory Univ 1958; **Resid:** Anatomic Pathology, Natl Heart Inst-NIH 1962; Internal Medicine, Johns Hopkins Hosp 1963; **Fellow:** Cardiovascular Disease, Natl Heart Inst-NIH 1964

Silva, Elvio G MD [Path] - **Spec Exp:** Gynecologic Pathology; Gynecologic Cancer; **Hospital:** UT MD Anderson Cancer Ctr, Cedars-Sinai Med Ctr; **Address:** MD Anderson Cancer Ctr, Dept Pathology, 1515 Holcombe Blvd, Unit 85, Houston, TX 77030; **Phone:** 713-792-3154; **Board Cert:** Anatomic Pathology 2007; **Med School:** Argentina 1969; **Resid:** Pathology, National Univ Med Ctr 1975; Anatomic Pathology, Univ Toronto 1978; **Fellow:** Surgical Pathology, MD Anderson Cancer Ctr 1979; **Fac Appt:** Prof Path

Walker, David H MD [Path] - **Spec Exp:** Infections-Emerging; Tropical Diseases; Biodefense; **Hospital:** UTMB - John Sealy Hospital; **Address:** UT Med Br Galveston, Dept Path, 301 University Blvd, Galveston, TX 77555-0609; **Phone:** 409-772-3989; **Board Cert:** Anatomic & Clinical Pathology 1974; **Med School:** Vanderbilt Univ 1969; **Resid:** Anatomic & Clinical Pathology, Peter Bent Brigham Hosp 1973; **Fellow:** Pathology, Harvard Univ 1973; **Fac Appt:** Prof Path, Univ Tex Med Br, Galveston

Wheeler, Thomas M MD [Path] - **Spec Exp:** Thyroid Disorders; Thyroid Cancer; **Hospital:** Ben Taub Genl Hosp; **Address:** Baylor Coll Med, Dept Pathology, One Baylor Plaza, rm T203, Houston, TX 77030; **Phone:** 713-798-4664; **Board Cert:** Anatomic & Clinical Pathology 1999; Cytopathology 1990; **Med School:** Baylor Coll Med 1977; **Resid:** Pathology, Baylor Coll Med 1981; **Fac Appt:** Prof Path, Baylor Coll Med

West Coast and Pacific

Amin, Mahul MD [Path] - **Spec Exp:** Genitourinary Pathology; Bladder Cancer; **Hospital:** Cedars-Sinai Med Ctr; **Address:** Cedars Sinai Hosp, 8700 Beverly Blvd, Ste 8728, Los Angeles, CA 90048; **Phone:** 310-423-6631; **Board Cert:** Anatomic & Clinical Pathology 1996; **Med School:** India 1983; **Resid:** Pathology, Henry Ford Hosp 1992; **Fellow:** Surgical Pathology, MD Anderson Cancer Ctr 1993; **Fac Appt:** Prof Path, Emory Univ

Arber, Daniel A MD [Path] - **Spec Exp:** Bone Marrow Pathology; Lymph Node Pathology; Spleen Pathology; **Hospital:** Stanford Univ Med Ctr, Lucile Packard Chldns Hosp/Stanford Univ Med Ctr; **Address:** Clinic Laboratories, Stanford Univ Med Ctr, 300 Pasteur Drive, rm H1507, MC 5627, Stanford, CA 94305; **Phone:** 650-725-5604; **Board Cert:** Anatomic & Clinical Pathology 1991; Hematology 1993; **Med School:** Univ Tex, San Antonio 1986; **Resid:** Anatomic & Clinical Pathology, Scott & White Meml Hosp 1991; **Fellow:** Hematopathology, City of Hope Natl Med Ctr 1993; **Fac Appt:** Prof Path, Stanford Univ

Bastian, Boris C MD [Path] - **Spec Exp:** Melanoma; Skin Cancer; **Hospital:** UCSF Med Ctr; **Address:** UCSF Comprehensive Cancer Center, Box 0808, San Francisco, CA 94143; **Phone:** 415-476-5132; **Med School:** Germany 1988; **Resid:** Dermatology, University of Wurzburg 1994; **Fellow:** Hematology, Ludwig-Maximilian-University 1989; **Fac Appt:** Asst Prof D, UCSF

Bollen, Andrew W MD [Path] - **Spec Exp:** Neuro-Pathology; Brain Tumors; Brain Infections; **Hospital:** UCSF Med Ctr, San Francisco Genl Hosp; **Address:** Dept Pathology/Neuropathology, 505 Parnassus Ave, M551, Box 0102, San Francisco, CA 94143-0511; **Phone:** 415-476-5236; **Board Cert:** Clinical Pathology 1993; Anatomic Pathology 1992; Neuropathology 1992; **Med School:** UCSD 1985; **Resid:** Anatomic Pathology, UCSF Med Ctr 1991; **Fellow:** Neuropathology, UCSF Med Ctr 1989; **Fac Appt:** Prof Path, UCSF

Chandrasoma, Parakrama T MD [Path] - **Spec Exp:** Gastrointestinal Pathology; Gastrointestinal Cancer; Neuro-Pathology; **Hospital:** LAC & USC Med Ctr; **Address:** LAC-USC Med Ctr, Dept Path, 1200 N State St, rm 16-905, Los Angeles, CA 90033; **Phone:** 323-226-4600; **Board Cert:** Anatomic Pathology 1982; **Med School:** Sri Lanka 1971; **Resid:** Anatomic Pathology, Univ Sri Lanka 1978; Anatomic Pathology, LAC-USC Med Ctr 1982; **Fac Appt:** Prof Path, USC Sch Med

Cochran, Alistair J MD [Path] - **Spec Exp:** Melanoma; Dermatopathology; **Hospital:** Ronald Reagan UCLA Med Ctr; **Address:** UCLA Med Ctr, Dept Path & Med, 10833 Le Conte Ave, rm 13145CHS, MC 173216, Los Angeles, CA 90095-1713; **Phone:** 310-825-2743; **Med School:** Scotland 1959; **Resid:** Dermatopathology, Western Infirmary 1968; **Fellow:** Immunology, Karolinska Inst 1970; **Fac Appt:** Prof Path, UCLA

Cote, Richard J MD [Path] - **Spec Exp:** Lymph Node Pathology; Bladder Cancer; Breast Cancer; **Hospital:** USC Norris Comp Cancer Ctr, USC Univ Hosp - R K Eamer Med Plz; **Address:** 1441 Eastlake Ave, rm 2424, Los Angeles, CA 90033; **Phone:** 323-865-0212; **Board Cert:** Anatomic Pathology 1987; **Med School:** Univ Chicago-Pritzker Sch Med 1980; **Resid:** Pathology, New York Hosp-Cornell 1987; **Fellow:** Pathology, Meml Sloan-Kettering Cancer Ctr 1990; **Fac Appt:** Prof Path, USC-Keck School of Medicine

Dubeau, Louis MD/PhD [Path] - **Spec Exp:** Ovarian Cancer; Breast Cancer; **Hospital:** USC Norris Comp Cancer Ctr; **Address:** USC Norris Cancer Ctr, Dept Pathology, 1441 Eastlake Ave, rm 6338, Los Angeles, CA 90033-1048; **Phone:** 323-865-0720; **Board Cert:** Anatomic Pathology 1984; **Med School:** McGill Univ 1979; **Resid:** Anatomic Pathology, McGill Univ Med Ctr 1984; **Fac Appt:** Prof Path, USC Sch Med

Ferrell, Linda MD [Path] - **Spec Exp:** Liver Pathology; **Hospital:** UCSF Med Ctr; **Address:** UCSF Med Ctr, Dept Pathology, 505 Parnassus Ave, rm M590, Box 0102, San Francisco, CA 94143-0102; **Phone:** 415-353-1090; **Board Cert:** Anatomic Pathology 1982; **Med School:** Univ Kans 1977; **Resid:** Anatomic Pathology, Univ Kansas Med Ctr 1979; Anatomic Pathology, UCSF Med Ctr 1981; **Fac Appt:** Prof Path, UCSF

Fishbein, Michael C MD [Path] - **Spec Exp:** Cardiovascular Pathology; Pulmonary Pathology; **Hospital:** Ronald Reagan UCLA Med Ctr; **Address:** 10833 Le Conte Ave, Los Angeles, CA 90095-1732; **Phone:** 310-825-9731; **Board Cert:** Anatomic & Clinical Pathology 1975; **Med School:** Univ IL Coll Med 1971; **Resid:** Anatomic & Clinical Pathology, UCLA-Harbor General Hosp 1975; **Fellow:** Pathology, Heart Lung Inst-NIH 1975; **Fac Appt:** Prof Path, UCLA

Govindarajan, Sugantha MD [Path] - **Spec Exp:** Liver Pathology; **Hospital:** Rancho Los Amigos Natl Rehab Ctr; **Address:** Rancho Los Amigos Natl Rehab Ctr, 7601 E Imperial Hwy, Bldg JPI - rm B170, Dept Pathology, Downey, CA 90242; **Phone:** 562-401-8996; **Board Cert:** Anatomic Pathology 1976; **Med School:** India 1969; **Resid:** Pathology, St Lukes Hosp 1976; **Fellow:** Pathology, Cleveland Clinic 1977; **Fac Appt:** Prof Path, USC Sch Med

Pathology

Hammar, Samuel P MD [Path] - **Spec Exp:** Lung Cancer; Pulmonary Pathology; **Hospital:** Harrison Meml Hosp; **Address:** Diagnostic Specialties Laboratory, 700 Lebo Blvd, Bremerton, WA 98310; **Phone:** 360-479-7707; **Board Cert:** Anatomic & Clinical Pathology 1975; **Med School:** Univ Wash 1970

Hendrickson, Michael MD [Path] - **Spec Exp:** Gynecologic Cancer; Gynecologic Pathology; **Hospital:** Stanford Univ Med Ctr; **Address:** Stanford Univ Med Ctr, Surg Path Lab, 300 Pasteur Drive, rm L230, MC 5324, Stanford, CA 94305; **Phone:** 650-725-5169; **Board Cert:** Anatomic Pathology 1975; **Med School:** Stanford Univ 1971; **Resid:** Anatomic Pathology, Stanford Univ Med Sch 1974; **Fac Appt:** Prof Path, Stanford Univ

Kanel, Gary MD [Path] - **Spec Exp:** Liver Disease; **Hospital:** USC Univ Hosp - R K Eamer Med Plz; **Address:** USC Univ Hosp, Dept Pathology, 1500 San Pablo St Fl 2, Los Angeles, CA 90033; **Phone:** 323-226-7127; **Board Cert:** Anatomic & Clinical Pathology 1979; **Med School:** Tufts Univ 1974; **Resid:** Pathology, Tufts-New England Med Ctr 1976; Pathology, Univ Chicago Hosp 1977; **Fellow:** Pathology, Tufts-New England Med Ctr 1979; **Fac Appt:** Prof Path, USC Sch Med

Kempson, Richard L MD [Path] - **Spec Exp:** Breast Pathology; Gynecologic Pathology; **Hospital:** Stanford Univ Med Ctr; **Address:** 300 Pasteur Drive, Ste H2110, Stanford, CA 94305-5243; **Phone:** 650-723-7211; **Board Cert:** Anatomic Pathology 1963; **Med School:** Tulane Univ 1955; **Resid:** Surgical Pathology, Barnes Hosp 1963; **Fellow:** Anatomic Pathology, Tulane Univ Med Ctr 1962; **Fac Appt:** Prof Path, Stanford Univ

Koss, Michael N MD [Path] - **Spec Exp:** Pulmonary Pathology; Lung Cancer; Mediastinal Tumors; **Hospital:** USC Norris Comp Cancer Ctr, USC Univ Hosp - R K Eamer Med Plz; **Address:** 2222 Ocean View Ave, Ste 212, 2011 Zonal Ave, Los Angeles, CA 90057; **Phone:** 323-226-6507; **Board Cert:** Anatomic Pathology 1979; **Med School:** Stanford Univ 1970; **Resid:** Pathology, Columbia Presby Med Ctr 1974; **Fellow:** Renal Pathology, Columbia Presby Med Ctr 1975; Pulmonary Pathology, Armed Forces Inst Path 1978; **Fac Appt:** Prof Path, USC Sch Med

Le Boit, Philip E MD [Path] - **Spec Exp:** Cutaneous Lymphoma; Skin Cancer; Dermatopathology; **Hospital:** UCSF Med Ctr; **Address:** UCSF - Dermatopathology Section, 1701 Divisadero St, Ste 350, San Francisco, CA 94115; **Phone:** 415-353-7546; **Board Cert:** Anatomic Pathology 1983; Clinical Pathology 1986; Dermatopathology 1983; **Med School:** Albany Med Coll 1979; **Resid:** Anatomic Pathology, UCSF Med Ctr 1981; Clinical Pathology, Mt Sinai Hosp 1982; **Fellow:** Dermatopathology, New York Hosp-Cornell Med Ctr 1983; **Fac Appt:** Prof Path, UCSF

Ljung, Britt-Marie E MD [Path] - **Spec Exp:** Breast Cancer; Cytopathology; Fine Needle Aspiration Biopsy; **Hospital:** UCSF - Mt Zion Med Ctr; **Address:** UCSF - Dept Pathology, 1600 Divisadero St, Box 1785, rm r-200, San Francisco, CA 94143-1785; **Phone:** 415-353-7320; **Board Cert:** Anatomic Pathology 1985; Cytopathology 1989; **Med School:** Sweden 1975; **Resid:** Pathology, Karolinska Hosp 1979; Anatomic Pathology, UCLA Med Ctr 1983; **Fac Appt:** Prof Path, UCSF

Mischel, Paul MD [Path] - **Spec Exp:** Neuro-Pathology; Brain Tumors; **Hospital:** Ronald Reagan UCLA Med Ctr; **Address:** UCLA Med Ctr, Div Neuropathology, 10833 Le Conte Ave, rm 13-317 CHS, Los Angeles, CA 90095-1732; **Phone:** 310-825-0377; **Board Cert:** Anatomic Pathology 1997; Neuropathology 1997; **Med School:** Cornell Univ-Weill Med Coll 1991; **Resid:** Anatomic & Clinical Pathology, UCLA Med Sch 1996; **Fellow:** Neurological Pathology, UCLA Med Sch 1995; Research, Howard Hughes Med Inst/UCSF 1998; **Fac Appt:** Assoc Prof Path, UCLA

Nathwani, Bharat N MD [Path] - **Spec Exp:** Hematopathology; Leukemia; Lymphoma; **Hospital:** LAC & USC Med Ctr; **Address:** LAC & USC Med Ctr, Dept Pathology, 1200 N State St, rm 2422, Los Angeles, CA 90033-4526; **Phone:** 323-226-7064; **Board Cert:** Anatomic Pathology 1977; **Med School:** India 1969; **Resid:** Pathology, JJ Group-Grant Med Ctr 1972; Pathology, Rush-Presby-St Lukes Med Ctr 1974; **Fellow:** Hematopathology, City Hope Natl Med Ctr 1975; **Fac Appt:** Prof Path, USC Sch Med

Rutgers, Joanne MD [Path] - **Spec Exp:** Gynecologic Cancer; Cytopathology; Gastrointestinal Pathology; **Hospital:** Long Beach Meml Med Ctr; **Address:** 2801 Atlantic Ave, Dept of Pathology, Long Beach, CA 90806; **Phone:** 562-933-0717; **Board Cert:** Clinical Pathology 1992; Anatomic Pathology 1985; Cytopathology 1997; **Med School:** UCSD 1981; **Resid:** Pathology, Montefiore Med Ctr 1983; Pathology, NYU Med Ctr 1985; **Fellow:** Gynecologic Pathology, Mass Genl Hosp 1989; **Fac Appt:** Assoc Clin Prof Path, UCLA

Sibley, Richard K MD [Path] - **Spec Exp:** Kidney Pathology; Breast Pathology; Liver Pathology; **Hospital:** Stanford Univ Med Ctr; **Address:** Stanford Univ Med Ctr, Dept Pathology, 300 Pasteur Drive, rm H2110, MC 5243, Stanford, CA 94305; **Phone:** 650-723-7211; **Board Cert:** Anatomic Pathology 1975; **Med School:** Univ Tex SW, Dallas 1971; **Resid:** Anatomic Pathology, Univ Chicago Hosps 1974; **Fellow:** Stanford Univ Med Ctr 1975; **Fac Appt:** Prof Path, Stanford Univ

Triche, Timothy J MD/PhD [Path] - **Spec Exp:** Pediatric Pathology; Pediatric Cancers; Sarcoma; **Hospital:** Chldns Hosp - Los Angeles; **Address:** Chldns Hosp of Los Angeles, Dept Path, 4650 Sunset Blvd, MS 43, Los Angeles, CA 90027; **Phone:** 323-361-4516; **Board Cert:** Anatomic Pathology 1975; **Med School:** Tulane Univ 1971; **Resid:** Anatomic Pathology, Barnes Hosp-Wash Univ 1973; Surgical Pathology, Barnes Hosp 1974; **Fellow:** Pathology, Natl Cancer Inst 1975; **Fac Appt:** Prof Path, USC Sch Med

True, Lawrence D MD [Path] - **Spec Exp:** Urologic Pathology; Prostate Cancer; Bladder Cancer; **Hospital:** Univ Wash Med Ctr; **Address:** Univ Wash Med Ctr, Dept Anatomic Path, 1959 NE Pacific St, rm BB220, Box 356100, Seattle, WA 98195-6100; **Phone:** 206-598-6400; **Board Cert:** Anatomic Pathology 1981; **Med School:** Tulane Univ 1971; **Resid:** Pathology, Univ Colo Hlth Sci Ctr 1980; **Fac Appt:** Prof Path, Univ Wash

Warnke, Roger A MD [Path] - **Spec Exp:** Lymphoma; Hematopathology; **Hospital:** Stanford Univ Med Ctr; **Address:** Stanford Univ, Dept Pathology, 300 Pasteur Drive, Ste L235, Stanford, CA 94305-5324; **Phone:** 650-725-5167; **Board Cert:** Anatomic Pathology 1975; **Med School:** Washington Univ, St Louis 1971; **Resid:** Pathology, Stanford Univ Med Ctr 1974; **Fellow:** Surgical Pathology, Stanford Univ Med Ctr 1975; Immunology, Stanford Univ Med Ctr 1976; **Fac Appt:** Prof Path, Stanford Univ

Weiss, Lawrence M MD [Path] - **Spec Exp:** Lymphoma; Hematopathology; Adrenal Pathology; **Hospital:** City of Hope Natl Med Ctr & Beckman Rsch; **Address:** City of Hope Natl Med Ctr, Div Pathology, 1500 E Duarte Rd, Duarte, CA 91010-0269; **Phone:** 626-359-8111 x62456; **Board Cert:** Anatomic Pathology 1985; **Med School:** Univ MD Sch Med 1981; **Resid:** Pathology, Brigham & Women's Hosp 1983; **Fellow:** Pathology, Stanford Univ Hosp 1984

Wilczynski, Sharon P MD/PhD [Path] - **Spec Exp:** Gynecologic Cancer; Breast Cancer; Ovarian Cancer; Clinical Trials; **Hospital:** City of Hope Natl Med Ctr & Beckman Rsch; **Address:** City Hope Natl Med Ctr-Dept of Pathology, 1500 E Duarte Blvd, Duarte, CA 91010; **Phone:** 626-256-4673 x62456; **Board Cert:** Anatomic & Clinical Pathology 1985; Cytopathology 1991; **Med School:** Med Coll PA Hahnemann 1981; **Resid:** Pathology, Hosp Univ Penn 1983; Anatomic & Clinical Pathology, Long Beach Meml Hosp 1985; **Fac Appt:** Prof Path, USC-Keck School of Medicine

Pediatrics

A pediatrician is concerned with the physical, emotional and social health of children from birth to young adulthood. Care encompasses a broad spectrum of health services ranging from preventive health-care to the diagnosis and treatment of acute and chronic diseases.

A pediatrician deals with biological, social and environmental influences on the developing child, and with the impact of disease and dysfunction on development.

Training Required: Three years

Pediatric Allergy and Immunology: An allergist-immunologist is trained in evaluation, physical and laboratory diagnosis and management of disorders involving the immune system. Selected examples of such conditions include asthma, anaphylaxis, rhinitis, eczema and adverse reactions to drugs, foods and insect stings as well as immune deficiency diseases (both acquired and congenital), defects in host defense and problems related to autoimmune disease, organ transplantation or malignancies of the immune system. As our understanding of the immune system develops, the scope of this specialty is widening.

Training Required: Prior certification in pediatrics *plus* two years in allergy/immunology. (Training programs are available at some medical centers to provide individuals with expertise in both allergy/immunology and pediatric pulmonology. Such individuals are candidates for dual certification.)

(continued on next page)

Certification in one of the following subspecialties requires additional training and examination.

Pediatric Cardiology: A pediatric cardiologist provides comprehensive care to patients with cardiovascular problems. This specialist is skilled in selecting, performing and evaluating the structural and functional assessment of the heart and blood vessels and the clinical evaluation of cardiovascular disease.

Pediatric Critical Care Medicine: A pediatrician who cares for children who are victims of life threatening disorders such as severe accidents, shock and diabetic acidosis.

Pediatric Endocrinology: A pediatrician who provides expert care to infants, children and adolescents who have diseases that result from an abnormality in the endocrine glands (glands which secrete hormones). These diseases include diabetes mellitus, growth failure, unusual size for age, early or late pubertal development, birth defects, the genital anomalies and disorders of the thyroid, the adrenal and pituitary glands.

Pediatric Gastroenterology: A pediatrician who specializes in the diagnosis and treatment of diseases of the digestive systems of infants, children and adolescents. This specialist treats conditions such as abdominal pain, ulcers, diarrhea, cancer and jaundice and performs complex diagnostic and therapeutic procedures using lighted scopes to see internal organs.

Pediatric Hematology-Oncology: A pediatrician trained in the combination of pediatrics, hematology and oncology to recognize and manage pediatric blood disorders and cancerous diseases.

Pediatric Infectious Diseases: A pediatrician trained to care for children in the diagnosis, treatment and prevention of infectious diseases. This specialist can apply specific knowledge to effect a better outcome for pediatric infections with complicated courses, underlying diseases that predispose to unusual or severe infections, unclear diagnoses, uncommon diseases and complex or investigational treatments.

Pediatric Nephrology: A pediatrician who deals with the normal and abnormal development and maturation of the kidney and urinary tract, the mechanisms by which the kidney can be damaged, the evaluation and treatment of renal diseases, fluid and electrolyte abnormalities, hypertension and renal replacement therapy.

Pediatric Otolaryngology: A pediatric otolaryngologist has special expertise in the management of infants and children with disorders that include congenital and acquired conditions involving the aerodigestive tract, nose and paranasal sinuses, the ear and other areas of the head and neck. The pediatric otolaryngologist has special skills in the diagnosis, treatment and management of childhood disorders of voice, speech, language and hearing.

Pediatric Pulmonology: A pediatrician dedicated to the prevention and treatment of all respiratory diseases affecting infants, children and young adults. This specialist is knowledgeable about the growth and development of the lung, assessment of respiratory function in infants and children and experienced in a variety of invasive and noninvasive diagnostic techniques.

Pediatric Rheumatology: A pediatrician who treats diseases of joints, muscle, bones and tendons. A pediatric rheumatologist diagnoses and treats arthritis, back pain, muscle strains, common athletic injuries and "collagen" diseases.

Pediatric Surgery: A surgeon with expertise in the management of surgical conditions in premature and newborn infants, children and adolescents.

PEDIATRICS

New England

Palfrey, Judith S MD [Ped] - **Spec Exp:** Special Health Care Needs (CSHCN); Developmental Disorders; **Hospital:** Children's Hospital - Boston; **Address:** Children's Hospital, 300 Longwood Ave, Boston, MA 02115; **Phone:** 617-355-4662; **Board Cert:** Pediatrics 1976; Developmental-Behavioral Pediatrics 2002; **Med School:** Columbia P&S 1971; **Resid:** Pediatrics, Montefiore Med Ctr 1974; **Fac Appt:** Prof Ped, Harvard Med Sch

Rappaport, Leonard MD [Ped] - **Spec Exp:** Developmental & Behavioral Disorders; **Hospital:** Children's Hospital - Boston; **Address:** Childrens Hosp Fegan 10, 300 Longwood Ave, Boston, MA 02115; **Phone:** 617-355-4683; **Board Cert:** Pediatrics 1983; Developmental-Behavioral Pediatrics 2002; **Med School:** Yale Univ 1977; **Resid:** Pediatrics, Chldns Hosp 1980; **Fellow:** Developmental-Behavioral Pediatrics, Chldns Hosp 1982; **Fac Appt:** Assoc Prof Ped, Harvard Med Sch

Shaywitz, Sally E MD [Ped] - **Spec Exp:** Learning Disorders-Studies Only; Dyslexia-Studies Only; **Hospital:** Yale-New Haven Hosp; **Address:** Yale Univ Sch Med, Dept Peds, 333 Cedar St, rm LMP-3089, New Haven, CT 06520; **Phone:** 203-785-4641; **Board Cert:** Pediatrics 1971; **Med School:** Albert Einstein Coll Med 1966; **Resid:** Pediatrics, Albert Einstein Coll Med 1970; **Fellow:** Pediatrics, Bronx Muni Hosp Ctr 1968; Behavioral Pediatrics, Albert Einstein Coll Med 1970; **Fac Appt:** Prof Ped, Yale Univ

Mid Atlantic

Berlin Jr, Cheston M MD [Ped] - **Spec Exp:** Phenylketonuria (PKU); Tourette's Syndrome; **Hospital:** Penn State Milton S Hershey Med Ctr; **Address:** Penn State Univ Coll Med, Pediatrics, PO Box 850, Hershey, PA 17033; **Phone:** 717-531-8006; **Board Cert:** Pediatrics 1982; **Med School:** Harvard Med Sch 1962; **Resid:** Pediatrics, Children's Hosp 1967; **Fac Appt:** Prof Ped, Penn State Univ-Hershey Med Ctr

Burgess, David B MD [Ped] - **Spec Exp:** Developmental & Behavioral Disorders; ADD/ADHD; Autism; **Hospital:** Chldns Hosp of Philadelphia, The; **Address:** Children's Hosp Philadelphia, Specialty Care Ctr, 4009 Black Horse Pike, Mays Landing, NJ 08330; **Phone:** 609-677-7895; **Board Cert:** Pediatrics 1978; Developmental-Behavioral Pediatrics 2004; **Med School:** Univ Wisc 1973; **Resid:** Pediatrics, Charity Hosp 1977; **Fellow:** Child Development, JFK Child Dev Ctr, Univ Colorado 1980; **Fac Appt:** Assoc Clin Prof Ped, Univ Pennsylvania

Cohen, William I MD [Ped] - **Spec Exp:** Down Syndrome; **Hospital:** Chldns Hosp of Pittsburgh - UPMC; **Address:** Children's Hosp Pittsburgh, Pediatrics, Child Development Unit, 3705 Fifth Ave, Pittsburgh, PA 15213; **Phone:** 412-692-5560; **Board Cert:** Pediatrics 1979; Developmental-Behavioral Pediatrics 2002; **Med School:** SUNY Buffalo 1975; **Resid:** Pediatrics, Children's Hosp 1978; **Fellow:** Developmental-Behavioral Pediatrics, Children's Hosp 1980; **Fac Appt:** Prof Ped, Univ Pittsburgh

Gartner Jr, J Carlton MD [Ped] - **Spec Exp:** Diagnostic Problems; Multisystem Disorders; **Hospital:** Alfred I duPont Hosp for Children; **Address:** Alfred I duPont Hosp for Children, 1600 Rockland Rd, rm 3D 245, Wilmington, DE 19899; **Phone:** 302-651-5946; **Board Cert:** Pediatrics 2000; **Med School:** Johns Hopkins Univ 1971; **Fac Appt:** Prof Ped, Thomas Jefferson Univ

Hofkosh, Dena MD [Ped] - **Spec Exp:** Developmental & Behavioral Disorders; Developmental Disorders; **Hospital:** Chldns Hosp of Pittsburgh - UPMC; **Address:** Childrens Hosp Pittsburgh, Dept Pediatrics, 3705 Fifth Ave, Pittsburgh, PA 15213; **Phone:** 412-692-6541; **Board Cert:** Pediatrics 1984; Neurodevelopmental Disabilities 2001; **Med School:** NYU Sch Med 1979; **Resid:** Pediatrics, Univ Pittsburgh Med Ctr 1982; **Fellow:** Ambulatory Pediatrics, Univ Pittsburgh Med Ctr 1984; **Fac Appt:** Prof Ped, Univ Pittsburgh

Morton, D Holmes MD [Ped] - **Spec Exp:** Genetic Disorders; Rare Disorders; **Hospital:** Lancaster Genl Hosp; **Address:** Clinic For Special Children, 535 Bunker Hill Rd, PO Box 128, Strasburg, PA 17579; **Phone:** 717-687-9407; **Board Cert:** Pediatrics 1987; **Med School:** Harvard Med Sch 1983; **Resid:** Pediatrics, Childrens Hosp 1986; **Fellow:** Research, Childrens Hosp 1988

Oeffinger, Kevin MD [Ped] - **Spec Exp:** Cancer Survivors-Late Effects of Therapy; **Hospital:** Meml Sloan-Kettering Cancer Ctr; **Address:** 1275 York Avenue, New York, NY 10065; **Phone:** 800-525-2225; **Board Cert:** Family Medicine 2000; **Med School:** Univ Tex, San Antonio 1984; **Resid:** Family Medicine, Baylor Coll Med 1985; **Fellow:** Family Medicine, Fam Practice Faculty Dev Ctr 1999; Natl Cancer Inst 2000

Vining, Eileen P MD [Ped] - **Spec Exp:** Pediatric Neurology; Epilepsy; Rasmussen's Syndrome; **Hospital:** Johns Hopkins Hosp - Baltimore (page 61); **Address:** Johns Hopkins Hospital, 600 N Wolfe St Meyer Bldg - rm 2-147, Baltimore, MD 21287; **Phone:** 410-955-9100; **Board Cert:** Pediatrics 1977; **Med School:** Johns Hopkins Univ 1972; **Resid:** Pediatrics, Children's Hosp 1974; **Fellow:** Developmental-Behavioral Pediatrics, JFK Inst/Johns Hopkins Hosp 1976; **Fac Appt:** Assoc Prof Ped, Johns Hopkins Univ

Zitelli, Basil MD [Ped] - **Hospital:** Chldns Hosp of Pittsburgh - UPMC; **Address:** Childrens Hosp Pittsburgh, Pittsburgh, PA 15213; **Board Cert:** Pediatrics 1976; **Med School:** Univ Pittsburgh 1971; **Resid:** Pediatrics, Johns Hopkins Hospital 1976; **Fellow:** Pediatrics, Johns Hopkins Hospital 1978; **Fac Appt:** Prof Ped, Univ Pittsburgh

Midwest

Berman, Brian W MD [Ped] - **Spec Exp:** Sickle Cell Disease; Thrombotic Disorders; Hemophilia; **Hospital:** Rainbow Babies & Chldns Hosp; **Address:** Rainbow Babies & Chldn's Hosp, 11100 Euclid Ave, MS RBC6019, Cleveland, OH 44106-6019; **Phone:** 216-844-3752; **Board Cert:** Pediatrics 1989; Pediatric Hematology-Oncology 1989; **Med School:** Temple Univ 1975; **Resid:** Pediatrics, St Chris Hosp for Chldn 1978; **Fellow:** Pediatric Hematology-Oncology, Yale-New Haven Hosp 1980; **Fac Appt:** Prof Ped, Case West Res Univ

Bull, Marilyn J MD [Ped] - **Spec Exp:** Developmental Disorders; Down Syndrome; Birth Defects; **Hospital:** Riley Hosp for Children; **Address:** 702 Barnhill Drive, rm 1601, Indianapolis, IN 46202; **Phone:** 317-274-4846; **Board Cert:** Pediatrics 1973; Clinical Genetics 1982; Neurodevelopmental Disabilities 2001; **Med School:** Univ Mich Med Sch 1968; **Resid:** Pediatrics, Children's Meml Hosp 1972; **Fellow:** Genetics, Boston Floating Hosp 1973; **Fac Appt:** Prof Ped, Indiana Univ

Fost, Norman C MD [Ped] - **Spec Exp:** Ethics; **Hospital:** Univ WI Hosp & Clins; **Address:** Univ Wisconsin Chldns Hosp, 600 Highland Ave, Madison, WI 53792-4108; **Phone:** 608-265-6050; **Board Cert:** Pediatrics 1970; **Med School:** Yale Univ 1964; **Resid:** Pediatrics, Johns Hopkins Hosp 1971; **Fellow:** Pediatrics, Harvard Sch Public Hlth 1973; **Fac Appt:** Prof Ped, Univ Wisc

Pediatrics

Jacob, Molly MD [Ped] - **Spec Exp:** Asthma; ADD/ADHD; Nutrition; **Hospital:** Children's Mem Hosp, Adv Illinois Masonic Med Ctr; **Address:** 3000 N Halstead Ave, Ste 825, Chicago, IL 60657; **Phone:** 773-528-3403; **Board Cert:** Pediatrics 1980; **Med School:** India 1968; **Resid:** Pediatrics, Ill Masonic Med Ctr 1979; **Fellow:** Ambulatory Pediatrics, Ill Masonic Med Ctr 1979; **Fac Appt:** Asst Clin Prof Ped, Univ IL Coll Med

Lantos, John MD [Ped] - **Spec Exp:** Chronic Illness; Palliative Care; Ethics; **Hospital:** La Rabida Chlds Hosp, Univ of Chicago Hosps; **Address:** 5841 S Maryland Ave, MC 6082, Chicago, IL 60637; **Phone:** 773-702-6602; **Board Cert:** Pediatrics 1986; **Med School:** Univ Pittsburgh 1981; **Resid:** Pediatrics, Chldns Natl Med Ctr 1984; **Fellow:** Clinical Ethics, Univ Chicago Hosps; **Fac Appt:** Prof Ped, Univ Chicago-Pritzker Sch Med

Southwest

Kleinerman, Eugenie S MD [Ped] - **Spec Exp:** Ewing's Sarcoma; Cancer Survivors-Late Effects of Therapy; **Hospital:** UT MD Anderson Cancer Ctr; **Address:** MD Anderson Cancer Ctr, Dept Pediatrics, 1515 Holcombe Blvd, Unit 87, Houston, TX 77030; **Phone:** 713-792-8110; **Board Cert:** Pediatrics 1980; **Med School:** Duke Univ 1975; **Resid:** Pediatrics, Children's Hosp-Natl Med Ctr 1978; **Fellow:** Immunology, Natl Cancer Inst 1981; **Fac Appt:** Prof Ped, Univ Tex, Houston

West Coast and Pacific

Berkowitz, Carol D MD [Ped] - **Spec Exp:** Child Abuse; **Hospital:** LAC - Harbor - UCLA Med Ctr; **Address:** LAC-Harbor-UCLA Med Ctr, 1000 W Carson St, Box 437, Torrance, CA 90509-2910; **Phone:** 310-222-3091; **Board Cert:** Pediatrics 2000; Pediatric Emergency Medicine 2006; **Med School:** Columbia P&S 1969; **Resid:** Pediatrics, Roosevelt Hosp 1972; **Fac Appt:** Clin Prof Ped, UCLA

Feldman, Kenneth W MD [Ped] - **Spec Exp:** Child Abuse; **Hospital:** Chldns Hosp and Regl Med Ctr - Seattle; **Address:** Odessa Brown Chldns Clin, 2101 E Yesler Way, Ste 100, Seattle, WA 98122; **Phone:** 206-987-7225; **Board Cert:** Pediatrics 1975; **Med School:** Univ Wisc 1970; **Resid:** Pediatrics, Chldns Regl Med Ctr 1974; **Fac Appt:** Clin Prof Ped, Univ Wash

Jones, Kenneth Lyons MD [Ped] - **Spec Exp:** Genetic Disorders; Dysmorphology; **Hospital:** UCSD Med Ctr; **Address:** 9500 Gilman Drive, San Diego, CA 92093-0828; **Phone:** 858-246-0047; **Board Cert:** Pediatrics 1971; **Med School:** Hahnemann Univ 1966; **Resid:** Pediatrics, Chldns Ortho Hosp 1969; **Fac Appt:** Prof Ped, UCSD

Zeltzer, Lonnie K MD [Ped] - **Spec Exp:** Pain Management; Complementary Medicine; **Hospital:** Mattel Chldns Hosp at UCLA; **Address:** UCLA Pediatric Pain Program, 10833 Le Conte Ave, #22-464 MDCC, Los Angeles, CA 90095-1752; **Phone:** 310-825-0731; **Board Cert:** Pediatrics 1976; **Med School:** Univ Cincinnati 1970; **Resid:** Pediatrics, Univ Ariz Hosp 1973; **Fellow:** Adolescent Medicine, Chldns Hosp 1976; **Fac Appt:** Prof Ped, UCLA

PEDIATRIC ALLERGY & IMMUNOLOGY

New England

Klein, Robert B MD [PA&I] - **Spec Exp:** Asthma; **Hospital:** Rhode Island Hosp; **Address:** Rhode Island Hosp, Dept of Pediatrics, 593 Eddy St, Providence, RI 02903; **Phone:** 401-444-8639; **Board Cert:** Pediatrics 1976; Allergy & Immunology 1977; **Med School:** Switzerland 1971; **Resid:** Pediatrics, Dartmouth/Hitchcock Med Ctr 1974; **Fellow:** Allergy & Immunology, UCLA 1976; **Fac Appt:** Prof Ped, Brown Univ

Mid Atlantic

Josephs, Shelby H MD [PA&I] - **Spec Exp:** Food Allergy; **Hospital:** Georgetown Univ Hosp; **Address:** 6410 Rockledge Drive, Ste 304, Bethesda, MD 20871; **Phone:** 301-530-7907; **Board Cert:** Pediatrics 1979; Allergy & Immunology 1985; **Med School:** Duke Univ 1975; **Resid:** Pediatrics, Children's Hosp 1977; Allergy & Immunology, Duke Univ Med Ctr 1979; **Fac Appt:** Assoc Clin Prof Ped, Georgetown Univ

Kamani, Naynesh R MD [PA&I] - **Spec Exp:** Stem Cell Transplant; Immunotherapy; Bone Marrow Transplant; **Hospital:** Chldns Natl Med Ctr; **Address:** Chldns Natl Med Ctr, Div Hematology, 111 Michigan Ave NW, Washington, DC 20010; **Phone:** 202-476-2800; **Board Cert:** Pediatrics 1983; Pediatric Allergy & Immunology 1983; **Med School:** Ethiopia 1975; **Resid:** Pediatrics, Downstate Med Ctr-Kings Co Hosp 1981; **Fellow:** Pediatric Allergy & Immunology, Children's Hosp 1983; **Fac Appt:** Prof Ped, Geo Wash Univ

Sampson, Hugh MD [PA&I] - **Spec Exp:** Food Allergy; Anaphylaxis; Eczema; **Hospital:** Mount Sinai Med Ctr (page 64); **Address:** Mt Sinai Sch Med, Dept Peds, 1 Gustave Levy Pl, Box 1198, New York, NY 10029-6500; **Phone:** 212-241-5548; **Board Cert:** Pediatrics 1980; Allergy & Immunology 1981; **Med School:** SUNY Buffalo 1975; **Resid:** Pediatrics, Chldns Meml Hosp 1979; **Fellow:** Allergy & Immunology, Duke Univ Med Ctr 1980; **Fac Appt:** Prof Ped, Mount Sinai Sch Med

Schuberth, Kenneth Charles MD [PA&I] - **Spec Exp:** Allergy; Asthma; **Hospital:** Johns Hopkins Hosp - Baltimore (page 61), Greater Baltimore Med Ctr; **Address:** 10807 Falls Rd, Ste 200, Lutherville, MD 21093; **Phone:** 410-321-9393; **Board Cert:** Pediatrics 1979; Allergy & Immunology 1983; **Med School:** Johns Hopkins Univ 1973; **Resid:** Pediatrics, Johns Hopkins Hosp 1978; **Fellow:** Allergy & Immunology, Johns Hopkins Hosp 1980; **Fac Appt:** Assoc Prof Ped, Johns Hopkins Univ

Skoner, David Peter MD [PA&I] - **Spec Exp:** Asthma & Allergy; Rhinitis; **Hospital:** Allegheny General Hosp; **Address:** Allegheny Genl Hosp, Div Asthma Allergy & Immunology, 320 E North Ave, Fl 7 - South Tower, Pittsburgh, PA 15212; **Phone:** 412-359-6640; **Board Cert:** Pediatrics 1985; Allergy & Immunology 1985; **Med School:** Temple Univ 1980; **Resid:** Pediatrics, Chldns Hosp Med Ctr 1983; **Fellow:** Allergy & Immunology, Chldns Hosp 1985; **Fac Appt:** Prof Ped, Drexel Univ Coll Med

Sly, R Michael MD [PA&I] - **Spec Exp:** Asthma; Allergy; Atopic Dermatitis; **Hospital:** Chldns Natl Med Ctr; **Address:** Children's Natl Med Ctr, Dept Allergy & Immunology, 111 Michigan Ave NW, Ste 1030, Washington, DC 20010-2970; **Phone:** 301-424-1755; **Board Cert:** Pediatrics 1980; Allergy & Immunology 1987; **Med School:** Washington Univ, St Louis 1960; **Resid:** Pediatrics, St Louis Chldns Hosp 1962; Pediatrics, Univ Kentucky Med Ctr 1963; **Fellow:** Pediatric Allergy & Immunology, UCLA Med Ctr 1967; **Fac Appt:** Prof Ped, Geo Wash Univ

Pediatric Allergy & Immunology

Wood, Robert A MD [PA&I] - **Spec Exp:** Food Allergy; Asthma; **Hospital:** Johns Hopkins Hosp - Baltimore (page 61); **Address:** 600 N Wolfe St, CMSC-1102, Baltimore, MD 21287; **Phone:** 410-955-5883; **Board Cert:** Pediatrics 1987; Allergy & Immunology 1997; **Med School:** Univ Rochester 1982; **Resid:** Pediatrics, Johns Hopkins Hosp 1985; **Fellow:** Allergy & Immunology, Johns Hopkins Hosp 1988; **Fac Appt:** Prof Ped, Johns Hopkins Univ

Southeast

Burks Jr, Arvil Wesley MD [PA&I] - **Spec Exp:** Asthma; Allergic Rhinitis; Food Allergy; Anaphylaxis; **Hospital:** Duke Univ Med Ctr; **Address:** Duke Univ Med Ctr, Box 2644, Durham, NC 27710; **Phone:** 919-684-9914; **Board Cert:** Pediatrics 1985; Allergy & Immunology 1985; **Med School:** Univ Ark 1980; **Resid:** Pediatrics, Ark Chldns Hosp 1983; **Fellow:** Allergy & Immunology, Duke Univ Med Ctr 1985; **Fac Appt:** Prof Ped, Duke Univ

Kelly, Cynthia S MD [PA&I] - **Spec Exp:** Asthma; Rhinitis; Sinusitis; **Hospital:** Chldns Hosp of King's Daughters; **Address:** Chlds Hosp of The Kings Daughters, 601 Childrens Lane, Norfolk, VA 23507; **Phone:** 757-668-8255; **Board Cert:** Pediatrics 2004; Allergy & Immunology 1997; **Med School:** Wayne State Univ 1985; **Resid:** Pediatrics, Univ Mich 1987; **Fellow:** Allergy & Immunology, UCLA 1988; Pediatric Infectious Disease, Vanderbilt Univ 1989; **Fac Appt:** Assoc Prof Ped, Eastern VA Med Sch

Ownby, Dennis R MD [PA&I] - **Spec Exp:** Food Allergy; Anaphylaxis; **Hospital:** Med Coll of GA Hosp and Clin; **Address:** Allergy & Immunology, 1120 15th St Bldg BG - rm 1019, Augusta, GA 30912-0004; **Phone:** 706-721-2390; **Board Cert:** Pediatrics 1977; Pediatric Allergy & Immunology 2006; Clinical & Laboratory Immunology 1986; **Med School:** Med Coll OH 1972; **Resid:** Pediatrics, Duke Med Ctr 1974; **Fellow:** Pediatric Allergy & Immunology, Duke Med Ctr 1977; **Fac Appt:** Prof Ped, Med Coll GA

Midwest

Lemanske Jr, Robert F MD [PA&I] - **Spec Exp:** Asthma; Allergy; Immune Deficiency; **Hospital:** Univ WI Hosp & Clins; **Address:** 600 Highland Ave, rm K4/916 CSC, Madison, WI 53792; **Phone:** 608-265-2206; **Board Cert:** Pediatrics 1980; Allergy & Immunology 1981; **Med School:** Univ Wisc 1975; **Resid:** Pediatrics, Univ Wisc Hosp 1978; **Fellow:** Allergy & Immunology, Univ Wisc Hosp 1980; Allergy & Immunology, Natl Inst Health 1983; **Fac Appt:** Prof Ped, Univ Wisc

Pongracic, Jacqueline MD [PA&I] - **Spec Exp:** Latex Allergy; Asthma; Food Allergy; **Hospital:** Children's Mem Hosp, Northwestern Meml Hosp; **Address:** 2300 Children's Plaza, Box 60, Chicago, IL 60614; **Phone:** 773-327-3710; **Board Cert:** Internal Medicine 1988; Allergy & Immunology 2001; **Med School:** Northwestern Univ 1985; **Resid:** Internal Medicine, North Shore Univ Hosp 1988; **Fellow:** Allergy & Immunology, Johns Hopkins Hosp 1991; **Fac Appt:** Asst Prof Ped, Northwestern Univ

Strunk, Robert MD [PA&I] - **Spec Exp:** Asthma; **Hospital:** St Louis Chldns Hosp; **Address:** 660 S Euclid Ave, Box 8116, St Louis, MO 63110; **Phone:** 314-454-2694; **Board Cert:** Pediatrics 1974; Allergy & Immunology 1987; **Med School:** Northwestern Univ 1968; **Resid:** Pediatrics, Cincinnati Chldns Hosp 1970; **Fellow:** Pediatric Allergy & Immunology, Boston Chldns Hosp 1974; **Fac Appt:** Prof Ped, Washington Univ, St Louis

Wolf, Raoul MD [PA&I] - **Spec Exp:** Asthma; Allergy; Immune Deficiency; **Hospital:** Univ of Chicago Hosps, La Rabida Chlds Hosp; **Address:** La Rabida Chldns Hosp, Dept A&I, E 65th St at Lake Michigan, Chicago, IL 60649; **Phone:** 773-753-8637; **Board Cert:** Pediatrics 1980; Allergy & Immunology 1983; **Med School:** South Africa 1969; **Resid:** Pediatrics, Baragwanath Hosp 1973; Pediatrics, Transvaal Meml Hosp Chldn 1976; **Fellow:** Allergy & Immunology, Chldns Hosp Med Ctr 1979; **Fac Appt:** Prof Ped, Univ Chicago-Pritzker Sch Med

Great Plains and Mountains

Bock, S Allan MD [PA&I] - **Spec Exp:** Asthma up to age 50; Allergy up to age 50; Food Allergy; **Hospital:** Boulder Community Hospital, Natl Jewish Med & Rsch Ctr; **Address:** Boulder Asthma & Allergy Clinics, 3950 Broadway, Boulder, CO 80304; **Phone:** 303-444-5991; **Board Cert:** Pediatrics 1977; Allergy & Immunology 1977; **Med School:** Univ MD Sch Med 1972; **Resid:** Pediatrics, Colo Med Ctr/Natl Jewish Med Ctr 1974; **Fellow:** Allergy & Immunology, Colo Med Ctr/Natl Jewish Med Ctr 1976; **Fac Appt:** Clin Prof Ped, Univ Colorado

Gelfand, Erwin W MD [PA&I] - **Spec Exp:** Immune Deficiency; Asthma; Allergy; **Hospital:** Natl Jewish Med & Rsch Ctr, Chldn's Hosp - Aurora, The; **Address:** National Jewish Med & Research Ctr, 1400 Jackson St, Denver, CO 80206; **Phone:** 303-398-1196; **Board Cert:** Pediatrics 1972; **Med School:** McGill Univ 1966; **Resid:** Pediatrics, Montreal Children's Hosp 1968; Pediatrics, Children's Hosp Med Ctr 1969; **Fellow:** Immunology, Children's Hosp Med Ctr 1971; **Fac Appt:** Prof Ped, Univ Colorado

Leung, Donald YM MD/PhD [PA&I] - **Spec Exp:** Atopic Dermatitis; Asthma; **Hospital:** Natl Jewish Med & Rsch Ctr, Chldn's Hosp - Aurora, The; **Address:** 1400 Jackson St, Bldg K - Ste 926I, Denver, CO 80206; **Phone:** 303-398-1379; **Board Cert:** Pediatrics 1982; Allergy & Immunology 1983; Clinical & Laboratory Immunology 1990; **Med School:** Univ Chicago-Pritzker Sch Med 1977; **Resid:** Pediatrics, Childrens Hosp 1979; **Fellow:** Allergy & Immunology, Childrens Hosp 1981; **Fac Appt:** Prof Ped, Univ Colorado

Southwest

Bahna, Sami L MD [PA&I] - **Spec Exp:** Food Allergy; Asthma; Eczema; **Hospital:** Louisiana State Univ Hosp; **Address:** LSU Hlth Scis Ctr, Dept Pediatrics, 1501 Kings Hwy, Shreveport, LA 71103; **Phone:** 318-675-7625; **Board Cert:** Pediatrics 1980; Allergy & Immunology 1981; **Med School:** Egypt 1964; **Resid:** Pediatrics, Univ Maryland Hosp 1975; **Fellow:** Allergy & Immunology, Harbor-UCLA Med Ctr 1978; **Fac Appt:** Prof Ped, Louisiana State U, New Orleans

Shearer, William T MD [PA&I] - **Spec Exp:** AIDS/HIV; Immune Deficiency; **Hospital:** Texas Chldns Hosp - Houston; **Address:** Tex Chldns Hosp, Div A&I, 6621 Fannin, St Fl 3, MC FC 330.01, Houston, TX 77030-2399; **Phone:** 832-824-1319; **Board Cert:** Pediatrics 1986; Allergy & Immunology 1989; Clinical & Laboratory Immunology 1986; **Med School:** Washington Univ, St Louis 1970; **Resid:** Pediatrics, Chldns Hosp-Wash Univ 1972; **Fellow:** Allergy & Immunology, Barnes Hosp-Wash Univ 1974; **Fac Appt:** Prof Ped, Baylor Coll Med

West Coast and Pacific

Church, Joseph MD [PA&I] - **Spec Exp:** AIDS/HIV; Immune Deficiency; **Hospital:** Chldns Hosp - Los Angeles; **Address:** Immunology and Allergy, MS 75, 4650 Sunset Blvd, Los Angeles, CA 90027; **Phone:** 323-361-2501; **Board Cert:** Pediatrics 1977; Allergy & Immunology 1977; **Med School:** UMDNJ-NJ Med Sch, Newark 1972; **Resid:** Pediatrics, Chldns Hosp/Natl Med Ctr 1974; **Fellow:** Allergy & Immunology, Georgetown Med Ctr 1976; **Fac Appt:** Prof Ped, USC Sch Med

Pediatric Allergy & Immunology

Cowan, Morton J MD [PA&I] - **Spec Exp:** Immunodeficiency Disorders; Stem Cell Transplant-Fetal; Bone Marrow Transplant; **Hospital:** UCSF Med Ctr; **Address:** UCSF Med Ctr, Peds BMT Program, 505 Parnassus Ave, rm M659, San Francisco, CA 94143-1278; **Phone:** 415-476-2188; **Board Cert:** Pediatrics 1981; Allergy & Immunology 1983; **Med School:** Univ Pennsylvania 1970; **Resid:** Surgery, Duke Univ Med Ctr 1972; Pediatrics, UCSF Med Ctr 1977; **Fellow:** Research, Natl Inst Hlth 1975; Immunology, UCSF Med Ctr; **Fac Appt:** Prof Ped, UCSF

Epstein, Stuart MD [PA&I] - **Spec Exp:** Asthma & Allergy; Food Allergy; **Hospital:** Cedars-Sinai Med Ctr; **Address:** 9735 Wilshire Blvd, Ste 121, Beverly Hills, CA 90212-2101; **Phone:** 310-274-6853; **Board Cert:** Allergy & Immunology 1999; **Med School:** Univ IL Coll Med 1978; **Resid:** Pediatrics, Cedars Sinai Med Ctr 1980; **Fellow:** Pediatrics, UC Irvine 1981; Pediatrics, USC Med Ctr 1982; **Fac Appt:** Assoc Clin Prof Ped, UCLA

Fanous, Yvonne F MD [PA&I] - **Spec Exp:** Asthma & Allergy; Cystic Fibrosis; Immune Deficiency; **Hospital:** Loma Linda Univ Med Ctr; **Address:** 11370 Anderson St, Ste B-100, Loma Linda, CA 92354; **Phone:** 909-558-2388; **Board Cert:** Pediatrics 1983; Allergy & Immunology 1985; **Med School:** Egypt 1973; **Resid:** Pediatrics, Texas Tech Univ Hosp 1980; Pediatrics, Loma Linda Univ 1981; **Fellow:** Allergy & Immunology, UC Irvine 1983; **Fac Appt:** Assoc Prof A&I, Loma Linda Univ

Stiehm, E Richard MD [PA&I] - **Spec Exp:** Immune Deficiency; Allergy; Pediatric Rheumatology; **Hospital:** Ronald Reagan UCLA Med Ctr; **Address:** UCLA Children's Hosp, 22-387 MDCC, 10833 Le Conte Ave, Los Angeles, CA 90095-3075; **Phone:** 310-825-6481; **Board Cert:** Pediatrics 1964; Allergy & Immunology 1974; Diagnostic Lab Immunology 1986; **Med School:** Univ Wisc 1957; **Resid:** Pediatrics, Babies Hosp 1963; **Fellow:** Allergy & Immunology, Univ Wisc 1959; Allergy & Immunology, UCSF 1965; **Fac Appt:** Prof Ped, UCLA

Wara, Diane W MD [PA&I] - **Spec Exp:** AIDS/HIV; Immune Deficiency; **Hospital:** UCSF Med Ctr; **Address:** 505 Parnassus Ave, Box 0107, San Francisco, CA 94143; **Phone:** 415-476-2865; **Board Cert:** Pediatrics 1974; Allergy & Immunology 1975; **Med School:** UC Irvine 1969; **Resid:** Pediatrics, UCSF Med Ctr 1972; **Fellow:** Immunology, UCSF Med Ctr 1975; **Fac Appt:** Prof Ped, UCSF

PEDIATRIC CARDIOLOGY

New England

Lock, James E MD [PCd] - **Spec Exp:** Interventional Cardiology; Angioplasty-Pulmonary Artery; Cardiac Catheterization; Fetal Surgery; **Hospital:** Children's Hospital - Boston; **Address:** Chldns Hosp, Dept Cardiology, 300 Longwood Ave, Farley 2, Boston, MA 02115-5724; **Phone:** 617-355-7313; **Board Cert:** Pediatrics 1978; Pediatric Cardiology 1981; **Med School:** Stanford Univ 1973; **Resid:** Pediatrics, Univ Minn Hosp 1975; Pediatric Cardiology, Univ Minn Hosp 1977; **Fellow:** Cardiovascular Disease, Hosp Sick Chldn 1979; **Fac Appt:** Prof Ped, Harvard Med Sch

Newburger, Jane MD [PCd] - **Spec Exp:** Kawasaki Disease; Cholesterol/Lipid Disorders; Congenital Heart Disease; **Hospital:** Children's Hospital - Boston, Brigham & Women's Hosp; **Address:** Chldns Hosp, Dept Ped Cardiology, 300 Longwood Ave, Farley Bldg Fl 2, Boston, MA 02115-5724; **Phone:** 617-355-5427; **Board Cert:** Pediatrics 1979; Pediatric Cardiology 1983; **Med School:** Harvard Med Sch 1974; **Resid:** Pediatrics, Chldns Hosp Med Ctr 1976; **Fellow:** Pediatric Cardiology, Chldns Hosp Med Ctr 1979; **Fac Appt:** Prof Ped, Harvard Med Sch

Walsh, Edward P MD [PCd] - **Spec Exp:** Cardiac Electrophysiology; Arrhythmias; **Hospital:** Children's Hospital - Boston; **Address:** Chldns Hosp, Dept Cardiology, 300 Longwood Ave, Bader 2, Boston, MA 02115; **Phone:** 617-355-6328; **Board Cert:** Pediatrics 1985; Pediatric Cardiology 1985; **Med School:** Univ Pennsylvania 1979; **Resid:** Pediatrics, Chldns Hosp 1982; **Fellow:** Pediatric Cardiology, Chldns Hosp 1985; **Fac Appt:** Assoc Prof Ped, Harvard Med Sch

Mid Atlantic

Beerman, Lee B MD [PCd] - **Spec Exp:** Congenital Heart Disease-Adult & Child; Arrhythmias; **Hospital:** Chldns Hosp of Pittsburgh - UPMC; **Address:** Chldns Hosp-Heart Ctr, 3705 5th Ave, Fl 2 - rm 2820, Pittsburgh, PA 15213-2524; **Phone:** 412-692-5540; **Board Cert:** Pediatrics 1979; Pediatric Cardiology 1979; **Med School:** Univ Pittsburgh 1974; **Resid:** Pediatrics, Chldns Hosp 1977; **Fellow:** Pediatric Cardiology, Chldns Hosp 1979; **Fac Appt:** Prof Ped, Univ Pittsburgh

Biancaniello, Thomas MD [PCd] - **Spec Exp:** Congenital Heart Disease; Fetal Echocardiography; Interventional Cardiology; Cardiac Catheterization; **Hospital:** Stony Brook Univ Med Ctr; **Address:** Stony Brook Univ Hosp, Dept Pediatrics, HSC T11, 040, Stony Brook, NY 11794-8111; **Phone:** 631-444-5437; **Board Cert:** Pediatrics 1979; Pediatric Cardiology 1981; **Med School:** NY Med Coll 1975; **Resid:** Pediatrics, North Shore Univ Hosp 1977; **Fellow:** Pediatric Cardiology, Cincinnati Chldns Hosp 1980; **Fac Appt:** Prof Ped, SUNY Stony Brook

Bierman, Fredrick MD [PCd] - **Spec Exp:** Fetal Echocardiography; Kawasaki Disease; Congenital Heart Disease; **Hospital:** Schneider Chldn's Hosp; **Address:** Chldns Heart Ctr, Schneider Chldns Hosp, 269-01 76th Ave, rm 139, New Hyde Park, NY 11040; **Phone:** 718-470-7350; **Board Cert:** Pediatrics 1978; Pediatric Cardiology 1981; **Med School:** SUNY Downstate 1973; **Resid:** Pediatrics, Mount Sinai Med Ctr 1976; **Fellow:** Pediatric Cardiology, Harvard Chldns Hosp 1979; **Fac Appt:** Prof Ped, Albert Einstein Coll Med

Brenner, Joel I MD [PCd] - **Spec Exp:** Congenital Heart Disease; **Hospital:** Johns Hopkins Hosp - Baltimore (page 61), Greater Baltimore Med Ctr; **Address:** Johns Hopkins Hosp, Pediatric Cardiology, 600 N Wolfe St, Brady 522, Baltimore, MD 21287; **Phone:** 410-955-5987; **Board Cert:** Pediatrics 1975; Pediatric Cardiology 1977; **Med School:** NY Med Coll 1970; **Resid:** Pediatrics, New York Hosp 1972; **Fellow:** Pediatric Cardiology, Yale-New Haven Hosp 1974; **Fac Appt:** Assoc Prof Ped, Johns Hopkins Univ

Cooper, Rubin MD [PCd] - **Spec Exp:** Congenital Heart Disease; Rheumatic Heart Disease; Kawasaki Disease; **Hospital:** NYPresby-Morgan Stanley Children's Hosp (page 66), NY Hosp Queens; **Address:** 525 E 68th St, Ste F695B, New York, NY 10021; **Phone:** 212-746-3561; **Board Cert:** Pediatrics 1976; Pediatric Cardiology 1979; **Med School:** NY Med Coll 1971; **Resid:** Pediatrics, Strong Meml Hosp 1973; **Fellow:** Pediatric Cardiology, Strong Meml Hosp 1975; **Fac Appt:** Prof Ped, Cornell Univ-Weill Med Coll

Gewitz, Michael MD [PCd] - **Spec Exp:** Neonatal Cardiology; Kawasaki Disease; Echocardiography; Heart Failure; **Hospital:** Westchester Med Ctr, Vassar Bros Med Ctr; **Address:** Maria Fareri Chldns Hosp/NY Med Coll, Rte 100, Munger Pavillion, Ste 618, Valhalla, NY 10595; **Phone:** 914-594-4370; **Board Cert:** Pediatrics 1979; Pediatric Cardiology 1981; **Med School:** Hahnemann Univ 1974; **Resid:** Pediatrics, Chldns Hosp 1976; Pediatrics, Hosp Sick Chldn 1977; **Fellow:** Pediatric Cardiology, Yale-New Haven Hosp 1979; **Fac Appt:** Prof Ped, NY Med Coll

Pediatric Cardiology

Hellenbrand, William E MD [PCd] - **Spec Exp:** Interventional Cardiology; **Hospital:** NYPresby-Morgan Stanley Children's Hosp (page 66), Robert Wood Johnson Univ Hosp - New Brunswick; **Address:** Morgan Stanley Chlds Hosp of NY-Presby, 3959 Broadway Fl 2N - Ste 255, New York, NY 10032; **Phone:** 212-305-6069; **Board Cert:** Pediatrics 1975; Pediatric Cardiology 1977; **Med School:** SUNY Downstate 1970; **Resid:** Pediatrics, Yale-New Haven Hosp 1972; **Fellow:** Pediatric Cardiology, Yale-New Haven Hosp 1976; **Fac Appt:** Prof Ped, Columbia P&S

Parness, Ira A MD [PCd] - **Spec Exp:** Echocardiography; Congenital Heart Disease; Fetal Echocardiography; **Hospital:** Mount Sinai Med Ctr (page 64); **Address:** 1 Gustave Levy Pl, Box 1201, New York, NY 10029-6500; **Phone:** 212-241-8662; **Board Cert:** Pediatrics 1984; Pediatric Cardiology 1985; **Med School:** SUNY Downstate 1979; **Resid:** Pediatrics, Brookdale Hosp 1982; **Fellow:** Pediatric Cardiology, Children's Hosp 1985; **Fac Appt:** Assoc Prof Ped, Mount Sinai Sch Med

Radtke, Wolfgang MD [PCd] - **Spec Exp:** Interventional Cardiology; Cardiac Catheterization; Congenital Heart Disease-Adult & Child; **Hospital:** Alfred I duPont Hosp for Children; **Address:** Nemours Cardiac Ctr, 1600 Rockland Rd, Wilmington, DE 19803; **Phone:** 302-651-6600; **Board Cert:** Pediatrics 2002; Pediatric Cardiology 2004; **Med School:** Germany 1980; **Resid:** Pediatrics, Kiel Univ Chldns Hosp 1985; **Fellow:** Pediatric Cardiology, Chldns Hosp 1988; **Fac Appt:** Prof Ped, Jefferson Med Coll

Steinherz, Laurel MD [PCd] - **Spec Exp:** Cardiac Effects of Cancer/Cancer Therapy; **Hospital:** Meml Sloan-Kettering Cancer Ctr, NY-Presby Hosp/Weill Cornell (page 66); **Address:** 1275 York Avenue, New York, NY 10065; **Phone:** 800-525-2225; **Board Cert:** Pediatrics 1976; Pediatric Cardiology 1978; **Med School:** Albert Einstein Coll Med 1970; **Resid:** Pediatrics, Childrens Hosp 1972; **Fellow:** Pediatric Cardiology, NY Hosp-Cornell Med Ctr 1975; **Fac Appt:** Prof Ped, Cornell Univ-Weill Med Coll

Velvis, Harm MD [PCd] - **Spec Exp:** Cardiac Catheterization; Congenital Heart Disease; Heart Disease in Down Syndrome; **Hospital:** Albany Med Ctr, St Peter's Hosp - Albany; **Address:** Capital Dist Ped Cardio Assoc, 319 S Manning Blvd, Ste 203, Albany, NY 12208-1743; **Phone:** 518-489-3292; **Board Cert:** Pediatric Cardiology 2002; **Med School:** Netherlands 1980; **Resid:** Pediatrics, Albany Med Ctr 1987; **Fellow:** Pediatric Cardiology, UCSF Med Ctr 1990; **Fac Appt:** Assoc Clin Prof Ped, Albany Med Coll

Walsh, Christine A MD [PCd] - **Spec Exp:** Arrhythmias; Congenital Heart Disease; Syncope; **Hospital:** Montefiore Med Ctr, Montefiore Med Ctr - Weiler-Einstein Div; **Address:** 3415 Bainbridge Ave, Bronx, NY 10467-2401; **Phone:** 718-741-2310; **Board Cert:** Pediatrics 1978; Pediatric Cardiology 1983; Pediatric Critical Care Medicine 2003; **Med School:** Yale Univ 1973; **Resid:** Pediatrics, Columbia-Presby Med Ctr 1976; **Fellow:** Pediatric Cardiology, Columbia-Presby Med Ctr 1978; Pharmacology, Columbia P&S 1980; **Fac Appt:** Prof Ped, Albert Einstein Coll Med

Weinberg, Paul M MD [PCd] - **Spec Exp:** Cardiac Pathology; Cardiac MRI; **Hospital:** Chldns Hosp of Philadelphia, The; **Address:** Chldns Hosp, Div Cardiology, 34th St & Civic Ctr Blvd, Philadelphia, PA 19104; **Phone:** 215-590-3274; **Board Cert:** Pediatrics 1974; Pediatric Cardiology 1975; **Med School:** Jefferson Med Coll 1969; **Resid:** Pediatrics, Chldns Hosp 1971; Cardiology & Pathology, Chldns Hosp Med Ctr 1977; **Fellow:** Pediatric Cardiology, Chldns Hosp 1973; **Fac Appt:** Prof Ped, Univ Pennsylvania

America's Top Doctors® 8th Edition

Southeast

Boucek, Mark M MD [PCd] - **Spec Exp:** Transplant Medicine-Heart; Cardiac Catheterization; Heart Failure; Interventional Cardiology; **Hospital:** Joe Di Maggio Chldns Hosp; **Address:** J Dimaggio Chldns Hosp, Dept Ped Cardiology, 1150 N 35th Ave, Ste 575, Hollywood, FL 33021; **Phone:** 954-985-6939; **Board Cert:** Pediatrics 1982; Pediatric Cardiology 1983; **Med School:** Univ Miami Sch Med 1977; **Resid:** Pediatrics, Vanderbilt Univ Hosp 1979; **Fellow:** Pediatric Cardiology, Univ Utah Hlth Sci Ctr 1981; **Fac Appt:** Clin Prof Ped, Univ Hlth Sci, Coll Osteo Med

Bricker, John MD [PCd] - **Spec Exp:** Transplant Medicine-Heart; Congenital Heart Disease-Adult; **Hospital:** Univ of Kentucky Chandler Hosp; **Address:** 800 Rose St, MN 150, Lexington, KY 40536; **Phone:** 859-323-5481 x297; **Board Cert:** Pediatrics 1981; Pediatric Cardiology 1997; **Med School:** Ohio State Univ 1976; **Resid:** Pediatrics, Tex Chldns Hosp 1980; **Fellow:** Pediatric Cardiology, Tex Chldns Hosp 1983; **Fac Appt:** Prof Ped, Univ KY Coll Med

Colvin, Edward V MD [PCd] - **Spec Exp:** Congenital Heart Disease-Adult & Child; Fetal Echocardiography; Transplant Medicine-Heart; **Hospital:** Univ of Ala Hosp at Birmingham, Children's Hospital - Birmingham; **Address:** 320 Hillman Bldg, 620 20th St S, Birmingham, AL 35233; **Phone:** 205-934-3460; **Board Cert:** Pediatrics 1982; Pediatric Cardiology 1985; **Med School:** Univ Ala 1977; **Resid:** Pediatrics, Chldns Hosp 1980; **Fellow:** Pediatric Cardiology, Baylor Coll Med 1983; **Fac Appt:** Prof Ped, Univ Ala

Epstein, Michael L MD [PCd] - **Spec Exp:** Congenital Heart Disease; **Hospital:** All Children's Hosp; **Address:** All Children's Hosp, 801 Sixth St S, St Petersburg, FL 33701; **Phone:** 727-767-6941; **Board Cert:** Pediatrics 1976; Pediatric Cardiology 1981; **Med School:** Univ Tex Med Br, Galveston 1971; **Resid:** Pediatrics, Univ Ariz Hlth Sci Ctr 1974; **Fellow:** Pediatric Cardiology, Univ Minn Hosp 1979; **Fac Appt:** Prof Ped, Wayne State Univ

Fish, Frank A MD [PCd] - **Spec Exp:** Arrhythmias-Pediatric & Adult; Congenital Heart Disease-Adult; Pacemakers; **Hospital:** Vanderbilt Children's Hosp, Vanderbilt Univ Med Ctr; **Address:** Vanderbilt Chldns Hosp, Div Pediatric Cardiology, 2200 Children's Way, 5230 DOT, Nashville, TN 37232-9119; **Phone:** 615-322-7447; **Board Cert:** Pediatrics 1987; Pediatric Cardiology 2006; **Med School:** Indiana Univ 1983; **Resid:** Pediatrics, Indiana Univ Hosp 1986; **Fellow:** Pediatric Cardiology, Vanderbilt Univ Med Ctr 1989; Cardiac Electrophysiology, Chldns Meml Hosp 1990; **Fac Appt:** Assoc Prof Ped, Vanderbilt Univ

Fricker, Frederick Jay MD [PCd] - **Spec Exp:** Transplant Medicine-Heart; **Hospital:** Shands at Univ of FL; **Address:** Shands Hlthcre, Div Pediatric Cardiology, 1600 SW Archer Rd, Box 100296, Gainesville, FL 32610-0296; **Phone:** 352-273-7770; **Board Cert:** Pediatrics 1975; Pediatric Cardiology 1981; **Med School:** Loyola Univ-Stritch Sch Med 1970; **Resid:** Pediatrics, Children's Hosp 1973; **Fellow:** Pediatric Cardiology, Children's Hosp 1977; **Fac Appt:** Prof Ped, Univ Fla Coll Med

Moskowitz, William B MD [PCd] - **Spec Exp:** Patent Foramen Ovale; **Hospital:** Med Coll of VA Hosp; **Address:** Childrens Heart Ctr, Med Coll Virginia, 1200 E Broad St, PO Box 980543, Richmond, VA 23298; **Phone:** 804-828-9143; **Board Cert:** Pediatrics 1983; Pediatric Cardiology 1985; **Med School:** Univ S Fla Coll Med 1978; **Resid:** Pediatrics, Childrens Hosp 1981; **Fellow:** Pediatric Cardiology, Childrens Hosp 1984; **Fac Appt:** Prof Ped, Med Coll VA

Tamer, Dolores MD [PCd] - **Spec Exp:** Kawasaki Disease; **Hospital:** Jackson Meml Hosp, Univ of Miami Hosp & Clins/Sylvester Comp Canc Ctr; **Address:** Univ Miami, Dept Peds, PO Box 016960 (R-76), Miami, FL 33101-6960; **Phone:** 305-243-5430; **Board Cert:** Pediatrics 1966; Pediatric Cardiology 1967; **Med School:** SUNY Buffalo 1961; **Resid:** Pediatrics, Chldns Hosp 1963; Pediatrics, Chldns Hosp 1964; **Fellow:** Pediatrics, Chldns Hosp 1965; **Fac Appt:** Prof Ped, Univ Miami Sch Med

Pediatric Cardiology

Young, Ming-Lon MD [PCd] - **Spec Exp:** Cardiac Electrophysiology; Arrhythmias; **Hospital:** Jackson Meml Hosp, Univ of Miami Hosp & Clins/Sylvester Comp Canc Ctr; **Address:** Univ Miami, Dept Peds, PO Box 016960 (R-76), Miami, FL 33101-6960; **Phone:** 305-585-6683; **Board Cert:** Pediatric Cardiology 1985; Pediatrics 1985; **Med School:** Taiwan 1976; **Resid:** Preventive Medicine, Johns Hopkins Hosp 1979; Pediatrics, St Agnes Hosp 1981; **Fellow:** Pediatric Cardiology, Univ Miami Hosps 1985; **Fac Appt:** Prof Ped, Univ Miami Sch Med

Zahn, Evan M MD [PCd] - **Spec Exp:** Interventional Cardiology; Ventricular Septal Defect (Amplatzer R); Congenital Heart Disease; **Hospital:** Miami Children's Hosp, Baptist Hosp of Miami; **Address:** 3100 SW 62nd Ave Ambulatory Bldg Fl 2, Miami, FL 33155-4045; **Phone:** 305-666-6511 x4285; **Board Cert:** Pediatric Cardiology 2000; Pediatrics 1989; **Med School:** NY Med Coll 1986; **Resid:** Pediatrics, Univ Colorado Hosp 1989; **Fellow:** Interventional Cardiology, Hosp for Sick Children 1992

Midwest

Ackerman, Michael J MD [PCd] - **Spec Exp:** Long QT Interval Syndrome; Sudden Infant Death Syndrome (SIDS); Hypertrophic Cardiomyopathy (HCM); **Hospital:** Mayo Med Ctr & Clin - Rochester; **Address:** Mayo Clinic, Dept Ped Cardiology, 200 First St SW, Rochester, MN 55905; **Phone:** 507-284-0101; **Board Cert:** Pediatric Cardiology 2002; **Med School:** Mayo Med Sch 1995; **Resid:** Pediatric & Adolescent Medicine, Mayo Clinic 1998; **Fellow:** Pediatric Cardiology, Mayo Clinic 2000; **Fac Appt:** Assoc Prof Ped, Mayo Med Sch

Agarwala, Brojendra MD [PCd] - **Spec Exp:** Congenital Heart Disease; **Hospital:** Univ of Chicago Hosps; **Address:** 5841 S Maryland Ave, rm C-104, MC 405, Chicago, IL 60637; **Phone:** 773-702-6172; **Board Cert:** Pediatrics 1970; Pediatric Cardiology 1978; **Med School:** India 1965; **Resid:** Pediatrics, St Vincent Hosp Med Ctr 1969; **Fellow:** Pediatric Cardiology, NYU Med Ctr 1972; **Fac Appt:** Prof Ped, Univ Chicago-Pritzker Sch Med

Beekman III, Robert H MD [PCd] - **Spec Exp:** Interventional Cardiology; Cardiac Catheterization; **Hospital:** Cincinnati Chldns Hosp Med Ctr; **Address:** Cincinnati Chldns Hosp Med Ctr, Div Cardiology, 3333 Burnet Ave, MC 2003, Cincinnati, OH 45229-3026; **Phone:** 513-636-7072; **Board Cert:** Pediatrics 1981; Pediatric Cardiology 1983; **Med School:** Duke Univ 1976; **Resid:** Pediatrics, UCLA Med Ctr 1979; **Fellow:** Pediatric Cardiology, Univ Mich Hosp 1981; **Fac Appt:** Prof Ped, Univ Cincinnati

Caldwell, Randall MD [PCd] - **Spec Exp:** Transplant Medicine-Heart; Echocardiography; **Hospital:** Riley Hosp for Children, Clarian Hlth Ptrs; **Address:** 702 Barnhill Drive, RR-127, Indianapolis, IN 46202-5128; **Phone:** 317-274-8906; **Board Cert:** Pediatrics 1976; Pediatric Cardiology 1978; **Med School:** Indiana Univ 1971; **Resid:** Pediatrics, Indiana Med Ctr 1975; **Fellow:** Pediatric Cardiology, Indiana Med Ctr 1978; **Fac Appt:** Prof Ped, Indiana Univ

Cetta Jr, Frank MD [PCd] - **Spec Exp:** Congenital Heart Disease-Adult; Congenital Heart Disease; **Hospital:** Mayo Med Ctr & Clin - Rochester; **Address:** Mayo Clinic, Gonda 6-138 NW, 200 First St SW, Rochester, MN 55905; **Phone:** 507-266-0676; **Board Cert:** Pediatric Cardiology 2004; **Med School:** Loyola Univ-Stritch Sch Med 1987; **Resid:** Internal Medicine & Pediatrics, Loyola Medical Ctr 1991; **Fac Appt:** Assoc Prof Ped, Mayo Med Sch

Dick, Macdonald MD [PCd] - **Spec Exp:** Cardiac Electrophysiology; **Hospital:** Mott Chldns Hosp; **Address:** C.S. Motts Chldns Hosp, Dept Ped Cardio, 1500 E Med Ctr Drive, rm L1242, Box 0204, Ann Arbor, MI 48109; **Phone:** 734-936-7418; **Board Cert:** Pediatrics 1989; Pediatric Cardiology 2007; **Med School:** Univ VA Sch Med 1967; **Resid:** Pediatrics, Univ Va Hosp 1971; **Fellow:** Pediatric Cardiology, Chldns Hosp Med Ctr 1974; **Fac Appt:** Prof Ped, Univ Mich Med Sch

Driscoll, David J MD [PCd] - **Spec Exp:** Exercise Physiology; Klippel-Trenaunay Syndrome; Cardiomyopathy; **Hospital:** Mayo Med Ctr & Clin - Rochester; **Address:** Mayo Clinic - Pediatric Cardiology, 200 First St SW, Rochester, MN 55905-0001; **Phone:** 507-284-3297; **Board Cert:** Pediatrics 1976; Pediatric Cardiology 2006; **Med School:** Marquette Sch Med 1970; **Resid:** Pediatrics, Milwaukee Chldns Hosp 1972; Pediatrics, Milwaukee Chldns Hosp 1975; **Fellow:** Pediatric Cardiology, Baylor Coll Med 1978; **Fac Appt:** Prof Ped, Mayo Med Sch

Hijazi, Ziyad M MD [PCd] - **Spec Exp:** Interventional Cardiology; Congenital Heart Disease; Coarctation of the Aorta; **Hospital:** Univ of Chicago Hosps; **Address:** Rush Univ Med Ctr, 1653 W Congress Pkwy, Ste 770 Jones, Chicago, IL 60612; **Phone:** 312-942-8941; **Board Cert:** Pediatrics 2000; Pediatric Cardiology 2000; **Med School:** Jordan 1982; **Resid:** Pediatrics, Yale-New Haven Hosp 1988; **Fellow:** Pediatric Cardiology, Yale-New Haven Hosp 1991; **Fac Appt:** Prof Ped, Univ Chicago-Pritzker Sch Med

Latson, Larry A MD [PCd] - **Spec Exp:** Congenital Heart Disease; Interventional Cardiology; **Hospital:** Cleveland Clin Fdn (page 56); **Address:** Ped Cardiology, 9500 Euclid Ave, Desk M41, Cleveland, OH 44195; **Phone:** 216-445-6532; **Board Cert:** Pediatrics 1981; Pediatric Cardiology 1983; Pediatric Critical Care Medicine 2003; **Med School:** Baylor Coll Med 1976; **Resid:** Pediatrics, Baylor Coll Med 1978; **Fellow:** Pediatric Cardiology, Baylor Coll Med 1981; **Fac Appt:** Prof Ped, Case West Res Univ

O'Laughlin, Martin P MD [PCd] - **Spec Exp:** Cardiac Catheterization; Congenital Heart Disease-Adult & Child; Interventional Cardiology; **Hospital:** Chldns Mercy Hosps & Clinics, St Luke's Hosp of Kansas City; **Address:** 4400 Broadway, Ste 400, Kansas City, MO 64111; **Phone:** 816-931-5440; **Board Cert:** Pediatrics 1985; Pediatric Cardiology 2003; **Med School:** Columbia P&S 1980; **Resid:** Pediatrics, Baylor Coll Med 1984; **Fellow:** Pediatric Cardiology, Texas Chldns Hosp/Baylor 1987

Pahl, Elfriede MD [PCd] - **Spec Exp:** Transplant Medicine-Heart; Heart Failure; Congenital Heart Disease; Kawasaki Disease; **Hospital:** Children's Mem Hosp; **Address:** Children's Memorial Hosp, Ped Cardiology, 2300 Children's Plaza, Box 21, Chicago, IL 60614-3394; **Phone:** 773-880-6388; **Board Cert:** Pediatrics 1987; Pediatric Cardiology 2003; **Med School:** Northwestern Univ 1983; **Resid:** Pediatrics, Children's Meml Hosp 1986; **Fellow:** Pediatric Cardiology, Children's Hosp of Pittsburgh 1988; **Fac Appt:** Prof Ped, Northwestern Univ

Perry, James C MD [PCd] - **Spec Exp:** Congenital Heart Disease-Adult; Cardiac Electrophysiology; **Hospital:** Chldns Hosp and Clinics - Minneapolis; **Address:** Minnesota Children's Heart Clinic, 2545 Chicago Ave S, Ste 106, Minneapolis, MN 55404; **Phone:** 612-813-8800; **Board Cert:** Pediatric Cardiology 2006; Pediatric Cardiology 2006; **Med School:** Univ Rochester 1983; **Resid:** Pediatrics, Chldns Hosp 1986; **Fellow:** Pediatric Cardiology, Texas Chldns Hosp 1989; **Fac Appt:** Prof Ped, Yale Univ

Porter, Co-burn MD [PCd] - **Spec Exp:** Arrhythmias; Arrhythmias-Fetal; Transplant Medicine-Heart; **Hospital:** St Mary's Hosp - Rochester; **Address:** Mayo Clinic, Dept Ped Cardiology, 200 First St SW, Rochester, MN 55905-0001; **Phone:** 507-284-3297; **Board Cert:** Pediatrics 1977; Pediatric Cardiology 1983; **Med School:** Creighton Univ 1972; **Resid:** Pediatrics, Univ Colo Hlth Sci Ctr 1975; **Fellow:** Pediatric Cardiology, Baylor Coll Med 1977; Pediatric Cardiology, Baylor Coll Med 1981; **Fac Appt:** Prof Ped, Mayo Med Sch

Rocchini, Albert P MD [PCd] - **Spec Exp:** Congenital Heart Disease; Interventional Cardiology; Hypertension in Obesity; **Hospital:** Univ Michigan Hlth Sys; **Address:** Mott Chldns Hosp, Dept Ped Cardiology, 1500 E Med Ctr Drive, rm L1242, Box 0204, Ann Arbor, MI 48109-0204; **Phone:** 734-936-8993; **Board Cert:** Pediatrics 1989; Pediatric Cardiology 1989; **Med School:** Univ Pittsburgh 1972; **Resid:** Pediatrics, Univ Minn 1974; **Fellow:** Pediatric Cardiology, Chldns Hosp 1977; **Fac Appt:** Prof Ped, Univ Mich Med Sch

Pediatric Cardiology

Rosenthal, Amnon MD [PCd] - **Spec Exp:** Congenital Heart Disease; Congenital Heart Disease-Young Adult; **Hospital:** Univ Michigan Hlth Sys; **Address:** Mott Chldns Hosp, Dept Ped Cardiology, 1500 E Medical Ctr, rm L1242, Box 0204, Ann Arbor, MI 48109-0204; **Phone:** 734-936-8993; **Board Cert:** Pediatrics 1986; Pediatric Cardiology 1986; **Med School:** Albany Med Coll 1959; **Resid:** Pediatrics, Boston Chldns Hosp 1962; **Fellow:** Cardiovascular Disease, Boston Chldns Hosp 1968; **Fac Appt:** Prof Ped, Univ Mich Med Sch

Great Plains and Mountains

Minich, Lois LuAnn MD [PCd] - **Spec Exp:** Echocardiography; **Hospital:** Primary Children's Med Ctr; **Address:** Primary Chlds Med Ctr, Dept Ped Cardiology, 100 N Medical, Ste 1500, Salt Lake City, UT 84113; **Phone:** 801-662-5400; **Board Cert:** Pediatrics 2000; Pediatric Cardiology 2000; **Med School:** W VA Univ 1986; **Resid:** Pediatrics, Fletcher Allen Health Care 1989; **Fellow:** Pediatric Cardiology, Univ Michigan Hosps 1992

Southwest

Dreyer, William J MD [PCd] - **Spec Exp:** Congenital Heart Disease; Transplant Medicine-Heart; Cardiomyopathy; **Hospital:** Texas Chldns Hosp - Houston; **Address:** Texas Chldns Hosp, 6621 Fannin St, MS 19345C, Houston, TX 77030; **Phone:** 832-826-5659; **Board Cert:** Pediatrics 1987; Pediatric Cardiology 2006; **Med School:** Univ Fla Coll Med 1981; **Resid:** Pediatrics, UCSF Med Ctr 1984; **Fellow:** Pediatric Cardiology, Baylor Coll Med 1988; **Fac Appt:** Assoc Prof Ped, Baylor Coll Med

Friedman, Richard A MD [PCd] - **Spec Exp:** Cardiac Electrophysiology; **Hospital:** Texas Chldns Hosp - Houston; **Address:** Texas Children's Hospital, 6621 Fannin St, MC 19345-C, Houston, TX 77030-2303; **Phone:** 832-826-5600; **Board Cert:** Pediatrics 1986; Pediatric Cardiology 2003; **Med School:** Univ Pittsburgh 1980; **Resid:** Pediatrics, Baylor Affil Hosps 1983; **Fellow:** Pediatric Cardiology, Baylor Affil Hosps 1985; **Fac Appt:** Assoc Prof Ped, Baylor Coll Med

Gillette, Paul C MD [PCd] - **Spec Exp:** Arrhythmias; **Hospital:** Cook Chldns Med Ctr, Harris Methodist Hosp - Fort Worth; **Address:** Pediatric Cardiology, 209 Bonnie Brae St, Ste 100, Denton, TX 76201; **Phone:** 940-243-0104; **Board Cert:** Pediatrics 1974; Pediatric Cardiology 1975; **Med School:** Med Univ SC 1969; **Resid:** Pediatrics, Baylor Coll Med 1972; **Fellow:** Pediatric Cardiology, Baylor Coll Med 1974

Mahony, Lynn MD [PCd] - **Spec Exp:** Congenital Heart Disease; Marfan's Syndrome; Congestive Heart Failure; **Hospital:** Chldns Med Ctr of Dallas; **Address:** 1935 Motor District Drive, Dallas, TX 75235; **Phone:** 214-456-2333; **Board Cert:** Pediatrics 1979; Pediatric Cardiology 1997; **Med School:** Stanford Univ 1975; **Resid:** Pediatrics, Stanford Univ 1978; **Fellow:** Pediatric Cardiology, UCSF Med Ctr 1981; **Fac Appt:** Assoc Prof Ped, Univ Tex SW, Dallas

Moodie, Douglas S MD [PCd] - **Spec Exp:** Marfan's Syndrome; Congenital Heart Disease-Adult & Child; **Hospital:** Ochsner Fdn Hosp; **Address:** Ochsner Chldns Health Ctr, 1315 Jefferson Hwy, New Orleans, LA 70121; **Phone:** 504-842-4827; **Board Cert:** Pediatrics 1977; Pediatric Cardiology 1977; **Med School:** Med Coll Wisc 1972; **Resid:** Pediatrics, Mayo Clinic 1974; **Fellow:** Pediatric Cardiology, Mayo Clinic 1977

Rogers Jr, James H MD [PCd] - **Spec Exp:** Congenital Heart Disease; **Hospital:** Christus Santa Rosa Children's Hosp, Univ Hlth Sys - Univ Hosp (San Antonio, TX); **Address:** Childrens Heart Network, 1901 Babcock Rd, Ste 301, San Antonio, TX 78229; **Phone:** 210-341-7722; **Board Cert:** Pediatrics 1976; Pediatric Cardiology 1977; **Med School:** Med Coll GA 1971; **Resid:** Pediatrics, Wilford Hall USAF Med Ctr 1974; **Fellow:** Pediatric Cardiology, Med Coll Georgia 1976; **Fac Appt:** Clin Prof Ped, Univ Tex, San Antonio

West Coast and Pacific

Bernstein, Daniel MD [PCd] - **Spec Exp:** Transplant Medicine-Heart; Cardiomyopathy; **Hospital:** Lucile Packard Chldns Hosp/Stanford Univ Med Ctr, Stanford Univ Med Ctr; **Address:** Lucile Packard Chldns Hosp, Div Ped Card, 750 Welch Rd, Ste 305, Palo Alto, CA 94304-1510; **Phone:** 650-723-7913; **Board Cert:** Pediatrics 1984; Pediatric Cardiology 1985; **Med School:** NYU Sch Med 1978; **Resid:** Pediatrics, Montefiore Hosp-Einstein 1982; **Fellow:** Pediatric Cardiology, UCSF 1986; **Fac Appt:** Prof Ped, Stanford Univ

Boucek Jr, Robert J MD [PCd] - **Spec Exp:** Congenital Heart Disease; Cardiomyopathy; Transplant Medicine-Heart; **Hospital:** Chldns Hosp and Regl Med Ctr - Seattle; **Address:** 4800 Sand Point Way NE, MS G0035, Seattle, WA 98105; **Phone:** 206-987-2015; **Board Cert:** Pediatrics 1974; Pediatric Cardiology 1977; **Med School:** Tulane Univ 1969; **Resid:** Pediatrics, Duke Univ Med Ctr 1971; **Fellow:** Ambulatory Pediatrics, US Naval Hosp 1973; Pediatric Cardiology, Vanderbilt Med Ctr 1976; **Fac Appt:** Prof Ped, Univ Wash

Hohn, Arno R MD [PCd] - **Spec Exp:** Hypertension; Preventive Cardiology; **Hospital:** Chldns Hosp - Los Angeles, LAC & USC Med Ctr; **Address:** Chldns Hosp, Div Cardiology, 4650 Sunset Blvd, MS 34, Los Angeles, CA 90027; **Phone:** 323-361-2535; **Board Cert:** Pediatrics 1986; Pediatric Cardiology 1986; **Med School:** NY Med Coll 1956; **Resid:** Pediatrics, Chldns Hosp 1958; Pediatrics, Chldns Hosp 1962; **Fellow:** Pediatric Cardiology, Chldns Hosp 1963; **Fac Appt:** Prof Ped, USC Sch Med

Perry, Stanton Bruce MD [PCd] - **Spec Exp:** Interventional Cardiology; **Hospital:** Lucile Packard Chldns Hosp/Stanford Univ Med Ctr; **Address:** L Packard Chldns Hosp, Ped Cardiology, 750 Welch Rd, Ste 305, Palo Alto, CA 94304; **Phone:** 650-723-7913; **Board Cert:** Pediatrics 1986; Pediatric Cardiology 1988; **Med School:** Iceland 1978; **Resid:** Pediatrics, St Louis Chldns Hosp 1983; **Fellow:** Pediatric Cardiology, Chldns Hosp 1984; **Fac Appt:** Assoc Prof Ped, Stanford Univ

Takahashi, Masato MD [PCd] - **Spec Exp:** Kawasaki Disease; Cardiac Catheterization; Congenital Heart Disease-Adult; **Hospital:** Chldns Hosp - Los Angeles, USC Univ Hosp - R K Eamer Med Plz; **Address:** Chldns Hosp-LA, Div Cardiology, 4650 Sunset Blvd, MS 34, Los Angeles, CA 90027-6062; **Phone:** 323-361-2461; **Board Cert:** Pediatrics 1966; Pediatric Cardiology 1992; **Med School:** Indiana Univ 1960; **Resid:** Pediatrics, Ind Med Ctr 1963; **Fellow:** Pediatric Cardiology, UCLA Med Ctr 1967; **Fac Appt:** Prof Ped, USC Sch Med

Teitel, David F MD [PCd] - **Hospital:** UCSF Med Ctr; **Address:** UCSF, Dept Ped Cardiology, 505 Parnassus Ave, rm M1235, San Francisco, CA 94143-0544; **Phone:** 415-353-2008; **Board Cert:** Pediatrics 1980; Pediatric Cardiology 2004; **Med School:** Univ Toronto 1975; **Resid:** Pediatrics, Childrens Hosp 1980; **Fellow:** Pediatric Cardiology, UCSF Med Ctr 1982; **Fac Appt:** Prof Ped, UCSF

PEDIATRIC CRITICAL CARE MEDICINE

New England

Fleisher, Gary R MD [PCCM] - **Spec Exp:** Infectious Disease; Trauma; **Hospital:** Children's Hospital - Boston; **Address:** Chldns Hosp, Dept Med, 300 Longwood Ave, Hunnewell 258, Boston, MA 02115-5724; **Phone:** 617-355-5022; **Board Cert:** Emergency Medicine 2001; Pediatrics 1992; Pediatric Emergency Medicine 2007; **Med School:** Jefferson Med Coll 1973; **Resid:** Pediatrics, Chldns Hosp 1976; Pediatrics, Chldns Hosp 1977; **Fellow:** Infectious Disease, Chldns Hosp 1979; **Fac Appt:** Prof Ped, Harvard Med Sch

Mid Atlantic

Fuhrman, Bradley P MD [PCCM] - **Hospital:** Women's & Chldn's Hosp of Buffalo, The; **Address:** Chldns Hosp Buffalo, Dept Ped Critical Care, 219 Bryant St, Buffalo, NY 14222-2006; **Phone:** 716-878-7442; **Board Cert:** Pediatrics 1992; Pediatric Critical Care Medicine 2003; Neonatal-Perinatal Medicine 1979; Pediatric Cardiology 1979; **Med School:** NYU Sch Med 1971; **Resid:** Pediatrics, Univ Minnesota Med Ctr 1973; **Fellow:** Pediatric Cardiology, Univ Minnesota 1974; Neonatal-Perinatal Medicine, Univ Minnesota 1979; **Fac Appt:** Prof Ped, SUNY Buffalo

Nichols, David G MD [PCCM] - **Spec Exp:** Respiratory Failure; Mechanical Ventilation; **Hospital:** Johns Hopkins Hosp - Baltimore (page 61); **Address:** Johns Hopkins Hosp - Pediatric CCM, 733 N Broadway, Ste 115, Baltimore, MD 21205; **Phone:** 410-955-8401; **Board Cert:** Pediatrics 1982; Anesthesiology 1984; Pediatric Critical Care Medicine 2003; **Med School:** Mount Sinai Sch Med 1977; **Resid:** Pediatrics, Childrens Hosp 1980; Anesthesiology, Hosp Univ Penn 1983; **Fellow:** Critical Care Anesthesiology, Childrens Hosp 1983; **Fac Appt:** Prof Ped, Johns Hopkins Univ

Thompson, Ann Ellen MD [PCCM] - **Spec Exp:** Mechanical Ventilation; Critical Care; Respiratory Failure; **Hospital:** Chldns Hosp of Pittsburgh - UPMC; **Address:** Chldns Hosp, Dept Ped Crit Care, 3705 Fifth Ave Bldg Main Tower - rm 6840, Pittsburgh, PA 15213-2584; **Phone:** 412-692-5164; **Board Cert:** Anesthesiology 1980; Pediatrics 1992; Pediatric Critical Care Medicine 2003; **Med School:** Tufts Univ 1974; **Resid:** Pediatrics, Chldns Hosp 1977; Anesthesiology, Hosp Univ Penn 1980; **Fellow:** Pediatric Critical Care Medicine, Chldns Hosp 1979; **Fac Appt:** Prof Ped, Univ Pittsburgh

Midwest

Sarnaik, Ashok P MD [PCCM] - **Spec Exp:** Critical Care; Perinatal Medicine; **Hospital:** Chldns Hosp of Michigan; **Address:** Chldns Hosp, Div Crit Care Med, 3901 Beaubien St, Carl's Bldg - Ste 4134, Detroit, MI 48201-2119; **Phone:** 313-745-5629; **Board Cert:** Pediatrics 1975; Neonatal-Perinatal Medicine 1979; Pediatric Critical Care Medicine 2003; **Med School:** India 1969; **Resid:** Pediatrics, JJ Hosp-Bombay Univ 1971; Pediatrics, Chldns Hosp Mich 1974; **Fellow:** Neonatal-Perinatal Medicine, Chldns Hosp Mich 1975; **Fac Appt:** Prof Ped, Wayne State Univ

Great Plains and Mountains

Dean, Jonathan M MD [PCCM] - **Hospital:** Primary Children's Med Ctr; **Address:** Primary Chlds Med Ctr, Pediatric ICU, 100 N Medical Drive, Salt Lake City, UT 84113; **Phone:** 801-587-7572; **Board Cert:** Pediatrics 1981; Pediatric Critical Care Medicine 2003; **Med School:** Northwestern Univ 1977; **Resid:** Pediatrics, Children's Hosp 1981; **Fellow:** Pediatric Critical Care Medicine, Johns Hopkins Hosp 1983; **Fac Appt:** Prof Ped, Univ Utah

Southwest

Anand, Kanwaljeet Singh MD/PhD [PCCM] - **Spec Exp:** Pain Management; Critical Care; **Hospital:** Arkansas Chldns Hosp; **Address:** Arkansas Chldns Hosp, Div CCM, 800 Marshall St, Sturg-slot 512-12, Little Rock, AR 72202-3591; **Phone:** 501-364-3568; **Board Cert:** Pediatric Critical Care Medicine 2004; **Med School:** India 1981; **Resid:** Pediatrics, Chldns Hosp 1991; Neonatal-Perinatal Medicine, John Radcliffe Hosp 1985; **Fellow:** Pediatric Critical Care Medicine, Mass Genl Hosp 1993; **Fac Appt:** Prof Ped, Univ Ark

Perez Fontan, J Julio MD [PCCM] - **Spec Exp:** Respiratory Failure; **Hospital:** UT Southwestern Med Ctr - Dallas, Chldns Med Ctr of Dallas; **Address:** UT SW Med Ctr, Dept Peds, 5323 Harry Hines Blvd, Dallas, TX 75390-9063; **Phone:** 214-648-9618; **Board Cert:** Pediatrics 1987; Pediatric Critical Care Medicine 2003; **Med School:** Spain 1977; **Resid:** Pediatrics, Chldns Hosp/Univ Barcelona 1981; **Fellow:** Critical Care Medicine, UCSF Med Ctr 1984; **Fac Appt:** Prof Ped, Univ Tex SW, Dallas

Taylor, Richard P MD [PCCM] - **Hospital:** Univ Hlth Sys - Univ Hosp (San Antonio, TX); **Address:** Univ Texas HSC, Dept Ped Critical Care, 7703 Floyd Curl Drive, Box 7829, San Antonio, TX 78229; **Phone:** 210-567-5314; **Board Cert:** Internal Medicine 1988; Pediatrics 1989; Pediatric Critical Care Medicine 2004; **Med School:** Univ Tex Med Br, Galveston 1984; **Resid:** Internal Medicine, St Joseph Mercy Hosp 1988; Pediatrics, UNiv Michigan Med Ctr 1988; **Fellow:** Pediatric Critical Care Medicine, Univ Michigan Med Ctr 1995; **Fac Appt:** Assoc Prof Ped

Thomas, James A MD [PCCM] - **Hospital:** Chldns Med Ctr of Dallas; **Address:** Children's Medical Ctr of Dallas, PICU, 1935 Medical District Drive, Dallas, TX 75235; **Phone:** 214-456-5095; **Board Cert:** Pediatric Critical Care Medicine 2004; Pediatrics 2007; **Med School:** Stanford Univ 1989; **Resid:** Pediatrics, Children's Hosp 1992; **Fellow:** Pediatric Critical Care Medicine, U Texas SW Med Ctr 1996

West Coast and Pacific

Schwarz, Adam J MD [PCCM] - **Hospital:** Chldns Hosp Orange Co - CHOC; **Address:** Chldns Hosp of Orange, 455 S Main St, Orange, CA 92868; **Phone:** 714-532-8620; **Board Cert:** Pediatrics 2001; Pediatric Critical Care Medicine 2004; **Med School:** Stanford Univ 1990; **Resid:** Pediatrics, Stanford Med Ctr 1993; **Fellow:** Pediatric Critical Care Medicine, Harbor-UCLA Med Ctr 1996; **Fac Appt:** Assoc Clin Prof Ped

Zimmerman, Jerry John MD [PCCM] - **Spec Exp:** Inflammation in Critical Illness; Sepsis; Septic Shock; **Hospital:** Chldns Hosp and Regl Med Ctr - Seattle, Harborview Med Ctr; **Address:** Children's Hosp & Regl Med Ctr, 4800 Sand Point Way NE, MS W8866, Seattle, WA 98105-0371; **Phone:** 206-987-2170; **Board Cert:** Pediatrics 1992; Pediatric Critical Care Medicine 2003; **Med School:** Univ Wisc 1979; **Resid:** Pediatrics, Univ Wisconsin Hosp 1982; **Fellow:** Pediatric Critical Care Medicine, Childrens Natl Med Ctr 1984; **Fac Appt:** Prof Ped, Univ Wash

PEDIATRIC ENDOCRINOLOGY

New England

Casella, Samuel Joseph MD [PEn] - **Spec Exp:** Thyroid Disorders; Growth/Development Disorders; **Hospital:** Dartmouth - Hitchcock Med Ctr; **Address:** Dartmouth-Hitchcock Med Ctr, Ped Endocrinology, One Medical Center Drive, Lebanon, NH 03756; **Phone:** 603-653-9877; **Board Cert:** Pediatrics 1985; Pediatric Endocrinology 1986; **Med School:** SUNY Upstate Med Univ 1981; **Resid:** Pediatrics, Upstate Med Ctr 1984; **Fellow:** Pediatric Endocrinology, NC Meml Hosp-Univ NC 1986; **Fac Appt:** Assoc Prof Ped, Johns Hopkins Univ

Gordon, Catherine M MD [PEn] - **Spec Exp:** Bone Disorders-Metabolic; **Hospital:** Children's Hospital - Boston; **Address:** Children's Hospital, Ped Endocrinology, 300 Longwood Ave, Boston, MA 02115; **Phone:** 617-355-7476; **Board Cert:** Pediatric Endocrinology 2007; Adolescent Medicine 2001; **Med School:** Univ NC Sch Med 1991; **Resid:** Pediatrics, Children's Hosp 1994; **Fellow:** Pediatric Endocrinology, Children's Hosp 1996; **Fac Appt:** Assoc Prof Ped, Harvard Med Sch

Levitsky, Lynne Lipton MD [PEn] - **Spec Exp:** Diabetes; Growth/Development Disorders; Cushing's Syndrome; **Hospital:** Mass Genl Hosp; **Address:** Mass Genl Hosp, Ped Endo, 55 Fruit St, YAW-6800, Boston, MA 02114-2696; **Phone:** 617-726-2909; **Board Cert:** Pediatrics 1971; Pediatric Endocrinology 1978; **Med School:** Yale Univ 1966; **Resid:** Pediatrics, Children's Hosp 1968; **Fellow:** Pediatric Endocrinology, Univ Maryland Hosp 1970; **Fac Appt:** Assoc Prof Ped, Harvard Med Sch

Ludwig, David S MD/PhD [PEn] - **Spec Exp:** Obesity; Nutrition; **Hospital:** Children's Hospital - Boston; **Address:** Chldns Hosp, Div Endocrinology, 333 Longwood Ave Fl 6 - rm 624, Boston, MA 02115; **Phone:** 617-355-7476; **Board Cert:** Pediatric Endocrinology 2003; **Med School:** Stanford Univ 1990; **Resid:** Pediatrics, Chldns Hosp 1993; **Fellow:** Pediatric Endocrinology, Chldns Hosp 1995; **Fac Appt:** Asst Prof Ped, Harvard Med Sch

Rivkees, Scott MD [PEn] - **Spec Exp:** Thyroid Disorders; **Hospital:** Yale-New Haven Hosp; **Address:** Yale Child Hlth Rsch Ctr, 464 Congress Ave, PO Box 208081, New Haven, CT 06520; **Phone:** 203-764-9199; **Board Cert:** Pediatrics 1987; Pediatric Endocrinology 2005; **Med School:** UMDNJ-NJ Med Sch, Newark 1982; **Resid:** Pediatrics, Mass Genl Hosp 1985; **Fellow:** Pediatric Endocrinology, Mass Genl Hosp 1986; **Fac Appt:** Prof Ped, Yale Univ

Tamborlane, William V MD [PEn] - **Spec Exp:** Diabetes; **Hospital:** Yale-New Haven Hosp; **Address:** Yale Pediatric Endocrinology, 333 Cedar St, rm 3091-LMP, New Haven, CT 06510-3289; **Phone:** 203-764-6747; **Board Cert:** Pediatrics 1978; Pediatric Endocrinology 1986; **Med School:** Georgetown Univ 1972; **Resid:** Pediatrics, Georgetown Univ Hosp 1975; **Fellow:** Pediatric Endocrinology, Yale-NewHaven Hosp 1977; **Fac Appt:** Prof Ped, Yale Univ

Mid Atlantic

Alter, Craig A MD [PEn] - **Spec Exp:** Diabetes; Growth Disorders; Thyroid Disorders; Pubertal Disorders; **Hospital:** Chldns Hosp of Philadelphia, The; **Address:** Children's Hosp of Philadelphia, Dept Pediatric Endocrinology, 34th & Civic Ctr Blvd, Philadelphia, PA 19104; **Phone:** 215-590-3174; **Board Cert:** Pediatrics 2005; Pediatric Endocrinology 2003; **Med School:** Harvard Med Sch 1987; **Resid:** Pediatrics, Boston Children's Hosp 1990; **Fellow:** Pediatric Endocrinology, Chidren's Hosp 1993; **Fac Appt:** Assoc Prof Ped, Univ Pennsylvania

Arslanian, Silva MD [PEn] - **Spec Exp:** Diabetes; Obesity; **Hospital:** Chldns Hosp of Pittsburgh - UPMC; **Address:** Chldns Hosp Pittsburgh, Div Endocrinology, 3705 5th Ave, DeSoto Wing, rm 4A 400-11, Pittsburgh, PA 15213; **Phone:** 412-692-6935; **Board Cert:** Pediatrics 1983; Pediatric Endocrinology 1983; **Med School:** Lebanon 1978; **Resid:** Pediatrics, American Univ Hosp 1980; **Fellow:** Pediatric Endocrinology, Chldns Hosp 1983; **Fac Appt:** Prof Ped, Univ Pittsburgh

Becker, Dorothy J MD [PEn] - **Spec Exp:** Diabetes; **Hospital:** Chldns Hosp of Pittsburgh - UPMC; **Address:** Children's Hosp Pittsburgh, Div Endocrinology, 3705 5th Ave, 4A-400 DeSoto, Pittsburgh, PA 15213; **Phone:** 412-692-5172; **Board Cert:** Pediatrics 1978; Pediatric Endocrinology 1978; **Med School:** South Africa 1964; **Resid:** Pediatrics, Univ Capetown 1972; Endocrinology, Diabetes & Metabolism, Univ Capetown 1974; **Fellow:** Pediatric Endocrinology, Univ Pittsburgh 1976; **Fac Appt:** Prof Ped, Univ Pittsburgh

De Luca, Francesco MD [PEn] - **Spec Exp:** Growth Disorders; Metabolic Syndrome; Osteoporosis; **Hospital:** St Christopher's Hosp for Chldn; **Address:** St Christophers Hosp for Children, Endocrinology Section, Ste 3303, Erie Ave & Front St, Philadelphia, PA 19134; **Phone:** 215-427-8100; **Board Cert:** Pediatrics 2002; Pediatric Endocrinology 2003; **Med School:** Italy 1983; **Resid:** Pediatrics, Cath Univ Sacred Heart Affil Hosp; Pediatrics, Albert Einstein Med Ctr; **Fellow:** Pediatric Endocrinology, St Christophers Hosp; Pediatric Endocrinology, Natl Inst Hlth; **Fac Appt:** Assoc Prof Ped, Drexel Univ Coll Med

New, Maria I MD [PEn] - **Spec Exp:** Adrenal Disorders; **Hospital:** Mount Sinai Med Ctr (page 64); **Address:** Mount Sinai Medical Ctr, 1 Gustave L Levy Pl, Box 1198, New York, NY 10029; **Phone:** 212-241-8210; **Board Cert:** Pediatrics 1960; **Med School:** Univ Pennsylvania 1954; **Resid:** Pediatrics, New York Hosp 1957; **Fellow:** Pediatric Endocrinology, New York Hosp 1958; Endocrinology, Diabetes & Metabolism, New York Hosp 1964; **Fac Appt:** Prof Ped, Cornell Univ-Weill Med Coll

Oberfield, Sharon E MD [PEn] - **Spec Exp:** Adrenal Disorders; Neuroendocrine Growth Disorders; Growth Disorders; **Hospital:** NYPresby-Morgan Stanley Children's Hosp (page 66); **Address:** 630 W 168th St PH East Bldg - Ste 522, New York, NY 10032; **Phone:** 212-305-6559; **Board Cert:** Pediatrics 1979; Pediatric Endocrinology 2000; **Med School:** Cornell Univ-Weill Med Coll 1974; **Resid:** Pediatrics, NY Hosp-Cornell 1976; **Fellow:** Pediatric Endocrinology, NY Hosp-Cornell 1979; **Fac Appt:** Prof Ped, Columbia P&S

Plotnick, Leslie Parker MD [PEn] - **Spec Exp:** Diabetes; Growth Disorders; Thyroid Disorders; **Hospital:** Johns Hopkins Hosp - Baltimore (page 61); **Address:** Johns Hopkins Hospital, Dept Pediatric Endocrinology, Baltimore, MD 21287; **Phone:** 410-955-6463; **Board Cert:** Pediatrics 1975; Pediatric Endocrinology 1978; **Med School:** Univ MD Sch Med 1970; **Resid:** Pediatrics, Johns Hopkins Hosp 1972; **Fellow:** Pediatric Endocrinology, Johns Hopkins Hosp 1974; **Fac Appt:** Prof Ped, Johns Hopkins Univ

Sklar, Charles A MD [PEn] - **Spec Exp:** Cancer Survivors-Late Effects of Therapy; Growth Disorders in Childhood Cancer; Pituitary Disorders; **Hospital:** Meml Sloan-Kettering Cancer Ctr; **Address:** 1275 York Avenue, New York, NY 10065; **Phone:** 800-525-2225; **Board Cert:** Pediatrics 1979; Pediatric Endocrinology 1980; **Med School:** USC Sch Med 1974; **Resid:** Pediatrics, Childrens Hosp 1976; **Fellow:** Pediatric Endocrinology, UCSF Med Ctr 1979; **Fac Appt:** Assoc Prof Ped, Cornell Univ-Weill Med Coll

Pediatric Endocrinology

Sperling, Mark A MD [PEn] - **Spec Exp:** Diabetes; Growth/Development Disorders; Hypoglycemia; **Hospital:** Chldns Hosp of Pittsburgh - UPMC, UPMC Presby, Pittsburgh; **Address:** Chldns Hosp Pittsburgh, Endocrinology, 3705 5th Ave DeSoto Bldg Fl 4A - Ste 400, Pittsburgh, PA 15213-2524; **Phone:** 412-692-5172; **Board Cert:** Pediatrics 1986; Pediatric Endocrinology 1986; **Med School:** Australia 1962; **Resid:** Internal Medicine, Prince Henry Hosp 1964; Pediatrics, Royal Chldns Hosp 1968; **Fellow:** Pediatric Endocrinology, Chldns Hosp 1970; **Fac Appt:** Prof Ped, Univ Pittsburgh

Stanley, Charles MD [PEn] - **Spec Exp:** Hyperinsulinism-Congenital; Hypoglycemia; **Hospital:** Chldns Hosp of Philadelphia, The; **Address:** Chldns Hosp, Div Endocrinology, 34th St & Civic Ctr Blvd, rm 8416, Philadelphia, PA 19104; **Phone:** 215-590-3174; **Board Cert:** Pediatrics 1976; Pediatric Endocrinology 1978; **Med School:** Univ VA Sch Med 1970; **Resid:** Pediatrics, Chldns Hosp 1972; **Fellow:** Pediatric Endocrinology, Chldns Hosp 1976; **Fac Appt:** Prof Ped, Univ Pennsylvania

Southeast

Diamond, Frank MD [PEn] - **Spec Exp:** Growth Disorders; Obesity; Calcium Disorders in Newborn; **Hospital:** All Children's Hosp, Tampa Genl Hosp; **Address:** 801 6th St S, ACH Box 6900, St Petersburg, FL 33701; **Phone:** 727-767-4237; **Board Cert:** Pediatrics 1979; Pediatric Endocrinology 1980; **Med School:** Penn State Univ-Hershey Med Ctr 1974; **Resid:** Pediatrics, Chldns Hosp-Univ Alabama 1976; **Fellow:** Pediatric Endocrinology, Chldns Hosp-Univ Penn 1978; **Fac Appt:** Prof Ped, Univ S Fla Coll Med

Freemark, Michael S MD [PEn] - **Spec Exp:** Thyroid Disorders; Neuroendocrine Growth Disorders; Diabetes; **Hospital:** Duke Univ Med Ctr, Durham Regional Hosp; **Address:** DUMC, Box 3080, 3000 Erwin Rd, Lenox Baker Bldg, Ste 200, Durham, NC 27705; **Phone:** 919-684-8350; **Board Cert:** Pediatrics 1980; Pediatric Endocrinology 1983; **Med School:** Duke Univ 1976; **Resid:** Pediatrics, Duke Univ Med Ctr 1979; **Fellow:** Pediatric Endocrinology, Duke Univ Med Ctr 1983; Pediatric Endocrinology, Hospital Necker Enfants Malades 1993; **Fac Appt:** Prof Ped, Duke Univ

Friedman, Nancy E MD [PEn] - **Spec Exp:** Calcium Disorders; Bone Disorders-Metabolic; Growth/Development Disorders; Cancer Survivors-Late Effects of Therapy; **Hospital:** Duke Univ Med Ctr; **Address:** Duke Consultative Services, 3713 Benson Drive, Ste 202, Durham, NC 27609; **Phone:** 919-684-3772; **Board Cert:** Pediatrics 1979; Pediatric Endocrinology 2003; **Med School:** Med Coll VA 1975; **Resid:** Pediatrics, Childrens Hosp Med Ctr 1977; Pediatrics, Childrens Meml Hosp 1978; **Fellow:** Endocrinology, Diabetes & Metabolism, Michael Reese Hosp 1980; **Fac Appt:** Asst Clin Prof Ped, Duke Univ

Key Jr, L Lyndon MD [PEn] - **Spec Exp:** Osteopetrosis; Osteoporosis-Juvenile; **Hospital:** MUSC Med Ctr; **Address:** MUSC Med Ctr, Dept Pediatrics, 135 Rutledge Ave, Box 250561, Charleston, SC 29425; **Phone:** 843-792-6807; **Board Cert:** Pediatrics 1983; Pediatric Endocrinology 1983; **Med School:** Univ NC Sch Med 1977; **Resid:** Pediatrics, Duke Univ Med Ctr 1980; **Fellow:** Endocrinology, Chldns Hosp 1983; **Fac Appt:** Prof Ped, Med Univ SC

Meacham, Lillian R MD [PEn] - **Spec Exp:** Growth Disorders in Childhood Cancer; Cancer Survivors-Late Effects of Therapy; **Hospital:** Emory Univ Hosp; **Address:** Emory Childrens Ctr, 2015 Uppergate Drive, Atlanta, GA 30322; **Phone:** 404-727-5753; **Board Cert:** Pediatrics 2006; Pediatric Endocrinology 2006; **Med School:** Emory Univ 1984; **Resid:** Pediatrics, Emory Univ Hosp 1987; **Fellow:** Pediatric Endocrinology, Emory Univ Hosp 1990; **Fac Appt:** Assoc Prof Ped, Emory Univ

Schwartz, Robert P MD [PEn] - **Hospital:** Wake Forest Univ Baptist Med Ctr (page 73); **Address:** Wake Forest Univ Sch Med-Dept Pediatrics, Med Ctr Blvd, Winston-Salem, NC 27157-0001; **Phone:** 336-716-3199; **Board Cert:** Pediatrics 1994; Pediatric Endocrinology 2002; **Med School:** Univ Fla Coll Med 1968; **Resid:** Pediatrics, Charlotte Meml Hosp 1970; Pediatrics, Duke Univ Med Ctr 1971; **Fellow:** Pediatric Endocrinology, Duke Univ Med Ctr 1971; Pediatric Endocrinology, Duke Univ Med Ctr 1974; **Fac Appt:** Prof Ped, Wake Forest Univ

Silverstein, Janet H MD [PEn] - **Spec Exp:** Diabetes; Growth/Development Disorders; **Hospital:** Shands at Univ of FL, Shands at Alachua Gen Hosp; **Address:** Univ Florida - Shands Hlthcare, 1600 SW Archer Rd, Box 100296, Gainesville, FL 32610-3003; **Phone:** 352-334-1390; **Board Cert:** Pediatrics 1975; Pediatric Endocrinology 2004; **Med School:** Univ Pennsylvania 1970; **Resid:** Pediatrics, Chldns Hosp 1972; Pediatrics, Chldns Hosp 1975; **Fellow:** Pediatric Endocrinology, Duke Univ Med Ctr 1977; **Fac Appt:** Prof Ped, Univ Fla Coll Med

Midwest

Allen, David Bruce MD [PEn] - **Spec Exp:** Growth Disorders; Pubertal Disorders; Diabetes; **Hospital:** Univ WI Hosp & Clins; **Address:** Univ Wisc American Fam Chldn's Hosp, H4/448 CSC-Pediatrics, 600 Highland Ave, Madison, WI 53792-4108; **Phone:** 608-263-5835; **Board Cert:** Pediatrics 1986; Pediatric Endocrinology 2004; **Med School:** Duke Univ 1980; **Resid:** Pediatrics, Univ Wisc Hosp 1985; **Fellow:** Pediatric Endocrinology, Univ Wisc Hosp 1988; **Fac Appt:** Prof Ped, Univ Wisc

Eugster, Erica MD [PEn] - **Spec Exp:** Pubertal Disorders; Turner Syndrome; **Hospital:** Riley Hosp for Children; **Address:** Riley Chldns Hosp, 702 Barnhill Drive, rm 5960, Indianapolis, IN 46202; **Phone:** 317-274-3889; **Board Cert:** Pediatrics 2002; Pediatric Endocrinology 2005; **Med School:** Med Coll PA 1990; **Resid:** Pediatrics, Marshfield Clin-St Josephs Hosp 1994; **Fellow:** Pediatric Endocrinology, Univ Minn Hosp 1994; **Fac Appt:** Prof Ped, Indiana Univ

Gutai, James MD [PEn] - **Hospital:** Chldns Hosp of Michigan, Marquette Genl Hosp; **Address:** Morris J Hood Comp Diabetes Ctr, 4201 St Antoine St, Univ Hlth Ctr, Box 247, Detroit, MI 48201; **Phone:** 313-577-0133; **Board Cert:** Pediatrics 1977; Pediatric Endocrinology 1980; **Med School:** Temple Univ 1970; **Resid:** Pediatrics, Johns Hopkins Hosp 1976; **Fellow:** Pediatric Endocrinology, Johns Hopkins Hosp 1976; **Fac Appt:** Prof Ped, Wayne State Univ

Levy, Richard Alshuler MD [PEn] - **Spec Exp:** Growth Disorders; Pituitary Disorders; Thyroid Disorders; **Hospital:** Rush - Copley Med Ctr, Ingalls Meml Hosp; **Address:** 1725 W Harrison St, Ste 328, Chicago, IL 60612-3863; **Phone:** 312-942-8989; **Board Cert:** Internal Medicine 1976; Pediatrics 1983; Endocrinology 1985; Pediatric Endocrinology 1986; **Med School:** Louisiana State U, New Orleans 1971; **Resid:** Internal Medicine, U Mass Med Ctr 1977; Pediatrics, Beth Israel Hosp 1978; **Fellow:** Endocrinology, Diabetes & Metabolism, Barnes Jewish Hosp 1982; **Fac Appt:** Asst Prof Ped, Rush Med Coll

Menon, Ram K MD [PEn] - **Spec Exp:** Growth/Development Disorders; Diabetes; **Hospital:** Univ Michigan Hlth Sys; **Address:** Univ Mich Med Ctr, MPB SPC5178, 1500 E Medical Ctr Drive, Ann Arbor, MI 48109; **Phone:** 734-764-5175; **Board Cert:** Pediatrics 2002; Pediatric Endocrinology 2003; **Med School:** India 1979; **Resid:** Pediatrics, All India Inst of Medical Science 1984; **Fellow:** Pediatric Endocrinology, Children's Hosp 1989; **Fac Appt:** Assoc Prof Ped, Univ Mich Med Sch

Pediatric Endocrinology

Rogers, Douglas G MD [PEn] - **Spec Exp:** Diabetes; Growth/Development Disorders; Thyroid Disorders; **Hospital:** Cleveland Clin Fdn (page 56); **Address:** Div Pediatric Endocrinology, 9500 Euclid Ave, Box A120, Cleveland, OH 44195-0001; **Phone:** 216-445-8048; **Board Cert:** Pediatrics 1984; Pediatric Endocrinology 1986; **Med School:** Ros Franklin Univ/Chicago Med Sch 1978; **Resid:** Pediatrics, Cardinal Glennon Chldns Hosp 1981; **Fellow:** Endocrinology, Diabetes & Metabolism, St Louis Chldns Hosp 1985

Rosenfield, Robert L MD [PEn] - **Spec Exp:** Polycystic Ovarian Syndrome; Pubertal Disorders; Menstrual Disorders; **Hospital:** Univ of Chicago Hosps; **Address:** 5841 S Maryland Ave, MC 5053, Chicago, IL 60637-1463; **Phone:** 773-702-6169; **Board Cert:** Pediatrics 1986; Pediatric Endocrinology 1986; **Med School:** Northwestern Univ 1960; **Resid:** Pediatrics, Chldns Hosp 1963; **Fellow:** Pediatric Endocrinology, Chldns Hosp 1968; **Fac Appt:** Prof Ped, Univ Chicago-Pritzker Sch Med

White, Neil H MD [PEn] - **Spec Exp:** Diabetes; Hypoglycemia; **Hospital:** St Louis Chldns Hosp; **Address:** St Louis Chldn's Hosp, One Children's Pl, CB 8116, St Louis, MO 63110-1010; **Phone:** 314-454-6051; **Board Cert:** Pediatrics 1981; Pediatric Endocrinology 1983; **Med School:** Albert Einstein Coll Med 1975; **Resid:** Pediatrics, St Louis Chldns Hosp 1977; **Fellow:** Endocrinology, Diabetes & Metabolism, Washington Univ 1979; **Fac Appt:** Prof Ped, Washington Univ, St Louis

Zimmerman, Donald MD [PEn] - **Spec Exp:** Growth Disorders in Childhood Cancer; Thyroid Cancer; Thyroid Disorders; Growth/Development Disorders; **Hospital:** Children's Mem Hosp; **Address:** Children's Memorial Hosp, 2300 Children's Plaza, Div Endocrinology, Box 54, Chicago, IL 60614; **Phone:** 773-327-7740; **Board Cert:** Internal Medicine 1977; Endocrinology 1979; Pediatrics 1983; Pediatric Endocrinology 2001; **Med School:** Univ IL Coll Med 1974; **Resid:** Internal Medicine, Johns Hopkins Hosp 1977; Pediatrics, Mayo Clinic 1981; **Fellow:** Endocrinology, Diabetes & Metabolism, Mayo Clinic 1980; **Fac Appt:** Prof Ped, Northwestern Univ

Great Plains and Mountains

Foster, Carol M MD [PEn] - **Spec Exp:** Diabetes; Growth/Development Disorders; Pubertal Disorders; **Hospital:** Primary Children's Med Ctr, Univ Utah Hosps and Clins; **Address:** Utah Diabetes Ctr, 615 Arapeen Drive, Ste 100, Salt Lake City, UT 84108; **Phone:** 801-581-7761; **Board Cert:** Pediatrics 1983; Pediatric Endocrinology 1983; **Med School:** Washington Univ, St Louis 1978; **Resid:** Pediatrics, Univ Utah Hlth Scis Ctr 1981; **Fellow:** Pediatric Endocrinology, Natl Inst Hlth 1984; **Fac Appt:** Prof Med, Univ Utah

Kappy, Michael S MD/PhD [PEn] - **Spec Exp:** Growth/Development Disorders; Thyroid Disorders; Pubertal Disorders; **Hospital:** Chldn's Hosp - Aurora, The; **Address:** Childrens Hosp, Dept Ped Endocrinology, 13123 E 16th Ave, Box B265, Aurora, CO 80045; **Phone:** 720-777-6128; **Board Cert:** Pediatrics 1973; Pediatric Endocrinology 1980; **Med School:** Univ Wisc 1967; **Resid:** Pediatrics, Univ Colorado Med Ctr 1972; **Fellow:** Pediatric Endocrinology, Johns Hopkins Hosp 1980; **Fac Appt:** Prof Ped, Univ Colorado

Klingensmith, Georgeanna MD [PEn] - **Spec Exp:** Diabetes; **Hospital:** Chldn's Hosp - Aurora, The; **Address:** Barbara Davis Ctr for Childhood Diabetes, MS B140, PO Box 6511, Aurora, CO 80045-0511; **Phone:** 303-724-2323; **Board Cert:** Pediatrics 1976; Pediatric Endocrinology 2000; **Med School:** Duke Univ 1971; **Resid:** Pediatrics, Childrens Hosp 1973; **Fellow:** Pediatric Endocrinology, Johns Hopkins Hosp 1976; Pediatric Endocrinology, Childrens Hosp 1974; **Fac Appt:** Prof Ped, Univ Colorado

West Coast and Pacific

Geffner, Mitchell Eugene MD [PEn] - **Spec Exp:** Growth Disorders; Pubertal Disorders; Thyroid Disorders; **Hospital:** Chldns Hosp - Los Angeles; **Address:** Chlds Hosp LA, Div Endocrinology, 4650 Sunset Blvd, MS 61, Los Angeles, CA 90027; **Phone:** 323-669-4606; **Board Cert:** Pediatrics 1980; Pediatric Endocrinology 2006; **Med School:** Albert Einstein Coll Med 1975; **Resid:** Pediatrics, LAC-USC Med Ctr 1979; **Fellow:** Pediatric Endocrinology, UCLA Med Ctr 1982; **Fac Appt:** Prof Ped, USC Sch Med

Kaufman, Francine R MD [PEn] - **Spec Exp:** Diabetes; Growth/Development Disorders; **Hospital:** Chldns Hosp - Los Angeles, USC Univ Hosp - R K Eamer Med Plz; **Address:** Chldns Hosp, Div Endocrinology, 4650 W Sunset Blvd, MS 61, Los Angeles, CA 90027; **Phone:** 323-669-4606; **Board Cert:** Pediatrics 1981; Pediatric Endocrinology 1983; **Med School:** Ros Franklin Univ/Chicago Med Sch 1976; **Resid:** Pediatrics, Children's Hosp 1978; **Fellow:** Pediatric Endocrinology, Children's Hosp 1980; **Fac Appt:** Prof Ped, USC Sch Med

Wilson, Darrell M MD [PEn] - **Spec Exp:** Diabetes; Growth Disorders; **Hospital:** Stanford Univ Med Ctr, Lucile Packard Chldns Hosp/Stanford Univ Med Ctr; **Address:** Stanford Univ Med Ctr - Pediatrics, 300 Pasteur Rd, Ste G-313, MC 5208, Stanford, CA 94305-5208; **Phone:** 650-723-5791; **Board Cert:** Pediatrics 1982; Pediatric Endocrinology 2003; **Med School:** UCSD 1977; **Resid:** Pediatrics, Stanford Univ Med Ctr 1980; **Fellow:** Endocrinology, Diabetes & Metabolism, Stanford Univ Med Ctr 1984; **Fac Appt:** Prof Ped, Stanford Univ

PEDIATRIC GASTROENTEROLOGY

New England

Kleinman, Ronald E MD [PGe] - **Spec Exp:** Transplant Medicine-Liver; Nutrition; **Hospital:** Mass Genl Hosp, N Shore Children's Hosp; **Address:** Mass Genl Hosp, Div Ped GI/Nutrition, 55 Fruit St, VBK 107, Boston, MA 02114; **Phone:** 617-726-8705; **Board Cert:** Pediatrics 1992; Pediatric Gastroenterology 2005; **Med School:** NY Med Coll 1972; **Resid:** Pediatrics, Albert Einstein Coll Med 1977; **Fellow:** Pediatric Gastroenterology, Mass Genl Hosp 1980; **Fac Appt:** Prof Ped, Harvard Med Sch

Mid Atlantic

Baker Jr, Robert D MD/PhD [PGe] - **Spec Exp:** Gastroesophageal Reflux Disease (GERD); Cystic Fibrosis; Nutrition; **Hospital:** Women's & Chldn's Hosp of Buffalo, The; **Address:** Childrens Hospital, Div Gastroenterology, 219 Bryant St, Buffalo, NY 14222-2006; **Phone:** 716-878-7793; **Board Cert:** Pediatrics 1978; Pediatric Gastroenterology 2005; **Med School:** Temple Univ 1972; **Resid:** Pediatrics, Buffalo Chldns Hosp 1975; **Fellow:** Gastroenterology, Mass Genl Hosp/Chldns Hosp Med Ctr 1983; Nutritional Biochemistry, MIT 1984; **Fac Appt:** Prof Ped, SUNY Buffalo

Baker, Susan S MD/PhD [PGe] - **Spec Exp:** Nutrition; Obesity; Liver Disease; **Hospital:** Women's & Chldn's Hosp of Buffalo, The; **Address:** Childrens Hospital, Div Gastroenterology, 219 Bryant St, Buffalo, NY 14201-2099; **Phone:** 716-878-7793; **Board Cert:** Pediatrics 1978; Pediatric Gastroenterology 2005; **Med School:** Temple Univ 1972; **Resid:** Pediatrics, Buffalo Chldns Hosp 1975; **Fellow:** Nutrition, MIT 1981; Gastroenterology, Mass Genl Hosp 1984; **Fac Appt:** Prof Ped, SUNY Buffalo

Pediatric Gastroenterology

Baldassano, Robert N MD [PGe] - **Spec Exp:** Inflammatory Bowel Disease; Ulcerative Colitis; Crohn's Disease; **Hospital:** Chldns Hosp of Philadelphia, The; **Address:** Chldns Hosp of Philadelphia, GI/Nutrition, 324 S 34th St, Philadelphia, PA 19104-4399; **Phone:** 215-590-3630; **Board Cert:** Pediatrics 1989; Pediatric Gastroenterology 2000; **Med School:** SUNY Downstate 1984; **Resid:** Pediatrics, Childrens Hosp 1988; **Fellow:** Pediatric Gastroenterology, Childrens Hosp 1991; **Fac Appt:** Assoc Prof Ped, Univ Pennsylvania

Benkov, Keith J MD [PGe] - **Spec Exp:** Inflammatory Bowel Disease/Crohn's; Liver Disease; Celiac Disease; **Hospital:** Mount Sinai Med Ctr (page 64), Englewood Hosp & Med Ctr; **Address:** 5 E 98th St, Box 1656, New York, NY 10029; **Phone:** 212-241-5415; **Board Cert:** Pediatrics 1984; Pediatric Gastroenterology 1998; **Med School:** Mount Sinai Sch Med 1979; **Resid:** Pediatrics, Mount Sinai Hosp 1982; **Fellow:** Pediatric Gastroenterology, Mount Sinai Hosp 1984; **Fac Appt:** Assoc Prof Ped, Mount Sinai Sch Med

Fasano, Alessio MD [PGe] - **Spec Exp:** Celiac Disease; Diarrheal Diseases; Nutrition; **Hospital:** Univ of MD Med Sys; **Address:** 20 Penn St, rm 351, Baltimore, MD 21201; **Phone:** 410-706-5501; **Med School:** Italy ; **Resid:** Pediatrics, Univ Naples; **Fellow:** Univ Naples; **Fac Appt:** Prof Ped, Univ MD Sch Med

Hillemeier, A Craig MD [PGe] - **Spec Exp:** Gastroesophageal Reflux Disease (GERD); Inflammatory Bowel Disease/Crohn's; **Hospital:** Penn State Milton S Hershey Med Ctr, Penn State Chldns Hosp; **Address:** Hershey Medical Ctr, 500 University Drive, MC H085, Hershey, PA 17033-0850; **Phone:** 717-531-6700; **Board Cert:** Pediatrics 1981; Pediatric Gastroenterology 2005; **Med School:** Loyola Univ-Stritch Sch Med 1976; **Resid:** Pediatrics, Loyola Univ Stritch 1978; **Fellow:** Pediatric Gastroenterology, Yale New Haven Med Ctr 1982; **Fac Appt:** Prof Ped, Penn State Univ-Hershey Med Ctr

Levy, Joseph MD [PGe] - **Spec Exp:** Celiac Disease; Irritable Bowel Syndrome; Gastroesophageal Reflux Disease (GERD); Nutrition in Autism; **Hospital:** NYU Med Ctr (page 68); **Address:** 160 E 32nd St Fl 2, New York, NY 10016; **Phone:** 212-263-5407; **Board Cert:** Pediatrics 1981; Pediatric Gastroenterology 2004; **Med School:** Israel 1973; **Resid:** Pediatrics, Beth Israel Med Ctr 1977; **Fellow:** Research, Columbia-Presby Med Ctr 1975; Pediatric Gastroenterology, Columbia-Presby Med Ctr 1979; **Fac Appt:** Prof Ped, NYU Sch Med

Newman, Leonard MD [PGe] - **Spec Exp:** Inflammatory Bowel Disease; Celiac Disease; **Hospital:** Westchester Med Ctr, Our Lady of Mercy Med Ctr; **Address:** NY Med College, Dept Ped, Munger Pavillion - rm 123, Valhalla, NY 10595; **Phone:** 914-594-4610; **Board Cert:** Pediatrics 1975; Pediatric Gastroenterology 1990; **Med School:** NY Med Coll 1970; **Resid:** Pediatrics, UCSD Med Ctr 1972; Pediatrics, NY Med Coll 1973; **Fellow:** Gastroenterology, Bronx Lebanon Hosp/Einstein 1974; **Fac Appt:** Prof Ped, NY Med Coll

Oliva-Hemker, Maria M MD [PGe] - **Spec Exp:** Inflammatory Bowel Disease/Crohn's; Ulcerative Colitis; Malabsorption Syndrome; **Hospital:** Johns Hopkins Hosp - Baltimore (page 61); **Address:** Johns Hopkins Hosp, Ped GI & Nutrition, 600 N Wolfe St, Brady 320, Baltimore, MD 21287-2631; **Phone:** 410-955-8765; **Board Cert:** Pediatrics 2007; Pediatric Gastroenterology 2007; **Med School:** Johns Hopkins Univ 1986; **Resid:** Pediatrics, Johns Hopkins Hosp 1989; **Fellow:** Gastroenterology, Johns Hopkins Hosp 1992; **Fac Appt:** Assoc Prof Ped, Johns Hopkins Univ

Piccoli, David A MD [PGe] - **Spec Exp:** Liver Disease; Alagille Syndrome; **Hospital:** Chldns Hosp of Philadelphia, The; **Address:** Chlds Hosp of Philadelphia, Div Gastroenterology/Nutrition, 34th St and Civic Ctr Blvd, Ste 9S20C, Philadelphia, PA 19104; **Phone:** 215-590-1678; **Board Cert:** Pediatrics 1984; Pediatric Gastroenterology 2005; **Med School:** Harvard Med Sch 1979; **Resid:** Pediatrics, Chldns Hosp Med Ctr 1983; **Fellow:** Gastroenterology, Chldns Hosp 1986; **Fac Appt:** Prof Ped, Univ Pennsylvania

Schwarz, Kathleen B MD [PGe] - **Spec Exp:** Hepatitis B & C; Transplant Medicine-Liver; Liver Disease; **Hospital:** Johns Hopkins Hosp - Baltimore (page 61); **Address:** Johns Hopkins Pediatric GI, 600 N Wolfe St, Brady 320, Baltimore, MD 21287-0005; **Phone:** 410-955-8769; **Board Cert:** Pediatrics 1977; Pediatric Gastroenterology 2005; Pediatric Transplant Hepatology 2006; **Med School:** Washington Univ, St Louis 1972; **Resid:** Pediatrics, St Louis Chldns Hosp 1974; **Fellow:** Pediatric Gastroenterology, St Louis Chldns Hosp 1976; **Fac Appt:** Prof Ped, Johns Hopkins Univ

Schwarz, Steven M MD [PGe] - **Spec Exp:** Gastroesophageal Reflux Disease (GERD); Nutrition; Endoscopy; **Hospital:** SUNY Downstate Med Ctr; **Address:** Children's Hosp at SUNY Downstate, 445 Lenox Rd, Box 49, Brooklyn, NY 11203; **Phone:** 718-270-4714; **Board Cert:** Pediatrics 1979; Pediatric Gastroenterology 1998; **Med School:** Columbia P&S 1974; **Resid:** Pediatrics, Columbia-Presby Med Ctr 1977; **Fellow:** Pediatric Gastroenterology, Stanford Univ Med Ctr 1978; Pediatric Gastroenterology, Columbia-Presby Med Ctr 1980; **Fac Appt:** Prof Ped, SUNY Downstate

Spivak, William MD [PGe] - **Spec Exp:** Inflammatory Bowel Disease/Crohn's; Ulcerative Colitis; Gastroesophageal Reflux Disease (GERD); **Hospital:** Lenox Hill Hosp (page 62); **Address:** 177 E 87th St, Ste 305, New York, NY 10128; **Phone:** 212-369-7700; **Board Cert:** Pediatrics 1981; Pediatric Gastroenterology 2005; **Med School:** Albert Einstein Coll Med 1976; **Resid:** Pediatrics, Jacobi Med Ctr 1979; **Fellow:** Gastroenterology, Childrens Hosp 1982; Research, Brigham & Womens Hosp 1982; **Fac Appt:** Clin Prof Ped, Cornell Univ-Weill Med Coll

Squires, Robert H MD [PGe] - **Spec Exp:** Liver Disease; **Hospital:** Chldns Hosp of Pittsburgh - UPMC; **Address:** Children's Hosp Pittsburgh, Hepatology, 3705 Fifth Ave, Pittsburgh, PA 15213; **Phone:** 412-692-5180; **Board Cert:** Pediatrics 1981; Pediatric Gastroenterology 2005; **Med School:** Univ Tex Med Br, Galveston 1977; **Resid:** Pediatrics, Children's Hosp 1979; **Fellow:** Pediatric Gastroenterology, Children's Hosp 1982; **Fac Appt:** Prof Ped, Univ Pittsburgh

Suchy, Frederick J MD [PGe] - **Spec Exp:** Hepatitis; Liver Disease; Neonatal Cholestasis; **Hospital:** Mount Sinai Med Ctr (page 64); **Address:** Mount Sinai Medical Ctr, 1 Gustave Levy Pl, Box 1198, New York, NY 10029; **Phone:** 212-241-6933; **Board Cert:** Pediatrics 1982; Pediatric Gastroenterology 2004; Pediatric Transplant Hepatology 2006; **Med School:** Univ Cincinnati 1974; **Resid:** Pediatrics, Chidren's Hosp Med Ctr 1978; **Fellow:** Pediatric Gastroenterology, Chidren's Hosp Med Ctr 1981; **Fac Appt:** Prof Ped, Mount Sinai Sch Med

Treem, William R MD [PGe] - **Spec Exp:** Liver Disease; Inflammatory Bowel Disease; Celiac Disease; **Hospital:** SUNY Downstate Med Ctr, Long Island Coll Hosp (page 57); **Address:** SUNY Downstate Med Ctr, Dept Peds, 445 Lennox Rd, Box 49, Brooklyn, NY 11203; **Phone:** 718-270-4714; **Board Cert:** Pediatrics 1982; Pediatric Gastroenterology 2005; **Med School:** Stanford Univ 1977; **Resid:** Pediatrics, Children's Hosp 1980; **Fellow:** Pediatric Gastroenterology, Univ Penn Hosp 1985; **Fac Appt:** Prof Ped, SUNY Downstate

Southeast

Hill, Ivor D MD [PGe] - **Spec Exp:** Celiac Disease; Inflammatory Bowel Disease; Diarrheal Diseases; **Hospital:** Wake Forest Univ Baptist Med Ctr (page 73); **Address:** Wake Forest Univ Sch Med, Div Ped Gastro, Medical Center Blvd, Winston-Salem, NC 27157; **Phone:** 336-716-3009; **Board Cert:** Pediatrics 2007; Pediatric Gastroenterology 2003; **Med School:** South Africa 1972; **Resid:** Pediatrics, Addington Hosp 1976; Pediatrics, Red Cross Chldns Hosp 1977; **Fellow:** Pediatric Gastroenterology, Red Cross Chlds Hosp 1980; **Fac Appt:** Prof Ped, Wake Forest Univ

Pediatric Gastroenterology

Novak, Donald A MD [PGe] - **Spec Exp:** Liver Disease; **Hospital:** Shands at Univ of FL; **Address:** Shands @ Univ Florida, Div Ped Gastro, 1600 SW Archer Rd, Box 100296, Gainesville, FL 32610-0296; **Phone:** 352-392-6410; **Board Cert:** Pediatrics 1987; Pediatric Gastroenterology 1990; **Med School:** Univ S Fla Coll Med 1981; **Resid:** Pediatrics, Univ South Fla 1984; **Fellow:** Pediatric Gastroenterology, Childrens Hosp 1987; **Fac Appt:** Prof Ped, Univ Fla Coll Med

Thompson, John F MD [PGe] - **Spec Exp:** Inflammatory Bowel Disease/Crohn's; Short Bowel Syndrome; Transplant Medicine-Bowel; **Hospital:** Jackson Meml Hosp; **Address:** Jackson Meml Hospital, Dept Pediatrics, Div GI & Nutrition, 1601 NW 12th Ave, rm 3005A, MC D820, Miami, FL 33136; **Phone:** 305-243-6426; **Board Cert:** Pediatrics 1983; Pediatric Gastroenterology 2005; **Med School:** Loyola Univ-Stritch Sch Med 1977; **Resid:** Pediatrics, Wylers Chldns Hosp-Univ Chicago 1980; **Fellow:** Pediatric Gastroenterology, Babies Hosp-Columbia Univ 1985; **Fac Appt:** Prof Ped, Univ Miami Sch Med

Ulshen, Martin H MD [PGe] - **Spec Exp:** Liver Disease; Inflammatory Bowel Disease; Irritable Bowel Syndrome; **Hospital:** Duke Univ Med Ctr; **Address:** Duke Univ Med Ctr, Box 3009, Durham, NC 27710; **Phone:** 919-684-5068; **Board Cert:** Pediatrics 1993; Pediatric Gastroenterology 2005; **Med School:** Univ Rochester 1969; **Resid:** Pediatrics, Univ Colorado Med Ctr 1974; **Fellow:** Pediatric Gastroenterology, Univ Colorado Med Ctr 1975; Pediatric Gastroenterology, Chldns Hosp 1977; **Fac Appt:** Prof Ped, Duke Univ

Midwest

Berman, James MD [PGe] - **Spec Exp:** Inflammatory Bowel Disease/Crohn's; Nutrition; Ulcerative Colitis; **Hospital:** Loyola Univ Med Ctr, Adv Luth Genl Hosp; **Address:** Loyola Univ Med Ctr, Dept Ped Gastro, 2160 S 1st Ave Bldg 105 - rm 3346, Maywood, IL 60153-3304; **Phone:** 708-327-9073; **Board Cert:** Pediatrics 1986; Pediatric Gastroenterology 2005; **Med School:** Univ Pittsburgh 1981; **Resid:** Pediatrics, Chldns Hosp 1984; **Fellow:** Pediatric Gastroenterology, Mass Genl Hosp/Chldns Hosp 1987; **Fac Appt:** Asst Prof Ped, Loyola Univ-Stritch Sch Med

Cohen, Mitchell B MD [PGe] - **Spec Exp:** Inflammatory Bowel Disease; Diarrheal Diseases; Celiac Disease; **Hospital:** Cincinnati Chldns Hosp Med Ctr; **Address:** Chldns Hosp Med Ctr, 3333 Burnet Ave, (MLC 2010), Cincinnati, OH 45229; **Phone:** 513-636-4415; **Board Cert:** Pediatrics 1981; Pediatric Gastroenterology 2005; **Med School:** Mount Sinai Sch Med 1977; **Resid:** Pediatrics, Johns Hopkins Hosp 1980; **Fellow:** Pediatric Gastroenterology, Chldns Hosp Med Ctr 1986; **Fac Appt:** Prof Ped, Univ Cincinnati

El-Youssef, Mounif MD [PGe] - **Spec Exp:** Liver Disease; **Hospital:** Mayo Med Ctr & Clin - Rochester; **Address:** Mayo Clinic, Div Ped Gastroenterology, 200 First St SW, Rochester, MN 55905; **Phone:** 507-284-2141; **Board Cert:** Pediatric Gastroenterology 2005; **Med School:** Belgium 1982; **Resid:** Pediatrics, Cleveland Clinic 1987; **Fellow:** Pediatric Gastroenterology, Harvard Med Sch 1990

Gunasekaran, T S MD [PGe] - **Spec Exp:** Gastroesophageal Reflux Disease (GERD); Esophageal Disorders; Inflammatory Bowel Disease; Pain-Abdominal Recurrent; **Hospital:** Adv Luth Genl Hosp, Loyola Univ Med Ctr; **Address:** Lutheran Genl Chldns Hosp, Dept Ped GI, 1675 Dempster St, Park Ridge, IL 60068; **Phone:** 847-723-7700; **Board Cert:** Pediatrics 2000; Pediatric Gastroenterology 2000; **Med School:** India 1977; **Resid:** Pediatrics 1982; Pediatrics 1987; **Fellow:** Pediatric Gastroenterology, BC Childrens Hosp 1992; **Fac Appt:** Assoc Clin Prof Ped, Loyola Univ-Stritch Sch Med

Kirschner, Barbara S MD [PGe] - **Spec Exp:** Ulcerative Colitis; Pain-Abdominal Recurrent; Inflammatory Bowel Disease/Crohn's; **Hospital:** Univ of Chicago Hosps; **Address:** Univ Chicago Comer Childrens Hosp, 5839 S Maryland Ave, Ste C-474, MC 4085, Chicago, IL 60637; **Phone:** 773-702-6418; **Board Cert:** Pediatrics 1972; Pediatric Gastroenterology 2004; **Med School:** Med Coll PA Hahnemann 1967; **Resid:** Pediatrics, Univ Chicago Hosps 1970; **Fellow:** Pediatric Gastroenterology, Univ Chicago 1977; **Fac Appt:** Prof Ped, Univ Chicago-Pritzker Sch Med

Molleston, Jean P MD [PGe] - **Spec Exp:** Liver Disease; Inflammatory Bowel Disease/Crohn's; **Hospital:** Riley Hosp for Children; **Address:** Indiana Univ-Riley Chldns Hosp, Div Ped Gastroenterology, 702 Barnhill Drive, rm ROC 4210, Indianapolis, IN 46202-5225; **Phone:** 317-274-3774; **Board Cert:** Pediatric Gastroenterology 2003; **Med School:** Washington Univ, St Louis 1986; **Resid:** Pediatrics, Chldns Hosp 1988; **Fellow:** Pediatric Gastroenterology, Washington Univ Med Ctr 1991; **Fac Appt:** Assoc Clin Prof Ped, Indiana Univ

Rothbaum, Robert J MD [PGe] - **Spec Exp:** Inflammatory Bowel Disease; **Hospital:** St Louis Chldns Hosp, Barnes-Jewish Hosp; **Address:** 1 Children's Pl, NWT Bldg Fl 9, Box 8116, St Louis, MO 63110; **Phone:** 314-454-6173; **Board Cert:** Pediatrics 1981; Pediatric Gastroenterology 2005; **Med School:** Univ Chicago-Pritzker Sch Med 1976; **Resid:** Pediatrics, St Louis Chldns Hosp 1978; **Fellow:** Ambulatory Pediatrics, St Louis Chldns Hosp 1979; Pediatric Gastroenterology, Chldns Hosp Med Ctr 1982; **Fac Appt:** Prof Ped, Washington Univ, St Louis

Rudolph, Colin D MD [PGe] - **Spec Exp:** Feeding Disorders; Nutrition; Gastrointestinal Motility Disorders; Gastrointestinal Functional Disorders; **Hospital:** Chldns Hosp - Wisconsin; **Address:** Children's Hospital of Wisconsin, 9000 W Wisconsin Ave, Ste 604, Milwaukee, WI 53226; **Phone:** 414-266-3690; **Board Cert:** Pediatrics 1987; Pediatric Gastroenterology 2005; **Med School:** Case West Res Univ 1982; **Resid:** Pediatrics, Children's Hosp 1984; **Fellow:** Pediatric Gastroenterology, UCSF Med Ctr 1986; **Fac Appt:** Assoc Prof Ped, Univ Wisc

Whitington, Peter F MD [PGe] - **Spec Exp:** Transplant Medicine-Liver; Liver Disease; **Hospital:** Children's Mem Hosp; **Address:** Chldns Meml Hosp, Div Ped Gastro, 2300 Children's Plaza, Box 57, Chicago, IL 60614; **Phone:** 773-880-4643; **Board Cert:** Pediatrics 1977; Pediatric Gastroenterology 2005; Pediatric Transplant Hepatology 2006; **Med School:** Univ Tenn Coll Med, Memphis 1971; **Resid:** Pediatrics, Univ Tenn Hosp 1975; **Fellow:** Gastroenterology, Johns Hopkins Hosp 1977; Gastroenterology, Univ Wisconsin 1978; **Fac Appt:** Prof Ped, Northwestern Univ

Wyllie, Robert MD [PGe] - **Spec Exp:** Inflammatory Bowel Disease/Crohn's; Ulcerative Colitis; **Hospital:** Cleveland Clin Fdn (page 56); **Address:** Cleveland Clinic, 9500 Euclid Ave, Desk A111, Cleveland, OH 44195; **Phone:** 216-444-2237; **Board Cert:** Pediatrics 1982; Pediatric Gastroenterology 1997; **Med School:** Indiana Univ 1976; **Resid:** Pediatrics, Indiana Univ Med Ctr 1979; **Fellow:** Pediatric Gastroenterology, Indiana Univ Med Ctr 1980

Great Plains and Mountains

Hoffenberg, Edward J MD [PGe] - **Spec Exp:** Inflammatory Bowel Disease/Crohn's; Celiac Disease; **Hospital:** Chldn's Hosp - Aurora, The, Univ Colorado Hosp; **Address:** Chldns Hosp, Div Gastroenterology, 13123 E 16th Ave, Box B290, Denver, CO 80218; **Phone:** 303-861-6669; **Board Cert:** Pediatrics 1989; Pediatric Gastroenterology 2000; **Med School:** Case West Res Univ ; **Resid:** Pediatrics, Rainbow Babies & Chldns Hosp; **Fellow:** Pediatric Gastroenterology, Chldns Hosp; **Fac Appt:** Assoc Prof Ped, Univ Colorado

Pediatric Gastroenterology

Krebs, Nancy F MD [PGe] - **Spec Exp:** Obesity; Nutrition; **Hospital:** Chldn's Hosp - Aurora, The; **Address:** Children's Hospital, Health Ctr, 13123 E 16th Ave, Box B270, Aurora, CO 80045; **Phone:** 303-724-3260; **Board Cert:** Pediatrics 1999; Pediatric Gastroenterology 2003; **Med School:** Univ Colorado 1987; **Resid:** Pediatrics, Univ Colorado Health Sci Ctr 1990; **Fellow:** Pediatric Gastroenterology, Univ Colorado Health Sci Ctr 1992; Nutrition, Univ Colorado Health Sci Ctr 1993; **Fac Appt:** Prof Ped, Univ Colorado

Vanderhoof, Jon A MD [PGe] - **Spec Exp:** Nutrition; Short Bowel Syndrome; Probiotics; **Hospital:** Boys Town Natl Rsch Hosp, Children's Hosp - Omaha; **Address:** Boystown Hospital & Clinic, 14040 Boys Town Hospital Rd, Boystown, NE 68010; **Phone:** 402-778-6820; **Board Cert:** Pediatrics 1993; Pediatric Gastroenterology 2005; **Med School:** Univ Nebr Coll Med 1972; **Resid:** Pediatrics, Univ Nebr Coll Med 1974; **Fellow:** Pediatric Gastroenterology, UCLA Med Ctr 1976; **Fac Appt:** Prof Ped, Univ Nebr Coll Med

Southwest

Rhoads, J Marc MD [PGe] - **Spec Exp:** Diarrheal Diseases; Inflammatory Bowel Disease; Intestinal Disorders; **Hospital:** Meml Hermann Hosp - Texas Med Ctr; **Address:** Univ Texas Hlth Sci Ctr, Dept Pediatrics-Gastroenterology, 6410 Fannin St Fl 5 - Ste 500, Houston, TX 77030; **Phone:** 832-325-6516; **Board Cert:** Pediatrics 1986; Pediatric Gastroenterology 2005; **Med School:** Johns Hopkins Univ 1980; **Resid:** Pediatrics, UCLA Med Ctr 1983; **Fellow:** Pediatric Gastroenterology, Hosp for Sick Children 1986; **Fac Appt:** Prof Ped, Univ Tex, Houston

West Coast and Pacific

Christie, Dennis L MD [PGe] - **Hospital:** Chldns Hosp and Regl Med Ctr - Seattle; **Address:** Chldns Hosp Med Ctr, Div Gastroenterology, 4800 Sand Point Way NE, MS 7830, Seattle, WA 98105-3901; **Phone:** 206-987-2521; **Board Cert:** Pediatrics 1992; Pediatric Gastroenterology 2005; **Med School:** Northwestern Univ 1968; **Resid:** Pediatrics, Univ Wash Med Ctr 1971; **Fellow:** Pediatric Gastroenterology, UCLA Ctr Hlth Sci 1976; **Fac Appt:** Prof Ped, Univ Wash

Heyman, Melvin Bernard MD [PGe] - **Spec Exp:** Inflammatory Bowel Disease/Crohn's; Short Bowel Syndrome; Gastroesophageal Reflux Disease (GERD); **Hospital:** UCSF Med Ctr; **Address:** UCSF, Dept Ped Gastroenterology, 400 Parnassus Ave Fl 2, San Francisco, CA 94143-0136; **Phone:** 415-476-5892; **Board Cert:** Pediatrics 1981; Pediatric Gastroenterology 2005; **Med School:** UCLA 1976; **Resid:** Pediatrics, LAC-USC Med Ctr 1979; **Fellow:** Gastroenterology, UCLA Med Ctr 1981; Nutrition, Human Nutrition Res Ctr 1990; **Fac Appt:** Prof Ped, UCSF

McDiarmid, Suzanne V MD [PGe] - **Spec Exp:** Transplant Medicine-Liver; Transplant Medicine-Intestine; Transplant Immunology; **Hospital:** Ronald Reagan UCLA Med Ctr; **Address:** UCLA Med Ctr, 18033 Leconte Ave, Room MDCC 12-328, Los Angeles, CA 90095; **Phone:** 310-206-6134; **Board Cert:** Pediatrics 1984; Pediatric Gastroenterology 2000; **Med School:** New Zealand 1976; **Resid:** Pediatrics, UCLA Med Center 1980; **Fac Appt:** Prof Ped, UCLA

Sinatra, Frank R MD [PGe] - **Spec Exp:** Liver Disease; **Hospital:** Women & Children's Hosp - LA, Chldns Hosp - Los Angeles; **Address:** Women's & Children's Hospital, 1240 N Mission Rd, rm L902, Los Angeles, CA 90033; **Phone:** 323-226-3691; **Board Cert:** Pediatrics 1992; Pediatric Gastroenterology 2005; **Med School:** USC Sch Med 1971; **Resid:** Pediatrics, Children's Hosp 1974; **Fellow:** Gastroenterology, Stanford Univ Med Ctr 1976; **Fac Appt:** Prof Ped, USC Sch Med

PEDIATRIC HEMATOLOGY-ONCOLOGY

New England

Albritton, Karen H MD [PHO] - **Spec Exp:** Sarcoma; Adolescent/Young Adult Cancers; **Hospital:** Dana-Farber Cancer Inst; **Address:** Dana Farber Cancer Inst, 44 Binney St, Smith 338, Boston, MA 02115; **Phone:** 617-582-7976; **Board Cert:** Pediatric Hematology-Oncology 2002; Medical Oncology 2001; **Med School:** Univ Tex, San Antonio 1992; **Resid:** Internal Medicine & Pediatrics, Univ NC Hosps 1996; **Fellow:** Hematology & Oncology, Univ NC Hosps 2000

Altman, Arnold MD [PHO] - **Spec Exp:** Leukemia; **Hospital:** CT Chldns Med Ctr; **Address:** CT Childrens Med Ctr, Hematology/Oncology, 282 Washington St, Ste 2J, Hartford, CT 06106; **Phone:** 860-545-9630; **Board Cert:** Pediatrics 1971; Pediatric Hematology-Oncology 1974; **Med School:** Johns Hopkins Univ 1965; **Resid:** Pediatrics, Chldns Hosp Med Ctr 1970; **Fellow:** Pediatric Hematology-Oncology, Chldns Hosp Med Ctr 1972; **Fac Appt:** Prof Ped, Univ Conn

Diller, Lisa R MD [PHO] - **Spec Exp:** Neuroblastoma; Cancer Survivors-Late Effects of Therapy; **Hospital:** Dana-Farber Cancer Inst; **Address:** Dana-Farber Cancer Inst, 44 Binney St, Shields Warren 312, Boston, MA 02115; **Phone:** 617-632-5642; **Board Cert:** Pediatric Hematology-Oncology 2007; **Med School:** UCSD 1985; **Resid:** Pediatrics, Chldns Hosp 1988; **Fellow:** Pediatric Hematology-Oncology, Chldns Hosp-Dana Farber Cancer Inst 1991; **Fac Appt:** Assoc Prof Ped, Harvard Med Sch

Grier, Holcombe E MD [PHO] - **Spec Exp:** Bone Cancer; Ewing's Sarcoma; **Hospital:** Dana-Farber Cancer Inst, Children's Hospital - Boston; **Address:** Dana Farber Cancer Inst, 44 Binney St, G350, Boston, MA 02115; **Phone:** 617-632-3971; **Board Cert:** Pediatrics 1983; Internal Medicine 1980; Pediatric Hematology-Oncology 2005; **Med School:** Univ Pennsylvania 1976; **Resid:** Pediatrics, NC Meml Hosp 1980; Internal Medicine, NC Meml Hosp 1980; **Fellow:** Pediatric Oncology, Dana Farber Chldn's Hosp 1984; **Fac Appt:** Assoc Prof Ped, Harvard Med Sch

Homans, Alan C MD [PHO] - **Spec Exp:** Leukemia; **Hospital:** FAHC - Med Ctr Campus; **Address:** Vermont Childrens Hosp, 111 Colchester Ave, Smith 5-rm 559, Burlington, VT 05401; **Phone:** 802-847-2850; **Board Cert:** Pediatrics 1985; Pediatric Hematology-Oncology 1987; **Med School:** Ohio State Univ 1979; **Resid:** Pediatrics, Med Ctr Hosp 1981; Pediatrics, Univ Massachusetts Med Ctr 1981; **Fellow:** Pediatric Hematology-Oncology, Rhode Island Hosp 1985; **Fac Appt:** Prof Ped, Univ VT Coll Med

Israel, Mark A MD [PHO] - **Spec Exp:** Neuro-Oncology; Brain Tumors; Neuroblastoma; **Hospital:** Dartmouth - Hitchcock Med Ctr; **Address:** Norris Cotton Cancer Ctr, One Medical Center Drive, Lebanon, NH 03756; **Phone:** 603-653-3611; **Board Cert:** Pediatrics 1982; **Med School:** Albert Einstein Coll Med 1973; **Resid:** Pediatrics, Chldns Hosp Med Ctr 1975; **Fellow:** Pediatric Hematology-Oncology, Natl Cancer Inst 1981; **Fac Appt:** Prof Ped, Dartmouth Med Sch

Kieran, Mark MD/PhD [PHO] - **Spec Exp:** Brain Tumors; Neuro-Oncology; **Hospital:** Children's Hospital - Boston, Dana-Farber Cancer Inst; **Address:** Dana Farber Cancer Inst, 44 Binney St, Shields Warren Ste 331, Boston, MA 02115; **Phone:** 617-632-2680; **Board Cert:** Pediatric Hematology-Oncology 2004; **Med School:** Univ Calgary 1986; **Resid:** Pediatrics, Montreal Chldns Hosp 1992; **Fellow:** Pediatric Hematology-Oncology, Chldns Hosp 1995; **Fac Appt:** Asst Prof Ped, Harvard Med Sch

Pediatric Hematology-Oncology

Kretschmar, Cynthia S MD [PHO] - **Spec Exp:** Brain Tumors; Neuroblastoma; Drug Discovery & Development; **Hospital:** Tufts Med Ctr; **Address:** Floating Hosp, Div Pediatric Hem/Onc, 750 Washington St, NEMC 14, Boston, MA 02111; **Phone:** 617-636-5535; **Board Cert:** Pediatrics 1984; Pediatric Hematology-Oncology 1987; **Med School:** Yale Univ 1978; **Resid:** Pediatrics, Yale-New Haven Hosp 1981; **Fellow:** Pediatric Hematology-Oncology, Dana Farber Cancer Inst 1984; **Fac Appt:** Prof Ped, Tufts Univ

Sallan, Stephen MD [PHO] - **Spec Exp:** Pediatric Cancers; Leukemia; **Hospital:** Children's Hospital - Boston; **Address:** Dana Farber Cancer Inst, Dept Ped Oncology, 44 Binney St, Ste 1642, Boston, MA 02115; **Phone:** 617-632-3316; **Board Cert:** Pediatrics 1972; **Med School:** Wayne State Univ 1967; **Resid:** Pediatrics, Chldns Hosp 1969; Pediatrics, Hosp Sick Chldn 1970; **Fellow:** Pediatric Oncology, Chldns Hosp Med Ctr 1975; **Fac Appt:** Prof Ped, Harvard Med Sch

Schwartz, Cindy Lee MD [PHO] - **Spec Exp:** Hodgkin's Disease; Bone Cancer; Cancer Survivors-Late Effects of Therapy; **Hospital:** Rhode Island Hosp; **Address:** RI Hospital, Dept Ped-Div Ped Hem/Onc, 593 Eddy St, MPS, rm 117, Providence, RI 02903-4923; **Phone:** 401-444-5171; **Board Cert:** Pediatrics 1985; Pediatric Hematology-Oncology 2002; **Med School:** Brown Univ 1979; **Resid:** Pediatrics, Johns Hopkins Hosp 1982; **Fellow:** Pediatric Hematology-Oncology, Johns Hopkins Hosp 1985; **Fac Appt:** Prof Med, Brown Univ

Weinstein, Howard J MD [PHO] - **Spec Exp:** Bone Marrow Transplant; Leukemia; Lymphoma; **Hospital:** Mass Genl Hosp; **Address:** 55 Fruit St, Yawkey 8B-8893, Boston, MA 02114-2622; **Phone:** 617-724-3315; **Board Cert:** Pediatrics 1977; **Med School:** Univ MD Sch Med 1972; **Resid:** Pediatrics, Mass Genl Hosp 1974; **Fellow:** Pediatric Hematology-Oncology, Dana Farber Cancer Inst/Chldns Hosp 1977; **Fac Appt:** Prof Ped, Harvard Med Sch

Wolfe, Lawrence C MD [PHO] - **Spec Exp:** Leukemia; Neuro-Oncology; Cancer Survivors-Late Effects of Therapy; Transfusion Medicine; **Hospital:** Tufts Med Ctr, St Anne's Hosp; **Address:** Floating Hosp, Div Pediatric Hem/Onc, 750 Washington St, NEMC 014, Boston, MA 02111; **Phone:** 617-636-5535; **Board Cert:** Pediatrics 1981; Pediatric Hematology-Oncology 1987; **Med School:** Harvard Med Sch 1976; **Resid:** Pediatrics, Chldns Hosp 1978; **Fellow:** Pediatric Hematology-Oncology, Chldns Hosp 1991; **Fac Appt:** Prof Ped, Tulane Univ

Mid Atlantic

Adamson, Peter C MD [PHO] - **Spec Exp:** Drug Development; Clinical Trials; Rhabdomyosarcoma; Pediatric Cancers; **Hospital:** Chldns Hosp of Philadelphia, The; **Address:** Chldns Hosp of Philadelphia, 34th St & Civic Ctr Blvd Abramson Bldg, Philadelphia, PA 19104; **Phone:** 215-590-2299; **Board Cert:** Pediatrics 1988; Pediatric Hematology-Oncology 2005; **Med School:** Cornell Univ-Weill Med Coll 1984; **Resid:** Pediatrics, Children's Hosp 1987; **Fellow:** Pediatric Hematology-Oncology, Natl Cancer Inst 1990; **Fac Appt:** Assoc Prof Pharm, Univ Pennsylvania

Arceci, Robert J MD/PhD [PHO] - **Spec Exp:** Leukemia; Histiocytoma; Bone Marrow Transplant; **Hospital:** Johns Hopkins Hosp - Baltimore (page 61); **Address:** Kimmel Cancer Ctr, Bunting-Blaustein Bldg, 1650 Orleans St, I-207, Baltimore, MD 21231-1000; **Phone:** 410-502-7519; **Board Cert:** Pediatrics 1987; Pediatric Hematology-Oncology 2005; **Med School:** Univ Rochester 1981; **Resid:** Pediatrics, Chldns Hosp 1983; **Fellow:** Pediatric Hematology-Oncology, Chldns Hosp/Dana Farber Cancer Ctr 1986; **Fac Appt:** Prof Ped, Johns Hopkins Univ

Brecher, Martin L MD [PHO] - **Spec Exp:** Brain Tumors; Lymphoma; Hodgkin's Disease; Leukemia; **Hospital:** Roswell Park Cancer Inst, Women's & Chldn's Hosp of Buffalo, The; **Address:** Roswell Park Cancer Inst, Dept Pediatrics, Elm & Carlton Sts, Buffalo, NY 14263; **Phone:** 716-845-2333; **Board Cert:** Pediatrics 1977; Pediatric Hematology-Oncology 1978; **Med School:** SUNY Buffalo 1972; **Resid:** Pediatrics, Buffalo Chldns Hosp 1975; **Fellow:** Hematology & Oncology, Buffalo Chldns Hosp/Roswell Park Cancer Inst 1977; **Fac Appt:** Prof Ped, SUNY Buffalo

Brodeur, Garrett MD [PHO] - **Spec Exp:** Neuroblastoma; **Hospital:** Chldns Hosp of Philadelphia, The; **Address:** Chldns Hosp Philadelphia, 34th St & Civic Ctr Blvd Abramson Bldg, Philadelphia, PA 19104; **Phone:** 215-590-2817; **Board Cert:** Pediatrics 1980; Pediatric Hematology-Oncology 1980; **Med School:** Washington Univ, St Louis 1975; **Resid:** Pediatrics, St Louis Childrens Hosp 1977; **Fellow:** Pediatric Hematology-Oncology, St Jude Childrens Rsch Hosp 1979; **Fac Appt:** Prof Ped, Univ Pennsylvania

Bussel, James MD [PHO] - **Spec Exp:** Autoimmune Disease; Bleeding/Coagulation Disorders; **Hospital:** NY-Presby Hosp/Weill Cornell (page 66), Lenox Hill Hosp (page 62); **Address:** 525 E 68th St, rm P-695, New York, NY 10021; **Phone:** 212-746-3474; **Board Cert:** Pediatrics 1979; Pediatric Hematology-Oncology 1981; **Med School:** Columbia P&S 1975; **Resid:** Pediatrics, Chldns Hosp 1978; **Fellow:** Pediatric Hematology-Oncology, NY Hosp 1981; **Fac Appt:** Prof Ped, Cornell Univ-Weill Med Coll

Cairo, Mitchell S MD [PHO] - **Spec Exp:** Bone Marrow Transplant; Leukemia; Lymphoma; **Hospital:** NYPresby-Morgan Stanley Children's Hosp (page 66); **Address:** Babies/Chldns Hosp-Presby Med Ctr, 3959 Broadway, CHN 10-03, New York, NY 10032; **Phone:** 212-305-8316; **Board Cert:** Pediatrics 1980; Pediatric Hematology-Oncology 1982; **Med School:** UCSF 1976; **Resid:** Pediatrics, UCLA Med Ctr 1978; **Fellow:** Pediatric Hematology-Oncology, Indiana Univ Med Ctr 1981; **Fac Appt:** Prof Ped, Columbia P&S

Carroll, William L MD [PHO] - **Spec Exp:** Pediatric Cancers; Leukemia; **Hospital:** NYU Med Ctr (page 68); **Address:** NYU Med Ctr, Div Ped Hem/Onc, 160 E 32nd St Fl 2, New York, NY 10016; **Phone:** 212-263-9947; **Board Cert:** Pediatrics 1984; Pediatric Hematology-Oncology 1987; **Med School:** UC Irvine 1978; **Resid:** Pediatrics, Chldns Hosp Med Ctr 1981; **Fellow:** Pediatric Hematology-Oncology, Stanford Univ 1987; **Fac Appt:** Prof Ped, NYU Sch Med

Chen, Allen R MD/PhD [PHO] - **Spec Exp:** Bone Marrow Transplant; Hodgkin's Disease; Immunotherapy; Graft vs Host Disease; **Hospital:** Johns Hopkins Hosp - Baltimore (page 61); **Address:** Johns Hopkins Hosp, Div Peds Oncology, 1650 Orleans St, CRB 2M53, Baltimore, MD 21231; **Phone:** 410-955-7385; **Board Cert:** Pediatrics 2002; **Med School:** Duke Univ 1986; **Resid:** Pediatrics, Chldns Hosp Med Ctr 1989; **Fellow:** Pediatric Hematology-Oncology, Fred Hutchinson Canc Ctr 1993; Bone Marrow Transplant, Fred Hutchinson Canc Ctr 1994; **Fac Appt:** Assoc Prof Ped, Johns Hopkins Univ

Civin, Curt Ingraham MD [PHO] - **Spec Exp:** Pediatric Cancers; Leukemia; Bone Marrow Transplant; **Hospital:** Johns Hopkins Hosp - Baltimore (page 61); **Address:** 1650 Orleans St, rm CRB-2M44, Baltimore, MD 21231-1000; **Phone:** 410-955-8816; **Board Cert:** Pediatrics 1979; Pediatric Hematology-Oncology 1980; **Med School:** Harvard Med Sch 1974; **Resid:** Pediatrics, Chldns Hosp 1976; **Fellow:** Pediatric Hematology-Oncology, Natl Cancer Inst 1979; **Fac Appt:** Prof Ped, Johns Hopkins Univ

Drachtman, Richard A MD [PHO] - **Spec Exp:** Pediatric Cancers; Sickle Cell Disease; **Hospital:** Robert Wood Johnson Univ Hosp - New Brunswick, Jersey Shore Univ Med Ctr; **Address:** Cancer Inst of New Jersey, 195 Little Albany St, New Brunswick, NJ 08903-2681; **Phone:** 732-235-5437; **Board Cert:** Pediatric Hematology-Oncology 2007; **Med School:** Ros Franklin Univ/Chicago Med Sch 1984; **Resid:** Pediatrics, N Shore Univ Hosp 1988; **Fellow:** Pediatric Hematology-Oncology, Mount Sinai Hosp 1991; **Fac Appt:** Assoc Prof Ped, UMDNJ-RW Johnson Med Sch

Pediatric Hematology-Oncology

Dunkel, Ira J MD [PHO] - **Spec Exp:** Retinoblastoma; Brain & Spinal Cord Tumors; Brain Tumors; Pediatric Cancers; **Hospital:** Meml Sloan-Kettering Cancer Ctr; **Address:** 1275 York Avenue, New York, NY 10065; **Phone:** 800-525-2225; **Board Cert:** Pediatric Hematology-Oncology 2007; **Med School:** Duke Univ 1985; **Resid:** Pediatrics, Duke Univ Med Ctr 1988; **Fellow:** Pediatric Hematology-Oncology, Memorial-Sloan Kettering 1992; **Fac Appt:** Asst Prof Ped, Cornell Univ-Weill Med Coll

Felix, Carolyn A MD [PHO] - **Spec Exp:** Leukemia; Leukemia in Infants; **Hospital:** Chldns Hosp of Philadelphia, The; **Address:** Chldns Hosp of Philadelphia, 34th St & Civic Ctr Blvd Abramson Bldg, Philadelphia, PA 19104; **Phone:** 215-590-2831; **Board Cert:** Pediatrics 1987; Pediatric Hematology-Oncology 1987; **Med School:** Boston Univ 1981; **Resid:** Pediatrics, Chldns Hosp 1984; **Fellow:** Pediatric Hematology-Oncology, Natl Cancer Inst-Pediatric Br 1987; **Fac Appt:** Assoc Prof Ped, Univ Pennsylvania

Frantz, Christopher N MD [PHO] - **Spec Exp:** Solid Tumors; Neuroblastoma; Leukemia; **Hospital:** Alfred I duPont Hosp for Children, Christiana Care Hlth Svs; **Address:** Alfred I duPont Hosp for Chldn, 1600 Rockland Rd, Box 269, Wilmington, DE 19899; **Phone:** 302-651-5500; **Board Cert:** Pediatrics 1977; Pediatric Hematology-Oncology 2005; **Med School:** Albert Einstein Coll Med 1971; **Resid:** Pediatrics, Chldns Hosp 1976; **Fellow:** Pediatric Hematology-Oncology, Chldns Hosp/Dana Farber Cancer Inst 1979

Garvin, James MD/PhD [PHO] - **Spec Exp:** Brain Tumors; Pediatric Cancers; Bone Marrow Transplant; **Hospital:** NYPresby-Morgan Stanley Children's Hosp (page 66); **Address:** 161 Fort Washington Ave Fl 7 - rm 708, New York, NY 10032-3729; **Phone:** 212-305-8685; **Board Cert:** Pediatrics 1982; Pediatric Hematology-Oncology 1984; **Med School:** Jefferson Med Coll 1976; **Resid:** Pediatrics, Chldns Hosp 1978; Pediatrics, Middlesex Hosp 1979; **Fellow:** Pediatric Hematology-Oncology, Dana Farber Cancer Inst/Childrens Hosp 1982; **Fac Appt:** Clin Prof Ped, Columbia P&S

Giardina, Patricia MD [PHO] - **Spec Exp:** Thalassemia; **Hospital:** NY-Presby Hosp/Weill Cornell (page 66); **Address:** 525 E 68th St, rm P 695, New York, NY 10065; **Phone:** 212-746-3400; **Board Cert:** Pediatrics 1974; Pediatric Hematology-Oncology 1974; **Med School:** NY Med Coll 1968; **Resid:** Pediatrics, Lenox Hill Hosp; Pediatrics, NY Hosp-Cornell Med Ctr

Grupp, Stephan A MD [PHO] - **Spec Exp:** Stem Cell Transplant; Neuroblastoma; Bone Marrow Transplant; **Hospital:** Chldns Hosp of Philadelphia, The; **Address:** Childrens Hosp - Oncology, 34th St & Civic Ctr Blvd Abramson Bldg, Philadelphia, PA 19104; **Phone:** 215-590-2821; **Board Cert:** Pediatric Hematology-Oncology 2002; **Med School:** Univ Cincinnati 1987; **Resid:** Pediatrics, Chldns Hosp 1990; **Fellow:** Pediatric Hematology-Oncology, Dana Farber Cancer Inst/Chldns Hosp 1992; **Fac Appt:** Asst Prof Ped, Univ Pennsylvania

Halpern, Steven MD [PHO] - **Spec Exp:** Leukemia & Lymphoma; Brain Tumors; Hodgkin's Disease; Hemophilia; **Hospital:** Hackensack Univ Med Ctr, Overlook Hosp; **Address:** 30 Prospect Ave, Ste TCI, Hackensack, NJ 07601; **Phone:** 201-996-5437; **Board Cert:** Pediatrics 1981; Pediatric Hematology-Oncology 1982; **Med School:** Ros Franklin Univ/Chicago Med Sch 1976; **Resid:** Pediatrics, St Christopher's Hosp for Children 1979; **Fellow:** Pediatric Hematology-Oncology, Childrens Hosp 1982; **Fac Appt:** Asst Prof Ped, UMDNJ-NJ Med Sch, Newark

Harris, Michael B MD [PHO] - **Spec Exp:** Leukemia & Lymphoma; Bone Tumors; Cancer Survivors-Late Effects of Therapy; **Hospital:** Hackensack Univ Med Ctr; **Address:** Tomorrows Chldns Inst, JM Sanzari Chldns Hosp, 30 Prospect Ave, Imus 1-TCI, rm PC116, Hackensack, NJ 07601; **Phone:** 201-996-5437; **Board Cert:** Pediatrics 1974; Pediatric Hematology-Oncology 1974; **Med School:** Albert Einstein Coll Med 1969; **Resid:** Pediatrics, Chldns Hosp 1971; **Fellow:** Pediatric Hematology-Oncology, Chldns Hosp 1974; **Fac Appt:** Prof Ped, UMDNJ-NJ Med Sch, Newark

Helman, Lee Jay MD [PHO] - **Spec Exp:** Solid Tumors; **Hospital:** Natl Inst of Hlth - Clin Ctr; **Address:** National Cancer Inst, NIH, 31 Center Drive, rm 3A11, Bethesda, MD 20892-2440; **Phone:** 301-496-4257; **Board Cert:** Internal Medicine 1983; Medical Oncology 1985; **Med School:** Univ MD Sch Med 1980; **Resid:** Internal Medicine, Barnes Hosp 1983; **Fellow:** Oncology, Natl Inst Hlth 1986

Hinkle, Andrea S MD [PHO] - **Spec Exp:** Cancer Survivors-Late Effects of Therapy; **Hospital:** Univ of Rochester Strong Meml Hosp; **Address:** Golisano Childrens Hosp at Strong, 601 Elmwood Ave, Box 667, Rochester, NY 14642; **Phone:** 585-275-8138; **Board Cert:** Pediatrics 2006; Pediatric Hematology-Oncology 2000; **Med School:** Brown Univ 1987; **Resid:** Pediatrics, Boston City Hosp 1991; **Fellow:** Pediatric Hematology-Oncology, Chldns Natl Med Ctr 1994; **Fac Appt:** Asst Prof Ped, Univ Rochester

Jakacki, Regina MD [PHO] - **Spec Exp:** Neuro-Oncology; Clinical Trials; Palliative Care; **Hospital:** Chldns Hosp of Pittsburgh - UPMC; **Address:** Children's Hospital Pittsburgh, 3705 Fifth Ave, rm 4B 220, Pittsburgh, PA 15213; **Phone:** 412-692-7056; **Board Cert:** Pediatric Hematology-Oncology 2007; **Med School:** Univ Pennsylvania 1985; **Resid:** Pediatrics, Childrens Hosp 1988; **Fellow:** Pediatric Hematology-Oncology, Childrens Hosp 1991; **Fac Appt:** Assoc Prof Ped, Univ Pittsburgh

Jayabose, Somasundaram MD [PHO] - **Spec Exp:** Sickle Cell Disease; Leukemia; Lymphoma; **Hospital:** Westchester Med Ctr, Good Samaritan Hosp - Suffern; **Address:** NY Med Coll, Dept Pediatrics, Munger Pavilion, rm 110, Valhalla, NY 10595; **Phone:** 914-493-7997; **Board Cert:** Pediatrics 1975; Pediatric Hematology-Oncology 1976; **Med School:** India 1969; **Resid:** Pediatrics, Metropolitan Hosp Ctr 1974; **Fellow:** Pediatric Hematology-Oncology, LI Jewish Med Ctr 1976; **Fac Appt:** Prof Ped, NY Med Coll

Kamen, Barton A MD/PhD [PHO] - **Spec Exp:** Drug Development; Leukemia; **Hospital:** Robert Wood Johnson Univ Hosp - New Brunswick; **Address:** Cancer Inst of New Jersey, 195 Little Albany St, rm 3507, New Brunswick, NJ 08903; **Phone:** 732-235-8864; **Board Cert:** Pediatrics 1981; Pediatric Hematology-Oncology 1987; **Med School:** Case West Res Univ 1976; **Resid:** Pediatrics, Yale-New Haven Hosp 1978; **Fellow:** Pediatric Hematology-Oncology, Yale-New Haven Hosp 1980; **Fac Appt:** Prof Ped, UMDNJ-RW Johnson Med Sch

Korones, David N MD [PHO] - **Spec Exp:** Brain Tumors; Palliative Care; Pediatric Cancers; **Hospital:** Univ of Rochester Strong Meml Hosp; **Address:** Golisano Childrens Hosp at Strong, 601 Elmwood Ave, Box 777, Rochester, NY 14642-8777; **Phone:** 585-275-2981; **Board Cert:** Pediatrics 1987; Pediatric Hematology-Oncology 2006; Hospice & Palliative Medicine 2002; **Med School:** Vanderbilt Univ 1983; **Resid:** Pediatrics, Strong Meml Hosp 1986; **Fellow:** Pediatrics, Yale Univ 1988; Pediatric Hematology-Oncology, Strong Meml Hosp 1991; **Fac Appt:** Assoc Prof Ped, Univ Rochester

Kushner, Brian H MD [PHO] - **Spec Exp:** Neuroblastoma; Bone Marrow Transplant; Immunotherapy; **Hospital:** Meml Sloan-Kettering Cancer Ctr; **Address:** 1275 York Avenue, New York, NY 10065; **Phone:** 800-525-2225; **Board Cert:** Pediatrics 1983; Pediatric Hematology-Oncology 1987; **Med School:** Johns Hopkins Univ 1976; **Resid:** Pediatrics, Columbia-Presby Med Ctr 1978; Pediatrics, New York Hosp 1979; **Fellow:** Pediatric Hematology-Oncology, Boston Chldns Hosp 1980; Pediatric Hematology-Oncology, Meml Sloan Kettering Cancer Ctr 1986; **Fac Appt:** Prof Ped, Cornell Univ-Weill Med Coll

Pediatric Hematology-Oncology

Lange, Beverly J MD [PHO] - **Spec Exp:** Leukemia; Brain & Spinal Cord Tumors; **Hospital:** Chldns Hosp of Philadelphia, The; **Address:** Chldns Hosp Phila, Medical Oncology, 34th St & Civic Ctr Blvd, Wood Center, 4th Fl, Philadelphia, PA 19104; **Phone:** 215-590-2249; **Board Cert:** Pediatrics 1976; Pediatric Hematology-Oncology 1997; **Med School:** Temple Univ 1971; **Resid:** Pediatrics, Philadelphia Genl Hosp 1973; **Fellow:** Pediatric Oncology, Chldns Hosp; **Fac Appt:** Prof Ped, Univ Pennsylvania

Lipton, Jeffrey M MD/PhD [PHO] - **Spec Exp:** Bone Marrow Failure Disorders; Stem Cell Transplant; Bone Marrow Transplant; **Hospital:** Schneider Chldn's Hosp; **Address:** Div Hem-Onc & Stem Cell Transplant, 269-01 76th Ave, rm 255, MC-07670, New Hyde Park, NY 11040-1433; **Phone:** 718-470-3460; **Board Cert:** Pediatrics 1981; **Med School:** St Louis Univ 1975; **Resid:** Pediatrics, Boston Chldns Hosp 1977; **Fellow:** Pediatric Hematology-Oncology, Boston Chldns Hosp/Dana Farber Cancer Inst 1979; **Fac Appt:** Prof Ped, Albert Einstein Coll Med

Luchtman-Jones, Lori MD [PHO] - **Spec Exp:** Leukemia; Bleeding/Coagulation Disorders; **Hospital:** Chldns Natl Med Ctr; **Address:** Chldn's Natl Med Ctr, 111 Michigan Ave NW Fl 4 - Ste 4043, Washington, DC 20010; **Phone:** 202-476-2140; **Board Cert:** Pediatrics 1999; Pediatric Hematology-Oncology 2004; **Med School:** UCSD 1987; **Resid:** Pediatrics, UCSD School Med 1990; **Fellow:** Pediatric Hematology-Oncology, Washington Univ 1995; **Fac Appt:** Asst Prof Ped, Washington Univ, St Louis

Maris, John M MD [PHO] - **Spec Exp:** Neuroblastoma; Clinical Trials; **Hospital:** Chldns Hosp of Philadelphia, The; **Address:** Chldns Hosp Philadelphia - Oncology, 34th St & Civic Ctr Blvd Abramson Bldg, Philadelphia, PA 19104-4318; **Phone:** 215-590-5244; **Board Cert:** Pediatric Hematology-Oncology 2004; **Med School:** Univ Pennsylvania 1989; **Resid:** Pediatrics, Chldns Hosp 1992; **Fellow:** Pediatric Hematology-Oncology, Chldns Hosp 1996

Meadows, Anna T MD [PHO] - **Spec Exp:** Cancer Survivors-Late Effects of Therapy; Clinical Trials; Retinoblastoma; **Hospital:** Chldns Hosp of Philadelphia, The; **Address:** Childrens Hospital, Div Oncology, 34th St & Civic Center Blvd, Philadelphia, PA 19104; **Phone:** 215-590-2804; **Board Cert:** Pediatrics 1974; Pediatric Hematology-Oncology 1974; **Med School:** Med Coll PA 1969; **Resid:** Pediatrics, St Christopher's Hosp 1971; **Fellow:** Pediatric Hematology-Oncology, St Christopher's Hosp 1972; **Fac Appt:** Prof Ped, Univ Pennsylvania

Meek, Rita S MD [PHO] - **Hospital:** Alfred I duPont Hosp for Children, Christiana Care Hlth Svs; **Address:** Dupont Hosp for Children, Div Hem-Onc, 1600 Rockland Rd, Wilmington, DE 19899; **Phone:** 302-651-5500; **Board Cert:** Pediatrics 1979; Pediatric Hematology-Oncology 1980; **Med School:** Geo Wash Univ 1974; **Resid:** Pediatrics, Childns Hosp Natl Med Ctr 1977; **Fellow:** Pediatric Hematology-Oncology, Chldns Hosp Natl Med Ctr 1979; **Fac Appt:** Assoc Clin Prof Ped, Jefferson Med Coll

Meyers, Paul MD [PHO] - **Spec Exp:** Pediatric Cancers; Bone Tumors; Sarcoma; **Hospital:** Meml Sloan-Kettering Cancer Ctr, NY-Presby Hosp/Weill Cornell (page 66); **Address:** 1275 York Avenue, New York, NY 10065; **Phone:** 800-525-2225; **Board Cert:** Pediatrics 1978; Pediatric Hematology-Oncology 1978; **Med School:** Mount Sinai Sch Med 1973; **Resid:** Pediatrics, Mt Sinai Hosp 1976; **Fellow:** Pediatric Hematology-Oncology, NY Hosp-Cornell Med Ctr 1979; **Fac Appt:** Prof Ped, Cornell Univ-Weill Med Coll

O'Reilly, Richard MD [PHO] - **Spec Exp:** Bone Marrow Transplant; **Hospital:** Meml Sloan-Kettering Cancer Ctr, NY-Presby Hosp/Weill Cornell (page 66); **Address:** 1275 York Avenue, New York, NY 10065; **Phone:** 800-525-2225; **Board Cert:** Pediatrics 1974; **Med School:** Univ Rochester 1968; **Resid:** Pediatrics, Chldrns Hosp 1972; **Fellow:** Infectious Disease, Chldrns Hosp 1973; **Fac Appt:** Prof Ped, Cornell Univ-Weill Med Coll

Parker, Robert MD [PHO] - **Spec Exp:** Pediatric Cancers; Bleeding/Coagulation Disorders; Platelet Disorders; Lymphoma; **Hospital:** Stony Brook Univ Med Ctr; **Address:** Stony Brook Univ Hosp, Dept Peds, HSC T-11, Rm 029, Stony Brook, NY 11794-8111; **Phone:** 631-444-7720; **Board Cert:** Pediatrics 1983; Pediatric Hematology-Oncology 1984; **Med School:** Brown Univ 1976; **Resid:** Internal Medicine, Roger Williams Med Ctr 1977; Pediatrics, Rhode Island Hosp 1979; **Fellow:** Pediatric Hematology-Oncology, Natl Cancer Inst 1981; Hematology, Natl Cancer Inst 1984; **Fac Appt:** Prof Ped, SUNY Stony Brook

Rausen, Aaron R MD [PHO] - **Spec Exp:** Leukemia & Lymphoma; Bone Tumors; Retinoblastoma; **Hospital:** NYU Med Ctr (page 68), Lenox Hill Hosp (page 62); **Address:** NYU Medical Ctr, 160 E 32nd St Fl 2, New York, NY 10016; **Phone:** 212-263-7144; **Board Cert:** Pediatrics 1960; Pediatric Hematology-Oncology 1974; **Med School:** SUNY Downstate 1954; **Resid:** Pediatrics, Bellevue Hosp 1956; Pediatrics, Mount Sinai 1959; **Fellow:** Hematology, Chldns Hosp 1961; **Fac Appt:** Prof Ped, NYU Sch Med

Reaman, Gregory MD [PHO] - **Spec Exp:** Leukemia; Lymphoma; Cancer Survivors-Late Effects of Therapy; **Hospital:** Chldns Natl Med Ctr; **Address:** 111 Michigan Ave NW, Washington, DC 20010-2916; **Phone:** 202-476-2800; **Board Cert:** Pediatrics 1978; Pediatric Hematology-Oncology 1978; **Med School:** Loyola Univ-Stritch Sch Med 1973; **Resid:** Hematology, Montreal Chldns Hosp 1975; Pediatrics, Montreal Chldns Hosp 1976; **Fellow:** Pediatric Oncology, Natl Cancer Inst 1979; **Fac Appt:** Prof Ped, Geo Wash Univ

Rheingold, Susan R MD [PHO] - **Spec Exp:** Leukemia; Clinical Trials; **Hospital:** Chldns Hosp of Philadelphia, The; **Address:** Chldns Hosp Phila - Div Oncology, 34th & Civic Ctr Blvd, Philadelphia, PA 19104; **Phone:** 215-590-3025; **Board Cert:** Pediatrics 2003; Pediatric Hematology-Oncology 2000; **Med School:** Univ Pennsylvania 1992; **Resid:** Pediatrics, Johns Hopkins Hosp 1995; **Fellow:** Pediatric Hematology-Oncology, Chldns Hosp 1999; **Fac Appt:** Asst Prof Ped, Univ Pennsylvania

Ritchey, Arthur MD [PHO] - **Spec Exp:** Leukemia; Bleeding/Coagulation Disorders; **Hospital:** Chldns Hosp of Pittsburgh - UPMC; **Address:** Chldns Hosp, Div Hematology/Oncology, 3705 Fifth Ave, Desoto Wing 4B, Ste 385, Pittsburgh, PA 15213; **Phone:** 412-692-5055; **Board Cert:** Pediatrics 1977; Pediatric Hematology-Oncology 2000; **Med School:** Univ Cincinnati 1972; **Resid:** Pediatrics, Johns Hopkins Hosp 1975; **Fellow:** Pediatric Hematology-Oncology, Yale-New Haven Hosp 1980; **Fac Appt:** Prof Ped, Univ Pittsburgh

Shafer, Frank E MD [PHO] - **Spec Exp:** Bleeding/Coagulation Disorders; Anemia; Thrombotic Disorders; Hemophilia; **Hospital:** St Christopher's Hosp for Chldn, St Luke's Hosp - Bethlehem; **Address:** St Christophers Hosp, Hematology, Erie Ave at Front St Fl 2, Philadelphia, PA 19134-1095; **Phone:** 215-427-5096; **Board Cert:** Pediatrics 2007; Pediatric Hematology-Oncology 2007; **Med School:** Creighton Univ 1983; **Resid:** Pediatrics, Univ Colo HSC 1986; **Fellow:** Pediatric Hematology-Oncology, Chldns Natl Med Ctr 1990; **Fac Appt:** Assoc Prof Ped, Drexel Univ Coll Med

Steinherz, Peter G MD [PHO] - **Spec Exp:** Leukemia & Lymphoma; Pediatric Cancers; Wilms' Tumor; **Hospital:** Meml Sloan-Kettering Cancer Ctr, NY-Presby Hosp/Weill Cornell (page 66); **Address:** 1275 York Avenue, New York, NY 10065; **Phone:** 800-525-2225; **Board Cert:** Pediatrics 1973; Pediatric Hematology-Oncology 1978; **Med School:** Albert Einstein Coll Med 1968; **Resid:** Pediatrics, New York Hosp-Cornell 1971; **Fellow:** Pediatric Hematology-Oncology, New York Hosp-Cornell 1975; **Fac Appt:** Prof Ped, Cornell Univ-Weill Med Coll

Pediatric Hematology-Oncology

Weinblatt, Mark E MD [PHO] - **Spec Exp:** Leukemia & Lymphoma; Sickle Cell Disease/Anemia; Bleeding/Coagulation Disorders; Thalassemia; **Hospital:** Winthrop - Univ Hosp; **Address:** Winthrop Univ Hosp, 200 Old Country Rd, Mineola, NY 11501; **Phone:** 516-663-9400; **Board Cert:** Pediatrics 1980; Pediatric Hematology-Oncology 1982; **Med School:** Albert Einstein Coll Med 1976; **Resid:** Pediatrics, Jacobi Med Ctr 1979; **Fellow:** Pediatric Hematology-Oncology, Children's Hosp 1981; **Fac Appt:** Prof Ped, SUNY Stony Brook

Weiner, Michael MD [PHO] - **Spec Exp:** Hodgkin's Disease; Lymphoma; Leukemia; **Hospital:** NY-Presby Hosp/Columbia (page 66), St Joseph's Regl Med Ctr - Paterson; **Address:** 161 Fort Washington Ave, Irving Pavilion-FL 7, New York, NY 10032-3710; **Phone:** 212-305-9770; **Board Cert:** Pediatrics 1980; Pediatric Hematology-Oncology 1980; **Med School:** SUNY Hlth Sci Ctr 1972; **Resid:** Pediatrics, Montefiore Med Ctr 1974; **Fellow:** Pediatric Hematology-Oncology, NYU Med Ctr 1976; Pediatric Hematology-Oncology, Johns Hopkins Hosp 1977; **Fac Appt:** Prof Ped, Columbia P&S

Wexler, Leonard MD [PHO] - **Spec Exp:** Rhabdomyosarcoma; Bone Cancer; Gastrointestinal Stromal Tumors; Sarcoma-Soft Tissue; **Hospital:** Meml Sloan-Kettering Cancer Ctr; **Address:** 1275 York Avenue, New York, NY 10065; **Phone:** 800-525-2225; **Board Cert:** Pediatrics 2000; Pediatric Hematology-Oncology 2000; **Med School:** Boston Univ 1985; **Resid:** Pediatrics, Montefiore Med Ctr 1988; **Fellow:** Pediatric Hematology-Oncology, National Cancer Inst 1991; **Fac Appt:** Assoc Prof Ped, Columbia P&S

Southeast

Barredo, Julio C MD [PHO] - **Spec Exp:** Cancer Survivors-Late Effects of Therapy; Clinical Trials; **Hospital:** Univ of Miami Hosp & Clins/Sylvester Comp Canc Ctr; **Address:** Dept Pediatrics, R131 PO Box 016960, Miami, FL 33136; **Phone:** 305-585-5635; **Board Cert:** Pediatric Hematology-Oncology 2007; **Med School:** Peru 1982; **Resid:** Pediatrics, Kings Co Hosp 1987; **Fellow:** Pediatric Hematology-Oncology, Chldns Hosp/USC 1988; **Fac Appt:** Prof Ped, Med Univ SC

Bertolone, Salvatore MD [PHO] - **Spec Exp:** Bone Marrow Transplant; Kasabach-Merritt Syndrome (KMS); Sickle Cell Disease; **Hospital:** Kosair Chldn's Hosp, Norton Hosp; **Address:** Kosair Childrens Hosp, Dept Ped Hem/Onc, 571 S Floyd St, rm 445, Louisville, KY 40202-3820; **Phone:** 502-852-8450; **Board Cert:** Pediatrics 1975; Pediatric Hematology-Oncology 1976; **Med School:** Univ Louisville Sch Med 1970; **Resid:** Pediatrics, Univ Louisville 1972; **Fellow:** Pediatric Hematology-Oncology, Univ Colorado 1974; **Fac Appt:** Prof Ped, Univ Louisville Sch Med

Blatt, Julie MD [PHO] - **Spec Exp:** Neuroblastoma; Cancer Survivors-Late Effects of Therapy; **Hospital:** Univ NC Hosps; **Address:** UNC, Dept Ped Hematology Oncology, CB 7220, Chapel Hill, NC 27599-7220; **Phone:** 919-966-1178; **Board Cert:** Pediatrics 1981; Pediatric Hematology-Oncology 1982; **Med School:** Johns Hopkins Univ 1976; **Resid:** Pediatrics, Columbia-Presby Hosp 1978; **Fellow:** Pediatric Oncology, Natl Cancer Inst 1982; **Fac Appt:** Prof Ped, Univ NC Sch Med

Frangoul, Haydar A MD [PHO] - **Spec Exp:** Stem Cell Transplant; **Hospital:** Vanderbilt Univ Med Ctr; **Address:** Ped Hem/Onc Clinic, 1215 21st Ave S, 397 PRB, Nashville, TN 37232-6310; **Phone:** 615-936-1762; **Board Cert:** Pediatrics 2001; Pediatric Hematology-Oncology 2000; **Med School:** Amer Univ Beirut 1990; **Resid:** Pediatrics, Duke Univ Med Ctr 1993; **Fellow:** Pediatric Hematology-Oncology, Duke Univ Med Ctr 1994; **Fac Appt:** Assoc Prof Ped, Vanderbilt Univ

Friedman, Henry S MD [PHO] - **Spec Exp:** Neuro-Oncology; Brain & Spinal Cord Tumors; **Hospital:** Duke Univ Med Ctr; **Address:** Preston Robert Tisch, Brain Tumor Ctr at Duke, DUMC, rm 3624, Durham, NC 27710; **Phone:** 919-684-5301; **Board Cert:** Pediatrics 1982; Pediatric Hematology-Oncology 1982; **Med School:** SUNY Upstate Med Univ 1977; **Resid:** Pediatrics, SUNY Upstate Med Ctr 1980; **Fellow:** Pediatric Hematology-Oncology, Duke Univ Med Ctr 1983; **Fac Appt:** Prof Ped, Duke Univ

Furman, Wayne L MD [PHO] - **Spec Exp:** Neuroblastoma; Liver Cancer; Drug Development; **Hospital:** St Jude Children's Research Hosp; **Address:** St Jude Children's Research Hospital, 332 N Lauderdale St, MS 260, Memphis, TN 38105; **Phone:** 901-495-2800; **Board Cert:** Pediatrics 1985; Pediatric Hematology-Oncology 1987; **Med School:** Ohio State Univ 1979; **Resid:** Pediatrics, Children's Hosp 1983; **Fellow:** Pediatric Hematology-Oncology, St Jude Children's Rsch Hosp 1985; **Fac Appt:** Prof Ped, Univ Tenn Coll Med, Memphis

Gajjar, Amar MD [PHO] - **Spec Exp:** Brain Tumors; Medulloblastoma; Neuro-Oncology; Drug Development; **Hospital:** St Jude Children's Research Hosp; **Address:** St Judes Children's Hosp, Dept Oncology, 332 N Lauderdale, rm C6024, MS 260, Memphis, TN 38105-2794; **Phone:** 901-495-4599; **Board Cert:** Pediatrics 1989; Pediatric Hematology-Oncology 2000; **Med School:** India 1984; **Resid:** Pediatrics, All Children's Hosp 1989; **Fellow:** Hematology & Oncology, St Jude Children's Hosp 1990; **Fac Appt:** Prof Ped, Univ Tenn Coll Med, Memphis

Godder, Kamar MD/PhD [PHO] - **Spec Exp:** Stem Cell Transplant; Leukemia; Palliative Care; **Hospital:** Med Coll of VA Hosp; **Address:** PO Box 980121, Richmond, VA 23219; **Phone:** 804-828-9605; **Board Cert:** Pediatric Hematology-Oncology 2005; **Med School:** Israel 1980; **Resid:** Pediatrics, Hadassah-Mt Scopus 1984; **Fellow:** Pediatric Hematology-Oncology, Meml Sloan Kettering Cancer Ctr 1988; **Fac Appt:** Prof Ped, Va Commonwealth Univ Sch Med

Gold, Stuart H MD [PHO] - **Spec Exp:** Leukemia; Brain Tumors; Cancer Survivors-Late Effects of Therapy; **Hospital:** Univ NC Hosps; **Address:** UNC, Dept Ped Hematology Oncology, Univ of NC at Chapel Hill, CB# 7236, Chapel Hill, NC 27599-7220; **Phone:** 919-966-1178; **Board Cert:** Pediatrics 1986; Pediatric Hematology-Oncology 1987; **Med School:** Vanderbilt Univ 1981; **Resid:** Pediatrics, Univ Colorado Hlth Sci Ctr 1984; **Fellow:** Pediatric Hematology-Oncology, Univ Colorado Hlth Sci Ctr 1989; **Fac Appt:** Prof Ped, Univ NC Sch Med

Green, Daniel M MD [PHO] - **Spec Exp:** Wilms' Tumor; Fertility in Cancer Survivors; Cancer Survivors-Late Effects of Therapy; **Hospital:** St Jude Children's Research Hosp; **Address:** Dept Epidemiology & Cancer Control, St Jude Chldn's Rsch Hosp, 332 N Lauderdale St, MS 735, Memphis, TN 38105-2794; **Phone:** 901-495-5915; **Board Cert:** Pediatrics 1986; Pediatric Hematology-Oncology 1997; **Med School:** St Louis Univ 1973; **Resid:** Pediatrics, Boston City Hosp 1975; **Fellow:** Pediatric Hematology-Oncology, Chldn's Hosp Med Ctr 1978; **Fac Appt:** Prof Ped, Univ Tenn Coll Med, Memphis

Hudson, Melissa MD [PHO] - **Spec Exp:** Cancer Survivors-Late Effects of Therapy; Hodgkin's Disease; **Hospital:** St Jude Children's Research Hosp; **Address:** St Jude Children's Research Hosp, 332 N Lauderdale St, MS 735, Memphis, TN 38105; **Phone:** 901-495-3384; **Board Cert:** Pediatrics 1988; Pediatric Hematology-Oncology 2006; **Med School:** Univ Tex SW, Dallas 1983; **Resid:** Pediatrics, Univ Texas Affil Hosps 1986; **Fellow:** Pediatric Hematology-Oncology, MD Anderson Cancer Ctr 1989

Johnston, J Martin MD [PHO] - **Spec Exp:** Leukemia; Lymphoma; Hemophilia; **Hospital:** Meml Hlth Univ Med Ctr - Savannah; **Address:** Backus Children's Hosp Outpatient Ctr, 4700 Waters Ave, PO Box 23089, Savannah, GA 31403-3089; **Phone:** 912-350-8194; **Board Cert:** Pediatric Hematology-Oncology 2002; **Med School:** Duke Univ 1984; **Resid:** Pediatrics, Univ Utah Med Ctr 1988; **Fellow:** Pediatric Hematology-Oncology, Barnes Jewish Hosp 1991

Pediatric Hematology-Oncology

Kane, Javier R MD [PHO] - **Spec Exp:** Palliative Care; **Hospital:** St Jude Children's Research Hosp; **Address:** St Jude Chldns Rsch Hosp, Dept Oncology, 332 N Lauderdale St, rm C6040, MS 260, Memphis, TN 38105-2794; **Phone:** 901-495-4152; **Board Cert:** Pediatrics 2007; Pediatric Hematology-Oncology 2004; **Med School:** Mexico 1986; **Resid:** Pediatrics, Austin Med Ed Prog 1992; **Fellow:** Pediatric Hematology-Oncology, Univ Tennessee

Keller Jr, Frank G MD [PHO] - **Spec Exp:** Leukemia; Hodgkin's Disease; **Hospital:** Emory Univ Hosp; **Address:** Emory Healthcare Pediatrics Dept, 2015 Uppergate Drive NE Fl 4, Atlanta, GA 30322; **Phone:** 404-727-5740; **Board Cert:** Pediatric Hematology-Oncology 2002; **Med School:** Univ NC Sch Med 1986; **Resid:** Pediatrics, Vanderbilt Univ Med Ctr 1990; **Fellow:** Pediatric Hematology-Oncology, Duke Univ Med Ctr 1993; **Fac Appt:** Assoc Prof Ped, Emory Univ

Kreissman, Susan G MD [PHO] - **Spec Exp:** Neuroblastoma; Clinical Trials; **Hospital:** Duke Univ Med Ctr; **Address:** Duke Univ Med Ctr, Box 2916, Durham, NC 27710; **Phone:** 919-684-3401; **Board Cert:** Pediatric Hematology-Oncology 2004; **Med School:** Mount Sinai Sch Med 1985; **Resid:** Pediatrics, Chldns Hosp 1988; **Fellow:** Pediatric Hematology-Oncology, Chldns Hosp/Dana Farber Cancer Inst 1991; **Fac Appt:** Assoc Prof Ped, Duke Univ

Kurtzberg, Joanne MD [PHO] - **Spec Exp:** Stem Cell Transplant; Bone Marrow Transplant; **Hospital:** Duke Univ Med Ctr; **Address:** Duke Univ Med Ctr, Box 3350, Durham, NC 27710; **Phone:** 919-668-1100; **Board Cert:** Pediatrics 1982; Pediatric Hematology-Oncology 1982; **Med School:** NY Med Coll 1976; **Resid:** Pediatrics, Dartmouth Med Ctr 1977; Pediatrics, Upstate Med Ctr 1979; **Fellow:** Pediatric Hematology-Oncology, Upstate Med Ctr 1980; Pediatric Hematology-Oncology, Duke Med Ctr 1983; **Fac Appt:** Prof Ped, Duke Univ

Kuttesch, John F MD [PHO] - **Spec Exp:** Brain Tumors; Brain Tumors-Recurrent; **Hospital:** Vanderbilt Children's Hosp; **Address:** Vanderbilt Pediatric Hem/Oncology, 2220 Pierce Ave, Rm 397 PRB, Nashville, TN 37232-6310; **Phone:** 615-936-1762; **Board Cert:** Pediatric Hematology-Oncology 2007; **Med School:** Univ Tex, Houston 1985; **Resid:** Pediatrics, Vanderbilt Univ Med Ctr 1988; **Fellow:** Pediatric Hematology-Oncology, St Judes Chldns Hosp 1992; **Fac Appt:** Assoc Prof Ped, Vanderbilt Univ

Moscow, Jeffrey A MD [PHO] - **Spec Exp:** Pediatric Cancers; **Hospital:** Univ of Kentucky Chandler Hosp; **Address:** Univ Kentucky - Kentucky Clinic, 740 S Limestone, rm J457, Lexington, KY 40536-0001; **Phone:** 859-257-4554; **Board Cert:** Pediatrics 1988; Pediatric Hematology-Oncology 2006; **Med School:** Dartmouth Med Sch 1982; **Resid:** Pediatrics, Univ Texas SW Med Ctr 1985; **Fellow:** Pediatric Hematology-Oncology, Natl Cancer Inst 1986; **Fac Appt:** Prof Ped, Univ KY Coll Med

Neuberg, Ronnie W MD [PHO] - **Spec Exp:** Pediatric Cancers; Gene Therapy; Clinical Trials; Brain Tumors; **Hospital:** Palmetto Richland Mem Hosp; **Address:** Palmetto Health Richland, 7 Richland Medical Park Drive, Ste 203, Columbia, SC 29203; **Phone:** 803-434-3533; **Board Cert:** Pediatrics 1982; Pediatric Hematology-Oncology 1982; **Med School:** SUNY Buffalo 1977; **Resid:** Pediatrics, Childrens Hosp 1980; **Fellow:** Pediatric Hematology-Oncology, SUNY Upstate Med Ctr 1982; **Fac Appt:** Assoc Prof Ped, Univ SC Sch Med

Nieder, Michael L MD [PHO] - **Spec Exp:** Bone Marrow Transplant; **Hospital:** All Children's Hosp; **Address:** 801 6th St S, Dept 7865, St Petersburg, FL 33701-4816; **Phone:** 727-767-6856; **Board Cert:** Pediatrics 1986; Pediatric Hematology-Oncology 1987; **Med School:** Univ IL Coll Med 1982; **Resid:** Pediatrics, Children's Meml Hosp 1985; **Fellow:** Pediatric Hematology-Oncology, Children's Meml Hosp 1988; **Fac Appt:** Prof Ped, Univ S Fla Coll Med

Olson, Thomas A MD [PHO] - **Spec Exp:** Platelet Disorders; Sarcoma; Brain Tumors; **Hospital:** Emory Univ Hosp; **Address:** Aflac Cancer & Blood Disorders Ctr, Outpatient Clinic, 1405 Clifton Rd NE, Atlanta, GA 30322; **Phone:** 404-785-1200; **Board Cert:** Pediatrics 1982; Pediatric Hematology-Oncology 1984; **Med School:** Loyola Univ-Stritch Sch Med 1978; **Resid:** Pediatrics, Walter Reed AMC 1981; **Fellow:** Pediatric Hematology-Oncology, Walter Reed AMC 1983; **Fac Appt:** Assoc Prof Ped, Emory Univ

Pui, Ching Hon MD [PHO] - **Spec Exp:** Leukemia; Lymphoma; **Hospital:** St Jude Children's Research Hosp; **Address:** St Jude Chldns Rsch Hosp, 332 N Lauderdale St, Memphis, TN 38105; **Phone:** 901-495-3335; **Board Cert:** Pediatrics 1980; Pediatric Hematology-Oncology 1982; **Med School:** Taiwan 1976; **Resid:** Pediatrics, St Jude Chldns Rsch Hosp 1979; **Fellow:** Hematology & Oncology, St Jude Chldns Rsch Hosp 1981; **Fac Appt:** Prof Ped, Univ Tenn Coll Med, Memphis

Rosoff, Philip M MD [PHO] - **Spec Exp:** Cancer Survivors-Late Effects of Therapy; Down Syndrome; Leukemia; **Hospital:** Duke Univ Med Ctr; **Address:** Duke Univ Med Ctr, Box 2916, Durham, NC 27710-0001; **Phone:** 919-684-3401; **Board Cert:** Pediatrics 1984; Pediatric Hematology-Oncology 2002; **Med School:** Case West Res Univ 1978; **Resid:** Pediatrics, Chldns Hosp 1980; **Fellow:** Pediatric Hematology-Oncology, Chldns Hosp/Dana Farber Cancer Inst 1984; **Fac Appt:** Assoc Prof Ped, Duke Univ

Sandler, Eric MD [PHO] - **Spec Exp:** Bone Marrow Transplant; Leukemia; Clinical Trials; **Hospital:** Wolfson Chldns Hosp; **Address:** 807 Childrens Way, Jacksonville, FL 32207; **Phone:** 904-390-3793; **Board Cert:** Pediatric Hematology-Oncology 2007; **Med School:** Univ VT Coll Med 1985; **Resid:** Pediatrics, UCSF Med Ctr 1988; **Fellow:** Pediatric Hematology-Oncology, Univ Fla Med Sch 1991; **Fac Appt:** Assoc Prof Ped, Mayo Med Sch

Sandlund Jr, John T MD [PHO] - **Spec Exp:** Lymphoma, Non-Hodgkin's; Leukemia & Lymphoma; Ataxia Telangiectasia; **Hospital:** St Jude Children's Research Hosp; **Address:** St Jude Children's Research Hosp, 332 N Lauderdale St, MS 260, Memphis, TN 38105; **Phone:** 901-495-3300; **Board Cert:** Pediatrics 1986; Pediatric Hematology-Oncology 1987; **Med School:** Ohio State Univ 1980; **Resid:** Pediatrics, Columbus Chldns Hosp 1983; **Fellow:** Hematology, Natl Cancer Inst 1986; Research, Natl Cancer Inst 1987

Santana, Victor M MD [PHO] - **Spec Exp:** Solid Tumors; **Hospital:** St Jude Children's Research Hosp; **Address:** St Jude Chldn's Rsch Hosp, Dept Oncology, 332 N Lauderdale, rm C6017, MS 260, Memphis, TN 38105-2794; **Phone:** 901-495-2424; **Board Cert:** Pediatrics 1982; Pediatric Hematology-Oncology 1984; **Med School:** Puerto Rico 1978; **Resid:** Pediatrics, Johns Hopkins Hosp 1981; **Fellow:** Pediatric Hematology-Oncology, Johns Hopkins Hosp 1984

Shearer, Patricia C MD [PHO] - **Spec Exp:** Wilms' Tumor; Cancer Survivors-Late Effects of Therapy; **Hospital:** Shands at Univ of FL; **Address:** Univ Florida HSC, Div Ped Hem/Oncology, PO Box 100296, Gainesville, FL 32610; **Phone:** 352-392-5633; **Board Cert:** Pediatric Hematology-Oncology 2007; **Med School:** Louisiana State U, New Orleans 1986; **Resid:** Pediatrics, Johns Hopkins Hosp 1989; **Fellow:** Hematology & Oncology, St Jude Chldns Rsch Hosp 1992

Tebbi, Cameron MD [PHO] - **Spec Exp:** Adolescent/Young Adult Cancers; Hemophilia; Hodgkin's Disease; Leukemia; **Hospital:** St Josephs Chldns Hosp, Tampa Genl Hosp; **Address:** 3001 W Martin Luther King Jr Blvd, Tampa, FL 33607; **Phone:** 813-870-4824; **Board Cert:** Pediatrics 1974; Pediatric Hematology-Oncology 1980; **Med School:** Iran 1968; **Resid:** Pediatrics, Cincinnati Chldns Hosp 1972; Pediatric Hematology-Oncology, MD Anderson Cancer Inst 1972; **Fellow:** Pediatric Hematology-Oncology, St Louis Chldns Hosp 1973; Medical Oncology, Ontario Cancer Inst 1974

Pediatric Hematology-Oncology

Wang, Winfred C MD [PHO] - **Spec Exp:** Sickle Cell Disease; Bone Marrow Failure Disorders; Anemia-Aplastic; **Hospital:** St Jude Children's Research Hosp, Le Bonheur Chldns Med Ctr; **Address:** St Jude Chldn Rsch Hosp, 262 Danny Thomas Pl, rm R5036, Memphis, TN 38105-2729; **Phone:** 901-595-3497; **Board Cert:** Pediatrics 1972; Pediatric Hematology-Oncology 1974; **Med School:** Univ Chicago-Pritzker Sch Med 1967; **Resid:** Pediatrics, Montefiore Med Ctr 1969; Pediatrics, Kauike-olani Chldn's Hosp 1970; **Fellow:** Pediatric Hematology-Oncology, UCSF 1975; **Fac Appt:** Prof Ped, Univ Tenn Coll Med, Memphis

Whitlock, James A MD [PHO] - **Spec Exp:** Leukemia; Drug Development; **Hospital:** Vander-bilt Children's Hosp, Vanderbilt Univ Med Ctr; **Address:** Vanderbilt Univ Med Ctr, Dept Peds, 2220 Pierce Ave, rm 397 PRB, Nashville, TN 37232-6310; **Phone:** 615-936-1762; **Board Cert:** Pediatric Hematology-Oncology 2007; **Med School:** Vanderbilt Univ 1984; **Resid:** Pediatrics, Vanderbilt Univ Med Ctr 1987; **Fellow:** Pediatric Hematology-Oncology, Vanderbilt Univ Med Ctr 1990; **Fac Appt:** Assoc Prof Ped, Vanderbilt Univ

Woods, William G MD [PHO] - **Spec Exp:** Leukemia; Neuroblastoma; **Hospital:** Chldns Hlth-care Atlanta - Egleston, Chldns Hlthcare Atlanta - Scottish Rite; **Address:** AFLAC Cancer Ctr & Blood Disorders Svc, 2015 Uppergate Drive, rm 404, Atlanta, GA 30322; **Phone:** 404-785-6170; **Board Cert:** Pediatrics 1976; Pediatric Hematology-Oncology 1978; **Med School:** Univ Pennsylvania 1972; **Resid:** Pediatrics, Univ Minnesota Hosps 1975; **Fellow:** Hematology, Univ Minnesota Hosps 1977; **Fac Appt:** Prof Ped, Emory Univ

Midwest

Arndt, Carola A MD [PHO] - **Spec Exp:** Sarcoma; Brain Tumors; Stem Cell Transplant; **Hospital:** Mayo Med Ctr & Clin - Rochester; **Address:** Mayo Clinic, Dept Pediatrics, 200 1st St SW, Rochester, MN 55905; **Phone:** 507-284-2652; **Board Cert:** Pediatrics 1982; Pediatric Hematology-Oncology 1987; **Med School:** Boston Univ 1978; **Resid:** Pediatrics, Naval Reg Med Ctr 1981; **Fellow:** Pediatric Hematology-Oncology, Natl Inst Hlth 1984

Boxer, Laurence MD [PHO] - **Spec Exp:** Congenital Neutropenia-Severe; Anemias & Red Cell Disorders; Thrombotic Disorders; Anemia-Aplastic; **Hospital:** Univ Michigan Hlth Sys; **Address:** Univ Michigan, L-2110 Womens Hosp, 1500 E Medical Ctr Dr, Box 0238, Ann Arbor, MI 48109-0238; **Phone:** 734-764-7127; **Board Cert:** Pediatrics 1971; Pediatric Hematology-Oncology 1974; **Med School:** Stanford Univ 1966; **Resid:** Pediatrics, Yale-New Haven Hosp 1968; Pediatrics, Stanford Univ Hosp 1969; **Fellow:** Hematology, Childrens Hosp-Harvard 1974; **Fac Appt:** Prof Ped, Univ Mich Med Sch

Camitta, Bruce M MD [PHO] - **Spec Exp:** Anemia-Aplastic; Leukemia; Bone Marrow Trans-plant; **Hospital:** Chldns Hosp - Wisconsin; **Address:** Midwest Childrens Cancer Ctr, 8701 Water-town Plank Rd, Ste 3018, Milwaukee, WI 53226; **Phone:** 414-456-4170; **Board Cert:** Pediatrics 1971; Pediatric Hematology-Oncology 1976; **Med School:** Johns Hopkins Univ 1966; **Resid:** Pedi-atrics, Children's Hosp 1968; Pediatrics, Johns Hopkins Hosp 1969; **Fellow:** Pediatric Hematology-Oncology, Children's Hosp 1973; **Fac Appt:** Prof Ped, Med Coll Wisc

Castle, Valerie MD [PHO] - **Spec Exp:** Neuroblastoma; Bleeding/Coagulation Disorders; Can-cer Survivors-Late Effects of Therapy; **Hospital:** Univ Michigan Hlth Sys; **Address:** Univ Mich Comp Cancer Ctr & Geriatric Ctr, 1500 E Med Ctr Drive, Desk B1-358, Ann Arbor, MI 48109-0911; **Phone:** 734-736-6336; **Board Cert:** Pediatric Hematology-Oncology 2006; **Med School:** McMas-ter Univ 1983; **Resid:** Pediatrics, McMaster Univ Med Ctr 1986; **Fellow:** Pediatric Hematology-On-cology, Univ Mich Hosps 1989; **Fac Appt:** Prof Ped, Univ Mich Med Sch

Cohn, Susan L MD [PHO] - **Spec Exp:** Neuroblastoma; **Hospital:** Univ of Chicago Hosps; **Address:** Univ Chicago, 5841 S Maryland Ave, MC 4060, Chicago, IL 60637-1470; **Phone:** 773-702-2571; **Board Cert:** Pediatrics 1985; Pediatric Hematology-Oncology 1987; **Med School:** Univ IL Coll Med 1980; **Resid:** Pediatrics, Michael Reese Hosp 1984; **Fellow:** Hematology & Oncology, Children's Memorial Hosp 1985; **Fac Appt:** Prof Ped, Univ Chicago-Pritzker Sch Med

Corey, Seth J MD [PHO] - **Spec Exp:** Bone Marrow Failure Disorders; Leukemia; Myelodysplastic Syndromes; Ataxia Telangiectasia; **Hospital:** Children's Mem Hosp; **Address:** Robert Lurie Comp Cancer Ctr, Lurie 5-107, 303 E Superior St, Chicago, IL 60611; **Phone:** 312-503-6694; **Board Cert:** Pediatrics 1986; Pediatric Hematology-Oncology 2004; **Med School:** Tulane Univ 1982; **Resid:** Pediatrics, St Louis Chldns Hosp 1985; **Fellow:** Hematology & Oncology, Tufts Med Sch 1992; Research, Boston Chldns-Dana Farber Ctr 1989; **Fac Appt:** Prof Ped, Northwestern Univ-Feinberg Sch Med

Croop, James M MD/PhD [PHO] - **Spec Exp:** Rhabdomyosarcoma; Clinical Trials; **Hospital:** Riley Hosp for Children; **Address:** Riley Hosp for Children, Hem/Oncology, 202 Barnhill Drive, ROC 4340, Indianapolis, IN 46202; **Phone:** 317-274-8784; **Board Cert:** Pediatrics 1985; Pediatric Hematology-Oncology 2005; **Med School:** Univ Pennsylvania 1980; **Resid:** Pediatrics, Children's Hosp 1983; **Fellow:** Pediatric Hematology-Oncology, Children's Hosp 1985; **Fac Appt:** Prof Ped, Indiana Univ

Davies, Stella M MD/PhD [PHO] - **Spec Exp:** Leukemia; Bone Marrow Transplant; Stem Cell Transplant; **Hospital:** Cincinnati Chldns Hosp Med Ctr; **Address:** Cincinnati Chldns Hosp Med Ctr, 3333 Burnet Ave, MLC 7015, Cincinnati, OH 45229-3039; **Phone:** 513-636-2469; **Med School:** England 1981; **Resid:** Pediatrics, Univ Newcastle Med Ctr 1985; **Fellow:** Pediatric Hematology-Oncology, Univ Minn Med Ctr 1993; **Fac Appt:** Prof Ped, Univ Cincinnati

DeBaun, Michael R MD [PHO] - **Spec Exp:** Sickle Cell Disease; **Hospital:** St Louis Chldns Hosp; **Address:** St Louis Children's Hospital, One Children's Pl Fl 9S, St Louis, MO 63110; **Phone:** 314-454-6018; **Board Cert:** Pediatrics 2008; Pediatric Hematology-Oncology 2002; **Med School:** Stanford Univ 1987; **Resid:** Pediatrics, St Louis Children's Hosp 1990; **Fellow:** Pediatric Hematology-Oncology, St Louis Children's Hosp 1993; **Fac Appt:** Assoc Prof Ped, Washington Univ, St Louis

Fallon, Robert J MD/PhD [PHO] - **Spec Exp:** Lymphoma; Hodgkin's Disease; Stem Cell Transplant; **Hospital:** Riley Hosp for Children; **Address:** Riley Childrens Hospital, 702 Barnhill Drive, rm Riley 4340, Indianapolis, IN 46202; **Phone:** 317-274-8784; **Board Cert:** Internal Medicine 1983; Medical Oncology 1985; **Med School:** NYU Sch Med 1980; **Resid:** Internal Medicine, Brigham & Womens Hosp 1983; **Fellow:** Hematology & Oncology, Brigham & Womens Hosp/Dana Farber Cancer Inst 1985; **Fac Appt:** Prof Ped, Indiana Univ

Ferrara, James MD [PHO] - **Spec Exp:** Bone Marrow Transplant; Graft vs Host Disease; Inflammatory Cytokines; **Hospital:** Univ Michigan Hlth Sys; **Address:** Univ Michigan Comprehensive Cancer Ctr, 1500 E Medical Center Drive, Ste 6308, Ann Arbor, MI 48109-0942; **Phone:** 734-615-1340; **Board Cert:** Pediatrics 2004; Pediatric Hematology-Oncology 2005; **Med School:** Georgetown Univ 1980; **Resid:** Pediatrics, Children's Hosp 1982; **Fellow:** Pediatric Hematology-Oncology, Children's Hosp 1985; **Fac Appt:** Prof Ped, Univ Mich Med Sch

Friebert, Sarah E MD [PHO] - **Spec Exp:** Palliative Care; Cancer Survivors-Late Effects of Therapy; **Hospital:** Children's Hosp & Med Ctr- Akron; **Address:** Children's Hosp Med Ctr of Akron, One Perkins Sq Fl 5, Akron, OH 44308; **Phone:** 330-543-8730; **Board Cert:** Pediatrics 2004; Pediatric Hematology-Oncology 2008; **Med School:** Case West Res Univ 1993; **Resid:** Pediatrics, Chldns Hosp 1996; **Fellow:** Pediatric Hematology-Oncology, Rainbow Babies-Chldns Hosp 1999; **Fac Appt:** Asst Prof Ped, NE Ohio Univ

Pediatric Hematology-Oncology

Goldman, Stewart MD [PHO] - **Spec Exp:** Neuro-Oncology; Brain Tumors; Clinical Trials; **Hospital:** Children's Mem Hosp; **Address:** Childrens Meml Hosp, Div Hem/Onc, 2300 Childrens Plaza, Box 30, Chicago, IL 60614; **Phone:** 773-880-4562; **Board Cert:** Pediatric Hematology-Oncology 2004; **Med School:** Loyola Univ-Stritch Sch Med 1985; **Resid:** Pediatrics, Univ Chicago Hosps 1988; **Fellow:** Pediatric Hematology-Oncology, Univ Chicago Hosps 1991

Haut, Paul R MD [PHO] - **Spec Exp:** Stem Cell Transplant; Bone Marrow Transplant; Leukemia; **Hospital:** Riley Hosp for Children; **Address:** Riley Hospital for Children, 702 Barnhill Drive, rm 4340, Indianapolis, IN 46202; **Phone:** 317-274-2143; **Board Cert:** Pediatrics 2001; Pediatric Hematology-Oncology 2000; **Med School:** Univ Ark 1990; **Resid:** Pediatrics, Arkansas Children's Hosp 1994; **Fellow:** Pediatric Hematology-Oncology, Children's Meml Hosp 1997; **Fac Appt:** Assoc Prof Ped, Indiana Univ

Hayani, Ammar MD [PHO] - **Spec Exp:** Leukemia; Solid Tumors; **Hospital:** Adv Christ Med Ctr, Central DuPage Hosp; **Address:** Hope Children's Hospital, 4440 W 95th St, Oak Lawn, IL 60453-2600; **Phone:** 708-684-4094; **Board Cert:** Pediatric Hematology-Oncology 2005; **Med School:** Syria 1982; **Resid:** Pediatrics, Louisiana State Univ 1987; **Fellow:** Pediatric Hematology-Oncology, Baylor Coll Med 1991

Hayashi, Robert J MD [PHO] - **Spec Exp:** Bone Marrow Transplant; Cancer Survivors-Late Effects of Therapy; Leukemia; **Hospital:** St Louis Chldns Hosp; **Address:** St Louis Chldns Hosp, Div Ped Hem Onc, One Children's Pl, Ste 9 South, Campus Box 8116, St Louis, MO 63110; **Phone:** 314-454-6018; **Board Cert:** Pediatrics 2007; Pediatric Hematology-Oncology 2007; **Med School:** Washington Univ, St Louis 1986; **Resid:** Pediatrics, St Louis Children's Hosp 1989; **Fellow:** Pediatric Hematology-Oncology, Johns Hopkins Hosp 1992; **Fac Appt:** Asst Prof Ped, Washington Univ, St Louis

Hetherington, Maxine MD [PHO] - **Spec Exp:** Brain Tumors; **Hospital:** Chldns Mercy Hosps & Clinics; **Address:** Childrens Mercy Hosptial, 2401 Gillham Rd, Kansas City, MO 64108; **Phone:** 816-234-3265; **Board Cert:** Pediatrics 1983; Pediatric Hematology-Oncology 1987; **Med School:** Univ Tenn Coll Med, Memphis 1978; **Resid:** Pediatrics, Childrens Med Ctr 1981; **Fellow:** Pediatric Hematology-Oncology, Univ Texas Hlth Sci Ctr 1987; **Fac Appt:** Assoc Prof Ped, Univ MO-Kansas City

Hilden, Joanne M MD [PHO] - **Spec Exp:** Brain Tumors; Leukemia & Lymphoma; Bone Tumors; Soft Tissue Tumors; **Hospital:** St Vincent Hosp & Hlth Svcs - Indianapolis; **Address:** Peyton Manning Children's Hospital, at St Vincent, 8402 Harcourt Rd, Ste 603, Indianapolis, IN 46260; **Phone:** 317-338-3466; **Board Cert:** Pediatrics 2006; Pediatric Hematology-Oncology 2002; **Med School:** Univ Minn 1988; **Resid:** Pediatrics, Univ Minn Med Ctr 1991; **Fellow:** Pediatric Hematology-Oncology, Univ Minn Med Ctr 1994; **Fac Appt:** Assoc Prof Ped, Indiana Univ

Hord, Jeffrey D MD [PHO] - **Spec Exp:** Hematologic Malignancies; Bone Marrow Failure Disorders; Sickle Cell Disease; **Hospital:** Children's Hosp & Med Ctr- Akron; **Address:** Akron Childrens Hosp, Hematology/Oncology, One Perkins Square, Akron, OH 44308; **Phone:** 330-543-8580; **Board Cert:** Pediatric Hematology-Oncology 2004; **Med School:** Univ KY Coll Med 1989; **Resid:** Pediatrics, Children's Hosp 1992; **Fellow:** Pediatric Hematology-Oncology, Vanderbilt Univ Med Ctr 1995; **Fac Appt:** Assoc Prof Ped, NE Ohio Univ

Hutchinson, Raymond MD [PHO] - **Spec Exp:** Leukemia; Hodgkin's Disease; **Hospital:** Univ Michigan Hlth Sys; **Address:** Univ Michigan Hosp, 1500 E Med Ctr Drive, rm L2110, Ann Arbor, MI 48109-5238; **Phone:** 734-764-7126; **Board Cert:** Pediatrics 1979; Pediatric Hematology-Oncology 1980; **Med School:** Harvard Med Sch 1973; **Resid:** Pediatrics, New England Med Ctr 1975; **Fellow:** Pediatric Hematology-Oncology, Childrens Hosp 1978; **Fac Appt:** Prof Ped, Univ Mich Med Sch

Lusher, Jeanne M MD [PHO] - **Hospital:** Chldns Hosp of Michigan; **Address:** Children's Hospital Michigan, Div Hem/Onc, 3901 Beaubien Blvd, Detroit, MI 48201; **Phone:** 313-745-5515; **Board Cert:** Pediatrics 1986; Pediatric Hematology-Oncology 1986; **Med School:** Univ Cincinnati 1960; **Resid:** Pediatrics, Charity Hosp/Tulane Univ 1963; **Fellow:** Hematology & Oncology, Charity Hosp/Tulane Univ 1965; Hematology & Oncology, Saint Louis Children's Hosp 1966; **Fac Appt:** Prof Ped, Wayne State Univ

Manera, Ricarchito MD [PHO] - **Spec Exp:** Leukemia; Brain Tumors; Lymphoma; **Hospital:** Loyola Univ Med Ctr; **Address:** Loyola University Med Ctr, 2160 S First Ave, Maywood, IL 60611; **Phone:** 708-327-9136; **Board Cert:** Pediatrics 2003; Pediatric Hematology-Oncology 2004; **Med School:** Philippines 1984; **Resid:** Pediatrics, Bronx-Lebanon Hosp Ctr 1995; **Fellow:** Pediatric Hematology-Oncology, MD Anderson Cancer Ctr 1994; Pediatric Hematology-Oncology, Columbia-Presby Med Ctr 1996; **Fac Appt:** Assoc Prof Ped, Loyola Univ-Stritch Sch Med

Morgan, Elaine MD [PHO] - **Spec Exp:** Leukemia; Palliative Care; Ethics; **Hospital:** Children's Mem Hosp; **Address:** Children's Meml Hosp, Div Hem/Onc, 2300 Children's Plaza, Box 30, Chicago, IL 60614; **Phone:** 773-880-4562; **Board Cert:** Pediatrics 1976; Pediatric Hematology-Oncology 1978; Hospice & Palliative Medicine 2005; **Med School:** Univ Pennsylvania 1971; **Resid:** Pediatrics, Chldns Hosp 1974; **Fellow:** Pediatric Hematology-Oncology, Chldns Hosp Med Ctr 1975; Pediatric Hematology-Oncology, Chldns Meml Med Ctr 1976; **Fac Appt:** Prof Ped, Northwestern Univ-Feinberg Sch Med

Nachman, James MD [PHO] - **Spec Exp:** Leukemia & Lymphoma; Bone Tumors; Hodgkin's Disease; **Hospital:** Univ of Chicago Hosps; **Address:** Univ Chicago Hosps, 5841 S Maryland Ave, rm C-429, MC 4060, Chicago, IL 60637; **Phone:** 773-702-6808; **Board Cert:** Pediatrics 1979; Pediatric Hematology-Oncology 1980; **Med School:** Johns Hopkins Univ 1974; **Resid:** Pediatrics, Chldns Meml Hosp 1977; Pediatrics, Fell-Wylers Chldns Hosp 1980; **Fellow:** Pediatric Hematology-Oncology, Chldns Meml Hosp 1979; **Fac Appt:** Prof Ped, Univ Chicago-Pritzker Sch Med

Neglia, Joseph MD [PHO] - **Spec Exp:** Cancer Survivors-Late Effects of Therapy; **Hospital:** Univ Minn Med Ctr, Fairview - Univ Campus; **Address:** Univ Minnesota-Div Ped Hem/Oncology, 420 Delaware St SE, MMC 484, Minneapolis, MN 55455; **Phone:** 612-626-2778; **Board Cert:** Pediatrics 1986; Pediatric Hematology-Oncology 1987; **Med School:** Loma Linda Univ 1981; **Resid:** Pediatrics, Baylor Coll Med 1984; **Fellow:** Pediatric Hematology-Oncology, Univ Minn Hosp 1987; **Fac Appt:** Prof Ped, Univ Minn

Puccetti, Diane MD [PHO] - **Spec Exp:** Brain Tumors; Neuro-Oncology; Cancer Survivors-Late Effects of Therapy; **Hospital:** Univ WI Hosp & Clins; **Address:** Univ Wisconsin Childrens Hosp, 600 Highland Ave, MC 4116, Madison, WI 53792; **Phone:** 608-263-6420; **Board Cert:** Pediatric Hematology-Oncology 2007; **Med School:** Med Coll OH 1985; **Resid:** Pediatrics, UC-Irvine Med Ctr 1986; Pediatrics, Med Coll Ohio 1988; **Fellow:** Pediatric Hematology-Oncology, Riley Hosp Chldn 1991; **Fac Appt:** Assoc Clin Prof Ped, Univ Wisc

Razzouk, Bassem I MD [PHO] - **Spec Exp:** Leukemia; Clinical Trials; **Hospital:** St Vincent Hosp & Hlth Svcs - Indianapolis; **Address:** St Vincent Hosp & Hlth Services, Center for Cancer & Blood Diseases, 2001 W 86th St, Indianapolis, IN 46260; **Phone:** 317-388-4673; **Board Cert:** Pediatric Hematology-Oncology 2004; **Med School:** Lebanon 1987; **Resid:** Pediatrics, American Univ Med Ctr 1990; Pediatrics, SUNY Hlth Sci Ctr 1992; **Fellow:** Hematology & Oncology, St Jude Children's Rsch Hosp 1995

Salvi, Sharad MD [PHO] - **Spec Exp:** Leukemia; Bleeding/Coagulation Disorders; Anemia; **Hospital:** Adv Christ Med Ctr, Central DuPage Hosp; **Address:** Hope Chldns Hosp, 4440 W 95th St, Oak Lawn, IL 60453; **Phone:** 708-684-4094; **Board Cert:** Pediatrics 1982; Pediatric Hematology-Oncology 1982; **Med School:** India 1974; **Resid:** Pediatrics, Lincoln Meml Hosp 1979; **Fellow:** Pediatric Hematology-Oncology, Chldns Hosp/Roswell Park Meml Cancer Inst 1981

Pediatric Hematology-Oncology

Sencer, Susan F MD [PHO] - **Spec Exp:** Pediatric Cancers; Complementary Medicine; **Hospital:** Chldns Hosp and Clinics - Minneapolis; **Address:** Chldns Specialty Clinic, Hem/Onc Clin, 2525 Chicago Ave S, Fl 4 - Ste 4150, Minneapolis, MN 55404; **Phone:** 612-813-5940; **Board Cert:** Pediatric Hematology-Oncology 2007; **Med School:** Univ Minn 1984; **Resid:** Pediatrics, Univ Minn 1988; **Fellow:** Pediatric Hematology-Oncology, Univ Minn 1991

Shapiro, Amy D MD [PHO] - **Spec Exp:** Hemophilia; **Hospital:** St Vincent Hosp & Hlth Svcs - Indianapolis; **Address:** Indiana Hemophilia & Thrombosis Ctr, 8402 Harcourt Rd, Ste 500, Indianapolis, IN 46260; **Phone:** 317-871-0000; **Board Cert:** Pediatrics 1986; Pediatric Hematology-Oncology 1987; **Med School:** NYU Sch Med 1980; **Resid:** Pediatrics, Univ Colo Hlth Sci Ctr 1982; **Fellow:** Pediatric Hematology-Oncology, Univ Colo Hlth Sci Ctr 1983

Sondel, Paul M MD [PHO] - **Spec Exp:** Immunotherapy; Stem Cell Transplant; Pediatric Cancers; **Hospital:** Univ WI Hosp & Clins; **Address:** Univ Wisconsin-American Fam Chldns Hosp, 600 Highland Ave, K4-448 Clin Sci Ctr, Madison, WI 53792-4672; **Phone:** 608-263-6200; **Board Cert:** Pediatrics 1981; **Med School:** Harvard Med Sch 1977; **Resid:** Pediatrics, Univ Wisconsin Hosp 1980; **Fellow:** Research, Sidney Farber Cancer Inst/Harvard 1974; **Fac Appt:** Prof Ped, Univ Wisc

Tannous, Raymond MD [PHO] - **Spec Exp:** Wilms' Tumor; Leukemia & Lymphoma; Pain-Cancer; **Hospital:** Univ Iowa Hosp & Clinics; **Address:** Univ Iowa Hosps & Clinics, Dept Peds, 200 Hawkins Drive, rm 2528 JCP, Iowa City, IA 52242; **Phone:** 319-356-1905; **Board Cert:** Pediatrics 1976; Pediatric Hematology-Oncology 1978; **Med School:** France 1972; **Resid:** Pediatrics, St Jude Chldns Rsch Hosp 1976; **Fellow:** Pediatric Hematology-Oncology, St Jude Chldns Rsch Hosp 1977; **Fac Appt:** Assoc Prof Ped, Univ Iowa Coll Med

Valentino, Leonard Anthony MD [PHO] - **Spec Exp:** Bleeding/Coagulation Disorders; Thrombotic Disorders; Hemophilia; **Hospital:** Rush Univ Med Ctr, Rush - Copley Med Ctr; **Address:** Rush Univ Med Ctr, 1725 W Harrison St, Ste 710, Chicago, IL 60612-3828; **Phone:** 312-942-5983; **Board Cert:** Pediatrics 2000; Pediatric Hematology-Oncology 1998; **Med School:** Creighton Univ 1984; **Resid:** Pediatrics, Univ Illinios Med Ctr 1987; **Fellow:** Pediatric Hematology-Oncology, UCLA Med Ctr 1990; **Fac Appt:** Assoc Prof Ped, Rush Med Coll

Vik, Terry A MD [PHO] - **Spec Exp:** Neuroblastoma; Clinical Trials; Cancer Survivors-Late Effects of Therapy; Leukemia; **Hospital:** Riley Hosp for Children; **Address:** Riley Hosp Children, 702 Barnhill Drive, Riley 4340, Indianapolis, IN 46202; **Phone:** 317-274-2143; **Board Cert:** Pediatrics 1987; Pediatric Hematology-Oncology 2004; **Med School:** Johns Hopkins Univ 1983; **Resid:** Pediatrics, UCLA Med Ctr 1986; **Fellow:** Pediatric Hematology-Oncology, Chldns Hosp 1989; **Fac Appt:** Assoc Prof Ped, Indiana Univ

Yaddanapudi, Ravindranath MD [PHO] - **Spec Exp:** Leukemia; **Hospital:** Chldns Hosp of Michigan; **Address:** Children's Hospital Michigan, Div Hem/Onc, 3901 Beaubien Blvd, Detroit, MI 48201; **Phone:** 313-745-5515; **Board Cert:** Pediatrics 1970; Pediatric Hematology-Oncology 1974; **Med School:** India 1964; **Resid:** Pathology, Western Penn Hosp 1967; Pediatrics, Children's Hosp 1969; **Fellow:** Pediatric Hematology-Oncology, Children's Hosp Michigan 1971; **Fac Appt:** Prof Ped, Wayne State Univ

Great Plains and Mountains

Abromowitch, Minnie MD [PHO] - **Hospital:** Children's Hosp - Omaha; **Address:** Children's Hosp-Dept Ped Hem Oncology, 8200 Dodge St, Omaha, NE 68114; **Phone:** 402-955-3950; **Board Cert:** Pediatrics 1980; Pediatric Hematology-Oncology 1982; **Med School:** Canada 1972; **Resid:** Pediatrics, Hospital for Sick Children 1976; **Fellow:** Pediatric Hematology-Oncology, Univ Manitoba 1978; Pediatric Hematology-Oncology, St Jude Chldns Research Hosp 1980; **Fac Appt:** Assoc Prof Ped, Univ Nebr Coll Med

Bruggers, Carol S MD [PHO] - **Spec Exp:** Brain Tumors; Clinical Trials; **Hospital:** Primary Children's Med Ctr; **Address:** Primary Children's Medical Ctr, 100 N Medical Drive, Salt Lake City, UT 84113; **Phone:** 801-662-4700; **Board Cert:** Pediatrics 2000; Pediatric Hematology-Oncology 2000; **Med School:** Mich State Univ 1984; **Resid:** Pediatrics, Univ Colorado Health Sci Ctr 1987; **Fellow:** Pediatric Hematology-Oncology, Duke Univ Med Ctr 1991; **Fac Appt:** Assoc Prof Med, Univ Utah

Coccia, Peter MD [PHO] - **Spec Exp:** Bone Marrow Transplant; Leukemia & Lymphoma; Solid Tumors; **Hospital:** Nebraska Med Ctr, Children's Hosp - Omaha; **Address:** Univ Nebr Med Ctr, Dept Pediatrics, 982168 Nebraska Med Ctr, Omaha, NE 68198-2168; **Phone:** 402-559-7257; **Board Cert:** Clinical Pathology 1972; Hematology 1975; Pediatrics 1976; Pediatric Hematology-Oncology 1976; **Med School:** SUNY Upstate Med Univ 1968; **Resid:** Pathology, Upstate Med Ctr 1970; Pediatrics, Univ Minn 1973; **Fellow:** Pediatric Hematology-Oncology, Univ Minn 1974; **Fac Appt:** Prof Ped, Univ Nebr Coll Med

Manco-Johnson, Marilyn MD [PHO] - **Spec Exp:** Hemophilia; Thrombotic Disorders; **Hospital:** Chldn's Hosp - Aurora, The, Univ Colorado Hosp; **Address:** Univ Colorado, Hemophilia Ctr, Box 6507, MS F416, Aurora, CO 80045-0507; **Phone:** 303-724-0365; **Board Cert:** Pediatrics 1979; Pediatric Hematology-Oncology 1980; **Med School:** Jefferson Med Coll 1974; **Resid:** Pediatrics, Univ Colorado Affil Hosps 1977; **Fellow:** Pediatric Hematology-Oncology, Chldn's Hosp/Colorado Med Ctr 1981; **Fac Appt:** Prof Ped, Univ Colorado

Odom, Lorrie F MD [PHO] - **Spec Exp:** Leukemia; Solid Tumors; Cancer Survivors-Late Effects of Therapy; **Hospital:** Presby - St Luke's Med Ctr, Chldn's Hosp - Aurora, The; **Address:** Rocky Mountain Ped Hem Onc, 1601 E 19th Ave, Ste 6600, Denver, CO 80218; **Phone:** 303-832-2344; **Board Cert:** Pediatrics 1974; Pediatric Hematology-Oncology 1976; **Med School:** Univ Colorado 1969; **Resid:** Pediatrics, Childrens Hosp 1972; **Fellow:** Pediatric Hematology-Oncology, Dana-Farber Cancer Inst 1974; Pediatric Hematology-Oncology, Univ Colorado Med Ctr 1975; **Fac Appt:** Clin Prof Ped, Univ Colorado

Southwest

Abella, Esteban MD [PHO] - **Spec Exp:** Leukemia; Anemia-Aplastic; Neuroblastoma; Bone Marrow Transplant; **Hospital:** Banner Desert Med Ctr, St Joseph's Hosp & Med Ctr - Phoenix; **Address:** 1432 S Dobson, Ste 107, Mesa, AZ 85202; **Phone:** 480-833-1123; **Board Cert:** Pediatric Hematology-Oncology 2002; **Med School:** Dominican Republic 1985; **Resid:** Pediatrics, Chldns Hosp Michigan 1988; **Fellow:** Pediatric Hematology-Oncology, Chldns Hosp Michigan/Wayne St Univ 1991

Berg, Stacey MD [PHO] - **Hospital:** Texas Chldns Hosp - Houston; **Address:** Texas Chldns Cancer Ctr, Ped Hem-Onc, 6621 Fannin St, MC 3-3320, Houston, TX 77030; **Phone:** 832-824-4240; **Board Cert:** Pediatrics 2007; Pediatric Hematology-Oncology 2007; **Med School:** Univ Pittsburgh 1985; **Resid:** Pediatrics, Chldns Hosp 1988; **Fellow:** Pediatric Hematology-Oncology, Natl Inst Hlth 1991; **Fac Appt:** Prof Ped, Baylor Coll Med

Pediatric Hematology-Oncology

Blaney, Susan MD [PHO] - **Spec Exp:** Brain Tumors; Neuro-Oncology; Drug Development; Clinical Trials; **Hospital:** Texas Chldns Hosp - Houston; **Address:** 6621 Fannin St #CC 1410.00, Houston, TX 77030; **Phone:** 832-822-1482; **Board Cert:** Pediatrics 1998; Pediatric Hematology-Oncology 2005; **Med School:** Med Coll OH 1984; **Resid:** Pediatrics, Letterman AMC 1987; **Fellow:** Pediatric Oncology, Walter Reed AMC 1990; **Fac Appt:** Prof Ped, Baylor Coll Med

Buchanan, George R MD [PHO] - **Spec Exp:** Sickle Cell Disease; Thrombotic Disorders; Hemophilia; Leukemia; **Hospital:** Chldns Med Ctr of Dallas; **Address:** Univ Texas SW Med Ctr, Peds Hem Onc, 5323 Harry Hines Blvd, MC 9063, Dallas, TX 75390-9063; **Phone:** 214-456-2382; **Board Cert:** Pediatrics 1975; Pediatric Hematology-Oncology 2000; **Med School:** Univ Chicago-Pritzker Sch Med 1970; **Resid:** Pediatrics, Chldn's Meml Hosp 1973; **Fellow:** Hematology & Oncology, Chldn's Meml Hosp 1975; **Fac Appt:** Prof Ped, Univ Tex SW, Dallas

Dreyer, ZoAnn E MD [PHO] - **Spec Exp:** Cancer Survivors-Late Effects of Therapy; Leukemia in Infants; **Hospital:** Texas Chldns Hosp - Houston; **Address:** Texas Childrens Hosp, Clinical Care Ctr, 6701 Fannin Fl 14, MC CC1400, Houston, TX 77030; **Phone:** 832-822-4242; **Board Cert:** Pediatrics 1988; Pediatric Hematology-Oncology 2005; **Med School:** UC Davis 1982; **Resid:** Pediatrics, Baylor Affil Hosps 1985; **Fellow:** Pediatric Hematology-Oncology, Baylor Coll Med 1988; **Fac Appt:** Assoc Prof Ped, Baylor Coll Med

Goldman, Stanton C MD [PHO] - **Spec Exp:** Leukemia; Lymphoma; Stem Cell Transplant; **Hospital:** Med City Dallas Hosp; **Address:** 7777 Forest Ln, Ste D400, Dallas, TX 75230; **Phone:** 972-566-6647; **Board Cert:** Pediatrics 2001; Pediatric Hematology-Oncology 2004; **Med School:** Boston Univ 1990; **Resid:** Pediatrics, Chldns Natl Med Ctr; **Fellow:** Pediatric Hematology-Oncology, Johns Hopkins Hosp

Graham, Michael L MD [PHO] - **Spec Exp:** Bone Marrow Transplant; Leukemia; Stem Cell Transplant; **Hospital:** Univ Med Ctr - Tucson; **Address:** Univ Arizona Hlth Science Ctr, 1501 N Campbell Ave, rm 4341, Box 245073, Tucson, AZ 85724-5073; **Phone:** 520-626-6527; **Board Cert:** Pediatrics 1980; Pediatric Hematology-Oncology 1984; **Med School:** Brown Univ 1975; **Resid:** Pediatrics, Johns Hopkins Hosp 1978; Pediatric Hematology-Oncology, Johns Hopkins Hosp 1980; **Fellow:** Medical Oncology, Yale-New Haven Hosp 1982; **Fac Appt:** Assoc Prof Ped, Univ Ariz Coll Med

Hoots, William K MD [PHO] - **Spec Exp:** Hemophilia; **Hospital:** UT MD Anderson Cancer Ctr; **Address:** Gulf States, Hemophilia & Thrombophilia Ctr, 6655 Travis, Ste 400 HMC, Houston, TX 77030; **Phone:** 713-500-8360; **Board Cert:** Pediatrics 1980; Pediatric Hematology-Oncology 1980; **Med School:** Univ NC Sch Med 1975; **Resid:** Pediatrics, Chldns Med Ctr 1978; **Fellow:** Pediatric Hematology-Oncology, Univ NC Med Ctr 1980; **Fac Appt:** Prof Ped, Univ Tex, Houston

Murphy, Sharon B MD [PHO] - **Spec Exp:** Lymphoma, Non-Hodgkin's; Leukemia; **Address:** UTHSCSA - Children's Cancer Research Inst, 8403 Floyd Curl Drive, MS 7784, San Antonio, TX 78229-3900; **Phone:** 210-562-9000; **Board Cert:** Pediatrics 1990; Pediatric Hematology-Oncology 1990; **Med School:** Harvard Med Sch 1969; **Resid:** Pediatrics, Univ Colorado Med Ctr 1971; **Fellow:** Pediatric Hematology-Oncology, Chldns Hosp 1973; **Fac Appt:** Prof Ped, Univ Tex, San Antonio

Scher, Charles D MD [PHO] - **Spec Exp:** Sickle Cell Disease; Leukemia; **Hospital:** Tulane Univ Hosp & Clin; **Address:** Tulane Univ Hosp, Dept Pediatrics, 1430 Tulane Ave, Box SL-37, New Orleans, LA 70112; **Phone:** 504-988-5412; **Board Cert:** Pediatrics 1972; **Med School:** Univ Pennsylvania 1965; **Resid:** Pediatrics, Bronx Muni Hosp Ctr 1967; Pediatrics, Chldns Hosp Med Ctr 1972; **Fellow:** Pediatric Hematology-Oncology, Chldns Hosp Med Ctr 1974; **Fac Appt:** Prof Ped, Tulane Univ

Tomlinson, Gail E MD [PHO] - **Spec Exp:** Cancer Survivors-Late Effects of Therapy; Cancer Genetics; Liver Cancer; Kidney Cancer; **Hospital:** Chldns Med Ctr of Dallas, UT Southwestern Med Ctr - Dallas; **Address:** UT Southwestern Med Ctr, 5323 Harry Hines Blvd, Dallas, TX 75390-8593; **Phone:** 214-648-4907; **Board Cert:** Pediatrics 2001; Pediatric Hematology-Oncology 2002; **Med School:** Geo Wash Univ 1984; **Resid:** Pediatrics, Chldns Hosp Natl Med Ctr 1987; **Fellow:** Pediatric Hematology-Oncology, MD Anderson Cancer Ctr 1989; Pediatric Hematology-Oncology, Univ Texas SW Med Ctr 1992; **Fac Appt:** Assoc Prof Ped, Univ Tex SW, Dallas

Wall, Donna A MD [PHO] - **Spec Exp:** Bone Marrow & Stem Cell Transplant; Immunotherapy; **Hospital:** Methodist Chldns Hosp of South Texas, Christus Santa Rosa Children's Hosp; **Address:** Texas Transplant Inst, 7711 Louis Pasteur, Ste 708, San Antonio, TX 78229; **Phone:** 210-575-7268; **Board Cert:** Pediatrics 1986; Pediatric Hematology-Oncology 1987; **Med School:** Canada 1981; **Resid:** Pediatrics, NY Presby-Columbia Med Ctr 1983; Pediatrics, New England Med Ctr 1985; **Fellow:** Pediatric Hematology-Oncology, Dana Farber Cancer Inst 1986

Winick, Naomi J MD [PHO] - **Spec Exp:** Leukemia; **Hospital:** Chldns Med Ctr of Dallas; **Address:** Ctr for Cancer & Blood Disorders, 1935 Motor St, Dallas, TX 75235-7794; **Phone:** 214-456-2382; **Board Cert:** Pediatrics 1984; Pediatric Hematology-Oncology 1987; **Med School:** Northwestern Univ 1978; **Resid:** Pediatrics, Babies Hosp-Columbia Presbyterian Med Ctr 1981; **Fellow:** Pediatric Hematology-Oncology, Sloan-Kettering Cancer Ctr 1983; **Fac Appt:** Prof Ped, Univ Tex SW, Dallas

West Coast and Pacific

Andrews, Robert G MD [PHO] - **Spec Exp:** Bone Marrow Transplant; Leukemia; Lymphoma; **Hospital:** Chldns Hosp and Regl Med Ctr - Seattle; **Address:** Seattle Cancer Care Alliance, 825 Eastlake Ave E, PO Box 19023, Seattle, WA 98109-1024; **Phone:** 206-288-1024; **Board Cert:** Pediatrics 1984; Pediatric Hematology-Oncology 1984; **Med School:** Univ Minn 1976; **Resid:** Pediatrics, New England Med Ctr 1979; **Fellow:** Pediatric Hematology-Oncology, Children's Hosp Med Ctr 1983; **Fac Appt:** Assoc Prof Ped, Univ Wash

Ducore, Jonathan M MD [PHO] - **Spec Exp:** Brain Tumors; Bone & Soft Tissue Tumors; Bleeding/Coagulation Disorders; **Hospital:** UC Davis Med Ctr; **Address:** UC Davis Med Ctr, Dept Pediatrics, Div Pediatric Hematology/Oncology, 2516 Stockton Blvd, Sacramento, CA 95817; **Phone:** 916-734-2781; **Board Cert:** Pediatrics 1978; Pediatric Hematology-Oncology 1978; **Med School:** Duke Univ 1973; **Resid:** Pediatrics, Chldns Med Ctr 1975; **Fellow:** Pediatric Hematology-Oncology, Univ Colorado Med Ctr 1977; Cancer Research, Natl Cancer Inst 1980; **Fac Appt:** Assoc Prof Ped, UC Davis

Finklestein, Jerry Z MD [PHO] - **Spec Exp:** Cancer Survivors-Late Effects of Therapy; Anemias & Red Cell Disorders; **Hospital:** Long Beach Meml Med Ctr, LAC - Harbor - UCLA Med Ctr; **Address:** 2653 Elm Ave, Ste 200, Long Beach, CA 90806-1652; **Phone:** 562-492-1062; **Board Cert:** Pediatrics 1980; Pediatric Hematology-Oncology 1974; **Med School:** McGill Univ 1963; **Resid:** Pediatrics, Montreal Chldns Hosp 1966; **Fellow:** Pediatric Hematology-Oncology, LA Chldns Hosp 1968; **Fac Appt:** Clin Prof Ped, UCLA

Finlay, Jonathan MD [PHO] - **Spec Exp:** Brain Tumors; **Hospital:** Chldns Hosp - Los Angeles; **Address:** Chldns Hosp-LA, Ped Hematology/Oncology, 4650 Sunset Blvd, MS 54, Los Angeles, CA 90027-6016; **Phone:** 323-361-8147; **Board Cert:** Pediatrics 1984; Pediatric Hematology-Oncology 1987; **Med School:** England 1973; **Resid:** Pediatrics, Univ Birmingham 1975; Pediatrics, Christie Hosp 1976; **Fellow:** Pediatric Allergy & Immunology, Univ Wisconsin Hosp 1978; Pediatric Hematology-Oncology, Univ Wisconsin Hosp 1980; **Fac Appt:** Prof Ped, USC-Keck School of Medicine

Pediatric Hematology-Oncology

Friedman, Debra L MD [PHO] - **Spec Exp:** Cancer Survivors-Late Effects of Therapy; Hodgkin's Disease; Retinoblastoma; **Hospital:** Chldns Hosp and Regl Med Ctr - Seattle, Univ Wash Med Ctr; **Address:** Fred Hutchinson Research Ctr, 1100 Fairview Ave N, Ste D5-280, Seattle, WA 98109; **Phone:** 206-667-5935; **Board Cert:** Pediatric Hematology-Oncology 1998; **Med School:** UMDNJ-RW Johnson Med Sch 1991; **Resid:** Pediatrics, Chldns Hosp 1994; **Fellow:** Pediatric Hematology-Oncology, Chldns Hosp 1997; **Fac Appt:** Asst Prof Ped, Univ Wash

Geyer, J Russell MD [PHO] - **Spec Exp:** Brain Tumors; **Hospital:** Chldns Hosp and Regl Med Ctr - Seattle, Providence Alaska Med Ctr; **Address:** Chldns Hosp & Reg Med Ctr - Div Hem/Onc, 4800 Sands Point Way NE, MS B-6553, Seattle, WA 98105; **Phone:** 206-987-2106; **Board Cert:** Pediatrics 1983; Pediatric Hematology-Oncology 1987; **Med School:** Wayne State Univ 1977; **Resid:** Pediatrics, Chldns Hosp Michigan 1980; **Fellow:** Pediatric Hematology-Oncology, Univ Michigan Med Ctr 1981; **Fac Appt:** Prof Ped, Univ Wash

Glader, Bertil MD/PhD [PHO] - **Spec Exp:** Genetic Blood Disorders; Hemophilia; **Hospital:** Lucile Packard Chldns Hosp/Stanford Univ Med Ctr; **Address:** 770 Welch Rd Fl 2 - rm 261, Palo Alto, CA 94304; **Phone:** 650-497-8953; **Board Cert:** Pediatrics 1982; Pediatric Hematology-Oncology 2005; Hematology 1983; **Med School:** Northwestern Univ 1968; **Resid:** Pediatrics, Chldns Hosp Med Ctr 1973; **Fellow:** Hematology, Chldns Hosp Med Ctr 1975; **Fac Appt:** Prof Ped, Stanford Univ

Hawkins, Douglas MD [PHO] - **Spec Exp:** Bone Tumors; Ewing's Sarcoma; Leukemia; Rhabdomyosarcoma; **Hospital:** Chldns Hosp and Regl Med Ctr - Seattle; **Address:** Children's Hosp & Regl Med Ctr, 4800 Sand Point Way NE, Box 5371, MS B6553, Seattle, WA 98105; **Phone:** 206-987-2106; **Board Cert:** Pediatrics 2001; Pediatric Hematology-Oncology 2004; **Med School:** Harvard Med Sch 1990; **Resid:** Pediatrics, Univ Washington Med Ctr 1993; **Fellow:** Pediatric Hematology-Oncology, Fred Hutchinson Cancer Research Ctr 1996

Horn, Biljana N MD [PHO] - **Spec Exp:** Bone Marrow Transplant; Brain Tumors; Stem Cell Transplant; Immunotherapy; **Hospital:** UCSF Med Ctr; **Address:** UCSF Med Ctr, Pediatric BMT Program, 505 Parnassus Ave, rm M-659, San Francisco, CA 94143; **Phone:** 415-476-2188; **Board Cert:** Pediatrics 2005; Pediatric Hematology-Oncology 2004; **Med School:** Croatia 1983; **Resid:** Pediatrics, Rainbow Babies & Chldns Hosp 1991; **Fellow:** Pediatric Hematology-Oncology, Natl Cancer Inst 1994; Pediatric Neuro-Oncology, UCSF 1998; **Fac Appt:** Assoc Prof Ped, UCSF

Kadota, Richard P MD [PHO] - **Spec Exp:** Bone Marrow Transplant; Brain Tumors; Clinical Trials; **Hospital:** Rady Children's Hosp - San Diego; **Address:** Children's Hospital San Diego, 3020 Children's Way, MC 5035, San Diego, CA 92123; **Phone:** 858-966-5811; **Board Cert:** Pediatrics 1984; Pediatric Hematology-Oncology 1984; **Med School:** Northwestern Univ 1979; **Resid:** Pediatrics, Mayo Clinic 1983; **Fellow:** Pediatric Hematology-Oncology, Mayo Clinic 1985; **Fac Appt:** Clin Prof Ped, UCSD

Kapoor, Neena MD [PHO] - **Spec Exp:** Bone Marrow Transplant; **Hospital:** Chldns Hosp - Los Angeles; **Address:** Chlds Hosp LA-Rsch Immunology/BMT, 4650 Sunset Blvd, MS 62, Los Angeles, CA 90027; **Phone:** 323-361-2546; **Board Cert:** Pediatrics 1978; Pediatric Hematology-Oncology 1996; **Med School:** India 1972; **Resid:** Pediatrics, Rhode Island Hosp 1976; **Fellow:** Pediatric Hematology-Oncology, Meml Sloan-Kettering Cancer Ctr 1978; **Fac Appt:** Prof Ped, USC Sch Med

Link, Michael P MD [PHO] - **Spec Exp:** Stem Cell Transplant; **Hospital:** Lucile Packard Chldns Hosp/Stanford Univ Med Ctr, Stanford Univ Med Ctr; **Address:** 1000 Welch Rd, Ste 300, Palo Alto, CA 94304; **Phone:** 650-723-5535; **Board Cert:** Pediatrics 1979; Pediatric Hematology-Oncology 1980; **Med School:** Stanford Univ 1974; **Resid:** Pediatrics, Chldns Hosp Med Ctr 1976; **Fellow:** Hematology & Oncology, Dana Farber Cancer Inst 1979; **Fac Appt:** Prof Ped, Stanford Univ

Marina, Neyssa MD [PHO] - **Spec Exp:** Sarcoma; Cancer Survivors-Late Effects of Therapy; Germ Cell Tumors; **Hospital:** Lucile Packard Chldns Hosp/Stanford Univ Med Ctr; **Address:** Pediatric Hematology & Oncology, 725 Walsh Rd-Clinic E, Palo Alto, CA 94304; **Phone:** 650-497-8953; **Board Cert:** Pediatrics 1987; Pediatric Hematology-Oncology 2005; **Med School:** Puerto Rico 1983; **Resid:** Pediatrics, Univ Pediatric Hosp 1986; **Fellow:** Pediatric Hematology-Oncology, St Jude Children's Hosp 1989; **Fac Appt:** Prof Ped, Stanford Univ

Matthay, Katherine K MD [PHO] - **Spec Exp:** Neuroblastoma; Bone Marrow & Stem Cell Transplant; **Hospital:** UCSF Med Ctr; **Address:** UCSF, Dept Ped Onc, 505 Parnassus Ave, Box 0106, San Francisco, CA 94143; **Phone:** 415-476-0603; **Board Cert:** Pediatrics 1979; Pediatric Hematology-Oncology 1980; **Med School:** Univ Pennsylvania 1973; **Resid:** Pediatrics, Univ Colorado 1976; **Fellow:** Pediatric Hematology-Oncology, UCSF 1979; **Fac Appt:** Prof Ped, UCSF

Nicholson, Henry Stacy MD [PHO] - **Spec Exp:** Brain Tumors; Cancer Survivors-Late Effects of Therapy; **Hospital:** Doernbecher Chldns Hosp/OHSU, OR Hlth & Sci Univ; **Address:** OR Hlth Scis Univ, 707 SW Gaines Rd, Portland, OR 97239; **Phone:** 503-494-4265; **Board Cert:** Pediatric Hematology-Oncology 2007; **Med School:** Med Coll GA 1985; **Resid:** Pediatrics, Chldns National Med Ctr 1988; **Fellow:** Pediatric Hematology-Oncology, Chldns National Med Ctr 1991; **Fac Appt:** Prof Ped, Oregon Hlth Sci Univ

Pendergrass, Thomas W MD [PHO] - **Spec Exp:** Sarcoma; Leukemia & Lymphoma; Retinoblastoma; **Hospital:** Chldns Hosp and Regl Med Ctr - Seattle, Univ Wash Med Ctr; **Address:** Children's Hosp Regional Med Ctr, 4800 Sandpoint Way NE, Box 5371, MS B6553, Seattle, WA 98105; **Phone:** 206-987-2106; **Board Cert:** Pediatrics 1978; **Med School:** Univ Tenn Coll Med, Memphis 1971; **Resid:** Pediatrics, Children's Memorial Hosp 1973; **Fellow:** Pediatric Hematology-Oncology, Children's Hosp Med Ctr 1977; **Fac Appt:** Prof Ped, Univ Wash

Rosenthal, Joseph MD [PHO] - **Spec Exp:** Bone Marrow Transplant; Clinical Trials; **Hospital:** City of Hope Natl Med Ctr & Beckman Rsch; **Address:** City of Hope Med Ctr, 1500 E Duarte Rd, Duarte, CA 91010; **Phone:** 626-256-4673 x68442; **Board Cert:** Pediatrics 2003; Pediatric Hematology-Oncology 2004; **Med School:** Israel 1984; **Resid:** Pediatrics, Soroka MC 1988; Pediatrics, Chldrn Hosp 1995; **Fellow:** Pediatric Hematology-Oncology, Univ Colorado 1991; Pediatric Hematology-Oncology, Chldrn Hosp 1994; **Fac Appt:** Assoc Prof Ped, USC-Keck School of Medicine

Russo, Carolyn MD [PHO] - **Spec Exp:** Brain Tumors; Cancer Survivors-Late Effects of Therapy; Palliative Care; **Hospital:** Kaiser Permanente Santa Clara Med Ctr; **Address:** 710 Lawrence Expwy, Dept 190, Santa Clara, CA 95051; **Phone:** 408-554-9810; **Board Cert:** Pediatric Hematology-Oncology 2005; **Med School:** UCLA 1984; **Resid:** Pediatrics, Harbor-UCLA Med Ctr 1987; **Fellow:** Pediatric Hematology-Oncology, Stanford Med Ctr 1990

Sakamoto, Kathleen M MD [PHO] - **Spec Exp:** Fanconi's Anemia; **Hospital:** Chldns Hosp - Los Angeles; **Address:** Mattel Chldns Hosp UCLA, Div Hem-Onc, 10833 Le Conte Ave, Los Angeles, CA 90095-1752; **Phone:** 310-825-6708; **Board Cert:** Pediatrics 2007; Pediatric Hematology-Oncology 2007; **Med School:** Univ Cincinnati 1985; **Resid:** Pediatrics, Children's Hosp 1988; **Fellow:** Pediatric Hematology-Oncology, Children's Hosp 1991; **Fac Appt:** Prof Ped, UCLA

Siegel, Stuart E MD [PHO] - **Spec Exp:** Leukemia; Infections in Cancer Patients; Psychiatry in Childhood Cancer; Solid Tumors; **Hospital:** Chldns Hosp - Los Angeles, Ventura Cnty Med Ctr; **Address:** Children's Hospital, 4650 Sunset Blvd, MS 54, Los Angeles, CA 90027-6062; **Phone:** 323-361-2205; **Board Cert:** Pediatrics 1973; Pediatric Hematology-Oncology 1976; **Med School:** Boston Univ 1967; **Resid:** Pediatrics, Univ Minnesota Hosps 1969; **Fellow:** Pediatric Hematology-Oncology, Natl Cancer Inst 1972; **Fac Appt:** Prof Ped, USC Sch Med

Pediatric Hematology-Oncology

Wilkinson, Robert W MD [PHO] - **Hospital:** Kapiolani Med Ctr for Women & Chldn; **Address:** Kapiolani Med Ctr for Women & Children, 1319 Punahou St, Ste 1050, Honolulu, HI 96826; **Phone:** 808-942-8144; **Board Cert:** Pediatrics 1986; Pediatric Hematology-Oncology 1986; **Med School:** Tulane Univ 1967; **Resid:** Pediatrics, Los Angeles Co-USC Med Ctr 1971; **Fellow:** Pediatric Hematology-Oncology, Los Angeles Co-USC Med Ctr 1972; **Fac Appt:** Assoc Prof Ped, Univ Hawaii JA Burns Sch Med

PEDIATRIC INFECTIOUS DISEASE

New England

Andiman, Warren A MD [PInf] - **Spec Exp:** AIDS/HIV; Viral Infections; Lyme Disease; Infectious Mononucleosis; **Hospital:** Yale-New Haven Hosp; **Address:** 333 Cedar St, rm 418 LSOG, Box 208064, New Haven, CT 06520-8064; **Phone:** 203-785-4730; **Board Cert:** Pediatrics 1975; **Med School:** Albert Einstein Coll Med 1969; **Resid:** Pediatrics, Babies Hosp-Columbia Presby 1971; **Fellow:** Pediatric Infectious Disease, Yale Univ Sch Med 1973; **Fac Appt:** Prof Ped, Yale Univ

Baltimore, Robert MD [PInf] - **Spec Exp:** Neonatal Infections; Hospital Acquired Infections; Tuberculosis; **Hospital:** Yale-New Haven Hosp; **Address:** Yale Univ Sch Med, Dept Pediatrics, 333 Cedar St, Box 208064, New Haven, CT 06520-8064; **Phone:** 203-785-4655; **Board Cert:** Pediatrics 1975; Pediatric Infectious Disease 2002; **Med School:** SUNY Buffalo 1968; **Resid:** Pediatrics, Univ Chicago Hosps 1971; **Fellow:** Infectious Disease, Boston City Hosp-Harvard 1976; **Fac Appt:** Prof Ped, Yale Univ

Durbin Jr, William Applebee MD [PInf] - **Hospital:** UMass Meml - Univ Campus; **Address:** 55 Lake Ave N, Worcester, MA 01655; **Phone:** 508-856-2650; **Board Cert:** Pediatrics 1978; Pediatric Infectious Disease 2002; **Med School:** Columbia P&S 1972; **Resid:** Pediatrics, Boston Chlns Hosp 1977; **Fellow:** Infectious Disease, Boston Chldns Hosp/Beth Israel 1979; **Fac Appt:** Prof Ped, Univ Mass Sch Med

Jenson, Hal B MD [PInf] - **Spec Exp:** Viral Infections; Tumor Virology; Vaccines; **Hospital:** Baystate Med Ctr; **Address:** 759 Chestnut St, Springfield, MA 01199; **Phone:** 419-794-5588; **Board Cert:** Pediatrics 1985; Pediatric Infectious Disease 2002; **Med School:** Geo Wash Univ 1979; **Resid:** Pediatrics, Rainbow Babies-Chldns Hosp. 1983; **Fellow:** Pediatric Infectious Disease, Yale Univ Sch Med 1985; **Fac Appt:** Prof Ped, Tufts Univ

Shapiro, Eugene D MD [PInf] - **Spec Exp:** Lyme Disease; Vaccines; **Hospital:** Yale-New Haven Hosp; **Address:** Yale Univ, Dept Pediatrics, 333 Cedar St, Box 208064, New Haven, CT 06520-8064; **Phone:** 203-688-4518; **Board Cert:** Pediatrics 1980; Pediatric Infectious Disease 2002; **Med School:** UCSF 1976; **Resid:** Pediatrics, Chldns Hosp 1979; **Fellow:** Pediatric Infectious Disease, Chldns Hosp 1981; Research, Yale Univ 1983; **Fac Appt:** Prof Ped, Yale Univ

Mid Atlantic

Borkowsky, William MD [PInf] - **Spec Exp:** AIDS/HIV; **Hospital:** NYU Med Ctr (page 68), Bellevue Hosp Ctr; **Address:** 550 1st Ave, Dept Pediatrics, New York, NY 10016; **Phone:** 212-263-6513; **Board Cert:** Pediatrics 1979; Pediatric Infectious Disease 2002; **Med School:** NYU Sch Med 1972; **Resid:** Pediatrics, Bellevue Hosp Ctr 1975; **Fellow:** Infectious Disease, Bellevue Hosp Ctr-NYU 1978; **Fac Appt:** Prof Ped, NYU Sch Med

Krilov, Leonard MD [PInf] - **Spec Exp:** Infections-Respiratory; Infections in Int'l Adopted Children; Chronic Fatigue Syndrome; Lyme Disease; **Hospital:** Winthrop - Univ Hosp; **Address:** 120 Mineola Blvd, Ste 210, Mineola, NY 11501; **Phone:** 516-663-9570; **Board Cert:** Pediatrics 1983; Pediatric Infectious Disease 2001; **Med School:** Columbia P&S 1978; **Resid:** Pediatrics, Johns Hopkins Hosp 1981; **Fellow:** Pediatric Infectious Disease, Chldns Hosp 1984; **Fac Appt:** Prof Ped, SUNY Stony Brook

Long, Sarah S MD [PInf] - **Spec Exp:** Whooping Cough; Vaccines; Antibiotic Resistance; **Hospital:** St Christopher's Hosp for Chldn; **Address:** St Christopher's Hosp for Children, Erie Ave at Front St, Ste 1112, Philadelphia, PA 19134; **Phone:** 215-427-5201; **Board Cert:** Pediatrics 2002; Pediatric Infectious Disease 2002; **Med School:** Jefferson Med Coll 1970; **Resid:** Pediatrics, St Christophers Hosp Chldn 1973; **Fellow:** Pediatric Infectious Disease, Temple Univ Sch Med 1975; **Fac Appt:** Prof Ped, Drexel Univ Coll Med

Michaels, Marian G MD [PInf] - **Hospital:** Chldns Hosp of Pittsburgh - UPMC; **Address:** Children's Hosp Pittsburgh, Div Infectious Disease, 3705 Firth Ave, Pittsburgh, PA 15213; **Phone:** 412-692-7438; **Board Cert:** Pediatrics 2005; Pediatric Infectious Disease 2002; **Med School:** Univ Pennsylvania 1985; **Resid:** Pediatrics, Children's Hosp 1988; Pediatrics, Hosp for Sick Children 1989; **Fellow:** Pediatric Infectious Disease, Univ Pittsburgh 1992; **Fac Appt:** Assoc Prof Ped, Univ Pittsburgh

Munoz, Jose Luis MD [PInf] - **Spec Exp:** Lyme Disease; Immune Deficiency; AIDS/HIV; **Hospital:** Westchester Med Ctr; **Address:** Pediatric Infectious Disease, 19 Bradhurst Ave, Ste 1400, Hawthorne, NY 10532; **Phone:** 914-493-8333; **Board Cert:** Pediatrics 1989; Pediatric Infectious Disease 2002; **Med School:** Yale Univ 1978; **Resid:** Pediatrics, Yale New Haven Hosp 1981; **Fellow:** Pediatric Infectious Disease, Univ Rochester 1984; **Fac Appt:** Assoc Prof Ped, NY Med Coll

Offit, Paul A MD [PInf] - **Spec Exp:** Vaccines; **Hospital:** Chldns Hosp of Philadelphia, The; **Address:** Children's Hospital of Philadelphia, Abramson Bldg, 34th St & Civic Center Blvd, Ste 1202D, Philadelphia, PA 19104; **Phone:** 215-590-2017; **Board Cert:** Pediatrics 1982; **Med School:** Univ MD Sch Med 1977; **Resid:** Pediatrics, Children's Hosp 1980; **Fac Appt:** Assoc Clin Prof Ped, Univ Pennsylvania

Saiman, Lisa MD [PInf] - **Spec Exp:** Cystic Fibrosis Infection; Fungal Infections; Hospital Acquired Infections; Tuberculosis; **Hospital:** NYPresby-Morgan Stanley Children's Hosp (page 66); **Address:** Columbia University, 650 W 168th St Fl 4 PH4 W - rm 470, New York, NY 10032; **Phone:** 212-305-9446; **Board Cert:** Pediatrics 1987; Pediatric Infectious Disease 2002; **Med School:** Albert Einstein Coll Med 1983; **Resid:** Pediatrics, Babies Hosp/NY Presbyterian 1986; **Fellow:** Infectious Disease, Babies Hosp/NY Prebyterian 1989; **Fac Appt:** Assoc Clin Prof Ped, Columbia P&S

Singh, Nalini MD [PInf] - **Hospital:** Chldns Natl Med Ctr; **Address:** Div Infectious Disease, 111 Michigan Ave NW, Ste 35 West Wing, rm 100, Washington, DC 20010; **Phone:** 202-476-5051; **Board Cert:** Pediatrics 1982; Pediatric Infectious Disease 2005; **Med School:** India 1973; **Resid:** Pediatrics, Univ Mass Med Ctr 1979; **Fellow:** Infectious Disease, Natl Inst Hlth 1981; **Fac Appt:** Assoc Prof Ped, Geo Wash Univ

Southeast

Clements III, Dennis A MD/PhD [PInf] - **Hospital:** Duke Univ Med Ctr; **Address:** Duke Univ Med Center, Box 2802, Durham, NC 27710; **Phone:** 919-681-7714; **Board Cert:** Pediatrics 1978; **Med School:** Univ Rochester 1973; **Resid:** Pediatrics, Duke Univ Med Ctr 1976; **Fellow:** Pediatric Infectious Disease, Duke Univ Med Ctr 1988; **Fac Appt:** Assoc Prof Ped, Duke Univ

Pediatric Infectious Disease

Edwards, Kathryn M MD [PInf] - **Spec Exp:** Vaccines; Clinical Trials; **Hospital:** Vanderbilt Univ Med Ctr; **Address:** Vanderbilt Univ, Peds Infectious Disease, 1161 21st Ave S, CCC-5311, Med Ctr N, Nashville, TN 37232-2581; **Phone:** 615-322-8299; **Board Cert:** Pediatrics 1978; Pediatric Infectious Disease 2005; **Med School:** Univ Iowa Coll Med 1973; **Resid:** Pediatrics, Childrens Meml Hosp 1976; **Fellow:** Pediatric Infectious Disease, Childrens Meml Hosp 1980; **Fac Appt:** Prof Ped, Vanderbilt Univ

Emmanuel, Patricia MD [PInf] - **Spec Exp:** Infections in Immunocompromised Patients; AIDS/HIV; Congenital Infections; **Hospital:** Tampa Genl Hosp, All Children's Hosp; **Address:** 17 Davis Blvd, Ste 200, Tampa, FL 33606; **Phone:** 813-259-8800; **Board Cert:** Pediatrics 2004; Pediatric Infectious Disease 2002; **Med School:** Univ Fla Coll Med 1986; **Resid:** Pediatrics, Univ So Fla 1989; **Fellow:** Infectious Disease, Univ So Fla 1993; **Fac Appt:** Assoc Prof Ped, Univ S Fla Coll Med

Givner, Laurence B MD [PInf] - **Spec Exp:** Streptococcal Infections; Rocky Mountain Spotted Fever; **Hospital:** Wake Forest Univ Baptist Med Ctr (page 73), Brenner Chldrn's Hosp; **Address:** Wake Forest Univ Sch Med, Dept Ped, Medical Center Blvd, Winston-Salem, NC 27157-0001; **Phone:** 336-716-6568; **Board Cert:** Pediatrics 1984; Pediatric Infectious Disease 2002; **Med School:** Univ MD Sch Med 1978; **Resid:** Pediatrics, Univ Maryland 1982; **Fellow:** Infectious Disease, Baylor Coll Med 1984; **Fac Appt:** Prof Ped, Wake Forest Univ

Ingram, David MD [PInf] - **Hospital:** WakeMed New Bern; **Address:** WakeMed - Andrews Ctr, 3024 New Bern Ave, Ste 307, Raleigh, NC 27610; **Phone:** 919-350-2800; **Board Cert:** Pediatrics 1980; Pediatric Infectious Disease 2002; **Med School:** Yale Univ 1967; **Resid:** Pediatrics, Yale-New Haven Hosp 1971; **Fellow:** Pediatric Infectious Disease, Chldns Hosp Med Ctr 1973; **Fac Appt:** Prof Ped, Univ NC Sch Med

McKinney Jr, Ross E MD [PInf] - **Spec Exp:** Infections in Immunocompromised Patients; **Hospital:** Duke Univ Med Ctr; **Address:** Duke Univ Med Ctr, Box 3461, Durham, NC 27710; **Phone:** 919-668-9000; **Board Cert:** Pediatrics 1983; Pediatric Infectious Disease 2002; **Med School:** Univ Rochester 1979; **Resid:** Pediatrics, Duke Univ Med Ctr 1982; **Fellow:** Pediatric Infectious Disease, Duke Univ Med Ctr 1985; **Fac Appt:** Assoc Prof Ped, Duke Univ

Mitchell, Charles D MD [PInf] - **Spec Exp:** AIDS/HIV; Viral Infections; **Hospital:** Jackson Meml Hosp; **Address:** Miller Sch Med, Div Infectious Disease, PO Box 016960, Miami, FL 33101; **Phone:** 305-243-2700; **Board Cert:** Pediatric Infectious Disease 2002; Pediatrics 1986; **Med School:** Univ Tex Med Br, Galveston 1977; **Resid:** Pediatrics, Univ Minn Hosp 1981; **Fellow:** Pediatric Infectious Disease, Univ Minn Hosp 1984; **Fac Appt:** Asst Prof Ped, Univ Miami Sch Med

Scott, Gwendolyn MD [PInf] - **Spec Exp:** AIDS/HIV; **Hospital:** Jackson Meml Hosp, Univ of Miami Hosp & Clins/Sylvester Comp Canc Ctr; **Address:** Univ Miami, Peds-Inf Dis/Immun Div, Batchelor Chldn's Res Inst (D4-4), 1580 NW 10th Ave, rm 286, Miami, FL 33136; **Phone:** 305-243-6522; **Board Cert:** Pediatrics 1978; Pediatric Infectious Disease 2002; **Med School:** UCSF 1972; **Resid:** Pediatrics, San Francisco Genl Hosp 1973; Pediatrics, Univ Maryland Hosp 1975; **Fellow:** Pediatric Infectious Disease, Univ Miami 1978; **Fac Appt:** Prof Ped, Univ Miami Sch Med

Midwest

Kleiman, Martin B MD [PInf] - **Spec Exp:** Histoplasmosis; Blastomycosis; Meningitis; AIDS/HIV; **Hospital:** Riley Hosp for Children; **Address:** 702 Barnhill Drive, Ste ROC4380, Indianapolis, IN 46202; **Phone:** 317-274-7260; **Board Cert:** Pediatrics 1973; Pediatric Infectious Disease 2002; **Med School:** SUNY Upstate Med Univ 1968; **Resid:** Pediatrics, Upstate Med Ctr 1971; **Fellow:** Infectious Disease, Johns Hopkins Hosp 1976; **Fac Appt:** Prof Ped, Indiana Univ

McAuley, James B MD [PInf] - **Spec Exp:** Tuberculosis; **Hospital:** Rush Univ Med Ctr; **Address:** 1725 W Harrison St, Ste 718, Chicago, IL 60612; **Phone:** 312-563-2683; **Board Cert:** Pediatric Infectious Disease 2004; Internal Medicine 1989; Pediatric Infectious Disease 2002; **Med School:** Northwestern Univ 1989; **Resid:** Internal Medicine, Univ Chicago Hosp 1987; Pediatrics, Univ Chicago Hosp 1989; **Fellow:** Infectious Disease, Univ Chicago Hosp 1990; **Fac Appt:** Assoc Prof Ped, Rush Med Coll

Shulman, Stanford MD [PInf] - **Spec Exp:** Kawasaki Disease; Streptococcal Infections; **Hospital:** Children's Mem Hosp, Northwestern Meml Hosp; **Address:** Children's Meml Hosp, 2515 Clarke St, Ste 900, Chicago, IL 60614-3318; **Phone:** 773-880-4187; **Board Cert:** Pediatrics 1972; Pediatric Infectious Disease 2002; **Med School:** Univ Chicago-Pritzker Sch Med 1967; **Resid:** Pediatrics, Univ Chicago Hosps 1970; **Fellow:** Infectious Disease, Shands Hosp 1973; **Fac Appt:** Prof Ped, Northwestern Univ

Wald, Ellen MD [PInf] - **Spec Exp:** Urinary Tract Infections; Infections-Respiratory; Meningitis; **Hospital:** Univ WI Hosp & Clins; **Address:** Univ Wisconsin Chldns Hosp, 600 Highland Ave, Box 4108, Madison, WI 57392; **Phone:** 608-263-8558; **Board Cert:** Pediatrics 1973; Pediatric Infectious Disease 2002; **Med School:** SUNY Downstate 1968; **Resid:** Pediatrics, Kings Co Hosp 1971; **Fellow:** Infectious Disease, Univ Maryland Hosp 1973; **Fac Appt:** Prof Ped, Univ Wisc

Southwest

Baker, Carol J MD [PInf] - **Spec Exp:** Streptococcal Infections; Neonatal Infections; Vaccines; **Hospital:** Texas Chldns Hosp - Houston, Ben Taub Genl Hosp; **Address:** Baylor Coll Med, Dept Peds, One Baylor Plaza, rm 302 A, MC BCM320, Houston, TX 77030; **Phone:** 713-798-4790; **Board Cert:** Pediatrics 1973; Pediatric Infectious Disease 2002; **Med School:** Baylor Coll Med 1968; **Resid:** Pediatrics, Baylor Coll Med 1971; **Fellow:** Pediatric Infectious Disease, Baylor Coll Med 1973; Infectious Disease, Boston City Hosp/Harvard Med Sch 1974; **Fac Appt:** Prof Ped, Baylor Coll Med

Jacobs, Richard F MD [PInf] - **Spec Exp:** Tuberculosis; Viral Infections; Drug Discovery & Development; **Hospital:** Arkansas Chldns Hosp, UAMS Med Ctr; **Address:** 800 Marshall St, Slot 512-11, Little Rock, AR 72202-3591; **Phone:** 501-364-1416; **Board Cert:** Pediatrics 1982; Pediatric Infectious Disease 2002; **Med School:** Univ Ark 1977; **Resid:** Pediatrics, Ark Chldns Hosp 1980; **Fellow:** Infectious Disease, Univ Washington 1982; **Fac Appt:** Prof Ped, Univ Ark

Kaplan, Sheldon MD [PInf] - **Spec Exp:** Pneumococcal Infections; Meningitis; **Hospital:** Texas Chldns Hosp - Houston; **Address:** Texas Chldns Hosp, Div Infectious Disease, 6621 Fannin St, MC 3-2371, Houston, TX 77030; **Phone:** 832-824-4330; **Board Cert:** Pediatrics 1978; Pediatric Infectious Disease 2002; **Med School:** Univ MO-Columbia Sch Med 1973; **Resid:** Pediatrics, St Louis Chldns Hosp 1975; **Fellow:** Pediatric Infectious Disease, St Louis Chldns Hosp 1977; **Fac Appt:** Prof Ped, Baylor Coll Med

Kline, Mark MD [PInf] - **Spec Exp:** AIDS/HIV; **Hospital:** Texas Chldns Hosp - Houston; **Address:** Texas Children's Hosp, 6621 Fannin St, MC CCC1210, Houston, TX 77030; **Phone:** 832-822-1038; **Board Cert:** Pediatrics 1987; Pediatric Infectious Disease 2002; **Med School:** Baylor Coll Med 1981; **Resid:** Pediatrics, Baylor Coll Med 1985; **Fellow:** Pediatric Infectious Disease, Baylor Coll Med 1987; **Fac Appt:** Prof Ped, Baylor Coll Med

McCracken Jr, George H MD [PInf] - **Spec Exp:** Meningitis; Antibiotic Resistance; **Hospital:** UT Southwestern Med Ctr - Dallas; **Address:** Univ Texas SW Med Ctr, Dept Peds, 5323 Harry Hines Blvd, Ste F3-202, MC 9063, Dallas, TX 75390-9063; **Phone:** 214-456-6500; **Board Cert:** Pediatrics 1967; Pediatric Infectious Disease 2002; **Med School:** Cornell Univ-Weill Med Coll 1962; **Resid:** Pediatrics, NY-Cornell Med Ctr 1965; Pediatrics, Univ Texas SW Med Ctr 1966

Pediatric Infectious Disease

West Coast and Pacific

Bradley, John S MD [PInf] - **Spec Exp:** Meningitis; Brain Infections; **Hospital:** Rady Children's Hosp - San Diego; **Address:** 3020 Children's Way, MC 5041, San Diego, CA 92123; **Phone:** 858-966-7785; **Board Cert:** Pediatrics 1981; Pediatric Infectious Disease 2002; **Med School:** UC Davis 1976; **Resid:** Pediatrics, UC Davis Med Ctr 1980; **Fellow:** Pediatric Infectious Disease, Stanford Univ Hosp 1981; **Fac Appt:** Assoc Clin Prof Ped, UCSD

Bryson, Yvonne J MD [PInf] - **Spec Exp:** AIDS/HIV; Herpes Simplex; **Hospital:** Ronald Reagan UCLA Med Ctr; **Address:** 10833 Le Conte Ave, MDCC, rm 22-442, Los Angeles, CA 90095-1752; **Phone:** 310-825-5235; **Board Cert:** Pediatrics 1976; **Med School:** Univ Tex SW, Dallas 1970; **Resid:** Pediatrics, UCSD Med Ctr 1974; **Fellow:** Infectious Disease, UCSD Med Ctr 1976; **Fac Appt:** Prof Ped, UCLA

Mason, Wilbert Henry MD [PInf] - **Spec Exp:** Kawasaki Disease; **Hospital:** Chldns Hosp - Los Angeles, USC Univ Hosp - R K Eamer Med Plz; **Address:** Chldns Hosp, Div Inf Dis, 4650 Sunset Blvd, MS 51, Los Angeles, CA 90027-6062; **Phone:** 323-361-2509; **Board Cert:** Pediatrics 1975; Pediatric Infectious Disease 2002; **Med School:** UC Irvine 1970; **Resid:** Pediatrics, Chldns Hosp 1973; **Fellow:** Infectious Disease, Chldns Hosp 1974; **Fac Appt:** Assoc Clin Prof Ped, USC Sch Med

Petru, Ann MD [PInf] - **Spec Exp:** AIDS/HIV; **Hospital:** Chldns Hosp - Oakland; **Address:** Childrens Hosp, Div Infectious Disease, 747 52nd St, Oakland, CA 94609; **Phone:** 510-428-3336; **Board Cert:** Pediatrics 1983; Pediatric Infectious Disease 2002; **Med School:** UCSF 1978; **Resid:** Pediatrics, Chldns Hosp Med Ctr 1982; **Fellow:** Pediatric Infectious Disease, Chldns Hosp Med Ctr 1983; **Fac Appt:** Asst Clin Prof Med, UCSF

PEDIATRIC NEPHROLOGY

Mid Atlantic

Dabbagh, Shermine MD [PNep] - **Spec Exp:** Kidney Disease; Kidney Failure-Chronic; Transplant Medicine-Kidney; **Hospital:** Alfred I duPont Hosp for Children; **Address:** Dupont Hosp for Children, Div Nephrology, 1600 Rockland Rd, PO Box 269, Wilmington, DE 19899; **Phone:** 302-651-4426; **Board Cert:** Pediatrics 1985; Pediatric Nephrology 1985; **Med School:** Lebanon 1979; **Resid:** Pediatrics, Univ Virginia Hosp 1981; **Fellow:** Pediatric Nephrology, Univ Wisconsin 1984

Ellis, Demetrius MD [PNep] - **Spec Exp:** Transplant Medicine-Kidney; Hypertension; **Hospital:** Chldns Hosp of Pittsburgh - UPMC; **Address:** Children's Hospital, Dept Nephrology, 3705 Fifth Ave, 4B, rm 412, Pittsburgh, PA 15213; **Phone:** 412-692-5182; **Board Cert:** Pediatrics 1978; Pediatric Nephrology 1979; **Med School:** SUNY Buffalo 1973; **Resid:** Pediatrics, Chldns Hosp 1975; **Fellow:** Pediatric Nephrology, Chldns Hosp-Natl Med Ctr 1977; **Fac Appt:** Prof Ped, Univ Pittsburgh

Fivush, Barbara A MD [PNep] - **Spec Exp:** Transplant Medicine-Kidney; **Hospital:** Johns Hopkins Hosp - Baltimore (page 61); **Address:** Johns Hopkins Hosp-Div. Nephrology, 200 N Wolfe St, rm 3055, Baltimore, MD 21287; **Phone:** 410-955-2467; **Board Cert:** Pediatrics 1984; Pediatric Nephrology 2003; **Med School:** Boston Univ 1978; **Resid:** Pediatrics, Johns Hopkins Hosp 1981; **Fellow:** Pediatric Nephrology, Johns Hopkins Hosp 1983; Pediatric Nephrology, Childs Hosp Natl Med Ctr 1984; **Fac Appt:** Assoc Prof Ped, Johns Hopkins Univ

Kaplan, Bernard S MD [PNep] - **Spec Exp:** Hemolytic Uremic Syndrome; Polycystic Kidney Disease; **Hospital:** Chldns Hosp of Philadelphia, The; **Address:** Chldns Hosp of Philadelphia, Div Nephrology, 34 St & Civic Ctr Blvd, rm 2143, Philadelphia, PA 19104; **Phone:** 215-590-2449; **Board Cert:** Pediatrics 1972; Pediatric Nephrology 1974; **Med School:** South Africa 1964; **Resid:** Pediatrics, Baragwanath Hosp, Transvaal Meml Hosp 1970; Nephrology, Royal Victoria Hosp 1973; **Fellow:** Nephrology, Montreal Chldns Hosp 1972; **Fac Appt:** Prof Ped, Univ Pennsylvania

Mendley, Susan MD [PNep] - **Spec Exp:** Transplant Medicine-Kidney; Hypertension; Dialysis Care; **Hospital:** Univ of MD Med Sys; **Address:** Univ Maryland Med System, 22 S Greene St, Pediatric Nephrol N5W67, Baltimore, MD 21201; **Phone:** 410-328-5303; **Board Cert:** Internal Medicine 1988; Nephrology 2000; **Med School:** Boston Univ 1984; **Resid:** Internal Medicine, Univ Chicago Hosps 1987; **Fellow:** Nephrology, Univ Chicago 1990; Pediatric Nephrology, Chldns Meml Hosp/Northwestern Univ 1991; **Fac Appt:** Asst Prof Ped, Univ MD Sch Med

Nash, Martin MD [PNep] - **Spec Exp:** Nephrotic Syndrome; Kidney Failure; Urinary Abnormalities; **Hospital:** NYPresby-Morgan Stanley Children's Hosp (page 66); **Address:** Morgan Stanley Chlds Hosp of NY-Presby, 3959 Broadway, rm 701, New York, NY 10032-1559; **Phone:** 212-305-5825; **Board Cert:** Pediatrics 1969; Nephrology 1974; **Med School:** Duke Univ 1964; **Resid:** Internal Medicine, Georgetown Univ Hosp 1965; Pediatrics, Columbia-Presby Med Ctr 1967; **Fellow:** Pediatric Nephrology, Montefiore Med Ctr 1971; **Fac Appt:** Clin Prof Ped, Columbia P&S

Roskes, Saul David MD [PNep] - **Hospital:** Johns Hopkins Hosp - Baltimore (page 61); **Address:** 10807 Falls Rd, Ste 200, Lutherville, MD 21093; **Phone:** 410-321-9393; **Board Cert:** Pediatrics 1970; Pediatric Nephrology 1976; **Med School:** Johns Hopkins Univ 1963; **Resid:** Pediatrics, Bronx Muni Hosp Ctr 1965; Pediatrics, Johns Hopkins Hosp 1968; **Fac Appt:** Assoc Prof Ped, Johns Hopkins Univ

Southeast

Chandar, Jayanthi J MD [PNep] - **Spec Exp:** Kidney Disease; Transplant Medicine-Kidney; Renal Replacement Therapy; **Hospital:** Jackson Meml Hosp; **Address:** Univ Miami, Dept Peds-Div Nephrology, PO Box 016960 (M-714), Miami, FL 33163; **Phone:** 305-585-6726; **Board Cert:** Pediatrics 2005; Pediatric Nephrology 2003; **Med School:** India 1983; **Resid:** Pediatrics, Jackson Memorial Hosp 1987; **Fellow:** Pediatric Nephrology, Jackson Memorial Hosp 1993; **Fac Appt:** Assoc Prof Ped, Univ Miami Sch Med

Garin, Eduardo Humberto MD [PNep] - **Hospital:** Shands at Univ of FL; **Address:** Shands Healthcare, Dept Ped Nephrology, 1600 SW Archer Rd, rm HD214, Box 100296, Gainesville, FL 32610; **Phone:** 352-392-4434; **Board Cert:** Pediatrics 1976; Pediatric Nephrology 1976; **Med School:** Chile 1970; **Resid:** Pediatrics, Univ Hosp and Clinics 1973; **Fellow:** Pediatric Nephrology, Shands Hosp Univ FL 1975; **Fac Appt:** Prof Ped, Univ S Fla Coll Med

Wyatt, Robert J MD [PNep] - **Spec Exp:** Kidney Disease-Autoimmune; Berger's Disease (IgA Nephropathy); **Hospital:** Le Bonheur Chldns Med Ctr; **Address:** Univ Tennessee, Dept Peds, 777 Washington Ave, Ste P110, Memphis, TN 38105; **Phone:** 901-448-2070; **Board Cert:** Pediatrics 1978; Pediatric Nephrology 1979; **Med School:** Med Coll GA 1973; **Resid:** Pediatrics, Kentucky Med Ctr 1976; **Fellow:** Pediatric Nephrology, Cincinnati Chldns Hosp 1979; **Fac Appt:** Prof Ped, Univ Tenn Coll Med, Memphis

Pediatric Nephrology

Zilleruelo, Gaston E MD [PNep] - **Spec Exp:** Transplant Medicine-Kidney; Nephrotic Syndrome; Congenital Anomalies-Genitourinary; **Hospital:** Jackson Meml Hosp, Broward General Med Ctr; **Address:** Univ Miami, Dept Peds-Div Nephrology, PO Box 016960 (M-714), Miami, FL 33136; **Phone:** 305-585-6726; **Board Cert:** Pediatrics 1979; Pediatric Nephrology 1991; **Med School:** Chile 1969; **Resid:** Pediatrics, L Calvo-Mackenna Chldns Hosp 1972; Pediatrics, Jackson Meml Hosp 1977; **Fellow:** Pediatric Nephrology, Jackson Meml Hosp 1979; **Fac Appt:** Prof Ped, Univ Miami Sch Med

Midwest

Andreoli, Sharon MD [PNep] - **Spec Exp:** Kidney Disease; Hypertension; **Hospital:** Riley Hosp for Children, Indiana Univ Hosp; **Address:** 699 West Drive, rm 213, Indianapolis, IN 46202; **Phone:** 317-278-0854; **Board Cert:** Pediatrics 1983; Pediatric Nephrology 1985; **Med School:** Indiana Univ 1978; **Resid:** Pediatrics, James W Riley Hosp 1981; **Fellow:** Pediatric Nephrology, Univ Minnesota 1981; Pediatric Nephrology, James W Riley Hosp/Indiana Univ 1984; **Fac Appt:** Prof Ped, Indiana Univ

Avner, Ellis D MD [PNep] - **Spec Exp:** Polycystic Kidney Disease; Kidney Disease-Genetic; **Hospital:** Chldns Hosp - Wisconsin; **Address:** Medical Coll Wisconsin, 999 92nd Ave, Milwaukee, WI 53226; **Phone:** 414-337-7702; **Board Cert:** Pediatrics 1980; Pediatric Nephrology 1982; **Med School:** Univ Pennsylvania 1975; **Resid:** Pediatrics, Chldns Hosp Med Ctr 1978; **Fellow:** Pediatric Nephrology, Chldns Hosp Med Ctr 1980; **Fac Appt:** Prof Ped, Med Coll Wisc

Bunchman, Timothy E MD [PNep] - **Spec Exp:** Lupus/SLE; **Hospital:** DeVos Children's Hosp; **Address:** DeVos Ped Nephrology/Transplant, 221 Michigan Ave NE, MC 083, Grand Rapids, MI 49503; **Phone:** 616-391-3788; **Board Cert:** Pediatrics 1986; Pediatric Nephrology 2003; **Med School:** Loyola Univ-Stritch Sch Med 1981; **Resid:** Internal Medicine & Pediatrics, St Louis Univ 1982; Pediatrics, St Louis Univ 1984; **Fellow:** Pediatric Nephrology, Mayo Clinic 1986; Pediatric Nephrology, Univ Minn 1987; **Fac Appt:** Prof Ped, Univ Mich Med Sch

Cohn, Richard MD [PNep] - **Spec Exp:** Transplant Medicine-Kidney; Nephrotic Syndrome; Kidney Disease-Chronic; **Hospital:** Children's Mem Hosp; **Address:** Childrens Meml Hosp, 2300 Children's Plaza, MC-37, Chicago, IL 60614-3394; **Phone:** 773-327-3930; **Board Cert:** Pediatrics 1978; Pediatric Nephrology 1979; **Med School:** Albert Einstein Coll Med 1972; **Resid:** Pediatrics, Johns Hopkins Hosp 1975; **Fellow:** Pediatric Nephrology, Univ Minn 1978; **Fac Appt:** Prof Ped, Northwestern Univ

Friedman, Aaron L MD [PNep] - **Spec Exp:** Hypertension; Transplant Medicine-Kidney; Growth Disorders; **Hospital:** Univ Minn Med Ctr, Fairview - Univ Campus; **Address:** Univ Minnesota Chldns Hosp Fairview, MMC 391, 420 Delaware St SE, Minneapolis, MN 55455; **Phone:** 612-626-2802; **Board Cert:** Pediatrics 1979; Pediatric Nephrology 2003; **Med School:** SUNY Upstate Med Univ 1974; **Resid:** Pediatrics, Univ Wisconsin Med Ctr 1976; **Fellow:** Pediatric Nephrology, Univ Wisconsin 1980; **Fac Appt:** Prof Ped, Univ Minn

Kashtan, Clifford E MD [PNep] - **Spec Exp:** Transplant Medicine-Kidney; Kidney Disease-Genetic; **Hospital:** Univ Minn Med Ctr, Fairview - Univ Campus; **Address:** Univ Minn Chldns Hosp Fairview, 420 Delaware St SEd, MMC 491, Minneapolis, MN 55455; **Phone:** 612-626-2922; **Board Cert:** Pediatrics 1983; Pediatric Nephrology 2003; **Med School:** Wayne State Univ 1978; **Resid:** Pediatrics, Boston City Hosp 1981; **Fellow:** Pediatric Nephrology, Mass Genl Hosp 1984; Pediatric Nephrology, Univ Minnesota Hosp 1987; **Fac Appt:** Prof Ped, Univ Minn

Langman, Craig MD [PNep] - **Spec Exp:** Kidney Stones; Osteoporosis-Juvenile; Oxalosis; **Hospital:** Children's Mem Hosp, Evanston Hosp; **Address:** Children's Meml Hosp, 2300 N Children's Plaza, Box 37, Chicago, IL 60614-3394; **Phone:** 773-327-3930; **Board Cert:** Pediatrics 1982; Pediatric Nephrology 1982; **Med School:** Hahnemann Univ 1977; **Resid:** Pediatrics, Chldns Hosp 1979; **Fellow:** Pediatric Nephrology, Chldns Hosp 1981; **Fac Appt:** Prof Ped, Northwestern Univ

Nevins, Thomas E MD [PNep] - **Spec Exp:** Kidney Failure-Chronic; Transplant Medicine-Kidney; Hypertension; **Hospital:** Univ Minn Med Ctr, Fairview - Univ Campus; **Address:** Fairview Univ Med Ctr, Dept Peds, 420 Delaware St SE, MMC-491, Minneapolis, MN 55455-0374; **Phone:** 612-626-2922; **Board Cert:** Pediatrics 1975; Pediatric Nephrology 1992; **Med School:** Washington Univ, St Louis 1969; **Resid:** Pediatrics, Univ Minnesota Hosps 1972; **Fellow:** Nephrology, Univ Minnesota Hosps 1978; **Fac Appt:** Prof Ped, Univ Minn

Warady, Bradley MD [PNep] - **Spec Exp:** Dialysis Care; Transplant Medicine-Kidney; Kidney Disease-Chronic; **Hospital:** Chldns Mercy Hosps & Clinics; **Address:** Chldns Mercy Hosps & Clins, Dept Ped Nephrology, 2401 Gillham Rd, Kansas City, MO 64108; **Phone:** 816-234-3010; **Board Cert:** Pediatrics 1984; Pediatric Nephrology 1985; **Med School:** Univ IL Coll Med 1979; **Resid:** Pediatrics, Chldns Mercy Hosp 1982; **Fellow:** Pediatric Nephrology, Colorado Univ Med Ctr 1984

West Coast and Pacific

Alexander, Steven R MD [PNep] - **Spec Exp:** Kidney Failure; Transplant Medicine-Kidney; Nephrotic Syndrome; **Hospital:** Lucile Packard Chldns Hosp/Stanford Univ Med Ctr; **Address:** Stanford Univ Med Ctr, Dept Peds, 300 Pasteur Drive, rm G306, Stanford, CA 94305-5208; **Phone:** 650-723-7903; **Board Cert:** Pediatrics 1986; Pediatric Nephrology 1986; **Med School:** Baylor Coll Med 1971; **Resid:** Pediatrics, Baylor Affil Hosps 1976; **Fellow:** Pediatric Nephrology, Baylor Affil Hosps 1978; **Fac Appt:** Prof Ped, Stanford Univ

Ettenger, Robert B MD [PNep] - **Spec Exp:** Transplant Medicine-Kidney; Hypertension in Children; Urinary Tract Infections; Kidney Disease; **Hospital:** Ronald Reagan UCLA Med Ctr, Mattel Chldns Hosp at UCLA; **Address:** Mattel Chldns Hosp, Dept Ped Nephrology, 10833 Le Conte Ave, Box 951752, Los Angeles, CA 90095; **Phone:** 310-206-6987; **Board Cert:** Pediatrics 1986; Pediatric Nephrology 1986; **Med School:** Univ Pennsylvania 1968; **Resid:** Pediatrics, St Christophers Hosp Chldn 1971; **Fellow:** Pediatric Nephrology, Chldns Hosp 1975; **Fac Appt:** Prof Ped, UCLA

Flynn, Joseph T MD [PNep] - **Spec Exp:** Hypertension; Dialysis Care; **Hospital:** Chldns Hosp and Regl Med Ctr - Seattle; **Address:** Children's Hospital, Ped Nephrology, PO Box 5371, rm A-7931, Seattle, WA 98105; **Phone:** 206-987-2524; **Board Cert:** Pediatrics ; Pediatric Nephrology 2008; **Med School:** SUNY Upstate Med Univ 1987; **Resid:** Pediatrics, St Christophers Hosp 1990; **Fellow:** Pediatric Nephrology, St Christophers Hosp 1993; **Fac Appt:** Prof Ped, Univ Wash

Jordan, Stanley C MD [PNep] - **Spec Exp:** Transplant Medicine-Kidney; **Hospital:** Cedars-Sinai Med Ctr; **Address:** Cedars Sinai Med Ctr, Div Ped Nephrology, 8635 W 3rd St, Ste 590W, Los Angeles, CA 90048; **Phone:** 310-423-2624; **Board Cert:** Pediatrics 1978; Pediatric Nephrology 1979; Clinical & Laboratory Immunology 1988; **Med School:** Univ NC Sch Med 1973; **Resid:** Pediatrics, UCLA Med Ctr 1976; Pediatric Nephrology, UCLA Med Ctr 1977; **Fellow:** Renal Immunology, Scripps Clinic 1978; Dialysis & Tranplantation, Chldns Hosp 1980; **Fac Appt:** Prof Ped, UCLA

McDonald, Ruth A MD [PNep] - **Spec Exp:** Transplant Medicine-Kidney; Kidney Disease; **Hospital:** Chldns Hosp and Regl Med Ctr - Seattle; **Address:** 4800 Sand Point Way NE, rm A-7931, Seattle, WA 98105; **Phone:** 206-987-2524; **Board Cert:** Pediatric Nephrology 2005; **Med School:** Univ Minn 1987; **Resid:** Pediatrics, Chldns Hosp & Med Ctr 1990; **Fellow:** Pediatric Nephrology, Chldns Hosp & Med Ctr 1993; **Fac Appt:** Assoc Prof Ped, Univ Wash

Pediatric Nephrology

Watkins, Sandra MD [PNep] - **Spec Exp:** Kidney Failure-Chronic; Hemolytic Uremic Syndrome; **Hospital:** Chldns Hosp and Regl Med Ctr - Seattle; **Address:** 4800 Sand Point Way NE, rm A-7931, Seattle, WA 98105; **Phone:** 206-987-2524; **Board Cert:** Pediatrics 1987; Pediatric Nephrology 1988; **Med School:** Univ Tex, Houston 1981; **Resid:** Pediatrics, Univ Wash Chldns Hosp 1984; **Fellow:** Nephrology, Univ Wash Sch Med 1986; **Fac Appt:** Prof Ped, Univ Wash

PEDIATRIC OTOLARYNGOLOGY

New England

Cunningham, Michael MD [PO] - **Spec Exp:** Head & Neck Tumors; Sinus Disorders; Hemangiomas; **Hospital:** Mass Eye & Ear Infirmary, Mass Genl Hosp; **Address:** Mass Eye & Ear Infirmary, 243 Charles St, Boston, MA 02114; **Phone:** 617-573-4250; **Board Cert:** Otolaryngology 1988; **Med School:** Univ Rochester 1981; **Resid:** Pediatrics, Mass General Hosp 1983; Otolaryngology, U Pittsburgh Eye & Ear Hosp 1988; **Fellow:** Pediatric Otolaryngology, Mass Eye & Ear Infirm 1989; **Fac Appt:** Assoc Prof Oto, Harvard Med Sch

Eavey, Roland D MD [PO] - **Spec Exp:** Ear Reconstruction/Microtia; Ear Disorders/Surgery; **Hospital:** Mass Eye & Ear Infirmary; **Address:** Mass Eye & Ear Infirmary, 243 Charles St, Boston, MA 02114-3002; **Phone:** 617-573-3190; **Board Cert:** Pediatrics 1982; Otolaryngology 1981; **Med School:** Univ Pennsylvania 1975; **Resid:** Pediatrics, Chldns Hosp 1977; Surgery, Kaiser Hosp 1978; **Fellow:** Otolaryngology, Mass EE Infirm 1981; **Fac Appt:** Assoc Prof Oto, Harvard Med Sch

Healy, Gerald MD [PO] - **Hospital:** Children's Hospital - Boston; **Address:** Chldns Hosp, Dept Otolaryngology, 300 Longwood Ave, LO-367, Boston, MA 02115; **Phone:** 617-355-5064; **Board Cert:** Otolaryngology 1972; **Med School:** Boston Univ 1967; **Resid:** Surgery, Boston Univ Hosps 1969; Otolaryngology, Boston Univ Hosps 1972; **Fac Appt:** Prof Oto, Harvard Med Sch

McGill, Trevor MD [PO] - **Spec Exp:** Head & Neck Tumors; Cholesteatoma; Lymphatic Malformations-Head & Neck; Hemangiomas; **Hospital:** Children's Hospital - Boston; **Address:** Childrens Hosp, Dept Otolaryngology, 300 Longwood Ave, MS LO-367, Boston, MA 02115; **Phone:** 617-355-6460; **Board Cert:** Otolaryngology 1988; **Med School:** Ireland 1967; **Resid:** Otolaryngology, Royal Natl Throat Nose & Ear Hosp 1974; **Fellow:** Otolaryngology, Mass Eye & Ear Infirmary 1976; **Fac Appt:** Prof Oto, Harvard Med Sch

Mid Atlantic

April, Max M MD [PO] - **Spec Exp:** Sinus Disorders; Neck Masses; Laryngeal Disorders; Tonsil/Adenoid Disorders; **Hospital:** NY-Presby Hosp/Weill Cornell (page 66), Long Island Jewish Med Ctr; **Address:** Weill-Cornell Medical Ctr, Dept Otolaryngology, 1305 York Ave Fl 5, New York, NY 10021; **Phone:** 646-962-2225; **Board Cert:** Otolaryngology 1990; **Med School:** Boston Univ 1985; **Resid:** Otolaryngology, Boston Univ Med Ctr 1990; **Fellow:** Pediatric Otolaryngology, Johns Hopkins Hosp 1991; **Fac Appt:** Clin Prof Oto, Cornell Univ-Weill Med Coll

Casselbrant, Margaretha L MD/PhD [PO] - **Spec Exp:** Ear Infections; **Hospital:** Chldns Hosp of Pittsburgh - UPMC; **Address:** Children's Hospital, Dept Otolaryngology, 3705 Fifth Ave Fl 3, Pittsburgh, PA 15213; **Phone:** 412-692-5460; **Board Cert:** Otolaryngology 1992; **Med School:** Sweden 1973; **Resid:** Otolaryngology, Malmo Genl Hosp-Univ of Lund 1978; **Fellow:** Otolaryngology, Univ Pittsburgh 1982; **Fac Appt:** Prof Oto, Univ Pittsburgh

Dolitsky, Jay MD [PO] - **Spec Exp:** Ear Infections; Neck Masses; Tonsil/Adenoid Disorders; Sleep Disorders; **Hospital:** New York Eye & Ear Infirm (page 65), St Vincent Cath Med Ctrs - Manhattan; **Address:** 404 Park Ave S Fl 12, New York, NY 10016; **Phone:** 212-679-3499; **Board Cert:** Otolaryngology 1990; **Med School:** SUNY Downstate 1981; **Resid:** Otolaryngology, Manhattan EET Hosp 1990; **Fellow:** Pediatric Otolaryngology, Children's Hosp 1992; **Fac Appt:** Assoc Prof Oto, NY Med Coll

Goldsmith, Ari J MD [PO] - **Spec Exp:** Voice Disorders; Airway Disorders; Hearing Loss; Sleep Apnea; **Hospital:** Long Island Coll Hosp (page 57); **Address:** 97 Amity St, Brooklyn, NY 11201; **Phone:** 718-780-1498; **Board Cert:** Otolaryngology 1994; **Med School:** Albert Einstein Coll Med 1988; **Resid:** Otolaryngology, LI Jewish Hosp 1993; **Fellow:** Pediatric Otolaryngology, Children's Hospital 1994; **Fac Appt:** Assoc Prof Oto, SUNY Hlth Sci Ctr

Haddad Jr, Joseph MD [PO] - **Spec Exp:** Ear Infections; Sinus Disorders; Cleft Palate/Lip; **Hospital:** NYPresby-Morgan Stanley Children's Hosp (page 66); **Address:** Morgan Stanley Chldns Hosp of NY-Presby, 3959 Broadway, Ste 501N, New York, NY 10032-1559; **Phone:** 212-305-8933; **Board Cert:** Otolaryngology 1988; **Med School:** NYU Sch Med 1983; **Resid:** Surgery, Columbia-Presby Hosp 1985; Otolaryngology, Columbia-Presby Hosp 1988; **Fellow:** Pediatric Otolaryngology, Childrens Hosp 1990; **Fac Appt:** Clin Prof Oto, Columbia P&S

Harley, Earl H MD [PO] - **Spec Exp:** Infectious Disease; **Hospital:** Georgetown Univ Hosp; **Address:** Georgetown Univ Hosp, 3800 Reservoir Rd NW, Gorman Bldg Fl 1, Washington, DC 20007; **Phone:** 202-444-8186; **Board Cert:** Otolaryngology 1984; **Med School:** Howard Univ 1971; **Resid:** Pediatrics, San Diego Naval Hosp 1973; Otolaryngology, Oakland Naval Hosp 1984; **Fellow:** Pediatric Otolaryngology, Chldn's Hosp Natl Med Ctr 1988; Pediatric Otolaryngology, Mass EE Infirm/Harvard Med Sch 1989; **Fac Appt:** Asst Prof Oto, Georgetown Univ

Jones, Jacqueline MD [PO] - **Spec Exp:** Sinus Disorders/Surgery; Ear Infections; **Hospital:** NY-Presby Hosp/Weill Cornell (page 66), Lenox Hill Hosp (page 62); **Address:** 1175 Park Ave, Ste 1A, New York, NY 10128; **Phone:** 212-996-2559; **Board Cert:** Otolaryngology 1989; **Med School:** Cornell Univ-Weill Med Coll 1984; **Resid:** Otolaryngology, Hosp Univ Penn 1989; **Fellow:** Pediatric Otolaryngology, Chldns Hosp 1990; **Fac Appt:** Assoc Prof Oto, Cornell Univ-Weill Med Coll

Kazahaya, Ken MD [PO] - **Spec Exp:** Cochlear Implants; Skull Base Surgery; Otology; Sinus Disorders; **Hospital:** Chldns Hosp of Philadelphia, The, Hosp Univ Penn - UPHS (page 60); **Address:** Children's Hosp of Philadelphia, Div Pediatric Otolaryngology, 34th St & Civic Ctr Blvd Wood Bldg Fl 1, Philadelphia, PA 19104; **Phone:** 215-590-3440; **Board Cert:** Otolaryngology 1999; **Med School:** Univ Pennsylvania 1993; **Resid:** Otolaryngology, Hosp U Penn 1998; **Fellow:** Pediatric Otolaryngology, Children's Hosp 2000; **Fac Appt:** Asst Prof Oto, Univ Pennsylvania

Rosenfeld, Richard M MD [PO] - **Spec Exp:** Sinus Disorders/Surgery; Head & Neck Surgery; Ear Disorders/Surgery; Ear Disorders/Surgery; **Hospital:** Long Island Coll Hosp (page 57), SUNY Downstate Med Ctr; **Address:** Univ Otolaryngologists, 134 Atlantic Ave, Brooklyn, NY 11201; **Phone:** 718-780-1498; **Board Cert:** Otolaryngology 1989; **Med School:** SUNY Buffalo 1984; **Resid:** Otolaryngology, Mount Sinai Med Ctr 1989; **Fellow:** Pediatric Otolaryngology, Chldn's Hosp 1991; **Fac Appt:** Prof Oto, SUNY Downstate

Tunkel, David E MD [PO] - **Spec Exp:** Laryngeal Disorders; Otology; Head & Neck Surgery; **Hospital:** Johns Hopkins Hosp - Baltimore (page 61); **Address:** 601 N Caroline St, rm 6161, Baltimore, MD 21287; **Phone:** 410-955-1559; **Board Cert:** Otolaryngology 1990; **Med School:** Johns Hopkins Univ 1984; **Resid:** Surgery, Johns Hopkins Hosp 1986; Otolaryngology, Johns Hopkins Hosp 1990; **Fellow:** Pediatric Otolaryngology, Childrens Natl Med Ctr 1991; **Fac Appt:** Assoc Prof Oto, Johns Hopkins Univ

Pediatric Otolaryngology

Ward, Robert MD [PO] - **Spec Exp:** Airway Disorders; Sinus Disorders/Surgery; Choanal Atresia; **Hospital:** NY-Presby Hosp/Weill Cornell (page 66), Manhattan Eye, Ear & Throat Hosp; **Address:** 1305 York Ave Fl 5, New York, NY 10021; **Phone:** 646-962-2224; **Board Cert:** Otolaryngology 1986; **Med School:** Cornell Univ-Weill Med Coll 1981; **Resid:** Surgery, New York Hosp 1983; Otolaryngology, New York Hosp 1986; **Fellow:** Pediatric Otolaryngology, Chldns Hosp 1986; **Fac Appt:** Assoc Clin Prof Oto, Cornell Univ-Weill Med Coll

Southeast

Darrow, David H MD/DDS [PO] - **Spec Exp:** Airway Disorders; Sinus Disorders; Otology; Neck Masses; **Hospital:** Chldns Hosp of King's Daughters; **Address:** Chldns Hosp of Kings Daughters, Div Otolaryngology, 601 Childrens Lane, Norfolk, VA 23507; **Phone:** 757-668-9327; **Board Cert:** Otolaryngology 1994; **Med School:** Duke Univ 1987; **Resid:** Otolaryngology, UCSD Med Ctr 1993; **Fellow:** Pediatric Otolaryngology, Chldns Meml Hosp 1994; **Fac Appt:** Assoc Prof Oto, Eastern VA Med Sch

Drake, Amelia F MD [PO] - **Spec Exp:** Head & Neck Surgery; **Hospital:** Univ NC Hosps; **Address:** 170 Manning Drive, Physicians Bldg, Box CB 7070, Chapel Hill, NC 27599; **Phone:** 919-966-8926; **Board Cert:** Otolaryngology 1987; **Med School:** Univ NC Sch Med 1981; **Resid:** Otolaryngology, Univ Michigan Hosps 1986

Orobello Jr, Peter W MD [PO] - ; **Address:** 801 6th St S, Ste 7535, St Petersburg, FL 33701; **Phone:** 727-329-5400; **Board Cert:** Otolaryngology 1988; **Med School:** Univ Cincinnati 1983; **Resid:** Surgery, Univ Cincinnati Med Ctr 1984; Otolaryngology, Univ Cincinnati Med Ctr 1988; **Fellow:** Pediatric Otolaryngology, Johns Hopkins Hosp 1989; **Fac Appt:** Asst Clin Prof Ped, Univ S Fla Coll Med

Midwest

Arjmand, Ellis MD/PhD [PO] - **Spec Exp:** Hearing Loss; Cochlear Implants; **Hospital:** Cincinnati Chldns Hosp Med Ctr; **Address:** Children's Hospital, Dept Otolaryngology, 3333 Burnet Ave, MS 2018, Cincinnati, OH 45229; **Phone:** 513-636-4355; **Board Cert:** Otolaryngology 1994; **Med School:** Northwestern Univ 1986; **Resid:** Otolaryngology, Barnes Jewish Hosp 1993; **Fellow:** Pediatric Otolaryngology, Barnes Jewish Hosp 1994; **Fac Appt:** Assoc Prof Oto, Univ Cincinnati

Arnold, James E MD [PO] - **Spec Exp:** Airway Disorders; Otology; Ear Tumors; **Hospital:** Rainbow Babies & Chldns Hosp, Univ Hosps Case Med Ctr; **Address:** 11100 Euclid Ave, Lakeside Bldg Fl 4, Cleveland, OH 44106-2602; **Phone:** 216-844-5031; **Board Cert:** Otolaryngology 1982; **Med School:** Univ Tex, San Antonio 1977; **Resid:** Otolaryngology, Fitzsimons Army Med Ctr 1982; **Fellow:** Pediatric Otolaryngology, Childrens Hosp 1987; **Fac Appt:** Prof Oto, Case West Res Univ

Belenky, Walter MD [PO] - **Spec Exp:** Cochlear Implants; Airway Disorders; **Hospital:** Chldns Hosp of Michigan; **Address:** Chldns Hosp, Dept Ped Oto, 3901 Beaubien Fl 3, Detroit, MI 48201; **Phone:** 313-745-9048; **Board Cert:** Otolaryngology 1970; **Med School:** Univ Mich Med Sch 1963; **Resid:** Surgery, William Beaumont Hosps 1965; Otolaryngology, Wayne Affil Hosp 1968

Cotton, Robin MD [PO] - **Spec Exp:** Tracheal Surgery; Head & Neck Surgery; Airway Reconstruction; **Hospital:** Cincinnati Chldns Hosp Med Ctr; **Address:** Cincinnati Chldns Hosp, 3333 Burnet Ave, ML 2018, Cincinnati, OH 45229-3039; **Phone:** 513-636-4355; **Board Cert:** Otolaryngology 1972; **Med School:** England 1965; **Resid:** Otolaryngology, Univ Birmingham 1968; Otolaryngology, Univ Toronto Med Ctr 1972; **Fellow:** Head and Neck Surgery, Univ Cincinnati Med Ctr 1973; **Fac Appt:** Prof Oto, Univ Cincinnati

Holinger, Lauren D MD [PO] - **Spec Exp:** Airway Disorders; Swallowing Disorders; Cough-Chronic; **Hospital:** Children's Mem Hosp; **Address:** Chldns Meml Hosp, Dept Otolaryngology, 2300 N Childrens Plaza, Box 25, Chicago, IL 60614-3394; **Phone:** 773-880-4457; **Board Cert:** Otolaryngology 1975; **Med School:** Ros Franklin Univ/Chicago Med Sch 1971; **Resid:** Surgery, Univ Colorado Affil Hosp 1972; Otolaryngology, Univ Colorado Affil Hosp 1975; **Fellow:** Pediatric Otolaryngology, Chldns Meml Hosp 1976; **Fac Appt:** Prof Oto, Northwestern Univ

Katz, Robert L MD [PO] - **Spec Exp:** Ear Infections; Sinus Disorders/Surgery; Hearing Loss; **Hospital:** Cleveland Clin Fdn (page 56); **Address:** 29800 Bainbridge Rd, Solon, OH 44139-2202; **Phone:** 440-519-6950; **Board Cert:** Otolaryngology 1968; **Med School:** Case West Res Univ 1963; **Resid:** Surgery, Mount Sinai Hosp 1965; Otolaryngology, Mass EE Infirm/Chldns Hosp 1968; **Fac Appt:** Clin Prof Oto, Case West Res Univ

Miller, Robert P MD [PO] - **Spec Exp:** Ear Disorders/Surgery; Airway Disorders; Sinus Disorders; **Hospital:** Adv Luth Genl Hosp, Children's Mem Hosp; **Address:** 8780 W Golf Rd, Ste 200, Niles, IL 60714; **Phone:** 847-674-5585; **Board Cert:** Otolaryngology 1978; **Med School:** Loyola Univ-Stritch Sch Med 1974; **Resid:** Otolaryngology, Univ Illinois Hosps 1978; **Fellow:** Pediatric Otolaryngology, Chldns Hosp Med Ctr 1987; **Fac Appt:** Asst Clin Prof Oto, Univ IL Coll Med

Myer III, Charles M MD [PO] - **Spec Exp:** Airway Disorders; Head & Neck Tumors; Neck Masses; **Hospital:** Cincinnati Chldns Hosp Med Ctr; **Address:** Cincinnati Chldns Hosp, Dept Oto, 3333 Burnet Ave Bldg C Fl 3 - Ste 375, Cincinnati, OH 45229; **Phone:** 513-636-4355; **Board Cert:** Otolaryngology 1984; **Med School:** Univ Ala 1978; **Resid:** Otolaryngology, Univ Cincinnati 1984; **Fellow:** Otolaryngology, Chldns Hosp 1985; **Fac Appt:** Prof Oto, Univ Cincinnati

Great Plains and Mountains

Chan, Kenny H MD [PO] - **Spec Exp:** Ear Infections; Sinusitis; **Hospital:** Chldn's Hosp - Aurora, The, Porter Adventist Hosp; **Address:** Chldns Hosp, Dept Otolaryngology, 13123 E 16th Ave, Box B455, Aurora, CO 80045; **Phone:** 720-777-4776; **Board Cert:** Otolaryngology 1984; **Med School:** Loma Linda Univ 1977; **Resid:** Surgery, Oregon Hlth Sci Univ 1978; Otolaryngology, Loma Linda Univ Hosp 1983; **Fellow:** Pediatric Otolaryngology, Chldns Hosp 1987; **Fac Appt:** Prof Oto, Univ Colorado

Lusk, Rodney P MD [PO] - **Spec Exp:** Cochlear Implants; Sinus Disorders/Surgery; Sleep Disorders/Apnea; **Hospital:** Boys Town Natl Rsch Hosp, Children's Hosp - Omaha; **Address:** Boystown National Research Hosp, 555 N 30th St, Omaha, NE 68131; **Phone:** 402-498-6502; **Board Cert:** Otolaryngology 1982; **Med School:** Univ MO-Columbia Sch Med 1977; **Resid:** Head and Neck Surgery, Univ Iowa Hosp & Clinics 1982; **Fellow:** Pediatric Otolaryngology, Chldns Hosp 1983

Southwest

Bower, Charles MD [PO] - **Spec Exp:** Airway Disorders; Sleep Disorders/Apnea; Sinus Disorders/Surgery; **Hospital:** Arkansas Chldns Hosp; **Address:** Arkansas Chldns Hosp, Dept Ped Oto, 800 Marshall St, Slot 836, Little Rock, AR 72202-3510; **Phone:** 501-364-1047; **Board Cert:** Otolaryngology 1990; **Med School:** Univ Ark 1985; **Resid:** Otolaryngology, Univ Ark Med Ctr 1991; **Fellow:** Pediatric Otolaryngology, Chldns Hosp 1992; **Fac Appt:** Assoc Prof Oto, Univ Ark

Pediatric Otolaryngology

Duncan III, Newton O MD [PO] - **Spec Exp:** Sinus Disorders; Airway Disorders; Head & Neck Surgery; **Hospital:** Texas Chldns Hosp - Houston, Methodist Hosp - Houston; **Address:** Childrens Ear Nose & Throat, 6550 Fannin St, Ste 2001, Houston, TX 77030-2709; **Phone:** 713-796-2001; **Board Cert:** Otolaryngology 1986; **Med School:** Baylor Coll Med 1978; **Resid:** Surgery, Baylor Coll Med 1983; Otolaryngology, Baylor Coll Med 1986; **Fellow:** Pediatric Otolaryngology, Univ Wash 1991; Pediatric Otolaryngology, Royal Alexandra Hosp Chld 1992; **Fac Appt:** Asst Clin Prof Oto, Baylor Coll Med

Friedman, Ellen M MD [PO] - **Spec Exp:** Airway Disorders; Lymphatic Malformations-Head & Neck; **Hospital:** Texas Chldns Hosp - Houston; **Address:** 67010 Fannin, Ste 540, MC CC6102, Houston, TX 77030; **Phone:** 832-822-3250; **Board Cert:** Otolaryngology 1981; **Med School:** Albert Einstein Coll Med 1975; **Resid:** Surgery, Montefiore Hosp 1976; Otolaryngology, Washington Hosp Ctr 1979; **Fellow:** Pediatric Otolaryngology, Boston Chldns Hosp; **Fac Appt:** Prof Oto, Baylor Coll Med

West Coast and Pacific

Crockett, Dennis M MD [PO] - **Spec Exp:** Head & Neck Cancer; Airway Disorders; **Hospital:** Chldns Hosp - Los Angeles, USC Univ Hosp - R K Eamer Med Plz; **Address:** USC Health Consultation Ctr #2, 1420 San Pablo St, Ste 4600, Los Angeles, CA 90033; **Phone:** 323-442-5790; **Board Cert:** Otolaryngology 1985; **Med School:** USC Sch Med 1979; **Resid:** Otolaryngology, LAC-USC Med Ctr 1984; **Fellow:** Pediatrics, Boston Chldns Hosp 1985; **Fac Appt:** Assoc Prof Oto, USC Sch Med

Geller, Kenneth Allen MD [PO] - **Spec Exp:** Airway Disorders; Sinus Disorders/Surgery; Head & Neck Cancer; **Hospital:** Chldns Hosp - Los Angeles, Huntington Memorial Hosp; **Address:** Chldns Hosp, Div Otolaryngology, 4650 Sunset Blvd, MS 58, Los Angeles, CA 90027; **Phone:** 323-361-2145; **Board Cert:** Otolaryngology 1978; **Med School:** USC Sch Med 1972; **Resid:** Surgery, Wadsworth VA Hosp 1975; Otolaryngology, UCLA Hlth Scis Ctr 1978; **Fellow:** Pediatric Otolaryngology, Chldns Hosp 1979; **Fac Appt:** Assoc Clin Prof Oto, USC Sch Med

Inglis, Andrew MD [PO] - **Spec Exp:** Airway Disorders; Voice Disorders; **Hospital:** Chldns Hosp and Regl Med Ctr - Seattle; **Address:** Children's Hospital & Medical Ctr, 4800 Sand Point Way NE, MS W6640, Seattle, WA 98105-0371; **Phone:** 206-987-2105; **Board Cert:** Otolaryngology 1987; **Med School:** Med Coll PA Hahnemann 1981; **Resid:** Surgery, Virginia Mason Hosp 1983; Otolaryngology, Univ Washington Hosps 1987; **Fellow:** Pediatric Otolaryngology, Royal Alexandria Hosp Chldn 1987; **Fac Appt:** Assoc Prof Oto, Univ Wash

Richardson, Mark A MD [PO] - **Spec Exp:** Sinus Disorders; Airway Disorders; Lymphatic Malformations-Head & Neck; **Hospital:** Doernbecher Chldns Hosp/OHSU, Providence St Vincent Med Ctr; **Address:** 3181 SW Sam Jackson Park Rd, MC PV01, Dept Otolaryngology/Head & Neck Surgery, Portland, OR 97239; **Phone:** 503-494-5350; **Board Cert:** Otolaryngology 1979; **Med School:** Med Univ SC 1975; **Resid:** Otolaryngology, Med Univ Hosp 1979; **Fellow:** Pediatric Otolaryngology, Chldns Hosp Med Ctr 1980; **Fac Appt:** Prof Oto, Oregon Hlth Sci Univ

Rosbe, Kristina W MD [PO] - **Spec Exp:** Airway Disorders; Sinus Disorders/Surgery; Cochlear Implants; Neck Masses; **Hospital:** UCSF Med Ctr; **Address:** UCSF Med Ctr, Dept Otolaryngology, 400 Parnassus Ave, Box 0342, San Francisco, CA 94143-0342; **Phone:** 415-353-2757; **Board Cert:** Orthopaedic Surgery 1999; **Med School:** Dartmouth Med Sch 1993; **Resid:** Surgery, Univ N Carolina Hosps 1994; Otolaryngology, Univ N Carolina Hosps 1998; **Fellow:** Pediatric Otolaryngology, Chldns Hosp 2000; **Fac Appt:** Assoc Prof Ped, UCSF

PEDIATRIC PULMONOLOGY

New England

Lapey, Allen MD [PPul] - **Spec Exp:** Cystic Fibrosis; Asthma; Food Allergy; **Hospital:** Mass Genl Hosp; **Address:** 15 Parkman St, POB 101, Boston, MA 02114; **Phone:** 617-726-8707; **Board Cert:** Pediatrics 1972; Allergy & Immunology 1978; Pediatric Pulmonology 2003; **Med School:** Univ Rochester 1966; **Resid:** Pediatrics, Chldns Hosp 1968; **Fellow:** Pediatric Pulmonology, Mass Genl Hosp 1972; Allergy & Immunology, Mass Genl Hosp 1972; **Fac Appt:** Asst Clin Prof Ped, Harvard Med Sch

Mid Atlantic

Borowitz, Drucy S MD [PPul] - **Spec Exp:** Cystic Fibrosis; **Hospital:** Women's & Chldn's Hosp of Buffalo, The; **Address:** Women & Childrens Hospital, 219 Bryant St, Buffalo, NY 14222; **Phone:** 716-878-7561; **Board Cert:** Pediatrics 1984; Pediatric Gastroenterology 2007; **Med School:** Cornell Univ-Weill Med Coll 1979; **Resid:** Pediatrics, UCSF Med Ctr 1982; **Fellow:** Nutrition, UCSF Med Ctr 1983; **Fac Appt:** Clin Prof Ped, SUNY Buffalo

Dozor, Allen J MD [PPul] - **Spec Exp:** Asthma; Cystic Fibrosis; **Hospital:** Westchester Med Ctr; **Address:** NY Med College, Munger Pavilion, Pediatric Pulmonology, Ste 106, Valhalla, NY 10595-1600; **Phone:** 914-493-7585; **Board Cert:** Pediatrics 1981; Pediatric Pulmonology 2003; **Med School:** Penn State Univ-Hershey Med Ctr 1977; **Resid:** Pediatrics, St Vincent's Hosp & Med Ctr 1980; **Fellow:** Pediatric Pulmonology, Chldns Hosp 1982; **Fac Appt:** Prof Ped, NY Med Coll

Kattan, Meyer MD [PPul] - **Spec Exp:** Asthma; Cystic Fibrosis; Chronic Lung Disease; **Hospital:** NY-Presby Hosp/Columbia (page 66), Englewood Hosp & Med Ctr; **Address:** 3959 Broadway, CHC 7-701, New York, NY 10032; **Phone:** 212-305-5122; **Board Cert:** Pediatrics 1980; Pediatric Pulmonology 2003; **Med School:** McGill Univ 1973; **Resid:** Pediatrics, Chldns Hosp 1975; Pediatrics, Hosp for Sick Children 1976; **Fellow:** Pulmonary Disease, Hosp for Sick Children 1978; **Fac Appt:** Prof Ped, Columbia P&S

Kurland, Geoffrey MD [PPul] - **Spec Exp:** Transplant Medicine-Lung; **Hospital:** Chldns Hosp of Pittsburgh - UPMC; **Address:** Children's Hospital, Ped Pulmonology, 3705 Fifth Ave, Pittsburgh, PA 15213; **Phone:** 412-692-5630; **Board Cert:** Pediatrics 1978; Allergy & Immunology 1979; Pediatric Pulmonology 2003; **Med School:** Stanford Univ 1973; **Resid:** Pediatrics, Stanford Affil Hosps 1976; **Fellow:** Allergy & Immunology, Stanford Affil Hosps 1978; **Fac Appt:** Prof Ped, Univ Pittsburgh

Loughlin, Gerald M MD [PPul] - **Spec Exp:** Sleep Disorders/Apnea; Swallowing Disorders; Asthma & Chronic Lung Disease; Breathing Disorders; **Hospital:** NY-Presby Hosp/Weill Cornell (page 66); **Address:** Cornell Med Coll, Dept Peds, 525 E 68th St, rm M-622, New York, NY 10021-4870; **Phone:** 212-746-4111; **Board Cert:** Pediatrics 1993; Pediatric Pulmonology 2003; **Med School:** Univ Rochester 1973; **Resid:** Pediatrics, Univ Ariz Med Ctr 1973; **Fellow:** Pediatric Pulmonology, Univ Ariz Med Ctr 1977; **Fac Appt:** Prof Ped, Cornell Univ-Weill Med Coll

Marcus, Carole L MD [PPul] - **Spec Exp:** Sleep Disorders/Apnea; **Hospital:** Chldns Hosp of Philadelphia, The; **Address:** Chldns Hosp of Philadelphia, Wood Bldg 5FL, 34th St & Civic Ctr Blvd, Philadelphia, PA 19104; **Phone:** 215-590-3749; **Board Cert:** Pediatrics 2000; Pediatric Pulmonology 2000; **Med School:** South Africa 1982; **Resid:** Pediatrics, LIJ/SUNY Brooklyn Med Ctr 1986; **Fellow:** Pediatric Pulmonology, Chldns Hosp 1991; **Fac Appt:** Assoc Prof Ped, Univ Pennsylvania

Pediatric Pulmonology

Orenstein, David M MD [PPul] - **Spec Exp:** Cystic Fibrosis; **Hospital:** Chldns Hosp of Pittsburgh - UPMC; **Address:** Children's Hospital, Ped Pulmonology, 3705 Fifth Ave, Pittsburgh, PA 15213; **Phone:** 412-692-5630; **Board Cert:** Pediatrics 1979; Pediatric Pulmonology 2004; **Med School:** Case West Res Univ 1973; **Resid:** Pediatrics, Rainbow Babies & Chldn's Hosp 1976; **Fellow:** Pediatric Pulmonology, Rainbow Babies & Chldn's Hosp 1978; **Fac Appt:** Prof Ped, Univ Pittsburgh

Panitch, Howard B MD [PPul] - **Spec Exp:** Chronic Obstructive Lung Disease (COPD); Cystic Fibrosis; **Hospital:** Chldns Hosp of Philadelphia, The; **Address:** Chldns Hosp Of Philadelphia - Div Pulmonology, 34th St & Civic Blvd, Wood Bldg - 5th Fl, Philadelphia, PA 19104; **Phone:** 215-590-3749; **Board Cert:** Pediatrics 1987; Pediatric Pulmonology 1997; **Med School:** Univ Pittsburgh 1982; **Resid:** Pediatrics, Children's Hosp 1985; **Fellow:** Pediatric Pulmonology, St Christopher's Hosp 1988; **Fac Appt:** Assoc Prof Ped, Univ Pennsylvania

Quittell, Lynne MD [PPul] - **Spec Exp:** Cystic Fibrosis; Asthma; **Hospital:** NYPresby-Morgan Stanley Children's Hosp (page 66); **Address:** Morgan Stanley Chlds Hosp of NY-Presby, 3959 Broadway Fl 7, New York, NY 10032-1551; **Phone:** 212-305-5122; **Board Cert:** Pediatrics 1986; Pediatric Pulmonology 2004; **Med School:** Israel 1981; **Resid:** Pediatrics, Schneider Chldns Hosp 1984; **Fellow:** Pediatric Pulmonology, St Christopher's Hosp 1988; **Fac Appt:** Assoc Prof Ped, Columbia P&S

Zeitlin, Pamela L MD [PPul] - **Spec Exp:** Cystic Fibrosis; **Hospital:** Johns Hopkins Hosp - Baltimore (page 61), Mt Washington Ped Hosp; **Address:** 200 N Wolfe St, Baltimore, MD 21287; **Phone:** 410-955-2035; **Board Cert:** Pediatrics 1988; Pediatric Pulmonology 2000; **Med School:** Yale Univ 1983; **Resid:** Pediatrics, Johns Hopkins Hosp 1986; **Fellow:** Pediatric Pulmonology, Johns Hopkins Hosp 1989; **Fac Appt:** Prof Ped, Johns Hopkins Univ

Southeast

Murphy, Thomas M MD [PPul] - **Spec Exp:** Cystic Fibrosis; Asthma; Pneumonia; **Hospital:** Duke Univ Med Ctr; **Address:** Duke Univ Med Ctr, Box 2994, Durham, NC 27710; **Phone:** 919-684-3364; **Board Cert:** Internal Medicine 1976; Pediatrics 2003; Pediatric Pulmonology 2004; **Med School:** Univ Rochester 1973; **Resid:** Internal Medicine, Georgetown Univ Hosp 1976; **Fellow:** Pediatric Pulmonology, Georgetown Univ Hosp 1978; **Fac Appt:** Assoc Prof Ped, Duke Univ

Rubin, Bruce MD [PPul] - **Spec Exp:** Asthma; Cystic Fibrosis; Mucus Clearance Disorders; **Hospital:** Wake Forest Univ Baptist Med Ctr (page 73); **Address:** Dept of Pediatrics-Wake Forest Univ Med Sch, Medical Center Blvd, Winston-Salem, NC 27157; **Phone:** 336-713-4500; **Board Cert:** Pediatrics 1984; Pediatric Pulmonology 2005; **Med School:** Tulane Univ 1979; **Resid:** Pediatrics, Tulane Univ 1981; **Fellow:** Pediatric Pulmonary & Critical Care, Hosp for Sick Children 1983; **Fac Appt:** Prof Ped, Wake Forest Univ

Sallent, Jorge A MD [PPul] - **Spec Exp:** Chronic Lung Disease of Infancy; Asthma & Chronic Lung Disease; Lung Injuries - RSV Related; **Hospital:** St Mary's Med Ctr - W Palm Bch, Palms - West Hosp; **Address:** Pediatric Respiratory Ctr, 500 US Highway 1, Lake Park, FL 33403-3598; **Phone:** 561-863-0105; **Board Cert:** Pediatrics 1984; Pediatric Pulmonology 2003; **Med School:** Dominican Republic 1978; **Resid:** Pediatrics, Orlando Regional Med Ctr 1983; **Fellow:** Pediatric Pulmonology, Univ Florida 1986; **Fac Appt:** Asst Prof Ped, Univ Fla Coll Med

Sherman, James MD [PPul] - **Spec Exp:** Asthma; Airway Disorders; Cough-Chronic; **Hospital:** Carilion Roanoke Meml Hosp; **Address:** 102 Highland Ave, Ste 203, Roanoke, VA 24013; **Phone:** 540-985-9835; **Board Cert:** Pediatrics 1981; Pediatric Pulmonology 2003; **Med School:** Univ S Fla Coll Med 1975; **Resid:** Pediatrics, SUNY Upstate Med Ctr 1977; Pediatrics, Tampa Genl Hosp- Univ So Florida 1978; **Fellow:** Pediatric Pulmonology, Rainbow Babies & Children's Hosp 1981; **Fac Appt:** Prof Ped, Univ Fla Coll Med

Midwest

Green, Thomas P MD [PPul] - **Spec Exp:** Respiratory Failure; Breathing Disorders; **Hospital:** Children's Mem Hosp, Evanston Hosp; **Address:** Chldns Meml Hosp, Dept Pulm-Crit Care Med, 2300 Chldns Pl, Box 86, Chicago, IL 60614; **Phone:** 773-880-8150; **Board Cert:** Pediatrics 1992; Pulmonary Disease 2002; Pediatric Critical Care Medicine 2003; **Med School:** Stanford Univ 1974; **Resid:** Pediatrics, Univ Minn Med Ctr 1977; **Fellow:** Pharmacology, Univ Minn Med Ctr 1979; Pediatric Pulmonology, Univ Minn Med Ctr 1994; **Fac Appt:** Prof Ped, Northwestern Univ

Kemp, James S MD [PPul] - **Spec Exp:** Sudden Infant Death Syndrome (SIDS); Breathing Disorders; **Hospital:** St Louis Chldns Hosp; **Address:** One Children's Place, Ste 2C, St Louis, MO 63141; **Phone:** 314-454-2694; **Board Cert:** Pediatrics 1981; Pediatric Pulmonology 2000; **Med School:** Creighton Univ 1976; **Resid:** Pediatrics, Cardinal Glennon Chldns Hosp 1978; Pediatrics, Baylor Univ 1979; **Fellow:** Pediatric Pulmonology, Texas Chldns Hosp 1988; **Fac Appt:** Assoc Prof Ped, St Louis Univ

Kim, Young-Jee MD [PPul] - **Spec Exp:** Asthma; Chest Wall Deformities-Pediatric; Rare Lung Disease-Pediatric; **Hospital:** Riley Hosp for Children; **Address:** Riley Chldns Hosp - Dept Ped Pulm, 702 Barnhill Rd, ROC-rm 4270, Indianapolis, IN 46202-5128; **Phone:** 317-274-7208; **Board Cert:** Pediatric Pulmonology 2006; **Med School:** South Korea 1986; **Resid:** Pediatrics, Duke Univ Med Ctr 1995; **Fellow:** Pediatric Pulmonology, Yale Univ Med Sch 1991; Pediatric Pulmonology, Riley Hosp Chldn 1998; **Fac Appt:** Assoc Prof Ped, Indiana Univ

Konstan, Michael W MD [PPul] - **Spec Exp:** Cystic Fibrosis; **Hospital:** Rainbow Babies & Chldns Hosp; **Address:** Div Ped Pulmonology, 11100 Euclid Ave, Ste 3001, MS 6006, Cleveland, OH 44106-2624; **Phone:** 216-844-1997; **Board Cert:** Pediatrics 1986; Pediatric Pulmonology 2004; **Med School:** Case West Res Univ 1982; **Resid:** Pediatrics, Chldn's Hosp 1985; **Fellow:** Pediatric Pulmonology, Rainbow Babies & Chldns Hosp 1988; **Fac Appt:** Prof Ped, Case West Res Univ

Kurachek, Stephen MD [PPul] - **Spec Exp:** Critical Care; Asthma; **Hospital:** Chldns Hosp and Clinics - Minneapolis; **Address:** 2545 Chicago Ave S, Ste 617, Minneapolis, MN 55404; **Phone:** 612-863-3226; **Board Cert:** Pediatrics 1985; Pediatric Pulmonology 2004; Pediatric Critical Care Medicine 2003; **Med School:** Univ Miami Sch Med 1978; **Resid:** Pediatrics, Univ Hosp 1981; **Fellow:** Pulmonary Disease, Boston Chldns Hosp 1984; **Fac Appt:** Asst Clin Prof Ped, Univ Minn

Stern, Robert C MD [PPul] - **Spec Exp:** Cystic Fibrosis; Lung Disease; **Hospital:** Rainbow Babies & Chldns Hosp; **Address:** Div Pediatric Pulmonology, 11100 Euclid Ave, rm 3001, Cleveland, OH 44106-1736; **Phone:** 216-844-3267; **Board Cert:** Pediatrics 1968; Pediatric Pulmonology 2002; **Med School:** Albert Einstein Coll Med 1963; **Resid:** Pediatrics, Univ Hosp 1965; Pediatrics, Bronx Muni Hosp Ctr 1966; **Fellow:** Pediatric Pulmonology, Univ Hosp; **Fac Appt:** Prof Ped, Case West Res Univ

Pediatric Pulmonology

Great Plains and Mountains

Accurso, Frank J MD [PPul] - **Spec Exp:** Cystic Fibrosis; **Hospital:** Chldn's Hosp - Aurora, The; **Address:** Childrens Hosp, 13123 E 16th Ave, Box B395, Aurora, CO 80045; **Phone:** 303-837-2522; **Board Cert:** Pediatrics 1980; Pediatric Pulmonology 2003; **Med School:** Albert Einstein Coll Med 1974; **Resid:** Pediatrics, Univ Colo Hlth Sci Ctr 1977; **Fellow:** Pulmonary Disease, Univ Colo Hlth Sci Ctr 1980; **Fac Appt:** Prof Ped, Univ Colorado

Larsen, Gary L MD [PPul] - **Hospital:** Natl Jewish Med & Rsch Ctr, Chldn's Hosp - Aurora, The; **Address:** Natl Jewish Med & Rsrch Ctr, 1400 Jackson St, rm J303, Denver, CO 80206-2761; **Phone:** 303-398-1617; **Board Cert:** Pediatrics 1976; Pediatric Pulmonology 2003; **Med School:** Columbia P&S 1971; **Resid:** Pediatrics, Univ Colorado Med Ctr 1974; **Fellow:** Pediatric Pulmonology, Univ Colorado Med Ctr 1978; **Fac Appt:** Prof Ped, Univ Colorado

Southwest

Fan, Leland Lane MD [PPul] - **Spec Exp:** Interstitial Lung Disease; **Hospital:** Texas Chldns Hosp - Houston; **Address:** 6701 Fannin St, MC CCC 1040.01, Houston, TX 77030; **Phone:** 832-822-3300; **Board Cert:** Pediatrics 1978; Pediatric Pulmonology 2002; Pediatric Critical Care Medicine 2003; **Med School:** Baylor Coll Med 1973; **Resid:** Pediatrics, UCSF Med Ctr 1975; Pediatrics, Univ Colo Hlth Sci Ctr 1976; **Fellow:** Pediatric Pulmonary & Critical Care, Univ Colo Hlth Sci Ctr 1978; **Fac Appt:** Prof Ped, Baylor Coll Med

Morgan, Wayne J MD [PPul] - **Spec Exp:** Cystic Fibrosis; Asthma; **Hospital:** Univ Med Ctr - Tucson, Tucson Med Ctr; **Address:** Univ Arizona Hlth Sci Ctr, Div Pediatric Pulmonology, 1501 N Campbell Ave, Box 245073, Tucson, AZ 85724; **Phone:** 520-626-7780; **Board Cert:** Pediatrics 1982; Pediatric Pulmonology 2003; **Med School:** McGill Univ 1976; **Resid:** Pediatrics, Montreal Chldns Hosp 1980; **Fellow:** Pediatric Pulmonology, Univ Ariz Hlth Sci 1982; **Fac Appt:** Prof Ped, Univ Ariz Coll Med

Warren, Robert H MD [PPul] - **Spec Exp:** Muscular Dystrophy; Pulmonary Rehabilitation; **Hospital:** Arkansas Chldns Hosp; **Address:** Arkansas Chldns Hosp, Pulmonary Med, 800 Marshall St, Slot 512-17, Little Rock, AR 72202; **Phone:** 501-364-1006; **Board Cert:** Pediatrics 1973; Pediatric Pulmonology 2003; **Med School:** Univ Ark 1967; **Resid:** Pediatrics, LSU Med Ctr 1971; **Fellow:** Pediatric Pulmonology, Tulane Univ Sch Med; **Fac Appt:** Assoc Prof Ped, Univ Ark

West Coast and Pacific

Cooper, Dan M MD [PPul] - **Hospital:** UC Irvine Med Ctr; **Address:** UCI Medical Center, Department of Pediatrics, 101 The City Drive S ZC Bldg, MC 4482, Orange, CA 92868; **Phone:** 714-532-7983; **Board Cert:** Pediatrics 1980; Pediatric Pulmonology 1994; **Med School:** UCSF 1974; **Resid:** Internal Medicine, Hadassah Hosp; Pediatrics, Children's Hosp Med Ctr; **Fellow:** Pediatric Pulmonology, Babies' Hosp-Columbia Univ; **Fac Appt:** Prof Ped, UC Irvine

Keens, Thomas G MD [PPul] - **Spec Exp:** Sudden Infant Death Syndrome (SIDS); Breathing Disorders; **Hospital:** Chldns Hosp - Los Angeles; **Address:** Chldns Hosp, Div Pulmonology, 4650 W Sunset Blvd, Box 83, Los Angeles, CA 90027-6062; **Phone:** 323-361-2101; **Board Cert:** Pediatrics 1978; Neonatal-Perinatal Medicine 1983; Pediatric Pulmonology 2003; **Med School:** UCSD 1972; **Resid:** Pediatrics, Chldns Hosp 1975; **Fellow:** Pediatric Pulmonology, Hosp Sick Chldn 1977; **Fac Appt:** Prof Ped, USC Sch Med

Platzker, Arnold CG MD [PPul] - **Spec Exp:** Asthma; Chronic Lung Disease; Cystic Fibrosis; **Hospital:** Chldns Hosp - Los Angeles, Mattel Chldns Hosp at UCLA; **Address:** Chldns Hosp, Div Ped Pulmonology, 4650 Sunset Blvd, Box 83, Los Angeles, CA 90027-6062; **Phone:** 323-361-2101; **Board Cert:** Pediatrics 1967; Neonatal-Perinatal Medicine 1975; Pediatric Pulmonology 2002; **Med School:** Tufts Univ 1962; **Resid:** Pediatrics, City Hosp 1964; Pediatrics, Stanford Univ Med Ctr 1966; **Fellow:** Pediatric Pulmonology, UCSF Med Ctr 1971; Neonatal-Perinatal Medicine, UCSF Med Ctr 1971; **Fac Appt:** Prof Ped, USC Sch Med

Ramsey, Bonnie W MD [PPul] - **Spec Exp:** Cystic Fibrosis; **Hospital:** Chldns Hosp and Regl Med Ctr - Seattle; **Address:** Chldns Hosp & Regl Med Ctr, 1100 Olive Way, Ste 500, MS MPW 5-4, Seattle, WA 98101; **Board Cert:** Pediatrics 1981; Pediatric Pulmonology 2007; **Med School:** Harvard Med Sch 1976; **Resid:** Pediatrics, Chldns Hosp 1978; Pediatrics, Chldns Hosp 1979; **Fellow:** Pediatric Critical Care Medicine, Chldns Hosp 1981; **Fac Appt:** Prof Ped, Univ Wash

Redding, Gregory MD [PPul] - **Spec Exp:** Asthma; Chest Wall Deformities-Pediatric; Interstitial Lung Disease; **Hospital:** Chldns Hosp and Regl Med Ctr - Seattle; **Address:** Pulmonary Div, Chlds Hosp & Regl Med Ctr, 4800 Sand Point Way NE, MS A-5937, Seattle, WA 98105; **Phone:** 206-987-2174; **Board Cert:** Pediatrics 1992; Pediatric Pulmonology 2003; **Med School:** Stanford Univ 1974; **Resid:** Pediatrics, Harbor-UCLA Affil Hosps 1977; **Fellow:** Pediatric Pulmonology, Univ Colo Affil Hosps 1979; **Fac Appt:** Prof Ped, Univ Wash

PEDIATRIC RHEUMATOLOGY

New England

McCarthy, Paul L MD [PRhu] - **Spec Exp:** Lupus/SLE; Juvenile Arthritis; Dermatomyositis; Vasculitis; **Hospital:** Yale-New Haven Hosp; **Address:** Yale Schl Med, 333 Cedar St, Box 208064, New Haven, CT 06520-3206; **Phone:** 203-688-2475; **Board Cert:** Pediatrics 1974; Pediatric Rheumatology 2007; **Med School:** Georgetown Univ 1969; **Resid:** Pediatrics, Chldns Hosp 1972; **Fellow:** Pediatrics, Chldns Hosp 1974; **Fac Appt:** Prof Ped, Yale Univ

Mid Atlantic

Finkel, Terri H MD [PRhu] - **Spec Exp:** Juvenile Arthritis; Lupus/SLE; Vasculitis; **Hospital:** Chldns Hosp of Philadelphia, The; **Address:** Chldns Hosp of Philadelphia, Div Rheum, 34th St & Civic Ctr Blvd, Chldns Seashore House, rm 236, Philadelphia, PA 19104; **Phone:** 215-590-2547; **Board Cert:** Pediatrics 1988; Pediatric Rheumatology 2002; **Med School:** Stanford Univ 1982; **Resid:** Pediatrics, Univ Colorado Med Ctr 1985; **Fellow:** Pediatric Rheumatology, Natl Jewish Med Ctr 1990; **Fac Appt:** Assoc Prof Ped, Univ Pennsylvania

Goldsmith, Donald P MD [PRhu] - **Spec Exp:** Arthritis; Juvenile Arthritis; **Hospital:** St Christopher's Hosp for Chldn; **Address:** St Christophers Hosp for Children, Rheumatology Section, Erie Ave at Front St, Philadelphia, PA 19134; **Phone:** 215-427-5051; **Board Cert:** Pediatrics 1974; Allergy & Immunology 1975; Pediatric Rheumatology 2007; **Med School:** Univ VT Coll Med 1967; **Resid:** Pediatrics, St Christophers Hosp for Chldn 1973; **Fellow:** Allergy Immunology & Rheumatology, St Christophers Hosp for Chldn 1975; **Fac Appt:** Prof Ped, Drexel Univ Coll Med

Pediatric Rheumatology

Haines, Kathleen A MD [PRhu] - **Spec Exp:** Juvenile Arthritis; Lupus/SLE; Immune Deficiency; **Hospital:** Hackensack Univ Med Ctr, NYU Med Ctr (page 68); **Address:** Hackensack Univ Med Ctr, Don Imus Ped Ctr, 30 Prospect Ave Fl 3, Hackensack, NJ 07601; **Phone:** 201-996-5306; **Board Cert:** Pediatrics 1980; Allergy & Immunology 1981; Pediatric Rheumatology 2007; **Med School:** Albert Einstein Coll Med 1975; **Resid:** Pediatrics, New York Hosp 1977; **Fellow:** Allergy & Immunology, New York Hosp 1980; Rheumatology, NYU Med Sch 1982; **Fac Appt:** Assoc Prof Ped, UMDNJ-NJ Med Sch, Newark

Ilowite, Norman T MD [PRhu] - **Spec Exp:** Juvenile Arthritis; Lyme Disease; Lupus/SLE; Vasculitis; **Hospital:** Montefiore Med Ctr; **Address:** Montefiore Children's Hosp, Rheumatology, 3415 Bainbridge Ave, Bronx, NY 10467; **Phone:** 718-741-2456; **Board Cert:** Pediatrics 1985; Clinical & Laboratory Immunology 1990; Pediatric Rheumatology 2007; **Med School:** SUNY Downstate 1979; **Resid:** Pediatrics, Chldns Hosp Natl Med Ctr 1982; **Fellow:** Pediatric Rheumatology, Univ WA Med Ctr 1984; **Fac Appt:** Prof Ped, Albert Einstein Coll Med

Lehman, Thomas MD [PRhu] - **Spec Exp:** Arthritis; Scleroderma; Lupus/SLE; Rheumatoid Arthritis; **Hospital:** Hosp For Special Surgery (page 59), NY-Presby Hosp/Weill Cornell (page 66); **Address:** 535 E 70th St, New York, NY 10021-4872; **Phone:** 212-606-1151; **Board Cert:** Pediatrics 1979; Pediatric Rheumatology 2007; **Med School:** Jefferson Med Coll 1974; **Resid:** Pediatrics, Chldns Hosp 1976; Pediatrics, UCSF Med Ctr 1977; **Fellow:** Pediatric Rheumatology, Chldns Hosp 1979; Rheumatology, Natl Inst Hlth 1983; **Fac Appt:** Prof Ped, Cornell Univ-Weill Med Coll

Sherry, David D MD [PRhu] - **Spec Exp:** Pain-Musculoskeletal; Reflex Sympathetic Dystrophy (RSD); Juvenile Arthritis; Lupus/SLE; **Hospital:** Chldns Hosp of Philadelphia, The; **Address:** Chldns Hosp of Phildelphia, Div Rheum, 34th St & Civic Ctr Blvd, rm 236, Chldns Seashore House, Philadelphia, PA 19104; **Phone:** 215-590-2547; **Board Cert:** Pediatrics 1981; Pediatric Rheumatology 2000; **Med School:** Texas Tech Univ 1977; **Resid:** Pediatrics, Duke Univ Med Ctr 1980; **Fellow:** Pediatric Rheumatology, Univ British Columbia 1982; **Fac Appt:** Prof Ped, Univ Pennsylvania

Sills, Edward M MD [PRhu] - **Spec Exp:** Juvenile Arthritis; Lupus/SLE; Dermatomyositis; **Hospital:** Johns Hopkins Hosp - Baltimore (page 61); **Address:** Johns Hopkins Hosp, 200 N Wolfe St, Ste 2-127, Baltimore, MD 21205; **Phone:** 410-955-6145; **Board Cert:** Pediatrics 1968; Pediatric Rheumatology 2000; **Med School:** NYU Sch Med 1963; **Resid:** Pediatrics, Bronx Muni Hosp 1967; **Fac Appt:** Assoc Prof Ped, Johns Hopkins Univ

Southeast

Passo, Murray H MD [PRhu] - **Hospital:** MUSC Med Ctr; **Address:** MUSC, Dept Pediatrics, Div Pediatric Rheumatology, 135 Rutledge Ave, MSC 561, Charleston, SC 29425-5610; **Phone:** 843-792-5696; **Board Cert:** Pediatrics 1979; Pediatric Rheumatology 2007; **Med School:** Indiana Univ 1974; **Resid:** Pediatrics, Riley Chldns Hosp 1977; **Fellow:** Rheumatology, Indiana Univ Hosps 1979

Schanberg, Laura E MD [PRhu] - **Spec Exp:** Rheumatic Diseases of Childhood; Fibromyalgia; **Hospital:** Duke Univ Med Ctr; **Address:** Duke Univ Med Ctr, Box 3212, Durham, NC 27710; **Phone:** 919-684-6575; **Board Cert:** Pediatric Rheumatology 2007; **Med School:** Duke Univ 1984; **Resid:** Pediatrics, Duke Univ Med Ctr 1987; **Fellow:** Pediatric Rheumatology, Duke Univ Med Ctr 1991; **Fac Appt:** Asst Prof Ped, Duke Univ

Sleasman, John W MD [PRhu] - **Spec Exp:** Infectious Disease; Immunodeficiency Disorders; **Hospital:** All Children's Hosp; **Address:** All Childrens Hosp, Div Ped Immun/Rheumatology, 801 6th St S, Box 9350, St Petersburg, FL 33701; **Phone:** 727-553-1257; **Board Cert:** Pediatrics 1988; Diagnostic Lab Immunology 1990; **Med School:** Univ Tenn Coll Med, Memphis 1981; **Resid:** Pediatrics, Shands Hosp 1984; **Fellow:** Pediatric Infectious Disease, Shands Hosp 1987; Immunology, Dana Farber Cancer Inst 1988

Midwest

Klein-Gitelman, Marisa MD [PRhu] - **Spec Exp:** Lupus/SLE; Arthritis-Juvenile; **Hospital:** Children's Mem Hosp; **Address:** Chldns Meml Hosp, 2300 Children's Plaza, Box 50, Chicago, IL 60614; **Phone:** 773-880-4360; **Board Cert:** Pediatrics 2006; Pediatric Rheumatology 2002; **Med School:** Washington Univ, St Louis 1985; **Resid:** Pediatrics, Columbia-Presby Med Ctr 1989; **Fellow:** Pediatric Rheumatology, New England Med Ctr 1993; **Fac Appt:** Assoc Prof Ped, Northwestern Univ

Wagner-Weiner, Linda MD [PRhu] - **Spec Exp:** Lupus/SLE; Juvenile Arthritis; Vasculitis; **Hospital:** La Rabida Chlds Hosp, Univ of Chicago Hosps; **Address:** La Rabida Chldns Hosp, East 65th Street at Lake Michigan, Chicago, IL 60649; **Phone:** 773-753-8644; **Board Cert:** Pediatrics 1984; Pediatric Rheumatology 2000; **Med School:** Rush Med Coll 1979; **Resid:** Pediatrics, Univ Chicago Hosps 1982; **Fellow:** Pediatric Rheumatology, Univ Chicago/La Rabida Chldns Hosp 1984; **Fac Appt:** Asst Prof Ped, Univ Chicago-Pritzker Sch Med

Southwest

Myones, Barry Lee MD [PRhu] - **Spec Exp:** Vasculitis; Kawasaki Disease; Dermatomyositis; Scleroderma; **Hospital:** Texas Chldns Hosp - Houston; **Address:** Tex Chldns Hosp, Ped Rheum Ctr, 6701 Fannin St Fl 11, Houston, TX 77030; **Phone:** 832-824-3830; **Board Cert:** Pediatrics 1983; Pediatric Rheumatology 2000; **Med School:** Albany Med Coll 1977; **Resid:** Pediatrics, Duke Univ Med Ctr 1980; **Fellow:** Pediatric Rheumatology, Chldns Hosp-Stanford 1983; Rheumatology, Univ N Carolina 1988; **Fac Appt:** Assoc Clin Prof Ped, Baylor Coll Med

Warren, Robert W MD [PRhu] - **Spec Exp:** Juvenile Arthritis; Lupus/SLE; **Hospital:** Texas Chldns Hosp - Houston; **Address:** Texas Childrens Hosp, Pediatric Rheumatology Ctr, 6701 Fannin St Fl 11, Houston, TX 77030-2303; **Phone:** 832-824-3830; **Board Cert:** Pediatrics 1983; Allergy & Immunology 1983; Pediatric Rheumatology 2007; **Med School:** Washington Univ, St Louis 1978; **Resid:** Pediatrics, Duke Univ Med Ctr 1980; **Fellow:** Rheumatology, Duke Univ Med Ctr 1983; **Fac Appt:** Assoc Prof Ped, Baylor Coll Med

Wilking, Andrew MD [PRhu] - **Spec Exp:** Arthritis; Lupus/SLE; Dermatomyositis; **Hospital:** Texas Chldns Hosp - Houston; **Address:** Tex Chldns Hosp, Ped Rheum Ctr, 6701 Fannin St Fl 11, Houston, TX 77030; **Phone:** 832-824-3830; **Board Cert:** Pediatrics 1985; **Med School:** Columbia P&S 1978; **Resid:** Pediatrics, Babies Hosp 1981; **Fellow:** Pediatric Rheumatology, Tex Chldns Hosp 1983; **Fac Appt:** Assoc Prof Ped, Baylor Coll Med

West Coast and Pacific

Emery, Helen M MD [PRhu] - **Spec Exp:** Rheumatic Diseases of Childhood; **Hospital:** Chldns Hosp and Regl Med Ctr - Seattle, Univ Wash Med Ctr; **Address:** Chldns Hosp & Regl Med Ctr, Ped Rheum, 4800 Sand Point Way NE, MS M1-8, Seattle, WA 98105; **Phone:** 206-987-2057; **Board Cert:** Pediatrics 1992; Pediatric Rheumatology 2007; **Med School:** Australia 1971; **Resid:** Pediatrics, Chldns Orth Hosp-Univ Wash 1975; **Fellow:** Pediatric Rheumatology, Chldns Orth Hosp-Univ Wash 1977; **Fac Appt:** Prof Ped, Univ Wash

Sandborg, Christy I MD [PRhu] - **Spec Exp:** Lupus/SLE; **Hospital:** Lucile Packard Chldns Hosp/Stanford Univ Med Ctr; **Address:** 300 Pasteur Drive, Stanford, CA 94305; **Phone:** 650-736-7642; **Board Cert:** Pediatrics 1984; Pediatric Rheumatology 2007; **Med School:** UCLA 1977; **Resid:** Pediatrics, Chldns Hosp 1979; **Fellow:** Pediatric Rheumatology, Chldns Hosp 1981; **Fac Appt:** Prof Ped, Stanford Univ

PEDIATRIC SURGERY

New England

Jennings, Russell W MD [PS] - **Spec Exp:** Fetal Surgery; Pediatric Cardiac Surgery; Robotic Surgery; **Hospital:** Children's Hospital - Boston, Brigham & Women's Hosp; **Address:** Chldns Hosp, Fegan 3, 300 Longwood Ave, Boston, MA 02115; **Phone:** 617-355-3038; **Board Cert:** Surgery 1995; Pediatric Surgery 1998; **Med School:** UCSF 1986; **Resid:** Surgery, UCSF Med Ctr 1991; **Fellow:** Fetal Surgery, Fetal Trmt Ctr/UCSF Med Ctr 1994; Pediatric Surgery, Chldns Hosp 1996; **Fac Appt:** Asst Prof S, Harvard Med Sch

Latchaw, Laurie MD [PS] - **Spec Exp:** Thoracic Surgery; Cancer Surgery; Lung Disease in Newborns; Neonatal Surgery; **Hospital:** Dartmouth - Hitchcock Med Ctr; **Address:** Dartmouth-Hitchcock Med Ctr, Dept Ped Surg, One Medical Center Drive, Labanon, NH 03756; **Phone:** 603-653-9883; **Board Cert:** Surgery 2001; Pediatric Surgery 2003; **Med School:** Rush Med Coll 1976; **Resid:** Surgery, Univ Texas 1981; **Fellow:** Pediatric Surgery, Montreal Chldns Hosp 1983; **Fac Appt:** Assoc Prof S, Dartmouth Med Sch

Mayer Jr, John E MD [PS] - **Spec Exp:** Pediatric Cardiothoracic Surgery; **Hospital:** Children's Hospital - Boston; **Address:** Chldns Hosp, Dept Cardiac Surg, 300 Longwood Ave, Bader 273, Boston, MA 02115; **Phone:** 617-355-8258; **Board Cert:** Thoracic Surgery 2001; **Med School:** Yale Univ 1972; **Resid:** Surgery, Univ Minn Med Ctr 1979; **Fellow:** Cardiothoracic Surgery, Univ Minn Med Ctr 1981; **Fac Appt:** Prof S, Harvard Med Sch

Moss, R Lawrence MD [PS] - **Spec Exp:** Congenital Anomalies; Cancer Surgery; Minimally Invasive Surgery; **Hospital:** Yale-New Haven Hosp; **Address:** Dept Surgery-Ped Surgery, PO Box 208062, rm FMB132, New Haven, CT 06520-8062; **Phone:** 203-785-2701; **Board Cert:** Surgery 1999; Pediatric Surgery 2003; Surgical Critical Care 2000; **Med School:** UCSD 1986; **Resid:** Surgery, Virginia Mason Med Ctr 1991; Surgical Critical Care, Chldns Mem Hosp 1992; **Fellow:** Pediatric Surgery, Chldns Mem Hosp 1994; **Fac Appt:** Prof S, Yale Univ

Shamberger, Robert MD [PS] - **Spec Exp:** Inflammatory Bowel Disease; Critical Care; Cancer Surgery; **Hospital:** Children's Hospital - Boston; **Address:** Children's Hosp-Dept Surgery, 300 Longwood Ave, Fegan - 3, Boston, MA 02115; **Phone:** 617-355-8326; **Board Cert:** Surgery 2002; Surgical Critical Care 1999; Pediatric Surgery 2003; **Med School:** Harvard Med Sch 1975; **Resid:** Surgery, Massachusetts Genl Hosp 1978; Pediatric Surgery, Children's Hosp 1985; **Fellow:** Surgical Oncology, NCI-Surgical Branch 1980; **Fac Appt:** Prof S, Harvard Med Sch

Tracy Jr, Thomas F MD [PS] - **Spec Exp:** Thoracic Surgery; Endoscopic Surgery; Fetal Surgery; Hirschsprung's Disease; **Hospital:** Rhode Island Hosp; **Address:** 2 Dudley St, Ste 180, Providence, RI 02905; **Phone:** 401-421-1939; **Board Cert:** Surgery 2006; Pediatric Surgery 2006; **Med School:** Israel 1981; **Resid:** Surgery, Med Coll Virginia 1986; **Fellow:** Pediatric Surgery, Columbia Presby Med Ctr 1988; **Fac Appt:** Prof S, Brown Univ

Vacanti, Joseph P MD [PS] - **Spec Exp:** Transplant-Liver; **Hospital:** Mass Genl Hosp; **Address:** Mass General Hospital Warren Bldg, 55 Fruit St, rm 1157, Boston, MA 02114-2696; **Phone:** 617-724-1725; **Board Cert:** Pediatric Surgery 1997; **Med School:** Univ Nebr Coll Med 1974; **Resid:** Surgery, Mass Genl Hosp 1980; Pediatric Surgery, Children's Hosp 1983; **Fac Appt:** Prof S, Harvard Med Sch

Mid Atlantic

Adzick, N Scott MD [PS] - **Spec Exp:** Fetal Surgery; Congenital Hyperinsulinism; Neonatal Surgery; Twin to Twin Transfusion Syndrome (TTTS); **Hospital:** Chldns Hosp of Philadelphia, The; **Address:** St 5113 Wood Bldg, Chldns Hosp-Philadelphia, 34th St & Civic Ctr Blvd, Philadelphia, PA 19104-4399; **Phone:** 215-590-2727; **Board Cert:** Surgery 2006; Pediatric Surgery 1999; **Med School:** Harvard Med Sch 1979; **Resid:** Surgery, Mass Genl Hosp 1986; Pediatric Surgery, Chldns Hosp 1988; **Fellow:** Research, UCSF Med Ctr 1985; **Fac Appt:** Prof S, Univ Pennsylvania

Alexander, Frederick MD [PS] - **Spec Exp:** Inflammatory Bowel Disease; Solid Tumors; Congenital Anomalies-Gastrointestinal; **Hospital:** Hackensack Univ Med Ctr; **Address:** Joseph M Sanzari Chldns Hosp-HUMC, 30 Prospect Ave, Ste PC331, Hackensack, NJ 07601; **Phone:** 201-996-2921; **Board Cert:** Pediatric Surgery 1999; **Med School:** Columbia P&S 1976; **Resid:** Surgery, Brigham-Womens Hosp 1984; **Fellow:** Pediatric Surgery, Chldns Hosp 1986; **Fac Appt:** Clin Prof S

Colombani, Paul M MD [PS] - **Spec Exp:** Thoracic Surgery; Transplant-Kidney; Transplant-Liver; Cancer Surgery; **Hospital:** Johns Hopkins Hosp - Baltimore (page 61); **Address:** 600 N Wolfe St, Harvey 319, Baltimore, MD 21287; **Phone:** 410-955-2717; **Board Cert:** Surgery 2003; Pediatric Surgery 2003; **Med School:** Univ KY Coll Med 1976; **Resid:** Surgery, Geo Wash Univ Hosp 1981; **Fellow:** Pediatric Surgery, Johns Hopkins Hosp 1983; **Fac Appt:** Prof S, Johns Hopkins Univ

Dolgin, Stephen MD [PS] - **Spec Exp:** Neonatal Surgery; Ulcerative Colitis; Laparoscopy & Thoracostomy; Inflammatory Bowel Disease/Crohn's; **Hospital:** Schneider Chldn's Hosp, N Shore Univ Hosp; **Address:** Schneider Children's Hosp, Pediatric Surgery, 269-01 76th Ave, New Hyde Park, NY 11040; **Phone:** 718-470-3636; **Board Cert:** Surgery 2000; Pediatric Surgery 2003; Surgical Critical Care 2000; **Med School:** NYU Sch Med 1977; **Resid:** Surgery, Peter Bent Brigham Hosp 1982; Pediatric Surgery, Chldns Meml Hosp 1984; **Fac Appt:** Prof S, Albert Einstein Coll Med

Eichelberger, Martin R MD [PS] - **Spec Exp:** Trauma; **Hospital:** Chldns Natl Med Ctr; **Address:** Childrens National Med Ctr, 111 Michigan Ave NW, Washington, DC 20010; **Phone:** 202-476-2778; **Board Cert:** Pediatric Surgery 2003; **Med School:** Hahnemann Univ 1971; **Resid:** Surgery, Case-Western Res Hosp 1978; **Fellow:** Pediatric Surgery, Childrens Hosp 1980; **Fac Appt:** Prof S, Geo Wash Univ

Flake, Alan W MD [PS] - **Spec Exp:** Fetal Surgery; Stem Cell Transplant-Fetal; Neonatal Surgery; **Hospital:** Chldns Hosp of Philadelphia, The; **Address:** Children's Hosp, Dept Surgery, 34th St & Civic Center Blvd, Abramson 1116, Philadelphia, PA 19104; **Phone:** 215-590-2727; **Board Cert:** Surgery 2000; Pediatric Surgery 1999; **Med School:** Univ Ark 1981; **Resid:** Surgery, UCSF Med Ctr 1988; **Fellow:** Pediatric Surgery, Chldns Hosp Med Ctr 1990; **Fac Appt:** Prof S, Univ Pennsylvania

Ginsburg, Howard B MD [PS] - **Spec Exp:** Neonatal Surgery; Tumor Surgery; Pediatric Urology; Gastrointestinal Surgery; **Hospital:** NYU Med Ctr (page 68), Bellevue Hosp Ctr; **Address:** NYU Medical Ctr, Div Pediatric Surgery, 530 1st Ave, Ste 10W, New York, NY 10016-6402; **Phone:** 212-263-7391; **Board Cert:** Surgery 1978; Pediatric Surgery 2001; **Med School:** Univ Cincinnati 1972; **Resid:** Surgery, NYU-Bellvue Hosp 1977; Pediatric Surgery, Columbia-Presby Med Ctr 1979; **Fellow:** Pediatric Surgery, Mass Genl Hosp 1980; **Fac Appt:** Assoc Prof S, NYU Sch Med

Gittes, George K MD [PS] - **Spec Exp:** Gastrointestinal Surgery; **Hospital:** Chldns Hosp of Pittsburgh - UPMC; **Address:** Childrens Hosp Pittsburgh, Dept Surgery, 3705 Fifth Ave, Ste 4A-485, Pittsburgh, PA 15213; **Phone:** 412-692-7280; **Board Cert:** Surgery 2003; Pediatric Surgery 1998; **Med School:** Harvard Med Sch 1987; **Resid:** Surgery, UCSF Med Ctr 1994; **Fellow:** Pediatric Surgery, Childrens Mercy Hosp 1995; **Fac Appt:** Prof S, Univ Pittsburgh

Pediatric Surgery

Glick, Philip L MD [PS] - **Spec Exp:** Robotic Surgery; Neonatal Surgery; Pediatric Cancers; Chest Wall Deformities; **Hospital:** Women's & Chldn's Hosp of Buffalo, The, Roswell Park Cancer Inst; **Address:** Childrens Hospital, Dept Pediatric Surg, 219 Bryant St, Buffalo, NY 14222-2006; **Phone:** 716-878-7449; **Board Cert:** Surgery 2006; Pediatric Surgery 1997; Surgical Critical Care 1999; **Med School:** UCSF 1979; **Resid:** Surgery, UCSF Med Ctr 1985; **Fellow:** Fetal Surgery, UCSF Med Ctr 1984; Pediatric Surgery, Chldns Hosp Med Ctr 1988; **Fac Appt:** Prof S, SUNY Buffalo

Kane, Timothy D MD [PS] - **Spec Exp:** Minimally Invasive Surgery; Chest Wall Repair; Neonatal Surgery; **Hospital:** Chldns Hosp of Pittsburgh - UPMC; **Address:** Chldns Hosp Pittsburgh - Dept Surg, 3705 Fifth Ave 4A485, Pittsburgh, PA 15213; **Phone:** 412-692-7280; **Board Cert:** Surgery 2001; Pediatric Surgery 2004; **Med School:** SUNY Upstate Med Univ 1992; **Resid:** Surgery, Univ Cincinnati Hosp 1999; **Fellow:** Pediatric Surgery, UAB Chldns Hosp 2001; **Fac Appt:** Asst Prof S, Univ Pittsburgh

La Quaglia, Michael MD [PS] - **Spec Exp:** Cancer Surgery; Neuroblastoma; Liver Tumors; Colon & Rectal Cancer; **Hospital:** Meml Sloan-Kettering Cancer Ctr, NY-Presby Hosp/Weill Cornell (page 66); **Address:** 1275 York Avenue, New York, NY 10065; **Phone:** 800-525-2225; **Board Cert:** Surgery 2003; Pediatric Surgery 2007; **Med School:** UMDNJ-NJ Med Sch, Newark 1976; **Resid:** Surgery, Mass Genl Hosp 1983; **Fellow:** Cardiothoracic Surgery, Broadgreen Ctr 1984; Pediatric Surgery, Chldns Hosp 1985; **Fac Appt:** Prof S, Cornell Univ-Weill Med Coll

Nance, Michael L MD [PS] - **Spec Exp:** Trauma; Critical Care; Brain Injury; Congenital Anomalies; **Hospital:** Chldns Hosp of Philadelphia, The; **Address:** Chldns Hosp of Philadelphia, Dept Surgery, 34th & Civic Ctr Blvd, Philadelphia, PA 19104; **Phone:** 215-590-5932; **Board Cert:** Surgery 2005; Pediatric Surgery 2007; **Med School:** Louisiana State U, New Orleans 1988; **Resid:** Surgery, Hosp U Penn 1995; **Fellow:** Surgical Critical Care, Hosp U Penn 1996; Pediatric Surgery, Chldns Hosp Philadelphia 1997; **Fac Appt:** Assoc Prof PS, Univ Pennsylvania

Quaegebeur, Jan M MD [PS] - **Spec Exp:** Arterial Switch; Heart Valve Surgery; Congenital Heart Surgery; Pediatric Cardiac Surgery; **Hospital:** NYPresby-Morgan Stanley Children's Hosp (page 66); **Address:** Morgan Stanley Chlds Hosp of NY-Presby, 3959 Broadway, Ste 276, New York, NY 10032; **Phone:** 212-305-5975; **Med School:** Belgium 1969; **Resid:** Surgery, St Michel Clinic 1973; **Fellow:** Thoracic Surgery, Baylor Coll Med 1974; Thoracic Surgery, Univ Hosp 1978; **Fac Appt:** Prof S, Columbia P&S

Schwartz, Marshall Z MD [PS] - **Spec Exp:** Gastrointestinal Surgery; Neonatal Surgery; Transplant-Kidney; **Hospital:** St Christopher's Hosp for Chldn, St Luke's Hosp - Bethlehem; **Address:** St Christopher's Hosp for Chldn, Dept of Surgery, Erie at Front St, Ste 2204, Philadelphia, PA 19134; **Phone:** 215-427-5446; **Board Cert:** Surgery 1998; Pediatric Surgery 1999; **Med School:** Univ Minn 1970; **Resid:** Surgery, Univ Minnesota Hosp 1972; Pediatric Surgery, Chldns Hosp Med Ctr - Harvard Med Sch 1974; **Fellow:** Surgery, Univ Minnesota Hosp 1975; **Fac Appt:** Prof S, Jefferson Med Coll

Shlasko, Edward MD [PS] - **Spec Exp:** Laparoscopic Surgery; Robotic Surgery; **Hospital:** Maimonides Med Ctr (page 63), Mount Sinai Med Ctr (page 64); **Address:** Dept Ped Surg, 921 49th St, Brooklyn, NY 11219-2923; **Phone:** 718-283-7384; **Board Cert:** Surgery 1999; Pediatric Surgery 2001; **Med School:** Columbia P&S 1985; **Resid:** Surgery, Mount Sinai Hosp 1991; **Fellow:** Surgical Oncology, NIH-NCI Surg Branch 1989; Pediatric Surgery, SUNY Hlth Sci Ctr 1993; **Fac Appt:** Assoc Prof S, Mount Sinai Sch Med

Spray, Thomas L MD [PS] - **Spec Exp:** Cardiac Surgery-Adult & Pediatric; Transplant-Heart & Lung; Neonatal & Infant Cardiac Surgery; Congenital Heart Disease-Adult; **Hospital:** Chldns Hosp of Philadelphia, The, Hosp Univ Penn - UPHS (page 60); **Address:** Children's Hosp of Philadelphia, Surgery, 34th St & Civic Center Blvd, Ste 8527, Philadelphia, PA 19104; **Phone:** 215-590-2708; **Board Cert:** Thoracic Surgery 2004; **Med School:** Duke Univ 1973; **Resid:** Surgery, Duke Univ Med Ctr 1975; Cardiothoracic Surgery, Duke Univ Med Ctr 1983; **Fac Appt:** Prof S, Univ Pennsylvania

Stolar, Charles J H MD [PS] - **Spec Exp:** Pediatric Cancers; Neonatal Surgery; Diaphragmatic hernia; **Hospital:** NYPresby-Morgan Stanley Children's Hosp (page 66); **Address:** Morgan Stanley Chldns Hosp NY-Presby, 3959 Broadway, Fl 2 - rm 215 North, New York, NY 10032; **Phone:** 212-342-8586; **Board Cert:** Surgery 2001; Pediatric Surgery 1996; **Med School:** Georgetown Univ 1974; **Resid:** Surgery, Univ Illinois Hosp 1980; **Fellow:** Pediatric Surgery, Chldns Hosp Natl Med Ctr 1982; **Fac Appt:** Prof S, Columbia P&S

Velcek, Francisca MD [PS] - **Spec Exp:** Anorectal Malformations; Pediatric Gynecology; Neonatal Surgery; Hernia; **Hospital:** Lenox Hill Hosp (page 62), Long Island Coll Hosp (page 57); **Address:** 965 5th Ave, New York, NY 10021; **Phone:** 212-744-9396; **Board Cert:** Surgery 1974; Pediatric Surgery 2007; **Med School:** Philippines 1966; **Resid:** Surgery, St Clares Hosp 1971; Pediatric Surgery, SUNY Downstate Med Ctr 1975; **Fellow:** Pediatric Surgery, SUNY Downstate Med Ctr 1973; **Fac Appt:** Prof S, SUNY Hlth Sci Ctr

Weber, Thomas K MD [PS] - **Hospital:** Albany Med Ctr; **Address:** Albany Medical Ctr, 47 New Scotland Ave, MC 61, Albany, NY 12208; **Phone:** 518-262-5831; **Board Cert:** Surgery 2005; **Med School:** Ohio State Univ 1971; **Resid:** Surgery, Univ MI Hosp & Hlth Ctr 1977; **Fellow:** Pediatric Surgery, Chldns Natl Med Ctr 1979; **Fac Appt:** Prof S, Albany Med Coll

Southeast

Bond, Sheldon J MD [PS] - **Spec Exp:** Pediatric Cancers; Fetal Surgery; Trauma; **Hospital:** Kosair Chldn's Hosp; **Address:** University Pediatric Surgery Assocs, 234 E Gray St, Ste 766, Louisville, KY 40202; **Phone:** 502-583-7337; **Board Cert:** Surgery 1998; Pediatric Surgery 1999; Surgical Critical Care 2001; **Med School:** Med Coll Wisc 1983; **Resid:** Surgery, Univ Louisville Med Ctr 1989; **Fellow:** Fetal Surgery, UCSF Med Ctr; Pediatric Surgery, Chldns Natl Med Ctr 1991; **Fac Appt:** Prof S, Univ Louisville Sch Med

Davidoff, Andrew M MD [PS] - **Spec Exp:** Neuroblastoma; Cancer Surgery; **Hospital:** St Jude Children's Research Hosp, Le Bonheur Chldns Med Ctr; **Address:** St Jude Chldns Rsch Hosp, Dept Surg, 332 N Lauderdale St, Memphis, TN 38105; **Phone:** 901-495-4060; **Board Cert:** Surgery 1995; Pediatric Surgery 1998; **Med School:** Univ Pennsylvania 1987; **Resid:** Surgery, Duke Med Ctr 1994; **Fellow:** Pediatric Surgery, Chldns Hosp 1996; **Fac Appt:** Assoc Prof S, Univ Tenn Coll Med, Memphis

Fallat, Mary E MD [PS] - **Spec Exp:** Trauma; Burn Care; **Hospital:** Kosair Chldn's Hosp, Univ of Louisville Hosp; **Address:** University Pediatric Surgery Assocs, 234 E Gray St, Ste 766, Louisville, KY 40202; **Phone:** 502-583-7337; **Board Cert:** Surgery 1995; Pediatric Surgery 1997; **Med School:** SUNY Upstate Med Univ 1979; **Resid:** Surgery, Univ Louisville Med Ctr 1985; **Fellow:** Research, Mass Genl Hosp 1983; Pediatric Surgery, Chldns Natl Med Ctr 1987; **Fac Appt:** Prof S, Univ Louisville Sch Med

Pediatric Surgery

Georgeson, Keith E MD [PS] - **Spec Exp:** Hirschsprung's Disease; Minimally Invasive Surgery; Gastroesophageal Reflux Disease (GERD); **Hospital:** Children's Hospital - Birmingham; **Address:** Chlds Hosp of Alabama, Dept Ped Surgery, 1600 7th Ave S, Ste ACC300, Birmingham, AL 35233-1711; **Phone:** 205-939-9688; **Board Cert:** Surgery 2000; Pediatric Surgery 2007; **Med School:** Loma Linda Univ 1969; **Resid:** Surgery, Loma Linda Univ Med Ctr 1973; Pediatric Surgery, Chldn's Hosp Mich 1975; **Fac Appt:** Prof S, Univ Ala

Morgan III, Walter M MD [PS] - **Spec Exp:** Germ Cell Tumors; Neuroblastoma; Bone Cancer; Congenital Anomalies; **Hospital:** Vanderbilt Children's Hosp, Vanderbilt Univ Med Ctr; **Address:** Vanderbilt Children's Hosp-Dept Ped Surgery, 2200 Children's Way, Ste 4150, Nashville, TN 37232-9780; **Phone:** 615-936-1050; **Board Cert:** Pediatric Surgery 2001; **Med School:** Vanderbilt Univ 1982; **Resid:** Surgery, Johns Hopkins Hosp 1988; **Fellow:** Pediatric Surgery, Johns Hopkins Hosp 1990; **Fac Appt:** Asst Prof S, Vanderbilt Univ

Nakayama, Don K MD [PS] - **Spec Exp:** Neonatal Surgery; Minimally Invasive Surgery; **Hospital:** Med Ctr of Central GA; **Address:** 777 Hemlock St, Hospital Box 140, Macon, GA 31201; **Phone:** 478-633-1367; **Board Cert:** Surgery 2003; Pediatric Surgery 2005; **Med School:** UCSF 1978; **Resid:** Surgery, UCSF Hosps 1984; **Fellow:** Pediatric Surgery, Childrens Hosp 1986; **Fac Appt:** Prof S, Mercer Univ Sch Med

Nuss, Donald MD [PS] - **Spec Exp:** Chest Wall Deformities; Minimally Invasive Surgery; **Hospital:** Chldns Hosp of King's Daughters; **Address:** Chldns Surg Specialty Grp, 601 Childrens Ln, Ste Pectus, Norfolk, VA 23507; **Phone:** 757-668-7703; **Board Cert:** Surgery 1973; Pediatric Surgery 1997; **Med School:** South Africa 1963; **Resid:** Surgery, Mayo Clinic 1971; Pediatric Surgery, Red Cross Chldns Hosp 1973; **Fac Appt:** Prof S, Eastern VA Med Sch

Paidas, Charles N MD [PS] - **Spec Exp:** Pediatric Cancers; Chest Wall Deformities; Pediatric Transplant Surgery; Hernia; **Hospital:** Tampa Genl Hosp, Univ of S FL - Tampa; **Address:** Tampa Genl Hosp, Div Ped Surgery, 2 Columbia Drive, rm 6441, Tampa, FL 33606; **Phone:** 813-259-0929; **Board Cert:** Surgery 1999; Pediatric Surgery 2001; Surgical Critical Care 2002; **Med School:** NY Med Coll 1981; **Resid:** Surgery, NY Med Coll Affil Hosps 1987; **Fellow:** Pediatric Surgery, Johns Hopkins Hosp 1991; **Fac Appt:** Prof S, Univ S Fla Coll Med

Rice, Henry MD [PS] - **Spec Exp:** Neonatal Surgery; Cancer Surgery; **Hospital:** Duke Univ Med Ctr; **Address:** Duke Univ Med Ctr, Dept Ped Surg, DUMC, Box 3815, Durham, NC 27710; **Phone:** 919-681-5077; **Board Cert:** Surgery 1997; Pediatric Surgery 2000; **Med School:** Yale Univ 1988; **Resid:** Surgery, Univ Wash Affil Hosps 1996; **Fellow:** Pediatric Surgery, Chldns Hosp of Buffalo 1998; **Fac Appt:** Assoc Prof S, Duke Univ

Ricketts, Richard R MD [PS] - **Spec Exp:** Neonatal Surgery; Cancer Surgery; Gastrointestinal Surgery; **Hospital:** Chldns Hlthcare Atlanta - Egleston; **Address:** 1975 Century Blvd, Ste 6, Atlanta, GA 30345; **Phone:** 404-982-9938; **Board Cert:** Surgery 2004; Pediatric Surgery 2001; **Med School:** Northwestern Univ 1973; **Resid:** Surgery, LAC-USC Med Ctr 1978; **Fellow:** Pediatric Surgery, Chldns Meml Hosp 1980; **Fac Appt:** Prof S, Emory Univ

Rodgers, Bradley M MD [PS] - **Spec Exp:** Thoracic Surgery; Neonatal Surgery; Minimally Invasive Surgery; **Hospital:** Univ Virginia Med Ctr; **Address:** U VA Chldns Hosp, Dept Surgery, PO Box 800709, Charlottesville, VA 22908; **Phone:** 434-924-2673; **Board Cert:** Surgery 1997; Pediatric Surgery 2005; Thoracic Surgery 1975; **Med School:** Johns Hopkins Univ 1966; **Resid:** Surgery, Duke Univ Med Ctr 1968; Cardiothoracic Surgery, Duke Univ Med Ctr 1973; **Fellow:** Pediatric Surgery, Chldns Hosp 1974; **Fac Appt:** Prof S, Univ VA Sch Med

Shochat, Stephen J MD [PS] - **Spec Exp:** Cancer Surgery; Chest Wall Deformities; **Hospital:** St Jude Children's Research Hosp; **Address:** St Jude Childrens Research Hosp, Dept Surgery, 332 N Lauderdale St, Memphis, TN 38105; **Phone:** 901-495-2911; **Board Cert:** Surgery 1969; Thoracic Surgery 1975; Pediatric Surgery 2005; **Med School:** Med Coll VA 1963; **Resid:** Surgery, Barnes Hosp 1964; Pediatric Surgery, Boston Children's Hosp 1968; **Fellow:** Thoracic Surgery, George Washington Univ Med Ctr 1974; **Fac Appt:** Prof S, Univ Tenn Coll Med, Memphis

Stylianos, Steven MD [PS] - **Spec Exp:** Trauma; Neonatal Surgery; Chest Wall Deformities; **Hospital:** Miami Children's Hosp; **Address:** Miami Childrens Hosp, 3200 SW 60th Court, Ste 201, Miami, FL 33155; **Phone:** 305-662-8320; **Board Cert:** Surgery 2002; Pediatric Surgery 2003; **Med School:** NYU Sch Med 1983; **Resid:** Surgery, Columbia-Presby Med Ctr 1988; Pediatric Surgery, Chldns Hosp 1992; **Fellow:** Pediatric Trauma, New England Med Ctr 1990; **Fac Appt:** Assoc Prof S, Univ Miami Sch Med

Midwest

Aiken, John Judson MD [PS] - **Spec Exp:** Tumor Surgery; Chest Wall Deformities; Hernia; Solid Tumors; **Hospital:** Chldns Hosp - Wisconsin; **Address:** 999 N 92nd St, Ste C-320, Milwaukee, WI 53226-4875; **Phone:** 414-266-6550; **Board Cert:** Surgery 2004; Pediatric Surgery 2000; **Med School:** Univ Cincinnati 1984; **Resid:** Surgery, Mass Genl Hosp 1991; **Fellow:** Pediatric Surgery, Chldns Hosp 1993; **Fac Appt:** Assoc Prof S, Med Coll Wisc

Barksdale Jr, Edward M MD [PS] - **Spec Exp:** Gastrointestinal Surgery; Nutrition in Bowel Disorders; Neuroblastoma; Minimally Invasive Surgery; **Hospital:** Rainbow Babies & Chldns Hosp; **Address:** Rainbow Babies & Children's Hosp, 11100 Euclid Ave, rm 122, Cleveland, OH 44106; **Phone:** 216-844-8623; **Board Cert:** Surgery 2002; Pediatric Surgery 2003; **Med School:** Harvard Med Sch 1984; **Resid:** Surgery, Mass Genl Hosp 1992; **Fellow:** Surgical Research, Mass Genl Hosp 1989; Pediatric Surgery, Childrens Hosp 1994; **Fac Appt:** Prof S, Ohio State Univ

Bensard, Denis D MD [PS] - **Spec Exp:** Endoscopic Surgery; Trauma; Critical Care; **Hospital:** St Vincent Hosp & Hlth Svcs - Indianapolis; **Address:** St Vincent Pediatric Surgical Svcs, 2001 W 86th St, Indianapolis, IN 46260; **Phone:** 317-338-8857; **Board Cert:** Surgery 2002; Pediatric Surgery 2005; Surgical Critical Care 2003; **Med School:** Univ Colorado 1986; **Resid:** Surgery, Univ Colorado Med Ctr 1992; **Fellow:** Pediatric Surgery, Ohio State Univ 1995; **Fac Appt:** Assoc Prof S, Univ Colorado

Bove, Edward L MD [PS] - **Spec Exp:** Pediatric Cardiothoracic Surgery; Hypoplastic Left Heart Syndrome; Congenital Heart Surgery; **Hospital:** Univ Michigan Hlth Sys; **Address:** C.S. Mott Chldns Hosp, Dept Surg, 1500 E Med Ctr Drive, rm F7830, Box 0223, Ann Arbor, MI 48109-0223; **Phone:** 734-936-4980; **Board Cert:** Thoracic Surgery 1998; **Med School:** Albany Med Coll 1972; **Resid:** Surgery, Univ Mich Med Ctr 1976; Thoracic Surgery, Univ Mich Med Ctr 1979; **Fellow:** Pediatric Cardiac Surgery, Hosp Sick Chldn 1980; **Fac Appt:** Prof S, Univ Mich Med Sch

Caniano, Donna MD [PS] - **Hospital:** Nationwide Chldn's Hosp; **Address:** Children's Surgical Assocs Corp, 700 Children's Drive, Columbus, OH 43205; **Phone:** 614-722-3900; **Board Cert:** Surgery 2001; Pediatric Surgery 1993; **Med School:** Albany Med Coll 1976; **Resid:** Surgery, Albany Med Ctr 1981; **Fellow:** Pediatric Surgery, Columbus Chldn's Hosp 1983; **Fac Appt:** Prof S, Ohio State Univ

Pediatric Surgery

Crombleholme, Timothy M MD [PS] - **Spec Exp:** Fetal Surgery; Twin to Twin Transfusion Syndrome (TTTS); **Hospital:** Cincinnati Chldns Hosp Med Ctr, Univ Hosp - Cincinnati; **Address:** Fetal Care Center of Cincinnati, 3333 Burnet Ave, MC 11020, Cincinnati, OH 45229; **Phone:** 513-636-9608; **Board Cert:** Surgery 2003; Pediatric Surgery 2007; **Med School:** Tufts Univ 1984; **Resid:** Surgery, UCSF Med Ctr 1991; **Fellow:** Pediatric Surgery, Tufts-New England Med Ctr 1993; **Fac Appt:** Prof S, Univ Cincinnati

Duncan, Brian W MD [PS] - **Spec Exp:** Pediatric Cardiac Surgery; Neonatal & Infant Cardiac Surgery; Transplant-Heart-Pediatric; **Hospital:** Cleveland Clin Fdn (page 56); **Address:** 9500 Euclid Ave, MC M41, Cleveland, OH 44195; **Phone:** 216-444-9365; **Board Cert:** Surgery 2004; Thoracic Surgery 2006; **Med School:** Indiana Univ 1985; **Resid:** Surgery, Mass General Hosp 1992; Thoracic Surgery, Mass General Hosp 1995; **Fellow:** Surgical Research, UCSF Med Ctr; **Fac Appt:** Prof S, Cleveland Cl Coll Med/Case West Res

Ehrlich, Peter F MD [PS] - **Spec Exp:** Pediatric Cancers; Wilms' Tumor; Thyroid Cancer; **Hospital:** Mott Chldns Hosp, Mich State Univ-Hurley Med Ctr; **Address:** Mott Children's Hospital, 1500 E Medical Center Drive, rm F3970, Ann Arbor, MI 48109-0245; **Phone:** 734-764-4151; **Board Cert:** Surgery 1997; Pediatric Surgery 2000; **Med School:** Canada 1989; **Resid:** Surgery, Univ Toronto Med Ctr 1996; **Fellow:** Pediatric Surgery, Children's Natl Med Ctr 1998; **Fac Appt:** Assoc Clin Prof S, Univ Mich Med Sch

Holterman, Mark J MD [PS] - **Spec Exp:** Minimally Invasive Surgery; Neonatal Surgery; Transplant-Liver; Transplant-Bowel; **Hospital:** Univ of IL Med Ctr at Chicago; **Address:** Univ of Illinos, Pediatric Surgery, 840 S Wood St, Ste 416, MC 958, Chicago, IL 60612; **Phone:** 312-413-7707; **Board Cert:** Surgery 2001; Pediatric Surgery 2007; **Med School:** Univ VA Sch Med 1985; **Resid:** Surgery, Univ Virginia Hosp 1993; **Fellow:** Pediatric Surgery, Childrens Hosp & Med Ctr 1993; **Fac Appt:** Assoc Prof S, Univ IL Coll Med

Ilbawi, Michel MD [PS] - **Spec Exp:** Cardiac Surgery; Congenital Anomalies; Cardiovascular Surgery; **Hospital:** Adv Christ Med Ctr, Adv Luth Genl Hosp; **Address:** Hope Chldns Hosp at Adv Christ Med Ctr, 4440 W 95th St, Oak Lawn, IL 60453; **Phone:** 708-684-3029; **Board Cert:** Thoracic Surgery 1998; **Med School:** Lebanon 1971; **Resid:** Surgery, American Univ Hosp 1975; Thoracic Surgery, Univ Hosps 1977; **Fellow:** Thoracic Surgery, Chldns Meml Hosp 1978; **Fac Appt:** Clin Prof S, Univ IL Coll Med

Lobe, Thom E MD [PS] - **Spec Exp:** Minimally Invasive Surgery; Robotic Surgery; Pediatric Urology; **Hospital:** Iowa Methodist Med Ctr; **Address:** Blank Children's Hospital, 1212 Pleasant St, Ste 300, Des Moines, IA 50309; **Phone:** 515-241-6000; **Board Cert:** Surgery 1989; Pediatric Surgery 1989; **Med School:** Univ MD Sch Med 1975; **Resid:** Surgery, Ohio State Univ Med Ctr 1979; Pediatric Surgery, Childrens Hosp 1981

Mavroudis, Constantine MD [PS] - **Spec Exp:** Congenital Heart Disease; Transplant-Heart & Lung; Coronary Artery Surgery; **Hospital:** Cleveland Clin Fdn (page 56); **Address:** 9500 Euclid, Ped Cardiology, M41, Cleveland, OH 44195; **Phone:** 216-445-5015; **Board Cert:** Surgery 2000; Thoracic Surgery 2000; **Med School:** Univ VA Sch Med 1973; **Resid:** Surgery, UCSF Med Ctr 1979; **Fellow:** Thoracic Surgery, UCSF Med Ctr 1977; **Fac Appt:** Prof S, Northwestern Univ

Oldham, Keith T MD [PS] - **Spec Exp:** Neonatal Surgery; Thoracic Surgery; Gastrointestinal Surgery; **Hospital:** Chldns Hosp - Wisconsin; **Address:** 999 N 92nd St, Ste 320, Milwaukee, WI 53226; **Phone:** 414-266-6550; **Board Cert:** Surgery 2000; Pediatric Surgery 1991; Surgical Critical Care 1995; **Med School:** Med Coll VA 1976; **Resid:** Surgery, Univ Wash Med Ctr 1981; **Fellow:** Pediatric Surgery, Univ Cincinnati Chldns Hosp 1983; **Fac Appt:** Prof S, Med Coll Wisc

Pena, Alberto MD [PS] - **Spec Exp:** Imperforate Anus; Anorectal Malformations; Colon & Rectal Surgery; **Hospital:** Cincinnati Chldns Hosp Med Ctr; **Address:** Cincinnati Chlds Hosp Med Ctr, 3333 Burnet Ave, MLC 2023, Cincinnati, OH 45229; **Phone:** 513-636-3240; **Med School:** Mexico 1962; **Resid:** Surgery, Military Hosp 1966; **Fellow:** Pediatric Surgery, Childrens Hosp 1971; Cardiovascular Surgery, Childrens Hosp 1969

Reynolds, Marleta MD [PS] - **Spec Exp:** Critical Care; Trauma; Congenital Anomalies; **Hospital:** Children's Mem Hosp; **Address:** Chldns Meml Hosp, Dept Ped Surg, 2300 Children's Plaza, Box 63, Chicago, IL 60614; **Phone:** 773-880-4292; **Board Cert:** Surgery 1991; Thoracic Surgery 1995; Pediatric Surgery 1993; **Med School:** Tulane Univ 1976; **Resid:** Surgery, Tulane Univ Affil Hosp 1981; Pediatric Surgery, Chldns Meml Hosp 1983; **Fellow:** Cardiothoracic Surgery, Northwestern Univ 1985; **Fac Appt:** Asst Prof S, Northwestern Univ

Sato, Thomas T MD [PS] - **Spec Exp:** Neonatal Surgery; Congenital Anomalies; Laparoscopy & Thoracostomy; **Hospital:** Chldns Hosp - Wisconsin; **Address:** 999 N 92nd St, Ste C320, Milwaukee, WI 53226; **Phone:** 414-266-6550; **Board Cert:** Surgery 2006; Pediatric Surgery 2007; **Med School:** USC Sch Med 1988; **Resid:** Surgery, Univ Wash Med Ctr 1995; **Fellow:** Surgery, Harborview Med Ctr 1993; Pediatric Surgery, Chldns Natl Med Ctr 1997; **Fac Appt:** Assoc Prof S, Med Coll Wisc

Sheldon, Curtis A MD [PS] - **Spec Exp:** Pediatric Urology; Genitourinary Reconstruction; Transplant-Kidney-Pediatric; **Hospital:** Cincinnati Chldns Hosp Med Ctr; **Address:** Childrens Hosp, Div Pediatric Urology, 3333 Burnet Ave, MC 5037, Cincinnati, OH 45229; **Phone:** 513-636-4975; **Board Cert:** Urology 1993; Pediatric Surgery 1997; **Med School:** UCSD 1976; **Resid:** Urology, Univ Minnesota Affil Hosp 1981; Surgery, Univ Minnesota Affil Hosp 1983; **Fellow:** Pediatric Surgery, Chldns Hosp Med Ctr 1985; Pediatric Urology, Hosp for Sick Chldn 1986; **Fac Appt:** Prof S, Univ Cincinnati

Warner, Brad MD [PS] - **Spec Exp:** Gastrointestinal Surgery; Neonatal Surgery; Cancer Surgery; **Hospital:** St Louis Chldns Hosp; **Address:** 1 Children's Pl, Ste 5S60, St. Louis, MO 63110; **Phone:** 314-454-6066; **Board Cert:** Surgery 1998; Pediatric Surgery 2001; **Med School:** Univ MO-Kansas City 1982; **Resid:** Surgery, Univ Cincinnati Med Ctr 1989; **Fellow:** Pediatric Surgery, Chldns Hosp Med Ctr 1991; **Fac Appt:** Prof S, Univ Cincinnati

Great Plains and Mountains

Karrer, Frederick M MD [PS] - **Spec Exp:** Liver Surgery; Transplant-Liver; Critical Care; **Hospital:** Chldn's Hosp - Aurora, The, Denver Health Med Ctr; **Address:** Children's Hospital, Dept Surgery, 13123 E 16th Ave, Box B323, Aurora, CO 80045; **Phone:** 720-777-6571; **Board Cert:** Surgery 1996; Pediatric Surgery 1997; Surgical Critical Care 1998; **Med School:** Univ Nebr Coll Med 1979; **Resid:** Surgery, Univ Ariz Med Ctr 1984; Pediatric Surgery, Children's Meml Hosp 1988; **Fellow:** Transplant Surgery, Univ Pittsburgh 1986; **Fac Appt:** Prof S, Univ Colorado

Meyers, Rebecka L MD [PS] - **Spec Exp:** Transplant-Liver; Tumor Surgery-Pediatric; Biliary Surgery; Pancreatic Surgery; **Hospital:** Primary Children's Med Ctr, Univ Utah Hosps and Clins; **Address:** Primary Chlds Med Ctr, Dept Ped Surg, 100 N Medical Drive, Ste 2600, Salt Lake City, UT 84113; **Phone:** 801-662-2950; **Board Cert:** Surgery 2003; Pediatric Surgery 1996; **Med School:** Oregon Hlth Sci Univ 1985; **Resid:** Surgery, UCSF Med Ctr 1990; **Fellow:** Research, Cardio Rsch Inst-UCSF 1992; Pediatric Surgery, St Christopher's Hosp for Chldn 1994; **Fac Appt:** Assoc Prof S, Univ Utah

Pediatric Surgery

Ziegler, Moritz M MD [PS] - **Spec Exp:** Hirschsprung's Disease; Gastrointestinal Surgery; Neuroblastoma; Tumor Surgery-Pediatric; **Hospital:** Chldn's Hosp - Aurora, The; **Address:** Chldns Hosp, Dept Surgery, 13123 E 16th Ave, Box 323, Aurora, CO 80045; **Phone:** 720-777-6524; **Board Cert:** Surgery 1975; Pediatric Surgery 1995; **Med School:** Univ Mich Med Sch 1968; **Resid:** Surgery, Univ Penn Hosp 1975; Pediatric Surgery, Chldns Hosp 1977; **Fellow:** Surgical Oncology, Amer Oncologic Hosp 1975; **Fac Appt:** Prof S, Univ Colorado

Southwest

Arensman, Robert MD [PS] - **Spec Exp:** Congenital Anomalies; **Hospital:** Ochsner Fdn Hosp, Tulane Univ Hosp & Clin; **Address:** 1514 Jefferson Hwy, New Orleans, LA 70121; **Phone:** 504-842-3907; **Board Cert:** Surgery 1979; Pediatric Surgery 1989; **Med School:** Univ IL Coll Med 1969; **Resid:** Surgery, Univ Illinois Med Ctr 1972; Surgery, Univ Illinois Med Ctr 1976; **Fellow:** Pediatric Surgery, Chldns Natl Med Ctr 1978

Foglia, Robert P MD [PS] - **Spec Exp:** Congenital Anomalies; Burn Care; **Hospital:** Chldns Med Ctr of Dallas; **Address:** 1935 Medical District Drive, Dallas, TX 75235; **Phone:** 214-456-6040; **Board Cert:** Surgery 2002; Pediatric Surgery 1995; Surgical Critical Care 1993; **Med School:** Georgetown Univ 1974; **Resid:** Surgery, UCLA Med Ctr 1981; **Fellow:** Pediatric Surgery, Chldns Hosp Natl Med Ctr 1983; **Fac Appt:** Prof S, Univ Tex SW, Dallas

Jackson, Richard J MD [PS] - **Spec Exp:** Cancer Surgery; Neonatal Surgery; Robotic Surgery; **Hospital:** Arkansas Chldns Hosp; **Address:** Arkansas Chldns Hosp - Ped Surgery, 800 Marshall St, MS 837, Little Rock, AR 72202; **Phone:** 501-364-1446; **Board Cert:** Surgery 1997; Pediatric Surgery 2001; Surgical Critical Care 1998; **Med School:** W VA Univ 1983; **Resid:** Surgery, W Va Univ Hosps 1988; Pediatric Surgery, Chldns Hosp 1989; **Fellow:** Pediatric Critical Care Medicine, Chldns Hosp-Univ Pittsburgh 1990; Pediatric Surgery, Chldns Hosp-Univ Pittsburgh 1992; **Fac Appt:** Assoc Prof S, Univ Ark

Nuchtern, Jed MD [PS] - **Spec Exp:** Thoracic Surgery; Cancer Surgery; Laparoscopic Surgery; **Hospital:** Texas Chldns Hosp - Houston, Ben Taub Genl Hosp; **Address:** Texas Children's Hosp, 6621 Fannin St, MC CC650, Houston, TX 77030; **Phone:** 832-822-3135; **Board Cert:** Surgery 2003; Surgical Critical Care 2002; Pediatric Surgery 1998; **Med School:** Harvard Med Sch 1985; **Resid:** Surgery, Univ Washington 1992; Pediatric Surgery, Baylor Coll Med 1995; **Fellow:** Cellular Molecular Biology, Natl Inst Hlth 1990; **Fac Appt:** Prof S, Baylor Coll Med

Skinner, Michael A MD [PS] - **Spec Exp:** Endocrine Cancers; Thyroid Cancer; **Hospital:** UT Southwestern Med Ctr - Dallas; **Address:** UT Southwestern Med Ctr at Dallas, 5323 Harry Hines Blvd, Dallas, TX 75390; **Phone:** 214-456-6040; **Board Cert:** Surgery 2000; Pediatric Surgery 2003; **Med School:** Rush Med Coll 1984; **Resid:** Surgery, Duke Univ Med Ctr 1991; **Fellow:** Pediatric Surgery, Indiana Univ 1993; **Fac Appt:** Assoc Prof S, Univ Tex SW, Dallas

West Coast and Pacific

Albanese, Craig T MD [PS] - **Spec Exp:** Fetal Surgery; Laparoscopic Surgery; Twin to Twin Transfusion Syndrome (TTTS); **Hospital:** Lucile Packard Chldns Hosp/Stanford Univ Med Ctr; **Address:** 780 Welch Rd, Ste 206, MC 5733, Palo Alto, CA 94304; **Phone:** 650-723-6439; **Board Cert:** Surgery 2000; Pediatric Surgery 2003; **Med School:** SUNY Hlth Sci Ctr 1986; **Resid:** Surgery, Mt Sinai Med Ctr 1991; **Fellow:** Pediatric Surgery, Chldns Hosp 1994; **Fac Appt:** Prof S, Stanford Univ

America's Top Doctors® 8th Edition

Ford, Henri R MD [PS] - **Spec Exp:** Minimally Invasive Surgery; Trauma; **Hospital:** Chldns Hosp - Los Angeles; **Address:** 4650 Sunset Blvd, MS 100, Los Angeles, CA 90027; **Phone:** 323-361-2104; **Board Cert:** Surgery 2002; Pediatric Surgery 2005; **Med School:** Harvard Med Sch 1984; **Resid:** Surgery, New York Hosp 1991; **Fellow:** Pediatric Surgery, Chldns Hosp Pittsburgh 1995

Hilfiker, Mary L MD/PhD [PS] - **Hospital:** UCSD Med Ctr; **Address:** 8010 Frost St, Ste 414, San Diego, CA 92123; **Phone:** 858-966-7711; **Board Cert:** Surgery 2004; Pediatric Surgery 2007; **Med School:** Wright State Univ 1988; **Resid:** Surgery, U New Mexico Med Ctr 1993; **Fellow:** Pediatric Surgery, SUNY-Children's Hosp 1995; **Fac Appt:** Assoc Clin Prof S, UCSD

Krummel, Thomas M MD [PS] - **Spec Exp:** Minimally Invasive Surgery; Robotic Surgery; Fetal Surgery; **Hospital:** Lucile Packard Chldns Hosp/Stanford Univ Med Ctr, Stanford Univ Med Ctr; **Address:** Dept Surgery, 701B Welch Rd, Ste 225, MC 5784, Stanford, CA 94305-5784; **Phone:** 650-498-4292; **Board Cert:** Surgery 2004; Pediatric Surgery 2007; **Med School:** Univ Wisc 1977; **Resid:** Surgery, Med Coll Va Hosp 1983; Pediatric Surgery, Chldns Hosp 1985; **Fellow:** Fetal Surgery, UCSF Med Ctr 1985; **Fac Appt:** Prof S, Stanford Univ

Sawin, Robert S MD [PS] - **Spec Exp:** Pediatric Cancers; Thoracic Surgery; Neonatal Surgery-Gastrointestinal; **Hospital:** Chldns Hosp and Regl Med Ctr - Seattle; **Address:** Chldns Hosp & Regl Med Ctr, PO Box 5371, MS W7724, Seattle, WA 98105-0371; **Phone:** 206-987-2039; **Board Cert:** Surgery 1999; Surgical Critical Care 2001; Pediatric Surgery 1999; **Med School:** Univ Pittsburgh 1982; **Resid:** Surgery, Brigham Women's Hosp 1987; **Fellow:** Pediatric Surgery, Chldns Hosp 1989; **Fac Appt:** Prof S, Univ Wash

Stein, James E MD [PS] - **Hospital:** Chldns Hosp - Los Angeles; **Address:** Children's Hospital of LA, 4650 Sunset Blvd, MS 100, Los Angeles, CA 90027; **Phone:** 323-361-2491; **Board Cert:** Surgery 2004; Pediatric Surgery 2005; **Med School:** Tufts Univ 1986; **Resid:** Surgery, Tufts New England Med Ctr 1993; **Fellow:** Pediatric Surgery, Royal Chldns Hosp 1994; Pediatric Surgery, Babies Hosp/Columbia Presby 1996; **Fac Appt:** Assoc Prof S, USC Sch Med

Bascom Palmer
EYE INSTITUTE

⊔ UNIVERSITY OF MIAMI HEALTH SYSTEM

www.bascompalmer.org
800-329-7000

Miami:
900 NW 17th Street, Miami, FL 33136 • 305-326-6000
Palm Beach Gardens:
7101 Fairway Drive, Palm Beach Gardens, FL 33418 • 561-515-1500
Naples:
311 9th Street North, Naples, FL 34102 • 239-659-3937
Plantation:
1000 South Pine Island Road, Plantation, FL 33324 • 954-465-2700

INTERNATIONALLY ACCLAIMED

Bascom Palmer Eye Institute is committed to the protection and preservation of the treasured gift of sight. The Institute's full-time faculty of internationally-respected physicians and scientists are skilled in every ophthalmic subspecialty. Bascom Palmer Eye Institute, which serves as the Department of Ophthalmology for the University of Miami Miller School of Medicine in Miami, Florida, is recognized as one of the world's finest and most progressive centers for ophthalmic care, research and education.

BASCOM PALMER EYE INSTITUTE EARNS TOP RATINGS

Bascom Palmer Eye Institute continues to be ranked the nation's best ophthalmic hospital by board-certified ophthalmologists from across the United States. In 2008, Bascom Palmer was named the #1 eye hospital in the United States by *U.S. News & World Report* for the fifth year in a row. Bascom Palmer has also received the #1 ranking for its Clinical (Patient Care) and Residency programs by *Ophthalmology Times*, which annually ranks the top ophthalmology programs in the United States.

PEDIATRIC OPHTHALMOLOGISTS DIAGNOSE AND TREAT CHILDHOOD EYE DISEASE AND DISORDERS

Bascom Palmer Eye Institute is one of only a few centers giving special attention to the diverse ophthalmic needs of children from infancy through adolescence- a critical time when clear vision plays an important role in mental, physical and social development. As a major referral center serving the southeastern United States, the Caribbean and South America, the Institute treats approximately 7,000 children annually in its William and Norma Horvitz Children's Clinic, an outstanding ophthalmic facility designed specifically for pediatric care.Our spacious outpatient clinic is specifically designed to meet the unique ophthalmic and social needs of children with visual deficiencies as well as adults and children with strabismus. The clinic's diagnostic and treatment services encompass the common eye disorders of childhood, such as amblyopia and strabismus, as well as rare disorders affecting infants and children. With the support of the extensive resources of the entire Bascom Palmer Eye Institute, the Horvitz Clinic specializes in the blinding and visually-impairing diseases of childhood including congenital cataracts, congenital glaucoma, retinopathy of prematurity, detached retinas, ocular infections, hereditary disorders and tumors.

Cleveland Clinic

Children's Hospital

Cleveland Clinic Children's Hospital is ranked among the top pediatric hospitals in the United States, with more that 80 pediatricians recognized as "Best Doctors in America." Our specialists are nationally recognized for sophisticated diagnosis and innovative care of complex or chronic medical conditions affecting infants, children and adolescents as well as nationally funded research initiatives that are leading to advanced treatments for young patients.

- Our Center for Pediatric and Congenital Heart Disease is known for groundbreaking catheter and surgical treatments.

- As part of Cleveland Clinic's Neurological Institute, our pediatric epilepsy specialists offer highly specialized diagnosis and surgery for different seizure disorders.

- Our pediatric digestive disease specialists utilize breakthrough technology to diagnose and treat gastrointestinal problems.

- Children's Hospital oncologists are national leaders in the treatment of childhood leukemia and other cancers.

- A comprehensive Fetal Care Center with maternal-fetal medicine specialists who diagnose fetal problems and treat them in the womb or immediately after birth.

In addition, Cleveland Clinic Children's Hospital has the only comprehensive pediatric transplant center in Northern Ohio, offering heart, lung, liver and kidney transplantation and follow-up.

Our Pediatric ICU offers outstanding outcomes, saving many more young lives than similar centers, largely due to the 24-hour presence of seasoned critical care specialists. Our Pediatric Critical Care Transport Service transferred over 1,300 patients to our Children's Hospital from Ohio and surrounding states in 2007.

Our expertise in specialty pediatrics extends into the realm of long-term care for developmental, behavioral and rehabilitation needs. The Cleveland Clinic Children's Hospital for Rehabilitation, Shaker Campus, serves pediatric patients with chronic or complex medical conditions as one of just a handful of freestanding accredited pediatric rehabilitation hospitals in the country, and the only one in Ohio.

For more information about the Cleveland Clinic Children's Hospital, to schedule a second opinion or to learn about assistance for out-of-town patients, call 800.890.2467 or visit www.clevelandclinic.org/childrenstopdocs.

Children's Hospital | 9500 Euclid Avenue / AC311 | Cleveland OH 44195

Cleveland Clinic Children's Hospital

More than 200 Cleveland Clinic pediatricians and pediatric specialists offer advanced specialty and subspecialty care and rehabilitation for acute illnesses and injuries, as well as chronic and disabling conditions. Children with serious or complex medical problems such as congenital heart disease, cancer, epilepsy and digestive disorders are treated at our Main Campus. Our Shaker Campus is home to the Cleveland Clinic Children's Hospital for Rehabilitation, The Center for Autism and developmental, behavioral, therapeutic and rehabilitation programs that promote functional independence in children.

Maimonides Medical Center
MAIMONIDES INFANTS & CHILDREN'S HOSPITAL

4802 Tenth Avenue • Brooklyn, New York 11219
Phone: (718) 283-7500 • Fax: (718) 635-6149
http://www.maimonidesmed.org

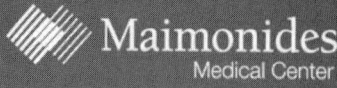

Maimonides
Medical Center

The Maimonides Infants & Children's Hospital is a NACHRI-certified children's hospital-within-a-hospital. Offering over 30 sub-specialty divisions as well as primary care, the Pediatrics program is unrivaled in the region and serves one of the largest pediatric populations in the nation.

Steven Shelov, MD, head of the Children's Hospital and author of several bestselling books on childrearing, has built a family-centered pediatrics program in a state-of-the-art medical environment, where babies, children and adolescents receive the best and most appropriate care. For most children, this involves preventing illness and promoting healthy growth. For those whose problems are more complicated, Maimonides specialists can treat every manner of childhood disorder no matter how rare or complex. The level and quality of critical care provided is evidenced by the demand for the Maimonides Pediatric Transport Program, through which critically ill children from other hospitals are transferred to Maimonides.

In recognition of its excellence in obstetrics and pediatrics, Maimonides was designated a Regional Perinatal Center by the New York State Department of Health.

Pediatric Specialties include:

Allergy	Infectious Disease
Behavioral & Developmental Pediatrics	Neonatology
	Nephrology
Cardiology	Neurology
Critical Care Medicine	Ophthalmology
Dentistry & Dental Surgery	Orthopedic Surgery
Emergency Medicine	Otolaryngology
Endocrinology	Psychiatry/Psychology
Gastroenterology	Pulmonology
Genetics	Rheumatology
Hematology/Oncology	Surgery
Immunology	Urology

Physicians at Maimonides are among the ten percent in the US who use computers to enter patient orders, thereby reducing the risk of errors, increasing efficiency, and speeding the healing process. Maimonides has appeared on the American Hospital Association's "Most Wired" and "Most Wireless" lists more often than any other healthcare institution in the metropolitan area. Advanced technology allows our doctors to focus more attention on caring for their patients.

Maimonides Medical Center – Passionate about medicine, compassionate about people.

www.maimonidesmed.org/pediatrics

NewYork-Presbyterian
The University Hospital of Columbia and Cornell

Morgan Stanley Children's Hospital of NewYork-Presbyterian
Columbia University Medical Center

3959 Broadway, New York, NY 10032

Komansky Center for Children's Health
NewYork-Presbyterian Hospital
Weill Cornell Medical Center

525 East 68th Street, New York, NY 10021

Sponsorship:	Voluntary Not-for-Profit
Beds:	387
Accreditation:	Joint Commission on Accreditation of Healthcare Organizations (JCAHO)

OVERVIEW:

NewYork-Presbyterian brings together the outstanding pediatric services and resources of the Morgan Stanley Children's Hospital and the Komansky Center for Children's Health to create one of the largest, most comprehensive children's hospital in the world.

With more than 1,000 pediatricians and medical and surgical subspecialists on staff, and teams of specially trained pediatric health professionals, NewYork-Presbyterian provides the highest level of care from infancy to adolescence. The Hospital's expertise in addressing simple and complex medical conditions and the psychological and emotional issues that accompany them is unparalleled. The Hospital offers:

- Adolescent Medicine
- Allergy
- Anesthesiology and Pain Management
- Cardiology
- Child Development and Behavioral Medicine
- Critical Care
- Dermatology
- Diabetes and Endocrinology
- Gastroenterology
- Genetics
- Hematology
- Infectious Disease
- Neonatal-Perinatal Medicine
- Nephrology
- Neurology
- Neurosurgery
- Oncology
- Primary Care
- Psychiatry and Mental Health
- Rheumatology
- Laboratory and Radiology Diagnostic Services
- Pediatric Emergency Care in emergency medicine, burn and trauma
- Surgical Services in cardiac, dental, oral and maxillofacial, general neurosurgery, ophthalmology, orthopedics, otolaryngology, plastic surgery, transplantation and urology

Physician Referral: For a physician referral or for information, call **1-800-245-KIDS** (1-800-245-5437) or visit our website at **www.childrensnyp.org**

CHILDREN'S HOSPITAL HIGHLIGHTS INCLUDE:

- One of the country's largest and most successful pediatric cardiology and cardiac surgery programs.

- Only provider in the region to offer three major transplant surgeries – heart, liver and kidney.

- One of three Level 1-designated Pediatric Trauma Centers in New York State and only one in New York City.

- Nationally recognized pediatric oncologists. Bone marrow transplantation program is one of the largest in the nation.

- Sophisticated neonatal intensive care that sets standards nationwide.

- Referral center and regional resource for hospitals needing expertise of our pediatric intensive care units. Seriously ill children can be transferred to NewYork-Presbyterian through the Pediatric Critical Care Transport Program.

NYU Cancer Institute

NYU LANGONE MEDICAL CENTER

Looking for information on our expert physicians?
1-212-731-5000

NYU Clinical Cancer Center
160 East 34th Street
New York, New York 10016
www.nyuci.org/atcd

NYU Langone Medical Center
550 First Avenue
(at 31st Street)
New York, New York 10016
www.nyumc.org/atcd

Stephen D. Hassenfeld Children's Center for Cancer and Blood Disorders
160 East 32nd Street
New York, New York 10016
www.nyumc.org/hassenfeld

A Collaborative Approach
The NYU Cancer Institute, an NCI designated center, is a "matrix cancer center" without walls operating within the larger NYU Langone Medical Center. With over 175 members and a research funding base of over $81 million, this structure strengthens our capabilities to forge collaborations across medical and scientific disciplines, which translates to comprehensive care for our patients and discoveries that will influence the future of this disease.

Renowned Expertise
Team members' compassion and expertise help patients better manage the symptoms of their disease as well as their special needs. Our highly skilled Magnet™ nursing team not only plays a pivotal role in coordinating direct patient care, but is also a source of invaluable patient education.

A Patient-Focused Setting
The NYU Clinical Cancer Center, with over 70 faculty members from various disciplines at the New York University School of Medicine, is the principal outpatient facility of the Cancer Institute and serves as home for our patients and their caregivers. The center and its multidisciplinary team of experts provide access to the latest treatment options and clinical trials along with a variety of programs in cancer prevention, screening, diagnostics, genetic counseling, and supportive services. When it comes to kids and cancer, the Stephen D. Hassenfeld Children's Center for Cancer and Blood Disorders offers not just innovation but insight. As a leading member of the NCI-sponsored Children's Oncology Group, our physicians are known for developing new ways to treat childhood cancer. Our affiliation with Bellevue Hospital, the oldest public hospital in the country, affords clinically distinctive opportunities to learn and care for patients with cancer by observing its presentation and behavior in a variety of patient groups.

Sponsored Page

NYU Child Study Center
NYU LANGONE MEDICAL CENTER

577 First Avenue
New York, NY 10016
212.263.6622
www.AboutOurKids.org

CHILD AND ADOLESCENT PSYCHIATRY

The New York University Child Study Center is dedicated to increasing the awareness of child and adolescent psychiatric disorders and improving the research necessary to advance the prevention, identification, and treatment of these disorders on a national scale. The NYU Child Study Center was named the Department of Child and Adolescent Psychiatry within the NYU School of Medicine, making it the second independent department of child and adolescent psychiatry in the country.

The NYU Child Study Center is built around seven research-driven Institutes focused on key mental health problems facing children and adolescents. The Center's premiere clinicians implement the knowledge gained from research, resulting in care that incorporates the most up-to-date information about the causes, symptoms, and treatments of mental disorders. The treatment options include Cognitive Behavioral Therapy, behavioral therapy, family and couples therapy, parent training, group sessions, and medication. School consultations and academic remediation are also available.

The CSC's research institutes and clinical arms include:
The Anita Saltz Institute for Anxiety and Mood Disorders
The Asperger Institute
The Institute for Attention Deficit and Hyperactivity and Behavior Disorders (ADHD)
The Phyllis Green and Randolph Cōwen Institute for Pediatric Neuroscience
The Institute for Prevention Science
The Institute for Tourette and Tic Disorders
The Institute for Trauma and Resilience

A key goal of the NYU Child Study Center is to increase the body of scientific knowledge of child and adolescent mental illness. Since its founding in 1997, the Child Study Center has published over 400 articles in peer-reviewed journals and its faculty has made thousands of presentations at national and international scientific meetings.

NYU **Langone Medical Center**

550 First Avenue (at 31St Street)
New York, NY 10016
Physician Referral:
(888)7-NYU-MED (888-769-8633)
www.nyumc.org

NYU CHILDREN'S HEALTH

NYU Langone Medical Center's Children's Health Team is comprised of some of the best clinical specialists in the country. Among the programs they offer are:

Apnea/SIDS Program —identifying and treating of infants with apnea and infants who are at increased risk for 5105

Center for Child and Adolescent Sports Medicine — developmentally sensitive and comprehensive evaluation and treatment of sports-related injuries in children

NYU- Hospital for Joint Diseases Center for Children — holistic outpatient treatment of children and adolescents with a wide range of orthopaedic and neurological conditions

Child Study Center — advancing the field of mental health for children and adolescents through evidence-based practice, science, and education

Cochlear Implant Program — restoring hearing to profoundly deaf children

Craniofacial Program — treating facial deformities discovered at birth Epilepsy Program — state-of-the-art evaluation and multidisciplinary treatment of children with epilepsy

Familial Dysautonomia Program — the only center in the U.S. providing care to individuals affected with this genetic disorder

Hassenfeld Children c Center — comprehensive outpatient care for children with cancer and blood disorders

Headache Center — thorough diagnosis and evaluation to help pediatric patients manage frequency and severity of chronic headaches

Hemangiomas and Vascular Malformation Program —
multidisciplinary care for children with hemangiomas and vascular malformations

Orthopaedic Immediate Care Center at the Hosp ital for Joint Diseases— evaluation and treatment of urgent pediatric and adult orthopaedic problems, such as fractures

Pediatric Rehabilitation Service — multi-disciplinary pediatric rehabilitation for a variety of congenital and acquired disabilities on an inpatient and outpatient basis

Preschool and Early Intervention Program — individualized educational and early intervention services for children under five Stem Cell Transplant Program — Using stem cell transplant to treat brain and other solid tumors, under the auspices of the Hassenfeld Children's Center, which was the site of much of the original stem cell harvest and transplantation research.

NYU Langone Medical Center

550 First Avenue (at 31St Street)
New York, NY 10016
Physician Referral:
(888)7-NYU-MED (888-769-8633)
www.nyumc.org

PEDIATRIC ALLERGY AND IMMUNOLOGY

NYU Langone Medical Center's Children's Health Team is comprised of some of the best clinical specialists in the country. Among the programs they offer are:

Apnea/SIDS Program —identifying and treating of infants with apnea and infants who are at increased risk for SIDS.

Center for Child and Adolescent Sports Medicine — developmentally sensitive and comprehensive evaluation and treatment of sports-related injuries in children.

NYU- Hospital for Joint Diseases Center for Children — holistic outpatient treatment of children and adolescents with a wide range of orthopaedic and neurological conditions.

Child Study Center — advancing the field of mental health for children and adolescents through evidence-based practice, science, and education.

Cochlear Implant Program — restoring hearing to profoundly deaf children.

Craniofacial Program — treating facial deformities discovered at birth.

Epilepsy Program — state-of-the-art evaluation and multidisciplinary treatment of children with epilepsy.

Familial Dysautonomia Program — the only center in the U.S. providing care to individuals affected with this genetic disorder.

Hassenfeld Children's Center — comprehensive outpatient care for children with cancer and blood disorders.

Headache Center— thorough diagnosis and evaluation to help pediatric patients manage frequency and severity of chronic headaches.

Hemangiomas and Vascular Malformation Program — multidisciplinary care for children with hernangiomas and vascular malformations.

Orthopaedic Immediate Care Center at the Hospital for Joint Diseases Orthopaedic Institute — evaluation and treatment of urgent pediatric and adult orthopaedic problems, such as fractures.

Pediatric Rehabilitation Service — multi-disciplinary pediatric rehabilitation for a variety of congenital and acquired disabilities on an inpatient and outpatient basis.

Preschool and Early Intervention Program — individualized educational and early intervention services for children under five.

Stem Cell Transplant Program — Using stem cell transplant to treat brain and other solid tumors, under the auspices of the Hassenfeld Children's Center, which was the site of much of the original stem cell harvest and transplantation research.

NYU Langone Medical Center

550 First Avenue (at 31St Street)
New York, NY 10016
Physician Referral:
(888)7-NYU-MED (888-769-8633)
www.nyumc.org

PEDIATRIC CARDIOLOGY

NYU's Pediatric Cardiology Program is motivated by an academic approach to patient care. A leader for more than three decades, the Pediatric Cardiology Program remains at the forefront of innovation in both research and clinical care. It is also an outstanding training ground for future pediatricians dedicated to the heart health of children.

There is a long list of recent advances that are benefiting infants, children, and young adults with a wide range of heart problems. First, a growing emphasis on minimally invasive surgical techniques allows for quicker recoveries and shorter hospital stays. Various clinical sub-disciplines further support the Pediatric Cardiology Program, including:

Cardiothoracic Surgery — corrective procedures for all types of congenital and acquired heart disease.

Pediatric Cardiac Critical Care — intensive care for children with heart disease, provided capably and compassionately by a staff of pediatric cardiologists, neonatologists, cardiac anesthesiologists, respiratory therapists, and pediatric intensive care nurses.

Pediatric Non-Invasive Cardiac Imaging — the use of echocardiography and magnetic resonance imaging (MM) to diagnose and monitor a wide range of cardiac abnormalities.

Pediatric Cardiac Electrophysiology — a wide array of diagnostic and therapeutic services, including arrhythmia detection and pacemaker placement.

Pediatric Interventional Cardiac Catheterization —the treatment of serious heart conditions in a nonsurgical setting, sometimes used in combination with open-heart surgery.

Pediatric Cardiopulmonary Exercise Laboratory — assesses the cardiorespiratory response of exercise in children as young as three and four years old. The Lab features some of the most sophisticated equipment in the region for measuring oxygen consumption, cardiac output, and lung capacity.

At NYU Langone Medical Center, a child's heart health is a family affair.

The Pediatric Cardiology staff at NYU is vigilant in helping children stay in contact with their parents during a stay at the medical center.

Whenever possible, parents are welcome to stay overnight in their child's room on the pediatric floor. Social workers and child life experts are always on hand to give families the information and support they need to cope with their child's disease during and after their hospital stay.

NYU Langone Medical Center

550 First Avenue (at 31St Street)
New York, NY 10016
Physician Referral:
(888)7-NYU-MED (888-769-8633)
www.nyumc.org

PEDIATRIC CRITICAL CARE

When children experience medical problems, they deserve the most compassionate, state-of-the-art medical care possible. Yet, pediatric patients have needs, medical and emotional, that are unique and different from those of adults. To better meet these needs, Tisch Hospital at NYU Langone Medical Center has recently completed a major expansion and improvement of its Pediatric Intensive Care Unit (PICU).

In most hospitals, pediatric patients recover in specialized areas annexed to the adult units for their particular ailment. For example, children recovering from neurosurgery would have awakened in a pediatric section of the neurosurgery unit to find a crowded and noisy recovery room that did not cater to their unique physical and emotional needs. At NYU, they recover in an environment developed especially for them, with a multidisciplinary staff assembled just for them.

The PICU at NYU Langone Medical Center has the added advantage of being a real resource to referring physicians, providing them with the technology, expertise and time-saving procedures that can help them save lives.

At NYU Langone Medical Center, parents are viewed as integral members of the healthcare team because each child's recovery is strongly influenced by continued family involvement. In recognition of this, each room has a roll-away sofa or chair so one parent can spend the night in close proximity to the child for the duration of their stay. In addition, there is a special family room that was created to give families a quiet place to gather together. Of course, the PICU staff also strives to keep children in contact with their parents and to keep parents informed throughout their child's stay.

NYU Langone Medical Center

550 First Avenue (at 31St Street)
New York, NY 10016
Physician Referral:
(888)7-NYU-MED (888-769-8633)
www.nyumc.org

PEDIATRIC GASTROENTEROLOGY

The Section of Gastroenterology in the Department of Pediatrics at NYU Langone Medical Center is dedicated to providing the highest quality medical care and state-of-the-art techniques in the evaluation and management of gastrointestinal, liver, and nutritional disorders from infancy to young adulthood. With access to the latest in endoscopic procedures performed at one of the country's leading academic hospitals, patients can receive comprehensive and multidisciplinary treatments for a vast range of conditions. Below are just some of the disorders NYU's pediatric gastroenterologists evaluate and treat.

- Abdominal pain
- Celiac sprue
- Congenital bowel dysfunction
- Congenital liver disorders and chronic liver disease
- ConstipationIhncopresis
- Diarrhea
- Feeding problems in infants
- Failure to thrive
- Food allergy
- Lactose intolerance
- Gastrointestinal bleeding
- Gastroesophageal reflux
- Hepatitis
- Malabsorption
- Pancreatitis
- Peptic disease
- Ulcerative colitis and Crohn's disease
- Vomiting

Among common disorders are chronic abdominal pain, diarrhea, constipation, and vomiting. Most children will occasionally experience one or more of these symptoms during their childhood years. Some children, however, develop recurrent symptoms, which interrupt their normal life, inhibit their development, disrupt their school performance and affect their emotional well being and self-esteem. It is these children who often need the pediatric gastroenterologist's expertise to pinpoint the problem and determine the most effective therapy. At NYU Langone Medical Center, a whole range of therapeutic services is available, as well as access to clinical rehabilitation and some of the country's finest surgeons.

NYU Langone Medical Center

550 First Avenue (at 31St Street)
New York, NY 10016
Physician Referral:
(888)7-NYU-MED (888-769-8633)
www.nyumc.org

PEDIATRIC HEMATOLOGY PROGRAM

For decades, children with chronic blood diseases have come to NYU Langone Medical Center's Pediatric Hematology Program for comprehensive medical care, including a full range of psychosocial support services to meet every need. Members of t he program's expert staff are guided by a patient- and family-centered approach to care, with all the advantages of a leading academic medical center at their fingertips.

The Program addresses the needs of patients with red blood cell disorders, including a variety of anemias and thalassemias — problems of hemoglobin metabolism — as well as vascular problems and malformations, coagulation disorders, and numerous other hemostatic abnormalities.

Patients requiring hospitalization are treated on the pediatric floor of Tisch Hospital, where they benefit from its advanced diagnostic and therapeutic expertise and the support of all pediatric subspecialties. Families are actively encouraged to become knowledgeable about their children's disease and its management. Our multidisciplinary team works closely with the patient's primary care physician to coordinate both medical and psychosocial care.

PSYCHOSOCIAL SERVICES

To help children and families cope with their disease and to prevent later psychological trauma, our behavioral health professionals are committed to a holistic approach to patient care. Among the services we provide are art therapy, relaxation training, play therapy, psychiatric evaluation, neuropsychological assessment, individual and group counseling, and patient education.

THE PEDIATRIC SPECIAL HEMATOLOGY LABORATORY

As a service to clinicians, the Pediatric Special Hematology Laboratory provides comprehensive hemostasis and red cell testing. Tests have been adapted so that small quantities of blood can be drawn from pediatric patients. The Laboratory's repertoire of test procedures is routinely upgraded to incorporate the latest developments in the field. It strives to provide fast, precise test information that leads to effective treatments while maintaining rigorous quality control standards.

NYU | **Langone Medical Center**

550 First Avenue (at 31St Street)
New York, NY 10016
Physician Referral:
(888)7-NYU-MED (888-769-8633)
www.nyumc.org

PEDIATRIC INFECTIOUS DISEASES
Pediatric Infectious Diseases Clinic

One major provider of health care services for mothers and children with HIV infection in Manhattan is the Pediatric Infectious Diseases (PID) Family Clinic at Bellevue Hospital, which follows over 300 families, including more than 120 children who are HIV-positive. Initiated in 1982 with the aid of private philanthropy and now funded in large part by federal support, this program has made major contributions to the understanding of the transmission of HIV from mothers to children and has contributed to their improved care and longevity.

The PID multidisciplinary health care team maintains a close relationship with patients and follows them closely, providing the majority of medical and psychosocial care for HIV-infected children on an outpatient basis. Thus far, the team has proved successful, as indicated by the average daily census of less than one HIV-infected child.

ADOLESCENT HIV CLINIC
The Bellevue Adolescent Clinic provides free, confidential HIV testing, pre- and post-test counseling, complete medical evaluations, comprehensive medical care, and referral to clinical trials for HIV positive teens. NYU Langone Medical Center was recently designated a Reaching for Excellence in Adolescent Care and Health (REACH) site, an NIH/HRSA-funded project. REACH's primary goal is to increase understanding of the natural history of HIV in teens.

DAY HOSPITAL PROGRAM
In addition to the outpatient program, children requiring intravenous infusions during the course of their illness are seen in the Pediatric AIDS Day Hospital. Candidates for infusion include patients receiving intravenous gammaglobulin or those with vomiting, diarrhea and/or decreased oral intake who would benefit from intravenous hydration. While these children do not routinely require hospitalization, they do require 4-6 hour periods of observation with adequate nursing and physician supervision. The Pediatric AIDS Day Hospital provides the medical, nursing, psychological, and social support services these patients require, maintaining an organized and efficient delivery of care, as well as providing a facility in which innovative treatments can be developed and implemented. Pediatric patients can also use the new Day Hospital for non-acute care outside of regular clinic hours.

Medical services are provided for the children by Pediatric Infectious Disease attendings, post-doctoral fellows, a pediatrician, with a dermatologist and a pedondontist available on call. Psychologist provide developmental testing. Medical care for parents is provided in the same clinic by adult infectious disease specialist and an obstetrician/gynecologist, who see parents while their children are being seen. In addition to nursing, staff also include public health advisors who screen mothers for risk factors, counsel, and initiate testing, as well as provide follow-up for mothers in prenatal care, a counselor who makes home visits, provides emotional support, and aids in the follow-up effort; and a full range of clinical social work and child life services.

NYU Langone Medical Center

550 First Avenue (at 31St Street)
New York, NY 10016
Physician Referral:
(888)7-NYU-MED (888-769-8633)
www.nyumc.org

PEDIATRIC PULMONOLOGY

On the forefront of technology, NYU pediatric lung care specialists utilize minimally invasive techniques, providing complete pediatric general surgical and thoracic services for infants, children and adolescents. This includes surgery for congenital and acquired problems, surgery in premature infants, tumor surgery, and surgery on the lungs, esophageal surgery and repair of chest wall deformities. With over a decade of experience in using minimally invasive techniques to treat these problems and state-of-the-art instruments and techniques, the team of pediatricians can perform these procedures with minimal discomfort, little scarring, and limited hospitalization. Consultation requests for conditions prenatally diagnosed are welcome.

Because NYU Langone Medical Center is committed to comprehensive care through an interdisciplinary approach, its pediatric lung specialists are able to join forces with other centers, departments, and divisions within the medical center. Pulmonary care at the NYU Infant Apnea/SIDS Program of Neonatology, within the Department Pediatrics, for example, is specially designed and dedicated to the identification and treatment of infants with apnea and infants who are at an increased risk for sudden infant death syndrome (SIDS). The program consists of physicians and nurses specially trained in this area, and it provides testing and treatment for apnea and identification of high risk infants. Physicians and nurses also supply extensive education to the surrounding community and around-the-clock support to families of high risk infants.

NYU Langone Medical Center

550 First Avenue (at 31St Street)
New York, NY 10016
Physician Referral:
(888)7-NYU-MED (888-769-8633)
www.nyumc.org

PEDIATRIC RHEUMATOLOGY

CAUSES OF ARTHRITIS IN CHILDREN

Arthritis is the term used to describe inflammation and swelling of the tissues in a joint. Perhaps surprisingly, viruses are the most common cause of arthritis in children. This type of arthritis is usually temporary and passes quickly without permanent damage. However, a bacterial joint infection is a more urgent matter. Called septic arthritis, this painful condition requires urgent care to prevent the spread of infection and the possibility of permanent damage to the joint. At its first sign, NYU's expert medical staff are quick to take steps to fight the infection at its source. Normally, septic arthritis is completely cured with antibiotics.

JUVENILE IDIOPATHIC ARTHRITIS

An umbrella term for several different patterns of arthritis in children, Juvenile Idiopathic Arthritis (JIA) refers to arthritic disorders caused by an autoimmune reaction. Autoimmune disease occurs when the body begins to attack its own tissues as if they were foreign substances. NYU's pediatric rheumatologists are expert in diagnosing and treating at least seven different types of JIA. These are diagnosed by putting together a total picture that includes the age of the child and the presence of associated arthritis in the family. The physician also considers which joints have been tender and swollen and for how long, and which laboratory tests are abnormal.

Although JIA is not curable at present, rheumatologists have learned that aggressive, early treatment with methotrexate and injections of corticosteroids into the joints can usually prevent significant damage. The increased use of methotrexate in combination with newly discovered biologic agents, such as Etanercept and Infliximab, gives even greater reason for optimism. Juvenile arthritis, once a crippler of children, is fast becoming a highly manageable disease.

NYU Langone Medical Center

PEDIATRIC SURGERY

When it comes to surgery, children are not just smaller versions of adults. NYU Langone Medical Center provides comprehensive pediatric surgical care that starts even before the child is admitted and may continue long after patient discharge. In addition to its top-quality surgeons and surgical nurses, the Medical Center offers a wide array of Child Life Services to help children and their families become familiar with the hospital environment and allay fears that often accompany a hospital stay.

SURGICAL EXPERTISE
Besides general surgical services, NYU is renowned for its achievements in the full spectrum of pediatric surgical specialties, including transplant, neurosurgery, thoracic surgery, cancer surgery, abdominal surgery, and reconstructive surgery, among others. With more than a decade of experience using minimally invasive techniques to treat a broad range of medical problems, NYU surgeons strive to cut pain and scarring down to size and keep children as safe and comfortable as humanly possible. Shorter hospital stays and faster recovery — both benefits associated with minimally invasive surgery — mean that children can return home and resume their lives far sooner than in the recent past.

CHILD LIFE SERVICES
The pediatric unit at Tisch Hospital is home to a Child Life Program that focuses on creating a supportive environment for children undergoing surgery. The Program comprises many small services that add up to a total approach to caring for the whole child and supporting families in the process. Just a few examples of these services are:
• Pre-Admission Orientation and Information — Informational packets are available for families through pre-admission testing and doctors' offices. Parents and their children are also encouraged to attend an orientation session with a member of the Child Life staff.
• Therapeutic Play — To help children face the challenges they may encounter during their hospital stay, therapists use arts and crafts, music, horticulture, games, and cooking.
• Pediatric Library and Computer Center — A great variety of children's books, videos, and audiotapes are available in the pediatric library, which also houses two computers with Internet access.
• Teen Esteem Workshop Series — In cooperation with the Social Work Department, this workshop series was developed to address the special needs of teenagers who are living with chronic or life-threatening illnesses.

Warmth, contact, and caring make all the difference in the world when a youngster is recovering from surgery. At every point, Child Life staff and volunteers reach out to each child in many different ways. Too sick to visit the playroom? A volunteer will make an individual bedside visit to make sure the young patient's needs are being met. Just a little bit lonely? Foster grandparents are on hand to comfort, console, and entertain children whose parents may be unable to be present during the day. And since everyone knows happiness is a warm puppy, a group of specially trained dogs and their owners volunteer regularly for special visits with eligible children.

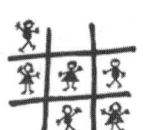

Wake Forest University Baptist
MEDICAL CENTER®

Brenner Children's Hospital
Wake Forest University Baptist Medical Center

Medical Center Boulevard • Winston-Salem, NC 27157
336-716-2011
Health On-Call® (Patient access) 1-800-446-2255
Physician Inquiries (PAL®) 1-877-716-1999
www.brennerchildrens.org

AN OPTIMAL PLACE FOR HEALING

Building on its tradition of excellence, Brenner Children's Hospital is housed in a state-of-the-art, 160-bed pediatric facility — an innovative environment designed to meet the complex needs of young patients and their families. Brenner Children's holistic care approach, outstanding facility, medical excellence and depth of pediatric subspecialty expertise – including western North Carolina's only Level IV neonatal intensive care nursery — have made it the resource for children's health in this region.

FAMILY-CENTERED

The pediatric tower exemplifies the gold standard for quality care and comfort, with spacious private rooms that encourage parents to room-in, a rooftop garden and play area, soothing quiet areas and interactive play centers. A Ronald McDonald Family Room –one of the first in the world—offers parents a comfortable place for respite and refreshment.

HOLISTIC CARE

Brenner Children's Hospital reflects a "whole child" philosophy. Every effort is made to meet emotional, spiritual and social needs as children receive expert medical care. Child Life specialists help patients and families cope with issues of hospitalization and illness.

COMMITTED TO CHILDREN'S HEALTH

Staffed by Wake Forest University School of Medicine faculty, Brenner Children's Hospital is committed to children's health research. Examples include the National Institutes of Health (NIH) Pediatric Heart Network. Brenner Children's Hospital joins other children's hospitals in the nation conducting clinical trials on patients with heart defects.

To make an appointment or find a specialist at Brenner Children's Hospital, call Health On-Call® at 1-800-446-2255.

PEDIATRIC EXPERTISE

- Brenner Children's Hospital is the region's only full service pediatric facility. More than 120 pediatric specialists and subspecialists provide expert care for critically ill children from N.C., W.V., TN, VA and S.C.

- Brenner Children's Hospital offers children highly specialized, minimally invasive procedures often not available elsewhere in the Southeast, such as outpatient heart surgery for patent ductus arteriosus. Pediatric specialists manage every aspect of care.

- The neonatal intensive care nursery (the region's only Level IV nursery) at Brenner Children's Hospital participates in research to find new therapies and treatments.

- Brenner Children's houses the area's only pediatric Emergency Department, where children receive emergency care designed specifically for them.

- The Wake Forest Baptist ECMO (heart/lung) unit is one of only a few centers in the U.S. that supports newborns and children.

- Brenner Children's is one of eight centers in the United States participating in the National Institutes of Health (NIH) Pediatric Heart Network, which searches for the best ways to care for patients with heart defects.

- Our pediatric oncologists and nurses participate in a national Children's Oncology Group, a group of national researchers who evaluate current therapies used in treating children with cancer. This ensures that our children have access to the best cancer treatments available.

KNOWLEDGE MAKES ALL THE DIFFERENCE.

Physical Medicine & Rehabilitation

Physical medicine and rehabilitation, also referred to as rehabilitation medicine, is the medical specialty concerned with diagnosing, evaluating and treating patients with physical disabilities. These disabilities may arise from conditions affecting the musculoskeletal system such as neck and back pain, sports injuries, or other painful conditions affecting the limbs, for example carpal tunnel syndrome. Alternatively, the disabilities may result from neurological trauma or disease such as spinal cord injury, head injury or stroke.

A physician certified in physical medicine and rehabilitation is often called a physiatrist. The primary goal of the physiatrist is to achieve maximal restoration of physical, psychological, social and vocational function through comprehensive rehabilitation. Pain management is often an important part of the role of the physiatrist. For diagnosis and evaluation, a physiatrist may include the techniques of electromyography to supplement the standard history, physical, X-ray and laboratory examinations. The physiatrist has expertise in the appropriate use of therapeutic exercise, prosthetics (artificial limbs), orthotics and mechanical and electrical devices.

Training Required: Four years *plus* one year clinical practice.

Certification in the following subspecialty requires additional training and examination.

Spinal Cord Injury Medicine: A physician who addresses the prevention, diagnosis, treatment and management of traumatic spinal cord injury and non-traumatic etiologies of spinal cord dysfunction by working in an interdisciplinary manner. Care is provided to patients of all ages on a lifelong basis and covers related medical, physical, psychological and vocational disabilities and complications.

PHYSICAL MEDICINE & REHABILITATION

New England

Richter, Edwin MD [PMR] - **Hospital:** Stamford Hosp; **Address:** 32 Strawberry Hill Ct Fl 4 - Ste 9, Stamford, CT 06902; **Phone:** 203-316-0610; **Board Cert:** Physical Medicine & Rehabilitation 1992; **Med School:** NYU Sch Med 1987; **Resid:** Physical Medicine & Rehabilitation, NYU Med Ctr 1991

Silver, Julie K MD [PMR] - **Spec Exp:** Post Polio Syndrome/Rehabilitation; **Hospital:** Spaulding Rehab Hosp; **Address:** Spaulding Rehabilitation Outpatient Ctr, 570 Worcester Rd, Framingham, MA 01702; **Phone:** 508-872-2200; **Board Cert:** Physical Medicine & Rehabilitation 2006; **Med School:** Georgetown Univ 1991; **Resid:** Physical Medicine & Rehabilitation, Natl Rehab Hosp 1995; **Fac Appt:** Asst Prof PMR, Harvard Med Sch

Zafonte, Ross DO [PMR] - **Spec Exp:** Brain Injury Rehabilitation; Spinal Cord Injury; **Hospital:** Spaulding Rehab Hosp; **Address:** Spaulding Rehab Hospital, 125 Nashua St, rm A55, Boston, MA 02114; **Phone:** 617-573-2754; **Board Cert:** Physical Medicine & Rehabilitation 1990; **Med School:** Nova SE Univ, Coll Osteo Med 1985; **Resid:** Physical Medicine & Rehabilitation, Mt Sinai Med Ctr 1989; **Fac Appt:** Clin Prof PMR, Boston Univ

Mid Atlantic

Ahn, Jung Hwan MD [PMR] - **Spec Exp:** Spinal Cord Injury; Stroke Rehabilitation; Neurologic Rehabilitation; **Hospital:** NYU Med Ctr (page 68); **Address:** 400 E 34th St, rm 421, New York, NY 10016-4901; **Phone:** 212-263-6122; **Board Cert:** Physical Medicine & Rehabilitation 1980; Spinal Cord Injury Medicine 1998; **Med School:** South Korea 1970; **Resid:** Obstetrics & Gynecology, Elmhurst City Hosp - Mt Sinai 1976; Physical Medicine & Rehabilitation, NYU Med Ctr 1979; **Fellow:** Spinal Cord Injury Medicine, NYU Med Ctr 1980; **Fac Appt:** Clin Prof PMR, NYU Sch Med

Aseff, John N MD [PMR] - **Spec Exp:** Electrodiagnosis; Pain-Soft Tissue; **Hospital:** Natl Rehab Hosp, Washington Hosp Ctr; **Address:** National Rehabilitation Hosp, 102 Irving St NW, Washington, DC 20010; **Phone:** 202-877-1916; **Board Cert:** Physical Medicine & Rehabilitation 1978; **Med School:** Ohio State Univ 1973; **Resid:** Surgery, Univ Hosps Cleveland 1975; Physical Medicine & Rehabilitation, Ohio State Univ Hosps 1977; **Fac Appt:** Assoc Clin Prof PMR, Georgetown Univ

Bach, John MD [PMR] - **Spec Exp:** Respiratory Disorders; Neuromuscular Disorders; Amyotrophic Lateral Sclerosis (ALS); Post Polio Syndrome/Rehabilitation; **Hospital:** UMDNJ-Univ Hosp-Newark; **Address:** 150 Bergen St, Ste B403, Newark, NJ 07103; **Phone:** 973-972-7195; **Board Cert:** Physical Medicine & Rehabilitation 1986; **Med School:** UMDNJ-NJ Med Sch, Newark 1976; **Resid:** Physical Medicine & Rehabilitation, NYU Med Ctr 1980; **Fellow:** Neurological Muscular Disease, Univ Hosp 1983; **Fac Appt:** Prof PMR, UMDNJ-NJ Med Sch, Newark

Ballard, Pamela H MD [PMR] - **Spec Exp:** Spinal Cord Injury; Spasticity Management; Neuromuscular Disorders; **Hospital:** Natl Rehab Hosp; **Address:** 102 Irving St NW, Ste 2164, Washington, DC 20010; **Phone:** 202-877-1621; **Board Cert:** Physical Medicine & Rehabilitation 1991; Spinal Cord Injury Medicine 1999; **Med School:** Howard Univ 1986; **Resid:** Physical Medicine & Rehabilitation, Sinai Hosp 1990

Braddom, Randall L MD [PMR] - **Spec Exp:** Electromyography; Pain-Neck; Pain-Low Back; Musculoskeletal Disorders; **Hospital:** Riverview Med Ctr; **Address:** Orthopaedic, Sports Medicine & Rehab Ctr, 80 Oak Hill Rd, rm 368, Red Bank, NJ 07701; **Phone:** 732-741-2313; **Board Cert:** Physical Medicine & Rehabilitation 1974; **Med School:** Ohio State Univ 1968; **Resid:** Physical Medicine & Rehabilitation, Ohio State Univ Hosp 1973; **Fac Appt:** Clin Prof PMR, UMDNJ-NJ Med Sch, Newark

De Lateur, Barbara J MD [PMR] - **Spec Exp:** Frailty Syndrome; **Hospital:** Johns Hopkins Bayview Med Ctr (page 61); **Address:** Johns Hopkins Bayview Med Ctr, Rehab, AA Bldg Fl 01 - rm 1661, Baltimore, MD 21224; **Phone:** 410-550-5299; **Board Cert:** Physical Medicine & Rehabilitation 1970; **Med School:** Univ Wash 1963; **Resid:** Physical Medicine & Rehabilitation, Univ Wash Hosp 1968; **Fac Appt:** Prof PMR, Johns Hopkins Univ

Dillard, James N MD [PMR] - **Spec Exp:** Pain Management; Acupuncture; Complementary Medicine; Nutrition; **Hospital:** Stamford Hosp; **Address:** 110 E 59th St, Ste 10A, New York, NY 10022; **Phone:** 212-265-4038; **Board Cert:** Physical Medicine & Rehabilitation 2005; **Med School:** Rush Med Coll 1990; **Resid:** Physical Medicine & Rehabilitation, Columbia-Presby Med Ctr 1994; **Fac Appt:** Asst Clin Prof PMR, Columbia P&S

Esquenazi, Alberto M MD [PMR] - **Spec Exp:** Amputee Rehabilitation; Mobility Evaluation & Treatment; Post Polio Syndrome/Rehabilitation; **Hospital:** MossRehab Hosp; **Address:** Moss Rehab Hosp, 60 E Township Line Rd, Philadelphia, PA 19027; **Phone:** 215-663-6676; **Board Cert:** Physical Medicine & Rehabilitation 1986; **Med School:** Mexico 1981; **Resid:** Physical Medicine & Rehabilitation, Temple Univ 1985; **Fellow:** Gait and Prosthetics, Moss Rehab Hosp 1986; **Fac Appt:** Prof PMR, Jefferson Med Coll

Evans, Sarah Helen MD [PMR] - **Spec Exp:** Pediatric Rehabilitation; **Hospital:** Chldns Natl Med Ctr; **Address:** Children's National Medical Ctr, Pediatric Rehabilitation, 111 Michigan Ave NW, Washington, DC 20010; **Phone:** 202-476-3080; **Board Cert:** Physical Medicine & Rehabilitation 1992; Pediatrics 2002; Pediatric Rehabilitation Medicine 2003; **Med School:** Univ MD Sch Med 1984; **Resid:** Pediatrics, Univ Colorado Hlth Sci Ctr 1987; **Fellow:** Physical Medicine & Rehabilitation, Univ Colorado Hlth Sci Ctr 1988; Pediatric Rehabilitation Medicine, Children's Hosp 1989; **Fac Appt:** Assoc Prof PMR, Univ Colorado

Feinberg, Joseph Hunt MD [PMR] - **Spec Exp:** Peripheral Neuropathy; Spinal Rehabilitation; Electrodiagnosis; Sports Medicine; **Hospital:** Hosp For Special Surgery (page 59), Kessler Inst for Rehab - W Orange; **Address:** 523 E 72nd St Fl 2, New York, NY 10021-4872; **Phone:** 212-606-1568; **Board Cert:** Physical Medicine & Rehabilitation 1991; **Med School:** Albany Med Coll 1983; **Resid:** Surgery, Mt Sinai Hosp 1985; Physical Medicine & Rehabilitation, Rusk Inst Rehab 1990; **Fellow:** Orthopaedic Pathology, Hosp Spec Surg 1986; Orthopaedic Biomechanics, Univ Iowa Hosp & Clins 1987; **Fac Appt:** Assoc Prof PMR, Cornell Univ-Weill Med Coll

Fried, Guy W MD [PMR] - **Spec Exp:** Brain Injury Rehabilitation; Spinal Cord Injury; Neurogenic Bladder; **Hospital:** Magee Rehab Hosp; **Address:** Magee Hospital, 1513 Race St, Philadelphia, PA 19102-1177; **Phone:** 215-587-3394; **Board Cert:** Physical Medicine & Rehabilitation 1990; Spinal Cord Injury Medicine 1999; Pain Medicine 2000; **Med School:** Yale Univ 1985; **Resid:** Physical Medicine & Rehabilitation, Thos Jefferson Univ Hosp 1989; **Fac Appt:** Asst Prof PMR, Thomas Jefferson Univ

Kirshblum, Steven C MD [PMR] - **Spec Exp:** Spinal Cord Injury; **Hospital:** Kessler Inst for Rehab - W Orange, St Barnabas Med Ctr; **Address:** Kessley Institute, 1199 Pleasant Valley Way, West Orange, NJ 07052-1424; **Phone:** 973-731-3600 x2258; **Board Cert:** Physical Medicine & Rehabilitation 1991; Spinal Cord Injury Medicine 1998; **Med School:** Ros Franklin Univ/Chicago Med Sch 1986; **Resid:** Physical Medicine & Rehabilitation, Mount Sinai Med Ctr 1990; **Fac Appt:** Prof PMR, UMDNJ-NJ Med Sch, Newark

Physical Medicine & Rehabilitation

Lutz, Gregory MD [PMR] - **Spec Exp:** Spinal Rehabilitation; Sports Medicine; Pain-Low Back; **Hospital:** Hosp For Special Surgery (page 59), Univ Med Ctr - Princeton; **Address:** 523 E 72nd St Fl 2, New York, NY 10021-4898; **Phone:** 212-606-1648; **Board Cert:** Physical Medicine & Rehabilitation 2003; **Med School:** Georgetown Univ 1988; **Resid:** Physical Medicine & Rehabilitation, Mayo Clinic 1992; **Fellow:** Sports Medicine, Hosp For Spec Surg 1993; **Fac Appt:** Assoc Prof PMR, Cornell Univ-Weill Med Coll

Ma, Dong M MD [PMR] - **Spec Exp:** Electromyography; Musculoskeletal Disorders; **Hospital:** Rusk Inst of Rehab Med (page 71), NYU Med Ctr (page 68); **Address:** 400 E 34th St, rm 211, New York, NY 10016; **Phone:** 212-263-6338; **Board Cert:** Physical Medicine & Rehabilitation 1979; **Med School:** South Korea 1968; **Resid:** Physical Medicine & Rehabilitation, NYU Med Ctr 1975; **Fellow:** Physical Medicine & Rehabilitation, NYU Med Ctr 1977; **Fac Appt:** Clin Prof PMR, NYU Sch Med

Marino, Ralph J MD [PMR] - **Spec Exp:** Spinal Cord Injury; **Hospital:** Thomas Jefferson Univ Hosp; **Address:** 132 S 10th St, 375 Main Bldg, Philadelphia, PA 19107; **Phone:** 215-955-1200; **Board Cert:** Physical Medicine & Rehabilitation 1988; Spinal Cord Injury Medicine 2000; **Med School:** Jefferson Med Coll 1982; **Resid:** Physical Medicine & Rehabilitation, Thos Jefferson Univ Hosp 1987; **Fac Appt:** Assoc Prof PMR, Jefferson Med Coll

Mayer, Nathaniel MD [PMR] - **Spec Exp:** Motor Control Analysis; Spasticity Management; Brain Injury Rehabilitation; **Hospital:** MossRehab Hosp; **Address:** Moss Rehab Hosp, Drucker Brain Injury Ctr, 60 E Township Line Rd, Elkins Park, PA 19027; **Phone:** 215-663-6681; **Board Cert:** Physical Medicine & Rehabilitation 1976; **Med School:** Albert Einstein Coll Med 1968; **Resid:** Physical Medicine & Rehabilitation, Temple Univ Hosp 1973; **Fac Appt:** Prof PMR, Temple Univ

Munin, Michael C MD [PMR] - **Spec Exp:** Spasticity Management; Amputee Rehabilitation; Hip Surgery Rehabilitation; Electrodiagnosis; **Hospital:** UPMC Presby, Pittsburgh, UPMC Inst Rehab & Rsch; **Address:** Univ Pittsburgh Physicians, 3471 Fifth Ave, Kaufman Bldg Ste 1103, Pittsburgh, PA 15213; **Phone:** 412-648-6979; **Board Cert:** Physical Medicine & Rehabilitation 1993; **Med School:** Jefferson Med Coll 1988; **Resid:** Physical Medicine & Rehabilitation, Thomas Jefferson Univ Hosp 1992; **Fac Appt:** Assoc Prof PMR, Univ Pittsburgh

Ragnarsson, Kristjan T MD [PMR] - **Spec Exp:** Spinal Cord Injury; Brain Injury Rehabilitation; Pain-Back & Neck; **Hospital:** Mount Sinai Med Ctr (page 64); **Address:** 5 E 98th St Fl 6, New York, NY 10029-6501; **Phone:** 212-659-9370; **Board Cert:** Physical Medicine & Rehabilitation 1976; **Med School:** Iceland 1969; **Resid:** Physical Medicine & Rehabilitation, NYU Med Ctr 1974; **Fellow:** Spinal Cord & Brain Injury Rehab, NYU Med Ctr 1975; **Fac Appt:** Prof PMR, Mount Sinai Sch Med

Ried, Stephanie R MD [PMR] - **Spec Exp:** Pediatric Rehabilitation; **Hospital:** Shriners Hosp for Chldn-Phila; **Address:** Shriners Hosp for Children, Dept Physical Med & Rehab, 3551 N Broad St, Philadelphia, PA 19140; **Phone:** 215-430-4000; **Board Cert:** Pediatrics 1989; Physical Medicine & Rehabilitation 2006; Pediatric Rehabilitation Medicine 2006; **Med School:** Univ Mich Med Sch 1986; **Resid:** Pediatrics, Baylor Affil Hosps 1989; Physical Medicine & Rehabilitation, Univ Michigan Med Ctr 1992; **Fac Appt:** Asst Prof PMR, Temple Univ

Schwartz, L Matthew MD [PMR] - **Spec Exp:** Lymphedema; Head & Neck Cancer; Pain-Cancer; Pain Management; **Hospital:** Montgomery Rehab Hosp; **Address:** Montgomery Rehab Hosp, Medical Office, 8601 Stenton Ave, Wyndmoor, PA 19038; **Phone:** 215-233-6226; **Board Cert:** Physical Medicine & Rehabilitation 1992; Pain Medicine 2003; **Med School:** UMDNJ-NJ Med Sch, Newark 1987; **Resid:** Physical Medicine & Rehabilitation, Hosp U Penn 1989; Physical Medicine & Rehabilitation, Thos Jefferson Univ Hosp 1991; **Fac Appt:** Clin Prof PMR, Univ Pennsylvania

Slipman, Curtis W MD [PMR] - **Spec Exp:** Spinal Rehabilitation; Pain Management; Musculoskeletal Disorders; **Hospital:** Hosp Univ Penn - UPHS (page 60); **Address:** Hosp Univ Penn, Dept Rehab Med, 3400 Spruce St White Bldg Fl Ground, Philadelphia, PA 19104; **Phone:** 215-662-3259; **Board Cert:** Physical Medicine & Rehabilitation 1987; **Med School:** Baylor Coll Med 1983; **Resid:** Physical Medicine & Rehabilitation, Columbia-Presby Med Ctr 1986; **Fac Appt:** Assoc Prof PMR, Univ Pennsylvania

Stubblefield, Michael MD [PMR] - **Spec Exp:** Cancer Rehabilitation; Pain-Cancer; Pain-Musculoskeletal; Electrodiagnosis; **Hospital:** Meml Sloan-Kettering Cancer Ctr; **Address:** 1275 York Avenue, New York, NY 10065; **Phone:** 800-525-2225; **Board Cert:** Internal Medicine 2001; Physical Medicine & Rehabilitation 2002; Electrodiagnostic Medicine 2003; **Med School:** Columbia P&S 1996; **Resid:** Internal Medicine, Columbia Presby Med Ctr 2001; Physical Medicine & Rehabilitation, Columbia Presby Med Ctr 2001; **Fac Appt:** Asst Prof PMR, Cornell Univ-Weill Med Coll

Southeast

Cardenas, Diana D MD [PMR] - **Spec Exp:** Spinal Cord Injury; Spina Bifida; **Hospital:** Univ of Miami Hosp & Clins/Sylvester Comp Canc Ctr, Jackson Meml Hosp; **Address:** Univ Miami, Dept Rehab Medicine, PO Box 016960 (C-206), Miami, FL 33101; **Phone:** 305-243-9516; **Board Cert:** Physical Medicine & Rehabilitation 1977; **Med School:** Univ Tex SW, Dallas 1973; **Resid:** Physical Medicine & Rehabilitation, Univ Wash Affil Hosps 1976; **Fac Appt:** Prof PMR, Univ Miami Sch Med

Creamer, Michael DO [PMR] - **Spec Exp:** Spinal Cord Injury; Pain Management; Electrodiagnosis; **Hospital:** Orlando Regl Med Ctr, Florida Hosp - Orlando; **Address:** 100 W Gore St, Ste 203, Orlando, FL 32806-1041; **Phone:** 407-649-8707; **Board Cert:** Physical Medicine & Rehabilitation 1992; Spinal Cord Injury Medicine 1998; Pain Medicine 2000; **Med School:** Chicago Coll Osteo Med 1987; **Resid:** Physical Medicine & Rehabilitation, Rehab Inst Chicago 1991; **Fac Appt:** Asst Prof Med, Univ Fla Coll Med

Diamond, Paul T MD [PMR] - **Spec Exp:** Neurorehabilitation; Geriatric Rehabilitation; **Hospital:** Univ Virginia Med Ctr; **Address:** Univ of Virginia Hlth Sci Ctr, Dept Rehabilitation, 545 Ray C Hunt Drive, Ste 240, Charlottesville, VA 22903; **Phone:** 434-243-5622; **Board Cert:** Internal Medicine 1989; Physical Medicine & Rehabilitation 2003; **Med School:** Univ VA Sch Med 1986; **Resid:** Internal Medicine, Johns Hospkins Bayview Hosp 1989; Physical Medicine & Rehabilitation, Sinai/Johns Hopkins Hosp 1992; **Fac Appt:** Assoc Prof PMR, Univ VA Sch Med

Gater Jr, David R MD/PhD [PMR] - **Spec Exp:** Spinal Cord Injury; Exercise Physiology; Electrodiagnosis; **Hospital:** Hunter Holmes McGuire VA Med Ctr, VCU Med Ctr; **Address:** 1201 Broadrock Blvd, Richmond, VA 23249; **Phone:** 804-675-5000 x5455; **Board Cert:** Physical Medicine & Rehabilitation 2007; Spinal Cord Injury Medicine 1999; Electrodiagnostic Medicine 1998; **Med School:** Univ Ariz Coll Med 1992; **Resid:** Physical Medicine & Rehabilitation, UC Davis Med Ctr 1994; **Fac Appt:** Prof PMR, Va Commonwealth Univ Sch Med

Jackson, Amie Brown MD [PMR] - **Spec Exp:** Spinal Cord Injury; **Hospital:** Univ of Ala Hosp at Birmingham, Children's Hospital - Birmingham; **Address:** Univ Alabama-Spine Rehab Ctr, 619 19th St S, Ste 190, Birmingham, AL 35249; **Phone:** 205-934-4131; **Board Cert:** Physical Medicine & Rehabilitation 1990; **Med School:** Univ Ala 1984; **Resid:** Physical Medicine & Rehabilitation, Univ Alabama Med Ctr 1987; **Fac Appt:** Prof PMR, Univ Ala

Kerrigan, D Casey MD [PMR] - **Spec Exp:** Gait Disorders; **Hospital:** Univ Virginia Med Ctr; **Address:** Univ Va, Dept Physical Med Rehab, 545 Ray C Hunt Drive, Ste 240, Charlottesville, VA 22908-1004; **Phone:** 434-243-0378; **Board Cert:** Physical Medicine & Rehabilitation 1992; **Med School:** Harvard Med Sch 1987; **Resid:** Physical Medicine & Rehabilitation, UCLA Med Ctr 1991; **Fac Appt:** Prof PMR, Univ VA Sch Med

Physical Medicine & Rehabilitation

King Jr, Richard W MD [PMR] - **Spec Exp:** Cancer Rehabilitation; Lymphedema; Soft Tissue Radiation Necrosis; Soft Tissue Radiation Necrosis-Breast; **Hospital:** WellStar Windy Hill Hosp, WellStar Cobb Hosp; **Address:** HyOx Medical Treatment Ctr, 2550 Windy Hill Rd, Ste 110, Marietta, GA 30067; **Phone:** 678-303-3200; **Board Cert:** Physical Medicine & Rehabilitation 1988; Undersea & Hyperbaric Medicine 2002; **Med School:** Emory Univ 1979; **Resid:** Physical Medicine & Rehabilitation, Emory Univ Hosp 1987; **Fac Appt:** Asst Clin Prof PMR, Emory Univ

Lipkin, David L MD [PMR] - **Spec Exp:** Geriatric Rehabilitation; Pain-Back; Rheumatology; **Hospital:** Mount Sinai Med Ctr - Miami; **Address:** PO Box 630127, Miami, FL 33163-0127; **Phone:** 305-672-1256; **Board Cert:** Physical Medicine & Rehabilitation 1971; **Med School:** Belgium 1964; **Resid:** Pediatrics, Jersey City Med Ctr 1966; Physical Medicine & Rehabilitation, Bronx Muni Hosp 1969; **Fellow:** Research, Natl Inst Hlth-Einstein Coll Med 1969; **Fac Appt:** Assoc Clin Prof PMR, Univ Miami Sch Med

Nelson, Maureen R MD [PMR] - **Spec Exp:** Pediatric Rehabilitation; Brachial Plexus Palsy; Electrodiagnosis; **Hospital:** Carolinas Med Ctr, Levine Chldns Hosp; **Address:** Carolinas Rehab, Dept PM&R, 1100 Blythe Blvd, Charlotte, NC 28203; **Phone:** 704-355-4330; **Board Cert:** Physical Medicine & Rehabilitation 1990; Pediatric Rehabilitation Medicine 2003; **Med School:** Univ IL Coll Med 1985; **Resid:** Physical Medicine & Rehabilitation, Univ Tex Hlth Scis Ctr 1989; **Fellow:** Pediatric Rehabilitation Medicine, Alfred I Dupont Inst 1990; **Fac Appt:** Assoc Clin Prof PMR, Univ NC Sch Med

Stewart, Paula JB MD [PMR] - **Spec Exp:** Lymphedema; Brain Tumors; Spinal Cord Tumors; Cancer Rehabilitation; **Hospital:** Healthsouth Lakeshore Rehab Hosp; **Address:** Healthsouth Lakeshore Rehab Hosp, 3800 Ridgeway Drive, Birmingham, AL 35209; **Phone:** 205-868-2347; **Board Cert:** Physical Medicine & Rehabilitation 1996; Spinal Cord Injury Medicine 2000; **Med School:** Univ Minn 1987; **Resid:** Physical Medicine & Rehabilitation, Mayo Clinic 1991

Midwest

Chen, David MD [PMR] - **Spec Exp:** Spinal Cord Injury; **Hospital:** Rehab Inst - Chicago; **Address:** 345 E Superior St, Ste 1146, Chicago, IL 60611; **Phone:** 312-238-0764; **Board Cert:** Physical Medicine & Rehabilitation 1992; Spinal Cord Injury Medicine 1998; **Med School:** Univ IL Coll Med 1987; **Resid:** Physical Medicine & Rehabilitation, Northwestern Med Sch 1991; **Fac Appt:** Asst Prof PMR, Northwestern Univ

Cheville, Andrea MD [PMR] - **Spec Exp:** Lymphedema; Cancer Rehabilitation; Pain-Cancer; **Hospital:** Mayo Med Ctr & Clin - Rochester; **Address:** Mayo Clinic, Dept Physical Med & Rehab, 200 1st St SW, Rochester, MN 55905; **Phone:** 507-266-8913; **Board Cert:** Physical Medicine & Rehabilitation 1998; **Med School:** Harvard Med Sch 1993; **Resid:** Physical Medicine & Rehabilitation, UMDNJ Med Ctr 1997; **Fellow:** Pain & Palliative Care, Meml Sloan Kettering Cancer Ctr 1999; **Fac Appt:** Asst Prof PMR, Mayo Med Sch

Clairmont, Albert C MD [PMR] - **Spec Exp:** Spasticity Management; Electrodiagnosis; **Hospital:** Ohio St Univ Med Ctr; **Address:** Dodd Hall - Davis Center, 480 Medical Center Drive, Columbus, OH 43210; **Phone:** 614-293-4837; **Board Cert:** Physical Medicine & Rehabilitation 1985; Pediatrics 1985; **Med School:** Jamaica 1974; **Resid:** Pediatrics, Columbus Chldns Hosp 1981; Physical Medicine & Rehabilitation, Ohio St Univ Hosps 1983; **Fac Appt:** Assoc Clin Prof PMR, Ohio State Univ

Colachis III, Samuel C MD [PMR] - **Spec Exp:** Spinal Cord Injury; Electrodiagnosis; **Hospital:** Ohio St Univ Med Ctr; **Address:** Dodd Hall - Davis Center, 480 Medical Center Drive, Columbus, OH 43210; **Phone:** 614-293-4837; **Board Cert:** Physical Medicine & Rehabilitation 1988; Spinal Cord Injury Medicine 2003; **Med School:** USC Sch Med 1984; **Resid:** Physical Medicine & Rehabilitation, Ohio State Univ Hosps 1987; **Fellow:** Electrodiagnosis, Ohio State Univ Hosps 1988; **Fac Appt:** Assoc Prof PMR, Ohio State Univ

DePompolo, Robert W MD [PMR] - **Spec Exp:** Cancer Rehabilitation; Lymphedema; **Hospital:** St Mary's Hosp - Rochester, Mayo Med Ctr & Clin - Rochester; **Address:** Mayo Clinic, Dept Phys Med & Rehab, 200 1st St SW, Rochester, MN 55905; **Phone:** 507-255-8972; **Board Cert:** Physical Medicine & Rehabilitation 1981; **Med School:** Wayne State Univ 1977; **Resid:** Physical Medicine & Rehabilitation, Univ Minnesota 1980

Dillingham, Timothy R MD [PMR] - **Spec Exp:** Electrodiagnosis; Electromyography; Amputee Rehabilitation; **Hospital:** Froedtert Meml Lutheran Hosp; **Address:** Froedtert Memorial Hospital, 9200 W Wisconsin Ave, rm 2183, Milwaukee, WI 53226; **Phone:** 414-805-7343; **Board Cert:** Physical Medicine & Rehabilitation 1991; **Med School:** Univ Wash 1986; **Resid:** Physical Medicine & Rehabilitation, Univ Wash Affil Hosps 1990; **Fac Appt:** Prof PMR, Med Coll Wisc

Feldman, Joseph L MD [PMR] - **Spec Exp:** Lymphedema; **Hospital:** NorthShore Univ Hlth-Sys; **Address:** 2650 Ridge Ave, rm 2204, Evanston, IL 60201-1718; **Phone:** 847-570-2066; **Board Cert:** Physical Medicine & Rehabilitation 1971; **Med School:** Univ IL Coll Med 1965; **Resid:** Physical Medicine & Rehabilitation, Univ of Ilinois 1969; **Fac Appt:** Asst Prof PMR, Northwestern Univ

Frost, Frederick S MD [PMR] - **Spec Exp:** Spinal Cord Injury; Stroke Rehabilitation; Geriatric Rehabilitation; **Hospital:** Cleveland Clin Fdn (page 56); **Address:** Cleveland Clinic Fdn, 9500 Euclid Ave, MC C21, Cleveland, OH 44195; **Phone:** 216-445-2006; **Board Cert:** Physical Medicine & Rehabilitation 1988; Spinal Cord Injury Medicine 1998; **Med School:** Northwestern Univ 1983; **Resid:** Physical Medicine & Rehabilitation, Northwestern Meml Hosp 1987; **Fellow:** Spinal Cord Injury Medicine, Rehab Inst Chicago; **Fac Appt:** Asst Prof PMR, Cleveland Cl Coll Med/Case West Res

Gamble, Gail L MD [PMR] - **Spec Exp:** Lymphedema; Head & Neck Cancer; Bone Tumors-Metastatic; **Hospital:** Rehab Inst - Chicago; **Address:** Rehab Inst of Chicabo, 345 E Superior St, Chicago, IL 60611; **Phone:** 312-238-7670; **Board Cert:** Physical Medicine & Rehabilitation 1985; **Med School:** Mayo Med Sch 1979; **Resid:** Physical Medicine & Rehabilitation, Mayo Clinic 1983

Gittler, Michelle MD [PMR] - **Spec Exp:** Spinal Cord Injury; Amputee Rehabilitation; **Hospital:** Schwab Rehab Hosp, Univ of Chicago Hosps; **Address:** 1401 S California Blvd, Chicago, IL 60608; **Phone:** 773-522-5853; **Board Cert:** Physical Medicine & Rehabilitation 2003; Spinal Cord Injury Medicine 1998; **Med School:** Univ IL Coll Med 1988; **Resid:** Physical Medicine & Rehabilitation, Rehab Inst Chicago 1992; **Fac Appt:** Assoc Clin Prof S, Univ Chicago-Pritzker Sch Med

Haig, Andrew MD [PMR] - **Spec Exp:** International Health; Pain-Back & Neck; Electrodiagnosis; **Hospital:** Univ Michigan Hlth Sys, VA Med Ctr - Ann Arbor; **Address:** Univ Michigan Spine Program, 325 E Eisenhower, Burlington Bldg - Ste 100, Ann Arbor, MI 48108-3346; **Phone:** 734-763-4200; **Board Cert:** Physical Medicine & Rehabilitation 1987; Pain Medicine 2002; **Med School:** Med Coll Wisc 1983; **Resid:** Physical Medicine & Rehabilitation, Northwestern Univ 1986; **Fac Appt:** Assoc Prof PMR, Univ Mich Med Sch

Physical Medicine & Rehabilitation

Keen, Mary MD [PMR] - **Spec Exp:** Pediatric Rehabilitation; Spasticity Management; Neurodevelopmental Disability; Autism; **Hospital:** Marianjoy Rehab Hosp, Central DuPage Hosp; **Address:** Marianjoy Rehab Medical Clinic, 26 W 171 Roosevelt Rd, Wheaton, IL 60187; **Phone:** 630-909-7005; **Board Cert:** Physical Medicine & Rehabilitation 1984; Pediatrics 1998; Neurodevelopmental Disabilities 2001; **Med School:** Northwestern Univ 1979; **Resid:** Physical Medicine & Rehabilitation, Univ Wash Med Ctr 1983; Pediatrics, Loyola Univ Med Ctr 1990; **Fac Appt:** Assoc Clin Prof Ped, Loyola Univ-Stritch Sch Med

Kirschner, Kristi MD [PMR] - **Spec Exp:** Brain Injury; Spinal Cord Injury; Women's Health/Disabilities; **Hospital:** Rehab Inst - Chicago; **Address:** Rehab Inst of Chicago, 345 E Superior St Fl 11, Chicago, IL 60611-2654; **Phone:** 312-238-4744; **Board Cert:** Physical Medicine & Rehabilitation 1991; **Med School:** Univ Chicago-Pritzker Sch Med 1986; **Resid:** Physical Medicine & Rehabilitation, Northwestern Meml Hosp 1990; **Fellow:** Clinical Ethics, Maclean Ctr/ Univ Chicago 1995; **Fac Appt:** Assoc Prof PMR, Northwestern Univ

Kuiken, Todd A MD/PhD [PMR] - **Spec Exp:** Amputee Rehabilitation; Prosthesis Control; Gait Disorders; **Hospital:** Rehab Inst - Chicago; **Address:** Rehab Inst of Chicago, 345 E Superior St, rm 1309, Chicago, IL 60611; **Phone:** 312-238-8072; **Board Cert:** Physical Medicine & Rehabilitation 2006; **Med School:** Northwestern Univ 1990; **Resid:** Physical Medicine & Rehabilitation, Rehab Inst Chicago 1995; **Fac Appt:** Assoc Prof PMR, Northwestern Univ

La Ban, Myron M MD [PMR] - **Spec Exp:** Pain-Back; Electromyography; **Hospital:** William Beaumont Hosp; **Address:** 3535 W Thirteen Mile Rd, Ste 437, Royal Oak, MI 48073; **Phone:** 248-288-2237; **Board Cert:** Physical Medicine & Rehabilitation 1967; **Med School:** Univ Mich Med Sch 1961; **Resid:** Physical Medicine & Rehabilitation, Univ Ohio Hosps 1965; **Fac Appt:** Clin Prof PMR, Ohio State Univ

Leonard Jr, James A MD [PMR] - **Spec Exp:** Amputee Rehabilitation; Electrodiagnosis; **Hospital:** Univ Michigan Hlth Sys; **Address:** Univ Michigan, Dept Physical Med & Rehab, 325 E Eisenhower Pkwy, Ste 100, Ann Arbor, MI 48108; **Phone:** 734-936-7175; **Board Cert:** Physical Medicine & Rehabilitation 1977; **Med School:** Univ Mich Med Sch 1972; **Resid:** Physical Medicine & Rehabilitation, Univ Mich Med Ctr 1975; **Fac Appt:** Clin Prof PMR, Univ Mich Med Sch

Mysiw, W Jerry MD [PMR] - **Spec Exp:** Brain Injury Rehabilitation; **Hospital:** Ohio St Univ Med Ctr; **Address:** Dodd Hall - Davis Center, 480 Medical Center Drive, rm 1011, Columbus, OH 43210-1245; **Phone:** 614-293-7604; **Board Cert:** Physical Medicine & Rehabilitation 1985; **Med School:** Ohio State Univ 1981; **Resid:** Physical Medicine & Rehabilitation, Ohio State Univ Med Ctr 1984; **Fac Appt:** Assoc Prof PMR, Ohio State Univ

Nobunaga, Austin MD [PMR] - **Spec Exp:** Spinal Cord Injury; Electrodiagnosis; **Hospital:** Univ Hosp - Cincinnati; **Address:** Drake Center, 151 W Galbraith Rd, South Pavillion, Cincinnati, OH 45216; **Phone:** 513-418-2707; **Board Cert:** Physical Medicine & Rehabilitation 1990; Spinal Cord Injury Medicine 1999; **Med School:** Univ Mich Med Sch 1985; **Resid:** Physical Medicine & Rehabilitation, Rehab Inst Chicago 1989

Press, Joel MD [PMR] - **Spec Exp:** Sports Medicine; Pain-Back; Musculoskeletal Injuries; **Hospital:** Rehab Inst - Chicago; **Address:** Ctr for Spine, Sports & Occup Rehab, 1030 N Clark St, Ste 500, Chicago, IL 60610; **Phone:** 312-238-7767; **Board Cert:** Physical Medicine & Rehabilitation 1989; **Med School:** Univ IL Coll Med 1984; **Resid:** Physical Medicine & Rehabilitation, Northwestern Meml Hosp 1988; **Fac Appt:** Assoc Clin Prof PMR, Northwestern Univ

Roth, Elliot MD [PMR] - **Spec Exp:** Stroke Rehabilitation; Neurologic Rehabilitation; Geriatric Rehabilitation; **Hospital:** Rehab Inst - Chicago, Northwestern Meml Hosp; **Address:** Rehab Inst Chicago, 345 E Superior St, Chicago, IL 60611-2654; **Phone:** 312-238-4637; **Board Cert:** Physical Medicine & Rehabilitation 1987; **Med School:** Northwestern Univ 1982; **Resid:** Physical Medicine & Rehabilitation, Northwestern Univ 1985; **Fellow:** Physical Medicine & Rehabilitation, Rehab Inst Chicago 1986; **Fac Appt:** Prof PMR, Northwestern Univ

Sisung, Charles MD [PMR] - **Spec Exp:** Rheumatic Diseases of Childhood; Trauma Rehabilitation; Burn Care; **Hospital:** Rehab Inst - Chicago; **Address:** 345 E Superior St, rm 1158, Chicago, IL 60611; **Phone:** 312-238-1246; **Board Cert:** Pediatrics 2004; Physical Medicine & Rehabilitation 1991; Pediatric Rehabilitation Medicine 2003; **Med School:** Univ Mich Med Sch 1981; **Resid:** Pediatrics, Mott Chldns Hosp/Univ Mich 1984; Physical Medicine & Rehabilitation, Schwab Rehab Hosp 1989; **Fellow:** Pediatric Rheumatology, Univ Chicago Hosps 1991; **Fac Appt:** Asst Prof PMR, Northwestern Univ

Sliwa, James A DO [PMR] - **Spec Exp:** Post Polio Syndrome/Rehabilitation; Multiple Sclerosis; Pain-Back; **Hospital:** Rehab Inst - Chicago; **Address:** Rehab Inst Chicago, 345 E Superior St, rm 1108, Chicago, IL 60611-3015; **Phone:** 312-238-4093; **Board Cert:** Physical Medicine & Rehabilitation 2005; **Med School:** Chicago Coll Osteo Med 1980; **Resid:** Physical Medicine & Rehabilitation, Rehab Inst 1984; **Fac Appt:** Prof PMR, Northwestern Univ

Smith, Joanne MD [PMR] - **Spec Exp:** Pain-Pelvic; Pain-Back; **Hospital:** Rehab Inst - Chicago, Northwestern Meml Hosp; **Address:** Rehab Inst of Chicago, 345 E Superior St, Ste 1507, Chicago, IL 60611; **Phone:** 312-238-0815; **Board Cert:** Physical Medicine & Rehabilitation 2003; **Med School:** Mich State Univ 1988; **Resid:** Physical Medicine & Rehabilitation, Northwestern Univ 1992; **Fac Appt:** Asst Prof PMR, Northwestern Univ

Volshteyn, Oksana MD [PMR] - **Spec Exp:** Spinal Cord Injury; **Hospital:** Rehab Inst St. Louis, Barnes-Jewish Hosp; **Address:** 4444 Forest Park, Box 8518, St Louis, MO 63108; **Phone:** 314-658-3887; **Board Cert:** Physical Medicine & Rehabilitation 1986; Spinal Cord Injury Medicine 1999; **Med School:** Russia 1976; **Resid:** Physical Medicine & Rehabilitation, Barnes Jewish Hosp 1985; **Fac Appt:** Assoc Prof N, Washington Univ, St Louis

Great Plains and Mountains

Lammertse, Daniel MD [PMR] - **Spec Exp:** Spinal Cord Injury; **Hospital:** Craig Hosp; **Address:** CNS Med Grp, 3425 S Clarkson St, Engelwood, CO 80113; **Phone:** 303-789-8220; **Board Cert:** Physical Medicine & Rehabilitation 1980; Spinal Cord Injury Medicine 1998; **Med School:** Ohio State Univ 1976; **Resid:** Physical Medicine & Rehabilitation, Ohio State Univ Hosp 1979; **Fac Appt:** Assoc Clin Prof PMR, Univ Colorado

Mason, Kristin D MD [PMR] - **Spec Exp:** Neurologic Rehabilitation; Electrodiagnosis; Musculoskeletal Injuries; **Hospital:** Swedish Med Ctr - Englewood; **Address:** Rehabilitation Assocs of Colorado, 8515 Pearl St, Ste 100, Thornton, CO 80229; **Phone:** 303-286-2888; **Board Cert:** Physical Medicine & Rehabilitation 2003; **Med School:** Baylor Coll Med 1988; **Resid:** Physical Medicine & Rehabilitation, Rehab Inst Chicago 1992

Matthews, Dennis J MD [PMR] - **Spec Exp:** Brain Injury Rehabilitation; Neuromuscular Disorders; Cerebral Palsy; **Hospital:** Chldn's Hosp - Aurora, The; **Address:** Chldns Hosp, Dept Rehabilitation, 13123 E 16th Ave, Box 285, Aurora, CO 80045; **Phone:** 720-777-3907; **Board Cert:** Physical Medicine & Rehabilitation 1979; Pediatric Rehabilitation Medicine 2003; **Med School:** Univ Colorado 1975; **Resid:** Physical Medicine & Rehabilitation, Univ Minnesota Hosps 1978; **Fellow:** Research, Univ Minnesota Hosps 1978; **Fac Appt:** Assoc Prof PMR, Univ Colorado

Physical Medicine & Rehabilitation

Southwest

Barber, Douglas B MD [PMR] - **Spec Exp:** Spinal Cord Injury; **Hospital:** VA Med Ctr N TX Hlth Sys; **Address:** Univ Hlth Sci Ctr, Dept of Rehab Med, 7703 Floyd Curl Drive, MC 7798, San Antonio, TX 78229-3900; **Phone:** 210-567-5353; **Board Cert:** Physical Medicine & Rehabilitation 1992; Spinal Cord Injury Medicine 1999; **Med School:** Univ Tex, Houston 1987; **Resid:** Physical Medicine & Rehabilitation, Univ TX Hlth Scis Ctr 1991; **Fac Appt:** Assoc Prof PMR, Univ Tex, San Antonio

Dumitru, Daniel MD/PhD [PMR] - **Spec Exp:** Electrodiagnosis; **Hospital:** Univ Hlth Sys - Univ Hosp (San Antonio, TX); **Address:** Univ Tex Hlth Sci Ctr, Dept Rehab Med, 7703 Floyd Curl Drive, San Antonio, TX 78229-3900; **Phone:** 210-358-0770; **Board Cert:** Physical Medicine & Rehabilitation 1984; **Med School:** Univ Cincinnati 1980; **Resid:** Physical Medicine & Rehabilitation, VA Hosp/Univ Hosp 1983; **Fac Appt:** Prof PMR, Univ Tex, San Antonio

Francisco, Gerard E MD [PMR] - **Spec Exp:** Spasticity Management; Brain Injury Rehabilitation; Stroke Rehabilitation; **Hospital:** TIRR; **Address:** The Inst of Rehab & Research, 1333 Moursund St, Houston, TX 77030-3405; **Phone:** 713-797-5246; **Board Cert:** Physical Medicine & Rehabilitation 1995; **Med School:** Philippines 1989; **Resid:** Physical Medicine & Rehabilitation, UMDNJ-Univ Hosp 1994; **Fellow:** Physical Medicine & Rehabilitation, Baylor Coll Med 1995; **Fac Appt:** Assoc Clin Prof PMR, Univ Tex, Houston

Harris, David K MD [PMR] - **Spec Exp:** Spinal Rehabilitation; Spinal Cord Injury; Pain-Back; Pain-Spine; **Hospital:** St Davids Medical Center - Austin, Seton Med Ctr; **Address:** Spine Austin, 3001 Bee Cave Rd, Ste 200, Austin, TX 78746; **Phone:** 512-454-1234; **Board Cert:** Physical Medicine & Rehabilitation 2004; Spinal Cord Injury Medicine 1998; Pain Medicine 2004; **Med School:** Univ Tex SW, Dallas 1988; **Resid:** Physical Medicine & Rehabilitation, Univ Colorado Hlth Sci Ctr 1992

Ivanhoe, Cindy MD [PMR] - **Spec Exp:** Brain Injury Rehabilitation; **Hospital:** TIRR; **Address:** 1333 Moursund St, Ste D-110, Houston, TX 77030-3405; **Phone:** 713-942-7300; **Board Cert:** Physical Medicine & Rehabilitation 1993; **Med School:** Mexico 1984; **Resid:** Physical Medicine & Rehabilitation, Univ Ill Coll Med 1992; **Fellow:** Brain Injury, Baylor Coll Med 1993; **Fac Appt:** Asst Prof PMR, Baylor Coll Med

Kevorkian, Charles G MD [PMR] - **Spec Exp:** Stroke Rehabilitation; Neuromuscular Disorders; Electrodiagnosis; **Hospital:** St Luke's Episcopal Hosp - Houston; **Address:** Baylor Coll Med, Dept PMR, 6624 Fannin St, Ste 2330, Houston, TX 77030-2335; **Phone:** 713-798-4061; **Board Cert:** Physical Medicine & Rehabilitation 1980; **Med School:** Australia 1972; **Resid:** Physical Medicine & Rehabilitation, Prince Henry Hosp 1976; Physical Medicine & Rehabilitation, Mayo Clinic 1979; **Fac Appt:** Assoc Prof PMR, Baylor Coll Med

King, John Chandler MD [PMR] - **Spec Exp:** Stroke Rehabilitation; Electrodiagnosis; Pain-Chronic; **Hospital:** Univ Hlth Sys - Univ Hosp (San Antonio, TX); **Address:** Univ Tex Hlth Sci Ctr, Dept Rehab Med, 7703 Floyd Curl Drive, MC 7798, San Antonio, TX 78229-3900; **Phone:** 210-567-5345; **Board Cert:** Physical Medicine & Rehabilitation 1987; Spinal Cord Injury Medicine 2000; **Med School:** Oral Roberts Sch Med 1983; **Resid:** Physical Medicine & Rehabilitation, Baylor Coll Med 1986; **Fac Appt:** Prof PMR, Univ Tex, San Antonio

West Coast and Pacific

Carter, Gregory T MD [PMR] - **Spec Exp:** Neuromuscular Disorders; Muscular Dystrophy; Amyotrophic Lateral Sclerosis (ALS); Charcot Marie Tooth Disease; **Hospital:** Providence Centralia Hosp, Univ Wash Med Ctr; **Address:** 1800 Cooks Hill Rd, Ste E, Centralia, WA 98531; **Phone:** 360-330-8626; **Board Cert:** Physical Medicine & Rehabilitation 1991; Neuromuscular Medicine 2006; **Med School:** Loyola Univ-Stritch Sch Med 1986; **Resid:** Physical Medicine & Rehabilitation, UC Davis Med Ctr 1990; **Fellow:** Neuromuscular Medicine, UC Davis Med Ctr 1991; **Fac Appt:** Clin Prof PMR, Univ Wash

Herring, Stanley A MD [PMR] - **Spec Exp:** Sports Medicine; Pain-Back; Spinal Rehabilitation; **Hospital:** Harborview Med Ctr; **Address:** 325 9th Ave, Box 359721, Seattle, WA 98104; **Phone:** 206-744-0401; **Board Cert:** Physical Medicine & Rehabilitation 1983; **Med School:** Univ Tex SW, Dallas 1979; **Resid:** Physical Medicine & Rehabilitation, Univ Washington Med Ctr 1982; **Fac Appt:** Clin Prof PMR, Univ Wash

Jaffe, Kenneth M MD [PMR] - **Spec Exp:** Brain Injury; Spinal Cord Injury; Limb Deficiency-Arthrogryposis; **Hospital:** Chldns Hosp and Regl Med Ctr - Seattle; **Address:** 4800 Sand Point Way NE, Seattle, WA 98105; **Phone:** 206-987-2114; **Board Cert:** Pediatrics 1980; Physical Medicine & Rehabilitation 1982; **Med School:** Harvard Med Sch 1975; **Resid:** Pediatrics, Univ Wash-Chldns Hosp 1980; Physical Medicine & Rehabilitation, Univ Wash Affil Hosp 1982; **Fac Appt:** Prof PMR, Univ Wash

Kraft, George H MD [PMR] - **Spec Exp:** Multiple Sclerosis; Spinal Cord Injury; Electrodiagnosis; **Hospital:** Univ Wash Med Ctr; **Address:** 1959 NE Pacific St, Box 356490, Seattle, WA 98195; **Phone:** 206-598-3344; **Board Cert:** Physical Medicine & Rehabilitation 1969; Spinal Cord Injury Medicine 1998; **Med School:** Ohio State Univ 1963; **Resid:** Physical Medicine & Rehabilitation, UCSF-Moffitt Hosp 1965; Physical Medicine & Rehabilitation, Ohio State Univ Med Ctr 1967; **Fac Appt:** Prof PMR, Univ Wash

Massagli, Teresa Luisa MD [PMR] - **Spec Exp:** Spinal Cord Injury-Pediatric; Brain Injury Rehabiliation-Pediatric; **Hospital:** Chldns Hosp and Regl Med Ctr - Seattle; **Address:** Chldns Hosp & Regl Med Ctr, 4800 Sandy Point Way NE, PO Box 5371, MS W6847, Seattle, WA 98105-3916; **Phone:** 206-987-2180; **Board Cert:** Pediatrics 1987; Physical Medicine & Rehabilitation 1989; Spinal Cord Injury Medicine 1998; **Med School:** Yale Univ 1982; **Resid:** Pediatrics, Yale-New Haven Hosp 1985; **Fellow:** Physical Medicine & Rehabilitation, Univ Washington 1988; **Fac Appt:** Prof PMR, Univ Wash

Robinson, Lawrence R MD [PMR] - **Spec Exp:** Electrodiagnosis; Electromyography; Botox Therapy; **Hospital:** Harborview Med Ctr, Univ Wash Med Ctr; **Address:** 325 9th Ave, Box 359898, Harborview Med Ctr, Seattle, WA 98104; **Phone:** 206-744-2523; **Board Cert:** Physical Medicine & Rehabilitation 1987; **Med School:** Baylor Coll Med 1982; **Resid:** Physical Medicine & Rehabilitation, Northwestern Meml Hosp 1985; **Fac Appt:** Prof PMR, Univ Wash

Saal, Jeffrey A MD [PMR] - **Spec Exp:** Pain-Lower Back (IDET procedure); Spinal Rehabilitation; Sports Medicine; **Address:** 500 Arguello St, Ste 100, Redwood City, CA 94063; **Phone:** 650-851-4900; **Board Cert:** Internal Medicine 1978; Physical Medicine & Rehabilitation 1982; **Med School:** Tulane Univ 1975; **Resid:** Internal Medicine, VA Med Ctr 1978; Physical Medicine & Rehabilitation, Stanford Univ Affil Hosps 1981; **Fac Appt:** Assoc Clin Prof PMR, UC Irvine

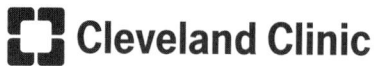
Cleveland Clinic

Physical Medicine and Rehabilitation

A strong, comprehensive rehabilitation program can help patients regain lost skills, improve function, relearn tasks and maximize independence. Cleveland Clinic Department of Physical Medicine and Rehabilitation, part of the Rehabilitation Institute, offers patients several competitive edges – high quality physical, occupational and speech therapy programs, innovative treatments and interdisciplinary teamwork. Cleveland Clinic rehabilitation professionals work with patients who have suffered a variety of injuries or who have neuromuscular diseases or other conditions that greatly influence quality of life.

Cleveland Clinic rehabilitation therapists are trained in Neuro-Developmental Treatment (NDT), an advanced therapeutic approach designed for people with neurological challenges, such as stroke. Cleveland Clinic has more NDT-trained therapists than any other center in the region.

Rehabilitation physicians are highly regarded and provide medical directorship service to more than 55 acute inpatient rehabilitation beds throughout Greater Cleveland. Consulting services are provided to inpatient, outpatient and sub-acute settings. If the need arises, patients have quick access to any number of Cleveland Clinic medical specialists, an important benefit to patients with multiple or complex medical problems.

For more information about the Cleveland Clinic Department of Physical Medicine and Rehabilitation, to schedule a second opinion or to learn about assistance for out-of-town patients, call 800.890.2467 or visit www.clevelandclinic.org/rehabtopdocs.

Physical Medicine and Rehabilitation
9500 Euclid Avenue / AC311 | Cleveland OH 44195

Primary Conditions We Treat:
- Brain injury, brain tumors, stroke, and aneurysms
- Spinal cord injury
- Cancer
- Parkinson's Disease
- Post-Heart Transplant
- MS and Transverse Myelitis

We also offer:
- Return-to-Work Services
- Drivers Evaluation & Rehabilitation
- Orthotic and Prosthetic Services
- Golf Performance Assessment
- Low Vision Assistance
- Hand and Upper Extremity Rehabilitation
- Chronic Pain Rehabilitation
- Aquatic Rehabilitation
- Vestibular Rehabilitation
- Custom Orthotic and Prosthetic Fabrication

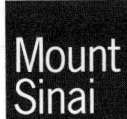
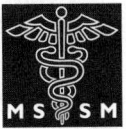

**MOUNT SINAI
SCHOOL OF
MEDICINE**

THE MOUNT SINAI MEDICAL CENTER
REHABILITATION MEDICINE
One Gustave L. Levy Place
Fifth Avenue and 100th Street
New York, NY 10029-6574
Physician Referral: 1-800-MD-SINAI (637-4624)
www.mountsinai.org

The Department of Rehabilitation Medicine at The Mount Sinai Medical Center is a Center of Excellence in the delivery of complete care for people with disabilities. A wide range of comprehensive patient care services is available for individuals with spinal cord injuries, brain injuries, and a variety of neuromuscular, musculoskeletal, and chronic conditions. We are accredited by CARF (Commission on Accreditation of Rehabilitation Facilities) for our inpatient spinal cord and brain injury programs—the only such accredited programs at non-VA hospitals in New York City—as well as for our comprehensive rehabilitation medicine program.

Our Team-Oriented Approach is pivotal to successful rehabilitation. The interdisciplinary team approach at Mount Sinai takes advantage of each discipline's expertise to provide the highest quality coordinated care. Our experienced professionals evaluate each patient and meet regularly to develop and implement individualized treatment plans in partnership with patients and their families. Our goal is to make each individual with a disability maximally self-sufficient and mobile, and able to return to community life.

The Mount Sinai Rehabilitation Center team is led by Kristjan T. Ragnarsson, MD, whose leadership and innovative approach to patient care has had a major impact in the field of rehabilitation medicine. The Center includes physicians, primary rehabilitation nurses, nurse practitioners, and professional staff in physical therapy, occupational therapy, speech therapy, nutrition, social work, psychology, therapeutic recreation, and vocational counseling. Special rehabilitation medicine programs include the following:

• **The Spinal Cord Injury Rehabilitation Program** provides comprehensive care to individuals with spinal cord injuries. This includes a full range of innovative medical and rehabilitation services. For example, our "Do It" program is a unique outpatient program that facilitates community integration.

• **The Brain Injury Rehabilitation Program** provides comprehensive care to individuals with brain injuries. It is well recognized that the treatment of individuals with cognitive and behavioral challenges is critical to community integration. Our Program contains specialists uniquely qualified to meet these challenges.

• **The Sports Therapy Center** is a comprehensive outpatient physical and occupational therapy facility offering individualized treatments for people with a variety of musculoskeletal conditions. It is conveniently located in midtown Manhattan.

MODEL SYSTEMS OF CARE

• Consistently ranked among the top rehabilitation centers by *U.S. News & World Report*

• One of fourteen programs designated by the National Institute of Disability and Rehabilitation Research (NIDRR) as a Model System of Care for Spinal Cord Injury, the only such designated program in New York State

• One of fourteen programs designated by NIDRR as a Model System of Care for Traumatic Brain Injury, the only such designated program in New York State

• The only NIDRR-designated Research and Training Center for Traumatic Brain Injury Intervention

NYU Langone Medical Center

550 First Avenue (at 31St Street)
New York, NY 10016
Physician Referral:
(888)7-NYU-MED (888-769-8633)
www.nyumc.org

PHYSICAL MEDICINE AND REHABILITATION

Founded by Dr. Howard A. Rusk in 1948, the Rusk institute of Rehabilitation Medicine is the world's first and one of the largest university centers for the treatment of adults and children with disabilities. Every year since 1989 when US. News & World Report initiated its hospital rankings, the Rusk Institute has ranked the number one rehabilitation center in New York and one of the top ten in the nation. It treats adults and children with neurologic, orthopaedic, and a wide variety of physical disabilities on both an inpatient and outpatient basis.

These include:
Aphasia
Amputation
Arthritis
Back Pain
Brain Injury
Brain Tumor Related Disabilities
Cardiac Dysfunction
Cerebral Palsy
Hand Disabilities
Hip and Lower Extremity Fractures
Joint Replacements
Lymphedema
Multiple Sclerosis
Neurological Disorders
Neuromuscular Diseases
Orthopaedic Surgery
Osteoporosis
Pain (acute and chronic)

Parkinson's Disease
Pediatric Rehabilitation
Pulmonary Diseases
     (Asthma, Bronchitis, Emphysema)
Rhizotomy
Scoliosis
Spasticity
Spina Bifida
Spinal Cord Injury
Sports Injuries
Stroke
Swallowing Disorders
Traumatic Injuries
Urinary Incontinence
Vestibular (balance) Disorders

The Hospital for Joint Diseases Rehabilitation Services Programs provide comprehensive inpatient (72 beds) rehabilitation care for ortho-rehab and neuro-rehab patients. Both programs are CARF (Commission on the Accreditation of Rehabilitation Facilities) accredited. There are five outpatient centers to serve patients as well:

Plastic Surgery

A plastic surgeon deals with the repair, reconstruction or replacement of physical defects of form or function involving the skin, musculoskeletal system, craniomaxillofacial structures, hand, extremities, breast and trunk and external genitalia. He/she uses aesthetic surgical principles not only to improve undesirable qualities of normal structures (commonly called "cosmetic surgery") but in all reconstructive procedures as well.

A plastic surgeon possesses special knowledge and skill in the design and surgery of grafts, flaps, free tissue transfer and replantation. Competence in the management of complex wounds, the use of implantable materials, and in tumor surgery is required.

Training Required: Five to seven years

Certification in one of the following subspecialties requires additional training and examination.

Plastic Surgery within the Head and Neck: A plastic surgeon with additional training in plastic and reconstructive procedures within the head, face, neck and associated structures, including cutaneous head and neck oncology and reconstruction, management of maxillofacial trauma, soft tissue repair and neural surgery.

The field is diverse and involves a wide age range of patients, from the newborn to the aged. While both cosmetic and reconstructive surgery are practiced, there are many additional procedures which interface with them.

Surgery of the Hand (see Hand Surgery)

PLASTIC SURGERY

New England

Collins, Dale MD [PlS] - **Spec Exp:** Breast Cancer; Breast Reconstruction; **Hospital:** Dartmouth - Hitchcock Med Ctr; **Address:** Div Plastic Surgery, 1 Medical Center Drive, Lebanon, NH 03756; **Phone:** 603-653-3500; **Board Cert:** Plastic Surgery 2007; **Med School:** Emory Univ 1989; **Resid:** Plastic Surgery, Washington Univ Med Ctr 1994; **Fellow:** Microsurgery, Washington Univ Med Ctr 1995; **Fac Appt:** Assoc Prof PlS, Dartmouth Med Sch

Constantian, Mark B MD [PlS] - **Spec Exp:** Rhinoplasty; Rhinoplasty Revision; Nasal Reconstruction; **Hospital:** St Joseph Hosp, Southern NH Med Ctr; **Address:** 19 Tyler St, Ste 302, Nashua, NH 03060-2951; **Phone:** 603-880-7700; **Board Cert:** Plastic Surgery 1979; **Med School:** Univ VA Sch Med 1972; **Resid:** Surgery, Boston Univ Med Ctr 1976; **Fellow:** Plastic Reconstructive Surgery, Medical Coll VA 1978

Eriksson, Elof MD/PhD [PlS] - **Spec Exp:** Abdominoplasty; Cosmetic Surgery-Breast; Skin Laser Surgery; **Hospital:** Brigham & Women's Hosp; **Address:** Brigham & Women's Hosp, Div Plas Surg, 75 Francis St, Boston, MA 02115; **Phone:** 617-732-5093; **Board Cert:** Plastic Surgery 1980; **Med School:** Sweden 1969; **Resid:** Surgery, Chicago Affil Hosps 1977; **Fellow:** Plastic Surgery, Med Coll Va 1979; **Fac Appt:** Prof PlS, Harvard Med Sch

Feldman, Joel MD [PlS] - **Spec Exp:** Cosmetic Surgery-Face; Burns-Reconstructive Plastic Surgery; **Hospital:** Mount Auburn Hosp, Mass Genl Hosp; **Address:** 300 Mt Auburn St, Ste 304, Cambridge, MA 02138; **Phone:** 617-661-5998; **Board Cert:** Surgery 1975; Plastic Surgery 1977; **Med School:** Harvard Med Sch 1969; **Resid:** Surgery, Mass Genl Hosp 1974; Plastic Surgery, Johns Hopkins Hosp 1976; **Fac Appt:** Assoc Clin Prof PlS, Harvard Med Sch

Gallico, G Gregory MD [PlS] - **Spec Exp:** Liposuction & Body Contouring; **Hospital:** Mass Genl Hosp; **Address:** 170 Commonwealth Ave, Boston, MA 02116; **Phone:** 617-267-5553; **Board Cert:** Plastic Surgery 1982; **Med School:** Harvard Med Sch 1973; **Resid:** Surgery, Mass Genl Hosp 1980; Plastic Surgery, Mass Genl Hosp 1981; **Fellow:** Immunology, Oxford Univ Med Sch 1977; **Fac Appt:** Assoc Clin Prof S, Harvard Med Sch

May Jr, James W MD [PlS] - **Spec Exp:** Cosmetic Surgery; Breast Reconstruction; Hand Surgery; **Hospital:** Mass Genl Hosp; **Address:** Mass Genl Hosp, 15 Parkman St, WACC 435, Boston, MA 02114; **Phone:** 617-726-8220; **Board Cert:** Surgery 1975; Plastic Surgery 1977; **Med School:** Northwestern Univ 1969; **Resid:** Plastic Surgery, Mass Genl Hosp 1975; **Fellow:** Hand Surgery, Univ Louisville 1975; **Fac Appt:** Prof S, Harvard Med Sch

Meara, John MD/DMD [PlS] - **Spec Exp:** Cleft Palate/Lip; Craniofacial Surgery-Pediatric; **Hospital:** Children's Hospital - Boston; **Address:** Department of Plastic Surgery, 300 Longwood Ave, Hunnewell 158, Boston, MA 02115; **Phone:** 617-355-4401; **Board Cert:** Plastic Surgery 2001; Otolaryngology 1998; **Med School:** Univ Mich Med Sch 1990; **Resid:** Plastic Surgery, Brigham & Womens & The Chldns Hosps 1999; Otolaryngology, Mass Eye & Ear Infirmary 1997; **Fellow:** Craniofacial Surgery, Royal Chldns Hosp 2000; **Fac Appt:** Assoc Prof PlS, Harvard Med Sch

Mulliken, John B MD [PlS] - **Spec Exp:** Pediatric Plastic Surgery; Cleft Palate/Lip; Vascular Malformations; **Hospital:** Children's Hospital - Boston; **Address:** Chldns Hosp, Div Plas Surg, 300 Longwood Ave, Hunnewell-1, Boston, MA 02115-5724; **Phone:** 617-355-7686; **Board Cert:** Surgery 1972; Plastic Surgery 1975; **Med School:** Columbia P&S 1964; **Resid:** Surgery, Mass Genl Hosp 1970; Plastic Surgery, Johns Hopkins Hosp 1974; **Fac Appt:** Prof S, Harvard Med Sch

Orgill, Dennis MD [PlS] - **Spec Exp:** Wound Healing/Care; Burns-Reconstructive Plastic Surgery; **Hospital:** Brigham & Women's Hosp; **Address:** Brigham & Women's Hosp, Dept Plas Surg, 75 Francis St, Boston, MA 02115; **Phone:** 617-732-5456; **Board Cert:** Surgery 2000; Plastic Surgery 1994; **Med School:** Harvard Med Sch 1985; **Resid:** Surgery, Brigham & Women's Hosp 1990; **Fellow:** Plastic Surgery, Brigham & Women's Hosp 1992; **Fac Appt:** Assoc Prof S, Harvard Med Sch

Persing, John A MD [PlS] - **Spec Exp:** Craniofacial Surgery; Vascular Malformations; Cosmetic Surgery; Cosmetic Surgery; **Hospital:** Yale-New Haven Hosp; **Address:** Yale Plastic Surgery, 330 Cedar St Boardroom Bldg Fl 3, New Haven, CT 06519-3218; **Phone:** 203-785-2570; **Board Cert:** Plastic Surgery 1985; Neurological Surgery 1986; **Med School:** Univ VT Coll Med 1974; **Resid:** Surgery, Univ Arizona Med Ctr 1976; Neurological Surgery, Univ Virginia Med Ctr 1982; **Fellow:** Plastic Surgery, Univ Virginia Med Ctr 1984; **Fac Appt:** Prof PlS, Yale Univ

Stadelmann, Wayne K MD [PlS] - **Spec Exp:** Melanoma-Head & Neck; Breast Reconstruction; Breast Augmentation; **Hospital:** Concord Hospital, Elliot Hosp; **Address:** 248 Pleasant St, Ste 201, Concord, NH 03301; **Phone:** 603-224-5200; **Board Cert:** Plastic Surgery 1999; **Med School:** Univ Chicago-Pritzker Sch Med 1990; **Resid:** Surgery, Univ Chicago Hosps 1994; Plastic Surgery, Univ S Florida/H Lee Moffit Cancer Ctr 1997

Stahl, Richard S MD [PlS] - **Spec Exp:** Breast Cosmetic & Reconstructive Surgery; Chest Wall Reconstruction; Abdominal Wall Reconstruction; **Hospital:** Yale-New Haven Hosp, Hosp of St Raphael; **Address:** 5 Durham Rd, Guilford, CT 06437; **Phone:** 203-458-4440; **Board Cert:** Surgery 2001; Plastic Surgery 1984; **Med School:** Vanderbilt Univ 1976; **Resid:** Surgery, Yale New Haven Hosp 1981; **Fellow:** Plastic Surgery, Emory Univ Med Ctr 1983; **Fac Appt:** Clin Prof S, Yale Univ

Sullivan, Patrick K MD [PlS] - **Spec Exp:** Cosmetic Surgery-Face; Cosmetic Surgery-Breast; Rhinoplasty; **Hospital:** Rhode Island Hosp; **Address:** 235 Plain St, Ste 502, Providence, RI 02905; **Phone:** 401-831-8300; **Board Cert:** Otolaryngology 1985; Plastic Surgery 1989; **Med School:** Mayo Med Sch 1979; **Resid:** Otolaryngology, Univ Colo Hlth Scis Ctr 1984; Plastic Surgery, Rhode Island Hosp 1986; **Fellow:** Craniofacial Surgery, Dr Paul Tessier & Dr Hugo Obwegeser 1987; **Fac Appt:** Assoc Prof PlS, Brown Univ

Mid Atlantic

Aston, Sherrell MD [PlS] - **Spec Exp:** Cosmetic Surgery-Face; Rhinoplasty; Cosmetic Surgery-Breast; Liposuction & Body Contouring; **Hospital:** Manhattan Eye, Ear & Throat Hosp, NYU Med Ctr (page 68); **Address:** 728 Park Ave, New York, NY 10021; **Phone:** 212-249-6000; **Board Cert:** Surgery 1974; Plastic Surgery 1978; **Med School:** Univ VA Sch Med 1968; **Resid:** Surgery, UCLA Med Ctr 1973; Plastic Surgery, New York Univ 1975; **Fellow:** Surgery, Johns Hopkins Hosp 1970; **Fac Appt:** Prof PlS, NYU Sch Med

Attinger, Christopher E MD [PlS] - **Spec Exp:** Limb Surgery/Reconstruction; Diabetic Leg/Foot; Wound Healing/Care; Lower Limb Reconstruction; **Hospital:** Georgetown Univ Hosp; **Address:** Georgetown Univ Hosp-Wound Healing Ctr, 3800 Resorvoir Rd NW 1 Bles Bldg, Washington, DC 20007; **Phone:** 202-444-5462; **Board Cert:** Plastic Surgery 1992; **Med School:** Yale Univ 1981; **Resid:** Surgery, Brigham & Women's Hosp 1986; Plastic Surgery, NYU Med Ctr 1989; **Fellow:** Vascular Surgery, Brigham & Women's Hosp 1987; Hand Surgery, NYU Med Ctr 1990; **Fac Appt:** Prof PlS, Georgetown Univ

Plastic Surgery

Baker, Daniel MD [PlS] - **Spec Exp:** Cosmetic Surgery-Face; Reconstructive Surgery-Face; Rhinoplasty; **Hospital:** Manhattan Eye, Ear & Throat Hosp; **Address:** 65 E 66th St, New York, NY 10021; **Phone:** 212-734-9695; **Board Cert:** Plastic Surgery 1978; **Med School:** Columbia P&S 1968; **Resid:** Surgery, UCSF Med Ctr 1975; Plastic Surgery, NYU Med Ctr 1977; **Fellow:** Head and Neck Surgery, NYU Med Ctr/St Vincents Hosp 1978; **Fac Appt:** Assoc Prof PlS, NYU Sch Med

Bartlett, Scott P MD [PlS] - **Spec Exp:** Craniofacial Surgery/Reconstruction; Pediatric Plastic Surgery; Facial Plastic & Reconstructive Surgery; **Hospital:** Hosp Univ Penn - UPHS (page 60), Chldns Hosp of Philadelphia, The; **Address:** Hosp Univ Penn, 3400 Spruce St, Philadelphia, PA 19104-4227; **Phone:** 215-662-2096; **Board Cert:** Plastic Surgery 1987; **Med School:** Washington Univ, St Louis 1975; **Resid:** Surgery, Mass Genl Hosp 1983; Plastic Surgery, Mass Genl Hosp 1985; **Fellow:** Craniofacial Surgery, Hosp U Penn 1986; **Fac Appt:** Prof PlS, Univ Pennsylvania

Boyajian, Michael J MD [PlS] - **Spec Exp:** Pediatric Plastic Surgery; **Hospital:** Chldns Natl Med Ctr; **Address:** 111 Michigan Ave NW, Ste 4W-100, Washington, DC 20010-2978; **Phone:** 202-476-2150; **Board Cert:** Plastic Surgery 1984; **Med School:** NYU Sch Med 1976; **Resid:** Surgery, Univ Colo Med Ctr 1979; Surgery, Univ Cincinnati Hosp 1981; **Fellow:** Plastic Surgery, Brigham & Women's Hosp 1983; Craniofacial Surgery, Chldns Hosp 1983; **Fac Appt:** Asst Prof PlS, Geo Wash Univ

Bucky, Louis P MD [PlS] - **Spec Exp:** Cosmetic Surgery-Face; Botox Therapy; Cosmetic Surgery-Breast; Liposuction & Body Contouring; **Hospital:** Pennsylvania Hosp (page 60), Hosp Univ Penn - UPHS (page 60); **Address:** 230 W Washington Square, Ste 101, Philadelphia, PA 19106; **Phone:** 215-829-6320; **Board Cert:** Plastic Surgery 1997; **Med School:** Harvard Med Sch 1986; **Resid:** Surgery, Mass Genl Hosp 1992; Plastic Surgery, Mass Genl Hosp 1994; **Fellow:** Microsurgery, Meml Sloan Kettering Cancer Ctr 1995; Craniofacial Surgery, Miami Chldns Hosp 1996; **Fac Appt:** Assoc Prof S, Univ Pennsylvania

Chiu, David T.W. MD [PlS] - **Spec Exp:** Hand & Microvascular Surgery; Cosmetic Surgery-Face; Peripheral Nerve Surgery; **Hospital:** NYU Med Ctr (page 68), Lenox Hill Hosp (page 62); **Address:** 900 Park Ave, New York, NY 10021-0231; **Phone:** 212-879-8880; **Board Cert:** Plastic Surgery 1982; Hand Surgery 2000; **Med School:** Columbia P&S 1973; **Resid:** Surgery, Barnes Jewish Hosp 1977; Plastic Surgery, Columbia-Presby Med Ctr 1979; **Fellow:** Hand Surgery, NYU Med Ctr 1980; **Fac Appt:** Prof S, NYU Sch Med

Cordeiro, Peter G MD [PlS] - **Spec Exp:** Reconstructive Surgery; Breast Reconstruction; Facial Plastic & Reconstructive Surgery; **Hospital:** Meml Sloan-Kettering Cancer Ctr, Manhattan Eye, Ear & Throat Hosp; **Address:** 1275 York Avenue, New York, NY 10065; **Phone:** 800-525-2225; **Board Cert:** Surgery 1998; Plastic Surgery 1994; **Med School:** Harvard Med Sch 1983; **Resid:** Surgery, New Eng Deaconess Hosp-Harvard 1989; Plastic Surgery, NYU Med Ctr 1991; **Fellow:** Microsurgery, Meml Sloan-Kettering Cancer Ctr. 1992; Craniofacial Surgery, Univ Miami 1992; **Fac Appt:** Prof S, Cornell Univ-Weill Med Coll

Cutting, Court MD [PlS] - **Spec Exp:** Cleft Palate/Lip; Reconstructive Plastic Surgery; Rhinoplasty; Craniofacial Surgery/Reconstruction; **Hospital:** NYU Med Ctr (page 68); **Address:** 333 E 34th St, Ste 1K, New York, NY 10016-6481; **Phone:** 212-447-6229; **Board Cert:** Otolaryngology 1980; Plastic Surgery 1986; **Med School:** Univ Chicago-Pritzker Sch Med 1975; **Resid:** Otolaryngology, Univ Iowa Hosps 1980; Plastic Surgery, NYU Med Ctr 1983; **Fellow:** Craniofacial Surgery, NYU Med Ctr 1984; **Fac Appt:** Prof PlS, NYU Sch Med

Dagum, Alexander B MD [PlS] - **Spec Exp:** Reconstructive Plastic Surgery; Microvascular Surgery; Hand Surgery; **Hospital:** Stony Brook Univ Med Ctr; **Address:** SUNY Health Science Ctr, T19-060, Box 8191, Stony Brook, NY 11794-8191; **Phone:** 631-444-8210; **Board Cert:** Plastic Surgery 2003; Hand Surgery 2004; **Med School:** Canada 1987; **Resid:** Surgery, Univ Ottawa Civic Hosp 1988; Plastic Surgery, Univ Toronto Med Ctr 1993; **Fellow:** Microsurgery, Univ Toronto Med Ctr 1984; Hand Surgery, Stony Brook Univ Hosp 1995; **Fac Appt:** Assoc Prof S, SUNY Stony Brook

Deleyiannis, Frederic W B MD [PlS] - **Spec Exp:** Head & Neck Reconstruction; Maxillofacial Surgery; Craniofacial Surgery; Pediatric Plastic Surgery; **Hospital:** UPMC Presby, Pittsburgh, Chldns Hosp of Pittsburgh - UPMC; **Address:** Falk Medical Bldg, 3601 Fifth Ave, Ste 6B, Pittsburgh, PA 15213; **Phone:** 412-648-9670; **Board Cert:** Otolaryngology 2000; Plastic Surgery 2003; **Med School:** Yale Univ 1992; **Resid:** Otolaryngology, Univ Washington Med Ctr 1999; Plastic Surgery, Univ Pittsburgh Med Ctr 2003; **Fellow:** Head and Neck Surgery, Univ Oviedo Med Ctr 2000; Reconstructive Microsurgery, Univ Pittsburgh Med Ctr 2000; **Fac Appt:** Asst Prof PlS, Univ Pittsburgh

Dufresne, Craig R MD [PlS] - **Spec Exp:** Craniofacial Surgery; Cosmetic Surgery; **Hospital:** Inova Fairfax Hosp; **Address:** 5530 Wisconsin Ave, Ste 1235, Chevy Chase, MD 20815; **Phone:** 301-654-9151; **Board Cert:** Plastic Surgery 1986; **Med School:** Columbia P&S 1977; **Resid:** Surgery, Johns Hopkins Hosp 1982; Plastic Surgery, NYU Med Ctr 1984; **Fellow:** Craniofacial Surgery, NYU Med Ctr 1985; **Fac Appt:** Clin Prof PlS, Georgetown Univ

Glat, Paul M MD [PlS] - **Spec Exp:** Pediatric & Adult Plastic Surgery; Burns-Reconstructive Plastic Surgery; Craniofacial Surgery; Cleft Palate/Lip; **Hospital:** St Christopher's Hosp for Chldn, Bryn Mawr Hosp; **Address:** St Christopher's Hosp for Children, Eire Ave at Font St, Ste 2204, Philadelphia, PA 19134; **Phone:** 215-427-5191; **Board Cert:** Surgery 1995; Plastic Surgery 1999; **Med School:** NYU Sch Med 1988; **Resid:** Surgery, NYU Med Ctr 1994; Plastic Surgery, NYU Med Ctr 1996; **Fellow:** Craniofacial Surgery, Univ Penn 1997; **Fac Appt:** Assoc Prof PlS, Drexel Univ Coll Med

Gold, Alan MD [PlS] - **Spec Exp:** Cosmetic Surgery; Cosmetic Surgery-Face & Eyes; Nasal Surgery; **Hospital:** N Shore Univ Hosp, Glen Cove Hosp; **Address:** 833 Northern Blvd, Ste 240, Great Neck, NY 11021-5308; **Phone:** 516-498-2800; **Board Cert:** Plastic Surgery 1979; **Med School:** SUNY Downstate 1971; **Resid:** Surgery, N Shore Univ Hosp 1975; Plastic Surgery, Kings County-Suny Med Ctr 1978; **Fellow:** Hand Surgery, Nassau County Med Ctr 1976; **Fac Appt:** Assoc Clin Prof S, Cornell Univ-Weill Med Coll

Hidalgo, David MD [PlS] - **Spec Exp:** Cosmetic Surgery-Face; Cosmetic Surgery-Breast; Rhinoplasty; Reconstructive Surgery; **Hospital:** Manhattan Eye, Ear & Throat Hosp, NY-Presby Hosp/Weill Cornell (page 66); **Address:** 655 Park Ave Fl 1, New York, NY 10021-5937; **Phone:** 212-517-9777; **Board Cert:** Plastic Surgery 1987; **Med School:** Georgetown Univ 1978; **Resid:** Surgery, NYU Med Ctr 1983; Plastic Surgery, NYU Med Ctr 1985; **Fellow:** Microsurgery, NYU Med Ctr 1986; **Fac Appt:** Clin Prof S, Cornell Univ-Weill Med Coll

Hoffman, Lloyd MD [PlS] - **Spec Exp:** Cosmetic Surgery-Face; Liposuction; Breast Reconstruction; **Hospital:** NY-Presby Hosp/Columbia (page 66), Lenox Hill Hosp (page 62); **Address:** 12A E 68th St, New York, NY 10021; **Phone:** 212-861-1640; **Board Cert:** Plastic Surgery 1989; **Med School:** Northwestern Univ 1978; **Resid:** Surgery, New York Hosp 1983; Plastic Surgery, NYU Med Ctr 1986; **Fellow:** Hand Surgery, NYU Med Ctr 1987; **Fac Appt:** Assoc Prof PlS, Cornell Univ-Weill Med Coll

Plastic Surgery

Hurwitz, Dennis J MD [PlS] - **Spec Exp:** Body Contouring; Cosmetic Surgery-Face; Rhinoplasty; **Hospital:** Magee-Womens Hosp - UPMC, Chldns Hosp of Pittsburgh - UPMC; **Address:** 3109 Forbes Ave, Ste 500, Pittsburgh, PA 15213; **Phone:** 412-802-6100; **Board Cert:** Plastic Surgery 2005; **Med School:** Univ MD Sch Med 1970; **Resid:** Surgery, Dartmouth Med Ctr 1975; Plastic Surgery, Univ Pittsburgh Med Ctr 1977; **Fac Appt:** Prof S, Univ Pittsburgh

Imber, Gerald MD [PlS] - **Spec Exp:** Cosmetic Surgery-Face; Eyelid Surgery; **Hospital:** NY-Presby Hosp/Weill Cornell (page 66); **Address:** 1009 5th Ave, Lower Level, New York, NY 10028; **Phone:** 212-472-1800; **Board Cert:** Plastic Surgery 1976; **Med School:** SUNY Downstate 1966; **Resid:** Surgery, LI Jewish Med Ctr 1972; Plastic Surgery, NY Hosp 1974; **Fac Appt:** Asst Clin Prof S, Cornell Univ-Weill Med Coll

Leipziger, Lyle S MD [PlS] - **Spec Exp:** Cosmetic Surgery-Face & Eyes; Cosmetic Surgery-Breast; Breast Reconstruction; Liposuction & Body Contouring; **Hospital:** N Shore Univ Hosp, Long Island Jewish Med Ctr; **Address:** 825 Northern Blvd Fl 3, Great Neck, NY 11021; **Phone:** 516-465-8787; **Board Cert:** Plastic Surgery 1994; **Med School:** Cornell Univ-Weill Med Coll 1985; **Resid:** Plastic Surgery, New York Hosp 1990; **Fellow:** Craniofacial Surgery, Johns Hopkins Hosp 1991; **Fac Appt:** Asst Prof S, Albert Einstein Coll Med

Little, John W MD [PlS] - **Spec Exp:** Cosmetic Surgery-Face; **Hospital:** Georgetown Univ Hosp; **Address:** 1145 19th St NW, Ste 802, Washington, DC 20036; **Phone:** 202-467-6700; **Board Cert:** Surgery 1975; Plastic Surgery 1977; **Med School:** Harvard Med Sch 1969; **Resid:** Surgery, Case Western Reserve Affil Hosps 1974; Plastic Surgery, Case Western Reserve Affil Hosps 1975; **Fellow:** Plastic Surgery, Jackson Meml Hosp 1977; **Fac Appt:** Clin Prof PlS, Georgetown Univ

Loree, Thom R MD [PlS] - **Spec Exp:** Head & Neck Cancer; Thyroid Cancer; Reconstructive Surgery; **Hospital:** Roswell Park Cancer Inst, Millard Fillmore Gates Cir Hosp; **Address:** Roswell Park Cancer Inst, Dept Head & Neck Surgery, Elm & Carlton Sts, Buffalo, NY 14263; **Phone:** 716-845-3158; **Board Cert:** Surgery 1997; Plastic Surgery 2004; **Med School:** Geo Wash Univ 1982; **Resid:** Surgery, St Lukes-Roosevelt Hosp 1987; Plastic Surgery, St Lukes-Roosevelt Hosp 1989; **Fellow:** Head & Neck Surgical Oncology, Meml Sloan-Kettering Cancer Ctr 1990; **Fac Appt:** Assoc Prof S, SUNY Buffalo

Low, David W MD [PlS] - **Spec Exp:** Microsurgery; Cosmetic & Reconstructive Surgery; Vascular Malformations; Cleft Palate/Lip; **Hospital:** Hosp Univ Penn - UPHS (page 60), Chldns Hosp of Philadelphia, The; **Address:** Hosp Univ Penn - Div Plastic Surg, 3400 Spruce St, 10 Penn Tower, Philadelphia, PA 19104; **Phone:** 215-662-2040; **Board Cert:** Plastic Surgery 1991; **Med School:** Harvard Med Sch 1980; **Resid:** Surgery, Hosp U Penn 1986; **Fellow:** Plastic Reconstructive Surgery, Hosp U Penn 1989; **Fac Appt:** Assoc Prof S, Univ Pennsylvania

Mackay, Donald R MD/DDS [PlS] - **Spec Exp:** Craniofacial Surgery; Cleft Lip/Palate; Cosmetic Surgery-Face & Breast; Reconstructive Surgery; **Hospital:** Penn State Milton S Hershey Med Ctr; **Address:** MS Hershey Med Ctr Plastic Surgery, 500 University Drive, PO Box 850, Hershey, PA 17033; **Phone:** 717-531-8952; **Board Cert:** Plastic Surgery 2006; **Med School:** South Africa 1980; **Resid:** Plastic Surgery, Univ Teaching Hosps 1984; Plastic Surgery, MS Hershey Med Ctr 1995; **Fac Appt:** Prof PlS, Penn State Univ-Hershey Med Ctr

Manders, Ernest K MD [PlS] - **Spec Exp:** Facial Nerve Disorders; **Hospital:** UPMC Presby, Pittsburgh, Magee-Womens Hosp - UPMC; **Address:** 3550 Terrace St, Ste 668, Scaife Hall, Div Plastic Surgery, Pittsburgh, PA 15261; **Phone:** 412-648-9670; **Board Cert:** Surgery 1998; Plastic Surgery 1982; **Med School:** Harvard Med Sch 1972; **Resid:** Surgery, Univ Michigan Med Ctr 1979; Plastic Surgery, Univ Michigan Med Ctr 1981; **Fellow:** Viral Oncology, Natl Insts of Allergy-Infectious Disease 1975; **Fac Appt:** Prof S, Univ Pittsburgh

Manson, Paul MD [PlS] - **Spec Exp:** Cosmetic Surgery; Facial Trauma/Fractures; Skin Cancer; **Hospital:** Johns Hopkins Hosp - Baltimore (page 61), Univ of MD Med Sys; **Address:** 601 N Caroline St, McElderry-8152F, Baltimore, MD 21287; **Phone:** 410-955-9470; **Board Cert:** Plastic Surgery 1979; **Med School:** Northwestern Univ 1968; **Resid:** Surgery, New Eng Deaconess Hosp 1971; Plastic Surgery, Johns Hopkins Hosp 1978; **Fellow:** Surgery, Lahey Clinic 1974; **Fac Appt:** Prof PlS, Johns Hopkins Univ

Matarasso, Alan MD [PlS] - **Spec Exp:** Cosmetic Surgery-Face & Eyes; Rhinoplasty; Liposuction; Abdominoplasty; **Hospital:** Manhattan Eye, Ear & Throat Hosp, New York Eye & Ear Infirm (page 65); **Address:** 1009 Park Ave, New York, NY 10028-0936; **Phone:** 212-249-7500; **Board Cert:** Plastic Surgery 1986; **Med School:** Univ Miami Sch Med 1979; **Resid:** Surgery, Montefiore Med Ctr 1983; Plastic Surgery, Montefiore Med Ctr 1985; **Fellow:** Plastic Surgery, Manhattan EET Hosp/NYU 1985; **Fac Appt:** Clin Prof PlS, Albert Einstein Coll Med

McCarthy, Joseph G MD [PlS] - **Spec Exp:** Craniofacial Surgery-Pediatric; Reconstructive Surgery-Face; Cosmetic Surgery-Face; **Hospital:** NYU Med Ctr (page 68), Manhattan Eye, Ear & Throat Hosp; **Address:** 722 Park Ave, New York, NY 10021-4954; **Phone:** 212-628-4420; **Board Cert:** Surgery 1972; Plastic Surgery 1974; **Med School:** Columbia P&S 1964; **Resid:** Surgery, Columbia-Presby Med Ctr 1971; Plastic Surgery, NYU Med Ctr 1973; **Fac Appt:** Prof S, NYU Sch Med

Napoli, Joseph A MD/DDS [PlS] - **Spec Exp:** Cleft Palate/Lip; Maxillofacial Surgery; Craniofacial Surgery-Pediatric; **Hospital:** Alfred I duPont Hosp for Children; **Address:** Al duPont Hosp for Children, 1600 Rockland Rd, Wilmington, DE 19803; **Phone:** 302-651-4200; **Board Cert:** Plastic Surgery 2004; **Med School:** Columbia P&S 1987; **Resid:** Oral & Maxillofacial Surgery, Columbia-Presby Med Ctr 1985; Plastic Reconstructive Surgery, Dartmouth-Hitchcock Med Ctr 2001; **Fellow:** Craniofacial Surgery, Royal Chldns Hosp 2002; Pediatric Plastic Surgery, Royal Chldns Hosp 2002

Noone, R Barrett MD [PlS] - **Spec Exp:** Breast Reconstruction; Cosmetic Surgery; **Hospital:** Bryn Mawr Hosp, Lankenau Hosp; **Address:** 888 Glenbrook Ave, Bryn Mawr, PA 19010-2506; **Phone:** 610-527-4833; **Board Cert:** Surgery 1972; Plastic Surgery 1974; **Med School:** Univ Pennsylvania 1965; **Resid:** Surgery, Hosp Univ Penn 1971; Plastic Surgery, Hosp Univ Penn 1973; **Fac Appt:** Clin Prof S, Univ Pennsylvania

Pitman, Gerald H MD [PlS] - **Spec Exp:** Cosmetic Surgery-Face; Liposuction; Abdominoplasty; **Hospital:** Manhattan Eye, Ear & Throat Hosp, NYU Med Ctr (page 68); **Address:** 170 E 73rd St, New York, NY 10021-4352; **Phone:** 212-517-2600; **Board Cert:** Plastic Surgery 1978; **Med School:** Univ Pennsylvania 1968; **Resid:** Surgery, Columbia-Presby Hosp 1975; Plastic Surgery, NYU Med Ctr 1977; **Fellow:** Microsurgery, NYU Med Ctr 1981; **Fac Appt:** Clin Prof PlS, NYU Sch Med

Posnick, Jeffrey C MD/DMD [PlS] - **Spec Exp:** Cosmetic Surgery-Face; Craniofacial Surgery/Reconstruction; Maxillofacial Surgery; **Hospital:** Georgetown Univ Hosp; **Address:** 5530 Wisconsin Ave, Ste 1250, Chevy Chase, MD 20815; **Phone:** 301-986-9475; **Board Cert:** Plastic Surgery 1988; **Med School:** Vanderbilt Univ 1979; **Resid:** Surgery, Mass Genl Hosp 1983; Plastic Surgery, Eastern Virginia Med Sch 1986; **Fellow:** Craniofacial Surgery, Hosp Univ Penn/Chldns Hosp 1983; **Fac Appt:** Clin Prof PlS, Georgetown Univ

Ramirez, Oscar M MD [PlS] - **Spec Exp:** Cosmetic Surgery-Face; Facial Implants (Endoscopic); Breast Reduction; **Hospital:** Greater Baltimore Med Ctr; **Address:** 2219 York Rd, Ste 100, Timonium, MD 21093; **Phone:** 410-560-7090; **Board Cert:** Plastic Surgery 1985; **Med School:** Peru 1976; **Resid:** Surgery, Franklin Sq Hosp 1982; Plastic Surgery, Univ Pittsburgh Affil Hosps 1984; **Fellow:** Craniofacial Surgery, Manuel Gea Gonzalez Hosp 1984; **Fac Appt:** Asst Clin Prof S, Johns Hopkins Univ

Plastic Surgery

Serletti, Joseph M MD [PlS] - **Spec Exp:** Breast Reconstruction; Reconstructive Surgery; Cosmetic Surgery; **Hospital:** Hosp Univ Penn - UPHS (page 60); **Address:** Hosp Univ Penn, 3400 Spruce St, 10 Penn Tower, Philadelphia, PA 19104; **Phone:** 215-662-3743; **Board Cert:** Plastic Surgery 2003; **Med School:** Univ Rochester 1982; **Resid:** Surgery, U Rochester Med Ctr 1986; Plastic Surgery, U Rochester Med Ctr 1988; **Fellow:** Reconstructive Surgery, Johns Hopkins Hosp 1990; **Fac Appt:** Prof PlS, Univ Pennsylvania

Seyfer, Alan MD [PlS] - **Spec Exp:** Chest Wall Reconstruction; Cleft Palate/Lip; Hand Surgery; **Hospital:** W Reed Army Med Ctr; **Address:** USUHS-School of Medicine, 4301 Jones Bridge Rd, Bethesda, MD 20814; **Phone:** 301-295-0441; **Board Cert:** Hand Surgery 1999; Plastic Surgery 1982; **Med School:** Louisiana State U, New Orleans 1973; **Resid:** Surgery, Fitzsimons AMC 1978; Plastic Surgery, Walter Reed AMC 1981; **Fellow:** Hand Surgery, Duke Univ Med Ctr 1980; **Fac Appt:** Prof S, Uniformed Srvs Univ, Bethesda

Siebert, John W MD [PlS] - **Spec Exp:** Facial Plastic & Reconstructive Surgery; Microsurgery; Cosmetic Surgery-Face; **Hospital:** NYU Med Ctr (page 68), Manhattan Eye, Ear & Throat Hosp; **Address:** 50 E 71 St, New York, NY 10021; **Phone:** 212-737-8300; **Board Cert:** Plastic Surgery 1991; **Med School:** Univ Wisc 1981; **Resid:** Surgery, Mass Genl Hosp 1986; Plastic Surgery, NYU Med Ctr 1988; **Fellow:** Microsurgery, NYU Med Ctr 1989; **Fac Appt:** Assoc Prof S, NYU Sch Med

Slezak, Sheri MD [PlS] - **Spec Exp:** Breast Reconstruction; **Hospital:** Univ of MD Med Sys; **Address:** Univ Maryland, Dept Plastic Surgery, 22 S Greene St, rm S8D12, Baltimore, MD 21201; **Phone:** 410-328-2360; **Board Cert:** Plastic Surgery 1991; **Med School:** Harvard Med Sch 1980; **Resid:** Surgery, Columbia-Presby Med Ctr 1985; Plastic Surgery, Johns Hopkins Hosp 1989; **Fac Appt:** Assoc Prof PlS, Univ MD Sch Med

Spence, Robert J MD [PlS] - **Spec Exp:** Burns-Reconstructive Plastic Surgery; Scleroderma; Tissue Banking; **Hospital:** Good Samaritan Hosp; **Address:** 5601 Loch Raven Blvd, Baltimore, MD 21239; **Phone:** 443-444-2876; **Board Cert:** Plastic Surgery 1981; **Med School:** Johns Hopkins Univ 1972; **Resid:** Surgery, Johns Hopkins Hops 1974; Surgery, Hershey Med Ctr 1978; **Fellow:** Plastic Surgery, Johns Hopkins Hosp 1980; **Fac Appt:** Assoc Prof S, Johns Hopkins Univ

Spinelli, Henry M MD [PlS] - **Spec Exp:** Cosmetic Surgery-Face; Craniofacial Surgery/Reconstruction; Oculoplastic & Orbital Surgery; **Hospital:** NY-Presby Hosp/Weill Cornell (page 66), Manhattan Eye, Ear & Throat Hosp; **Address:** 875 Fifth Ave, New York, NY 10021-4952; **Phone:** 212-570-6235; **Board Cert:** Ophthalmology 1987; Plastic Surgery 1993; **Med School:** NYU Sch Med 1981; **Resid:** Ophthalmology, Manhattan EET Hosp 1985; Plastic Reconstructive Surgery, NYU-Bellevue Hosp 1990; **Fellow:** Craniofacial Surgery, NYU Med Ctr 1991; **Fac Appt:** Clin Prof S, Cornell Univ-Weill Med Coll

Staffenberg, David A MD [PlS] - **Spec Exp:** Craniofacial Surgery/Reconstruction; Pediatric Plastic Surgery; Facial Plastic & Reconstructive Surgery; Cosmetic Surgery-Face; **Hospital:** Montefiore Med Ctr; **Address:** 1625 Poplar St, Bronx, NY 10467; **Phone:** 718-920-4462; **Board Cert:** Plastic Surgery 1999; **Med School:** NY Med Coll 1989; **Resid:** Surgery, Maimonides Med Ctr 1995; Plastic Surgery, Emory Univ Med Ctr 1997; **Fellow:** Craniofacial Surgery, UCLA Med Ctr 1998; **Fac Appt:** Assoc Prof PlS, Albert Einstein Coll Med

Sultan, Mark MD [PlS] - **Spec Exp:** Breast Reconstruction; Cosmetic Surgery-Breast; Cosmetic Surgery-Face; **Hospital:** St Luke's - Roosevelt Hosp Ctr - Roosevelt Div (page 57), Beth Israel Med Ctr - Petrie Division (page 57); **Address:** 1100 Park Ave, New York, NY 10128; **Phone:** 212-360-0700; **Board Cert:** Plastic Surgery 1992; **Med School:** Columbia P&S 1982; **Resid:** Surgery, Columbia-Presby Hosp 1987; Plastic Surgery, Columbia-Presby Hosp 1990; **Fellow:** Head and Neck Surgery, Emory Univ Hosp 1989; **Fac Appt:** Assoc Prof S, Columbia P&S

Tabbal, Nicolas MD [PlS] - **Spec Exp:** Rhinoplasty; Cosmetic Surgery-Face; Eyelid Surgery; **Hospital:** Manhattan Eye, Ear & Throat Hosp, NYU Med Ctr (page 68); **Address:** 521 Park Ave, New York, NY 10021-8140; **Phone:** 212-644-5800; **Board Cert:** Plastic Surgery 1980; **Med School:** Lebanon 1972; **Resid:** Surgery, Am Univ Med Ctr 1976; Plastic Surgery, Akron City Hosp 1979; **Fellow:** Surgery, Upstate Med Ctr 1977; Reconstructive Microsurgery, NYU Med Ctr 1980

Thorne, Charles MD [PlS] - **Spec Exp:** Cosmetic Surgery-Face & Breast; Ear Reconstruction/Microtia; Craniofacial Surgery; Pediatric Plastic Surgery; **Hospital:** NYU Med Ctr (page 68), Manhattan Eye, Ear & Throat Hosp; **Address:** 812 Park Ave, New York, NY 10021-2759; **Phone:** 212-794-0044; **Board Cert:** Plastic Surgery 1991; **Med School:** UCLA 1981; **Resid:** Surgery, Mass Genl Hosp 1986; Plastic Surgery, NYU Med Ctr 1988; **Fellow:** Craniofacial Surgery, NYU Med Ctr 1989; **Fac Appt:** Assoc Prof PlS, NYU Sch Med

Vander Kolk, Craig Alan MD [PlS] - **Spec Exp:** Cosmetic Surgery; Cleft Palate/Lip; Craniofacial Surgery/Reconstruction; **Hospital:** Johns Hopkins Hosp - Baltimore (page 61); **Address:** Johns Hopkins Outpatient Ctr, 601 N Caroline St Fl 8, Baltimore, MD 21287; **Phone:** 410-955-6897; **Board Cert:** Plastic Surgery 1989; **Med School:** Univ Mich Med Sch 1980; **Resid:** Surgery, Univ Mich Med Ctr 1983; Plastic Surgery, Univ Mich Med Ctr 1986; **Fellow:** Hand Surgery, St Vincents Hosp 1985; Craniofacial Surgery, Chldns Hosp 1987; **Fac Appt:** Assoc Prof PlS, Johns Hopkins Univ

Whitaker, Linton A MD [PlS] - **Spec Exp:** Cosmetic Surgery-Face; Craniofacial Surgery/Reconstruction; Facial Tumors; Eyelid Surgery; **Hospital:** Hosp Univ Penn - UPHS (page 60), Chldns Hosp of Philadelphia, The; **Address:** Hosp Univ Penn -10 Penn Tower, 3400 Spruce St, Philadelphia, PA 19104; **Phone:** 215-662-2048; **Board Cert:** Surgery 1970; Plastic Surgery 1978; **Med School:** Tulane Univ 1962; **Resid:** Surgery, Dartmouth Affl Hosp 1969; Plastic Surgery, Hosp Univ Penn 1971; **Fac Appt:** Prof PlS, Univ Pennsylvania

Zide, Barry M MD/DMD [PlS] - **Spec Exp:** Facial Surgery-Chin & Lip; Hemangiomas/Birthmarks; Facial Reconstruction-Cancer; Craniofacial Surgery-Pediatric; **Hospital:** NYU Med Ctr (page 68), Lenox Hill Hosp (page 62); **Address:** 420 E 55th St, Ste 1D, New York, NY 10022-5140; **Phone:** 212-421-2424; **Board Cert:** Plastic Surgery 1981; **Med School:** Tufts Univ 1973; **Resid:** Surgery, Stanford Med Ctr 1976; Plastic Surgery, U NC Hosp 1978; **Fellow:** Head and Neck Oncology, Roswell Park Cancer Inst 1979; Craniofacial Surgery, NYU Med Ctr 1980; **Fac Appt:** Prof PlS, NYU Sch Med

Southeast

Allen, Robert J MD [PlS] - **Spec Exp:** Breast Reconstruction; **Hospital:** Roper Hosp, New York Eye & Ear Infirm (page 65); **Address:** 125 Doughty St, Ste 590, Charleston, SC 29403; **Phone:** 888-890-3437; **Board Cert:** Plastic Surgery 1985; **Med School:** Med Univ SC 1976; **Resid:** Surgery, LSU Med Ctr 1982; Plastic Surgery, LSU Med Ctr 1981; **Fellow:** Microsurgery, NYU Med Ctr 1983; **Fac Appt:** Assoc Clin Prof PlS, Louisiana State U, New Orleans

Argenta, Louis C MD [PlS] - **Spec Exp:** Pediatric Plastic Surgery; Craniofacial Surgery; Wound Healing/Care; **Hospital:** Wake Forest Univ Baptist Med Ctr (page 73); **Address:** WFU Bapt Med Ctr, Dept Plastic Surg, Medical Center Blvd, Winston-Salem, NC 27157-1075; **Phone:** 336-716-4171; **Board Cert:** Plastic Surgery 1982; **Med School:** Univ Mich Med Sch 1969; **Resid:** Surgery, Univ Mich Hosp 1977; Plastic Surgery, Univ Mich Hosp 1979; **Fellow:** Craniofacial Surgery, Hosp Foch 1982; **Fac Appt:** Prof PlS, Wake Forest Univ

Plastic Surgery

Beasley, Michael MD [PlS] - **Spec Exp:** Breast Reconstruction & Augmentation; Liposuction; Body Contouring; **Hospital:** Presby Hosp - Charlotte; **Address:** 2215 Randolph Rd, Charlotte, NC 28207-1523; **Phone:** 704-372-6846; **Board Cert:** Plastic Surgery 1989; **Med School:** Univ NC Sch Med 1980; **Resid:** Surgery, NC Meml Hosp 1985; Plastic Surgery, Emory Univ Hosp 1987; **Fellow:** Plastic Surgery, St. Joseph Hospital 1987; **Fac Appt:** Assoc Clin Prof PlS, Univ NC Sch Med

Bermant, Michael A MD [PlS] - **Spec Exp:** Gynecomastia & Cosmetic Breast Surgery; Ear Reshaping (Otoplasty) & Rhinoplasty; Liposuction & Body Contouring; Abdominoplasty; **Hospital:** CJW Med Ctr; **Address:** 11601 Ironbridge Rd, Ste 201, Chester, VA 23831; **Phone:** 804-748-7737; **Board Cert:** Plastic Surgery 1991; **Med School:** Northwestern Univ 1978; **Resid:** Surgery, St Vincents Hosp 1982; Plastic Surgery, St Louis Univ Med Ctr 1984; **Fellow:** Microsurgery, NYU Med Ctr 1985

Carraway, James Howard MD [PlS] - **Spec Exp:** Oculoplastic Surgery; Cosmetic Surgery-Face; Eyelid Surgery; **Hospital:** Sentara Leigh Hosp; **Address:** 5589 Greenwich Rd, Ste 100, Virginia Beach, VA 23462; **Phone:** 757-557-0300; **Board Cert:** Surgery 1972; Plastic Surgery 1974; **Med School:** Univ VA Sch Med 1962; **Resid:** Surgery, Norfolk Med Ctr 1970; Plastic Surgery, Eastern VA Med Ctr 1973; **Fellow:** Plastic Surgery, Glasgow Royal Infirmary 1970; **Fac Appt:** Prof PlS, Eastern VA Med Sch

Cruse, C Wayne MD [PlS] - **Spec Exp:** Burns-Reconstructive Plastic Surgery; Cancer Reconstruction; **Hospital:** Tampa Genl Hosp, H Lee Moffitt Cancer Ctr & Research Inst; **Address:** 12902 Magnolia Dr, Ste 4035, Tampa, FL 33612; **Phone:** 813-972-8414; **Board Cert:** Plastic Surgery 1981; **Med School:** Univ Louisville Sch Med 1972; **Resid:** Surgery, Univ S Fla Hosp 1977; Plastic Surgery, Univ KY Hosp-Chandler Med Ctr 1979; **Fac Appt:** Prof S, Univ S Fla Coll Med

Fix, R Jobe MD [PlS] - **Spec Exp:** Breast Reconstruction; Hand Surgery; Microsurgery; **Hospital:** Univ of Ala Hosp at Birmingham, Children's Hospital - Birmingham; **Address:** Univ of Alabama Hosp, Div Plastic Surg, 510 S 20th St, FOT-Ste 1102, Birmingham, AL 35294; **Phone:** 205-934-3358; **Board Cert:** Surgery 1997; Hand Surgery 2001; Plastic Surgery 1991; **Med School:** Univ Nebr Coll Med 1982; **Resid:** Surgery, Valley Med Ctr 1987; Plastic Surgery, Univ Ala Hosp 1989; **Fac Appt:** Prof PlS, Univ Ala

Georgiade, Gregory MD [PlS] - **Spec Exp:** Breast Reconstruction; Cleft Palate/Lip; **Hospital:** Duke Univ Med Ctr; **Address:** Duke Univ Med Ctr, Box 3960, Durham, NC 27710; **Phone:** 919-684-3039; **Board Cert:** Plastic Surgery 1981; Surgery 2001; **Med School:** Duke Univ 1973; **Resid:** Surgery, Duke Univ Med Ctr 1978; Plastic Surgery, Duke Univ Med Ctr 1980; **Fac Appt:** Prof S, Duke Univ

Gregory, Richard O MD [PlS] - **Spec Exp:** Skin Laser Surgery; Cosmetic Surgery-Face; Facial Rejuvenation; **Hospital:** Florida Hosp Celebration Hlth, Florida Hosp - Orlando; **Address:** 400 Celebration Pl, Ste A320, Celebration, FL 34747; **Phone:** 407-303-4250; **Board Cert:** Plastic Surgery 1981; **Med School:** Indiana Univ 1971; **Resid:** Surgery, Duke Univ Med Ctr 1977; Plastic Surgery, Duke Univ Med Ctr 1979; **Fellow:** Hand Surgery, Univ Louisville Hlth Sci Ctr 1979; **Fac Appt:** Assoc Clin Prof PlS, Univ S Fla Coll Med

Grotting, James S MD [PlS] - **Spec Exp:** Cosmetic Surgery-Face & Body; Cosmetic Surgery-Breast; Breast Reconstruction; **Hospital:** UAB Highlands Hosp; **Address:** One Inverness Center Pkwy, Ste 100, Birmingham, AL 35242-4865; **Phone:** 205-930-1600; **Board Cert:** Plastic Surgery 1986; **Med School:** Univ Minn 1978; **Resid:** Surgery, Univ Wash Affil Hosp 1983; Plastic Surgery, UCSF Med Ctr 1985; **Fac Appt:** Clin Prof PlS, Univ Ala

Hagan, Kevin Francis MD [PlS] - **Spec Exp:** Reconstructive Surgery; Breast Surgery; Cosmetic Surgery; **Hospital:** Vanderbilt Univ Med Ctr; **Address:** Vanderbilt Univ Med Ctr, Dept Plastic Surg, D-4207 Med Ctr N, Nashville, TN 37232; **Phone:** 615-936-3574; **Board Cert:** Plastic Surgery 1983; **Med School:** Johns Hopkins Univ 1974; **Resid:** Surgery, Med Coll VA Hosps 1979; Plastic Surgery, UCSF Med Ctr 1982; **Fellow:** Microsurgery, Dr Harry Buncke Med Clinic 1980; **Fac Appt:** Assoc Prof PlS, Vanderbilt Univ

Hester Jr, T Roderick MD [PlS] - **Spec Exp:** Cosmetic Surgery-Face; Breast Reconstruction; **Hospital:** Emory Univ Hosp; **Address:** 3200 Downwood Cir, Ste 6340, Atlanta, GA 30327-1610; **Phone:** 404-351-0051; **Board Cert:** Plastic Surgery 1980; Surgery 1973; **Med School:** Emory Univ 1967; **Resid:** Surgery, Emory Affil Hosps 1972; Plastic Reconstructive Surgery, Emory Affil Hosps 1978; **Fac Appt:** Assoc Prof PlS, Emory Univ

Hunstad, Joseph P MD [PlS] - **Spec Exp:** Cosmetic Surgery-Face & Body; Cosmetic Dermatology; **Hospital:** Carolinas Med Ctr-Univ; **Address:** 8605 Cliff Cameron Drive, Ste 100, Charlotte, NC 28269; **Phone:** 704-549-0500; **Board Cert:** Plastic Surgery 1989; **Med School:** Mich State Univ 1981; **Resid:** Surgery, Butterworth Hosp 1984; Plastic Surgery, Grand Rapids Area Med Ed Ct 1986; **Fellow:** Reconstructive Microsurgery, MECOM MicSurg Inst 1987

Kelly, Kevin J MD/DDS [PlS] - **Spec Exp:** Craniofacial Surgery; Cosmetic Surgery; Maxillofacial Surgery; **Hospital:** Vanderbilt Univ Med Ctr; **Address:** Vanderbilt Univ Med Ctr, Dept Plastic Surgery, 1161 21st Ave S, rm D4207, Nashville, TN 37232-2345; **Phone:** 615-322-2350; **Board Cert:** Plastic Surgery 1991; **Med School:** SUNY Downstate 1982; **Resid:** Surgery, Albany Med Ctr 1986; Plastic Surgery, Albany Med Ctr 1988; **Fellow:** Craniofacial Surgery, Johns Hopkins Med Ctr 1989; **Fac Appt:** Assoc Prof PlS, Vanderbilt Univ

Levin, L Scott MD [PlS] - **Spec Exp:** Toe-to-Hand Transfer; Reconstructive Microvascular Surgery; Microsurgery; **Hospital:** Duke Univ Med Ctr; **Address:** Duke Univ Med Ctr, Baker Bldg - rm 134, Box 3945, Durham, NC 27710; **Phone:** 919-613-7797; **Board Cert:** Plastic Surgery 1993; Hand Surgery 2004; Orthopaedic Surgery 2004; **Med School:** Temple Univ 1982; **Resid:** Orthopaedic Surgery, Duke Univ Med Ctr 1988; Plastic Surgery, Duke Univ Med Ctr 1989; **Fac Appt:** Prof S, Duke Univ

Matthews, David C MD [PlS] - **Spec Exp:** Craniofacial Surgery/Reconstruction; **Hospital:** Carolinas Med Ctr, Presby Hosp - Charlotte; **Address:** 1719 South Blvd, Ste B, Charlotte, NC 28203-2747; **Phone:** 704-375-2955; **Board Cert:** Plastic Surgery 1983; **Med School:** Univ Cincinnati 1974; **Resid:** Surgery, Hosp Univ Penn 1980; Plastic Surgery, Hosp Univ Penn 1982; **Fellow:** Craniofacial Surgery, Royal Melbourne Hosp; **Fac Appt:** Clin Prof PlS, Univ NC Sch Med

Maxwell, G Patrick MD [PlS] - **Spec Exp:** Cosmetic Surgery-Breast; Cosmetic Surgery-Face; Breast Reconstruction; **Hospital:** Baptist Hosp - Nashville, Centennial Med Ctr; **Address:** Nashville Plastic Surgery, 2021 Church St, Medical Plaza II, Ste 310, Nashville, TN 37203; **Phone:** 615-284-8200; **Board Cert:** Plastic Surgery 1981; **Med School:** Vanderbilt Univ 1972; **Resid:** Surgery, Johns Hopkins Hosp 1976; Plastic Surgery, Johns Hopkins Hosp 1979; **Fellow:** Microsurgery, Davies Med Ctr 1975; **Fac Appt:** Asst Clin Prof PlS, Vanderbilt Univ

McCraw, John MD [PlS] - **Spec Exp:** Breast Reconstruction; **Hospital:** Univ Hosps & Clins - Jackson; **Address:** Univ Mississippi Med Ctr, Div Plastic Surg, 2500 N State St, Jackson, MS 39216; **Phone:** 601-815-1343; **Board Cert:** Surgery 1972; Plastic Surgery 1974; **Med School:** Univ MO-Columbia Sch Med 1966; **Resid:** Orthopaedic Surgery, Duke U Med Ctr 1969; Surgery, Univ Florida Med Ctr 1971; **Fellow:** Plastic Surgery, Univ Florida Med Ctr 1973; **Fac Appt:** Prof PlS, Univ Miss

Plastic Surgery

Molnar, Joseph MD/PhD [PlS] - **Spec Exp:** Burns-Reconstructive Plastic Surgery; Reconstructive Microvascular Surgery; Hand Surgery; **Hospital:** Wake Forest Univ Baptist Med Ctr (page 73); **Address:** Wake Forest Univ Sch Med, Dept Plastic Surg, Medical Ctr Blvd, Winston-Salem, NC 27157-1075; **Phone:** 336-716-0432; **Board Cert:** Plastic Surgery 2005; Hand Surgery 2000; **Med School:** Ohio State Univ 1977; **Resid:** Surgery, Univ Wash Med Ctr 1989; Plastic Surgery, Med Coll VA 1992; **Fellow:** Microsurgery, Med Coll Wisc 1199; Hand Surgery, Med Coll Wisc 1994; **Fac Appt:** Asst Prof PlS, Wake Forest Univ

Morgan, Raymond F MD [PlS] - **Spec Exp:** Cosmetic Surgery; Laser Surgery; Hand Surgery; **Hospital:** Univ Virginia Med Ctr; **Address:** Univ VA Hlth Sys, Dept Plas Surg, PO Box 800376, Charlottesville, VA 22908; **Phone:** 434-924-2413; **Board Cert:** Plastic Surgery 1983; Hand Surgery 2005; **Med School:** W VA Univ 1976; **Resid:** Surgery, Johns Hopkins Hosp 1980; Plastic Surgery, Johns Hopkins Hosp 1982; **Fellow:** Hand Surgery, Union Meml Hosp; **Fac Appt:** Prof PlS, Univ VA Sch Med

Smith Jr, David J MD [PlS] - **Spec Exp:** Breast Reconstruction; Burns-Reconstructive Plastic Surgery; **Hospital:** Univ of S FL - Tampa; **Address:** Div Plastic Surg, 4 Columbia Drive, Ste 650, Tampa, FL 33606; **Phone:** 813-259-0929; **Board Cert:** Plastic Surgery 1981; **Med School:** Indiana Univ 1973; **Resid:** Surgery, Emory Univ-Grady Hosp 1988; Plastic Surgery, Inidana Univ 1980; **Fellow:** Hand Surgery, Univ Louisville 1979; **Fac Appt:** Prof S, Univ S Fla Coll Med

Stuzin, James M MD [PlS] - **Spec Exp:** Cosmetic Surgery-Face; Eyelid Surgery; Skin Laser Surgery-Resurfacing; **Hospital:** Mercy Hosp; **Address:** 3225 Aviation Ave, Ste 100-200, Coconut Grove, FL 33133; **Phone:** 305-854-8828; **Board Cert:** Plastic Surgery 1989; **Med School:** Univ Fla Coll Med 1978; **Resid:** Surgery, Univ Wash Affil Hosp 1983; Plastic Surgery, NYU Med Ctr 1986; **Fellow:** Craniofacial Surgery, UCLA Med Ctr 1987

Tobin, Gordon R MD [PlS] - **Spec Exp:** Reconstructive Plastic Surgery; Transplant-Hand; Cosmetic Surgery; **Hospital:** Univ of Louisville Hosp, Jewish Hosp HlthCre Svcs Inc; **Address:** 601 S Floyd St, Ste 700, Louisville, KY 40202; **Phone:** 502-583-8303; **Board Cert:** Plastic Surgery 1978; **Med School:** UCSF 1969; **Resid:** Surgery, Univ Ariz Affil Hosps 1975; Plastic Surgery, Univ Ariz Affil Hosps 1976; **Fellow:** Pediatric Plastic Surgery, Univ Miami 1973; Cosmetic Plastic Surgery, Univ Miami 1973; **Fac Appt:** Prof PlS, Univ Louisville Sch Med

Vasconez, Luis O MD [PlS] - **Spec Exp:** Cosmetic Surgery-Face; Breast Reconstruction; **Hospital:** Univ of Ala Hosp at Birmingham; **Address:** 510 20th St S, FOT 1102, Birmingham, AL 35294-3411; **Phone:** 205-934-3245; **Board Cert:** Surgery 1970; Plastic Surgery 1971; **Med School:** Washington Univ, St Louis 1962; **Resid:** Surgery, Strong Meml Hosp 1970; Plastic Surgery, Shands Hosp-Univ FL 1969; **Fac Appt:** Prof S, Univ Ala

Wolfe, S Anthony MD [PlS] - **Spec Exp:** Craniofacial Surgery/Reconstruction; Maxillofacial Surgery; Cosmetic Surgery; **Hospital:** South Miami Hosp, Miami Children's Hosp; **Address:** 6280 Sunset Drive, Ste 400, Miami, FL 33143; **Phone:** 305-662-4111; **Board Cert:** Surgery 1973; Plastic Surgery 1978; **Med School:** Harvard Med Sch 1965; **Resid:** Surgery, Peter Bent Brigham Hosp 1972; Plastic Surgery, Jackson Meml Hosp 1974; **Fac Appt:** Assoc Clin Prof PlS, Univ Miami Sch Med

Midwest

Bauer, Bruce MD [PlS] - **Spec Exp:** Cleft Palate/Lip; Vascular Birthmarks; Ear Reconstruction/Microtia; Pigmented Lesions; **Hospital:** Children's Mem Hosp, NorthShore Univ Hlth-Sys; **Address:** Chldns Meml Hosp Outpatient Ctr, 467 West Deming, Chicago, IL 60614; **Phone:** 773-327-2440; **Board Cert:** Plastic Surgery 1980; **Med School:** Northwestern Univ 1974; **Resid:** Surgery, Northwestern Meml Hosp 1977; Plastic Surgery, Northwestern Meml Hosp 1979; **Fac Appt:** Prof S, Northwestern Univ

Bentz, Michael L MD [PlS] - **Spec Exp:** Pediatric Plastic Surgery; Facial Deformities/Reconstruction; Hand Surgery; Hand Reconstruction; **Hospital:** Univ WI Hosp & Clins, Meriter Hosp; **Address:** Univ Wisconsin Hosp, 600 Highland Ave, CSC, rm G5-361, Madison, WI 53792-3236; **Phone:** 608-263-1367; **Board Cert:** Surgery 1998; Plastic Surgery 1994; **Med School:** Temple Univ 1984; **Resid:** Surgery, Temple Univ Hosp 1989; Plastic Surgery, Univ Pittsburgh Med Ctr 1992; **Fellow:** Research, Univ Pittsburgh 1990; **Fac Appt:** Prof S, Univ Wisc

Billmire, David A MD [PlS] - **Spec Exp:** Cleft Palate/Lip; Reconstructive Plastic Surgery; **Hospital:** Cincinnati Chldns Hosp Med Ctr, Univ Hosp - Cincinnati; **Address:** 3333 Burnet Ave, MC 2020, Cincinnati, OH 45229; **Phone:** 513-636-7181; **Board Cert:** Plastic Surgery 1985; **Med School:** Ohio State Univ 1975; **Resid:** Surgery, Univ Hosp 1982; Plastic Surgery, Univ Hosp 1984; **Fellow:** Craniofacial Surgery, Texas Craniofacial Fdn; **Fac Appt:** Assoc Clin Prof S, Univ Cincinnati

Brandt, Keith MD [PlS] - **Spec Exp:** Breast Reconstruction; Reconstructive Surgery; Microsurgery; Hand & Wrist Surgery; **Hospital:** Barnes-Jewish Hosp, St Louis Chldns Hosp; **Address:** 660 S Euclid, Box 8238, St Louis, MO 63110-1010; **Phone:** 314-747-0541; **Board Cert:** Surgery 1999; Plastic Surgery 2003; Hand Surgery 2005; **Med School:** Univ Tex, Houston 1983; **Resid:** Surgery, Univ Nebraska Med Ctr 1989; Plastic Surgery, Univ Tennessee 1991; **Fellow:** Hand Surgery, Wash Univ 1992; Microsurgery, Wash Univ 1993; **Fac Appt:** Prof S, Washington Univ, St Louis

Buchman, Steven R MD [PlS] - **Spec Exp:** Pediatric Plastic Surgery; Craniofacial Surgery-Pediatric; Craniofacial Surgery; **Hospital:** Mott Chldns Hosp, Univ Michigan Hlth Sys; **Address:** Mott Children's Hospital, 1500 E Med Ctr Drive, rm 7894, Ann Arbor, MI 48109-5219; **Phone:** 734-763-8063; **Board Cert:** Plastic Surgery 2005; **Med School:** Univ VA Sch Med 1985; **Resid:** Surgery, Hosp Univ Penn 1990; Plastic Surgery, Hosp Univ Penn 1992; **Fellow:** Craniofacial Surgery, UCLA Med Ctr 1993; **Fac Appt:** Prof PlS, Univ Mich Med Sch

Canady, John MD [PlS] - **Spec Exp:** Cleft Palate/Lip; Craniofacial Surgery; Pediatric Plastic Surgery; **Hospital:** Univ Iowa Hosp & Clinics; **Address:** Univ Iowa Hosp, Dept Plastic Surg & Otolaryngology, 200 Hawkins Drive, rm 21262 PFP, Iowa City, IA 52240; **Phone:** 319-356-2168; **Board Cert:** Otolaryngology 1988; Plastic Surgery 1992; **Med School:** Univ Iowa Coll Med 1983; **Resid:** Otolaryngology, Univ Iowa Hosp 1988; Plastic Surgery, Univ Kansas Med Ctr 1990; **Fac Appt:** Prof PlS, Univ Iowa Coll Med

Coleman, John J MD [PlS] - **Spec Exp:** Cancer Reconstruction; Breast Reconstruction; Head & Neck Surgery; Pediatric Plastic Surgery; **Hospital:** Indiana Univ Hosp, Riley Hosp for Children; **Address:** 545 Barnhill Dr, Emerson Hall, Ste 232, Indianapolis, IN 46202-5120; **Phone:** 317-274-8106; **Board Cert:** Surgery 1998; Plastic Surgery 1981; **Med School:** Harvard Med Sch 1973; **Resid:** Surgery, Emory Univ Affil Hosp 1978; Plastic Surgery, Emory Univ Affil Hosp 1979; **Fellow:** Surgical Oncology, Univ Maryland Med Ctr 1981; **Fac Appt:** Prof S, Indiana Univ

Plastic Surgery

Hammond, Dennis C MD [PlS] - **Spec Exp:** Breast Surgery; Breast Reduction; **Hospital:** Spectrum Hlth Blodgett Campus; **Address:** 4070 Lake Drive SE, Ste 202, Grand Rapids, MI 49546; **Phone:** 616-464-4420; **Board Cert:** Plastic Surgery 1994; **Med School:** Univ Mich Med Sch 1985; **Resid:** Surgery, Blodgett Meml Med Ctr 1988; Plastic Reconstructive Surgery, Grand Rapids Area Med Educ Ctr 1990; **Fellow:** Plastic Surgery, Baptist Hosp 1991; Hand & Microvascular Surgery, Med Coll Wisconsin 1992

Kane, Alex A MD [PlS] - **Spec Exp:** Pediatric Plastic Surgery; Craniofacial Surgery; Cleft Palate/Lip; **Hospital:** St Louis Chldns Hosp, Barnes-Jewish Hosp; **Address:** St Louis Children's Hospital, 6600 S Euclid, Box 8283, St Louis, MO 63110; **Phone:** 314-454-4894; **Board Cert:** Plastic Surgery 2001; **Med School:** Dartmouth Med Sch 1991; **Resid:** Surgery, Barnes Jewish Hosp 1994; Plastic Surgery, Barnes Jewish Hosp 1998; **Fellow:** Craniofacial Surgery, Chang-Gung Meml Hosp 1999; Craniofacial Imaging, Natl Lab for Diagnostic Research 1999; **Fac Appt:** Asst Prof S, Washington Univ, St Louis

Kuzon Jr, William M MD/PhD [PlS] - **Spec Exp:** Facial Paralysis Reconstruction; Abdominal Wall Reconstruction; Gender Reassignment Surgery; **Hospital:** Univ Michigan Hlth Sys, VA Med Ctr; **Address:** Univ Michigan, Dept Surgery, Taubman Ctr, 1500 E Medical Center Drive, rm 2130, Ann Arbor, MI 48109-0340; **Phone:** 734-936-5890; **Board Cert:** Plastic Surgery 2006; **Med School:** Univ Rochester 1981; **Resid:** Plastic Surgery, Univ Toronto Med Ctr 1990; **Fellow:** Microvascular Surgery, Univ Toronto Med Ctr 1991; Hand & Microvascular Surgery, Univ Pittsburgh Med Ctr 1992; **Fac Appt:** Prof PlS, Univ Mich Med Sch

MacKinnon, Susan E MD [PlS] - **Spec Exp:** Nerve Surgery & Transplantation; Hand Surgery; Reconstructive Surgery; Peripheral Nerve Surgery; **Hospital:** Barnes-Jewish Hosp; **Address:** Washington Univ Sch Med, 660 S Euclid Ave, Box 8238, St Louis, MO 63110; **Phone:** 314-362-4586; **Med School:** Canada 1975; **Resid:** Surgery, Queens Univ-Kingston 1978; Plastic Surgery, Univ Toronto Med Ctr 1980; **Fellow:** Neurological Surgery, Univ Toronto Med Ctr 1981; Hand Surgery, Union Meml Hosp 1982; **Fac Appt:** Prof S, Washington Univ, St Louis

Marsh, Jeffrey L MD [PlS] - **Spec Exp:** Cleft Palate/Lip; Craniofacial Surgery/Reconstruction; Pediatric Plastic Surgery; **Hospital:** St John's Mercy Med Ctr - St Louis; **Address:** 621 S New Ballas Rd, Ste 260A, St Louis, MO 63141; **Phone:** 314-251-4772; **Board Cert:** Plastic Surgery 1979; **Med School:** Johns Hopkins Univ 1970; **Resid:** Surgery, UCLA Med Ctr 1975; Plastic Surgery, Univ Va Hosp 1977; **Fellow:** Craniofacial Surgery, Cannisburn Hosp; Craniofacial Surgery, Clinic Belvedere Hosp; **Fac Appt:** Clin Prof PlS, St Louis Univ

Mustoe, Thomas A MD [PlS] - **Spec Exp:** Cosmetic Surgery-Face; Cosmetic Surgery-Breast; Rhinoplasty; **Hospital:** Northwestern Meml Hosp, Evanston Hosp; **Address:** NW Med Faculty Fdn-Plastic Surgery, 675 North St Clair St Fl 19 - Ste 250, Chicago, IL 60611-5975; **Phone:** 312-695-6022; **Board Cert:** Otolaryngology 1983; Plastic Surgery 1987; **Med School:** Harvard Med Sch 1978; **Resid:** Surgery, Brigham & Womens Hosp 1980; Otolaryngology, Mass Eye & Ear Infirmary 1983; **Fellow:** Plastic Surgery, Brigham & Womens Hosp 1985; **Fac Appt:** Prof S, Northwestern Univ

Polley, John W MD [PlS] - **Spec Exp:** Craniofacial Surgery; Pediatric Plastic Surgery; Maxillofacial Surgery; **Hospital:** Rush Univ Med Ctr; **Address:** Rush U Med Ctr, Plastic Surgery, 1725 W Harrison St, Ste 425, Professional Bldg, Chicago, IL 60612-3841; **Phone:** 312-563-3000; **Board Cert:** Plastic Surgery 1992; **Med School:** Northwestern Univ 1983; **Resid:** Surgery, Mich State Univ 1986; Plastic Surgery, Mich State Univ 1988; **Fellow:** Craniofacial Surgery, Chang Gung Meml Hosp 1989; Hosp for Sick Chldn 1990; **Fac Appt:** Prof PlS, Rush Med Coll

Puckett, Charles L MD [PlS] - **Spec Exp:** Cosmetic & Reconstructive Surgery; Breast Surgery; **Hospital:** Univ of Missouri Hosp & Clins, Columbia Regional Hosp; **Address:** 1 Hospital Drive, Ste M349, Columbia, MO 65212-5276; **Phone:** 573-882-2275; **Board Cert:** Surgery 1972; Plastic Surgery 1977; **Med School:** Wake Forest Univ 1966; **Resid:** Surgery, Duke Univ Med Ctr 1971; Plastic Surgery, Duke Univ Med Ctr 1976; **Fac Appt:** Prof S, Univ MO-Columbia Sch Med

Rees, Riley S MD [PlS] - **Spec Exp:** Wound Healing/Care; Melanoma; **Hospital:** Univ Michigan Hlth Sys, VA Med Ctr - Ann Arbor; **Address:** University of Michigan, 2130 Taubman Ctr, 1500 E Medical Center Drive, Box 0340, Ann Arbor, MI 48109-0340; **Phone:** 734-615-3435; **Board Cert:** Plastic Surgery 1981; **Med School:** Univ Utah 1972; **Resid:** Surgery, LSU Med Ctr 1978; Plastic Surgery, Vanderbilt Univ Med Ctr 1980; **Fac Appt:** Prof S, Univ Mich Med Sch

Sanger, James R MD [PlS] - **Spec Exp:** Reconstructive Surgery; Hand Surgery; Microsurgery; **Hospital:** Froedtert Meml Lutheran Hosp, Chldns Hosp - Wisconsin; **Address:** Med Coll Wisc, Dept Plastic Surg, 8700 Watertown Plank Rd, Milwaukee, WI 53226; **Phone:** 414-805-5451; **Board Cert:** Plastic Surgery 1982; Hand Surgery 1999; **Med School:** Univ Wisc 1974; **Resid:** Surgery, LAC-Harbor UCLA Med Ctr 1979; Plastic Surgery, Med Coll Wisc Affil Hosps 1981; **Fellow:** Hand Surgery, Med Coll Wisc Affil Hosps 1982; **Fac Appt:** Prof PlS, Med Coll Wisc

Siemionow, Maria MD/PhD [PlS] - **Spec Exp:** Microsurgery; Peripheral Nerve Surgery; Reconstructive Plastic Surgery; Transplant Surgery; **Hospital:** Cleveland Clin Fdn (page 56); **Address:** Cleveland Clin Fdn, 9500 Euclid Ave, MC A60, Cleveland, OH 44195; **Phone:** 216-445-2405; **Med School:** Poland 1974; **Resid:** Surgery, Inst Orth & Rehab Med; **Fellow:** Plastic Surgery, Univ Hosp; Microsurgery, Univ Louisville Hosp

Sood, Rajiv MD [PlS] - **Spec Exp:** Burns-Reconstructive Plastic Surgery; Pediatric Hand Surgery; **Hospital:** Wishard Hlth Srvs, Riley Hosp for Children; **Address:** Indiana Univ School Med, Plastic Surgery, 1001 W 10th St Fl D-4, Indianapolis, IN 46202; **Phone:** 317-278-1022; **Board Cert:** Plastic Surgery 1994; Hand Surgery 2006; **Med School:** Albany Med Coll 1984; **Resid:** Surgery, Temple Univ Hosp 1989; **Fellow:** Plastic Surgery, Cleveland Clinic Fdn 1991; Hand Surgery, Union Meml Hosp 1992; **Fac Appt:** Prof S, Indiana Univ

Vogt, Peter MD [PlS] - **Spec Exp:** Cosmetic Surgery; **Hospital:** Mercy Hosp - Coon Rapids, Unity Hosp - Fridley; **Address:** 319 Barry Ave S, Ste 300, Wayzata, MN 55391; **Phone:** 952-473-1111; **Board Cert:** Plastic Surgery 1974; **Med School:** Univ Manitoba 1965; **Resid:** Surgery, Montreal Genl Hosp 1970; Plastic Surgery, Winnipeg Hlth Scis Ctr 1973

Walton Jr, Robert L MD [PlS] - **Spec Exp:** Cosmetic Surgery-Face; Nasal Reconstruction; Breast Reconstruction; **Hospital:** Univ of Chicago Hosps, Resurrection Hlth Care St Joseph Hosp; **Address:** 60 E Delaware, Ste 1430, Chicago, IL 60611-1495; **Phone:** 312-337-7795; **Board Cert:** Plastic Surgery 1980; **Med School:** Univ Kans 1972; **Resid:** Surgery, Johns Hopkins Hosp 1974; Plastic Surgery, Yale-New Haven Hosp 1978; **Fellow:** Hand Surgery, Hartford Hosp 1978

Wilkins, Edwin G MD [PlS] - **Spec Exp:** Breast Reconstruction; Lower Limb Reconstruction; Microsurgery; **Hospital:** Univ Michigan Hlth Sys; **Address:** Univ Mich, Div Plastic Surg, 1500 E Med Ctr Drive, rm 2130 Taubman Ctr, Ann Arbor, MI 48109-5340; **Phone:** 734-998-6022; **Board Cert:** Plastic Surgery 1991; **Med School:** Wake Forest Univ 1981; **Resid:** Surgery, Charlotte Meml Hosp 1986; Plastic Surgery, Vanderbilt Univ Med Ctr 1988; **Fellow:** Reconstructive Microsurgery, Univ Louisville Sch Med 1989; **Fac Appt:** Assoc Prof PlS, Univ Mich Med Sch

Yetman, Randall MD [PlS] - **Spec Exp:** Breast Reconstruction; Melanoma; **Hospital:** Cleveland Clin Fdn (page 56); **Address:** 9500 Euclid Ave, Desk A60, Cleveland, OH 44195; **Phone:** 216-444-6908; **Board Cert:** Plastic Surgery 1984; **Med School:** Univ Miami Sch Med 1975; **Resid:** Surgery, Montefiore Med Ctr 1979; Plastic Surgery, NY Cornell Med Ctr 1981; **Fellow:** Plastic Surgery, Cleveland Clin Fdn 1982

Plastic Surgery

Young, Vernon Leroy MD [PlS] - **Spec Exp:** Breast Augmentation; Skin Laser Surgery-Resurfacing; Body Contouring after Weight Loss; **Address:** 969 N Mason Rd, Ste 170, St Louis, MO 63141; **Phone:** 314-628-8200; **Board Cert:** Plastic Surgery 1981; **Med School:** Univ KY Coll Med 1970; **Resid:** Surgery, Univ KY Med Ctr 1977; Plastic Surgery, Barnes Hosp-Wash Univ 1979; **Fac Appt:** Prof S, Washington Univ, St Louis

Zins, James MD [PlS] - **Spec Exp:** Cosmetic Surgery-Face; Maxillofacial Surgery; Craniofacial Surgery; **Hospital:** Cleveland Clin Fdn (page 56); **Address:** Department of Plastic Surgery, 9500 Euclid Ave, Desk A-60, Cleveland, OH 44195; **Phone:** 216-444-6901; **Board Cert:** Plastic Surgery 1985; **Med School:** Univ Pennsylvania 1974; **Resid:** Surgery, Hosp Univ Penn 1980; Plastic Surgery, Hosp Univ Penn 1982; **Fellow:** Craniofacial Surgery, Hosp Univ Penn 1978; Maxillofacial Surgery, Hosp Sick Chldn 1983

Great Plains and Mountains

Grossman, John A MD [PlS] - **Spec Exp:** Cosmetic Surgery; **Hospital:** Rose Med Ctr, Cedars-Sinai Med Ctr; **Address:** 4600 Hale Pkwy, Ste 100, Denver, CO 80220; **Phone:** 303-320-5566; **Board Cert:** Surgery 1974; Plastic Surgery 1976; **Med School:** Cornell Univ-Weill Med Coll 1967; **Resid:** Surgery, Boston City Hosp 1973; Plastic Surgery, Univ Colo Hlth Scis Ctr 1975; **Fellow:** Surgery, Harvard Med Sch 1973

Ketch, Lawrence L MD [PlS] - **Spec Exp:** Pediatric Plastic Surgery; Craniofacial Surgery; Cleft Palate/Lip; **Hospital:** Univ Colorado Hosp, Chldn's Hosp - Aurora, The; **Address:** 13123 E 16th Ave, Box B467, Aurora, CO 80045; **Phone:** 720-777-3880; **Board Cert:** Plastic Surgery 1982; Hand Surgery 1992; **Med School:** Univ Colorado 1974; **Resid:** Surgery, Univ Colo Affil Hosp 1979; **Fellow:** Plastic Surgery, Univ Miami 1981; **Fac Appt:** Prof S, Univ Colorado

Southwest

Barone, Constance M MD [PlS] - **Spec Exp:** Craniofacial Surgery; Craniosynostosis; Cosmetic Surgery; Breast Augmentation; **Hospital:** Univ Hlth Sys - Univ Hosp (San Antonio, TX), Christus Santa Rosa Hosp; **Address:** 2829 Babcock Rd, Ste 615, San Antonio, TX 78229; **Phone:** 210-614-0400; **Board Cert:** Plastic Surgery 1991; **Med School:** Mount Sinai Sch Med 1982; **Resid:** Surgery, Temple Univ Hosp 1987; Plastic Surgery, NYU Med Ctr 1989; **Fellow:** Craniofacial Surgery, Montefiore/Einstein Coll Med 1992; **Fac Appt:** Prof PlS, Univ Tex, San Antonio

Barton Jr, Fritz MD [PlS] - **Spec Exp:** Cosmetic Surgery-Face; Liposuction & Body Contouring; **Hospital:** Baylor Univ Medical Ctr; **Address:** Dallas Plastic Surgery Institute, 9101 N Central Expresswy Ave, Ste 600, Dallas, TX 75231; **Phone:** 214-821-9355; **Board Cert:** Surgery 1975; Plastic Surgery 1977; **Med School:** Univ Tex SW, Dallas 1967; **Resid:** Surgery, Parkland Meml Hosp 1974; NYU Med Ctr 1976; **Fac Appt:** Prof PlS, Univ Tex SW, Dallas

Beals, Stephen P MD [PlS] - **Spec Exp:** Craniofacial Surgery; Pediatric Plastic Surgery; Cosmetic Surgery-Face; **Hospital:** St Joseph's Hosp & Med Ctr - Phoenix, Phoenix Children's Hosp; **Address:** 500 W Thomas Rd, Ste 960, Phoenix, AZ 85013-4223; **Phone:** 602-266-9066; **Board Cert:** Plastic Surgery 1986; **Med School:** Wayne State Univ 1978; **Resid:** Surgery, William Beaumont Hospital 1983; Plastic Surgery, Phoenix Plastic Surgery Inst 1985; **Fellow:** Craniofacial Surgery, Hospital for Sick Children 1985; **Fac Appt:** Asst Prof PlS, Mayo Med Sch

Burns, Alton J MD [PlS] - **Spec Exp:** Cosmetic Surgery; Skin Laser Surgery; Vascular Birthmarks; **Hospital:** Baylor Univ Medical Ctr, Chldns Med Ctr of Dallas; **Address:** 9101 N Central Expresswy St, Ste 600, Dallas, TX 75231; **Phone:** 214-823-1978; **Board Cert:** Plastic Surgery 1990; **Med School:** Univ Tex SW, Dallas 1981; **Resid:** Surgery, Univ Utah Hosp 1986; Plastic Surgery, Univ Tex SW Med Ctr 1988; **Fellow:** Vascular Anomalies, Chldns Hosp 1988; **Fac Appt:** Asst Prof PlS, Univ Tex SW, Dallas

Byrd, H Stephenson MD [PlS] - **Spec Exp:** Cosmetic Surgery-Face; Craniofacial Surgery; Pediatric Plastic Surgery; **Hospital:** Baylor Univ Medical Ctr; **Address:** 9101 N Central Expressway Ave, Ste 600, Dallas, TX 75231; **Phone:** 214-821-9662; **Board Cert:** Plastic Surgery 1980; **Med School:** Univ Tex Med Br, Galveston 1972; **Resid:** Surgery, Univ Utah Med Ctr 1977; Plastic Surgery, Dallas Co Hosp-Parkland Meml 1979; **Fac Appt:** Clin Prof PlS, Univ Tex SW, Dallas

Friedland, Jack A MD [PlS] - **Spec Exp:** Cleft Palate/Lip; Cosmetic Surgery-Face & Body; Cosmetic Surgery-Breast; Rhinoplasty; **Hospital:** St Joseph's Hosp & Med Ctr - Phoenix, Scottsdale Hlthcare - Shea; **Address:** 7425 E Shea Blvd, Ste 103, Scottsdale, AZ 85260-6411; **Phone:** 480-905-1700; **Board Cert:** Surgery 1971; Plastic Surgery 1975; **Med School:** Northwestern Univ 1965; **Resid:** Surgery, NYU Med Ctr & Bellevue Hosp-NYU 1970; Plastic Reconstructive Surgery, NYU Medical Ctr 1974; **Fac Appt:** Assoc Prof PlS, Mayo Med Sch

Gunter, Jack MD [PlS] - **Spec Exp:** Rhinoplasty; Rhinoplasty Revision; **Hospital:** Presby Hosp of Dallas; **Address:** 8144 Walnut Hill Lane, Ste 170, Dallas, TX 75231-4218; **Phone:** 214-369-8123; **Board Cert:** Otolaryngology 1969; Plastic Surgery 1981; **Med School:** Univ Okla Coll Med 1963; **Resid:** Surgery, Univ Ark Med Ctr 1965; Otolaryngology, Tulane Univ Hosp 1968; **Fellow:** Mercy Hosp 1969; Plastic Surgery, Univ Mich Hosp 1980; **Fac Appt:** Clin Prof PlS, Univ Tex SW, Dallas

Hamra, Sameer T MD [PlS] - **Spec Exp:** Cosmetic Surgery-Face; Rhinoplasty; **Hospital:** Mary Shiels Hosp; **Address:** 9301 N Central Expresswy, Ste 551, Tower 2, Dallas, TX 75231; **Phone:** 214-754-9001; **Board Cert:** Surgery 1970; Plastic Surgery 1977; **Med School:** Univ Okla Coll Med 1963; **Resid:** Plastic Surgery, NYU Med Ctr 1973; Surgery, Univ Okla 1968; **Fellow:** Surgery, Univ Lausanne 1966; **Fac Appt:** Asst Clin Prof S, Univ Tex SW, Dallas

Kelly, John M MD [PlS] - **Spec Exp:** Cosmetic Surgery-Face; Breast Surgery; Liposuction; **Hospital:** Integris Baptist Med Ctr - OK; **Address:** 3301 NW 63rd St, Oklahoma City, OK 73116-3705; **Phone:** 405-842-9732; **Board Cert:** Surgery 1970; Plastic Surgery 1978; **Med School:** Univ Ark 1963; **Resid:** Surgery, Univ Virginia Hosp 1969; Plastic Surgery, Johns Hopkins Hosp 1971; **Fac Appt:** Clin Prof S, Univ Okla Coll Med

Meltzer, Toby R MD [PlS] - **Spec Exp:** Gender Reassignment Surgery; Penile Inversion Technique; Breast Augmentation; **Hospital:** Scottsdale Hlthcare - Osborn; **Address:** 7025 N Scottsdale Rd, Ste 302, Scottsdale, AZ 85253; **Phone:** 866-876-6329; **Board Cert:** Plastic Surgery 1992; **Med School:** Louisiana State U, New Orleans 1983; **Resid:** Surgery, Charity Hosp Louisiana 1988; Plastic Surgery, Univ Michigan Med Ctr 1990; **Fellow:** Burn Surgery, Wayne State Univ 1987; **Fac Appt:** Asst Clin Prof S, Univ Ariz Coll Med

Menick, Frederick J MD [PlS] - **Spec Exp:** Reconstructive Surgery-Face; Breast Reconstruction; Cancer Reconstruction; Cosmetic Surgery; **Hospital:** St Joseph's Hosp - Tucson; **Address:** 1102 N Eldorado Pl, Tucson, AZ 85712; **Phone:** 520-881-4525; **Board Cert:** Plastic Surgery 1983; **Med School:** Yale Univ 1970; **Resid:** Surgery, Stanford Med Ctr; Surgery, Univ Ariz Med Ctr 1979; **Fellow:** Plastic Surgery, Queen Victoria Hosp/UC Irvine 1982; **Fac Appt:** Assoc Clin Prof S, Univ Ariz Coll Med

Plastic Surgery

Nath, Rahul Kumar MD [PlS] - **Spec Exp:** Brachial Plexus Palsy; Peripheral Nerve Surgery; **Hospital:** Meml Hermann Hosp - Texas Med Ctr, Methodist Hosp - Houston; **Address:** Texas Nerve & Paralysis Inst, 6400 Fannin St, Ste 2420, Houston, TX 77030; **Phone:** 713-592-9900; **Board Cert:** Plastic Surgery 1998; **Med School:** Northwestern Univ 1988; **Resid:** Surgery, Northwestern Med Ctr 1991; Plastic Surgery, Washington Univ 1994

Robb, Geoffrey L MD [PlS] - **Spec Exp:** Breast Reconstruction; Head & Neck Cancer Reconstruction; Facial Plastic & Reconstructive Surgery; **Hospital:** UT MD Anderson Cancer Ctr, St Luke's Episcopal Hosp - Houston; **Address:** 1515 Holcombe Blvd, Unit 443, Houston, TX 77030; **Phone:** 713-794-1247; **Board Cert:** Otolaryngology 1979; Plastic Surgery 1986; **Med School:** Univ Miami Sch Med 1974; **Resid:** Otolaryngology, Naval Reg Med Ctr 1979; Plastic Surgery, Univ Pittsburgh 1985; **Fellow:** Microvascular Surgery, Univ Pittsburgh 1986; **Fac Appt:** Prof PlS, Univ Tex, Houston

Rohrich, Rod J MD [PlS] - **Spec Exp:** Nasal Surgery; Rhinoplasty; Breast Reconstruction; Wound Healing/Care; **Hospital:** UT Southwestern Med Ctr - Dallas, Baylor Univ Medical Ctr; **Address:** Univ Tex SW Med Ctr, Plastic Surgery, 1801 Inwood Rd, Dallas, TX 75390-9132; **Phone:** 214-645-3119; **Board Cert:** Plastic Surgery 1987; Hand Surgery 1990; **Med School:** Baylor Coll Med 1979; **Resid:** Plastic Surgery, Univ Mich Hosp 1985; Plastic Surgery, Radcliffe Infirm/Oxford 1983; **Fellow:** Hand Surgery, Mass Genl Hosp-Harvard 1987; **Fac Appt:** Prof PlS, Univ Tex SW, Dallas

Schusterman, Mark A MD [PlS] - **Spec Exp:** Breast Reconstruction; Cancer Reconstruction; Cosmetic Surgery-Face & Breast; **Hospital:** St Luke's Episcopal Hosp - Houston, Park Plaza Hosp; **Address:** 6624 Fannin St, Ste 1420, Houston, TX 77030; **Phone:** 713-794-0368; **Board Cert:** Plastic Surgery 1989; **Med School:** Univ Louisville Sch Med 1980; **Resid:** Surgery, Univ Hosp 1985; Pediatric Surgery, Univ Pittsburgh Med Ctr 1987; **Fellow:** Microsurgery, Univ Pittsburgh Med Ctr 1988; **Fac Appt:** Clin Prof PlS, Baylor Coll Med

Stal, Samuel MD [PlS] - **Spec Exp:** Pediatric Plastic Surgery; Craniofacial Surgery; Cleft Palate/Lip; Maxillofacial Surgery; **Hospital:** Texas Chldns Hosp - Houston; **Address:** Texas Children's Hosp, 6621 Fannin St, MC CCC 620.10, Houston, TX 77030; **Phone:** 832-822-3180; **Board Cert:** Otolaryngology 1981; Plastic Surgery 1982; **Med School:** Loyola Univ-Stritch Sch Med 1974; **Resid:** Otolaryngology, Univ Chicago Hosps 1979; Plastic Surgery, Baylor College Med 1981; **Fellow:** Craniofacial Surgery, Enfant Malade Hosp 1982; **Fac Appt:** Prof Oto, Baylor Coll Med

Tebbetts, John B MD [PlS] - **Spec Exp:** Breast Augmentation; Rhinoplasty; Liposuction; **Hospital:** Mary Shiels Hosp, Baylor Univ Medical Ctr; **Address:** 2801 Lemmon Ave W, Ste 300, Dallas, TX 75204-2398; **Phone:** 214-220-2712; **Board Cert:** Surgery 1978; Plastic Surgery 1980; **Med School:** Univ Tex Med Br, Galveston 1972; **Resid:** Surgery, Univ Utah Med Ctr 1977; Plastic Surgery, Dallas Co Hospital-Parkland Meml Hosp 1979; **Fac Appt:** Asst Clin Prof PlS, Univ Tex SW, Dallas

Yuen, James C MD [PlS] - **Spec Exp:** Hand Reconstruction; Breast Reconstruction; Head & Neck Cancer Reconstruction; Chest Wall Reconstruction; **Hospital:** UAMS Med Ctr; **Address:** Univ Aransas for Med Scis, Plastic Surgery, 4301 W Markham, Ste 720, Little Rock, AR 72205; **Phone:** 501-686-8711; **Board Cert:** Surgery 1991; Plastic Surgery 1995; **Med School:** Med Coll VA 1985; **Resid:** Surgery, W Virginia Med Ctr 1990; Plastic Reconstructive Surgery, Duke Univ Med Ctr 1993; **Fellow:** Hand & Microvascular Surgery, Kleinert Inst of Hand & Microsurgery 1991; **Fac Appt:** Assoc Prof S, Univ Ark

West Coast and Pacific

Alter, Gary J MD [PlS] - **Spec Exp:** Genitourinary Reconstruction; Gender Reassignment Surgery; **Hospital:** Cedars-Sinai Med Ctr, Ronald Reagan UCLA Med Ctr; **Address:** 416 N Bedford Drive, Ste 400, Beverly Hills, CA 90210-4318; **Phone:** 310-275-5566; **Board Cert:** Urology 1981; Plastic Surgery 2007; **Med School:** UCLA 1973; **Resid:** Urology, Baylor Med Ctr 1979; Plastic Surgery, Mayo Clinic 1992; **Fellow:** Genitourinary Surgery, Eastern Va Med Sch 1992; **Fac Appt:** Clin Prof PlS, UCLA

Andersen, James S MD [PlS] - **Spec Exp:** Cancer Reconstruction; Breast Reconstruction; Head & Neck Reconstruction; **Hospital:** City of Hope Natl Med Ctr & Beckman Rsch; **Address:** City of Hope National Cancer Ctr, Div Plastic Surgery, 1500 E Duarte Rd, Duarte, CA 91010; **Phone:** 626-471-7100; **Board Cert:** Plastic Surgery 1994; **Med School:** Jefferson Med Coll 1983; **Resid:** Surgery, Hosp U Penn 1989; Plastic Surgery, Hosp U Penn 1991; **Fellow:** Microsurgery, USC Med Ctr 1992; **Fac Appt:** Assoc Clin Prof S, USC Sch Med

Brent, Burton D MD [PlS] - **Spec Exp:** Ear Reconstruction/Microtia; **Hospital:** El Camino Hosp/Camino Hlthcare Sys; **Address:** 2995 Woodside Rd, Ste 300, Woodside, CA 94062-2401; **Phone:** 650-851-5300; **Board Cert:** Plastic Surgery 1974; **Med School:** Ros Franklin Univ/Chicago Med Sch 1963; **Resid:** Surgery, University Hosp 1970; Plastic Surgery, Loyola Univ Med Ctr 1973; **Fellow:** Plastic Surgery, Canniesburn Hosp; **Fac Appt:** Assoc Clin Prof PlS, Stanford Univ

Brink, Robert Ross MD [PlS] - **Spec Exp:** Cosmetic Surgery; **Hospital:** Mills - Peninsula Hlth Svcs; **Address:** 66 Bovet Rd, Ste 101, San Mateo, CA 94402-3126; **Phone:** 650-570-6066; **Board Cert:** Plastic Surgery 1980; **Med School:** Univ Mich Med Sch 1970; **Resid:** Surgery, UC Davis Med Ctr 1977; Plastic Surgery, UCSF Med Ctr 1979

Carstens, Michael H MD [PlS] - **Spec Exp:** Pediatric Plastic Surgery; Cleft Palate/Lip; Vascular Birthmarks; Ear Reconstruction/Microtia; **Hospital:** Cardinal Glennon Mem Children's Hosp; **Address:** 3635 Vista Ave Fl 3, Plastic Surgery, St Louis, CA 63110; **Phone:** 314-268-4010; **Board Cert:** Plastic Surgery 2006; **Med School:** Stanford Univ 1981; **Resid:** Surgery, Boston Univ Med Ctr 1987; **Fellow:** Plastic Reconstructive Surgery, Univ Pittsburgh 1989; Craniofacial Surgery, Univ Pittsburgh 1990; **Fac Appt:** Prof PlS, Univ MO-Columbia Sch Med

Cohen, Steven R MD [PlS] - **Spec Exp:** Craniofacial Surgery-Pediatric; Craniofacial Surgery/Reconstruction; **Hospital:** Rady Children's Hosp - San Diego, UCSD Med Ctr; **Address:** 8899 Univ Center Ln, Ste 350, San Diego, CA 92122; **Phone:** 858-453-7224; **Board Cert:** Plastic Surgery 1992; **Med School:** Geo Wash Univ 1980; **Resid:** Surgery, Columbia-Presby Med Ctr 1982; Surgery, Dartmouth-Hitchcock Med Ctr 1987; **Fellow:** Plastic Surgery, Hosp Univ Penn 1989; Craniofacial Surgery, UCLA Med Ctr 1990

Daniel, Rollin K MD [PlS] - **Spec Exp:** Cosmetic Surgery-Face; Rhinoplasty; **Hospital:** Hoag Meml Hosp Presby; **Address:** 1441 Avocado Ave, Ste 308, Newport Beach, CA 92660; **Phone:** 949-721-0494; **Board Cert:** Plastic Surgery 1977; **Med School:** Columbia P&S 1972; **Resid:** Plastic Surgery, McGill Univ Affil Hosps 1975; Hand Surgery, Univ Louisville Hosp 1976; **Fellow:** Craniofacial Surgery, Toronto Genl Hosp

Fisher, Garth MD [PlS] - **Spec Exp:** Cosmetic Surgery-Face; Cosmetic Surgery-Breast; Rhinoplasty; **Hospital:** St John's Hlth Ctr, Santa Monica; **Address:** 120 S Spalding Drive, Ste 222, Beverly Hills, CA 90212; **Phone:** 310-273-5995; **Board Cert:** Plastic Surgery 1993; **Med School:** Univ Miss 1984; **Resid:** Surgery, UC Irvine Medical Ctr 1989; Plastic Surgery, UC Irvine Medical Ctr 1991

Plastic Surgery

Fodor, Peter B MD [PlS] - **Spec Exp:** Cosmetic Surgery; Liposuction & Body Contouring; **Hospital:** Olympia Med Ctr, Century City Hosp; **Address:** 2080 Century Park E, Ste 710, Century City, CA 90067; **Phone:** 310-203-9818; **Board Cert:** Plastic Surgery 1977; **Med School:** Univ Wisc 1966; **Resid:** Surgery, Columbia-Presby Med Ctr 1968; Plastic Surgery, St Luke's Hosp 1976; **Fac Appt:** Assoc Clin Prof S, UCLA

Garner, Warren L MD [PlS] - **Spec Exp:** Burns-Reconstructive Plastic Surgery; Wound Healing/Care; Skin Healing; **Hospital:** LAC & USC Med Ctr, USC Univ Hosp - R K Eamer Med Plz; **Address:** 1510 San Pablo St, Ste 415, Los Angeles, CA 90033; **Phone:** 323-442-6470; **Board Cert:** Plastic Surgery 1991; Surgical Critical Care 2001; **Med School:** Univ Kans 1978; **Resid:** Surgery, Ohio State Univ Hosp 1985; Plastic Surgery, Wash Univ Hosp 1989; **Fellow:** Critical Care Medicine, Ohio State Univ Hosp 1986; **Fac Appt:** Assoc Prof S, USC Sch Med

Gruss, Joseph MD [PlS] - **Spec Exp:** Maxillofacial & Craniofacial Surgery; Facial Trauma/Fractures; Cleft Palate/Lip; Pediatric Plastic Surgery; **Hospital:** Chldns Hosp and Regl Med Ctr - Seattle, Harborview Med Ctr; **Address:** Childrens Hosp & Regional Med Ctr, 4800 Sand Point Way NE, Box 5371, Seattle, WA 98105-3901; **Phone:** 206-987-2039; **Med School:** South Africa 1969; **Resid:** Plastic Surgery, Toronto Western Hosp 1976; Plastic Surgery, Hosp for Sick Children 1976; **Fellow:** Surgical Oncology, Princess Margaret Hosp 1977; Head and Neck Surgery, Princess Margaret Hosp 1977; **Fac Appt:** Prof PlS, Univ Wash

Hardesty, Robert MD [PlS] - **Spec Exp:** Cosmetic Surgery-Face & Body; Cosmetic & Reconstructive Surgery; Body Contouring; Cosmetic Surgery-Breast; **Hospital:** Riverside Comm Hosp, Loma Linda Univ Med Ctr; **Address:** 4646 Brockton Ave, Ste 302, Riverside, CA 92506; **Phone:** 951-686-7600; **Board Cert:** Surgery 1984; Plastic Surgery 1989; **Med School:** Loma Linda Univ 1978; **Resid:** Surgery, Loma Linda Univ Med Ctr 1983; Plastic Surgery, Univ Pittsburgh 1986; **Fellow:** Pediatric Plastic Surgery, Washington Univ Chldns Hosp 1987; **Fac Appt:** Clin Prof PlS, Loma Linda Univ

Hoefflin, Steven M MD [PlS] - **Spec Exp:** Cosmetic Surgery-Face; Reconstructive Surgery; **Hospital:** St John's Hlth Ctr, Santa Monica; **Address:** 1530 Arizona Ave, Santa Monica, CA 90404-1234; **Phone:** 310-451-4733; **Board Cert:** Plastic Surgery 1978; **Med School:** UCLA 1972; **Resid:** Surgery, UCLA Med Ctr 1974; Plastic Reconstructive Surgery, UCLA Med Ctr 1977; **Fac Appt:** Assoc Clin Prof PlS, UCLA

Horowitz, Jed H MD [PlS] - **Spec Exp:** Cosmetic Surgery-Breast; Cosmetic Surgery-Face; **Hospital:** Hoag Meml Hosp Presby, Orange Coast Memorial Med Ctr; **Address:** 7677 Center Ave, Ste 401, Huntington Beach, CA 92647-3098; **Phone:** 714-902-1100; **Board Cert:** Plastic Surgery 1986; **Med School:** SUNY Buffalo 1977; **Resid:** Surgery, Grady Meml Hosp 1983; **Fellow:** Plastic Surgery, Univ Virginia 1985; **Fac Appt:** Asst Clin Prof PlS, USC Sch Med

Isik, Ferda Frank MD [PlS] - **Spec Exp:** Cosmetic Surgery-Face & Body; Breast Reconstruction; **Hospital:** Swedish Med Ctr - Seattle; **Address:** The Polyclinic, 1145 Broadway, Seattle, WA 98122; **Phone:** 206-860-4566; **Board Cert:** Surgery 2001; Plastic Surgery 2007; **Med School:** Mount Sinai Sch Med 1985; **Resid:** Surgery, Boston Univ Hosps 1990; Plastic Surgery, Univ Wash 1995; **Fellow:** Pathology, NIH / Univ Wash 1992

Jewell, Mark L MD [PlS] - **Spec Exp:** Liposuction & Body Contouring; Cosmetic Surgery-Face; Breast Reconstruction; Cosmetic Surgery-Breast; **Address:** 630 E 13th Ave, Eugene, OR 97401; **Phone:** 541-683-3234; **Board Cert:** Plastic Surgery 1981; **Med School:** Univ Kans 1973; **Resid:** Surgery, LAC-Harbor Med Ctr 1976; Plastic Surgery, Erlanger Hosp 1979; **Fellow:** Burn Surgery, LAC-USC Med Ctr 1977; **Fac Appt:** Asst Clin Prof PlS, Oregon Hlth Sci Univ

Kawamoto Jr, Henry K MD [PlS] - **Spec Exp:** Cosmetic Surgery; Craniofacial Surgery; Maxillofacial Surgery; **Hospital:** Ronald Reagan UCLA Med Ctr, St John's Hlth Ctr, Santa Monica; **Address:** 1301 20th St, Ste 460, Santa Monica, CA 90404; **Phone:** 310-829-0391; **Board Cert:** Surgery 1972; Plastic Surgery 1976; **Med School:** USC Sch Med 1964; **Resid:** Surgery, Columbia-Presby Med Ctr 1971; Plastic Surgery, NYU Med Ctr 1973; **Fellow:** Craniofacial Surgery, Dr Paul Tessier 1974; **Fac Appt:** Clin Prof PlS, UCLA

Koplin, Lawrence M MD [PlS] - **Spec Exp:** Cosmetic Surgery-Face; **Hospital:** Cedars-Sinai Med Ctr; **Address:** 465 N Roxbury Drive, Ste 800, Beverly Hills, CA 90210; **Phone:** 310-277-3223; **Board Cert:** Plastic Surgery 1985; **Med School:** Baylor Coll Med 1976; **Resid:** Surgery, Kaiser Fdn Hosp 1981; Plastic Surgery, St Joseph Hosp 1983

Leaf, Norman MD [PlS] - **Spec Exp:** Cosmetic Surgery-Face; Cosmetic Surgery-Breast; **Hospital:** Cedars-Sinai Med Ctr, Ronald Reagan UCLA Med Ctr; **Address:** 436 N Bedford, Ste 103, Beverly Hills, CA 90210-4310; **Phone:** 310-274-8001; **Board Cert:** Surgery 1973; Plastic Surgery 1974; **Med School:** Univ Chicago-Pritzker Sch Med 1966; **Resid:** Surgery, Univ Chicago Hosps 1972; Plastic Surgery, Univ Chicago Hosps 1973; **Fellow:** Research, Univ Chicago Hosp-US Pub Hlth Svc-NIH 1969; **Fac Appt:** Asst Clin Prof PlS, UCLA

Lesavoy, Malcolm A MD [PlS] - **Spec Exp:** Reconstructive Surgery; Cosmetic Surgery; Hand Surgery; **Hospital:** Ronald Reagan UCLA Med Ctr; **Address:** 16311 Ventura Blvd, Ste 555, Encino, CA 91436-4314; **Phone:** 818-986-8270; **Board Cert:** Plastic Surgery 1977; **Med School:** Ros Franklin Univ/Chicago Med Sch 1969; **Resid:** Surgery, Univ Chicago Hosps 1974; Plastic Surgery, Univ Miami Hosp/Clinics 1976; **Fac Appt:** Clin Prof PlS, UCLA

Markowitz, Bernard Lloyd MD [PlS] - **Spec Exp:** Cosmetic Surgery-Face; Craniofacial Surgery/Reconstruction; **Hospital:** Ronald Reagan UCLA Med Ctr, Cedars-Sinai Med Ctr; **Address:** 9675 Brighton Way, Ste 350, Beverly Hills, CA 90210; **Phone:** 310-205-5557; **Board Cert:** Plastic Surgery 1989; **Med School:** NYU Sch Med 1979; **Resid:** Surgery, NYU Med Ctr 1984; Plastic Surgery, NYU Med Ctr 1986; **Fellow:** Maxillofacial Surgery, Johns Hopkins Hosp 1987; Microvascular Surgery, Johns Hopkins Hosp 1987; **Fac Appt:** Clin Prof PlS, UCLA

Marten, Timothy Ja MD [PlS] - **Spec Exp:** Cosmetic Surgery-Face; Facial Rejuvenation; **Hospital:** CA Pacific Med Ctr, St Mary's Med Ctr - San Fran; **Address:** Marten Clinic of Plastic Surgery, 450 Sutter St, Ste 2222, San Francisco, CA 94108-4207; **Phone:** 415-677-9937; **Board Cert:** Plastic Surgery 1993; **Med School:** UC Davis 1982; **Resid:** Surgery, Kaiser Fdn Hosp 1987; Plastic Surgery, Univ Illinois Chicago Hosp 1989; **Fellow:** Cosmetic Plastic Surgery, Connell Aesthetic Network 1990; Cosmetic Plastic Surgery, Baker, Gordon, & Stuzin

Miller, Timothy A MD [PlS] - **Spec Exp:** Cosmetic Surgery-Face; Eyelid Cancer & Reconstruction; Skin Cancer; Nasal Reconstruction; **Hospital:** Ronald Reagan UCLA Med Ctr; **Address:** UCLA Med Ctr, Div Plastic Surg, 200 UCLA Med Plaza, Ste 465, Los Angeles, CA 90095-8344; **Phone:** 310-825-5644; **Board Cert:** Surgery 1971; Plastic Surgery 1973; **Med School:** UCLA 1963; **Resid:** Surgery, Johns Hopkins Hosp; Thoracic Surgery, UCLA Med Ctr 1969; **Fellow:** Plastic Surgery, Univ Pittsburgh 1971; **Fac Appt:** Prof S, UCLA

Nichter, Larry S MD [PlS] - **Spec Exp:** Breast Reconstruction & Augmentation; Cosmetic Surgery-Face; Liposuction & Body Contouring; Hand Surgery; **Hospital:** Hoag Meml Hosp Presby, Orange Coast Memorial Med Ctr; **Address:** 7677 Center Ave, Ste 401, Huntington Beach, CA 92647-3098; **Phone:** 714-902-1100; **Board Cert:** Plastic Surgery 1986; **Med School:** Boston Univ 1978; **Resid:** Surgery, UCLA Medical Ctr 1982; Plastic Surgery, Univ Virginia Med Ctr 1985; **Fellow:** Hand & Microvascular Surgery, Univ Virginia 1983; Craniofacial Surgery, Univ Virginia 1985; **Fac Appt:** Clin Prof PlS, Univ SC Sch Med

Plastic Surgery

Paul, Malcolm D MD [PIS] - **Spec Exp:** Cosmetic Surgery-Face; Cosmetic Surgery-Breast; Liposuction & Body Contouring; **Hospital:** Hoag Meml Hosp Presby; **Address:** 1401 Avocado Ave, Ste 810, Newport Beach, CA 92660-8708; **Phone:** 949-760-5047; **Board Cert:** Plastic Surgery 1976; **Med School:** Univ MD Sch Med 1969; **Resid:** Surgery, Geo Wash Med Ctr 1973; Plastic Surgery, Geo Wash Med Ctr 1975; **Fac Appt:** Clin Prof S, UC Irvine

Rand, Richard Pierce MD [PIS] - **Spec Exp:** Cosmetic Surgery-Face; Cosmetic Surgery-Breast; Abdominoplasty; **Hospital:** Overlake Hosp Med Ctr; **Address:** 1135 116th Ave NE, Ste 630, Bellevue, WA 98004-4623; **Phone:** 425-688-8828; **Board Cert:** Surgery 1998; Plastic Surgery 1991; **Med School:** Univ Mich Med Sch 1981; **Resid:** Surgery, Tufts-New England Med Ctr 1986; Plastic Surgery, Emory Univ Hosp 1989; **Fellow:** Craniofacial Surgery, Univ Miami 1989; **Fac Appt:** Assoc Prof S, Univ Wash

Reinisch, John F MD [PIS] - **Spec Exp:** Ear Reconstruction/Microtia; Cleft Palate/Lip; Craniofacial Surgery/Reconstruction; **Hospital:** Cedars-Sinai Med Ctr; **Address:** 250 N Robertson Blvd, Ste 506, Beverly Hills, CA 90211; **Phone:** 310-385-6090; **Board Cert:** Plastic Surgery 1980; **Med School:** Harvard Med Sch 1970; **Resid:** Surgery, Univ Mich Med Ctr 1975; Plastic Surgery, Univ Virginia Hosp 1978; **Fac Appt:** Prof S, USC Sch Med

Ristow, Brunno MD [PIS] - **Spec Exp:** Cosmetic Surgery-Face; Facial Plastic & Reconstructive Surgery; Rhinoplasty; Nasal Reconstruction; **Hospital:** CA Pacific Med Ctr - Pacific Campus; **Address:** 2100 Webster St, Ste 501, San Francisco, CA 94115-2381; **Phone:** 415-202-1507; **Board Cert:** Plastic Surgery 1975; **Med School:** Brazil 1966; **Resid:** Surgery, NY Hosp-Cornell Med Ctr 1971; Plastic Surgery, NYU Med Ctr 1973; **Fellow:** Plastic Surgery, NYU Med Ctr 1968

Romano, James John MD [PIS] - **Spec Exp:** Cosmetic Surgery; Cosmetic Surgery-Breast; Rhinoplasty; **Hospital:** Seton Med Ctr, CA Pacific Med Ctr - CA Campus; **Address:** 126 Post St, Ste 618, San Francisco, CA 94108; **Phone:** 415-981-3911; **Board Cert:** Plastic Surgery 1990; **Med School:** Eastern VA Med Sch 1980; **Resid:** Surgery, Georgetown Univ Hosp 1985; Plastic Surgery, Johns Hopkins Hosp 1988; **Fac Appt:** Asst Prof PIS, USC Sch Med

Rosenberg, Howard L MD [PIS] - **Spec Exp:** Cosmetic Surgery-Breast; Cosmetic Surgery-Face; Liposuction; **Hospital:** El Camino Hosp/Camino Hlthcare Sys; **Address:** 2204 Grant Rd, Ste 201, Mountain View, CA 94040; **Phone:** 650-961-2652; **Board Cert:** Surgery 1975; Plastic Surgery 1977; **Med School:** Johns Hopkins Univ 1969; **Resid:** Surgery, UCLA Med Ctr 1974; Plastic Surgery, Stanford Univ Med Ctr 1976; **Fac Appt:** Asst Clin Prof PIS, Stanford Univ

Sherman, Randolph MD [PIS] - **Spec Exp:** Facial Paralysis; Breast Reconstruction; Limb Surgery/Reconstruction; **Hospital:** USC Univ Hosp - R K Eamer Med Plz, Cedars-Sinai Med Ctr; **Address:** 1510 San Pablo St, Ste 415, Los Angeles, CA 90033; **Phone:** 323-442-6482; **Board Cert:** Surgery 2004; Plastic Surgery 1986; Hand Surgery 2000; **Med School:** Univ MO-Columbia Sch Med 1977; **Resid:** Surgery, UCSF Hosps 1981; Surgery, State Univ of New York 1983; **Fellow:** Plastic Surgery, USC Med Ctr 1985; **Fac Appt:** Prof S, USC Sch Med

Singer, Robert MD [PIS] - **Spec Exp:** Cosmetic Surgery-Face; Cosmetic Surgery-Breast; Liposuction & Body Contouring; **Hospital:** Scripps Meml Hosp - La Jolla; **Address:** 9834 Genesee Ave, Ste 100, La Jolla, CA 92037-1214; **Phone:** 858-455-0290; **Board Cert:** Plastic Surgery 1977; **Med School:** SUNY Buffalo 1967; **Resid:** Surgery, Stanford Med Ctr 1969; Plastic Surgery, Vanderbilt Univ Hosp 1976; **Fellow:** Neurological Surgery, Rigs Hosp-Kommunes Hosp 1976

Stevenson, Thomas R MD [PIS] - **Spec Exp:** Breast Reconstruction; Cosmetic Surgery-Face; Cosmetic Surgery-Breast; **Hospital:** UC Davis Med Ctr, Sutter Gen Hosp; **Address:** 3301 C St, Ste 1100, Sacramento, CA 95816; **Phone:** 916-734-4323; **Board Cert:** Plastic Surgery 1983; Hand Surgery 1994; Surgery 2003; **Med School:** Univ Kans 1972; **Resid:** Surgery, Univ Virginia Hosp 1978; Plastic Surgery, Emory Univ Hosp 1982; **Fac Appt:** Prof PIS, UC Davis

Wells, James H MD [PlS] - **Spec Exp:** Cleft Palate/Lip; Breast Surgery; **Hospital:** Long Beach Meml Med Ctr; **Address:** 2880 Atlantic Ave, Ste 290, Long Beach, CA 90806; **Phone:** 562-595-6543; **Board Cert:** Plastic Surgery 1978; **Med School:** Univ Tex Med Br, Galveston 1966; **Resid:** Surgery, Ochsner Fdn Hosp 1971; Plastic Surgery, Univ Virginia Hosp 1975

Cleveland Clinic

Plastic Surgery

Cleveland Clinic Department of Plastic Surgery, part of the Dermatology and Plastic Surgery Institute, offers a full array of subspecialized care for adult and pediatric patients.

The department has focused on minimally invasive techniques in facial cosmetic surgery. This includes alternatives to face and necklift surgery, short-scar facelifts and minimally invasive facelift techniques. Cleveland Clinic plastic surgeons offer numerous methods of breast reconstruction that can be performed either at the time of mastectomy or as a secondary procedure. These techniques include breast implants and expanders; pedicled transverse rectus abdominis myocutaneous (TRAM) flaps (using abdominal skin and muscle); and free-tissue transfers such as deep inferior epigastric perforator (DIEP) flap. The DIEP flap minimizes injury to the abdominal wall while providing an ideal breast reconstruction using the patient's own tissue.

Cleveland Clinic plastic surgeons offer expert diagnostic and management options including:

- Facial cosmetic surgery
- Reconstructive breast surgery
- Reconstruction after cancer
- Cosmetic breast surgery
- Body Contouring
- Liposuction
- Hand surgery
- Pediatric surgery and craniofacial surgery
- Microsurgery
- Complex wound repair

In addition to standard body contouring techniques including abdominoplasty and a wide variety of liposuction techniques, the department is particularly interested in plastic surgery after significant weight loss.

The department also includes a team of surgeons adept at handling all types of traumatic, congenital and work-related hand, peripheral nerve and upper-extremity problems.

Pediatric surgery and craniofacial surgery are strong specialties in this department.

For more information about the Cleveland Clinic Department of Plastic Surgery, to schedule a second opinion or to learn about assistance for out-of-town patients, call 800.890.2467 or visit clevelandclinic.org/plasticstopdocs.

Cleveland Clinic Department of Plastic Surgery
9500 Euclid Avenue / AC311 | Cleveland OH 44195

Preventive & Occupational Medicine

A preventive medicine specialist focuses on the health of individuals and defined populations in order to protect, promote and maintain health and well-being, and to prevent disease, disability and premature death. A preventive medicine physician may be a specialist in general preventive medicine, public health, occupational medicine, or aerospace medicine. This specialist works with large population groups as well as with individual patients to promote health and understand the risks of disease, injury, disability, and death, seeking to modify and eliminate these risks.

Training Required: Three years

OCCUPATIONAL MEDICINE

New England

Cullen, Mark R MD [OM] - **Spec Exp:** Mesothelioma; **Hospital:** Yale-New Haven Hosp; **Address:** 135 College St, Ste 392, New Haven, CT 06510; **Phone:** 203-785-6434; **Board Cert:** Internal Medicine 1979; Occupational Medicine 1986; **Med School:** Yale Univ 1976; **Resid:** Internal Medicine, Yale-New Haven Hosp 1979; **Fac Appt:** Prof Med, Yale Univ

Mid Atlantic

Brandt-Rauf, Paul W MD [OM] - **Spec Exp:** Occupational Medicine; Environmental Medicine; **Address:** Columbia Univ Sch Public Hlth, Dept Env Hlth Sci, 60 Haven Ave, Ste B1 - rm 106, New York, NY 10032-2604; **Phone:** 212-305-3464; **Board Cert:** Internal Medicine 1984; Occupational Medicine 1986; **Med School:** Columbia P&S 1979; **Resid:** Pathology, Columbia Presby Hosp 1981; Internal Medicine, Georgetown Univ Hosp 1983; **Fellow:** Occupational Medicine, Columbia Presby Hosp 1984; **Fac Appt:** Prof OM, Columbia P&S

Gochfeld, Michael MD/PhD [OM] - **Spec Exp:** Environmental Medicine; Chemical Exposure; Mercury Toxic Exposure; **Hospital:** Robert Wood Johnson Univ Hosp - New Brunswick; **Address:** Enviro & Occupational Health - EOHSI, 170 Frelinghuysen Rd, Ste 200, Piscataway, NJ 08854; **Phone:** 732-445-0123 x627; **Board Cert:** Occupational Medicine 1983; **Med School:** Albert Einstein Coll Med 1965; **Resid:** Behavioral Medicine, Rockefeller Univ 1977; **Fac Appt:** Prof OM, UMDNJ-RW Johnson Med Sch

Landrigan, Philip MD [OM] - **Spec Exp:** Environmental Health in Children; **Hospital:** Mount Sinai Med Ctr (page 64); **Address:** Dept of Comm & Prev Med, One Gustave L Levy Pl, Box 1057, New York, NY 10029-6500; **Phone:** 212-824-7018; **Board Cert:** Pediatrics 1973; Public Health & Genl Preventive Med 1979; Occupational Medicine 1983; **Med School:** Harvard Med Sch 1967; **Resid:** Internal Medicine, Metro Genl Hosp 1968; Pediatrics, Chldns Hosp 1970; **Fellow:** Epidemiology, Ctrs for Disease Control 1973; Occupational Medicine, Univ London 1977; **Fac Appt:** Prof Ped, Mount Sinai Sch Med

West Coast and Pacific

Harber, Philip I MD [OM] - **Spec Exp:** Occupational Medicine; Environmental Medicine; **Hospital:** Ronald Reagan UCLA Med Ctr; **Address:** UCLA Med Ctr, Dept Occupational Med, 10880 Wilshire Blvd, Ste 1800, Los Angeles, CA 90024; **Phone:** 310-794-8144; **Board Cert:** Internal Medicine 1979; Pulmonary Disease 1980; Occupational Medicine 1982; **Med School:** Univ Pennsylvania 1972; **Resid:** Internal Medicine, Georgetown Univ Med Ctr 1978; Occupational Medicine, Johns Hopkins Hosp 1980; **Fellow:** Pulmonary Disease, Johns Hopkins Hosp 1980; **Fac Appt:** Assoc Prof Med, UCLA

PREVENTIVE MEDICINE

Mid Atlantic

Cahill, John MD [PrM] - **Spec Exp:** Tropical Diseases; International Health; Disaster Relief Medicine; **Hospital:** St Luke's - Roosevelt Hosp Ctr - Roosevelt Div (page 57), St Luke's - Roosevelt Hosp Ctr - St Luke's Hosp (page 57); **Address:** 425 W 59th St, Ste 8A, New York, NY 10019; **Phone:** 212-492-5500; **Board Cert:** Emergency Medicine 2001; **Med School:** Mount Sinai Sch Med 1996; **Resid:** Emergency Medicine, Rhode Island Hosp 1997; Emergency Medicine, Rhode Island Hosp 2000; **Fellow:** Tropical Medicine, Royal Coll Surgeons 1998; **Fac Appt:** Asst Clin Prof Med, Columbia P&S

Hoffman, Robert S MD [PrM] - **Spec Exp:** Poison Control; Bioterrorism Preparedness; **Hospital:** NYU Med Ctr (page 68), Bellevue Hosp Ctr; **Address:** NY Poison Control Ctr, 455 1st Ave, rm 123, New York, NY 10016; **Phone:** 212-340-4494; **Board Cert:** Internal Medicine 1987; Emergency Medicine 2005; Medical Toxicology 1999; **Med School:** NYU Sch Med 1984; **Resid:** Internal Medicine, NYU Med Ctr 1987; **Fellow:** Medical Toxicology, NYU Med Ctr 1989; **Fac Appt:** Asst Clin Prof EM, NYU Sch Med

Lane, Dorothy S MD [PrM] - **Spec Exp:** Women's Health; Cancer Prevention; Health Promotion & Disease Prevention; **Hospital:** Stony Brook Univ Med Ctr; **Address:** Stony Brook Univ Sch Med, HSC L2, rm 142, Stony Brook, NY 11794-8222; **Phone:** 631-444-2094; **Board Cert:** Public Health & Genl Preventive Med 1970; Family Medicine 2000; **Med School:** Columbia P&S 1965; **Resid:** Public Health & Genl Preventive Med, NY Health Dept 1968; **Fac Appt:** Prof PrM, SUNY Stony Brook

Pearson, Thomas A MD/PhD [PrM] - **Spec Exp:** Preventive Cardiology; Cholesterol/Lipid Disorders; **Hospital:** Univ of Rochester Strong Meml Hosp; **Address:** 601 Elmwood Ave, Box 644, Rochester, NY 14642; **Phone:** 585-341-7100; **Board Cert:** Internal Medicine 1983; Preventive Medicine 1986; **Med School:** Johns Hopkins Univ 1976; **Resid:** Preventive Medicine, Johns Hopkins Hosp 1979; Internal Medicine, Johns Hopkins Hosp 1980; **Fellow:** Cardiovascular Disease, Johns Hopkins Hosp 1983; **Fac Appt:** Prof PrM, Univ Rochester

Weiss, Stanley H MD [PrM] - **Spec Exp:** Cancer Epidemiology & Control; AIDS Related Infections; Bioterrorism Preparedness; Infections in Cancer Patients; **Hospital:** UMDNJ-Univ Hosp-Newark; **Address:** NJ Medical School-UMDNJ, 30 Bergen St, ADMC16, Ste 1614, Newark, NJ 07107-3000; **Phone:** 973-972-4623; **Board Cert:** Internal Medicine 1981; Medical Oncology 1985; **Med School:** Harvard Med Sch 1978; **Resid:** Internal Medicine, Montefiore Med Ctr 1981; **Fellow:** Medical Oncology, National Cancer Inst 1985; Epidemiology, National Cancer Inst 1987; **Fac Appt:** Prof PrM, UMDNJ-NJ Med Sch, Newark

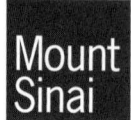
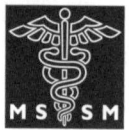

Psychiatry

A psychiatrist specializes in the prevention, diagnosis and treatment of mental, addictive and emotional disorders such as schizophrenia and other psychotic disorders, mood disorders, anxiety disorders, substance-related disorders, sexual and gender identity disorders and adjustment disorders. The psychiatrist is able to understand the biologic, psychologic and social components of illness, and therefore is uniquely prepared to treat the whole person. A psychiatrist is qualified to order diagnostic laboratory tests and to prescribe medications, evaluate and treat psychologic and interpersonal problems and to intervene with families who are coping with stress, crises and other problems in living.

Training Required: Four years

Certification in one of the following subspecialties requires additional training and examination.

Addiction Psychiatry: A psychiatrist who focuses on the evaluation and treatment of individuals with alcohol, drug, or other substance-related disorders and of individuals with the dual diagnosis of substance-related and other psychiatric disorders.

Child and Adolescent Psychiatry: A psychiatrist with additional training in the diagnosis and treatment of developmental, behavioral, emotional and mental disorders of childhood and adolescence.

Geriatric Psychiatry: A psychiatrist with expertise in the prevention, evaluation, diagnosis and treatment of mental and emotional disorders in the elderly. The geriatric psychiatrist seeks to improve the psychiatric care of the elderly both in health and in disease.

PSYCHIATRY

New England

Block, Susan D MD [Psyc] - **Spec Exp:** Psychiatry in Cancer; **Hospital:** Dana-Farber Cancer Inst; **Address:** Dana Farber Cancer Inst, 44 Binney St, SW 411, Boston, MA 02115; **Phone:** 617-632-6181; **Board Cert:** Psychiatry 1984; Internal Medicine 1981; **Med School:** Case West Res Univ 1977; **Resid:** Internal Medicine, Beth Israel Hosp 1980; Psychiatry, Beth Israel Hosp 1982; **Fac Appt:** Assoc Prof Psyc, Harvard Med Sch

Friedman, Matthew J MD/PhD [Psyc] - **Spec Exp:** Post Traumatic Stress Disorder; Psychopharmacology; Anxiety & Mood Disorders; **Hospital:** VA Aff Med Ctr - White River Junction, Dartmouth - Hitchcock Med Ctr; **Address:** National Center for PTSD, VA Medical Ctr, 215 N Main St, White River Junction, VT 05009; **Phone:** 802-296-5132; **Board Cert:** Psychiatry 1976; **Med School:** Univ KY Coll Med 1976; **Resid:** Psychiatry, Mass Genl Hosp 1972; Psychiatry, Dartmouth Hitchcock Med Ctr 1973; **Fac Appt:** Prof Psyc, Dartmouth Med Sch

Goff, Donald C MD [Psyc] - **Spec Exp:** Schizophrenia; Psychopharmacology; **Hospital:** Mass Genl Hosp; **Address:** Erich Lindemann Mental Health Ctr, Freedom Trail Clinic, 25 Staniford St, Boston, MA 02114; **Phone:** 617-912-7800; **Board Cert:** Psychiatry 1986; **Med School:** UCLA 1980; **Resid:** Psychiatry, Mass Genl Hosp 1984; **Fellow:** Psychopharmacology, Tufts New Engl Med Ctr 1985; **Fac Appt:** Assoc Prof Psyc, Harvard Med Sch

Greenberg, Donna B MD [Psyc] - **Spec Exp:** Psychiatry in Cancer; **Hospital:** Mass Genl Hosp; **Address:** Mass General Hospital, Warren 605, 55 Fruit St, Boston, MA 02114-2696; **Phone:** 617-726-2984; **Board Cert:** Internal Medicine 1978; Psychiatry 1990; **Med School:** Univ Rochester 1975; **Resid:** Internal Medicine, Boston City Hosp 1978; Psychiatry, Mass Genl Hosp 1989; **Fellow:** Psychiatry, Mass Genl Hosp 1979; **Fac Appt:** Assoc Prof Psyc, Harvard Med Sch

Gunderson, John G MD [Psyc] - **Spec Exp:** Personality Disorders; Personality Disorders-Borderline; Psychotherapy; **Hospital:** McLean Hosp; **Address:** McLean Hospital, 115 Mill St, Belmont, MA 02478-9106; **Phone:** 617-855-2293; **Board Cert:** Psychiatry 1974; **Med School:** Harvard Med Sch 1967; **Resid:** Psychiatry, Mass Mental Hlth Ctr 1971; **Fac Appt:** Prof Psyc, Harvard Med Sch

Herman, John B MD [Psyc] - **Spec Exp:** Depression; Anxiety Disorders; **Hospital:** Mass Genl Hosp; **Address:** Mass Genl Hosp, Dept Psychiatry, 55 Fruit St, Bulfinch 351, Boston, MA 02114-3139; **Phone:** 617-726-2993; **Board Cert:** Psychiatry 1987; **Med School:** Univ Wisc 1980; **Resid:** Psychiatry, Mass Genl Hosp 1984; **Fac Appt:** Asst Prof Psyc, Harvard Med Sch

Jacobson, Alan M MD [Psyc] - **Spec Exp:** Depression in Diabetes; **Hospital:** Beth Israel Deaconess Med Ctr - Boston; **Address:** Joslin Diabetes Center/Joslin Clinic, One Joslin Pl, Boston, MA 02215; **Phone:** 617-732-2440; **Board Cert:** Psychiatry 1975; **Med School:** Univ Chicago-Pritzker Sch Med 1969; **Resid:** Psychiatry, Mass Genl Hosp 1973; **Fac Appt:** Prof Psyc, Harvard Med Sch

Jenike, Michael Andrew MD [Psyc] - **Spec Exp:** Obsessive-Compulsive Disorder; Geriatric Psychiatry; **Hospital:** Mass Genl Hosp; **Address:** Obsessive Compulsive Disorders Unit, 185 Cambridge St, Ste 2200, Boston, MA 02114; **Phone:** 617-726-6766; **Board Cert:** Psychiatry 1984; **Med School:** Univ Okla Coll Med 1978; **Resid:** Psychiatry, Mass Genl Hosp 1982; **Fellow:** Psychiatry, Harvard Med Sch; Psychiatry, Mass Genl Hosp; **Fac Appt:** Prof Psyc, Harvard Med Sch

McGlashan, Thomas MD [Psyc] - **Spec Exp:** Schizophrenia-Early Detection/Treatment; Personality Disorders; **Hospital:** Connecticut Mental Hlth Ctr, Yale-New Haven Hosp; **Address:** Yale Univ Sch Med, Dept Psychiatry, 301 Cedar St, New Haven, CT 06519; **Phone:** 203-737-2077; **Board Cert:** Psychiatry 1973; **Med School:** Univ Pennsylvania 1967; **Resid:** Psychiatry, Mass Mental Hlth Ctr 1971; **Fac Appt:** Prof Psyc, Yale Univ

Phillips, Katharine A MD [Psyc] - **Spec Exp:** Body Dysmorphic Disorder (BDD); Eating Disorders; **Hospital:** Butler Hosp; **Address:** Butler Hosp, The Body Image Prgm, 345 Blackstone Blvd, Providence, RI 02906; **Phone:** 401-455-6490; **Board Cert:** Psychiatry 1992; **Med School:** Dartmouth Med Sch 1987; **Resid:** Psychiatry, McLean Hosp 1991; **Fac Appt:** Prof Psyc, Brown Univ

Pitman, Roger Keith MD [Psyc] - **Spec Exp:** Post Traumatic Stress Disorder; **Hospital:** Mass Genl Hosp; **Address:** Mass Genl Hosp, Rm 2616, Bldg 149, 13th St, Charlestown, MA 02129; **Phone:** 617-726-5333; **Board Cert:** Psychiatry 1975; Forensic Psychiatry 2004; **Med School:** Univ VT Coll Med 1969; **Resid:** Psychiatry, Tufts-New England Med Ctr/VA Med Ctr 1973; **Fellow:** Behavioral Neurology, Beth Israel Hosp/Harvard; **Fac Appt:** Prof Psyc, Harvard Med Sch

Price, Lawrence H MD [Psyc] - **Spec Exp:** Mood Disorders; Anxiety Disorders; Depression; **Hospital:** Butler Hosp; **Address:** Butler Hospital, Dept Psychiatry, 345 Blackstone Blvd, Providence, RI 02906; **Phone:** 401-455-6533; **Board Cert:** Psychiatry 1983; **Med School:** Univ Mich Med Sch 1978; **Resid:** Psychiatry, Yale-New Haven Hosp 1982; **Fellow:** Psychiatry, Yale-New Haven Hosp 1983; **Fac Appt:** Prof Psyc, Brown Univ

Rasmussen, Steven A MD [Psyc] - **Spec Exp:** Obsessive-Compulsive Disorder; **Hospital:** Butler Hosp; **Address:** Butler Hosp, 345 Blackstone Blvd, Providence, RI 02906; **Phone:** 401-455-6209; **Board Cert:** Psychiatry 1983; **Med School:** Brown Univ 1977; **Resid:** Psychiatry, Yale Univ 1981; **Fac Appt:** Assoc Prof Psyc, Brown Univ

Rauch, Paula K MD [Psyc] - **Spec Exp:** Psychiatry in Childhood Cancer; Children/Families facing Severe Illness; Parent Guidance in Parental Cancer; **Hospital:** Mass Genl Hosp; **Address:** Mass General Hosp, Dept Child Psychiatry, 32 Fruit St, Yawkey 6, Boston, MA 02114; **Phone:** 617-724-5600; **Board Cert:** Psychiatry 1990; Child & Adolescent Psychiatry 1991; **Med School:** Univ Cincinnati 1981; **Resid:** Psychiatry, Mass Genl Hosp 1984; **Fac Appt:** Asst Prof Psyc, Harvard Med Sch

Rosenbaum, Jerrold F MD [Psyc] - **Spec Exp:** Anxiety & Mood Disorders; **Hospital:** Mass Genl Hosp; **Address:** 55 Fruit St, Bulfinch 351, Boston, MA 02114; **Phone:** 617-726-3482; **Board Cert:** Psychiatry 1978; **Med School:** Yale Univ 1973; **Resid:** Psychiatry, Mass Genl Hosp 1977; **Fac Appt:** Prof Psyc, Harvard Med Sch

Salzman, Carl MD [Psyc] - **Spec Exp:** Psychopharmacology; Geriatric Psychiatry; Psychotherapy; **Hospital:** MA Mental Hlth Ctr, Beth Israel Deaconess Med Ctr - Boston; **Address:** Havard Medical School, Dept Psychiatry, 25 Shattuck St, Boston, MA 02115; **Phone:** 617-998-5006; **Board Cert:** Psychiatry 1970; **Med School:** SUNY Upstate Med Univ 1963; **Resid:** Psychiatry, Mass Mental Hlth Ctr 1967; Psychiatry, Natl Inst Mental Hlth 1969; **Fac Appt:** Prof Psyc, Harvard Med Sch

Shapiro, Edward R MD [Psyc] - **Spec Exp:** Psychoanalysis; **Hospital:** Austen Riggs Ctr; **Address:** Austen Riggs Ctr, 25 Main St, PO Box 962, Stockbridge, MA 01262; **Phone:** 413-298-5511; **Board Cert:** Psychiatry 1974; **Med School:** Harvard Med Sch 1968; **Resid:** Psychiatry, Mass Mental Hlth Ctr 1972; **Fellow:** Natl Inst Mental Hlth 1974; **Fac Appt:** Assoc Clin Prof Psyc, Harvard Med Sch

Psychiatry

van der Kolk, Bessel MD [Psyc] - **Spec Exp:** Post Traumatic Stress Disorder; Child Abuse; **Hospital:** Boston Med Ctr, Arbour Hospital - Boston; **Address:** 16 Braddock Park, Boston, MA 02116-5804; **Phone:** 617-247-1720; **Board Cert:** Psychiatry 1976; **Med School:** Univ Chicago-Pritzker Sch Med 1970; **Resid:** Psychiatry, Harvard Med Sch 1974; **Fac Appt:** Prof Psyc, Boston Univ

Mid Atlantic

Akhtar, Salman MD [Psyc] - **Spec Exp:** Psychoanalysis; **Hospital:** Thomas Jefferson Univ Hosp; **Address:** Jefferson Med College, Dept Psychiatry, 833 Chestnut St, Ste 210, Philadelphia, PA 19107; **Phone:** 215-955-2547; **Board Cert:** Psychiatry 1977; **Med School:** India 1968; **Resid:** Psychiatry, UMDNJ Med Ctr 1974; Psychiatry, Univ Virginia Med Ctr 1976; **Fellow:** Psychoanalysis, Philadelphia Psych Inst 1986

Appelbaum, Paul S MD [Psyc] - **Spec Exp:** Forensic Psychiatry; Depression; Anxiety & Mood Disorders; **Hospital:** NY-Presby Hosp/Columbia (page 66); **Address:** NY State Psychiatric Inst, 1051 Riverside Drive, rm 6714, Box 122, New York, NY 10032; **Phone:** 212-543-4184; **Board Cert:** Psychiatry 1981; Forensic Psychiatry 2004; **Med School:** Harvard Med Sch 1976; **Resid:** Psychiatry, Mass Mental Health Ctr 1980; **Fac Appt:** Prof Psyc, Columbia P&S

Basch, Samuel MD [Psyc] - **Spec Exp:** Psychopharmacology; Psychiatry in Physical Illness; Psychiatry in Cancer; Psychoanalysis; **Hospital:** Mount Sinai Med Ctr (page 64); **Address:** 10 E 85th St, Ste 1B, New York, NY 10028-0412; **Phone:** 212-427-0344; **Board Cert:** Psychiatry 1970; **Med School:** Hahnemann Univ 1961; **Resid:** Psychiatry, Mount Sinai Hosp 1965; **Fellow:** Psychoanalysis, Columbia Presby Hosp 1976; **Fac Appt:** Clin Prof Psyc, Mount Sinai Sch Med

Boronow, John Joseph MD [Psyc] - **Spec Exp:** Psychotic Disorders; Schizophrenia; **Hospital:** Sheppard Pratt Hlth Sys; **Address:** 6501 N Charles St, rm TJ-113, Towson, MD 21284; **Phone:** 410-938-4306; **Board Cert:** Psychiatry 1983; **Med School:** Yale Univ 1977; **Resid:** Psychiatry, New York Hosp 1981; **Fellow:** Psychopharmacology, Natl Inst Mntl Hlth 1983; **Fac Appt:** Assoc Clin Prof Psyc, Univ MD Sch Med

Brandt, Harry A MD [Psyc] - **Spec Exp:** Eating Disorders; **Hospital:** St Joseph Med Ctr, Sheppard Pratt Hlth Sys; **Address:** Ctr Eating Disorders, 6535 N Charles St, Ste 300, Baltimore, MD 21204; **Phone:** 410-938-5252; **Board Cert:** Psychiatry 1989; **Med School:** Univ MD Sch Med 1983; **Resid:** Psychiatry, Univ Maryland Hosp 1986; **Fellow:** Biological Psychiatry, Natl Inst Mental Hlth 1988; **Fac Appt:** Assoc Clin Prof Psyc, Univ MD Sch Med

Breitbart, William MD [Psyc] - **Spec Exp:** Psychiatry in Cancer; AIDS Related Cancers; Pain-Cancer; Palliative Care; **Hospital:** Meml Sloan-Kettering Cancer Ctr; **Address:** 1275 York Avenue, New York, NY 10065; **Phone:** 800-525-2225; **Board Cert:** Internal Medicine 1982; Psychiatry 1986; Psychosomatic Medicine 2005; **Med School:** Albert Einstein Coll Med 1978; **Resid:** Internal Medicine, Bronx Muni Hosp Ctr 1982; Psychiatry, Bronx Muni Hosp Ctr 1984; **Fellow:** Psychiatric Oncology, Meml Sloan Kettering Cancer Ctr 1986; **Fac Appt:** Prof Psyc, Cornell Univ-Weill Med Coll

Brodkin, Edward S MD [Psyc] - **Spec Exp:** Autism; Learning Disorders (Social); Asperger's Syndrome; **Hospital:** Hosp Univ Penn - UPHS (page 60); **Address:** Univ Penn Sch Med, Translational Rsch Lab, 125 S 31st St, rm 2220, Philadelphia, PA 19104-3403; **Phone:** 215-746-0118; **Board Cert:** Psychiatry 2006; **Med School:** Harvard Med Sch 1992; **Resid:** Psychiatry, Yale-New Haven Hosp 1996; **Fellow:** Neurological Biology, Yale Univ Sch Med 1998; Genetics, Princeton Univ 2002; **Fac Appt:** Asst Prof Psyc, Univ Pennsylvania

America's Top Doctors® 8th Edition

Bronheim, Harold MD [Psyc] - **Spec Exp:** Psychiatry in Body Image Awareness; Relationship Problems; Psychiatry in Physical Illness; Liaison Psychiatry; **Hospital:** Mount Sinai Med Ctr (page 64); **Address:** 1155 Park Ave, New York, NY 10128-1209; **Phone:** 212-996-5777; **Board Cert:** Psychiatry 1985; Internal Medicine 1986; Psychosomatic Medicine 2005; Geriatric Psychiatry 2001; **Med School:** SUNY Hlth Sci Ctr 1980; **Resid:** Psychiatry, Mount Sinai Hosp 1984; **Fellow:** Internal Medicine, Beth Israel Hosp 1985; **Fac Appt:** Clin Prof Psyc, Mount Sinai Sch Med

Buysse, Daniel J MD [Psyc] - **Spec Exp:** Sleep Disorders; **Hospital:** UPMC Presby, Pittsburgh; **Address:** 3811 O'Hara St, rm E-1127, Pittsburgh, PA 15213; **Phone:** 412-246-6413; **Board Cert:** Psychiatry 1988; Sleep Medicine 2007; **Med School:** Univ Mich Med Sch 1983; **Resid:** Psychiatry, Western Psych Inst 1987; **Fellow:** Sleep Medicine, Univ of Pittsburgh; **Fac Appt:** Asst Prof Psyc, Univ Pittsburgh

Cohen, Mitchell Joseph MD [Psyc] - **Spec Exp:** Pain-Chronic; Psychiatry in Physical Illness; Anxiety Disorders; **Hospital:** Thomas Jefferson Univ Hosp; **Address:** 833 Chestnut St E, Ste 210B, Philadelphia, PA 19107; **Phone:** 215-955-6592; **Board Cert:** Psychiatry 1989; Pain Medicine 2002; **Med School:** Med Coll PA 1984; **Resid:** Psychiatry, Johns Hopkins Hosp 1988; **Fac Appt:** Prof Psyc, Thomas Jefferson Univ

DePaulo Jr, J Raymond MD [Psyc] - **Spec Exp:** Bipolar/Mood Disorders; Depression; **Hospital:** Johns Hopkins Hosp - Baltimore (page 61); **Address:** Johns Hopkins Hosp, Dept Psychiatry, 600 N Wolfe St, Meyer 4-113, Baltimore, MD 21287-7413; **Phone:** 410-955-3130; **Board Cert:** Psychiatry 1977; **Med School:** Johns Hopkins Univ 1972; **Resid:** Psychiatry, Johns Hopkins Hosp 1977; **Fac Appt:** Prof Psyc, Johns Hopkins Univ

Doghramji, Karl MD [Psyc] - **Spec Exp:** Sleep Disorders/Apnea; Narcolepsy; **Hospital:** Thomas Jefferson Univ Hosp; **Address:** 1015 Walnut St, Curtis Bldg Fl 3 - rm 319, Philadelphia, PA 19107; **Phone:** 215-955-6175; **Board Cert:** Psychiatry 1986; **Med School:** Thomas Jefferson Univ 1980; **Resid:** Psychiatry, Thomas Jefferson Univ Hosp 1984; **Fellow:** Sleep Medicine, Montefiore Med Ctr; **Fac Appt:** Prof Psyc, Thomas Jefferson Univ

Eaton Jr, James S MD [Psyc] - **Spec Exp:** Anxiety Disorders; Sexual Identity Issues; Depression; Diagnostic Second Opinions; **Hospital:** Georgetown Univ Hosp, G Washington Univ Hosp; **Address:** 4214 50th St NW, Washington, DC 20016; **Phone:** 202-333-5796; **Board Cert:** Psychiatry 1976; **Med School:** Tulane Univ 1962; **Resid:** Internal Medicine, Tulane Univ Med Ctr 1966; Psychiatry, Tulane Univ Med Ctr 1968; **Fellow:** Psychoanalysis, Tulane Univ Med Ctr 1973; **Fac Appt:** Clin Prof Psyc, Georgetown Univ

Eth, Spencer MD [Psyc] - **Spec Exp:** Forensic Psychiatry; Post Traumatic Stress Disorder; **Hospital:** St Vincent Cath Med Ctrs - Manhattan; **Address:** 144 W 12th St, rm 174, New York, NY 10011-8202; **Phone:** 212-604-8196; **Board Cert:** Child & Adolescent Psychiatry 1982; Geriatric Psychiatry 2000; Forensic Psychiatry 2005; Addiction Psychiatry 1998; **Med School:** UCLA 1976; **Resid:** Psychiatry, NY Cornell Med Ctr 1979; **Fellow:** Child & Adolescent Psychiatry, Cedars -Sinai Med Ctr 1981; **Fac Appt:** Prof Psyc, NY Med Coll

Fallon, Brian MD [Psyc] - **Spec Exp:** Lyme Disease; Hypochondria; Obsessive-Compulsive Disorder; Psychiatry in Physical Illness; **Hospital:** NY-Presby Hosp/Columbia (page 66); **Address:** 1051 Riverside Drive, Unit #69, New York, NY 10032; **Phone:** 212-543-5487; **Board Cert:** Psychiatry 1991; **Med School:** Columbia P&S 1985; **Resid:** Psychiatry, NY Presby-Columbia Univ 1989; **Fellow:** New York State Psychiatric Institute 1992; **Fac Appt:** Assoc Prof Psyc, Columbia P&S

Psychiatry

First, Michael B MD [Psyc] - **Spec Exp:** Psychotherapy; Psychopharmacology; Forensic Psychiatry; **Hospital:** NY-Presby Hosp/Columbia (page 66); **Address:** NY State Psychiatric Inst, Unit 60, 1051 Riverside Drive, New York, NY 10032; **Phone:** 212-543-5531; **Board Cert:** Psychiatry 1989; **Med School:** Univ Pittsburgh 1983; **Resid:** Psychiatry, NY State Psych Inst 1987; **Fellow:** Psychiatric Research, NY State Psych Inst 1988; **Fac Appt:** Clin Prof Psyc, Columbia P&S

Ganguli, Rohan MD [Psyc] - **Spec Exp:** Schizophrenia; **Hospital:** Western Psych Inst & Clin - UPMC; **Address:** Western Psychiatric Inst & Clinic, 3811 O'Hara St, Pittsburgh, PA 15213; **Phone:** 412-246-5006; **Board Cert:** Psychiatry 1980; **Med School:** India 1973; **Resid:** Psychiatry, Memorial Univ 1978; Psychiatry, Univ Pittsburgh Med Ctr 1978; **Fac Appt:** Prof Psyc, Univ Pittsburgh

Guarda, Angela S MD [Psyc] - **Spec Exp:** Eating Disorders; **Hospital:** Johns Hopkins Hosp - Baltimore (page 61); **Address:** Johns Hopkins Hosp, Eating Disorder Program, Meyer 101, 600 N Wolfe St, Baltimore, MD 21287; **Phone:** 410-614-4624; **Board Cert:** Psychiatry 2006; **Med School:** Univ MD Sch Med 1991; **Resid:** Psychiatry, Johns Hopkins Hosp 1995; **Fac Appt:** Assoc Prof Psyc, Johns Hopkins Univ

Halmi, Katherine MD [Psyc] - **Spec Exp:** Eating Disorders; **Hospital:** NY-Presby Hosp/Westchester Div (page 66); **Address:** NY Presby Hosp - Westchester Div, 21 Bloomingdale Rd, White Plains, NY 10605; **Phone:** 914-997-5875; **Board Cert:** Pediatrics 1970; Psychiatry 1977; **Med School:** Univ Iowa Coll Med 1965; **Resid:** Pediatrics, Univ Iowa Hosp 1968; Psychiatry, Univ Iowa Hosp 1972; **Fellow:** Child Development, Univ Iowa Hosp 1969; **Fac Appt:** Prof Psyc, Cornell Univ-Weill Med Coll

Haskett, Roger F MD [Psyc] - **Spec Exp:** Depression; Mood Disorders; Anxiety Disorders; **Hospital:** Western Psych Inst & Clin - UPMC; **Address:** Western Psychiatric Inst, 3811 O'Hara St, Pittsburgh, PA 15213; **Phone:** 412-586-9207; **Board Cert:** Psychiatry 1984; **Med School:** Australia 1968; **Resid:** Psychiatry, Royal Melbourne Hosp 1977; **Fellow:** Psychiatric Research, UNic Bichigan 1979; **Fac Appt:** Prof Psyc, Univ Pittsburgh

Hollander, Eric MD [Psyc] - **Spec Exp:** Obsessive-Compulsive Disorder; Anxiety Disorders; Autism; **Hospital:** Mount Sinai Med Ctr (page 64); **Address:** 300 Central Park West, Ste 1C, New York, NY 10024-1513; **Phone:** 212-873-4051; **Board Cert:** Psychiatry 1987; **Med School:** SUNY Hlth Sci Ctr 1982; **Resid:** Internal Medicine, Mount Sinai Hosp 1983; Psychiatry, Mount Sinai Hosp 1986; **Fellow:** Psychiatry, Columbia-Presby Med Ctr 1988; **Fac Appt:** Prof Psyc, Mount Sinai Sch Med

Kavey, Neil B MD [Psyc] - **Spec Exp:** Narcolepsy; Sleep Disorders/Apnea; **Hospital:** NY-Presby Hosp/Columbia (page 66); **Address:** Columbia Presby Med Ctr, Sleep Disorders Ctr, 161 Ft Washington Ave Fl 3 - rm 342, New York, NY 10032; **Phone:** 212-305-1860; **Board Cert:** Psychiatry 1976; Sleep Medicine 2003; **Med School:** Columbia P&S 1969; **Resid:** Psychiatry, Columbia Presby Med Ctr 1973; **Fac Appt:** Clin Prof Psyc, Columbia P&S

Klagsbrun, Samuel C MD [Psyc] - **Spec Exp:** Psychiatry in Cancer; Psychiatry in Terminal Illness; **Hospital:** Four Winds Hosp; **Address:** Four Winds Hospital, 800 Cross River Rd, Katonah, NY 10536; **Phone:** 914-763-8151; **Board Cert:** Psychiatry 1977; **Med School:** Ros Franklin Univ/Chicago Med Sch 1962; **Resid:** Psychiatry, Yale-New Haven Hosp 1966; **Fac Appt:** Clin Prof Psyc, Albert Einstein Coll Med

Kunkel, Elisabeth J MD [Psyc] - **Spec Exp:** Psychiatry in Cancer; Psychiatry in Physical Illness; **Hospital:** Thomas Jefferson Univ Hosp; **Address:** Thomas Jefferson Univ, 1020 Samson St, Thompson Bldg, Ste 1652, Philadelphia, PA 19107; **Phone:** 215-955-9545; **Board Cert:** Psychiatry 1989; Addiction Psychiatry 1998; Psychosomatic Medicine 2005; **Med School:** McGill Univ 1983; **Resid:** Psychiatry, NYU Med Ctr 1987; **Fellow:** Liaison Psychiatry, Meml Sloan Kettering Cancer Ctr 1989; **Fac Appt:** Prof Psyc, Jefferson Med Coll

Kupfer, David J MD [Psyc] - **Spec Exp:** Bipolar/Mood Disorders; **Hospital:** Western Psych Inst & Clin - UPMC; **Address:** Western Psychiatric Inst & Clinic, 3811 O'Hara St, Pittsburgh, PA 15213-2593; **Phone:** 412-246-6777; **Board Cert:** Psychiatry 1978; **Med School:** Yale Univ 1965; **Resid:** Psychiatry, Yale-New Haven Hosp 1970; Psychiatry, Natl Inst Mental Hlth 1969; **Fellow:** Psychiatry, Yale-New Haven Hosp 1967; **Fac Appt:** Prof Psyc, Univ Pittsburgh

Lawson, William B MD [Psyc] - **Spec Exp:** Bipolar/Mood Disorders; Addiction/Substance Abuse; Dual Diagnosis; **Hospital:** Howard Univ Hosp; **Address:** Howard Univ Hosp, Dept Psychiatry, 2041 Georgia Ave NW, Ste 5B01, Washington, DC 20060; **Phone:** 202-865-6611; **Board Cert:** Psychiatry 1984; Addiction Psychiatry 2006; **Med School:** Univ Chicago-Pritzker Sch Med 1978; **Resid:** Psychiatry, Stanford Univ Med Ctr 1981; Psychiatry, Natl Inst Mental Hlth 1982; **Fellow:** Neuropsychiatry, Natl Inst Mental Hlth 1984; **Fac Appt:** Prof Psyc, Howard Univ

Loewenstein, Richard MD [Psyc] - **Spec Exp:** Trauma Psychiatry; Dissociative Disorders; Child Abuse; **Hospital:** Sheppard Pratt Hlth Sys; **Address:** 6501 N Charles St, Ste A305, Box 6815, Baltimore, MD 21204; **Phone:** 410-938-5070; **Board Cert:** Psychiatry 1980; **Med School:** Yale Univ 1975; **Resid:** Psychiatry, Yale Affil Hosps 1979; **Fellow:** Psychiatry, NIH,NIMH-Biol Psych Br 1982; **Fac Appt:** Assoc Clin Prof Psyc, Univ MD Sch Med

Manevitz, Alan MD [Psyc] - **Spec Exp:** Marital/Family/Sex Therapy; Fibromyalgia Syndrome (FMS); Post Traumatic Stress Disorder; ADD/ADHD; **Hospital:** NY-Presby Hosp/Weill Cornell (page 66), Lenox Hill Hosp (page 62); **Address:** 60 Sutton Place South, Ste 1CN, New York, NY 10022; **Phone:** 212-751-5072; **Board Cert:** Psychiatry 1987; **Med School:** Columbia P&S 1980; **Resid:** Psychiatry, New York Hosp 1984; **Fellow:** Psychopharmacology, New York Hosp 1985; **Fac Appt:** Assoc Clin Prof Psyc, Cornell Univ-Weill Med Coll

Mann, J John MD/PhD [Psyc] - **Spec Exp:** Mood Disorders; Clinical Trials; **Hospital:** NY-Presby Hosp/Columbia (page 66); **Address:** NYS Psychiatric Institute, 1051 Riverside Drive, New York, NY 10032; **Phone:** 212-543-5571; **Board Cert:** Psychiatry 1980; **Med School:** Australia 1978; **Resid:** Psychiatry, Royal Melbourne Hosp 1976; **Fac Appt:** Prof Psyc, Columbia P&S

Marin, Deborah B MD [Psyc] - **Spec Exp:** Alzheimer's Disease; **Hospital:** Mount Sinai Med Ctr (page 64); **Address:** Mount Sinai Hospital, One Gustave L Levy Pl, Box 1068, New York, NY 10029; **Phone:** 212-241-7139; **Board Cert:** Psychiatry 1990; **Med School:** Mount Sinai Sch Med 1984; **Resid:** Psychiatry, Mount Sinai Hosp 1988; **Fellow:** Psychiatry, New York Hosp-Cornell Med Ctr 1991; **Fac Appt:** Prof Psyc, Mount Sinai Sch Med

McCann, Merle C MD [Psyc] - **Hospital:** Sheppard Pratt Hlth Sys; **Address:** Sheppard & Enoch Pratt Hosp, 6501 N Charles St,, rm PJ-111, Baltimore, MD 21204; **Phone:** 410-938-3000; **Board Cert:** Psychiatry 1986; **Med School:** Med Coll VA 1981; **Resid:** Psychiatry, Geo Wash Univ Hosp 1985; **Fac Appt:** Asst Clin Prof Psyc, Univ MD Sch Med

Oquendo, Maria A MD [Psyc] - **Spec Exp:** Bipolar/Mood Disorders-Consult; Depression-Consult; Suicidal Behavior-Consult; Cross Cultural Psychiatry; **Hospital:** NY State Psychiatric Inst; **Address:** 300 W 72nd St, Ste 1F, New York, NY 10023-2661; **Phone:** 212-721-2805; **Board Cert:** Psychiatry 1989; **Med School:** Columbia P&S 1984; **Resid:** Psychiatry, Payne Whitney Clinic 1988; **Fac Appt:** Clin Prof Psyc, Columbia P&S

Roose, Steven MD [Psyc] - **Spec Exp:** Depression in the Elderly; **Hospital:** NY-Presby Hosp/Columbia (page 66); **Address:** NY State Psychiatric Institute, 1051 Riverside Drive, New York, NY 10032; **Phone:** 212-831-8644; **Board Cert:** Psychiatry 1979; **Med School:** Mount Sinai Sch Med 1974; **Resid:** Psychiatry, NY Psychiatric Inst 1978; **Fellow:** Research, Columbia-Presby Med Ctr 1981; **Fac Appt:** Clin Prof Psyc, Columbia P&S

Psychiatry

Rosenthal, Richard N MD [Psyc] - **Spec Exp:** Anxiety & Mood Disorders; Addiction/Substance Abuse; **Hospital:** St Luke's - Roosevelt Hosp Ctr - Roosevelt Div (page 57), Beth Israel Med Ctr - Petrie Division (page 57); **Address:** 1090 Amerstdam Ave Fl 16 - Ste G, New York, NY 10025; **Phone:** 212-523-5366; **Board Cert:** Psychiatry 1985; Addiction Psychiatry 2003; **Med School:** SUNY Hlth Sci Ctr 1980; **Resid:** Psychiatry, Mount Sinai Hosp 1984; **Fac Appt:** Prof Psyc, Columbia P&S

Rosse, Richard B MD [Psyc] - **Hospital:** VA Med Ctr - Washington; **Address:** Mental Health Dept (116A), 50 Irving St NW, Washington, DC 20422-0001; **Phone:** 202-745-8156; **Board Cert:** Psychiatry 1986; **Med School:** Univ MD Sch Med 1980; **Resid:** Psychiatry, Georgetown Univ Med Ctr 1984; **Fac Appt:** Prof Psyc, Howard Univ

Roth, Andrew J MD [Psyc] - **Spec Exp:** Psychiatry of Prostate Cancer; Bereavement/Traumatic Grief; **Hospital:** Meml Sloan-Kettering Cancer Ctr; **Address:** 641 Lexington Ave Fl 7, New York, NY 10022; **Phone:** 646-888-0024; **Board Cert:** Psychiatry 1993; Psychosomatic Medicine 2005; **Med School:** NY Med Coll 1988; **Resid:** Psychiatry, Mt Sinai Med Ctr 1992; **Fellow:** Liaison Psychiatry, Meml Sloan-Kettering Canc Ctr 1994

Sadock, Virginia MD [Psyc] - **Spec Exp:** Psychotherapy; Sexual Dysfunction; Anxiety & Depression; Marital/Family/Sex Therapy; **Hospital:** NYU Med Ctr (page 68); **Address:** 4 E 89th St, Ste 1E, New York, NY 10128; **Phone:** 212-427-0885; **Board Cert:** Psychiatry 1975; **Med School:** NY Med Coll 1970; **Resid:** Psychiatry, Metropolitan Hosp 1973; **Fac Appt:** Clin Prof Psyc, NYU Sch Med

Samberg, Eslee MD [Psyc] - **Spec Exp:** Psychoanalysis; **Hospital:** NY-Presby Hosp/Weill Cornell (page 66); **Address:** 2211 Broadway, Ste 1H, New York, NY 10024-6263; **Phone:** 212-874-7725; **Board Cert:** Psychiatry 1983; **Med School:** Cornell Univ-Weill Med Coll 1978; **Resid:** Psychiatry, NY Hosp-Cornell Med Ctr 1982; **Fac Appt:** Assoc Clin Prof Psyc, Cornell Univ-Weill Med Coll

Shear, M Katherine MD [Psyc] - **Spec Exp:** Panic Disorder; Anxiety Disorders; Bereavement/Traumatic Grief; Phobias; **Hospital:** NY-Presby Hosp/Columbia (page 66); **Address:** 1255 Amsterdam Ave, New York, NY 10027; **Phone:** 412-897-7449; **Board Cert:** Internal Medicine 1975; Psychiatry 1981; **Med School:** Tufts Univ 1972; **Resid:** Internal Medicine, Mt Sinai Hosp 1976; Psychiatry, Payne Whitney Clin 1979; **Fellow:** Psychosomatic Medicine, Montefiore Hosp 1980; **Fac Appt:** Prof Psyc, Colombia

Stone, Michael H MD [Psyc] - **Spec Exp:** Personality Disorders; Psychoanalysis; Forensic Psychiatry; **Hospital:** NY-Presby Hosp/Columbia (page 66); **Address:** 225 Central Park West, Ste 114, New York, NY 10024-6027; **Phone:** 212-758-2000; **Board Cert:** Psychiatry 1971; **Med School:** Cornell Univ-Weill Med Coll 1958; **Resid:** Internal Medicine, Bellevue Hosp 1961; Psychiatry, NYS Psych Inst 1966; **Fellow:** Hematology, Meml Sloan Kettering Cancer Ctr 1962; Medical Oncology, Meml Sloan Kettering Cancer Ctr 1963; **Fac Appt:** Clin Prof Psyc, Columbia P&S

Sussman, Norman MD [Psyc] - **Spec Exp:** Psychopharmacology; Anxiety & Mood Disorders; Bipolar/Mood Disorders; **Hospital:** NYU Med Ctr (page 68); **Address:** 150 E 58th St, Fl 27, New York, NY 10155; **Phone:** 212-588-9722; **Board Cert:** Psychiatry 1980; **Med School:** NY Med Coll 1975; **Resid:** Psychiatry, Metropolitan Hosp Ctr 1977; Psychiatry, Westchester Co Med Ctr 1978; **Fac Appt:** Clin Prof Psyc, NYU Sch Med

Thase, Michael E MD [Psyc] - **Spec Exp:** Anxiety & Mood Disorders; Psychopharmacology; Depression; **Hospital:** Hosp Univ Penn - UPHS (page 60); **Address:** Univ Penn, dept Psychiatry, 3535 Market St, Ste 670, Piladelphia, PA 19104; **Phone:** 215-746-6680; **Board Cert:** Psychiatry 1984; **Med School:** Ohio State Univ 1979; **Resid:** Psychiatry, Western Psych Inst 1983; **Fellow:** Research, Univ Pittsburgh Sch Med 1984; **Fac Appt:** Prof Psyc, Univ Pennsylvania

Wait, Susan B MD [Psyc] - **Spec Exp:** Post Traumatic Stress Disorder; Dissociative Disorders; Anxiety & Mood Disorders; Dialectical Behavioral Therapy; **Hospital:** Sheppard Pratt Hlth Sys; **Address:** Sheppard Pratt Hlth System, 6501 N Charles St, Baltimore, MD 21285; **Phone:** 410-938-5076; **Board Cert:** Psychiatry 1993; **Med School:** Med Coll PA Hahnemann 1987; **Resid:** Psychiatry, Sheppard Pratt Hosp 1991; **Fac Appt:** Assoc Clin Prof Psyc, Univ MD Sch Med

Walsh, B Timothy MD [Psyc] - **Spec Exp:** Eating Disorders; **Hospital:** NY State Psychiatric Inst, NY-Presby Hosp/Columbia (page 66); **Address:** NY State Psychiatric Inst-Unit 98, 1051 Riverside Dr, New York, NY 10032-2695; **Phone:** 212-543-5739; **Board Cert:** Psychiatry 1978; **Med School:** Harvard Med Sch 1972; **Resid:** Internal Medicine, Dartmouth Affil Hosps 1973; Psychiatry, Bronx Muni Hosp Ctr 1977; **Fac Appt:** Prof Psyc, Columbia P&S

Southeast

Blazer II, Dan G MD/PhD [Psyc] - **Spec Exp:** Geriatric Psychiatry; Mood Disorders; **Hospital:** Duke Univ Med Ctr; **Address:** Duke Univ Med Ctr, Dept Psychiatary, 3521 Hospital S, Box 3003, Durham, NC 27710-3003; **Phone:** 919-684-4128; **Board Cert:** Psychiatry 1977; Geriatric Psychiatry 2000; **Med School:** Univ Tenn Coll Med, Memphis 1969; **Resid:** Psychiatry, Duke Univ Med Ctr 1975; **Fellow:** Liaison Psychiatry, Montefiore Hosp 1976; **Fac Appt:** Prof Psyc, Duke Univ

Canterbury II, Randolph J MD [Psyc] - **Spec Exp:** Panic Disorder; Depression; Substance Abuse; **Hospital:** Univ Virginia Med Ctr; **Address:** Univ Virginia Dept Psychiatry, Div Outpatient Psychiatry, Box 800623, Charlottesville, VA 22908-0623; **Phone:** 434-243-5719; **Board Cert:** Internal Medicine 1983; Psychiatry 1985; Psychosomatic Medicine 2005; **Med School:** W VA Univ 1979; **Resid:** Internal Medicine, Univ Va Hosp 1983; Psychiatry, Univ Va Hosp 1985; **Fac Appt:** Prof Psyc, Univ VA Sch Med

Dell, Diana L MD [Psyc] - **Spec Exp:** Postpartum Depression; Menstrual Disorders (PMS); Pregnancy & Mental Health Issues; Women's Health-Mental & Reproductive; **Hospital:** Duke Univ Med Ctr; **Address:** Duke University Medical Ctr, Box 3263, Durham, NC 27710; **Phone:** 919-668-2570; **Board Cert:** Psychiatry 2001; Obstetrics & Gynecology 1998; **Med School:** Louisiana State U, New Orleans 1982; **Resid:** Obstetrics & Gynecology, Charity Hosp 1986; Psychiatry, Univ N Carolina Hosps 1998; **Fellow:** Psychosomatic Medicine, Univ Toronto 1999; **Fac Appt:** Prof Psyc, Duke Univ

Giustra Jr, Lawrence J MD [Psyc] - **Spec Exp:** Psychotherapy; Marital/Family/Sex Therapy; **Hospital:** Emory Univ Hosp; **Address:** 1945 Cliff Valley Way NE, Ste 202, Atlanta, GA 30329; **Phone:** 404-325-2139; **Board Cert:** Psychiatry 1982; **Med School:** Johns Hopkins Univ 1976; **Resid:** Psychiatry, Mass General Hosp 1980; **Fac Appt:** Asst Prof Psyc, Emory Univ

Kendler, Kenneth S MD [Psyc] - **Spec Exp:** Schizophrenia; Mood Disorders; **Hospital:** Med Coll of VA Hosp; **Address:** Med Coll VA, Dept Psyc, PO Box 980126, Richmond, VA 23298-0126; **Phone:** 804-828-8590; **Board Cert:** Psychiatry 1981; **Med School:** Stanford Univ 1976; **Resid:** Psychiatry, Yale-New Haven Hosp 1980; **Fac Appt:** Prof Psyc, Med Coll VA

Klapheke, Martin M MD [Psyc] - **Spec Exp:** Transplantation Psychiatry; Psychoanalysis; **Hospital:** Univ of Louisville Hosp; **Address:** 2010 Cherokee Pkwy, Ste 3, Louisville, KY 40204; **Phone:** 502-456-1770; **Board Cert:** Psychiatry 1985; **Med School:** Univ KY Coll Med 1979; **Resid:** Psychiatry, Mayo Grad Sch Med 1982; **Fellow:** Child & Adolescent Psychiatry, Mayo Grad Sch Med 1984; Psychoanalysis, Topeka Inst Psychoanalysis 1994; **Fac Appt:** Clin Prof Psyc, Univ Louisville Sch Med

Psychiatry

Levy, Steven T MD [Psyc] - **Spec Exp:** Depression; Anxiety & Mood Disorders; Bipolar/Mood Disorders; **Hospital:** Emory Univ Hosp; **Address:** Emory Univ Dept Psychiatry, 2004 Ridgewood Drive, Ste 300, Atlanta, GA 30322; **Phone:** 404-727-0397; **Board Cert:** Psychiatry 1976; **Med School:** Duke Univ 1969; **Resid:** Psychiatry, Yale-New Haven Hosp 1973; **Fac Appt:** Prof Psyc, Emory Univ

McCall, William V MD [Psyc] - **Spec Exp:** Sleep Disorders; Electroconvulsive Therapy (ECT); Depression; **Hospital:** Wake Forest Univ Baptist Med Ctr (page 73); **Address:** Wake Forest U Sch of Med, Dept Psychiatry, Medical Center Blvd, Winston-Salem, NC 27157; **Phone:** 336-716-2911; **Board Cert:** Psychiatry 1990; Geriatric Psychiatry 2005; Sleep Medicine 2007; **Med School:** Duke Univ 1984; **Resid:** Psychiatry, Duke Univ Med Ctr 1987; **Fellow:** Sleep Medicine, Duke Univ Med Ctr 1988; **Fac Appt:** Prof Psyc, Wake Forest Univ

Powers, Pauline MD [Psyc] - **Spec Exp:** Eating Disorders; **Hospital:** Tampa Genl Hosp; **Address:** University S Fla, 3515 E Fletcher Ave, Tampa, FL 33613-4706; **Phone:** 813-974-2926; **Board Cert:** Psychiatry 1977; **Med School:** Univ Iowa Coll Med 1971; **Resid:** Psychiatry, Univ Iowa Med Ctr 1974; Psychiatry, Univ Calif-Davis Med Ctr 1975; **Fac Appt:** Prof Psyc, Univ S Fla Coll Med

Weiner, Richard D MD/PhD [Psyc] - **Spec Exp:** Bipolar/Mood Disorders; Electroconvulsive Therapy (ECT); Depression; Schizophrenia; **Hospital:** Duke Univ Med Ctr, VA Med Ctr - Durham; **Address:** Duke Univ Medical Ctr, Dept Psychiatry, Box 3309, Durham, NC 27710; **Phone:** 919-681-8742; **Board Cert:** Psychiatry 1979; Clinical Neurophysiology 2003; **Med School:** Duke Univ 1973; **Resid:** Psychiatry, Duke Univ Med Ctr 1976; **Fellow:** Electroencephalography, Duke Univ Med Ctr 1977; **Fac Appt:** Prof Psyc, Duke Univ

Weisler, Richard H MD [Psyc] - **Spec Exp:** Depression; Bipolar/Mood Disorders; **Hospital:** Duke Univ Med Ctr, Univ NC Hosps; **Address:** 700 Spring Forest Rd, Ste 125, Raleigh, NC 27609; **Phone:** 919-872-5900; **Board Cert:** Psychiatry 1982; **Med School:** Univ NC Sch Med 1977; **Resid:** Psychiatry, Duke Univ Med Ctr 1982; **Fac Appt:** Assoc Prof Psyc, Duke Univ

Midwest

Andersen, Arnold MD [Psyc] - **Spec Exp:** Eating Disorders; **Hospital:** Univ Iowa Hosp & Clinics; **Address:** Univ Iowa, Dept Psychiatry, 200 Hawkins Drive, rm 2880-JPP, Iowa City, IA 52242; **Phone:** 319-356-1354; **Board Cert:** Psychiatry 1980; **Med School:** Cornell Univ-Weill Med Coll 1968; **Resid:** Psychiatry, New York Hosp 1970; Psychiatry, Johns Hopkins Hosp 1976; **Fellow:** Psychiatry, Natl Inst Mental Hlth 1975; **Fac Appt:** Prof Psyc, Univ Iowa Coll Med

Calabrese, Joseph R MD [Psyc] - **Spec Exp:** Bipolar/Mood Disorders; **Hospital:** Univ Hosps Case Med Ctr; **Address:** Case Western Reserve Univ, 11400 Euclid Ave, Ste 200, Cleveland, OH 44106; **Phone:** 216-844-2865; **Board Cert:** Psychiatry 1989; **Med School:** Ohio State Univ 1980; **Resid:** Psychiatry, Cleveland Clinic 1984; **Fellow:** Biological Psychiatry, Natl Inst Mental Hlth 1986; **Fac Appt:** Prof Psyc, Case West Res Univ

Cloninger, C Robert MD [Psyc] - **Spec Exp:** Personality Disorders; **Hospital:** Barnes-Jewish Hosp; **Address:** Wash Univ Sch Med, Dept Psyc, 660 S Euclid Ave, Box 8134, St Louis, MO 63110; **Phone:** 314-362-7005; **Board Cert:** Psychiatry 1975; **Med School:** Washington Univ, St Louis 1970; **Resid:** Psychiatry, Barnes Hosp 1973; Psychiatry, Renard Hosp-Wash Univ 1973; **Fac Appt:** Prof Psyc, Washington Univ, St Louis

Crow, Scott J MD [Psyc] - **Spec Exp:** Eating Disorders; Obesity; **Hospital:** Univ Minn Med Ctr, Fairview - Univ Campus; **Address:** Univ Minn, Dept Psychiatry, 2450 Riverside Ave, F282/2A West, Minneapolis, MN 55454; **Phone:** 612-273-9807; **Board Cert:** Psychiatry 1994; **Med School:** Univ Minn 1988; **Resid:** Psychiatry, Univ Minn 1992; **Fellow:** Psychiatry, Univ Minn 1992; **Fac Appt:** Prof Psyc, Univ Minn

Greden, John F MD [Psyc] - **Spec Exp:** Anxiety & Mood Disorders; Depression; **Hospital:** Univ Michigan Hlth Sys; **Address:** Univ Michigan Comp Depression Ctr, Rachel Upjohn Bldg, 4250 Plymouth Rd, Ann Arbor, MI 48109-2700; **Phone:** 734-763-9629; **Board Cert:** Psychiatry 1975; **Med School:** Univ Minn 1967; **Resid:** Psychiatry, Univ Minn Med Ctr 1969; Psychiatry, Walter Reed AMC 1972; **Fac Appt:** Prof Psyc, Univ Mich Med Sch

Janicak, Philip G MD [Psyc] - **Spec Exp:** Psychopharmacology; Mood Disorders; Psychotic Disorders; **Hospital:** Rush Univ Med Ctr; **Address:** Rush Univ Med Ctr, Dept Psych, 1720 W Polk St, M Field Bldg, rm 107, Chicago, IL 60612-4328; **Phone:** 312-942-7287; **Board Cert:** Psychiatry 1978; **Med School:** Loyola Univ-Stritch Sch Med 1973; **Resid:** Psychiatry, McGaw Hosp/Loyola Med Ctr 1976; **Fac Appt:** Prof Psyc, Rush Med Coll

Levine, Stephen B MD [Psyc] - **Spec Exp:** Sexual Dysfunction; Relationship Problems; Sexual Identity Issues; **Hospital:** Univ Hosps Case Med Ctr; **Address:** 23230 Chagrin Blvd, Ste 350, Beach-wood, OH 44122-5446; **Phone:** 216-831-2900; **Board Cert:** Psychiatry 1976; **Med School:** Case West Res Univ 1967; **Resid:** Psychiatry, Univ Hosps Cleveland 1973; **Fac Appt:** Clin Prof Psyc, Case West Res Univ

Locala, Joseph MD [Psyc] - **Spec Exp:** Psychiatry in Transplant Patients; Mood Disorders; Anxiety Disorders; **Hospital:** Cleveland Clin Fdn (page 56); **Address:** Cleveland Clinic, WO Walker Ctr, 10524 Euclid Ave Fl 13, Cleveland, OH 44106; **Phone:** 216-844-2400; **Board Cert:** Psychiatry 2006; Psychosomatic Medicine 2006; **Med School:** Temple Univ 1989; **Resid:** Psychiatry, Medical Ctr Hosp 1993; **Fellow:** Cleveland Clinic 1994

McCallum, Kimberli E MD [Psyc] - **Spec Exp:** Eating Disorders; **Hospital:** St Luke's Hosp - Chesterfield, MO; **Address:** McCallum Place, 231 W Lockwood Ave, Ste 201, St. Louis, MO 63119; **Phone:** 314-968-1900; **Board Cert:** Psychiatry 1993; Child & Adolescent Psychiatry 1994; **Med School:** Yale Univ 1986; **Resid:** Psychiatry, UCLA Neuropsyc Inst 1991; **Fellow:** Child Psychiatry, Washington Univ 1993; **Fac Appt:** Assoc Clin Prof Psyc, Washington Univ, St Louis

Nurnberger Jr, John I MD/PhD [Psyc] - **Spec Exp:** Bipolar/Mood Disorders; Depression; **Hospital:** Indiana Univ Hosp; **Address:** Institute Psychiatric Research-IUMC, 791 Union Dr, Indianapolis, IN 46202; **Phone:** 317-278-4344; **Board Cert:** Psychiatry 1981; **Med School:** Indiana Univ 1975; **Resid:** Psychiatry, Columbia-Presby Med Ctr 1978; **Fac Appt:** Prof Psyc, Indiana Univ

Renshaw, Domeena MD [Psyc] - **Spec Exp:** Sexual Dysfunction; Sexual Problems in Children; **Hospital:** Loyola Univ Med Ctr; **Address:** Loyola Univ Hosp, Dept Psychiatry, 2160 S 1st Ave, Maywood, IL 60153; **Phone:** 708-216-3752; **Board Cert:** Psychiatry 1972; **Med School:** South Africa 1960; **Resid:** Pediatrics, Chldns Hosp/Harvard 1963; Psychiatry, Loyola Univ Med Ctr 1968; **Fac Appt:** Prof Psyc, Loyola Univ-Stritch Sch Med

Riba, Michelle B MD [Psyc] - **Spec Exp:** Psychiatry in Cancer; **Hospital:** Univ Michigan Hlth Sys; **Address:** Univ Mich Med Ctr, Dept Psychiatry, 1500 E Medical Center Dr, MCHC, rm F6236, Ann Arbor, MI 48109-0295; **Phone:** 734-764-6879; **Board Cert:** Psychiatry 1991; Psychosomatic Medicine 2005; **Med School:** Univ Conn 1985; **Resid:** Psychiatry, Univ Connecticut 1988; **Fac Appt:** Clin Prof Psyc, Univ Mich Med Sch

Psychiatry

Strakowski, Stephen M MD [Psyc] - **Spec Exp:** Bipolar/Mood Disorders; Psychotic Disorders; Dual Diagnosis; Addiction/Substance Abuse; **Hospital:** Univ Hosp - Cincinnati; **Address:** Univ Cincinnati Coll Med, Dept Psychiatry, 231 Albert Sabin Way, Cincinnati, OH 45267-0559; **Phone:** 513-558-4274; **Board Cert:** Psychiatry 1993; **Med School:** Vanderbilt Univ 1988; **Resid:** Psychiatry, McLean Hosp-Harvard Med Sch 1992; **Fac Appt:** Prof Psyc, Univ Cincinnati

Wooten, Virgil D MD [Psyc] - **Spec Exp:** Sleep Disorders; **Hospital:** Bethesda North Hosp, Good Samaritan Hosp - Cincinnati; **Address:** Bethesda Sleep Ctr, 10475 Montgomery Rd, Ste 1D, Cincinnati, OH 45242; **Phone:** 513-745-1690; **Board Cert:** Psychiatry 1985; Sleep Medicine 2007; **Med School:** Univ Ark 1980; **Resid:** Psychiatry, Univ Hosp-VA Hosp 1984; **Fellow:** Sleep Medicine, Univ Hosp 1985

Zorumski, Charles F MD [Psyc] - **Spec Exp:** Neuro-Psychiatry; Psychopharmacology; **Hospital:** Barnes-Jewish Hosp; **Address:** 660 S Euclid Ave, CB8134 Ave, St Louis, MO 63110-1010; **Phone:** 314-747-2680; **Board Cert:** Psychiatry 1984; **Med School:** St Louis Univ 1978; **Resid:** Psychiatry, Barnes-Jewish Hosp 1982; **Fac Appt:** Prof Psyc, Washington Univ, St Louis

Great Plains and Mountains

Freedman, Robert MD [Psyc] - **Spec Exp:** Schizophrenia; **Hospital:** Univ Colorado Hosp; **Address:** Univ Colorado, Dept Psychiatry, 13001 E 17th Ave, Box E2351, Aurora, CO 80045; **Phone:** 303-724-4940; **Board Cert:** Psychiatry 1980; **Med School:** Harvard Med Sch 1972; **Resid:** Psychiatry, Univ Chicago Hosps & Clins 1978; **Fellow:** Neuropharmacology, NIMH-Neuropharm Lab / St Elizabeth's Hosp; **Fac Appt:** Prof Psyc, Univ Colorado

Greiner, Carl B MD [Psyc] - **Spec Exp:** Psychiatry in Cancer; Psychiatry in Physical Illness; Palliative Care; Post Traumatic Stress Disorder; **Hospital:** Nebraska Med Ctr; **Address:** UNMC, dept Psychiatry, 985575 Nebraska Medical Ctr, Omaha, NE 68198-5575; **Phone:** 402-552-6002; **Board Cert:** Psychiatry 1984; Forensic Psychiatry 1999; **Med School:** Univ Cincinnati 1978; **Resid:** Psychiatry, Univ Cincinnati Med Ctr 1982; **Fac Appt:** Prof Psyc, Univ Nebr Coll Med

Hoffman, Daniel A MD [Psyc] - **Spec Exp:** ADD/ADHD-Neurofeedback Treatment; **Hospital:** Rose Med Ctr; **Address:** Neuro-Therapy Clinic, Orchard Falls Bldg, 7800 E Orchard Rd, Ste 340, Greenwood Village, CO 80111; **Phone:** 303-741-4800; **Board Cert:** Psychiatry 1981; **Med School:** Wayne State Univ 1974; **Resid:** Psychiatry, Univ Colo Hlth Sci Ctr 1977; **Fac Appt:** Asst Clin Prof Psyc, Univ Colorado

Mitchell, James E MD [Psyc] - **Spec Exp:** Eating Disorders; **Hospital:** MeritCare Hosp; **Address:** NeuroPsychiatric Research Inst, 120 S 8th St, 2nd Fl, Fargo, ND 58103; **Phone:** 701-293-1335; **Board Cert:** Psychiatry 1979; **Med School:** Northwestern Univ 1972; **Resid:** Psychiatry, Fairview-Univ Med Ctr 1976; **Fac Appt:** Prof Psyc, Univ ND Sch Med

Weiner, Kenneth L MD [Psyc] - **Spec Exp:** Eating Disorders; **Address:** 1830 Franklin St, Ste 500, Denver, CO 80218; **Phone:** 303-220-1655; **Board Cert:** Psychiatry 1983; **Med School:** Tufts Univ 1977; **Resid:** Psychiatry, Univ Colorado Hlth Sci Ctr 1981; **Fac Appt:** Asst Clin Prof Psyc, Univ Colorado

Wilson, Daniel R MD/PhD [Psyc] - **Spec Exp:** Psychopharmacology; Forensic Psychiatry; **Hospital:** Creighton Univ Med Ctr; **Address:** 3528 Dodge St, Omaha, NE 68131; **Phone:** 402-345-8828; **Board Cert:** Psychiatry 1989; Forensic Psychiatry 1998; **Med School:** Univ Iowa Coll Med 1983; **Resid:** Psychiatry, McLean Hosp 1987; **Fellow:** Geriatric Psychiatry, McLean Hosp 1987; Genetics, Cambridge Univ 1993; **Fac Appt:** Prof Psyc, Creighton Univ

America's Top Doctors® 8th Edition

Southwest

Avery, Eric N MD [Psyc] - **Spec Exp:** Depression; Dementia; Arts in the Healing Process; AIDS/HIV Liaison Psychiatry; **Hospital:** UT Med Br Hosp at Galveston; **Address:** Univ Texas Medical Branch, Dept Psychiatry, 301 University Blvd, Route 186, Galveston, TX 77555; **Phone:** 409-747-5784; **Board Cert:** Psychiatry 2003; **Med School:** Univ Tex Med Br, Galveston 1974; **Resid:** Psychiatry, NY State Psych Inst 1978; **Fellow:** Liaison Psychiatry for AIDS/HIV, NY State Psych Inst 1994; **Fac Appt:** Asst Prof Psyc, Univ Tex Med Br, Galveston

Bowden, Charles L MD [Psyc] - **Spec Exp:** Bipolar/Mood Disorders; **Hospital:** Univ Hlth Sys - Univ Hosp (San Antonio, TX); **Address:** Univ Tex Hlth Sci Ctr, Dept Psychiatry, 7526 Louis Pasteur, San Antonio, TX 78229-3900; **Phone:** 210-567-5555; **Board Cert:** Psychiatry 1970; **Med School:** Baylor Coll Med 1964; **Resid:** Psychiatry, NY State Psyc Inst/Columbia-Presby Med Ctr 1968; **Fac Appt:** Prof Psyc, Univ Tex, San Antonio

Davidson, Joyce E MD [Psyc] - **Spec Exp:** Obsessive-Compulsive Disorder; Bipolar/Mood Disorders; Schizophrenia; **Hospital:** Menninger Clinic; **Address:** 2801 Gessner Drive, Houston, TX 77080; **Phone:** 713-275-5419; **Board Cert:** Psychiatry 1988; **Med School:** Univ MO-Kansas City 1979; **Resid:** Psychiatry, Karl Menninger Sch Psyc 1982; **Fellow:** Child & Adolescent Psychiatry, Karl Menninger Sch Psyc 1984

Gabbard, Glen O MD [Psyc] - **Spec Exp:** Personality Disorders-Borderline; Cognitive Psychotherapy; Psychoanalysis; **Hospital:** Baylor Univ Medical Ctr; **Address:** 6655 Travis, Ste 500, Houston, TX 77030; **Phone:** 713-798-6397; **Board Cert:** Psychiatry 1979; **Med School:** Rush Med Coll 1975; **Resid:** Psychiatry, Menninger Sch Psyc 1978; **Fellow:** Psychoanalysis, Topeka Inst Psychoanalysis 1984; **Fac Appt:** Clin Prof Psyc, Univ Kans

Gelenberg, Alan MD [Psyc] - **Spec Exp:** Psychopharmacology; Mood Disorders; Depression; **Hospital:** Univ Med Ctr - Tucson; **Address:** Healthcare Tech System, 7917 Mineral Point, Ste 300, Madison, AZ 35717; **Phone:** 608-827-2440; **Board Cert:** Psychiatry 1975; **Med School:** Univ Pennsylvania 1969; **Resid:** Psychiatry, Mass General Hosp 1973; **Fac Appt:** Clin Prof Psyc, Med Coll Wisc

Haque, Waheedul MD [Psyc] - **Spec Exp:** Depression; Panic Disorder; **Hospital:** UT Med Br Hosp at Galveston; **Address:** Univ Texas Med Branch, Dept Psychiatry, 301 University Blvd, Route 0190, Galveston, TX 77555; **Phone:** 409-747-9722; **Board Cert:** Psychiatry 1970; **Med School:** India 1962; **Resid:** Psychiatry, Barnes Jewish Med Ctr 1969; **Fac Appt:** Prof Psyc, Univ Tex Med Br, Galveston

Hirschfeld, Robert M A MD [Psyc] - **Spec Exp:** Bipolar/Mood Disorders; Schizophrenia; Depression; Suicide; **Hospital:** UT Med Br Hosp at Galveston; **Address:** Univ Texas Med Branch, Dept Psychiatry, 301 University Blvd, 1.302 Rebecca Sealy Hosp, Galveston, TX 77555-0188; **Phone:** 409-747-9791; **Board Cert:** Psychiatry 1975; **Med School:** Univ Mich Med Sch 1968; **Resid:** Psychiatry, Stanford Univ Med Ctr 1972; **Fac Appt:** Prof Psyc, Univ Tex Med Br, Galveston

Mohl, Paul C MD [Psyc] - **Spec Exp:** Psychopharmacology; Psychotherapy; **Hospital:** UT Southwestern Med Ctr - Dallas; **Address:** 5323 Harry Hines Blvd, Dallas, TX 75390-9070; **Phone:** 214-648-7312; **Board Cert:** Psychiatry 1977; **Med School:** Duke Univ 1971; **Resid:** Psychiatry, Duke Univ Hosp 1974; **Fac Appt:** Prof Psyc, Univ Tex SW, Dallas

Valentine, Alan D MD [Psyc] - **Spec Exp:** Psychiatry in Cancer; Palliative Care; **Hospital:** UT MD Anderson Cancer Ctr; **Address:** MD Anderson Cancer Center, Dept Psychiatry Unit 453, PO Box 301402, Houston, TX 77230-1402; **Phone:** 713-745-3344; **Board Cert:** Psychiatry 1992; Geriatric Psychiatry 2006; Psychosomatic Medicine 2005; **Med School:** Univ Tex, Houston 1986; **Resid:** Psychiatry, Univ Texas Affil Hosps; **Fac Appt:** Assoc Prof Psyc, Univ Tex, Houston

Psychiatry

Weiner, Myron MD [Psyc] - **Spec Exp:** Psychiatry-Geriatric; Alzheimer's Disease; **Hospital:** UT Southwestern Med Ctr - Dallas; **Address:** Univ Texas SW Med Ctr, 5323 Harry Hines Blvd, Dallas, TX 75390-9129; **Phone:** 214-648-5555; **Board Cert:** Psychiatry 1966; Geriatric Psychiatry 2001; **Med School:** Tulane Univ 1957; **Resid:** Psychiatry, Parkland Hosp 1963; **Fellow:** Geriatric Psychiatry, Mt Sinai Med Ctr 1985; **Fac Appt:** Prof Psyc, Univ Tex SW, Dallas

West Coast and Pacific

Blumenfield, Michael MD [Psyc] - **Spec Exp:** Psychotherapy; Psychopharmacology; Psychosomatic Disorders; Disaster Psychiatry; **Address:** 5901 Nita Ave, Woodland Hills, CA 91367; **Phone:** 818-716-1143; **Board Cert:** Psychiatry 1970; Psychosomatic Medicine 2005; **Med School:** SUNY Downstate 1964; **Resid:** Psychiatry, Kings County Hosp 1968; **Fellow:** Psychosomatic Medicine, Kings County Hosp 1971; **Fac Appt:** Prof Emeritus Psyc, NY Med Coll

Burt, Vivien K MD/PhD [Psyc] - **Spec Exp:** Women's Health-Mental Health; Impulse-Control Disorders; Psychiatric Disorders in Pregnancy; Postpartum Depression; **Hospital:** UCLA Neuropsychiatric Hosp, VA Med Ctr - W Los Angeles; **Address:** 300 UCLA Medical Plaza, Ste 2337, Los Angeles, CA 90095; **Phone:** 310-562-4942; **Board Cert:** Psychiatry 1990; **Med School:** McGill Univ 1984; **Resid:** Psychiatry, UCLA-Neurpsyc Inst 1988; **Fac Appt:** Assoc Prof Psyc, UCLA

Bystritsky, Alexander MD/PhD [Psyc] - **Spec Exp:** Obsessive-Compulsive Disorder; Anxiety Disorders; Psychopharmacology; **Hospital:** UCLA Neuropsychiatric Hosp; **Address:** 300 UCLA Med Plaza, Ste 2200, Box 956968, Los Angeles, CA 90095-6968; **Phone:** 310-206-5133; **Board Cert:** Psychiatry 1988; **Med School:** Russia 1977; **Resid:** Psychiatry, NYU Med Ctr 1985; **Fellow:** Psychiatry, UCLA 1987; **Fac Appt:** Prof Psyc, UCLA

Eisendrath, Stuart J MD [Psyc] - **Spec Exp:** Depression; Munchausen Syndrome; Cognitive Psychotherapy; **Hospital:** UCSF Med Ctr; **Address:** UCSF Med Ctr, 401 Parnassus Ave, MC-0984, San Francisco, CA 94143-0984; **Phone:** 415-476-7868; **Board Cert:** Psychiatry 1980; **Med School:** Med Coll Wisc 1974; **Resid:** Psychiatry, Langley Porter NPI 1978; **Fellow:** Liaison Psychiatry, Langley Porter NPI 1979; **Fac Appt:** Prof Psyc, UCSF

Fann, Jesse R MD [Psyc] - **Spec Exp:** Psychiatry in Physical Illness; Psychiatry in Neurologic Disorders; Psychiatry in Cancer; **Hospital:** Univ Wash Med Ctr, Harborview Med Ctr; **Address:** Univ Washington Med Ctr, Psychiatry-Box 356560, 1959 NE Pacific St, Seattle, WA 98195-6560; **Phone:** 206-685-4280; **Board Cert:** Psychiatry 2005; **Med School:** Northwestern Univ 1989; **Resid:** Psychiatry, Univ Washington Med Ctr 1993; **Fellow:** Liaison Psychiatry, Univ Washington Med Ctr 1995; **Fac Appt:** Asst Prof Psyc, Univ Wash

Friedman, Barry MD [Psyc] - **Spec Exp:** Psychopharmacology; Psychoanalysis; **Address:** 435 N Bedford Dr, Ste 112, Beverly Hills, CA 90210; **Phone:** 310-274-4372; **Board Cert:** Psychiatry 1974; **Med School:** UCSF 1965; **Resid:** Psychiatry, UCLA Med Ctr 1971; **Fellow:** Psychoanalysis, Los Angeles Psychoanalytic Inst 1992; **Fac Appt:** Assoc Clin Prof Psyc, UCLA

Gitlin, Michael Jay MD [Psyc] - **Spec Exp:** Mood Disorders; **Hospital:** UCLA Neuropsychiatric Hosp; **Address:** UCLA NPI-Mood Disorders Clinic, 300 Medical Plaza, Ste 2200, Los Angeles, CA 90095-6968; **Phone:** 310-206-3654; **Board Cert:** Psychiatry 1981; **Med School:** Univ Pennsylvania 1975; **Resid:** Psychiatry, UCLA Med Ctr 1979; **Fac Appt:** Prof Psyc, UCLA

Guilleminault, Christian MD [Psyc] - **Spec Exp:** Sleep Disorders/Apnea; **Hospital:** Stanford Univ Med Ctr; **Address:** 401 Quarry Rd, Ste 3301A, Stanford, CA 94305; **Phone:** 650-723-6601; **Med School:** France 1968; **Fac Appt:** Prof Psyc, Stanford Univ

Keepers, George MD [Psyc] - **Spec Exp:** Neuro-Psychiatry; ADD/ADHD; **Hospital:** OR Hlth & Sci Univ; **Address:** 3181 SW Sam Jackson Park Rd, MC UHN80, Portland, OR 97239; **Phone:** 503-494-8144; **Board Cert:** Psychiatry 1984; **Med School:** Baylor Coll Med 1977; **Resid:** Psychiatry, Oregon Hlth Sci Univ 1981; **Fac Appt:** Prof Psyc, Oregon Hlth Sci Univ

Leuchter, Andrew Francis MD [Psyc] - **Spec Exp:** Depression; **Hospital:** UCLA Neuropsychiatric Hosp; **Address:** 760 Westwood Pl, rm 37-452, Los Angeles, CA 90024; **Phone:** 310-825-0207; **Board Cert:** Psychiatry 1986; Geriatric Psychiatry 2001; **Med School:** Baylor Coll Med 1980; **Resid:** Psychiatry, UCLA-Neuro Psyc Inst & Hosp 1984; **Fellow:** Geriatric Psychiatry, UCLA Med Ctr 1986; **Fac Appt:** Prof Psyc, UCLA

Liberman, Robert Paul MD [Psyc] - **Spec Exp:** Schizophrenia; Psychotic Disorders; Psychiatric Rehabilitation; **Hospital:** UCLA Neuropsychiatric Hosp; **Address:** UCLA Neuropsychiatric Institute, 760 Westwood Plaza, Los Angeles, CA 90095; **Phone:** 310-206-1616; **Board Cert:** Psychiatry 1969; **Med School:** Johns Hopkins Univ 1963; **Resid:** Psychiatry, Mass Mntl Hlth Ctr 1967; **Fellow:** Pharmacology, UCSF Med Ctr 1961; Research, Harvard Med Sch 1968; **Fac Appt:** Prof Psyc, UCLA

Marder, Stephen Robert MD [Psyc] - **Spec Exp:** Schizophrenia; Psychopharmacology; **Hospital:** VA Med Ctr - W Los Angeles, Ronald Reagan UCLA Med Ctr; **Address:** West Los Angeles VA - Gr LA Hlth Svcs, 11301 Wilshire Blvd, Bldg MIRECC 210A, Los Angeles, CA 90073; **Phone:** 310-268-3647; **Board Cert:** Psychiatry 1977; **Med School:** SUNY Buffalo 1971; **Resid:** Psychiatry, LAC-USC Med Ctr 1975; **Fac Appt:** Prof Psyc, UCLA

Marmar, Charles MD [Psyc] - **Spec Exp:** Post Traumatic Stress Disorder; Bereavement/Traumatic Grief; **Hospital:** VA Med Ctr - San Francisco; **Address:** 4150 Clement St Bldg 8 - rm 320-1, Mental Hlth Svc 116A, San Francisco, CA 94941; **Phone:** 415-221-4810 x3436; **Board Cert:** Psychiatry 1982; **Med School:** Univ Manitoba 1970; **Resid:** Psychiatry, Univ Toronto Hosp 1976; **Fellow:** Anxiety Disorder, Langley Porter Inst-UCSF 1978; **Fac Appt:** Prof Psyc, UCSF

Nelson, J Craig MD [Psyc] - **Spec Exp:** Geriatric Psychiatry; Psychopharmacology; Mood Disorders; **Hospital:** UCSF Med Ctr; **Address:** UCSF-Langley Porter Psychiatric Inst, 401 Parnassus Ave, Box 0984, San Francisco, CA 94143-0984; **Phone:** 415-476-7500; **Board Cert:** Psychiatry 1974; Geriatric Psychiatry 2002; **Med School:** Univ Wisc 1968; **Resid:** Psychiatry, Yale-New Haven Hosp 1970; Psychiatry, Yale-New Haven Hosp 1974; **Fac Appt:** Prof Psyc, UCSF

Neppe, Vernon M MD/PhD [Psyc] - **Spec Exp:** Neuro-Psychiatry; Psychopharmacology; Forensic Psychiatry; **Hospital:** Overlake Hosp Med Ctr; **Address:** Pacific Neuropsychiatric Inst, 6300 Meridian Ave NE, Ste 353, Seattle, WA 98115; **Phone:** 206- 52-76289; **Board Cert:** Psychiatry 1988; Geriatric Psychiatry 2001; **Med School:** South Africa 1973; **Resid:** Neurology, Univ Witwatersrand 1979; Psychiatry, Univ Witwatersrand 1980; **Fellow:** Psychopharmacology, NY Hosp/Cornell Med Ctr 1983; Neuropsychiatry, NY Hosp/Cornell Med Ctr 1983

Norman, Kim Peter MD [Psyc] - **Spec Exp:** Eating Disorders/Obesity; Personality Disorders; Dual Diagnosis; **Hospital:** UCSF Med Ctr; **Address:** UCSF-Langley Porter Psyc Inst, 401 Parnassus Ave, rm 250, Box A-221, San Francisco, CA 94143; **Phone:** 415-476-7402; **Board Cert:** Psychiatry 1983; **Med School:** Albert Einstein Coll Med 1977; **Resid:** Psychiatry, Langley Porter Psyc Inst 1981; **Fac Appt:** Clin Prof Psyc, UCSF

Pi, Edmond H MD [Psyc] - **Spec Exp:** Psychopharmacology; Cross Cultural Psychiatry; Anxiety Disorders; **Hospital:** LAC & USC Med Ctr; **Address:** LAC USC Healthcare Network, 1200 N State St, rm 10-621, Los Angeles, CA 90033; **Phone:** 323-226-7975; **Board Cert:** Psychiatry 1980; **Med School:** South Korea 1972; **Resid:** Psychiatry, SUNY-Stony Brook Affil Hosp 1977; Psychiatry, Univ Kentucky Hosp-Chandler Med Ctr 1978; **Fac Appt:** Prof Psyc, USC Sch Med

Pynoos, Robert S MD [Psyc] - **Spec Exp:** Post Traumatic Stress Clinical Trials; **Hospital:** UCLA Neuropsychiatric Hosp; **Address:** Natl Ctr for Child Traumatic Stress-UCLA, 11150 W Olympic Blvd, Ste 650, Los Angeles, CA 90064; **Phone:** 310-235-2633; **Board Cert:** Psychiatry 1980; **Med School:** Columbia P&S 1972; **Resid:** Pediatrics, Mt Sinai Hosp; Psychiatry, NY Presby-Cornell Med Ctr; **Fac Appt:** Prof Psyc, UCLA

Raskind, Murray MD [Psyc] - **Spec Exp:** Geriatric Psychiatry; Alzheimer's Disease; Post Traumatic Stress Disorder; **Hospital:** VA Puget Sound Hlth Care Sys, Univ Wash Med Ctr; **Address:** VA Puget Sound Health Care System, Mental Hlth Svc 116, 1660 S Columbia Way, Seattle, WA 98108; **Phone:** 206-768-5375; **Board Cert:** Psychiatry 1976; Geriatric Psychiatry 2001; **Med School:** Columbia P&S 1968; **Resid:** Internal Medicine, Harlem Hosp Ctr 1970; Psychiatry, Univ Wash Affil Hosps 1973; **Fac Appt:** Prof Psyc, Univ Wash

Reus, Victor I MD [Psyc] - **Spec Exp:** Psychopharmacology; Bipolar/Mood Disorders; Behavioral Disorders; **Hospital:** UCSF Med Ctr; **Address:** 401 Parnassus Ave, San Francisco, CA 94143-0984; **Phone:** 415-476-7478; **Board Cert:** Psychiatry 1977; Geriatric Psychiatry 2000; **Med School:** Univ MD Sch Med 1973; **Resid:** Psychiatry, Univ Wisc Med Ctr 1976; **Fellow:** Biological Psychiatry, Natl Inst Mntl Hlth 1978; **Fac Appt:** Prof Psyc, UCSF

Roy-Byrne, Peter P MD [Psyc] - **Spec Exp:** Anxiety & Mood Disorders; Panic Disorder; Bipolar/Mood Disorders; Post Traumatic Stress Disorder; **Hospital:** Harborview Med Ctr, Univ Wash Med Ctr; **Address:** 325 9th Ave, Box 359911, Seattle, WA 98104; **Phone:** 206-341-4200; **Board Cert:** Psychiatry 1983; **Med School:** Tufts Univ 1978; **Resid:** Psychiatry, UCLA Neuropsych Inst 1982; **Fellow:** Biological Psychiatry, Natl Inst Hlth - NIMH 1984; **Fac Appt:** Prof Psyc, Univ Wash

Saxena, Sanjaya MD [Psyc] - **Spec Exp:** Obsessive-Compulsive Disorder; **Hospital:** UCSD Med Ctr; **Address:** La Jolla Professional Building, 8950 Via La Jolla Drive, La Jolla, CA 92037; **Phone:** 858-534-6200; **Board Cert:** Psychiatry 2006; **Med School:** Univ Minn 1990; **Resid:** Psychiatry, UCLA Neuropsychiatric Hosp 1994; **Fellow:** Neuroimaging, Charles A. Dana Fdn 1996; **Fac Appt:** Asst Prof Psyc, UCSD

Schatzberg, Alan F MD [Psyc] - **Spec Exp:** Depression; Anxiety & Mood Disorders; Psychopharmacology; **Hospital:** Stanford Univ Med Ctr; **Address:** Stanford Univ, Dept Psychiatry, 401 Quarry Rd, Ste 3301A, Stanford, CA 94305-5717; **Phone:** 650-723-6811; **Board Cert:** Psychiatry 1975; **Med School:** NYU Sch Med 1968; **Resid:** Psychiatry, Mass Mental Hlth Ctr 1972; **Fellow:** Psychiatry, Mass Mental Hlth Ctr/Harvard 1972; **Fac Appt:** Prof Psyc, Stanford Univ

Spiegel, David MD [Psyc] - **Spec Exp:** Hypnosis; Psychiatry in Cancer; Post Traumatic Stress Disorder; **Hospital:** Stanford Univ Med Ctr; **Address:** Stanford Univ Sch Medicine, Dept Psychiatry & Behavioral Sciences, 401 Quarry Rd, rm 2325, Stanford, CA 94305-5718; **Phone:** 650-723-6421; **Board Cert:** Psychiatry 1976; **Med School:** Harvard Med Sch 1971; **Resid:** Psychiatry, Mass Mental Hlth Ctr 1974; Psychiatry, Cambridge Hosp-Harvard Med Sch 1974; **Fellow:** Community Psychiatry, Harvard Med Sch 1974; **Fac Appt:** Prof Psyc, Stanford Univ

Stein, Murray B MD [Psyc] - **Spec Exp:** Anxiety Disorders; Panic Disorder; Post Traumatic Stress Disorder; **Hospital:** UCSD Med Ctr, VA San Diego Hlthcre Sys; **Address:** UCSD Dept Psychiatry, 8950 Villa La Jolla Drive, Ste B218, La Jolla, CA 92037; **Phone:** 858-534-6400; **Board Cert:** Psychiatry 1989; **Med School:** Univ Manitoba 1983; **Resid:** Psychiatry, Univ Toronto Hosp 1986; Psychiatry, Natl Inst Mental Hlth-NIH 1987; **Fellow:** Anxiety Disorder, Natl Inst Mental Hlth-NIH 1990; **Fac Appt:** Prof Psyc, UCSD

Strouse, Thomas B MD [Psyc] - **Spec Exp:** Psychiatry in Cancer; Pain-Cancer; Psychiatry in Physical Illness; Psychopharmacology; **Hospital:** Ronald Reagan UCLA Med Ctr, Cedars-Sinai Med Ctr; **Address:** Resnick Neuropsychiatric Hosp at UCLA, 150 Westwood Plaza, Ste 4230B, Los Angeles, CA 90024; **Phone:** 310-267-9159; **Board Cert:** Psychiatry 1993; Pain Medicine 2000; Hospice & Palliative Medicine 1998; **Med School:** Case West Res Univ 1987; **Resid:** Psychiatry, UCLA Med Ctr 1991; **Fac Appt:** Clin Prof Psyc, UCLA

Sullivan, Mark MD/PhD [Psyc] - **Spec Exp:** Psychiatry in Heart Disease Patients; Pain-Chronic; Psychiatry in Terminal Illness; **Hospital:** Univ Wash Med Ctr; **Address:** Univ Washington, Dept Psych, 1959 NE Pacific St, Box 356560, Seattle, WA 98195; **Phone:** 206-543-3925; **Board Cert:** Psychiatry 1991; **Med School:** Vanderbilt Univ 1984; **Resid:** Psychiatry, Univ Washington Med Ctr 1988; **Fac Appt:** Assoc Prof Psyc, Univ Wash

Weinstock, Robert MD [Psyc] - **Spec Exp:** Adolescent Psychiatry; Addiction/Substance Abuse; **Hospital:** Cedars-Sinai Med Ctr; **Address:** 1823 Sawtelle Blvd, Los Angeles, CA 90025; **Phone:** 310-477-9933; **Board Cert:** Psychiatry 1975; Forensic Psychiatry 2004; **Med School:** NYU Sch Med 1966; **Resid:** Psychiatry, McLean Hosp 1970; McLean Hosp 1972; **Fellow:** Psychiatric Research, Boston Univ 1974; **Fac Appt:** Clin Prof Psyc, UCLA

Zerbe, Kathryn J MD [Psyc] - **Spec Exp:** Eating Disorders; Women's Health-Mental Health; Psychoanalysis; **Hospital:** OR Hlth & Sci Univ; **Address:** 3181 SW Sam Jackson Park Rd, MC OP02, Portland, OR 97239; **Phone:** 503-494-1009; **Board Cert:** Psychiatry 1984; **Med School:** Temple Univ 1978; **Resid:** Psychiatry, Menninger Clin 1982; Psychoanalysis, Topeka Inst for Psychoanalysis 1992; **Fac Appt:** Prof Psyc, Oregon Hlth Sci Univ

Zisook, Sidney MD [Psyc] - **Spec Exp:** Bereavement/Traumatic Grief; Depression; Suicide; **Hospital:** VA San Diego Hlthcre Sys, UCSD Med Ctr; **Address:** UCSD, Dept Psychiatry, 9500 Gilman Drive, MS 9116A, La Jolla, CA 92093; **Phone:** 858-534-4040; **Board Cert:** Psychiatry 1975; **Med School:** Loyola Univ-Stritch Sch Med 1969; **Resid:** Psychiatry, Mass Genl Hosp 1973; **Fellow:** Psychiatry, Harvard 1973; **Fac Appt:** Prof Psyc, UCSD

ADDICTION PSYCHIATRY

New England

Schottenfeld, Richard MD [AdP] - **Spec Exp:** Drug Abuse-Consultation; Alcohol Abuse-Consultation; **Hospital:** Yale-New Haven Hosp; **Address:** Connecticut Mental Health Ctr, 34 Park St, rm S-204, New Haven, CT 06519; **Phone:** 203-974-7349; **Board Cert:** Psychiatry 1984; **Med School:** Yale Univ 1976; **Resid:** Psychiatry, Yale Psych Inst 1982; **Fellow:** Epidemiology, Yale Univ 1984; **Fac Appt:** Assoc Prof Psyc, Yale Univ

Ziedonis, Douglas M MD [AdP] - **Spec Exp:** Tobacco Abuse; **Hospital:** UMass Memorial Med Ctr; **Address:** Univ Mass Medical School, Dept Psychiatry, 55 Lake Ave N, Worcester, MA 01655; **Phone:** 508-856-3066; **Board Cert:** Psychiatry 1994; Addiction Psychiatry 2006; **Med School:** Penn State Univ-Hershey Med Ctr 1985; **Resid:** Psychiatry, UCLA Med Ctr 1989; **Fellow:** Addiction Psychiatry, UCLA Med Ctr 1990; **Fac Appt:** Prof Psyc, Univ Mass Sch Med

Addiction Psychiatry

Mid Atlantic

Frances, Richard J MD [AdP] - **Spec Exp:** Alcohol Abuse; Substance Abuse; Forensic Psychiatry; Addiction/Substance Abuse; **Hospital:** Silver Hill Hosp, NYU Med Ctr (page 68); **Address:** 510 E 86th St, Ste 1D, New York, NY 10028; **Phone:** 212-861-0570; **Board Cert:** Psychiatry 1976; Addiction Psychiatry 2002; **Med School:** NYU Sch Med 1971; **Resid:** Psychiatry, Bronx Meml Hosp 1974; **Fellow:** Psychoanalysis, NY Psychoanalitic Inst 1978; **Fac Appt:** Clin Prof Psyc, NYU Sch Med

Galanter, Marc MD [AdP] - **Spec Exp:** Alcohol Abuse; Drug Abuse; **Hospital:** NYU Med Ctr (page 68), Bellevue Hosp Ctr; **Address:** 285 Central Park West, New York, NY 10024-3006; **Phone:** 212-877-4093; **Board Cert:** Psychiatry 1974; Addiction Psychiatry 2002; **Med School:** Albert Einstein Coll Med 1967; **Resid:** Psychiatry, Bronx Muni Hosp-Einstein 1971; **Fac Appt:** Prof Psyc, NYU Sch Med

Kampman, Kyle M MD [AdP] - **Spec Exp:** Addiction/Substance Abuse; Cocaine Addiction; Opiate Addiction; **Hospital:** Hosp Univ Penn - UPHS (page 60); **Address:** Charles O'Brien Treatment Ctr, 3900 Chestnut St, Philadelphia, PA 19104; **Phone:** 215-222-3815; **Board Cert:** Psychiatry 2004; Addiction Psychiatry 2006; **Med School:** Tulane Univ 1985; **Resid:** Psychiatry, Univ Penn 1993; **Fellow:** Substance Abuse, Univ Penn 1994; **Fac Appt:** Assoc Prof Psyc, Univ Pennsylvania

Kleber, Herbert MD [AdP] - **Spec Exp:** Opiate Addiction; Cocaine Addiction; Drug Abuse; **Hospital:** NY-Presby Hosp/Columbia (page 66), NY State Psychiatric Inst; **Address:** 1051 Riverside Dr, New York, NY 10032-1007; **Phone:** 212-543-5570; **Med School:** Jefferson Med Coll 1960; **Resid:** Psychiatry, Yale-New Haven Hosp 1964; **Fac Appt:** Prof Psyc, Columbia P&S

Strain, Eric C MD [AdP] - **Spec Exp:** Addiction/Substance Abuse; Dual Diagnosis; Opiate Addiction; **Hospital:** Johns Hopkins Bayview Med Ctr (page 61); **Address:** 4940 Eastern Ave, Baltimore, MD 21224; **Phone:** 410-550-0016; **Board Cert:** Psychiatry 1989; Addiction Psychiatry 2002; **Med School:** Ohio State Univ 1984; **Resid:** Psychiatry, Johns Hopkins Hosp 1988; **Fellow:** Addiction Psychiatry, Johns Hopkins Hosp 1990; **Fac Appt:** Prof Psyc, Johns Hopkins Univ

Southeast

Anton, Raymond F MD [AdP] - **Spec Exp:** Alcohol Abuse; Clinical Trials; **Hospital:** MUSC Med Ctr; **Address:** MUSC Dept Psychiatry, 67 President St, Box 250861, Charleston, SC 29425; **Phone:** 843-792-1226; **Board Cert:** Psychiatry 1982; Addiction Psychiatry 1997; **Med School:** UMDNJ-Rutgers Med Sch 1976; **Resid:** Psychiatry, Yale-New Haven Hosp/CT Mental Health Ctr 1980; **Fac Appt:** Prof Psyc, Med Univ SC

Brady, Kathleen T MD/PhD [AdP] - **Spec Exp:** Addiction/Substance Abuse; Dual Diagnosis; **Hospital:** MUSC Med Ctr; **Address:** MUSC Inst of Psychiatry, 67 President St, Box 250861, Charleston, SC 29425; **Phone:** 843-792-9888; **Board Cert:** Psychiatry 1992; Addiction Psychiatry 2002; **Med School:** Med Univ SC 1985; **Resid:** Psychiatry, Med Univ SC 1989; **Fellow:** Addiction Psychiatry, Med Univ SC 1989; **Fac Appt:** Prof Psyc, Med Univ SC

Midwest

Stine, Susan M MD/PhD [AdP] - **Spec Exp:** Addiction/Substance Abuse; Opiate Addiction; **Hospital:** Detroit Med Ctr; **Address:** Wayne State Univ Sch Med, Dept Psychiatry, 2761 E Jefferson Ave, Detroit, MI 48201; **Phone:** 313-993-9879; **Board Cert:** Psychiatry 1993; Addiction Psychiatry 2002; **Med School:** Univ Miami Sch Med 1983; **Resid:** Psychiatry, Yale-New Haven Hosp 1987; **Fac Appt:** Assoc Prof Psyc, Wayne State Univ

Great Plains and Mountains

Howell, Elizabeth F MD [AdP] - **Spec Exp:** Opiate Addiction; Alcohol Abuse; Addiction/Substance Abuse; Pain Management; **Hospital:** Univ Utah Hosps and Clins; **Address:** Univ Utah Neuropsychiatric Inst, 501 Chipeta Way, Salt Lake City, UT 84108; **Phone:** 801-585-1575; **Board Cert:** Psychiatry 1985; Addiction Psychiatry 2003; **Med School:** Med Univ SC 1980; **Resid:** Psychiatry, Med Univ South Carolina 1984; **Fellow:** Psychiatric Research, Med Univ South Carolina 1985; **Fac Appt:** Assoc Clin Prof Psyc, Univ Utah

Southwest

Kosten, Thomas MD [AdP] - **Spec Exp:** Cocaine Addiction; Alcohol Abuse; Psychopharmacology; Opiate Addiction; **Hospital:** DeBakey VA Med Ctr-Houston, UT MD Anderson Cancer Ctr; **Address:** Michael DeBakey VA Medical Ctr, 2002 Holcombe Blvd, Research - Building 110, Houston, TX 77030; **Phone:** 713-794-7032; **Board Cert:** Psychiatry 1984; Addiction Psychiatry 2002; **Med School:** Cornell Univ-Weill Med Coll 1977; **Resid:** Psychiatry, Yale-New Haven Hosp 1981; **Fellow:** Epidemiology, Yale-New Haven Hosp 1983; **Fac Appt:** Prof Psyc, Baylor Coll Med

West Coast and Pacific

McCance-Katz, Elinore F MD/PhD [AdP] - **Spec Exp:** Addiction/Substance Abuse; Psychopharmacology; **Hospital:** UCSF Med Ctr; **Address:** UCSF Dept Psychiatry, 1001 Potrero Ave, Ste 7M-WD93, San Francisco, CA 94110; **Phone:** 415-206-4010; **Board Cert:** Psychiatry 1993; Addiction Psychiatry 2002; **Med School:** Univ Conn 1987; **Resid:** Psychiatry, Inst of Living 1990; Psychiatry, Yale Univ 1991; **Fellow:** Neuropsychopharmacology, Yale Univ Sch Med 1991; **Fac Appt:** Prof Psyc, UCSF

Schuckit, Marc A MD [AdP] - **Spec Exp:** Alcohol Abuse; Psychopharmacology; **Hospital:** VA San Diego Hlthcre Sys; **Address:** VA San Diego Healthcare System, Dept Psychiatry (116A), 3350 La Jolla Village Drive, San Diego, CA 92161-2002; **Phone:** 858-552-8585 x7978; **Board Cert:** Psychiatry 1974; **Med School:** Washington Univ, St Louis 1968; **Resid:** Psychiatry, Washington Univ 1971; Psychiatry, UC San Diego 1972; **Fac Appt:** Prof Psyc, UCSD

Walker, R Dale MD [AdP] - **Spec Exp:** Alcohol Abuse-Consultation; Drug Abuse-Consultation; Substance Abuse-Consultation; **Hospital:** OR Hlth & Sci Univ; **Address:** Oregon Hlth & Sci Univ, 3181 SW Sam Jackson Pk Rd, MC GH151, Portland, OR 97239; **Phone:** 503-494-3703; **Board Cert:** Psychiatry 1982; **Med School:** Univ Okla Coll Med 1972; **Resid:** Psychiatry, Univ Oklahoma Med Ctr 1973; Psychiatry, UCSD Med Ctr 1977; **Fellow:** Public Health & Genl Preventive Med, Andriga Stampur; **Fac Appt:** Prof Psyc, Oregon Hlth Sci Univ

CHILD & ADOLESCENT PSYCHIATRY

New England

Biederman, Joseph MD [ChAP] - **Spec Exp:** ADD/ADHD; Anxiety & Mood Disorders; Psychopharmacology; **Hospital:** Mass Genl Hosp; **Address:** 55 Fruit St Yawkey Bldg - rm 6900, Boston, MA 02114; **Phone:** 617-726-1743; **Board Cert:** Psychiatry 1983; Child & Adolescent Psychiatry 1984; **Med School:** Argentina 1971; **Resid:** Psychiatry, Hadassah Univ Hosp 1977; Psychiatry, Mass Genl Hosp 1981; **Fellow:** Child Psychiatry, Childrens Hosp 1979; **Fac Appt:** Prof Psyc, Harvard Med Sch

Child & Adolescent Psychiatry

Coyle, Joseph MD [ChAP] - **Spec Exp:** Neuro-Psychiatry; Psychiatric Genetics; Mental Retardation; **Hospital:** McLean Hosp; **Address:** McLean Hospital, 115 Mill St, Belmont, MA 02478-1048; **Phone:** 617-855-2101; **Board Cert:** Psychiatry 1980; **Med School:** Johns Hopkins Univ 1969; **Resid:** Psychiatry, Johns Hopkins Hosp 1976; **Fellow:** Psychopharmacology, NIMH 1973; **Fac Appt:** Prof Psyc, Harvard Med Sch

Fritz, Gregory K MD [ChAP] - **Spec Exp:** Asthma; Psychosomatic Disorders; **Hospital:** Rhode Island Hosp; **Address:** RI Hosp, Child & Family Psychiatry, 1 Hoppin St Fl 2, Providence, RI 02903; **Phone:** 401-444-7573; **Board Cert:** Psychiatry 1977; Child & Adolescent Psychiatry 1978; **Med School:** Tufts Univ 1971; **Resid:** Psychiatry, San Mateo Co Hosp 1974; Child Psychiatry, Stanford Univ Med Ctr 1977; **Fac Appt:** Prof Psyc, Brown Univ

Herzog, David B MD [ChAP] - **Spec Exp:** Eating Disorders; Somatic Disorders-Adolescent; **Hospital:** Mass Genl Hosp; **Address:** 2 Longfellow Place, Ste 200, Boston, MA 02114; **Phone:** 617-724-0799; **Board Cert:** Pediatrics 1980; Psychiatry 1982; Child & Adolescent Psychiatry 1986; **Med School:** Mexico 1973; **Resid:** Pediatrics, Univ Wisc 1975; Pediatrics, Boston City Hosp 1976; **Fellow:** Child & Adolescent Psychiatry, Chldns Hosp 1978; Psychiatry, Mass Genl Hosp 1980; **Fac Appt:** Prof Psyc, Harvard Med Sch

Hudziak, James MD [ChAP] - **Spec Exp:** ADD/ADHD; Obsessive-Compulsive Disorder; Psychopharmacology; **Hospital:** FAHC - Med Ctr Campus; **Address:** Univ Vermont Med Sch, Dept Psychiatry, 1 S Prospect Dr, MCHS-Arnold 6-UHC Campus, Burlington, VT 05401; **Phone:** 802-847-4560; **Board Cert:** Psychiatry 2005; Child & Adolescent Psychiatry 2005; **Med School:** Univ Minn 1988; **Resid:** St Louis Chldns Hosp 1991; **Fac Appt:** Assoc Prof Psyc, Univ VT Coll Med

King, Robert A MD [ChAP] - **Spec Exp:** Tourette's Syndrome; Obsessive-Compulsive Disorder; Psychoanalysis; **Hospital:** Yale-New Haven Hosp; **Address:** Yale Child Study Ctr, 230 S Frontage Rd, Box 207900, New Haven, CT 06519-1124; **Phone:** 203-785-5880; **Board Cert:** Psychiatry 1974; Child & Adolescent Psychiatry 1981; **Med School:** Harvard Med Sch 1968; **Resid:** Pediatrics, Chldns Hosp 1969; Psychiatry, Mass Mental Hlth Ctr 1971; **Fellow:** Child Psychiatry, Chldns Hosp 1972; Child Psychiatry, Chldns Hosp Natl Med Ctr 1974; **Fac Appt:** Prof Psyc, Yale Univ

Leckman, James F MD [ChAP] - **Spec Exp:** Tourette's Syndrome; Obsessive-Compulsive Disorder; Autism; **Hospital:** Yale-New Haven Hosp; **Address:** Yale Child Study Ctr, 230 S Frontage Rd, Box 207900, New Haven, CT 06520-7900; **Phone:** 203-785-7971; **Board Cert:** Psychiatry 1980; Child & Adolescent Psychiatry 1982; **Med School:** Univ New Mexico 1973; **Resid:** Psychiatry, Yale Univ 1979; Child & Adolescent Psychiatry, Yale Chld Stdy Ctr 1980; **Fellow:** Psychiatry, Natl Inst Mental Hlth 1976; **Fac Appt:** Prof Psyc, Yale Univ

Spencer, Thomas MD [ChAP] - **Spec Exp:** ADD/ADHD; **Hospital:** Mass Genl Hosp; **Address:** Mass General Hospital, 55 Fruit St, Ste YAW 6A, Boston, MA 02114; **Phone:** 617-724-5600; **Board Cert:** Psychiatry 1984; Child & Adolescent Psychiatry 1993; **Med School:** Univ Wisc 1978; **Resid:** Psychiatry, New England Med Ctr 1984; **Fellow:** Child & Adolescent Psychiatry, Mass General Hosp 1992; **Fac Appt:** Assoc Prof Psyc, Harvard Med Sch

Volkmar, Fred R MD [ChAP] - **Spec Exp:** Autism; Asperger's Syndrome; Developmental Disorders; Mental Retardation; **Hospital:** Yale-New Haven Hosp; **Address:** Yale Child Study Ctr, 230 S Frontage Rd, Box 207900, New Haven, CT 06519-1124; **Phone:** 203-785-5759; **Board Cert:** Psychiatry 1981; Child & Adolescent Psychiatry 1988; **Med School:** Stanford Univ 1976; **Resid:** Psychiatry, Stanford Univ 1980; Child & Adolescent Psychiatry, Yale Univ Child Study Ctr 1982; **Fac Appt:** Prof Psyc, Yale Univ

Wilens, Timothy MD [ChAP] - **Spec Exp:** ADD/ADHD; Bipolar/Mood Disorders; Addiction/Substance Abuse; **Hospital:** Mass Genl Hosp; **Address:** Mass Genl Hosp, Dept Psyc, 55 Fruit St Yawkey Bldg - Ste 6A, Boston, MA 02114; **Phone:** 617-724-5600; **Board Cert:** Psychiatry 1990; Child & Adolescent Psychiatry 1991; Addiction Psychiatry 1994; **Med School:** Univ Mich Med Sch 1985; **Resid:** Internal Medicine, Henry Ford Hosp 1986; Psychiatry, Mass Genl Hosp 1988; **Fellow:** Child & Adolescent Psychiatry, Mass Genl Hosp 1990; **Fac Appt:** Assoc Prof Psyc, Harvard Med Sch

Mid Atlantic

Abright, Arthur R MD [ChAP] - **Spec Exp:** Bipolar/Mood Disorders; ADD/ADHD; Post Traumatic Stress Disorder; **Hospital:** St Vincent Cath Med Ctrs - Manhattan; **Address:** 144 W 12th St, New York, NY 10011-8202; **Phone:** 212-604-8213; **Board Cert:** Psychiatry 1978; Child & Adolescent Psychiatry 1981; **Med School:** Univ Tex SW, Dallas 1973; **Resid:** Psychiatry, St Vincent's Hosp 1974; Psychiatry, NY Hosp-Cornell Med Ctr 1977; **Fellow:** Child & Adolescent Psychiatry, NY Hosp-Cornell Med Ctr 1979; **Fac Appt:** Clin Prof Psyc, NY Med Coll

Bird, Hector MD [ChAP] - **Spec Exp:** ADD/ADHD; Anxiety & Depression; Personality Disorders; **Hospital:** NY-Presby Hosp/Columbia (page 66); **Address:** 300 W 72nd St, Ste 1F, New York, NY 10023-2004; **Phone:** 212-874-5311; **Board Cert:** Psychiatry 1975; Child & Adolescent Psychiatry 1977; **Med School:** Yale Univ 1965; **Resid:** Psychiatry, NY State Psych Inst 1971; NY State Psych Inst 1972; **Fellow:** Psychoanalysis, WA White Institute 1977; **Fac Appt:** Prof Emeritus Psyc, Columbia P&S

Bogrov, Michael MD [ChAP] - **Spec Exp:** ADD/ADHD; Mood Disorders; **Hospital:** Sheppard Pratt Hlth Sys, Johns Hopkins Hosp - Baltimore (page 61); **Address:** 6501 N Charles St, P.O. Box 6815, Towson, MD 21204-6815; **Phone:** 410-938-4913; **Board Cert:** Psychiatry 1993; Child & Adolescent Psychiatry 1994; **Med School:** Emory Univ 1987; **Resid:** Psychiatry, Univ Maryland 1990; Johns Hopkins Hosp 1992; **Fac Appt:** Asst Prof Psyc, Johns Hopkins Univ

Brent, David A MD [ChAP] - **Spec Exp:** Suicide; **Hospital:** Western Psych Inst & Clin - UPMC; **Address:** Western Psych Inst & Clinic, 3811 O'Hara St, Ste 315 BFT, Pittsburgh, PA 15213-2593; **Phone:** 412-246-5596; **Board Cert:** Pediatrics 1981; Psychiatry 1982; Child & Adolescent Psychiatry 1983; **Med School:** Jefferson Med Coll 1974; **Resid:** Psychiatry, Western Psych Inst 1982; **Fellow:** Psychiatry, Univ Colorado Med Ctr 1976; **Fac Appt:** Prof Psyc, Univ Pittsburgh

Coffey, Barbara J MD [ChAP] - **Spec Exp:** Tourette's Syndrome; ADD/ADHD; Obsessive-Compulsive Disorder; **Hospital:** NYU Med Ctr (page 68); **Address:** NYU Child Study Ctr, 577 1st Ave, New York, NY 10016; **Phone:** 212-263-3926; **Board Cert:** Psychiatry 1981; Child & Adolescent Psychiatry 1986; **Med School:** Tufts Univ 1975; **Resid:** Psychiatry, Boston Univ 1978; Child & Adolescent Psychiatry, Tufts Univ 1980; **Fac Appt:** Assoc Prof Psyc, NYU Sch Med

Foley, Carmel MD [ChAP] - **Spec Exp:** Mood Disorders; **Hospital:** Schneider Chldn's Hosp; **Address:** Schneider Chldns Hosp, 269-01 76th Ave Fl 4, New Hyde Park, NY 11040; **Phone:** 718-470-3550; **Board Cert:** Psychiatry 1979; Child & Adolescent Psychiatry 1981; Addiction Psychiatry 1997; Forensic Psychiatry 1999; **Med School:** Ireland 1972; **Resid:** Psychiatry, St Patrick's Hosp 1976; Psychiatry, Lafayette Clinic 1977; **Fellow:** Child & Adolescent Psychiatry, Lafayette Clinic 1979; **Fac Appt:** Assoc Prof Psyc, Albert Einstein Coll Med

Fornari, Victor MD [ChAP] - **Spec Exp:** Eating Disorders; Trauma Psychiatry; Post Traumatic Stress Disorder; **Hospital:** Zucker Hillside Hosp; **Address:** Zucker Hillside Hospital, Ambulatory Care Pavilion Lower Level, 75-59 263rd St, Glen Oaks, NY 11004; **Phone:** 718-470-3510; **Board Cert:** Psychiatry 1984; Child & Adolescent Psychiatry 1985; **Med School:** SUNY Downstate 1979; **Resid:** Psychiatry, Hosp Univ Penn 1982; **Fellow:** Child & Adolescent Psychiatry, LIJ Med Ctr 1984; **Fac Appt:** Assoc Prof Psyc, NYU Sch Med

Child & Adolescent Psychiatry

Greenspan, Stanley MD [ChAP] - **Spec Exp:** Autism; Infant/Toddler Psychiatry; **Hospital:** G Washington Univ Hosp; **Address:** 7201 Glenbrook Rd, Bethesda, MD 20814; **Phone:** 301-657-2348; **Board Cert:** Psychiatry 1972; **Med School:** Yale Univ 1966; **Resid:** Psychiatry, Columbia-Presby Psych Inst 1969; **Fellow:** Child & Adolescent Psychiatry, Childrens Hosp Natl Med Ctr 1971; **Fac Appt:** Clin Prof Psyc, Geo Wash Univ

Hertzig, Margaret MD [ChAP] - **Spec Exp:** Developmental Disorders; ADD/ADHD; **Hospital:** NY-Presby Hosp/Weill Cornell (page 66); **Address:** 525 E 68th St, Box 140, New York, NY 10021-4870; **Phone:** 212-746-5712; **Board Cert:** Psychiatry 1968; Child & Adolescent Psychiatry 1975; **Med School:** NYU Sch Med 1960; **Resid:** Pediatrics, Jewish Hosp 1962; Psychiatry, Bellevue Psych Hosp 1964; **Fellow:** Psychiatric Research, NYU Sch Med 1966; **Fac Appt:** Prof Psyc, Cornell Univ-Weill Med Coll

Pomeroy, John C MD [ChAP] - **Spec Exp:** Autism; Mental Retardation; Developmental Disorders; **Hospital:** Stony Brook Univ Med Ctr; **Address:** The Cody Center for Autism, 5 Medical Drive, Port Jefferson Stn, NY 11776; **Phone:** 631-632-3070; **Board Cert:** Psychiatry 1984; Child & Adolescent Psychiatry 1988; **Med School:** England 1973; **Resid:** Psychiatry, St Mary's Hosp 1979; **Fellow:** Child & Adolescent Psychiatry, Univ Iowa Hosps 1981; **Fac Appt:** Assoc Prof Psyc, SUNY Stony Brook

Pruitt, David B MD [ChAP] - **Hospital:** Univ of MD Med Sys; **Address:** Univ Maryland, Div Child & Adolescent Psychiatry, 701 W Pratt St, Ste 429, Baltimore, MD 21201; **Phone:** 410-328-3522; **Board Cert:** Psychiatry 1979; Child & Adolescent Psychiatry 1981; **Med School:** Univ Tex, Houston 1974; **Resid:** Psychiatry, Hosp Univ Penn 1978; Child Guidance Ctr 1979; **Fac Appt:** Prof Psyc, Univ MD Sch Med

Rapoport, Judith MD [ChAP] - **Spec Exp:** Schizophrenia; Obsessive-Compulsive Disorder; **Hospital:** Natl Inst of Hlth - Clin Ctr; **Address:** 3010 44th Place NW, Washington, DC 20016; **Phone:** 202-966-7355; **Board Cert:** Psychiatry 1969; Child & Adolescent Psychiatry 1969; **Med School:** Harvard Med Sch 1959; **Resid:** Psychiatry, Mass Mental Hlth Ctr 1961; Psychiatry, St Elizabeth Hosp 1962; **Fellow:** Psychiatry, Karolinska Inst 1964; Child & Adolescent Psychiatry, Childns Hosp 1966

Riddle, Mark A MD [ChAP] - **Spec Exp:** Psychopharmacology; Anxiety Disorders; Mood Disorders; **Hospital:** Johns Hopkins Hosp - Baltimore (page 61); **Address:** 600 N Wolfe St, CMSC-346, Baltimore, MD 21287-3325; **Phone:** 410-955-2320; **Board Cert:** Psychiatry 1982; Child & Adolescent Psychiatry 1986; **Med School:** Indiana Univ 1977; **Resid:** Psychiatry, Yale-New Haven Hosp 1981; **Fellow:** Child & Adolescent Psychiatry, Yale Child Study Ctr 1983; **Fac Appt:** Prof Psyc, Johns Hopkins Univ

Rostain, Anthony L MD [ChAP] - **Spec Exp:** ADD/ADHD; Autism; Tourette's Syndrome; Asperger's Syndrome; **Hospital:** Chldns Hosp of Philadelphia, The, Penn Presby Med Ctr - UPHS (page 60); **Address:** Hosp U Penn, Dept Psychiatry, 3535 Market St Fl 2, Philadelphia, PA 19104; **Phone:** 215-746-7210; **Board Cert:** Pediatrics 1985; Psychiatry 1988; Child & Adolescent Psychiatry 1989; **Med School:** NYU Sch Med 1980; **Resid:** Pediatrics, Children's Hosp 1983; Psychiatry, Hosp U Penn 1987; **Fellow:** Child Psychiatry, Philadelphia Child Guidance Clin 1988; **Fac Appt:** Assoc Prof Psyc, Univ Pennsylvania

Turecki, Stanley K MD [ChAP] - **Spec Exp:** Temperamentally Difficult Child; ADD/ADHD; Parenting Issues; **Hospital:** Lenox Hill Hosp (page 62), Beth Israel Med Ctr - Petrie Division (page 57); **Address:** 136 E 64th St, Ste 1B, New York, NY 10021-2137; **Phone:** 212-355-2535; **Board Cert:** Psychiatry 1978; Child & Adolescent Psychiatry 1981; **Med School:** South Africa 1961; **Resid:** Psychiatry, Tara Hospital 1969; Child & Adolescent Psychiatry, Mt Sinai Hosp 1971

Walkup, John MD [ChAP] - **Spec Exp:** Anxiety Disorders; **Hospital:** Johns Hopkins Hosp - Baltimore (page 61); **Address:** Johns Hopkins Hosp, Dept Child Psyc, 600 N Wolfe St, CMSC 314, Baltimore, MD 21287; **Phone:** 410-955-5823 x1; **Board Cert:** Psychiatry 1987; Child & Adolescent Psychiatry 1992; **Med School:** Univ Minn 1982; **Resid:** Psychiatry, Yale Univ Med Sch 1985; Yale Chld Study Ctr 1988; **Fac Appt:** Asst Prof Psyc, Johns Hopkins Univ

Weller, Elizabeth B MD [ChAP] - **Spec Exp:** Anxiety & Mood Disorders; Bipolar/Mood Disorders; ADD/ADHD; Aggression Disorders; **Hospital:** Chldns Hosp of Philadelphia, The; **Address:** Children's Hosp of Philadelphia, Mood & Anxiety Ctr, 34th & Civic Center Blvd, Philadelphia, PA 19104; **Phone:** 215-590-7573; **Board Cert:** Psychiatry 1981; Child & Adolescent Psychiatry 1982; **Med School:** Lebanon 1975; **Resid:** Psychiatry, Renard Hosp-Wash Univ 1978; **Fellow:** Child & Adolescent Psychiatry, Univ Kansas Med Ctr 1979; **Fac Appt:** Prof Psyc

Southeast

Deas, Deborah V MD [ChAP] - **Spec Exp:** Addiction/Substance Abuse; Dual Diagnosis; Substance Abuse in ADHD Patients; **Hospital:** MUSC Med Ctr; **Address:** MUSC, Ctr for Drug & Alcohol Programs, 67 President St, Charleston, SC 29425; **Phone:** 843-792-5214; **Board Cert:** Psychiatry 2005; Child & Adolescent Psychiatry 2007; Addiction Psychiatry 1997; **Med School:** Med Univ SC 1989; **Resid:** Psychiatry, MUSC Med Ctr 1992; **Fellow:** Child & Adolescent Psychiatry, MUSC Med Ctr 1994; Addiction Psychiatry, MUSC/Natl Inst Alcohol Abuse & Alcoholism 1994; **Fac Appt:** Prof Psyc, Med Univ SC

Heston, Jerry D MD [ChAP] - **Hospital:** Le Bonheur Chldns Med Ctr, St Jude Children's Research Hosp; **Address:** Child & Adolescent Psychiatric Assocs, 1135 Cully Rd, Ste 100, Cordova, TN 38106; **Phone:** 901-752-1980; **Board Cert:** Psychiatry 1988; Pediatrics 2004; Child & Adolescent Psychiatry 1989; **Med School:** Univ S Fla Coll Med 1981; **Resid:** Pediatrics, LeBonheur Chldns Hosp 1984; Psychiatry, Univ Tennessee 1986; **Fellow:** Child & Adolescent Psychiatry, Univ Tennessee 1988

Sexson, Sandra G B MD [ChAP] - **Spec Exp:** Psychiatry in Transplant Patients; Death & Dying; **Hospital:** Med Coll of GA Hosp and Clin; **Address:** Medical College Georgia, 997 St Sebastian Way, Augusta, GA 30912; **Phone:** 706-721-6699; **Board Cert:** Psychiatry 1980; Child & Adolescent Psychiatry 1981; **Med School:** Univ Miss 1971; **Resid:** Psychiatry, Tex Hlth Sci Ctr 1974; Washington Univ 1978; **Fellow:** Child & Adolescent Psychiatry, Washington Univ 1978; **Fac Appt:** Prof Psyc, Med Coll GA

Wright, Harry H MD [ChAP] - **Spec Exp:** Infant/Toddler Psychiatry; Autism & Developmental Disorders; Anxiety Disorders; **Hospital:** William S Hall Psyc Inst, Richland Mem Hosp; **Address:** 3555 Harden St Ext, Ste 301, Columbia, SC 29203-6894; **Phone:** 803-434-4250; **Board Cert:** Psychiatry 1982; Child & Adolescent Psychiatry 1984; **Med School:** Univ Pennsylvania 1976; **Resid:** Psychiatry, Wm S Hall Psyc Inst 1979; **Fellow:** Child & Adolescent Psychiatry, Wm S Hall Psyc Inst-Univ S Carolina 1981; **Fac Appt:** Prof Psyc, Univ SC Sch Med

Midwest

Alessi, Norman E MD [ChAP] - **Spec Exp:** Mood Disorders; Telepsychiatry; Psychopharmacology; **Hospital:** Univ Michigan Hlth Sys; **Address:** 825 Victors Way, Ste 310, Ann Arbor, MI 48108-2830; **Phone:** 734-222-6222; **Board Cert:** Psychiatry 1982; Child & Adolescent Psychiatry 1985; **Med School:** Emory Univ 1976; **Resid:** Psychiatry, Univ Mich Med Ctr 1980; Child Psychiatry, Univ Mich Med Ctr 1981; **Fellow:** Child & Adolescent Psychiatry, Univ Mich Med Ctr 1983; **Fac Appt:** Prof Emeritus Psyc, Univ Mich Med Sch

Child & Adolescent Psychiatry

Boxer, Gary H MD [ChAP] - **Spec Exp:** ADD/ADHD; Parenting Issues; Mood Disorders; **Hospital:** St Louis Chldns Hosp; **Address:** St Louis Chldns Hosp, Dept Psychiatry, 24 S Kingshighway Blvd, St Louis, MO 63108; **Phone:** 314-286-1740; **Board Cert:** Psychiatry 1986; Child & Adolescent Psychiatry 1988; **Med School:** Univ Colorado 1980; **Resid:** Psychiatry, Univ Michigan Med Ctr 1983; **Fellow:** Child Psychiatry, Univ Colorado 1985; **Fac Appt:** Assoc Prof Psyc, Washington Univ, St Louis

Campo, John V MD [ChAP] - **Spec Exp:** Psychosomatic Disorders; Psychiatry in Physical Illness; **Hospital:** Nationwide Chldn's Hosp, Ohio St Univ Med Ctr; **Address:** Columbus Chldn's Hosp, 700 Childrens Drive, Timken Hall H2K, Columbus, OH 43205; **Phone:** 614-722-2291; **Board Cert:** Pediatrics 1986; Psychiatry 1989; Child & Adolescent Psychiatry 1993; **Med School:** Univ Pennsylvania 1982; **Resid:** Pediatrics, Childrens Hosp 1985; Psychiatry, West Psych Inst Clin 1989

Dulcan, Mina K MD [ChAP] - **Spec Exp:** ADD/ADHD; **Hospital:** Children's Mem Hosp; **Address:** Chldns Meml Hosp, Dept Psyc, 2300 Children's Plaza, Box 10, Chicago, IL 60614; **Phone:** 773-880-4811; **Board Cert:** Psychiatry 1978; Child & Adolescent Psychiatry 1979; **Med School:** Penn State Univ-Hershey Med Ctr 1974; **Resid:** Psychiatry, Western Psych Inst/Clinic 1977; **Fellow:** Child Psychiatry, Western Psych Inst 1978; **Fac Appt:** Prof Psyc, Northwestern Univ

Leventhal, Bennett MD [ChAP] - **Spec Exp:** Autism; ADD/ADHD; Psychopharmacology; **Hospital:** Univ of IL Med Ctr at Chicago; **Address:** Univ Illinois, Dept Psychiatry, 1747 W Roosevelt Rd, MC 747, Chicago, IL 60608; **Phone:** 312-355-3026; **Board Cert:** Psychiatry 1979; Child & Adolescent Psychiatry 1980; **Med School:** Louisiana State U, New Orleans 1974; **Resid:** Psychiatry, Duke Univ Med Ctr 1978; **Fellow:** Child & Adolescent Psychiatry, Duke Univ Med Ctr 1977; **Fac Appt:** Prof Psyc, Univ IL Coll Med

Luby, Joan L MD [ChAP] - **Spec Exp:** Mood Disorders; **Hospital:** Barnes-Jewish Hosp; **Address:** Wash Univ Sch Med, Dept Psychiatry, 660 S Euclid Ave, Box 8134, St Louis, MO 63110; **Phone:** 314-286-2730; **Board Cert:** Psychiatry 1993; Child & Adolescent Psychiatry 1993; **Med School:** Wayne State Univ 1985; **Resid:** Psychiatry, Stanford Univ Sch Med 1988; **Fellow:** Child & Adolescent Psychiatry, Stanford Univ Sch Med 1990; **Fac Appt:** Assoc Prof Psyc, Washington Univ, St Louis

Martini, D Richard MD [ChAP] - **Spec Exp:** Psychiatry in Physical Illness; Post Traumatic Stress Disorder; ADD/ADHD; Brain Injury; **Hospital:** Children's Mem Hosp; **Address:** Children's Meml Hospital, Psychiatry, 2300 Children's Plaza, Box 10, Chicago, IL 60614-3394; **Phone:** 773-880-4825; **Board Cert:** Psychiatry 1987; Child & Adolescent Psychiatry 1990; **Med School:** Univ Nebr Coll Med 1982; **Resid:** Psychiatry, Univ Pittsburgh Med Ctr 1985; Child & Adolescent Psychiatry, Univ Pittsburgh Med Ctr 1987; **Fac Appt:** Assoc Prof Psyc, Northwestern Univ

McDougle, Christopher J MD [ChAP] - **Spec Exp:** Autism & Developmental Disorders; Obsessive-Compulsive Disorder; Tourette's Syndrome; **Hospital:** Riley Hosp for Children, Methodist Hosp - Indianapolis; **Address:** 1111 W 10th St, Psychiatry Bldg - rm A-305, Indianapolis, IN 46202-4800; **Phone:** 317-274-8162; **Board Cert:** Psychiatry 1992; Child & Adolescent Psychiatry 2006; **Med School:** Indiana Univ 1986; **Resid:** Psychiatry, Yale Univ 1990; **Fellow:** Child & Adolescent Psychiatry, Yale Child Study Ctr 1995; **Fac Appt:** Prof Psyc, Indiana Univ

Slomowitz, Marcia MD [ChAP] - **Spec Exp:** ADD/ADHD; Bipolar/Mood Disorders; Depression; Obsessive-Compulsive Disorder; **Hospital:** Northwestern Meml Hosp; **Address:** 333 N Michigan Ave, Ste 1125, Chicago, IL 60601; **Phone:** 312-726-1083; **Board Cert:** Psychiatry 1982; Child & Adolescent Psychiatry 1983; **Med School:** Univ Wisc 1977; **Resid:** Psychiatry, Univ Cincinnati 1980; **Fellow:** Child & Adolescent Psychiatry, Univ Cincinnati 1982; **Fac Appt:** Asst Prof Psyc, Northwestern Univ

Southwest

Bleiberg, Efrain MD [ChAP] - **Spec Exp:** Trauma Psychiatry; Personality Disorders; **Hospital:** Menninger Clinic; **Address:** Menninger Hosp & Clinic, 2801 Gessner Drive, Box 809045, Houston, TX 77280-9045; **Phone:** 713-275-5213; **Board Cert:** Psychiatry 1985; Child & Adolescent Psychiatry 1986; **Med School:** Mexico 1976; **Resid:** Psychiatry, Menninger Fdn 1980; **Fellow:** Child & Adolescent Psychiatry, Menninger Fdn 1981

Emslie, Graham J MD [ChAP] - **Spec Exp:** Depression; **Hospital:** Chldns Med Ctr of Dallas; **Address:** UT SW Med Ctr at Dallas, 5323 Harry Hines Blvd, Dallas, TX 75390-8589; **Phone:** 214-456-5921; **Board Cert:** Psychiatry 1981; **Med School:** Scotland 1974; **Resid:** Psychiatry, Univ Rochester 1978; Child Psychiatry, Stanford Med Ctr 1981; **Fac Appt:** Prof Psyc, Univ Tex SW, Dallas

Sargent III, A John MD [ChAP] - **Spec Exp:** Eating Disorders; Suicide; Family Therapy; Trauma Psychiatry; **Hospital:** Ben Taub Genl Hosp, Texas Chldns Hosp - Houston; **Address:** Baylor Coll Med, Dept Psychiatry, One Baylor Plaza, Houston, TX 77030-3411; **Phone:** 713-798-7889; **Board Cert:** Pediatrics 1979; Psychiatry 1988; Child & Adolescent Psychiatry 1989; **Med School:** Univ Rochester 1973; **Resid:** Pediatrics, Univ Wisc Hosp 1977; Phila Child Guidance Ctr 1980; **Fellow:** Ambulatory Pediatrics, Univ Wisc Hosp 1976; **Fac Appt:** Prof Psyc, Baylor Coll Med

Zeanah Jr, Charles H MD [ChAP] - **Spec Exp:** Attachment Disorders; Abuse/Neglect; Adoption-International; **Hospital:** Tulane Univ Hosp & Clin; **Address:** Tulane Univ Sch Med, Dept Psych & Neurology, 1440 Canal St, TB-52, New Orleans, LA 70112-2715; **Phone:** 504-988-5402; **Board Cert:** Psychiatry 1983; Child & Adolescent Psychiatry 1983; **Med School:** Tulane Univ 1977; **Resid:** Psychiatry, Duke Univ Med Ctr 1980; Stanford Univ Med Ctr 1982; **Fellow:** Research, Stanford Univ Med ctr 1984; **Fac Appt:** Prof Psyc, Tulane Univ

West Coast and Pacific

King, Bryan H MD [ChAP] - **Spec Exp:** Mental Retardation; Autism; Self-Injurious Behavior (SIB); **Hospital:** Chldns Hosp and Regl Med Ctr - Seattle; **Address:** Chldns Hosp & Regl Med Ctr, Dept Psych, 4800 Sand Point Way NE, MS W3636, Seattle, WA 98105; **Phone:** 206-987-4080; **Board Cert:** Psychiatry 1991; Child & Adolescent Psychiatry 2004; **Med School:** Med Coll Wisc 1983; **Resid:** Psychiatry, UCLA Neuropsych Inst 1987; **Fellow:** Child & Adolescent Psychiatry, UCLA Neuropsych Inst 1990; **Fac Appt:** Prof Psyc, Univ Wash

McCracken, James T MD [ChAP] - **Spec Exp:** Obsessive-Compulsive Disorder; Tourette's Syndrome; **Hospital:** UCLA Neuropsychiatric Hosp; **Address:** UCLA Neuropsychiatric Inst, 760 Westwood Plaza, Ste 48-270, Los Angeles, CA 90027; **Phone:** 310-825-0470; **Board Cert:** Psychiatry 1986; Child & Adolescent Psychiatry 1988; **Med School:** Baylor Coll Med 1980; **Resid:** Psychiatry, Duke Univ Med Ctr 1984; **Fellow:** Child & Adolescent Psychiatry, UCLA Neuropsych Inst 1985; **Fac Appt:** Prof Psyc, UCLA

McKelvey, Robert S MD [ChAP] - **Spec Exp:** Suicide; Depression; Cross Cultural Psychiatry; **Hospital:** Doernbecher Chldns Hosp/OHSU; **Address:** Oregon Hlth Sci Univ, 3181 SW Sam Jackson Park Rd, MC DC7P, Portland, OR 97239; **Phone:** 503-418-5775; **Board Cert:** Psychiatry 1980; Child & Adolescent Psychiatry 1982; **Med School:** Dartmouth Med Sch 1974; **Resid:** Psychiatry, Cambridge Hosp 1977; 1979; **Fellow:** Child Psychiatry, McLean Hosp 1979; **Fac Appt:** Prof Psyc, Oregon Hlth Sci Univ

Child & Adolescent Psychiatry

Ponton, Lynn Elisabeth MD [ChAP] - **Spec Exp:** Behavioral Disorders; Eating Disorders; **Hospital:** UCSF Med Ctr; **Address:** 201 Edgewood Ave, San Francisco, CA 94117; **Phone:** 415-664-3039; **Board Cert:** Psychiatry 1985; Child & Adolescent Psychiatry 1985; **Med School:** Univ Wisc 1978; **Resid:** Psychiatry, Hosp Univ Penn 1980; Psychiatry, UCSF Med Ctr 1981; **Fellow:** Child & Adolescent Psychiatry, UCSF Med Ctr 1983; **Fac Appt:** Prof Psyc, UCSF

Russell, Andrew T MD [ChAP] - **Spec Exp:** ADD/ADHD; Schizophrenia; Developmental Disorders; **Hospital:** UCLA Neuropsychiatric Hosp; **Address:** Neuropsych Inst - UCLA, 760 Westwood Plaza, Los Angeles, CA 90024; **Phone:** 310-825-0389; **Board Cert:** Psychiatry 1980; Child & Adolescent Psychiatry 2004; **Med School:** Univ Colorado 1970; **Resid:** Psychiatry, UCLA Med Ctr 1973; **Fellow:** Child & Adolescent Psychiatry, UCLA Med Ctr 1977; **Fac Appt:** Prof Psyc, UCLA

Steiner, Hans MD [ChAP] - **Spec Exp:** Aggression Disorders; Eating Disorders; Trauma Psychiatry; **Hospital:** Stanford Univ Med Ctr; **Address:** Division Child Psych & Child Devlp, 401 Quarry Rd, Ste MC 5719, Stanford, CA 94305-5719; **Phone:** 650-723-5511; **Board Cert:** Psychiatry 1979; Child & Adolescent Psychiatry 1981; **Med School:** Austria 1972; **Resid:** Psychiatry, SUNY Syracuse Med Ctr 1976; **Fellow:** Child & Adolescent Psychiatry, Univ Mich Hosps 1978; **Fac Appt:** Prof Psyc, Stanford Univ

Terr, Lenore MD [ChAP] - **Spec Exp:** Trauma Psychiatry; Forensic Psychiatry; Psychotherapy; **Hospital:** UCSF Med Ctr; **Address:** 450 Sutter St, Ste 1336, San Francisco, CA 94108-4204; **Phone:** 415-433-7800; **Board Cert:** Psychiatry 1968; Child & Adolescent Psychiatry 1969; **Med School:** Univ Mich Med Sch 1961; **Resid:** Psychiatry, Univ Mich Med Ctr 1964; **Fellow:** Child & Adolescent Psychiatry, Univ Mich 1966; **Fac Appt:** Clin Prof Psyc, UCSF

GERIATRIC PSYCHIATRY

Mid Atlantic

Greenwald, Blaine MD [GerPsy] - **Spec Exp:** Depression; Dementia; **Hospital:** Long Island Jewish Med Ctr, Forest Hills Hosp; **Address:** 75-59 263rd St, Div Geriatric Psychiatry, Glen Oaks, NY 11004; **Phone:** 718-470-8159; **Board Cert:** Psychiatry 1983; Geriatric Psychiatry 2000; **Med School:** NY Med Coll 1978; **Resid:** Psychiatry, Mount Sinai Hosp 1982; **Fellow:** Geriatric Psychiatry, Mount Sinai Hosp/Bronx VA Hosp 1983; **Fac Appt:** Assoc Prof Psyc, Albert Einstein Coll Med

Kennedy, Gary MD [GerPsy] - **Spec Exp:** Alzheimer's Disease; Dementia; Depression; **Hospital:** Montefiore Med Ctr; **Address:** Dept Psyc & Behav Science, Montefiore Medical Center, 111 E 210th St, Bronx, NY 10467; **Phone:** 718-920-4236; **Board Cert:** Psychiatry 1980; Geriatric Psychiatry 2000; Psychosomatic Medicine 2005; **Med School:** Univ Tex, San Antonio 1975; **Resid:** Psychiatry, VA Hosp-Univ Texas 1979; **Fellow:** Geriatric Psychiatry, Montefiore Hosp 1984; **Fac Appt:** Prof Psyc, Albert Einstein Coll Med

Lyketsos, Constantine G MD [GerPsy] - **Spec Exp:** Alzheimer's Disease; Neuro-Psychiatry; Depression; **Hospital:** Johns Hopkins Bayview Med Ctr (page 61); **Address:** JHU Bayview Med Ctr, 5300 Alpha Commons Drive Fl 4th, Baltimore, MD 21224; **Phone:** 410-550-0062; **Board Cert:** Psychiatry 1994; Geriatric Psychiatry 1995; Psychosomatic Medicine 2005; **Med School:** Washington Univ, St Louis 1988; **Resid:** Psychiatry, Johns Hopkins Hosp 1992; **Fellow:** Neuropsychiatry, Johns Hopkins Hosp 1994; **Fac Appt:** Prof Psyc, Johns Hopkins Univ

Reisberg, Barry MD [GerPsy] - **Spec Exp:** Alzheimer's Disease; Dementia; Depression; **Hospital:** NYU Med Ctr (page 68); **Address:** Aging & Dementia Rsch Ctr - NYU, 550 First Ave, THN 316, New York, NY 10016; **Phone:** 212-263-8550; **Board Cert:** Psychiatry 1976; Geriatric Psychiatry 2000; **Med School:** NY Med Coll 1972; **Resid:** Psychiatry, Metropolitan Hosp 1975; **Fellow:** Psychiatric Research, Univ London 1975; **Fac Appt:** Prof Psyc, NYU Sch Med

Rosen, Jules MD [GerPsy] - **Spec Exp:** Alzheimer's Disease; Dementia; **Hospital:** Western Psych Inst & Clin - UPMC, UPMC Presby, Pittsburgh; **Address:** Western Psych Inst & Clin, 3811 O'Hara St, Pittsburgh, PA 15213; **Phone:** 412-692-4200; **Board Cert:** Psychiatry 1984; Geriatric Psychiatry 2003; **Med School:** Univ Cincinnati 1978; **Resid:** Psychiatry, Univ Mich Med Ctr 1982; **Fac Appt:** Prof Psyc, Univ Pittsburgh

Rovner, Barry W MD [GerPsy] - **Spec Exp:** Alzheimer's Disease; Behavioral Problems & Dementia; Depression; **Hospital:** Thomas Jefferson Univ Hosp; **Address:** Jefferson Hospital for Neuroscience, 900 Walnut St Fl 4, Philadelphia, PA 19107; **Phone:** 215-503-1254; **Board Cert:** Psychiatry 1985; Geriatric Psychiatry 2000; **Med School:** Jefferson Med Coll 1980; **Resid:** Psychiatry, Johns Hopkins Hosp 1984; **Fac Appt:** Assoc Prof Psyc, Jefferson Med Coll

Streim, Joel E MD [GerPsy] - **Spec Exp:** Psychiatry in Physical Illness; Psychiatric Barriers to Physical Rehab; Alzheimer's Disease; **Hospital:** Hosp Univ Penn - UPHS (page 60), VA Med Ctr; **Address:** Univ Penn, Dept Geriatric Psychiatry, 3535 Market St Fl 3, Philadelphia, PA 19104; **Phone:** 215-615-3086; **Board Cert:** Psychiatry 1988; Geriatric Psychiatry 2000; **Med School:** Univ Rochester 1978; **Resid:** Psychiatry, Univ Wisconsin 1985; **Fellow:** Liaison Psychiatry, Univ Rochester/Strong Mem 1981; Geriatric Psychiatry, VA Med Ctr 1988; **Fac Appt:** Prof Psyc, Univ Pennsylvania

Southeast

Holroyd, Suzanne MD [GerPsy] - **Spec Exp:** Dementia; Psychoses-Late Onset; Mood Disorders; **Hospital:** Univ Virginia Med Ctr; **Address:** Univ of Virginia Health Sys, Dept Psych, Box 800623, Chalottesville, VA 22908; **Phone:** 434-924-2241; **Board Cert:** Psychiatry 1992; Geriatric Psychiatry 2004; **Med School:** Univ VA Sch Med 1986; **Resid:** Psychiatry, Johns Hopkins Hosp 1990; **Fellow:** Geriatric Psychiatry, Johns Hopkins Hosp 1991; **Fac Appt:** Prof Psyc, Univ VA Sch Med

Stein, Elliott M MD [GerPsy] - **Spec Exp:** Anxiety & Depression; Memory Disorders; Dementia; Stress Management; **Hospital:** Mount Sinai Med Ctr - Miami; **Address:** Mount Sinai Med Ctr, 4300 Alton Rd, Warner Bldg, Ste 360, Miami Beach, FL 33140; **Phone:** 305-534-3636; **Board Cert:** Psychiatry 1979; Geriatric Psychiatry 2001; **Med School:** Univ Miami Sch Med 1973; **Resid:** Psychiatry, Herrick Meml Hosp 1976; **Fac Appt:** Assoc Clin Prof Psyc, Univ Miami Sch Med

Tune, Larry MD [GerPsy] - **Spec Exp:** Alzheimer's Disease; Dementia; Psychopharmacology; Psychoses-Late Onset; **Hospital:** Wesley Woods Ger Hosp; **Address:** Wesley Woods Health Ctr, Dept Psychiatry, 1841 Clifton Rd NE, Atlanta, GA 30329; **Phone:** 404-728-4969; **Board Cert:** Psychiatry 1991; Geriatric Psychiatry 2004; **Med School:** Univ VA Sch Med 1975; **Resid:** Psychiatry, Johns Hopkins Hosp 1979; Neurology, Johns Hopkins Hosp 1983; **Fellow:** Psychopharmacology, Johns Hopkins Univ 1981; **Fac Appt:** Prof Psyc, Emory Univ

Geriatric Psychiatry

Midwest

Grossberg, George MD [GerPsy] - **Spec Exp:** Alzheimer's Disease; Depression; Behavioral Problems & Dementia; **Hospital:** St Louis Univ Hosp; **Address:** St Louis Univ Sch Med, Dept Psychiatry, 1438 S Grand Blvd, St Louis, MO 63104; **Phone:** 314-977-4850; **Board Cert:** Psychiatry 1982; Geriatric Psychiatry 2001; **Med School:** St Louis Univ 1975; **Resid:** Psychiatry, St Louis Univ Med Ctr 1979; **Fac Appt:** Prof Psyc, St Louis Univ

Mellow, Alan M MD/PhD [GerPsy] - **Spec Exp:** Dementia; Depression; **Hospital:** Univ Michigan Hlth Sys; **Address:** Univ Mich, Dept Geriatric Psyc, 1500 E Med Ctr Drive, rm 1127, Box 0920, Ann Arbor, MI 48109; **Phone:** 734-222-4350; **Board Cert:** Psychiatry 1988; Geriatric Psychiatry 1991; **Med School:** Northwestern Univ 1981; **Resid:** Internal Medicine, Univ Chicago Hosp 1982; Psychiatry, McLean Hosp-Harvard 1985; **Fellow:** Psychiatry, Natl Inst Mental Hlth 1988; **Fac Appt:** Prof Psyc, Univ Mich Med Sch

Great Plains and Mountains

Burke, William J MD [GerPsy] - **Spec Exp:** Depression; Dementia; Alzheimer's Disease; Panic Disorder; **Hospital:** Nebraska Med Ctr; **Address:** Nebraska Medical Ctr, Dept Psychiatry, 985580 Nebraska Medical Ctr, Omaha, NE 68198-5580; **Phone:** 402-552-6002; **Board Cert:** Psychiatry 1986; Geriatric Psychiatry 2001; **Med School:** Univ Nebr Coll Med 1980; **Resid:** Internal Medicine, Univ Nebraska Med Ctr 1981; Psychiatry, Wash Univ Barnes Hosp 1984; **Fac Appt:** Prof Psyc, Univ Nebr Coll Med

West Coast and Pacific

Borson, Soo MD [GerPsy] - **Spec Exp:** Alzheimer's Disease; Psychiatry in Physical Illness; Dementia; Memory Disorders; **Hospital:** Univ Wash Med Ctr; **Address:** Univ Washington Hlth Sciences Ctr, 1959 NE Pacific St, CB 356560, Seattle, WA 98105-6008; **Phone:** 206-598-7792; **Board Cert:** Psychiatry 1985; Geriatric Psychiatry 2000; **Med School:** Stanford Univ 1969; **Resid:** Psychiatry, Univ Wash 1979; **Fellow:** Geriatric Psychiatry, Univ Wash 1981; **Fac Appt:** Prof Psyc, Univ Wash

Kramer, Barry Alan MD [GerPsy] - **Spec Exp:** Electroconvulsive Therapy (ECT); Depression; **Hospital:** Cedars-Sinai Med Ctr, Kaiser Permanente LA Med Ctr; **Address:** PO Box 5792, Beverly Hills, CA 90209; **Phone:** 310-423-4014; **Board Cert:** Psychiatry 1978; Geriatric Psychiatry 2001; **Med School:** Hahnemann Univ 1974; **Resid:** Psychiatry, Montefiore Hosp & Med Ctr 1977; **Fellow:** Geriatric Psychiatry, UCLA-USC Long Term Gero Ctr 1986

Small, Gary W MD [GerPsy] - **Spec Exp:** Dementia; Alzheimer's Disease; Memory Disorders; Memory & Longevity; **Hospital:** Ronald Reagan UCLA Med Ctr; **Address:** UCLA, Neuropsych Inst, 760 Westwood Plaza, 88-201 NPI, Los Angeles, CA 90095; **Phone:** 310-825-0291; **Board Cert:** Psychiatry 1983; Geriatric Psychiatry 2001; **Med School:** USC Sch Med 1977; **Resid:** Psychiatry, Mass Genl Hosp 1981; **Fellow:** Psychiatry, UCLA Med Ctr 1983; **Fac Appt:** Prof Psyc, UCLA

Veith, Richard C MD [GerPsy] - **Spec Exp:** Depression in Cardiovascular Disease; **Hospital:** Univ Wash Med Ctr; **Address:** Univ Washington Health Sciences Ctr, BB 1644, Box 356560, 1959 NE Pacific St, Seattle, WA 98195; **Phone:** 206-543-3752; **Board Cert:** Psychiatry 1979; Geriatric Psychiatry 2000; **Med School:** Univ Wash 1973; **Resid:** Psychiatry, Univ Wash Med Ctr 1977; **Fac Appt:** Prof Psyc, Univ Wash

Cleveland Clinic

Psychiatry and Psychology

The Cleveland Clinic Department of Psychiatry and Psychology offers the full range of mental health and behavioral services for children, adolescents and adults. Our highly trained staff, offering expert clinical evaluation and treatment, includes psychiatrists, psychologists, clinical nurse specialists, social workers, counselors and therapists. In addition to evaluating and treating patients, our staff educates trainees, professionals and the public on the latest developments in psychiatry and the behavioral sciences.

We are ranked among the top 25 psychiatric programs in the country and are ranked best in Ohio, according to *U.S.News and World Report's* survey of "America's Best Hospitals."

The Department of Psychiatry and Psychology includes Adult Psychiatry, Child and Adolescent Psychiatry, Chemical Dependency, General Psychology, Habit Management, Neuropsychology, Psychosomatic Medicine and Psychiatric Occupational Therapy.

The department is part of the Cleveland Clinic Neurological Institute, a fully integrated entity with a disease-specific focus, combining all physicians and other healthcare providers in neurology, neurosurgery, neuroradiology, the behavioral sciences and nursing who treat children and adults with neurological and neurobehavioral disorders. Our staff of more than 100 specialists sees one of the largest and most diverse patient populations in the country. Because of our clinical expertise, academic achievement and innovative research, the Cleveland Clinic Neurological Institute has earned an international reputation for excellence.

Our staff treats a wide range of symptoms and problems involving personal or family crises. Among the types of problems for which children and adults seek our professional help:

- Attention Deficit Disorder
- Disruptive Behavior
- Eating Disorders
- Mood and Anxiety Disorders
- Schizophrenia
- Sleeping Problems
- Stress
- Substance Abuse
- Work/Life/Family Problems

Our staff provides individualized assessments, medication management and counseling for individuals, couples, groups and families. The department offers care through outpatient, urgent care and routine visits, as well as inpatient treatment programs.

Our staff also serves as consultants for patients admitted to Cleveland Clinic medical and surgical units, and are key team members in the treatment of many conditions including epilepsy, movement disorders, organ transplantation, morbid obesity, chronic pain, headaches and cancer. Through the Psychiatric Neuromodulation Center, we offer both traditional and novel treatments to patients with psychiatric disorders resistant to common therapies.

For more information about the Cleveland Clinic Department of Psychiatry and Psychology, to schedule a second opinion or to learn about assistance for out-of-town patients, call 800.890.2467 or visit www.clevelandclinic.org/psychtopdocs.

Department of Psychiatry and Psychology
9500 Euclid Avenue / AC311 | Cleveland OH 44195

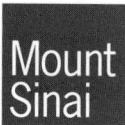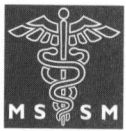

THE MOUNT SINAI MEDICAL CENTER
PSYCHIATRY
One Gustave L. Levy Place
Fifth Avenue and 100th Street
New York, NY 10029-6574
Physician Referral: 1-800-MD-SINAI (637-4624)
www.mountsinai.org

The Department of Psychiatry at Mount Sinai strives to rapidly bring tomorrow's breakthrough treatments from clinical neuroscience research to clinical care today.

We serve infants, children, adolescents, adults, and seniors, offering mental health evaluation and treatment for such conditions as autism, attention-deficit hyperactivity disorder (ADHD), behavioral disorders, care of children after trauma, schizophrenia, Alzheimer's disease, mood and anxiety disorders, obsessive-compulsive disorder (OCD), substance abuse (with co-occurring disorders), posttraumatic stress disorder (PTSD), eating disorders, reproductive psychiatry, impulse control disorders, and personality disorders.

CLINICAL SERVICES

The Department of Psychiatry is organized around key Centers of Excellence that link academic thought leaders to clinicians throughout the Department in a diagnosis-based system. We offer a full range of diagnostic and treatment services, including brain imaging, psychotherapy, psychopharmacology, crisis intervention and emergency services, electroconvulsive therapy (ECT), psychological and neuropsychological testing, and a new clinical initiative that focuses on the management of difficult clinical cases. The Department of Psychiatry has also been deeply engaged in Mount Sinai's World Trade Center Worker and Volunteer Screening Program, which has screened thousands of people for 9/11-related physical and mental health problems. We also offer special programs for Holocaust survivors and children of Holocaust survivors.

NEW AND EXPANDING PROGRAMS

The Seaver and New York Autism Center of Excellence has specialized training and unique expertise working with children, adolescents, and adults on the autism spectrum. We offer comprehensive assessment and evaluation services, innovative treatment approaches, including social skills therapy groups, and a Community Outreach Program for parent groups, agencies, and schools.

We have recently created a new Center for Eating and Weight Disorders that serves adults and children, offering innovative, proven-effective treatment for anorexia nervosa, bulimia nervosa, binge eating disorder, and obesity.

The Mood and Anxiety Disorders Program is applying brain imaging techniques to aid in diagnosis, and offering the latest treatment strategies for patients who suffer from panic attacks, generalized anxiety disorder, social phobia, depression, and related conditions.

The Compulsive and Impulsive Disorders Center of Excellence provides state-of-the-art diagnostic evaluation and treatment for obsessive-compulsive disorder and related conditions and impulsive disorders (such as pathological gambling) using a team-based approach.

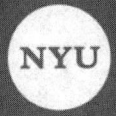
NYU **Langone Medical Center**

550 First Avenue (at 31St Street)
New York, NY 10016
Physician Referral:
(888)7-NYU-MED (888-769-8633)
www.nyumc.org

BEHAVIORAL HEALTH

Treating Mental Illness and Emotional Disorders

The Behavioral Health Program at NYU Medical Center offers the most up-to-date, scientifically validated treatments available for a wide range of disorders, including: stress/anxiety, schizophrenia, depression, shyness, insomnia, low self-esteem, women's issues, sexual difficulties, panic attacks and phobias, manic-depression, obsessions and compulsions, and attention deficit/hyperactivity disorder.

The Program serves its patients through a variety of approaches, including career counseling, assertiveness training, marital/couples counseling, and individual, group, or family therapy.

BEHAVIORAL HEALTH AT NYU
COMPRISES THREE COMPONENTS:

• A 22 bed inpatient unit services an adult population including a Young Adult Program. The service combines comprehensive diagnostic assessment and treatment including psychopharma-cology, neuropsychology, psychotherapies, and electroconvulsive therapy. A multidisciplinary team approach provides a continuum of behavioral and therapeutic modalities.

• The Outpatient Psychiatry Program provides treatment to adults suffering from a broad range of mental disorders including anxiety, depression, bipolar disorder, schizoaffective disorder, schizophrenia, insomnia, adult attention-deficit hyperactivity disorder (ADHD), and personality disorders. Treatment options include individual psychotherapy, medication, or the combination.

• The Program in Human Sexuality provides a comprehensive and in-depth examination of a full range of sexual disorders, such as erectile disorder, premature ejaculation, male orgasmic disorder, female orgasmic and arousal disorders, vaginisumus, dyspareunia, lack of desire, the unconsummated marriage and sexual incompatibility between partners. Developed over the years to include the most recent advances in the field, the Program ensures that couples and individuals who seek treatment receive individualized care appropriate to their condition.

PEACE OF MIND

At NYU Langone Medical Center, scientific innovation goes hand in hand with patient care. Our physician-scientists continue to lead the way in the burgeoning field of psychopharmacology. With the rapid pace of scientific discovery at NYU, people with mood disorders and their families stand to reap the benefits of medical research sooner rather than later. A number of clinical studies are currently ender way to test new treatments for depression and bipolar disorder, with potentially lifealtering results for the millions who suffer from these debilitating illnesses.

NYU Langone Medical Center

550 First Avenue (at 31St Street)
New York, NY 10016
Physician Referral
(888)7-NYU-MED (888-769-8633)
www.nyumc.org

PSYCHIATRY

In close collaboration with the NYU School of Medicine, which has one of the largest and most distinguished psychiatry faculties in the United States, the NYU Medical Center Department of Psychiatry offers these special services:

The Inpatient Unit is an academic service which combines comprehensive diagnostic assessment and treatment including psychopharmacology, neuropsychology, psychotherapies, and electroconvulsive therapy (ECT). For more information please call 212-263-5 567.

Behavioral Health Program is the outpatient psychiatric service including licensed psychiatrists, psychologists and social workers. It offers a variety of the most up-to-date and scientifically validated treatments including psychotherapy, medication management or a combination. For more information, please call 212-263-7419.

NYU LANGONE MEDICAL CENTER

NYU Langone Medical Center is a national training center for mental health professionals, offering a fully-accredited graduate program whose goal is to train and prepare the next generation of mental health professionals to meet the demands of a complex and expanding field and to translate research into advanced clinical care and effective treatments.

Committed to patient care, research, and training, the Department of Psychiatry at NYU Langone Medical Center is home to some of the nations' most respected clinical psychiatrists and psychologists, with specialties in psychoanalysis, psychopharmacology, behavioral therapy, child psychiatry, geriatric psychiatry, neuropsychiatry, and positron emission tomography

Pulmonary Disease
a subspecialty of Internal Medicine

An internist who treats diseases of the lungs and airways. The pulmonologist diagnoses and treats cancer, pneumonia, pleurisy, asthma, occupational diseases, bronchitis, sleep disorders, emphysema and other complex disorders of the lungs.

Training Required: Three years in internal medicine *plus* additional training and examination for certification in pulmonary disease.

PULMONARY DISEASE

New England

Beamis, John MD [Pul] - **Spec Exp:** Interventional Pulmonology; Bronchoscopy; **Hospital:** Lahey Clin; **Address:** Lahey Clinic, 41 Mall Rd, Burlington, MA 01805; **Phone:** 781-744-3240; **Board Cert:** Internal Medicine 1974; Pulmonary Disease 1978; Critical Care Medicine 1999; **Med School:** Univ VT Coll Med 1970; **Resid:** Internal Medicine, New Eng Deacones Hosp 1973; **Fellow:** Pulmonary Disease, New Eng Deacones Hosp 1974; Pulmonary Disease, Naval Hosp 1977; **Fac Appt:** Assoc Prof Med, Tufts Univ

Braman, Sidney MD [Pul] - **Spec Exp:** Asthma; Chronic Obstructive Lung Disease (COPD); **Hospital:** Rhode Island Hosp; **Address:** Rhode Island Hosp, Div Pulmonology, 593 Eddy St, APC Bldg Fl 7, Providence, RI 02903; **Phone:** 401-444-3567; **Board Cert:** Internal Medicine 1971; Pulmonary Disease 1972; **Med School:** Temple Univ 1967; **Resid:** Internal Medicine, Philadelphia Genl Hosp 1969; **Fellow:** Pulmonary Disease, Hosp Univ Penn 1970; Pulmonary Disease, Walter Reed AMC 1971; **Fac Appt:** Prof Med, Brown Univ

Celli, Bartolome MD [Pul] - **Spec Exp:** Chronic Obstructive Lung Disease (COPD); Mechanical Ventilation; Respiratory Failure; **Hospital:** St Elizabeth's Med Ctr; **Address:** St Elizabeth's Med Ctr, Dept Pulmonary Disease, 736 Cambridge St, Boston, MA 02135; **Phone:** 617-789-2545; **Board Cert:** Internal Medicine 1975; Pulmonary Disease 1978; **Med School:** Venezuela 1971; **Resid:** Internal Medicine, St Vincent Hosp 1973; Internal Medicine, Boston City Hosp 1976; **Fellow:** Pulmonary Disease, Boston Univ Med Ctr 1977; **Fac Appt:** Prof Med, Tufts Univ

Christiani, David MD [Pul] - **Spec Exp:** Occupational Lung Disease; **Hospital:** Mass Genl Hosp, MA Respiratory Hosp; **Address:** Mass Genl Hosp, Pulmonary Assocs, 55 Fruit St Cox 201B Bldg, Boston, MA 02114; **Phone:** 617-726-1721; **Board Cert:** Internal Medicine 1979; Occupational Medicine 1984; Pulmonary Disease 1988; **Med School:** Tufts Univ 1976; **Resid:** Internal Medicine, Boston City Hosp 1979; Occupational Medicine, Harvard Sch Public Health 1981; **Fellow:** Pulmonary Disease, Mass Genl Hosp 1987; **Fac Appt:** Prof Med, Harvard Med Sch

Enelow, Richard Ian MD [Pul] - **Spec Exp:** Interstitial Lung Disease; Lung Disease; **Hospital:** Dartmouth - Hitchcock Med Ctr; **Address:** Chief of Pulmonary & Critical Care, Dartmouth-Hitchcock Medical Ctr, 1 Medical Center Drive, Lebanon, NH 03756; **Phone:** 603-650-5383; **Board Cert:** Internal Medicine 1986; Pulmonary Disease 2002; **Med School:** Boston Univ 1983; **Resid:** Internal Medicine, New England Deaconess Med Ctr 1986; **Fellow:** Pulmonary Disease, Univ VA Hlth Scis Ctr 1992; **Fac Appt:** Prof Med, Dartmouth Med Sch

Ernst, Armin MD [Pul] - **Spec Exp:** Interventional Pulmonology; Tracheal Stenosis; Airway Disorders; **Hospital:** Beth Israel Deaconess Med Ctr - Boston; **Address:** Beth Israel Deaconess Med Ctr, 185 Pilgrim Rd, Deaconess Bldg - Ste 201, Boston, MA 02215; **Phone:** 617-632-8252; **Board Cert:** Internal Medicine 2003; Pulmonary Disease 2006; Critical Care Medicine 2007; **Med School:** Germany 1988; **Resid:** Internal Medicine, Thoraxklinik-Univ Heidelberg; Internal Medicine, Univ Tex Hlth Sci Ctr 1993; **Fellow:** Pulmonary Critical Care Medicine, Deaconess Med Ctr/Brigham & Women's 1996; Interventional Pulmonology, Thoraxklinik-Univ Heidelberg; **Fac Appt:** Assoc Prof Med, Harvard Med Sch

Fanta, Christopher MD [Pul] - **Spec Exp:** Asthma; Chronic Obstructive Lung Disease (COPD); Bronchiectasis; **Hospital:** Brigham & Women's Hosp, Faulkner Hosp; **Address:** 75 Francis St, Boston, MA 02115; **Phone:** 617-732-6770; **Board Cert:** Internal Medicine 1978; Pulmonary Disease 1980; **Med School:** Harvard Med Sch 1975; **Resid:** Internal Medicine, Peter Bent Brigham Hosp 1978; **Fellow:** Pulmonary Disease, Peter Bent Brigham Hosp 1980; **Fac Appt:** Assoc Prof Med, Harvard Med Sch

Friedman, Lloyd Neal MD [Pul] - **Spec Exp:** Tuberculosis; **Hospital:** Milford Hosp, Yale-New Haven Hosp; **Address:** Milford Hospital, 300 Seaside Ave, Milford, CT 06460; **Phone:** 203-876-4288; **Board Cert:** Internal Medicine 1983; Pulmonary Disease 1988; Critical Care Medicine 1999; **Med School:** Yale Univ 1979; **Resid:** Internal Medicine, Beth Israel Med Ctr 1980; Internal Medicine, Oregon Hlth Scis Univ 1983; **Fellow:** Pulmonary Intensive Care, Yale-New Haven Hosp 1988; **Fac Appt:** Clin Prof Med, Yale Univ

Irwin, Richard S MD [Pul] - **Spec Exp:** Cough; Asthma; Chronic Obstructive Lung Disease (COPD); Critical Care; **Hospital:** UMass Meml - Univ Campus; **Address:** 55 Lake Ave N, Worcester, MA 01655-0002; **Phone:** 508-856-1919; **Board Cert:** Internal Medicine 1972; Pulmonary Disease 1974; Critical Care Medicine 2007; **Med School:** Tufts Univ 1968; **Resid:** Internal Medicine, Tufts-New England Med Ctr 1970; **Fellow:** Pulmonary Disease, Columbia-Presby Hosp 1972; **Fac Appt:** Prof Med, Univ Mass Sch Med

Mahler, Donald A MD [Pul] - **Spec Exp:** Chronic Obstructive Lung Disease (COPD); Asthma; Breathing Disorders; **Hospital:** Dartmouth - Hitchcock Med Ctr; **Address:** Dartmouth-Hitchcock Med Ctr, Div Pulmonary Med, One Medical Center Drive, Lebanon, NH 03756-0001; **Phone:** 603-650-5533; **Board Cert:** Internal Medicine 1978; Pulmonary Disease 1980; **Med School:** Loyola Univ-Stritch Sch Med 1972; **Resid:** Internal Medicine, Dartmouth-Hitchcock Med Ctr 1977; **Fellow:** Pulmonary Disease, Yale-New Haven Hosp 1980; **Fac Appt:** Prof Med, Dartmouth Med Sch

Metersky, Mark L MD [Pul] - **Spec Exp:** Pulmonary Infections; Asthma; Pulmonary Hypertension; **Hospital:** Univ of Conn Hlth Ctr, John Dempsey Hosp; **Address:** Univ Conn Hlth Ctr, 263 Farmington Ave, Farmington, CT 06030-1321; **Phone:** 860-679-3343; **Board Cert:** Internal Medicine 1988; Pulmonary Disease 2003; Critical Care Medicine 2003; **Med School:** NYU Sch Med 1985; **Resid:** Internal Medicine, Boston City Hosp 1988; **Fellow:** Pulmonary Critical Care Medicine, UCSD Med Ctr 1992; **Fac Appt:** Assoc Prof Med, Univ Conn

Millman, Richard P MD [Pul] - **Spec Exp:** Sleep Disorders/Apnea; **Hospital:** Rhode Island Hosp, Miriam Hosp; **Address:** RI Hosp, Div Pulm, Crit Care & Sleep Med, 593 Eddy St, APC 701, Providence, RI 02903-4923; **Phone:** 401-444-2670; **Board Cert:** Internal Medicine 1979; Pulmonary Disease 1982; Critical Care Medicine 1999; **Med School:** Univ Pennsylvania 1976; **Resid:** Internal Medicine, Univ Mich Hosp 1979; **Fellow:** Pulmonary Disease, Univ Penn 1981; **Fac Appt:** Prof Med, Brown Univ

Nardell, Edward MD [Pul] - **Spec Exp:** Tuberculosis; **Hospital:** Brigham & Women's Hosp; **Address:** Center for Health and Human Rights, 651 Huntington Ave, Boston, MA 02120; **Phone:** 617-432-6937; **Board Cert:** Internal Medicine 1975; Pulmonary Disease 1982; **Med School:** Hahnemann Univ 1972; **Resid:** Internal Medicine, Hahnemann Univ Hosp 1975; **Fellow:** Pulmonary Disease, Mass Genl Hosp 1977; **Fac Appt:** Assoc Prof Med, Harvard Med Sch

Parsons, Polly E MD [Pul] - **Spec Exp:** Critical Care; Lung Injury-Acute; **Hospital:** FAHC - UHC Campus; **Address:** Fletcher Allen Health Care, 111 Colchester Ave, Fletcher 311, Burlington, VT 05401; **Phone:** 802-847-6177; **Board Cert:** Internal Medicine 1981; Pulmonary Disease 1986; Critical Care Medicine 2005; **Med School:** Univ Ariz Coll Med 1978; **Resid:** Internal Medicine, Univ Colorado Hosp 1981; **Fellow:** Pulmonary Disease, Univ Colorado Hosp 1985; **Fac Appt:** Prof Med, Univ VT Coll Med

Pulmonary Disease

Redlich, Carrie MD [Pul] - **Spec Exp:** Occupational Lung Disease; **Hospital:** Yale-New Haven Hosp; **Address:** Yale Occupational & Environmental Med, 135 College St Fl 3 - Ste 392, New Haven, CT 06510; **Phone:** 203-785-4197; **Board Cert:** Internal Medicine 1986; Occupational Medicine 1990; Pulmonary Disease 2002; **Med School:** Yale Univ 1982; **Resid:** Internal Medicine, Yale-New Haven Hosp 1986; Occupational Medicine, Yale-New Haven Hosp 1987; **Fellow:** Pulmonary Disease, Univ Washington 1989; **Fac Appt:** Assoc Prof Med, Yale Univ

Rochester, Carolyn MD [Pul] - **Spec Exp:** Chronic Obstructive Lung Disease (COPD); **Hospital:** VA Conn Hlthcre Sys, Yale-New Haven Hosp; **Address:** Yale Univ Sch Med, Pulm & Crit Care Sect, 300 Cedar St, Box 208057, New Haven, CT 06520-8057; **Phone:** 203-785-3207; **Board Cert:** Internal Medicine 1986; Pulmonary Disease 2002; **Med School:** Columbia P&S 1983; **Resid:** Internal Medicine, Columbia Presby Med Ctr 1986; **Fellow:** Pulmonary Disease, Columbia Presby Med Ctr 1988; **Fac Appt:** Asst Prof Med, Yale Univ

White, David P MD [Pul] - **Spec Exp:** Sleep Disorders/Apnea; **Hospital:** Brigham & Women's Hosp; **Address:** Brigham & Women's Hosp, Division of Sleep Med, 75 Francis St, Boston, MA 02115; **Phone:** 617-732-5778; **Board Cert:** Internal Medicine 1978; Pulmonary Disease 1982; Critical Care Medicine 1997; **Med School:** Emory Univ 1975; **Resid:** Internal Medicine, Univ Colo Med Ctr 1978; **Fellow:** Pulmonary Disease, Univ Colo Med Ctr 1982; **Fac Appt:** Assoc Prof Med, Harvard Med Sch

Mid Atlantic

Arcasoy, Selim M MD [Pul] - **Spec Exp:** Transplant Medicine-Lung; Chronic Obstructive Lung Disease (COPD); Interstitial Lung Disease; **Hospital:** NY-Presby Hosp/Columbia (page 66); **Address:** Ctr for Advanced Lung Dis/Transp, 622 W 168th St PH Bldg Fl 14E - rm 104, New York, NY 10032-3720; **Phone:** 212-305-6589; **Board Cert:** Internal Medicine 2003; Pulmonary Disease 2006; Critical Care Medicine 2007; **Med School:** Turkey 1990; **Resid:** Internal Medicine, SUNY Downstate Med Ctr 1994; **Fellow:** Pulmonary Critical Care Medicine, Univ Pittsburgh Med Ctr 1998; **Fac Appt:** Assoc Prof Med, Columbia P&S

Bascom, Rebecca MD [Pul] - **Spec Exp:** Environmental Diseases; Chemical Exposure; **Hospital:** Penn State Milton S Hershey Med Ctr; **Address:** Hershey Med Ctr, PO Box 850, MC HO41, Hershey, PA 17033-0850; **Phone:** 717-531-6525; **Board Cert:** Internal Medicine 1982; Occupational Medicine 1987; Pulmonary Disease 1988; Critical Care Medicine 1998; **Med School:** Oregon Hlth Sci Univ 1979; **Resid:** Internal Medicine, Johns Hopkins Hosp 1982; Occupational Medicine, Johns Hopkins 1985; **Fellow:** Pulmonary Disease, Johns Hopkins 1985; **Fac Appt:** Prof Med, Penn State Univ-Hershey Med Ctr

Criner, Gerard J MD [Pul] - **Spec Exp:** Chronic Obstructive Lung Disease (COPD); Pulmonary Fibrosis; Pulmonary Hypertension; Critical Care; **Hospital:** Temple Univ Hosp; **Address:** Temple Univ Hosp, Pulmonary Med, 3401 N Broad St Fl 7, Philadelphia, PA 19140; **Phone:** 215-707-5555; **Board Cert:** Internal Medicine 1982; Critical Care Medicine 2007; Pulmonary Disease 1986; **Med School:** Temple Univ 1979; **Resid:** Internal Medicine, Temple Univ Hosp 1983; **Fellow:** Pulmonary Disease, Boston Univ 1986; **Fac Appt:** Prof Med, Temple Univ

Deitz, Joel L MD [Pul] - **Spec Exp:** Respiratory Failure; Chronic Obstructive Lung Disease (COPD); Cough; **Hospital:** Penn Presby Med Ctr - UPHS (page 60), Hosp Univ Penn - UPHS (page 60); **Address:** Penn-Presby Med Ctr, Pulmonology, 51 N 39th St, Philadelphia Heart Inst Fl 1 Rear, Philadelphia, PA 19104; **Phone:** 215-662-8766; **Board Cert:** Internal Medicine 1980; Pulmonary Disease 1984; Critical Care Medicine 1997; **Med School:** Tufts Univ 1977; **Resid:** Internal Medicine, Med Coll Va Med Ctr 1980; **Fellow:** Pulmonary Disease, Duke Univ Med Ctr 1984; **Fac Appt:** Assoc Clin Prof Med, Univ Pennsylvania

Greenberg, Harly MD [Pul] - **Spec Exp:** Sleep Disorders/Apnea; Lung Disease; Critical Care; **Hospital:** Long Island Jewish Med Ctr, N Shore Univ Hosp; **Address:** North Shore LIJ Sleep Disorders Ctr, 410 Lakeville Rd, Ste 105, New Hyde Park, NY 11040; **Phone:** 516-465-3899; **Board Cert:** Internal Medicine 1985; Pulmonary Disease 1988; **Med School:** NYU Sch Med 1982; **Resid:** Internal Medicine, North Shore Univ Hosp 1985; **Fellow:** Pulmonary Disease, NYU-Bellevue Hosp Ctr 1987; **Fac Appt:** Assoc Prof Med, Albert Einstein Coll Med

Hansen-Flaschen, John MD [Pul] - **Spec Exp:** Interstitial Lung Disease; Diagnostic Problems; Chronic Obstructive Lung Disease (COPD); **Hospital:** Hosp Univ Penn - UPHS (page 60); **Address:** Hosp Univ Penn, Div Pulm, Allergy and Crit Care, 3400 Spruce St Radvin Bldg Fl 3 - Ste F, Philadelphia, PA 19104; **Phone:** 215-662-3202; **Board Cert:** Pulmonary Disease 1982; Critical Care Medicine 1988; Internal Medicine 1979; **Med School:** NYU Sch Med 1976; **Resid:** Internal Medicine, Hosp Univ Penn 1979; **Fellow:** Pulmonary Disease, Hosp Univ Penn 1981; Critical Care Medicine, Hosp Univ Penn 1982; **Fac Appt:** Prof Med, Univ Pennsylvania

Kamholz, Stephan MD [Pul] - **Spec Exp:** Pulmonary Disease-Second Opinion Only; **Hospital:** N Shore Univ Hosp, Long Island Jewish Med Ctr; **Address:** 300 Community Drive, Dept Medicine, 4DSU, Manhasset, NY 11030; **Phone:** 516-562-4310; **Board Cert:** Internal Medicine 1987; Pulmonary Disease 1978; Critical Care Medicine 1997; **Med School:** NY Med Coll 1972; **Resid:** Internal Medicine, Montefiore Hosp Med Ctr 1975; **Fellow:** Pulmonary Disease, Montefiore Hosp Med Ctr 1977; **Fac Appt:** Prof Med, NYU Sch Med

King, Earl D MD [Pul] - **Spec Exp:** Lung Cancer; **Hospital:** Fox Chase Cancer Ctr (page 58); **Address:** Fox Chase Cancer Center, 333 Cottman Ave, Philadelphia, PA 19111; **Phone:** 215-728-5703; **Board Cert:** Internal Medicine 1989; Pulmonary Disease 2002; Critical Care Medicine 2003; **Med School:** Penn State Univ-Hershey Med Ctr 1986; **Resid:** Internal Medicine, Temple Univ Med Ctr 1989; **Fellow:** Pulmonary Disease, Johns Hopkins Hosp 1993; Sleep Medicine, Johns Hopkins Hosp 1993

Kotloff, Robert M MD [Pul] - **Spec Exp:** Transplant Medicine-Lung; Lung Disease-Complex; **Hospital:** Hosp Univ Penn - UPHS (page 60); **Address:** Hospital University of Pensylvania, Penn Lung Ctr, 3400 Spruce St, 838W Gates, Philadelphia, PA 19104; **Phone:** 215-662-3202; **Board Cert:** Internal Medicine 1986; Pulmonary Disease 1990; Critical Care Medicine 1991; **Med School:** Yale Univ 1983; **Resid:** Internal Medicine, Temple Univ Hosp 1986; **Fellow:** Pulmonary Disease, Hosp Univ Penn 1990; **Fac Appt:** Assoc Prof Med, Univ Pennsylvania

Libby, Daniel MD [Pul] - **Spec Exp:** Asthma; Lung Cancer; Interstitial Lung Disease; **Hospital:** NY-Presby Hosp/Weill Cornell (page 66); **Address:** 635 Madison Ave, Ste 1101, New York, NY 10021; **Phone:** 212-628-6611; **Board Cert:** Internal Medicine 1977; Pulmonary Disease 1980; **Med School:** Baylor Coll Med 1974; **Resid:** Internal Medicine, New York Hosp 1977; **Fellow:** Pulmonary Disease, New York Hosp 1979; **Fac Appt:** Clin Prof Med, Cornell Univ-Weill Med Coll

Nash, Thomas MD [Pul] - **Spec Exp:** Asthma; Cough; Pneumonia; **Hospital:** NY-Presby Hosp/Weill Cornell (page 66); **Address:** 310 E 72nd St, New York, NY 10021-4726; **Phone:** 212-734-6612; **Board Cert:** Internal Medicine 1981; Infectious Disease 1984; Pulmonary Disease 1988; **Med School:** NYU Sch Med 1978; **Resid:** Internal Medicine, New York Hosp-Cornell 1981; **Fellow:** Infectious Disease, New York Hosp-Cornell 1985; Pulmonary Disease, Meml Sloan Kettering Cancer Ctr 1985; **Fac Appt:** Assoc Clin Prof Med, NYU Sch Med

Niederman, Michael MD [Pul] - **Spec Exp:** Infections-Respiratory; Emphysema; Respiratory Failure; Pneumonia; **Hospital:** Winthrop - Univ Hosp; **Address:** 222 Station Plaza N, Ste 400, Mineola, NY 11501-3893; **Phone:** 516-663-2834; **Board Cert:** Internal Medicine 1980; Pulmonary Disease 1983; Critical Care Medicine 2007; **Med School:** Boston Univ 1977; **Resid:** Internal Medicine, Northwestern Univ Med Ctr 1980; **Fellow:** Pulmonary Disease, Yale-New Haven Hosp 1983; **Fac Appt:** Prof Med, SUNY Stony Brook

Pulmonary Disease

Pack, Allan MD/PhD [Pul] - **Spec Exp:** Sleep Disorders/Apnea; **Hospital:** Hosp Univ Penn - UPHS (page 60); **Address:** Penn Sleep Center, 3624 Market St, Ste 201, Philadelphia, PA 19104; **Phone:** 215-615-3669; **Med School:** Scotland 1967; **Resid:** Internal Medicine, Univ Glasgow Med Ctr 1972; **Fellow:** Pulmonary Disease, Univ Glasgow Med Ctr 1975; **Fac Appt:** Prof Med, Univ Pennsylvania

Palevsky, Harold I MD [Pul] - **Spec Exp:** Pulmonary Hypertension; Pulmonary Vascular Disease; Thromboembolic Disorders; Pulmonary Embolism; **Hospital:** Penn Presby Med Ctr - UPHS (page 60), Hosp Univ Penn - UPHS (page 60); **Address:** Penn Presbyterian Medical Ctr, 39th & Market Sts, Philadelphia Heart Inst Fl 1 Rear, Philadelphia, PA 19104; **Phone:** 215-662-8717; **Board Cert:** Internal Medicine 2007; Pulmonary Disease 2007; Critical Care Medicine 2007; **Med School:** Med Coll VA 1978; **Resid:** Internal Medicine, Hosp Univ Penn 1981; **Fellow:** Pulmonary Critical Care Medicine, Hosp Univ Penn 1984; **Fac Appt:** Prof Med, Univ Pennsylvania

Reilly Jr, John Joseph MD [Pul] - **Spec Exp:** Transplant Medicine-Lung; Emphysema; Chronic Obstructive Lung Disease (COPD); **Hospital:** UPMC Presby, Pittsburgh; **Address:** 1220 Scaife Hall, 3550 Terrace St, Pittsburgh, PA 15261; **Phone:** 412-648-9091; **Board Cert:** Internal Medicine 1984; Pulmonary Disease 1986; Critical Care Medicine 1997; **Med School:** Harvard Med Sch 1981; **Resid:** Internal Medicine, Brigham & Women's Hosp 1984; **Fellow:** Pulmonary Disease, Brigham & Women's Hosp 1987; **Fac Appt:** Assoc Prof Med, Harvard Med Sch

Rossman, Milton D MD [Pul] - **Spec Exp:** Beryllium-induced Lung Disease; Sarcoidosis; Interstitial Lung Disease; **Hospital:** Hosp Univ Penn - UPHS (page 60); **Address:** Hosp of Univ Penn, 3400 Spruce St, 834W Gates Bldg, Philadelphia, PA 19104-4283; **Phone:** 215-662-6413; **Board Cert:** Internal Medicine 1975; Pulmonary Disease 1978; **Med School:** Jefferson Med Coll 1970; **Resid:** Internal Medicine, Univ Hosps 1975; **Fellow:** Pulmonary Disease, Hosp Univ Penn 1977; **Fac Appt:** Prof Med, Univ Pennsylvania

Schluger, Neil MD [Pul] - **Spec Exp:** Tuberculosis; Pulmonary Infections; Chronic Obstructive Lung Disease (COPD); **Hospital:** NY-Presby Hosp/Columbia (page 66); **Address:** Div Pulm, Allergy & Crit Care Med, 630 W 168th St, PH-8 East, Rm 101, New York, NY 10032; **Phone:** 212-305-9817; **Board Cert:** Internal Medicine 1988; Pulmonary Disease 2003; **Med School:** Univ Pennsylvania 1985; **Resid:** Internal Medicine, St Lukes Hosp 1989; **Fellow:** Pulmonary Critical Care Medicine, NY Hosp-Cornell 1992; **Fac Appt:** Prof Med, Columbia P&S

Schwab, Richard MD [Pul] - **Spec Exp:** Sleep Disorders/Apnea; **Hospital:** Hosp Univ Penn - UPHS (page 60); **Address:** Penn Sleep Center, 3624 Market St Fl 2 - Ste 201, Philadelphia, PA 19104; **Phone:** 215-662-7772; **Board Cert:** Internal Medicine 1986; Pulmonary Disease 2000; Critical Care Medicine 2000; **Med School:** Univ Pennsylvania 1983; **Resid:** Internal Medicine, Hosp Univ Penn 1986; **Fellow:** Pulmonary Critical Care Medicine, Hosp Univ Penn 1991; **Fac Appt:** Asst Prof Med, Univ Pennsylvania

Steiger, David MD [Pul] - **Spec Exp:** Rheumatologic Diseases of the Lung; Thromboembolic Disorders; Pulmonary Hypertension; Critical Care; **Hospital:** Hosp For Joint Diseases (page 70), NYU Med Ctr (page 68); **Address:** 305 2nd Ave, Ste 16, New York, NY 10003; **Phone:** 212-598-6091; **Board Cert:** Internal Medicine 1987; Pulmonary Disease 2002; Critical Care Medicine 2005; **Med School:** England 1981; **Resid:** Internal Medicine, St Thomas's Hosp 1984; Internal Medicine, St Lukes Hosp 1989; **Fellow:** Pulmonary Disease, UCSF Med Ctr 1994; **Fac Appt:** Asst Prof Med, NYU Sch Med

Steinberg, Harry MD [Pul] - **Spec Exp:** Asthma; Emphysema; Lung Cancer; **Hospital:** Long Island Jewish Med Ctr, N Shore Univ Hosp; **Address:** LI Jewish Med Ctr, Dept Med, 270-05 76th Ave, New Hyde Park, NY 11040-1433; **Phone:** 516-465-5400; **Med School:** Temple Univ 1966; **Resid:** Internal Medicine, LI Jewish Med Ctr 1969; Pulmonary Critical Care Medicine, LI Jewish Med Ctr 1970; **Fellow:** Pulmonary Disease, Hosp U Penn 1974; **Fac Appt:** Clin Prof Med, Albert Einstein Coll Med

Stover-Pepe, Diane E MD [Pul] - **Spec Exp:** Interstitial Lung Disease; Pulmonary Infections; Pulmonary Disease/Immunocompromised; **Hospital:** Meml Sloan-Kettering Cancer Ctr; **Address:** 1275 York Avenue, New York, NY 10065; **Phone:** 800-525-2225; **Board Cert:** Internal Medicine 1975; Pulmonary Disease 1978; **Med School:** Albert Einstein Coll Med 1970; **Resid:** Internal Medicine, Harlem Hosp Ctr 1972; Internal Medicine, NY Hosp-Cornell Med Ctr 1975; **Fellow:** Pulmonary Disease, Albert Einstein Med Ctr 1977; **Fac Appt:** Prof Med, Cornell Univ-Weill Med Coll

Strollo, Patrick J MD [Pul] - **Spec Exp:** Sleep Disorders/Apnea; **Hospital:** UPMC Montefiore, UPMC Presby, Pittsburgh; **Address:** Montefiore Univ Hospital, 3459 5th Ave, Ste S639.11, Pittsburgh, PA 15213; **Phone:** 412-692-2880; **Board Cert:** Internal Medicine 1984; Pulmonary Disease 1988; Sleep Medicine 2007; **Med School:** Uniformed Srvs Univ, Bethesda 1981; **Resid:** Internal Medicine, Wilford Hall Med Ctr 1984; **Fellow:** Pulmonary Disease, Wilford Hall Med Ctr 1987; **Fac Appt:** Assoc Prof Med, Univ Pittsburgh

Teirstein, Alvin MD [Pul] - **Spec Exp:** Sarcoidosis; Interstitial Lung Disease; Occupational Lung Disease; Lung Cancer; **Hospital:** Mount Sinai Med Ctr (page 64), VA Med Ctr - Bronx; **Address:** Mount Sinai Med Ctr, 1 Gustave Levy Pl, Box 1232, New York, NY 10029; **Phone:** 212-241-5656; **Board Cert:** Internal Medicine 1961; Pulmonary Disease 1969; **Med School:** SUNY Downstate 1953; **Resid:** Internal Medicine, Mt Sinai Med Ctr 1957; **Fellow:** Pulmonary Disease, Mt Sinai Med Ctr 1954; Pulmonary Disease, VA Med Ctr 1956; **Fac Appt:** Prof Med, Mount Sinai Sch Med

Terry, Peter Browne MD [Pul] - **Hospital:** Johns Hopkins Hosp - Baltimore (page 61); **Address:** 1830 E Monument St Fl 5, Baltimore, MD 21205; **Phone:** 410-955-3467; **Board Cert:** Internal Medicine 1973; Pulmonary Disease 1976; **Med School:** St Louis Univ 1968; **Resid:** Internal Medicine, Univ Conn Hlth Ctr 1970; Internal Medicine, Johns Hopkins Hosp 1973; **Fellow:** Pulmonary Disease, Johns Hopkins Hosp 1974; Pulmonary Disease, Mayo Clinic 1975; **Fac Appt:** Prof Med, Johns Hopkins Univ

Thomashow, Byron MD [Pul] - **Spec Exp:** Emphysema; Asthma; Respiratory Failure; Chronic Obstructive Lung Disease (COPD); **Hospital:** NY-Presby Hosp/Columbia (page 66); **Address:** 161 Fort Washington Ave, rm 311, New York, NY 10032; **Phone:** 212-305-5261; **Board Cert:** Internal Medicine 1977; Pulmonary Disease 1980; **Med School:** Columbia P&S 1974; **Resid:** Internal Medicine, Roosevelt Hosp 1977; Pulmonary Disease, Roosevelt Hosp 1978; **Fellow:** Pulmonary Disease, Harlem Hosp Ctr 1979; **Fac Appt:** Clin Prof Med, Columbia P&S

Tino, Gregory MD [Pul] - **Spec Exp:** Emphysema-Lung Volume Reduction; Interstitial Lung Disease; Bronchiectasis; Chronic Obstructive Lung Disease (COPD); **Hospital:** Hosp Univ Penn - UPHS (page 60); **Address:** Hosp Univ Penn, Div Pulmonary & Critical Care, 3400 Spruce St Radvin Bldg Fl 3 - Ste F, Philadelphia, PA 19104; **Phone:** 215-349-5303; **Board Cert:** Internal Medicine 1989; **Med School:** Mount Sinai Sch Med 1986; **Resid:** Internal Medicine, Hosp Univ Penn 1989; **Fellow:** Pulmonary Disease, Hosp Univ Penn 1992; **Fac Appt:** Assoc Prof Med, Univ Pennsylvania

Unger, Michael MD [Pul] - **Spec Exp:** Lung Cancer; Bronchoscopy; Cancer Prevention; **Hospital:** Fox Chase Cancer Ctr (page 58); **Address:** Fox Chase Cancer Center, 7701 Burholme Ave, Philadelphia, PA 19111; **Phone:** 215-728-6900; **Board Cert:** Internal Medicine 1977; Pulmonary Disease 1978; **Med School:** France 1971; **Resid:** Internal Medicine, Mt Sinai Hosp 1974; **Fellow:** Pulmonary Disease, New York Hosp-Cornell 1976; **Fac Appt:** Clin Prof Med, Thomas Jefferson Univ

Pulmonary Disease

Wenzel, Sally E MD [Pul] - **Spec Exp:** Asthma; Bronchiolitis Obliterans; Allergy; Inflammatory Pulmonary Diseases; **Hospital:** UPMC Montefiore; **Address:** UPMC Montefiore, 3601 Fifth Ave, Falk Medical Bldg Fl 4, Pittsburgh, PA 15213; **Phone:** 412-692-2210; **Board Cert:** Internal Medicine 1984; Pulmonary Disease 1986; **Med School:** Univ Fla Coll Med 1981; **Resid:** Internal Medicine, NC Baptist Hosp 1984; **Fellow:** Pulmonary Disease, Med Coll VA Hosp 1986; **Fac Appt:** Prof Med, Univ Colorado

White, Dorothy MD [Pul] - **Spec Exp:** Lung Cancer; Lung Disease(Drug-Induced); Lung Disease(Immunocompromised); **Hospital:** Meml Sloan-Kettering Cancer Ctr; **Address:** 1275 York Avenue, New York, NY 10065; **Phone:** 800-525-2225; **Board Cert:** Internal Medicine 1980; Pulmonary Disease 1984; **Med School:** SUNY Hlth Sci Ctr 1977; **Resid:** Internal Medicine, New York Hosp 1980; Internal Medicine, Meml Sloan Kettering Cancer Ctr 1981; **Fellow:** Pulmonary Disease, Yale-New Haven Hosp 1984; **Fac Appt:** Prof Med, Cornell Univ-Weill Med Coll

Southeast

Alberts, W Michael MD [Pul] - **Spec Exp:** Lung Cancer; **Hospital:** H Lee Moffitt Cancer Ctr & Research Inst; **Address:** H Lee Moffitt Cancer Ctr, Thoracic Onc, 12902 Magnolia Drive, Tampa, FL 33612; **Phone:** 813-979-3067; **Board Cert:** Internal Medicine 1980; Pulmonary Disease 1982; **Med School:** Univ IL Coll Med 1977; **Resid:** Internal Medicine, Ohio State Univ Hosp 1980; **Fellow:** Pulmonary Critical Care Medicine, UCSD Med Ctr 1983; **Fac Appt:** Prof Med, Univ S Fla Coll Med

Antony, Veena B MD [Pul] - **Spec Exp:** Pleural Disease; **Hospital:** Shands at Univ of FL; **Address:** Shands at the Univ of Florida, 1600 SW Archer Rd, Box 100225, Gainesville, FL 32610-0225; **Phone:** 352-392-2666; **Board Cert:** Internal Medicine 1979; Pulmonary Disease 1982; **Med School:** India 1974; **Resid:** Internal Medicine, Kingsbrook Jewish Med Ctr; **Fellow:** Pulmonary Disease, Univ Co Hlth Sci Ctr; Pulmonary Disease, Natl Jewish Hosp-Asthma Ctr

Brooks, Stuart M MD [Pul] - **Spec Exp:** Occupational Lung Disease; Asthma; Lung Injuries-Inhalation Induced; **Hospital:** Tampa Genl Hosp, H Lee Moffitt Cancer Ctr & Research Inst; **Address:** USF College of Public Health, 12901 Bruce B Downs Blvd, Box 56 MDC, Tampa, FL 33612-3805; **Phone:** 813-389-6000; **Board Cert:** Internal Medicine 1977; Pulmonary Disease 1969; Occupational Medicine 1987; **Med School:** Univ Cincinnati 1962; **Resid:** Internal Medicine, Boston City Hosp 1967; **Fellow:** Pulmonary Disease, Boston City Hosp 1969; **Fac Appt:** Prof Med, Univ S Fla Coll Med

Campbell, G Douglas MD [Pul] - **Spec Exp:** Infectious Disease-Lung; **Hospital:** Univ Hosps & Clins - Jackson, VA Med Ctr; **Address:** Univ Mississippi Med Ctr, Div Pulm, 2500 N State St, Jackson, MS 39216-4505; **Phone:** 601-984-5650; **Board Cert:** Internal Medicine 1979; Pulmonary Disease 1986; **Med School:** Univ Miss 1976; **Resid:** Internal Medicine, Univ Miss Hosp 1979; **Fellow:** Pulmonary Disease, Univ Tex Hlth Sci Ctr 1983; Infectious Disease, Univ Calgary HSC 1985; **Fac Appt:** Prof Med, Univ Miss

Christman, Brian W MD [Pul] - **Spec Exp:** Chronic Obstructive Lung Disease (COPD); Sepsis; Critical Care; **Hospital:** VA Med Ctr - Nashville, Vanderbilt Univ Med Ctr; **Address:** VA Tennessee Valley Hlth Care System, 1310 24th Ave S, MC 111, Nashville, TN 37212; **Phone:** 615-327-4751 x5349; **Board Cert:** Internal Medicine 1984; Pulmonary Disease 1986; Critical Care Medicine 1999; **Med School:** Univ Okla Coll Med 1981; **Resid:** Internal Medicine, Vanderbilt Univ Med Ctr 1984; **Fellow:** Pulmonary Disease, Vanderbilt Univ Med Ctr 1987

Cooper, John Allen D MD [Pul] - **Spec Exp:** Drug Induced Lung Disease; Chronic Obstructive Lung Disease (COPD); **Hospital:** Univ of Ala Hosp at Birmingham, VA Med Ctr; **Address:** 215 Tinsley Harrison Tower, 1900 University Blvd, Birmingham, AL 35294; **Phone:** 205-975-6770; **Board Cert:** Internal Medicine 1981; Pulmonary Disease 1984; **Med School:** Duke Univ 1978; **Resid:** Internal Medicine, Univ Virginia Hosp 1981; **Fellow:** Pulmonary Disease, Yale Univ 1985; **Fac Appt:** Prof Med, Univ Ala

Cooper, William R MD [Pul] - **Spec Exp:** Critical Care; Asthma; Chronic Obstructive Lung Disease (COPD); **Hospital:** Sentara VA Beach Genl Hosp; **Address:** 1008 First Colonial Rd, Ste 103, Virginia Beach, VA 23454-3071; **Phone:** 757-481-2515; **Board Cert:** Internal Medicine 1972; Pulmonary Disease 1974; Critical Care Medicine 1999; **Med School:** Univ VA Sch Med 1969; **Resid:** Internal Medicine, Cleveland Metro Genl Hosp 1971; Pulmonary Disease, Univ Va Hosp 1973; **Fellow:** Pulmonary Disease, Mount Sinai Med Ctr 1974

Doherty, Dennis E MD [Pul] - **Spec Exp:** Asthma; Chronic Obstructive Lung Disease (COPD); Interstitial Lung Disease; **Hospital:** Univ of Kentucky Chandler Hosp, VA Med Ctr - Lexington; **Address:** Univ Kentucky Med Ctr, Div Pulm & Crit Care, 740 S Limestone, rm L-543, Lexington, KY 40536-0284; **Phone:** 859-323-5045; **Board Cert:** Internal Medicine 1985; Pulmonary Disease 1988; **Med School:** Ohio State Univ 1980; **Resid:** Internal Medicine, Ohio State Univ Hosp 1983; **Fellow:** Pulmonary Disease, Univ Colorado Hlth Sci Ctr 1986; **Fac Appt:** Prof Med, Univ KY Coll Med

Donohue, James Francis MD [Pul] - **Spec Exp:** Asthma; Chronic Obstructive Lung Disease (COPD); Sarcoidosis; **Hospital:** Univ NC Hosps; **Address:** Univ NC, Div Pulmonary Disease, 4125 Bio-informatics Bldg. CB 7020, Chapel Hill, NC 27599-7020; **Phone:** 919-966-2531; **Board Cert:** Internal Medicine 1975; Pulmonary Disease 1976; **Med School:** UMDNJ-NJ Med Sch, Newark 1969; **Resid:** Internal Medicine, UMDNJ-Newark 1971; Internal Medicine, NC Meml Hosp 1974; **Fellow:** Pulmonary Disease, Univ North Carolina 1976; **Fac Appt:** Prof Med, Univ NC Sch Med

Dunlap, Nancy E MD/PhD [Pul] - **Spec Exp:** Tubercolosis-non infectious; **Hospital:** Univ of Ala Hosp at Birmingham; **Address:** 2000 6th Ave S Fl 3/Admin, Birmingham, AL 35233; **Phone:** 205-801-7900; **Board Cert:** Internal Medicine 1984; Pulmonary Disease 1988; Critical Care Medicine 1999; **Med School:** Duke Univ 1981; **Resid:** Internal Medicine, Univ Alabama Med Ctr 1984; **Fellow:** Pulmonary Disease, Univ Alabama 1987; **Fac Appt:** Prof Med, Univ Ala

Fulkerson Jr, William J MD [Pul] - **Spec Exp:** Respiratory Failure; Thromboembolic Disorders; **Hospital:** Duke Univ Med Ctr; **Address:** Duke Univ Med Ctr, Trent Drive, Box 3121, Durham, NC 27710; **Phone:** 919-684-1860; **Board Cert:** Internal Medicine 1981; Pulmonary Disease 1984; Critical Care Medicine 1996; **Med School:** Univ NC Sch Med 1977; **Resid:** Internal Medicine, Vanderbilt Univ Hosp 1980; **Fellow:** Pulmonary Disease, Vanderbilt Univ Hosp 1983; **Fac Appt:** Prof Med, Duke Univ

Garver Jr, Robert MD [Pul] - **Spec Exp:** Lung Cancer; Lung Disease; **Hospital:** Univ of Ala Hosp at Birmingham; **Address:** 1900 University Blvd, THT 215, Birmingham, AL 35294; **Phone:** 205-934-7556; **Board Cert:** Internal Medicine 1984; Pulmonary Disease 1986; **Med School:** Johns Hopkins Univ 1981; **Resid:** Internal Medicine, Johns Hopkins Hosp 1984; **Fellow:** Pulmonary Disease, NHLBI 1985; **Fac Appt:** Prof Med, Univ Ala

Goldman, Allan L MD [Pul] - **Spec Exp:** Occupational Lung Disease; Airway Disorders; Lung Cancer; **Hospital:** Tampa Genl Hosp, James A Haley VA Hosp; **Address:** USF Coll Med, Dept Internal Medicine, 12901 Bruce B Downs Blvd, Box MDC19, Tampa, FL 33612-4742; **Phone:** 813-974-2271; **Board Cert:** Internal Medicine 1972; Pulmonary Disease 1972; **Med School:** Univ Minn 1968; **Resid:** Internal Medicine, Brooke Army Hosp 1970; **Fellow:** Pulmonary Disease, Walter Reed Army Hosp 1972; **Fac Appt:** Prof Med, Univ S Fla Coll Med

Pulmonary Disease

Harman, Eloise M MD [Pul] - **Hospital:** Shands at Univ of FL; **Address:** Shands at Univ of Florida, 1600 SW Archer Rd, Box 100225, Gainesville, FL 32610-0225; **Phone:** 352-392-2666; **Board Cert:** Internal Medicine 1973; Pulmonary Disease 1976; Critical Care Medicine 1997; **Med School:** Johns Hopkins Univ 1970; **Resid:** Internal Medicine, Johns Hopkins Hosp 1972; **Fellow:** Pulmonary Disease, NY Hosp-Cornell Med Ctr 1974; **Fac Appt:** Prof Med, Univ Fla Coll Med

Haynes Jr, Johnson MD [Pul] - **Spec Exp:** Sickle Cell Disease-Lung; Chronic Obstructive Lung Disease (COPD); **Hospital:** Univ of S AL Med Ctr; **Address:** Univ S Alabama Medical Ctr, 2451 Fillingim St, MCSB 1530, Mobile, AL 36617; **Phone:** 251-471-7847; **Board Cert:** Internal Medicine 1983; Pulmonary Disease 1986; **Med School:** Univ S Ala Coll Med 1980; **Resid:** Internal Medicine, Univ S Alabama Med Ctr 1983; **Fellow:** Pulmonary Disease, Univ S Alabama Med Ctr 1986; **Fac Appt:** Prof Med, Univ S Ala Coll Med

Henke, David C MD [Pul] - **Spec Exp:** Asthma; Chronic Obstructive Lung Disease (COPD); Vasculitis; **Hospital:** Univ NC Hosps; **Address:** Univ NC Med Sch, Div Pulm Dis & Crit Care Med, 130 Mason Farm Rd, Box 7705, Chapel Hill, NC 27599-7020; **Phone:** 919-966-6838; **Board Cert:** Internal Medicine 1980; Dermatology 1983; Pulmonary Disease 1988; **Med School:** Univ NC Sch Med 1977; **Resid:** Internal Medicine, NC Memorial Hosp 1980; Dermatology, NC Meml NIEHS 1984; **Fellow:** Pulmonary Disease, NC Memorial Hosp 1987; **Fac Appt:** Assoc Prof Med, Univ NC Sch Med

Johnson, Bruce Ellsworth MD [Pul] - **Spec Exp:** Sleep Disorders/Apnea; **Hospital:** Sentara VA Beach Genl Hosp; **Address:** 1008 First Colonial Rd, Ste 103, Virginia Beach, VA 23454-3002; **Phone:** 757-481-2515; **Board Cert:** Internal Medicine 1981; Pulmonary Disease 1986; Critical Care Medicine 2001; **Med School:** Med Coll GA 1978; **Resid:** Internal Medicine, Univ VA Med Ctr 1981; **Fellow:** Pulmonary Disease, Univ VA Med Ctr 1983

Koenig, Steven M MD [Pul] - **Spec Exp:** Sleep Disorders/Apnea; Occupational Lung Disease; Asthma; **Hospital:** Univ Virginia Med Ctr; **Address:** Univ Va Hlth System, Dept Med, Pulmonary Div, Box 800546, Charlottesville, VA 22908-0546; **Phone:** 434-243-9212; **Board Cert:** Internal Medicine 1987; Pulmonary Disease 2000; Critical Care Medicine 2001; **Med School:** Univ Pennsylvania 1984; **Resid:** Internal Medicine, Univ Chicago Hosps 1987; **Fellow:** Pulmonary Critical Care Medicine, Univ Chicago 1990; Sleep Medicine, Deaconess Hosp 1994; **Fac Appt:** Prof Med, Univ VA Sch Med

Light, Richard W MD [Pul] - **Spec Exp:** Pleural Disease; **Hospital:** Vanderbilt Univ Med Ctr; **Address:** Vanderbilt Univ Med Ctr-Pulmonary Medicine, 1161 21st Ave S, T1218 MCN, Nashville, TN 37232-2650; **Phone:** 615-322-3412; **Board Cert:** Internal Medicine 1972; Pulmonary Disease 1974; **Med School:** Johns Hopkins Univ 1968; **Resid:** Internal Medicine, Johns Hopkins Hosp 1970; **Fellow:** Pulmonary Disease, Johns Hopkins Hosp 1972; **Fac Appt:** Prof Med, Vanderbilt Univ

LoRusso, Thomas J MD [Pul] - **Spec Exp:** Critical Care; Sleep Disorders/Apnea; **Hospital:** Inova Fairfax Hosp; **Address:** 1800 Town Ctr Drive, Ste 419, Reston, VA 20190; **Phone:** 703-620-3926; **Board Cert:** Internal Medicine 2003; Pulmonary Disease 2002; Critical Care Medicine 2001; **Med School:** SUNY Upstate Med Univ 1987; **Resid:** Internal Medicine, Univ Hosp-SUNY 1990; **Fellow:** Pulmonary Disease, Cedars Sinai Med Ctr 1993

Loyd, James E MD [Pul] - **Spec Exp:** Pulmonary Fibrosis; Interstitial Lung Disease; Transplant Medicine-Lung; Pulmonary Hypertension; **Hospital:** Vanderbilt Univ Med Ctr; **Address:** Vanderbilt Univ Med Ctr, Div Pulmonary Medicine, 1161 21st Ave S, rm T-1218 MCN, Nashville, TN 37232-2650; **Phone:** 615-322-4752; **Board Cert:** Internal Medicine 1978; Pulmonary Disease 1984; Critical Care Medicine 1997; **Med School:** W VA Univ 1973; **Resid:** Internal Medicine, Vanderbilt Univ Hosp 1976; **Fellow:** Pulmonary Disease, Vanderbilt Univ Hosp 1978; **Fac Appt:** Prof Med, Vanderbilt Univ

Sahn, Steven A MD [Pul] - **Spec Exp:** Pleural Disease; Interstitial Lung Disease; Chronic Obstructive Lung Disease (COPD); Pulmonary Fibrosis; **Hospital:** MUSC Med Ctr; **Address:** MUSC, Div Pulm & Crit Care Med, 96 Jonathan Lucas St, Box 250630, Charleston, SC 29425-8900; **Phone:** 843-792-3167; **Board Cert:** Internal Medicine 1974; Pulmonary Disease 1974; **Med School:** Univ Louisville Sch Med 1968; **Resid:** Internal Medicine, Univ Iowa Hosp 1971; **Fellow:** Pulmonary Disease, Univ CO Hlth Sci Ctr 1973; **Fac Appt:** Prof Med, Med Univ SC

Staton Jr, Gerald W MD [Pul] - **Spec Exp:** Asthma; Chronic Obstructive Lung Disease (COPD); Interstitial Lung Disease; Sarcoidosis; **Hospital:** Wesley Woods Ger Hosp, Crawford Long Hosp of Emory Univ; **Address:** 550 Peachtree St NE Fl 6, Atlanta, GA 30308; **Phone:** 404-686-2505; **Board Cert:** Internal Medicine 1978; Pulmonary Disease 1982; Critical Care Medicine 2007; **Med School:** Med Coll GA 1976; **Resid:** Internal Medicine, Stanford Univ Med Ctr 1979; **Fellow:** Pulmonary Disease, Mass Genl Hosp 1981; **Fac Appt:** Prof Med, Emory Univ

Tapson, Victor MD [Pul] - **Spec Exp:** Pulmonary Hypertension; Chronic Obstructive Lung Disease (COPD); Emphysema; **Hospital:** Duke Univ Med Ctr; **Address:** Duke Univ Med Ctr, Dept Pulm Critical Care Med, Box 31175, Durham, NC 27710; **Phone:** 919-684-6237; **Board Cert:** Internal Medicine 1986; Pulmonary Disease 2000; **Med School:** Hahnemann Univ 1982; **Resid:** Internal Medicine, Duke Univ Med Ctr 1986; **Fellow:** Pulmonary Disease, Boston Univ 1989; **Fac Appt:** Prof Med, Duke Univ

Vaughey, Ellen MD [Pul] - **Spec Exp:** Critical Care; Sleep Disorders/Apnea; **Hospital:** Inova Fairfax Hosp, Virginia Hosp Ctr - Arlington; **Address:** 3289 Woodburn Rd, Ste 350, Annandale, VA 22003; **Phone:** 703-641-8616; **Board Cert:** Internal Medicine 2001; Pulmonary Disease 2002; Critical Care Medicine 2003; **Med School:** Georgetown Univ 1987; **Resid:** Internal Medicine, Thomas Jefferson Univ Hosp 1990; **Fellow:** Pulmonary Disease, Roger Williams Hosp-Brown Univ 1993

Voelkel, Norbert F MD [Pul] - **Spec Exp:** Pulmonary Hypertension; Asthma; Emphysema; **Hospital:** Med Coll of VA Hosp; **Address:** Med Coll of VA Hosp, Box 980456, Richmond, VA 23298; **Phone:** 804-628-9614; **Med School:** Germany 1972; **Resid:** Internal Medicine, Univ Hamburg 1977; **Fellow:** Research, Univ Colorado 1978; Pulmonary Disease, Univ Colorado 1981; **Fac Appt:** Prof Med, Univ Colorado

Wanner, Adam MD [Pul] - **Spec Exp:** Asthma; **Hospital:** Jackson Meml Hosp; **Address:** Univ Miami Sch Med, Div Pulm & Crit Care, Box 016960 (R-47), Miami, FL 33101; **Phone:** 305-243-3045; **Board Cert:** Internal Medicine 1973; Pulmonary Disease 1974; **Med School:** Switzerland 1966; **Resid:** Internal Medicine, Kantonsspital Aarau 1970; **Fellow:** Pulmonary Disease, Mt Sinai Med Ctr 1972; **Fac Appt:** Prof Med, Univ Miami Sch Med

Wheeler, Arthur P MD [Pul] - **Spec Exp:** Critical Care; Sepsis; Respiratory Distress Syndrome (ARDS); **Hospital:** Vanderbilt Univ Med Ctr; **Address:** Vanderbilt Univ Medical Ctr, 1161 21st Ave S, rm T-1217 MCN, Nashville, TN 37232-2650; **Phone:** 615-322-3412; **Board Cert:** Internal Medicine 1985; Pulmonary Disease 1988; Critical Care Medicine 1999; **Med School:** Univ MD Sch Med 1982; **Resid:** Internal Medicine, Vanderbilt Univ Med Ctr 1985; **Fellow:** Pulmonary Disease, Vanderbilt Univ Med Ctr 1986; **Fac Appt:** Assoc Prof Med, Vanderbilt Univ

Young Jr, K Randall MD [Pul] - **Spec Exp:** Transplant Medicine-Lung; Cystic Fibrosis; **Hospital:** Univ of Ala Hosp at Birmingham; **Address:** 422 Tinsley Harrison Tower, 1900 University Blvd, Birmingham, AL 35294; **Phone:** 205-934-5400; **Board Cert:** Internal Medicine 1982; Pulmonary Disease 1986; Allergy & Immunology 1987; **Med School:** Jefferson Med Coll 1978; **Resid:** Internal Medicine, Yale-New Haven Hosp 1982; Pulmonary Critical Care Medicine, Yale-New Haven Hosp 1985; **Fellow:** Allergy & Immunology, Nat Inst Hlth 1988; **Fac Appt:** Prof Med, Univ Ala

Pulmonary Disease

Midwest

Balk, Robert A MD [Pul] - **Spec Exp:** Asthma; Cystic Fibrosis; Respiratory Failure; **Hospital:** Rush Univ Med Ctr, Rush Oak Park Hosp; **Address:** 1725 W Harrison St, Ste 054, Chicago, IL 60612; **Phone:** 312-942-6744; **Board Cert:** Internal Medicine 1981; Pulmonary Disease 1986; Critical Care Medicine 1997; **Med School:** Univ MO-Kansas City 1978; **Resid:** Internal Medicine, Univ MO-Kansas City Affil Hosps 1981; **Fellow:** Pulmonary Critical Care Medicine, Univ Ark Hosp 1983; **Fac Appt:** Prof Med, Rush Med Coll

Fahey, Patrick J MD [Pul] - **Hospital:** Loyola Univ Med Ctr, Hines VA Hosp; **Address:** Loyola Univ Med Ctr, 2160 1st Ave Bldg 102 - rm 7606, Maywood, IL 60153-3304; **Phone:** 708-216-3300; **Board Cert:** Internal Medicine 1976; Pulmonary Disease 1978; **Med School:** Univ Wisc 1973; **Resid:** Internal Medicine, St Elizabeth's Hosp 1976; **Fellow:** Pulmonary Disease, Strong Meml Hosp 1980; **Fac Appt:** Prof Med, Loyola Univ-Stritch Sch Med

Fletcher, Eugene MD [Pul] - **Spec Exp:** Chronic Obstructive Lung Disease (COPD); Sleep Disorders/Apnea; **Hospital:** Floyd Meml Hosp & Hlth Svcs; **Address:** 428 Vincennes St, New Albany, IN 47150; **Phone:** 812-948-5841; **Board Cert:** Internal Medicine 1974; Pulmonary Disease 1980; **Med School:** Temple Univ 1971; **Resid:** Internal Medicine, Univ Colo Affil Hosp 1973; Internal Medicine, Fitzsimons Army Med Ctr 1974; **Fellow:** Pulmonary Disease, Univ Okla Hlth Scis Ctr 1974

Garrity Jr, Edward MD [Pul] - **Spec Exp:** Transplant Medicine-Lung; Pulmonary Vascular Disease; Asthma; Cystic Fibrosis; **Hospital:** Univ of Chicago Hosps; **Address:** Univ of Chicago Hospitals, 5841 S Maryland Ave, MC 0999, Chicago, IL 60637; **Phone:** 773-702-9660; **Board Cert:** Internal Medicine 1979; Pulmonary Disease 1998; Critical Care Medicine 1998; **Med School:** Loyola Univ-Stritch Sch Med 1976; **Resid:** Internal Medicine, Loyola Univ Med Ctr 1979; **Fellow:** Pulmonary Disease, Univ Chicago Hosps 1983; **Fac Appt:** Prof Med, Univ Chicago-Pritzker Sch Med

Grum, Cyril M MD [Pul] - **Spec Exp:** Asthma; Cystic Fibrosis; **Hospital:** Univ Michigan Hlth Sys; **Address:** Univ Mich, Div Pulm & Crit Care Med, 1500 E Med Ctr Drive, rm 3110, Taubman Ctr, Ann Arbor, MI 48109-0368; **Phone:** 734-647-9342; **Board Cert:** Internal Medicine 1980; Pulmonary Disease 1982; **Med School:** Med Coll Wisc 1977; **Resid:** Internal Medicine, Cleveland Clinic; **Fellow:** Pulmonary Disease, Univ Mich Hosps; **Fac Appt:** Prof Med, Univ Mich Med Sch

Hall, Jesse MD [Pul] - **Spec Exp:** Respiratory Failure; Critical Care; Sleep Disorders/Apnea; **Hospital:** Univ of Chicago Hosps; **Address:** 5841 S Maryland Ave, MC 6026, Chicago, IL 60637; **Phone:** 773-702-1454; **Board Cert:** Internal Medicine 1980; Critical Care Medicine 1998; **Med School:** Univ Chicago-Pritzker Sch Med 1977; **Resid:** Internal Medicine, Univ Chicago Hosps 1982; **Fac Appt:** Prof Med, Univ Chicago-Pritzker Sch Med

Hertz, Marshall MD [Pul] - **Spec Exp:** Transplant Medicine-Lung; Transplant Medicine-Heart & Lung; Pulmonary Hypertension; **Hospital:** Univ Minn Med Ctr, Fairview - Univ Campus; **Address:** Pulmonary, Allergy & Critical Care Med, 420 Delaware St SE, MMC 276, Minneapolis, MN 55455; **Phone:** 612-624-0999; **Board Cert:** Internal Medicine 1981; Pulmonary Disease 1984; **Med School:** Univ Mich Med Sch 1978; **Resid:** Internal Medicine, Univ Minn Med Ctr 1982; **Fellow:** Pulmonary Critical Care Medicine, Univ Minn Med Ctr 1984; **Fac Appt:** Prof Med, Univ Minn

Hunninghake, Gary MD [Pul] - **Spec Exp:** Sarcoidosis; Interstitial Lung Disease; **Hospital:** Univ Iowa Hosp & Clinics; **Address:** Univ Iowa, Div Pulmonary Disease, 200 Hawkins Drive W319DGH, Iowa City, IA 52242-1081; **Phone:** 319-356-4187; **Board Cert:** Internal Medicine 1975; Pulmonary Disease 1980; Allergy & Immunology 1977; **Med School:** Univ Kans 1972; **Resid:** Internal Medicine, Univ Kansas Med Ctr 1974; Pulmonary Disease, Natl Inst Hlth 1976; **Fac Appt:** Prof Med, Univ Iowa Coll Med

Hyers, Thomas M MD [Pul] - **Spec Exp:** Thromboembolic Disorders; Chronic Obstructive Lung Disease (COPD); Occupational Medicine; **Hospital:** SSM St Joseph Hosp of Kirkwood; **Address:** CARE Clinical Research, 533 Couch Ave, Ste 140, St Louis, MO 63122; **Phone:** 314-909-9779; **Board Cert:** Internal Medicine 1974; Pulmonary Disease 1980; Critical Care Medicine 1999; **Med School:** Duke Univ 1968; **Resid:** Internal Medicine, Univ Wash Med Ctr 1975; Pulmonary Disease, Univ Colorado Hosp 1977; **Fellow:** Pulmonary Disease, Natl Inst Hlth 1972; **Fac Appt:** Clin Prof Med, St Louis Univ

Jett, James R MD [Pul] - **Spec Exp:** Lung Cancer; Mesothelioma; Thymoma; **Hospital:** Mayo Med Ctr & Clin - Rochester; **Address:** Mayo Clinic, Thoracic Diseases, 200 First St SW, Rochester, MN 55905; **Phone:** 507-284-5398; **Board Cert:** Internal Medicine 1976; Pulmonary Disease 1978; **Med School:** Univ MO-Columbia Sch Med 1973; **Resid:** Internal Medicine, Mayo Clinic 1976; **Fellow:** Pulmonary Disease, Mayo Clinic 1978; **Fac Appt:** Prof Med, Mayo Med Sch

Kaye, Mitchell MD [Pul] - **Spec Exp:** Chronic Obstructive Lung Disease (COPD); Asthma; **Hospital:** Univ Minn Med Ctr, Fairview - Univ Campus; **Address:** Minn Lung Ctr, 920 E 28th St, Ste 700, Minneapolis, MN 55407; **Phone:** 612-863-3750; **Board Cert:** Internal Medicine 1987; Pulmonary Disease 2000; Critical Care Medicine 2001; **Med School:** Univ Minn 1984; **Resid:** Internal Medicine, Univ Ill Hosps & Clins 1987; **Fellow:** Pulmonary Disease, Northwestern Univ Med Sch 1989

Kovitz, Kevin L MD [Pul] - **Spec Exp:** Interventional Pulmonology; **Hospital:** Central DuPage Hosp, Alexian Brothers Med Ctr; **Address:** Chicago Chest Ctr/Suburban Lung Assocs, 800 Biesterfield Rd, Ste 510, Elk Grove Village, IL 60007; **Phone:** 847-981-3660; **Board Cert:** Internal Medicine 1988; Pulmonary Disease 2002; Critical Care Medicine 2005; **Med School:** Israel 1985; **Resid:** Internal Medicine, Univ Maryland Hosps 1988; **Fellow:** Pulmonary Disease, Johns Hopkins Hosp 1992; Interventional Pulmonology, Sainte Marguerite Hosp 1993

Krowka, Michael J MD [Pul] - **Spec Exp:** Hepatopulmonary Syndrome; Pulmonary Hypertension; Chronic Obstructive Lung Disease (COPD); **Hospital:** Mayo Med Ctr & Clin - Rochester; **Address:** Mayo Clinic, Div Pulm & Crit Care Med, 200 First St SW, Rochester, MN 55905; **Phone:** 507-284-3764; **Board Cert:** Internal Medicine 1983; Pulmonary Disease 1986; **Med School:** Univ Nevada 1980; **Resid:** Internal Medicine, Evanston Hosp 1983; **Fellow:** Pulmonary Disease, Mayo Clinic 1986; **Fac Appt:** Prof Med, Mayo Med Sch

Lefrak, Stephen MD [Pul] - **Spec Exp:** Emphysema-Lung Volume Reduction; Critical Care; **Hospital:** Barnes-Jewish Hosp; **Address:** Wash Univ Sch Med, Div Pulm & Crit Care Med, 660 S Euclid Ave, Box 8052, St Louis, MO 63110; **Phone:** 314-362-6044; **Board Cert:** Internal Medicine 1972; Pulmonary Disease 1972; **Med School:** SUNY Downstate 1965; **Resid:** Internal Medicine, Boston Univ Hosp 1968; Pulmonary Disease, Kings Co Hosp Ctr 1969; **Fellow:** Cardiopulmonary Disease, Columbia-Presby Hosp 1970; **Fac Appt:** Prof Med, Washington Univ, St Louis

Lem, Vincent M MD [Pul] - **Spec Exp:** Asthma; **Hospital:** St Luke's Hosp of Kansas City; **Address:** 4321 Washington St, Ste 6000, Kansas City, MO 64111; **Phone:** 816-756-2255; **Board Cert:** Internal Medicine 1982; Pulmonary Disease 1984; Critical Care Medicine 2004; **Med School:** Univ Kans 1978; **Resid:** Internal Medicine, St Luke's Hosp 1982; **Fellow:** Pulmonary Disease, Univ Texas Hlth Sci Ctr 1984; **Fac Appt:** Assoc Clin Prof Med, Univ MO-Kansas City

Marini, John Joseph MD [Pul] - **Spec Exp:** Critical Care; Mechanical Ventilation; Chronic Obstructive Lung Disease (COPD); **Hospital:** Regions Hosp - St Paul; **Address:** 640 Jackson St, MS 11203B, St Paul, MN 55101; **Phone:** 651-254-3456; **Board Cert:** Internal Medicine 2004; Pulmonary Disease 2003; Critical Care Medicine 2002; **Med School:** Johns Hopkins Univ 1973; **Resid:** Internal Medicine, Univ Washington Med Ctr 1976; **Fellow:** Pulmonary Disease, Univ Washington Med Ctr 1978; **Fac Appt:** Prof Med, Univ Minn

Pulmonary Disease

Martinez, Fernando J MD [Pul] - **Spec Exp:** Lung Disease; Critical Care; **Hospital:** Univ Michigan Hlth Sys; **Address:** 1500 E Med Ctr Dr Taubman Bldg - rm 3916, Ann Arbor, MI 48109-0360; **Phone:** 734-763-7668; **Board Cert:** Internal Medicine 1986; Pulmonary Disease 1988; Critical Care Medicine 2000; **Med School:** Univ Fla Coll Med 1983; **Resid:** Internal Medicine, Beth Israel Hosp 1986; **Fellow:** Pulmonary Disease, Boston Univ 1989; **Fac Appt:** Prof Med, Univ Mich Med Sch

McLennan, Geoffrey MD [Pul] - **Spec Exp:** Lung Cancer; Emphysema; Chronic Obstructive Lung Disease (COPD); Bronchoscopy; **Hospital:** Univ Iowa Hosp & Clinics; **Address:** Univ Iowa Hosp, 200 Hawkins Drive, Ste 4900JPP, Iowa City, IA 52242; **Phone:** 319-353-8201; **Med School:** Australia ; **Resid:** Internal Medicine, Royal Adelaide Medical Sch; **Fellow:** Pulmonary Disease, Queen Elizabeth Hosp; **Fac Appt:** Prof Med, Univ Iowa Coll Med

Mehta, Atul MD [Pul] - **Spec Exp:** Transplant Medicine-Lung; Emphysema-Lung Volume Reduction; Interventional Pulmonology; **Hospital:** Cleveland Clin Fdn (page 56); **Address:** Cleveland Clin Fdn, 9500 Euclid Ave, Ste A-90, Cleveland, OH 44195-0001; **Phone:** 216-444-2911; **Board Cert:** Internal Medicine 1981; Pulmonary Disease 1984; **Med School:** India 1976; **Resid:** Internal Medicine, St Francis Med Ctr 1980; Internal Medicine, Easton Hosp 1981; **Fellow:** Pulmonary Disease, Cleveland Clin 1983

Popovich Jr, John MD [Pul] - **Spec Exp:** Lung Disease; Pulmonary Embolism; Interstitial Lung Disease; Critical Care; **Hospital:** Henry Ford Hosp; **Address:** Henry Ford Hosp, Dept Int Med, 2799 W Grand Blvd, Detroit, MI 48202; **Phone:** 313-916-1828; **Board Cert:** Internal Medicine 1978; Pulmonary Disease 1980; Critical Care Medicine 1996; **Med School:** Univ Mich Med Sch 1975; **Resid:** Internal Medicine, Henry Ford Hosp 1978; **Fellow:** Pulmonary Disease, Henry Ford Hosp 1980; **Fac Appt:** Prof Med, Wayne State Univ

Prakash, Udaya MD [Pul] - **Spec Exp:** Bronchoscopy; **Hospital:** Mayo Med Ctr & Clin - Rochester; **Address:** Mayo Clinic, Div Pulm & Crit Care Med, 200 First St SW, Rochester, MN 55905; **Phone:** 507-284-4162; **Board Cert:** Internal Medicine 1987; Pulmonary Disease 1976; **Med School:** India 1969; **Resid:** Internal Medicine, Mayo Clinic 1973; **Fellow:** Pulmonary Disease, Mayo Clinic 1976; **Fac Appt:** Prof Med, Mayo Med Sch

Shore, Bernard L MD [Pul] - **Spec Exp:** Lung Disease; Palliative Care; Pain Management; **Hospital:** Barnes-Jewish Hosp; **Address:** 1110 Highland Plaza Drive E, Ste 375, St Louis, MO 63110; **Phone:** 314-367-3113; **Board Cert:** Internal Medicine 1980; Pulmonary Disease 1982; **Med School:** Washington Univ, St Louis 1977; **Resid:** Internal Medicine, Barnes Hosp 1980; **Fellow:** Pulmonary Disease, Wash Univ Med Ctr 1982; **Fac Appt:** Assoc Clin Prof Med, Washington Univ, St Louis

Silver, Michael R MD [Pul] - **Spec Exp:** Chronic Obstructive Lung Disease (COPD); Lung Cancer; Asthma; **Hospital:** Rush Univ Med Ctr, Rush Oak Park Hosp; **Address:** Rush Univ Med Ctr, Professional Office Bldg 3, 1725 W Harrison St, Ste 054, Chicago, IL 60612; **Phone:** 312-942-6744; **Board Cert:** Internal Medicine 1984; Pulmonary Disease 1988; Critical Care Medicine 1999; **Med School:** Albany Med Coll 1981; **Resid:** Internal Medicine, Rush-Presby-St Luke's Med Ctr 1985; **Fellow:** Pulmonary Critical Care Medicine, Rush-Presby-St Luke's Med Ctr 1987; **Fac Appt:** Assoc Prof Med, Rush Med Coll

Simon, Richard H MD [Pul] - **Spec Exp:** Cystic Fibrosis; **Hospital:** Univ Michigan Hlth Sys; **Address:** Univ Michigan Div Pulmonary Medicine, 6301 MSRB III, 1150 W Medical Center Drive, Ann Arbor, MI 48109; **Phone:** 734-647-9342; **Board Cert:** Internal Medicine 1976; Pulmonary Disease 1980; **Med School:** Duke Univ 1972; **Resid:** Internal Medicine, UCSF Med Ctr 1975; Internal Medicine, Univ Colorado Affil Hosps 1976; **Fellow:** Pulmonary Disease, Univ Colorado 1981; **Fac Appt:** Prof Med, Univ Mich Med Sch

America's Top Doctors® 8th Edition

Stoller, James MD [Pul] - **Spec Exp:** Emphysema/Alpha-1 Antitrypsin Deficiency; **Hospital:** Cleveland Clin Fdn (page 56); **Address:** Cleveland Clinic Fdn, Div Pulmonary Med, 9500 Euclid Ave, Desk A90, Cleveland, OH 44195; **Phone:** 216-444-1960; **Board Cert:** Internal Medicine 1982; Pulmonary Disease 1984; Critical Care Medicine 2007; **Med School:** Yale Univ 1979; **Resid:** Internal Medicine, Peter Bent Brigham Hosp 1982; **Fellow:** Pulmonary Disease, Brigham & Women's Hosp 1983; Critical Care Medicine, Mass Genl Hosp 1985; **Fac Appt:** Prof Med, Cleveland Cl Coll Med/Case West Res

Tobin, Martin MD [Pul] - **Spec Exp:** Mechanical Ventilation; Chronic Obstructive Lung Disease (COPD); **Hospital:** Loyola Univ Med Ctr, Hines VA Hosp; **Address:** Hines VA Hosp (111N), Fifth Ave and Roosevelt Rd, Bldg 1 - rm E438, Hines, IL 60141; **Phone:** 708-202-2705; **Board Cert:** Internal Medicine 1983; Pulmonary Disease 1984; **Med School:** Ireland 1975; **Resid:** Internal Medicine, Trinity Coll Hosps 1979; Pulmonary Disease, Kings Coll Hosp 1980; **Fellow:** Pulmonary Critical Care Medicine, Mount Sinai Hosp 1983; Pulmonary Critical Care Medicine, Univ Pittsburgh 1983; **Fac Appt:** Prof Med, Loyola Univ-Stritch Sch Med

Trulock, Elbert MD [Pul] - **Spec Exp:** Transplant Medicine-Lung; Emphysema-Lung Volume Reduction; Pulmonary Hypertension; Cystic Fibrosis; **Hospital:** Barnes-Jewish Hosp; **Address:** Wash Univ Sch Med, Dept Pulm, 660 S Euclid Ave, Box 8052, St Louis, MO 63110; **Phone:** 314-454-8766; **Board Cert:** Internal Medicine 1981; Pulmonary Disease 1984; **Med School:** Emory Univ 1978; **Resid:** Internal Medicine, Barnes Hosp 1981; **Fellow:** Pulmonary Disease, Wash Univ Med Ctr 1983; **Fac Appt:** Prof Med, Washington Univ, St Louis

Wiedemann, Herbert P MD [Pul] - **Spec Exp:** Respiratory Distress Syndrome (ARDS); Asthma; Emphysema; **Hospital:** Cleveland Clin Fdn (page 56); **Address:** Cleveland Clinic-Pulmonary & Allergy, 9500 Euclid Ave, Desk A90, Cleveland, OH 44195; **Phone:** 216-444-8335; **Board Cert:** Internal Medicine 1980; Pulmonary Disease 1984; Critical Care Medicine 1997; **Med School:** Cornell Univ 1977; **Resid:** Internal Medicine, Univ Wash Hosps 1980; Internal Medicine, Harborview Hosp 1981; **Fellow:** Pulmonary Disease, Yale Univ 1984

Wunderink, Richard MD [Pul] - **Spec Exp:** Infectious Disease-Lung; Pneumonia; Sepsis; **Hospital:** Northwestern Meml Hosp; **Address:** 675 N St Clair Galter Bldg - rm 18-250, Chicago, IL 60611; **Phone:** 312-695-1800; **Board Cert:** Internal Medicine 1983; Pulmonary Disease 1986; **Med School:** Indiana Univ 1980; **Resid:** Internal Medicine, Butterworth Hosp 1983; **Fellow:** Pulmonary Disease, Henry Ford Hosp 1985; **Fac Appt:** Prof Med, Northwestern Univ

Great Plains and Mountains

Brown, Kevin K MD [Pul] - **Spec Exp:** Pulmonary Fibrosis; Interstitial Lung Disease; Autoimmune Lung Disease; **Hospital:** Natl Jewish Med & Rsch Ctr, Univ Colorado Hosp; **Address:** Natl Jewish Health, 1400 Jackson St, Denver, CO 80206-2762; **Phone:** 303-398-1621; **Board Cert:** Internal Medicine 1989; Pulmonary Disease 2005; **Med School:** Univ Minn 1984; **Resid:** Internal Medicine, Providence Med Ctr 1989; **Fellow:** Pulmonary Disease, Maine Med Ctr 1992; Pulmonary Disease, Univ Colo Hlth Scis Ctr 1994; **Fac Appt:** Assoc Prof Med, Univ Colorado

Elliott, C Gregory MD [Pul] - **Spec Exp:** Pulmonary Hypertension; Thromboembolic Disorders; **Hospital:** Intermountain Med Ctr, LDS Hosp; **Address:** Intermountain Med Ctr, Dept Medicine, 5121 S Cottonwood St, Murray, UT 84157; **Phone:** 801-507-4609; **Board Cert:** Internal Medicine 1976; Pulmonary Disease 1978; **Med School:** Univ MD Sch Med 1973; **Resid:** Internal Medicine, Univ Maryland Hosp 1976; **Fellow:** Pulmonary Disease, Univ Utah 1978; **Fac Appt:** Prof Med, Univ Utah

Pulmonary Disease

Iseman, Michael MD [Pul] - **Spec Exp:** Tuberculosis; Mycobacterial Infections; **Hospital:** Natl Jewish Med & Rsch Ctr; **Address:** Natl Jewish Med & Rsch Ctr, 1400 Jackson St, rm J223, Denver, CO 80206; **Phone:** 303-398-1667; **Board Cert:** Internal Medicine 1972; Pulmonary Disease 1976; **Med School:** Columbia P&S 1965; **Resid:** Internal Medicine, Bellevue Hosp 1967; Internal Medicine, Harlem Hosp 1970; **Fellow:** Pulmonary Disease, Harlem Hosp 1972; **Fac Appt:** Prof Med, Univ Colorado

Kaplan, James MD [Pul] - **Spec Exp:** Critical Care; Sleep Disorders/Apnea; **Hospital:** Overland Pk Regl Med Ctr, Providence Med Ctr; **Address:** 10550 Quivira, Ste 335, Overland Park, KS 66215-2304; **Phone:** 913-599-3800; **Board Cert:** Internal Medicine 1987; Pulmonary Disease 2000; Critical Care Medicine 2003; **Med School:** Univ MO-Kansas City 1984; **Resid:** Internal Medicine, Barnes Hosp 1987; **Fellow:** Pulmonary Disease, Barnes Hosp-Wash Univ 1987

Make, Barry J MD [Pul] - **Spec Exp:** Chronic Obstructive Lung Disease (COPD); Emphysema; Asthma; **Hospital:** Natl Jewish Med & Rsch Ctr, Rose Med Ctr; **Address:** Natl Jewish Health, 1400 Jackson St, rm K729, Denver, CO 80206-2762; **Phone:** 303-398-1703; **Board Cert:** Internal Medicine 1973; **Med School:** Jefferson Med Coll 1970; **Resid:** Internal Medicine, Univ Michigan Med Ctr 1973; **Fellow:** Pulmonary Disease, West Virginia Med Ctr 1974; Pulmonary Disease, Boston Univ Med Ctr 1976; **Fac Appt:** Prof Med, Univ Colorado

Martin, Richard J MD [Pul] - **Spec Exp:** Asthma; Vocal Cord Disorders; Chronic Obstructive Lung Disease (COPD); **Hospital:** Natl Jewish Med & Rsch Ctr, Univ Colorado Hosp; **Address:** Natl Jewish Med & Research Ctr, 1400 Jackson St, Denver, CO 80206-2762; **Phone:** 303-398-1847; **Board Cert:** Internal Medicine 1976; Pulmonary Disease 1978; **Med School:** Univ Mich Med Sch 1971; **Resid:** Internal Medicine, Tulane Univ Affil Hosp 1976; **Fellow:** Pulmonary Disease, Univ Oklahoma 1978; **Fac Appt:** Prof Med, Univ Colorado

Newman, Lee S MD [Pul] - **Spec Exp:** Occupational Lung Disease; Sarcoidosis; Lung Disease; **Hospital:** Univ Colorado Hosp; **Address:** Univ Colorado Hlth Science Ctr, 4200 E 9th Ave, rm B-164, Denver, CO 80262; **Phone:** 303-315-6124; **Board Cert:** Internal Medicine 1983; Pulmonary Disease 1986; **Med School:** Vanderbilt Univ 1980; **Resid:** Internal Medicine, Emory Univ Affil Prgm 1984; **Fellow:** Pulmonary Disease, Univ Colorado 1987; **Fac Appt:** Prof Med, Univ Colorado

Pingleton, Susan MD [Pul] - **Spec Exp:** Critical Care; Hospital Acquired Infections; **Hospital:** Univ of Kansas Hosp; **Address:** 3901 Rainbow Blvd, MS 1022, Kansas City, KS 66160; **Phone:** 913-588-6000; **Board Cert:** Internal Medicine 1977; Pulmonary Disease 1978; Critical Care Medicine 1991; **Med School:** Univ Kans 1972; **Resid:** Internal Medicine, Univ Kansas Med Ctr 1975; **Fac Appt:** Prof Med, Univ Kans

Rennard, Stephen I MD [Pul] - **Spec Exp:** Chronic Obstructive Lung Disease (COPD); Emphysema; **Address:** University of Nebraska Medical Ctr, 985885 Nebrasaka Medical Center, Omaha, NE 68198-5885; **Phone:** 402-559-7313; **Board Cert:** Internal Medicine 1978; Pulmonary Disease 1982; **Med School:** Baylor Coll Med 1975; **Resid:** Internal Medicine, Barnes Hosp-Washington Univ 1977; **Fac Appt:** Prof Med, Univ Nebr Coll Med

Rose, Cecile MD [Pul] - **Spec Exp:** Occupational Lung Disease; Sarcoidosis; Pneumonia; **Hospital:** Natl Jewish Med & Rsch Ctr; **Address:** 1400 Jackson St, rm G-211, Denver, CO 80206-2761; **Phone:** 303-398-1520; **Board Cert:** Internal Medicine 1983; Pulmonary Disease 1986; Occupational Medicine 1987; **Med School:** Univ IL Coll Med 1980; **Resid:** Internal Medicine, Med Coll Virginia Hosp 1983; **Fellow:** Pulmonary Disease, Med Coll Virginia Hosp 1985; **Fac Appt:** Assoc Prof Med, Univ Colorado

Schwarz, Marvin I MD [Pul] - **Spec Exp:** Interstitial Lung Disease; Pulmonary Vascular Disease; Lung Hemorrhage; **Hospital:** Univ Colorado Hosp, Natl Jewish Med & Rsch Ctr; **Address:** Div Pulmonary Science & Critical Care, 4200 Ninth Ave, Denver, CO 80262-0001; **Phone:** 303-315-4211; **Board Cert:** Internal Medicine 1970; Pulmonary Disease 1971; **Med School:** Tulane Univ 1964; **Resid:** Internal Medicine, Charity Hosp 1967; **Fellow:** Pulmonary Disease, Charity Hosp/Tulane Univ 1969; **Fac Appt:** Prof Med, Univ Colorado

Southwest

Arroliga, Alejandro C MD [Pul] - **Spec Exp:** Pulmonary Hypertension; Respiratory Distress Syndrome (ARDS); Critical Care; **Hospital:** Scott & White Mem Hosp; **Address:** 2401 S 31st St, Temple, TX 76508; **Phone:** 254-724-9887; **Board Cert:** Internal Medicine 2000; Pulmonary Disease 2000; Critical Care Medicine 2003; **Med School:** Mexico 1984; **Resid:** Internal Medicine, Coney Island Hosp 1990; **Fellow:** Pulmonary Critical Care Medicine, Yale-New Haven Hosp 1993; **Fac Appt:** Prof Med, Cleveland Cl Coll Med/Case West Res

Guidry, George Gary MD [Pul] - **Spec Exp:** Chronic Obstructive Lung Disease (COPD); Asthma; Pneumonia; Lung Cancer; **Hospital:** Lafayette Genl Med Ctr, Our Lady of Lourdes Reg Med Ctr - Lafayette; **Address:** 155 Hospital Drive, Ste 206, Lafayette, LA 70503-2852; **Phone:** 337-234-3204; **Board Cert:** Internal Medicine 1988; Pulmonary Disease 1999; **Med School:** Louisiana State U, New Orleans 1985; **Resid:** Internal Medicine, LSU Med Ctr 1988; **Fellow:** Pulmonary Disease, LSU Med Ctr; **Fac Appt:** Assoc Clin Prof Med, Louisiana State U, New Orleans

Levin, David C MD [Pul] - **Spec Exp:** Asthma; Chronic Obstructive Lung Disease (COPD); **Hospital:** OU Med Ctr, VA Med Ctr - Oklahoma City; **Address:** OU Physicians Building, 825 NE 10th St, Ste 2500, Oklahoma City, OK 73104; **Phone:** 405-271-7001; **Board Cert:** Internal Medicine 1973; Pulmonary Disease 1976; **Med School:** Case West Res Univ 1970; **Resid:** Internal Medicine, Univ Colorado Hlth Sci Ctr 1974; **Fellow:** Pulmonary Disease, Univ Colorado Hlth Sci Ctr 1975; **Fac Appt:** Prof Med, Univ Okla Coll Med

Perret, Philip S MD [Pul] - **Spec Exp:** Chronic Obstructive Lung Disease (COPD); **Hospital:** Our Lady of Lourdes Reg Med Ctr - Lafayette; **Address:** 614 W St Mary Blvd, Lafayette, LA 70506; **Phone:** 337-232-6435; **Board Cert:** Internal Medicine 1978; Pulmonary Disease 1980; Critical Care Medicine 1997; **Med School:** Emory Univ 1974; **Resid:** Internal Medicine, Emory Univ Hosp 1977; **Fellow:** Pulmonary Disease, Emory Univ Hosp 1979

Shellito, Judd E MD [Pul] - **Spec Exp:** Pulmonary Infections; Occupational Lung Disease; **Hospital:** L Boggs Med Ctr; **Address:** 3600 Prytania St, Ste 35, New Orleans, LA 70115; **Phone:** 504-895-5748; **Board Cert:** Internal Medicine 1977; Pulmonary Disease 1980; **Med School:** Tulane Univ 1974; **Resid:** Internal Medicine, Evanston Hosp 1978; **Fellow:** Pulmonary Critical Care Medicine, Univ New Mexico Hosp 1980; **Fac Appt:** Prof Med, Louisiana State U, New Orleans

Summer, Warren MD [Pul] - **Spec Exp:** Chronic Obstructive Lung Disease (COPD); Asthma; Respiratory Distress Syndrome (ARDS); **Hospital:** L Boggs Med Ctr; **Address:** 3600 Prytania St, Ste 35, New Orleans, LA 70115; **Phone:** 504-895-5748; **Board Cert:** Internal Medicine 1972; Pulmonary Disease 1972; **Med School:** Georgetown Univ 1965; **Resid:** Internal Medicine, Maimonides Med Ctr 1968; **Fellow:** Pulmonary Disease, Georgetown Univ Hosp 1969; **Fac Appt:** Prof Med, Louisiana State U, New Orleans

Pulmonary Disease

Weissler, Jonathan C MD [Pul] - **Spec Exp:** Interstitial Lung Disease; Asthma; **Hospital:** UT Southwestern Med Ctr - Dallas, Parkland Meml Hosp - Dallas; **Address:** 5323 Harry Hines Blvd, Dallas, TX 75390-9034; **Phone:** 214-645-1825; **Board Cert:** Internal Medicine 1982; Pulmonary Disease 1984; Critical Care Medicine 2007; **Med School:** NYU Sch Med 1979; **Resid:** Internal Medicine, Univ Texas Hlth Sci Ctr 1982; **Fellow:** Pulmonary Disease, Univ Texas Hlth Sci Ctr 1985; **Fac Appt:** Prof Med, Univ Tex SW, Dallas

West Coast and Pacific

Albertson, Timothy MD/PhD [Pul] - **Spec Exp:** Critical Care; Transplant Medicine-Lung; **Hospital:** UC Davis Med Ctr; **Address:** UC Davis, Div Pulm Crit Care, 4150 V St, Ste 3400, Patient Support Svcs Bldg, Sacramento, CA 95817-9002; **Phone:** 916-734-3564; **Board Cert:** Pulmonary Disease 1984; Critical Care Medicine 1996; Emergency Medicine 1997; Medical Toxicology 2005; **Med School:** UC Davis 1977; **Resid:** Internal Medicine, Univ Arizona 1980; Internal Medicine, UC Davis Med Ctr 1981; **Fellow:** Pulmonary Critical Care Medicine, UC Davis Med Ctr 1983; **Fac Appt:** Prof Med, UC Davis

Balmes, John Randolph MD [Pul] - **Spec Exp:** Occupational Lung Disease; **Hospital:** San Francisco Genl Hosp, UCSF Med Ctr; **Address:** UCSF, Division Occup & Envr Med, Campus Box 0843, San Francisco, CA 94143-0843; **Phone:** 415-206-8314; **Board Cert:** Internal Medicine 1979; Pulmonary Disease 1984; **Med School:** Mount Sinai Sch Med 1976; **Resid:** Internal Medicine, Mount Sinai Hosp 1979; **Fellow:** Pulmonary Disease, Yale-New Haven Hosp 1981; **Fac Appt:** Prof Med, UCSF

Bellamy, Paul E MD [Pul] - **Spec Exp:** Critical Care; **Hospital:** KFH Woodland Hills Med Ctr; **Address:** Kaiser Woodland Hills Med Ctr, Pulm Div, 5601 De Soto Ave, Med Office Twr, Fl 4, Woodland Hills, CA 91367; **Phone:** 818-719-3530; **Board Cert:** Internal Medicine 1978; Pulmonary Disease 1980; Critical Care Medicine 2007; **Med School:** SUNY Buffalo 1975; **Resid:** Internal Medicine, Univ Hosps-Case West Res 1978; **Fellow:** Pulmonary Disease, UCLA Med Ctr 1980; **Fac Appt:** Clin Prof Med, UCLA

Boushey Jr, Homer A MD [Pul] - **Spec Exp:** Asthma; **Hospital:** UCSF Med Ctr; **Address:** UCSF Med Ctr, Dept Med, 400 Parnassus Ave, Box 0359, San Francisco, CA 94143; **Phone:** 415-353-2961; **Board Cert:** Internal Medicine 1972; Pulmonary Disease 1974; **Med School:** UCSF 1968; **Resid:** Internal Medicine, UCSF Med Ctr 1970; Internal Medicine, Beth Israel Hosp 1971; **Fellow:** Pulmonary Disease, Oxford Univ 1972; Pulmonary Disease, UCSF Hosp 1973; **Fac Appt:** Prof Med, UCSF

Catanzaro, Antonino MD [Pul] - **Spec Exp:** Tuberculosis; Coccidioidomycosis; Mycobacterial Infections; **Hospital:** UCSD Med Ctr; **Address:** 200 W Arbor Drive, MC 8374, San Diego, CA 92103; **Phone:** 619-543-5550; **Board Cert:** Internal Medicine 1972; Pulmonary Disease 1976; **Med School:** SUNY Buffalo 1965; **Resid:** Internal Medicine, Georgetown Univ Hosp 1970; **Fellow:** Pulmonary Critical Care Medicine, UCSD Med Ctr 1972; Research, Scripps Clin Rsch Fdn 1972; **Fac Appt:** Prof Med, UCSD

Heffner, John E MD [Pul] - **Spec Exp:** Critical Care; Respiratory Failure; **Hospital:** Providence Portland Med Ctr; **Address:** 1111 NE 99th Ave, Ste 200, Portland, OR 97220; **Phone:** 503-963-3030; **Board Cert:** Internal Medicine 1977; Pulmonary Disease 1982; Critical Care Medicine 2005; **Med School:** UCLA 1974; **Resid:** Internal Medicine, Univ Colo Med Ctr 1978; **Fac Appt:** Prof Med, Med Univ SC

Hopewell, Philip MD [Pul] - **Spec Exp:** AIDS/HIV; Tuberculosis; Infectious Disease-Lung; **Hospital:** San Francisco Genl Hosp; **Address:** 1001 Potrero Ave, Ste 5K1, San Francisco, CA 94110; **Phone:** 415-206-8313; **Board Cert:** Internal Medicine 1973; Pulmonary Disease 1974; **Med School:** W VA Univ 1965; **Resid:** Internal Medicine, UCSF Med Ctr 1971; **Fellow:** Pulmonary Disease, UCSF Med Ctr 1973; **Fac Appt:** Prof Med, UCSF

Huang, Laurence MD [Pul] - **Spec Exp:** AIDS/HIV; Pneumocystis Carinii Pneumonia (PCP); **Hospital:** San Francisco Genl Hosp; **Address:** UCSF Positive Health Program - SFGH, 995 Potrero Ave, Bldg 80-Ward 84, San Francisco, CA 94110; **Phone:** 415-206-2400; **Board Cert:** Internal Medicine 2003; Pulmonary Disease 2006; Critical Care Medicine 2007; **Med School:** Columbia P&S 1989; **Resid:** Internal Medicine, Columbia-Presby Hosp 1992; Pulmonary Critical Care Medicine, UCSF Med Ctr 1995; **Fac Appt:** Assoc Clin Prof Med, UCSF

Hudson, Leonard MD [Pul] - **Spec Exp:** Critical Care; Lung Injury-Acute; Respiratory Failure; **Hospital:** Harborview Med Ctr; **Address:** Harborview Medical Ctr, 325 9th Ave, Box 359762, Seattle, WA 98104; **Phone:** 206-744-3123; **Board Cert:** Internal Medicine 1973; Pulmonary Disease 1974; **Med School:** Univ Wash 1964; **Resid:** Internal Medicine, New York Hosp 1966; Internal Medicine, Univ Wash Hosps 1969; **Fellow:** Pulmonary Disease, Univ Colo Med Ctr 1971; **Fac Appt:** Prof Med, Univ Wash

Jacoby, David MD [Pul] - **Hospital:** OR Hlth & Sci Univ; **Address:** 3181 SW Sam Jackson Park Rd, MC UHN67, Dept Pulmonary/Crit Care, Portland, OR 97239; **Phone:** 503-494-6158; **Board Cert:** Internal Medicine 1983; Pulmonary Disease 1986; **Med School:** NY Med Coll 1980; **Resid:** Internal Medicine, Temple Univ Hosp 1983; **Fellow:** Pulmonary Critical Care Medicine, UCSF Hosp 1987; **Fac Appt:** Prof Med, Oregon Hlth Sci Univ

King Jr, Talmadge E MD [Pul] - **Spec Exp:** Interstitial Lung Disease; Sarcoidosis; Asthma; **Hospital:** UCSF Med Ctr; **Address:** 505 Parnassus Ave, Ste 5H22, San Francisco, CA 94143-0120; **Phone:** 415-476-0909; **Board Cert:** Internal Medicine 1977; Pulmonary Disease 1982; **Med School:** Harvard Med Sch 1974; **Resid:** Internal Medicine, Grady-Emory Univ Affil Hosp 1977; **Fellow:** Pulmonary Critical Care Medicine, Univ Colo Hlth Sci Ctr 1979; **Fac Appt:** Prof Med, UCSF

Lynch, Joseph P MD [Pul] - **Spec Exp:** Transplant Medicine-Lung; Interstitial Lung Disease; Pulmonary Fibrosis; **Hospital:** Ronald Reagan UCLA Med Ctr; **Address:** UCLA - Div Pulmonary Med, 10833 Le Conte Ave, CHS Bldg - rm 37-131, Los Angeles, CA 90095-1690; **Phone:** 310-825-8599; **Board Cert:** Internal Medicine 1976; Pulmonary Disease 1980; **Med School:** Harvard Med Sch 1973; **Resid:** Internal Medicine, Univ Mich Med Ctr 1976; **Fellow:** Pulmonary Disease, Univ Mich Med Ctr 1978; **Fac Appt:** Prof Med, UCLA

Martin, Thomas R MD [Pul] - **Spec Exp:** Respiratory Distress Syndrome (ARDS); Critical Care; **Hospital:** VA Puget Sound Hlth Care Sys; **Address:** Seattle VA Hosp - Pulmonary Rsch 151L, 1660 S Columbian Way, Seattle, WA 98108; **Phone:** 206-764-2345; **Board Cert:** Internal Medicine 1976; Pulmonary Disease 1980; **Med School:** Univ Pennsylvania 1973; **Resid:** Internal Medicine, Univ Washington Med Ctr 1977; **Fellow:** Pulmonary Disease, Univ Washington 1980; **Fac Appt:** Prof Med, Univ Wash

Matthay, Michael Anthony MD [Pul] - **Spec Exp:** Critical Care; Respiratory Distress Syndrome (ARDS); **Hospital:** UCSF Med Ctr; **Address:** UCSF Med Ctr, 505 Parnasas Ave, rm M-917, San Francisco, CA 94143-0624; **Phone:** 415-353-1206; **Board Cert:** Internal Medicine 1976; Pulmonary Disease 1980; Critical Care Medicine 1987; **Med School:** Univ Pennsylvania 1973; **Resid:** Internal Medicine, Univ Colo Med Ctr 1976; **Fellow:** Surgery, UCLA Med Ctr 1979; **Fac Appt:** Prof Med, UCSF

Pulmonary Disease

Mosenifar, Zab MD [Pul] - **Spec Exp:** Chronic Obstructive Lung Disease (COPD); Interstitial Lung Disease; Asthma; Pulmonary Hypertension; **Hospital:** Cedars-Sinai Med Ctr; **Address:** Cedars-Sinai Med Ctr, Div Pulmonary Med, 8700 Beverly Blvd, rm 6732 South Twr, Los Angeles, CA 90048-1804; **Phone:** 310-423-4685; **Board Cert:** Internal Medicine 1978; Pulmonary Disease 1980; **Med School:** Iran 1973; **Resid:** Internal Medicine, Thomas Jefferson Univ Hosp; Internal Medicine, UCLA Med Ctr; **Fellow:** Pulmonary Disease, UCLA Med Ctr; **Fac Appt:** Prof Med, UCLA

Patterson, James R MD [Pul] - **Spec Exp:** Sleep Disorders/Apnea; **Hospital:** Providence Portland Med Ctr; **Address:** 1111 NE 99th Ave, Ste 200, Portland, OR 97220; **Phone:** 503-963-3030; **Board Cert:** Internal Medicine 1972; Pulmonary Disease 2001; **Med School:** Columbia P&S 1968; **Resid:** Internal Medicine, Columbia-Presby Med Ctr 1970; **Fellow:** Pulmonary Disease, Fitzsimons Army Med Ctr 1973; **Fac Appt:** Clin Prof Med, Oregon Hlth Sci Univ

Raghu, Ganesh MD [Pul] - **Spec Exp:** Interstitial Lung Disease; Pulmonary Fibrosis; Sarcoidosis; Transplant-Lung; **Hospital:** Univ Wash Med Ctr; **Address:** 1959 NE Pacific St, Box 356166, Seattle, WA 98195; **Phone:** 206-598-4615; **Board Cert:** Internal Medicine 1982; **Med School:** India 1974; **Resid:** Internal Medicine, Univ Rochester-Strong Meml Hosp 1978; Internal Medicine, SUNY Buffalo Med Ctr 1981; **Fellow:** Pulmonary Critical Care Medicine, Univ Washington 1984; **Fac Appt:** Prof Med, Univ Wash

Rizk, Norman W MD [Pul] - **Spec Exp:** Critical Care; Asthma; **Hospital:** Stanford Univ Med Ctr; **Address:** 300 Pasteur Drive, Ste H3142, Stanford, CA 94305-5236; **Phone:** 650-725-7061; **Board Cert:** Internal Medicine 1979; Pulmonary Disease 1984; Critical Care Medicine 1996; **Med School:** Yale Univ 1976; **Resid:** Internal Medicine, San Fran Genl Hosp 1980; **Fellow:** Pulmonary Disease, Moffitt Hosp-UCSF 1983; **Fac Appt:** Prof Med, Stanford Univ

Rubin, Lewis MD [Pul] - **Spec Exp:** Pulmonary Hypertension; Pulmonary Vascular Disease; **Hospital:** UCSD Med Ctr; **Address:** UCSD Med Ctr, Pulmonary & Critical Care, 9300 Campus Point Drive, MC 7381, La Jolla, CA 92037-7381; **Phone:** 858-657-8700; **Board Cert:** Internal Medicine 1978; Pulmonary Disease 1980; **Med School:** Albert Einstein Coll Med 1975; **Resid:** Internal Medicine, Duke Univ Med Ctr 1978; **Fellow:** Pulmonary Disease, Duke Univ Med Ctr 1979; **Fac Appt:** Prof Med, UCSD

Sharma, Om Prakash MD [Pul] - **Spec Exp:** Sarcoidosis; Interstitial Lung Disease; Hypersensitivity Pneumonitis; **Hospital:** LAC & USC Med Ctr, USC Univ Hosp - R K Eamer Med Plz; **Address:** 1200 N State St GNH Bldg - rm 11900, Los Angeles, CA 90033; **Phone:** 323-226-7923; **Board Cert:** Internal Medicine 1987; **Med School:** India 1959; **Resid:** Internal Medicine, Norwalk Hosp 1963; Internal Medicine, Einstein Med Coll Hosp 1965; **Fellow:** Pulmonary Disease, Einstein Med Coll Hosp 1966; Research, Royal Coll Physicians 1969; **Fac Appt:** Prof Med, USC Sch Med

Tharratt, Robert S MD [Pul] - **Spec Exp:** Bioterrorism Preparedness; Toxicology; **Hospital:** UC Davis Med Ctr; **Address:** UC Davis Med Ctr, Div Pulm Crit Care, 4150 V St, Ste 3400-Pt Support Services Bldg, Sacramento, CA 95817-2214; **Phone:** 916-734-3564; **Board Cert:** Pulmonary Disease 1988; Critical Care Medicine 1999; Medical Toxicology 2004; Emergency Medicine 2007; **Med School:** UCLA 1983; **Resid:** Internal Medicine, UC Davis Med Ctr 1986; **Fellow:** Pulmonary Critical Care Medicine, UC Davis Med Ctr 1989; **Fac Appt:** Prof Med, UC Davis

Wallace, Jeanne M MD [Pul] - **Spec Exp:** Pulmonary Infections; Sleep Disorders/Apnea; Asthma; **Hospital:** Olive View Med Ctr; **Address:** Olive View UCLA Med Ctr, 14445 Olive View Dr, Sylmar, CA 91342-1437; **Phone:** 818-364-3205; **Board Cert:** Internal Medicine 1977; Pulmonary Disease 1980; Sleep Medicine 2007; **Med School:** UCLA 1974; **Resid:** Internal Medicine, UCSF Med Ctr 1977; **Fellow:** Pulmonary Disease, UCSD Med Ctr 1980; **Fac Appt:** Assoc Prof Med, UCLA

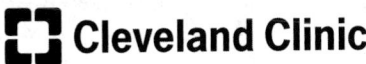
Cleveland Clinic

Pulmonary, Allergy and Critical Care Medicine

Individuals with all types of acute or chronic lung diseases, as well as sleep disordered breathing (sleep apnea) can access specialty care at Cleveland Clinic. In 2007, physicians in the Department of Pulmonary, Allergy and Critical Care Medicine provided over 54,000 outpatient visits and cared for more than 1,400 hospital admissions.

In collaboration with thoracic surgery colleagues, we evaluate patients for:

- Lung transplantation
- Lung-volume reduction surgery (LVRS) for emphysema
- Pulmonary thomboednarterectomy (for chronic pulmonary hypertension secondary to thromboemboli)

Lung Transplantation

Cleveland Clinic's Lung Transplant Program is the largest in Ohio and among the largest in the United States. Since the program began, it has grown to include dozens of single lung, double lung, and heart/lung transplants every year. The average wait time for a lung transplantation at Cleveland Clinic is significantly lower than the national average.

Sarcoidosis Center of Excellence

In January 2003, Cleveland Clinic was awarded a $2 million grant from the Department of Health and Human Services to establish a Sarcoidosis Center of Excellence. The only such center in Northeastern Ohio, the center aims to raise awareness of pulmonary sarcoidosis, improve the quality of sarcoidosis care and minimize the degree to which it can affect quality of life.

Areas of Expertise

Acute respiratory distress syndrome (ARDS), Allergy rhinitis, Allergies (drug and food; latex), Aspirin desensitization, Asthma, Beryllium-induced lung disease, Chronic obstructive pulmonary disease (COPD), Including alpha-1 antitrypsin deficiency, Interstitial lung disease, Interventional bronchology, Lung cancer, Lymphangioleiomyomatosis (LAM), Pulmonary alveolar proteinosis (PAP), Pulmonary vascular disease, Sarcoidosis, Sepsis, Sleep-disordered breathing, Urticaria, Weaning from mechanical ventilation

For more information about the Cleveland Clinic Department of Pulmonary, Allergy and Critical Care Medicine, to schedule a second opinion or to learn about assistance for out-of-town patients, call 800.890.2467 or visit www. clevelandclinic.org/pulmonarytopdocs.

Department of Pulmonology, Allergy and Critical Care Medicine
9500 Euclid Avenue / AC311 | Cleveland OH 44195

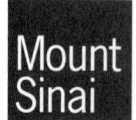
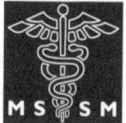

Mount Sinai

M S ⚕ S M

MOUNT SINAI
SCHOOL OF
MEDICINE

The mission of Mount Sinai's Division of Pulmonary, Critical Care, and Sleep Medicine is to offer state-of-the-art patient care, cutting-edge translational research, and hands-on teaching. In fulfillment of this philosophy, each faculty member is charged with the success of a specific program.

Mount Sinai's Sarcoidosis Service, the largest of its kind in the world, is a Center of Excellence for research in sarcoidosis. It is the only site in the United States that performs the diagnostic Kveim-Siltzbach skin test for sarcoidosis, which eliminates the need for more invasive, uncomfortable, and expensive procedures. Through its Pulmonary Physiology Laboratory, Mount Sinai has been instrumental in establishing normal values for various pulmonary function tests and is currently conducting clinical studies of new tests for obesity, sarcoidosis, asthma, and lung cancer. Pulmonary specialists at Mount Sinai are investigating asthma and emphysema, lung cancer, collagen vascular diseases, pulmonary infections, occupational lung diseases, and critical care outcomes. Mount Sinai has the largest screening program for workers and general population exposed at the World Trade Center catastrophe site on 9/11 and thereafter. Programs and services offered include:

- **Asthma Program,** which uses a multidisciplinary team approach, focusing on patient education and skill building to foster self-management;

- **Chronic Obstructive Pulmonary Disease (COPD) Program,** offering—for one of the nation's most underdiagnosed conditions—a coordinated approach of exercise, treatment, and education that improves quality of life and clinical outlook;

- **Critical Care Medicine Program,** featuring state-of-the-art medical intensive care and respiratory care units;

- **Interventional Pulmonary Service,** which performs diagnostic and therapeutic procedures for patients with advanced pulmonary diseases;

- **Lung Transplant Program,** for patients with advanced lung disease that has progressed despite optimal medical therapy;

- **Occupational Lung Disorders Program,** specializing in diagnosis and management of occupational lung disorders, such as occupational asthma and bronchitis, asbestosis, silicosis, and heavy metal lung injury;

- **Pulmonary Fibrosis/Interstitial Lung Disease Program,** which treats patients with chronic inflammatory and scarring disorders of the lungs, including collagen vascular-associated pulmonary diseases;

- **Pulmonary Physiology Laboratory,** a service that has recently doubled in capacity and that performs the full range of physiological testing for lung disease;

- **Pulmonary Vascular Program,** offering diagnosis and management of pulmonary hypertension;

- **Pulmonary Rehabilitation Program,** which provides occupational, physical, and cardiopulmonary rehabilitation programs for patients with disabling lung disorders, as well as pre- and postoperative consultation and therapy;

- **Respiratory Care Unit,** recently opened for chronic ventilator-dependent patients and those with advanced lung disease;

- **Thoracic Oncology Service,** which provides multidisciplinary medical care for lung cancer, as a joint effort with the Department of Cardiothoracic Surgery;

- **Sarcoidosis Service,** which has passed its 20,000 enrollee count and offers standard care as well as the opportunity to participate in new clinical trials to sixty new enrollees per week.

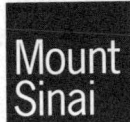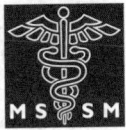

THE MOUNT SINAI MEDICAL CENTER
SLEEP MEDICINE

One Gustave L. Levy Place
Fifth Avenue and 100th Street
New York, NY 10029-6574
Physician Referral: 1-800-MD-SINAI (637-4624)
www.mountsinai.org

Mount Sinai's recently expanded Center for Sleep Medicine is a full-service program that specializes in the comprehensive, compassionate, personalized care of individuals with sleep disorders.

We use state-of-the-art equipment to diagnose and treat all aspects of sleep pathology, including breathing-related disorders, insomnia, restless leg syndrome, periodic limb movements, and narcolepsy. An initial consultation includes a clinical history and physical examination. In some cases, the diagnosis and treatment plan can be completed in a single visit. In other cases, the evaluation requires a sleep study (typically over one or two nights) or other tests. Overnight tests are completed by 7:00 am, so it is usually not necessary to miss a day of work. In rare instances, daytime studies are also recommended.

Services available at the Center for Sleep Medicine include:

- Consultations with board-certified sleep specialists;

- Overnight sleep testing and daytime testing provided by experienced physicians and technicians. During a sleep study, the patient is monitored by painless, noninvasive technology (PSG) that records breathing, heart rate, brain waves, oxygen levels, and eye and leg movement;

- Treatment for a sleep disorder that may include a device to aid the patient's breathing while sleeping (called CPAP or BiPAP), medication, or light therapy as well as neuropsychiatric interventions as needed. If indicated, consultations with other specialists are available to aid in diagnosis and therapy;

- Mechanical, behavioral, surgical, dental, and pharmacological therapies, as required. Consultations can also be arranged with pulmonologists, ear, nose, and throat surgeons, bariatric surgeons, dentists, and psychiatrists.

MOUNT SINAI SPECIALIZES IN TREATING OBSTRUCTIVE SLEEP APNEA

Approximately 20 million Americans suffer from obstructive sleep apnea (OSA), which occurs when muscles of the back of the mouth and the throat relax during sleep, causing a complete (apnea) or partial (hypopnea) blockage of the airway. Each time that happens, there can be an awakening and the oxygen level may fall, causing the heart to work harder. When untreated, this disorder can lead to hypertension, heart failure, and stroke, as well as to bouts of daytime sleepiness that increase the risk of motor vehicle and industrial accidents. In seniors, sleepiness is often misperceived as a natural consequence of aging. If you are overweight and snore, you may have sleep apnea or another sleep disorder. If you are concerned about your sleep, ask for an appointment with one of our board-certified sleep specialists by calling (212) 241-5098.

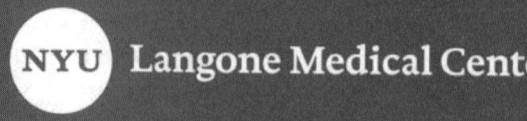

PULMONOLOGY

The Pulmonary and Critical Care Medicine Division at NYU Medical Center is characterized by its commitment to clinical excellence, teaching and clinical and basic science research.

PULMONOLOGY AND CRITICAL CARE MEDICINE

The NYU Langone Medical Center Pulmonology and Critical Care Medicine section has a full continuum of services available for diagnosis, treatment and research of both the inpatient and ambulatory patient. Available services include a state-of-the-art Pulmonary Function Laboratory (see right), a specialized inpatient pulmonary unit with a dedicated respiratory care unit, a specialized medical critical care unit staffed with dedicated pulmonary/critical care physicians and a multidisciplinary interventional bronchoscopy program integrated with thoracic radiology.

In addition to the clinical services, active research is being conducted at the clinical and basic science levels in the areas of asthma and chronic obstructive pulmonary diseases, lung physiology and sleep disorders, interventional bronchoscopy, lung cancer screening and treatment, environmental and occupational lung diseases, pulmonary fibrosis, tuberculosis, and sepsis.

LUNG SURGERY AT NYULANGONE MEDICAL CENTER

The department of cardiothoracic surgery provides complete adult and pediatric general surgical and thoracic services, including surgery for congenital and acquired problems, tumor surgery, surgery on the lungs, esophageal surgery, and repair of chest wall deformities. We have over a decade of experience in using minimally invasive techniques to treat these problems. By using state-of-the-art instruments and techniques, often we can perform these procedures with minimal discomfort, little scarring and limited hospitalization.

PULMONARY REHABILITATION

Housed in the Joan and Joel Smilow Cardiac Rehabilitation and Prevention Center of the Rusk Institute of Rehabilitation Medicine, the cardiopulmonary rehabilitation unit is fully staff and equipped to handle both the inpatient and outpatient needs of the respiratory patient. The unit has dedicated inpatient beds for the hospitalized patients staffed by a Pulmonary Rehabilitation Team, comprised of pulmonologists, cardiologists, nurses, physical therapists, occupational therapists, psychologists, nutritionists, and social workers. Our exercise gym is equipped with exercise, monitoring, and resuscitation equipment for the safe and comprehensive delivery of services.

NYU LANGONE MEDICAL CENTER

The Pulmonary Function Laboratory at NYU Langone Medical Center offers several standard and specialized pulmonary tests, including:

- Spirometry (timed vital capacity, FEV1/FVC)
- Bronchodilator responsiveness (spirometry before and after bronchodilator administration)
- Flow volume loop
- Lung volumes (helium dilution and/or plethysmography)
- Maximum voluntary ventilation
- Diffusing capacity (single-breath carbon monoxide)
- Arterial and capillary blood gas analysis
- Pulse oximetry
- Airway resistance
- Maximal inspiratory and expiratory pressures
- Airway hyperactivity evaluation
- Oxygen dosage determinations

Radiation Oncology
a subspecialty of Radiology

A radiation oncologist deals with the therapeutic applications of radiant energy and its modifiers and the study and management of disease, especially malignant tumors.

Training Required: Four years in radiology *plus* additional training and examination.

RADIATION ONCOLOGY

New England

Choi, Noah C MD [RadRO] - **Spec Exp:** Lung Cancer; Esophageal Cancer; Mesothelioma; **Hospital:** Mass Genl Hosp; **Address:** Mass Genl Hosp, Dept Rad Oncology, 100 Blossom St, Cox 307, Boston, MA 02114; **Phone:** 617-726-6050; **Board Cert:** Therapeutic Radiology 1970; **Med School:** South Korea 1963; **Resid:** Radiation Oncology, Princess Margaret Hosp 1970; **Fac Appt:** Prof RadRO, Harvard Med Sch

D'Amico, Anthony V MD/PhD [RadRO] - **Spec Exp:** Prostate Cancer; Brachytherapy; **Hospital:** Dana-Farber Cancer Inst, Brigham & Women's Hosp; **Address:** Brigham & Women's Hosp, Dept Rad Onc, 75 Francis St, Ste L2, Boston, MA 02115; **Phone:** 617-732-7936; **Board Cert:** Radiation Oncology 1999; **Med School:** Univ Pennsylvania 1990; **Resid:** Radiation Oncology, Hosp Univ Penn 1994; **Fac Appt:** Prof RadRO, Harvard Med Sch

DeLaney, Thomas Francis MD [RadRO] - **Spec Exp:** Sarcoma; Proton Beam Therapy; **Hospital:** Mass Genl Hosp; **Address:** Francis H. Burr Proton Therapy Ctr, 30 Fruit St, Bosont, MA 02114; **Phone:** 617-726-6876; **Board Cert:** Therapeutic Radiology 1986; Radiation Oncology 1999; **Med School:** Harvard Med Sch 1982; **Resid:** Therapeutic Radiology, Mass Genl Hosp 1986; **Fac Appt:** Assoc Prof RadRO, Harvard Med Sch

Harris, Jay R MD [RadRO] - **Spec Exp:** Breast Cancer; **Hospital:** Brigham & Women's Hosp, Dana-Farber Cancer Inst; **Address:** Dana Farber Cancer Inst, 44 Binney St, rm D1622, Boston, MA 02115; **Phone:** 617-632-2291; **Board Cert:** Therapeutic Radiology 1999; **Med School:** Stanford Univ 1970; **Resid:** Radiation Oncology, Joint Ctr Rad Ther 1976; **Fellow:** Radiation Therapy, Harvard Med Sch 1977; **Fac Appt:** Prof RadRO, Harvard Med Sch

Knisely, Jonathan MD [RadRO] - **Spec Exp:** Brain Tumors; Stereotactic Radiosurgery; Gastrointestinal Cancer; **Hospital:** Yale-New Haven Hosp; **Address:** Yale Univ Sch Med, Dept Therapeutic Radiology, 15 York St, Hunter Bldg-HRT 133, New Haven, CT 06520-8040; **Phone:** 203-785-2960; **Board Cert:** Internal Medicine 1989; Radiation Oncology 1993; **Med School:** Univ Pennsylvania 1986; **Resid:** Internal Medicine, Michael Reese Hosp 1989; Radiation Oncology, Univ Toronto Med Ctr 1992; **Fac Appt:** Assoc Prof, Yale Univ

Loeffler, Jay S MD [RadRO] - **Spec Exp:** Stereotactic Radiosurgery; Brain Tumors-Benign; Meningioma; Acoustic Neuroma; **Hospital:** Mass Genl Hosp; **Address:** Mass General Hosp, Radiation Oncology, 100 Blossom St, Boston, MA 02114; **Phone:** 617-724-1548; **Board Cert:** Therapeutic Radiology 1986; **Med School:** Brown Univ 1982; **Resid:** Radiation Oncology, Harvard Joint Ctr for Rad Ther 1986; **Fellow:** Cancer Biology, Harvard Sch Pub Hlth 1985; **Fac Appt:** Prof RadRO, Harvard Med Sch

Mauch, Peter M MD [RadRO] - **Spec Exp:** Lymphoma; Hodgkin's Disease; **Hospital:** Dana-Farber Cancer Inst; **Address:** Dana Farber Cancer Inst, 75 Francis St, Ste RadOnc L2, Boston, MA 02115; **Phone:** 617-632-4116; **Board Cert:** Therapeutic Radiology 1978; **Med School:** St Louis Univ 1974; **Resid:** Radiation Therapy, Harvard Joint Ctr 1978; **Fac Appt:** Prof, Harvard Med Sch

Peschel, Richard E MD [RadRO] - **Spec Exp:** Prostate Cancer; **Hospital:** Yale-New Haven Hosp; **Address:** Yale-New Haven Hosp, Dept Radiology, 15 York St, rm HRT 142, New Haven, CT 06510; **Phone:** 203-785-2958; **Board Cert:** Therapeutic Radiology 1982; **Med School:** Yale Univ 1977; **Resid:** Radiation Oncology, Yale-New Haven Hosp 1981; **Fac Appt:** Prof RadRO, Yale Univ

America's Top Doctors® 8th Edition

Recht, Abram MD [RadRO] - **Spec Exp:** Breast Cancer; Gastrointestinal Cancer; Gynecologic Cancer; **Hospital:** Beth Israel Deaconess Med Ctr - Boston; **Address:** Beth Israel Deaconess Med Ctr, 330 Brookline Ave, Boston, MA 02215; **Phone:** 617-667-2345; **Board Cert:** Therapeutic Radiology 1984; **Med School:** Johns Hopkins Univ 1980; **Resid:** Radiation Oncology, Joint Ctr Radiation Therapy 1984; **Fac Appt:** Assoc Prof RadRO, Harvard Med Sch

Roberts, Kenneth MD [RadRO] - **Spec Exp:** Pediatric Cancers; Lymphoma; Hodgkin's Disease; **Hospital:** Yale-New Haven Hosp, Backus Hosp, Norwich; **Address:** Yale Univ School of Medicine, Dept Radiation Therapy, 15 York St, New Haven, CT 06520-8040; **Phone:** 203-785-2957; **Board Cert:** Internal Medicine 1987; Medical Oncology 1989; Radiation Oncology 1995; **Med School:** Duke Univ 1984; **Resid:** Internal Medicine, Ohio State Univ Hosps 1987; Radiation Oncology, Duke Univ Med Ctr 1992; **Fellow:** Hematology & Oncology, Duke Univ Med Ctr 1989; **Fac Appt:** Assoc Prof Rad, Yale Univ

Shipley, William U MD [RadRO] - **Spec Exp:** Bladder Cancer; Prostate Cancer; **Hospital:** Mass Genl Hosp; **Address:** Mass Genl Hosp, Dept Rad Oncology, 100 Blossom St, Cox 347, Boston, MA 02114; **Phone:** 617-726-8146; **Board Cert:** Therapeutic Radiology 1975; **Med School:** Harvard Med Sch 1966; **Resid:** Surgery, Mass Genl Hosp 1971; Radiation Therapy, Harvard Joint Ctr Rad Therapy 1973; **Fellow:** Radiation Therapy, Royal Marsden Hosp 1974; **Fac Appt:** Prof RadRO, Harvard Med Sch

Tarbell, Nancy MD [RadRO] - **Spec Exp:** Brain Tumors-Pediatric; Proton Beam Therapy; **Hospital:** Mass Genl Hosp; **Address:** Massachusetts Genl Hosp BPTC107, 55 Fruit St, Boston, MA 02114; **Phone:** 617-724-1836; **Board Cert:** Therapeutic Radiology 1983; **Med School:** SUNY Upstate Med Univ 1979; **Resid:** Radiation Therapy, Harvard Med School 1983; **Fac Appt:** Prof RadRO, Harvard Med Sch

Wazer, David E MD [RadRO] - **Spec Exp:** Breast Cancer; Melanoma; **Hospital:** Rhode Island Hosp, Tufts Med Ctr; **Address:** 593 Eddy St, Providence, RI 02903; **Phone:** 401-444-8311; **Board Cert:** Radiation Oncology 1988; **Med School:** NYU Sch Med 1982; **Resid:** Radiation Oncology, Tufts New England Med Ctr 1988; **Fellow:** Neurological Chemistry, NYU Med Ctr 1984; **Fac Appt:** Prof RadRO, Tufts Univ

Wilson, Lynn D MD [RadRO] - **Spec Exp:** Lymphoma, Cutaneous T Cell (CTCL); Lymphoma, Cutaneous B Cell (CBCL); Lung Cancer; Head & Neck Cancer; **Hospital:** Yale-New Haven Hosp; **Address:** Yale Univ Sch Med, Dept Therapeutic Rad, PO Box 208040, New Haven, CT 06520-8040; **Phone:** 203-688-1861; **Board Cert:** Radiation Oncology 2004; **Med School:** Geo Wash Univ 1990; **Resid:** Therapeutic Radiology, Yale-New Haven Hosp 1994; **Fac Appt:** Prof RadRO, Yale Univ

Zietman, Anthony L MD [RadRO] - **Spec Exp:** Prostate Cancer; Urologic Cancer; Proton Beam Therapy; **Hospital:** Mass Genl Hosp; **Address:** Mass Genl Hosp, 100 Blossom St, Cox 3, Boston, MA 02114; **Phone:** 617-724-4000; **Board Cert:** Radiation Oncology 1994; **Med School:** England 1983; **Resid:** Internal Medicine, St Stephens & Westminster Hosp 1986; Radiation Oncology, Mass Genl Hosp 1989; **Fellow:** Radiation Oncology, Middlesex/Mt Vernon Hosps 1991; **Fac Appt:** Prof RadRO, Harvard Med Sch

Mid Atlantic

Berg, Christine D MD [RadRO] - **Spec Exp:** Breast Cancer-Early Detection; Breast Cancer-High Risk; **Hospital:** Natl Inst of Hlth - Clin Ctr; **Address:** 6130 Executive Blvd, Bethesda, MD 20892-7346; **Phone:** 301-496-8544; **Board Cert:** Internal Medicine 1980; Medical Oncology 1983; Therapeutic Radiology 1999; **Med School:** Northwestern Univ 1977; **Resid:** Internal Medicine, Northwestern Meml Hosp 1981; Radiation Oncology, Georgetown Univ Hosp 1986; **Fellow:** Medical Oncology, Natl Cancer Inst-NIH 1984

Radiation Oncology

Constine, Louis Sanders MD [RadRO] - **Spec Exp:** Pediatric Cancers; Lymphoma; Cancer Survivors-Late Effects of Therapy; Sarcoma; **Hospital:** Univ of Rochester Strong Meml Hosp; **Address:** 601 Elmwood Ave, Box 647, Rochester, NY 14642; **Phone:** 585-275-5622; **Board Cert:** Pediatrics 1978; Therapeutic Radiology 1981; Pediatric Hematology-Oncology 1978; **Med School:** Johns Hopkins Univ 1973; **Resid:** Pediatrics, Moffitt Hosp-UCSF Med Ctr 1975; Pediatrics, Stanford Hosp Med Ctr 1976; **Fellow:** Therapeutic Radiology, Stanford Hosp Med Ctr 1981; Pediatric Hematology-Oncology, Univ Wash/Chldns Ortho Hosp 1978; **Fac Appt:** Prof RadRO, Univ Rochester

DeWeese, Theodore L MD [RadRO] - **Spec Exp:** Urologic Cancer; Prostate Cancer; Testicular Cancer; **Hospital:** Johns Hopkins Hosp - Baltimore (page 61); **Address:** Johns Hopkins Hosp, Weinberg Bldg, 401 N Broadway, rm 1363, Baltimore, MD 21231; **Phone:** 410-955-8893; **Board Cert:** Radiation Oncology 1995; **Med School:** Univ Colorado 1990; **Resid:** Radiation Oncology, Johns Hopkins Hosp 1994; **Fellow:** Urologic Oncology, Johns Hopkins Hosp 1995; **Fac Appt:** Prof RadRO, Johns Hopkins Univ

Dicker, Adam P MD/PhD [RadRO] - **Spec Exp:** Prostate Cancer; **Hospital:** Thomas Jefferson Univ Hosp; **Address:** Bodine Cancer Treatment Ctr, 111 South 11th St, Philadelphia, PA 19107-5097; **Phone:** 215-955-6527; **Board Cert:** Radiation Oncology 2000; **Med School:** Cornell Univ-Weill Med Coll 1992; **Resid:** Surgery, Lenox Hill Hosp 1994; Radiation Oncology, Meml Sloan Kettering Cancer Ctr 1997; **Fac Appt:** Assoc Prof RadRO, Thomas Jefferson Univ

Dritschilo, Anatoly MD [RadRO] - **Spec Exp:** Prostate Cancer; **Hospital:** Georgetown Univ Hosp; **Address:** Georgetown Univ Hosp, Dept Radiation Medicine, LL-Bliss, 3800 Reservoir Rd NW, Washington, DC 20007; **Phone:** 202-687-2144; **Board Cert:** Therapeutic Radiology 1977; **Med School:** UMDNJ-NJ Med Sch, Newark 1973; **Resid:** Radiation Therapy, Harvard Joint Rad Ther Ctr 1977; **Fac Appt:** Prof Med, Georgetown Univ

Ennis, Ronald D MD [RadRO] - **Spec Exp:** Prostate Cancer; Brachytherapy; Gynecologic Cancer; **Hospital:** St Luke's - Roosevelt Hosp Ctr - Roosevelt Div (page 57), Beth Israel Med Ctr - Petrie Division (page 57); **Address:** St Luke's Roosevelt Hosp, Dept Rad Oncol, 1000 10th Ave, Lower Level, New York, NY 10019; **Phone:** 212-523-7165; **Board Cert:** Radiation Oncology 2005; **Med School:** Yale Univ 1990; **Resid:** Therapeutic Radiology, Yale-New Haven Hosp 1994

Flickinger, John C MD [RadRO] - **Spec Exp:** Neuro-Oncology; Brain & Spinal Tumors; **Hospital:** UPMC Presby, Pittsburgh; **Address:** UPMC Cancer Ctr, Radiation Oncology, 200 Lothrop St, Ste B 300, Pittsburgh, PA 15213; **Phone:** 412-647-3600; **Board Cert:** Therapeutic Radiology 1985; **Med School:** Univ Chicago-Pritzker Sch Med 1981; **Resid:** Radiation Therapy, Mass General Hosp 1985; **Fac Appt:** Prof RadRO, Univ Pittsburgh

Formenti, Silvia C MD [RadRO] - **Spec Exp:** Breast Cancer; Chemo-Radiation Combined Therapy; **Hospital:** NYU Med Ctr (page 68); **Address:** NYU Med Ctr, Dept Radiation Oncology, 160 E 34th St, New York, NY 10016; **Phone:** 212-263-2601; **Board Cert:** Radiation Oncology 1991; **Med School:** Italy 1980; **Resid:** Internal Medicine, San Carlo Borromeo Hosp 1983; Medical Oncology, Univ of Pavia Med Ctr 1985; **Fellow:** Radiation Oncology, USC Med Ctr 1990; **Fac Appt:** Asst Prof RadRO, NYU Sch Med

Freedman, Gary MD [RadRO] - **Spec Exp:** Breast Cancer; **Hospital:** Fox Chase Cancer Ctr (page 58); **Address:** Fox Chase Cancer Ctr-Radiation Onc Dept, 7701 Burholme Ave, Philadelphia, PA 19111; **Phone:** 215-728-3815; **Board Cert:** Radiation Oncology 2000; **Med School:** Temple Univ 1993; **Resid:** Radiation Oncology, Fox Chase Cancer Center 1998

Glassburn, John R MD [RadRO] - **Spec Exp:** Gynecologic Cancer; Prostate Cancer; Breast Cancer; **Hospital:** Pennsylvania Hosp (page 60); **Address:** Pennsylvania Hosp, Dept Radiation Oncology, 800 Spruce St, Philadelphia, PA 19107; **Phone:** 215-829-3873; **Board Cert:** Therapeutic Radiology 1973; **Med School:** Hahnemann Univ 1966; **Resid:** Radiation Oncology, Hahnemann Hosp 1972; **Fac Appt:** Clin Prof RadRO, Univ Pennsylvania

Glatstein, Eli MD [RadRO] - **Spec Exp:** Lymphoma; Lung Cancer; Photodynamic Therapy; Sarcoma; **Hospital:** Hosp Univ Penn - UPHS (page 60); **Address:** Hosp Univ Penn, Dept Rad Oncology, 3400 Spruce St, Donner Bldg Fl 2, Philadelphia, PA 19104; **Phone:** 215-662-3383; **Board Cert:** Therapeutic Radiology 1972; **Med School:** Stanford Univ 1964; **Resid:** Radiation Therapy, Stanford Med Ctr 1970; **Fellow:** Radiological Biology, Hammersmith Hosp 1972; **Fac Appt:** Prof RadRO, Univ Pennsylvania

Goodman, Robert L MD [RadRO] - **Spec Exp:** Breast Cancer; Lymphoma; Prostate Cancer; Brain Tumors; **Hospital:** St Barnabas Med Ctr; **Address:** St Barnabas Med Ctr, Dept Rad Oncology, 94 Old Short Hills Rd, Livingston, NJ 07039; **Phone:** 973-322-5133; **Board Cert:** Internal Medicine 1971; Therapeutic Radiology 1974; Medical Oncology 1975; **Med School:** Columbia P&S 1966; **Resid:** Internal Medicine, Beth Israel Hosp 1970; Radiation Therapy, Harvard Joint Ctr Rad Therapy 1974; **Fellow:** Hematology, NY-Presby Hosp 1969

Greenberger, Joel S MD [RadRO] - **Spec Exp:** Lung Cancer; Esophageal Cancer; **Hospital:** UPMC Presby, Pittsburgh; **Address:** UPMC Cancer Ctr, Radiation Oncology, 200 Lothrop St, Ste B300, Pittsburgh, PA 15232; **Phone:** 412-647-3600; **Board Cert:** Therapeutic Radiology 1977; **Med School:** Harvard Med Sch 1971; **Resid:** Radiation Therapy, Mass General Hosp 1977; **Fac Appt:** Prof RadRO, Univ Pittsburgh

Haffty, Bruce MD [RadRO] - **Spec Exp:** Breast Cancer; Head & Neck Cancer; Lung Cancer; **Hospital:** Robert Wood Johnson Univ Hosp - New Brunswick, Robert Wood Johnson Univ Hosp Hamilton; **Address:** The Cancer Institute of New Jersey, 195 Little Albany St, New Brunswick, NJ 08903; **Phone:** 732-253-3939; **Board Cert:** Radiation Oncology 1988; **Med School:** Yale Univ 1984; **Resid:** Radiation Oncology, Yale-New Haven Hosp 1988; **Fac Appt:** Prof RadRO, Robert W Johnson Med Sch

Hahn, Stephen M MD [RadRO] - **Spec Exp:** Lung Cancer; Prostate Cancer; Sarcoma; Photodynamic Therapy; **Hospital:** Hosp Univ Penn - UPHS (page 60), Penn Presby Med Ctr - UPHS (page 60); **Address:** Hosp of the Univ of Penn, 3400 Spruce St 2 Donner Bldg, Philadelphia, PA 19104; **Phone:** 215-662-7296; **Board Cert:** Radiation Oncology 2004; Internal Medicine 1987; Medical Oncology 2001; **Med School:** Temple Univ 1984; **Resid:** Internal Medicine, UCSF Med Ctr 1988; Medical Oncology, Natl Inst Hlth 1991; **Fellow:** Radiation Oncology, Natl Inst Hlth 1994; **Fac Appt:** Prof RadRO, Univ Pennsylvania

Harrison, Louis MD [RadRO] - **Spec Exp:** Brachytherapy; Head & Neck Cancer; Radiation Therapy-Intraoperative; **Hospital:** Beth Israel Med Ctr - Petrie Division (page 57), St Luke's - Roosevelt Hosp Ctr - Roosevelt Div (page 57); **Address:** Beth Israel Med Ctr, Dept Rad Onc, 10 Union Square East, Ste 4G, New York, NY 10003-3314; **Phone:** 212-844-8087; **Board Cert:** Therapeutic Radiology 1986; **Med School:** SUNY Downstate 1982; **Resid:** Therapeutic Radiology, Yale-New Haven Hosp 1986; **Fac Appt:** Prof RadRO, Albert Einstein Coll Med

Horwitz, Eric MD [RadRO] - **Spec Exp:** Prostate Cancer; Intensity Modulated Radiotherapy (IMRT); Brachytherapy; **Hospital:** Fox Chase Cancer Ctr (page 58); **Address:** Fox Chase Cancer Ctr, Dept Radiation Oncology, 333 Cottman Ave, Philadelphia, PA 19111; **Phone:** 215-728-2995; **Board Cert:** Radiation Oncology 1999; **Med School:** Albany Med Coll 1992; **Resid:** Radiation Oncology, William Beaumont Hosp 1997

Radiation Oncology

Isaacson, Steven MD [RadRO] - **Spec Exp:** Brain Tumors; Neuro-Oncology; Stereotactic Radiosurgery; **Hospital:** NY-Presby Hosp/Columbia (page 66); **Address:** Columbia Presby Med Ctr, Dept Rad Oncol, 622 W 168th St BHN Bldg - rm B11, New York, NY 10032-3720; **Phone:** 212-305-2611; **Board Cert:** Radiation Oncology 1988; Otolaryngology 1978; **Med School:** Jefferson Med Coll 1973; **Resid:** Otolaryngology, Hosp Univ Penn 1978; Radiation Oncology, SUNY Hlth Sci Ctr 1988; **Fac Appt:** Clin Prof RadRO, Columbia P&S

Kleinberg, Lawrence MD [RadRO] - **Spec Exp:** Brain & Spinal Cord Tumors; Brain Tumors-Metastatic; Stereotactic Radiosurgery; Esophageal Cancer; **Hospital:** Johns Hopkins Hosp - Baltimore (page 61); **Address:** Johns Hopkins Oncology Ctr Weinberg Bldg, 401 N Broadway, Ste 1440, Baltimore, MD 21231; **Phone:** 410-614-2597; **Board Cert:** Radiation Oncology 1994; **Med School:** Yale Univ 1989; **Resid:** Radiation Oncology, Meml Sloan-Kettering Canc Ctr 1993; **Fac Appt:** Assoc Prof RadRO, Johns Hopkins Univ

Konski, Andre MD [RadRO] - **Spec Exp:** Esophageal Cancer; Rectal Cancer; Pancreatic Cancer; Gastrointestinal Cancer; **Hospital:** Fox Chase Cancer Ctr (page 58), Jeanes Hosp; **Address:** Fox Chase Cancer Ctr, Dept Rad Onc, 333 Cottman Ave, Philadelphia, PA 19111; **Phone:** 215-728-2916; **Board Cert:** Radiation Oncology 2000; **Med School:** NY Med Coll 1984; **Resid:** Radiation Oncology, Stong Meml/Genesee Hosps 1988

Kuettel, Michael MD/PhD [RadRO] - **Spec Exp:** Prostate Cancer; **Hospital:** Roswell Park Cancer Inst; **Address:** Roswell Park Cancer Inst, Radiation Med, Elm and Carlton St, Buffalo, NY 14263; **Phone:** 716-845-1562; **Board Cert:** Radiation Oncology 1992; **Med School:** Northwestern Univ-Feinberg Sch Med 1985; **Resid:** Internal Medicine, Northwestern Hosp 1986; Radiation Oncology, Johns Hopkins Hosp 1990; **Fac Appt:** Prof Med, SUNY Buffalo

Lepanto, Philip B MD [RadRO] - **Hospital:** St Mary's Med Ctr - Huntington, Cabell Huntington Hosp; **Address:** St Mary's Med Ctr, Dept Radiation Oncology, 2900 First Ave, Huntington, WV 25702; **Phone:** 304-526-1143; **Board Cert:** Therapeutic Radiology 1975; **Med School:** Univ Louisville Sch Med 1970; **Resid:** Diagnostic Radiology, Graduate Hosp 1972; Radiation Therapy, Hosp Univ Penn 1975; **Fac Appt:** Clin Prof Rad, Marshall Univ

Machtay, Mitchell MD [RadRO] - **Spec Exp:** Head & Neck Cancer; Skin Cancer; Skull Base Tumors; **Hospital:** Thomas Jefferson Univ Hosp; **Address:** Bodine Ctr for Cancer Treatment, Dept Rad Onc, 111 S 11 St, Bodine Ctr, Philadelphia, PA 19107-5097; **Phone:** 215-955-6706; **Board Cert:** Radiation Oncology 1994; **Med School:** NYU Sch Med 1989; **Resid:** Radiation Oncology, Hosp Univ Penn 1993; **Fac Appt:** Assoc Prof RadRO, Jefferson Med Coll

McCormick, Beryl MD [RadRO] - **Spec Exp:** Breast Cancer; Eye Tumors/Cancer; **Hospital:** Meml Sloan-Kettering Cancer Ctr, NY-Presby Hosp/Weill Cornell (page 66); **Address:** 1275 York Avenue, New York, NY 10065; **Phone:** 800-525-2225; **Board Cert:** Therapeutic Radiology 1977; **Med School:** UMDNJ-NJ Med Sch, Newark 1973; **Resid:** Therapeutic Radiology, Meml Sloan Kettering Cancer Ctr 1977; **Fac Appt:** Prof RadRO, Cornell Univ-Weill Med Coll

Nicolaou, Nicos MD [RadRO] - **Spec Exp:** Lymphoma; Hodgkin's Disease; **Hospital:** Fox Chase Cancer Ctr (page 58); **Address:** 333 Cottman Avenue, Philadelphia, PA 19111-2497; **Phone:** 215-728-3815; **Board Cert:** Radiation Oncology 1999; **Med School:** Canada 1984; **Resid:** Radiation Oncology, British Columbia Cancer Agency 1989; **Fellow:** Radiation Oncology, Fox Chase Cancer Ctr 1990

Nori, Dattatreyudu MD [RadRO] - **Spec Exp:** Breast Cancer; Prostate Cancer; Gynecologic Cancer; **Hospital:** NY-Presby Hosp/Weill Cornell (page 66), NY Hosp Queens; **Address:** 525 E 68th St, Box 575, New York, NY 10021-4870; **Phone:** 212-746-3679; **Board Cert:** Therapeutic Radiology 1979; **Med School:** India 1970; **Resid:** Radiation Oncology, Meml Sloan Kettering Cancer Ctr 1975; **Fellow:** Radiation Oncology, Meml Sloan Kettering Cancer Ctr 1978; **Fac Appt:** Prof RadRO, Cornell Univ-Weill Med Coll

Pollack, Alan MD/PhD [RadRO] - **Spec Exp:** Prostate Cancer; Genitourinary Cancer; Sarcoma; **Hospital:** Fox Chase Cancer Ctr (page 58); **Address:** Fox Chase Cancer Ctr, Rad Oncology, 333 Cottman Ave, Philadelphia, PA 19111; **Phone:** 215-728-2940; **Board Cert:** Radiation Oncology 1993; **Med School:** Univ Miami Sch Med 1987; **Resid:** Radiation Oncology, MD Anderson Cancer Ctr 1992; **Fac Appt:** Prof RadRO, Temple Univ

Regine, William F MD [RadRO] - **Spec Exp:** Stereotactic Radiosurgery; Brain & Spinal Tumors; Gastrointestinal Cancer; **Hospital:** Univ of MD Med Sys; **Address:** Univ MD Med System-Greenbaum Cancer Ctr, 22 S Green St Guldelsky Bldg, Baltimore, MD 21201; **Phone:** 410-328-6080; **Board Cert:** Radiation Oncology 1992; **Med School:** SUNY Upstate Med Univ 1987; **Resid:** Radiation Oncology, Thomas Jefferson Univ Hosp 1991; **Fellow:** Radiation Oncology, Thomas Jefferson Univ Hosp 1992; **Fac Appt:** Prof RadRO, Univ MD Sch Med

Rotman, Marvin MD [RadRO] - **Spec Exp:** Bladder Cancer; Gynecologic Cancer; Breast Cancer; Prostate Cancer; **Hospital:** SUNY Downstate Med Ctr, Long Island Coll Hosp (page 57); **Address:** 450 Clarkson Ave, Box 1211, Brooklyn, NY 11203-2056; **Phone:** 718-270-2181; **Board Cert:** Diagnostic Radiology 1966; Radiation Oncology 1999; **Med School:** Jefferson Med Coll 1958; **Resid:** Internal Medicine, Albert Einstein Med Ctr 1960; Radiation Oncology, Montefiore Hosp Med Ctr 1965; **Fac Appt:** Prof RadRO, SUNY Downstate

Schiff, Peter B MD/PhD [RadRO] - **Spec Exp:** Prostate Cancer; Gynecologic Cancer; Breast Cancer; **Hospital:** NY-Presby Hosp/Columbia (page 66); **Address:** Columbia Univ Med Ctr, Dept Rad Oncology, 622 W 168th St, New York, NY 10032-3720; **Phone:** 212-305-2991; **Board Cert:** Radiation Oncology 1990; **Med School:** Albert Einstein Coll Med 1984; **Resid:** Radiation Oncology, Meml Sloan Kettering Cancer Ctr 1988; **Fac Appt:** Prof RadRO, Columbia P&S

Solin, Lawrence J MD [RadRO] - **Spec Exp:** Breast Cancer; **Hospital:** Hosp Univ Penn - UPHS (page 60); **Address:** Univ Penn Med Ctr, Dept Rad Oncology, 3400 Spruce St, 2 Donner Bldg, Philadelphia, PA 19104; **Phone:** 215-662-7267; **Board Cert:** Radiation Oncology 1999; Therapeutic Radiology 1984; **Med School:** Brown Univ 1978; **Resid:** Surgery, Thos Jefferson Univ Hosp 1981; Radiation Oncology, Thos Jefferson Univ Hosp 1984; **Fac Appt:** Prof RadRO, Univ Pennsylvania

Stock, Richard MD [RadRO] - **Spec Exp:** Prostate Cancer; **Hospital:** Mount Sinai Med Ctr (page 64); **Address:** 1184 5th Ave Fl 1 - rm P1-34, New York, NY 10029; **Phone:** 212-241-7502; **Board Cert:** Radiation Oncology 1993; **Med School:** Mount Sinai Sch Med 1988; **Resid:** Radiation Oncology, Meml Sloan Kettering Cancer Ctr 1992; **Fac Appt:** Prof RadRO, Mount Sinai Sch Med

Wharam Jr, Moody D MD [RadRO] - **Spec Exp:** Pediatric Cancers; Brain Tumors; Sarcoma-Soft Tissue; **Hospital:** Johns Hopkins Hosp - Baltimore (page 61); **Address:** Kimmel Cancer Ctr, Dept Rad Oncology, 401 N Broadway St, Ste 1440, Baltimore, MD 21231-1146; **Phone:** 410-955-7312; **Board Cert:** Therapeutic Radiology 1974; **Med School:** Univ VA Sch Med 1969; **Resid:** Radiation Oncology, UCSF Medical Ctr 1973; **Fac Appt:** Prof RadRO, Johns Hopkins Univ

Radiation Oncology

Yahalom, Joachim MD [RadRO] - **Spec Exp:** Lymphoma; Hodgkin's Disease; Multiple Myeloma; **Hospital:** Meml Sloan-Kettering Cancer Ctr; **Address:** 1275 York Avenue, New York, NY 10065; **Phone:** 800-525-2225; **Board Cert:** Radiation Oncology 1988; **Med School:** Israel 1976; **Resid:** Internal Medicine, Hadassah Hosp 1979; Radiation Oncology, Hadassah Hosp 1984; **Fellow:** Radiation Oncology, Meml Sloan Kettering Canc Ctr 1986; **Fac Appt:** Prof RadRO, Cornell Univ-Weill Med Coll

Zelefsky, Michael J MD [RadRO] - **Spec Exp:** Prostate Cancer; Brachytherapy; Bladder Cancer; **Hospital:** Meml Sloan-Kettering Cancer Ctr; **Address:** 1275 York Avenue, New York, NY 10065; **Phone:** 800-525-2225; **Board Cert:** Radiation Oncology 1991; **Med School:** Albert Einstein Coll Med 1986; **Resid:** Radiation Oncology, Meml Sloan Kettering Cancer Ctr 1990; **Fac Appt:** Prof RadRO, Cornell Univ-Weill Med Coll

Southeast

Anscher, Mitchell MD [RadRO] - **Spec Exp:** Prostate Cancer; Brachytherapy; **Hospital:** Med Coll of VA Hosp, Henrico Doctors Hosp; **Address:** Virginia Commonwealth Univ, Department of Radiation Oncology, Box 980058, Richmond, VA 23298-0058; **Phone:** 804-828-7238; **Board Cert:** Radiation Oncology 1987; Internal Medicine 1984; **Med School:** Med Coll VA 1981; **Resid:** Internal Medicine, St Marys Hosp 1984; Radiation Oncology, Duke Univ Med Ctr 1987; **Fac Appt:** Prof RadRO, Va Commonwealth Univ Sch Med

Bonner, James Alan MD [RadRO] - **Spec Exp:** Head & Neck Cancer; Lung Cancer; **Hospital:** Univ of Ala Hosp at Birmingham; **Address:** 1824 6th Ave S, WTI, rm 105, Birmingham, AL 35294; **Phone:** 205-934-2761; **Board Cert:** Radiation Oncology 1990; **Med School:** Wayne State Univ 1985; **Resid:** Radiation Oncology, Univ Michigan Med Ctr 1989; **Fac Appt:** Prof RadRO, Univ Ala

Brizel, David M MD [RadRO] - **Spec Exp:** Head & Neck Cancer; Sarcoma; Lymphoma; **Hospital:** Duke Univ Med Ctr; **Address:** Duke Univ Med Ctr, Dept Rad Onc, Box 3085, Durham, NC 27710-0001; **Phone:** 919-668-5637; **Board Cert:** Radiation Oncology 1987; **Med School:** Northwestern Univ 1983; **Resid:** Radiation Oncology, Harvard Joint Center 1987; **Fac Appt:** Prof RadRO, Duke Univ

Chakravarthy, Anuradha MD [RadRO] - **Spec Exp:** Breast Cancer; Gastrointestinal Cancer; **Hospital:** Vanderbilt Univ Med Ctr; **Address:** Vanderbilt Univ Med Ctr, Dept Rad Onc, 1301 22nd Ave S, Preston Research Bldg, Ste 1003, Nashville, TN 37232; **Phone:** 615-322-2555; **Board Cert:** Radiation Oncology 1994; Internal Medicine 1986; Medical Oncology 1989; **Med School:** Geo Wash Univ 1983; **Resid:** Internal Medicine, Mayo Clinic 1986; Medical Oncology, Univ MD Cancer Ctr 1989; **Fellow:** Radiation Oncology, Johns Hopkins Hosp; **Fac Appt:** Asst Prof RadRO, Vanderbilt Univ

Crocker, Ian MD [RadRO] - **Spec Exp:** Brain Tumors; Eye Tumors/Cancer; Vascular Brachytherapy; **Hospital:** Emory Univ Hosp, Crawford Long Hosp of Emory Univ; **Address:** Emory Univ Hosp-Dept Radiation Oncology, 1365 Clifton Rd NE, T Ste 104, Atlanta, GA 30322; **Phone:** 404-778-3473; **Board Cert:** Therapeutic Radiology 1999; Internal Medicine 1980; **Med School:** Univ Saskatchewan 1976; **Resid:** Internal Medicine, Univ Hosp-Univ West Ontario 1980; **Fellow:** Radiation Oncology, Princess Margaret Hosp-Univ Toronto 1983; **Fac Appt:** Prof RadRO, Emory Univ

Halle, Jan MD [RadRO] - **Spec Exp:** Breast Cancer; Lung Cancer; **Hospital:** Univ NC Hosps; **Address:** Univ North Carolina Sch Med, Dept Rad Onc, 101 Manning Drive, CB 7512, Gravely Bldg, Chapel Hill, NC 27599; **Phone:** 919-966-7700; **Board Cert:** Therapeutic Radiology 1982; **Med School:** Tufts Univ 1975; **Resid:** Radiation Oncology, North Carolina Meml Hosp 1981; **Fac Appt:** Assoc Prof RadRO, Univ NC Sch Med

America's Top Doctors® 8th Edition

Jose, Baby Oliapuram MD [RadRO] - **Spec Exp:** Head & Neck Cancer; Lung Cancer; Gynecologic Cancer; Prostate Cancer; **Hospital:** Univ of Louisville Hosp; **Address:** James G. Brown Cancer Center, 529 S Jackson St Fl 4, Louisville, KY 40202; **Phone:** 502-561-2700; **Board Cert:** Therapeutic Radiology 1978; **Med School:** India 1971; **Resid:** Surgery, CMC Hosp 1974; Radiation Oncology, CMC Hosp 1976; **Fellow:** Radiation Oncology, Brown Univ-RI Hosp 1979; **Fac Appt:** Prof RadRO, Univ Louisville Sch Med

Kun, Larry E MD [RadRO] - **Spec Exp:** Brain Tumors; Pediatric Cancers; **Hospital:** St Jude Children's Research Hosp, Le Bonheur Chldns Med Ctr; **Address:** St Jude Chldns Research Hosp-Dept Rad Onc, 332 N Lauderdale St, rm C2002F, MS 220, Memphis, TN 38105; **Phone:** 901-495-3565; **Board Cert:** Therapeutic Radiology 1973; **Med School:** Jefferson Med Coll 1968; **Resid:** Therapeutic Radiology, Penrose Cancer Hosp 1972; **Fellow:** Radiation Oncology, Natl Cancer Inst 1974; Radiation Oncology, Rotterdam Radiotherapy Inst 1975; **Fac Appt:** Prof, Univ Tenn Coll Med, Memphis

Landry, Jerome C MD [RadRO] - **Spec Exp:** Gastrointestinal Cancer; Stomach Cancer; Sarcoma; Breast Cancer; **Hospital:** Emory Univ Hosp, Grady Hlth Sys; **Address:** Emory Clinic, Dept Rad Oncology, 1365 Clifton Rd NE, Ste A-1304, Atlanta, GA 30322; **Phone:** 404-778-3651; **Board Cert:** Radiation Oncology 1988; **Med School:** Harvard Med Sch 1983; **Resid:** Radiation Oncology, Mass Genl Hosp 1987; **Fac Appt:** Prof RadRO, Emory Univ

Larner, James MD [RadRO] - **Spec Exp:** Neuro-Oncology; Brain Tumors; **Hospital:** Univ Virginia Med Ctr; **Address:** Univ Virginia Medical Ctr, Dept Radiation Oncology, PO Box 800383, Charlottesville, VA 22908; **Phone:** 434-924-5191; **Board Cert:** Radiation Oncology 1989; Internal Medicine 1983; Hematology 1988; Medical Oncology 1987; **Med School:** Univ VA Sch Med 1980; **Resid:** Internal Medicine, Thos Jefferson Univ Hosp 1983; Radiation Oncology, Montefiore-Einstein Med Ctr 1989; **Fellow:** Hematology & Oncology, Thos Jefferson Univ Hosp 1986; **Fac Appt:** Assoc Prof Med, Univ VA Sch Med

Lee, W Robert MD [RadRO] - **Spec Exp:** Prostate Cancer; Brachytherapy; Intensity Modulated Radiotherapy (IMRT); **Hospital:** Duke Univ Med Ctr; **Address:** Duke Univ Med Ctr, Div Radiation Oncology, Box 3085, Durham, NC 27710; **Phone:** 919-668-7342; **Board Cert:** Radiation Oncology 1994; **Med School:** Univ VA Sch Med 1989; **Resid:** Radiation Oncology, Univ Florida 1993; **Fac Appt:** Prof RadRO, Duke Univ

Lewin, Alan A MD [RadRO] - **Spec Exp:** Breast Cancer; Lung Cancer; Brain & Spinal Cord Tumors; **Hospital:** Baptist Hosp of Miami; **Address:** Baptist Hosp Cancer Treatment Ctr, Dept Rad Onc, 8900 N Kendall Drive, Miami, FL 33176-2118; **Phone:** 786-596-6566; **Board Cert:** Therapeutic Radiology 1982; Medical Oncology 1981; Hematology 1978; Internal Medicine 1976; **Med School:** Geo Wash Univ 1973; **Resid:** Internal Medicine, Mt Sinai Hosp 1976; **Fellow:** Hematology & Oncology, Beth Israel Med Ctr 1978; Radiation Oncology, Joint Ctr Radiation Therapy 1980; **Fac Appt:** Clin Prof RadRO, Univ Miami Sch Med

Marcus Jr, Robert B MD [RadRO] - **Spec Exp:** Pediatric Cancers; Sarcoma; Bone Cancer; Brain Tumors; **Hospital:** Emory Univ Hosp; **Address:** Emory Clinic, Dept Rad Oncology, 1365 Clifton Rd NE, Ste A-1302, Atlanta, GA 30322; **Phone:** 404-778-3473; **Board Cert:** Therapeutic Radiology 1980; **Med School:** Univ Fla Coll Med 1975; **Resid:** Radiation Oncology, Shands Hosp 1979; **Fac Appt:** Prof RadRO, Emory Univ

Markoe, Arnold M MD [RadRO] - **Spec Exp:** Eye Tumors/Cancer; Orbital Tumors/Cancer; Head & Neck Cancer; **Hospital:** Univ of Miami Hosp & Clins/Sylvester Comp Canc Ctr; **Address:** Univ of Miami Sylvester Comp Cancer Ctr, 1475 NW 12th Ave, Ste 024750, Box D31, Miami, FL 33101; **Phone:** 305-243-4319; **Board Cert:** Therapeutic Radiology 1983; **Med School:** Hahnemann Univ 1977; **Resid:** Radiation Oncology, Hahnemann Hosp 1981; **Fac Appt:** Prof RadRO, Univ Miami Sch Med

Radiation Oncology

Marks, Lawrence MD [RadRO] - **Spec Exp:** Breast Cancer; Lung Cancer; **Hospital:** Univ NC Hosps; **Address:** UNC Dept Rad Onc, Campus Box 7512, Chapel Hill, NC 27599-7512; **Phone:** 919-966-0400; **Board Cert:** Radiation Oncology 1989; **Med School:** Univ Rochester 1985; **Resid:** Radiation Oncology, Mass Genl Hosp 1989; **Fac Appt:** Prof RadRO, Univ NC Sch Med

McGarry, Ronald C MD/PhD [RadRO] - **Spec Exp:** Lung Cancer; Lymphoma; Clinical Trials; Stereotactic Radiosurgery; **Hospital:** Univ of Kentucky Chandler Hosp; **Address:** Chandler Medical Ctr, Radiation Medicine, 800 Rose St, rm C114C, Lexington, KY 40536; **Phone:** 859-323-6880; **Board Cert:** Radiation Oncology 1999; **Med School:** Canada 1992; **Resid:** Radiation Oncology, Univ W Ontario Regl Cancer Ctr 1997; **Fac Appt:** Prof RadRO, Univ KY Coll Med

Mendenhall, Nancy P MD [RadRO] - **Spec Exp:** Breast Cancer; Lymphoma; Hodgkin's Disease; **Hospital:** Shands at Univ of FL; **Address:** Univ Florida, Dept Radiation Oncology, Box 100385, Gainesville, FL 32610-0385; **Phone:** 352-265-0287; **Board Cert:** Therapeutic Radiology 1985; **Med School:** Univ Fla Coll Med 1980; **Resid:** Diagnostic Radiology, Shands-Univ of Florida 1984; **Fac Appt:** Prof RadRO, Univ Fla Coll Med

Mendenhall, William M MD [RadRO] - **Spec Exp:** Head & Neck Cancer; Stereotactic Radiosurgery; Colon Cancer; **Hospital:** Shands at Univ of FL; **Address:** Univ Florida, Dept Radiation Oncology, Box 100385, Gainesville, FL 32610-0385; **Phone:** 352-265-0287; **Board Cert:** Therapeutic Radiology 1983; **Med School:** Univ S Fla Coll Med 1978; **Resid:** Radiation Oncology, University of Florida 1983; **Fac Appt:** Prof RadRO, Univ Fla Coll Med

Merchant, Thomas DO [RadRO] - **Spec Exp:** Brain Tumors-Pediatric; **Hospital:** St Jude Children's Research Hosp; **Address:** St Jude Children's Research Hosp, 332 N Lauderdale St, Ste 2002, MS 220, Memphis, TN 38105; **Phone:** 901-495-3604; **Board Cert:** Radiation Oncology 1995; **Med School:** Chicago Coll Osteo Med 1989; **Resid:** Radiation Oncology, Meml Sloan Kettering Cancer Ctr 1994

Meredith, Ruby F MD [RadRO] - **Spec Exp:** Multiple Myeloma; Breast Cancer; **Hospital:** Univ of Ala Hosp at Birmingham; **Address:** Univ Alabama Hosps-Radiation Oncology, 619 19th St S, Birmingham, AL 35233; **Phone:** 205-934-2763; **Board Cert:** Radiation Oncology 1987; **Med School:** Ohio State Univ 1983; **Resid:** Radiation Oncology, Med Coll Va 1987; **Fac Appt:** Prof RadRO, Univ Ala

Prosnitz, Leonard MD [RadRO] - **Spec Exp:** Lymphoma; Breast Cancer; Hyperthermia Treatment of Cancer; Sarcoma; **Hospital:** Duke Univ Med Ctr; **Address:** Duke Univ Med Ctr, Dept Rad Onc, Box 3085, Durham, NC 27710; **Phone:** 919-668-5637; **Board Cert:** Therapeutic Radiology 1970; **Med School:** SUNY Downstate 1961; **Resid:** Internal Medicine, Dartmouth Affil Hosps 1963; Radiation Oncology, Yale-New Haven Hosp 1969; **Fellow:** Hematology & Oncology, Yale-New Haven Hosp 1967; **Fac Appt:** Prof RadRO, Duke Univ

Randall, Marcus MD [RadRO] - **Spec Exp:** Gynecologic Cancer; Stereotactic Radiosurgery; **Hospital:** Univ of Kentucky Chandler Hosp; **Address:** Univ Kentucky Medical Ctr, 800 Rose St, rm C114D, Lexington, KY 40536-0001; **Phone:** 859-257-7618; **Board Cert:** Therapeutic Radiology 1986; **Med School:** Univ NC Sch Med 1982; **Resid:** Radiation Oncology, Univ Va Med Ctr 1986; **Fellow:** Radiation Oncology, Univ Va Med Ctr 1986; **Fac Appt:** Prof RadRO, Univ KY Coll Med

Rich, Tyvin Andrew MD [RadRO] - **Spec Exp:** Colon & Rectal Cancer; Chemo-Radiation Combined Therapy; Esophageal Cancer; **Hospital:** Univ Virginia Med Ctr; **Address:** Univ Va Hlth Sys, Dept Rad Onc, Box 800383, Charlottesville, VA 22908-0383; **Phone:** 434-924-5191; **Board Cert:** Radiation Oncology 1978; **Med School:** Univ VA Sch Med 1973; **Resid:** Mass Genl Hosp 1978; **Fellow:** Radiation Oncology, Mt Vernon Hosp/Gray Lab; **Fac Appt:** Prof RadRO, Univ VA Sch Med

Rosenman, Julian MD/PhD [RadRO] - **Spec Exp:** Lung Cancer; Breast Cancer; Prostate Cancer; **Hospital:** Univ NC Hosps; **Address:** Univ North Carolina, Dept Rad Onc, 101 Manning Drive, CB 7512, Gravely Bldg, Chapel Hill, NC 27599-7512; **Phone:** 919-966-7700; **Board Cert:** Therapeutic Radiology 1981; **Med School:** Univ Tex SW, Dallas 1977; **Resid:** Therapeutic Radiology, Mass Genl Hosp 1981; **Fac Appt:** Prof RadRO, Univ NC Sch Med

Sailer, Scott MD [RadRO] - **Spec Exp:** Head & Neck Cancer; Genitourinary Cancer; Pediatric Cancers; Pediatric Radiology; **Hospital:** WakeMed Cary, WakeMed New Bern; **Address:** 300 Ashville Ave, Ste 110, Cary, NC 27511; **Phone:** 919-854-4588; **Board Cert:** Radiation Oncology 1988; **Med School:** Harvard Med Sch 1984; **Resid:** Radiation Therapy, Mass Genl Hosp 1988

Shaw, Edward G MD [RadRO] - **Spec Exp:** Stereotactic Radiosurgery; Brain Tumors; **Hospital:** Wake Forest Univ Baptist Med Ctr (page 73); **Address:** Wake Forest Med Ctr, Dept Rad Onc, Medical Center Blvd, Comp Cancer Ctr, Winston-Salem, NC 27157-1029; **Phone:** 336-713-6506; **Board Cert:** Radiation Oncology 1987; **Med School:** Rush Med Coll 1983; **Resid:** Radiation Oncology, Mayo Grad Sch Med 1987; **Fac Appt:** Prof RadRO, Wake Forest Univ

Tepper, Joel E MD [RadRO] - **Spec Exp:** Gastrointestinal Cancer; Sarcoma; Rectal Cancer; **Hospital:** Univ NC Hosps; **Address:** North Carolina Clin Cancer Ctr, Dept Rad Onc - CB#7512, Chapel Hill, NC 27599-7512; **Phone:** 919-966-0400; **Board Cert:** Therapeutic Radiology 1976; **Med School:** Washington Univ, St Louis 1972; **Resid:** Therapeutic Radiology, Mass Genl Hosp 1976; **Fellow:** Therapeutic Radiology, Mass Genl Hosp 1977; **Fac Appt:** Prof RadRO, Univ NC Sch Med

Toonkel, Leonard M MD [RadRO] - **Spec Exp:** Prostate Cancer; Breast Cancer; Brachytherapy; **Hospital:** Mount Sinai Med Ctr - Miami; **Address:** Dept Radiation Oncology, 4300 Alton Rd, Miami Beach, FL 33140; **Phone:** 305-535-3400; **Board Cert:** Therapeutic Radiology 1979; **Med School:** Univ Miami Sch Med 1975; **Resid:** Radiation Therapy, Jackson Meml Hosp 1977; Diagnostic Radiology, MD Anderson Hosp 1978; **Fellow:** Radiation Oncology, MD Anderson Hosp 1979; **Fac Appt:** Assoc Clin Prof Rad, Univ Miami Sch Med

Trotti III, Andrea MD [RadRO] - **Spec Exp:** Head & Neck Cancer; Gastrointestinal Cancer; Skin Cancer; **Hospital:** H Lee Moffitt Cancer Ctr & Research Inst; **Address:** H Lee Moffitt Cancer Ctr, Dept Rad Onc, 12902 Magnolia Drive, Tampa, FL 33612-9416; **Phone:** 813-972-8424; **Board Cert:** Radiation Oncology 1988; **Med School:** Univ Fla Coll Med 1984; **Resid:** Radiation Oncology, Univ Alabama 1988; **Fac Appt:** Prof RadRO, Univ S Fla Coll Med

Willett, Christopher MD [RadRO] - **Spec Exp:** Gastrointestinal Cancer; Clinical Trials; **Hospital:** Duke Univ Med Ctr; **Address:** Duke Univ Med Ctr, PO Box 3085, Durham, NC 27710; **Phone:** 919-668-5640; **Board Cert:** Therapeutic Radiology 1985; **Med School:** Tufts Univ 1981; **Resid:** Radiation Oncology, Mass Genl Hosp 1986; **Fac Appt:** Prof, Duke Univ

Wolfson, Aaron H MD [RadRO] - **Spec Exp:** Bone Tumors; Sarcoma-Soft Tissue; **Hospital:** Univ of Miami Hosp & Clins/Sylvester Comp Canc Ctr; **Address:** Univ of Miami Sylvester Comp Cancer Ctr, 1475 NW 12th Ave, Box D31, Miami, FL 33101; **Phone:** 305-243-4319; **Board Cert:** Radiation Oncology 1999; **Med School:** Univ Fla Coll Med 1982; **Resid:** Radiation Oncology, Med Coll of Virginia 1989; **Fac Appt:** Prof RadRO, Univ Miami Sch Med

Radiation Oncology

Midwest

Abrams, Ross A MD [RadRO] - **Spec Exp:** Gastrointestinal Cancer; Lymphoma; **Hospital:** Rush Univ Med Ctr; **Address:** Women's Center for Radiation Therapy, 500 S Paulina, Ground Floor Atrium, Chicago, IL 60612; **Phone:** 312-942-5751; **Board Cert:** Internal Medicine 1976; Medical Oncology 1979; Hematology 1982; Radiation Oncology 1987; **Med School:** Univ Pennsylvania 1973; **Resid:** Internal Medicine, Pennsylvania Hosp 1975; Hematology & Oncology, Hosp Univ Penn 1976; **Fellow:** Hematology & Oncology, Natl Cancer Inst 1978; Radiation Oncology, Med Coll Wisconsin 1987; **Fac Appt:** Prof RadRO, Rush Med Coll

Ben-Josef, Edgar MD [RadRO] - **Spec Exp:** Bone Cancer; Gastrointestinal Cancer; Pancreatic Cancer; Intensity Modulated Radiotherapy (IMRT); **Hospital:** Univ Michigan Hlth Sys; **Address:** Univ of Mich Hosp, 1500 E Medical Ctr Drive, rm UH B2C490, Ann Arbor, MI 48109-0010; **Phone:** 734-936-8207; **Board Cert:** Radiation Oncology 1994; **Med School:** Israel 1986; **Resid:** Radiation Oncology, Wayne State Univ Hosp 1994; **Fellow:** Cancer Biology, Wayne State Univ Hosp 1995; **Fac Appt:** Assoc Prof RadRO, Univ Mich Med Sch

Charboneau, J William MD [RadRO] - **Spec Exp:** Radiofrequency Tumor Ablation; Liver Cancer; Thyroid Cancer; **Hospital:** Mayo Med Ctr & Clin - Rochester; **Address:** Mayo Clinic, 200 First St SW, Rochester, MN 55905-0002; **Phone:** 507-284-2097; **Board Cert:** Diagnostic Radiology 1980; **Med School:** Univ Wisc 1976; **Resid:** Diagnostic Radiology, Mayo Clinic 1980; **Fac Appt:** Prof, Mayo Med Sch

Emami, Bahman MD [RadRO] - **Spec Exp:** Head & Neck Cancer; Lung Cancer; **Hospital:** Loyola Univ Med Ctr, Hines VA Hosp; **Address:** Loyola Univ Med Ctr, Dept Rad Onc, 2160 S First Ave Bldg 105 - rm 2932, Maywood, IL 60153-3328; **Phone:** 708-216-2729; **Board Cert:** Therapeutic Radiology 1976; **Med School:** Iran 1968; **Resid:** Radiation Therapy, St Vincents Hosp 1973; Radiation Therapy, New England Med Ctr 1976; **Fellow:** Radiation Therapy, New England Med Ctr 1977; **Fac Appt:** Prof RadRO, Loyola Univ-Stritch Sch Med

Forman, Jeffrey D MD [RadRO] - **Spec Exp:** Neutron Therapy for Advanced Cancer; Genitourinary Cancer; Prostate Cancer; **Address:** 70 Fulton St, Pontiac, MI 48341; **Phone:** 248-338-0300; **Board Cert:** Radiation Oncology 1986; **Med School:** NYU Sch Med 1982; **Resid:** Radiation Oncology, Johns Hopkins Hosp 1986; **Fellow:** Therapeutic Radiology, Johns Hopkins Hosp 1987; **Fac Appt:** Prof RadRO, Wayne State Univ

Grigsby, Perry W MD [RadRO] - **Spec Exp:** Gynecologic Cancer; Thyroid Cancer; **Hospital:** Barnes-Jewish Hosp, St Louis Chldns Hosp; **Address:** Washington Univ School Med, Dept Rad Onc, 4921 Parkview Pl, Box 9038635, St Louis, MO 63110; **Phone:** 314-747-7236; **Board Cert:** Radiation Oncology 1987; **Med School:** Univ KY Coll Med 1982; **Resid:** Radiation Oncology, Barnes Jewish Hosp 1985; **Fac Appt:** Prof, Washington Univ, St Louis

Halpern, Howard MD/PhD [RadRO] - **Spec Exp:** Breast Cancer; Esophageal Cancer; Gynecologic Cancer; **Hospital:** Univ of Chicago Hosps, Univ of IL Med Ctr at Chicago; **Address:** 1801 W Taylor St, rm C400, MC-933, Chicago, IL 60612; **Phone:** 312-996-3630; **Board Cert:** Therapeutic Radiology 1984; **Med School:** Univ Miami Sch Med 1980; **Resid:** Therapeutic Radiology, Jnt Ctr Rad Ther Harvard 1984; **Fellow:** Therapeutic Radiology, Jnt Ctr Rad Ther Harvard 1985; **Fac Appt:** Prof Rad, Univ Chicago-Pritzker Sch Med

Haraf, Daniel MD [RadRO] - **Spec Exp:** Head & Neck Cancer; Lung Cancer; Prostate Cancer; **Hospital:** Univ of Chicago Hosps; **Address:** Univ Chicago Hosps, Dept Rad Oncology, 5758 S Maryland, MS 9006, Chicago, IL 60637; **Phone:** 773-702-6870; **Board Cert:** Internal Medicine 1985; Radiation Oncology 1990; **Med School:** Ros Franklin Univ/Chicago Med Sch 1982; **Resid:** Internal Medicine, Michael Reese Hosp 1985; **Fellow:** Radiation Oncology, Michael Reese Hosp 1988; **Fac Appt:** Clin Prof RadRO, Univ Chicago-Pritzker Sch Med

Hayman, James A MD [RadRO] - **Spec Exp:** Breast Cancer; Stomach Cancer; Lung Cancer; Brain Tumors; **Hospital:** Univ Michigan Hlth Sys; **Address:** Univ of Mich Hosp, 1500 E Medical Ctr Drive, rm UH B2C490, Ann Arbor, MI 48109-0010; **Phone:** 734-936-4288; **Board Cert:** Radiation Oncology 2004; **Med School:** Univ Chicago-Pritzker Sch Med 1991; **Resid:** Radiation Therapy, Joint Ctr for Radiation Therapy 1996; **Fac Appt:** Assoc Prof RadRO, Univ Mich Med Sch

Kiel, Krystyna D MD [RadRO] - **Spec Exp:** Breast Cancer; Sarcoma; Gastrointestinal Cancer; Colon & Rectal Cancer; **Hospital:** Northwestern Meml Hosp; **Address:** Northwestern Meml Hosp, Radiation Oncology, 251 E Huron St Galter Bldg - Ste L178, Chicago, IL 60611-2914; **Phone:** 312-926-2520; **Board Cert:** Therapeutic Radiology 1983; Radiation Oncology 2000; **Med School:** Univ Mass Sch Med 1977; **Resid:** Radiation Oncology, Mass Genl Hosp 1982; **Fac Appt:** Assoc Prof Rad, Northwestern Univ

Kim, Jae Ho MD [RadRO] - **Spec Exp:** Brain Tumors; Spinal Cord Tumors; Breast Cancer; **Hospital:** Henry Ford Hosp; **Address:** Radiation Oncology, 2799 W Grand Blvd, Detroit, MI 48202; **Phone:** 313-916-1029; **Board Cert:** Therapeutic Radiology 1973; **Med School:** Korea 1959; **Resid:** Therapeutic Radiology, Meml-Sloan-Kettering 1972; **Fellow:** Diagnostic Radiology, Meml-Sloan-Kettering 1968; **Fac Appt:** Prof RadRO, Wayne State Univ

Lawrence, Theodore S MD/PhD [RadRO] - **Spec Exp:** Gastrointestinal Cancer; Liver Cancer; Pancreatic Cancer; **Hospital:** Univ Michigan Hlth Sys; **Address:** Univ of Mich Hosp, Dept Rad Onc, 1500 E Med Ctr Dr, B2C502, Box 5010, Ann Arbor, MI 48109-5010; **Phone:** 734-936-4300; **Board Cert:** Internal Medicine 1983; Medical Oncology 1985; Radiation Oncology 1987; **Med School:** Cornell Univ-Weill Med Coll 1980; **Resid:** Internal Medicine, Stanford Univ Hosp 1983; Radiation Oncology, Natl Cancer Inst 1987; **Fellow:** Medical Oncology, Natl Cancer Inst 1986; **Fac Appt:** Prof RadRO, Univ Mich Med Sch

Lee, Chung K MD [RadRO] - **Spec Exp:** Head & Neck Cancer; Breast Cancer; Lymphoma; Gastrointestinal Cancer; **Hospital:** Univ Minn Med Ctr, Fairview - Univ Campus; **Address:** Dept of Radiation Oncology, 420 Delaware St SE, MMC 400, Minneapolis, MN 55455; **Phone:** 612-273-6700; **Board Cert:** Therapeutic Radiology 1976; **Med School:** Korea 1965; **Resid:** Therapeutic Radiology, Univ of Minn Hosp 1976; Diagnostic Radiology, Yonsei Univ Hosp 1971; **Fac Appt:** Prof, Univ Minn

Macklis, Roger M MD [RadRO] - **Spec Exp:** Radioimmunotherapy of Cancer; Breast Cancer; Lymphoma; **Hospital:** Cleveland Clin Fdn (page 56); **Address:** Cleveland Cin Fdn, Dept Rad Onc, 9500 Euclid Ave, Desk T28, Cleveland, OH 44195; **Phone:** 216-444-5576; **Board Cert:** Radiation Oncology 1989; **Med School:** Harvard Med Sch 1983; **Resid:** Radiation Oncology, Joint Ctr Radiotherapy Inst 1987; **Fellow:** Research, Dana Farber Cancer Inst 1987; **Fac Appt:** Prof RadRO, Case West Res Univ

Martenson Jr, James A MD [RadRO] - **Spec Exp:** Mucositis; Esophageal Cancer; **Hospital:** Mayo Med Ctr & Clin - Rochester; **Address:** Mayo Clinic, Dept Rad/Onc, 200 First St SW, Rochester, MN 55905; **Phone:** 507-284-4561; **Board Cert:** Therapeutic Radiology 1985; **Med School:** Univ Wash 1981; **Resid:** Radiation Oncology, Mayo Clinic 1985; **Fac Appt:** Assoc Prof, Mayo Med Sch

Mehta, Minesh P MD [RadRO] - **Spec Exp:** Brain Tumors; Lung Cancer; Pediatric Cancers; **Hospital:** Univ WI Hosp & Clins; **Address:** Univ Wisconsin, Dept Rad Oncology, 600 Highland Ave, K4B-100, Madison, WI 53792; **Phone:** 608-263-8500; **Board Cert:** Radiation Oncology 1988; **Med School:** Zambia 1981; **Resid:** Internal Medicine, Ndola Central Hosp 1983; Radiation Oncology, Ndola Central Hosp 1988; **Fac Appt:** Prof RadRO, Univ Wisc

Radiation Oncology

Michalski, Jeff M MD [RadRO] - **Spec Exp:** Prostate Cancer; Sarcoma; Pediatric Cancers; **Hospital:** Barnes-Jewish Hosp, St Louis Chldns Hosp; **Address:** Washington Univ Sch Med, Dept Rad Oncology, 4921 Parkview Place, Lower Level, Box 8224, St Louis, MO 63110; **Phone:** 314-362-8566; **Board Cert:** Radiation Oncology 1991; **Med School:** Med Coll Wisc 1986; **Resid:** Radiation Oncology, Columbia Presby Med Ctr 1988; Radiation Oncology, Mallinckrodt Inst of Radiology 1990; **Fellow:** Radiation Oncology, Mallinckrodt Inst of Radiology 1991; **Fac Appt:** Assoc Prof RadRO, Washington Univ, St Louis

Mittal, Bharat MD [RadRO] - **Spec Exp:** Head & Neck Cancer; Lymphoma; Skin Cancer; **Hospital:** Northwestern Meml Hosp; **Address:** 251 E Huron St, Bldg LC-178, Chicago, IL 60611; **Phone:** 312-926-2520; **Board Cert:** Radiation Oncology 1981; **Med School:** India 1973; **Resid:** Internal Medicine, Christian Med Coll 1976; Radiation Oncology, Northwestern Meml Hosp 1980; **Fellow:** Radiation Oncology, Mallinckrodt Inst 1981; **Fac Appt:** Prof RadRO, Northwestern Univ

Movsas, Benjamin MD [RadRO] - **Spec Exp:** Lung Cancer; Brain Tumors; Prostate Cancer; Stereotactic Radiosurgery; **Hospital:** Henry Ford Hosp; **Address:** Henry Ford Health System, Radiation Oncology, 2799 W Grand Blvd, Detroit, MI 48202-2608; **Phone:** 313-916-5188; **Board Cert:** Radiation Oncology 1999; **Med School:** Washington Univ, St Louis 1990; **Resid:** Radiation Oncology, National Cancer Inst 1995

Myerson, Robert J MD [RadRO] - **Spec Exp:** Gastrointestinal Cancer; Breast Cancer; Hyperthermia Treatment of Cancer; **Hospital:** Barnes-Jewish Hosp; **Address:** Ctr for Advanced Med-Siteman Cancer Ctr, 4921 Parkview Pl, Box 9038635, St Louis, MO 63110; **Phone:** 314-747-7236; **Board Cert:** Therapeutic Radiology 1985; **Med School:** Univ Miami Sch Med 1980; **Resid:** Radiation Therapy, Hosp Univ Penn 1984; **Fac Appt:** Prof RadRO, Washington Univ, St Louis

Pierce, Lori J MD [RadRO] - **Spec Exp:** Breast Cancer; **Hospital:** Univ Michigan Hlth Sys; **Address:** Univ Hosp, Dept Rad Onc, 1500 E Med Ctr, rm B2C440, Box 5010, Ann Arbor, MI 48109-5099; **Phone:** 734-936-4300; **Board Cert:** Radiation Oncology 1989; **Med School:** Duke Univ 1985; **Resid:** Radiation Oncology, Hosp Univ Penn 1989; **Fac Appt:** Prof RadRO, Univ Mich Med Sch

Sandler, Howard M MD [RadRO] - **Spec Exp:** Prostate Cancer; Genitourinary Cancer; Brain Tumors; **Hospital:** Univ Michigan Hlth Sys; **Address:** Univ Michigan Med Ctr, Dept Rad Onc, 1500 E Med Ctr Dr. UH B2C502, Box 5010, Ann Arbor, MI 48109-5010; **Phone:** 734-936-9338; **Board Cert:** Radiation Oncology 1989; **Med School:** Univ Conn 1985; **Resid:** Radiation Oncology, Hosp Univ Penn 1989; **Fac Appt:** Prof RadRO, Univ Mich Med Sch

Schomberg, Paula J MD [RadRO] - **Spec Exp:** Brain Tumors; Pediatric Cancers; **Hospital:** Mayo Med Ctr & Clin - Rochester; **Address:** Mayo Clinic - Charlton Bldg, Desk R, 200 1st St SW, Rochester, MN 55905; **Phone:** 507-284-3551; **Board Cert:** Therapeutic Radiology 1984; **Med School:** Med Coll Wisc 1979; **Resid:** Radiation Therapy, Mayo Clinic 1983; **Fac Appt:** Prof RadRO, Mayo Med Sch

Small Jr, William MD [RadRO] - **Spec Exp:** Gynecologic Cancer; Gastrointestinal Cancer; Breast Cancer; Pancreatic Cancer; **Hospital:** Northwestern Meml Hosp; **Address:** Northwestern Meml Hosp, Rad Oncology, 251 E Huron St Galter Bldg - Ste L178, Chicago, IL 60611; **Phone:** 312-926-2520; **Board Cert:** Radiation Oncology 2004; **Med School:** Northwestern Univ 1990; **Resid:** Radiation Oncology, Northwestern Univ 1994; **Fac Appt:** Prof RadRO, Northwestern Univ

Taylor, Marie E MD [RadRO] - **Spec Exp:** Breast Cancer; **Hospital:** Barnes-Jewish Hosp, Barnes-Jewish West County Hosp; **Address:** Center for Advanced Med-Siteman Cancer Ctr, 4921 Parkview Pl, Box 8224, St Louis, MO 63110; **Phone:** 314-747-7236; **Board Cert:** Radiation Oncology 1987; **Med School:** Univ Wash 1982; **Resid:** Radiation Oncology, Univ Wash Med Ctr 1986

Thornton Jr, Allan F MD [RadRO] - **Spec Exp:** Proton Beam Therapy; **Address:** Midwest Proton Radiotherapy Institute, 2425 N Milo B Sampson Ln, Bloomington, IN 47408; **Phone:** 812-349-5074; **Board Cert:** Radiation Oncology 1999; **Med School:** Univ VA Sch Med 1981; **Resid:** Radiation Oncology, Princess Margaret Hosp 1986

Vicini, Frank A MD [RadRO] - **Spec Exp:** Breast Cancer; Prostate Cancer; Brachytherapy; **Hospital:** William Beaumont Hosp; **Address:** William Beaumont Hospital, 3601 W 13 Mile Rd, Royal Oak, MI 48073; **Phone:** 248-551-1219; **Board Cert:** Radiation Oncology 1999; **Med School:** Wayne State Univ 1985; **Resid:** Radiation Oncology, William Beaumont Hosp 1989; **Fellow:** Radiation Oncology, Harvard Med Sch/Joint Ctr for Rad Ther 1990; **Fac Appt:** Clin Prof RadRO, Univ Mich Med Sch

Weichselbaum, Ralph R MD [RadRO] - **Spec Exp:** Gene Targeted Radiotherapy; Head & Neck Cancer; Esophageal Cancer; **Hospital:** Univ of Chicago Hosps; **Address:** Univ Chicago, Dept Rad Onc, 5758 S Maryland Ave, MC-9006-DCAM-1D, Chicago, IL 60637; **Phone:** 773-702-0817; **Board Cert:** Therapeutic Radiology 1975; **Med School:** Univ IL Coll Med 1971; **Resid:** Therapeutic Radiology, Harvard Jt Ctr Rad Therapy 1975; **Fellow:** Diagnostic Radiology, Harvard Med Sch 1976; **Fac Appt:** Prof Rad, Univ Chicago-Pritzker Sch Med

Wilson, J Frank MD [RadRO] - **Spec Exp:** Breast Cancer; Skin Cancer; **Hospital:** Froedtert Meml Lutheran Hosp; **Address:** Dept Radiation Oncology, 9200 W Wisconsin Ave, Milwaukee, WI 53226; **Phone:** 414-805-4400; **Board Cert:** Therapeutic Radiology 1971; **Med School:** Univ MO-Columbia Sch Med 1965; **Resid:** Radiation Oncology, Penrose Cancer Hosp 1969; **Fellow:** Radiation Oncology, Natl Cancer Inst/NIH 1971; **Fac Appt:** Prof RadRO, Med Coll Wisc

Great Plains and Mountains

Gaffney, David K MD/PhD [RadRO] - **Spec Exp:** Breast Cancer; Gynecologic Cancer; **Hospital:** Univ Utah Hosps and Clins; **Address:** Huntsman Cancer Hosp, Dept Rad Oncology, 1950 Circle of Hope, rm 1440, Salt Lake City, UT 84112-5560; **Phone:** 801-581-2396; **Board Cert:** Radiation Oncology 1997; **Med School:** Med Coll Wisc 1992; **Resid:** Radiation Oncology, Univ Utah Hosps 1996; **Fac Appt:** Assoc Prof, Univ Utah

Rabinovitch, Rachel A MD [RadRO] - **Spec Exp:** Breast Cancer; Lymphoma; **Hospital:** Univ Colorado Hosp; **Address:** Anschutz Cancer Pavilion, Dept Rad Oncology, 1665 N Ursula St, PO Box 6510, MS F-706, Aurora, CO 80045; **Phone:** 720-848-0156; **Board Cert:** Radiation Oncology 1994; **Med School:** Albert Einstein Coll Med 1989; **Resid:** Radiation Oncology, Meml Sloan Kettering Cancer Ctr 1993; **Fac Appt:** Assoc Prof RadRO, Univ Colorado

Shrieve, Dennis C MD [RadRO] - **Spec Exp:** Brain Tumors-Adult & Pediatric; Genitourinary Cancer; Gastrointestinal Cancer; **Hospital:** Univ Utah Hosps and Clins, Primary Children's Med Ctr; **Address:** Huntsman Cancer Inst, Dept Rad Oncology, 1950 Circle of Hope, Salt Lake City, UT 84112; **Phone:** 801-581-2396; **Board Cert:** Radiation Oncology 1993; **Med School:** Univ Miami Sch Med 1989; **Resid:** Radiation Oncology, UCSF Med Ctr; **Fac Appt:** Prof RadRO, Univ Utah

Smalley, Stephen R MD [RadRO] - **Spec Exp:** Colon Cancer; Gastrointestinal Cancer; **Hospital:** Olathe Med Ctr; **Address:** Olathe Med Ctr, 20375 W 151st St, Doctors Bldg - Ste 180, Olathe, KS 66061-4575; **Phone:** 913-768-7200; **Board Cert:** Internal Medicine 1982; Radiation Oncology 1987; Medical Oncology 1985; **Med School:** Univ MO-Kansas City 1979; **Resid:** Internal Medicine, Mayo Clinic 1982; Radiation Oncology, Mayo Clinic 1986; **Fellow:** Medical Oncology, Mayo Clinic 1984; **Fac Appt:** Prof RadRO, Univ Kans

Radiation Oncology

Southwest

Ang, Kie-Kian MD/PhD [RadRO] - **Spec Exp:** Head & Neck Cancer; **Hospital:** UT MD Anderson Cancer Ctr; **Address:** UT MD Anderson Cancer Ctr, 1515 Holcombe Blvd, Box 97, Houston, TX 77030; **Phone:** 713-563-8400; **Board Cert:** Radiation Oncology 1987; **Med School:** Belgium 1975; **Resid:** Radiation Oncology, Univ Hosp Louvian 1980; **Fac Appt:** Prof, Univ Tex, Houston

Buchholz, Thomas A MD [RadRO] - **Spec Exp:** Breast Cancer; **Hospital:** UT MD Anderson Cancer Ctr; **Address:** Univ Texas MD Anderson Cancer Ctr, 1515 Holcombe Blvd, Unit 97, Houston, TX 77030-4000; **Phone:** 713-794-4892; **Board Cert:** Radiation Oncology 1993; **Med School:** Tufts Univ 1988; **Resid:** Radiation Oncology, Univ Washington Med Ctr 1993; **Fellow:** Research, Univ Washington Med Ctr 1994; **Fac Appt:** Prof RadRO, Univ Tex, Houston

Choy, Hak MD [RadRO] - **Spec Exp:** Lung Cancer; **Hospital:** UT Southwestern Med Ctr - Dallas; **Address:** UT SW Med Ctr - Dallas, Dept Rad-Onc, 5801 Forest Park Rd, Dallas, TX 75390-9183; **Phone:** 214-645-7600; **Board Cert:** Radiation Oncology 1993; **Med School:** Univ Tex Med Br, Galveston 1987; **Resid:** Radiation Oncology, Ohio State Univ Hosp 1989; Radiation Oncology, Univ Texas Hlth Sci Ctr 1991; **Fac Appt:** Prof RadRO, Univ Tex SW, Dallas

Cox, James D MD [RadRO] - **Spec Exp:** Lung Cancer; Esophageal Cancer; Thymoma; **Hospital:** UT MD Anderson Cancer Ctr; **Address:** Univ Tex MD Anderson Cancer Ctr, 1515 Holcombe Blvd, Unit 97, Houston, TX 77030; **Phone:** 713-563-2316; **Board Cert:** Radiation Oncology 1999; **Med School:** Univ Rochester 1965; **Resid:** Diagnostic Radiology, Penrose Cancer Hosp 1969; **Fellow:** Therapeutic Radiology, Inst Gustave-Roussy 1970; **Fac Appt:** Prof RadRO, Univ Tex, Houston

Eifel, Patricia J MD [RadRO] - **Spec Exp:** Cervical Cancer; Uterine Cancer; Vulvar Disease/Cancer; Vaginal Cancer; **Hospital:** UT MD Anderson Cancer Ctr; **Address:** MD Anderson Cancer Ctr, Dept Rad Onc, 1515 Holcombe Blvd, Unit 1202, Houston, TX 77030-4009; **Phone:** 713-563-6830; **Board Cert:** Therapeutic Radiology 1983; **Med School:** Stanford Univ 1977; **Resid:** Radiation Oncology, Stanford Univ Med Ctr 1981; **Fellow:** Therapeutic Radiology, Stanford Univ Med Ctr 1982

Grado, Gordon L MD [RadRO] - **Spec Exp:** Prostate Cancer; Brachytherapy; **Hospital:** Scottsdale Hlthcare - Shea; **Address:** 2926 N Civic Center Plaza, Scottsdale, AZ 85251; **Phone:** 480-614-6300; **Board Cert:** Therapeutic Radiology 1981; Radiation Oncology 1999; **Med School:** Southern IL Univ 1977; **Resid:** Therapeutic Radiology, Mayo Clinic 1981

Gunderson, Leonard MD [RadRO] - **Spec Exp:** Gastrointestinal Cancer; Brachytherapy; Sarcoma; **Hospital:** Mayo Clinic - Scottsdale; **Address:** Mayo Clinic, Dept Radiation Oncol, 5777 E Mayo Blvd, Phoenix, AZ 85054; **Phone:** 480-342-1262; **Board Cert:** Therapeutic Radiology 1975; **Med School:** Univ KY Coll Med 1969; **Resid:** Radiation Oncology, Latter Day Saints Hosp 1974; **Fac Appt:** Prof RadRO, Mayo Med Sch

Herman, Terence S MD [RadRO] - **Spec Exp:** Breast Cancer; Sarcoma; Brain Tumors; **Hospital:** OU Med Ctr; **Address:** Oklahoma Univ Health Sci Ctr, 825 NE 10th St, OUPB 1430, Oklahoma City, OK 73104-5417; **Phone:** 405-271-5641; **Board Cert:** Internal Medicine 1975; Medical Oncology 1977; Therapeutic Radiology 1985; **Med School:** Univ Conn 1972; **Resid:** Internal Medicine, Univ Arizona Med Ctr 1975; Radiation Oncology, Stanford Univ Med Ctr 1985; **Fellow:** Medical Oncology, Univ Arizona 1977; **Fac Appt:** Prof RadRO, Univ Okla Coll Med

Janjan, Nora Anita MD [RadRO] - **Spec Exp:** Gastrointestinal Cancer; Palliative Care; **Hospital:** UT MD Anderson Cancer Ctr; **Address:** Univ TX MD Anderson Cancer Ctr, 1515 Holcombe Blvd, Box 97, Houston, TX 77030; **Phone:** 713-563-2326; **Board Cert:** Radiation Oncology 2000; **Med School:** Univ Ariz Coll Med 1979; **Resid:** Internal Medicine, Baylor Affil Hosps 1981; Radiation Oncology, Baylor Affil Hosps 1984; **Fac Appt:** Prof RadRO, Univ Tex, Houston

Jhingran, Anuja MD [RadRO] - **Spec Exp:** Gynecologic Cancer; Brachytherapy; **Hospital:** UT MD Anderson Cancer Ctr; **Address:** MD Anderson Cancer Ctr, 1515 Holcombe Ave, Box 1202, Houston, TX 77030; **Phone:** 713-563-2300; **Board Cert:** Radiation Oncology 1993; **Med School:** Texas Tech Univ 1988; **Resid:** Radiation Oncology, Baylor College Med 1993; **Fac Appt:** Assoc Prof RadRO, Univ Tex, Houston

Komaki, Ritsuko U MD [RadRO] - **Spec Exp:** Lung Cancer; Thymoma; Esophageal Cancer; **Hospital:** UT MD Anderson Cancer Ctr; **Address:** UT-MD Anderson Cancer Ctr, Dept Rad Onc, 1515 Holcombe Blvd, Unit 97, Houston, TX 77030; **Phone:** 713-563-2300; **Board Cert:** Therapeutic Radiology 1977; Radiation Oncology 2001; **Med School:** Japan 1969; **Resid:** Radiation Oncology, Med Coll Wisc 1978; **Fac Appt:** Prof RadRO, Univ Tex, Houston

Kuske, Robert R MD [RadRO] - **Spec Exp:** Breast Cancer; **Hospital:** Scottsdale Hlthcare - Shea; **Address:** 8994 E Desert Cove Ave, Ste 100, Scottsdale, AZ 85260; **Phone:** 602-274-4484; **Board Cert:** Therapeutic Radiology 1985; **Med School:** Univ Cincinnati 1980; **Resid:** Radiation Oncology, Univ Cincinnati Med Ctr 1984

Lee, Andrew K MD [RadRO] - **Spec Exp:** Prostate Cancer; Proton Beam Therapy; Genitourinary Cancer; **Hospital:** UT MD Anderson Cancer Ctr; **Address:** MD Anderson Cancer Ctr, 1515 Holcombe Blvd, Unit 1202, Houston, TX 77030; **Phone:** 713-563-2443; **Board Cert:** Radiation Oncology 2001; **Med School:** Univ Minn 1996; **Resid:** Radiation Oncology, Joint Ctr for Radiation Therapy/Harvard 2001; **Fac Appt:** Assoc Prof RadRO, Univ Tex, Houston

Medbery, Clinton A MD [RadRO] - **Spec Exp:** Breast Cancer; Gynecologic Cancer; **Hospital:** St Anthony Hosp -Oklahoma City; **Address:** Southwest Radiation Oncology, 1011 N Dewey Ave, Oklahoma City, OK 73101; **Phone:** 405-272-7311; **Board Cert:** Internal Medicine 1980; Medical Oncology 1983; Radiation Oncology 1987; **Med School:** Med Univ SC 1976; **Resid:** Internal Medicine, Naval Hosp 1980; Radiation Oncology, Natl Cancer Inst 1987; **Fellow:** Medical Oncology, Naval Hosp 1982

Senzer, Neil N MD [RadRO] - **Spec Exp:** Clinical Trials; Gene Targeted Radiotherapy; Gene Therapy; **Hospital:** Baylor Univ Medical Ctr; **Address:** Mary Crowley Medical Research Ctr, 3535 Worth St, Ste 302, Dallas, TX 75246-2044; **Phone:** 214-370-1400; **Board Cert:** Pediatrics 1976; Pediatric Hematology-Oncology 1978; Therapeutic Radiology 1985; **Med School:** SUNY Buffalo 1971; **Resid:** Pediatrics, Johns Hopkins Hosp 1974; Radiation Oncology, St Barnabas Med Ctr 1985; **Fellow:** Pediatric Hematology-Oncology, St Jude Chldns Rsch Hosp 1978

Shina, Donald C MD [RadRO] - **Spec Exp:** Breast Cancer; **Hospital:** St Vincent Hosp - Santa Fe; **Address:** Santa Fe Cancer Ctr at St Vincent Hosp, 455 Saint Michael's Drive, Santa Fe, NM 87505; **Phone:** 505-820-5233; **Board Cert:** Internal Medicine 1977; Medical Oncology 1979; Therapeutic Radiology 1981; **Med School:** Case West Res Univ 1974; **Resid:** Internal Medicine, Univ Hosps 1977; **Fellow:** Radiation Oncology, Univ Hosps 1980; Medical Oncology, Univ Hosps 1980

Stea, Baldassarre MD/PhD [RadRO] - **Spec Exp:** Brain Tumors; Stereotactic Radiosurgery; Pediatric Cancers; **Hospital:** Univ Med Ctr - Tucson, Tucson Med Ctr; **Address:** Univ Hlth Scis Ctr, Dept Rad Onc, 1501 N Campbell Ave, Tucson, AZ 85724-0001; **Phone:** 520-626-6724; **Board Cert:** Radiation Oncology 1987; **Med School:** Geo Wash Univ 1983; **Resid:** Radiation Oncology, Natl Cancer Inst 1987; **Fac Appt:** Prof RadRO, Univ Ariz Coll Med

Radiation Oncology

Woo, Shiao Y MD [RadRO] - **Spec Exp:** Brain Tumors-Adult & Pediatric; Proton Beam Therapy; Stereotactic Radiosurgery; Pediatric Cancers; **Hospital:** UT MD Anderson Cancer Ctr, Texas Chldns Hosp - Houston; **Address:** UT-MD Anderson Cancer Ctr, 1515 Holcombe, Box 1150, Unit 97, Houston, TX 77030; **Phone:** 713-563-2324; **Board Cert:** Radiation Oncology 1988; Pediatrics 1980; **Med School:** Malaysia 1972; **Resid:** Pediatrics, Georgetown Univ Hosp 1978; **Fellow:** Pediatric Hematology-Oncology, Georgetown Univ Hosp 1980; Radiation Oncology, Georgetown Univ Hosp 1988; **Fac Appt:** Prof RadRO, Baylor Coll Med

West Coast and Pacific

Bahn, Duke K MD [RadRO] - **Spec Exp:** Prostate Cancer-Cryosurgery; **Hospital:** Comm Meml Hosp - Ventura; **Address:** Prostate Inst of America, 168 N Brent St, Ste 402, Ventura, CA 93003; **Phone:** 805-585-3082; **Board Cert:** Diagnostic Radiology 1978; **Med School:** Korea 1970; **Resid:** Diagnostic Radiology, Wayne State Univ Med Ctr 1978

Donaldson, Sarah S MD [RadRO] - **Spec Exp:** Pediatric Cancers; Hodgkin's Disease; **Hospital:** Stanford Univ Med Ctr; **Address:** 875 Blake Wilbur Drive, CC Bldg Fl G - rm 226, MC 5847, Stanford, CA 94305-5847; **Phone:** 650-723-6195; **Board Cert:** Therapeutic Radiology 1974; **Med School:** Harvard Med Sch 1968; **Resid:** Radiation Oncology, Stanford Univ Med Ctr 1972; **Fellow:** Pediatric Hematology-Oncology, Inst Gustave-Roussy 1973; Pediatric Hematology-Oncology, MD Anderson Cancer Ctr 1971; **Fac Appt:** Prof RadRO, Stanford Univ

Douglas, James G MD [RadRO] - **Spec Exp:** Pediatric Cancers; Head & Neck Cancer; Brain Tumors; **Hospital:** Univ Wash Med Ctr, Chldns Hosp and Regl Med Ctr - Seattle; **Address:** Univ Washington Med Ctr, Dept Radiation Onc, 1959 NE Pacific St, Box 356043, Seattle, WA 98195-6043; **Phone:** 206-598-4100; **Board Cert:** Pediatrics 1986; Radiation Oncology 1997; **Med School:** Case West Res Univ 1980; **Resid:** Pediatrics, Children's Hosp Med Ctr 1983; Radiation Oncology, Univ Washington Med Ctr 1996; **Fellow:** Pediatric Hematology-Oncology, Natl Inst Hlth 1986; **Fac Appt:** Assoc Prof RadRO, Univ Wash

Fowble, Barbara MD [RadRO] - **Spec Exp:** Breast Cancer; **Hospital:** UCSF Med Ctr; **Address:** 1600 Divisadero St, Ste H1031, 7701 Burholme Ave, San Francisco, CA 94143-1708; **Phone:** 415-353-7175; **Board Cert:** Therapeutic Radiology 1976; **Med School:** Jefferson Med Coll 1972; **Resid:** Therapeutic Radiology, Bellevue Hosp Ctr-NYU 1975; Therapeutic Radiology, Hahnemann 1976; **Fellow:** Radiation Therapy, Jefferson Hosp 1977; **Fac Appt:** Prof RadRO, UCSF

Halberg, Francine MD [RadRO] - **Spec Exp:** Breast Cancer; **Hospital:** Marin Genl Hosp, UCSF Med Ctr; **Address:** Marin Cancer Inst-Dept of Rad.Oncology, 1350 S Eliseo Drive, Ste 100, Greenbrae, CA 94904; **Phone:** 415-925-7326; **Board Cert:** Internal Medicine 1981; Therapeutic Radiology 1984; **Med School:** Cornell Univ-Weill Med Coll 1978; **Resid:** Internal Medicine, USPHS Hosp 1981; **Fellow:** Radiation Oncology, Stanford Univ Med Ctr 1984; **Fac Appt:** Assoc Prof RadRO, UCSF

Hancock, Steven MD [RadRO] - **Spec Exp:** Prostate Cancer; Breast Cancer; Cancer Survivors-Late Effects of Therapy; **Hospital:** Stanford Univ Med Ctr; **Address:** Stanford Cancer Center-Dept Rad Onc, 875 Blake Wilber Drive, MC 5847, Stanford, CA 94305; **Phone:** 650-723-6440; **Board Cert:** Therapeutic Radiology 1982; Internal Medicine 1980; **Med School:** Stanford Univ 1976; **Resid:** Radiation Therapy, Stanford Univ Med Ctr 1981; Internal Medicine, Stanford Univ Med Ctr 1979; **Fac Appt:** Prof RadRO, Stanford Univ

Hoppe, Richard T MD [RadRO] - **Spec Exp:** Lymphoma; Hodgkin's Disease; **Hospital:** Stanford Univ Med Ctr; **Address:** Stanford Med Ctr, Dept Rad Onc, 875 Blake Wilbur, MC 5847, Stanford, CA 94305-5847; **Phone:** 650-723-5510; **Board Cert:** Therapeutic Radiology 1976; **Med School:** Cornell Univ-Weill Med Coll 1971; **Resid:** Radiation Therapy, Stanford Univ Med Ctr 1976; **Fac Appt:** Prof, Stanford Univ

Koh, Wui-Jin MD [RadRO] - **Spec Exp:** Gynecologic Cancer; Brachytherapy; Clinical Trials; **Hospital:** Univ Wash Med Ctr; **Address:** Univ Washington Med Ctr, Dept of Radiation Oncology, Box 356043, Seattle, WA 98195; **Phone:** 206-598-4121; **Board Cert:** Radiation Oncology 1988; **Med School:** Loma Linda Univ 1984; **Resid:** Radiation Oncology, Univ Washington Med Ctr 1988; **Fellow:** Tumor Imaging, Univ Washington Med Ctr 1988; **Fac Appt:** Prof RadRO, Univ Wash

Laramore, George E MD/PhD [RadRO] - **Spec Exp:** Neutron Therapy for Advanced Cancer; Salivary Gland Tumors; Head & Neck Cancer; Skin Cancer; **Hospital:** Univ Wash Med Ctr; **Address:** Univ Washington Med Ctr, Dept Rad Onc Box 356043, Seattle, WA 98195; **Phone:** 206-598-4110; **Board Cert:** Therapeutic Radiology 1980; Radiation Oncology 2000; **Med School:** Univ Miami Sch Med 1976; **Resid:** Radiation Oncology, Univ Washington 1980; **Fac Appt:** Prof RadRO, Univ Wash

Larson, David A MD/PhD [RadRO] - **Spec Exp:** Neuro-Oncology; Brain Tumors; Stereotactic Radiosurgery; **Hospital:** UCSF Med Ctr; **Address:** UCSF Med Ctr, Dept Rad Onc, 505 Parnassus Ave, rm L-75, San Francisco, CA 94143-0226; **Phone:** 415-353-8900; **Board Cert:** Therapeutic Radiology 1986; **Med School:** Univ Miami Sch Med 1981; **Resid:** Radiation Therapy, Joint Ctr RadTherapy 1985; **Fac Appt:** Prof RadRO, UCSF

Le, Quynh-Thu Xuan MD [RadRO] - **Spec Exp:** Head & Neck Cancer; Lung Cancer; Thoracic Cancers; Clinical Trials; **Hospital:** Stanford Univ Med Ctr; **Address:** Stanford Univ, Dept Rad Oncology, 875 Blake Wilbur Drive, MC 5847, Stanford, CA 94305; **Phone:** 650-498-5032; **Board Cert:** Radiation Oncology 1998; **Med School:** UCSF 1993; **Resid:** Radiation Oncology, UCSF Med Ctr 1997; **Fac Appt:** Assoc Prof RadRO, Stanford Univ

Mundt, Arno J MD [RadRO] - **Spec Exp:** Gynecologic Cancer; Intensity Modulated Radiotherapy (IMRT); **Hospital:** UCSD Med Ctr; **Address:** Moores UCSD Cancer Ctr, Radiation Oncology Dept, 3855 Health Sciences Drive, MC 0843, La Jolla, CA 92093; **Phone:** 858-822-6046; **Board Cert:** Radiation Oncology 1994; **Med School:** Univ Mich Med Sch 1987; **Resid:** Physical Medicine & Rehabilitation, George Washington Univ Hosp 1990; Radiation Oncology, Univ Chicago Hosps 1993; **Fac Appt:** Assoc Prof RadRO, Univ Chicago-Pritzker Sch Med

Park, Catherine C MD [RadRO] - **Spec Exp:** Breast Cancer; Lymphoma; **Hospital:** UCSF Med Ctr; **Address:** 1600 Divisadero St, Ste H1031, Box 1708, San Francisco, CA 94115; **Phone:** 415-353-9807; **Board Cert:** Radiation Oncology 2000; **Med School:** UCLA 1995; **Resid:** Radiation Oncology, Harvard Med School 2000; **Fac Appt:** Assoc Prof RadRO, UCSF

Pezner, Richard D MD [RadRO] - **Spec Exp:** Brain Tumors; Breast Cancer; Stereotactic Radiosurgery; **Hospital:** City of Hope Natl Med Ctr & Beckman Rsch; **Address:** City of Hope Med Ctr-Div Radiation Onc, 1500 E Duarte Rd, Duarte, CA 91010-3000; **Phone:** 626-301-8247; **Board Cert:** Therapeutic Radiology 1979; **Med School:** Northwestern Univ 1975; **Resid:** Radiation Oncology, Oregon Health Sci Ctr 1979; **Fac Appt:** Clin Prof RadRO, UC Irvine

Quivey, Jeanne M MD [RadRO] - **Spec Exp:** Head & Neck Cancer; Breast Cancer; Eye Tumors/Cancer; Intensity Modulated Radiotherapy (IMRT); **Hospital:** UCSF Med Ctr; **Address:** UCSF Med Ctr @ Mt Zion, Radiation Oncology Dept, 1600 Divisadero St, Box 1708, San Francisco, CA 94115-3010; **Phone:** 415-353-7175; **Board Cert:** Therapeutic Radiology 1974; **Med School:** UCSF 1970; **Resid:** Radiation Therapy, UCSF Med Ctr 1974; **Fac Appt:** Prof RadRO, UCSF

Radiation Oncology

Roach III, Mack MD [RadRO] - **Spec Exp:** Prostate Cancer; Genitourinary Cancer; Lung Cancer; **Hospital:** UCSF - Mt Zion Med Ctr, UCSF Med Ctr; **Address:** UCSF Radiation Oncology, 1600 Divisadero St, Ste H1031, San Francisco, CA 94143-1708; **Phone:** 415-353-7181; **Board Cert:** Medical Oncology 1985; Radiation Oncology 1987; Internal Medicine 1984; **Med School:** Stanford Univ 1979; **Resid:** Internal Medicine, ML King Genl Hosp 1981; Radiation Oncology, Stanford Univ Med Ctr 1987; **Fellow:** Medical Oncology, UCSF Med Ctr 1983; **Fac Appt:** Prof RadRO, UCSF

Rose, Christopher M MD [RadRO] - **Spec Exp:** Prostate Cancer; Breast Cancer; Intensity Modulated Radiotherapy (IMRT); **Hospital:** Providence St Joseph Med Ctr; **Address:** Valley Radiotherapy Assocs, The Ctr for Radiation Therapy, 9229 Wilshire Blvd, Beverly Hills, CA 90210; **Phone:** 310-205-5777; **Board Cert:** Radiation Oncology 1999; **Med School:** Harvard Med Sch 1974; **Resid:** Internal Medicine, Beth Israel Deaconess 1976; Radiation Oncology, Joint Ctr Rad Therapy 1979; **Fellow:** Cancer Research, British Inst Cancer Rsch 1979; **Fac Appt:** Assoc Clin Prof RadRO, UCLA

Rossi, Carl John MD [RadRO] - **Spec Exp:** Prostate Cancer; Proton Beam Therapy; **Hospital:** Loma Linda Univ Med Ctr; **Address:** Loma Linda Univ Med Ctr, 11234 Anderson St, rm B124, Loma Linda, CA 92354; **Phone:** 909-558-4280; **Board Cert:** Radiation Oncology 1994; **Med School:** Loyola Univ-Stritch Sch Med 1988; **Resid:** Radiation Oncology, Loma Linda Univ Med Ctr 1992; **Fac Appt:** Asst Prof RadRO, Loma Linda Univ

Russell, Kenneth J MD [RadRO] - **Spec Exp:** Prostate Cancer; Lymphoma; Genitourinary Cancer; **Hospital:** Univ Wash Med Ctr; **Address:** Seattle Cancer Care Alliance, G1101, 825 Eastlake Ave E, Seattle, WA 98109; **Phone:** 206-288-7318; **Board Cert:** Therapeutic Radiology 1984; **Med School:** Harvard Med Sch 1979; **Resid:** Radiation Therapy, Stanford Univ Med Ctr 1983; **Fellow:** Radiological Biology, Stanford Univ Med Ctr 1985; **Fac Appt:** Prof, Univ Wash

Streeter Jr, Oscar E MD [RadRO] - **Spec Exp:** Lung Cancer; Head & Neck Cancer; **Hospital:** USC Norris Comp Cancer Ctr, USC Univ Hosp - R K Eamer Med Plz; **Address:** Norris Comp Cancer Ctr-Dept Rad Onc, 1441 Eastlake Ave Fl Ground, Los Angeles, CA 90033; **Phone:** 323-865-3051; **Board Cert:** Radiation Oncology 1989; **Med School:** Howard Univ 1982; **Resid:** Radiation Oncology, Howard Univ 1986; **Fac Appt:** Assoc Prof RadRO, USC Sch Med

Tripuraneni, Prabhakar MD [RadRO] - **Spec Exp:** Prostate Cancer; Head & Neck Cancer; Lymphoma; **Hospital:** Scripps Green Hosp, Scripps Meml Hosp - La Jolla; **Address:** Scripps Clinic, Div Radiation Oncology, 10666 N Torrey Pines Rd, MSB 1, La Jolla, CA 92037; **Phone:** 858-554-2000; **Board Cert:** Therapeutic Radiology 1983; **Med School:** India 1976; **Resid:** Radiation Oncology, Univ Alberta 1981; Radiation Oncology, UCSF Med Ctr 1983; **Fac Appt:** Clin Prof, UCSD

Wara, William M MD [RadRO] - **Spec Exp:** Brain & Spinal Tumors; Sarcomas; Pediatric Tumors; **Hospital:** UCSF Med Ctr; **Address:** UCSF Med Ctr, Div Radiation Oncology, 505 Parnassus Ave, rm L-08, San Francisco, CA 94143-0226; **Phone:** 415-353-8950; **Board Cert:** Therapeutic Radiology 1974; **Med School:** UC Irvine 1969; **Resid:** Therapeutic Radiology, UCSF Medical Ctr 1973; **Fac Appt:** Prof RadRO, UCSF

Wong, Jeffrey Y C MD [RadRO] - **Spec Exp:** Radioimmunotherapy of Cancer; Prostate Cancer; Multiple Myeloma; Leukemia; **Hospital:** City of Hope Natl Med Ctr & Beckman Rsch; **Address:** City of Hope Med Ctr-Dept Radiation Onc, 1500 E Duarte Rd, Duarte, CA 91768-3012; **Phone:** 626-359-8111 x62969; **Board Cert:** Therapeutic Radiology 1985; **Med School:** Johns Hopkins Univ 1981; **Resid:** Radiation Oncology, UCSF Med Ctr 1985; **Fac Appt:** Clin Prof RadRO, UC Irvine

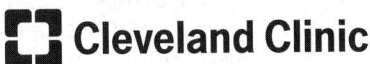 Cleveland Clinic

Radiation Oncology

The Department of Radiation Oncology at the Cleveland Clinic Taussig Cancer Institute is one of the busiest and most technologically advanced clinical radiotherapy programs in the country. Our specialists provide care at five additional facilities in Northeast Ohio and one in Florida.

Technology: Cleveland Clinic offers a full range of advanced technology equipment, including two simulators, six linear accelerators, two- and three-dimensional treatment planning computers, a high-dose-rate brachytherapy unit and a contact unit for early-stage rectal lesions. In addition, Cleveland Clinic is one of the few hospitals to offer treatment of intracranial and extracranial tumors using the Gamma Knife Perfexion and Novalis platforms. In addition, we offer the Calypso 4D Localization System for prostate cancer treatment and Hyperthermia therapy to treat a variety of tumors.

How do you measure quality?
Visit clevelandclinic.org/quality for information on the criteria most often used to measure quality in health care; data on how Cleveland Clinic compares with other health care centers; patient satisfaction data; and quality measures for numerous specific diseases and conditions, including cancer.

Innovation: Cleveland Clinic has one of the most active brachytherapy programs in the U.S. In addition to intracavitary and intraluminal treatments, Cleveland Clinic has developed many novel approaches to brachytherapy, especially with prostate cancer. Cleveland Clinic Radiation Oncology was also one of the first programs to implement intensity-modulated radiation therapy (IMRT), image-guided radiation therapy (IGRT) and radioimmunotherapy (RIT).

Patient Services: Cleveland Clinic offers free round-trip transportation for patients who have difficulty getting to daily treatments from their homes. In addition, our free wellness program, Reflections, offers a variety of complementary and aesthetic therapies, which allow patients the opportunity to be pampered, to regain a sense of control and to take some time for themselves. The treatments are designed to reduce anxiety, and include healing therapies such as Reiki, reflexology, guided imagery, facials, makeovers and massotherapy.

Research: Cleveland Clinic is active in a number of in-house, pharmaceutical and cooperative group trials. We have been one of the leading enrollers in many national studies and are a leader in combining novel agents such as radiation sensitizers with radiation therapy. In addition, our Department of Radiation Oncology houses one of the largest prostate cancer databases (>10,000 patients) in the nation.

For more information about the Cleveland Clinic Department of Radiation Oncology, to schedule a second opinion or to learn about assistance for out-of-town patients, call 800.890.2467 or visit www.clevelandclinic.org/radonctopdocs.

Department of Radiation Oncology | 9500 Euclid Avenue / AC311 | Cleveland OH 44195

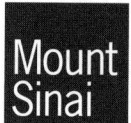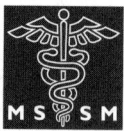

MOUNT SINAI
SCHOOL OF
MEDICINE

THE MOUNT SINAI MEDICAL CENTER
RADIOLOGY
One Gustave L. Levy Place
Fifth Avenue and 100th Street
New York, NY 10029-6574
Physician Referral: 1-800-MD-SINAI (637-4624)
www.mountsinai.org

Mount Sinai offers patients one of the world's most comprehensive and sophisticated arrays of diagnostic and interventional radiology services. Our Department of Radiology uses filmless digital technology that spans magnetic resonance imaging (MRI), multi-slice computed tomography (CT), positron emission tomography CT (PET-CT), single photon tomography CT (SPECT-CT), advanced ultrasound, conventional radiography, digital mammography, and state-of-the-art Picture Archiving Communication System (PACS) technology.

COMPREHENSIVE DIAGNOSTIC SERVICES
Mount Sinai provides the entire range of diagnostic radiology services in a patient-friendly environment. Its nationally renowned radiologic physicians specialize in every area of disease diagnosis, as well as disease prevention and innovative therapeutic approaches.

EARLY DETECTION PROGRAMS
We are committed to special screening approaches for early disease detection. Radiological screenings for colon cancer and Alzheimer's disease are joining those already in place for breast and lung cancer and atherosclerosis. The early detection programs use a variety of imaging techniques (for example, CT and MRI for atherosclerosis, CT for colon cancer, PET for oncology, and digital mammography, MRI, and computer-aided diagnosis for breast cancer).

MINIMALLY INVASIVE PROCEDURES
Radiology at Mount Sinai has moved beyond diagnosis to therapeutic intervention. Interventional radiologists at Mount Sinai perform biopsies, vascular therapies, and uterine artery embolization for fibroids (an alternative to hysterectomy), as well as treatments for aneurysms, atherosclerosis, and many types of cancer.

DEVELOPING NEW DIAGNOSTIC TOOLS
Radiology at Mount Sinai is an active center of imaging research and development. Mount Sinai physicians and scientists developed a special form of MRI to noninvasively diagnose heart disease and atherosclerosis and thereby identify patients at greatest risk for stroke and heart attack. We actively collaborate with other disciplines to develop and refine imaging tools that will make prevention, diagnosis, and prognosis increasingly effective. That is the case, for example, in neuroscience, where the imaging innovations impact on our understanding of neurodegenerative conditions such as Parkinson's disease, as well as multiple sclerosis, stroke, brain tumors, and various psychiatric disorders; cardiovascular disease, where studies are underway to predict the risk associated with atherosclerotic plaques and new therapies for aortic and cerebral artery aneurysms; and liver disease, where radiologists, transplant surgeons, and hepatologists collaborate closely to develop optimal therapeutic strategies.

NYU Cancer Institute

NYU LANGONE MEDICAL CENTER

A Collaborative Approach

The NYU Cancer Institute, an NCI designated center, is a "matrix cancer center" without walls operating within the larger NYU Langone Medical Center. With over 175 members and a research funding base of over $81 million, this structure strengthens our capabilities to forge collaborations across medical and scientific disciplines, which translates to comprehensive care for our patients and discoveries that will influence the future of this disease.

Renowned Expertise

Team members' compassion and expertise help patients better manage the symptoms of their disease as well as their special needs. Our highly skilled Magnet™ nursing team not only plays a pivotal role in coordinating direct patient care, but is also a source of invaluable patient education.

A Patient-Focused Setting

The NYU Clinical Cancer Center, with over 70 faculty members from various disciplines at the New York University School of Medicine, is the principal outpatient facility of the Cancer Institute and serves as home for our patients and their caregivers. The center and its multidisciplinary team of experts provide access to the latest treatment options and clinical trials along with a variety of programs in cancer prevention, screening, diagnostics, genetic counseling, and supportive services. When it comes to kids and cancer, the Stephen D. Hassenfeld Children's Center for Cancer and Blood Disorders offers not just innovation but insight. As a leading member of the NCI-sponsored Children's Oncology Group, our physicians are known for developing new ways to treat childhood cancer. Our affiliation with Bellevue Hospital, the oldest public hospital in the country, affords clinically distinctive opportunities to learn and care for patients with cancer by observing its presentation and behavior in a variety of patient groups.

Radiology

A radiologist utilizes radiologic methodologies to diagnose and treat disease. Physicians practicing in the field of radiology most often specialize in radiology, diagnostic radiology, radiation oncology or radiological physics.

Diagnostic Radiology: A radiologist who utilizes X-ray, radionuclides, ultrasound and electromagnetic radiation to diagnose and treat disease.

Training Required: Four years

Radiation Oncology: A radiologist who deals with the therapeutic applications of radiant energy and its modifiers and the study and management of disease, especially malignant tumors.

Certification in one of the following subspecialties requires additional training and examination.

Neuroradiology: A radiologist who diagnoses and treats diseases utilizing imaging procedures as they relate to the brain, spine and spinal cord, head, neck and organs of special sense in adults and children.

Pediatric Radiology: A radiologist who is proficient in all forms of diagnostic imaging as it pertains to the treatment of diseases in the newborn, infant, child and adolescent. This specialist has knowledge of both imaging and interventional procedures related to the care and management of diseases of children. A pediatric radiologist must be highly knowledgeable of all organ systems as they relate to growth and development, congenital malformations, diseases peculiar to infants and children and diseases that begin in childhood but cause substantial residual impairment in adulthood.

Vascular and Interventional Radiology: A radiologist who diagnoses and treats diseases by various radiologic imaging modalities. These include fluoroscopy, digital radiography, computed tomography, sonography and magnetic resonance imaging.

DIAGNOSTIC RADIOLOGY

New England

Benson, Carol MD [DR] - **Spec Exp:** Obstetric Ultrasound; Thyroid Ultrasound; Fetal Surgical Imaging; **Hospital:** Brigham & Women's Hosp; **Address:** Brigham & Women's Hospital, Dept Radiology, 75 Francis St, Boston, MA 02115; **Phone:** 617-732-6280; **Board Cert:** Diagnostic Radiology 1984; **Med School:** Univ Pennsylvania 1980; **Resid:** Diagnostic Radiology, New York Hosp-Cornell 1984; **Fellow:** Ultrasound, Brigham & Womens Hosp 1985; **Fac Appt:** Prof Rad, Harvard Med Sch

Black, William C MD [DR] - **Spec Exp:** Chest Radiology; Lung Cancer; CT Chest Scan; **Hospital:** Dartmouth - Hitchcock Med Ctr; **Address:** Dartmouth Hitchcock Med Ctr, Dept Radiology, 1 Medical Center Drive, Lebanon, NH 03756; **Phone:** 603-650-7443; **Board Cert:** Diagnostic Radiology 1983; **Med School:** Med Coll VA 1979; **Resid:** Diagnostic Radiology, Univ Virginia Hosp 1983; **Fellow:** Ultrasound/CT, Univ Virginia Hosp 1984; **Fac Appt:** Prof Rad, Dartmouth Med Sch

Kopans, Daniel B MD [DR] - **Spec Exp:** Breast Imaging; **Hospital:** Mass Genl Hosp; **Address:** Mass Genl Hosp, Avon Comprehensive Breast Ctr, 15 Parkman St, WAC 240, Boston, MA 02114-3117; **Phone:** 617-726-3093; **Board Cert:** Diagnostic Radiology 1977; **Med School:** Harvard Med Sch 1973; **Resid:** Diagnostic Radiology, Mass Genl Hosp 1977; **Fac Appt:** Prof Rad, Harvard Med Sch

McCarthy, Shirley M MD/PhD [DR] - **Spec Exp:** Gynecologic Cancer; Pelvic Imaging; **Hospital:** Yale-New Haven Hosp; **Address:** Yale-New Haven Hosp, 333 Cedar St, Ste TE2, New Haven, CT 06520-3206; **Phone:** 203-785-2384; **Board Cert:** Diagnostic Radiology 1983; **Med School:** Yale Univ 1979; **Resid:** Diagnostic Radiology, Yale-New Haven Hosp 1983; **Fellow:** Cross Sectional Imaging, UCSF Med Ctr 1984; **Fac Appt:** Prof Rad, Yale Univ

Palmer, William E MD [DR] - **Spec Exp:** Musculoskeletal Imaging; Pain-Vertebral Collapse/Osteoporosis; Sports Related Injuries; **Hospital:** Mass Genl Hosp; **Address:** 15 Parkman St, Wang Bldg, rm 515, Boston, MA 02114; **Phone:** 617-726-7717; **Board Cert:** Internal Medicine 1987; Diagnostic Radiology 1991; **Med School:** Yale Univ 1984; **Resid:** Internal Medicine, Hosp Univ Penn 1987; Diagnostic Radiology, Mass Genl Hosp 1991; **Fac Appt:** Assoc Prof Rad, Harvard Med Sch

Schepps, Barbara MD [DR] - **Spec Exp:** Breast Imaging; **Hospital:** Rhode Island Hosp; **Address:** Anne C Pappas Breast Imaging Ctr, 2 Dudley St, Ste G85, Providence, RI 02903; **Phone:** 401-444-6266; **Board Cert:** Diagnostic Radiology 1973; **Med School:** Hahnemann Univ 1968; **Resid:** Diagnostic Radiology, Boston City Hosp 1972; **Fac Appt:** Clin Prof Rad, Brown Univ

Weinreb, Jeffrey C MD [DR] - **Spec Exp:** MRI; Breast Cancer; Abdominal Imaging; Prostate Cancer; **Hospital:** Yale-New Haven Hosp; **Address:** Yale Univ Sch Medicine, Dept Radiology, 333 Cedar St, rm MRC147, Box 208042, New Haven, CT 06520-8042; **Phone:** 203-785-5913; **Board Cert:** Diagnostic Radiology 1983; **Med School:** Mount Sinai Sch Med 1978; **Resid:** Diagnostic Radiology, LI Jewish Med Ctr 1982; **Fellow:** Ultrasound/CT, Hosp Univ Penn 1983; **Fac Appt:** Prof Rad, Yale Univ

Diagnostic Radiology

Mid Atlantic

Adler, Ronald S MD/PhD [DR] - **Spec Exp:** Musculoskeletal Imaging; Ultrasound; Power Doppler Imaging; **Hospital:** Hosp For Special Surgery (page 59), NY-Presby Hosp/Weill Cornell (page 66); **Address:** Hospital for Special Surgery, 535 E 70th St, New York, NY 10021; **Phone:** 212-606-1635; **Board Cert:** Diagnostic Radiology 1988; **Med School:** Wayne State Univ 1984; **Resid:** Diagnostic Radiology, Univ Mich Med Ctr 1988; **Fellow:** Ultrasound/CT/MRI, Univ Mich Med Ctr 1989; **Fac Appt:** Prof Rad, Cornell Univ-Weill Med Coll

Austin, John H M MD [DR] - **Spec Exp:** Lung Cancer; Chest Radiology; **Hospital:** NY-Presby Hosp/Columbia (page 66); **Address:** Columbia Presby Hosp, Dept Radiology, 622 W 168th St, MHB 3-202C, New York, NY 10032-3784; **Phone:** 212-305-2986; **Board Cert:** Diagnostic Radiology 1970; **Med School:** Yale Univ 1965; **Resid:** Diagnostic Radiology, UCSF Med Ctr 1968; **Fellow:** Diagnostic Radiology, UCSF Med Ctr 1970; **Fac Appt:** Prof Rad, Columbia P&S

Berg, Wendie A MD/PhD [DR] - **Spec Exp:** Breast Imaging; Breast Cancer; **Hospital:** Johns Hopkins Hosp - Baltimore (page 61); **Address:** Johns Hopkins, Greenspring Station Breast Ctr, 10755 Falls Rd, Ste 440, Lutherville, MD 21093; **Phone:** 410-583-2700; **Board Cert:** Diagnostic Radiology 1992; **Med School:** Johns Hopkins Univ 1987; **Resid:** Diagnostic Radiology, Johns Hopkins Hosp 1992; **Fellow:** Abdominal Imaging, Johns Hopkins Univ 1992

Bluemke, David A MD/PhD [DR] - **Spec Exp:** Cardiac Imaging; MRI; **Hospital:** Natl Inst of Hlth - Clin Ctr; **Address:** 900 Rockville Pike, Bldg 10 - rm 1C 355X, Bethesda, MD 20892; **Phone:** 301-402-1854; **Board Cert:** Diagnostic Radiology 1993; **Med School:** Univ Chicago-Pritzker Sch Med 1989; **Resid:** Diagnostic Radiology, Johns Hopkins Hosp 1993; **Fellow:** Diagnostic Imaging, Johns Hopkins Hosp 1994; **Fac Appt:** Prof Rad, Johns Hopkins Univ

Brem, Rachel F MD [DR] - **Spec Exp:** Breast Imaging; **Hospital:** G Washington Univ Hosp; **Address:** GW Medical Faculty Assocs, 2150 Pennsylvania Ave NW, DC Level, Washington, DC 20037; **Phone:** 202-741-3036; **Board Cert:** Diagnostic Radiology 1990; **Med School:** Columbia P&S 1984; **Resid:** Diagnostic Radiology, Johns Hopkins Hosp 1989; **Fellow:** Mammography, Johns Hopkins Hosp 1990; **Fac Appt:** Prof, Geo Wash Univ

Cohen, Burton A MD [DR] - **Spec Exp:** CT Scan; MRI; Ovarian Cancer; PET Imaging; **Hospital:** Mount Sinai Med Ctr (page 64); **Address:** 165 E 84th St, New York, NY 10028; **Phone:** 212-535-9770; **Board Cert:** Diagnostic Radiology 1979; **Med School:** NY Med Coll 1975; **Resid:** Diagnostic Radiology, Mount Sinai Hosp 1979; **Fac Appt:** Assoc Clin Prof Rad, Mount Sinai Sch Med

Cohen, Harris L MD [DR] - **Spec Exp:** Pediatric Radiology; Fetal Ultrasound/Obstetrical Imaging; Obstetric Ultrasound; **Hospital:** Stony Brook Univ Med Ctr; **Address:** Stony Brook Univ Hosp, Dept Radiology, HCS level 4, rm 120, Stony Brook, NY 11794-8460; **Phone:** 631-444-8193; **Board Cert:** Diagnostic Radiology 1980; Pediatric Radiology 2005; **Med School:** SUNY Downstate 1976; **Resid:** Internal Medicine, Nassau County Med Ctr 1977; Diagnostic Radiology, Univ Hosp 1980; **Fellow:** Pediatric Radiology, Children's Hosp 1981; **Fac Appt:** Prof Rad, SUNY Stony Brook

Coleman, Beverly G MD [DR] - **Spec Exp:** Ultrasound; **Hospital:** Hosp Univ Penn - UPHS (page 60); **Address:** Univ Penn Radiology, Ground Dulles, 3400 Spruce St, Philadelphia, PA 19104; **Phone:** 215-662-3046; **Board Cert:** Diagnostic Radiology 1978; **Med School:** Harvard Med Sch 1974; **Resid:** Diagnostic Radiology, Univ Penn Hosp 1975; Diagnostic Radiology, Univ Mich Hosp 1977; **Fellow:** Ultrasound, Univ Penn Hosp 1979; **Fac Appt:** Prof Rad, Univ Pennsylvania

Conant, Emily F MD [DR] - **Spec Exp:** Breast Cancer; Breast Imaging; **Hospital:** Hosp Univ Penn - UPHS (page 60); **Address:** Hosp U Penn, Dept Radiology (Breast Imaging), 3400 Spruce St, 1 Silverstein, Philadelphia, PA 19104; **Phone:** 215-662-4032; **Board Cert:** Diagnostic Radiology 1989; **Med School:** Univ Pennsylvania 1983; **Resid:** Diagnostic Radiology, Hosp Univ Penn 1986; **Fellow:** Breast Imaging, Hosp Univ Penn 1989; **Fac Appt:** Prof Rad, Univ Pennsylvania

Dalinka, Murray MD [DR] - **Spec Exp:** Bone Disorders-Metabolic; Musculoskeletal Disorders; MRI; **Hospital:** Hosp Univ Penn - UPHS (page 60); **Address:** Hosp Univ Penn, Dept Radiology, 3400 Spruce St, Philadelphia, PA 19104; **Phone:** 215-662-3019; **Board Cert:** Diagnostic Radiology 1969; **Med School:** Univ Mich Med Sch 1964; **Resid:** Diagnostic Radiology, Montefiore Med Ctr 1968; **Fac Appt:** Prof Rad, Univ Pennsylvania

Dershaw, D David MD [DR] - **Spec Exp:** Breast Imaging; Breast Cancer; Mammography; **Hospital:** Meml Sloan-Kettering Cancer Ctr; **Address:** 1275 York Avenue, New York, NY 10065; **Phone:** 800-525-2225; **Board Cert:** Diagnostic Radiology 1978; **Med School:** Jefferson Med Coll 1974; **Resid:** Diagnostic Radiology, New York Hosp 1978; **Fellow:** Ultrasound, Thos Jefferson Univ Hosp 1979; **Fac Appt:** Prof Rad, Cornell Univ-Weill Med Coll

Edelstein, Barbara A MD [DR] - **Spec Exp:** Breast Cancer; Women's Imaging; **Address:** 1045 Park Ave, New York, NY 10028; **Phone:** 212-860-7700; **Board Cert:** Diagnostic Radiology 1983; **Med School:** NY Med Coll 1977; **Resid:** Diagnostic Radiology, Montefiore Hosp 1982

Evers, Kathryn MD [DR] - **Spec Exp:** Breast Cancer; Mammography; **Hospital:** Fox Chase Cancer Ctr (page 58); **Address:** Fox Chase Cancer Ctr, Diagnostic Imaging, 333 Cottman Ave, Philadelphia, PA 19111; **Phone:** 215-728-4316; **Board Cert:** Diagnostic Radiology 1980; **Med School:** NYU Sch Med 1975; **Resid:** Diagnostic Radiology, Hosp Univ Penn 1980; **Fellow:** Gastrointestinal Radiology, Hosp Univ Penn 1981; **Fac Appt:** Assoc Clin Prof Rad, Temple Univ

Fishman, Elliot MD [DR] - **Spec Exp:** CT Body Scan; Abdominal Imaging; Cardiac Imaging; Cancer Imaging; **Hospital:** Johns Hopkins Hosp - Baltimore (page 61); **Address:** Johns Hopkins Hosp, Dept Radiology, 601 N Caroline St, JHOC 3254, Baltimore, MD 21287-0006; **Phone:** 410-955-5173; **Board Cert:** Diagnostic Radiology 1981; **Med School:** Univ MD Sch Med 1977; **Resid:** Diagnostic Radiology, Sinai Hosp 1980; **Fellow:** Computerized Tomography, Johns Hopkins Hosp 1981; **Fac Appt:** Prof Rad, Johns Hopkins Univ

Fuhrman, Carl R MD [DR] - **Spec Exp:** Thoracic Imaging; **Hospital:** UPMC Presby, Pittsburgh; **Address:** UPMC-Dept Radiology, 200 Lothrop St, Ste E177 PUH, Pittsburgh, PA 15213; **Phone:** 412-647-7288; **Board Cert:** Diagnostic Radiology 1983; **Med School:** Univ Pittsburgh 1979; **Resid:** Diagnostic Radiology, Presbyterian Univ Hosp 1983; **Fac Appt:** Prof Rad, Univ Pittsburgh

Gefter, Warren B MD [DR] - **Spec Exp:** Thoracic Imaging; **Hospital:** Hosp Univ Penn - UPHS (page 60); **Address:** Hospital Univ of Pennsylvania, 1 Silverstein, 3400 Spruce St, Philadelphia, PA 19104; **Phone:** 215-662-6724; **Board Cert:** Diagnostic Radiology 1978; **Med School:** Univ Pennsylvania 1974; **Resid:** Diagnostic Radiology, Hosp U Penn 1978; **Fac Appt:** Prof Rad, Univ Pennsylvania

Hann, Lucy MD [DR] - **Spec Exp:** Liver & Biliary Cancer Ultrasound; Ovarian Cancer Ultrasound Diagnosis; Thyroid Ultrasound; **Hospital:** Meml Sloan-Kettering Cancer Ctr; **Address:** 1275 York Avenue, New York, NY 10065; **Phone:** 800-525-2225; **Board Cert:** Diagnostic Radiology 1977; **Med School:** Harvard Med Sch 1971; **Resid:** Diagnostic Radiology, Hosp Univ Penn 1974; Diagnostic Radiology, Mass General Hosp 1977; **Fellow:** Body Imaging, Mass General Hosp 1978; **Fac Appt:** Prof Rad, Cornell Univ-Weill Med Coll

Diagnostic Radiology

Henschke, Claudia L MD/PhD [DR] - **Spec Exp:** Lung Cancer; Lung Disease; Thoracic Imaging; **Hospital:** NY-Presby Hosp/Weill Cornell (page 66); **Address:** NY Weill Medical College, Dept Radiology, 525 E 68th St, Box 586, New York, NY 10021; **Phone:** 212-746-1325; **Board Cert:** Diagnostic Radiology 1981; **Med School:** Howard Univ 1977; **Resid:** Diagnostic Radiology, Brigham & Womens Hosp 1983; **Fac Appt:** Prof Rad, Cornell Univ-Weill Med Coll

Hricak, Hedvig MD/PhD [DR] - **Spec Exp:** Prostate Cancer-MR Spectroscopy (MRSI); Breast Imaging; Breast Cancer; **Hospital:** Meml Sloan-Kettering Cancer Ctr; **Address:** 1275 York Avenue, New York, NY 10065; **Phone:** 800-525-2225; **Board Cert:** Diagnostic Radiology 1978; **Med School:** Yugoslavia 1970; **Resid:** Diagnostic Radiology, St Joseph Mercy Hosp 1977; **Fellow:** Ultrasound/CT, Henry Ford Hosp 1978; **Fac Appt:** Prof Rad, Cornell Univ-Weill Med Coll

Jaramillo, Diego MD [DR] - **Spec Exp:** Pediatric Radiology; **Hospital:** Chldns Hosp of Philadelphia, The; **Address:** Children's Hosp of Philadelphia, Radiology, 34th & Civic Center Blvd, rm 3184, Philadelphia, PA 19104; **Phone:** 267-425-7110; **Board Cert:** Diagnostic Radiology 1987; Pediatric Radiology 2005; **Med School:** Colombia 1981; **Resid:** Diagnostic Radiology, U Texas 1987; **Fellow:** Pediatric Radiology, Children's Hosp 1989; **Fac Appt:** Assoc Prof Rad, Univ Pennsylvania

Kanal, Emanuel MD [DR] - **Spec Exp:** Neuroradiology; MRI; **Hospital:** UPMC Presby, Pittsburgh; **Address:** Univ Pittsburgh Med Ctr, Dept Radiology, 200 Lothrop St, rm D132, Pittsburgh, PA 15213-2582; **Phone:** 412-647-3540; **Board Cert:** Diagnostic Radiology 1985; Neuroradiology 1997; **Med School:** Univ Pittsburgh 1981; **Resid:** Diagnostic Radiology, Univ Pittsburgh Med Ctr 1985; **Fellow:** Magnetic Resonance Imaging, Pittsburgh NMR Inst 1986; Neurological Radiology, Univ Pittsburgh Med Ctr 1993; **Fac Appt:** Prof Rad, Univ Pittsburgh

Kurtz, Alfred B MD [DR] - **Spec Exp:** Obstetric Ultrasound; **Hospital:** Thomas Jefferson Univ Hosp; **Address:** Thomas Jefferson Univ Hosp, Dept Radiology, 111 S 11th St, Ste 3350A-B, Philadelphia, PA 19107; **Phone:** 215-955-6343; **Board Cert:** Diagnostic Radiology 1977; **Med School:** Stanford Univ 1972; **Resid:** Internal Medicine, Montefiore Med Ctr 1974; Diagnostic Radiology, Montefiore Med Ctr 1977; **Fellow:** Ultrasound, Thomas Jefferson Univ Hosp 1978; **Fac Appt:** Prof Rad, Jefferson Med Coll

Levy, Angela D MD [DR] - **Spec Exp:** Abdominal Imaging; **Hospital:** Unif Serv Univ of the Hlth Sci, Armed Forces Inst of Path; **Address:** Uniformed Services Univ of the Hlth Scis, Dept Radiology, 4301 Jones Bridge Rd, rm C1071, Bethesda, MD 20814; **Phone:** 301-295-3145; **Board Cert:** Diagnostic Radiology 1993; **Med School:** Uniformed Srvs Univ, Bethesda 1988; **Resid:** Diagnostic Radiology, Walter Reed Army Hosp 1992; **Fac Appt:** Assoc Prof Rad, Uniformed Srvs Univ, Bethesda

Megibow, Alec J MD [DR] - **Spec Exp:** Abdominal Imaging; Gastrointestinal Imaging; CT Body Scan; **Hospital:** NYU Med Ctr (page 68); **Address:** 550 1st Ave, HHC 232, New York, NY 10016; **Phone:** 212-263-5222; **Board Cert:** Diagnostic Radiology 1978; **Med School:** SUNY Upstate Med Univ 1974; **Resid:** Diagnostic Radiology, Bellevue/NYU Med Ctr 1978; **Fac Appt:** Prof Rad, NYU Sch Med

Mirvis, Stuart E MD [DR] - **Spec Exp:** Trauma Radiology; **Hospital:** Univ of MD Med Sys; **Address:** Univ Maryland Med Ctr, Dept Radiology, 22 S Greene St, Baltimore, MD 21201; **Phone:** 410-328-8845; **Board Cert:** Diagnostic Radiology 1984; **Med School:** Johns Hopkins Univ 1979; **Resid:** Diagnostic Radiology, Univ Maryland Med Ctr 1984; **Fellow:** Trauma Radiology, Univ Maryland Med Ctr 1985; **Fac Appt:** Prof Rad, Univ MD Sch Med

Mitnick, Julie MD [DR] - **Spec Exp:** Mammography; Breast Cancer; **Address:** 650 1st Ave, New York, NY 10016; **Phone:** 212-686-4440; **Board Cert:** Diagnostic Radiology 1977; **Med School:** NYU Sch Med 1973; **Resid:** Diagnostic Radiology, NYU Med Ctr 1977; **Fellow:** Pediatric Radiology, NYU Med Ctr 1978; **Fac Appt:** Assoc Clin Prof Rad, NYU Sch Med

America's Top Doctors® 8th Edition

Norton, Karen MD [DR] - **Spec Exp:** Pediatric Radiology; **Hospital:** Newark Beth Israel Med Ctr; **Address:** 201 Lyons Ave, Newark, NJ 07112; **Phone:** 973-926-7689; **Board Cert:** Diagnostic Radiology 1984; Pediatric Radiology 2005; **Med School:** Mount Sinai Sch Med 1980; **Resid:** Pediatrics, NYU Med Ctr 1981; Diagnostic Radiology, Mount Sinai Hosp 1984; **Fellow:** Pediatric Radiology, Mount Sinai Hosp 1985

Orel, Susan G MD [DR] - **Spec Exp:** Breast Imaging; Breast Cancer; **Hospital:** Hosp Univ Penn - UPHS (page 60); **Address:** Hosp Univ Penn, Dept Radiology, 3400 Spruce St, 1 Silverstein, Philadelphia, PA 19104; **Phone:** 215-662-3016; **Board Cert:** Diagnostic Radiology 1989; **Med School:** Univ Pennsylvania 1986; **Resid:** Diagnostic Radiology, Johns Hopkins Hosp 1989; **Fac Appt:** Prof Rad, Univ Pennsylvania

Panicek, David MD [DR] - **Spec Exp:** Bone Cancer; Soft Tissue Tumors; Musculoskeletal Imaging; **Hospital:** Meml Sloan-Kettering Cancer Ctr; **Address:** 1275 York Avenue, New York, NY 10065; **Phone:** 800-525-2225; **Board Cert:** Diagnostic Radiology 1984; **Med School:** Cornell Univ-Weill Med Coll 1980; **Resid:** Diagnostic Radiology, NY Hosp-Cornell Med Ctr 1984; **Fac Appt:** Prof Rad, Cornell Univ-Weill Med Coll

Potter, Hollis J MD [DR] - **Spec Exp:** Musculoskeletal Imaging; Cartilage Damage; Arthroplasty Imaging; **Hospital:** Hosp For Special Surgery (page 59); **Address:** Hosp for Special Surgery, MRI-basement, 535 E 70th St, New York, NY 10021-4892; **Phone:** 212-606-1882; **Board Cert:** Diagnostic Radiology 1990; **Med School:** NY Med Coll 1985; **Resid:** Diagnostic Radiology, North Shore Univ Hosp 1990; **Fellow:** Diagnostic Radiology, Hosp Special Surgery 1991; **Fac Appt:** Prof Rad, Cornell Univ-Weill Med Coll

Rao, Vijay M MD [DR] - **Spec Exp:** Head & Neck Tumors Imaging; TMJ Imaging; Ear Nose & Throat Imaging; **Hospital:** Thomas Jefferson Univ Hosp; **Address:** 132 S 10th St, 1087, Main Bldg, Philadelphia, PA 19107-4824; **Phone:** 215-955-4804; **Board Cert:** Diagnostic Radiology 1978; Neuroradiology 1997; **Med School:** India 1973; **Resid:** Diagnostic Radiology, Thomas Jefferson Univ Hosp 1978; **Fac Appt:** Prof Rad, Thomas Jefferson Univ

Reinus, William R MD [DR] - **Spec Exp:** Musculoskeletal Imaging; **Hospital:** Temple Univ Hosp; **Address:** Temple Univ Hospital, Dept Radiology, 3401 N Broad St, Philadelphia, PA 19140; **Phone:** 215-707-4264; **Board Cert:** Diagnostic Radiology 1983; **Med School:** NYU Sch Med 1979; **Resid:** Radiology, Mallinkradt Inst Rad 1983; **Fellow:** Musculoskeletal Imaging, Mallinkradt Inst Rad 1984; **Fac Appt:** Assoc Prof Rad, Temple Univ

Teal, James S MD [DR] - **Spec Exp:** Interventional Radiology; **Hospital:** Howard Univ Hosp; **Address:** Howard Univ Hosp, Dept Radiology, 2041 Georgia Ave NW, Washington, DC 20060-0001; **Phone:** 202-865-1571; **Board Cert:** Diagnostic Radiology 1970; **Med School:** Univ Tex Med Br, Galveston 1965; **Resid:** Diagnostic Radiology, Mt Zion Hosp 1969; **Fellow:** Neuroradiology, LAC-USC Med Ctr 1970; **Fac Appt:** Prof Rad, Howard Univ

White, Charles S MD [DR] - **Spec Exp:** Thoracic Imaging; **Hospital:** Univ of MD Med Sys; **Address:** Univ Maryland Med Ctr, Dept Radiology, 22 S Greene St, Baltimore, MD 21201; **Phone:** 410-328-3477; **Board Cert:** Diagnostic Radiology 1991; Internal Medicine 1987; **Med School:** SUNY Buffalo 1984; **Resid:** Internal Medicine, Columbia-Presby Hosp 1987; Diagnostic Radiology, Columbia-Presby Hosp 1991; **Fellow:** Thoracic Radiology, Columbia-Presby Med Ctr; **Fac Appt:** Prof, Univ MD Sch Med

Diagnostic Radiology

Yankelevitz, David MD [DR] - **Spec Exp:** Lung Cancer; Thoracic Imaging; **Hospital:** NY-Presby Hosp/Weill Cornell (page 66); **Address:** 520 E 70th St, Weill Cornell Starr Bldg, New York, NY 10021; **Phone:** 212-746-9729; **Board Cert:** Diagnostic Radiology 1987; Nuclear Medicine 1987; **Med School:** SUNY Hlth Sci Ctr 1981; **Resid:** Diagnostic Radiology, Long Island Coll Hosp 1984; Nuclear Medicine, NY-Cornell Med Ctr 1987; **Fellow:** Diagnostic Radiology, NY-Cornell Med Ctr 1987; **Fac Appt:** Prof Rad, Cornell Univ-Weill Med Coll

Southeast

Abbitt, Patricia L MD [DR] - **Spec Exp:** Ultrasound; Interventional Radiology; Breast Imaging; Breast Cancer; **Hospital:** Shands at Univ of FL; **Address:** Shands Healthcare, Dept Radiology, 1600 SW Archer Rd, PO Box 100374, Gainesville, FL 32610; **Phone:** 352-265-0291; **Board Cert:** Diagnostic Radiology 1986; **Med School:** Tufts Univ 1981; **Resid:** Diagnostic Radiology, Univ VA Med Ctr 1986; **Fellow:** Breast Imaging, Univ VA Med Ctr 1987; **Fac Appt:** Prof, Univ Fla Coll Med

Berland, Lincoln L MD [DR] - **Spec Exp:** Abdominal Imaging; Gastrointestinal Imaging; **Hospital:** Univ of Ala Hosp at Birmingham; **Address:** UAB Diagnositic Radiology, N348 Jefferson Tower Bldg, 619 19th St S, Birmingham, AL 35249-6830; **Phone:** 205-934-7978; **Board Cert:** Diagnostic Radiology 1980; **Med School:** Washington Univ, St Louis 1975; **Resid:** Diagnostic Radiology, Med Coll Wisconsin Hosps 1979; **Fellow:** Ultrasound/CT, Med Coll Wisconsin Hosps 1980; **Fac Appt:** Prof Rad, Univ Ala

Mancuso, Anthony MD [DR] - **Spec Exp:** Head & Neck Imaging; Neuroradiology; **Hospital:** Shands at Univ of FL; **Address:** Shands Hosp, Univ Florida, Dept Rad, 1600 SW Archer Rd, Gainesville, FL 32610; **Phone:** 352-265-0296; **Board Cert:** Diagnostic Radiology 1978; **Med School:** Univ Miami Sch Med 1973; **Resid:** Diagnostic Radiology, UCLA Med Ctr 1977; **Fellow:** Neuroradiology, UCLA Med Ctr 1978; **Fac Appt:** Prof, Univ Fla Coll Med

Partain, C Leon MD/PhD [DR] - **Spec Exp:** MRI; Nuclear Radiology; **Hospital:** Vanderbilt Univ Med Ctr; **Address:** Vanderbilt Univ Med Ctr, Dept Radiology, 1161 21st Ave S, rm RR1223 MCN, Nashville, TN 37232-2675; **Phone:** 615-343-3588; **Board Cert:** Nuclear Medicine 1979; Diagnostic Radiology 1980; Nuclear Radiology 1981; **Med School:** Washington Univ, St Louis 1975; **Resid:** Diagnostic Radiology, Univ North Carolina 1979; Nuclear Medicine, Univ North Carolina 1979; **Fac Appt:** Prof, Vanderbilt Univ

Patz, Edward F MD [DR] - **Spec Exp:** Thoracic Imaging; PET Imaging; Lung Cancer; **Hospital:** Duke Univ Med Ctr; **Address:** Duke Univ Med Ctr, Dept Radiology, Box 3808, Durham, NC 27710; **Phone:** 919-684-7311; **Board Cert:** Diagnostic Radiology 1990; **Med School:** Univ MD Sch Med 1985; **Resid:** Diagnostic Radiology, Brigham & Womens Hosp 1990; **Fellow:** Thoracic Radiology, Brigham & Womens Hosp 1990; **Fac Appt:** Prof, Duke Univ

Pisano, Etta D MD [DR] - **Spec Exp:** Breast Imaging; **Hospital:** Univ NC Hosps; **Address:** UNC Health Care, 101 Manning Dr, Box 7510, Chapel Hill, NC 27599; **Phone:** 919-966-1081; **Board Cert:** Diagnostic Radiology 1988; **Med School:** Duke Univ 1983; **Resid:** Diagnostic Radiology, Beth Israel Hosp 1988; **Fac Appt:** Prof, Univ NC Sch Med

White, Richard D MD [DR] - **Spec Exp:** Cardiovascular Imaging; **Hospital:** Shands Jacksonville; **Address:** Univ Florida Coll of Med, Radiology, 655 W 8th St Fl 2, Jacksonville, FL 32209; **Phone:** 904-244-4224; **Board Cert:** Diagnostic Radiology 1986; **Med School:** Duke Univ 1981; **Resid:** Diagnostic Radiology, UCSF Med Ctr 1985; **Fellow:** Cardiovascular Radiology, UCSF Med Ctr 1987; **Fac Appt:** Prof, Univ Fla Coll Med

Yoon, Sydney MD [DR] - **Spec Exp:** MRI; CT Body Scan; Uterine Fibroid Embolization; Interventional Radiology; **Address:** Sand Lake Imaging, 9350 Turkey Lake Rd, Orlando, FL 32819; **Phone:** 407-363-2772; **Board Cert:** Internal Medicine 1989; Diagnostic Radiology 1993; Vascular & Interventional Radiology 1998; Neuroradiology 2006; **Med School:** Univ Chicago-Pritzker Sch Med 1986; **Resid:** Internal Medicine, Johns Hopkins Hosp 1989; Diagnostic Radiology, UCLA Med Ctr 1993; **Fellow:** Neuroradiology, Columbia Presby Med Ctr 1995; Vascular & Interventional Radiology, UCLA Med Ctr 1997

Midwest

Edelman, Robert R MD [DR] - **Spec Exp:** MRI; Cardiac CT Angiography; **Hospital:** Evanston Hosp; **Address:** Evanston Hosp, Dept Radiology, 2650 Ridge Ave, rm 5108, Evanston, IL 60201; **Phone:** 847-570-2475; **Board Cert:** Diagnostic Radiology 1984; **Med School:** Boston Univ 1980; **Resid:** Diagnostic Radiology, Beth Israel Deaconess Med Ctr 1984; **Fac Appt:** Prof Rad, Northwestern Univ

Flamm, Scott D MD [DR] - **Spec Exp:** Cardiac MRI; Cardiovascular Imaging; Congenital Heart Disease; **Hospital:** Cleveland Clin Fdn (page 56); **Address:** Cleveland Clinic, 9500 Euclid Ave, MC Hb6, Cleveland, OH 44195; **Phone:** 216-444-2740; **Board Cert:** Diagnostic Radiology 1993; **Med School:** Geo Wash Univ 1988; **Resid:** Diagnostic Radiology, UCLA Med Ctr 1992; **Fellow:** Cardiovascular Disease, UCSF Med Ctr 1994; **Fac Appt:** Assoc Prof Rad, Case West Res Univ

Goodman, Lawrence R MD [DR] - **Spec Exp:** Thoracic Imaging; Pulmonary Embolism; Lung Disease; **Hospital:** Froedtert Meml Lutheran Hosp; **Address:** Froedtert Meml Lutheran Hosp, Dept Radiology, 9200 West Wisconsin Avenue, Milwaukee, WI 53226; **Phone:** 414-805-3120; **Board Cert:** Diagnostic Radiology 1973; **Med School:** SUNY Downstate 1968; **Resid:** Diagnostic Radiology, Boston Univ/City Hosp 1972; **Fellow:** Thoracic Radiology, UCSF Med Ctr 1973; **Fac Appt:** Prof Rad, Med Coll Wisc

Helvie, Mark A MD [DR] - **Spec Exp:** Breast Imaging; Breast Cancer; Mammography; **Hospital:** Univ Michigan Hlth Sys; **Address:** 2910N Taubman Univ Michigan Health Ctr, 1500 E Medical Ctr Drive, Ann Arbor, MI 48109-0326; **Phone:** 734-936-4367; **Board Cert:** Internal Medicine 1983; Diagnostic Radiology 1986; **Med School:** Univ NC Sch Med 1980; **Resid:** Internal Medicine, Univ Michigan Hosps 1983; Diagnostic Radiology, Univ Michigan Hosps 1986; **Fellow:** Breast Imaging, Univ Michigan Hosps 1987; **Fac Appt:** Prof, Univ Mich Med Sch

Jackson, Valerie P MD [DR] - **Spec Exp:** Breast Imaging; **Hospital:** Indiana Univ Hosp; **Address:** Indiana Univ Hosp, Dept Radiology, 550 N University Blvd, #0663, Indianapolis, IN 46202; **Phone:** 317-274-1866; **Board Cert:** Diagnostic Radiology 1982; **Med School:** Indiana Univ 1978; **Resid:** Diagnostic Radiology, Indiana Univ Med Ctr 1982; **Fac Appt:** Prof Rad, Indiana Univ

Monsees, Barbara MD [DR] - **Spec Exp:** Mammography; Breast Cancer; **Hospital:** Barnes-Jewish Hosp; **Address:** Ctr for Advanced Med, Campus Box 8131, 510 S Kingshighway Blvd, St Louis, MO 63110; **Phone:** 314-454-7500; **Board Cert:** Diagnostic Radiology 1980; **Med School:** Washington Univ, St Louis 1975; **Resid:** Pediatrics, St Louis Chldns Hosp 1977; Diagnostic Radiology, Mallinckrodt Inst Radiology 1980; **Fac Appt:** Prof, Washington Univ, St Louis

Sagel, Stuart S MD [DR] - **Spec Exp:** Lung Cancer; Occupational Lung Disease; Pulmonary Embolism; **Hospital:** Barnes-Jewish Hosp; **Address:** Mallinckrodt Inst Rad-Barnes Hosp, 510 S Kingshighway Blvd, Box 8131, St Louis, MO 63110-1016; **Phone:** 314-362-2927; **Board Cert:** Diagnostic Radiology 1970; **Med School:** Temple Univ 1965; **Resid:** Diagnostic Radiology, Yale New Haven Hosp 1968; Diagnostic Radiology, UCSF Med Ctr 1970; **Fac Appt:** Prof, Washington Univ, St Louis

Diagnostic Radiology

Sivit, Carlos MD [DR] - **Spec Exp:** Pediatric Radiology; Abdominal Imaging; **Hospital:** Rainbow Babies & Chldns Hosp; **Address:** Dept Radiology, 11100 Euclid Ave, Cleveland, OH 44106-1736; **Phone:** 216-844-1172; **Board Cert:** Pediatrics 1987; Diagnostic Radiology 1987; **Med School:** Univ VA Sch Med 1981; **Resid:** Pediatrics, Vanderbilt Univ Hosp 1984; Diagnostic Radiology, George Washington Univ Hosp 1987; **Fellow:** Pediatric Radiology, Chldns Natl Med Ctr 1989; **Fac Appt:** Prof Rad, Case West Res Univ

Strife, Janet L MD [DR] - **Spec Exp:** Pediatric Radiology; Cardiac Imaging; **Hospital:** Cincinnati Chldns Hosp Med Ctr; **Address:** Children's Hospital, Dept Radiology, 3333 Burnet Ave, MC 5031, Cincinnati, OH 45229; **Phone:** 513-636-7535; **Board Cert:** Diagnostic Radiology 1974; Pediatric Radiology 2004; **Med School:** UMDNJ-NJ Med Sch, Newark 1968; **Resid:** Diagnostic Radiology, Univ Cincinnati Med Ctr 1971; Diagnostic Radiology, Johns Hopkins Hosp 1973; **Fellow:** Pediatrics, Johns Hopkins Hosp; **Fac Appt:** Prof, Univ Cincinnati

Swensen, Stephen J MD [DR] - **Spec Exp:** Lung Cancer; Lung Disease; **Hospital:** Mayo Med Ctr & Clin - Rochester; **Address:** Mayo Clinic - Diagnostic Radiology, 200 1st St SW, Rochester, MN 55905; **Phone:** 507-538-3270; **Board Cert:** Diagnostic Radiology 1986; **Med School:** Univ Wisc 1981; **Resid:** Diagnostic Radiology, Mayo Clinic 1986; **Fellow:** Pulmonary Radiology, Brigham & Womens Hosp 1987; **Fac Appt:** Prof Rad, Mayo Med Sch

Wells, Robert G MD [DR] - **Spec Exp:** Pediatric Radiology; **Hospital:** Chldns Hosp - Wisconsin; **Address:** Pediatric Diagnostic Imaging, 8522 W Capitol Drive, Milwaukee, WI 53222; **Phone:** 414-847-1800; **Board Cert:** Diagnostic Radiology 1984; Pediatric Radiology 2004; Vascular & Interventional Radiology 2004; **Med School:** Med Coll Wisc 1980; **Resid:** Diagnostic Radiology, St Luke's Hosp 1984; **Fellow:** Pediatric Radiology, Milwaukee Chldn's Hosp 1985; **Fac Appt:** Assoc Prof Rad, Univ Wisc

Great Plains and Mountains

Dodd III, Gerald Dewey MD [DR] - **Spec Exp:** Ultrasound; **Hospital:** Univ Colorado Hosp; **Address:** 12401 E 17th Ave, MS L954, Aurora, CO 80045; **Phone:** 720-848-6608; **Board Cert:** Diagnostic Radiology 1987; **Med School:** Univ Tex, Houston 1983; **Resid:** Diagnostic Radiology, Univ Hosp 1987; **Fellow:** Abdominal Imaging & Angio-Interventional, Univ Hosp 1988; **Fac Appt:** Prof, Univ Tex, San Antonio

Southwest

Harolds, Jay A MD [DR] - **Hospital:** Integris Baptist Med Ctr - OK; **Address:** Integris Baptist Medical Ctr, Radiology, 3300 Northwest Expressway, Oklahoma City, OK 73112; **Phone:** 405-949-3202; **Board Cert:** Diagnostic Radiology 1975; Nuclear Radiology 1979; Nuclear Medicine 1980; **Med School:** SUNY Buffalo 1971; **Resid:** Diagnostic Radiology, Georgetown Univ Hosps 1975; Nuclear Medicine, Vanderbilt Univ Hosps 1980

Huynh, Phan Tuong MD [DR] - **Spec Exp:** Mammography; Breast Cancer; **Hospital:** St Luke's Episcopal Hosp - Houston; **Address:** 6624 Fannin St, St Luke's Tower, Women's Ctr Fl 10, Houston, TX 77030; **Phone:** 832-355-8130; **Board Cert:** Diagnostic Radiology 1994; **Med School:** Univ VA Sch Med 1989; **Resid:** Diagnostic Radiology, Univ Virginia Med Ctr 1994; **Fellow:** Mammography, Univ Virginia 1995; **Fac Appt:** Assoc Clin Prof Rad, Baylor Coll Med

Otto, Pamela MD [DR] - **Spec Exp:** Breast Imaging; **Hospital:** Univ Hlth Sys - Univ Hosp (San Antonio, TX), Audie L Murphy Meml Vets Hosp; **Address:** 7703 Floyd Curl Drive, MC 7800, San Antonio, TX 78229-3900; **Phone:** 210-450-5050; **Board Cert:** Diagnostic Radiology 1993; **Med School:** Univ MO-Columbia Sch Med 1988; **Resid:** Diagnostic Radiology, Univ Texas Hlth Sci Ctr 1993; **Fellow:** Breast Imaging, Univ Texas Hlth Sci Ctr 1993; **Fac Appt:** Assoc Prof Rad, Univ Tex, San Antonio

West Coast and Pacific

Bassett, Lawrence W MD [DR] - **Spec Exp:** Breast Imaging; **Hospital:** Ronald Reagan UCLA Med Ctr; **Address:** 200 UCLA Med Plaza, rm 165-47, Los Angeles, CA 90095; **Phone:** 310-206-9608; **Board Cert:** Diagnostic Radiology 1975; **Med School:** UC Irvine 1968; **Resid:** Diagnostic Radiology, UCLA Med Ctr 1972; **Fac Appt:** Prof, UCLA

Feig, Stephen A MD [DR] - **Spec Exp:** Breast Imaging; Breast Cancer; **Hospital:** UC Irvine Med Ctr; **Address:** 101 The City Drive S, Rte 140, Orange, CA 92868-3298; **Phone:** 714-456-6905; **Board Cert:** Diagnostic Radiology 1972; **Med School:** NYU Sch Med 1967; **Resid:** Radiology, Bronx Muni Hosp 1971; **Fac Appt:** Prof Rad, UC Irvine

Filly, Roy A MD [DR] - **Spec Exp:** Obstetric Ultrasound; **Hospital:** UCSF Med Ctr; **Address:** UCSF Med Ctr, Dept Diagnostic Radiology, 505 Parnassus Ave, Box 0628, San Francisco, CA 94143-0628; **Phone:** 415-353-1628; **Board Cert:** Diagnostic Radiology 1974; **Med School:** Ohio State Univ 1970; **Resid:** Diagnostic Radiology, Stanford Univ Med Ctr 1974; **Fac Appt:** Prof Rad, UCSF

Gilsanz, Vicente MD [DR] - **Spec Exp:** Pediatric Radiology; Bone Disorders-Metabolic; **Hospital:** Chldns Hosp - Los Angeles; **Address:** Children's Hospital, LA, 4650 Sunset Blvd, MS 81, Los Angeles, CA 90027; **Phone:** 323-361-4571; **Board Cert:** Internal Medicine 1973; Diagnostic Radiology 1976; Pediatric Radiology 2004; **Med School:** Spain 1969; **Resid:** Internal Medicine, Mayo Clinic 1973; Diagnostic Radiology, Mt Sinai Hosp 1976; **Fellow:** Pediatric Radiology, Childrens Hosp 1978; **Fac Appt:** Prof Rad, USC Sch Med

Lehman, Constance D MD/PhD [DR] - **Spec Exp:** Breast Imaging; **Hospital:** Univ Wash Med Ctr; **Address:** Seattle Cancer Care Alliance, 825 Eastlake Ave E, rm G2600, Seattle, WA 98109-1023; **Phone:** 206-288-2046; **Board Cert:** Diagnostic Radiology 1995; **Med School:** Yale Univ 1990; **Resid:** Diagnostic Radiology, Univ Wash Med Ctr 1995; **Fellow:** Diagnostic Radiology, Univ Wash Med Ctr 1996; **Fac Appt:** Prof Rad, Univ Wash

Rubin, Geoffrey D MD [DR] - **Spec Exp:** Cardiovascular Imaging; Cardiac Imaging; Thoracic Imaging; **Hospital:** Stanford Univ Med Ctr; **Address:** Stanford Univ Med Ctr, 300 Pasteur Drive, rm S 072, MC 5105, Stanford, CA 94305; **Phone:** 650-723-7647; **Board Cert:** Diagnostic Radiology 1992; **Med School:** UCSD 1987; **Resid:** Diagnostic Radiology, Stanford Univ Med Ctr 1992; **Fellow:** Body Imaging, Stanford Univ Med Ctr 1993; **Fac Appt:** Prof Rad, Stanford Univ

Thurmond, Amy S MD [DR] - **Spec Exp:** Women's Imaging; Infertility-Fallopian Tube Intervention; Women's Gynecological Health; **Hospital:** OR Hlth & Sci Univ; **Address:** 8950 SW Nimbus Ave, Beaverton, OR 97008; **Phone:** 503-643-7226; **Board Cert:** Diagnostic Radiology 1987; **Med School:** UCLA 1982; **Resid:** Cardiovascular Disease, St Vincent Hosp Med Ctr 1984; Diagnostic Radiology, Oreg Hlth Scis Univ 1987; **Fellow:** Interventional Radiology, Oreg Hlth Scis Univ 1988; **Fac Appt:** Assoc Prof, Oregon Hlth Sci Univ

Diagnostic Radiology

Wood, Beverly MD/PhD [DR] - **Spec Exp:** Pediatric Radiology; **Hospital:** LAC & USC Med Ctr, Loma Linda Chldns Hosp; **Address:** Loma Linda Univ Chldns Hosp, Div Pediatric Radiology, 11234 Anderson St, rm 2835, Loma Linda, CA 92354; **Phone:** 909-558-4281; **Board Cert:** Diagnostic Radiology 1972; Pediatric Radiology 2003; **Med School:** Univ Rochester 1965; **Resid:** Diagnostic Radiology, Strong Meml Hosp 1971; **Fellow:** Pediatric Radiology, Strong Meml Hosp 1972; **Fac Appt:** Prof Rad, USC Sch Med

NEURORADIOLOGY

New England

Curtin, Hugh D MD [NRad] - **Spec Exp:** Head & Neck Radiology; **Hospital:** Mass Eye & Ear Infirmary; **Address:** Mass Eye & Ear Infirmary, Dept Radiology, 243 Charles St Fl 6, Boston, MA 02114; **Phone:** 617-573-3563 x4; **Board Cert:** Diagnostic Radiology 1976; Neuroradiology 1999; **Med School:** SUNY Upstate Med Univ 1972; **Resid:** Diagnostic Radiology, Presbyterian Univ Hosp 1976; **Fellow:** Neuroradiology, Foundation Rothschild; **Fac Appt:** Prof, Harvard Med Sch

Hackney, David B MD [NRad] - **Hospital:** Beth Israel Deaconess Med Ctr - Boston; **Address:** BIDMC, Dept Radiology, 330 Brookline Ave, Boston, MA 02215; **Phone:** 617-754-2009; **Board Cert:** Diagnostic Radiology 1984; Neuroradiology 2005; **Med School:** Cornell Univ 1980; **Resid:** Diagnostic Radiology, UCSD Med Ctr 1983; **Fellow:** Neurological Radiology, Mass Genl Hosp 1985; **Fac Appt:** Prof Rad, Harvard Med Sch

Hirsch, Joshua A MD [NRad] - **Spec Exp:** Interventional Neuroradiology; Endovascular Surgery; Minimally Invasive Spinal Surgery; Osteoporosis Spine-Vertebroplasty; **Hospital:** Mass Genl Hosp; **Address:** Mass Genl Hospital, Interventional Neuroradiology, 55 Fruit St Gray Bldg - rm 241, Boston, MA 02114; **Phone:** 617-726-1767; **Board Cert:** Diagnostic Radiology 1996; **Med School:** Univ Pennsylvania 1991; **Resid:** Diagnostic Radiology, Hosp Univ Penn 1996; **Fellow:** Neuroradiology, Hosp Univ Penn 1995; Interventional Neuroradiology, Lahey Clinic 1998; **Fac Appt:** Asst Prof Rad, Harvard Med Sch

Norbash, Alexander M MD [NRad] - **Spec Exp:** Interventional Neuroradiology; Aneurysm-Cerebral; Osteoporosis Spine-Kyphoplasty; **Hospital:** Boston Med Ctr; **Address:** BMC, Dept Radiology, 88 E Newton St Fl 2, Boston, MA 02118; **Phone:** 617-638-6610; **Board Cert:** Diagnostic Radiology 1991; Neuroradiology 2004; **Med School:** Univ MO-Kansas City 1986; **Resid:** Diagnostic Radiology, St Francis Hosp 1990; Diagnostic Radiology, Presby Univ Hosp 1991; **Fellow:** Neurological Radiology, Stanford Univ Hosp 1993; Interventional Radiology, Stanford Univ Hosp 1994; **Fac Appt:** Prof, Boston Univ

Mid Atlantic

Berenstein, Alejandro MD [NRad] - **Spec Exp:** Interventional Neuroradiology; Aneurysm-Cerebral; Endovascular Surgery; **Hospital:** St Luke's - Roosevelt Hosp Ctr - Roosevelt Div (page 57); **Address:** Hyman-Newman Inst Neurolgy & Neuro Surg, 1000 10th Ave, rm GG16, New York, NY 10019; **Phone:** 212-636-3400; **Board Cert:** Diagnostic Radiology 1976; **Med School:** Mexico 1970; **Resid:** Diagnostic Radiology, Mount Sinai Med Ctr 1976; **Fellow:** Neuroradiology, NYU Med Ctr 1978; **Fac Appt:** Prof Rad, NYU Sch Med

Drayer, Burton P MD [NRad] - **Spec Exp:** Stroke; Parkinson's Disease/Aging Brain; MRI & CT of Brain & Spine; **Hospital:** Mount Sinai Med Ctr (page 64); **Address:** 1 Gustave Levy Pl, Box 1234, New York, NY 10029; **Phone:** 212-241-6403; **Board Cert:** Neurology 1976; Diagnostic Radiology 1978; Neuroradiology 2006; **Med School:** Ros Franklin Univ/Chicago Med Sch 1971; **Resid:** Neurology, Univ Vt Med Ctr 1975; Diagnostic Radiology, Univ Pitt Hlth Ctr 1977; **Fellow:** Neuroradiology, Univ Pitt Hlth Ctr 1978; **Fac Appt:** Prof Rad, Mount Sinai Sch Med

Flanders, Adam E MD [NRad] - **Spec Exp:** Spinal Trauma; Head Injury; **Hospital:** Thomas Jefferson Univ Hosp; **Address:** 132 10th St, 1072 Main Bldg, Philadelphia, PA 19107; **Phone:** 215-955-2430; **Board Cert:** Diagnostic Radiology 1987; Neuroradiology 1996; **Med School:** Rush Med Coll 1983; **Resid:** Diagnostic Radiology, Univ Illinois Hosps 1987; **Fellow:** Neuroradiology, Thos Jefferson Univ Hosp; **Fac Appt:** Prof Rad, Thomas Jefferson Univ

Grossman, Robert I MD [NRad] - **Spec Exp:** Multiple Sclerosis Imaging; Brain Injury; MRI; **Hospital:** NYU Med Ctr (page 68), Bellevue Hosp Ctr; **Address:** NYU Med Ctr, Dept Radiology, 560 First Ave, RUSK 229, New York, NY 10016; **Phone:** 212-263-3269; **Board Cert:** Diagnostic Radiology 1979; Neuroradiology 2005; **Med School:** Univ Pennsylvania 1973; **Resid:** Neurological Surgery, Hosp Univ Penn 1976; Diagnostic Radiology, Hosp Univ Penn 1979; **Fellow:** Neuroradiology, Mass Genl Hosp 1981; **Fac Appt:** Prof Rad, NYU Sch Med

Hurst, Robert W MD [NRad] - **Spec Exp:** Interventional Neuroradiology; Aneurysm; Carotid Artery Stent Placement; Intracranial Angioplasty & Stent; **Hospital:** Hosp Univ Penn - UPHS (page 60); **Address:** Dept Radiology/Neuroradiology, HUP, 3400 Spruce St, Ground FL, Founders Bldg, Philadelphia, PA 19104; **Phone:** 215-662-3572; **Board Cert:** Neurology 1986; Diagnostic Radiology 1989; Neuroradiology 2005; **Med School:** Univ Tex, Houston 1981; **Resid:** Neurology, Univ Virginia Hosp 1985; Diagnostic Radiology, Univ Virginia Hosp 1989; **Fellow:** Neurological Radiology, Hosp Univ Penn 1990; Interventional Radiology, NYU Med Ctr 1991; **Fac Appt:** Prof Rad, Univ Pennsylvania

Khandji, Alexander G MD [NRad] - **Spec Exp:** Pituitary Disorders; Spinal Imaging; MRI; Brain Tumors; **Hospital:** NY-Presby Hosp/Columbia (page 66); **Address:** 177 Ft Washington Ave, Ste 4-156, New York, NY 10032-3173; **Phone:** 212-305-7669; **Board Cert:** Diagnostic Radiology 1985; Neuroradiology 2006; **Med School:** SUNY Downstate 1980; **Resid:** Surgery, MS Hershey Med Ctr 1982; Diagnostic Radiology, Columbia-Presby Med Ctr 1985; **Fellow:** Neuroradiology, Columbia-Presby Med Ctr 1987; **Fac Appt:** Clin Prof Rad, Columbia P&S

Litt, Andrew W MD [NRad] - **Spec Exp:** Vascular Lesions of the CNS; Cerebrovascular Disease; Stroke; **Hospital:** NYU Med Ctr (page 68); **Address:** NYU Medical Ctr, Dept Radiology, 560 1st Ave, IRM 232, New York, NY 10016-6402; **Phone:** 212-263-8121; **Board Cert:** Diagnostic Radiology 1988; Neuroradiology 2005; **Med School:** NYU Sch Med 1983; **Resid:** Diagnostic Radiology, NYU Med Ctr 1987; **Fellow:** Neuroradiology, NYU Med Ctr 1988; **Fac Appt:** Prof Rad, NYU Sch Med

Loevner, Laurie A MD [NRad] - **Spec Exp:** Head & Neck Surgery; **Hospital:** Hosp Univ Penn - UPHS (page 60); **Address:** Univ Penn Med Ctr-Dept Rad, 3400 Spruce St, Philadelphia, PA 19104; **Phone:** 215-662-3020; **Board Cert:** Diagnostic Radiology 1993; Neuroradiology 2006; **Med School:** Univ Pennsylvania 1988; **Resid:** Univ Michigan Hosps 1993; **Fellow:** Neuroradiology, Univ Penn Med Ctr 1995; **Fac Appt:** Clin Prof Rad, Univ Pennsylvania

Pile-Spellman, John MD [NRad] - **Spec Exp:** Interventional Neuroradiology; Cerebrovascular Disease; Aneurysm; Arteriovenous Malformations; **Hospital:** NY-Presby Hosp/Columbia (page 66); **Address:** 177 Fort Washington Ave, MHB 8SK, New York, NY 10032-3713; **Phone:** 212-305-6515; **Board Cert:** Diagnostic Radiology 1984; **Med School:** Tufts Univ 1978; **Resid:** Neurological Surgery, New England Med Ctr 1981; Neurological Radiology, Mass Genl Hosp 1984; **Fellow:** Interventional Neuroradiology, NYU Med Ctr 1986; **Fac Appt:** Prof Rad, Columbia P&S

Neuroradiology

Tenner, Michael MD [NRad] - **Spec Exp:** Stroke; Aneurysm-Cerebral; Arteriovenous Malformations; Carotid Artery Stent Placement; **Hospital:** Westchester Med Ctr; **Address:** NY Med Coll, Dept Radiology, Route 100, Valhalla, NY 10595; **Phone:** 914-493-8158; **Board Cert:** Diagnostic Radiology 1967; Neuroradiology 2007; **Med School:** Univ MD Sch Med 1960; **Resid:** Diagnostic Radiology, Univ Maryland Hosp 1962; Diagnostic Radiology, Univ Maryland Hosp 1966; **Fellow:** Neuroradiology, Neurological Inst-Columbia Presby 1968; **Fac Appt:** Prof Rad, NY Med Coll

Vezina, L Gilbert MD [NRad] - **Spec Exp:** Pediatric Neuroradiology; Brain Tumors; Neurofibromatosis; **Hospital:** Chldns Natl Med Ctr; **Address:** Chldns Natl Med Ctr, Dept Radiology, 111 Michigan Ave NW, Washington, DC 20010-2970; **Phone:** 202-476-3651; **Board Cert:** Diagnostic Radiology 1987; Neuroradiology 1998; **Med School:** McGill Univ 1983; **Resid:** Diagnostic Radiology, Mass Genl Hosp 1987; **Fellow:** Neurological Radiology, Mass Genl Hosp 1989; Pediatric Neuroradiology, Chldns Natl Med Ctr 1991; **Fac Appt:** Prof, Geo Wash Univ

Yousem, David M MD [NRad] - **Hospital:** Johns Hopkins Hosp - Baltimore (page 61); **Address:** Johns Hopkins Hosp, Div Neuroradiology, 600 N Wolfe St Phipps Bldg - rm B-100, Baltimore, MD 21287; **Phone:** 410-955-2353; **Board Cert:** Diagnostic Radiology 1987; Neuroradiology 2005; **Med School:** Univ Mich Med Sch 1983; **Resid:** Diagnostic Radiology, Johns Hopkins Hosp 1987; **Fellow:** Neuroradiology, Hosp Univ Penn 1990; **Fac Appt:** Prof, Johns Hopkins Univ

Zimmerman, Robert A MD [NRad] - **Spec Exp:** Pediatric Neuroradiology; **Hospital:** Chldns Hosp of Philadelphia, The; **Address:** Childrens Hosp Philadelphia, Radiology, 34th St & Civic Center Blvd, Philadelphia, PA 19104; **Phone:** 215-590-2569; **Board Cert:** Diagnostic Radiology 1970; Neuroradiology 1995; **Med School:** Georgetown Univ 1964; **Resid:** Diagnostic Radiology, Hosp Univ Penn 1969; **Fac Appt:** Prof Rad, Univ Pennsylvania

Zinreich, S James MD [NRad] - **Spec Exp:** Head & Neck Radiology; **Hospital:** Johns Hopkins Hosp - Baltimore (page 61); **Address:** Johns Hopkins Hospital, 600 N Wolfe St Phipps Bldg - rm B-100, Baltimore, MD 21287; **Phone:** 410-614-3020; **Board Cert:** Diagnostic Radiology 1982; Neuroradiology 2006; **Med School:** Belgium 1976; **Resid:** Diagnostic Radiology, Sinai Hosp; **Fac Appt:** Prof Oto, Johns Hopkins Univ

Southeast

Dion, Jacques E MD [NRad] - **Spec Exp:** Stroke; Intracranial Angioplasty & Stent; Aneurysm-Cerebral; Osteoporosis Spine-Vertebroplasty; **Hospital:** Emory Univ Hosp; **Address:** Emory Univ Hosp, Dept Neuroradiology, 1364 Clifton Rd NE, rm A121, Atlanta, GA 30322; **Phone:** 404-712-4991; **Board Cert:** Diagnostic Radiology 1982; Neuroradiology 1998; **Med School:** Univ Ottawa 1978; **Resid:** Diagnostic Radiology, Harbor-UCLA Med Ctr 1981; Diagnostic Radiology, Notre Dame Hosp 1983; **Fellow:** Neuroradiology, Univ Hospital 1985; **Fac Appt:** Prof, Emory Univ

Jensen, Mary E MD [NRad] - **Spec Exp:** Interventional Neuroradiology; Osteoporosis Spine-Vertebroplasty; Aneurysm-Cerebral; **Hospital:** Univ Virginia Med Ctr; **Address:** Univ of Virginia Med Ctr, Dept Radiology, Box 800170, Charlottesville, VA 22908; **Phone:** 434-924-9719; **Board Cert:** Diagnostic Radiology 1987; **Med School:** Med Coll VA 1982; **Resid:** Diagnostic Radiology, Univ Virginia Med Ctr 1991; **Fellow:** Interventional Neuroradiology, UCLA Med Ctr 1992; **Fac Appt:** Assoc Prof, Univ VA Sch Med

Joseph, Gregory J MD [NRad] - **Spec Exp:** Stroke; Aneurysm-Cerebral; Intracranial Angioplasty & Stent; **Hospital:** Presby Hosp - Charlotte; **Address:** Presbyterian Hosp, Dept Radiology, 200 Hawthorne Ln, Charlotte, NC 28204; **Phone:** 704-384-9654; **Board Cert:** Diagnostic Radiology 1989; **Med School:** Georgetown Univ 1984; **Resid:** Diagnostic Radiology, Georgetown Univ Hosp 1989; Vascular & Interventional Radiology, Emory Univ Hosp 1990; **Fellow:** Neuroradiology, Emory Univ Hosp 1991

Murtagh, F Reed MD [NRad] - **Spec Exp:** Neuro-Oncology; Brain Tumor Imaging; Spinal Tumor Imaging; **Hospital:** H Lee Moffitt Cancer Ctr & Research Inst; **Address:** Univ Diagnostic Institute-USF, 3301 Alumni Drive, Tampa, FL 33612; **Phone:** 813-975-0725; **Board Cert:** Diagnostic Radiology 1978; Neuroradiology 2004; **Med School:** Temple Univ 1971; **Resid:** Diagnostic Radiology, Jackson Meml Hosp 1978; **Fellow:** Neurological Radiology, Univ Miami 1979; **Fac Appt:** Prof Rad, Univ S Fla Coll Med

Provenzale, James M MD [NRad] - **Spec Exp:** Brain Tumor Imaging; Multiple Sclerosis Imaging; Brain Imaging-Pediatric; **Hospital:** Duke Univ Med Ctr; **Address:** Duke University Medical Ctr, Dept Radiology, Box 3808, Durham, NC 27710; **Phone:** 919-684-7218; **Board Cert:** Neurology 1988; Diagnostic Radiology 1991; Neuroradiology 2001; **Med School:** Albany Med Coll 1983; **Resid:** Neurology, NC Memorial Hosp 1987; Diagnostic Radiology, Mass General Hosp 1991; **Fellow:** Neuroradiology, Mass General Hosp 1992; **Fac Appt:** Prof, Duke Univ

Quencer, Robert MD [NRad] - **Spec Exp:** Spinal Cord Injury; **Hospital:** Univ of Miami Hosp & Clins/Sylvester Comp Canc Ctr, Jackson Meml Hosp; **Address:** Univ Miami, Dept Radiology, 1150 NW 14th St, Ste 511, M828, Miami, FL 33136-2116; **Phone:** 305-243-4701; **Board Cert:** Diagnostic Radiology 1972; Neuroradiology 1995; **Med School:** SUNY Upstate Med Univ 1967; **Resid:** Diagnostic Radiology, Columbia-Presbyterian Med Ctr 1971; **Fellow:** Neuroradiology, Neurological Inst 1972; **Fac Appt:** Prof, Univ Miami Sch Med

Midwest

Ball Jr, William S MD [NRad] - **Spec Exp:** Pediatric Neuroradiology; **Hospital:** Cincinnati Chldns Hosp Med Ctr; **Address:** Cincinnati Chldns Hosp, Dept Neuroradiology, 3333 Burnet Ave, ML 5031, Cincinnati, OH 45229-3039; **Phone:** 513-636-8574; **Board Cert:** Diagnostic Radiology 1982; Pediatrics 1982; Neuroradiology 1999; **Med School:** Tulane Univ 1974; **Resid:** Pediatrics, Oschner Fdn Hosp 1977; Diagnostic Radiology, Univ New Mexico 1978; **Fellow:** Pediatric Radiology, Chldns Hosp Med Ctr 1981; Neuroradiology, Univ New Mexico Med Ctr 1979; **Fac Appt:** Prof, Univ Cincinnati

Cross III, DeWitte T MD [NRad] - **Spec Exp:** Interventional Neuroradiology; Aneurysm-Cerebral; Stroke; **Hospital:** Barnes-Jewish Hosp, St Louis Chldns Hosp; **Address:** Wash Univ, Dept Radiology, 510 S Kingshighway Blvd, Box 8131, St Louis, MO 63110-1016; **Phone:** 314-362-5580; **Board Cert:** Diagnostic Radiology 1985; Neuroradiology 2006; **Med School:** Univ Ala 1980; **Resid:** Diagnostic Radiology, Naval Hosp 1985; **Fellow:** Neuroradiology, NY Med Coll 1988; Neuroradiology, Columbia Univ 1989; **Fac Appt:** Assoc Prof Rad, Washington Univ, St Louis

Haughton III, Victor M MD [NRad] - **Spec Exp:** Spinal Imaging; **Hospital:** Univ WI Hosp & Clins; **Address:** Univ WI Hosps & Clins, Dept Radiology, 600 Highland Ave, MC 3252, Madison, WI 53792; **Phone:** 608-263-9179; **Board Cert:** Diagnostic Radiology 1974; Neuroradiology 1995; **Med School:** Yale Univ 1967; **Resid:** Diagnostic Radiology, Peter Bent Brigham Hosp 1973; **Fellow:** Neurological Radiology, Peter Bent Brigham Hosp 1974; **Fac Appt:** Prof Rad, Univ Wisc

Kallmes, David F MD [NRad] - **Spec Exp:** Aneurysm-Cerebral; Stroke; Osteoporosis Spine-Vertebroplasty; **Hospital:** Mayo Med Ctr & Clin - Rochester; **Address:** Mayo Clinic, Old Marion Hall, 200 First St SW, Rochester, MN 55905; **Phone:** 507-255-5032; **Board Cert:** Diagnostic Radiology 1994; Neuroradiology 1998; **Med School:** Univ Mass Sch Med 1989; **Resid:** Diagnostic Radiology, Duke Univ Med Ctr 1993; **Fellow:** Neuroradiology, Univ Virginia Med Ctr 1995; **Fac Appt:** Assoc Prof Rad, Mayo Med Sch

Neuroradiology

Koeller, Kelly K MD [NRad] - **Spec Exp:** Brain Tumor Imaging; Head & Neck Tumors; Spinal Tumor Imaging; **Hospital:** Mayo Med Ctr & Clin - Rochester; **Address:** Mayo Clinic, 200 First St SW Charlton Bldg - rm 2-290, Rochester, MN 55905; **Phone:** 507-266-3412; **Board Cert:** Diagnostic Radiology 1990; Neuroradiology 2004; **Med School:** Univ Tenn Coll Med, Memphis 1982; **Resid:** Diagnostic Radiology, Naval Hosp 1990; **Fellow:** Neuroradiology, UCSF Med Ctr 1992

Masaryk, Thomas MD [NRad] - **Spec Exp:** Cerebrovascular Disease; Aneurysm-Cerebral; Vascular Lesions of the CNS; Carotid Artery Stent Placement; **Hospital:** Cleveland Clin Fdn (page 56); **Address:** Dept Radiology, 9500 Euclid Ave, MS L10, Cleveland, OH 44195; **Phone:** 216-444-6653; **Board Cert:** Diagnostic Radiology 1985; Neuroradiology 2005; **Med School:** Med Coll OH 1981; **Resid:** Diagnostic Radiology, Cleveland Clinic 1984; **Fellow:** Neurological Radiology, Cleveland Clinic 1985

Modic, Michael MD [NRad] - **Spec Exp:** MRI; Spinal Imaging; **Hospital:** Cleveland Clin Fdn (page 56); **Address:** 9500 Euclid Ave, Desk P34, Cleveland, OH 44195; **Phone:** 216-444-9308; **Board Cert:** Diagnostic Radiology 1979; Neuroradiology 2003; **Med School:** Case West Res Univ 1975; **Resid:** Diagnostic Radiology, Cleveland Clinic 1978; **Fellow:** Neuroradiology, Cleveland Clinic 1979; **Fac Appt:** Prof Rad, Ohio State Univ

Moran, Christopher J MD [NRad] - **Spec Exp:** Aneurysm-Cerebral; Cerebrovascular Disease/Stroke; Carotid Artery Stent Placement; Interventional Neuroradiology; **Hospital:** Barnes-Jewish Hosp; **Address:** Mallinckrodt Inst Radiology, Wash Univ Sch Med, Campus Box 8131, 510 S Kings Highway Blvd, St Louis, MO 63110; **Phone:** 314-362-5949; **Board Cert:** Diagnostic Radiology 1978; Neuroradiology 2004; **Med School:** St Louis Univ 1974; **Resid:** Diagnostic Radiology, Mallinckrodt Inst Rad/Wash U 1978; **Fellow:** Neuroradiology, Mallinckrodt Inst Rad/Wash U 1979; **Fac Appt:** Prof, Washington Univ, St Louis

Mukherji, Suresh K MD [NRad] - **Spec Exp:** Head & Neck Imaging; Head & Neck Tumors Imaging; **Hospital:** Univ Michigan Hlth Sys; **Address:** Univ of Michigan-Dept Radiology, 1500 E Medical Ctr Drive, UH-B2A209B, Ann Arbor, MI 48109-0030; **Phone:** 734-936-8865; **Board Cert:** Diagnostic Radiology 1992; Neuroradiology 2006; **Med School:** Georgetown Univ 1987; **Resid:** Diagnostic Radiology, Brigham & Women's Hosp 1992; **Fellow:** Neuroradiology, Univ Florida 1994; **Fac Appt:** Prof Oto, Univ Mich Med Sch

Rowley, Howard A MD [NRad] - **Spec Exp:** Epilepsy; Cerebrovascular Disease/Stroke; **Hospital:** Univ WI Hosp & Clins; **Address:** Univ WI Hosp & Clins, Dept Rad, 600 Highland Ave, MC 3252, Madison, WI 53792; **Phone:** 608-263-9179; **Board Cert:** Neurology 1991; Diagnostic Radiology 1993; Neuroradiology 2007; **Med School:** Washington Univ, St Louis 1985; **Resid:** Neurology, UCSF Med Ctr 1989; Diagnostic Radiology, UCSF Med Ctr 1991; **Fellow:** Neurological Radiology, UCSF Med Ctr; **Fac Appt:** Prof, Univ Wisc

Great Plains and Mountains

Osborn, Anne G MD [NRad] - **Spec Exp:** Spinal Imaging; Brain Imaging; Head & Neck Radiology; **Hospital:** Univ Utah Hosps and Clins; **Address:** Univ Utah Med Ctr, Dept Radiology, 30 N 1900 E, rm 1A71, Salt Lake City, UT 84132-2140; **Phone:** 801-581-7553; **Board Cert:** Diagnostic Radiology 1974; Neuroradiology 2004; **Med School:** Stanford Univ 1970; **Resid:** Diagnostic Radiology, Stanford Univ Hosp 1974; **Fellow:** Diagnostic Radiology, Univ Utah Hosp 1977; **Fac Appt:** Prof, Univ Utah

Southwest

Hunter, Jill V MD [NRad] - **Spec Exp:** Pediatric Neuroradiology; Brain Injury-Pediatric; **Hospital:** Texas Chldns Hosp - Houston; **Address:** 6621 Fannin, West Twr, Ste B120, MC 2-2521, Houston, TX 77030; **Phone:** 832-822-5324; **Board Cert:** Diagnostic Radiology 1997; Neuroradiology 1998; **Med School:** England 1975; **Resid:** Diagnostic Radiology, Baylor Coll Med 1978; **Fellow:** Neuroradiology, Queen Square Hosp 1992; **Fac Appt:** Assoc Prof Rad, Baylor Coll Med

Mawad, Michel E MD [NRad] - **Spec Exp:** Interventional Neuroradiology; **Hospital:** St Luke's Episcopal Hosp - Houston; **Address:** BCM Neurovascular, 6720 Bertner Ave, MC 4267, Houston, TX 77030; **Phone:** 713-798-2200; **Board Cert:** Diagnostic Radiology 1980; Neuroradiology 1995; **Med School:** Lebanon 1976; **Resid:** Diagnostic Radiology, St Luke's-Roosevelt Hosp 1979; **Fellow:** Neurological Radiology, Columbia-Presby Med Ctr 1980; **Fac Appt:** Prof, Baylor Coll Med

West Coast and Pacific

Atlas, Scott W MD [NRad] - **Spec Exp:** Stroke; MRI; Brain Tumors; **Hospital:** Stanford Univ Med Ctr; **Address:** Stanford Univ Med Ctr, Dept Rad, 300 Pasteur Drive, rm S-047, Stanford, CA 94304-2204; **Phone:** 650-498-7152; **Board Cert:** Diagnostic Radiology 1985; Neuroradiology 2005; **Med School:** Univ Chicago-Pritzker Sch Med 1981; **Resid:** Diagnostic Radiology, Northwestern Univ Med Ctr 1985; **Fellow:** Neuroradiology, Hosp Univ Pennsylvania 1987; **Fac Appt:** Prof, Stanford Univ

Barkovich, A James MD [NRad] - **Spec Exp:** Pediatric Neuroradiology; MRI; Brain Development Abnormalities; **Hospital:** UCSF Med Ctr; **Address:** UCSF Med Ctr, Dept Neuroradiology, 505 Parnassus Ave, rm L361, Box 0628, San Francisco, CA 94143-0628; **Phone:** 415-353-1655; **Board Cert:** Diagnostic Radiology 1984; Neuroradiology 2006; **Med School:** Geo Wash Univ 1980; **Resid:** Diagnostic Radiology, Letterman AMC 1984; **Fellow:** Neuroradiology, Walter Reed AMC 1986; **Fac Appt:** Prof Rad, UCSF

Barnes, Patrick D MD [NRad] - **Spec Exp:** Pediatric Neuroradiology; Brain Injury-Pediatric; Brain Development Abnormalities; Fetal Neuroradiology; **Hospital:** Lucile Packard Chldns Hosp/Stanford Univ Med Ctr; **Address:** Lucile Packard Chldns Hosp, Pediatric Neuroradiology, 725 Welch Rd, Palo Alto, CA 94304; **Phone:** 650-497-8376; **Board Cert:** Diagnostic Radiology 1977; **Med School:** Univ Okla Coll Med 1973; **Resid:** Diagnostic Radiology, Univ Okla Coll Med 1976; **Fellow:** Pediatric Neuroradiology, Chldns Hosp/Harvard Med Sch 1977; **Fac Appt:** Assoc Prof, Stanford Univ

Dillon, William P MD [NRad] - **Spec Exp:** Brain Tumors; **Hospital:** UCSF Med Ctr; **Address:** 505 Parnassus Ave, rm L 371, San Francisco, CA 94143-0628; **Phone:** 415-353-1668; **Board Cert:** Diagnostic Radiology 1982; Neuroradiology 2006; **Med School:** Loyola Univ-Stritch Sch Med 1978; **Resid:** Diagnostic Radiology, Univ Utah Hosp 1982; **Fellow:** Neuroradiology, UCSF Med Ctr 1983; **Fac Appt:** Prof, UCSF

Higashida, Randall T MD [NRad] - **Spec Exp:** Aneurysm-Cerebral; Stroke; Intracranial Angioplasty & Stent; **Hospital:** UCSF Med Ctr; **Address:** UCSF Med Ctr, Dept Interven Neurorad, 505 Parnassus Ave, rm L352, San Francisco, CA 94143-0628; **Phone:** 415-353-1863; **Board Cert:** Diagnostic Radiology 1984; **Med School:** Tulane Univ 1980; **Resid:** Diagnostic Radiology, UCLA Med Ctr 1984; **Fellow:** Neuroradiology, UCLA Med Ctr 1985; **Fac Appt:** Clin Prof, UCSF

Neuroradiology

Norman, David MD [NRad] - **Hospital:** UCSF Med Ctr; **Address:** UCSF Med Ctr, Dept Neuroradiology, 505 Parnassus Ave, rm L358, Box 0628, San Francisco, CA 94143-0628; **Phone:** 415-353-1668; **Board Cert:** Diagnostic Radiology 1972; Neuroradiology 2006; **Med School:** Univ Pennsylvania 1967; **Resid:** Diagnostic Radiology, Columbia-Presby Hosp 1971; **Fellow:** Neuroradiology, UCSF Med Ctr 1975; **Fac Appt:** Prof, UCSF

Teitelbaum, George P MD [NRad] - **Spec Exp:** Interventional Neuroradiology; Aneurysm-Cerebral; Carotid Artery Stent Placement; **Hospital:** USC Univ Hosp - R K Eamer Med Plz; **Address:** 1520 San Pablo St, Ste 3800, Los Angeles, CA 90033; **Phone:** 626-351-3369; **Board Cert:** Diagnostic Radiology 1984; **Med School:** UCSD 1980; **Resid:** Diagnostic Radiology, UC Irvine Med Ctr 1984; Interventional Radiology, George Washington 1985; **Fellow:** Magnetic Resonance Imaging, Huntington Med Research Inst 1988; UCSF Med Ctr 1994; **Fac Appt:** Prof NS, USC Sch Med

Vinuela, Fernando MD [NRad] - **Spec Exp:** Stroke; Intracranial Angioplasty & Stent; Aneurysm-Cerebral; **Hospital:** Ronald Reagan UCLA Med Ctr; **Address:** 757 West Wood Plaza, MC 743730, Los Angeles, CA 90095; **Phone:** 310-267-8765; **Board Cert:** Diagnostic Radiology 1979; **Med School:** Uruguay 1970; **Resid:** Diagnostic Radiology, Westminster Hosp 1975; Diagnostic Radiology, Victoria Hosp 1977; **Fellow:** Neuroradiology, Univ Hosp 1979; **Fac Appt:** Prof, UCLA

VASCULAR & INTERVENTIONAL RADIOLOGY

New England

Hallisey, Michael J MD [VIR] - **Spec Exp:** Uterine Fibroid Embolization; Liver Cancer/Chemoembolization; **Hospital:** Hartford Hosp; **Address:** 85 Seymour St, Ste 200, Hartford, CT 06106; **Phone:** 860-246-6589; **Board Cert:** Diagnostic Radiology 1991; Vascular & Interventional Radiology 1998; **Med School:** Univ Conn 1987; **Resid:** Diagnostic Radiology, Hospital of St Raphael 1991

Murphy, Timothy P MD [VIR] - **Spec Exp:** Uterine Fibroid Embolization; Aneurysm-Aortic; Hypertension-Renovascular; **Hospital:** Rhode Island Hosp; **Address:** Rhode Island Hospital, Dept Radiology, 593 Eddy Street, Providence, RI 02903-4970; **Phone:** 401-444-5194; **Board Cert:** Diagnostic Radiology 1992; Vascular & Interventional Radiology 2005; **Med School:** Boston Univ 1987; **Resid:** Diagnostic Radiology, Rhode Island Hosp 1992; **Fellow:** Vascular & Interventional Radiology, Rhode Island Hosp 1993; **Fac Appt:** Prof Rad, Brown Univ

White, Robert I MD [VIR] - **Spec Exp:** Uterine Fibroid Embolization; Pelvic Congestion Syndrome; Varicocele Embolization; Vascular Malformations; **Hospital:** Yale-New Haven Hosp; **Address:** Yale Univ Sch Med, Vasc & Interventional Rad, PO Box 208042, New Haven, CT 06520-8042; **Phone:** 203-737-5395; **Board Cert:** Diagnostic Radiology 1970; **Med School:** Baylor Coll Med 1963; **Resid:** Diagnostic Radiology, Johns Hopkins Hosp 1969; **Fellow:** Cardiovascular Disease, Johns Hopkins Hospital 1958; Cardiovascular Radiology, Univ Minn Medical Ctr 1971; **Fac Appt:** Prof Rad, Yale Univ

Mid Atlantic

Geschwind, Jean-Francois H MD [VIR] - **Spec Exp:** Liver Cancer/Chemoembolization; Cancer Chemoembolization; Cancer Radiotherapy; **Hospital:** Johns Hopkins Hosp - Baltimore (page 61); **Address:** Interventional Radiology, 600 N Wolfe St Blalock Bldg - rm 545, Baltimore, MD 21287; **Phone:** 410-955-6358; **Board Cert:** Diagnostic Radiology 1998; **Med School:** Boston Univ 1991; **Resid:** Diagnostic Radiology, UCSF Med Ctr 1996; **Fellow:** Interventional Radiology, Johns Hopkins Hosp 1998; **Fac Appt:** Assoc Prof, Johns Hopkins Univ

Haskal, Ziv MD [VIR] - **Spec Exp:** Uterine Fibroid Embolization; Vascular Malformations; Liver Cancer/Chemoembolization; **Hospital:** NY-Presby Hosp/Columbia (page 66); **Address:** Director, Div Interventional Radiology, 177 Fort Washington Ave, Ste MHB 4-100, New York, NY 10032; **Phone:** 212-305-8070; **Board Cert:** Diagnostic Radiology 1991; Vascular & Interventional Radiology 1999; **Med School:** Boston Univ 1986; **Resid:** Diagnostic Radiology, UCSF Med Ctr 1991; **Fellow:** Vascular & Interventional Radiology, UCSF Med Ctr 1992; **Fac Appt:** Prof Rad, Columbia P&S

McLean, Gordon K MD [VIR] - **Spec Exp:** Uterine Fibroid Embolization; Angioplasty & Stent Placement; **Hospital:** Western Penn Hosp; **Address:** Western Pennsylvania Hosp, Dept Radiology, 4800 Friendship Ave, Pittsburgh, PA 15224-1722; **Phone:** 412-578-7412; **Board Cert:** Diagnostic Radiology 1979; Vascular & Interventional Radiology 2005; **Med School:** Dartmouth Med Sch 1975; **Resid:** Diagnostic Radiology, Hosp Univ Penn 1979; **Fellow:** Angiography, Hosp Univ Penn 1980; **Fac Appt:** Prof, Univ Pennsylvania

Shlansky-Goldberg, Richard MD [VIR] - **Spec Exp:** Uterine Fibroid Embolization; Varicocele Embolization; Pelvic Congestion Syndrome; **Hospital:** Hosp Univ Penn - UPHS (page 60); **Address:** Hosp U Penn, Dept Radiology, 3400 Spruce St, 1 Silverstein Bldg, Philadelphia, PA 19104; **Phone:** 215-615-3541; **Board Cert:** Diagnostic Radiology 1989; Vascular & Interventional Radiology 1997; **Med School:** Univ Rochester 1984; **Resid:** Diagnostic Radiology, Thomas Jefferson Univ Hosp 1988; **Fac Appt:** Assoc Prof Rad, Univ Pennsylvania

Soulen, Michael C MD [VIR] - **Spec Exp:** Liver Cancer/Chemoembolization; Kidney Cancer; Radiofrequency Tumor Ablation; **Hospital:** Hosp Univ Penn - UPHS (page 60); **Address:** Hosp U Penn, Interventional Radiology, 3400 Spruce St, Philadelphia, PA 19104; **Phone:** 215-662-6839; **Board Cert:** Diagnostic Radiology 1989; Vascular & Interventional Radiology 1995; **Med School:** Univ Pennsylvania 1984; **Resid:** Diagnostic Radiology, Johns Hopkins Med Inst 1989; **Fellow:** Vascular & Interventional Radiology, Thomas Jefferson Univ Hosp 1991; **Fac Appt:** Prof Rad, Univ Pennsylvania

Sullivan, Kevin L MD [VIR] - **Hospital:** Thomas Jefferson Univ Hosp; **Address:** Thomas Jefferson Univ Hospital, Gibbon Bldg - Ste 4200, 111 S 11th St, Philadelphia, PA 19107; **Phone:** 215-955-6609; **Board Cert:** Diagnostic Radiology 1986; Vascular & Interventional Radiology 2005; **Med School:** UMDNJ-Rutgers Med Sch 1981; **Resid:** Radiology, Thomas Jefferson Univ 1986; **Fellow:** Diagnostic Radiology, Johns Hopkins Hosp 1988; **Fac Appt:** Assoc Prof Rad, Jefferson Med Coll

Trerotola, Scott O MD [VIR] - **Spec Exp:** Uterine Fibroid Embolization; Hereditary Hemorrhagic Telangiectasia; Varicocele Embolization; **Hospital:** Hosp Univ Penn - UPHS (page 60), Penn Presby Med Ctr - UPHS (page 60); **Address:** Hosp Univ Penn, Div Interventional Rad, 3400 Spruce St, 1 Silverstein, Philadelphia, PA 19104; **Phone:** 215-615-3540; **Board Cert:** Diagnostic Radiology 1991; Vascular & Interventional Radiology 2005; **Med School:** Univ Pennsylvania 1986; **Resid:** Diagnostic Radiology, Johns Hopkins Hosp 1991; **Fellow:** Vascular & Interventional Radiology, Johns Hopkins Hosp 1992; **Fac Appt:** Prof Rad, Univ Pennsylvania

Vascular & Interventional Radiology

Wood, Bradford J MD [VIR] - **Spec Exp:** Radiofrequency Tumor Ablation; Liver Cancer; Kidney Cancer; Gene Therapy Delivery Systems; **Hospital:** Natl Inst of Hlth - Clin Ctr; **Address:** National Inst Health, Bldg 10, 9000 Rockville Pike, msc 1182, Bethesda, MD 20892; **Phone:** 301-594-4511; **Board Cert:** Diagnostic Radiology 1996; Vascular & Interventional Radiology 2000; **Med School:** Univ VA Sch Med 1991; **Resid:** Diagnostic Radiology, Georgetown Univ Med Ctr 1996; **Fellow:** Abdominal/Interventional Radiology, Mass General Hosp 1997; **Fac Appt:** Asst Clin Prof Rad, Georgetown Univ

Southeast

Benenati, James F MD [VIR] - **Spec Exp:** Uterine Fibroid Embolization; Aneurysm-Abdominal Aortic; Peripheral Vascular Disease; **Hospital:** Baptist Hosp of Miami; **Address:** 8900 N Kendall Drive Fl 3, MC BCBI, Miami, FL 33176; **Phone:** 786-596-5990; **Board Cert:** Diagnostic Radiology 1988; Vascular & Interventional Radiology 2005; **Med School:** Univ S Fla Coll Med 1984; **Resid:** Diagnostic Radiology, Indiana Univ Hosp 1988; **Fellow:** Vascular & Interventional Radiology, Johns Hopkins Hosp 1989; **Fac Appt:** Prof Rad, Univ S Fla Coll Med

Bettmann, Michael A MD [VIR] - **Spec Exp:** Uterine Fibroid Embolization; Chemoembolization & Tumor Ablation; Carotid Artery Stent Placement; **Hospital:** Wake Forest Univ Baptist Med Ctr (page 73), Davis Reg Med Ctr; **Address:** Wake Forest Univ Sch Md - Radiology, Medical Center Blvd, Winston-Salem, NC 27157; **Phone:** 336-716-2463; **Board Cert:** Diagnostic Radiology 1975; Vascular & Interventional Radiology 2005; **Med School:** Albert Einstein Coll Med 1969; **Resid:** Diagnostic Radiology, Beth Israel Med Ctr-Harvard 1975; **Fellow:** Cardiovascular Radiology, Peter Bent Brigham Hosp-Harvard 1977; **Fac Appt:** Prof Rad, Wake Forest Univ

Hawkins Jr, Irvin MD [VIR] - **Hospital:** Shands at Univ of FL; **Address:** Shands at Univ of Florida, 1600 SW Archer Rd, Box 100374, Gainesville, FL 32608; **Phone:** 352-265-0116; **Board Cert:** Diagnostic Radiology 1969; **Med School:** Univ MD Sch Med 1962; **Resid:** Diagnostic Radiology, Ohio State Univ 1968; **Fellow:** Cardiovascular Radiology, Shands Tchg Hosps 1970; **Fac Appt:** Prof, Univ Fla Coll Med

Katzen, Barry T MD [VIR] - **Spec Exp:** Peripheral Vascular Disease; Aneurysm-Aortic; Carotid Artery Disease; **Hospital:** Baptist Hosp of Miami; **Address:** Baptist Cardiac & Vascular Inst, 8900 N Kendall Drive, Miami, FL 33176-2118; **Phone:** 786-596-5990; **Board Cert:** Diagnostic Radiology 1974; Vascular & Interventional Radiology 2004; **Med School:** Univ Miami Sch Med 1970; **Resid:** Diagnostic Radiology, New York Hosp-Cornell Med Ctr 1974

Lewis, Curtis A MD [VIR] - **Hospital:** Grady Hlth Sys, Emory Univ Hosp; **Address:** Grady Meml Hosp, Dept Rad, 56 Butler St SE, PO Box 26010, Atlanta, GA 30303; **Phone:** 404-616-6753; **Board Cert:** Diagnostic Radiology 1991; Vascular & Interventional Radiology 2007; **Med School:** Emory Univ 1986; **Resid:** Diagnostic Radiology, Emory Univ Affil Hosps 1991; **Fellow:** Interventional Radiology, Emory Univ Affil Hosps 1992; **Fac Appt:** Asst Prof Rad, Emory Univ

Mauro, Matthew MD [VIR] - **Spec Exp:** Cancer Chemoembolization; Cancer Radiotherapy; Gastrointestinal Cancer; **Hospital:** Univ NC Hosps; **Address:** University NC Hosps, Dept Radiology, CB 7510, 2006 Old Clinic Bldg, Chapel Hill, NC 27514; **Phone:** 919-966-4238; **Board Cert:** Diagnostic Radiology 1981; Vascular & Interventional Radiology 2003; **Med School:** Cornell Univ-Weill Med Coll 1977; **Resid:** Diagnostic Radiology, Univ NC Hosps 1981; **Fellow:** Interventional Radiology, Mallinckrodt Inst 1982; **Fac Appt:** Prof Rad, Univ NC Sch Med

Midwest

Cho, Kyung J MD [VIR] - **Spec Exp:** Chemoembolization & Tumor Ablation; Vascular Malformations; Peripheral Vascular Disease; **Hospital:** Univ Michigan Hlth Sys; **Address:** Univ Michigan Med Ctr, Dept Radiology, 1500 E Med Ctr Drive, CVC 5582, Ann Arbor, MI 48109-5868; **Phone:** 734-936-4466; **Board Cert:** Diagnostic Radiology 1974; Vascular & Interventional Radiology 2005; **Med School:** Korea 1966; **Resid:** Diagnostic Radiology, Wayne Med Ctr 1973; **Fellow:** Cardiovascular Radiology, Univ Michigan 1975; **Fac Appt:** Prof, Univ Mich Med Sch

Cragg, Andrew H MD [VIR] - **Spec Exp:** Uterine Fibroid Embolization; Aortic Stent Grafts; Endovascular Stent Grafts; **Hospital:** Univ Minn Med Ctr, Fairview - Riverside Campus, Fairview Southdale Hosp; **Address:** Minneapolis Vascular Clinic, 6405 France Ave S, Ste W440, Edina, MN 55435; **Phone:** 952-345-4179; **Board Cert:** Diagnostic Radiology 1986; Vascular & Interventional Radiology 1990; **Med School:** Univ Minn 1982; **Resid:** Diagnostic Radiology, Univ Minn Hosp 1986; **Fellow:** Interventional Radiology, Univ Minn Hosp 1987; **Fac Appt:** Prof, Univ Minn

Darcy, Michael MD [VIR] - **Spec Exp:** Portal Hypertension; Chemoembolization & Tumor Ablation; **Hospital:** Barnes-Jewish Hosp; **Address:** Washington Univ, Mallinckrodt Inst Radiology, 510 S Kingshighway Blvd, St Louis, MO 63110; **Phone:** 314-362-2900; **Board Cert:** Diagnostic Radiology 1985; Vascular & Interventional Radiology 2004; **Med School:** Ohio State Univ 1979; **Resid:** Surgery, Univ Minn Hosps 1982; Diagnostic Radiology, Univ Minn Hosps 1985; **Fellow:** Interventional Radiology, Univ Minn Hosps 1987; **Fac Appt:** Prof, Washington Univ, St Louis

Johnson, Matthew S MD [VIR] - **Spec Exp:** Vascular Disease; Uterine Fibroid Embolization; **Hospital:** Indiana Univ Hosp, Methodist Hosp - Indianapolis; **Address:** Indiana Univ Sch Med Dept Radiology, University Hosp, rm 0276, 550 N University Blvd, Indianapolis, IN 46202-5253; **Phone:** 317-274-1840; **Board Cert:** Diagnostic Radiology 1992; Vascular & Interventional Radiology 2006; **Med School:** Univ Mich Med Sch 1986; **Resid:** Surgery, Loyola Univ Med Ctr 1988; Diagnostic Radiology, Loyola Univ Med Ctr 1992; **Fellow:** Interventional Radiology, Johns Hopkins 1994; **Fac Appt:** Assoc Prof, Indiana Univ

Ketcham, Douglas B MD [VIR] - **Spec Exp:** Uterine Fibroid Embolization; Varicocele Embolization; Osteoporosis Spine-Vertebroplasty; **Hospital:** United Hosp, Regions Hosp - St Paul; **Address:** United Hospital, Dept Radiology, 333 N Smith Ave, St Paul, MN 55102; **Phone:** 651-241-8404; **Board Cert:** Diagnostic Radiology 1972; Vascular & Interventional Radiology 2005; **Med School:** Univ Wisc 1965; **Resid:** Diagnostic Radiology, Univ Minn Hosp 1971; **Fellow:** Neuroradiology, Univ Minn Hosp 1972

Nemcek, Albert A MD [VIR] - **Spec Exp:** Uterine Fibroid Embolization; Vascular Disease; **Hospital:** Northwestern Meml Hosp; **Address:** Northwestern Meml Hosp, 676 N St Clair St, Ste 800, Chicago, IL 60611; **Phone:** 312-926-5302; **Board Cert:** Diagnostic Radiology 1986; Vascular & Interventional Radiology 2005; **Med School:** UCSD 1982; **Resid:** Diagnostic Radiology, UCSD Med Ctr 1986; **Fellow:** Interventional Radiology, Northwestern Meml Hosp 1987; **Fac Appt:** Assoc Prof Rad, Northwestern Univ

Rilling, William S MD [VIR] - **Spec Exp:** Liver Cancer/Chemoembolization; Arteriovenous Malformations; Uterine Fibroid Embolization; **Hospital:** Froedtert Meml Lutheran Hosp; **Address:** Froedtert Hosp, Dept Radiology, 9200 W Wisconsin Ave, Milwaukee, WI 53226; **Phone:** 414-805-3028; **Board Cert:** Diagnostic Radiology 1995; Vascular & Interventional Radiology 1997; **Med School:** Univ Wisc 1990; **Resid:** Diagnostic Radiology, Univ Wisc Affil Hosps 1995; **Fellow:** Vascular & Interventional Radiology, Northwestern Meml Hosp 1996; **Fac Appt:** Assoc Prof, Univ Wisc

Vascular & Interventional Radiology

Salem, Riad MD [VIR] - **Spec Exp:** Cancer Radiotherapy; Cancer Chemoembolization; Liver Cancer/Chemoembolization; **Hospital:** Northwestern Meml Hosp; **Address:** Northwestern Univ Med Sch, Dept Radiology, 676 N St Clair St, Ste 800, Chicago, IL 60611; **Phone:** 312-695-0517; **Board Cert:** Diagnostic Radiology 1997; Vascular & Interventional Radiology 1999; **Med School:** McGill Univ 1993; **Resid:** Diagnostic Radiology, Geo Washington Univ Hosp 1997; **Fellow:** Interventional Radiology, Children's Hosp 1998; Interventional Radiology, Hosp U Penn 1998; **Fac Appt:** Asst Prof Rad, Northwestern Univ

Smith, Steven J MD [VIR] - **Spec Exp:** Angioplasty-Peripheral; Uterine Fibroid Embolization; Varicocele Embolization; **Hospital:** La Grange Meml Hosp; **Address:** 333 Chestnut St, Hinsdale, IL 60521; **Phone:** 630-856-7460; **Board Cert:** Diagnostic Radiology 1983; Vascular & Interventional Radiology 2006; **Med School:** Wayne State Univ 1979; **Resid:** Diagnostic Radiology, Henry Ford Hosp 1983; **Fellow:** Vascular & Interventional Radiology, Northwestern Meml Hosp 1984; **Fac Appt:** Assoc Clin Prof Rad, Northwestern Univ

Vogelzang, Robert MD [VIR] - **Spec Exp:** Uterine Fibroid Embolization; Varicocele Embolization; Vascular Malformations; **Hospital:** Northwestern Meml Hosp; **Address:** Northwestern Meml Hosp, Dept Rad, 251 E Huron, Chicago, IL 60611; **Phone:** 312-926-5113; **Board Cert:** Diagnostic Radiology 1981; Vascular & Interventional Radiology 2005; **Med School:** Ros Franklin Univ/Chicago Med Sch 1977; **Resid:** Diagnostic Radiology, Northwestern Meml Hosp 1982; **Fellow:** Interventional Radiology, Northwestern Meml Hosp; **Fac Appt:** Prof Rad, Northwestern Univ

Great Plains and Mountains

Durham, Janette D MD [VIR] - **Spec Exp:** Uterine Fibroid Embolization; Peripheral Vascular Disease; **Hospital:** Univ Colorado Hosp; **Address:** Univ Hosp, Dept Radiology, 4200 E Ninth Ave, Box A030, Denver, CO 80262; **Phone:** 720-848-7630; **Board Cert:** Diagnostic Radiology 1987; Vascular & Interventional Radiology 2006; **Med School:** Indiana Univ 1983; **Resid:** Diagnostic Radiology, Indiana Univ Hosp 1987; **Fellow:** Vascular & Interventional Radiology, Mass General Hosp 1988; **Fac Appt:** Assoc Prof, Univ Colorado

Kumpe, David A MD [VIR] - **Spec Exp:** Aneurysm-Cerebral; Stroke; Arterial & Venous Stents; Interventional Neuroradiology; **Hospital:** Univ Colorado Hosp; **Address:** Univ Hosp, Dept Radiology, 4200 E 9th Ave, Box A030, Denver, CO 80262; **Phone:** 720-848-7630; **Board Cert:** Diagnostic Radiology 1972; Vascular & Interventional Radiology 2005; **Med School:** Harvard Med Sch 1967; **Resid:** Diagnostic Radiology, Mass Genl Hosp 1971; **Fellow:** Neurological Radiology, Kantonsspital 1975; Angiography, Kantonsspital 1976; **Fac Appt:** Prof, Univ Colorado

Yakes, Wayne MD [VIR] - **Spec Exp:** Vascular Malformations; Interventional Neuroradiology; **Hospital:** Swedish Med Ctr - Englewood; **Address:** CNI, Vasc Malformation Ctr, 501 E Hampden Ave, Ste 4600, Englewood, CO 80113; **Phone:** 303-788-4280; **Board Cert:** Diagnostic Radiology 1983; Vascular & Interventional Radiology 1998; Neuroradiology 1999; **Med School:** Creighton Univ 1979; **Resid:** Diagnostic Radiology, Fitzsimons Med Ctr 1983; **Fellow:** Angiography, Walter Reed Med Ctr 1984; Interventional Neuroradiology, Baptist Hosp 1992; **Fac Appt:** Clin Prof, Univ Colorado

Southwest

Kay, Dennis MD [VIR] - **Spec Exp:** Diagnostic Radiology; **Hospital:** Ochsner Fdn Hosp; **Address:** Ochsner Clin, Dept Interventional Radiology, 1514 Jefferson Hwy, New Orleans, LA 70121-2429; **Phone:** 504-842-3470; **Board Cert:** Diagnostic Radiology 1986; Vascular & Interventional Radiology 2004; **Med School:** Tulane Univ 1981; **Resid:** Diagnostic Radiology, Ochsner Fdn Hosp 1985; **Fellow:** Vascular & Interventional Radiology, Beth Israel Hosp 1986; **Fac Appt:** Assoc Clin Prof, Tulane Univ

West Coast and Pacific

Dake, Michael D MD [VIR] - **Spec Exp:** Aortic Stent Grafts; Endovascular Stent Grafts; Vascular Disease; Aneurysm; **Hospital:** Stanford Univ Med Ctr; **Address:** Stanford Univ Cardiothoracic Surg, 300 Pasteur Drive, Falk Bldg, 2nd Fl, Stanford, CA 94305-5407; **Phone:** 605-724-0831; **Board Cert:** Internal Medicine 1981; Pulmonary Disease 1986; Vascular & Interventional Radiology 2006; **Med School:** Baylor Coll Med 1978; **Resid:** Internal Medicine, Baylor Hosp 1982; Diagnostic Radiology, UCSF Med Ctr 1986; **Fellow:** Pulmonary Disease, UCSF 1983; Interventional Radiology, UCSF 1987; **Fac Appt:** Prof TS, Stanford Univ

Gomes, Antoinette S MD [VIR] - **Spec Exp:** Cardiovascular Interventional Radiology; **Hospital:** Ronald Reagan UCLA Med Ctr; **Address:** Dept Radiological Sciences, Ronald Reagan UCLA Med Ctr, 757 Westwood Plaza, Ste 2125, Los Angeles, CA 90095; **Phone:** 310-267-8769; **Board Cert:** Diagnostic Radiology 1975; Vascular & Interventional Radiology 2004; **Med School:** Med Coll PA Hahnemann 1969; **Resid:** Internal Medicine, LAC-USC Med Ctr 1972; Diagnostic Radiology, Stanford Univ Med Ctr 1975; **Fellow:** Cardiovascular Radiology, UCLA Med Ctr 1976; Cardiovascular Radiology, Univ Minn 1978; **Fac Appt:** Prof Rad, UCLA

Goodwin, Scott C MD [VIR] - **Spec Exp:** Uterine Fibroid Embolization; Liver Cancer/Chemoembolization; **Hospital:** UC Irvine Med Ctr; **Address:** 101 The City Drive S, MC 5005, Route 140, Orange, CA 92868; **Phone:** 714-456-5033; **Board Cert:** Diagnostic Radiology 1989; Vascular & Interventional Radiology 1996; **Med School:** Harvard Med Sch 1984; **Resid:** Diagnostic Radiology, UCLA Medical Ctr 1988; **Fellow:** Vascular & Interventional Radiology, UCLA Medical Ctr 1989; **Fac Appt:** Prof, UCLA

Hovsepian, David M MD [VIR] - **Spec Exp:** Uterine Fibroid Embolization; Aneurysm-Aortic; Vascular Malformations-Pediatric; **Hospital:** Stanford Univ Med Ctr; **Address:** Interventional Radiology, 300 Pasteur Drive, rm H3651, Stanford, CA 94305-5642; **Phone:** 650-498-6022; **Board Cert:** Diagnostic Radiology 1991; Vascular & Interventional Radiology 2006; **Med School:** Columbia P&S 1986; **Resid:** Diagnostic Radiology, Columbia Presby Hosp 1991; **Fellow:** Interventional Radiology, Thomas Jefferson Univ Med Ctr 1993; **Fac Appt:** Prof Rad, Stanford Univ

Kaufman, John MD [VIR] - **Spec Exp:** Uterine Fibroid Embolization; Angioplasty & Stent Placement; **Hospital:** Dotter Institute - OHSU; **Address:** Dotter Interven Inst-OHSU Hosps & Clins, 3181 SW Sam Jackson Park Rd, MC L605, Portland, OR 97239; **Phone:** 503-494-7660; **Board Cert:** Diagnostic Radiology 1990; Vascular & Interventional Radiology 2005; **Med School:** Boston Univ 1982; **Resid:** Diagnostic Radiology, Boston Univ Med Ctr 1990; **Fellow:** Vascular & Interventional Radiology, Boston Univ Med Ctr 1991; **Fac Appt:** Prof Rad, Oregon Hlth Sci Univ

Keller, Frederick S MD [VIR] - **Spec Exp:** Uterine Fibroid Embolization; Arterial & Venous Stents; Urinary Tract Interventions; **Hospital:** OR Hlth & Sci Univ; **Address:** Dotter Interventional Inst, L-605, 3181 SW Sam Jackson Park Rd, Portland, OR 97239; **Phone:** 503-494-7660; **Board Cert:** Diagnostic Radiology 1977; Vascular & Interventional Radiology 2003; **Med School:** Univ Pennsylvania 1968; **Resid:** Diagnostic Radiology, Univ Oreg Hlth Scis Ctr 1977; **Fac Appt:** Prof, Oregon Hlth Sci Univ

Vascular & Interventional Radiology

McGahan, John P MD [VIR] - **Spec Exp:** Radiofrequency Tumor Ablation; Liver Cancer; Kidney Cancer; **Hospital:** UC Davis Med Ctr; **Address:** UC Davis Medical Ctr, Dept Radiology, 4860 Y St, Ste 3100, Sacramento, CA 95817; **Phone:** 916-734-3606; **Board Cert:** Diagnostic Radiology 1979; Vascular & Interventional Radiology 1995; **Med School:** Oregon Hlth Sci Univ 1974; **Resid:** Surgery, UC Davis Med Ctr 1976; Diagnostic Radiology, UC Davis Med Ctr 1979; **Fac Appt:** Prof Rad, UC Davis

Valji, Karim MD [VIR] - **Spec Exp:** Dialysis Access; **Hospital:** Univ Wash Med Ctr; **Address:** Univ of WA Med Ctr-Dept Rad, 1959 NE Pacific St, Box 375115, Seattle, WA 98195; **Phone:** 206-543-3320; **Board Cert:** Diagnostic Radiology 1989; Vascular & Interventional Radiology 1998; **Med School:** Harvard Med Sch 1982; **Resid:** Internal Medicine, UCSF Med Ctr 1984; Diagnostic Radiology, UCSD Med Ctr 1988; **Fellow:** Angiography, UCSD Med Ctr 1989; **Fac Appt:** Prof, Univ SD Sch Med

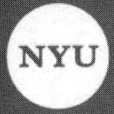
RADIOLOGY

The Diagnostic Core of Modern Medicine

LEADING EDGE TECHNOLOGY

The Department of Radiology at NYU Langone Medical Center is at the forefront of academic medicine and has some of the most advanced imaging equipment in the world, including:

-Dual source, dual energy multi-detector 64 slice CT
-Coronary Artery Disease and Virtual Colonoscopy screening programs
-Multi-channel MRI technology including two advanced state-of-the-art multi-channel 1.5 Tesla clinical scanners, two clinical/research 3-Tesla scanners and one 7-Tesla research scanner
-Advanced breast MR imaging
-High resolution I high sensitivity PET-CT
-Digital radiography
-Digital fluoroscopy
-Digital mammography
-Sterotactic biopsy capability
-Advanced digital subtraction angiography with 3D capability
-Minimally invasive techniques including radiofrequency ablation and chemoembolization
-State-of-the-art SPECT CT and SPECT gamma cameras
-Radioimmunotherapy
-Bone densitometry
-Cutting edge Medical Imaging Informatics and Radiology Information Systems

ON THE HORIZON

NYU Radiology is a leader in clinical care, research and education. Among Radiology Departments within Medical Schools, NYU is the 10th largest recipient of NIH research funding in the U.S. and first in New York.

A DRIVER OF CROSS-DISCIPLINARY CLINICAL EXCELLENCE

Radiology plays an increasingly pivotal role in medial, clinical, and translational research. With an explosion of imaging technologies, researchers at NYU are making rapid strides in the understanding of complex diseases. No longer merely a supportive discipline, radiology has been transformed into a dynamic driver of medical knowledge itself. For example, the new imaging technologies allow physicians to observe minute changes in tumor activity during cancer treatment, adjust the dosage accordingly, and monitor the disease process with a depth and precision that would have previously been unimaginable.

Reproductive Endocrinology
a subspecialty of Obstetrics & Gynecology

An obstetrician/gynecologist who is capable of managing complex problems relating to reproductive endocrinology and infertility.

Training Required: Four years *plus* two years in clinical practice before certification in obstetrics and gynecology is complete *plus* additional training and examination in reproductive endocrinology.

REPRODUCTIVE ENDOCRINOLOGY

New England

Carson, Sandra A MD [RE] - **Spec Exp:** Infertility-IVF; Laparoscopic Surgery; Endometriosis; Sexual Dysfunction; **Hospital:** Women & Infants Hosp of RI; **Address:** Women & Infants Hosp of RI, 101 Dudley St Fl 1, Providence, RI 02905; **Phone:** 401-274-1122 x8167; **Board Cert:** Obstetrics & Gynecology 2005; Reproductive Endocrinology 2005; **Med School:** Northwestern Univ 1977; **Resid:** Obstetrics & Gynecology, Prentice Womens Hosp 1981; **Fellow:** Reproductive Endocrinology, Michael Reese Hosp 1983; **Fac Appt:** Prof ObG, Brown Univ

Crowley, William F MD [RE] - **Spec Exp:** Pituitary Disorders; Kallmann's Syndrome; Fertility Preservation in Cancer; **Hospital:** Mass Genl Hosp; **Address:** Mass Genl Hosp, Reproductive Sci Ctr, 55 Fruit St, Bartlett Hall-Ext 5, Boston, MA 02114; **Phone:** 617-726-5390; **Board Cert:** Internal Medicine 1974; Endocrinology 1977; **Med School:** Tufts Univ 1969; **Resid:** Internal Medicine, Mass Genl Hosp 1971; Internal Medicine, Mass Genl Hosp 1974; **Fellow:** Endocrinology, Mass Genl Hosp 1976; **Fac Appt:** Prof Med, Harvard Med Sch

Ginsburg, Elizabeth MD [RE] - **Spec Exp:** Infertility-IVF; Fertility Preservation in Cancer; **Hospital:** Brigham & Women's Hosp, Dana-Farber Cancer Inst; **Address:** Brigham & Womens Hosp, Reproductive Med, 75 Francis St, Boston, MA 02115; **Phone:** 617-732-4222; **Board Cert:** Obstetrics & Gynecology 2006; Reproductive Endocrinology 2006; **Med School:** Mount Sinai Sch Med 1985; **Resid:** Obstetrics & Gynecology, Brigham & Womens Hosp 1989; **Fellow:** Reproductive Endocrinology, Brigham & Womens Hosp 1991

Hill III, Joseph A MD [RE] - **Spec Exp:** Miscarriage-Recurrent; Infertility-Female; Gynecology; **Hospital:** Portsmouth Regl Hosp, Winchester Hosp; **Address:** Fertility Ctr of New England, 330 Borthwick Ave, Ste 201, Portsmouth, NH 03801; **Phone:** 781-942-7000 x601; **Board Cert:** Obstetrics & Gynecology 2007; Reproductive Endocrinology 2007; **Med School:** Med Coll GA 1981; **Resid:** Obstetrics & Gynecology, Med Coll Ga 1985; **Fellow:** Reproductive Endocrinology, Brigham-Womens Hosp/Harvard 1987; Reproductive Immunology, Brigham-Womens Hosp/Harvard 1988; **Fac Appt:** Prof ObG, Harvard Med Sch

Hornstein, Mark D MD [RE] - **Spec Exp:** Infertility-IVF; Endometriosis; Laparoscopic Surgery; **Hospital:** Brigham & Women's Hosp, Newton - Wellesley Hosp; **Address:** Brigham & Women's Hospital, Center for Reproductive Medicine, 75 Francis St, Boston, MA 02115; **Phone:** 617-732-4222; **Board Cert:** Obstetrics & Gynecology 2007; Reproductive Endocrinology 2007; **Med School:** Univ Cincinnati 1982; **Resid:** Obstetrics & Gynecology, Brigham & Women's Hosp 1986; **Fellow:** Reproductive Endocrinology, Brigham & Women's Hosp 1988; **Fac Appt:** Assoc Prof ObG, Harvard Med Sch

Isaacson, Keith B MD [RE] - **Spec Exp:** Infertility; Endometriosis; Minimally Invasive Surgery; **Hospital:** Newton - Wellesley Hosp, Mass Genl Hosp; **Address:** 2014 Washington St Fl 2 West, Newton, MA 02462; **Phone:** 617-243-5205; **Board Cert:** Obstetrics & Gynecology 2001; Reproductive Endocrinology 2001; **Med School:** Med Coll GA 1983; **Resid:** Obstetrics & Gynecology, Ochsner Fdn Hosp 1987; **Fellow:** Reproductive Endocrinology, Hosp U Penn 1989; **Fac Appt:** Assoc Prof ObG, Harvard Med Sch

Luciano, Anthony A MD [RE] - **Spec Exp:** Infertility; Endometriosis; Menopause Problems; Osteoporosis; **Hospital:** Hosp of Central CT at New Britain, Hartford Hosp; **Address:** 100 Grand St, Ste E3, New Britain, CT 06050; **Phone:** 860-224-5467; **Board Cert:** Obstetrics & Gynecology 1980; Reproductive Endocrinology 1981; **Med School:** Univ Conn 1973; **Resid:** Obstetrics & Gynecology, Univ Connecticut Hosp 1977; **Fellow:** Reproductive Endocrinology, Univ Connecticut Hosp 1979; **Fac Appt:** Prof ObG, Univ Conn

Manganiello, Paul D MD [RE] - **Spec Exp:** Infertility; Menopause Problems; **Hospital:** Dartmouth - Hitchcock Med Ctr; **Address:** Dartmouth-Hitchcock Med Ctr, Dept Ob/Gyn, One Medical Center Drive, Lebanon, NH 03756; **Phone:** 603-653-9240; **Board Cert:** Obstetrics & Gynecology 1980; Reproductive Endocrinology 1984; **Med School:** Jefferson Med Coll 1973; **Resid:** Obstetrics & Gynecology, Thomas Jefferson Univ Hosp 1977; **Fellow:** Reproductive Endocrinology, Med Coll Ga Hosp 1979; **Fac Appt:** Assoc Prof ObG, Dartmouth Med Sch

Patrizio, Pasquale MD [RE] - **Spec Exp:** Infertility-IVF; Fertility Preservation in Cancer; **Hospital:** Yale-New Haven Hosp; **Address:** Yale Fertility Ctr, Dept OB/GYN, 150 Sargent Drive, New Haven, CT 06511; **Phone:** 203-785-4708; **Board Cert:** Obstetrics & Gynecology 2006; Reproductive Endocrinology 2006; **Med School:** Italy 1983; **Resid:** Obstetrics & Gynecology, Univ Naples 1987; Reproductive Endocrinology, Univ Pisa 1990; **Fellow:** Infertility, UC Irvine 1995; **Fac Appt:** Prof ObG, Yale Univ

Zinaman, Michael J MD [RE] - **Spec Exp:** Endometriosis; Infertility; Uterine Fibroids; **Hospital:** St Elizabeth's Med Ctr; **Address:** Caritas St Elizabeth's Med Ctr SMC5, 736 Cambridge St, Boston, MA 02135; **Phone:** 617-562-7018; **Board Cert:** Obstetrics & Gynecology 1996; Reproductive Endocrinology 1996; **Med School:** SUNY Downstate 1981; **Resid:** Obstetrics & Gynecology, Univ Chicago Hosps 1985; **Fellow:** Reproductive Endocrinology, Georgetown Univ 1987

Mid Atlantic

Bieber, Eric J MD [RE] - **Spec Exp:** Uterine Fibroids; Infertility; Endometriosis; **Hospital:** Geisinger Med Ctr; **Address:** 100 N Academy, MC 29-20, Danville, PA 17821; **Phone:** 570-271-6296; **Board Cert:** Obstetrics & Gynecology 2007; Reproductive Endocrinology 2007; **Med School:** Loyola Univ-Stritch Sch Med 1986; **Resid:** Obstetrics & Gynecology, Rush Presby-St Lukes Med Ctr 1990; **Fellow:** Reproductive Endocrinology, Univ Chicago 1993

Copperman, Alan B MD [RE] - **Spec Exp:** Infertility-IVF; Endometriosis; Laparoscopic Surgery; Hysteroscopic Surgery; **Hospital:** Mount Sinai Med Ctr (page 64); **Address:** 635 Madison Ave Fl 10, New York, NY 10022; **Phone:** 212-756-5777; **Board Cert:** Obstetrics & Gynecology 1996; Reproductive Endocrinology 1999; **Med School:** NY Med Coll 1989; **Resid:** Obstetrics & Gynecology, Yale-New Haven Hosp 1993; **Fellow:** Reproductive Endocrinology, Mount Sinai Med Ctr 1995; **Fac Appt:** Assoc Clin Prof ObG, Mount Sinai Sch Med

Coutifaris, Christos MD/PhD [RE] - **Spec Exp:** Infertility-IVF; Fertility Preservation in Cancer; Polycystic Ovarian Syndrome; **Hospital:** Hosp Univ Penn - UPHS (page 60); **Address:** Penn Fertility Care, 3701 Market St Fl 8 - Ste 800, Philadelphia, PA 19104; **Phone:** 215-662-6100; **Board Cert:** Obstetrics & Gynecology 2006; Reproductive Endocrinology 2006; **Med School:** Univ Pennsylvania 1982; **Resid:** Obstetrics & Gynecology, Hosp Univ Penn 1986; **Fellow:** Reproductive Endocrinology, Univ Penn 1987; **Fac Appt:** Prof ObG, Univ Pennsylvania

Reproductive Endocrinology

Damewood, Marian D MD [RE] - **Spec Exp:** Infertility-IVF; **Hospital:** York Hosp, Hosp Univ Penn - UPHS (page 60); **Address:** York Hosp, Dept Ob/Gyn, 1001 S George St, York, PA 17403; **Phone:** 717-851-2349; **Board Cert:** Obstetrics & Gynecology 1985; Reproductive Endocrinology 1987; **Med School:** Johns Hopkins Univ 1978; **Resid:** Obstetrics & Gynecology, Johns Hopkins Hosp 1982; **Fellow:** Reproductive Endocrinology, Johns Hopkins Hosp 1984; **Fac Appt:** Clin Prof ObG, Univ Pennsylvania

Grazi, Richard MD [RE] - **Spec Exp:** Infertility-IVF; Preimplantation Genetic Diagnosis; Fertility Preservation in Cancer; **Hospital:** Maimonides Med Ctr (page 63), Richmond Univ Med Ctr; **Address:** 1355 84th St, Brooklyn, NY 11228-3030; **Phone:** 718-283-8600; **Board Cert:** Obstetrics & Gynecology 2006; Reproductive Endocrinology 2006; **Med School:** SUNY Buffalo 1981; **Resid:** Obstetrics & Gynecology, NYU Med Ctr 1985; **Fellow:** Reproductive Endocrinology, UMDNJ Med Ctr 1987; **Fac Appt:** Assoc Clin Prof ObG, Mount Sinai Sch Med

Grifo, James A MD/PhD [RE] - **Spec Exp:** Infertility-IVF; Prenatal Genetic Diagnosis; **Hospital:** NYU Med Ctr (page 68), Bellevue Hosp Ctr; **Address:** 660 1st Ave Fl 5, New York, NY 10016; **Phone:** 212-263-7978; **Board Cert:** Obstetrics & Gynecology 2005; Reproductive Endocrinology 2005; **Med School:** Case West Res Univ 1984; **Resid:** Obstetrics & Gynecology, NY Hosp-Cornell Med Ctr 1988; **Fellow:** Reproductive Endocrinology, Yale-New Haven Hosp 1990; **Fac Appt:** Prof ObG, NYU Sch Med

Grunfeld, Lawrence MD [RE] - **Spec Exp:** Infertility-IVF; Hysteroscopic Surgery; Laparoscopic Surgery; **Hospital:** Mount Sinai Med Ctr (page 64), Lenox Hill Hosp (page 62); **Address:** 635 Madison Ave Fl 10, New York, NY 10022-1009; **Phone:** 212-756-5777; **Board Cert:** Obstetrics & Gynecology 2006; Reproductive Endocrinology 2006; **Med School:** Mount Sinai Sch Med 1979; **Resid:** Obstetrics & Gynecology, Montefiore Med Ctr 1984; **Fellow:** Reproductive Endocrinology, Montefiore Med Ctr 1987; **Fac Appt:** Assoc Clin Prof ObG, Mount Sinai Sch Med

Legro, Richard S MD [RE] - **Spec Exp:** Ovarian Failure; Polycystic Ovarian Syndrome; Infertility-IVF; **Hospital:** Penn State Milton S Hershey Med Ctr; **Address:** Hershey Med Ctr, 500 University Drive, PO Box 850, MC H103, Hershey, PA 17033; **Phone:** 717-531-8478; **Board Cert:** Obstetrics & Gynecology 2006; Reproductive Endocrinology 2006; **Med School:** Mount Sinai Sch Med 1987; **Resid:** Obstetrics & Gynecology, Magee Womens Hosp 1991; **Fellow:** Reproductive Endocrinology, USC Women's Hosp 1993; **Fac Appt:** Prof ObG, Penn State Univ-Hershey Med Ctr

Licciardi, Frederick L MD [RE] - **Spec Exp:** Infertility-IVF; Infertility; Fertility Preservation in Cancer; **Hospital:** NYU Med Ctr (page 68); **Address:** NYU Medical Ctr, 660 First Ave, 5th Fl, New York, NY 10016; **Phone:** 212-263-7754; **Board Cert:** Obstetrics & Gynecology 2007; Reproductive Endocrinology 2007; **Med School:** UMDNJ-Rutgers Med Sch 1986; **Resid:** Obstetrics & Gynecology, St Barnabas Med Ctr 1990; **Fellow:** Reproductive Endocrinology, NY Hosp-Cornell Med Ctr 1992; **Fac Appt:** Assoc Prof ObG, NYU Sch Med

McClamrock, Howard D MD [RE] - **Spec Exp:** Infertility-IVF; Prenatal Genetic Diagnosis; **Hospital:** Univ of MD Med Sys, St Joseph Med Ctr; **Address:** Univ Maryland, Dept OB/GYN, 405 W Redwood St Fl 3, Baltimore, MD 21201; **Phone:** 410-328-2304; **Board Cert:** Obstetrics & Gynecology 1998; Reproductive Endocrinology 1998; **Med School:** Univ NC Sch Med 1981; **Resid:** Obstetrics & Gynecology, Univ Maryland Hosp 1986; **Fellow:** Reproductive Endocrinology, Univ Maryland 1988; **Fac Appt:** Assoc Prof ObG, Univ MD Sch Med

McGovern, Peter G MD [RE] - **Spec Exp:** Infertility-IVF; Polycystic Ovarian Syndrome; Minimally Invasive Surgery; **Hospital:** UMDNJ-Univ Hosp-Newark, Hackensack Univ Med Ctr; **Address:** University Reproductive Assocs, 214 Terrace Ave, Hasbrouck Heights, NJ 07604; **Phone:** 201-288-6330; **Board Cert:** Obstetrics & Gynecology 2007; Reproductive Endocrinology 2007; **Med School:** NYU Sch Med 1986; **Resid:** Obstetrics & Gynecology, NYU-Bellevue Hosp Ctr 1990; **Fellow:** Reproductive Endocrinology, UMDNJ-Newark 1992; **Fac Appt:** Assoc Prof ObG, UMDNJ-NJ Med Sch, Newark

Noyes, Nicole MD [RE] - **Spec Exp:** Infertility-IVF; Fertility Preservation in Cancer; Reproductive Surgery; **Hospital:** NYU Med Ctr (page 68); **Address:** NYU Medical Ctr, 660 First Ave, 5th FL, New York, NY 10016; **Phone:** 212-263-7981; **Board Cert:** Obstetrics & Gynecology 2006; Reproductive Endocrinology 2006; **Med School:** Univ VT Coll Med 1986; **Resid:** Obstetrics & Gynecology, NY Hosp-Cornell Med Ctr 1990; **Fellow:** Reproductive Endocrinology, NY Hosp-Cornell Med Ctr 1992; **Fac Appt:** Assoc Prof ObG, NYU Sch Med

Pfeifer, Samantha MD [RE] - **Spec Exp:** Infertility-Female; Endometriosis; Turner Syndrome; **Hospital:** Hosp Univ Penn - UPHS (page 60); **Address:** Penn Health for Women, 250 King of Prussia Rd, Radnor, PA 19087; **Phone:** 610-902-2500; **Board Cert:** Obstetrics & Gynecology 2006; Reproductive Endocrinology 2006; **Med School:** Univ Pennsylvania 1986; **Resid:** Obstetrics & Gynecology, Hosp Univ Penn 1990; **Fellow:** Reproductive Endocrinology, Hosp Univ Penn 1993; **Fac Appt:** Asst Prof ObG, Univ Pennsylvania

Rosenwaks, Zev MD [RE] - **Spec Exp:** Infertility-IVF; Genetic Disorders; Fertility Preservation in Cancer; **Hospital:** NY-Presby Hosp/Weill Cornell (page 66); **Address:** Ctr For Reproductive Medicine & Infertility, 1305 York Ave Fl 6, New York, NY 10021-4872; **Phone:** 646-962-3743; **Board Cert:** Obstetrics & Gynecology 1978; Reproductive Endocrinology 1981; **Med School:** SUNY Downstate 1972; **Resid:** Obstetrics & Gynecology, LI Jewish Med Ctr 1976; **Fellow:** Reproductive Endocrinology, Johns Hopkins Hosp 1978; **Fac Appt:** Prof ObG, Cornell Univ-Weill Med Coll

Sanfilippo, Joseph MD [RE] - **Spec Exp:** Adolescent Gynecology; Infertility; Minimally Invasive Surgery; Menopause Problems; **Hospital:** Magee-Womens Hosp - UPMC; **Address:** Ctr for Fertility & Repro Endo-Magee Hosp, 300 Halket St, Ste 2309, Pittsburgh, PA 15213; **Phone:** 412-641-1204; **Board Cert:** Obstetrics & Gynecology 2001; Reproductive Endocrinology 2001; **Med School:** Ros Franklin Univ/Chicago Med Sch 1973; **Resid:** Obstetrics & Gynecology, SUNY Upstate 1977; **Fellow:** Reproductive Endocrinology, Univ of Louisville 1979; **Fac Appt:** Prof ObG, Univ Pittsburgh

Sauer, Mark MD [RE] - **Spec Exp:** Infertility-IVF; **Hospital:** NY-Presby Hosp/Columbia (page 66); **Address:** 1790 Broadway Fl 2, New York, NY 10019; **Phone:** 646-756-8282; **Board Cert:** Obstetrics & Gynecology 2008; Reproductive Endocrinology 2008; **Med School:** Univ IL Coll Med 1980; **Resid:** Obstetrics & Gynecology, Univ Illinois Med Ctr 1984; **Fellow:** Reproductive Endocrinology, Harbor-UCLA Med Ctr 1986; **Fac Appt:** Prof ObG, Columbia P&S

Seifer, David B MD [RE] - **Spec Exp:** Infertility; Infertility-Advanced Maternal Age; Fertility Preservation in Cancer; **Hospital:** Maimonides Med Ctr (page 63), Richmond Univ Med Ctr; **Address:** 1355 84th St, Brooklyn, NY 11228; **Phone:** 718-283-8600; **Board Cert:** Obstetrics & Gynecology 1998; Reproductive Endocrinology/Infertility 1998; **Med School:** Univ IL Coll Med 1981; **Resid:** Obstetrics & Gynecology, Stanford Univ Hosp 1985; **Fellow:** Reproductive Endocrinology, Yale-New Haven Hosp 1991; **Fac Appt:** Prof ObG, Mount Sinai Sch Med

Simon, James A MD [RE] - **Spec Exp:** Infertility; Menopause Problems; Osteoporosis; **Hospital:** G Washington Univ Hosp, Sibley Mem Hosp; **Address:** 1850 M St NW, Ste 450, Washington, DC 20036; **Phone:** 202-293-1000; **Board Cert:** Obstetrics & Gynecology 1998; Reproductive Endocrinology 1998; **Med School:** Rush Med Coll 1978; **Resid:** Obstetrics & Gynecology, George Washington Univ Hosp 1982; **Fellow:** Reproductive Endocrinology, Harbor-UCLA Medical Ctr 1985; **Fac Appt:** Clin Prof ObG, Geo Wash Univ

Reproductive Endocrinology

Sondheimer, Steven MD [RE] - **Spec Exp:** Infertility; **Hospital:** Hosp Univ Penn - UPHS (page 60); **Address:** Penn Fertility Care, 3701 Market St Fl 8, Philadelphia, PA 19104; **Phone:** 215-662-6100; **Board Cert:** Obstetrics & Gynecology 2005; Reproductive Endocrinology 2005; **Med School:** Univ Pennsylvania 1974; **Resid:** Obstetrics & Gynecology, Hosp Univ Penn 1978; **Fellow:** Endocrinology, Hosp Univ Penn 1980; **Fac Appt:** Prof ObG, Univ Pennsylvania

Tureck, Richard W MD [RE] - **Spec Exp:** Reproductive Surgery; Infertility; **Hospital:** Hosp Univ Penn - UPHS (page 60); **Address:** Penn Fertility Care, 3701 Market St Fl 8 - Ste 800, Philadelphia, PA 19104; **Phone:** 215-662-6100; **Board Cert:** Obstetrics & Gynecology 1982; **Med School:** Cornell Univ-Weill Med Coll 1975; **Resid:** Obstetrics & Gynecology, Roosevelt Hosp/Columbia Presby Med Ctr 1979; **Fellow:** Reproductive Endocrinology, Hosp U Penn 1981; **Fac Appt:** Prof ObG, Univ Pennsylvania

Wallach, Edward E MD [RE] - **Spec Exp:** Uterine Fibroids; Infertility-IVF; **Hospital:** Johns Hopkins Hosp - Baltimore (page 61); **Address:** Johns Hopkins at Greenspring Station, 2330 W Joppa Rd, Ste 301, Lutherville, MD 21093; **Phone:** 410-583-2751; **Board Cert:** Obstetrics & Gynecology 1979; Reproductive Endocrinology 1975; **Med School:** Cornell Univ-Weill Med Coll 1958; **Resid:** Obstetrics & Gynecology, Kings Co Hosp 1963; **Fellow:** Reproductive Endocrinology, Worcester Fdn Exper Biol 1962; **Fac Appt:** Prof ObG, Johns Hopkins Univ

Weiss, Gerson MD [RE] - **Spec Exp:** Infertility; Menopause Problems; **Hospital:** Hackensack Univ Med Ctr, UMDNJ-Univ Hosp-Newark; **Address:** 214 Terrace Ave, Hasbrouck Heights, NJ 07604-1815; **Phone:** 201-288-6330; **Board Cert:** Obstetrics & Gynecology 1993; Reproductive Endocrinology 1974; **Med School:** NYU Sch Med 1964; **Resid:** Obstetrics & Gynecology, Bellevue Hosp Ctr 1969; **Fellow:** Reproductive Endocrinology, Univ Pittsburgh 1973; **Fac Appt:** Prof ObG, UMDNJ-NJ Med Sch, Newark

Zacur, Howard A MD/PhD [RE] - **Spec Exp:** Prolactin Disorders; Uterine Fibroids; Hormonal Disorders; **Hospital:** Johns Hopkins Hosp - Baltimore (page 61); **Address:** Johns Hopkins at Green Spring Station, 10755 Falls Rd, Pavilion 2, Ste 335, Lutherville, MD 21093; **Phone:** 410-616-7140; **Board Cert:** Obstetrics & Gynecology 1994; Reproductive Endocrinology 1984; **Med School:** Univ Miami Sch Med 1973; **Resid:** Obstetrics & Gynecology, Johns Hopkins Hosp 1980; **Fellow:** Reproductive Endocrinology, Johns Hopkins Hosp 1982; **Fac Appt:** Prof ObG, Johns Hopkins Univ

Southeast

Berga, Sarah L MD [RE] - **Spec Exp:** Infertility-IVF; Hormonal Disorders; Menstrual Disorders; **Hospital:** Emory Univ Hosp, Crawford Long Hosp of Emory Univ; **Address:** Dept Gynecology & Obstetrics, 1639 Pierce Drive, rm 4208-WMB, Atlanta, GA 30322; **Phone:** 404-727-8600; **Board Cert:** Obstetrics & Gynecology 1998; Reproductive Endocrinology 1998; **Med School:** Univ VA Sch Med 1980; **Resid:** Obstetrics & Gynecology, Mass Genl Hosp 1984; **Fellow:** Reproductive Endocrinology, UCSD Med Ctr 1986; **Fac Appt:** Prof ObG, Emory Univ

Blackwell, Richard E MD/PhD [RE] - **Spec Exp:** Infertility-Female; Reproductive Medicine; Women's Health; **Hospital:** Univ of Ala Hosp at Birmingham, St Vincent's Hosp - Birmingham; **Address:** 618 S 20th St, Birmingham, AL 35294; **Phone:** 205-934-6090; **Board Cert:** Obstetrics & Gynecology 1982; Reproductive Endocrinology 1987; **Med School:** Baylor Coll Med 1975; **Resid:** Obstetrics & Gynecology, Univ Alabama Hosp 1979; **Fellow:** Reproductive Endocrinology, Univ Alabama Hosp 1981; Reproductive Endocrinology, The Salk Institute 1982; **Fac Appt:** Prof ObG, Univ Ala

Cowan, Bryan D MD [RE] - **Spec Exp:** Infertility-IVF; Uterine Fibroids; **Hospital:** Univ Hosps & Clins - Jackson; **Address:** University Hosp & Clinics, Dept Ob/Gyn, 2500 N State St, Jackson, MS 39216; **Phone:** 601-984-5300; **Board Cert:** Obstetrics & Gynecology 2006; Reproductive Endocrinology 2006; **Med School:** Univ Colorado 1975; **Resid:** Obstetrics & Gynecology, Portsmouth Naval Hosp 1979; **Fellow:** Reproductive Endocrinology, WRAH/NIH 1981; **Fac Appt:** Prof ObG, Univ Miss

DeVane, Gary W MD [RE] - **Spec Exp:** Infertility-IVF; Miscarriage-Recurrent; Endometriosis; **Hospital:** Florida Hosp - Orlando, Arnold Palmer Hosp for Chldn; **Address:** 3435 Pinehurst Ave, Orlando, FL 32804-4049; **Phone:** 407-740-0909; **Board Cert:** Obstetrics & Gynecology 1977; Reproductive Endocrinology 1982; **Med School:** Baylor Coll Med 1971; **Resid:** Obstetrics & Gynecology, UCSD Hosp 1975; **Fellow:** Reproductive Endocrinology, Univ Texas SW Hosp 1980

Fritz, Marc A MD [RE] - **Spec Exp:** Infertility; Menopause Problems; Menstrual Disorders; **Hospital:** Univ NC Hosps; **Address:** Univ NC Sch Med, Dept Ob/Gyn, CB 7570, 4001 Old Clinic, Chapel Hill, NC 27599-7570; **Phone:** 919-966-5283; **Board Cert:** Obstetrics & Gynecology 1996; Reproductive Endocrinology 1996; **Med School:** Tulane Univ 1977; **Resid:** Obstetrics & Gynecology, Wright State Univ 1981; **Fellow:** Reproductive Endocrinology, Oregon Hlth Sci Univ 1983; **Fac Appt:** Prof ObG, Univ NC Sch Med

Goodman, Neil MD [RE] - **Spec Exp:** Polycystic Ovarian Syndrome; Hormonal Disorders; Infertility; **Hospital:** Baptist Hosp of Miami, South Miami Hosp; **Address:** 9150 SW 87th Ave, Ste 210, Miami, FL 33176-2313; **Phone:** 305-595-6855; **Board Cert:** Internal Medicine 1973; Endocrinology, Diabetes & Metabolism 1975; **Med School:** Columbia P&S 1970; **Resid:** Internal Medicine, Beth Israel Hosp 1972; **Fellow:** Endocrinology, Mass Genl Hosp 1974; **Fac Appt:** Clin Prof Med, Univ Miami Sch Med

Hammond, Charles B MD [RE] - **Spec Exp:** Menopause Problems; Trophoblastic Disease; **Hospital:** Duke Univ Med Ctr; **Address:** Duke Univ Med Ctr, Box 3853, Durham, NC 27710-0001; **Phone:** 919-684-3008; **Board Cert:** Obstetrics & Gynecology 1972; Reproductive Endocrinology 1974; **Med School:** Duke Univ 1961; **Resid:** Obstetrics & Gynecology, Duke Med Ctr 1963; Obstetrics & Gynecology, Duke Med Ctr 1968; **Fellow:** Gynecology, Duke Med Ctr 1964; Reproductive Endocrinology, Natl Inst Hlth 1966; **Fac Appt:** Prof ObG, Duke Univ

Keefe, David Lawrence MD [RE] - **Spec Exp:** Infertility-IVF; Infertility-Advanced Maternal Age; **Hospital:** Univ of S FL - Tampa; **Address:** 2 A Columbia Drive, Tampa, FL 33606; **Phone:** 813-259-8500; **Board Cert:** Obstetrics & Gynecology 1993; Reproductive Endocrinology 1995; **Med School:** Georgetown Univ 1980; **Resid:** Psychiatry, Harvard Psych Srv/Camb Hosp 1983; Obstetrics & Gynecology, Yale New Haven Hosp 1989; **Fellow:** Psychiatry, Univ Chicago Hosp & Clins 1985; Reproductive Endocrinology, Yale New Haven Hosp 1991; **Fac Appt:** Prof ObG, Univ S Fla Coll Med

Murphy, Ana A MD [RE] - **Spec Exp:** Infertility; Endometriosis; Pelvic Surgery; **Hospital:** Med Coll of GA Hosp and Clin; **Address:** Med Coll Ga - Dept Ob/Gyn, BA-7313, 1120 15th St, Agusta, GA 30912; **Phone:** 706-722-4434; **Board Cert:** Obstetrics & Gynecology 2007; Reproductive Endocrinology 2007; **Med School:** Univ Mich Med Sch 1980; **Resid:** Obstetrics & Gynecology, Johns Hopkins Univ 1984; **Fellow:** Reproductive Endocrinology, Johns Hopkins Univ 1986; **Fac Appt:** Prof ObG, Med Coll GA

Ory, Steven J MD [RE] - **Spec Exp:** Infertility; Hormonal Disorders; Endometriosis; **Hospital:** Northwest Med Ctr, Meml Regl Hosp; **Address:** 2960 N State Road 7, Ste 300, Margate, FL 33063-5737; **Phone:** 954-247-6200; **Board Cert:** Obstetrics & Gynecology 2006; Reproductive Endocrinology 2006; **Med School:** Baylor Coll Med 1976; **Resid:** Obstetrics & Gynecology, Mayo Clinic 1980; **Fellow:** Reproductive Endocrinology, Duke Univ 1982; **Fac Appt:** Assoc Clin Prof ObG, Univ Miami Sch Med

Reproductive Endocrinology

Rock, John A MD [RE] - **Spec Exp:** Infertility-Female; Endometriosis; Vaginal/Uterine Abnormalities; Pelvic Reconstruction; **Hospital:** Baptist Hosp of Miami, Jackson N Med Ctr; **Address:** Florida Intl Univ, Univ Park, HLS 693, 11200 SW 8th St, Miami, FL 33146; **Phone:** 305-348-0283; **Board Cert:** Obstetrics & Gynecology 2005; Reproductive Endocrinology 2005; **Med School:** Louisiana State U, New Orleans 1972; **Resid:** Obstetrics & Gynecology, Duke Univ Med Ctr 1976; **Fellow:** Reproductive Endocrinology, Johns Hopkins Hosp 1978

Session, Donna R MD [RE] - **Spec Exp:** Ultrasound Guided Surgery; Infertility-Female; **Hospital:** Emory Univ Hosp; **Address:** Emory Reproductive Endocrinology, 550 Peachtree St, Ste 1800 MOT, Atlanta, GA 30308; **Phone:** 404-778-3401; **Board Cert:** Obstetrics & Gynecology 2004; Reproductive Endocrinology 2004; **Med School:** Eastern VA Med Sch 1986; **Resid:** Obstetrics & Gynecology, Winthrop Hosp 1990; **Fellow:** Reproductive Endocrinology, Columbia Presby Med Ctr 1993

Steinkampf, Michael MD [RE] - **Spec Exp:** Infertility; **Hospital:** Brookwood Med Ctr; **Address:** 2700 Highway 280, Ste 370 East, East Birmingham, AL 35223; **Phone:** 205-874-0000; **Board Cert:** Obstetrics & Gynecology 1997; Reproductive Endocrinology 1997; **Med School:** Louisiana State U, New Orleans 1981; **Resid:** Obstetrics & Gynecology, Parkland Meml Hosp 1985; **Fellow:** Reproductive Endocrinology, Univ Texas SW Med Ctr 1987; **Fac Appt:** Prof ObG, Univ Ala

Walmer, David K MD/PhD [RE] - **Spec Exp:** Infertility; Miscarriage-Recurrent; DES-Exposed Females; Endometriosis; **Hospital:** Duke Univ Med Ctr; **Address:** Duke Fertility Center, 5704 Fayetteville Rd, Durham, NC 27713; **Phone:** 919-572-4673; **Board Cert:** Obstetrics & Gynecology 2006; Reproductive Endocrinology 2006; **Med School:** Univ NC Sch Med 1982; **Resid:** Obstetrics & Gynecology, Univ Texas Health Sci Ctr 1987; **Fellow:** Reproductive Endocrinology, Duke Univ Med Ctr 1989; **Fac Appt:** Assoc Prof ObG, Duke Univ

Midwest

Barnes, Randall B MD [RE] - **Spec Exp:** Infertility-IVF; Polycystic Ovarian Syndrome; Miscarriage-Recurrent; **Hospital:** Northwestern Meml Hosp; **Address:** 675 N St Clair St, Ste 14-200, Chicago, IL 60611; **Phone:** 312-695-7269; **Board Cert:** Obstetrics & Gynecology 2006; Reproductive Endocrinology 2006; **Med School:** Johns Hopkins Univ 1979; **Resid:** Obstetrics & Gynecology, LAC-USC Med Ctr 1983; **Fellow:** Reproductive Endocrinology, LAC-USC Med Ctr 1985; **Fac Appt:** Assoc Prof ObG, Northwestern Univ

Christman, Gregory MD [RE] - **Spec Exp:** Infertility-IVF; Uterine Fibroids; **Hospital:** Univ Michigan Hlth Sys; **Address:** 475 Market Pl, Ste B, Ann Arbor, MI 48108; **Phone:** 734-763-4323; **Board Cert:** Obstetrics & Gynecology 2002; Reproductive Endocrinology 2002; **Med School:** Univ Wisc 1983; **Resid:** Obstetrics & Gynecology, Univ Wisconsin Med Sch 1987; **Fellow:** Reproductive Endocrinology, Univ North Carolina 1992; **Fac Appt:** Assoc Prof ObG, Univ Mich Med Sch

Diamond, Michael P MD [RE] - **Spec Exp:** Infertility-IVF; Infertility-Female; Polycystic Ovarian Syndrome; **Hospital:** Hutzel Hosp - Detroit, Harper Univ Hosp; **Address:** Univ Ctr for Women's Medicine, 26400 W 12 Mile Rd, Southfield, MI 48034; **Phone:** 248-352-8200; **Board Cert:** Obstetrics & Gynecology 2007; Reproductive Endocrinology 2007; **Med School:** Vanderbilt Univ 1981; **Resid:** Obstetrics & Gynecology, Vanderbilt Univ Med Ctr 1985; **Fellow:** Reproductive Endocrinology, Yale-New Haven Hosp 1987; Univ Penn 1996; **Fac Appt:** Prof ObG, Wayne State Univ

Dodds, William G MD [RE] - **Spec Exp:** Infertility; Endometriosis; Infertility-IVF; **Hospital:** Spectrum Hlth Butterworth Campus, Bronson Meth Hosp; **Address:** 3230 Eagle Park Drive NE, Grand Rapids, MI 49525; **Phone:** 616-988-2229; **Board Cert:** Obstetrics & Gynecology 2007; Reproductive Endocrinology 2007; **Med School:** Ohio State Univ 1982; **Resid:** Obstetrics & Gynecology, Ohio State Univ Med Ctr 1986; **Fellow:** Reproductive Endocrinology, Ohio State Univ 1988; **Fac Appt:** Assoc Prof ObG, Univ Mich Med Sch

Dumesic, Daniel Anthony MD [RE] - **Spec Exp:** Infertility-Female; Hormonal Disorders; Endometriosis; **Address:** Reproductive Med & Infertility Assocs, 2101 Woodwinds Drive, Ste 100, Woodbury, MN 55125; **Phone:** 651-222-6050; **Board Cert:** Obstetrics & Gynecology 1995; Reproductive Endocrinology 1995; **Med School:** Univ Wisc 1978; **Resid:** Obstetrics & Gynecology, UCSF Med Ctr 1982; **Fellow:** Reproductive Endocrinology, UCSF Med Ctr 1987

Falcone, Tommaso MD [RE] - **Spec Exp:** Minimally Invasive Surgery; Infertility-IVF; Endometriosis; **Hospital:** Cleveland Clin Fdn (page 56); **Address:** Cleveland Clin, Dept Ob/Gyn, 9500 Euclid Ave, Desk A81, Cleveland, OH 44195-0001; **Phone:** 216-444-1758; **Board Cert:** Obstetrics & Gynecology 1998; Reproductive Endocrinology 1998; **Med School:** McGill Univ 1981; **Resid:** Obstetrics & Gynecology, McGill Univ 1986; **Fellow:** Reproductive Endocrinology, McGill Univ 1989

Haney, Arthur F MD [RE] - **Spec Exp:** Infertility-Female; DES-Exposed Females; **Hospital:** Univ of Chicago Hosps; **Address:** 5841 S Maryland Ave, MC 2050, Chicago, IL 60637; **Phone:** 773-702-6127; **Board Cert:** Obstetrics & Gynecology 2007; Reproductive Endocrinology 2007; **Med School:** Univ Ariz Coll Med 1972; **Resid:** Obstetrics & Gynecology, Duke Univ Med Ctr 1976; **Fellow:** Reproductive Endocrinology, Duke Univ Med Ctr 1978; **Fac Appt:** Prof ObG, Univ Chicago-Pritzker Sch Med

Kazer, Ralph MD [RE] - **Spec Exp:** Polycystic Ovarian Syndrome; Infertility-IVF; **Hospital:** Northwestern Meml Hosp; **Address:** Northwestern Meml Hospital, 675 N St Clair St Fl 14 - Ste 200, Chicago, IL 60611; **Phone:** 312-695-7269; **Board Cert:** Obstetrics & Gynecology 2007; Reproductive Endocrinology 2007; **Med School:** Tufts Univ 1979; **Resid:** Obstetrics & Gynecology, Tufts Univ Med Ctr 1983; **Fellow:** Reproductive Endocrinology, UC San Diego Med Ctr 1986; **Fac Appt:** Assoc Prof ObG, Northwestern Univ

Milad, Magdy P MD [RE] - **Spec Exp:** Reproductive Surgery; Infertility; Uterine Fibroids; **Hospital:** Northwestern Meml Hosp, Children's Mem Hosp; **Address:** Northwestern Med Fac Fdn, 675 North St Clair, Fl 14 - Ste 200, Chicago, IL 60611-5975; **Phone:** 312-695-7269; **Board Cert:** Obstetrics & Gynecology 1994; Reproductive Endocrinology 1996; **Med School:** Wayne State Univ 1987; **Resid:** Obstetrics & Gynecology, William Beaumont Hosp 1991; **Fellow:** Reproductive Endocrinology, Mayo Clinic 1993; **Fac Appt:** Prof ObG, Northwestern Univ

Molo, Mary Wood MD [RE] - **Spec Exp:** Infertility-IVF; Uterine Fibroids; Fertility Preservation in Cancer; **Hospital:** Rush Univ Med Ctr; **Address:** 1725 W Harrison St, Ste 408 East, Chicago, IL 60612; **Phone:** 312-997-2229; **Board Cert:** Obstetrics & Gynecology 2006; Reproductive Endocrinology 2006; **Med School:** Southern IL Univ 1982; **Resid:** Obstetrics & Gynecology, Southern Illinois Affil Hosps 1984; Obstetrics & Gynecology, Rush Presby St Lukes Hosp 1987; **Fellow:** Reproductive Endocrinology, Rush Presby St Lukes Hosp 1989; **Fac Appt:** Asst Prof ObG, Rush Med Coll

Nagel, Theodore C MD [RE] - **Spec Exp:** Infertility-IVF; Hysteroscopic Surgery; Vaginal/Uterine Abnormalities; Laparoscopic Surgery; **Hospital:** Univ Minn Med Ctr, Fairview - Riverside Campus; **Address:** Reproductive Med Ctr, Univ Minnesota, 606 24th Ave S, Ste 500, Minnneapolis, MN 55454; **Phone:** 612-627-4564; **Board Cert:** Internal Medicine 1970; Endocrinology 1975; Obstetrics & Gynecology 1981; Reproductive Endocrinology 1983; **Med School:** Cornell Univ-Weill Med Coll 1963; **Resid:** Internal Medicine, Bellevue Hosp Ctr 1968; Obstetrics & Gynecology, Univ Minn Hosps 1977; **Fellow:** Endocrinology, Diabetes & Metabolism, Northwestern Univ Med Sch 1972; Reproductive Endocrinology, Univ Minnesota 1980; **Fac Appt:** Assoc Clin Prof ObG, Univ Minn

Odem, Randall R MD [RE] - **Spec Exp:** Infertility; Reproductive Surgery; Miscarriage-Recurrent; **Hospital:** Barnes-Jewish Hosp; **Address:** 4444 Forest Park Ave, Ste 3100, St Louis, MO 63108-2212; **Phone:** 314-286-2421; **Board Cert:** Obstetrics & Gynecology 2007; Reproductive Endocrinology 2007; **Med School:** Univ Iowa Coll Med 1981; **Resid:** Obstetrics & Gynecology, Univ Illinois Hosps 1985; **Fellow:** Reproductive Endocrinology, Wash Univ Sch Med 1987; **Fac Appt:** Prof ObG, Washington Univ, St Louis

Reproductive Endocrinology

Ratts, Valerie S MD [RE] - **Spec Exp:** Polycystic Ovarian Syndrome; Uterine Fibroids; Infertility-IVF; **Hospital:** Barnes-Jewish Hosp; **Address:** Washington Univ, Ctr for Reproductive Med/Infertility, 4444 Forest Park Ave, Ste 3100, St Louis, MO 63108; **Phone:** 314-286-2400; **Board Cert:** Obstetrics & Gynecology 2006; Reproductive Endocrinology 2006; **Med School:** Johns Hopkins Univ 1987; **Resid:** Obstetrics & Gynecology, Johns Hopkins Hosp 1991; **Fellow:** Reproductive Endocrinology, Johns Hopkins Hosp 1993; **Fac Appt:** Assoc Prof ObG, Washington Univ, St Louis

Smith, Yolanda R MD [RE] - **Spec Exp:** Infertility; Polycystic Ovarian Syndrome; **Hospital:** Univ Michigan Hlth Sys; **Address:** Women's Hospital, 1500 E Med Ctr Drive, rm L4100, Box 0276, Ann Arbor, MI 48109-0276; **Phone:** 734-763-4323; **Board Cert:** Obstetrics & Gynecology 2006; Reproductive Endocrinology 2006; **Med School:** Wake Forest Univ 1989; **Resid:** Obstetrics & Gynecology, Univ Mich Hosp 1993; **Fellow:** Reproductive Endocrinology, Johns Hopkins Hosp 1995; **Fac Appt:** Assoc Prof ObG, Univ Mich Med Sch

Great Plains and Mountains

Richardson, Marilyn MD [RE] - **Spec Exp:** Menopause Problems; Infertility; Polycystic Ovarian Syndrome; **Hospital:** Univ of Kansas Hosp; **Address:** 12616 W 62nd Terr, Ste 111, Shawnee, KS 66216; **Phone:** 913-631-0277; **Board Cert:** Obstetrics & Gynecology 2007; **Med School:** Univ Kans 1979; **Resid:** Obstetrics & Gynecology, Truman Med Ctr 1983; **Fellow:** Reproductive Endocrinology, Univ Texas Hlth Scis Ctr 1985; **Fac Appt:** Asst Clin Prof ObG, Univ Kans

Schlaff, William D MD [RE] - **Spec Exp:** Infertility; Endometriosis; Vaginal/Uterine Abnormalities; **Hospital:** Univ Colorado Hosp; **Address:** Dept of OB & Gyn, MS 8198-3, 12631 E 17th Ave, Aurora, CO 80045; **Phone:** 720-848-1690; **Board Cert:** Obstetrics & Gynecology 1995; Reproductive Endocrinology 1995; **Med School:** Univ Mich Med Sch 1977; **Resid:** Obstetrics & Gynecology, Univ Mich Hosps 1981; **Fellow:** Reproductive Endocrinology, Johns Hopkins Med Ctr 1985; **Fac Appt:** Prof ObG, Univ Colorado

Surrey, Eric S MD [RE] - **Spec Exp:** Infertility-IVF; Endometriosis; **Hospital:** Swedish Med Ctr - Englewood, Sky Ridge Med Ctr; **Address:** 10290 RidgeGate Circle, Lone Tree, CO 80124; **Phone:** 303-788-8300; **Board Cert:** Obstetrics & Gynecology 1998; Reproductive Endocrinology 1998; **Med School:** Univ Pennsylvania 1981; **Resid:** Obstetrics & Gynecology, UCLA Med Ctr 1986; **Fellow:** Reproductive Endocrinology, UCLA Med Ctr 1988

Southwest

Dickey, Richard P MD/PhD [RE] - **Spec Exp:** Infertility-IVF; **Hospital:** Tulane-Lakeside Hosp; **Address:** The Fertility Institute, 800 N Causeway Blvd, Ste 2C, Mandeville, LA 70448; **Phone:** 985-892-7621; **Board Cert:** Obstetrics & Gynecology 1967; Reproductive Endocrinology/Infertility 1976; **Med School:** Case West Res Univ 1960; **Fac Appt:** Clin Prof ObG, Louisiana State U, New Orleans

Schenken, Robert S MD [RE] - **Spec Exp:** Infertility-Female; Endometriosis; **Hospital:** Univ Hlth Sys - Univ Hosp (San Antonio, TX), Baptist Hlth Sys; **Address:** Univ Texas Med Sch, Dept OB/GYN, 7703 Floyd Curl Dr, MSC 7836, San Antonio, TX 78229-3900; **Phone:** 210-567-4950; **Board Cert:** Obstetrics & Gynecology 1995; Reproductive Endocrinology 1995; **Med School:** Baylor Coll Med 1977; **Resid:** Obstetrics & Gynecology, Bexar Co Hosp 1981; **Fellow:** Reproductive Endocrinology, Natl Inst Hlth 1982; Reproductive Endocrinology, Univ Tex Hlth Sci Ctr 1983; **Fac Appt:** Prof ObG, Univ Tex, San Antonio

West Coast and Pacific

Adamson, G David MD [RE] - **Spec Exp:** Infertility-Female; Endometriosis; Infertility-IVF; **Hospital:** Good Samaritan Hosp - San Jose, Stanford Univ Med Ctr; **Address:** 540 University Ave, Ste 200, Palo Alto, CA 94301; **Phone:** 650-322-1900; **Board Cert:** Obstetrics & Gynecology 1980; Reproductive Endocrinology 1982; **Med School:** Univ Toronto 1973; **Resid:** Obstetrics & Gynecology, Toronto Genl Hosp 1977; **Fellow:** Obstetrics & Gynecology, Toronto Genl Hosp 1978; Reproductive Endocrinology, Stanford Univ Hosp 1980; **Fac Appt:** Clin Prof ObG, Stanford Univ

Azziz, Ricardo MD [RE] - **Spec Exp:** Infertility-Female; Reproductive Surgery; Polycystic Ovarian Syndrome; **Hospital:** Cedars-Sinai Med Ctr; **Address:** Cedars Sinai-Ctr Fertility & Reproductive Med, 8700 Beverly Blvd, Ste 3611, Los Angeles, CA 90048; **Phone:** 310-423-9964; **Board Cert:** Obstetrics & Gynecology 1996; Reproductive Endocrinology 1996; **Med School:** Penn State Univ-Hershey Med Ctr 1981; **Resid:** Obstetrics & Gynecology, Georgetown Univ Hosp 1985; **Fellow:** Reproductive Endocrinology, Johns Hopkins Hosp 1987; **Fac Appt:** Prof ObG, UCLA

Marrs, Richard P MD [RE] - **Spec Exp:** Infertility-Female; Endometriosis; Uterine Fibroids; **Hospital:** Santa Monica - UCLA Med Ctr; **Address:** 11818 Wilshire Blvd, Ste 300, Los Angeles, CA 90025; **Phone:** 310-828-4008; **Board Cert:** Obstetrics & Gynecology 1980; Reproductive Endocrinology 1983; **Med School:** Univ Tex Med Br, Galveston 1974; **Resid:** Obstetrics & Gynecology, Univ Tex Hosps 1977; **Fellow:** Reproductive Endocrinology, USC Med Ctr 1979

Paulson, Richard J MD [RE] - **Spec Exp:** Infertility-IVF; Infertility-Advanced Maternal Age; **Hospital:** LAC & USC Med Ctr, Good Samaritan Hosp - Los Angeles; **Address:** USC Fertility, 1127 Wilshire Blvd, Ste 1400, Los Angeles, CA 90017; **Phone:** 213-975-9990; **Board Cert:** Obstetrics & Gynecology 2006; Reproductive Endocrinology 2006; **Med School:** UCLA 1980; **Resid:** Obstetrics & Gynecology, Harbor-UCLA Med Ctr 1984; **Fellow:** Reproductive Endocrinology, LAC-USC Med Ctr 1986; **Fac Appt:** Prof ObG, USC Sch Med

Soules, Michael R MD [RE] - **Spec Exp:** Reproductive Medicine; Infertility-Female; Infertility-IVF; **Hospital:** Northwest Hosp; **Address:** 1505 Westlake Ave N, Ste 400, Seattle, WA 98109; **Phone:** 206-301-5000; **Board Cert:** Obstetrics & Gynecology 2002; Reproductive Endocrinology 2002; **Med School:** UCLA 1972; **Resid:** Obstetrics & Gynecology, Univ Colorado Med Ctr 1976; **Fellow:** Reproductive Endocrinology, Duke Univ Hosp 1978; **Fac Appt:** Prof ObG, Univ Wash

Winer, Sharon A MD [RE] - **Spec Exp:** Hormonal Disorders; Infertility-Female; Vaginitis; Gynecology; **Hospital:** Cedars-Sinai Med Ctr, USC Univ Hosp - R K Eamer Med Plz; **Address:** 9400 Brighton Way, Ste 206, Beverly Hills, CA 90210-4709; **Phone:** 310-274-9100; **Board Cert:** Obstetrics & Gynecology 2005; Reproductive Endocrinology 2005; **Med School:** USC Sch Med 1978; **Resid:** Obstetrics & Gynecology, LAC-USC Med Ctr 1982; **Fellow:** Microsurgery, Hammersmith Hosp 1983; Reproductive Endocrinology, LAC-USC Med Ctr 1985; **Fac Appt:** Clin Prof ObG, USC Sch Med

Yee, Billy MD [RE] - **Spec Exp:** Infertility-IVF; **Hospital:** Long Beach Meml Med Ctr, Little Company of Mary Hosp; **Address:** 13950 Milton Ave, Ste 100, Westminster, CA 92683; **Phone:** 714-702-3001; **Board Cert:** Obstetrics & Gynecology 2007; Reproductive Endocrinology 2007; **Med School:** UC Davis 1978; **Resid:** Obstetrics & Gynecology, LAC-USC Med Ctr 1982; **Fellow:** Reproductive Endocrinology, LAC-USC Med Ctr 1985; **Fac Appt:** Assoc Clin Prof ObG, UC Irvine

NYU Langone Medical Center

550 First Avenue (at 31St Street)
New York, NY 10016
Physician Referral:
(888)7-NYU-MED (888-769-8633)
www.nyumc.org

PROGRAM FOR IVF REPRODUCTIVE SURGERYAND INFERTILITY

Today, thanks to promising new options in the treatment of infertility, specialists at NYU Langone Medical Center can help more patients realize their dreams of parenthood. With unique expertise in all aspects of reproductive endocrinology, including the diagnosis and treatment of endometriosis, fibroids, problems with ovulation or sperm function, and recurrent pregnancy loss, NYU Langone Medical Center uses the most advanced technology to assist infertile women and men who wish to conceive children.

From the initial diagnosis through all stages of treatment, couples receive state-of-the-art compassionate care based on their specific needs. After a comprehensive evaluation to determine the cause of infertility, couples are counseled on whether assisted reproduction is necessary. (Often, surgery can correct disorders that lead to infertility, like fibroids or endometriosis. Similarly, stimulation of a woman's ovaries with medication often results in pregnancy.) When the physician and couple agree that assisted reproduction is appropriate, the program offers:

In Vitro Fertilization
Donor Oocyte (Egg) and Sperm Services
Intracytoplasmic Sperm Injection (injection of a single sperm directly into an egg)
Assisted Hatching (creating an entry point in oocytes surrounded by tough tissue to assist sperm penetration)
Preimplantation Genetic Diagnosis (for couples with a high risk of bearing children with specific genetic disorders)
Cyropreservation (freezing embryos in liquid nitrogen to preserve them for future use) and several male infertility treatments:
Comprehensive evaluation of sperm health and fertility
Testicular Biopsy
Vasectomy Reversal
Epididymal Repair (surgery to clear sperm pathways within penis)
Microsurgical Sperm Aspiration (retrieval of sperm from inside the testes, when it is not present in the semen)
Varicocele Repair (surgical reduction of enlarged veins around penis to reduce high temperature in groin area, which adversely impacts on fertility)

Rheumatology

a subspecialty of Internal Medicine

An internist who treats diseases of joints, muscle, bones and tendons. This specialist diagnoses and treats arthritis, back pain, muscle strains, common athletic injuries and "collagen" diseases.

Training Required: Three years in internal medicine *plus* additional training and examination for certification in rheumatology.

RHEUMATOLOGY

New England

Albert, Daniel A MD [Rhu] - **Spec Exp:** Juvenile Arthritis; Rheumatology-Adult & Pediatric; **Hospital:** Dartmouth - Hitchcock Med Ctr; **Address:** Dartmouth-Hitchcock Med Ctr Rheumatology, One Medical Center Drive, Lebanon, NH 03756; **Phone:** 603-650-8622; **Board Cert:** Internal Medicine 1977; Rheumatology 1980; **Med School:** NYU Sch Med 1974; **Resid:** Internal Medicine, NC Meml Hosp 1977; **Fellow:** Rheumatology, UCSD 1981; **Fac Appt:** Prof Med, Univ Pennsylvania

Brenner, Michael B MD [Rhu] - **Spec Exp:** Gout; Rheumatoid Arthritis; Lupus/SLE; **Hospital:** Brigham & Women's Hosp; **Address:** Div Rheumatology Smith Bldg - rm 552, 1 Jimmy Fund Way, Boston, MA 02115; **Phone:** 617-525-1000; **Board Cert:** Internal Medicine 1978; Rheumatology 1982; **Med School:** Vanderbilt Univ 1975; **Resid:** Internal Medicine, Vanderbilt Univ Hosp 1979; **Fellow:** Rheumatology, UCLA Med Ctr 1981; **Fac Appt:** Prof Med, Harvard Med Sch

Kay, Jonathan MD [Rhu] - **Spec Exp:** Rheumatoid Arthritis; Psoriatic Arthritis; Ankylosing Spondylitis; Nephrogenic Fibrosing Dermopathy; **Hospital:** Mass Genl Hosp; **Address:** Rheumatology Assocs-MGH,, 55 Fruit St Yawkey Bldg - Ste 2C, Boston, MA 02114; **Phone:** 617-726-7938; **Board Cert:** Internal Medicine 1986; Rheumatology 1988; **Med School:** UCSF 1983; **Resid:** Internal Medicine, Hosp Univ Penn 1986; **Fellow:** Rheumatology/Immunology, Brigham & Womens Hosp 1989; **Fac Appt:** Assoc Clin Prof Med, Harvard Med Sch

Merkel, Peter MD [Rhu] - **Spec Exp:** Vasculitis; Scleroderma; **Hospital:** Boston Med Ctr; **Address:** Boston Univ Vasculitis Ctr, 72 E Concord St, E 533, Boston, MA 02118; **Phone:** 617-414-2500; **Board Cert:** Internal Medicine 2000; Rheumatology 2000; **Med School:** Yale Univ 1988; **Resid:** Internal Medicine, Hosp Univ Penn 1991; **Fellow:** Rheumatology, Mass General Hosp 1994

Polisson, Richard P MD [Rhu] - **Spec Exp:** Rheumatoid Arthritis; Lupus/SLE; **Hospital:** Mass Genl Hosp; **Address:** 55 Fruit St Yawkey Bldg - Ste 2C, Boston, MA 02114; **Phone:** 617-726-7938; **Board Cert:** Internal Medicine 1979; Rheumatology 1984; **Med School:** Duke Univ 1976; **Resid:** Internal Medicine, Duke Univ Med Ctr 1978; Internal Medicine, Natl Inst Hlth/NCI 1980; **Fellow:** Rheumatology, Mass Genl Hosp 1982; **Fac Appt:** Assoc Prof Med, Harvard Med Sch

Schoen, Robert T MD [Rhu] - **Spec Exp:** Rheumatoid Arthritis; Lyme Disease; Osteoporosis; **Hospital:** Yale-New Haven Hosp, Hosp of St Raphael; **Address:** 60 Temple St, Ste 6A, New Haven, CT 06510-2716; **Phone:** 203-789-2255; **Board Cert:** Internal Medicine 1979; Rheumatology 1982; **Med School:** Columbia P&S 1976; **Resid:** Internal Medicine, Yale New Haven Hosp 1979; **Fellow:** Rheumatology, Brigham & Womens Hosp 1981; **Fac Appt:** Clin Prof Med, Yale Univ

Shadick, Nancy A MD [Rhu] - **Spec Exp:** Lyme Disease; Rheumatoid Arthritis; Osteoarthritis; **Hospital:** Brigham & Women's Hosp; **Address:** Brigham & Women's Hosp, Arthritis Ctr, Dept Rheumatology, 75 Francis St, Boston, MA 02115-6105; **Phone:** 617-732-5266; **Board Cert:** Internal Medicine 1989; Rheumatology 2002; **Med School:** NYU Sch Med 1986; **Resid:** Internal Medicine, Columbia-Presby Hosp 1989; **Fellow:** Rheumatology, Brigham & Womens Hosp 1992; **Fac Appt:** Asst Prof Med, Harvard Med Sch

Simms, Robert W MD [Rhu] - **Spec Exp:** Rheumatoid Arthritis; Scleroderma; Lyme Disease; **Hospital:** Boston Med Ctr; **Address:** Boston Univ Sch Med, Arthritis Ctr, 72 E Concord St, Evans-501, Boston, MA 02118; **Phone:** 617-638-4312; **Board Cert:** Internal Medicine 1985; Rheumatology 1988; **Med School:** Univ Rochester 1980; **Resid:** Internal Medicine, North Shore Hosp 1982; Internal Medicine, Brigham & Women's Hosp 1985; **Fellow:** Rheumatology, Boston Univ Med Ctr 1987; **Fac Appt:** Prof Med, Boston Univ

Tsokos, George MD [Rhu] - **Spec Exp:** Lupus/SLE; **Hospital:** Beth Israel Deaconess Med Ctr - Boston; **Address:** Beth Israel Deaconess Med Ctr, Dept Rheumatology, 110 Francis St, Ste 4B, Boston, MA 02215; **Phone:** 617-632-8658; **Board Cert:** Internal Medicine 1983; Diagnostic Lab Immunology 1986; Rheumatology 1984; **Med School:** Greece 1975; **Resid:** Internal Medicine, Natl Univ 1979; Immunology, NIH-NIADDK 1981; **Fellow:** Rheumatology, NIH-NIADDK 1983

Weinblatt, Michael E MD [Rhu] - **Spec Exp:** Rheumatoid Arthritis; **Hospital:** Brigham & Women's Hosp; **Address:** Brigham & Womens Hosp, Arthritis Ctr, 45 Francis St, Boston, MA 02115-6110; **Phone:** 617-732-5331; **Board Cert:** Internal Medicine 1978; Rheumatology 1980; **Med School:** Univ MD Sch Med 1975; **Resid:** Internal Medicine, Univ Maryland Hosp 1978; **Fellow:** Rheumatology, Peter Bent Brigham Hosp 1980; **Fac Appt:** Prof Med, Harvard Med Sch

Mid Atlantic

Abramson, Steven B MD [Rhu] - **Spec Exp:** Arthritis; Inflammatory Muscle Disease; Osteoarthritis; **Hospital:** Hosp For Joint Diseases (page 70), NYU Med Ctr (page 68); **Address:** Hosp for Joint Diseases, 301 E 17th St, rm 1410, New York, NY 10003; **Phone:** 212-598-6110; **Board Cert:** Internal Medicine 1977; Rheumatology 1980; **Med School:** Harvard Med Sch 1974; **Resid:** Internal Medicine, Bellevue Hosp/NYU Med Ctr 1978; **Fellow:** Rheumatology, Bellevue Hosp/NYU Med Ctr 1983; **Fac Appt:** Prof Med, NYU Sch Med

Belmont, Howard Michael MD [Rhu] - **Spec Exp:** Lupus/SLE; Rheumatoid Arthritis; Scleroderma; **Hospital:** Hosp For Joint Diseases (page 70), NYU Med Ctr (page 68); **Address:** 305 2nd Ave, Ste 16, New York, NY 10003-2739; **Phone:** 212-598-6516; **Board Cert:** Internal Medicine 1983; Rheumatology 1986; **Med School:** Univ Pittsburgh 1980; **Resid:** Internal Medicine, Mt Sinai Hosp 1983; **Fellow:** Rheumatology, NYU/Bellevue Hosp 1985; **Fac Appt:** Assoc Prof Med, NYU Sch Med

Blume, Ralph S MD [Rhu] - **Spec Exp:** Vasculitis; Lupus/SLE; Rheumatoid Arthritis; **Hospital:** NY-Presby Hosp/Columbia (page 66); **Address:** 161 Fort Washington Ave, Ste 537, New York, NY 10032-3713; **Phone:** 212-305-5512; **Board Cert:** Internal Medicine 1972; Rheumatology 1974; **Med School:** Columbia P&S 1964; **Resid:** Internal Medicine, Columbia-Presby Med Ctr 1968; **Fellow:** Rheumatology, Columbia-Presby Med Ctr 1970; **Fac Appt:** Clin Prof Med, Columbia P&S

Bunning, Robert D MD [Rhu] - **Spec Exp:** Exercise Physiology; Rheumatoid Arthritis; Musculoskeletal Disorders; **Hospital:** Natl Rehab Hosp; **Address:** National Rehab Hosp, 102 Irving St NW Fl 2, Washington, DC 20010; **Phone:** 202-877-1660; **Board Cert:** Internal Medicine 1984; Rheumatology 1986; **Med School:** Univ Cincinnati 1979; **Resid:** Internal Medicine, Wash Hosp Ctr 1984; **Fellow:** Rheumatology, Wash Hosp Ctr 1983; **Fac Appt:** Asst Clin Prof Med, Geo Wash Univ

Buyon, Jill P MD [Rhu] - **Spec Exp:** Lupus/SLE in Pregnancy; Lupus/SLE in Menopause; **Hospital:** Hosp For Joint Diseases (page 70), NYU Med Ctr (page 68); **Address:** 246 E 20th St, New York, NY 10003; **Phone:** 646-356-9400; **Board Cert:** Internal Medicine 1981; Rheumatology 1984; **Med School:** Albert Einstein Coll Med 1978; **Resid:** Internal Medicine, Albert Einstein 1981; **Fellow:** Rheumatology, NYU Med Ctr 1983; **Fac Appt:** Prof Med, NYU Sch Med

Cupps, Thomas R MD [Rhu] - **Spec Exp:** Vasculitis; Hepatitis B-Immune Response; **Hospital:** Georgetown Univ Hosp; **Address:** 3800 Resevoir Rd NW, GUMC - Lower Level, Kober Cogan Bldg, Ste B100, Washington, DC 20007; **Phone:** 202-687-8233; **Board Cert:** Internal Medicine 1978; Allergy & Immunology 1981; **Med School:** Stanford Univ 1975; **Resid:** Internal Medicine, Strong Meml Hosp 1978; **Fellow:** Allergy & Immunology, Natl Inst Allergy & Inf Dis 1980; **Fac Appt:** Assoc Prof Med, Georgetown Univ

Rheumatology

Farber, Martin Stuart MD/PhD [Rhu] - **Hospital:** Sunnyview Hosp, Albany Med Ctr; **Address:** Sunnyview Hospital, 124 Rosa Rd, Schenectady, NY 12308-2198; **Phone:** 518-386-3644; **Board Cert:** Internal Medicine 1982; Rheumatology 1984; **Med School:** Albert Einstein Coll Med 1979; **Resid:** Internal Medicine, Boston City Hosp 1982; **Fellow:** Rheumatology, Boston Univ Sch Med 1984; **Fac Appt:** Asst Clin Prof Med, Albany Med Coll

Ginzler, Ellen MD [Rhu] - **Spec Exp:** Lupus/SLE; **Hospital:** SUNY Downstate Med Ctr, Kings County Hosp Ctr; **Address:** SUNY Downstate, Dept Rheumatology, 450 Clarkson Ave, Box 42, Brooklyn, NY 11203-0042; **Phone:** 718-270-1662; **Board Cert:** Internal Medicine 1972; Rheumatology 1974; **Med School:** Case West Res Univ 1969; **Resid:** Internal Medicine, Kings Co Hosp 1971; Internal Medicine, Bellevue Hosp 1972; **Fellow:** Rheumatology, Univ Hosp 1974; **Fac Appt:** Prof Med, SUNY Downstate

Gorevic, Peter D MD [Rhu] - **Spec Exp:** Autoimmune Disease; Amyloidosis/Joint Disease; Cryoglobulinemia; **Hospital:** Mount Sinai Med Ctr (page 64), Huntington Hosp; **Address:** Mount Sinai Medical Ctr, 1 Gustave L Levy Pl, New York, NY 10029; **Phone:** 212-241-1671; **Board Cert:** Allergy & Immunology 1977; Rheumatology 1976; Diagnostic Lab Immunology 1986; Internal Medicine 1973; **Med School:** NYU Sch Med 1970; **Resid:** Internal Medicine, NYU Med Ctr 1974; **Fellow:** Rheumatology, NYU Med Ctr 1976; Allergy & Immunology, NYU Med Ctr 1977; **Fac Appt:** Prof Med, Mount Sinai Sch Med

Gourley, Mark F MD [Rhu] - **Spec Exp:** Autoimmune Disease; Lupus/SLE; **Hospital:** Natl Inst of Hlth - Clin Ctr; **Address:** Natl Inst Hlth, 10 Center Drive Bldg 10 - rm 10/6N216F, Bethesda, MD 20892-1616; **Phone:** 301-451-6269; **Board Cert:** Internal Medicine 1988; Rheumatology 2002; **Med School:** Tulane Univ 1985; **Resid:** Internal Medicine, Univ Wisconsin Hosps 1988; **Fellow:** Rheumatology, Natl Inst Hlth 1996

Hochberg, Marc C MD [Rhu] - **Spec Exp:** Osteoporosis; Osteoarthritis; Rheumatoid Arthritis; **Hospital:** Univ of MD Med Sys; **Address:** Univ MD Sch Med, Div Rheum, 10 S Pine St, MSTF 8-34, Baltimore, MD 21201; **Phone:** 410-706-6474; **Board Cert:** Internal Medicine 1976; Rheumatology 1978; **Med School:** Johns Hopkins Univ 1973; **Resid:** Internal Medicine, Johns Hopkins Hosp 1975; **Fellow:** Rheumatology, Johns Hopkins Hosp 1977; **Fac Appt:** Prof Med, Univ MD Sch Med

Lahita, Robert G MD/PhD [Rhu] - **Spec Exp:** Lupus/SLE; Endocrinology & Joint Disorders; Immunodeficiency Disorders; **Hospital:** Newark Beth Israel Med Ctr, St Vincent Cath Med Ctrs - Manhattan; **Address:** 201 Lyons Ave, Newark, NJ 07112; **Phone:** 201-222-1266; **Board Cert:** Internal Medicine 2004; Rheumatology 2007; **Med School:** Jefferson Med Coll 1973; **Resid:** Internal Medicine, New York Hosp-Cornell 1976; **Fellow:** Rheumatology, Rockefeller Hosp 1978; **Fac Appt:** Prof Med, Mount Sinai Sch Med

Lockshin, Michael D MD [Rhu] - **Spec Exp:** Lupus/SLE; Antiphospholipid Syndrome (APS); Pregnancy & Rheumatic Disease; Lupus/SLE in Pregnancy; **Hospital:** Hosp For Special Surgery (page 59), NY-Presby Hosp/Weill Cornell (page 66); **Address:** 535 E 70th St, rm 661, New York, NY 10021-4872; **Phone:** 212-606-1461; **Board Cert:** Internal Medicine 1969; Rheumatology 1972; **Med School:** Harvard Med Sch 1963; **Resid:** Internal Medicine, Bellevue Hosp 1968; **Fellow:** Rheumatology, Columbia-Presby Hosp 1970; **Fac Appt:** Prof Med, Cornell Univ-Weill Med Coll

Medsger Jr, Thomas A MD [Rhu] - **Spec Exp:** Scleroderma; Raynaud's Disease; Polymyositis; Dermatomyocitis; **Hospital:** UPMC Presby, Pittsburgh; **Address:** Arthritis & Autoimmunity Ctr, 3601 Fifth Ave, 3B Falk Med Bldg, Pittsburgh, PA 15213; **Phone:** 412-647-6700; **Board Cert:** Internal Medicine 1972; Rheumatology 1972; **Med School:** Univ Pennsylvania 1962; **Resid:** Internal Medicine, Univ Pittsburgh 1968; **Fellow:** Rheumatology, Univ Pittsburgh 1966; Rheumatology, Univ Tenn Coll Med 1969; **Fac Appt:** Prof Med, Univ Pittsburgh

Mitnick, Hal J MD [Rhu] - **Spec Exp:** Rheumatoid Arthritis; Psoriatic Arthritis; Osteoporosis; **Hospital:** NYU Med Ctr (page 68); **Address:** 333 E 34th St, Ste 1C, New York, NY 10016-4977; **Phone:** 212-889-7217; **Board Cert:** Internal Medicine 1976; Rheumatology 1978; **Med School:** NYU Sch Med 1972; **Resid:** Internal Medicine, Bellevue Hosp 1976; **Fellow:** Rheumatology, NYU Med Ctr 1978; **Fac Appt:** Clin Prof Med, NYU Sch Med

Oddis, Chester MD [Rhu] - **Spec Exp:** Polymyositis; Dermatomyositis; Connective Tissue Disorders; **Hospital:** UPMC Presby, Pittsburgh, Penn State Milton S Hershey Med Ctr; **Address:** Univ Pittsburgh-Div Rheumatology, 3500 Terrace St, S 703 BST, Pittsburgh, PA 15261; **Phone:** 412-647-6700; **Board Cert:** Internal Medicine 1983; Rheumatology 1986; **Med School:** Penn State Univ-Hershey Med Ctr 1980; **Resid:** Internal Medicine, Hershey Med Ctr 1984; **Fellow:** Rheumatology, Univ Pittsburgh 1986; **Fac Appt:** Prof Med, Univ Pittsburgh

Paget, Stephen MD [Rhu] - **Spec Exp:** Rheumatoid Arthritis; Lupus/SLE; **Hospital:** Hosp For Special Surgery (page 59); **Address:** 535 E 70th St, rm 721 West, New York, NY 10021; **Phone:** 212-606-1845; **Board Cert:** Internal Medicine 1974; Rheumatology 1976; **Med School:** SUNY Downstate 1971; **Resid:** Internal Medicine, Johns Hopkins Hosp 1973; **Fellow:** Rheumatology, Hosp Special Surg 1975; **Fac Appt:** Clin Prof Med, Cornell Univ-Weill Med Coll

Petri, Michelle A MD [Rhu] - **Spec Exp:** Lupus/SLE; Antiphospholipid Syndrome (APS); **Hospital:** Johns Hopkins Hosp - Baltimore (page 61); **Address:** Div of Rheumatology, 1830 E Monument St, Ste 7500, Baltimore, MD 21205-2100; **Phone:** 410-955-9114; **Board Cert:** Internal Medicine 1983; Allergy & Immunology 1985; Rheumatology 1986; **Med School:** Harvard Med Sch 1980; **Resid:** Internal Medicine, Mass Genl Hosp 1983; **Fellow:** Allergy & Immunology, UCSF Med Ctr 1985; Rheumatology, UCSF Med Ctr 1986; **Fac Appt:** Prof Med, Johns Hopkins Univ

Plotz, Paul MD [Rhu] - **Hospital:** Natl Inst of Hlth - Clin Ctr; **Address:** Bldg 50 - rm 1503, 50 South Drive, MC 8023, Bethesda, MD 20892-1820; **Phone:** 301-496-9904; **Board Cert:** Internal Medicine 1970; **Med School:** Harvard Med Sch 1963; **Resid:** Internal Medicine, Beth Israel Hosp 1965; **Fellow:** Rheumatology, Clin Ctr- NIH 1968

Rosen, Antony MD [Rhu] - **Spec Exp:** Arthritis; Vasculitis; Musculoskeletal Disorders; **Hospital:** Johns Hopkins Hosp - Baltimore (page 61); **Address:** Johns Hopkins School of Medicine, Mason Lord Bldg, Center Toweer, 5200 Eastern Ave, rm 412, Baltimore, MD 21224; **Phone:** 410-550-1894; **Board Cert:** Internal Medicine 2003; Rheumatology 1996; **Med School:** South Africa 1984; **Resid:** Internal Medicine, Johns Hopkins Hosp 1992; **Fellow:** Rheumatology, Johns Hopkins Hosp 1994; Immunological Biology, Rockefeller Inst 1990; **Fac Appt:** Prof Med, Johns Hopkins Univ

Rothenberg, Russell R MD [Rhu] - **Spec Exp:** Fibromyalgia; Lupus/SLE; Rheumatoid Arthritis; **Hospital:** G Washington Univ Hosp; **Address:** 10215 Fernwood Rd, Ste 401, Bethesda, MD 20817; **Phone:** 301-571-2273; **Board Cert:** Internal Medicine 1980; Rheumatology 1982; **Med School:** Albany Med Coll 1977; **Resid:** Internal Medicine, LIJ Medical Ctr 1980; **Fellow:** Rheumatology, Mt Sinai Medical Ctr 1982; **Fac Appt:** Assoc Prof Med, Geo Wash Univ

Solomon, Gary MD [Rhu] - **Spec Exp:** Psoriatic Arthritis; Rheumatoid Arthritis; Autoimmune Disease; **Hospital:** Hosp For Joint Diseases (page 70), NYU Med Ctr (page 68); **Address:** Hosp Joint Diseases, Dept Rheumatology, 305 2nd Ave, Ste 16, New York, NY 10003-2747; **Phone:** 212-598-6516; **Board Cert:** Internal Medicine 1980; Rheumatology 1982; **Med School:** Mount Sinai Sch Med 1977; **Resid:** Internal Medicine, Mount Sinai Med Ctr 1980; **Fellow:** Rheumatology, Montefiore Med Ctr 1982; **Fac Appt:** Assoc Clin Prof Med, NYU Sch Med

Rheumatology

Spiera, Harry MD [Rhu] - **Spec Exp:** Lupus/SLE; Scleroderma; Vasculitis; **Hospital:** Mount Sinai Med Ctr (page 64), NY-Presby Hosp/Weill Cornell (page 66); **Address:** 1088 Park Ave, New York, NY 10128-1132; **Phone:** 212-860-4000 x36; **Board Cert:** Internal Medicine 1965; Rheumatology 1972; **Med School:** NYU Sch Med 1958; **Resid:** Internal Medicine, VA Med Ctr 1960; Internal Medicine, Mount Sinai Hosp 1961; **Fellow:** Rheumatology, Columbia-Presby Med Ctr 1963; **Fac Appt:** Clin Prof Med, Mount Sinai Sch Med

Starz, Terence W MD [Rhu] - **Spec Exp:** Arthritis; **Hospital:** UPMC St Margaret; **Address:** Arthritis & Int Medicine Assocs-UPMC, 3500 Fifth Ave Hieber Bldg Fl 4, Pittsburgh, PA 15213; **Phone:** 412-682-2434; **Board Cert:** Internal Medicine 1975; Rheumatology 1978; **Med School:** Jefferson Med Coll 1971; **Resid:** Internal Medicine, Presby-Univ Hosp 1975; **Fellow:** Rheumatology, Presby-Univ Hosp 1977; **Fac Appt:** Clin Prof Med, Univ Pittsburgh

Steen, Virginia MD [Rhu] - **Spec Exp:** Scleroderma; Lupus/SLE; Polymyositis; **Hospital:** Georgetown Univ Hosp; **Address:** 3800 Reservoir Rd, LL - Kober Cogan Bldg - Ste B100, Washington, DC 20007; **Phone:** 202-687-8233; **Board Cert:** Internal Medicine 1978; Rheumatology 1980; **Med School:** Univ Pittsburgh 1975; **Resid:** Internal Medicine, Hosp Univ Penn 1978; **Fellow:** Rheumatology, Presby Hosp 1980; **Fac Appt:** Prof Med, Georgetown Univ

Vivino, Frederick B MD [Rhu] - **Spec Exp:** Sjogren's Syndrome; **Hospital:** Penn Presby Med Ctr - UPHS (page 60); **Address:** Presbyterian Medical Ctr, 39th & Filberts Sts, PHI-2B, Philadelphia, PA 19104; **Phone:** 215-662-4333; **Board Cert:** Internal Medicine 1986; Rheumatology 1988; **Med School:** Temple Univ 1983; **Resid:** Internal Medicine, Hosp U Penn 1986; **Fellow:** Rheumatology, Hosp U Penn 1989; **Fac Appt:** Asst Clin Prof Med, Univ Pennsylvania

Weinstein, Arthur MD [Rhu] - **Spec Exp:** Lyme Disease; Lupus/SLE; **Hospital:** Washington Hosp Ctr, Georgetown Univ Hosp; **Address:** Washington Hosp Ctr, Div Rheumatology, 110 Irving St NW, rm 2A-66, Washington, DC 20010; **Phone:** 202-877-0333; **Board Cert:** Rheumatology 1976; Diagnostic Lab Immunology 1986; **Med School:** Univ Toronto 1967; **Resid:** Internal Medicine, Toronto Wellesley Hosp 1972; Rheumatology, Hammersmith Hosp 1971; **Fellow:** Rheumatology, Toronto Wellesley Hosp 1973; **Fac Appt:** Prof Med, Georgetown Univ

Wigley, Frederick M MD [Rhu] - **Spec Exp:** Scleroderma; Raynaud's Disease; **Hospital:** Johns Hopkins Bayview Med Ctr (page 61), Johns Hopkins Hosp - Baltimore (page 61); **Address:** 5501 Hopkins Bayview Cir, Ste 1B32, Baltimore, MD 21224; **Phone:** 410-550-7715; **Board Cert:** Internal Medicine 1975; Rheumatology 1980; **Med School:** Univ Fla Coll Med 1972; **Resid:** Internal Medicine, Johns Hopkins Hosp 1975; **Fellow:** Rheumatology, Johns Hopkins Hosp 1979; **Fac Appt:** Prof Med, Johns Hopkins Univ

Southeast

Allen, Nancy B MD [Rhu] - **Spec Exp:** Vasculitis; Wegener's Granulomatosis; Lupus/SLE; **Hospital:** Duke Univ Med Ctr; **Address:** Duke Univ Med Ctr, Box 3440, Durham, NC 27710; **Phone:** 919-684-2965; **Board Cert:** Internal Medicine 1981; Rheumatology 1984; **Med School:** Tufts Univ 1978; **Resid:** Internal Medicine, Duke Univ Med Ctr 1981; **Fellow:** Rheumatology, Duke Univ Med Ctr 1983; **Fac Appt:** Prof Med, Duke Univ

Chatham, Walter W MD [Rhu] - **Spec Exp:** Lupus/SLE; Connective Tissue Disorders; Rheumatoid Arthritis; **Hospital:** Univ of Ala Hosp at Birmingham; **Address:** Univ Alabama Birmingham Med Ctr, FOT 802, 1530 3rd Ave S, Birmingham, AL 35294-3408; **Phone:** 205-934-4212; **Board Cert:** Internal Medicine 1983; Rheumatology 1988; **Med School:** Vanderbilt Univ 1980; **Resid:** Internal Medicine, North Carolina Meml Hosp 1983; **Fellow:** Rheumatology, Univ Alabama Birmingham 1988; **Fac Appt:** Assoc Prof Med, Univ Ala

Crofford, Leslie J MD [Rhu] - **Spec Exp:** Fibromyalgia; Rheumatoid Arthritis; Lupus/SLE; **Hospital:** Univ of Kentucky Chandler Hosp; **Address:** 740 S Limestone St, rm J509, Lexington, KY 40536-0284; **Phone:** 859-323-4939; **Board Cert:** Internal Medicine 1987; Rheumatology 2003; **Med School:** Univ Tenn Coll Med, Memphis 1984; **Resid:** Internal Medicine, Barnes/Wash Univ 1987; **Fellow:** Rheumatology, Natl Inst Hlth Clin Ctr 1992; **Fac Appt:** Prof Med, Univ KY Coll Med

Hadler, Nortin MD [Rhu] - **Spec Exp:** Occupational Musculoskeletal Disorders; Musculoskeletal Disorders; Spondylitis-Back Pain; **Hospital:** Univ NC Hosps; **Address:** Univ North Carolina, Dept Medicine, 3300 Thurston Building, Box 7280, Chapel Hill, NC 27599-7280; **Phone:** 919-966-0566; **Board Cert:** Rheumatology 1974; Allergy & Immunology 1975; Internal Medicine 1987; **Med School:** Harvard Med Sch 1968; **Resid:** Internal Medicine, Mass Genl Hosp 1973; **Fellow:** Rheumatology, Natl Inst Hlth 1972; Allergy & Immunology, Clin Res Ctr 1974; **Fac Appt:** Prof Med, Univ NC Sch Med

Moore, Walter J MD [Rhu] - **Spec Exp:** Rheumatoid Arthritis; Lupus/SLE; **Hospital:** Med Coll of GA Hosp and Clin; **Address:** Medical College of Georgia, 1120 15th St, rm BI 5083, Augusta, GA 30912; **Phone:** 706-721-1450; **Board Cert:** Internal Medicine 1980; Rheumatology 1984; **Med School:** Georgetown Univ 1977; **Resid:** Internal Medicine, Walter Reed AMC 1980; **Fellow:** Rheumatology, Walter Reed AMC 1983; **Fac Appt:** Assoc Prof Med, Med Coll GA

Sergent, John S MD [Rhu] - **Spec Exp:** Vasculitis; **Hospital:** Vanderbilt Univ Med Ctr; **Address:** Vanderbilt Univ Med Ctr - Dept Medicine, D3100 Medical Ctr North, 1161 21st Ave S, Nashville, TN 37232-2358; **Phone:** 615-322-1900; **Board Cert:** Internal Medicine 1972; Rheumatology 1974; **Med School:** Vanderbilt Univ 1966; **Resid:** Internal Medicine, Johns Hopkins Hosp 1968; Internal Medicine, Vanderbilt Univ Hosp 1972; **Fellow:** Rheumatology, Hosp Special Surgery 1974; **Fac Appt:** Prof Med, Vanderbilt Univ

Silver, Richard M MD [Rhu] - **Spec Exp:** Scleroderma & Lung Disease; Pediatric Rheumatology; Connective Tissue Disorders; **Hospital:** MUSC Med Ctr; **Address:** MUSC Med Ctr, PO Box 250623, 96 Jonathan Lucas St, Ste 912, Charleston, SC 29425; **Phone:** 843-876-0500; **Board Cert:** Internal Medicine 1978; Rheumatology 1982; **Med School:** Vanderbilt Univ 1975; **Resid:** Internal Medicine, Univ NC Hosps 1978; **Fellow:** Rheumatology, UCSD Med Ctr 1981; **Fac Appt:** Prof Med, Med Univ SC

Sundy, John S MD/PhD [Rhu] - **Spec Exp:** Rheumatoid Arthritis; Gout; Lupus/SLE; **Hospital:** Duke Univ Med Ctr, Durham Regional Hosp; **Address:** 4309 Medical Park Drive, Ste 100, Durham, NC 27710; **Phone:** 919-668-2169; **Board Cert:** Rheumatology 1998; Allergy & Immunology 1999; Internal Medicine 2006; **Med School:** Hahnemann Univ 1991; **Resid:** Internal Medicine, Duke Univ Med Ctr 1993; **Fellow:** Rheumatology, Duke Univ Med Ctr 1996; Allergy & Immunology, Duke Univ Med Ctr 1998; **Fac Appt:** Asst Prof Med, Duke Univ

Wise, Christopher M MD [Rhu] - **Spec Exp:** Gout; Sjogren's Syndrome; Rheumatoid Arthritis; **Hospital:** Med Coll of VA Hosp; **Address:** Virginia Commonwealth Univ/MCV Campus, Box 980647, Richmond, VA 23298; **Phone:** 804-828-9341; **Board Cert:** Internal Medicine 1980; Rheumatology 1982; **Med School:** Univ NC Sch Med 1977; **Resid:** Internal Medicine, Med Coll Virginia Hosp 1980; **Fellow:** Rheumatology, Med Coll Virginia Hosp 1982; **Fac Appt:** Prof Med, Va Commonwealth Univ Sch Med

Rheumatology

Midwest

Adams, Elaine MD [Rhu] - **Spec Exp:** Rheumatoid Arthritis; Lupus/SLE; Spondyloarthropathies; **Hospital:** Loyola Univ Med Ctr, Hines VA Hosp; **Address:** Loyola Univ Med Ctr, Dept Rheumatology, 2160 S 1st Ave, Bldg 54 - rm 121, Maywood, IL 60153-5590; **Phone:** 708-216-8563; **Board Cert:** Internal Medicine 1981; Rheumatology 1984; **Med School:** Loyola Univ-Stritch Sch Med 1978; **Resid:** Internal Medicine, Loyola Univ Med Ctr 1981; **Fellow:** Rheumatology, Univ Wisconsin Med Ctr 1983; **Fac Appt:** Assoc Prof Med, Loyola Univ-Stritch Sch Med

Ashman, Robert F MD [Rhu] - **Spec Exp:** Lupus/SLE; Rheumatoid Arthritis; Inflammatory Muscle Disease; **Hospital:** Univ Iowa Hosp & Clinics; **Address:** Univ Iowa Hosp & Clinics, Div Rheumatology, 200 Hawkins Drive, rm C31-P GH, Iowa City, IA 52242-1081; **Phone:** 319-356-2287; **Board Cert:** Internal Medicine 1974; Rheumatology 1976; **Med School:** Columbia P&S 1966; **Resid:** Internal Medicine, Peter Bent Brigham Hosp 1970; **Fellow:** Rheumatology, UCLA Med Ctr 1973; **Fac Appt:** Prof Med, Univ Iowa Coll Med

Barr, Walter Gerard MD [Rhu] - **Spec Exp:** Scleroderma; Vasculitis; Stem Cell Transplant/Autoimmune Disease; **Hospital:** Northwestern Meml Hosp; **Address:** 675 N St Clair St, Ste 14-100, Chicago, IL 60611-5972; **Phone:** 312-695-8628; **Board Cert:** Internal Medicine 1978; Rheumatology 1982; **Med School:** Loyola Univ-Stritch Sch Med 1975; **Resid:** Internal Medicine, Loyola Univ Med Ctr 1978; **Fellow:** Rheumatology, Loyola Univ Med Ctr 1979; Rheumatology, Mayo Clinic 1982; **Fac Appt:** Assoc Prof Med, Northwestern Univ

Brasington, Richard MD [Rhu] - **Hospital:** Barnes-Jewish Hosp; **Address:** 4921 Parkview Pl Fl 5CAM - Ste C, Rheumatology CB 8045, St Louis, MO 63110; **Phone:** 314-286-2635; **Board Cert:** Internal Medicine 1985; Rheumatology 1986; **Med School:** Duke Univ 1980; **Resid:** Internal Medicine, Univ Iowa Med Ctr 1982; Internal Medicine, Univ Iowa Med Ctr 1985; **Fellow:** Rheumatology, Univ Iowa 1986; **Fac Appt:** Assoc Prof Med, Washington Univ, St Louis

Chang, Rowland W MD [Rhu] - **Spec Exp:** Rheumatoid Arthritis; Arthritis; Ankylosing Spondylitis; **Hospital:** Northwestern Meml Hosp, Rehab Inst - Chicago; **Address:** Rehab Inst of Chicago Arthritis Ctr, 345 E Superior St Fl 9, Chicago, IL 60611-2654; **Phone:** 312-238-2784; **Board Cert:** Internal Medicine 1979; Rheumatology 1982; **Med School:** Tufts Univ 1976; **Resid:** Internal Medicine, Mt Auburn Hosp 1979; **Fellow:** Rheumatology, Hammersmith Hosp 1980; Rheumatology, Brigham & Womens Hosp 1982; **Fac Appt:** Prof Med, Northwestern Univ

Curran, James J MD [Rhu] - **Spec Exp:** Rheumatoid Arthritis; Lupus/SLE; Sjogren's Syndrome; Polymyositis; **Hospital:** Univ of Chicago Hosps; **Address:** 5841 S Maryland Ave, MC-0930, Chicago, IL 60637-1463; **Phone:** 773-702-1232; **Board Cert:** Internal Medicine 1980; Rheumatology 1982; **Med School:** Univ IL Coll Med 1976; **Resid:** Internal Medicine, Bethesda Naval Hosp 1980; **Fellow:** Rheumatology, Univ Chicago Hosps 1982; **Fac Appt:** Prof Med, Univ Chicago-Pritzker Sch Med

Fischbein, Lewis C MD [Rhu] - **Spec Exp:** Rheumatoid Arthritis; Lupus/SLE; Hypertension; **Hospital:** Barnes-Jewish Hosp; **Address:** One Barnes-Jewish Hospital Plaza, Ste 16422, St Louis, MO 63110; **Phone:** 314-367-9595; **Board Cert:** Internal Medicine 1977; Rheumatology 1980; **Med School:** Washington Univ, St Louis 1974; **Resid:** Internal Medicine, Barnes Jewish Hosp 1977; **Fellow:** Rheumatology, Barnes Jewish Hosp 1979; **Fac Appt:** Assoc Prof Med, Washington Univ, St Louis

Katz, Robert S MD [Rhu] - **Spec Exp:** Rheumatoid Arthritis; Lupus/SLE; Fibromyalgia; **Hospital:** Rush Univ Med Ctr, Northwestern Meml Hosp; **Address:** 1725 W Harrison St, Ste 1039, Chicago, IL 60612-3841; **Phone:** 312-942-2159; **Board Cert:** Internal Medicine 1975; Rheumatology 1976; **Med School:** Univ MD Sch Med 1970; **Resid:** Internal Medicine, Washington Univ Med Ctr 1972; **Fellow:** Rheumatology, Johns Hopkins Hosp 1976; **Fac Appt:** Assoc Prof Med, Rush Med Coll

Klearman, Micki MD [Rhu] - **Spec Exp:** Arthritis; Lupus/SLE; Vasculitis; **Hospital:** Barnes-Jewish Hosp; **Address:** One Barnes-Jewish Hospital Plaza, Ste 16422, St Louis, MO 63110; **Phone:** 314-367-9595; **Board Cert:** Internal Medicine 1985; Rheumatology 1988; **Med School:** Washington Univ, St Louis 1981; **Resid:** Internal Medicine, Jewish Hosp 1985; **Fellow:** Rheumatology, Wash Univ 1987; **Fac Appt:** Assoc Clin Prof Med, Washington Univ, St Louis

Langford, Carol MD [Rhu] - **Spec Exp:** Vasculitis; **Hospital:** Cleveland Clin Fdn (page 56); **Address:** Cleveland Clinic Main Campus, MC A50, 9500 Euclid Ave, Cleveland, OH 44195; **Phone:** 216-445-6056; **Board Cert:** Internal Medicine 2000; Rheumatology 2000; **Med School:** UCLA 1987; **Resid:** Internal Medicine, Univ Mich 1990; **Fellow:** Rheumatology, Duke Univ Med Ctr 1991

Lawry, George V MD [Rhu] - **Hospital:** Univ Iowa Hosp & Clinics; **Address:** Univ Iowa Hosp & Clins, Dept Rheumatology, 200 Hawkins Drive, rm C31-GGH, Iowa City, IA 52242-1009; **Phone:** 319-356-1777; **Board Cert:** Internal Medicine 1978; Rheumatology 1982; **Med School:** Johns Hopkins Univ 1975; **Resid:** Internal Medicine, Mass Genl Hosp 1977; Internal Medicine, Stanford Hosp 1978; **Fellow:** Rheumatology, Wadsworth VA-UCLA Med Ctr 1981; **Fac Appt:** Clin Prof Med, Univ Iowa Coll Med

Luggen, Michael MD [Rhu] - **Hospital:** Univ Hosp - Cincinnati, Christ Hospital; **Address:** Christ Hosp Office Bldg, 2123 Auburn Ave, Ste 630, Cincinnati, OH 45219; **Phone:** 513-585-1970; **Board Cert:** Internal Medicine 1978; Rheumatology 1982; **Med School:** Columbia P&S 1974; **Resid:** Internal Medicine, Cinn Genl Hosp 1977; **Fellow:** Rheumatology, Univ Cincinnati 1982; **Fac Appt:** Prof Med, Univ Cincinnati

Luthra, Harvinder Singh MD [Rhu] - **Spec Exp:** Rheumatoid Arthritis; Ankylosing Spondylitis; Relapsing Polychondritis; **Hospital:** St Mary's Hosp - Rochester, Rochester Methodist Hosp; **Address:** Mayo Clinic, 200 First St SW, Rochester, MN 55905-0002; **Phone:** 507-266-4439; **Board Cert:** Internal Medicine 1973; Rheumatology 2002; **Med School:** India 1967; **Resid:** Ophthalmology, Christian Med Coll; Internal Medicine, Mount Sinai Hosp 1972; **Fellow:** Rheumatology, Mayo Grad Sch 1974; **Fac Appt:** Prof Med, Mayo Med Sch

McCune, W Joseph MD [Rhu] - **Spec Exp:** Lupus/SLE; Rheumatoid Arthritis; **Hospital:** Univ Michigan Hlth Sys; **Address:** Univ Mich, Dept Rheum, 1500 E Med Ctr, rm 3918 Taubman Ctr, Ann Arbor, MI 48109-0358; **Phone:** 734-647-5900; **Board Cert:** Internal Medicine 1978; Rheumatology 1982; **Med School:** Univ Cincinnati 1975; **Resid:** Internal Medicine, Univ Mich Hosps 1978; Rheumatology, Brigham Womens Hosp 1978; **Fellow:** Rheumatology, Brigham Womens Hosp 1981; **Fac Appt:** Prof Med, Univ Mich Med Sch

Michalska, Margaret MD [Rhu] - **Spec Exp:** Rheumatoid Arthritis; Connective Tissue Disorders; Osteoporosis; **Hospital:** Adv Illinois Masonic Med Ctr; **Address:** 3000 N Halsted St, Ste 409, Chicago, IL 60657; **Phone:** 773-296-7150; **Board Cert:** Internal Medicine 1988; Rheumatology 2000; **Med School:** Poland 1979; **Resid:** Internal Medicine, Hines VA Hosp 1988; **Fellow:** Biochemistry, Nortwestern Univ 1985; Rheumatology, Rush-Presby-St Lukes Med Ctr 1990; **Fac Appt:** Assoc Prof Med, Rush Med Coll

Rheumatology

Moder, Kevin G MD [Rhu] - **Spec Exp:** Rheumatoid Arthritis; Lupus/SLE; **Hospital:** Mayo Med Ctr & Clin - Rochester; **Address:** Mayo Clinic, Div Rheumatology, 200 First St SW, Rochester, MN 55905-0002; **Phone:** 507-284-4550; **Board Cert:** Internal Medicine 2000; Rheumatology 2000; **Med School:** Univ MO-Columbia Sch Med 1987; **Resid:** Internal Medicine, Mayo Clinic 1990; **Fellow:** Rheumatology, Mayo Clinic 1993; **Fac Appt:** Asst Prof Med, Mayo Med Sch

Pope, Richard M MD [Rhu] - **Spec Exp:** Rheumatoid Arthritis; Sjogren's Syndrome; Psoriatic Arthritis; **Hospital:** Northwestern Meml Hosp; **Address:** 675 N St Clair, Ste 14-100, Chicago, IL 60611-5966; **Phone:** 312-695-8628; **Board Cert:** Internal Medicine 1973; Clinical & Laboratory Immunology 1986; **Med School:** Loyola Univ-Stritch Sch Med 1970; **Resid:** Internal Medicine, Michael Reese Hosp 1972; **Fellow:** Rheumatology, Univ Wash Med Ctr 1974; **Fac Appt:** Prof Med, Northwestern Univ

Warner, Ann E MD [Rhu] - **Hospital:** St Luke's Hosp of Kansas City; **Address:** 4330 Wornall St, Ste 40, Kansas City, MO 64111-3210; **Phone:** 816-531-0930; **Board Cert:** Internal Medicine 1986; Rheumatology 1988; Allergy & Immunology 1999; **Med School:** Univ Kans 1983; **Resid:** Internal Medicine, St Luke's Hosp 1986; **Fellow:** Rheumatology, Univ Kansas Med Ctr 1989; **Fac Appt:** Asst Clin Prof Med, Univ MO-Kansas City

Great Plains and Mountains

Arend, William P MD [Rhu] - **Spec Exp:** Arthritis; Rheumatoid Arthritis; **Hospital:** Univ Colorado Hosp; **Address:** 1775 N Ursula St, Box 6511, MC b115, Univ of Colo, Dept of Rheumatology, Aurora, CO 80045; **Phone:** 720-848-1940; **Board Cert:** Internal Medicine 1971; Rheumatology 1980; **Med School:** Columbia P&S 1964; **Resid:** Internal Medicine, Univ Washington Hosp 1969; **Fellow:** Rheumatology, Univ Washington Hosp 1971; **Fac Appt:** Prof Med, Univ Colorado

O'Dell, James R MD [Rhu] - **Spec Exp:** Osteoarthritis; Rheumatoid Arthritis; **Address:** 983025 Nebraska Med Ctr, Omaha, NE 68198-3025; **Phone:** 402-559-4015; **Board Cert:** Internal Medicine 1980; Rheumatology 1984; **Med School:** Univ Nebr Coll Med 1977; **Resid:** Internal Medicine, Univ Nebraska Med Ctr 1981; **Fellow:** Rheumatology, Univ Colorado 1984; **Fac Appt:** Prof Med, Univ Nebr Coll Med

West, Sterling MD [Rhu] - **Spec Exp:** Lupus/SLE; Vasculitis; Osteoporosis; **Hospital:** Univ Colorado Hosp; **Address:** Barbara Davis Center, 1775 N Ursula St, Box B115, Aurora, CO 80045; **Phone:** 720-848-1940; **Board Cert:** Internal Medicine 1979; Rheumatology 1982; **Med School:** Emory Univ 1976; **Resid:** Internal Medicine, Fitzsimons Army Med Ctr 1979; **Fellow:** Rheumatology, Walter Reed Army Med Ctr 1981; **Fac Appt:** Prof Med, Univ Colorado

Southwest

Arnett Jr, Frank C MD [Rhu] - **Spec Exp:** Reiter's Syndrome; Spondylitis; Scleroderma; **Hospital:** Meml Hermann Hosp - Texas Med Ctr; **Address:** Hermann Prof Bldg, 6410 Fannin St, Ste 1100, Houston, TX 77030-5302; **Phone:** 832-325-7191; **Board Cert:** Internal Medicine 1972; Rheumatology 1976; Clinical & Laboratory Immunology 1990; **Med School:** Univ Cincinnati 1968; **Resid:** Internal Medicine, Johns Hopkins Hosp 1970; **Fellow:** Rheumatology, Johns Hopkins Hosp 1972; **Fac Appt:** Prof Med, Univ Tex, Houston

Chang-Miller, April MD [Rhu] - **Spec Exp:** Connective Tissue Disorders; Spondyloarthropathies; **Hospital:** Mayo Clinic - Scottsdale; **Address:** Mayo Clinic, Div Rheumatology, 13400 E Shea Blvd, Scottsdale, AZ 85259; **Phone:** 480-301-4342; **Board Cert:** Internal Medicine 1986; Rheumatology 2000; **Med School:** Yale Univ 1983; **Resid:** Internal Medicine, Mayo Clinic 1985; **Fellow:** Rheumatology, Mayo Clinic 1989; Biochemical and Molecular Biology, Mayo Clinic 1990; **Fac Appt:** Asst Prof Med, Mayo Med Sch

Davis, William Eugene MD [Rhu] - **Spec Exp:** Lupus/SLE; Rheumatoid Arthritis; Gout; **Hospital:** Ochsner Fdn Hosp; **Address:** Ochsner Clinic, Rheum, 1514 Jefferson Hwy, CA5, New Orleans, LA 70121-2483; **Phone:** 504-842-3920; **Board Cert:** Internal Medicine 1987; Rheumatology 1988; **Med School:** Louisiana State U, New Orleans 1983; **Resid:** Internal Medicine, Ochsner Fdn Hosp 1986; **Fellow:** Rheumatology, Univ Michigan 1988

Lindsey, Stephen M MD [Rhu] - **Spec Exp:** Osteoporosis; Lupus/SLE; **Hospital:** Baton Rouge Gen Med Ctr; **Address:** 9001 Summa Ave, Baton Rouge, LA 70809; **Phone:** 225-761-5500; **Board Cert:** Internal Medicine 1975; Rheumatology 1980; **Med School:** Louisiana State U, New Orleans 1972; **Resid:** Internal Medicine, Letterman AMC 1975; **Fellow:** Rheumatology, Walter Reed AMC 1979

Lipstate, James M MD [Rhu] - **Spec Exp:** Arthritis; Osteoporosis; **Hospital:** Our Lady of Lourdes Reg Med Ctr - Lafayette, Lafayette Genl Med Ctr; **Address:** 401 Audubon Blvd, Ste 102B, Lafayette, LA 70503; **Phone:** 337-237-7801; **Board Cert:** Internal Medicine 1983; Rheumatology 1986; **Med School:** Tulane Univ 1980; **Resid:** Internal Medicine, Univ Alabama Hosp 1983; **Fellow:** Rheumatology, Univ Alabama Hosp 1986; **Fac Appt:** Asst Clin Prof Med, Louisiana State U, New Orleans

Mayes, Maureen D MD/PhD [Rhu] - **Spec Exp:** Scleroderma; **Hospital:** Meml Hermann Hosp - Texas Med Ctr, LBJ General Hosp; **Address:** Univ Tex Hlth Sci Ctr, Div Rheum, 6410 Fannin St, Ste 600, Houston, TX 77030-1501; **Phone:** 832-325-7191; **Board Cert:** Internal Medicine 1980; Rheumatology 1982; **Med School:** Eastern VA Med Sch 1976; **Resid:** Internal Medicine, Cleveland Clinic Fnd 1979; **Fellow:** Rheumatology, Cleveland Clinic Fnd 1981; **Fac Appt:** Prof Med, Univ Tex, Houston

Sessoms, Sandra Lee MD [Rhu] - **Spec Exp:** Arthritis; Lupus/SLE; Autoimmune Disease; **Hospital:** Methodist Hosp - Houston, St Luke's Episcopal Hosp - Houston; **Address:** Meth Hosp, Div Rheum, 6550 Fannin St, Smith Twr, Ste 2500, Houston, TX 77030; **Phone:** 713-441-9000; **Board Cert:** Internal Medicine 1981; Rheumatology 1984; **Med School:** Baylor Coll Med 1978; **Resid:** Internal Medicine, Baylor Coll Med 1979; **Fellow:** Rheumatology, Baylor Coll Med 1983; **Fac Appt:** Assoc Prof Med, Baylor Coll Med

West Coast and Pacific

Bobrove, Arthur M MD [Rhu] - **Spec Exp:** Psoriatic Arthritis; Ankylosing Spondylitis; Sjogren's Syndrome; **Hospital:** Stanford Univ Med Ctr; **Address:** 795 El Camino Real, Palo Alto, CA 94301-2302; **Phone:** 650-853-2972; **Board Cert:** Internal Medicine 1972; Rheumatology 1976; **Med School:** Temple Univ 1967; **Resid:** Internal Medicine, Univ Mich Hosp 1969; Internal Medicine, Univ Mich Hosp 1972; **Fellow:** Immunology, Stanford Univ Hosp 1974; **Fac Appt:** Clin Prof Med, Stanford Univ

Clements, Philip J MD [Rhu] - **Spec Exp:** Scleroderma; Raynaud's Disease; **Hospital:** Ronald Reagan UCLA Med Ctr; **Address:** UCLA Sch Med, Rehab 32-59, 1000 Veteran Ave, Los Angeles, CA 90095-1670; **Phone:** 310-825-8414; **Board Cert:** Internal Medicine 1972; Rheumatology 1974; **Med School:** Indiana Univ 1965; **Resid:** Internal Medicine, Cedars-Sinai Med Ctr 1971; **Fellow:** Rheumatology, UCLA Med Ctr 1974; **Fac Appt:** Prof Med, UCLA

Rheumatology

Ehresmann, Glenn R MD [Rhu] - **Hospital:** USC Univ Hosp - R K Eamer Med Plz; **Address:** 1520 San Pablo St, Ste 1000, Los Angeles, CA 90033; **Phone:** 323-442-5100; **Board Cert:** Internal Medicine 1977; Rheumatology 1978; **Med School:** UC Irvine 1973; **Resid:** Internal Medicine, LAC-USC Med Ctr 1976; **Fellow:** Rheumatology, LAC-USC Med Ctr 1978; **Fac Appt:** Assoc Clin Prof Med, USC-Keck School of Medicine

Gershwin, Merrill Eric MD [Rhu] - **Spec Exp:** Allergy; Rheumatoid Arthritis; **Hospital:** UC Davis Med Ctr; **Address:** UC Davis Sch Med, Div Rheum, 451 E Health Sciences Drive, Ste 6510, Davis, CA 95616; **Phone:** 530-752-2884; **Board Cert:** Internal Medicine 1974; Rheumatology 1976; Allergy & Immunology 1979; **Med School:** Stanford Univ 1971; **Resid:** Internal Medicine, Tufts-New Eng Med Ctr 1972; Allergy & Immunology, Tufts-New Eng Med Ctr 1973; **Fellow:** Rheumatology, Natl Inst Hlth 1975; Allergy & Immunology, Natl Inst Hlth 1977; **Fac Appt:** Prof Med, UC Davis

Mease, Philip J MD [Rhu] - **Spec Exp:** Arthritis; Autoimmune Disease; Fibromyalgia; **Hospital:** Swedish Med Ctr - Seattle, Swedish Med Ctr Providence Campus; **Address:** 1101 Madison St, Ste 1000, Seattle, WA 98104; **Phone:** 206-386-2000; **Board Cert:** Internal Medicine 1980; Rheumatology 1982; **Med School:** Stanford Univ 1977; **Resid:** Internal Medicine, Univ Wash Med Ctr 1981; **Fellow:** Rheumatology, Univ Wash Med Ctr 1982; **Fac Appt:** Clin Prof Med, Univ Wash

Wallace, Daniel J MD [Rhu] - **Spec Exp:** Lupus/SLE; Rheumatoid Arthritis; Scleroderma; **Hospital:** Cedars-Sinai Med Ctr, Ronald Reagan UCLA Med Ctr; **Address:** 8737 Beverly Blvd, Ste 302, Los Angeles, CA 90048-1828; **Phone:** 310-652-0920; **Board Cert:** Internal Medicine 1978; Rheumatology 1982; **Med School:** USC Sch Med 1974; **Resid:** Internal Medicine, Cedars-Sinai Med Ctr 1977; **Fellow:** Rheumatology, UCLA Med Ctr 1979; **Fac Appt:** Clin Prof Med, UCLA

Wener, Mark MD [Rhu] - **Spec Exp:** Lupus/SLE; Vasculitis; Immunodeficiency Disorders; **Hospital:** Univ Wash Med Ctr; **Address:** Univ Washington Med Ctr, Div Rheumatology, 1959 NE Pacific St, Box 356166, Seattle, WA 98195; **Phone:** 206-598-4615; **Board Cert:** Internal Medicine 1978; Rheumatology 1980; Clinical & Laboratory Immunology 1986; **Med School:** Washington Univ, St Louis 1974; **Resid:** Internal Medicine, Univ Iowa Hosps 1978; **Fellow:** Rheumatology, Univ Iowa Hosp 1980; Immunology, Univ Wash 1981; **Fac Appt:** Assoc Prof Med, Univ Wash

Wofsy, David MD [Rhu] - **Spec Exp:** Lupus/SLE; **Hospital:** UCSF Med Ctr, VA Med Ctr - San Francisco; **Address:** 533 Parnassus Ave, Box 0633, San Francisco, CA 94143; **Phone:** 415-750-2104; **Board Cert:** Internal Medicine 1977; Rheumatology 1980; **Med School:** UCSD 1974; **Resid:** Internal Medicine, UCSF Hosps 1977; **Fellow:** Rheumatology, UCSF 1979; **Fac Appt:** Prof Med, UCSF

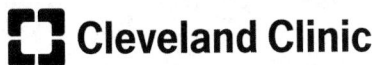
Cleveland Clinic

Rheumatic and Immunologic Diseases

Cleveland Clinic's Department of Rheumatic and Immunologic Diseases has a long-standing commitment to excellence and innovation in the research and care of patients with illnesses such as arthritis, osteoporosis and vasculitis. For the past several years, *U.S.News & World Report* has consistently ranked it among the nation's top five rheumatology programs.

Arthritis

Arthritis is a general term which describes inflammation in joints, characterized by redness, warmth, swelling and pain. Arthritis is a general term for more than 100 diseases. Some of the most commonly treated at the Department of Rheumatic and Immunologic Diseases include rheumatoid arthritis and osteoarthritis.

Osteoporosis

Cleveland Clinic's Center for Osteoporosis and Metabolic Bone Diseases is devoted to the evaluation and treatment of patients with osteoporosis and other forms of diseases that affect bones. The Center's goal is to evaluate patients at an early stage to prevent the complications of osteoporosis as well as additional disease manifestations.

Vasculitis

Cleveland Clinic's Center for Vasculitis Care and Research aims to ensure the best possible care for patients with vasculitis, discover the causes of these diseases and identify improved therapies. The department faculty has special expertise in vasculitis and has established extensive collaborations with other departments of Cleveland Clinic to bring complementary skills to both service and research.

Autoimmune Disease

The Department of Rheumatic and Immunologic Diseases also provides expert care for a variety of illnesses for which arthritis may not be a major feature. These include conditions for which the body's immune defense system, in part, turns on itself and damages one's own body, thus the term autoimmune. Examples of such disorders include systemic lupus, scleroderma, myositis, polychondritis and vasculitis.

For more information about the Cleveland Clinic Department of Rheumatic and Immunologic Disease, to schedule a second opinion or to learn about assistance for out-of-town patients, call 800.890.2467 or visit www. clevelandclinic.org/arthritistopdocs.

Department of Rheumatic and Immunologic Diseases
9500 Euclid Avenue / AC311 | Cleveland OH 44195

Sports Medicine

a subspecialty of Internal Medicine, Family Practice, Pediatrics, or Orthopaedics

A specialist trained to be responsible for continuous care in the field of sports medicine, not only for the enhancement of health and fitness, but also for the prevention of injury and illness. A sports medicine physician must have knowledge and experience in the promotion of wellness and the prevention of injury. Knowledge about special areas of medicine such as exercise physiology, biomechanics, nutrition, psychology, physical rehabilitation, epidemiology, physical evaluation, injuries (treatment and prevention and referral practice) and the role of exercise in promoting a healthy life style are essential to the practice of sports medicine. The sports medicine physician requires special education to provide the knowledge to improve the healthcare of the individual engaged in physical exercise (sports) whether as an individual or in team participation.

Training Required: Three years in internal medicine, family practice, or pediatrics or seven years in orthopaedics *plus* additional training and examination for certification in sports medicine.

For more information about the main specialties of these physicians, see **Internal Medicine, Family Practice, Pediatrics, Orthopaedics** section(s).

SPORTS MEDICINE

New England

Micheli, Lyle J MD [SM] - **Spec Exp:** Pediatric Sports Medicine; Dance/Ballet Injuries; **Hospital:** Beth Israel Deaconess Med Ctr - Boston, Children's Hospital - Boston; **Address:** Chldns Hosp, Div Sports Medicine, 319 Longwood Ave, Boston, MA 02115-5737; **Phone:** 617-355-3501; **Board Cert:** Orthopaedic Surgery 1973; **Med School:** Harvard Med Sch 1966; **Resid:** Surgery, Univ Hosps 1968; Orthopaedic Surgery, Mass Genl Hosp/Chldns Hosp 1972; **Fellow:** Pediatric Orthopaedic Surgery, Orth Rsch Soc-Traveling Fell 1973; **Fac Appt:** Assoc Clin Prof OrS, Harvard Med Sch

Scheller, Arnold D MD [SM] - **Spec Exp:** Sports Injuries; Ankle Surgery; Shoulder Surgery; Knee Surgery; **Hospital:** New England Bapt Hosp; **Address:** Pro Sports Orthopaedics, 235 Cypres St, Ste 300, Brookline, MA 02445; **Phone:** 617-738-8642; **Board Cert:** Orthopaedic Surgery 1980; **Med School:** Rush Med Coll 1980; **Resid:** Orthopaedic Surgery, New England Hosp 1983; **Fac Appt:** Asst Clin Prof OrS, Tufts Univ

Steiner, Mark E MD [SM] - **Spec Exp:** Shoulder Injuries; Knee Injuries; Arthroscopic Surgery; **Hospital:** New England Bapt Hosp; **Address:** 830 Boylston St, Ste 205, Chestnut Hill, MA 02467; **Phone:** 617-739-2003; **Board Cert:** Orthopaedic Surgery 1998; **Med School:** Columbia P&S 1978; **Resid:** Surgery, Mass General Hosp 1980; Orthopaedic Surgery, Mass General Hosp 1984; **Fellow:** Sports Medicine, U Oklahoma Med Ctr 1985

Mid Atlantic

Altchek, David MD [SM] - **Spec Exp:** Shoulder Surgery; Elbow Surgery; Knee Surgery; Arthroscopic Surgery; **Hospital:** Hosp For Special Surgery (page 59), NY-Presby Hosp/Weill Cornell (page 66); **Address:** Hospital for Special Surgery, 535 E 70th St, New York, NY 10021; **Phone:** 212-606-1909; **Board Cert:** Orthopaedic Surgery 2001; **Med School:** Cornell Univ-Weill Med Coll 1982; **Resid:** Orthopaedic Surgery, Hosp for Special Surg 1987; **Fellow:** Sports Medicine, Hosp for Special Surg 1988; **Fac Appt:** Assoc Prof OrS, Cornell Univ-Weill Med Coll

Bradley, James Phillip MD [SM] - **Spec Exp:** Reconstructive Surgery; Shoulder Surgery; Knee Surgery; **Hospital:** UPMC St Margaret, UPMC Shadyside; **Address:** 200 Delafield Ave, Ste 4010, Pittsburgh, PA 15215; **Phone:** 412-784-5783; **Board Cert:** Orthopaedic Surgery 2001; **Med School:** Georgetown Univ 1982; **Resid:** Surgery, Univ Tennessee 1984; Orthopaedic Surgery, Univ Hlth Ctr 1987; **Fellow:** Sports Medicine, Kerlan-Jobe Ortho Clinic 1988; **Fac Appt:** Assoc Prof OrS, Univ Pittsburgh

Ciccotti, Michael G MD [SM] - **Spec Exp:** Knee Reconstruction; Elbow Reconstruction; Shoulder Reconstruction; Arthroscopic Surgery; **Hospital:** Thomas Jefferson Univ Hosp, Bryn Mawr Hosp; **Address:** Rothman Institute, 925 Chestnut St Fl 5, Philadelphia, PA 19107; **Phone:** 267-339-3500; **Board Cert:** Orthopaedic Surgery 2005; **Med School:** Georgetown Univ 1986; **Resid:** Orthopaedic Surgery, Thos Jefferson Univ Med Ctr 1991; **Fellow:** Sports Medicine, Kerlan-Jobe Clinic/USC 1992; **Fac Appt:** Asst Clin Prof OrS, Jefferson Med Coll

Harner, Christopher D MD [SM] - **Spec Exp:** Knee Injuries; **Hospital:** UPMC South Side; **Address:** UPMC Center for Sports Medicine, 3200 S Water St, Pittsburgh, PA 15203; **Phone:** 412-432-3661; **Board Cert:** Orthopaedic Surgery 2008; **Med School:** Univ Mich Med Sch 1981; **Resid:** Orthopaedic Surgery, Univ Pittsburgh 1986; **Fellow:** Sports Medicine/Knee Surgery, Salt Lake City Knee & Sport 1987; **Fac Appt:** Prof OrS, Univ Pittsburgh

Hershman, Elliott MD [SM] - **Spec Exp:** Knee Injuries; Knee Surgery; Arthroscopic Surgery; Ligament Reconstruction; **Hospital:** Lenox Hill Hosp (page 62); **Address:** 130 E 77th St Fl 7, New York, NY 10021-1851; **Phone:** 212-744-8114; **Board Cert:** Orthopaedic Surgery 1998; **Med School:** Univ Rochester 1979; **Resid:** Orthopaedic Surgery, Lenox Hill Hosp 1984; **Fellow:** Sports Medicine, Cleveland Clinic 1985; **Fac Appt:** Asst Clin Prof OrS, Mount Sinai Sch Med

Levine, William MD [SM] - **Spec Exp:** Arthroscopic Surgery; Shoulder & Elbow Surgery; Knee Injuries; **Hospital:** NY-Presby Hosp/Columbia (page 66); **Address:** 622 W 168th St Fl PH-11, New York, NY 10032; **Phone:** 212-305-0762; **Board Cert:** Orthopaedic Surgery 1999; **Med School:** Case West Res Univ 1990; **Resid:** Surgery, Beth Israel Hosp 1991; Orthopaedic Surgery, New Eng Med Ctr Hosps 1995; **Fellow:** Shoulder Surgery, Columbia-Presby Med Ctr 1996; Sports Medicine, Univ MD Med Ctr 1998; **Fac Appt:** Assoc Prof OrS, Columbia P&S

Maharam, Lewis G MD [SM] - **Spec Exp:** Running Injuries; Primary Care Sports Medicine; Knee Injuries; Shoulder Injuries; **Hospital:** Hosp For Joint Diseases (page 70), NYU Med Ctr (page 68); **Address:** 24 W 57th St, New York, NY 10019-3918; **Phone:** 212-765-5763; **Med School:** Emory Univ 1985; **Resid:** Internal Medicine, Danbury Hosp 1987; Internal Medicine, NY Infirm/Beekman Downtown 1989; **Fellow:** Sports Medicine, Pascack Valley Hosp 1990; **Fac Appt:** Asst Clin Prof OrS, NYU Sch Med

Metzl, Jordan D MD [SM] - **Spec Exp:** Primary Care Sports Medicine; Adolescent Sports Medicine; Running Injuries; **Hospital:** Hosp For Special Surgery (page 59); **Address:** Hospital for Special Surgery, Sports Med, 535 E 70 St, New York, NY 10021-4872; **Phone:** 212-606-1678; **Board Cert:** Sports Medicine 2001; **Med School:** Univ MO-Columbia Sch Med 1993; **Resid:** Pediatrics, New England Med Ctr 1996; **Fellow:** Sports Medicine, Vanderbilt Univ Med Ctr 1996; Sports Medicine, Hosp Special Surgery 1997; **Fac Appt:** Asst Prof Ped, Cornell Univ-Weill Med Coll

Nisonson, Barton MD [SM] - **Spec Exp:** Knee Injuries; Shoulder & Knee Surgery; Sports Medicine; **Hospital:** Lenox Hill Hosp (page 62); **Address:** 130 E 77th St, New York, NY 10021-1851; **Phone:** 212-570-9120; **Board Cert:** Orthopaedic Surgery 1974; **Med School:** Columbia P&S 1966; **Resid:** Surgery, Columbia-Presby Med Ctr 1968; Orthopaedic Surgery, Columbia-Presby Med Ctr 1973

Plancher, Kevin D MD [SM] - **Spec Exp:** Shoulder Surgery; Elbow Surgery; Cartilage Damage & Transplant; Shoulder Replacement; **Hospital:** Beth Israel Med Ctr - Petrie Division (page 57), NY Westchester Sq Med Ctr; **Address:** 1160 Park Ave, New York, NY 10128; **Phone:** 212-876-5200; **Board Cert:** Orthopaedic Surgery 2007; Hand Surgery 2008; **Med School:** Georgetown Univ 1986; **Resid:** Orthopaedic Surgery, Mass Genl Hosp/Brigham & Womens Hosp 1991; **Fellow:** Hand Surgery, Indiana Hand Ctr 1993; Sports Medicine, Steadman-Hawkins Clinic 1994; **Fac Appt:** Assoc Clin Prof OrS, Albert Einstein Coll Med

Rodeo, Scott A MD [SM] - **Spec Exp:** Knee Injuries; Cartilage Damage; **Hospital:** Hosp For Special Surgery (page 59); **Address:** Hospital for Special Surgery, 535 E 70th St, New York, NY 10021; **Phone:** 212-606-1513; **Board Cert:** Orthopaedic Surgery 1998; **Med School:** Cornell Univ-Weill Med Coll 1989; **Resid:** Orthopaedic Surgery, Hosp Special Surgery 1994; **Fellow:** Sports Medicine, Hosp Special Surgery 1996; **Fac Appt:** Assoc Clin Prof OrS, Cornell Univ-Weill Med Coll

Sports Medicine

Southeast

Andrews, James R MD [SM] - **Spec Exp:** Shoulder Surgery; Elbow Surgery; Knee Surgery; **Hospital:** St Vincent's Hosp - Birmingham; **Address:** 806 St Vincents Drive, Women & Childrens Ctr, Ste 415, Birmingham, AL 35205; **Phone:** 205-939-3099; **Board Cert:** Orthopaedic Surgery 1974; **Med School:** Louisiana State U, New Orleans 1967; **Resid:** Orthopaedic Surgery, USPHS Hosp 1969; Orthopaedic Surgery, Touro Infirm-Tulane 1970; **Fellow:** Hand Surgery, VA Med Ctr; **Fac Appt:** Clin Prof OrS, Univ Ala

Garth Jr, William P MD [SM] - **Spec Exp:** Knee Ligament Reconstruction; Shoulder Reconstruction; **Hospital:** Univ of Ala Hosp at Birmingham, Children's Hospital - Birmingham; **Address:** Univ Alabama Birmingham - Sports Medicine, 1600 7th Ave S, Birmingham, AL 35233-1711; **Phone:** 205-934-1041; **Board Cert:** Orthopaedic Surgery 1980; Orthopaedic Sports Medicine 2007; **Med School:** Tulane Univ 1973; **Resid:** Surgery, Duke Univ Hosp 1975; Orthopaedic Surgery, Campbell Clinic 1979; **Fellow:** Sports Medicine, Sports Med Clinic 1984; **Fac Appt:** Prof OrS, Univ Ala

Speer, Kevin MD [SM] - **Spec Exp:** Shoulder Surgery; **Hospital:** Duke Health Raleigh; **Address:** 3404 Wake Forest Rd, Ste 201, Raleigh, NC 27609; **Phone:** 919-256-1511; **Board Cert:** Orthopaedic Surgery 2005; **Med School:** Johns Hopkins Univ 1985; **Resid:** Orthopaedic Surgery, Duke Univ Med Ctr 1991; **Fellow:** Sports Medicine, Hosp Special Surgery 1992; **Fac Appt:** Assoc Prof OrS, Duke Univ

Midwest

Cole, Brian J MD [SM] - **Spec Exp:** Cartilage Damage; Shoulder & Elbow Injuries; Knee Injuries; **Hospital:** Rush Univ Med Ctr; **Address:** 1725 W Harrison St, Ste 1063, Chicago, IL 60612-3841; **Phone:** 312-432-2381; **Board Cert:** Orthopaedic Surgery 1999; **Med School:** Univ Chicago-Pritzker Sch Med 1990; **Resid:** Orthopaedic Surgery, Hosp for Special Surgery 1996; **Fellow:** Sports Medicine, Univ Pittsburgh Med Ctr 1997; **Fac Appt:** Prof OrS, Rush Med Coll

Dimeff, Robert J MD [SM] - **Spec Exp:** Primary Care Sports Medicine; Nutrition; **Hospital:** Cleveland Clin Fdn (page 56); **Address:** 5555 Transportation Blvd, Garfield Heights, OH 44195; **Phone:** 216-444-2185; **Board Cert:** Family Medicine 2003; Sports Medicine 2003; **Med School:** NE Ohio Univ 1985; **Resid:** Family Medicine, Presbyterian-St Lukes Med Ctr 1989; **Fellow:** Sports Medicine, Cleveland Clinic 1990; **Fac Appt:** Assoc Prof FMed, Ohio State Univ

Ho, Sherwin S MD [SM] - **Spec Exp:** Shoulder & Knee Surgery; Arthroscopic Surgery; Cartilage Damage; **Hospital:** Univ of Chicago Hosps; **Address:** Univ Chicago, Dept Surgery, 5841 S Maryland Ave, MS 3079, Chicago, IL 60637-3079; **Phone:** 773-702-5978; **Board Cert:** Orthopaedic Surgery 1994; **Med School:** Univ Hawaii JA Burns Sch Med 1985; **Resid:** Orthopaedic Surgery, Univ Hawaii Med Ctr 1991; **Fellow:** Sports Medicine, Univ Chicago Hosp 1992; **Fac Appt:** Assoc Prof OrS, Univ Chicago-Pritzker Sch Med

McKeag, Douglas B MD [SM] - **Spec Exp:** Sports Medicine; Adolescent Sports Medicine; Preventive Medicine; **Hospital:** Indiana Univ Hosp, Methodist Hosp - Indianapolis; **Address:** Indiana Univ Dept Family Medicine, 1110 W Michigan St, Ste 200, Indianapolis, IN 46202-5209; **Phone:** 317-278-0360; **Board Cert:** Family Medicine 2005; Sports Medicine 1993; **Med School:** Mich State Univ 1973; **Resid:** Family Medicine, Grand Rapids Area Med Ctr 1976; **Fellow:** Family Medicine, Michigan St Univ 1977; Adolescent Medicine, Michigan St Univ 1977; **Fac Appt:** Prof FMed, Indiana Univ

Miniaci, Anthony MD [SM] - **Spec Exp:** Shoulder Reconstruction; Knee Reconstruction; Cartilage Damage; Knee Resurfacing; **Hospital:** Cleveland Clin Fdn (page 56); **Address:** Cleveland Clinic, 9500 Euclid Ave, Desk A41, Cleveland, OH 44195; **Phone:** 216-444-2625; **Med School:** Univ Western Ontario 1982; **Resid:** Orthopaedic Surgery, Univ Western Ontario 1987; **Fellow:** Sports Medicine, Kerlan-Jobe Orthopaedic Clin 1989; Orthopaedic Research, Univ Calgary 1990

Paletta, George A MD [SM] - **Spec Exp:** Ankle Surgery; Knee Surgery; **Address:** The Orthopaedic Ctr of St Louis, 14825 N Outer Forty Rd, Ste 200, Chesterfield, MO 63017; **Phone:** 314-336-2555; **Board Cert:** Orthopaedic Surgery 1998; **Med School:** Johns Hopkins Univ 1988; **Resid:** Orthopaedic Surgery, Cornell Univ Med Ctr 1994; **Fellow:** Orthopaedic Surgery, Cleveland Clin Fnd 1995; **Fac Appt:** Assoc Prof OrS, Washington Univ, St Louis

Great Plains and Mountains

Saint-Phard, Deborah MD [SM] - **Spec Exp:** Sports Medicine-Women; Spinal Rehabilitation; **Hospital:** Univ Colorado Hosp; **Address:** University Sports Medicine, 1745 S High St, Denver, CO 80210; **Phone:** 303-871-7752; **Board Cert:** Physical Medicine & Rehabilitation 2007; Pain Medicine 2004; **Med School:** Temple Univ 1992; **Resid:** Physical Medicine & Rehabilitation, Univ Colorado 1996; **Fellow:** Sports Medicine, Mayo Clinic 1997; **Fac Appt:** Assoc Prof PMR, Univ Colorado

West Coast and Pacific

Fronek, Jan MD [SM] - **Spec Exp:** Knee Injuries; Shoulder Injuries; Arthroscopic Surgery; Rotator Cuff Surgery; **Hospital:** Scripps Meml Hosp - La Jolla; **Address:** Scripps Clinic, 10666 N Torrey Pines Rd, MS B4, La Jolla, CA 92037; **Phone:** 858-554-9753; **Board Cert:** Orthopaedic Surgery 1999; **Med School:** Univ Rochester 1978; **Resid:** Orthopaedic Surgery, UCSD Med Ctr 1984; **Fellow:** Sports Medicine, Hosp Special Surgery 1985

Gambardella, Ralph A MD [SM] - **Spec Exp:** Cartilage Damage; Shoulder & Elbow Surgery; Knee Surgery; **Hospital:** Centinela Freeman Reg Med Ctr-Centinela, USC Univ Hosp - R K Eamer Med Plz; **Address:** Kerlan-Jobe Clinic, 6801 Park Terr, Ste 400, Los Angeles, CA 90045; **Phone:** 310-665-7200; **Board Cert:** Orthopaedic Surgery 1985; **Med School:** USC Sch Med 1977; **Resid:** Orthopaedic Surgery, USC Med Ctr 1982; **Fellow:** Sports Medicine, Southwestern Ortho Grp 1983; **Fac Appt:** Assoc Clin Prof S, USC Sch Med

Mirzayan, Raffy MD [SM] - **Spec Exp:** Fractures-Non Union; Cartilage Damage; Knee Injuries; **Hospital:** Kaiser Permanente Baldwin Pk Med Ctr; **Address:** Kaiser Permanente Med Ctr, Orthopaedics, 1011 Baldwin Park Blvd, Baldwin Park, CA 91706; **Phone:** 626-851-5256; **Board Cert:** Orthopaedic Surgery 2003; Sports Medicine 2007; **Med School:** USC Sch Med 1995; **Resid:** Orthopaedic Surgery, LAC/USC Med Ctr 2000; **Fellow:** Sports Medicine, Kerlan Jobe Ortho Clinic 2001

Schechter, David L MD [SM] - **Spec Exp:** Pain-Back; Sports Injuries; Muscle Pain-Stress Related; **Hospital:** Cedars-Sinai Med Ctr, Olympia Med Ctr; **Address:** 8500 Wilshire Blvd, Ste 705, Beverly Hills, CA 90211; **Phone:** 310-657-1022; **Board Cert:** Sports Medicine 2003; Family Medicine 2001; **Med School:** NYU Sch Med 1984; **Resid:** Family Medicine, UCLA/Santa Monica Hosp 1987; **Fac Appt:** Assoc Clin Prof FMed, USC Sch Med

Cleveland Clinic

Sports Health

Cleveland Clinic Sports Health brings together top orthopaedic surgeons, primary care sports physicians, physician assistants, nurses, physical therapists, athletic trainers, exercise physiologists, and strength and conditioning specialists to get athletes back in the game. Leaders in their specialties, our physicians work to diagnose, treat and rehabilitate injuries so athletes can perform at their best.

Cleveland Clinic Sports Health treats athletes of all sports, ages and skill levels. We have been chosen to care for the major professional sports teams in Cleveland because of our care and treatment that is focused, one-on-one and state-of-the-art. This involves conditioning to become stronger and faster, maximizing abilities, preventing and treating injuries, and improving future performance.

As one of the largest sports health practices in the nation, Cleveland Clinic Sports Health provides a host of services to many of the world's top professional and amateur athletes.

We've provided the physicians for Cleveland's professional teams for more than 25 years. Currently, we are the team physicians for the Cleveland Browns, Cleveland Cavaliers and Cleveland Indians. Our experienced staff has treated athletes from the AHL, EPL (English Premier League), NBA, NCAA, NFL, NHL, MLB, MLS, PBA, U.S.A. Boxing, U.S.A. Hockey, U.S. Olympic Team and WNBA.

Our world-renowned team of physicians is trained in diagnosing and treating the unique problems in amateur to high-performance athletes. They are involved in research every day to improve patient care and bring new treatments to the clinical setting.

For more information about the Cleveland Clinic Sports Health, to schedule a second opinion or to learn about assistance for out-of-town patients, call 800.890.2467 or visit www.clevelandclinic.org/ sportstopdocs.

Cleveland Clinic Sports Health offers specialized programs that focus on rehab, injury evaluation, injury prevention and strength and conditioning tailored to your sport. These programs include:

- Golf Performance Plus – designed for golfers of all ages and skill levels

- Jump Right – an eight week program designed to teach proper jumping and landing mechanics to help reduce the risk of serious knee injury.

- Optimal Runners Performance Program – Gait analysis, body comp testing, strength and flexibility testing, VO2 analysis, injury assessment, conditioning program

- Soccer Performance Program – conditioning programs, injury assessment and prevention

- Throw Right – A specialized baseball program designed to meet the needs of baseball athletes.

Sports Health | 9500 Euclid Avenue / AC311 | Cleveland OH 44195

Surgery

A surgeon manages a broad spectrum of surgical conditions affecting almost any area of the body. The surgeon establishes the diagnosis and provides the preoperative, operative and postoperative care to surgical patients and is usually responsible for the comprehensive management of the trauma victim and the critically ill surgical patient.

The surgeon uses a variety of diagnostic techniques, including endoscopy, for observing internal structures and may use specialized instruments during operative procedures. A general surgeon is expected to be familiar with the salient features of other surgical specialties in order to recognize problems in those areas and to know when to refer a patient to another specialist.

Training Required: Five years

For a description of the subspecialty **Hand Surgery**, **Pediatric Surgery** and **Vascular Surgery** see the corresponding section(s).

SURGERY

New England

Becker, James M MD [S] - **Spec Exp:** Inflammatory Bowel Disease; Gastrointestinal Cancer; Gastrointestinal Surgery; **Hospital:** Boston Med Ctr, Qunicy Med Ctr; **Address:** Boston Med Ctr, Dept Surg, 88 E Newton St, rm C500, Boston, MA 02118-2393; **Phone:** 617-638-8600; **Board Cert:** Surgery 1999; **Med School:** Case West Res Univ 1975; **Resid:** Surgery, Univ Utah Med Ctr 1980; **Fellow:** Research, Mayo Clinic 1982; **Fac Appt:** Prof S, Boston Univ

Brooks, David C MD [S] - **Spec Exp:** Gastrointestinal Surgery; **Hospital:** Brigham & Women's Hosp; **Address:** Brigham & Women's Hospital, Dept Surgery, 75 Francis St, ASB II Fl 3, Boston, MA 02115; **Phone:** 617-732-6337; **Board Cert:** Surgery 2003; **Med School:** Brown Univ 1976; **Resid:** Surgery, Brigham & Women's Hosp 1983; **Fac Appt:** Assoc Prof S, Harvard Med Sch

Cioffi, William MD [S] - **Spec Exp:** Trauma; Cancer Surgery; **Hospital:** Rhode Island Hosp; **Address:** Rhode Island Hosp, Dept Surg, 2 Dudley St, Ste 470, Providence, RI 02905; **Phone:** 401-553-8348; **Board Cert:** Surgery 1995; Surgical Critical Care 1997; **Med School:** Univ VT Coll Med 1981; **Resid:** Surgery, Med Ctr Hosp 1986; **Fac Appt:** Prof S, Brown Univ

Eisenberg, Burton L MD [S] - **Spec Exp:** Breast Cancer; Melanoma; Sarcoma; **Hospital:** Dartmouth - Hitchcock Med Ctr; **Address:** Dartmouth-Hitchcock Med Ctr, Dept Surgery, One Medical Center Drive, Lebanon, NH 03756; **Phone:** 603-650-9479; **Board Cert:** Surgery 1999; **Med School:** Univ Tenn Coll Med, Memphis 1974; **Resid:** Surgery, Wilford Hall USAF Med Ctr 1979; **Fellow:** Surgical Oncology, Meml Sloan-Kettering Cancer Ctr 1981; **Fac Appt:** Prof S, Dartmouth Med Sch

Emre, Sukru MD [S] - **Spec Exp:** Transplant-Liver-Adult & Pediatric; Hepatobiliary Surgery; Portal Hypertension; **Hospital:** Yale-New Haven Hosp; **Address:** 333 Cedar St, rm FMB112, Yale, CT 06520; **Phone:** 203-785-2565; **Med School:** Turkey 1977; **Resid:** Surgery, Univ Istanbul 1982; **Fellow:** Hepatobiliary Surgery, Univ Istanbul 1988; Transplant Surgery, Mount Sinai Med Ctr 1994; **Fac Appt:** Prof S, Mount Sinai Sch Med

Hebert, James C MD [S] - **Spec Exp:** Biliary Surgery; Colon & Rectal Surgery; **Hospital:** FAHC - Med Ctr Campus; **Address:** Fletcher Allen Hlth Care, 111 Colchester Ave, Burlington, VT 05401; **Phone:** 802-847-3344; **Board Cert:** Surgery 2000; **Med School:** Univ VT Coll Med 1977; **Resid:** Surgery, Med Ctr Hosp 1982; **Fac Appt:** Prof S, Univ VT Coll Med

Hughes, Kevin S MD [S] - **Spec Exp:** Breast Cancer; Ovarian Cancer; **Hospital:** Mass Genl Hosp; **Address:** Mass Genl Hosp, Dept Surgery, 55 Fruit St, Yawkey Center Fl 9 - Ste A, Boston, MA 02114; **Phone:** 617-724-4800; **Board Cert:** Surgery 2006; **Med School:** Dartmouth Med Sch 1979; **Resid:** Surgery, Mercy Hosp 1984; **Fellow:** Surgical Oncology, National Cancer Inst 1986; **Fac Appt:** Assoc Prof S, Harvard Med Sch

Iglehart, J Dirk MD [S] - **Spec Exp:** Breast Cancer; **Hospital:** Brigham & Women's Hosp, Dana-Farber Cancer Inst; **Address:** Brigham & Women's Hospital, 75 Francis St, Dept Surgery, Boston, MA 02115; **Phone:** 617-632-5178; **Board Cert:** Surgery 2005; **Med School:** Harvard Med Sch 1975; **Resid:** Surgery, Duke Univ Med Ctr 1981; Thoracic Surgery, Duke Univ Med Ctr 1984; **Fac Appt:** Prof S, Harvard Med Sch

Jenkins, Roger L MD [S] - **Spec Exp:** Transplant-Liver; Liver & Biliary Cancer; Pancreatic Cancer; **Hospital:** Lahey Clin, Children's Hospital - Boston; **Address:** Lahey Clin, Dept Hepatobiliary Surg, 41 Mall Rd, Burlington, MA 01805; **Phone:** 781-744-2500; **Board Cert:** Surgery 2005; **Med School:** Univ VT Coll Med 1977; **Resid:** Surgery, New Eng Deaconess Hosp 1982; **Fellow:** Cardiovascular Surgery, Deaconess Hosp 1983; Transplant Surgery, Univ Pittsburgh Hosp 1983; **Fac Appt:** Prof S, Tufts Univ

Kavanah, Maureen MD [S] - **Spec Exp:** Breast Cancer; Gynecologic Cancer; Melanoma; **Hospital:** Boston Med Ctr; **Address:** Boston Medical Ctr, 820 Harrison Ave, Bldg FGH, Boston, MA 02118; **Phone:** 617-638-8473; **Board Cert:** Surgery 1999; **Med School:** Tufts Univ 1975; **Resid:** Surgery, St Elizabeths Hosp 1979; **Fellow:** Surgical Oncology, Boston Univ Med Ctr 1981; **Fac Appt:** Assoc Prof S, Boston Univ

Krag, David MD [S] - **Spec Exp:** Sentinel Node Surgery; Breast Cancer; Cancer Surgery; Melanoma; **Hospital:** FAHC - UHC Campus; **Address:** Univ Vermont Coll Med, Dept Surgery, 89 Beaumont Ave, Given Bldg - E309C, Burlington, VT 05405; **Phone:** 802-656-5830; **Board Cert:** Surgery 20; **Med School:** Loyola Univ-Stritch Sch Med 1980; **Resid:** Surgery, UC Davis Med Ctr 1983; **Fellow:** Surgical Oncology, UCLA Med Ctr 1984; **Fac Appt:** Assoc Prof S, Univ VT Coll Med

Lipkowitz, George S MD [S] - **Spec Exp:** Transplant-Kidney; **Hospital:** Baystate Med Ctr; **Address:** 208 Ashley Ave, West Springfield, MA 01089; **Phone:** 413-747-4170 x151; **Board Cert:** Surgery 2006; **Med School:** SUNY Downstate 1980; **Resid:** Surgery, SUNY Kings Co Hosp 1985; **Fellow:** Transplant Surgery, SUNY Hlth Scis Ctr 1986; **Fac Appt:** Assoc Prof S, Tufts Univ

Ponn, Teresa MD [S] - **Spec Exp:** Breast Cancer; **Hospital:** Elliot Hosp; **Address:** Elliot Breast Health Center, 275 Mammoth Rd, Ste 1, Manchester, NH 03109; **Phone:** 603-668-3067; **Board Cert:** Surgery 2000; **Med School:** Univ Fla Coll Med 1976; **Resid:** Surgery, Stanford Univ Med Ctr 1982

Ryan, Colleen M MD [S] - **Spec Exp:** Burn Care; Toxic Epidermal Neurolysis; Wound Healing/Care; **Hospital:** Mass Genl Hosp, Boston Shriners Hosp; **Address:** MGH Burn Assocs, 55 Fruit St GRB Bldg - Ste 1303, Boston, MA 02114-2621; **Phone:** 617-726-3712; **Board Cert:** Surgery 1999; Surgical Critical Care 2003; **Med School:** Georgetown Univ 1982; **Resid:** Surgery, NE Deaconess Hosp 1988; **Fellow:** Hepatology, Hammersmith Hosp 1986; Burn Surgery, Mass Genl Hosp 1989; **Fac Appt:** Assoc Prof S, Harvard Med Sch

Salem, Ronald R MD [S] - **Spec Exp:** Cancer Surgery; Liver & Biliary Surgery; Gastrointestinal Cancer; **Hospital:** Yale-New Haven Hosp; **Address:** Yale Univ Sch Med, Dept Surg, 333 Cedar St, TMP 202, New Haven, CT 06520-8062; **Phone:** 203-785-3577; **Board Cert:** Surgery 2000; **Med School:** Zimbabwe 1978; **Resid:** Surgery, Hammersmith Hosp 1985; Surgery, New England Deaconess Hosp 1989; **Fac Appt:** Assoc Prof S, Yale Univ

Shikora, Scott A MD [S] - **Spec Exp:** Obesity/Bariatric Surgery; Laparoscopic Abdominal Surgery; **Hospital:** Tufts Med Ctr; **Address:** New England Medical Ctr, 800 Washington St, Box NEMC 900, Boston, MA 02111; **Phone:** 617-636-6093; **Board Cert:** Surgery 2001; **Med School:** Columbia P&S 1985; **Resid:** Surgery, New England Deaconess Hosp 1991; **Fellow:** Nutrition & Metabolism, New England Deaconess Hos 1989; **Fac Appt:** Prof S, Tufts Univ

Smith, Barbara Lynn MD/PhD [S] - **Spec Exp:** Breast Cancer; **Hospital:** Mass Genl Hosp; **Address:** Mass Genl Hosp, Dept Surgery, 55 Fruit St, Yawkey Center Fl 9 - Ste A, Boston, MA 02114; **Phone:** 617-724-4800; **Board Cert:** Surgery 2000; **Med School:** Harvard Med Sch 1983; **Resid:** Surgery, Brigham & Women's Hosp 1989; **Fac Appt:** Asst Prof S, Harvard Med Sch

Surgery

Sutton, John E MD [S] - **Spec Exp:** Esophageal Cancer; Liver & Biliary Surgery; Pancreatic Cancer; **Hospital:** Dartmouth - Hitchcock Med Ctr; **Address:** One Medical Center Drive, Lebanon, NH 03756; **Phone:** 603-650-8022; **Board Cert:** Surgery 2001; Surgical Critical Care 1995; **Med School:** Georgetown Univ 1974; **Resid:** Surgery, Dartmouth-Hitchcock Med Ctr 1981; **Fellow:** Surgical Critical Care, Dartmouth-Hitchcock Med Ctr 1983; **Fac Appt:** Prof S, Dartmouth Med Sch

Tanabe, Kenneth K MD [S] - **Spec Exp:** Liver Cancer; Colon & Rectal Cancer; Melanoma; **Hospital:** Mass Genl Hosp, Newton - Wellesley Hosp; **Address:** Mass General Hosp, Div Surgical Oncology, 55 Fruit St, Yawkey 7.924, Boston, MA 02114; **Phone:** 617-724-3868; **Board Cert:** Surgery 2000; **Med School:** UCSD 1985; **Resid:** Surgery, New York Hosp-Cornell 1990; **Fellow:** Surgical Oncology, MD Anderson Cancer Ctr 1993; **Fac Appt:** Assoc Prof S, Harvard Med Sch

Udelsman, Robert MD [S] - **Spec Exp:** Parathyroid Cancer; Adrenal Tumors; Thyroid Cancer; **Hospital:** Yale-New Haven Hosp; **Address:** Yale School Medicine, Chair of Surgery, 789 Howard Ave FMB Bldg - rm 102, New Haven, CT 06511; **Phone:** 203-785-2697; **Board Cert:** Surgery 1999; **Med School:** Geo Wash Univ 1981; **Resid:** Surgery, Natl Inst Hlth 1986; Surgery, Johns Hopkins Hosp 1989; **Fellow:** Gastrointestinal Surgery, Johns Hopkins Hosp 1990; **Fac Appt:** Prof S, Yale Univ

Ward, Barbara MD [S] - **Spec Exp:** Breast Cancer; Breast Disease; Breast Surgery; **Hospital:** Greenwich Hosp; **Address:** 77 Lafayette Pl, Ste 302, Greenwich, CT 06830-5426; **Phone:** 203-863-4250; **Board Cert:** Surgery 2002; **Med School:** Temple Univ 1983; **Resid:** Surgery, Yale-New Haven Hosp 1990; **Fellow:** Surgical Oncology, Natl Cancer Inst 1987; **Fac Appt:** Assoc Clin Prof S, Yale Univ

Warshaw, Andrew L MD [S] - **Spec Exp:** Pancreatic Cancer; Pancreatic Surgery; **Hospital:** Mass Genl Hosp; **Address:** Mass Genl Hosp, Dept Surg, 55 Fruit St, WHT 506, Boston, MA 02114-2696; **Phone:** 617-726-8254; **Board Cert:** Surgery 1971; **Med School:** Harvard Med Sch 1963; **Resid:** Surgery, Mass Genl Hosp 1971; **Fellow:** Internal Medicine, Mass Genl Hosp 1970; **Fac Appt:** Prof S, Harvard Med Sch

Zinner, Michael MD [S] - **Spec Exp:** Colon & Rectal Cancer; Gastrointestinal Surgery; Pancreatic Cancer; **Hospital:** Brigham & Women's Hosp, Dana-Farber Cancer Inst; **Address:** Brigham & Women's Hosp, Dept Surg, 75 Francis St, Twr 1, Ste 220, Boston, MA 02115; **Phone:** 617-732-8181; **Board Cert:** Surgery 2000; **Med School:** Univ Fla Coll Med 1971; **Resid:** Surgery, Johns Hopkins Hosp 1974; Surgery, Johns Hopkins Hosp 1979; **Fac Appt:** Prof S, Harvard Med Sch

Mid Atlantic

Alfonso, Antonio MD [S] - **Spec Exp:** Breast Cancer; Head & Neck Surgery; Thyroid Cancer; **Hospital:** Long Island Coll Hosp (page 57), SUNY Downstate Med Ctr; **Address:** Long Island Coll Hosp, 339 Hicks St, Brooklyn, NY 11201; **Phone:** 718-875-3244; **Board Cert:** Surgery 1973; **Med School:** Philippines 1968; **Resid:** Surgery, Temple Univ Hosp 1972; **Fellow:** Surgical Oncology, Meml Sloan Kettering Cancer Ctr 1974; **Fac Appt:** Prof S, SUNY Downstate

August, David MD [S] - **Spec Exp:** Cancer Surgery; Gastrointestinal Cancer; Breast Cancer; Sarcoma-Soft Tissue; **Hospital:** Robert Wood Johnson Univ Hosp - New Brunswick; **Address:** Canc Inst NJ, 195 Little Albany St, New Brunswick, NJ 08903-1914; **Phone:** 732-235-7701; **Board Cert:** Surgery 2005; **Med School:** Yale Univ 1980; **Resid:** Surgery, Yale-New Haven Hosp 1986; **Fellow:** Surgical Oncology, Natl Cancer Inst 1984; **Fac Appt:** Prof S, UMDNJ-RW Johnson Med Sch

Axelrod, Deborah MD [S] - **Spec Exp:** Breast Cancer; Breast Disease; **Hospital:** NYU Med Ctr (page 68), St Vincent Cath Med Ctrs - Manhattan; **Address:** NYU Clinical Cancer Ctr, 160 E 34th St, New York, NY 10016; **Phone:** 212-731-5366; **Board Cert:** Surgery 1997; **Med School:** Israel 1982; **Resid:** Surgery, Beth Israel Med Ctr 1988; **Fellow:** Surgical Oncology, Meml Sloan Kettering Cancer Ctr 1986; **Fac Appt:** Assoc Prof S, NYU Sch Med

Balch, Charles MD [S] - **Spec Exp:** Sentinel Node Surgery; Melanoma; Cancer Surgery; **Hospital:** Johns Hopkins Hosp - Baltimore (page 61); **Address:** 600 N Wolfe St Osler Bldg - Ste 624, Baltimore, MD 21287; **Phone:** 410-502-5977; **Board Cert:** Surgery 1997; **Med School:** Columbia P&S 1967; **Resid:** Surgery, Univ Alabama Med Ctr 1971; Surgery, Univ Alabama Med Ctr 1975; **Fellow:** Immunology, Scripps Clin-Rsch Fdn 1973; **Fac Appt:** Prof Surg & Onc, Johns Hopkins Univ

Ballantyne, Garth H MD [S] - **Spec Exp:** Laparoscopic Surgery; Gastroesophageal Reflux Disease (GERD); Colon Cancer; **Hospital:** Hackensack Univ Med Ctr; **Address:** 20 Prospect Ave, Ste 901, Hackensack, NJ 07601-1974; **Phone:** 201-996-2959; **Board Cert:** Surgery 2006; Colon & Rectal Surgery 1985; **Med School:** Columbia P&S 1977; **Resid:** Surgery, UCLA Med Ctr 1980; Surgery, Northwestern Univ 1982; **Fellow:** Colon & Rectal Surgery, Mayo Clinic 1984; **Fac Appt:** Prof S, UMDNJ-NJ Med Sch, Newark

Barie, Philip MD [S] - **Spec Exp:** Trauma; Critical Care; Hernia; **Hospital:** NY-Presby Hosp/Weill Cornell (page 66), Hosp For Special Surgery (page 59); **Address:** Weill Med College-Cornell Univ, 525 E 68th St, Ste P713A, New York, NY 10021-4873; **Phone:** 212-746-5401; **Board Cert:** Surgery 2004; Surgical Critical Care 2005; **Med School:** Boston Univ 1977; **Resid:** Surgery, NY Hosp-Cornell Med Ctr 1984; **Fellow:** Trauma, Albany Med Coll 1981; **Fac Appt:** Prof S, Cornell Univ-Weill Med Coll

Bartlett, David L MD [S] - **Spec Exp:** Peritoneal Carcinomatosis; Pancreatic Cancer; Liver Cancer; Appendix Cancer; **Hospital:** UPMC Shadyside; **Address:** UPMC Cancer Ctr, 5150 Centre Ave Fl 4 - rm 415, Pittsburgh, PA 15232; **Phone:** 412-692-2852; **Board Cert:** Surgery 2004; **Med School:** Univ Tex, Houston 1987; **Resid:** Surgery, Hosp Univ Penn 1993; **Fellow:** Surgical Oncology, Meml Sloan-Kettering Cancer Ctr 1995; **Fac Appt:** Assoc Prof S, Univ Pittsburgh

Bartlett, Stephen T MD [S] - **Spec Exp:** Transplant-Pancreas; Transplant-Kidney; **Hospital:** Univ of MD Med Sys; **Address:** 22 S Greene St, rm N4E40, Baltimore, MD 21201; **Phone:** 410-328-8407; **Board Cert:** Surgery 2004; Vascular Surgery 1996; **Med School:** Univ Chicago-Pritzker Sch Med 1979; **Resid:** Surgery, Hosp Univ Penn 1985; **Fellow:** Vascular Surgery, Northwestern Univ 1986; **Fac Appt:** Prof S, Univ MD Sch Med

Bessler, Marc MD [S] - **Spec Exp:** Obesity/Bariatric Surgery; Laparoscopic Surgery; **Hospital:** NY-Presby Hosp/Columbia (page 66); **Address:** NY Presby Med Ctr, Dept of Surgery, 161 Fort Washington Ave, rm 612, New York, NY 10032; **Phone:** 212-305-9506; **Board Cert:** Surgery 1997; **Med School:** NYU Sch Med 1989; **Resid:** Surgery, Columbia Presby Med Ctr 1995; **Fac Appt:** Assoc Prof S, Columbia P&S

Borgen, Patrick I MD [S] - **Spec Exp:** Breast Cancer; **Hospital:** Maimonides Med Ctr (page 63); **Address:** Maimonides Cancer Ctr, 6300 8th Ave, Brooklyn, NY 11220; **Phone:** 718-765-2570; **Board Cert:** Surgery 2002; **Med School:** Louisiana State U, New Orleans 1984; **Resid:** Surgery, Ochsner Fdn Hosp 1989; **Fellow:** Surgical Oncology, Meml Sloan Kettering Canc Ctr 1990; **Fac Appt:** Prof S, Cornell Univ-Weill Med Coll

Brennan, Murray MD [S] - **Spec Exp:** Sarcoma; Pancreatic Cancer; Stomach Cancer; Endocrine Cancers; **Hospital:** Meml Sloan-Kettering Cancer Ctr; **Address:** 1275 York Avenue, New York, NY 10065; **Phone:** 800-525-2225; **Board Cert:** Surgery 1975; **Med School:** New Zealand 1964; **Resid:** Surgery, Univ Otago Hosp 1969; **Fellow:** Surgery, Harvard Med Sch 1972; Surgery, Peter Bent Brigham Hosp 1975; **Fac Appt:** Prof S, Cornell Univ-Weill Med Coll

Surgery

Brody, Fred J MD [S] - **Spec Exp:** Gastrointestinal Surgery; Laparoscopic Surgery; Hernia; **Hospital:** G Washington Univ Hosp; **Address:** George Washington Univ Dept Surgery, 2150 Pennsylvania Ave NW, Ste 6B-412, Washington, DC 20037; **Phone:** 202-741-2587; **Board Cert:** Surgery 1998; **Med School:** Univ NC Sch Med 1991; **Resid:** Surgery, George Washington Univ Med Ctr 1997; **Fellow:** Laparoscopic Surgery, Duke Univ Med Ctr 1998; **Fac Appt:** Assoc Prof S, Geo Wash Univ

Bromberg, Jonathan S MD/PhD [S] - **Spec Exp:** Transplant-Kidney; Transplant-Pancreas; **Hospital:** Mount Sinai Med Ctr (page 64); **Address:** Mount Sinai Medical Ctr, One Gustave Levy Pl, Box 1104, New York, NY 10029-6500; **Phone:** 212-659-8086; **Board Cert:** Surgery 1997; **Med School:** Harvard Med Sch 1983; **Resid:** Surgery, Univ Washington Med Ctr 1988; **Fellow:** Transplant Surgery, Hosp U Penn 1990; **Fac Appt:** Prof S, Mount Sinai Sch Med

Cameron, John MD [S] - **Spec Exp:** Pancreatic Cancer; Pancreatic Surgery; Biliary Cancer; **Hospital:** Johns Hopkins Hosp - Baltimore (page 61); **Address:** 600 N Wolfe St Blalock Bldg - Ste 679, Baltimore, MD 21287; **Phone:** 410-955-5166; **Board Cert:** Surgery 1970; Thoracic Surgery 1971; **Med School:** Johns Hopkins Univ 1962; **Resid:** Surgery, Johns Hopkins Hosp 1970; **Fellow:** Thoracic Surgery, Johns Hopkins Hosp 1971; **Fac Appt:** Prof S, Johns Hopkins Univ

Carty, Sally E MD [S] - **Spec Exp:** Endocrine Tumors; Parathyroid Surgery; **Hospital:** UPMC Presby, Pittsburgh; **Address:** Univ Pittsburgh Med Ctr, Surgery, 497 Scaife Hall, 3550 Terrace St, Pittsburgh, PA 15261; **Phone:** 412-647-0467; **Board Cert:** Surgery 1999; **Med School:** Penn State Univ-Hershey Med Ctr 1984; **Resid:** Surgery, Penn State Hershey Med Ctr 1989; **Fellow:** Surgical Oncology, Natl Cancer Inst 1991; **Fac Appt:** Prof S, Univ Pittsburgh

Chabot, John A MD [S] - **Spec Exp:** Liver & Biliary Surgery; Pancreatic Cancer; Thyroid & Parathyroid Surgery; **Hospital:** NY-Presby Hosp/Columbia (page 66); **Address:** NY Presby-Columbia Medical Ctr, 161 Ft Washington Ave Fl 8 - Ste 819, New York, NY 10032; **Phone:** 212-305-9468; **Board Cert:** Surgery 2000; **Med School:** Dartmouth Med Sch 1983; **Resid:** Surgery, Columbia-Presby Med Ctr 1990; **Fac Appt:** Assoc Prof S, Columbia P&S

Choti, Michael A MD [S] - **Spec Exp:** Pancreatic Cancer; Liver Cancer-Metastatic; Carcinoid Tumors; Palliative Care; **Hospital:** Johns Hopkins Hosp - Baltimore (page 61); **Address:** Johns Hopkins Hosp., 600 N Wolfe St Blalock Bldg - rm 665, Baltimore, MD 21287; **Phone:** 410-955-7113; **Board Cert:** Surgery 1991; **Med School:** Yale Univ 1983; **Resid:** Surgery, Hosp Univ Penn 1990; **Fellow:** Surgical Oncology, Meml Sloan-Kettering Canc Ctr 1992; **Fac Appt:** Prof S, Johns Hopkins Univ

Coit, Daniel G MD [S] - **Spec Exp:** Melanoma; Pancreatic Cancer; Stomach Cancer; **Hospital:** Meml Sloan-Kettering Cancer Ctr; **Address:** 1275 York Avenue, New York, NY 10065; **Phone:** 800-525-2225; **Board Cert:** Surgery 2004; **Med School:** Univ Cincinnati 1976; **Resid:** Internal Medicine, New England Deaconess Hosp 1978; Surgery, New England Deaconess Hosp 1983; **Fellow:** Surgical Oncology, Meml Sloan Kettering Canc Ctr 1985; **Fac Appt:** Assoc Prof S, Cornell Univ-Weill Med Coll

Conti, David J MD [S] - **Spec Exp:** Transplant-Kidney; **Hospital:** Albany Med Ctr; **Address:** Albany Medical Center, 47 New Scotland Ave, MC 61GE, Albany, NY 12208; **Phone:** 518-262-5614; **Board Cert:** Surgery 1998; **Med School:** Northwestern Univ 1981; **Resid:** Surgery, Northwestern Meml Hosp 1987; **Fellow:** Transplant Surgery, Mass Genl Hosp 1989; **Fac Appt:** Prof S, Albany Med Coll

Cornwell III, Edward E MD [S] - **Spec Exp:** Trauma; **Hospital:** Howard Univ Hosp; **Address:** Howard Univ Hospital, 2041 Georgia Ave NW, Ste 4B02, Washington, DC 20060; **Phone:** 202-865-1441; **Board Cert:** Surgery 1996; Surgical Critical Care 1998; **Med School:** Howard Univ 1982; **Resid:** Surgery, LAC-USC Med Ctr 1987; **Fellow:** Trauma, Emer/Med Svcs System 1989; **Fac Appt:** Assoc Prof S, Johns Hopkins Univ

Courcoulas, Anita P MD [S] - **Spec Exp:** Obesity/Bariatric Surgery; Minimally Invasive Surgery; **Hospital:** Magee-Womens Hosp - UPMC; **Address:** Magee-Women's Hospital, 3380 Boulevard of the Allies, Ste 390, Pittsburgh, PA 15213; **Phone:** 412-641-3632; **Board Cert:** Surgery 2005; **Med School:** Boston Univ 1988; **Resid:** Surgery, Univ Pittsburgh Med Ctr 1996; **Fac Appt:** Assoc Prof S, Univ Pittsburgh

Curcillo, Paul G MD [S] - **Spec Exp:** Laparoscopic Surgery; Hernia; Robotic Surgery; **Hospital:** Hahnemann Univ Hosp; **Address:** 219 N Broad St Fl 10, Philadelphia, PA 19107; **Phone:** 215-762-5577; **Board Cert:** Surgery 2007; **Med School:** Univ Pennsylvania 1989; **Resid:** Surgery, Thos Jefferson Univ Hosp 1995; **Fac Appt:** Assoc Prof S, Drexel Univ Coll Med

Deitch, Edwin MD [S] - **Spec Exp:** Trauma; Burn Care; Critical Care; **Hospital:** UMDNJ-Univ Hosp-Newark; **Address:** 185 S Orange Ave, MSB, rm G506, Newark, NJ 07103; **Phone:** 973-972-5045; **Board Cert:** Surgery 1997; Surgical Critical Care 2006; **Med School:** Univ MD Sch Med 1973; **Resid:** Surgery, US Public Hlth Svc Hosp 1976; Surgery, US Public Hlth Svc Hosp 1978; **Fac Appt:** Prof S, UMDNJ-NJ Med Sch, Newark

Dempsey, Daniel MD [S] - **Spec Exp:** Gastrointestinal & Esophageal Surgery; Laparoscopic Surgery; Gastroesophageal Reflux Disease (GERD); **Hospital:** Temple Univ Hosp; **Address:** Temple Univ Hosp - Dept Surgery, 3401 N Broad St, 400 Parkinson Pavilion, Philadelphia, PA 19140; **Phone:** 215-707-5080; **Board Cert:** Surgery 2006; **Med School:** Univ Rochester 1979; **Resid:** Surgery, Hosp Univ Penn 1986; **Fac Appt:** Prof S, Temple Univ

Drebin, Jeffrey A MD/PhD [S] - **Spec Exp:** Pancreatic Cancer; Liver Cancer; Biliary Cancer; Gastrointestinal Cancer; **Hospital:** Hosp Univ Penn - UPHS (page 60); **Address:** Hosp Univ of Pennsylvania, 3400 Spruce St, 4 Silverstein Pavilion, Fl 4, Philadelphia, PA 19104; **Phone:** 215-662-2165; **Board Cert:** Surgery 2004; **Med School:** Harvard Med Sch 1987; **Resid:** Surgery, Johns Hopkins Hosp 1994; **Fellow:** Medical Oncology, Johns Hopkins Hosp 1991; Surgical Oncology, Johns Hopkins Hosp 1995; **Fac Appt:** Prof S, Univ Pennsylvania

Edge, Stephen B MD [S] - **Spec Exp:** Breast Cancer; **Hospital:** Roswell Park Cancer Inst; **Address:** Roswell Park Cancer Inst, Dept Surg Onc, Elm & Carlton Streets, Buffalo, NY 14263; **Phone:** 716-845-5789; **Board Cert:** Surgery 2006; **Med School:** Case West Res Univ 1979; **Resid:** Surgery, Univ Hosp 1986; **Fellow:** Surgical Oncology, Natl Cancer Inst 1984; **Fac Appt:** Prof S, SUNY Buffalo

Edington, Howard D MD [S] - **Spec Exp:** Melanoma; Breast Reconstruction; **Hospital:** Magee-Womens Hosp - UPMC; **Address:** Magee-Women's Hospital, Dept Surgery, 300 Halket St, rm 2502, Pittsburgh, PA 15213; **Phone:** 412-641-1342; **Board Cert:** Surgery 1998; Plastic Surgery 1993; **Med School:** Temple Univ 1983; **Resid:** Surgery, Univ Pittsburgh Med Ctr 1989; Plastic Surgery, Univ Pittsburgh Med Ctr 1990; **Fellow:** Hand Surgery, Univ Pittsburgh Med Ctr 1991; Surgical Oncology, National Cancer Inst 1993; **Fac Appt:** Assoc Prof S, Univ Pittsburgh

Edye, Michael MD [S] - **Spec Exp:** Laparoscopic Abdominal Surgery; Colon Cancer; Diverticulitis; Obesity/Bariatric Surgery; **Hospital:** Mount Sinai Med Ctr (page 64), Westchester Med Ctr; **Address:** 1060 Fifth Ave, New York, NY 10128; **Phone:** 212-426-9614; **Med School:** Australia 1977; **Resid:** Surgery, St Vincents Hosp 1980; Surgery, Royal N Shore Hosp 1984; **Fellow:** Laparoscopic Surgery, Univ Bordeaux 1992; **Fac Appt:** Assoc Clin Prof S, Mount Sinai Sch Med

Surgery

Emond, Jean C MD [S] - **Spec Exp:** Transplant-Liver; Liver Cancer; Liver & Biliary Cancer; **Hospital:** NY-Presby Hosp/Columbia (page 66), Holy Name Hosp; **Address:** 622 W 168th St, PH - Fl 14, New York, NY 10032; **Phone:** 212-305-9691; **Board Cert:** Surgery 2006; **Med School:** Univ Chicago-Pritzker Sch Med 1979; **Resid:** Surgery, Cook Cty Hosp 1984; **Fellow:** Surgery, Hopital P Brousse/Univ de Paris Sud 1985; Transplant Surgery, Univ Chicago Hosps 1987; **Fac Appt:** Prof S, Columbia P&S

Eng, Kenneth MD [S] - **Spec Exp:** Colon & Rectal Cancer & Surgery; Pancreatic Cancer; Inflammatory Bowel Disease; **Hospital:** NYU Med Ctr (page 68); **Address:** 530 1st Ave, Ste 6B, New York, NY 10016-6402; **Phone:** 212-263-7301; **Board Cert:** Surgery 1982; **Med School:** NYU Sch Med 1967; **Resid:** Surgery, NYU Med Ctr 1972; **Fac Appt:** Prof S, NYU Sch Med

Estabrook, Alison MD [S] - **Spec Exp:** Breast Cancer; Breast Disease; Breast Cancer-High Risk Women; **Hospital:** St Luke's - Roosevelt Hosp Ctr - Roosevelt Div (page 57); **Address:** 425 W 59th St, Ste 7A, New York, NY 10019-1104; **Phone:** 212-523-7500; **Board Cert:** Surgery 2004; **Med School:** NYU Sch Med 1978; **Resid:** Surgery, Columbia Presby Med Ctr 1984; **Fellow:** Surgical Oncology, Columbia Presby Med Ctr 1982; **Fac Appt:** Prof S, Columbia P&S

Fahey III, Thomas J MD [S] - **Spec Exp:** Endocrine Surgery; Pheochromocytoma; Pancreatic Cancer; **Hospital:** NY-Presby Hosp/Weill Cornell (page 66); **Address:** NY Presby Cornell Med Ctr, Dept Surgery, 525 E 68 St, rm F2024, Box 249, New York, NY 10065; **Phone:** 212-746-5130; **Board Cert:** Surgery 2002; **Med School:** Cornell Univ-Weill Med Coll 1986; **Resid:** Surgery, New York Hosp 1992; **Fellow:** Surgery, Royal North Shore Hosp 1993; **Fac Appt:** Assoc Prof S, Cornell Univ-Weill Med Coll

Fong, Yuman MD [S] - **Spec Exp:** Pancreatic Cancer; Liver & Biliary Cancer; Stomach Cancer; **Hospital:** Meml Sloan-Kettering Cancer Ctr, NY-Presby Hosp/Weill Cornell (page 66); **Address:** 1275 York Avenue, New York, NY 10065; **Phone:** 800-525-2225; **Board Cert:** Surgery 2002; **Med School:** Cornell Univ-Weill Med Coll 1984; **Resid:** Surgery, New York Hosp-Cornell Med Ctr 1992; **Fellow:** Surgical Oncology, Meml Sloan-Kettering Cancer Ctr 1994; **Fac Appt:** Prof S, Cornell Univ-Weill Med Coll

Fowler, Dennis MD [S] - **Spec Exp:** Minimally Invasive Surgery; **Hospital:** NY-Presby Hosp/Columbia (page 66); **Address:** 622 W 168th St Fl PH 12 - rm 126, New York, NY 10032; **Phone:** 212-305-0577; **Board Cert:** Surgery 1998; **Med School:** Univ Kans 1973; **Resid:** Surgery, St Lukes Hosp 1979; **Fellow:** Endoscopy, Mass Genl Hosp 1980; **Fac Appt:** Prof S, Columbia P&S

Fraker, Douglas L MD [S] - **Spec Exp:** Melanoma; Endocrine Tumors; Liver Cancer; Sarcoma; **Hospital:** Hosp Univ Penn - UPHS (page 60); **Address:** Hosp Univ Penn, Dept Surgery, 3400 Spruce St, 4 Silverstein Pavilion, Philadelphia, PA 19104; **Phone:** 215-662-7866; **Board Cert:** Surgery 2002; **Med School:** Harvard Med Sch 1983; **Resid:** Surgery, UCSF Med Ctr 1986; Surgery, UCSF Med Ctr 1991; **Fellow:** Surgical Oncology, National Cancer Inst 1989; **Fac Appt:** Prof S, Univ Pennsylvania

Frazier, Thomas MD [S] - **Spec Exp:** Breast Cancer; Breast Disease; **Hospital:** Bryn Mawr Hosp; **Address:** 101 S Bryn Mawr Ave, Ste 201, Bryn Mawr, PA 19010; **Phone:** 610-520-0700; **Board Cert:** Surgery 2004; **Med School:** Univ Pennsylvania 1968; **Resid:** Surgery, Hosp Univ Penn 1975; **Fellow:** Surgical Oncology, MD Anderson Cancer Ctr 1976; **Fac Appt:** Clin Prof S, Jefferson Med Coll

Gibbs, John F MD [S] - **Spec Exp:** Liver Cancer; Liver & Biliary Surgery; Pancreatic Cancer; **Hospital:** Roswell Park Cancer Inst; **Address:** Roswell Park Cancer Inst, Dept Surg Onc, Elm & Carlton Streets, Buffalo, NY 14263-0001; **Phone:** 716-845-5807; **Board Cert:** Surgery 2000; **Med School:** UCSD 1985; **Resid:** Surgery, Rush Presby-St Luke's Med Ctr 1990; **Fellow:** Transplant Surgery, Baylor Univ Med Ctr 1992; Surgical Oncology, Roswell Park Cancer Inst 1996; **Fac Appt:** Assoc Prof S, SUNY Buffalo

Hardy, Mark A MD [S] - **Spec Exp:** Transplant-Kidney; Parathyroid Surgery; Islet Cell Transplant; Immunotherapy; **Hospital:** NY-Presby Hosp/Columbia (page 66); **Address:** 177 Fort Washington Ave, New York, NY 10032; **Phone:** 212-305-5502; **Board Cert:** Surgery 1972; **Med School:** Albert Einstein Coll Med 1962; **Resid:** Surgery, Strong Meml Hosp 1964; Surgery, Bronx Muni Hosp Ctr/Einstein 1971; **Fellow:** Transplant Surgery, Harvard Med Sch 1969; **Fac Appt:** Prof S, Columbia P&S

Hoffman, John P MD [S] - **Spec Exp:** Pancreatic Cancer; Gastrointestinal Cancer; Breast Cancer; Pancreatic Surgery; **Hospital:** Fox Chase Cancer Ctr (page 58); **Address:** Fox Chase Cancer Ctr, 333 Cottman Ave, Philadelphia, PA 19111-2497; **Phone:** 215-728-3518; **Board Cert:** Surgery 1998; **Med School:** Case West Res Univ 1970; **Resid:** Surgery, Virginia Mason Hosp 1977; **Fellow:** Surgical Oncology, Meml Sloan Kettering Cancer Ctr 1980; **Fac Appt:** Prof S, Temple Univ

Jarnagin, William MD [S] - **Spec Exp:** Hepatobiliary Surgery; Liver Cancer; Pancreatic Cancer; **Hospital:** Meml Sloan-Kettering Cancer Ctr; **Address:** 1275 York Ave, New York, NY 10065; **Phone:** 212-639-7601; **Board Cert:** Surgery 2006; **Med School:** Rush Med Coll 1988; **Resid:** Surgery, Univ Calif San Francisco 1996; **Fellow:** Hepatopancreatobiliary Surgery, Meml Sloan-Kettering Cancer Ctr 1997

Johnson, Ronald R MD [S] - **Spec Exp:** Breast Cancer; **Hospital:** Magee-Womens Hosp - UPMC; **Address:** Magee-Womens Hosp - UPMC, 300 Halket St, Ste 2601, Pittsburgh, PA 15213; **Phone:** 412-641-1225; **Board Cert:** Surgery 1999; **Med School:** Univ Pittsburgh 1983; **Resid:** Surgery, Univ Pittsburgh Med Ctr 1989; **Fac Appt:** Asst Prof S, Univ Pittsburgh

Julian, Thomas B MD [S] - **Spec Exp:** Breast Cancer; Clinical Trials; **Hospital:** Allegheny General Hosp; **Address:** Allegheny Cancer Center, 320 E North Ave Fl 5, Pittsburgh, PA 15212; **Phone:** 412-359-8229; **Board Cert:** Surgery 2001; **Med School:** Univ Pittsburgh 1976; **Resid:** Surgery, Univ Pittsburgh Med Ctr 1982; **Fac Appt:** Assoc Prof S, Drexel Univ Coll Med

Kapur, Sandip MD [S] - **Spec Exp:** Transplant-Kidney; Islet Cell Transplant; Hepatobiliary Surgery; **Hospital:** NY-Presby Hosp/Weill Cornell (page 66); **Address:** 520 E 68th St, Ste F1919, New York, NY 10065; **Phone:** 212-746-5330; **Board Cert:** Surgery 2007; **Med School:** Cornell Univ-Weill Med Coll 1990; **Resid:** Surgery, Cornell Univ Med Ctr 1996; **Fellow:** Research, The Rogosin Institute 1994; Transplant Surgery, Thomas E. Starzl Transplant Inst 1998; **Fac Appt:** Assoc Prof S, Cornell Univ-Weill Med Coll

Karpeh Jr, Martin S MD [S] - **Spec Exp:** Gastrointestinal Cancer; Esophageal Cancer; Colon & Rectal Cancer; **Hospital:** Beth Israel Med Ctr - Petrie Division (page 57); **Address:** Beth Israel Med Ctr, Philips Ambulatory Ctr, 10 Union Square E, Ste 4C, New York, NY 10003; **Phone:** 212-420-4041; **Board Cert:** Surgery 1998; **Med School:** Penn State Univ-Hershey Med Ctr 1983; **Resid:** Surgery, Hosp Univ Penn 1989; **Fellow:** Surgical Oncology, Memorial Sloan Kettering Cancer Ctr 1991; **Fac Appt:** Prof S, Mount Sinai Sch Med

Kaufman, Howard L MD [S] - **Spec Exp:** Cancer Surgery; Vaccine Therapy; Melanoma; Immunotherapy; **Hospital:** NY-Presby Hosp/Columbia (page 66); **Address:** Columbia University, MHB-7SK, 177 Fort Washington Ave, New York, NY 10032-3733; **Phone:** 212-342-6042; **Board Cert:** Surgery 1996; **Med School:** Loyola Univ-Stritch Sch Med 1986; **Resid:** Surgery, Boston Univ Hosp 1995; **Fellow:** Surgical Oncology, Natl Cancer Inst 1996; **Fac Appt:** Assoc Prof S, Columbia P&S

Surgery

Lee, Kenneth K W MD [S] - **Spec Exp:** Pancreatic Cancer; Gastrointestinal Cancer & Surgery; **Hospital:** UPMC Presby, Pittsburgh, UPMC Shadyside; **Address:** UPMC Presbyterian, 200 Lothrop St, Ste 497, Scaife Hall, Pittsburgh, PA 15261; **Phone:** 412-647-0457; **Board Cert:** Surgery 1998; **Med School:** Univ Chicago-Pritzker Sch Med 1981; **Resid:** Surgery, Univ Chicago Hosps 1988; **Fac Appt:** Assoc Prof S, Univ Pittsburgh

Lentz, Christopher MD [S] - **Spec Exp:** Burn Care; Trauma; Critical Care; Wound Healing/Care; **Hospital:** Univ of Rochester Strong Meml Hosp; **Address:** Univ Rochester, Surgery Dept, 601 Elmwood Ave, Box SURG, Rochester, NY 14642; **Phone:** 585-275-2876; **Board Cert:** Surgery 1995; Surgical Critical Care 1996; **Med School:** Wayne State Univ 1988; **Resid:** Surgery, Med Coll Wisc 1994; **Fellow:** Surgical Critical Care, Shriners Burns Inst 1991; Burn Surgery, Univ N Carolina Med Ctr 1996; **Fac Appt:** Assoc Prof S, Univ Rochester

Libutti, Steven K MD [S] - **Spec Exp:** Liver Cancer; Pancreatic Cancer; Endocrine Tumors; Gastrointestinal Cancer; **Hospital:** Natl Inst of Hlth - Clin Ctr; **Address:** National Cancer Institute, Surgery Branch, 10 Center Drive Bldg 10 - rm 4W-5940, Bethesda, MD 20892-1201; **Phone:** 301-496-5049; **Board Cert:** Surgery 2004; **Med School:** Columbia P&S 1990; **Resid:** Surgery, Columbia Presby Med Ctr 1995; **Fellow:** Surgical Oncology, Natl Cancer Inst 1996

Manzarbeitia, Cosme Y MD [S] - **Spec Exp:** Transplant-Liver; Hepatobiliary Surgery; **Hospital:** Montgomery Hosp Med Ctr, Mercy Suburb Hosp; **Address:** Associated Surgeons, 1330 Powell St, Ste 100, Norristown, PA 19401; **Phone:** 610-272-3030; **Board Cert:** Surgery 1998; **Med School:** Spain 1982; **Resid:** Surgery, North Genl Hosp 1989; **Fellow:** Transplant Surgery, Mt Sinai Hosp 1991; **Fac Appt:** Assoc Prof S, Jefferson Med Coll

Marsh Jr, James W MD [S] - **Spec Exp:** Transplant-Liver; Liver Cancer; Pancreatic Cancer; **Hospital:** UPMC Presby, Pittsburgh; **Address:** UPMC, Starzl Transplant Inst, 3459 Fifth Ave 7 South, Pittsburgh, PA 15213; **Phone:** 412-692-2001; **Board Cert:** Surgery 2003; **Med School:** Univ Ark 1979; **Resid:** Surgery, St Paul Hosp 1984; **Fellow:** Transplant Surgery, Mayo Clinic 1985; Transplant Surgery, Univ Pittsburgh Hosps 1986; **Fac Appt:** Prof S, Univ Pittsburgh

Meyers, William C MD [S] - **Spec Exp:** Liver & Biliary Surgery; Liver Cancer; Hernia; **Hospital:** Hahnemann Univ Hosp; **Address:** 245 N 15th St, MS 413, Philadelphia, PA 19102; **Phone:** 215-762-1078; **Board Cert:** Surgery 2004; **Med School:** Columbia P&S 1975; **Resid:** Surgery, Duke U Med Ctr 1983; Surgery, Duke U Med Ctr 1982; **Fellow:** Gastroenterology, Duke U Med Ctr 1983; **Fac Appt:** Prof S, Drexel Univ Coll Med

Michelassi, Fabrizio MD [S] - **Spec Exp:** Gastrointestinal Cancer; Inflammatory Bowel Disease/Crohn's; Ulcerative Colitis; Colon & Rectal Cancer; **Hospital:** NY-Presby Hosp/Weill Cornell (page 66); **Address:** Weill Med College, Dept Surgery, 525 E 68th St, rm F-739, New York, NY 10021; **Phone:** 212-746-6006; **Board Cert:** Surgery 2002; **Med School:** Italy 1975; **Resid:** Surgery, NYU Med Ctr 1981; **Fellow:** Research, Mass Genl Hosp 1983; **Fac Appt:** Prof S, Cornell Univ-Weill Med Coll

Montgomery, Robert A MD/PhD [S] - **Spec Exp:** Transplant-Kidney; **Hospital:** Johns Hopkins Hosp - Baltimore (page 61); **Address:** Johns Hopkins Hosp, Transplant Surgery, 720 Rutland Ave Ross Bldg - Ste 765, Baltimore, MD 21205; **Phone:** 410-614-8297; **Board Cert:** Surgery 1997; **Med School:** Univ Rochester 1987; **Resid:** Surgery, Johns Hopkins Hosp 1995; **Fellow:** Transplant Surgery, Johns Hopkins Hosp 1997; **Fac Appt:** Assoc Prof S, Johns Hopkins Univ

Morrow, Monica MD [S] - **Spec Exp:** Breast Cancer; **Hospital:** Meml Sloan-Kettering Cancer Ctr; **Address:** 1275 York Avenue, New York, NY 10065; **Phone:** 800-525-2225; **Board Cert:** Surgery 2001; **Med School:** Jefferson Med Coll 1976; **Resid:** Surgery, Med Ctr Hosp Vermont 1981; **Fellow:** Surgical Oncology, Meml Sloan Kettering Cancer Ctr 1983; **Fac Appt:** Prof S, Cornell Univ-Weill Med Coll

Nava-Villarreal, Hector MD [S] - **Spec Exp:** Esophageal Cancer; Stomach Cancer; Barrett's Esophagus; **Hospital:** Roswell Park Cancer Inst; **Address:** Roswell Park Cancer Inst, Elm & Carlton Sts, Buffalo, NY 14263; **Phone:** 716-845-5915; **Board Cert:** Surgery 2001; **Med School:** Mexico 1967; **Resid:** Surgery, Buffalo Genl Hosp 1974; **Fellow:** Surgical Oncology, Roswell Park Cancer Inst 1976; **Fac Appt:** Assoc Prof S, SUNY Buffalo

Niederhuber, John E MD [S] - **Spec Exp:** Breast Cancer; Liver Cancer; Esophageal Cancer; Pancreatic Cancer; **Hospital:** Natl Inst of Hlth - Clin Ctr; **Address:** Natl Cancer Institute, 31 Center Drive Bldg 31, rm 11A48, MS 2590, Bethesda, MD 20892-2590; **Phone:** 301-594-6369; **Board Cert:** Surgery 1974; **Med School:** Ohio State Univ 1964; **Resid:** Surgery, Univ Mich Hosp 1973; **Fellow:** Immunology, Karolinska Inst 1971

Nowak, Eugene MD [S] - **Spec Exp:** Breast Cancer; Hernia; Gastrointestinal Surgery; Sentinel Node Surgery; **Hospital:** NY-Presby Hosp/Weill Cornell (page 66); **Address:** 325 E 79th St, New York, NY 10021-0954; **Phone:** 212-517-6693; **Board Cert:** Surgery 2002; **Med School:** UMDNJ-NJ Med Sch, Newark 1975; **Resid:** Surgery, NY Hosp-Cornell Med Ctr 1980; **Fac Appt:** Assoc Prof S, Cornell Univ-Weill Med Coll

O'Hea, Brian MD [S] - **Spec Exp:** Breast Cancer; Sentinel Node Surgery; **Hospital:** Stony Brook Univ Med Ctr; **Address:** SUNY Stony Brook, Dept Surg, HSC T-18, Rm 060, Stony Brook, NY 11794-8191; **Phone:** 631-444-1795; **Board Cert:** Surgery 2002; **Med School:** Georgetown Univ 1986; **Resid:** Surgery, St Vincent's Hosp 1991; **Fellow:** Breast Disease, Meml Sloan-Kettering Cancer Ctr 1996; **Fac Appt:** Asst Prof S, SUNY Stony Brook

Olthoff, Kim M MD [S] - **Spec Exp:** Transplant-Liver-Adult & Pediatric; Liver & Biliary Surgery; Liver Cancer; **Hospital:** Hosp Univ Penn - UPHS (page 60), Chldns Hosp of Philadelphia, The; **Address:** Hosp Univ Penn - Dept Surgery, 3400 Spruce St Dulles Bldg Fl 2, Philadelphia, PA 19104; **Phone:** 215-662-6136; **Board Cert:** Surgery 2003; **Med School:** Univ Chicago-Pritzker Sch Med 1986; **Resid:** Surgery, UCLA Med Ctr 1990; **Fellow:** Transplant Surgery, UCLA Med Ctr; **Fac Appt:** Assoc Prof S, Univ Pennsylvania

Osborne, Michael P MD [S] - **Spec Exp:** Breast Cancer; Breast Cancer-High Risk Women; Breast Disease; **Hospital:** Beth Israel Med Ctr - Petrie Division (page 57); **Address:** Philip Ambulatory Care Ctr, 10 Union Square E, Ste 4E, New York, NY 10003; **Phone:** 212-844-8770; **Med School:** England 1970; **Resid:** Surgery, Charing Cross Hosp 1977; Surgery, Royal Marsden Hosp 1980; **Fellow:** Surgical Oncology, Meml Sloan-Kettering Canc Ctr 1981; **Fac Appt:** Prof S, Cornell Univ-Weill Med Coll

Pachter, H Leon MD [S] - **Spec Exp:** Adrenal Surgery; Gastrointestinal Surgery; Pancreatic Cancer; Hernia; **Hospital:** NYU Med Ctr (page 68), Bellevue Hosp Ctr; **Address:** 530 1st Ave, Ste 6C, New York, NY 10016; **Phone:** 212-263-7302; **Board Cert:** Surgery 2000; **Med School:** NYU Sch Med 1971; **Resid:** Surgery, NYU Med Ctr 1976; **Fac Appt:** Prof S, NYU Sch Med

Park, Adrian E MD [S] - **Spec Exp:** Minimally Invasive Surgery; Gastrointestinal Surgery; Laparoscopic Surgery; **Hospital:** Univ of MD Med Sys; **Address:** Univ Maryland Dept Surgery, 22 S Greene St, S4B14, Baltimore, MD 21201; **Phone:** 410-328-7994; **Board Cert:** Surgery 2005; **Med School:** McMaster Univ 1987; **Resid:** Surgery, MC Master Univ 1992; **Fellow:** Laparoscopic Surgery, Hotel Dieu de Montreal 1993; **Fac Appt:** Prof S, Univ MD Sch Med

Paty, Philip B MD [S] - **Spec Exp:** Colon & Rectal Cancer; Pelvic Tumors; Appendix Cancer; **Hospital:** Meml Sloan-Kettering Cancer Ctr; **Address:** 1275 York Avenue, New York, NY 10065; **Phone:** 800-525-2225; **Board Cert:** Surgery 2001; **Med School:** Stanford Univ 1983; **Resid:** Surgery, UCSF Med Ctr 1990; **Fellow:** Surgical Oncology, Memorial Sloan Kettering Cancer Ctr 1992; **Fac Appt:** Prof S, Cornell Univ-Weill Med Coll

Surgery

Peitzman, Andrew B MD [S] - **Spec Exp:** Trauma; Gastrointestinal Surgery; Critical Care; **Hospital:** UPMC Presby, Pittsburgh, UPMC Shadyside; **Address:** Presbyterian Univ Hosp, Dept Surg - F 1281, 200 Lothrop St, Pittsburgh, PA 15213; **Phone:** 412-647-0635; **Board Cert:** Surgery 2004; Surgical Critical Care 1997; **Med School:** Univ Pittsburgh 1976; **Resid:** Surgery, Univ Pittsburgh Med Ctr 1979; Surgery, Univ Pittsburgh Med Ctr 1984; **Fellow:** Surgery, New York Hosp-Cornell Univ 1981; **Fac Appt:** Prof S, Univ Pittsburgh

Peters, Jeffrey H MD [S] - **Spec Exp:** Esophageal Surgery; Gastroesophageal Reflux Disease (GERD); **Hospital:** Univ of Rochester Strong Meml Hosp; **Address:** 601 Elmwood Ave, Box SURG, Rochester, NY 14642-8410; **Phone:** 585-275-2725; **Board Cert:** Surgery 1998; **Med School:** Ohio State Univ 1981; **Resid:** Surgery, Johns Hopkins Hosp 1988; **Fellow:** Allergy & Immunology, Johns Hopkins Hosp 1985; Esophageal Surgery, Creighton Univ; **Fac Appt:** Prof S, Univ Rochester

Petrelli, Nicholas J MD [S] - **Spec Exp:** Cancer Surgery; Gastrointestinal Cancer; **Hospital:** Christiana Care Hlth Svs; **Address:** Helen F Graham Cancer Ctr, 4701 Ogletown-Stanton Rd, Ste 1213, Newark, DE 19713; **Phone:** 302-623-4550; **Board Cert:** Surgery 1997; **Med School:** Tulane Univ 1973; **Resid:** Surgery, St Mary's Hosp-Med Ctr 1978; **Fellow:** Surgical Oncology, Roswell Park Cancer Inst 1980; **Fac Appt:** Prof S, Thomas Jefferson Univ

Ramanathan, Ramesh Chandran MD [S] - **Spec Exp:** Obesity/Bariatric Surgery; Minimally Invasive Surgery; Colon Cancer; Clinical Trials; **Hospital:** Magee-Womens Hosp - UPMC, UPMC Presby, Pittsburgh; **Address:** 3380 Boulevard of the Allies, Ste 390, Pittsburgh, PA 15213; **Phone:** 412-641-3668; **Board Cert:** Surgery 2004; **Med School:** India 1988; **Resid:** Surgery, Univ Hlth Ctr Univ Pitt Med Ctr 2003; **Fellow:** Surgical Oncology, Univ Pitt Med Ctr 1999; Minimally Invasive Surgery, Univ Pitt Med Ctr 2000; **Fac Appt:** Asst Prof S, Univ Pittsburgh

Reiner, Mark MD [S] - **Spec Exp:** Laparoscopic Surgery; Hernia; Esophageal Surgery; Pancreatic Surgery; **Hospital:** Mount Sinai Med Ctr (page 64), Lenox Hill Hosp (page 62); **Address:** 1010 5th Ave, New York, NY 10028-0130; **Phone:** 212-879-6677; **Board Cert:** Surgery 2001; **Med School:** SUNY Downstate 1974; **Resid:** Surgery, Mount Sinai Hosp 1979; **Fac Appt:** Clin Prof S, Mount Sinai Sch Med

Ridge, John Andrew MD/PhD [S] - **Spec Exp:** Head & Neck Cancer & Surgery; Thyroid Cancer & Surgery; Laryngeal Cancer; **Hospital:** Fox Chase Cancer Ctr (page 58); **Address:** Fox Chase Cancer Ctr, Dept Surgical Oncology, 333 Cottman Ave, Philadelphia, PA 19111; **Phone:** 215-728-3517; **Board Cert:** Surgery 2006; **Med School:** Stanford Univ 1981; **Resid:** Surgery, Univ Colorado Med Ctr 1987; **Fellow:** Surgical Oncology, Meml Sloan-Kettering Cancer Ctr 1989

Roh, Mark S MD [S] - **Spec Exp:** Liver Cancer; Cancer Surgery; **Hospital:** Allegheny General Hosp; **Address:** Allegheny General Hospital, Dept Surgery, 320 E North Ave, Pittsburgh, PA 15212; **Phone:** 412-359-6738; **Board Cert:** Surgery 2006; **Med School:** Ohio State Univ 1979; **Resid:** Surgery, Univ Pittsburgh Med Ctr 1982; Surgery, Univ Pittsburgh Med Ctr 1986; **Fellow:** Surgical Oncology, Meml Sloan-Kettering Cancer Ctr 1984; Surgical Oncology, Meml Sloan-Kettering Cancer Ctr 1987; **Fac Appt:** Prof S, Drexel Univ Coll Med

Rosato, Ernest F MD [S] - **Spec Exp:** Gastrointestinal Cancer & Surgery; Esophageal Cancer; Pancreatic Cancer; **Hospital:** Hosp Univ Penn - UPHS (page 60); **Address:** Hosp Univ Penn, Dept Surg, 3400 Spruce St, 4 Silverstein, Philadelphia, PA 19104; **Phone:** 215-662-2033; **Board Cert:** Surgery 1969; **Med School:** Univ Pennsylvania 1962; **Resid:** Surgery, Hosp Univ Penn 1968; **Fac Appt:** Prof S, Univ Pennsylvania

Rosenberg, Steven A MD [S] - **Spec Exp:** Melanoma; Kidney Cancer; **Hospital:** Natl Inst of Hlth - Clin Ctr; **Address:** National Cancer Institute, 9000 Rockville Pike CRC Bldg, rm 3W-3940, Bethesda, MD 20892; **Phone:** 301-496-4164; **Board Cert:** Surgery 1975; **Med School:** Johns Hopkins Univ 1964; **Resid:** Surgery, Peter Bent Brigham Hosp 1974

Roses, Daniel F MD [S] - **Spec Exp:** Breast Cancer; Melanoma; Thyroid Cancer; Parathyroid Surgery; **Hospital:** NYU Med Ctr (page 68); **Address:** 530 First Ave, Ste 6E, New York, NY 10016-6402; **Phone:** 212-263-7329; **Board Cert:** Surgery 1975; **Med School:** NYU Sch Med 1969; **Resid:** Surgery, NYU-Bellevue Hosp 1974; **Fellow:** Surgical Oncology, NYU-Bellevue Hosp 1978; **Fac Appt:** Prof Surg & Onc, NYU Sch Med

Rubino, Francesco MD [S] - **Spec Exp:** Gastrointestinal Metabolic Surgery; Diabetes Surgery-Rubino's Procedure; Obesity/Bariatric Surgery; **Hospital:** NY-Presby Hosp/Weill Cornell (page 66); **Address:** NY Presbyterian Hosp/Weill Cornell, 525 E 68th St, rm P714, New York, NY 10021; **Phone:** 212-746-5925; **Med School:** Italy ; **Resid:** Surgery, Catholic Univ/Policlinico Gemelli; **Fellow:** Laparoscopic Surgery, European Inst of Telesurgery; Research, Catholic Univ; **Fac Appt:** Asst Prof S, Cornell Univ-Weill Med Coll

Salky, Barry A MD [S] - **Spec Exp:** Laparoscopic Abdominal Surgery; Gastroesophageal Reflux Disease (GERD); Pancreatic Surgery; Ulcerative Colitis; **Hospital:** Mount Sinai Med Ctr (page 64); **Address:** Mt Sinai Medical Center, Div of Laparoscopic Surgery, 5 E 98th St, Box 1259, New York, NY 10029; **Phone:** 212-241-6156; **Board Cert:** Surgery 1998; **Med School:** Univ Tenn Coll Med, Memphis 1970; **Resid:** Surgery, Mount Sinai Hosp 1973; Surgery, Mount Sinai Hosp 1978; **Fac Appt:** Prof S, Mount Sinai Sch Med

Scantlebury, Velma P MD [S] - **Spec Exp:** Transplant-Kidney; Kidney Disease; **Hospital:** Christiana Care Hlth Svs; **Address:** 4735 Ogletown-Stanton Rd, Ste 2224, Map II, Newark, DE 19713; **Phone:** 302-623-3866; **Board Cert:** Surgery 2001; **Med School:** Columbia P&S 1981; **Resid:** Surgery, Harlem Hosp 1986; **Fellow:** Transplant Surgery, Univ Pittsburgh Med Ctr 1988

Schnabel, Freya MD [S] - **Spec Exp:** Breast Cancer; Breast Cancer-High Risk Women; **Hospital:** NYU Med Ctr (page 68); **Address:** 160 E 34th St Fl 3, New York, NY 10016; **Phone:** 212-731-5367; **Board Cert:** Surgery 1998; **Med School:** NYU Sch Med 1982; **Resid:** Surgery, NYU Med Ctr 1987; **Fellow:** Research, SUNY Hlth Sci Ctr 1988

Schraut, Wolfgang H MD [S] - **Spec Exp:** Inflammatory Bowel Disease; Gastrointestinal Surgery; Colon & Rectal Cancer & Surgery; Laparoscopic Surgery; **Hospital:** UPMC Presby, Pittsburgh, Magee-Womens Hosp - UPMC; **Address:** Univ Pittsburgh Med Ctr, Dept Surgery, 497 Scaife Hall, 3550 Terrace St, Pittsburgh, PA 15261; **Phone:** 412-647-0311; **Board Cert:** Surgery 1999; **Med School:** Germany 1970; **Resid:** Surgery, Univ Chicago Hosps 1978; **Fac Appt:** Prof S, Univ Pittsburgh

Shah, Jatin P MD [S] - **Spec Exp:** Head & Neck Cancer; Thyroid Cancer; Skull Base Tumors; **Hospital:** Meml Sloan-Kettering Cancer Ctr; **Address:** 1275 York Avenue, New York, NY 10065; **Phone:** 800-525-2225; **Board Cert:** Surgery 1975; **Med School:** India 1964; **Resid:** Surgery, SSG Hosp 1967; Surgery, New York Infirm 1974; **Fellow:** Head & Neck Surgical Oncology, Meml Sloan-Kettering Hosp 1972; **Fac Appt:** Prof S, Cornell Univ-Weill Med Coll

Shapiro, Ron MD [S] - **Spec Exp:** Transplant-Kidney; Transplant-Pancreas; Islet Cell Transplant; **Hospital:** UPMC Presby, Pittsburgh, Chldns Hosp of Pittsburgh - UPMC; **Address:** Starzl Transplantation Inst, UPMC_Montefiore - 7 South, 3459 Fifth Ave, Pittsburgh, PA 15213-2582; **Phone:** 412-647-5800; **Board Cert:** Surgery 2005; **Med School:** Stanford Univ 1980; **Resid:** Surgery, Mt Sinai Hosp 1986; **Fellow:** Transplant Surgery, Univ Pittsburgh 1988; **Fac Appt:** Prof S, Univ Pittsburgh

Sigurdson, Elin R MD [S] - **Spec Exp:** Breast Cancer; Colon & Rectal Cancer; Melanoma; Gastrointestinal Cancer; **Hospital:** Fox Chase Cancer Ctr (page 58); **Address:** 333 Cottman Ave, Philadelphia, PA 19111-2412; **Phone:** 215-728-3519; **Board Cert:** Surgery 1997; **Med School:** Canada 1980; **Resid:** Surgery, Univ Toronto Med Ctr 1984; **Fellow:** Surgical Oncology, Meml Sloan-Kettering Cancer Ctr 1987; **Fac Appt:** Assoc Prof S

Surgery

Singer, Samuel MD [S] - **Spec Exp:** Sarcoma-Soft Tissue; **Hospital:** Meml Sloan-Kettering Cancer Ctr; **Address:** 1275 York Avenue, New York, NY 10065; **Phone:** 800-525-2225; **Board Cert:** Surgery 1998; **Med School:** Harvard Med Sch 1982; **Resid:** Surgery, Brigham & Women's Hosp 1988; **Fellow:** Surgical Oncology, Dana Farber Cancer Inst 1990; **Fac Appt:** Assoc Prof S, Cornell Univ-Weill Med Coll

Skinner, Kristin A MD [S] - **Spec Exp:** Breast Cancer; Gastrointestinal Cancer; Melanoma; **Hospital:** Univ of Rochester Strong Meml Hosp; **Address:** Univ Rochester Med Ctr, 601 Elmwood Ave, Box SURG, Rochester, NY 14642; **Phone:** 585-276-3332; **Board Cert:** Surgery 2005; **Med School:** Johns Hopkins Univ 1988; **Resid:** Surgery, UCLA Med Ctr 1995; **Fellow:** Surgical Oncology, UCLA Med Ctr 1994; **Fac Appt:** Assoc Prof S, Univ Rochester

Sugarbaker, Paul H MD [S] - **Spec Exp:** Appendix Cancer; Peritoneal Carcinomatosis; Cystadenocarcinoma; Ovarian Cancer; **Hospital:** Washington Hosp Ctr; **Address:** Washington Hosp Ctr, 106 Irving St NW, Ste 3900N, Washington, DC 20010; **Phone:** 202-877-3908; **Board Cert:** Surgery 1973; **Med School:** Cornell Univ-Weill Med Coll 1967; **Resid:** Surgery, Peter Bent Brigham Hosp 1973; **Fellow:** Surgical Oncology, Mass Genl Hosp 1976; **Fac Appt:** Prof S, Univ Wash

Swistel, Alexander MD [S] - **Spec Exp:** Breast Cancer; Breast Disease; Sentinel Node Surgery; **Hospital:** NY-Presby Hosp/Weill Cornell (page 66), St Luke's - Roosevelt Hosp Ctr - Roosevelt Div (page 57); **Address:** 425 E 61st St Fl 8, New York, NY 10021; **Phone:** 212-821-0602; **Board Cert:** Surgery 2005; **Med School:** Brown Univ 1975; **Resid:** Surgery, St Luke's Roosevelt Hosp Ctr 1981; **Fellow:** Surgical Oncology, Meml Sloan Kettering Canc Ctr 1983; **Fac Appt:** Asst Prof S, Cornell Univ-Weill Med Coll

Tafra, Lorraine MD [S] - **Spec Exp:** Breast Cancer; **Hospital:** Anne Arundel Med Ctr; **Address:** 2001 Medical Parkway, Ste 120, Annapolis, MD 21401; **Phone:** 443-481-5300; **Board Cert:** Surgery 2005; **Med School:** Case West Res Univ 1986; **Resid:** Surgery, Rhode Island Hosp 1988; Surgery, Hosp Univ Penn 1992; **Fellow:** Surgical Oncology, John Wayne Cancer Inst 1994

Tartter, Paul MD [S] - **Spec Exp:** Breast Cancer; Breast Cancer in Elderly; Sentinel Node Surgery; **Hospital:** St Luke's - Roosevelt Hosp Ctr - Roosevelt Div (page 57), Mount Sinai Med Ctr (page 64); **Address:** 425 W 59th St, Ste 7A, New York, NY 10019-1104; **Phone:** 212-523-7500; **Board Cert:** Surgery 2003; **Med School:** Brown Univ 1977; **Resid:** Surgery, Mount Sinai Hosp 1982; **Fac Appt:** Assoc Prof S, Columbia P&S

Teperman, Lewis W MD [S] - **Spec Exp:** Transplant-Liver; Transplant-Kidney; Liver Tumors; **Hospital:** NYU Med Ctr (page 68); **Address:** 403 E 34th St Fl 3, New York, NY 10016; **Phone:** 212-263-8134; **Board Cert:** Surgery 1997; **Med School:** Mount Sinai Sch Med 1981; **Resid:** Surgery, Columbia Presby Med Ctr 1984; Surgery, LI Jewish Med Ctr 1986; **Fellow:** Transplant Surgery, Univ Pittsburgh 1988; **Fac Appt:** Assoc Prof S, NYU Sch Med

Tsangaris, Theodore N MD [S] - **Spec Exp:** Breast Cancer; **Hospital:** Johns Hopkins Hosp - Baltimore (page 61); **Address:** Johns Hopkins Hospital, 600 N Wolfe St, Carnegie 686, Baltimore, MD 21287; **Phone:** 410-955-2615; **Board Cert:** Surgery 2005; **Med School:** Geo Wash Univ 1983; **Resid:** Surgery, Geo Washington Univ Med Ctr 1989; **Fellow:** Surgical Oncology, Baylor Univ Med Ctr 1990; **Fac Appt:** Assoc Prof S, Johns Hopkins Univ

Willey, Shawna C MD [S] - **Spec Exp:** Breast Cancer; Clinical Trials; **Hospital:** Georgetown Univ Hosp; **Address:** 3800 Reservoir Rd NW, PHC Bldg Fl 4, Washington, DC 20007; **Phone:** 202-444-0241; **Board Cert:** Surgery 1998; **Med School:** Univ Iowa Coll Med 1982; **Resid:** Surgery, George Washington Univ Med Ctr 1988; **Fac Appt:** Asst Prof S, Georgetown Univ

Yang, James C MD [S] - **Spec Exp:** Kidney Cancer; Kidney Cancer Clinical Trials; Clinical Trials; Immunotherapy; **Hospital:** Natl Inst of Hlth - Clin Ctr; **Address:** National Cancer Institute, 9000 Rockville Pike CRC Bldg - rm 3-5952, Bethesda, MD 20892; **Phone:** 301-496-1574; **Board Cert:** Surgery 2005; **Med School:** UCSD 1978; **Resid:** Surgery, UCSD Med Ctr 1984; **Fellow:** Surgical Oncology, Natl Cancer Inst 1986

Yeo, Charles MD [S] - **Spec Exp:** Pancreatic Cancer; **Hospital:** Thomas Jefferson Univ Hosp; **Address:** 1015 Walnut St, Ste 620, Philadelphia, PA 19107; **Phone:** 215-955-9402; **Board Cert:** Surgery 2005; **Med School:** Johns Hopkins Univ 1979; **Resid:** Surgery, Johns Hopkins Hosp 1985; **Fellow:** Research, SUNY Downstate 1982; **Fac Appt:** Prof S, Thomas Jefferson Univ

Yurt, Roger W MD [S] - **Spec Exp:** Burn Care; Wound Healing/Care; Hyperbaric Medicine; **Hospital:** NY-Presby Hosp/Weill Cornell (page 66); **Address:** 525 E 68th St, rm L706, New York, NY 10021-4885; **Phone:** 212-746-5410; **Board Cert:** Surgery 1999; **Med School:** Univ Miami Sch Med 1972; **Resid:** Surgery, Parkland Meml Hosp 1974; Surgery, New York Hosp-Cornell Med Ctr 1980; **Fellow:** Internal Medicine, Brigham & Womens Hosp 1978; **Fac Appt:** Prof S, Cornell Univ-Weill Med Coll

Southeast

Adams, Reid MD [S] - **Spec Exp:** Hepatobiliary Surgery; Liver Cancer; Pancreatic & Biliary Surgery; **Hospital:** Univ Virginia Med Ctr; **Address:** UVA Health System, Dept Surgery, PO Box 800709, Charlottesville, VA 22908; **Phone:** 434-924-2839; **Board Cert:** Surgery 2003; **Med School:** Univ VA Sch Med 1987; **Resid:** Surgery, Univ Va Hlth Sci Ctr 1994; **Fellow:** Hepatopancreatobiliary Surgery, Univ Toronto Med Ctr 1995; **Fac Appt:** Assoc Prof S, Univ VA Sch Med

Albertson, David A MD [S] - **Spec Exp:** Endocrine Surgery; **Hospital:** Wake Forest Univ Baptist Med Ctr (page 73); **Address:** Wake Forest Univ Sch Med, Dept Surgery, Medical Center Blvd, Winston-Salem, NC 27157-1095; **Phone:** 336-716-0664; **Board Cert:** Surgery 1998; **Med School:** Univ VA Sch Med 1972; **Resid:** Surgery, NC Bapt Hosp 1977; **Fellow:** Endocrine Surgery, Boston Univ 1978; **Fac Appt:** Assoc Prof S, Wake Forest Univ

Bear, Harry D MD/PhD [S] - **Spec Exp:** Breast Cancer; Melanoma; Gastrointestinal Cancer; **Hospital:** Med Coll of VA Hosp; **Address:** Med Coll Virginia - VCU, PO Box 980011, Richmond, VA 23298; **Phone:** 804-828-9325; **Board Cert:** Surgery 2003; **Med School:** Med Coll VA 1975; **Resid:** Surgery, Brigham & Women's Hosp 1983; **Fellow:** Surgical Oncology, Med Coll Virgina 1984; **Fac Appt:** Prof Surg & Onc, Med Coll VA

Beauchamp, Robert D MD [S] - **Spec Exp:** Breast Cancer; Colon & Rectal Cancer; Pancreatic Cancer; **Hospital:** Vanderbilt Univ Med Ctr; **Address:** Medical Center North, rm D4316, 1161 21st Ave S, Nashville, TN 37232; **Phone:** 615-322-2363; **Board Cert:** Surgery 1997; **Med School:** Univ Tex Med Br, Galveston 1982; **Resid:** Surgery, Univ Tex Med Br 1987; **Fellow:** Cellular Molecular Biology, Vanderbilt Univ 1989; **Fac Appt:** Prof S, Vanderbilt Univ

Behrns, Kevin E MD [S] - **Spec Exp:** Pancreatic Cancer; Gastrointestinal Cancer & Surgery; **Hospital:** Shands at Univ of FL; **Address:** Shands Healthcare at Univ Florida, PO Box 100286, Gainesville, FL 32610-0286; **Phone:** 352-265-0761; **Board Cert:** Surgery 2005; **Med School:** Mayo Med Sch 1988; **Resid:** Surgery, Mayo Clinic 1995; **Fac Appt:** Prof S, Univ Fla Coll Med

Bland, Kirby MD [S] - **Spec Exp:** Breast Cancer; Colon Cancer; Thyroid & Parathyroid Cancer & Surgery; **Hospital:** Univ of Ala Hosp at Birmingham; **Address:** University of Alabama, Dept Surgery, 1530 3rd Ave S, BDB 502, Birmingham, AL 35294-0002; **Phone:** 205-975-2193; **Board Cert:** Surgery 2000; **Med School:** Univ Ala 1968; **Resid:** Surgery, Univ Fla Hosp 1970; Surgery, Univ Fla Hosp 1976; **Fellow:** Surgical Oncology, MD Anderson Cancer Ctr 1977; **Fac Appt:** Prof S, Univ Ala

Britt, L D MD [S] - **Spec Exp:** Trauma; Head Injury; **Hospital:** Sentara Norfolk Genl Hosp; **Address:** Eastern Virginia Med Sch, Dept Surgery, 825 Fairfax Ave, Ste 610, Norfolk, VA 23507; **Phone:** 757-446-8950; **Board Cert:** Surgery 2003; Surgical Critical Care 1997; **Med School:** Harvard Med Sch 1977; **Resid:** Surgery, Barnes Hosp-Wash Univ 1979; Surgery, Univ Illinois Chicago Med Ctr 1984; **Fellow:** Trauma, Md Inst Emer Med Serv Sys 1986; **Fac Appt:** Prof S, Eastern VA Med Sch

Calvo, Benjamin MD [S] - **Spec Exp:** Colon Cancer; Endocrine Cancers; Breast Cancer; **Hospital:** Univ NC Hosps; **Address:** Dept Surg CB 7213, Chapel Hill, NC 27599; **Phone:** 919-966-5221; **Board Cert:** Surgery 1999; **Med School:** Univ MD Sch Med 1981; **Resid:** Surgery, G Washington Univ Hosp 1988; Surgery, Natl Inst Hlth 1991; **Fellow:** Surgery, Meml Sloan Kettering Cancer Ctr 1993; **Fac Appt:** Assoc Prof S, Univ NC Sch Med

Cance, William George MD [S] - **Spec Exp:** Pancreatic Cancer; Colon & Rectal Cancer; Endocrine Cancers; **Hospital:** Shands at Univ of FL, Malcolm Randall VA Med Ctr; **Address:** Shands at Univ Florida-Dept Surgery, 1600 SW Archer Rd, PO Box 100286, Gainesville, FL 32610-0286; **Phone:** 352-265-0622; **Board Cert:** Surgery 1998; **Med School:** Duke Univ 1982; **Resid:** Surgery, Barnes Hosp-Wash Univ 1988; **Fellow:** Surgical Oncology, Meml Sloan Kettering Canc Ctr 1990; **Fac Appt:** Prof S, Univ Fla Coll Med

Chari, Ravi S MD [S] - **Spec Exp:** Liver Cancer; Biliary Cancer; Transplant-Liver; **Hospital:** Vanderbilt Univ Med Ctr; **Address:** Vanderbilt Univ Med Ctr, Hepatobillary Surg, 1313 21st Ave S, Ste 801 Oxford House, Nashville, TN 37232-4753; **Phone:** 615-936-2573; **Board Cert:** Surgery 2005; **Med School:** Canada 1989; **Resid:** Surgery, Duke Univ Med Ctr 1996; **Fellow:** Transplant Surgery, Univ Toronto-Toronto Hosp 1998; **Fac Appt:** Prof S, Vanderbilt Univ

Cole, David J MD [S] - **Spec Exp:** Breast Brachytherapy; Gastrointestinal Cancer; Vaccine Therapy; Gene Therapy; **Hospital:** MUSC Med Ctr; **Address:** 96 Jonathan Lucas St, PO BOX 250613, Charleston, SC 29425; **Phone:** 843-792-4638; **Board Cert:** Surgery 2000; **Med School:** Cornell Univ-Weill Med Coll 1986; **Resid:** Surgery, Emory Univ School Med 1991; **Fellow:** Surgical Oncology, Natl Cancer Institute 1994; **Fac Appt:** Prof S, Med Univ SC

Dilawari, Raza A MD [S] - **Spec Exp:** Liver & Biliary Cancer; Melanoma; Skin Cancer; Breast Cancer; **Hospital:** Methodist Univ Hosp - Memphis, St Francis Hosp - Memphis; **Address:** Methodist Univ Hosp, 1325 Eastmoreland Ave, Ste 410, Memphis, TN 38104; **Phone:** 901-725-1921; **Board Cert:** Surgery 1975; **Med School:** Pakistan 1968; **Resid:** Surgery, SUNY-Upstate Med Ctr 1974; **Fellow:** Surgical Oncology, Roswell Park Meml Hosp 1976; **Fac Appt:** Prof S, Univ Tenn Coll Med, Memphis

Eckhoff, Devin E MD [S] - **Spec Exp:** Transplant-Liver; Hepatobiliary Surgery; Transplant-Kidney; Hepatitis C; **Hospital:** Univ of Ala Hosp at Birmingham; **Address:** University of Alabama School of Medicine, 701 S 19th St LHRB Bldg - rm 710, Birmingham, AL 35294-0007; **Phone:** 205-975-7622; **Board Cert:** Surgery 2000; Surgical Critical Care 2001; **Med School:** Univ Minn 1986; **Resid:** Surgery, Univ Wisconsin Med Ctr 1992; **Fellow:** Transplant Surgery, Univ Wisconsin Med Ctr 1994; **Fac Appt:** Prof S, Univ Ala

Feliciano, David V MD [S] - **Spec Exp:** Vascular Surgery; Trauma; **Hospital:** Grady Hlth Sys; **Address:** Grady Memorial Hosp, Glenn Meml Bldg, 69 Jesse Hill Jr Dr SE, rm 304, Atlanta, GA 30303; **Phone:** 404-616-5456; **Board Cert:** Surgery 1998; Surgical Critical Care 1998; **Med School:** Georgetown Univ 1970; **Resid:** Surgery, Mayo Clinic 1977; **Fellow:** Cardiovascular Surgery, Texas Med Ctr/Baylor 1978; **Fac Appt:** Prof S, Emory Univ

Flynn, Michael B MD [S] - **Spec Exp:** Head & Neck Cancer; Head & Neck Surgery; **Hospital:** Univ of Louisville Hosp, Norton Hosp; **Address:** 601 S Floyd St, Ste 700, Louisville, KY 40202; **Phone:** 502-583-8303; **Board Cert:** Surgery 1972; **Med School:** Ireland 1962; **Resid:** Surgery, Univ Maryland Hosp 1969; **Fellow:** Surgical Oncology, MD Anderson Hosp 1971; **Fac Appt:** Prof S, Univ Louisville Sch Med

Gabram, Sheryl G A MD [S] - **Spec Exp:** Breast Cancer; Breast Disease; **Hospital:** Emory Univ Hosp, Grady Hlth Sys; **Address:** Winship Cancer Institute, 1365 Clifton Rd NE C Bldg Fl 2, Atlanta, GA 30322; **Phone:** 404-778-1230; **Board Cert:** Surgery 2006; **Med School:** Georgetown Univ 1982; **Resid:** Surgery, Washington Hosp Ctr 1987; **Fellow:** Trauma, Hartford Hosp 1988; **Fac Appt:** Prof S, Emory Univ

Gagner, Michel MD [S] - **Spec Exp:** Obesity/Bariatric Surgery; Adrenal Surgery; Pancreatic Surgery; Diabetes Surgery-Rubino's Procedure; **Hospital:** Mount Sinai Med Ctr - Miami; **Address:** Mount Sinai Medical Center, 4300 Alton Rd, Miami Beach, FL 33140; **Phone:** 212-746-5294; **Board Cert:** Surgery 2003; **Med School:** Canada 1982; **Resid:** Surgery, Royal Victoria Hosp/McGill 1988; **Fellow:** Hepatobiliary Surgery, Hosp Paul-Brousse 1989; Hepatobiliary Surgery, Lahey Clinic 1990; **Fac Appt:** Prof S, Cornell Univ-Weill Med Coll

Goldstein, Richard E MD/PhD [S] - **Spec Exp:** Endocrine Tumors; Thyroid Cancer & Surgery; Parathyroid Cancer; Parathyroid Surgery; **Hospital:** Univ of Louisville Hosp; **Address:** University Surgical Assocs, 601 S Floyd St, Ste 700, Louisville, KY 40202; **Phone:** 502-583-8303; **Board Cert:** Surgery 1999; **Med School:** Jefferson Med Coll 1982; **Resid:** Surgery, Vanderbilt Univ Hosp 1990; **Fac Appt:** Prof S, Univ Louisville Sch Med

Greene, Frederick L MD [S] - **Spec Exp:** Gastrointestinal Surgery; Gastrointestinal Cancer; Hernia; **Hospital:** Carolinas Med Ctr; **Address:** Carolinas Medical Ctr, 1025 Morehead Medical Drive, Ste 275, Charlotte, NC 28203; **Phone:** 704-355-1813; **Board Cert:** Surgery 1998; **Med School:** Univ VA Sch Med 1970; **Resid:** Surgery, Yale-New Haven Hosp 1976; **Fellow:** Surgical Oncology, Yale-New Haven Hosp 1973; **Fac Appt:** Prof S, Univ NC Sch Med

Hanks, John B MD [S] - **Spec Exp:** Endocrine Cancers; Breast Cancer; Thyroid Cancer & Surgery; Endocrine Surgery; **Hospital:** Univ Virginia Med Ctr; **Address:** Univ VA Hlth Sys, Dept Surg, PO Box 800709, Charlottesville, VA 22908-0709; **Phone:** 434-924-0376; **Board Cert:** Surgery 2001; **Med School:** Univ Rochester 1973; **Resid:** Surgery, Duke Univ Med Ctr 1982; **Fac Appt:** Prof S, Univ VA Sch Med

Hemming, Alan W MD [S] - **Spec Exp:** Liver Cancer; Transplant-Liver; Hepatobiliary Surgery; Pancreatic Cancer; **Hospital:** Shands at Univ of FL; **Address:** University of Florida, Dept Surgery, 1600 SW Archer Rd, rm 6142, Box 100286, Gainesville, FL 32610-3003; **Phone:** 352-265-0606; **Board Cert:** Surgery 2004; **Med School:** Canada 1987; **Resid:** Surgery, Univ British Columbia Med Ctr 1993; **Fellow:** Transplant Surgery, Univ Toronto/Hosp for Sick Children 1995; Hepatobiliary Surgery, Univ Toronto 1996; **Fac Appt:** Prof S, Univ Fla Coll Med

Herrmann, Virginia M MD [S] - **Spec Exp:** Breast Cancer; Nutrition & Cancer Prevention/Control; **Hospital:** MUSC Med Ctr; **Address:** MUSC Medical Ctr, Dept Surgery, 96 Jonathan Lucas St, Ste 420, PO Box 250613, Charleston, SC 29425; **Phone:** 843-792-1387; **Board Cert:** Surgery 2000; **Med School:** St Louis Univ 1974; **Resid:** Surgery, St Louis Univ Hosps 1979; **Fellow:** Surgery, Brigham & Women's Hosp 1980; **Fac Appt:** Prof S, Med Univ SC

Surgery

Heslin, Martin J MD [S] - **Spec Exp:** Gastrointestinal Cancer; Pancreatic Cancer; Biliary Cancer; Sarcoma-Soft Tissue; **Hospital:** Univ of Ala Hosp at Birmingham; **Address:** Univ Alabama, 1922 7th Ave S, Ste 321, Birmingham, AL 35294-0016; **Phone:** 205-934-3064; **Board Cert:** Surgery 1995; **Med School:** SUNY Upstate Med Univ 1987; **Resid:** Surgery, NYU Med Ctr 1994; Surgery, Meml Sloan-Kettering Canc Ctr 1991; **Fellow:** Surgical Oncology, Meml Sloan-Kettering Cancer Ctr 1996; **Fac Appt:** Prof S, Univ Ala

Howard, Richard J MD [S] - **Spec Exp:** Endocrine Surgery; Transplant-Kidney; Gastrointestinal Surgery; **Hospital:** Shands at Univ of FL; **Address:** Shands Healthcare Transplant Surgery, 1600 SW Archer Rd, Ste 6142, Gainesville, FL 32610; **Phone:** 352-265-0606; **Board Cert:** Surgery 2004; **Med School:** Yale Univ 1966; **Resid:** Surgery, Univ Minn Hosp 1975; **Fac Appt:** Prof S, Univ Fla Coll Med

Kelley, Mark C MD [S] - **Spec Exp:** Breast Cancer; Melanoma; **Hospital:** Vanderbilt Univ Med Ctr; **Address:** Div Surgical Oncology, 2220 Pierce Ave, 597 Preston Rsch Bldg, Nashville, TN 37232; **Phone:** 615-322-2391; **Board Cert:** Surgery 2005; **Med School:** Univ Fla Coll Med 1989; **Resid:** Surgery, Univ Fla-Shands Hosp 1995; **Fellow:** Surgical Oncology, John Wayne Cancer Inst-St Johns Hosp 1997; **Fac Appt:** Asst Prof Surg & Onc, Vanderbilt Univ

Koruda, Mark J MD [S] - **Spec Exp:** Gastrointestinal Surgery; Minimally Invasive Surgery; Inflammatory Bowel Disease; **Hospital:** Univ NC Hosps; **Address:** Univ NC Chapel Hill, Div Gastrointestinal Surgery, 320 Med Wing E, Campus Box 7081, Chapel Hill, NC 27599; **Phone:** 919-966-8436; **Board Cert:** Surgery 1999; **Med School:** Yale Univ 1981; **Resid:** Surgery, Hosp Univ Penn 1988; **Fac Appt:** Prof S, Univ NC Sch Med

Levi, Joe U MD [S] - **Spec Exp:** Pancreatic Cancer; Liver Disease; Liver Tumors; Biliary Surgery; **Hospital:** Jackson Meml Hosp; **Address:** 1475 NW 12th Ave, Ste 3524, Miami, FL 33136; **Phone:** 305-243-4211; **Board Cert:** Surgery 1975; **Med School:** Univ Fla Coll Med 1967; **Resid:** Surgery, Johns Hopkins Hosp 1969; Surgery, Jackson Meml Hosp 1974; **Fac Appt:** Prof S, Univ Miami Sch Med

Levine, Edward A MD [S] - **Spec Exp:** Breast Cancer; Esophageal Cancer; Peritoneal Carcinomatosis; **Hospital:** Wake Forest Univ Baptist Med Ctr (page 73); **Address:** Wake Forest Univ Baptist Med Ctr, Dept of Surgery, Medical Center Blvd, Winston-Salem, NC 27157; **Phone:** 336-716-4276; **Board Cert:** Surgery 1999; **Med School:** Ros Franklin Univ/Chicago Med Sch 1985; **Resid:** Surgery, Michael Reese Hosp 1990; **Fellow:** Surgical Oncology, Univ Illinois 1992; **Fac Appt:** Prof S, Wake Forest Univ

Lind, David Scott MD [S] - **Spec Exp:** Breast Cancer; Melanoma; Sarcoma; **Hospital:** Med Coll of GA Hosp and Clin; **Address:** MCG Health System-Dept Hem Onc, 1120 15th St, Augusta, GA 30912; **Phone:** 706-721-6744; **Board Cert:** Surgery 2000; **Med School:** Eastern VA Med Sch 1984; **Resid:** Surgery, Univ Texas 1989; **Fellow:** Medical Oncology, Med Coll Virginia 1992; **Fac Appt:** Prof Surg & Onc, Med Coll GA

Livingstone, Alan S MD [S] - **Spec Exp:** Liver & Biliary Cancer; Stomach Cancer; Esophageal Cancer; Pancreatic Cancer; **Hospital:** Jackson Meml Hosp, Univ of Miami Hosp & Clins/Sylvester Comp Canc Ctr; **Address:** Sylvester Comp Cancer Ctr, Dept Surgery (310T), 1475 NW 12th Ave, rm 3550, Miami, FL 33136-1002; **Phone:** 305-243-4902; **Board Cert:** Surgery 1995; **Med School:** McGill Univ 1971; **Resid:** Surgery, Montreal Genl Hosp 1976; Surgery, Jackson Meml Hosp 1975; **Fac Appt:** Prof S, Univ Miami Sch Med

Luterman, Arnold MD [S] - **Spec Exp:** Burn Care; Wound Healing/Care; Critical Care; **Hospital:** Univ of S AL Med Ctr; **Address:** Univ of S Alabama Med Ctr, Mastin Bldg, 2451 Fillingim St, rm 701, Mobile, AL 36617; **Phone:** 251-415-1475; **Board Cert:** Surgery 1996; Surgical Critical Care 1996; **Med School:** McGill Univ 1970; **Resid:** Surgery, Sinai Hospital 1973; Surgery, Jewish Gen Hosp. McGill U 1976; **Fellow:** Burn Surgery, Univ Washington Medical Ctr 1976; **Fac Appt:** Prof S, Univ S Ala Coll Med

Lyerly, H Kim MD [S] - **Spec Exp:** Breast Cancer; Immunotherapy; **Hospital:** Duke Univ Med Ctr, Durham Regional Hosp; **Address:** Duke Comprehensive Cancer Center, DUMC Box 2714, Durham, NC 27710; **Phone:** 919-684-5613; **Board Cert:** Surgery 2001; **Med School:** UCLA 1983; **Resid:** Surgery, Duke Univ Med Ctr 1990; **Fac Appt:** Prof S, Duke Univ

MacDonald Jr, Kenneth G MD [S] - **Spec Exp:** Gastrointestinal Surgery; Obesity/Bariatric Surgery; Pancreatic Surgery; **Hospital:** Pitt Cty Mem Hosp - Univ Med Ctr East Carolina; **Address:** Southern Surgical Assoc, PA, 2455 Emerald Pl, Greenville, NC 27834; **Phone:** 252-758-2224; **Board Cert:** Surgery 1998; **Med School:** W VA Univ 1981; **Resid:** Surgery, NC Baptist Hosp 1984; Surgery, Univ Med Ctr of E Carolina 1987; **Fac Appt:** Prof S, E Carolina Univ

MacFadyen Jr, Bruce V MD [S] - **Spec Exp:** Laparoscopic Surgery; Gastrointestinal Surgery; Endoscopy; **Hospital:** Med Coll of GA Hosp and Clin; **Address:** Medical College GA, Dept Surgery, 1120 15th St, Ste 4076, Augusta, GA 30912; **Phone:** 706-721-4651; **Board Cert:** Surgery 1975; **Med School:** Hahnemann Univ 1968; **Resid:** Surgery, Hosp Univ Penn 1972; Surgery, Hermann Hosp 1974; **Fellow:** MD Anderson Cancer Ctr 1978; **Fac Appt:** Prof S, Med Coll GA

McGrath, Patrick C MD [S] - **Spec Exp:** Breast Cancer; Cancer Surgery; **Hospital:** Univ of Kentucky Chandler Hosp; **Address:** Univ Kentucky Med Ctr, Dept Genl Surgery, 800 Rose St, rm C224, Lexington, KY 40536-0293; **Phone:** 859-323-6346 x233; **Board Cert:** Surgery 1996; **Med School:** Univ IL Coll Med 1980; **Resid:** Surgery, Med Coll Virginia Hosp 1986; **Fellow:** Surgical Oncology, Med Coll Virginia Hosp 1988; **Fac Appt:** Prof S, Univ KY Coll Med

McMasters, Kelly M MD [S] - **Spec Exp:** Melanoma; Breast Cancer; Liver Cancer; **Hospital:** Univ of Louisville Hosp; **Address:** 601 S Floyd St, Ste 700, Louisville, KY 40202; **Phone:** 502-583-8303; **Board Cert:** Surgery 2005; **Med School:** UMDNJ-RW Johnson Med Sch 1989; **Resid:** Surgery, Univ Louisville Sch Med 1994; **Fellow:** Surgical Oncology, Texas-MD Anderson Cancer Ctr 1995; **Fac Appt:** Prof S, Univ Louisville Sch Med

Meyer, Anthony A MD [S] - **Spec Exp:** Trauma/Critical Care; Burn Care; **Hospital:** Univ NC Hosps; **Address:** Univ NC-Sch Med, Dept Surgery, 4041 Burnett-Womack Bldg, CB7050, Chapel HIll, NC 27599-7050; **Phone:** 919-966-4321; **Board Cert:** Surgery 2001; Surgical Critical Care 2005; **Med School:** Univ Chicago-Pritzker Sch Med 1977; **Resid:** Surgery, UCSF Med Ctr 1982; **Fac Appt:** Prof S, Univ NC Sch Med

Neifeld, James MD [S] - **Spec Exp:** Melanoma; Head & Neck Cancer; Gastrointestinal Cancer; **Hospital:** Med Coll of VA Hosp; **Address:** Medical College of Virginia Hospital, PO Box 980645, Richmond, VA 23298-0645; **Phone:** 804-828-9324; **Board Cert:** Surgery 1998; **Med School:** Med Coll VA 1972; **Resid:** Surgery, Med Coll VA Hosp 1978; **Fac Appt:** Prof S, Va Commonwealth Univ Sch Med

Newell, Kenneth MD/PhD [S] - **Spec Exp:** Transplant-Kidney; Transplant-Pancreas; Transplant-Liver; **Hospital:** Emory Univ Hosp; **Address:** Emory Transplant Ctr, 101 Woodruff Cir, rm 5105 WMB, Atlanta, GA 30322; **Phone:** 404-727-2489; **Board Cert:** Surgery 1999; **Med School:** Univ Mich Med Sch 1984; **Resid:** Surgery, Loyola Univ Med Ctr 1989; **Fellow:** Transplant Surgery, Univ Chicago 1994; **Fac Appt:** Assoc Prof S, Emory Univ

Surgery

Pappas, Theodore N MD [S] - **Spec Exp:** Pancreatic Surgery; Laparoscopic Surgery; **Hospital:** Duke Univ Med Ctr; **Address:** Duke Univ Med Ctr, Dept Surgery, DUMC Box 3479, Durham, NC 27710-0001; **Phone:** 919-681-3442; **Board Cert:** Surgery 1997; **Med School:** Ohio State Univ 1981; **Resid:** Surgery, Brigham & Womens Hosp 1988; **Fellow:** Research, Wadworth VA Med Ctr 1985; **Fac Appt:** Prof S, Duke Univ

Pinson, C Wright MD [S] - **Spec Exp:** Transplant-Liver; Liver & Biliary Cancer; Pancreatic Cancer; Liver & Biliary Surgery; **Hospital:** Vanderbilt Univ Med Ctr; **Address:** Vanderbilt Univ Med Ctr, TVC 3810A, 1301 21st Ave S, Nashville, TN 37232-5545; **Phone:** 615-343-9324; **Board Cert:** Surgery 1996; Surgical Critical Care 1997; **Med School:** Vanderbilt Univ 1980; **Resid:** Surgery, Oregon Health Sci Ctr 1986; **Fellow:** Gastrointestinal Surgery, Lahey Clinic 1987; Transplant Surgery, Deaconess Hosp 1988; **Fac Appt:** Prof S, Vanderbilt Univ

Reintgen, Douglas S MD [S] - **Spec Exp:** Melanoma; Breast Cancer; Cancer Surgery; **Hospital:** Lakeland Regl Med Ctr; **Address:** 3525 Lakeland Hills Blvd, Lakeland, FL 33805-1965; **Phone:** 863-603-6565; **Board Cert:** Surgery 1997; **Med School:** Duke Univ 1979; **Resid:** Surgery, Duke Univ Med Ctr 1987; **Fac Appt:** Prof S, Univ S Fla Coll Med

Rosemurgy, Alexander S MD [S] - **Spec Exp:** Pancreatic Cancer; Gastrointestinal Surgery; **Hospital:** Tampa Genl Hosp; **Address:** Digestive Disorders Ctr, Tampa General Hospital, 2 Columbia Drive, rm F145, Tampa, FL 33601; **Phone:** 813-844-7393; **Board Cert:** Surgery 2005; **Med School:** Univ Mich Med Sch 1979; **Resid:** Surgery, Univ Chicago Hosps 1984; **Fac Appt:** Prof S, Univ S Fla Coll Med

Salo, Jonathan C MD [S] - **Spec Exp:** Gastrointestinal Cancer; Immunotherapy; **Hospital:** Carolinas Med Ctr; **Address:** Blumenthal Cancer Center, 1025 Morehead Medical Drive, Ste 600, Charlotte, NC 28204; **Phone:** 704-355-2884; **Board Cert:** Surgery 2005; **Med School:** UCSF 1981; **Resid:** Surgery, UCSF Med Ctr 1993; **Fellow:** Surgical Oncology, Natl Cancer Inst 1991; Surgical Oncology, Meml Sloan-Kettering Cancer Ctr 1998

Schirmer, Bruce D MD [S] - **Spec Exp:** Laparoscopic Surgery; Gastrointestinal Surgery; Pancreatic Surgery; Liver Surgery; **Hospital:** Univ Virginia Med Ctr; **Address:** Univ VA Hlth Sys, Dept Surgery, PO Box 800709, Charlottesville, VA 22908; **Phone:** 434-924-2104; **Board Cert:** Surgery 2005; **Med School:** Duke Univ 1978; **Resid:** Surgery, Duke Univ Med Ctr 1985; **Fac Appt:** Prof S, Univ VA Sch Med

Sharp, Kenneth MD [S] - **Spec Exp:** Gastrointestinal Surgery; Esophageal Disorders; Laparoscopic Surgery; Pancreatic Surgery; **Hospital:** Vanderbilt Univ Med Ctr; **Address:** Vanderbilt Univ Med Ctr, Div Gen Surgery, D-5203 Medical Center North, Nashville, TN 37232-2577; **Phone:** 615-322-0259; **Board Cert:** Surgery 2003; **Med School:** Johns Hopkins Univ 1977; **Resid:** Surgery, Johns Hopkins Univ Med Ctr 1984; **Fellow:** Hepatobiliary Surgery, Loch Raven VA Hosp 1981; Surgery, John Radcliffe Hosp 1982; **Fac Appt:** Prof S, Vanderbilt Univ

Slingluff Jr, Craig L MD [S] - **Spec Exp:** Melanoma; Immunotherapy; **Hospital:** Univ Virginia Med Ctr; **Address:** UVA Health System, Dept Surgery, PO Box 800709, Charlottesville, VA 22908; **Phone:** 434-924-1730; **Board Cert:** Surgery 2002; **Med School:** Univ VA Sch Med 1984; **Resid:** Surgery, Duke Univ Med Ctr 1991; **Fellow:** Surgical Research, Duke Univ Med Ctr 1992; **Fac Appt:** Prof S, Univ VA Sch Med

Sondak, Vernon K MD [S] - **Spec Exp:** Cancer Surgery; Melanoma; Sarcoma; **Hospital:** H Lee Moffitt Cancer Ctr & Research Inst; **Address:** H Lee Moffitt Cancer Ctr, Cutaneous Program, 12902 Magnolia Drive, Tampa, FL 33612; **Phone:** 813-745-1968; **Board Cert:** Surgery 1996; **Med School:** Boston Univ 1980; **Resid:** Surgery, UCLA Med Ctr 1987; **Fellow:** Surgical Oncology, UCLA Med Ctr 1984; **Fac Appt:** Prof S, Univ S Fla Coll Med

Stratta, Robert MD [S] - **Spec Exp:** Transplant-Pancreas; Transplant-Kidney; Gastrointestinal Surgery; **Hospital:** Wake Forest Univ Baptist Med Ctr (page 73); **Address:** Wake Forest Univ Baptist Med Ctr, Dept Surgery, Medical Center Blvd, Winston-Salem, NC 27157-1095; **Phone:** 336-716-6371; **Board Cert:** Surgery 2006; **Med School:** Univ Chicago-Pritzker Sch Med 1980; **Resid:** Surgery, Univ Utah Med Ctr 1986; **Fellow:** Transplant Surgery, Univ Wisc Hosps & Clins 1988; **Fac Appt:** Prof S, Wake Forest Univ

Sweeney, John F MD [S] - **Spec Exp:** Gastrointestinal Surgery; Robotic Surgery; **Hospital:** Emory Univ Hosp; **Address:** The Emory Clinic 'A', 1365 Clifton Rd NE, Atlanta, GA 30322; **Phone:** 404-778-3712; **Board Cert:** Surgery 2004; **Med School:** Rush Med Coll 1988; **Resid:** Surgery, Univ South Florida 1994; **Fellow:** Surgery, Univ South Florida 1995; **Fac Appt:** Prof S, Emory Univ

Tyler, Douglas S MD [S] - **Spec Exp:** Pancreatic Cancer; Colon & Rectal Cancer; Rectal Cancer/Sphincter Preservation; Melanoma; **Hospital:** Duke Univ Med Ctr; **Address:** Duke University Med Ctr, Box 3118, Durham, NC 27710; **Phone:** 919-684-6858; **Board Cert:** Surgery 2000; **Med School:** Dartmouth Med Sch 1985; **Resid:** Surgery, Duke Univ Med Ctr 1992; **Fellow:** Surgical Oncology, MD Anderson Cancer Ctr 1994; **Fac Appt:** Prof S, Duke Univ

Tzakis, Andreas MD [S] - **Spec Exp:** Transplant-Liver; Transplant-Bowel; **Hospital:** Jackson Meml Hosp; **Address:** 1801 NW 9th Ave, Ste 511, Miami, FL 33136; **Phone:** 305-355-5011; **Board Cert:** Surgery 2003; **Med School:** Greece 1974; **Resid:** Surgery, Mt Sinai Hosp 1979; Surgery, SUNY Stony Brook 1983; **Fellow:** Transplant Surgery, Univ Pittsburgh Med Ctr 1985; **Fac Appt:** Prof S, Univ Miami Sch Med

Urist, Marshall M MD [S] - **Spec Exp:** Cancer Surgery; Breast Cancer; Melanoma; **Hospital:** Univ of Ala Hosp at Birmingham; **Address:** Univ Alabama Sch Med, Dept Surgery, 1922 7th Ave S, Kracke Bldg, Ste 321, Birmingham, AL 35294; **Phone:** 205-934-3065; **Board Cert:** Surgery 2000; **Med School:** Univ Chicago-Pritzker Sch Med 1971; **Resid:** Surgery, Johns Hopkins Hosp 1978; **Fellow:** Surgical Oncology, UCLA Med Ctr 1976; **Fac Appt:** Prof S, Univ Ala

Vogel, Stephen Burton MD [S] - **Spec Exp:** Esophageal Cancer; Liver Cancer; **Hospital:** Shands at Univ of FL; **Address:** University of Florida, Dept Surgery, PO Box 100286, Gainesville, FL 32610-0286; **Phone:** 352-265-0604; **Board Cert:** Surgery 1995; **Med School:** Univ Fla Coll Med 1967; **Resid:** Surgery, Univ Minn Hosp 1975; **Fac Appt:** Prof S, Univ Fla Coll Med

White Jr, Richard L MD [S] - **Spec Exp:** Breast Cancer; Melanoma; Sarcoma; Immunotherapy; **Hospital:** Carolinas Med Ctr; **Address:** Carolinas Medical Center, 1000 Blythe Blvd, Box 32861, Charlotte, NC 28203; **Phone:** 704-355-2884; **Board Cert:** Surgery 2002; **Med School:** Columbia P&S 1986; **Resid:** Surgery, Georgetown Univ Hosp 1992; **Fellow:** Surgical Oncology, NIH-Natl Cancer Inst 1995; **Fac Appt:** Assoc Clin Prof S, Univ NC Sch Med

Whitworth, Pat W MD [S] - **Spec Exp:** Breast Cancer; **Hospital:** Baptist Hosp - Nashville, Centennial Med Ctr; **Address:** 300 20th Ave N, Ste 401, Nashville, TN 37203; **Phone:** 615-284-8229; **Board Cert:** Surgery 1999; **Med School:** Univ Tenn Coll Med, Memphis 1983; **Resid:** Surgery, Univ Louisville Med Ctr 1988; **Fellow:** Surgical Oncology, MD Anderson Cancer Ctr 1991; **Fac Appt:** Assoc Clin Prof S, Vanderbilt Univ

Willis, Irvin MD [S] - **Spec Exp:** Pancreatic Surgery; Cancer Surgery; Laparoscopic Surgery; **Hospital:** Mount Sinai Med Ctr - Miami; **Address:** 4302 Alton Rd, Ste 630, Miami Beach, FL 33140-2876; **Phone:** 305-534-6050; **Board Cert:** Surgery 1970; **Med School:** Univ Cincinnati 1964; **Resid:** Surgery, Univ Miami-Jackson Meml 1969

Surgery

Wood, William C MD [S] - **Spec Exp:** Breast Cancer; **Hospital:** Emory Univ Hosp; **Address:** Emory Univ Hosp, Dept Surgery, 1364 Clifton Rd NE, Ste B206, Atlanta, GA 30322; **Phone:** 404-727-5800; **Board Cert:** Surgery 1974; **Med School:** Harvard Med Sch 1966; **Resid:** Surgery, Mass Genl Hosp 1968; Surgery, Mass Genl Hosp 1974; **Fac Appt:** Prof S, Emory Univ

Yeatman, Timothy J MD [S] - **Spec Exp:** Liver Cancer; **Hospital:** H Lee Moffitt Cancer Ctr & Research Inst; **Address:** H Lee Moffitt Cancer Ctr, 12902 Magnolia Drive, Tampa, FL 33612-9497; **Phone:** 813-979-7292; **Board Cert:** Surgery 2000; **Med School:** Emory Univ 1984; **Resid:** Surgery, Univ Florida 1990; **Fellow:** Surgical Oncology, MD Anderson Cancer Ctr 1992; **Fac Appt:** Prof S, Univ S Fla Coll Med

Midwest

Angelos, Peter MD/PhD [S] - **Spec Exp:** Endocrine Tumors; Pheochromocytoma; Thyroid Disorders; Adrenal Tumors; **Hospital:** Univ of Chicago Hosps; **Address:** 5841 S Maryland Ave, MC 4052, Chicago, IL 60637; **Phone:** 773-702-4429; **Board Cert:** Surgery 2004; **Med School:** Boston Univ 1989; **Resid:** Surgery, Northwestern Univ 1995; **Fellow:** Medical Ethics, Univ of Chicago Hosps 1992; Endocrine Surgery, Univ of Michigan Med Sch 1996; **Fac Appt:** Prof S, Univ Chicago-Pritzker Sch Med

Aranha, Gerard MD [S] - **Spec Exp:** Pancreatic & Biliary Surgery; Stomach Cancer; Esophageal Cancer; **Hospital:** Loyola Univ Med Ctr, Hines VA Hosp; **Address:** Loyola Univ Med Ctr, Dept Surg, 2160 S First Ave Bldg 110 - rm 3236, Maywood, IL 60153-3328; **Phone:** 708-327-3430; **Board Cert:** Surgery 2006; **Med School:** India 1969; **Resid:** Surgery, Loyola Univ Med Ctr 1975; **Fellow:** Surgical Oncology, Univ Minn Hosp 1977; **Fac Appt:** Prof S, Loyola Univ-Stritch Sch Med

Averbook, Bruce J MD [S] - **Spec Exp:** Melanoma; Clinical Trials; **Hospital:** MetroHealth Med Ctr; **Address:** Metrohealth Medical Ctr, Surgical Oncology, 2500 Metrohealth Drive, rm C2110, Cleveland, OH 44109; **Phone:** 216-778-4795; **Board Cert:** Surgery 2000; **Med School:** Geo Wash Univ 1983; **Resid:** Surgery, UC Irvine Med Ctr 1990; **Fellow:** Surgical Oncology, NCI,NIH Surg Br 1993; **Fac Appt:** Assoc Prof S, Case West Res Univ

Benedetti, Enrico MD [S] - **Spec Exp:** Transplant-Liver; Transplant-Pancreas; Transplant-Kidney; Transplant-Bowel; **Hospital:** Univ of IL Med Ctr at Chicago, Adv Luth Genl Hosp; **Address:** Univ Illinois, Dept Surgery/Transplant, 840 S Wood St, rm 402, Chicago, IL 60612; **Phone:** 312-996-6771; **Board Cert:** Surgery 2003; **Med School:** Italy 1985; **Resid:** Surgery, Univ IL at Chicago Med Ctr 1993; **Fellow:** Transplant Surgery, Univ Minn Med Ctr 1994; **Fac Appt:** Prof S, Univ IL Coll Med

Blom, Dennis MD [S] - **Spec Exp:** Esophageal Cancer; Barrett's Esophagus; Esophageal Surgery; Gastroesophageal Reflux Disease (GERD); **Hospital:** Indiana Univ Hosp; **Address:** 545 Barnhill Drive, Emerson Hall Fl 5, Indianapolis, IN 46202; **Phone:** 317-278-7373; **Board Cert:** Surgery 2000; **Med School:** Albany Med Coll 1992; **Resid:** Surgery, Univ Rochester 1999; **Fellow:** Gastrointestinal Surgery, USC Univ Hosp 2001; **Fac Appt:** Assoc Prof S, Indiana Univ

Brems, John MD [S] - **Spec Exp:** Transplant-Liver; Pancreatic Cancer; Liver Cancer; **Hospital:** Loyola Univ Med Ctr; **Address:** 2160 S 1st Ave, MC-EMS-3268, Maywood, IL 60153-3328; **Phone:** 708-327-2539; **Board Cert:** Surgery 2004; Surgical Critical Care 2000; **Med School:** St Louis Univ 1981; **Resid:** Surgery, St Louis Univ 1986; **Fellow:** Transplant Surgery, UCLA Med Ctr 1987; **Fac Appt:** Prof S, Loyola Univ-Stritch Sch Med

Brunt, L Michael MD [S] - **Spec Exp:** Minimally Invasive Surgery; Adrenal Tumors; Hernia; **Hospital:** Barnes-Jewish Hosp; **Address:** Washington Univ Sch Medicine, Dept Surg, 660 S Euclid Ave, Box 8109, St Louis, MO 63110; **Phone:** 314-454-7194; **Board Cert:** Surgery 2006; **Med School:** Johns Hopkins Univ 1980; **Resid:** Surgery, Barnes Jewish Hosp 1987; **Fellow:** Surgery, Barnes Jewish Hosp 1984; **Fac Appt:** Prof S, Washington Univ, St Louis

Chang, Alfred E MD [S] - **Spec Exp:** Breast Cancer; Gastrointestinal Cancer; Melanoma; Sarcoma; **Hospital:** Univ Michigan Hlth Sys; **Address:** Univ Mich Comp Cancer Ctr, 1500 E Med Ctr Dr 3302 CGC, Ann Arbor, MI 48109-5932; **Phone:** 734-936-4392; **Board Cert:** Surgery 2001; **Med School:** Harvard Med Sch 1974; **Resid:** Surgery, Duke Univ Med Ctr 1976; Surgery, Hosp Univ Penn 1982; **Fellow:** Surgical Oncology, Natl Cancer Inst 1979; **Fac Appt:** Prof S, Univ Mich Med Sch

Chapman, William C MD [S] - **Spec Exp:** Transplant-Liver-Adult & Pediatric; Liver Cancer; Liver & Biliary Surgery; **Hospital:** Barnes-Jewish Hosp, St Louis Chldns Hosp; **Address:** Washington Univ Sch Med, 660 S Euclid Ave, Box 8604, St Louis, MO 63110; **Phone:** 314-362-7792; **Board Cert:** Surgery 2001; Surgical Critical Care 2001; **Med School:** Med Univ SC 1984; **Resid:** Surgery, Vanderbilt Univ Med Ctr 1991; **Fellow:** Hepatobiliary Surgery, Kings College Hosp 1992; **Fac Appt:** Prof S, Washington Univ, St Louis

Cronin II, David C MD/PhD [S] - **Spec Exp:** Transplant-Liver; Pediatric Transplant Surgery; Liver & Biliary Surgery; Pancreatic Surgery; **Hospital:** Froedtert Meml Lutheran Hosp; **Address:** Med Coll of Wisc, Div of Transplant Surg, 9200 W Wisconsin Ave, Ste 5700, Milwaukee, WI 53226; **Phone:** 414-955-6920; **Board Cert:** Surgery 2006; **Med School:** Mount Sinai Sch Med 1987; **Resid:** Surgery, Univ Chicago Hosps 1995; **Fellow:** Transplant Surgery, Univ Chicago Hosps 1997; Medical Ethics, Univ Chicago Hosps 2002; **Fac Appt:** Assoc Prof S, Univ Wisc

Crowe Jr, Joseph P MD [S] - **Spec Exp:** Breast Cancer; Tumor Surgery; **Hospital:** Cleveland Clin Fdn (page 56); **Address:** Cleveland Clinic Fdn, Dept Surg, 9500 Euclid Ave, Desk A10, Cleveland, OH 44195; **Phone:** 216-444-3024; **Board Cert:** Surgery 2004; **Med School:** Case West Res Univ 1978; **Resid:** Surgery, Univ Hosp-Case West Reserve 1983; **Fellow:** Surgical Oncology, Meml Sloan Kettering Cancer Ctr 1985

Deziel, Daniel J MD [S] - **Spec Exp:** Hepatobiliary Surgery; Pancreatic Surgery; Laparoscopic Surgery; **Hospital:** Rush Univ Med Ctr; **Address:** 1725 W Harrison, Ste 810, Chicago, IL 60612-3828; **Phone:** 312-942-6500; **Board Cert:** Surgery 2003; **Med School:** Univ Minn 1979; **Resid:** Surgery, Rush-Presby-St Luke's Med Ctr 1984; **Fellow:** Gastrointestinal Surgery, Lahey Clinic 1985; **Fac Appt:** Prof S, Rush Med Coll

Doherty, Gerard M MD [S] - **Spec Exp:** Endocrine Surgery; Adrenal Surgery; Laparoscopic Surgery; Thyroid Surgery; **Hospital:** Univ Michigan Hlth Sys; **Address:** A Taubman Hlth Care Center, 1500 E Medical Center Drive, rm 2920, Ann Arbor, MI 48109-5331; **Phone:** 734-615-4741; **Board Cert:** Surgery 2003; **Med School:** Yale Univ 1986; **Resid:** Surgery, UCSF Med Ctr 1993; **Fellow:** Medical Oncology, Natl Cancer Inst 1991; **Fac Appt:** Prof S, Univ Mich Med Sch

Donohue, John H MD [S] - **Spec Exp:** Gastrointestinal Cancer; Breast Cancer; Stomach Cancer; **Hospital:** Mayo Med Ctr & Clin - Rochester; **Address:** Mayo Clinic, Dept General Surgery, 200 First St SW, Rochester, MN 55905; **Phone:** 507-284-0362; **Board Cert:** Surgery 2005; **Med School:** Harvard Med Sch 1978; **Resid:** Surgery, UCSF Med Ctr 1981; Surgery, UCSF Med Ctr 1985; **Fellow:** Surgery, Natl Inst Hlth 1983; Surgical Oncology, Meml Sloan-Kettering Canc Ctr 1987; **Fac Appt:** Prof S, Mayo Med Sch

Eberlein, Timothy J MD [S] - **Spec Exp:** Breast Cancer; Melanoma; Immunotherapy; **Hospital:** Barnes-Jewish Hosp, St Louis Chldns Hosp; **Address:** Wash Univ School Med, Dept Surgery, 660 S Euclid Ave, Box 8109, St Louis, MO 63110-1093; **Phone:** 314-362-8020; **Board Cert:** Surgery 2006; **Med School:** Univ Pittsburgh 1977; **Resid:** Surgery, Peter Bent Brigham Hosp 1979; Surgery, Brigham-Womens Hosp 1985; **Fellow:** Allergy & Immunology, Natl Inst Hlth 1982; **Fac Appt:** Prof S, Washington Univ, St Louis

Edwards, Michael J MD [S] - **Spec Exp:** Breast Cancer; Melanoma; **Hospital:** Univ Hosp - Cincinnati; **Address:** 231 Albert Sabin Way, Box 670558, Cincinnati, OH 45267-0558; **Phone:** 513-558-4657; **Board Cert:** Surgery 1996; **Med School:** Emory Univ 1981; **Resid:** Surgery, Univ Louisville Hosp 1986; **Fellow:** Surgical Oncology, MD Anderson Cancer Ctr 1987; **Fac Appt:** Prof S, Univ Ark

Ellison, E Christopher MD [S] - **Spec Exp:** Biliary Surgery; Biliary Cancer; Pancreatic Cancer; **Hospital:** Ohio St Univ Med Ctr; **Address:** 1654 Upham Drive, Ste 327 Means Hall, Columbus, OH 43210-1236; **Phone:** 614-293-9722; **Board Cert:** Surgery 2001; **Med School:** Univ Wisc 1975; **Resid:** Surgery, Ohio State Univ 1981; **Fac Appt:** Prof S, Ohio State Univ

Farley, David R MD [S] - **Spec Exp:** Endocrine Surgery; Hepatobiliary Surgery; Laparoscopic Surgery; Hernia; **Hospital:** Mayo Med Ctr & Clin - Rochester; **Address:** Mayo Clinic, 200 First St SW, Mayo West 12, Rochester, MN 55905; **Phone:** 507-284-2644; **Board Cert:** Surgery 2002; **Med School:** Univ Wisc 1988; **Resid:** Surgery, Mayo Clinic 1994; **Fellow:** Endocrinology, Mayo Clinic 1995; **Fac Appt:** Assoc Prof S, Mayo Med Sch

Farrar, William B MD [S] - **Spec Exp:** Breast Cancer; Thyroid Cancer; **Hospital:** Arthur G James Cancer Hosp & Research Inst, Ohio St Univ Med Ctr; **Address:** 410 W 10th Ave, N924 Doan Hall, Columbus, OH 43210-1240; **Phone:** 614-293-8890; **Board Cert:** Surgery 2000; **Med School:** Univ VA Sch Med 1975; **Resid:** Surgery, Ohio State Univ Hosps 1980; **Fellow:** Surgical Oncology, Meml Sloan-Kettering Cancer Ctr 1982; **Fac Appt:** Prof S, Ohio State Univ

Ferguson, Ronald MD [S] - **Spec Exp:** Transplant-Kidney; **Hospital:** Ohio St Univ Med Ctr; **Address:** 1654 Upham Drive, Ste 363 Means, Columbus, OH 43210-1250; **Phone:** 614-293-6724; **Board Cert:** Surgery 2002; **Med School:** Washington Univ, St Louis 1971; **Resid:** Surgery, Univ Minn Hosp 1979; **Fellow:** Immunology, Univ Minn Hosp 1980; **Fac Appt:** Prof S, Ohio State Univ

Fung, John J MD/PhD [S] - **Spec Exp:** Transplant-Liver; Transplant-Kidney; Liver & Biliary Cancer; **Hospital:** Cleveland Clin Fdn (page 56); **Address:** Cleveland Clinic, Dept Surgery, 9500 Euclid Ave, Desk A80, Cleveland, OH 44195-0001; **Phone:** 216-444-3776; **Board Cert:** Surgery 1997; **Med School:** Univ Chicago-Pritzker Sch Med 1982; **Resid:** Surgery, Strong Memorial Hosp 1988; **Fellow:** Transplant Surgery, Univ Pittsburgh 1986; **Fac Appt:** Prof S, Cleveland Cl Coll Med/Case West Res

Gamelli, Richard L MD [S] - **Spec Exp:** Burn Care; Trauma/Critical Care; **Hospital:** Loyola Univ Med Ctr; **Address:** 2160 S First Ave EMS Bldg - rm 3244, Maywood, IL 60153; **Phone:** 708-216-8563; **Board Cert:** Surgery 1999; **Med School:** Univ VT Coll Med 1974; **Resid:** Surgery, Vermont Med Ctr Hosp 1979; **Fac Appt:** Prof S, Loyola Univ-Stritch Sch Med

Goulet Jr, Robert J MD [S] - **Spec Exp:** Breast Cancer; Breast Surgery; **Hospital:** Indiana Univ Hosp; **Address:** Indiana Cancer Pavilion, 535 Barnhill Drive, Ste 253, Indianapolis, IN 46202-5112; **Phone:** 317-274-9800; **Board Cert:** Surgery 2006; **Med School:** SUNY Downstate 1979; **Resid:** Surgery, SUNY-Downstate Med Ctr 1986; **Fellow:** Surgical Research, SUNY-Downstate Med Ctr 1983; **Fac Appt:** Assoc Prof S, Indiana Univ

Grant, Clive S MD [S] - **Spec Exp:** Thyroid & Parathyroid Cancer & Surgery; Adrenal Tumors; Breast Cancer; **Hospital:** Mayo Med Ctr & Clin - Rochester; **Address:** Mayo Clinic, Dept Surgery, 200 First St SW, Rochester, MN 55905-0001; **Phone:** 507-284-2644; **Board Cert:** Surgery 2001; **Med School:** Univ Colorado 1975; **Resid:** Surgery, Mayo Clinic 1980; **Fac Appt:** Prof S, Mayo Med Sch

Gruber, Scott A MD/PhD [S] - **Spec Exp:** Transplant-Kidney; Transplant-Pancreas; **Hospital:** Harper Univ Hosp, Chldns Hosp of Michigan; **Address:** Harper Professional Bldg, 4160 John R, Ste 400, Detroit, MI 48201; **Phone:** 313-745-7319; **Board Cert:** Surgery 2001; **Med School:** SUNY Downstate 1983; **Resid:** Surgery, Univ Minnesota Med Ctr 1986; **Fellow:** Surgery, Univ Minnesota Med Ctr 1989; Transplant Surgery, Univ Minnesota Med Ctr 1993; **Fac Appt:** Prof S, Wayne State Univ

Hansen, Nora M MD [S] - **Spec Exp:** Sentinel Node Surgery; Breast Cancer-High Risk Women; Breast Cancer Risk Assessment; **Hospital:** Northwestern Meml Hosp; **Address:** Lynn Sage Breast Surgery Ctr, 250 E Superior St Fl 4 - Ste 420, Chicago, IL 60611; **Phone:** 312-472-4720; **Board Cert:** Surgery 2006; **Med School:** NY Med Coll 1988; **Resid:** Surgery, Univ Chicago Hosps 1995; **Fellow:** Surgical Oncology, Univ Chicago Hosps 1996; **Fac Appt:** Assoc Prof S, Northwestern Univ

Harkema, James M MD [S] - **Spec Exp:** Breast Cancer; Thyroid Cancer; Parathyroid Cancer; **Hospital:** Mich State Univ-Sparrow Hos, Ingham Regl Med Ctr- Greenlawn Campus; **Address:** Sparrow Professional Bldg, 1200 E Michigan Ave, Ste 655, Lansing, MI 48912; **Phone:** 517-267-2461; **Board Cert:** Surgery 1975; **Med School:** Univ Mich Med Sch 1968; **Resid:** Surgery, Univ Mich Hosp 1974; **Fac Appt:** Prof S, Mich State Univ

Hinshaw, Daniel B MD [S] - **Spec Exp:** Palliative Care; **Hospital:** VA Med Ctr - Ann Arbor, Univ Michigan Hlth Sys; **Address:** VA Medical Ctr, 2215 Fuller Rd, rm 530, MS 112, Ann Arbor, MI 48105; **Phone:** 734-769-7100 x5939; **Board Cert:** Surgery 2003; **Med School:** Loma Linda Univ 1978; **Resid:** Surgery, Loma Linda U Med Ctr 1983; **Fellow:** Immunology, Scripps Clinic Rsch Fdn 1985; Cleveland Clinic 2001; **Fac Appt:** Clin Prof S, Univ Mich Med Sch

Howe, James MD [S] - **Spec Exp:** Endocrine Surgery; Gastrointestinal Cancer; Colon & Rectal Cancer; **Hospital:** Univ Iowa Hosp & Clinics; **Address:** Univ Iowa, Dept Surgery, 200 Hawkins Drive, 1504 John Colloton Pavilion, Iowa City, IA 52242-1086; **Phone:** 319-356-1727; **Board Cert:** Surgery 2006; **Med School:** Univ VT Coll Med 1987; **Resid:** Surgery, Barnes Hosp-Wash Univ 1994; **Fellow:** Research, Wash Univ-NCI 1991; Surgical Oncology, Meml Sloan Kettering Cancer Ctr 1996; **Fac Appt:** Prof S, Univ Iowa Coll Med

Kagan, Richard J MD [S] - **Spec Exp:** Burn Care; **Hospital:** Cincinnati Shriners Hosp, Univ Hosp - Cincinnati; **Address:** Cincinnati Shriners Hosp, 3229 Burnet Ave, Cincinnati, OH 45229; **Phone:** 513-872-6210; **Board Cert:** Surgery 2007; **Med School:** St Louis Univ 1974; **Resid:** Surgery, Univ IL Hosp 1980; **Fac Appt:** Prof S, Univ Cincinnati

Kim, Julian A MD [S] - **Spec Exp:** Melanoma; Breast Cancer; Gastrointestinal Cancer; Immunotherapy; **Hospital:** Univ Hosps Case Med Ctr; **Address:** Univ Hosps of Cleveland, LKS 5047, 11100 Euclid Ave, Cleveland, OH 44106-1716; **Phone:** 216-844-8247; **Board Cert:** Surgery 2002; **Med School:** Med Univ Ohio at Toledo 1986; **Resid:** Surgery, Univ Maryland Hosps 1991; **Fellow:** Surgical Oncology, Arthur James Cancer Hosp & Rsch Inst 1993; Immunotherapy, Ohio State Univ Comp Cancer Ctr 1994; **Fac Appt:** Assoc Prof S, Case West Res Univ

Kraybill Jr, William G MD [S] - **Spec Exp:** Sarcoma-Soft Tissue; Melanoma; Skin Cancer-Advanced; **Hospital:** St Luke's Hosp of Kansas City; **Address:** St Luke's Hosp, 4401 Wornall Rd, Ste 420, Kansas City, MO 64111; **Phone:** 816-932-5602; **Board Cert:** Surgery 2005; **Med School:** Univ Cincinnati 1969; **Resid:** Surgery, Univ Oregon Hlth Sci Ctr 1978; **Fellow:** Surgical Oncology, Meml Sloan Kettering Cancer Ctr 1980; **Fac Appt:** Prof S, Univ MO-Kansas City

Lillemoe, Keith D MD [S] - **Spec Exp:** Pancreatic Cancer; Colon Cancer; Pancreatic & Biliary Surgery; **Hospital:** Indiana Univ Hosp; **Address:** Indiana Univ, Dept Surgery, 545 Barnhill Drive, EH 203, Indianapolis, IN 46202-5112; **Phone:** 317-274-5707; **Board Cert:** Surgery 1995; **Med School:** Johns Hopkins Univ 1978; **Resid:** Surgery, Johns Hopkins Hosp 1985; **Fac Appt:** Prof S, Indiana Univ

Mamounas, Eleftherios P MD [S] - **Spec Exp:** Breast Cancer; **Hospital:** Aultman Hosp; **Address:** Aultman Cancer Ctr, 2600 6th St SW, Main 1, Clinical Trials Dept, Canton, OH 44710; **Phone:** 330-363-6281; **Board Cert:** Surgery 1999; **Med School:** Greece 1983; **Resid:** Surgery, McKeesport Hosp 1989; **Fellow:** Clinical Oncology, Univ Pittsburgh 1991; Surgical Oncology, Roswell Park Cancer Inst 1992; **Fac Appt:** Asst Clin Prof S, Case West Res Univ

Matas, Arthur J MD [S] - **Spec Exp:** Transplant-Kidney; **Hospital:** Univ Minn Med Ctr, Fairview - Univ Campus; **Address:** Dept Surgery, 420 Delaware St SE, MMC 328, Minneapolis, MN 55455; **Phone:** 612-625-6460; **Board Cert:** Surgery 2000; **Med School:** Univ Manitoba 1972; **Resid:** Surgery, Univ Minnesota Hosps 1979; **Fellow:** Transplant Surgery, Univ Minnesota Hosps 1980; **Fac Appt:** Prof S, Univ Minn

McHenry, Christopher R MD [S] - **Spec Exp:** Adrenal Surgery; Thyroid Surgery; Parathyroid Surgery; **Hospital:** MetroHealth Med Ctr; **Address:** MetroHealth Medical Ctr, Dept Surgery, 2500 Metro Health Drive, H917, Cleveland, OH 44109-1998; **Phone:** 216-778-4753; **Board Cert:** Surgery 1997; **Med School:** NE Ohio Univ 1984; **Resid:** Surgery, Loyola Univ Med Ctr 1989; **Fellow:** Endocrinology, Univ Toronto Med Ctr 1990; Head and Neck Surgery, Univ Toronto Med Ctr 1990; **Fac Appt:** Prof S, Case West Res Univ

Melvin, W Scott MD [S] - **Spec Exp:** Liver & Biliary Surgery; Pancreatic Cancer; Laparoscopic Surgery; **Hospital:** Ohio St Univ Med Ctr; **Address:** 410 W 10th Ave, Ste N729 Doan, Columbus, OH 43210; **Phone:** 614-293-4499; **Board Cert:** Surgery 2002; **Med School:** Med Coll OH 1987; **Resid:** Surgery, Univ Maryland 1992; **Fellow:** Gastrointestinal Surgery, Grant Med Ctr 1993; **Fac Appt:** Prof S, Ohio State Univ

Merrick III, Hollis W MD [S] - **Spec Exp:** Cancer Surgery; **Hospital:** Univ of Toledo Med Ctr; **Address:** 3065 Arlington Ave, Toledo, OH 43614-2570; **Phone:** 419-383-4421; **Board Cert:** Surgery 1997; **Med School:** McGill Univ 1964; **Resid:** Surgery, Royal Victoria Hosp 1972; **Fac Appt:** Prof S, Med Coll OH

Millis, J Michael MD [S] - **Spec Exp:** Transplant-Liver-Adult & Pediatric; Liver Cancer; Transplant-Pancreas; **Hospital:** Univ of Chicago Hosps; **Address:** Univ Chicago, Dept Surgery, 5841 S Maryland Ave, MC 5027, Chicago, IL 60637; **Phone:** 773-702-6319; **Board Cert:** Surgery 2001; Surgical Critical Care 2001; **Med School:** Univ Tenn Coll Med, Memphis 1985; **Resid:** Surgery, UCLA Med Ctr 1992; **Fellow:** Transplant Surgery, UCLA Med Ctr 1994; **Fac Appt:** Prof S, Univ Chicago-Pritzker Sch Med

Moley, Jeffrey F MD [S] - **Spec Exp:** Thyroid Cancer & Surgery; Endocrine Cancers; Melanoma; **Hospital:** Barnes-Jewish Hosp; **Address:** Washington Univ School Med, Dept Surgery, 660 S Euclid Ave, Box 8109, St Louis, MO 63110; **Phone:** 314-362-2280; **Board Cert:** Surgery 2005; **Med School:** Columbia P&S 1980; **Resid:** Surgery, Yale-New Haven Hosp 1985; **Fellow:** Surgical Oncology, National Cancer Inst 1987; **Fac Appt:** Prof S, Washington Univ, St Louis

Nagorney, David M MD [S] - **Spec Exp:** Pancreatic Cancer; Hepatobiliary Surgery; Gastrointestinal Cancer; **Hospital:** Mayo Med Ctr & Clin - Rochester; **Address:** Mayo Clinic, Dept Surgery, 200 1st St SW, Mayo E12, Rochester, MN 55905; **Phone:** 507-284-2644; **Board Cert:** Surgery 2001; **Med School:** Univ Kans 1975; **Resid:** Surgery, Mayo Clinic 1982; **Fellow:** Hepatobiliary Surgery, Hammersmith Hosp 1985; **Fac Appt:** Prof S, Mayo Med Sch

Nathanson, S David MD [S] - **Spec Exp:** Breast Cancer; Breast Cancer Risk Assessment; Melanoma; Sarcoma; **Hospital:** Henry Ford Hosp; **Address:** 2799 W Grand Blvd, Detroit, MI 48202; **Phone:** 313-916-2917; **Board Cert:** Surgery 2002; **Med School:** South Africa 1966; **Resid:** Surgery, Univ Witwaterstrand 1974; Surgical Oncology, UCLA Med Ctr 1980; **Fellow:** Surgery, UC Davis 1982; **Fac Appt:** Prof S, Case West Res Univ

Newman, Lisa A MD [S] - **Spec Exp:** Breast Cancer; **Hospital:** Univ Michigan Hlth Sys; **Address:** Univ Michigan Cancer Center, 1500 E Medical Center Drive, rm 3308-CGC, Ann Arbor, MI 48109; **Phone:** 734-936-8771; **Board Cert:** Surgery 2001; **Med School:** SUNY Downstate 1985; **Resid:** Surgery, Downstate Med Ctr 1990; **Fac Appt:** Assoc Prof S, Univ Mich Med Sch

Onders, Raymond P MD [S] - **Spec Exp:** Laparoscopic Surgery; Diaphragm Pacing via Laparoscopy; Gastrointestinal Cancer; **Hospital:** Univ Hosps Case Med Ctr; **Address:** University Hosps Cleveland, 11100 Euclid Ave, LKS 5047, Cleveland, OH 44106; **Phone:** 216-844-5797; **Board Cert:** Surgery 2001; **Med School:** NE Ohio Univ 1988; **Resid:** Surgery, Case Western Reserve Univ 1993; **Fac Appt:** Asst Prof S, Case West Res Univ

Ponsky, Jeffrey L MD [S] - **Spec Exp:** Minimally Invasive Surgery; Gastrointestinal Surgery; Endoscopy; **Hospital:** Univ Hosps Case Med Ctr; **Address:** Univ Hosps Cleveland, Dept Surgery, 11100 Euclid Ave, Cleveland, OH 44106; **Phone:** 216-844-3209; **Board Cert:** Surgery 2007; **Med School:** Case West Res Univ 1971; **Resid:** Surgery, Univ Hosps 1976; **Fac Appt:** Prof S, Case West Res Univ

Posner, Mitchell C MD [S] - **Spec Exp:** Pancreatic Cancer; Gastrointestinal Cancer; Esophageal Cancer; **Hospital:** Univ of Chicago Hosps; **Address:** Univ of Chicago Hospitals, 5841 S Maryland Ave, Ste G209, MC 5094, Chicago, IL 60637-1447; **Phone:** 773-834-0156; **Board Cert:** Surgery 2006; **Med School:** SUNY Buffalo 1981; **Resid:** Surgery, Univ Colorado Sch Med 1986; **Fellow:** Surgical Oncology, Meml Sloan Kettering Cancer Ctr 1988; **Fac Appt:** Prof S, Univ Chicago-Pritzker Sch Med

Prinz, Richard A MD [S] - **Spec Exp:** Adrenal Surgery; Thyroid & Parathyroid Surgery; Pancreatic & Biliary Surgery; **Hospital:** Rush Univ Med Ctr, Rush Oak Park Hosp; **Address:** 1725 W Harrison, Ste 818, Chicago, IL 60612-3841; **Phone:** 312-942-6511; **Board Cert:** Surgery 1994; **Med School:** Loyola Univ-Stritch Sch Med 1972; **Resid:** Surgery, Barnes Hosp 1974; Surgery, Loyola Univ Hosp 1977; **Fellow:** Endocrinology, Diabetes & Metabolism, Hammersmith Hosp 1980; **Fac Appt:** Prof S, Rush Med Coll

Rikkers, Layton F MD [S] - **Spec Exp:** Liver & Biliary Surgery; Pancreatic Cancer; Liver & Biliary Cancer; **Hospital:** Univ WI Hosp & Clins; **Address:** 600 Highland Ave, rm H4-710D, Madison, WI 53792; **Phone:** 608-265-8854; **Board Cert:** Surgery 1996; **Med School:** Stanford Univ 1970; **Resid:** Surgery, Univ Utah Hosp 1973; Surgery, Univ Utah Hosp 1976; **Fellow:** Hepatology, Royal Free Hosp 1974; **Fac Appt:** Prof S, Univ Wisc

Rosen, Charles B MD [S] - **Spec Exp:** Transplant-Liver; Transplant-Bile Duct; **Hospital:** Mayo Med Ctr & Clin - Rochester; **Address:** Dept Surg-Div Transplantation, 200 First St SW, Charlton 10A, Rochester, MN 55905-0001; **Phone:** 507-266-6640; **Board Cert:** Surgery 1999; **Med School:** Mayo Med Sch 1984; **Resid:** Surgery, Mayo Clinic 1989; **Fellow:** Transplant Surgery, Mayo Clinic 1991; **Fac Appt:** Assoc Prof S, Mayo Med Sch

Saha, Sukamal MD [S] - **Spec Exp:** Sentinel Node Surgery; Colon Cancer; Head & Neck Cancer & Surgery; **Hospital:** McLaren Reg Med Ctr, Genesys Reg Med Ctr - St Joseph Campus; **Address:** 3500 Calkins Rd, Ste A, Flint, MI 48532; **Phone:** 810-230-9600 x500; **Board Cert:** Surgery 2000; **Med School:** India 1977; **Resid:** Surgery, Hahnemann Univ Hosp 1985; Surgery, Easton Hosp 1987; **Fellow:** Surgical Oncology, Tulane Univ Med Ctr 1989; Head and Neck Surgery, Roswell Park Meml Hosp; **Fac Appt:** Asst Prof S, Mich State Univ

Surgery

Sarr, Michael G MD [S] - **Spec Exp:** Pancreatic Cancer; Gastrointestinal Cancer; Obesity/Bariatric Surgery; Gastrointestinal Motility Disorders; **Hospital:** Mayo Med Ctr & Clin - Rochester; **Address:** Mayo Clinic, Dept Surg, Desk West 6, Rochester, MN 55905; **Phone:** 507-284-2644; **Board Cert:** Surgery 2001; **Med School:** Johns Hopkins Univ 1976; **Resid:** Surgery, Johns Hopkins Hosp 1982; **Fellow:** Surgery, Mayo Clinic 1984; Surgery, Johns Hopkins Hosp 1985; **Fac Appt:** Prof S, Mayo Med Sch

Schulak, James A MD [S] - **Spec Exp:** Transplant-Kidney-Adult & Pediatric; Transplant-Pancreas & Liver; Pancreatic Surgery; **Hospital:** Univ Hosps Case Med Ctr; **Address:** Univ Hosps of Cleveland, Dept Surgery, 11100 Euclid Ave, MS 5047, Cleveland, OH 44106-5407; **Phone:** 216-844-0307; **Board Cert:** Surgery 2000; **Med School:** Univ Chicago-Pritzker Sch Med 1974; **Resid:** Surgery, Univ Chicago Hosp 1980; **Fellow:** Transplant Surgery, Univ Chicago Hosp 1981; **Fac Appt:** Prof S, Case West Res Univ

Schwartzentruber, Douglas J MD [S] - **Spec Exp:** Cancer Surgery; Melanoma; Kidney Cancer; **Hospital:** Goshen Genl Hosp; **Address:** Cancer Ctr at Goshen Health System, 200 High Park Ave, Goshen, IN 46526; **Phone:** 574-535-2888; **Board Cert:** Surgery 1997; **Med School:** Indiana Univ 1982; **Resid:** Surgery, Indiana Univ Med Ctr 1987; **Fellow:** Surgical Oncology, Natl Cancer Inst 1990; **Fac Appt:** Assoc Clin Prof S, Indiana Univ

Scott-Conner, Carol E H MD/PhD [S] - **Spec Exp:** Breast Cancer; Cancer Surgery; Laparoscopic Surgery; **Hospital:** Univ Iowa Hosp & Clinics, VA Med Ctr - Iowa City; **Address:** Univ Iowa, Dept Surg, 200 Hawkins Drive, rm 4601-JCP, Iowa City, IA 52242-1086; **Phone:** 319-356-0330; **Board Cert:** Surgery 2000; Surgical Critical Care 1998; **Med School:** NYU Sch Med 1976; **Resid:** Surgery, NYU Med Ctr 1981; **Fac Appt:** Prof S, Univ Iowa Coll Med

Sener, Stephen MD [S] - **Spec Exp:** Breast Cancer; Pancreatic Cancer; Lymphedema; Gastrointestinal Cancer & Surgery; **Hospital:** Evanston Hosp; **Address:** Evanston Hospital, Dept Surgery, 2650 Ridge Ave, rm 2507, Evanston, IL 60201-1718; **Phone:** 847-570-1328; **Board Cert:** Surgery 2001; **Med School:** Northwestern Univ 1977; **Resid:** Surgery, Northwestern Univ 1982; **Fellow:** Surgery, Meml Sloan Kettering Cancer Ctr 1984; **Fac Appt:** Prof S, Northwestern Univ

Shenk, Robert R MD [S] - **Spec Exp:** Breast Cancer; Melanoma; Pancreatic Cancer; Stomach Cancer; **Hospital:** Univ Hosps Case Med Ctr; **Address:** Univ Hosp Case Med Ctr, 11100 Euclid Ave, Dept General Surgery, Cleveland, OH 44106; **Phone:** 216-844-3026; **Board Cert:** Surgery 2004; **Med School:** Case West Res Univ 1978; **Resid:** Surgery, Univ Hosp 1985; Immunology, Natl Cancer Inst 1982; **Fellow:** Surgical Oncology, Anderson Hosp 1987; **Fac Appt:** Assoc Prof S, Case West Res Univ

Sielaff, Timothy D MD/PhD [S] - **Spec Exp:** Liver Cancer; Pancreatic Cancer; Gallbladder & Biliary Cancer; **Hospital:** Abbott - Northwestern Hosp; **Address:** Virginia Piper Cancer Inst, Liver and Pancreas Clinic, 800 E 28th St, Minneapolis, MN 55407; **Phone:** 612-863-7553; **Board Cert:** Surgery 1998; **Med School:** Med Coll VA 1989; **Resid:** Surgery, Univ Minn Hosps 1997; **Fellow:** Transplant Surgery, Univ Toronto 1998; **Fac Appt:** Assoc Prof S, Univ Minn

Simeone, Diane M MD [S] - **Spec Exp:** Pancreatic Cancer; Cancer Surgery; **Hospital:** Univ Michigan Hlth Sys; **Address:** Univ Michigan Health Systems, 1500 E Medical Center Drive, 2922D Taubman Center SPC 5331, Ann Arbor, MI 48109-5331; **Phone:** 734-936-5738; **Board Cert:** Surgery 2005; **Med School:** Duke Univ 1988; **Resid:** Surgery, Univ Mich 1995; **Fac Appt:** Prof S, Univ Mich Med Sch

Siperstein, Allan E MD [S] - **Spec Exp:** Laparoscopic Surgery; Endocrine Tumors; Thyroid & Parathyroid Cancer & Surgery; **Hospital:** Cleveland Clin Fdn (page 56); **Address:** Cleveland Clinic Fdn, Dept Genl Surg, 9500 Euclid Ave, Desk A80, Cleveland, OH 44195; **Phone:** 216-444-5664; **Board Cert:** Surgery 1997; **Med School:** Univ Tex SW, Dallas 1983; **Resid:** Surgery, UCSF Med Ctr 1990; **Fellow:** Research, UCSF Med Ctr 1988

Sollinger, Hans W MD/PhD [S] - **Spec Exp:** Transplant-Kidney; Transplant-Pancreas; **Hospital:** Univ WI Hosp & Clins; **Address:** 600 Highland Ave, rm H5-701, Madison, WI 53792; **Phone:** 608-262-8360; **Board Cert:** Surgery 1996; **Med School:** Germany 1974; **Resid:** Surgery, Univ Wisc Hosp 1980; **Fellow:** Immunological Biology, Univ Wisc Hosp 1977; **Fac Appt:** Prof S, Univ Wisc

Soper, Nathaniel MD [S] - **Spec Exp:** Laparoscopic Surgery; Gastroesophageal Reflux Disease (GERD); Biliary Surgery; **Hospital:** Northwestern Meml Hosp; **Address:** Northwestern Meml Hosp, Dept Surg, 251 E Huron St Galter Bldg - rm 3-150, Chicago, IL 60611; **Phone:** 312-926-4962; **Board Cert:** Surgery 2005; **Med School:** Univ Iowa Coll Med 1980; **Resid:** Surgery, Univ Utah Hosps 1986; **Fellow:** Digestive Dis, Mayo Clinic 1988; **Fac Appt:** Prof S, Northwestern Univ

Stahl, Donna L MD [S] - **Spec Exp:** Breast Cancer; Breast Surgery; **Hospital:** Good Samaritan Hosp - Cincinnati, Jewish Hosp - Kenwood - Cincinnati; **Address:** Donna Stahl & Assocs, 4850 Red Bank Expwy Fl 3, Cincinnati, OH 45227; **Phone:** 513-221-2544; **Board Cert:** Surgery 2000; **Med School:** Univ Iowa Coll Med 1971; **Resid:** Surgery, Univ Cincinnati Hosps 1978

Staren, Edgar MD/PhD [S] - **Spec Exp:** Breast Cancer; Endocrine Cancers; Liver Cancer; **Hospital:** Cancer Treatment Ctrs of Amer-Midwest Reg Med Ctr; **Address:** Cancer Treatment Centers of America, 2610 Sheridan Rd, Zion, IL 60099; **Phone:** 847-731-5805; **Board Cert:** Surgery 2006; **Med School:** Loyola Univ-Stritch Sch Med 1982; **Resid:** Surgery, Rush-Presby-St Lukes Med Ctr 1987; **Fellow:** Surgical Oncology, Rush-Presby-St Lukes Med Ctr 1988

Sutherland, David E MD/PhD [S] - **Spec Exp:** Transplant-Pancreas; Transplant-Kidney; Immunotherapy; **Hospital:** Univ Minn Med Ctr, Fairview - Univ Campus; **Address:** 420 Delaware St SE, MMC 280, Minneapolis, MN 55455-0341; **Phone:** 612-625-7600; **Board Cert:** Surgery 2007; **Med School:** Univ Minn 1966; **Resid:** Surgery, West Virginia Univ Hosp 1968; **Fellow:** Transplant Surgery, Univ Minn Hosps 1975; **Fac Appt:** Prof S, Univ Minn

Talamonti, Mark S MD [S] - **Spec Exp:** Pancreatic Cancer; Liver Cancer; Gastrointestinal Cancer & Surgery; Melanoma; **Hospital:** Evanston Hosp; **Address:** Evanston Hosp Hosp, 2560 Ridge Ave, Evanston, IL 60201; **Phone:** 847-570-1700; **Board Cert:** Surgery 1999; **Med School:** Northwestern Univ 1983; **Resid:** Surgery, Northwestern Meml Hosp 1989; **Fellow:** Surgical Oncology, MD Anderson Cancer Ctr 1991; **Fac Appt:** Assoc Prof S, Northwestern Univ

Thistlethwaite, J Richard MD/PhD [S] - **Spec Exp:** Transplant-Kidney; Transplant-Pancreas; Transplant-Liver; Pediatric Transplant Surgery; **Hospital:** Univ of Chicago Hosps; **Address:** 5841 S Maryland Ave, rm J-517, MC 5026, Chicago, IL 60637; **Phone:** 773-834-3537; **Board Cert:** Surgery 1996; **Med School:** Duke Univ 1977; **Resid:** Surgery, Mass Genl Hosp 1983; **Fellow:** Surgical Oncology, Natl Inst Hlth 1981; Transplant Surgery, Mass Genl Hosp 1984; **Fac Appt:** Prof S, Univ Chicago-Pritzker Sch Med

Tuttle, Todd M MD [S] - **Spec Exp:** Breast Cancer; Minimally Invasive Surgery; Cancer Surgery; **Hospital:** Univ Minn Med Ctr, Fairview - Univ Campus, Univ Minn Med Ctr, Fairview - Riverside Campus; **Address:** Univ Minn, Dept Surgery, 420 Delaware St SE, MMC 195, Minneapolis, MN 55455; **Phone:** 612-625-2991; **Board Cert:** Surgery 2004; **Med School:** Johns Hopkins Univ 1988; **Resid:** Surgery, Med Coll Virginia Hosps 1994; **Fellow:** Surgical Oncology, MD Anderson Cancer Ctr 1996; **Fac Appt:** Assoc Prof S

Vickers, Selwyn M MD [S] - **Spec Exp:** Pancreatic Cancer; Liver Tumors; Gastrointestinal Surgery; **Hospital:** Univ Minn Med Ctr, Fairview - Univ Campus; **Address:** University of Minnesota, 420 Delaware St SE, Phillips Wangensteen Bldg, MMC 88, Minneapolis, MN 55455; **Phone:** 612-625-5411; **Board Cert:** Surgery 2003; **Med School:** Johns Hopkins Univ 1986; **Resid:** Surgery, Johns Hopkins Hosp 1992; **Fac Appt:** Prof S, Johns Hopkins Univ

Wakefield, Thomas MD [S] - **Spec Exp:** Thrombotic Disorders; Bleeding/Coagulation Disorders; Pulmonary Embolism; **Hospital:** Univ Michigan Hlth Sys, VA Med Ctr - Ann Arbor; **Address:** Univ Mich, Dept Surg, Div Vasc Surg, 1500 E Medical Ctr Drive, CVC5179 SPC5867, Ann Arbor, MI 48109; **Phone:** 734-936-5820; **Board Cert:** Surgery 2002; Vascular Surgery 2005; Surgical Critical Care 2000; **Med School:** Med Coll OH 1978; **Resid:** Surgery, Univ Mich Med Ctr 1984; **Fellow:** Peripheral Vascular Surgery, Univ Mich Med Ctr 1986; **Fac Appt:** Prof S, Univ Mich Med Sch

Walker, Alonzo P MD [S] - **Spec Exp:** Breast Cancer; **Hospital:** Froedtert Meml Lutheran Hosp; **Address:** Dept Surgery, 9200 W Wisconsin Ave, Milwaukee, WI 53226-3522; **Phone:** 414-805-5737; **Board Cert:** Surgery 2004; **Med School:** Univ Fla Coll Med 1976; **Resid:** Surgery, Univ Maryland Hosps 1983; **Fac Appt:** Prof S, Med Coll Wisc

Walsh, R Matthew MD [S] - **Spec Exp:** Pancreatic Cancer; Gastrointestinal Surgery; Hepatobiliary Surgery; **Hospital:** Cleveland Clin Fdn (page 56); **Address:** Cleveland Clinic, Dept Surgery, Desk A80, 9500 Euclid Ave, Cleveland, OH 44195; **Phone:** 216-445-7576; **Board Cert:** Surgery 1999; **Med School:** Med Coll Wisc 1985; **Resid:** Surgery, Loyola Univ Hosp 1990; **Fellow:** Endoscopy, Mass General Hosp 1991; Hepatopancreatobiliary Surgery, Cleveland Clinic; **Fac Appt:** Assoc Prof S, Cleveland Cl Coll Med/Case West Res

Weigel, Ronald J MD/PhD [S] - **Spec Exp:** Breast Cancer; Endocrine Surgery; **Hospital:** Univ Iowa Hosp & Clinics; **Address:** Univ Iowa Carver Coll Med-Dept Surgery, 200 Hawkins Drive, 1516 JCP, Iowa City, IA 52242-1086; **Phone:** 319-356-4200; **Board Cert:** Surgery 2001; **Med School:** Yale Univ 1986; **Resid:** Surgery, Duke Univ Med Ctr 1992; **Fellow:** Immunology, Duke Univ Med Ctr; **Fac Appt:** Prof S, Univ Iowa Coll Med

Witt, Thomas MD [S] - **Spec Exp:** Breast Cancer; Breast Disease; **Hospital:** Rush Univ Med Ctr, Glenbrook Hosp; **Address:** 1725 W Harrison St, Ste 409, Chicago, IL 60612-3828; **Phone:** 312-942-2302; **Board Cert:** Surgery 2000; **Med School:** Northwestern Univ 1975; **Resid:** Surgery, Rush Presby-St Lukes Med Ctr 1980; **Fellow:** Surgical Oncology, Meml Sloan Kettering Cancer Ctr 1982; **Fac Appt:** Assoc Prof S, Rush Med Coll

Great Plains and Mountains

Edney, James A MD [S] - **Spec Exp:** Breast Cancer; Thyroid & Parathyroid Cancer & Surgery; Cancer Surgery; **Hospital:** Nebraska Med Ctr; **Address:** Univ Nebraska Med Ctr, Dept Surgery, 984030 Nebraska Medical Ctr, Omaha, NE 68198-4030; **Phone:** 402-559-7272; **Board Cert:** Surgery 2000; **Med School:** Univ Nebr Coll Med 1975; **Resid:** Surgery, Univ Nebraska Med Ctr 1980; **Fellow:** Surgical Oncology, Univ Colorado Med Ctr 1981; **Fac Appt:** Prof S, Univ Nebr Coll Med

Fitzgibbons Jr, Robert J MD [S] - **Spec Exp:** Hernia; Minimally Invasive Surgery; Gastrointestinal Surgery; **Hospital:** Creighton Univ Med Ctr, Archbishop Bergan Mercy Med Ctr; **Address:** Creighton Univ, Dept Surgery, 601 N 30th St, Ste 3700, Omaha, NE 68131-2100; **Phone:** 402-280-4503; **Board Cert:** Surgery 2002; **Med School:** Creighton Univ 1974; **Resid:** Surgery, Charity Hosp/LA State Univ 1979; **Fellow:** Surgery, Lahey Clinic 1980; **Fac Appt:** Prof S, Creighton Univ

McIntyre Jr, Robert C MD [S] - **Spec Exp:** Endocrine Surgery; Trauma; Critical Care; **Hospital:** Univ Colorado Hosp, Chldn's Hosp - Aurora, The; **Address:** Univ Colorado at Denver & Hlth Sci Ctr, 12631 E 17th Ave, PO Box 6511, MS C313, Aurora, CO 80045; **Phone:** 303-724-2724; **Board Cert:** Surgery 2002; Surgical Critical Care 2003; **Med School:** Tulane Univ 1987; **Resid:** Surgery, Univ Colorado 1992; **Fac Appt:** Assoc Prof S, Univ Colorado

Moore, Ernest E MD [S] - **Spec Exp:** Liver Trauma; Aortic Injuries; **Hospital:** Denver Health Med Ctr, Vail Valley Med Ctr; **Address:** Denver Hlth Med Ctr, 777 Bannock St, MC 0206, Denver, CO 80204-4597; **Phone:** 303-436-6558; **Board Cert:** Surgery 2006; Surgical Critical Care 2006; **Med School:** Univ Pittsburgh 1972; **Resid:** Surgery, Univ Vt Med Ctr 1976; **Fac Appt:** Prof S, Univ Colorado

Mulvihill, Sean J MD [S] - **Spec Exp:** Gastrointestinal Surgery; Liver & Biliary Cancer; Pancreatic Cancer; **Hospital:** Univ Utah Hosps and Clins; **Address:** Univ Utah, Dept Surgery, 30 N 1900 E, rm 3B110, Salt Lake City, UT 84132; **Phone:** 801-581-7304; **Board Cert:** Surgery 1999; **Med School:** USC Sch Med 1981; **Resid:** Surgery, UCLA Med Ctr 1987; **Fac Appt:** Prof S, Univ Utah

Nelson, Edward W MD [S] - **Spec Exp:** Breast Cancer; **Hospital:** Univ Utah Hosps and Clins; **Address:** University Utah Medical Ctr, Div Genl Surgery, 30 N 1900 E, Salt Lake City, UT 84132; **Phone:** 801-581-7738; **Board Cert:** Surgery 1999; **Med School:** Univ Utah 1974; **Resid:** Surgery, Univ Utah Medical Ctr 1979; **Fac Appt:** Prof S, Univ Utah

Pearlman, Nathan W MD [S] - **Spec Exp:** Gastrointestinal Cancer; Melanoma; Head & Neck Cancer; **Hospital:** Univ Colorado Hosp; **Address:** 12631 E 17th Ave L-15 Bldg - rm 6001, C-313, Aurora, CO 80045; **Phone:** 720-848-0168; **Board Cert:** Surgery 1974; **Med School:** Univ IL Coll Med 1966; **Resid:** Surgery, Univ Colorado Med Ctr 1973; **Fellow:** Surgical Oncology, Sloan-Kettering Cancer Ctr 1975; **Fac Appt:** Prof S, Univ Colorado

Petelin, Joseph B MD [S] - **Spec Exp:** Laparoscopic Abdominal Surgery; **Hospital:** Shawnee Mission Med Ctr; **Address:** 9119 W 74th St, Ste 255, Shawnee Mission, KS 66204; **Phone:** 913-432-5420; **Board Cert:** Surgery 1990; **Med School:** Univ Kans 1976; **Resid:** Surgery, Univ Kansas 1981; **Fac Appt:** Assoc Clin Prof S, Univ Kans

Saffle, Jeffrey MD [S] - **Spec Exp:** Burn Care; Wound Healing/Care; **Hospital:** Univ Utah Hosps and Clins; **Address:** Univ Utah, Dept Surgery, 30 N 1900 E, rm 3B306, Salt Lake City, UT 84132; **Phone:** 801-581-3595; **Board Cert:** Surgery 2002; Surgical Critical Care 1998; **Med School:** Univ Chicago-Pritzker Sch Med 1976; **Resid:** Surgery, Univ Utah Med Ctr 1982; **Fellow:** Burn Surgery, Univ Utah Med Ctr 1980; **Fac Appt:** Prof S, Univ Utah

Sasson, Aaron R MD [S] - **Spec Exp:** Gastrointestinal Cancer; Pancreatic Cancer; Liver Cancer; Biliary Cancer; **Address:** Univ Nebraska Med Ctr, Box 984030, Omaha, NE 68198-0001; **Phone:** 402-559-8941; **Board Cert:** Surgery 2000; **Med School:** UMDNJ-NJ Med Sch, Newark 1993; **Resid:** Surgery, Univ California-San Diego Med Ctr 1999; **Fellow:** Surgical Oncology, Fox Chase Cancer Ctr 2001; **Fac Appt:** Assoc Prof S, Univ Nebr Coll Med

Shaw Jr, Byers W MD [S] - **Spec Exp:** Transplant-Liver; Hepatobiliary Surgery; Liver Tumors; **Address:** 983285 Nebraska Med Ctr, Omaha, NE 68198-3285; **Phone:** 402-559-4076; **Board Cert:** Surgery 2003; Surgical Critical Care 1996; **Med School:** Case West Res Univ 1976; **Resid:** Surgery, Univ Utah Med Ctr 1981; **Fellow:** Transplant Surgery, Univ Pittsburgh 1983; **Fac Appt:** Prof S, Univ Nebr Coll Med

Southwest

Ames, Frederick C MD [S] - **Spec Exp:** Breast Cancer; **Hospital:** UT MD Anderson Cancer Ctr; **Address:** MD Anderson Cancer Ctr, Dept Surgery, 1515 Holcombe Blvd, Unit 444, Houston, TX 77030-4009; **Phone:** 713-792-6929; **Board Cert:** Surgery 1975; **Med School:** Univ Tex Med Br, Galveston 1969; **Resid:** Surgery, Univ Texas Hosp 1971; Surgery, St Joseph Hosp 1974; **Fellow:** Surgical Oncology, MD Anderson Cancer Ctr 1975; **Fac Appt:** Prof S, Univ Tex, Houston

Babiera, Gildy V MD [S] - **Spec Exp:** Breast Cancer; **Hospital:** UT MD Anderson Cancer Ctr, St Luke's Episcopal Hosp - Houston; **Address:** MD Anderson Cancer Ctr, 1515 Holcombe Blvd, Box 444, Houston, TX 77030-4009; **Phone:** 713-745-1563; **Board Cert:** Surgery 2000; **Med School:** NY Med Coll 1991; **Resid:** Surgery, NYU Med Ctr 1995; Surgery, NYU Med Ctr 1997; **Fellow:** Surgical Oncology, MD Anderson Cancer Ctr 1996; **Fac Appt:** Assoc Prof Surg & Onc, Univ Tex, Houston

Baker, Christopher C MD [S] - **Spec Exp:** Trauma/Critical Care; Colon & Rectal Surgery; Hernia; **Hospital:** Med Ctr LA @ New Orleans (Univ Hosp); **Address:** LSUHSC Sch Med, Dept Surg, CSRB Clinical Sci Rsch Bldg 508, 533 Blvd St, New Orleans, LA 70112; **Phone:** 504-568-4750; **Board Cert:** Surgery 2002; Surgical Critical Care 2007; **Med School:** Harvard Med Sch 1974; **Resid:** Surgery, UCSF Med Ctr 1981; **Fellow:** Trauma, San Francisco Genl Hosp 1979; **Fac Appt:** Prof S, Harvard Med Sch

Beitsch, Peter D MD [S] - **Spec Exp:** Breast Cancer; **Hospital:** Med City Dallas Hosp, Presby Hosp of Dallas; **Address:** 5920 Forrest Park Rd, Ste 500, Dallas, TX 75235; **Phone:** 214-956-6802; **Board Cert:** Surgery 2002; **Med School:** Univ Tex SW, Dallas 1986; **Resid:** Surgery, Univ TX SW Med Ctr 1993; **Fellow:** Surgical Oncology, MD Anderson Cancer Ctr 1990; Surgical Oncology, John Wayne Cancer Inst 1994

Bentley, Frederick R MD [S] - **Spec Exp:** Transplant Surgery; Transplant-Kidney; Transplant-Pancreas; **Hospital:** UAMS Med Ctr; **Address:** 4301 W Markham St, Slot 721-2, Little Rock, AR 72205; **Phone:** 501-686-8211; **Board Cert:** Surgery 1996; **Med School:** Louisiana State U, New Orleans 1977; **Resid:** Surgery, LSU Med Ctr 1983; **Fellow:** Research, Univ Minnesota 1982; Transplant Surgery, Univ Minnesota 1984; **Fac Appt:** Assoc Prof S, Univ Louisville Sch Med

Brunicardi, F Charles MD [S] - **Spec Exp:** Islet Cell Transplant; Pancreatic Cancer; Gastroesophageal Reflux Disease (GERD); **Hospital:** St Luke's Episcopal Hosp - Houston; **Address:** 1709 Dryden, Ste 1500, Houston, TX 77030; **Phone:** 713-798-8070; **Board Cert:** Surgery 1998; **Med School:** UMDNJ-Rutgers Med Sch 1980; **Resid:** Surgery, SUNY Brooklyn Hlth Sci Ctr 1989; **Fellow:** Pancreatic Physiology, SUNY Brooklyn Hlth Sci Ctr 1986; **Fac Appt:** Prof S, Baylor Coll Med

Curley, Steven A MD [S] - **Spec Exp:** Colon & Rectal Cancer; Liver Cancer; Hepatobiliary Surgery; **Hospital:** UT MD Anderson Cancer Ctr; **Address:** MD Anderson Cancer Ctr, Dept Surg Oncology, Unit 444, PO Box 301402, Houston, TX 77230-1402; **Phone:** 713-794-4957; **Board Cert:** Surgery 1997; **Med School:** Univ Tex, Houston 1982; **Resid:** Surgery, Univ New Mexico Hosps 1988; **Fellow:** Surgical Oncology, MD Anderson Cancer Ctr 1990; **Fac Appt:** Prof S, Univ Tex, Houston

Demarest III, Gerald B MD [S] - **Spec Exp:** Trauma; Burn Care; **Hospital:** Univ NM Hlth & Sci Ctr; **Address:** U New Mexico Health Science Ctr, 1 University New Mexico, MS 10-5610, Albuquerque, NM 83131-0001; **Phone:** 505-272-6441; **Board Cert:** Surgery 1999; Surgical Critical Care 2005; **Med School:** Columbia P&S 1973; **Resid:** Surgery, Univ Washington Med Ctr 1978; **Fellow:** Burn Surgery, Harborview Med Ctr 1979; Harborview Med Ctr 1980; **Fac Appt:** Assoc Prof S, Univ New Mexico

Dooley, William C MD [S] - **Spec Exp:** Breast Cancer; Tumors-Rare & Multiple; **Hospital:** OU Med Ctr, VA Med Ctr - Oklahoma City; **Address:** 825 NE 10th St, Ste 5200, Oklahoma City, OK 73104; **Phone:** 405-271-7867; **Board Cert:** Surgery 1997; **Med School:** Vanderbilt Univ 1982; **Resid:** Surgical Oncology, Oxford Univ 1986; Surgery, Johns Hopkins Hosp 1987; **Fellow:** Surgical Oncology, Johns Hopkins 1988; **Fac Appt:** Prof S, Univ Okla Coll Med

Ellis, Lee M MD [S] - **Spec Exp:** Liver Cancer; Colon & Rectal Cancer; Metastatic Cancer; **Hospital:** UT MD Anderson Cancer Ctr; **Address:** MD Anderson Cancer Ctr, Dept Surgery, 1515 Holcombe Blvd, Box 444, Houston, TX 77030; **Phone:** 713-792-6926; **Board Cert:** Surgery 1999; **Med School:** Univ VA Sch Med 1983; **Resid:** Surgery, Univ Fla-Shands Hosp 1990; **Fellow:** Surgical Oncology, MD Anderson Cancer Ctr 1992; **Fac Appt:** Prof S, Univ Tex, Houston

Euhus, David M MD [S] - **Spec Exp:** Breast Cancer; **Hospital:** UT Southwestern Med Ctr - Dallas; **Address:** Univ Texas SW Med Ctr - Div Surg Oncology, 5323 Harry Hines Blvd, MC 9155, Dallas, TX 75390-9155; **Phone:** 214-648-6467; **Board Cert:** Surgery 2001; **Med School:** St Louis Univ 1984; **Resid:** Surgery, UCLA Med Ctr 1991; **Fellow:** Surgical Oncology, UCLA Med Ctr 1988; Breast Disease, Queens Med Ctr 1990; **Fac Appt:** Assoc Prof S, Univ Tex SW, Dallas

Evans, Douglas B MD [S] - **Spec Exp:** Pancreatic Cancer; Thyroid Cancer; Endocrine Cancers; **Hospital:** UT MD Anderson Cancer Ctr; **Address:** Dept Surgery/Oncology, Unit 444, PO Box 301402, Houston, TX 77030-4095; **Phone:** 713-794-4324; **Board Cert:** Surgery 1996; **Med School:** Boston Univ 1983; **Resid:** Surgery, Dartmouth-Hitchcock Med Ctr 1988; **Fellow:** Surgical Oncology, MD Anderson Cancer Ctr 1990; **Fac Appt:** Prof S, Univ Tex, Houston

Feig, Barry W MD [S] - **Spec Exp:** Gastrointestinal Cancer; Sarcoma; Breast Cancer; **Hospital:** UT MD Anderson Cancer Ctr; **Address:** UT MD Anderson Cancer Ctr, Dept Surg Onc, Unit 444, PO Box 301402, Houston, TX 77230-1402; **Phone:** 713-794-1002; **Board Cert:** Surgery 1998; Surgical Critical Care 1996; **Med School:** SUNY Upstate Med Univ 1984; **Resid:** Surgery, Northwestern Univ Med Ctr 1990; **Fellow:** Trauma, Univ Minnesota 1991; Surgical Oncology, UT MD Anderson Cancer Ctr 1994; **Fac Appt:** Prof S, Univ Tex, Houston

Fisher, William E MD [S] - **Spec Exp:** Pancreatic Cancer; **Hospital:** St Luke's Episcopal Hosp - Houston; **Address:** Baylor College of Medicine, Dept Surgery, 1709 Dreyden, Ste 1500, Houston, TX 77030; **Phone:** 713-798-8070; **Board Cert:** Surgery 1999; **Med School:** Univ Cincinnati 1990; **Resid:** Surgery, Ohio State U Hosps 1996; **Fellow:** Cancer Research, Ohio State U Hosps 1998; **Fac Appt:** Asst Prof S, Baylor Coll Med

Franklin, Morris E MD [S] - **Spec Exp:** Laparoscopic Abdominal Surgery; Colon & Rectal Surgery; **Hospital:** Southeast Baptist Hosp, Baptist Med Ctr - San Antonio; **Address:** 4242 E Southcross Blvd, Ste 1, San Antonio, TX 78222; **Phone:** 210-333-7510; **Board Cert:** Surgery 1973; **Med School:** Univ Tex SW, Dallas 1967; **Resid:** Surgery, Bexar Co Hosp 1972; **Fac Appt:** Clin Prof S, Univ Tex, San Antonio

Grant, Michael D MD [S] - **Spec Exp:** Breast Cancer; **Hospital:** Baylor Univ Medical Ctr; **Address:** 3900 Junius, Ste 220, Baylor Medical Pavillion, Dallas, TX 75246; **Phone:** 214-826-7300; **Board Cert:** Surgery 2001; **Med School:** Univ Tex, Houston 1987; **Resid:** Surgery, Baylor Univ Med Ctr 1992; **Fellow:** Breast Cancer, Baylor Univ Med Ctr 1993

Gray, Richard J MD [S] - **Spec Exp:** Breast Cancer; Melanoma; **Hospital:** Mayo Clinic - Phoenix, Mayo Clinic - Scottsdale; **Address:** Mayo Clinic, 5777 E Mayo Blvd, Phoenix, AZ 85054; **Phone:** 480-342-2849; **Board Cert:** Surgery 2001; **Med School:** Mich State Univ 1995; **Resid:** Surgery, Mayo Clinic 2000; **Fellow:** Surgical Oncology, H Lee Moffitt Cancer Ctr 2001; **Fac Appt:** Assoc Prof S, Mayo Med Sch

Griswold, John A MD [S] - **Spec Exp:** Burn Care; **Hospital:** Univ Med Ctr - Lubbock; **Address:** Texas Tech Univ Hlth Scis Ctr, Dept Surg, 3601 4th St, MS 9905, Lubbock, TX 79430; **Phone:** 806-743-2373; **Board Cert:** Surgery 1999; Surgical Critical Care 2000; **Med School:** Creighton Univ 1981; **Resid:** Surgery, Texas Tech Univ Hlth Scis Ctr 1986; **Fellow:** Burn Surgery, Univ Washington 1988

Halff, Glenn A MD [S] - **Spec Exp:** Transplant-Liver; Liver Surgery; **Hospital:** Univ Hlth Sys - Univ Hosp (San Antonio, TX), Christus Santa Rosa Children's Hosp; **Address:** Univ TX Hlth Sci Ctr-Transplantation Ctr, 7703 Floyd Curl Drive, MC 785, San Antonio, TX 78229; **Phone:** 210-567-5777; **Board Cert:** Surgery 1998; Surgical Critical Care 2000; **Med School:** Univ Tex, Houston 1983; **Resid:** Surgery, NYU Med Ctr 1987; **Fellow:** Transplant Surgery, Univ Pittsburgh 1989; **Fac Appt:** Assoc Prof S, Univ Tex, San Antonio

Hunt, John L MD [S] - **Spec Exp:** Trauma; Burn Care; **Hospital:** UT Southwestern Med Ctr - Dallas; **Address:** UT Southwestern Med Ctr, Surgery, 5323 Harry Hines Blvd, MC 9158, Dallas, TX 75390-9158; **Phone:** 214-648-2152; **Board Cert:** Surgery 1972; Surgical Critical Care 1996; **Med School:** Univ Cincinnati 1964; **Resid:** Surgery, Cincinnati Genl Hosp 1971; **Fac Appt:** Prof S, Univ Tex SW, Dallas

Hunt, Kelly K MD [S] - **Spec Exp:** Breast Cancer; Sarcoma-Soft Tissue; Gene Therapy; **Hospital:** UT MD Anderson Cancer Ctr; **Address:** MD Anderson Cancer Ctr, 1515 Holcombe Blvd, Box 444, Houston, TX 77030-4000; **Phone:** 713-792-7216; **Board Cert:** Surgery 2001; **Med School:** Univ Tenn Coll Med, Memphis 1986; **Resid:** Surgery, UCLA Med Ctr 1993; **Fellow:** Surgical Oncology, MD Anderson Cancer Ctr 1996; **Fac Appt:** Prof S, Univ Tex, Houston

Jackson, Gilchrist MD [S] - **Spec Exp:** Thyroid & Parathyroid Surgery; Head & Neck Cancer & Surgery; Endocrine Tumors; Gastrointestinal Cancer & Surgery; **Hospital:** St Luke's Episcopal Hosp - Houston, Woman's Hosp TX, The; **Address:** 2727 W Holcombe Blvd Fl 3 A, Houston, TX 77027; **Phone:** 713-442-1132; **Board Cert:** Surgery 1998; **Med School:** Univ Louisville Sch Med 1974; **Resid:** Surgery, Parkland Hosp 1979; **Fellow:** Surgical Oncology, MD Anderson Hosp 1980; **Fac Appt:** Assoc Clin Prof S, Baylor Coll Med

Klimberg, Vicki S MD [S] - **Spec Exp:** Breast Cancer; Radiofrequency Tumor Ablation; **Hospital:** UAMS Med Ctr; **Address:** Univ Arkansas Medical Sciences, 4301 W Markham, MS 725, Little Rock, AR 72205-7199; **Phone:** 501-686-5669; **Board Cert:** Surgery 1999; **Med School:** Univ Fla Coll Med 1984; **Resid:** Surgery, Univ Fla 1990; **Fellow:** Clinical Oncology, Univ Fla 1991; Breast Disease, Univ Arkansas for Med Scis 1991; **Fac Appt:** Prof S, Univ Ark

Krouse, Robert S MD [S] - **Spec Exp:** Cancer Surgery; Gastrointestinal Cancer; Palliative Care; **Hospital:** VA Medical Center - Tucson; **Address:** Southern AZ VA Hosp Care System, Surg Care Line, 2-112, 3601 S 6th Ave, Tucson, AZ 85723; **Phone:** 520-792-1450 x6145; **Board Cert:** Surgery 1998; **Med School:** Hahnemann Univ 1991; **Resid:** Surgery, Univ Hawaii Integrated Surg Prog 1993; Immunotherapy, Natl Cancer Inst 1994; **Fellow:** Surgery, W Virginia Univ Sch Med 1997; Surgical Oncology, City of Hope Natl Med Ctr 2000; **Fac Appt:** Asst Prof S, Univ Ariz Coll Med

Kuhn, Joseph A MD [S] - **Spec Exp:** Liver Cancer; Peritoneal Carcinomatosis; Melanoma; **Hospital:** Baylor Univ Medical Ctr; **Address:** 3409 Worth St, Ste 420, Sammons Tower, Dallas, TX 75246; **Phone:** 214-824-9963; **Board Cert:** Surgery 1999; Surgical Critical Care 2003; **Med School:** Univ Tex Med Br, Galveston 1984; **Resid:** Surgery, Baylor Univ Med Ctr 1989; **Fellow:** Surgical Oncology, City Hosp Natl Med Ctr 1992

Lee, Jeffrey E MD [S] - **Spec Exp:** Melanoma; Pancreatic Cancer; Endocrine Tumors; **Hospital:** UT MD Anderson Cancer Ctr; **Address:** UT MD Anderson Cancer Ctr, 1400 Holcombe Blvd, Unit 444 Fl 12, Houston, TX 77030-4009; **Phone:** 713-792-7218; **Board Cert:** Surgery 1999; **Med School:** Stanford Univ 1984; **Resid:** Surgery, Stanford Univ Hosp 1987; Surgery, Stanford Univ Hosp 1991; **Fellow:** Immunology, Stanford Univ Sch Med 1989; Surgical Oncology, Univ Tex-MD Anderson Cancer Ctr 1993; **Fac Appt:** Prof S, Univ Tex, Houston

Leitch, A Marilyn MD [S] - **Spec Exp:** Breast Cancer & Surgery; Melanoma; Sarcoma; **Hospital:** UT Southwestern Med Ctr - Dallas; **Address:** UT Southwestern Med Ctr - Dept Surgery, 5323 Harry Hines Blvd, MC 9155, Dallas, TX 75390-9155; **Phone:** 214-648-3039; **Board Cert:** Surgery 2003; **Med School:** Univ Tex SW, Dallas 1978; **Resid:** Surgery, UCLA Med Ctr 1984; **Fellow:** Surgical Oncology, MD Anderson Cancer Ctr 1985; **Fac Appt:** Prof S, Univ Tex SW, Dallas

Li, Benjamin D L MD [S] - **Spec Exp:** Gastrointestinal Cancer; Sarcoma; Breast Cancer; **Hospital:** Louisiana State Univ Hosp, Willis Knighton Hlth Sys; **Address:** LSU Hlth Scis Ctr, Dept Surgery, 1501 Kings Hwy, Shreveport, LA 71130; **Phone:** 318-675-6123; **Board Cert:** Surgery 2002; **Med School:** Yale Univ 1986; **Resid:** Surgery, Northwestern Univ-McGraw Med Ctr 1992; **Fellow:** Surgical Oncology, Roswell Park Cancer Inst 1995; **Fac Appt:** Prof S, Louisiana State U, New Orleans

Livingston, Edward H MD [S] - **Spec Exp:** Gastrointestinal Surgery; Endocrine Surgery; Obesity/Bariatric Surgery; **Hospital:** UT Southwestern Med Ctr - Dallas; **Address:** UT Southwestern Medical Ctr, 5323 Harry Hines Blvd, MC 9156, Dallas, TX 75390-9156; **Phone:** 214-648-7956; **Board Cert:** Surgery 2003; **Med School:** UCLA 1985; **Resid:** Surgery, UCLA Med Ctr 1992; **Fac Appt:** Prof S, Univ Tex SW, Dallas

Mansfield, Paul F MD [S] - **Spec Exp:** Appendix Cancer; Stomach Cancer; Colon Cancer; Melanoma; **Hospital:** UT MD Anderson Cancer Ctr; **Address:** UT MD Anderson Cancer Ctr, 1516 Holcombe Blvd, rm 444, Houston, TX 77030; **Phone:** 713-794-5499; **Board Cert:** Surgery 2006; **Med School:** Jefferson Med Coll 1983; **Resid:** Surgery, Pennsylvania Hosp 1988; **Fellow:** Surgical Oncology, MD Anderson Cancer Ctr 1991; **Fac Appt:** Prof Surg & Onc, Univ Tex, Houston

Pisters, Peter MD [S] - **Spec Exp:** Pancreatic Cancer; Sarcoma-Soft Tissue; Gastrointestinal Cancer; **Hospital:** UT MD Anderson Cancer Ctr; **Address:** MD Anderson Cancer Ctr, PO Box 301402, Unit 444, Houston, TX 77230-1402; **Phone:** 713-794-1572; **Board Cert:** Surgery 2001; **Med School:** Univ Western Ontario 1985; **Resid:** Surgery, NYU/Bellevue Hosp 1992; **Fellow:** Surgical Research, Meml Sloan-Kettering Cancer Ctr 1989; Surgical Oncology, Meml Sloan-Kettering Cancer Ctr 1994; **Fac Appt:** Prof S, Univ Tex, Houston

Pockaj, Barbara A MD [S] - **Spec Exp:** Melanoma; Breast Cancer; Stomach Cancer; Clinical Trials; **Hospital:** Mayo Clinic - Scottsdale; **Address:** Mayo Clinic, Dept Surgery, 5777 E Mayo Blvd, Phoenix, AZ 85054; **Phone:** 480-342-1051; **Board Cert:** Surgery 2005; **Med School:** Vanderbilt Univ 1987; **Resid:** Surgery, Case Western Res Univ Affil Hosps 1995; **Fellow:** Surgical Oncology, Natl Inst Hlth 1992; **Fac Appt:** Assoc Prof S, Mayo Med Sch

Pollock, Raphael E MD/PhD [S] - **Spec Exp:** Sarcoma; **Hospital:** UT MD Anderson Cancer Ctr; **Address:** MD Anderson Cancer Ctr, Dept Surg Oncology, 1515 Holcombe Blvd, Unit 345, Houston, TX 77230; **Phone:** 713-792-8850; **Board Cert:** Surgery 2003; **Med School:** St Louis Univ 1977; **Resid:** Surgery, Univ Chicago 1979; Surgery, Rush Presby-St Lukes Hosp 1982; **Fellow:** Surgical Oncology, MD Anderson Cancer Ctr 1984; **Fac Appt:** Prof S, Univ Tex, Houston

Postier, Russell G MD [S] - **Spec Exp:** Pancreatic Cancer; Biliary Surgery; **Hospital:** OU Med Ctr; **Address:** Univ Oklahoma Dept Surgery, PO Box 26901, WP-2140, Oklahoma City, OK 73104; **Phone:** 405-271-3445; **Board Cert:** Surgery 2000; **Med School:** Univ Okla Coll Med 1975; **Resid:** Surgery, Johns Hopkins Hosp 1981; **Fac Appt:** Prof S, Univ Okla Coll Med

Surgery

Purdue, Gary F MD [S] - **Spec Exp:** Burn Care; **Hospital:** UT Southwestern Med Ctr - Dallas; **Address:** UT Southwestern Med Ctr, Surgery, 5323 Harry Hines Blvd, MC 9158, Dallas, TX 75390-9158; **Phone:** 214-648-2041; **Board Cert:** Surgery 1999; Surgical Critical Care 2006; **Med School:** Jefferson Med Coll 1976; **Resid:** Surgery, Mercy Hosp 1981; **Fellow:** Burn Surgery, Parkland Meml Hosp 1982; **Fac Appt:** Prof S, Univ Tex SW, Dallas

Ross, Merrick I MD [S] - **Spec Exp:** Sentinel Node Surgery; Breast Cancer; Melanoma; **Hospital:** UT MD Anderson Cancer Ctr; **Address:** UT MD Anderson Cancer Ctr, Dept Surg Onc, PO Box 301402, Unit 444, Houston, TX 77230-1402; **Phone:** 713-792-7217; **Board Cert:** Surgery 1997; **Med School:** Univ IL Coll Med 1980; **Resid:** Surgery, Univ Illinois Hosp & Clin 1982; Surgery, Univ Illinois Hosp & Clin 1987; **Fellow:** Research, Scripps Clin & Rsch 1984; Surgical Oncology, Univ TX-MD Anderson Cancer Ctr 1989; **Fac Appt:** Prof S, Univ Tex, Houston

Schlinkert, Richard T MD [S] - **Spec Exp:** Endocrine Surgery; Laparoscopic Surgery; Gastrointestinal Surgery; Adrenal Surgery; **Hospital:** Mayo Clinic - Scottsdale; **Address:** Mayo Clinic, Dept Surgery, 13400 E Shea Blvd, Scottsdale, AZ 85259-5404; **Phone:** 480-342-1051; **Board Cert:** Surgery 1996; **Med School:** Med Coll OH 1981; **Resid:** Surgery, Mayo Clinic 1986; **Fellow:** Hepatobiliary Surgery, Royal Infirmary 1987; **Fac Appt:** Prof S, Mayo Med Sch

Singletary, S Eva MD [S] - **Spec Exp:** Breast Cancer; **Hospital:** UT MD Anderson Cancer Ctr; **Address:** Univ Tex MD Anderson Cancer Ctr, 1515 Holcombe Blvd, Box 444, Houston, TX 77030-4009; **Phone:** 713-792-6937; **Board Cert:** Surgery 2003; **Med School:** Med Univ SC 1977; **Resid:** Surgery, Shands Hosp-Univ Florida 1983; **Fellow:** Surgery, UT MD Anderson Hosp 1985; **Fac Appt:** Prof S, Univ Tex, Houston

Skibber, John M MD [S] - **Spec Exp:** Rectal Cancer/Sphincter Preservation; Colon & Rectal Cancer-Familial Polyposis; **Hospital:** UT MD Anderson Cancer Ctr; **Address:** Unit 444 PO Box 301402, Houston, TX 77230-1402; **Phone:** 713-792-5165; **Board Cert:** Surgery 1998; **Med School:** Jefferson Med Coll 1981; **Resid:** Surgery, NYU Med Ctr 1989; **Fellow:** Surgical Oncology, Univ Texas-MD Anderson 1991; **Fac Appt:** Prof S, Univ Tex, Houston

Stewart, Ronald M MD [S] - **Spec Exp:** Trauma; **Hospital:** Univ Hlth Sys - Univ Hosp (San Antonio, TX); **Address:** Univ Tex Hlth Sci Ctr, Dept Surg-Trauma, 7703 Floyd Curl Drive, MC 7740, San Antonio, TX 78229-3900; **Phone:** 210-567-3623; **Board Cert:** Surgery 2000; Surgical Critical Care 2002; **Med School:** Univ Tex, San Antonio 1985; **Resid:** Surgery, Univ Tex Hlth Sci Ctr 1991; **Fellow:** Trauma, Univ Tenn Coll Med 1993; **Fac Appt:** Assoc Prof S, Univ Tex, San Antonio

Stolier, Alan J MD [S] - **Spec Exp:** Breast Cancer; **Hospital:** Ochsner Baptist Med Ctr, Louisiana State Univ Hosp; **Address:** 2525 Severn Ave, Metairie, LA 70002; **Phone:** 504-832-4200; **Board Cert:** Surgery 2006; **Med School:** Louisiana State U, New Orleans 1970; **Resid:** Surgery, Charity Hosp 1974; **Fellow:** Surgical Oncology, MD Anderson Hosp 1976

Vauthey, Jean Nicholas MD [S] - **Spec Exp:** Hepatobiliary Surgery; Liver Cancer; Gallbladder & Biliary Cancer; **Hospital:** UT MD Anderson Cancer Ctr; **Address:** UT MD Anderson Cancer Ctr -Surg Oncology, 1515 Holcombe Blvd, Unit 444, Houston, TX 77030; **Phone:** 713-792-2022; **Board Cert:** Surgery 2000; **Med School:** Switzerland 1979; **Resid:** Surgery, Ochsner Med Fdn 1989; **Fellow:** Hepatobiliary Surgery, Med Fac Univ Bern 1991; Surgical Oncology, Meml Sloan-Kettering Cancer Ctr 1993; **Fac Appt:** Prof S, Univ Tex, Houston

Woltering, Eugene MD [S] - **Spec Exp:** Carcinoid Tumors; **Hospital:** Kenner Reg Med Ctr; **Address:** 200 W Esplanade, Ste 200, Kenner, LA 70065; **Phone:** 504-464-8500; **Board Cert:** Surgery 2002; **Med School:** Ohio State Univ 1975; **Resid:** Surgery, Vanderbilt Med Ctr 1982; Surgical Oncology, Natl Inst Hlth 1979; **Fellow:** Surgical Oncology, Ohio State 1984

Wood, R Patrick MD [S] - **Spec Exp:** Liver Cancer; Liver Surgery; **Hospital:** St Luke's Episcopal Hosp - Houston; **Address:** 6624 Fannin St, Ste 1200, Houston, TX 77030; **Phone:** 713-795-8994; **Board Cert:** Surgery 2004; **Med School:** Univ Rochester 1979; **Resid:** Surgery, NYU/Bellevue Hosp Ctr 1984; **Fellow:** Transplant Surgery, Univ Pittsburgh 1985; **Fac Appt:** Clin Prof S, Univ Tex, Houston

Zannis, Victor J MD [S] - **Spec Exp:** Breast Cancer; **Hospital:** Phoenix Baptist Hosp & Med Ctr, J C Lincoln Hosp - North Mountain; **Address:** 2525 W Greenway Rd, Ste 130, Phoenix, AZ 85023; **Phone:** 602-942-8000; **Board Cert:** Surgery 2000; **Med School:** UCLA 1976; **Resid:** Surgery, Maricopa Med Ctr 1982

West Coast and Pacific

Anderson, Benjamin O MD [S] - **Spec Exp:** Breast Cancer & Surgery; **Hospital:** Univ Wash Med Ctr; **Address:** Univ Washington Dept Surgery, 1959 NE Pacific St, Box 356410, Seattle, WA 98195-6410; **Phone:** 206-288-6457; **Board Cert:** Surgery 2002; **Med School:** Albert Einstein Coll Med 1985; **Resid:** Surgery, Univ Colorado 1992; **Fellow:** Surgical Oncology, Meml Sloan Kettering Cancer Ctr 1994; **Fac Appt:** Prof S, Univ Wash

Ascher, Nancy L MD/PhD [S] - **Spec Exp:** Transplant-Liver; Transplant-Kidney; **Hospital:** UCSF Med Ctr; **Address:** 513 Parnassus Ave, Box 0104, San Francisco, CA 94143-0104; **Phone:** 415-476-1236; **Board Cert:** Surgery 2002; **Med School:** Univ Mich Med Sch 1974; **Resid:** Surgery, Univ Minn Hosp 1981; **Fellow:** Transplant Surgery, Univ Minn Hosp 1982; **Fac Appt:** Prof S, UCSF

Bilchik, Anton J MD [S] - **Spec Exp:** Gastrointestinal Cancer; Laparoscopic Surgery; **Hospital:** St John's Hlth Ctr, Santa Monica, Cedars-Sinai Med Ctr; **Address:** John Wayne Cancer Institute, 2200 Santa Monica Blvd, Santa Monica, CA 90404; **Phone:** 310-696-0716; **Board Cert:** Surgery 2004; **Med School:** South Africa 1985; **Resid:** Surgery, UCLA Med Ctr 1996; **Fellow:** John Wayne Cancer Inst. 1998; **Fac Appt:** Asst Clin Prof S, UCLA

Busuttil, Ronald W MD/PhD [S] - **Spec Exp:** Transplant-Liver; Liver Cancer; **Hospital:** Ronald Reagan UCLA Med Ctr; **Address:** UCLA Dept Surg, Transplant, 77-120 CHS Box 957054, Los Angeles, CA 90095-7054; **Phone:** 310-825-5318; **Board Cert:** Surgery 2007; **Med School:** Tulane Univ 1971; **Resid:** Surgery, UCLA Med Ctr 1976; **Fellow:** Surgery, UCLA Med Ctr 1975; **Fac Appt:** Prof S, UCLA

Butler, John A MD [S] - **Spec Exp:** Breast Cancer; Thyroid Cancer; Adrenal Tumors; Small Bowel Cancer; **Hospital:** UC Irvine Med Ctr; **Address:** UC-Irvine Medical Ctr, 101 City Drive S, Bldg 56 Office 252 Rt 81, Orange, CA 92868-3298; **Phone:** 714-456-8030; **Board Cert:** Surgery 2003; **Med School:** Loyola Univ-Stritch Sch Med 1976; **Resid:** Surgery, LAC-USC Med Ctr 1982; Surgery, Harbor-UCLA Med Ctr 1982; **Fellow:** Surgical Oncology, Meml Sloan-Kettering Cancer Ctr 1984; **Fac Appt:** Assoc Prof S, UC Irvine

Byrd, David MD [S] - **Spec Exp:** Tumor Surgery; Breast Cancer; Melanoma; **Hospital:** Univ Wash Med Ctr; **Address:** Univ Washington Med Ctr, Dept Surgical Specialites Center, 1959 NE Pacific St, Box 356165, Seattle, WA 98195; **Phone:** 206-598-4477; **Board Cert:** Surgery 1998; **Med School:** Tulane Univ 1982; **Resid:** Surgery, Univ Wash Med Ctr 1987; **Fellow:** Surgical Oncology, Univ Tex-MD Anderson Cancer Ctr 1992; **Fac Appt:** Assoc Prof S, Univ Wash

Surgery

Chang, Helena MD [S] - **Spec Exp:** Breast Cancer; Cancer Surgery; **Hospital:** Ronald Reagan UCLA Med Ctr; **Address:** 200 UCLA Medical Plaza, Ste B265-1, Revlon Breast Clinic, Los Angeles, CA 90095-8344; **Phone:** 310-825-2144; **Board Cert:** Surgery 1997; **Med School:** Temple Univ 1981; **Resid:** Surgery, Episcopal Hosp 1986; **Fellow:** Cellular Molecular Biology, Temple Univ 1977; Surgical Oncology, Meml Sloan-Kettering Cancer Ctr 1988; **Fac Appt:** Prof S, UCLA

Clark, Orlo H MD [S] - **Spec Exp:** Thyroid Cancer & Surgery; Neuroendocrine Tumors; Parathyroid Tumors; **Hospital:** UCSF - Mt Zion Med Ctr, UCSF Med Ctr; **Address:** UCSF Mt Zion Med Ctr, 1600 Divisadero St Fl 3, Box 1674, San Francisco, CA 94115-1926; **Phone:** 415-353-7687; **Board Cert:** Surgery 1974; **Med School:** Cornell Univ-Weill Med Coll 1967; **Resid:** Surgery, UCSF Med Ctr 1970; Surgery, UCSF Med Ctr 1973; **Fellow:** Surgery, Royal Med Sch London 1971; **Fac Appt:** Prof S, UCSF

Colquhoun, Steven D MD [S] - **Spec Exp:** Liver Cancer; Transplant-Liver; Pancreatic Cancer; Hepatobiliary Surgery; **Hospital:** Cedars-Sinai Med Ctr; **Address:** Cedars-Sinai Med Center, 8635 W 3rd St, Ste 590-W, Los Angeles, CA 90048; **Phone:** 310-423-2641; **Board Cert:** Surgery 2003; **Med School:** Loyola Univ-Stritch Sch Med 1984; **Resid:** Surgery, UCLA Med Ctr 1990; **Fellow:** Surgical Oncology, UCLA Med Ctr 1993; Transplant Surgery, UCLA Med Ctr 1994; **Fac Appt:** Assoc Clin Prof S, UCLA

Curet, Myriam MD [S] - **Spec Exp:** Obesity/Bariatric Surgery; Robotic Surgery; Minimally Invasive Surgery; **Hospital:** Stanford Univ Med Ctr; **Address:** 300 Pasteur Drive, rm H3680, Stanford, CA 94305-5655; **Phone:** 650-736-1613; **Board Cert:** Surgery 1997; **Med School:** Harvard Med Sch 1982; **Resid:** Surgery, Univ Chicago Hosps 1989; **Fellow:** Univ New Mexico 1994; **Fac Appt:** Prof S, Stanford Univ

Duh, Quan-Yang MD [S] - **Spec Exp:** Endocrine Surgery; Thyroid & Parathyroid Cancer & Surgery; Adrenal Tumors; Minimally Invasive Surgery; **Hospital:** UCSF Med Ctr, VA Med Ctr - San Francisco; **Address:** UCSF Medical Ctr, Box 1926, San Francisco, CA 94143-1926; **Phone:** 415-353-7789; **Board Cert:** Surgery 1997; **Med School:** UCSF 1981; **Resid:** Surgery, UCSF Med Ctr 1988; **Fellow:** Endocrine Surgery, UCSF Med Ctr 1987; **Fac Appt:** Prof S, UCSF

Eilber, Frederick R MD [S] - **Spec Exp:** Tumor Surgery; Sarcoma; **Hospital:** Ronald Reagan UCLA Med Ctr; **Address:** 200 UCLA Medical Plaza, Ste 120, Los Angeles, CA 90095-1718; **Phone:** 310-825-7086; **Board Cert:** Surgery 1973; **Med School:** Univ Mich Med Sch 1965; **Resid:** Surgery, Univ Maryland Hosp 1972; **Fellow:** Surgery, Univ Tex-MD Anderson Hosp 1973; **Fac Appt:** Prof S, UCLA

Ellenhorn, Joshua MD [S] - **Spec Exp:** Gastrointestinal Cancer; Pancreatic Surgery; Cancer Surgery; **Hospital:** City of Hope Natl Med Ctr & Beckman Rsch, Huntington Memorial Hosp; **Address:** City of Hope Med Ctr, 1500 E Duarte Rd, Duarte, CA 91010; **Phone:** 626-471-7100; **Board Cert:** Surgery 2000; **Med School:** Boston Univ 1984; **Resid:** Surgery, Univ Cincinnati Hosp 1991; **Fellow:** Surgical Oncology, Meml Sloan-Kettering Cancer Ctr 1993

Esquivel, Carlos O MD [S] - **Spec Exp:** Transplant-Liver; **Hospital:** Stanford Univ Med Ctr, Lucile Packard Chldns Hosp/Stanford Univ Med Ctr; **Address:** 750 Welch Rd, Ste 319, Palo Alto, CA 94304; **Phone:** 650-498-5689; **Board Cert:** Surgery 2003; Surgical Critical Care 1999; **Med School:** Costa Rica 1975; **Resid:** Surgery, UC- Davis Med Ctr 1984; **Fellow:** Transplant Surgery, Univ Hlth Ctr Pittsburgh 1985; **Fac Appt:** Prof S, Stanford Univ

Esserman, Laura J MD [S] - **Spec Exp:** Breast Cancer; **Hospital:** UCSF - Mt Zion Med Ctr, UCSF Med Ctr; **Address:** UCSF-Helen Diller Family Comp Cancer Ctr, 1600 Divisadero St Fl 2, Box 1710, San Francisco, CA 94115; **Phone:** 415-353-7070; **Board Cert:** Surgery 2001; **Med School:** Stanford Univ 1983; **Resid:** Surgery, Stanford Univ Med Ctr 1991; **Fellow:** Oncology, Stanford Univ Med Ctr 1988; **Fac Appt:** Assoc Prof S, UCSF

Essner, Richard MD [S] - **Spec Exp:** Sentinel Node Surgery; Melanoma; Gastrointestinal Surgery; **Hospital:** St John's Hlth Ctr, Santa Monica, Century City Hosp; **Address:** John Wayne Cancer Inst, 2103 Santa Monica Blvd, Fl 3rd, Santa Monica, CA 90404-2302; **Phone:** 310-998-3906; **Board Cert:** Surgery 1994; **Med School:** Emory Univ 1985; **Resid:** Surgery, Univ NC Hosps 1992; **Fac Appt:** Asst Clin Prof S, USC Sch Med

Giuliano, Armando E MD [S] - **Spec Exp:** Breast Cancer; Thyroid & Parathyroid Surgery; **Hospital:** St John's Hlth Ctr, Santa Monica, Ronald Reagan UCLA Med Ctr; **Address:** John Wayne Cancer Inst, 2200 Santa Monica Blvd, Santa Monica, CA 90404; **Phone:** 310-829-8089; **Board Cert:** Surgery 1999; **Med School:** Univ Chicago-Pritzker Sch Med 1973; **Resid:** Surgery, UCSF Med Ctr 1980; **Fellow:** Surgical Oncology, UCLA Med Ctr 1978; **Fac Appt:** Prof S, UCLA

Goodnight, James E MD [S] - **Spec Exp:** Melanoma; Breast Cancer; Bone & Soft Tissue Tumors; **Hospital:** UC Davis Med Ctr; **Address:** UC Davis Med Ctr, Dept Surgery, 2221 Stockton Blvd, rm 3112, Sacramento, CA 95817; **Phone:** 916-734-3190; **Board Cert:** Surgery 1997; **Med School:** Baylor Coll Med 1968; **Resid:** Surgery, Univ Utah Hosp 1976; **Fellow:** Surgical Oncology, UCLA Med Ctr 1978; **Fac Appt:** Prof S, UC Davis

Goodson III, William H MD [S] - **Spec Exp:** Breast Cancer; Breast Disease; **Hospital:** CA Pacific Med Ctr - Pacific Campus, UCSF - Mt Zion Med Ctr; **Address:** 2100 Webster St, Ste 401, San Francisco, CA 94115-2378; **Phone:** 415-923-3925; **Board Cert:** Surgery 2006; **Med School:** Harvard Med Sch 1971; **Resid:** Surgery, Univ Hosps 1976; Surgery, Children's Hosp 1977

Gower, Roland E MD [S] - **Spec Exp:** Breast Surgery; Biliary Surgery; Thyroid Surgery; **Hospital:** Providence Alaska Med Ctr, Alaska Regl Hosp; **Address:** 2841 De Barr Rd, Ste 41, Anchorage, AK 99508-2973; **Phone:** 907-279-3564; **Board Cert:** Surgery 1997; **Med School:** Vanderbilt Univ 1971; **Resid:** Surgery, Kansas Med Ctr 1975

Greenhalgh, David G MD [S] - **Spec Exp:** Burn Care; Nutrition; Wound Healing/Care; **Hospital:** Northern CA Shriners Hosp, UC Davis Med Ctr; **Address:** Shriners Hosp Chldn, 2425 Stockton Blvd, Sacramento, CA 95817; **Phone:** 916-453-2050; **Board Cert:** Surgery 2005; Surgical Critical Care 1998; **Med School:** SUNY Upstate Med Univ 1981; **Resid:** Surgery, MC Hosp of VT 1986; **Fellow:** Burn Surgery, Univ Wash Hosp 1989; **Fac Appt:** Prof S, UC Davis

Hoyt, David B MD [S] - **Spec Exp:** Trauma; Critical Care; Burn Care; **Hospital:** UC Irvine Med Ctr; **Address:** Univ California, Irvine-Dept Surgery, 333 City Blvd West, City Twr, Ste 700, Orange, CA 92868; **Phone:** 714-456-6262; **Board Cert:** Surgery 2004; Surgical Critical Care 2007; **Med School:** Case West Res Univ 1976; **Resid:** Surgery, UCSD Med Ctr 1984; **Fellow:** Immunopathology, Scripps Clin 1982; **Fac Appt:** Prof S, UC Irvine

Hunter, John G MD [S] - **Spec Exp:** Gastrointestinal & Esophageal Surgery; Laparoscopic Abdominal Surgery; Gastroesophageal Reflux Disease (GERD); **Hospital:** OR Hlth & Sci Univ; **Address:** Digestive Hlth Ctr, 3303 SW Bond Ave, MC CH6D, Portland, OR 97239; **Phone:** 503-494-4373; **Board Cert:** Surgery 2006; **Med School:** Univ Pennsylvania 1981; **Resid:** Surgery, Univ Utah Med Ctr 1987; **Fellow:** Gastrointestinal Surgery, Mass Genl Hosp 1988; Endoscopy, Univ West Ontario 1989; **Fac Appt:** Assoc Prof S, Oregon Hlth Sci Univ

Johnson, Denise L MD [S] - **Spec Exp:** Melanoma; Breast Cancer; **Hospital:** Stanford Univ Med Ctr; **Address:** Stanford Univ Med Ctr-Dept Surgery, 300 Pasteur Drive, Ste H3680, MC 5655, Stanford, CA 94305; **Phone:** 650-723-5672; **Board Cert:** Surgery 2001; **Med School:** Washington Univ, St Louis 1978; **Resid:** Surgery, Univ Illinois Med Ctr 1986; Immunology, Univ Texas SW Med Ctr 1982; **Fellow:** Surgical Oncology, City of Hope Med Ctr 1989; **Fac Appt:** Assoc Prof S, Stanford Univ

Surgery

Kaufman, Cary S MD [S] - **Spec Exp:** Breast Cancer; Breast Disease; **Hospital:** St Joseph Hosp - Bellingham; **Address:** 2940 Squalicum Pkwy, Ste 101, Bellingham, WA 98225; **Phone:** 360-671-9877; **Board Cert:** Surgery 2000; **Med School:** UCLA 1973; **Resid:** Surgery, Univ Wash Med Ctr 1975; Surgery, Harbor-UCLA Med Ctr 1979; **Fac Appt:** Asst Clin Prof S, Univ Wash

Klein, Andrew S MD [S] - **Spec Exp:** Transplant-Liver; Liver Cancer; Liver Failure; **Hospital:** Cedars-Sinai Med Ctr; **Address:** Cedars-Sinai Medical Center, 8635 W Third St, Ste 590W, Los Angeles, CA 90048; **Phone:** 310-423-2641; **Board Cert:** Surgery 2007; **Med School:** Johns Hopkins Univ 1979; **Resid:** Surgery, Johns Hopkins Hosp 1982; Surgery, Johns Hopkins Hosp 1986; **Fellow:** Transplant Surgery, UCLA-CHS 1988; **Fac Appt:** Clin Prof S, UCLA

Knudson, Mary Margaret MD [S] - **Spec Exp:** Breast Cancer; Trauma; **Hospital:** UCSF Med Ctr, San Francisco Genl Hosp; **Address:** 1001 Potrero Ave, Ste 3A, San Francisco, CA 94110; **Phone:** 415-206-3039; **Board Cert:** Surgery 1992; Surgical Critical Care 1998; **Med School:** Univ Mich Med Sch 1976; **Resid:** Surgery, Beth Israel Hosp 1979; Surgery, Univ Mich Med Ctr 1982; **Fellow:** Pediatric Surgery, Stanford Univ Hosps; **Fac Appt:** Assoc Prof S, UCSF

Moossa, AR MD [S] - **Spec Exp:** Pancreatic Cancer; Gastrointestinal Cancer; Hepatobiliary Surgery; **Hospital:** UCSD Med Ctr; **Address:** 9300 Campus Point Drive, MC 7212, La Jolla, CA 92037; **Phone:** 858-657-6113; **Med School:** England 1965; **Resid:** Surgery, Liverpool Univ Hosps 1970; **Fellow:** Surgical Oncology, Johns Hopkins Hosp 1972; **Fac Appt:** Prof S, UCSD

Nguyen, Ninh T MD [S] - **Spec Exp:** Laparoscopic Surgery; Obesity/Bariatric Surgery; Gastrointestinal Cancer & Surgery; **Hospital:** UC Irvine Med Ctr; **Address:** Div Gastrointestinal Surgery, 333 City Blvd W, Ste 850, Orange, CA 92868; **Phone:** 714-456-8598; **Board Cert:** Surgery 2006; **Med School:** Univ Tex, San Antonio 1990; **Resid:** Surgery, Mt Sinai Med Ctr 1995; **Fellow:** Surgical Oncology, Univ Pittsburgh Med Ctr 1997; Laparoscopic Surgery, Univ Pittsburgh Med Ctr 1998; **Fac Appt:** Assoc Prof S, UC Irvine

Nissen, Nicholas N MD [S] - **Spec Exp:** Liver Cancer; Transplant-Liver; Pancreatic Cancer; Minimally Invasive Surgery; **Hospital:** Cedars-Sinai Med Ctr; **Address:** Cedars-Sinai Medical Center, 8635 W 3rd St, Ste 590-W, Los Angeles, CA 90048; **Phone:** 310-423-2641; **Board Cert:** Surgery 1999; Surgical Critical Care 1999; **Med School:** Univ Minn 1991; **Resid:** Surgery, Loyola Univ Med Ctr 1998; **Fellow:** Surgical Critical Care, Univ Pittsburgh Med Ctr 1999; Hepatobiliary Surgery, UCLA Med Ctr 2001

Norton, Jeffrey A MD [S] - **Spec Exp:** Pancreatic Cancer; Gastrointestinal Cancer & Surgery; Endocrine Surgery; **Hospital:** Stanford Univ Med Ctr; **Address:** 875 Blake Wilbur Drive, Clinic F, Stanford, CA 94305; **Phone:** 650-723-5461; **Board Cert:** Surgery 2001; **Med School:** SUNY Upstate Med Univ 1973; **Resid:** Surgery, Duke Univ Med Ctr 1978; **Fellow:** Research, Natl Cancer Inst 1982; **Fac Appt:** Prof S, Stanford Univ

Pellegrini, Carlos MD [S] - **Spec Exp:** Esophageal Cancer; Esophageal Surgery; Barrett's Esophagus; Gastrointestinal Cancer & Surgery; **Hospital:** Univ Wash Med Ctr; **Address:** Univ Washington Medical Ctr, Dept Surgery, 1959 NE Pacific St, Box 356410, Seattle, WA 98195; **Phone:** 206-543-3106; **Board Cert:** Surgery 1998; **Med School:** Argentina 1971; **Resid:** Surgery, Granadero Hosp 1975; Surgery, Univ Chicago Hosps 1979; **Fac Appt:** Prof S, Univ Wash

Perkins, James D MD [S] - **Spec Exp:** Transplant-Pancreas; Transplant-Liver; Transplant-Kidney; **Hospital:** Univ Wash Med Ctr, Chldns Hosp and Regl Med Ctr - Seattle; **Address:** Univ Wash Med Ctr, Dept Surg, 1959 NE Pacific St, Box 356410, Seattle, WA 98195; **Phone:** 206-543-3825; **Board Cert:** Surgery 2004; **Med School:** Univ Ark 1979; **Resid:** Surgery, St Francis Regl Med Ctr 1984; **Fellow:** Transplant Surgery, Mayo Grad Sch; **Fac Appt:** Prof S, Univ Wash

Phillips, Edward H MD [S] - **Spec Exp:** Laparoscopic Surgery; Obesity/Bariatric Surgery; **Hospital:** Cedars-Sinai Med Ctr; **Address:** 8635 W 3rd St, Ste 795, Los Angeles, CA 90048-6101; **Phone:** 310-423-8350; **Board Cert:** Surgery 1998; **Med School:** USC Sch Med 1973; **Resid:** Surgery, USC Medical Ctr 1978; Vascular Surgery, Los Angeles Co-USC Medical Ctr 1979; **Fac Appt:** Assoc Clin Prof S, USC Sch Med

Rassman, William R MD [S] - **Spec Exp:** Hair Restoration/Transplant; **Address:** 2080 Century Park East, rm 607, Los Angeles, CA 90067; **Phone:** 310-553-9113; **Board Cert:** Surgery 1975; **Med School:** Med Coll VA 1966; **Resid:** Surgery, New York Hos -Cornell 1969; Surgery, Dartmouth Med Ctr 1973

Reber, Howard A MD [S] - **Spec Exp:** Pancreatic Cancer; Pancreatic Surgery; Gastrointestinal Cancer; **Hospital:** Ronald Reagan UCLA Med Ctr; **Address:** UCLA Medical Ctr, Dept Surgery, 10833 Le Conte Ave, Los Angeles, CA 90095-6904; **Phone:** 310-825-4976; **Board Cert:** Surgery 1971; **Med School:** Univ Pennsylvania 1964; **Resid:** Surgery, Hosp Univ Penn 1970; **Fac Appt:** Prof S, UCLA

Roberts, John P MD [S] - **Spec Exp:** Transplant-Liver; **Hospital:** UCSF Med Ctr, CA Pacific Med Ctr - Pacific Campus; **Address:** UCSF Medical Ctr, Div Transplant Surgery, 505 Parnassus Ave, rm M896, Box 0780, San Francisco, CA 94143-0780; **Phone:** 415-353-1888; **Board Cert:** Surgery 2006; **Med School:** UCSD 1980; **Resid:** Surgery, Univ Wash 1983; Surgery, Univ Wash 1987; **Fellow:** Surgery, Cornell-New York Hosp 1986; Transplant Surgery, Univ Minn Med Ctr 1988; **Fac Appt:** Prof S, UCSF

Rogers, Stanley J MD [S] - **Spec Exp:** Minimally Invasive Surgery; Gastrointestinal Surgery; Obesity/Bariatric Surgery; **Hospital:** San Francisco Genl Hosp, UCSF Med Ctr; **Address:** San Francisco General Hosp, Surgery, 1001 Potrero Ave, San Francisco, CA 94110; **Phone:** 415-206-6775; **Board Cert:** Surgery 2006; **Med School:** Univ Utah 1991; **Resid:** Surgery, UCSF Med Ctr 1997; **Fac Appt:** Assoc Prof S, UCSF

Satava, Richard M MD [S] - **Spec Exp:** Laparoscopic Abdominal Surgery; Gastrointestinal Surgery; **Hospital:** Univ Wash Med Ctr; **Address:** Univ Washington Med Ctr, Dept Surgery, 1959 NE Pacific St, Box 356410, Seattle, WA 98195; **Phone:** 206-685-0052; **Board Cert:** Surgery 2000; **Med School:** Hahnemann Univ 1968; **Resid:** Surgery, Mayo Clinic 1974; **Fellow:** Research, Mayo Clinic 1972

Selby, Robert R MD [S] - **Spec Exp:** Transplant-Liver; Transplant-Kidney; Transfusion Free Surgery; **Hospital:** USC Univ Hosp - R K Eamer Med Plz; **Address:** USC Univ Hosp, Organ Transplant, 1510 San Pablo St, Ste 200, Los Angeles, CA 90033-4612; **Phone:** 323-442-5908; **Board Cert:** Surgery 1999; Surgical Critical Care 2001; **Med School:** Univ MO-Columbia Sch Med 1979; **Resid:** Internal Medicine, Good Samaritan Hosp 1981; Surgery, Good Samaritan Hosp 1986; **Fellow:** Transplant Surgery, Presby Univ Hosp 1988; **Fac Appt:** Prof S, USC Sch Med

Silverstein, Melvin J MD [S] - **Spec Exp:** Breast Cancer; **Hospital:** Hoag Meml Hosp Presby; **Address:** 1 Hoag Drive, Box 6100, Newport Beach, CA 92658; **Phone:** 949-764-8281; **Board Cert:** Surgery 1971; **Med School:** Albany Med Coll 1965; **Resid:** Surgery, Boston City Hosp-Tufts Univ 1970; **Fellow:** Surgical Oncology, UCLA Med Ctr 1975

Sinanan, Mika N MD [S] - **Spec Exp:** Gastrointestinal Surgery; Gastrointestinal Cancer; Liver & Biliary Cancer; Laparoscopic Surgery; **Hospital:** Univ Wash Med Ctr; **Address:** Univ Washington, Dept Surgery, 1959 NE Pacific St, Box 356410, Seattle, WA 98195-6410; **Phone:** 206-543-5511; **Board Cert:** Surgery 1998; **Med School:** Johns Hopkins Univ 1980; **Resid:** Surgery, Univ Washington Hosp 1988; **Fellow:** Gastrointestinal Surgery, Univ Brit Columbia Med Ctr 1986; **Fac Appt:** Prof S, Univ Wash

Surgery

Sobel, Michael MD [S] - **Spec Exp:** Vein Disorders; **Hospital:** Univ Wash Med Ctr; **Address:** East Side Specialty Center, 1700 116th Ave NE, Bellevue, WA 98004; **Phone:** 425-646-7777; **Board Cert:** Surgery 2002; Vascular Surgery 1996; **Med School:** Albert Einstein Coll Med 1975; **Resid:** Surgery, Beth Israel Hosp 1982; **Fellow:** Vascular Surgery, NYU Med Ctr 1983; **Fac Appt:** Prof VascS, Univ Wash

Traverso, L William MD [S] - **Spec Exp:** Pancreatic Cancer; Laparoscopic Surgery; **Hospital:** Virginia Mason Med Ctr; **Address:** Virginia Mason Med Ctr, Dept Surg, 1100 9th Ave, Seattle, WA 98101; **Phone:** 206-223-8855; **Board Cert:** Surgery 1998; **Med School:** UCLA 1973; **Resid:** Surgery, UCLA Med Ctr 1978; **Fac Appt:** Clin Prof S, Univ Wash

Wagman, Lawrence D MD [S] - **Spec Exp:** Liver Cancer; Gastrointestinal Cancer; Breast Cancer; **Hospital:** City of Hope Natl Med Ctr & Beckman Rsch, San Dimas Comm Hosp; **Address:** City of Hope Natl Cancer Ctr, Dept Surgery, 1500 Duarte Rd, Duarte, CA 91010; **Phone:** 626-250-4673 x67100; **Board Cert:** Surgery 2005; **Med School:** Columbia P&S 1978; **Resid:** Surgery, Med Coll Virginia Hosp 1985; **Fellow:** Surgical Oncology, NIH/NCI 1982; **Fac Appt:** Assoc Clin Prof S, UCSD

Warren, Robert Samuel MD [S] - **Spec Exp:** Liver Cancer; **Hospital:** UCSF Med Ctr; **Address:** UCSF Comprehensive Cancer Center, 1600 Divisadero St Fl 4th, San Francisco, CA 94143-1932; **Phone:** 415-353-9846; **Board Cert:** Surgery 1998; **Med School:** Univ Minn 1980; **Resid:** Surgery, Univ Minn Hosps 1988; **Fellow:** Surgical Oncology, Meml Sloan-Kettering Cancer Ctr 1986; **Fac Appt:** Prof S, UCSF

Way, Lawrence W MD [S] - **Spec Exp:** Minimally Invasive Surgery; Liver Surgery; Pancreatic & Biliary Surgery; **Hospital:** UCSF Med Ctr; **Address:** 400 Parnassus Ave, Ste A655, Box 0338, San Francisco, CA 94143-0338; **Phone:** 415-353-2161; **Board Cert:** Surgery 1969; **Med School:** SUNY Buffalo 1959; **Resid:** Surgery, UCSF Med Ctr 1967; **Fellow:** Physiology, UCLA Med Ctr 1969; **Fac Appt:** Prof S, UCSF

Yeung, Raymond S W MD [S] - **Spec Exp:** Liver & Biliary Cancer; Liver Cancer; Melanoma; Breast Cancer; **Hospital:** Univ Wash Med Ctr; **Address:** Univ of Washington, Dept Surgery, 1959 NE Pacific St, Box 356410, Seattle, WA 98195-6410; **Phone:** 206-616-6408; **Board Cert:** Surgery 1999; **Med School:** Univ Toronto 1982; **Resid:** Surgery, University of Toronto 1987; **Fellow:** Surgical Oncology, Fox Chase Cancer Ctr 1992; **Fac Appt:** Prof S, Univ Wash

FOX CHASE
CANCER CENTER

333 Cottman Avenue
Philadelphia, PA 19111-2497
Phone: 1-888-FOX CHASE • Fax: 215-728-2702
www.fccc.edu

SURGICAL ONCOLOGY

The most experienced surgical oncologists have the best treatment outcomes. Fox Chase surgeons are highly specialized and focus solely on cancer care, including a wide variety of options ranging from minimally invasive approaches to complex plastic and reconstructive surgery.

Breast Cancer: We offer the most advanced diagnostic techniques, including digital mammography, stereotactic breast biopsy and sentinel lymph-node surgery. Treatment options include breast-preserving surgery with radiation therapy as well as skin-sparing mastectomy with cosmetic reconstructive surgery.

Gastrointestinal Cancers: Our gastrointestinal surgeons have extensive expertise with colorectal, pancreatic, gallbladder, liver and other bowel cancers and are the most experienced laparoscopic and robotic experts in the region. We also offer the most advanced endoscopic and minimally invasive techniques to avoid major surgery.

Genitourinary Cancers: Our urologic surgical oncologists have extensive expertise in the treatment of prostate, bladder, kidney, ureteral, adrenal, testicular and penile cancers. Our urologists emphasize organ preservation, quality of life and minimally invasive/robotic approaches to cancer surgery.

Gynecologic Cancers: Our gynecologic surgeons offer the most advanced laparoscopic and robotic techniques as well as complex open surgery for women with cancers of the uterus, ovary and cervix.

Head and Neck Cancers: The head and neck cancer center at Fox Chase provides patients with one-stop consultations with surgical, radiation and medical oncologists. Expertise includes otolaryngology, transoral laser surgery, plastic and microvascular reconstruction as well as robotic surgery.

Lung and Esophageal Cancers: Our thoracic surgeons offer a variety of minimally invasive techniques for patients with lung or esophageal cancers, including video-assisted thoracic surgery (VATS) and laparoscopic esophageal surgery. Fox Chase is one of only a few centers in the country offering these options.

Minimally Invasive Surgery

Our highly skilled surgeons are experts in minimally invasive procedures for cancer patients. Fox Chase is among the most experienced robotic centers in the region and use the most advanced robotic da Vinci S Surgical System for prostate, gynecologic, kidney and bladder, colon, lung and head and neck cancers.

Organ Preservation and Quality of Life

A major focus of surgical oncology at Fox Chase is preserving normal organ function and quality of life for cancer patients.

For more about Fox Chase physicians and services,
visit our web site, www.fccc.edu, or call 1-888-FOX CHASE.

Penn Medicine

Philadelphia, PA 19104
800.789.PENN
pennhealth.com

PENN ROBOTIC SURGERY

For more than 200 years, Penn has expanded the frontiers of medicine. Today, surgeons at Penn Medicine are leading the way in robotic-assisted surgery.

Most Comprehensive Program in the United States

Penn is home to five daVinci® Surgical Systems making it one of the largest robotic-assisted surgical programs in the United States. The equipment has been used for some time in urologic/prostate procedures, cardiac surgery, gastrointestinal and gynecological operations.

In addition, Penn surgeons have pioneered new procedures in head and neck surgery using the robotic-assisted technology. Penn was the first medical center in the world with an approved study to perform this surgery and many patients have benefited from transoral robotic surgery (TORS).

Benefits of Robotic Surgery

The advantages of robotic-assisted surgery include a tremendous enhancement in the surgeon's control of the instruments and the ability to perform more intricate procedures.

For patients, the benefits of robotic-assisted surgery may include:
- Less post-operative pain
- Less risk of infection
- Less anesthesia
- Less blood loss
- Shorter hospital stay
- Faster and more complete recovery
- Quicker return to normal daily activities

Experience Makes the Difference

Because of its many benefits, robotic-assisted surgery has gained increased popularity among the medical community in recent years. But technology is only as good as the hands that control it. Robotic technology is meant to be operated by skilled and experienced surgeons. The robotic surgery program at Penn is staffed by surgeons who far exceed the recommended level of experience required for its use.

Penn is also one of the largest, state-of-the-art surgical training centers in the country and the only training center on the East Coast for the new surgical system.

As the medical community embraces robotic-assisted surgery, our researchers, nurses, and surgeons remain at the forefront of this field by relentlessly advancing the application of this technology as well as educating the next generation of surgeons who will use it. The result is that Penn is the first place surgeons turn to learn the technology of tomorrow and the first place you should turn for answers.

Robotic Surgery Available at Penn:

- Cancer: Head and Neck, Throat, Mouth and Tongue, Prostate, Kidney, Heart, Uterus, Cervix

- Gastrointestinal: Bariatric LAP BAND®, Anti-reflux, Motility Disorders

- Gynecology: Pelvic Floor Reconstruction, Hysterectomy, Fibroid Removal, Myomectomy, Tubal Anastomosis

- Heart: Coronary Bypass, Mitral Valve Repair, Atrial Septal Defect Closure, Tumor Resection

- Urology: Prostatectomy, Nephrectomy, Pelvic Reconstruction

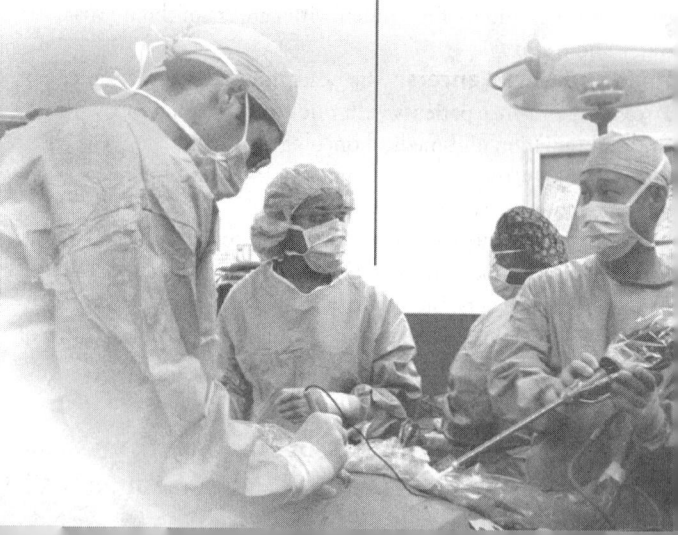

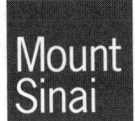
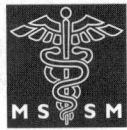

THE MOUNT SINAI MEDICAL CENTER
MINIMALLY INVASIVE SURGERY

One Gustave L. Levy Place
Fifth Avenue and 100th Street
New York, NY 10029-6574
Physician Referral: 1-800-MD-SINAI (637-4624)
www.mountsinai.org

The expert surgeons at Mount Sinai continue to be at the forefront of highly advanced, minimally invasive surgery. Using the latest instrumentation, Mount Sinai surgeons have applied these techniques to a broad spectrum of general and vascular surgical procedures, including aortic aneurysm repair, kidney transplantation, colon cancer resection, Crohn's disease surgery, robotic prostatectomy, and bariatric (weight loss) surgery.

Cardiac Surgeries
We perform many procedures using minimally invasive approaches, including aortic valve replacement, mitral valve replacement, mitral valve repair, and offpump coronary artery bypasses.

Weight Loss Surgeries
At Mount Sinai, we use the latest minimally invasive techniques to perform laparoscopic gastric bypass, lap band placement, duodenal switch, and sleeve gastrectomy. A full multidisciplinary team follows all aspects of pre- and postoperative care.

Urologic Surgeries
We can perform most traditional open surgeries laparoscopically, including nephrectomy, nephroureterectomy, radical prostatectomy, and cystectomy.

Transplant Surgeries
With laparoscopic kidney donation, we can remove kidneys from living donors using laparoscopic techniques.

Vascular Surgeries
Our vascular surgeons provide minimally invasive, durable treatments for vascular diseases such as aortic aneurysms, peripheral arterial occlusions, acute and chronic venous disease, and vascular trauma, as well as long-term vascular access for medical therapy or dialysis. Our surgeons were the first in the nation to perform minimally invasive aortic aneurysm repairs and are among the most experienced physicians in the world using this technique.

Abdominal Surgeries
We offer minimally invasive approaches for the treatment of diseases of the alimentary tract (esophagus, stomach) and gastrointestinal tract (small and large intestine, colon, rectum), as well as benign and malignant diseases of the hepatobiliary system.

Gynecologic Surgeries
We routinely treat endometriosis, uterine fibroids, ovarian cysts, and urinary incontinence laparoscopically. Surgeries for uterine, cervical, and ovarian cancers are also performed laparoscopically by our expert gynecologic oncologists.

ENT Surgeries
Top specialists in otolaryngologic surgery at Mount Sinai offer minimally invasive procedures and surgeries to treat many conditions involving the ear, nose, and throat, including cranial-based lesions, head and neck cancers, and nasal and sinus conditions.

TOP-RANKING MINIMALLY INVASIVE SURGEONS
In surveys of leading minimally invasive surgeons in a variety of specialties, Mount Sinai's physicians are consistently at the top of the lists in such areas as gynecologic oncology surgery, obstetrical surgery, colon and rectal surgery, liver and bilary surgery, thyroid surgery, hernia surgery, gastrointestinal surgery, thoracic surgery, and vascular surgery. Compared with traditional open surgery, minimally invasive procedures result in less tissue trauma, less scarring, and faster postoperative recovery time. Although the techniques vary from procedure to procedure and among different surgical subspecialties, minimally invasive surgical procedures typically employ video cameras and lens systems to provide anatomic visualization within a region of the body.

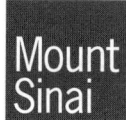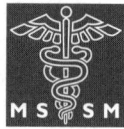

THE MOUNT SINAI MEDICAL CENTER
TRANSPLANTATION

One Gustave L. Levy Place
Fifth Avenue and 100th Street
New York, NY 10029-6574
Physician Referral: 1-800-MD-SINAI (637-4624)
www.mountsinai.org

Technological advances, along with improved medical therapies, continue to make hopes of a normal life after organ transplantation a reality. Today transplantation has become an accepted form of treatment for adults and children with a wide variety of diseases. Intensely committed to clinical and basic science research, members of Mount Sinai's Recanati/Miller Transplantation Institute investigate ways to improve organ preservation and reduce posttransplant complications and the side effects of immunosuppression. They also focus on the prevention of disease after a transplant and overall quality of life after this relatively new medical miracle.

A HISTORY OF ACHIEVEMENT

Mount Sinai surgeons were the first in New York State to perform liver transplantation, as well as the first in the state to perform living-donor liver transplantation.

CONTINUING THE TRADITION OF EXCELLENCE

Mount Sinai is one of the few hospitals in the country with expertise in small intestine/small bowel transplantation. Working closely with each patient's referring physician, our transplant specialists perform state-of-the-art procedures that profoundly affect patients' lives. Treatment at the Medical Center is not the end of the relationship. Caregivers at Mount Sinai continue to work with the referring physician to help maintain each patient's optimum health level.

A SAMPLING OF OUR INNOVATIVE PROGRAMS

The Kidney/Pancreas Transplant Program began more than thirty years ago, making Mount Sinai one of the first kidney transplant programs in the region. To date, the Medical Center has performed over 1,000 kidney transplants and approximately seventy pancreas transplants or combination kidney/pancreas procedures, for both adults and children. Although pancreas transplantation has gained widespread acceptance in the United States, Mount Sinai is one of the few centers in the greater New York area that performs the operation and is among the largest programs in the Northeast. Our Intestinal Transplant Program is one of the most established and respected in the nation. We offer a comprehensive approach to intestinal failure, and have developed a team approach that includes specialists from different fields working together to achieve the best possible result for each patient.

THE RECANATI/MILLER TRANSPLANTATION INSTITUTE

The Institute brings together clinical programs in adult and pediatric liver, kidney, pancreas, and intestine transplantation, and includes major research initiatives. In addition, heart and lung transplants are offered within the Department of Cardiothoracic Surgery. We are one of the largest transplant centers in the United States, performing more than 350 procedures annually. Patients from around the world come to Mount Sinai for transplants, including living-donor and traditional surgeries. The total volume of organ transplants at Mount Sinai places the hospital among the top academic medical centers nationally in this field.

NYU Langone Medical Center

550 First Avenue (at 31St Street)
New York, NY 10016
Physician Referral:
(888)7-NYU-MED (888-769-8633)
www.nyumc.org

MINIMALLY INVASIVE SURGERY

NYU Langone Medical Center has been at the forefront of minimally invasive surgery for two decades, treating conditions from heart disease, to prostate cancer, to obesity, to fetal anomalies in utero. Today, more patients are opting for minimally invasive procedures, a decision resulting in less pain, scarring, and surgical trauma. Post-operative recovery is also significantly reduced, allowing patients to resume their normal activities much sooner than with traditional surgery.

In 1996, surgeons at NYU Langone Medical Center performed the world's first minimally invasive valve repair and replacement, as well as the world's first triple cardiac bypass surgery. NYU vascular surgeons and radiologists helped pioneer minimally invasive aneurysm repair. In 1997, the Center installed the city's first Gamma Knife, a neurosurgical tool that allows surgeons to remove brain tumors that were once inoperable.

The Department of Surgery at New York University School of Medicine is a highly regarded and nationally recognized academic department. The department comprises divisions of:

Cardiothoracic Surgery

Minimally Invasive Surgery

Pediatric Surgery

Plastic Surgery (reconstructive and cosmetic) Surgical Oncology

Weight-Loss Surgery

Many faculty members receive national and international recognition for their work and hold leadership positions in both regional and national surgical societies. The department's goal is to develop leaders in clinical surgery and to provide the optimal academic surgical environment for patients, residents, and staff.

Thoracic Surgery

A thoracic surgeon provides the operative, perioperative care and critical care of patients with pathologic conditions within the chest. Included is the surgical care of coronary artery disease, cancers of the lung, esophagus and chest wall, abnormalities of the trachea, abnormalities of the great vessels and heart valves, congenital anomalies, tumors of the mediastinum and diseases of the diaphragm. The management of the airway and injuries of the chest is within the scope of the specialty.

Thoracic surgeons have the knowledge, experience and technical skills to accurately diagnose, operate upon safely and effectively manage patients with thoracic diseases of the chest. This requires substantial knowledge of cardiorespiratory physiology and oncology, as well as capability in the use of heart assist devices, management of abnormal heart rhythms and drainage of the chest cavity, respiratory support systems, endoscopy and invasive and noninvasive diagnostic techniques.

Training Required: Seven to eight years

THORACIC SURGERY

New England

Akins, Cary W MD [TS] - **Spec Exp:** Heart Valve Surgery; Coronary Artery Surgery; Aneurysm-Thoracic Aortic; **Hospital:** Mass Genl Hosp; **Address:** Mass Genl Hosp, Dept Surgery, Cox 648, Boston, MA 02114; **Phone:** 617-726-8218; **Board Cert:** Thoracic Surgery 2005; **Med School:** Harvard Med Sch 1970; **Resid:** Cardiovascular Surgery, Mass Genl Hosp 1975; **Fac Appt:** Clin Prof S, Harvard Med Sch

Bolman III, R Morton MD [TS] - **Spec Exp:** Heart Failure & Ventricular Containment; Ventricular Assist Device (LVAD); Mitral Valve Surgery; Aneurysm; **Hospital:** Brigham & Women's Hosp; **Address:** Brigham & Women's Hosp, Dept Cardiac Surg, 75 Francis St, rm CA211, Boston, MA 02115; **Phone:** 617-732-7678; **Board Cert:** Surgery 1991; Thoracic Surgery 2004; **Med School:** St Louis Univ 1973; **Resid:** Surgery, Duke Univ Med Ctr 1980; **Fellow:** Thoracic Surgery, Univ Minn Hosp 1982; **Fac Appt:** Prof S, Harvard Med Sch

Bueno, Raphael MD [TS] - **Spec Exp:** Lung Cancer; **Hospital:** Brigham & Women's Hosp; **Address:** Brigham and Women's Hospital, 75 Francis St, Division of Thoracic Surgery, Boston, MA 02115; **Phone:** 617-732-6824; **Board Cert:** Thoracic Surgery 2006; Surgery 2002; Surgical Critical Care 2003; **Med School:** Harvard Med Sch 1985; **Resid:** Surgery, Brigham & Women's Hosp 1992; **Fellow:** Surgical Critical Care, Brigham & Women's Hosp 1993; Cardiothoracic Surgery, Mass Genl Hosp 1997; **Fac Appt:** Assoc Prof S, Harvard Med Sch

DeCamp Jr, Malcolm M MD [TS] - **Spec Exp:** Lung Surgery; Esophageal Surgery; **Hospital:** Beth Israel Deaconess Med Ctr - Boston; **Address:** BIDMC-185 Pilgrim Rd, Deaconess Bldg - Ste 201, Boston, MA 02215; **Phone:** 617-632-8252; **Board Cert:** Surgery 2001; Thoracic Surgery 2003; **Med School:** Univ Louisville Sch Med 1983; **Resid:** Surgery, Brighams & Womens Hosp 1986; Surgery, Brighams & Womens Hosp 1990; **Fellow:** Cardiac Surgery, Brighams & Womens Hosp 1993; **Fac Appt:** Assoc Prof S, Harvard Med Sch

Elefteriades, John MD [TS] - **Spec Exp:** Aneurysm-Thoracic Aortic; Transplant-Heart; Ventricular Assist Device (LVAD); **Hospital:** Yale-New Haven Hosp; **Address:** Yale Sch of Medicine, Dept Cardiothoracic Surgery, PO Box 208039, New Haven, CT 06520; **Phone:** 203-785-2705; **Board Cert:** Thoracic Surgery 2004; **Med School:** Yale Univ 1976; **Resid:** Surgery, Yale-New Haven Hosp 1981; Cardiothoracic Surgery, Yale-New Haven Hosp 1983; **Fellow:** Cardiothoracic Surgery, Yale-New Haven Hosp 1983; **Fac Appt:** Prof S, Yale Univ

Gaissert, Henning A MD [TS] - **Spec Exp:** Esophageal Cancer; Tracheal Surgery; Lung Cancer; **Hospital:** Mass Genl Hosp; **Address:** Division of Thoracic Surgery, 55 Fruit St, BLK 1570, Boston, MA 02114; **Phone:** 617-726-5341; **Board Cert:** Surgery 2001; Thoracic Surgery 2004; **Med School:** Germany 1984; **Resid:** Surgery, Mass Genl Hosp 1989; Surgery, Barnes Jewish Hosp 1991; **Fellow:** Research, Harvard Med Sch 1993; Cardiothoracic Surgery, Barnes Jewish Hosp 1996; **Fac Appt:** Assoc Prof S, Harvard Med Sch

Kopf, Gary S MD [TS] - **Spec Exp:** Cardiac Surgery; Pediatric Cardiothoracic Surgery; Congenital Heart Disease; **Hospital:** Yale-New Haven Hosp; **Address:** Yale University School of Medicine, Dept of Surgery, Box 208039, New Haven, CT 06520-8039; **Phone:** 203-785-2702; **Board Cert:** Thoracic Surgery 2000; **Med School:** Harvard Med Sch 1970; **Resid:** Surgery, Peter Bent Brigham Hosp 1977; Cardiothoracic Surgery, Chldns Hosp Med Ctr 1980; **Fellow:** Cardiothoracic Surgery, Peter Bent Brigham Hosp 1980; **Fac Appt:** Prof S, Yale Univ

Mathisen, Douglas MD [TS] - **Spec Exp:** Tracheal Surgery; Lung Cancer; Esophageal Cancer; **Hospital:** Mass Genl Hosp, Newton - Wellesley Hosp; **Address:** Mass Genl Hosp, Dept Thor Surg, 55 Fruit St, Blake 1570, Boston, MA 02114; **Phone:** 617-726-6826; **Board Cert:** Thoracic Surgery 2002; **Med School:** Univ IL Coll Med 1974; **Resid:** Surgery, Mass Genl Hosp 1981; Thoracic Surgery, Mass Genl Hosp 1982; **Fellow:** Surgical Oncology, Natl Cancer Inst 1979; **Fac Appt:** Prof S, Harvard Med Sch

Nugent, William MD [TS] - **Spec Exp:** Thoracic Cancers; **Hospital:** Dartmouth - Hitchcock Med Ctr; **Address:** Dartmouth-Hitchcock Med Ctr, Dept Cardiothoracic Surgery, 1 Medical Center Drive, Lebanon, NH 03756-1000; **Phone:** 603-650-8572; **Board Cert:** Thoracic Surgery 2002; **Med School:** Albany Med Coll 1975; **Resid:** Surgery, Beth Israel Hosp 1980; Thoracic Surgery, Univ Michigan 1983; **Fellow:** Cardiothoracic Surgery, Mass Genl Hosp 1981; **Fac Appt:** Prof S, Dartmouth Med Sch

Sellke, Frank W MD [TS] - **Spec Exp:** Heart Valve Surgery; Angiogenesis; Coronary Artery Surgery; **Hospital:** Beth Israel Deaconess Med Ctr - Boston, Landmark Med Ctr; **Address:** Beth Israel Deaconess Med Ctr, Cardiac Surgery, 110 Francis St, Ste 2A, Boston, MA 02215; **Phone:** 617-632-8383; **Board Cert:** Surgery 2006; Thoracic Surgery 1999; **Med School:** Indiana Univ 1981; **Resid:** Surgery, Akron City Hosp 1987; Cardiothoracic Surgery, Univ Iowa Hosps & Clinics 1990; **Fac Appt:** Prof S, Harvard Med Sch

Singh, Arun K MD [TS] - **Spec Exp:** Cardiac Surgery; **Hospital:** Rhode Island Hosp; **Address:** CVT Surgical Group, 2 Dudley St, Ste 470, Providence, RI 02905-3248; **Phone:** 401-274-7546; **Board Cert:** Surgery 1973; Thoracic Surgery 1975; **Med School:** India 1967; **Resid:** Surgery, Columbia Presbyterian Med Ctr 1972; Cardiothoracic Surgery, Rhode Island Hosp 1974; **Fellow:** Cardiac Surgery, Hosp Sick Children 1975; **Fac Appt:** Clin Prof S, Brown Univ

Sugarbaker, David J MD [TS] - **Spec Exp:** Mesothelioma; Transplant-Lung; Esophageal Cancer; **Hospital:** Brigham & Women's Hosp, Dana-Farber Cancer Inst; **Address:** Brigham & Women's Hosp, 75 Francis St, Division of Thoracic Surgery, Boston, MA 02115-6110; **Phone:** 617-732-6824; **Board Cert:** Thoracic Surgery 1999; **Med School:** Cornell Univ-Weill Med Coll 1979; **Resid:** Surgery, Brigham & Women's Hosp 1982; Surgery, Brigham & Women's Hosp 1986; **Fellow:** Thoracic Surgery, Toronto Genl Hosp 1988; **Fac Appt:** Prof S, Harvard Med Sch

Swanson, Scott J MD [TS] - **Spec Exp:** Lung Cancer; Video Assisted Thoracic Surgery (VATS); Esophageal Cancer; **Hospital:** Brigham & Women's Hosp, Dana-Farber Cancer Inst; **Address:** Div Thoracic Surgery, Brigham & Women's Hosp, 75 Francis St, Boston, MA 02115; **Phone:** 617-525-7532; **Board Cert:** Surgery 2003; Thoracic Surgery 2006; **Med School:** Harvard Med Sch 1985; **Resid:** Surgery, Brigham & Womens Hosp 1990; **Fellow:** Cardiothoracic Surgery, Brigham & Womens Hosp 1994

Vander Salm, Thomas MD [TS] - **Spec Exp:** Heart Valve Surgery-Mitral; Cardiovascular Surgery; **Hospital:** N Shore Med Ctr - Salem Hosp; **Address:** Salem Hosp, Div Cardiac Surgery, 81 Highland Ave, Salem, MA 01970; **Phone:** 978-354-2500; **Board Cert:** Surgery 1974; Thoracic Surgery 2006; **Med School:** Johns Hopkins Univ 1966; **Resid:** Surgery, Mass Genl Hosp 1968; Surgery, Johns Hopkins Hosp 1969; **Fac Appt:** Prof S, Univ Mass Sch Med

Wain, John MD [TS] - **Spec Exp:** Transplant-Lung; Lung Cancer; Esophageal Cancer; **Hospital:** Mass Genl Hosp; **Address:** Mass Genl Hosp, Dept Thoracic Surg, 55 Fruit St, Blake 1570, Boston, MA 02114; **Phone:** 617-726-5200; **Board Cert:** Thoracic Surgery 2000; **Med School:** Jefferson Med Coll 1980; **Resid:** Surgery, Mass Genl Hosp 1985; **Fellow:** Cardiothoracic Surgery, Mass Genl Hosp 1988; **Fac Appt:** Asst Prof TS, Harvard Med Sch

Thoracic Surgery

Wright, Cameron D MD [TS] - **Spec Exp:** Lung Cancer; Esophageal Cancer; Tracheal Surgery; **Hospital:** Mass Genl Hosp; **Address:** Mass Genl Hosp, Div Thoracic Surg, 55 Fruit St, Blake 1570, Boston, MA 02114-2696; **Phone:** 617-726-5801; **Board Cert:** Surgery 2006; Thoracic Surgery 1997; **Med School:** Univ Mich Med Sch 1980; **Resid:** Surgery, Mass Genl Hosp 1986; Thoracic Surgery, Mass Genl Hosp 1988; **Fac Appt:** Assoc Prof S, Harvard Med Sch

Mid Atlantic

Acker, Michael A MD [TS] - **Spec Exp:** Transplant-Heart; Ventricular Assist Device (LVAD); Coronary Artery Surgery; Heart Valve Surgery; **Hospital:** Hosp Univ Penn - UPHS (page 60); **Address:** 3400 Spruce St, 4 Silverstein Pavillion, Philadelphia, PA 19104-4227; **Phone:** 215-349-8305; **Board Cert:** Surgery 2001; Thoracic Surgery 2001; **Med School:** Brown Univ 1981; **Resid:** Surgery, Hosp Univ Penn 1988; Cardiothoracic Surgery, Johns Hopkins Hosp 1991; **Fac Appt:** Assoc Prof S, Univ Pennsylvania

Adams, David H MD [TS] - **Spec Exp:** Mitral Valve Surgery; Heart Valve Surgery; Coronary Artery Surgery; **Hospital:** Mount Sinai Med Ctr (page 64); **Address:** Mt Sinai Hosp, Cardiac & Thoracic Surg, 1190 Fifth Ave, Box 1028, New York, NY 10029; **Phone:** 212-659-6820; **Board Cert:** Thoracic Surgery 2003; **Med School:** Duke Univ 1983; **Resid:** Surgery, Brigham & Women's Hosp 1988; Thoracic Surgery, Brigham & Women's Hosp 1990; **Fac Appt:** Prof TS, Mount Sinai Sch Med

Altorki, Nasser MD [TS] - **Spec Exp:** Esophageal Cancer; Lung Cancer; Gastroesophageal Reflux Disease (GERD); Thoracic Cancers; **Hospital:** NY-Presby Hosp/Weill Cornell (page 66); **Address:** 525 E 68th St, New York, NY 10021-4870; **Phone:** 212-746-5156; **Board Cert:** Surgery 2006; Thoracic Surgery 1998; **Med School:** Egypt 1978; **Resid:** Surgery, Univ Chicago Hosps 1985; **Fellow:** Cardiothoracic Surgery, Univ Chicago Hosps 1987; **Fac Appt:** Prof S, Cornell Univ-Weill Med Coll

Argenziano, Michael MD [TS] - **Spec Exp:** Robotic Cardiac Surgery; Coronary Artery Robotic Surgery; Maze Procedure for Atrial Fibrillation; **Hospital:** NY-Presby Hosp/Columbia (page 66); **Address:** Columbia Presby Med Ctr, Milstein Bldg, 177 Fort Washington Ave, rm 7-435, New York, NY 10032; **Phone:** 212-305-5888; **Board Cert:** Surgery 1999; Thoracic Surgery 2002; **Med School:** Columbia P&S 1992; **Resid:** Surgery, Columbia Presby Med Ctr 1998; **Fellow:** Cardiothoracic Surgery, Columbia Presby Med Ctr 1999; **Fac Appt:** Asst Prof S, Columbia P&S

Bains, Manjit MD [TS] - **Spec Exp:** Cardiothoracic Surgery; Esophageal Cancer; Lung Cancer; **Hospital:** Meml Sloan-Kettering Cancer Ctr; **Address:** 1275 York Avenue, New York, NY 10065; **Phone:** 800-525-2225; **Board Cert:** Surgery 1971; Thoracic Surgery 1972; **Med School:** India 1963; **Resid:** Surgery, Rochester Genl Hosp 1970; **Fellow:** Thoracic Surgery, Sloan Kettering Cancer Ctr 1972; **Fac Appt:** Clin Prof S, Cornell Univ-Weill Med Coll

Baumgartner, William MD [TS] - **Spec Exp:** Cardiac Surgery; **Hospital:** Johns Hopkins Hosp - Baltimore (page 61); **Address:** 600 N Wolfe St, Blalock Bldg, Ste 618, Baltimore, MD 21287; **Phone:** 410-955-5248; **Board Cert:** Thoracic Surgery 2001; **Med School:** Univ KY Coll Med 1973; **Resid:** Surgery, Stanford Univ Med Ctr 1975; Thoracic Surgery, Stanford Univ Med Ctr 1976; **Fac Appt:** Prof S, Johns Hopkins Univ

Bavaria, Joseph E MD [TS] - **Spec Exp:** Aortic Surgery; Transplant-Lung; Heart Valve Surgery; **Hospital:** Hosp Univ Penn - UPHS (page 60); **Address:** Hosp Univ Pennsylvania, 3400 Spruce St, 4 Silverstein, Philadelphia, PA 19104; **Phone:** 215-662-2017; **Board Cert:** Thoracic Surgery 2001; **Med School:** Tulane Univ 1983; **Resid:** Surgery, Hosp U Penn 1990; Cardiothoracic Surgery, Hosp U Penn/Children's Hosp 1992; **Fac Appt:** Prof S, Univ Pennsylvania

Bridges, Charles R MD [TS] - **Spec Exp:** Minimally Invasive Cardiac Surgery; Maze Procedure for Atrial Fibrillation; Aneurysm-Aortic; Heart Valve Surgery; **Hospital:** Pennsylvania Hosp (page 60), Hosp Univ Penn - UPHS (page 60); **Address:** 230 W Washington Square Fl 3, Farm Journal Bldg, Philadelphia, PA 19107; **Phone:** 215-829-8713; **Board Cert:** Surgery 2003; Thoracic Surgery 2004; **Med School:** Harvard Med Sch 1981; **Resid:** Internal Medicine, Brigham & Women's Hosp 1984; Surgery, Hosp U Penn 1991; **Fellow:** Cardiothoracic Surgery, Hosp U Penn 1993; **Fac Appt:** Assoc Prof S, Univ Pennsylvania

Conte Jr, John V MD [TS] - **Spec Exp:** Transplant-Heart; Transplant-Lung; Cardiac Surgery-Adult; **Hospital:** Johns Hopkins Hosp - Baltimore (page 61); **Address:** 600 N Wolfe St, Blalock 618, Baltimore, MD 21287-4618; **Phone:** 410-955-1753; **Board Cert:** Thoracic Surgery 1997; **Med School:** Georgetown Univ 1986; **Resid:** Surgery, Georgetown Univ Med Ctr 1992; Stanford Univ Med Ctr 1995

Cooper, Joel D MD [TS] - **Spec Exp:** Transplant-Lung; Emphysema-Lung Volume Reduction; Lung Surgery; **Hospital:** Hosp Univ Penn - UPHS (page 60); **Address:** Hosp Univ Penn, 3400 Spruce St, 4 Silverstein, Philadelphia, PA 19104; **Phone:** 215-662-2005; **Board Cert:** Surgery 1971; Thoracic Surgery 1972; **Med School:** Harvard Med Sch 1964; **Resid:** Surgery, Mass Genl Hosp 1968; Thoracic Surgery, Frenchay Hosp; **Fellow:** Research, Hammersmith Hosp; Thoracic Surgery, Mass Genl Hosp; **Fac Appt:** Prof S, Univ Pennsylvania

Demmy, Todd L MD [TS] - **Spec Exp:** Lung Cancer; Thoracic Cancers; Esophageal Cancer; **Hospital:** Roswell Park Cancer Inst, Buffalo General Hosp; **Address:** Roswell Park Cancer Inst, Carlton Bldg, Elm & Carlton Sts, rm 243, Buffalo, NY 14263; **Phone:** 716-845-5873; **Board Cert:** Surgery 1997; Thoracic Surgery 2000; Surgical Critical Care 2001; **Med School:** Jefferson Med Coll 1983; **Resid:** Surgery, Baylor Univ Medical Ctr 1988; Thoracic Surgery, Allegheny Genl Hosp 1991; **Fac Appt:** Assoc Prof S, SUNY Buffalo

Diehl, James T MD [TS] - **Spec Exp:** Cardiac Surgery-Adult; Aortic Surgery; **Hospital:** Thomas Jefferson Univ Hosp, Albert Einstein Med Ctr; **Address:** 1025 Walnut St, Ste 607, Philadelphia, PA 19107; **Phone:** 215-955-5654; **Board Cert:** Thoracic Surgery 2004; **Med School:** Albert Einstein Coll Med 1978; **Resid:** Surgery, Cleveland Clinic 1984; Cardiothoracic Surgery, Univ Toronto Med Ctr 1986; **Fac Appt:** Prof S, Thomas Jefferson Univ

Friedberg, Joseph MD [TS] - **Spec Exp:** Lung Cancer; Mesothelioma; Photodynamic Therapy; **Hospital:** Penn Presby Med Ctr - UPHS (page 60), Hosp Univ Penn - UPHS (page 60); **Address:** Penn-Presbyterian Medical Ctr, 51 N 39th St, rm W250, Philadelphia, PA 19104; **Phone:** 215-662-9195; **Board Cert:** Surgery 2006; Thoracic Surgery 2006; **Med School:** Harvard Med Sch 1986; **Resid:** Surgery, Mass General Hosp 1994; **Fellow:** Cardiothoracic Surgery, Brigham & Womens Hosp 1996

Furukawa, Satoshi MD [TS] - **Spec Exp:** Transplant-Heart & Lung; Cardiac Surgery-High Risk; Heart Valve Surgery; Minimally Invasive Cardiac Surgery; **Hospital:** Temple Univ Hosp; **Address:** 3401 N Broad St, Ste 300, Philadelphia, PA 19140; **Phone:** 215-707-3601; **Board Cert:** Surgery 2003; Thoracic Surgery 2005; **Med School:** Univ Pennsylvania 1984; **Resid:** Surgery, Hosp Univ Penn 1991; Thoracic Surgery, Hosp Univ Penn 1993; **Fac Appt:** Prof TS, Temple Univ

Galloway, Aubrey MD [TS] - **Spec Exp:** Minimally Invasive Heart Valve Surgery; Coronary Artery Surgery; Aneurysm-Thoracic Aortic; **Hospital:** NYU Med Ctr (page 68), Bellevue Hosp Ctr; **Address:** 530 1st Ave, Ste 9V, New York, NY 10016-6402; **Phone:** 212-263-7185; **Board Cert:** Thoracic Surgery 2006; **Med School:** Tulane Univ 1978; **Resid:** Surgery, Univ Colo Hlth Sci Ctr 1983; Cardiovascular Surgery, NYU Med Ctr 1985; **Fellow:** Research, Boston Children's Hosp 1981; Cardiothoracic Surgery, NYU Med Ctr 1985; **Fac Appt:** Prof TS, NYU Sch Med

Thoracic Surgery

Gharagozloo, Farid MD [TS] - **Spec Exp:** Video Assisted Thoracic Surgery (VATS); Lung Cancer; **Hospital:** G Washington Univ Hosp, Harbor Hosp Ctr; **Address:** 2175 K St NW, Ste 300, Washington, DC 20037; **Phone:** 202-775-8600; **Board Cert:** Thoracic Surgery 2001; **Med School:** Johns Hopkins Univ 1983; **Resid:** Surgery, Mayo Clinic 1989; Research, Harvard Med Sch 1986; **Fellow:** Cardiothoracic Surgery, Mayo Clinic 1992; **Fac Appt:** Prof S

Girardi Jr, Leonard N MD [TS] - **Spec Exp:** Aneurysm-Aortic; Cardiac Surgery; Marfan's Syndrome; Cardiothoracic Surgery; **Hospital:** NY-Presby Hosp/Weill Cornell (page 66); **Address:** 525 E 68th St, M404, New York, NY 10021; **Phone:** 212-746-5194; **Board Cert:** Surgery 2005; Thoracic Surgery 1998; **Med School:** Cornell Univ-Weill Med Coll 1989; **Resid:** Surgery, NY Presby-Cornell Med Ctr 1994; **Fellow:** Cardiothoracic Surgery, NY Presby Hosp 1996; Cardiothoracic Surgery, Baylor Coll Med 1997; **Fac Appt:** Assoc Prof TS, Cornell Univ-Weill Med Coll

Graver, L Michael MD [TS] - **Spec Exp:** Heart Valve Surgery-Aortic; Coronary Artery Surgery; Atrial Fibrillation; **Hospital:** Long Island Jewish Med Ctr, N Shore Univ Hosp; **Address:** 270-05 76th Ave, New Hyde Park, NY 11040-1433; **Phone:** 718-470-7460; **Board Cert:** Surgery 2003; Thoracic Surgery 2004; **Med School:** Albany Med Coll 1977; **Resid:** Surgery, St Luke's-Roosevelt Hosp Ctr 1982; Cardiovascular Surgery, Deaconness Hosp 1983; **Fellow:** Cardiovascular Pathology, NY Hosp-Cornell Med Ctr 1985; **Fac Appt:** Prof TS, Albert Einstein Coll Med

Griepp, Randall MD [TS] - **Spec Exp:** Aneurysm-Abdominal Aortic; Aneurysm-Thoracic Aortic; **Hospital:** Mount Sinai Med Ctr (page 64); **Address:** Mt Sinai Med Ctr, Dept Cardiothoracic Surg, 1190 5th Ave, New York, NY 10029; **Phone:** 212-659-9495; **Board Cert:** Thoracic Surgery 1997; **Med School:** Stanford Univ 1967; **Resid:** Surgery, Stanford Univ Hosp 1973; **Fellow:** Cardiothoracic Surgery, Stanford Univ Hosp 1972; **Fac Appt:** Prof TS, Mount Sinai Sch Med

Griffith, Bartley MD [TS] - **Spec Exp:** Transplant-Heart & Lung; Heart Valve Surgery; Aneurysm-Aortic; **Hospital:** Univ of MD Med Sys; **Address:** Univ Maryland, Div Cardiac Surg, N4W94, 22 S Greene St, Baltimore, MD 21201; **Phone:** 410-328-3822; **Board Cert:** Thoracic Surgery 2001; **Med School:** Jefferson Med Coll 1974; **Resid:** Surgery, Univ Hlth Ctr Hosps 1979; Thoracic Surgery, Univ Hlth Ctr Hosps 1981; **Fellow:** Research, Univ Hlth Ctr Hosps 1978; **Fac Appt:** Prof S, Univ MD Sch Med

Grossi, Eugene A MD [TS] - **Spec Exp:** Minimally Invasive Cardiac Surgery; Mitral Valve Surgery; Cardiac Tumors, Myxomas; **Hospital:** NYU Med Ctr (page 68); **Address:** NYU Med Ctr, 530 1st Ave, Ste 9V, New York, NY 10016-6402; **Phone:** 212-263-7452; **Board Cert:** Thoracic Surgery 2002; **Med School:** Columbia P&S 1981; **Resid:** Surgery, NYU Med Ctr 1987; Thoracic Surgery, NYU Med Ctr 1991; **Fac Appt:** Assoc Prof S, NYU Sch Med

Hargrove III, W Clark MD [TS] - **Spec Exp:** Mitral Valve Robotic Surgery; Heart Valve Surgery; Minimally Invasive Cardiac Surgery; **Hospital:** Penn Presby Med Ctr - UPHS (page 60); **Address:** Philadelphia Heart Inst, 51 N 39th St, Ste 2D, Philadelphia, PA 19104; **Phone:** 215-662-9595; **Board Cert:** Thoracic Surgery 2004; **Med School:** Wake Forest Univ 1973; **Resid:** Surgery, Hosp U Penn 1979; Cardiothoracic Surgery, Hosp U Penn 1984; **Fellow:** Vascular Surgery, Hosp U Penn 1981; **Fac Appt:** Clin Prof S, Univ Pennsylvania

Heitmiller, Richard F MD [TS] - **Spec Exp:** Esophageal Surgery; Esophageal Cancer; Lung Cancer; **Hospital:** Union Meml Hosp - Baltimore; **Address:** 3333 N Calvert St, Ste 610, Baltimore, MD 21218; **Phone:** 410-554-2063; **Board Cert:** Surgery 1997; Thoracic Surgery 1999; **Med School:** Johns Hopkins Univ 1979; **Resid:** Surgery, Mass Genl Hosp 1985; **Fellow:** Thoracic Surgery, Mass Genl Hosp 1987; **Fac Appt:** Assoc Prof Surg & Onc, Johns Hopkins Univ

Isom, O Wayne MD [TS] - **Spec Exp:** Cardiac Surgery; Coronary Artery Surgery; Heart Valve Surgery; **Hospital:** NY-Presby Hosp/Weill Cornell (page 66), NY Hosp Queens; **Address:** 525 E 68th St, rm M-404, New York, NY 10065; **Phone:** 212-746-5151; **Board Cert:** Surgery 1971; Thoracic Surgery 1972; **Med School:** Univ Tex, Houston 1965; **Resid:** Surgery, Parkland Meml Hosp 1970; **Fellow:** Thoracic Surgery, NYU Med Ctr 1972; **Fac Appt:** Prof TS, Cornell Univ-Weill Med Coll

Jonas, Richard A MD [TS] - **Spec Exp:** Pediatric Cardiothoracic Surgery; Congenital Heart Surgery; **Hospital:** Chldns Natl Med Ctr, Georgetown Univ Hosp; **Address:** 111 Michigan Ave NW, Washington, DC 20010; **Phone:** 202-884-2811; **Med School:** Australia 1974; **Resid:** Surgery, Royal Melbourne Hosp 1979; Thoracic Surgery, Green Lane Hosp 1982; **Fellow:** Thoracic Surgery, Brigham & Women's Hosp 1984

Kaiser, Larry R MD [TS] - **Spec Exp:** Lung Cancer; Esophageal Cancer; Mediastinal Tumors; **Hospital:** Hosp Univ Penn - UPHS (page 60), Pennsylvania Hosp (page 60); **Address:** Hosp Univ Pennsylvania, Dept Surgery, 3400 Spruce St, 4 Silverstein, Philadelphia, PA 19104-4219; **Phone:** 215-662-7538; **Board Cert:** Surgery 2005; Thoracic Surgery 2007; **Med School:** Tulane Univ 1977; **Resid:** Surgery, UCLA Med Ctr 1983; Cardiothoracic Surgery, Univ Toronto Hosps 1985; **Fellow:** Surgical Oncology, UCLA Med Ctr 1981; **Fac Appt:** Prof S, Univ Pennsylvania

Kanda, Louis T MD [TS] - **Spec Exp:** Heart Valve Surgery; **Hospital:** Washington Hosp Ctr; **Address:** Washington Regl Cardiac Surg, 110 Irving St NW, Ste 1E3, Washington, DC 20010; **Phone:** 202-877-5039; **Board Cert:** Thoracic Surgery 1991; **Med School:** Geo Wash Univ 1970; **Resid:** Surgery, Washington Hosp Ctr 1975; **Fellow:** Cardiothoracic Surgery, Cleveland Clin Fdn 1980; **Fac Appt:** Asst Prof S, Howard Univ

Katz, Nevin M MD [TS] - **Spec Exp:** Coronary Artery Surgery; Heart Valve Surgery; Critical Care; **Hospital:** G Washington Univ Hosp; **Address:** 2175 K St NW, Ste 300, Washington, DC 20037; **Phone:** 202-775-8600; **Board Cert:** Thoracic Surgery 2000; **Med School:** Case West Res Univ 1971; **Resid:** Surgery, Mass Genl Hosp 1976; Cardiothoracic Surgery, Univ Alabama Hosp 1980; **Fellow:** Cardiovascular Surgery, Univ Alabama 1978; **Fac Appt:** Clin Prof S, Geo Wash Univ

Keenan, Robert J MD [TS] - **Spec Exp:** Lung Cancer; Esophageal Cancer; Mediastinal Tumors; Emphysema-Lung Volume Reduction; **Hospital:** Allegheny General Hosp, Westmoreland Hosp; **Address:** Allegheny Genl Hosp, 14th Fl, 320 E North Ave, Pittsburgh, PA 15212; **Phone:** 412-359-6137; **Board Cert:** Surgery 2000; **Med School:** Canada 1984; **Resid:** Surgery, Univ Toronto Med Ctr 1989; **Fellow:** Thoracic Surgery, Univ Pittsburgh Med Ctr 1990; Thoracic Surgery, Univ Toronto Med Ctr 1991; **Fac Appt:** Prof TS, Drexel Univ Coll Med

Keller, Steven M MD [TS] - **Spec Exp:** Lung Cancer; Esophageal Cancer; Hyperhidrosis-Palmar; **Hospital:** Montefiore Med Ctr; **Address:** Greene Medical Arts Pavilion, 3400 Bainbridge Ave Fl 5 - Ste A, Bronx, NY 10467-2404; **Phone:** 718-920-7580; **Board Cert:** Surgery 1996; Thoracic Surgery 1996; **Med School:** Albany Med Coll 1977; **Resid:** Surgery, Mount Sinai Hosp 1985; Thoracic Surgery, Mem Sloan Kettering Cancer Ctr 1987; **Fellow:** Surgical Oncology, NIH/National Cancer Inst 1983; **Fac Appt:** Prof TS, Albert Einstein Coll Med

Kormos, Robert MD [TS] - **Spec Exp:** Transplant-Heart; Artificial Heart Devices; **Hospital:** UPMC Presby, Pittsburgh; **Address:** UPMC Presbyterian Hosp, 200 Lothrop St, Ste C700, Pittsburgh, PA 15213; **Phone:** 412-648-6259; **Med School:** Univ Western Ontario 1976; **Resid:** Surgery, Toronto Western Hosp 1978; Cardiothoracic Surgery, Toronto Genl Hosp/Hosp for Sick Chldn 1982; **Fellow:** Transplant Surgery, Univ Pittsburgh Med Ctr 1987; **Fac Appt:** Prof S, Univ Pittsburgh

Thoracic Surgery

Krasna, Mark MD [TS] - **Spec Exp:** Esophageal Cancer; Lung Cancer; Mesothelioma; **Hospital:** St Joseph Med Ctr, Univ of MD Med Sys; **Address:** 7505 Osler Drive Odea Bldg - Ste 303, Towson, MD 21204; **Phone:** 410-427-2220; **Board Cert:** Thoracic Surgery 2000; **Med School:** Israel 1982; **Resid:** Surgery, CMDNJ-Rutgers Med Sch 1988; **Fellow:** Cardiothoracic Surgery, New England Deaconess-Harvard 1990; **Fac Appt:** Prof S, Univ MD Sch Med

Krellenstein, Daniel J MD [TS] - **Spec Exp:** Lung Cancer; Minimally Invasive Thoracic Surgery; Asbestos-related Lung Disease; **Hospital:** Mount Sinai Med Ctr (page 64), Lenox Hill Hosp (page 62); **Address:** 16 E 98th St, Ste 1F, New York, NY 10029-6545; **Phone:** 212-423-9311; **Board Cert:** Surgery 1974; Thoracic Surgery 2006; **Med School:** SUNY Buffalo 1964; **Resid:** Surgery, SUNY Downstate Med Ctr 1972; **Fac Appt:** Assoc Clin Prof TS, Mount Sinai Sch Med

Krieger, Karl H MD [TS] - **Spec Exp:** Heart Valve Surgery; Coronary Artery Surgery; Cardiac Surgery-Adult; **Hospital:** NY-Presby Hosp/Weill Cornell (page 66), NY Hosp Queens; **Address:** Cardiothoracic Surgery Dept, 525 E 68th St, Ste M404, New York, NY 10021-4873; **Phone:** 212-746-5152; **Board Cert:** Thoracic Surgery 2004; **Med School:** Johns Hopkins Univ 1975; **Resid:** Surgery, Johns Hopkins 1976; Bellevue Hosp 1979; **Fellow:** Thoracic Surgery, NYU Med Ctr 1981; **Fac Appt:** Prof S, Cornell Univ-Weill Med Coll

Lang, Samuel MD [TS] - **Spec Exp:** Minimally Invasive Cardiac Surgery; Heart Valve Surgery; **Hospital:** St Vincent Cath Med Ctrs - Manhattan; **Address:** 170 W 12th St, Spellman-6, New York, NY 10011; **Phone:** 212-604-2488; **Board Cert:** Thoracic Surgery 2006; **Med School:** Univ Ala 1978; **Resid:** Surgery, UCLA Med Ctr 1982; Thoracic Surgery, NYU Med Ctr 1983; **Fellow:** Cardiothoracic Surgery, UCLA Med Ctr 1985; Pediatric Cardiac Surgery, Hosp for Sick Chldn 1986

Lansman, Steven MD/PhD [TS] - **Spec Exp:** Coronary Artery Surgery; Heart Valve Surgery; Ventricular Assist Device (LVAD); Transplant-Heart; **Hospital:** Westchester Med Ctr; **Address:** Westchester Medical Ctr, 95 Grasslands Rd, Macy Pavilion, rm 114W, Valhalla, NY 10595; **Phone:** 914-493-8793; **Board Cert:** Thoracic Surgery 2004; **Med School:** SUNY Hlth Sci Ctr 1977; **Resid:** Surgery, Montefiore Hosp Med Ctr 1982; **Fellow:** Thoracic Surgery, Univ Hosp 1984; **Fac Appt:** Prof S, NY Med Coll

Loulmet, Didier MD [TS] - **Spec Exp:** Heart Valve Surgery; Robotic Cardiac Surgery; Minimally Invasive Cardiac Surgery; **Hospital:** Lenox Hill Hosp (page 62); **Address:** Lenox Hill Hosp, William Black Hall, 130 E 77th St, Fl 4, New York, NY 10021; **Phone:** 212-434-3000; **Med School:** France 1984; **Resid:** Cardiothoracic Surgery, Paris Univ Hosp 1990; Cardiothoracic Surgery, Brigham & Women's Hosp 1991; **Fellow:** Pediatric Cardiac Surgery, Chldn's Hosp, Harvard Univ 1992

Magovern Jr, George J MD [TS] - **Spec Exp:** Cardiothoracic Surgery; Ventricular Assist Device (LVAD); **Hospital:** Allegheny General Hosp; **Address:** Cardiovascular Surgery Ctr, CVI-1, 320 E North Ave, NW Wing-Snyder Pavilion, Pittsburgh, PA 15212; **Phone:** 412-359-8820; **Board Cert:** Surgery 1993; Thoracic Surgery 1996; **Med School:** Univ Pittsburgh 1978; **Resid:** Surgery, Johns Hopkins Hosp 1981; Cardiovascular Surgery, Johns Hopkins Hosp 1985; **Fac Appt:** Prof S, Drexel Univ Coll Med

Marshall, Margaret Blair MD [TS] - **Spec Exp:** Lung Cancer; Esophageal Cancer; Thymoma; Mesothelioma; **Hospital:** Georgetown Univ Hosp, Sibley Mem Hosp; **Address:** Georgetown Univ Hosp, 3800 Reservoir Rd NW, 4PHC, Washington, DC 20007; **Phone:** 202-444-5045; **Board Cert:** Surgery 2000; Thoracic Surgery 2002; **Med School:** Georgetown Univ 1991; **Resid:** Surgery, Georgetown Univ Med Ctr 1995; Cardiothoracic Surgery, Hosp Univ Penn 2001; **Fellow:** Research, Children's Hosp 1998; **Fac Appt:** Assoc Prof S, Georgetown Univ

Michler, Robert E MD [TS] - **Spec Exp:** Heart Valve Surgery; Coronary Artery Surgery; Robotic Cardiac Surgery; Pediatric Cardiothoracic Surgery; **Hospital:** Montefiore Med Ctr, Montefiore Med Ctr - Weiler-Einstein Div; **Address:** Dept Cardiothoracic Surg, 3400 Bainbridge Ave Fl 5, Bronx, NY 10467; **Phone:** 718-920-2100; **Board Cert:** Surgery 1990; Thoracic Surgery 2000; **Med School:** Dartmouth Med Sch 1981; **Resid:** Surgery, Columbia Presby Med Ctr 1987; **Fellow:** Cardiothoracic Surgery, Columbia Presby Med Ctr 1989; Pediatric Surgery, Boston Children's Hosp 1990; **Fac Appt:** Prof S, Albert Einstein Coll Med

Morris, Rohinton J MD [TS] - **Spec Exp:** Transplant-Heart; Ventricular Assist Device (LVAD); Coronary Artery Surgery; **Hospital:** Hosp Univ Penn - UPHS (page 60), Penn Presby Med Ctr - UPHS (page 60); **Address:** Philadelphia Heart Inst, 51 N 39th St, Ste 2D, Philadelphia, PA 19104-4227; **Phone:** 215-349-8419; **Board Cert:** Thoracic Surgery 2003; **Med School:** Hahnemann Univ 1984; **Resid:** Surgery, Hahnemann Univ Hosp 1989; Thoracic Surgery, Hahnemann Univ Hosp 1992; **Fac Appt:** Assoc Clin Prof TS, Univ Pennsylvania

Naka, Yoshifumi MD/PhD [TS] - **Spec Exp:** Transplant-Heart & Lung; Ventricular Assist Device (LVAD); Heart Failure & Ventricular Containment; Mitral Valve Surgery; **Hospital:** NY-Presby Hosp/Columbia (page 66); **Address:** 177 Fort Washington Ave, MHB 7-435, New York, NY 10032; **Phone:** 212-305-0828; **Med School:** Japan 1984; **Resid:** Surgery, Osaka Police Hosp 1991; **Fellow:** Cardiovascular Surgery, Osaka Police Hosp 1993; Cardiothoracic Surgery, Columbia Univ 1998; **Fac Appt:** Asst Prof S, Columbia P&S

Oz, Mehmet C MD [TS] - **Spec Exp:** Transplant-Heart; Heart Valve Surgery; Minimally Invasive Cardiac Surgery; **Hospital:** NY-Presby Hosp/Columbia (page 66); **Address:** NY Presby Hosp, Dept Cardiothoracic Surg, 177 Ft Washington Ave, MHB- Rm 7, GN435, New York, NY 10032; **Phone:** 212-305-4434; **Board Cert:** Thoracic Surgery 2003; **Med School:** Univ Pennsylvania 1986; **Resid:** Surgery, Columbia Presby Med Ctr 1991; **Fellow:** Cardiothoracic Surgery, Columbia Presby Med Ctr 1993; **Fac Appt:** Prof S, Columbia P&S

Pass, Harvey MD [TS] - **Spec Exp:** Lung Cancer; Mesothelioma; Clinical Trials; **Hospital:** NYU Med Ctr (page 68); **Address:** NYU Cancer Ctr, 160 E 34th St Fl 8, New York, NY 10016; **Phone:** 212-731-5414; **Board Cert:** Thoracic Surgery 2001; **Med School:** Duke Univ 1973; **Resid:** Surgery, Duke Univ Med Ctr 1975; Surgery, Univ Miss Med Ctr 1980; **Fellow:** Cardiothoracic Surgery, MUSC Med Ctr 1982; **Fac Appt:** Prof S, NYU Sch Med

Pierson III, Richard N MD [TS] - **Spec Exp:** Transplant-Lung; Lung Cancer; Transplant-Heart; **Hospital:** Univ of MD Med Sys; **Address:** Univ Md Med Ctr, Dept Cardiothoracic Surg, 22 S Greene St, rm N4W94, Baltimore, MD 21201; **Phone:** 410-328-5842; **Board Cert:** Surgery 2000; Thoracic Surgery 2002; **Med School:** Columbia P&S 1983; **Resid:** Surgery, Univ Mich Med Ctr 1990; **Fellow:** Cardiothoracic Surgery, Mass General Hosp 1992; **Fac Appt:** Assoc Prof TS, Univ MD Sch Med

Pochettino, Alberto MD [TS] - **Spec Exp:** Aneurysm-Thoracic Aortic; Transplant-Lung; Left Ventricular Assist Device (LVAD); Heart Valve Disease; **Hospital:** Hosp Univ Penn - UPHS (page 60), Penn Presby Med Ctr - UPHS (page 60); **Address:** Hosp U Penn, 6 Silverstein Bldg, 3400 Spruce St, Philadelphia, PA 19104; **Phone:** 215-662-2957; **Board Cert:** Thoracic Surgery 2005; Surgery 2005; **Med School:** Northwestern Univ 1987; **Resid:** Surgery, SUNY-Upstate Med Ctr 1992; Thoracic Surgery, Hosp U Penn 1994; **Fac Appt:** Assoc Prof TS, Univ Pennsylvania

Thoracic Surgery

Rosengart, Todd MD [TS] - **Spec Exp:** Transfusion Free Surgery; Gene Therapy-Cardiac Angiogenesis; Minimally Invasive Surgery; Cardiac Surgery; **Hospital:** Stony Brook Univ Med Ctr; **Address:** Stonybrook Univ Hosp, Health Sci Ctr, Cardiothoracic Surgery, HSC-T19, rm 080, Stonybrook, NY 11794-0001; **Phone:** 631-444-1820; **Board Cert:** Surgery 1999; Thoracic Surgery 2002; **Med School:** Northwestern Univ 1983; **Resid:** Surgery, NYU Med Ctr 1985; Surgery, NYU Med Ctr 1989; **Fellow:** Thoracic Surgery, Natl Inst Hlth 1987; Cardiothoracic Surgery, NY-Cornell Med Ctr 1991; **Fac Appt:** Prof S, SUNY Stony Brook

Samuels, Louis MD [TS] - **Spec Exp:** Transplant-Heart; Artificial Heart Devices; Ventricular Assist Device (LVAD); **Hospital:** Lankenau Hosp; **Address:** 100 Lancaster Ave, 280 Lankenau Medical Science Bldg, Wynnwood, PA 19096; **Phone:** 610-896-9255; **Board Cert:** Surgery 1994; Thoracic Surgery 1996; **Med School:** Hahnemann Univ 1987; **Resid:** Surgery, Hahnemann Hosp 1992; Thoracic Surgery, Hahnemann Hosp 1995; **Fac Appt:** Prof S, Hahnemann Univ

Scott, Walter J MD [TS] - **Spec Exp:** Lung Cancer; Esophageal Cancer; Mediastinal Tumors; **Hospital:** Fox Chase Cancer Ctr (page 58); **Address:** Fox Chase Cancer Ctr, 333 Cottman Ave, rm C308, Philadelphia, PA 19111; **Phone:** 215-214-1427; **Board Cert:** Thoracic Surgery 1998; Surgery 1997; **Med School:** Univ Chicago-Pritzker Sch Med 1981; **Resid:** Surgery, Univ Chicago Med Ctr 1987; **Fellow:** Cardiothoracic Surgery, Univ Chicago Med Ctr 1989; **Fac Appt:** Assoc Prof TS, Temple Univ

Smith, Craig R MD [TS] - **Spec Exp:** Mitral Valve Surgery; Transplant-Heart; Minimally Invasive Cardiac Surgery; Robotic Cardiac Surgery; **Hospital:** NY-Presby Hosp/Columbia (page 66); **Address:** Columbia Presbyterian Med Ctr, 177 Fort Washington Ave, Ste 7-435, New York, NY 10032; **Phone:** 212-305-8312; **Board Cert:** Thoracic Surgery 2004; **Med School:** Case West Res Univ 1977; **Resid:** Surgery, Strong Meml Hosp 1982; **Fellow:** Cardiothoracic Surgery, Columbia Presby Med Ctr 1984; **Fac Appt:** Prof S, Columbia P&S

Sonett, Joshua R MD [TS] - **Spec Exp:** Minimally Invasive Thoracic Surgery; Transplant-Lung; Thoracic Cancers; **Hospital:** NY-Presby Hosp/Columbia (page 66); **Address:** 161 Fort Washington Ave, Ste 301, New York, NY 10032; **Phone:** 212-305-8086; **Board Cert:** Surgery 1994; Thoracic Surgery 1997; **Med School:** E Carolina Univ 1988; **Resid:** Surgery, Univ Mass Med Ctr 1993; **Fellow:** Cardiothoracic Surgery, Univ Pittsburgh Med Ctr 1994; Thoracic Surgery, Meml Sloan Kettering Cancer Ctr; **Fac Appt:** Assoc Prof S, Columbia P&S

Strong III, Michael D MD [TS] - **Spec Exp:** Coronary Artery Surgery; Heart Valve Surgery; Thoracic Aortic Surgery; **Hospital:** Hahnemann Univ Hosp; **Address:** Hahnemann Univ Hosp, Cardiothoracic Surg, 245 N 15th St, 744 N Tower, Philadelphia, PA 19102; **Phone:** 215-762-7802; **Board Cert:** Surgery 1974; Thoracic Surgery 2006; **Med School:** Jefferson Med Coll 1966; **Resid:** Surgery, Jefferson Hosp 1973; Thoracic Surgery, Temple Univ Hosp 1975; **Fac Appt:** Assoc Prof TS, Drexel Univ Coll Med

Tranbaugh, Robert MD [TS] - **Spec Exp:** Coronary Artery Surgery; Heart Valve Surgery; Aneurysm-Thoracic Aortic; **Hospital:** Beth Israel Med Ctr - Petrie Division (page 57); **Address:** 317 E 17th St Fl 11, New York, NY 10003; **Phone:** 212-420-2584; **Board Cert:** Thoracic Surgery 2004; **Med School:** Univ Pennsylvania 1976; **Resid:** Surgery, UCSF Med Ctr 1983; Cardiothoracic Surgery, UCSF Med Ctr 1985; **Fac Appt:** Assoc Prof TS, Albert Einstein Coll Med

Watson, Thomas J MD [TS] - **Spec Exp:** Esophageal Cancer; Gastroesophageal Reflux Disease (GERD); Lung Cancer; **Hospital:** Univ of Rochester Strong Meml Hosp, Highland Hosp - Rochester; **Address:** 601 Elmwood Ave, Box Surg, Rochester, NY 14642; **Phone:** 585-275-1509; **Board Cert:** Thoracic Surgery 1997; Surgery 2003; **Med School:** Univ SC Sch Med 1988; **Resid:** Surgery, LAC-USC Med Ctr 1993; Cardiothoracic Surgery, LAC-USC Med Ctr 1996; **Fellow:** Esophageal Surgery, LAC-USC Med Ctr 1994; **Fac Appt:** Assoc Prof S, Univ Rochester

Yang, Stephen C MD [TS] - **Spec Exp:** Mesothelioma; Lung Cancer; Esophageal Cancer; **Hospital:** Johns Hopkins Hosp - Baltimore (page 61), Johns Hopkins Bayview Med Ctr (page 61); **Address:** Johns Hopkins Hosp, 600 N Wolfe St Blalock Bldg - rm 240, Baltimore, MD 21287-5674; **Phone:** 410-614-3891; **Board Cert:** Surgery 2003; Thoracic Surgery 2005; **Med School:** Med Coll VA 1984; **Resid:** Surgery, Univ Tex Hlth Sci Ctr 1990; **Fellow:** Thoracic Surgery, MD Anderson Cancer Ctr 1992; Cardiothoracic Surgery, Med Coll Virginia 1994; **Fac Appt:** Assoc Prof TS, Johns Hopkins Univ

Southeast

Bichell, David P MD [TS] - **Spec Exp:** Cardiac Surgery-Neonatal; Cardiac Surgery-Pediatric; Congenital Heart Surgery; Minimally Invasive Cardiac Surgery; **Hospital:** Vanderbilt Children's Hosp, Vanderbilt Univ Med Ctr; **Address:** Vanderbilt Childrens Hosp, Div Pediatric Cardiac Surgery, 2200 Childrens Way, 5247 DOT, Nashville, TN 37232-9292; **Phone:** 615-343-6525; **Board Cert:** Thoracic Surgery 2006; **Med School:** Columbia P&S 1987; **Resid:** Surgery, Barnes Jewish Hosp 1994; Cardiothoracic Surgery, Brigham & Womens Hosp/Chldns Hosp 1996; **Fellow:** Cardiac Surgery, Brigham & Womens Hosp 1997; **Fac Appt:** Prof TS, Vanderbilt Univ

Boyd, W Douglas MD [TS] - **Spec Exp:** Robotic Cardiac Surgery; Ventricular Assist Device (LVAD); Minimally Invasive Cardiac Surgery; **Hospital:** Cleveland Clin - Weston; **Address:** Cleveland Clinic, Cardiothoracic Surgery, 2950 Cleveland Clinic Blvd, Weston, FL 33331; **Phone:** 954-659-5320; **Med School:** Univ Ottawa 1984; **Resid:** Surgery, Ottawa Civic Hospital 1990; Cardiothoracic Surgery, Ottowa Civic Hospital 1992; **Fellow:** Transplantation/Mechanical Assist Devices, Ottawa Heart Inst 1995; **Fac Appt:** Assoc Prof S, Univ S Fla Coll Med

Brunsting III, Louis A MD [TS] - **Spec Exp:** Coronary Artery Robotic Surgery; **Hospital:** Centennial Med Ctr, Baptist Hosp - Nashville; **Address:** Cardiothoracic Surgery Associates, 2400 Patterson St, Ste 223, Nashville, TN 37203; **Phone:** 615-329-1122; **Board Cert:** Thoracic Surgery 2001; **Med School:** UCSD 1983; **Resid:** Surgery, Univ Rochester 1985; Surgery, Univ Rochester 1989; **Fellow:** Surgery, Duke Univ 1987; Thoracic Surgery, Duke Univ 1991

Cerfolio, Robert J MD [TS] - **Spec Exp:** Lung Cancer; Tracheal Surgery; Chest Wall Tumors; Esophageal Cancer; **Hospital:** Univ of Ala Hosp at Birmingham; **Address:** 703 S 19th St, Ste 739, Birmingham, AL 35294; **Phone:** 205-934-5937; **Board Cert:** Thoracic Surgery 1997; Surgery 2003; **Med School:** Univ Rochester 1988; **Resid:** Surgery, Cornell-NY Hosp 1990; Surgery, Mayo Clinic 1993; **Fellow:** Cardiothoracic Surgery, Mayo Clinic 1996; **Fac Appt:** Prof TS, Univ Ala

Chitwood Jr, W Randolph MD [TS] - **Spec Exp:** Robotic Cardiac Surgery; Minimally Invasive Cardiac Surgery; Heart Valve Surgery; Mitral Valve Surgery; **Hospital:** Pitt Cty Mem Hosp - Univ Med Ctr East Carolina; **Address:** ECU Dept Surgery, 600 Moye Blvd, PCMH Teaching Annex, rm 277, Greenville, NC 27834; **Phone:** 252-744-4536; **Board Cert:** Thoracic Surgery 2005; **Med School:** Univ VA Sch Med 1974; **Resid:** Surgery, Duke Univ Med Ctr 1983; **Fellow:** Cardiovascular Surgery, Duke Univ Med Ctr 1984; **Fac Appt:** Prof S, E Carolina Univ

Christian, Karla G MD [TS] - **Spec Exp:** Congenital Heart Surgery; Transplant-Heart-Adult & Pediatric; Cardiac Surgery-Adult & Pediatric; **Hospital:** Vanderbilt Children's Hosp, Vanderbilt Univ Med Ctr; **Address:** Vanderbilt Chldns Hosp, Cardiac Surgery, 2200 Childrens Way, 5247 DOT, Nashville, TN 37232-9292; **Phone:** 615-936-5500; **Board Cert:** Surgery 2001; Thoracic Surgery 2003; **Med School:** Univ Wash 1985; **Resid:** Surgery, Univ Washington Med Ctr 1987; Surgery, Vanderbilt Univ Med Ctr 1991; **Fellow:** Cardiothoracic Surgery, Vanderbilt Univ Med Ctr 1994; **Fac Appt:** Assoc Prof S, Vanderbilt Univ

D'Amico, Thomas MD [TS] - **Spec Exp:** Lung Cancer; Esophageal Cancer; **Hospital:** Duke Univ Med Ctr; **Address:** Duke Univ Med Ctr, Dept Thoracic Surg, Box 3496, Durham, NC 27710; **Phone:** 919-684-4891; **Board Cert:** Surgery 2004; Thoracic Surgery 2006; **Med School:** Columbia P&S 1987; **Resid:** Surgery, Duke Univ Med Ctr 1989; Cardiothoracic Surgery, Duke Univ Med Ctr 1996; **Fellow:** Thoracic Oncology, Meml Sloan Kettering Cancer Ctr; **Fac Appt:** Assoc Prof S, Duke Univ

Dowling, Robert MD [TS] - **Spec Exp:** Cardiac Surgery; Transplant-Heart; **Hospital:** Jewish Hosp HlthCre Svcs Inc; **Address:** 201 Abraham Flexner Way, Ste 1200, Louisville, KY 40202; **Phone:** 502-583-8383; **Board Cert:** Surgery 1992; Thoracic Surgery 1995; **Med School:** Univ Pittsburgh 1985; **Resid:** Surgery, Presbyterian Hosp; **Fellow:** Thoracic Surgery, Univ Pittsburgh Med Ctr; **Fac Appt:** Prof S, Univ Louisville Sch Med

Drinkwater Jr, Davis C MD [TS] - **Spec Exp:** Transplant-Heart & Lung; Cardiac Surgery-Adult & Pediatric; **Hospital:** Centennial Med Ctr, Vanderbilt Children's Hosp; **Address:** 2400 Patterson St, Ste 400, Nashville, TN 37203; **Phone:** 615-342-5812; **Board Cert:** Surgery 1997; Thoracic Surgery 2005; **Med School:** Univ VT Coll Med 1976; **Resid:** Surgery, McGill Univ 1981; Cardiothoracic Surgery, McGill Univ 1983; **Fellow:** Cardiothoracic Surgery, Childrens Hosp 1984; **Fac Appt:** Clin Prof TS, Vanderbilt Univ

Glassford Jr, David M MD [TS] - **Spec Exp:** Cardiothoracic Surgery; **Hospital:** Saint Thomas Hosp - Nashville; **Address:** Cardiovascular Surgery Assocs, 4230 Harding Rd, Ste 202, Nashville, TN 37205; **Phone:** 615-385-4781; **Board Cert:** Surgery 1998; Surgical Critical Care 1999; Thoracic Surgery 2007; **Med School:** Univ Tex Med Br, Galveston 1970; **Resid:** Surgery, Univ Texas Med Br 1975; Thoracic Surgery, Ochsner Clinic 1977; **Fac Appt:** Asst Clin Prof TS, Vanderbilt Univ

Harpole Jr, David H MD [TS] - **Spec Exp:** Lung Cancer; Mesothelioma; Esophageal Cancer; **Hospital:** Duke Univ Med Ctr; **Address:** Duke Univ Med Ctr-Thoracic Surgery, 2424 Erwin Rd, Ste 403 - rm 4071, Durham, NC 27705; **Phone:** 919-668-8413; **Board Cert:** Surgery 2002; Thoracic Surgery 2003; **Med School:** Univ VA Sch Med 1984; **Resid:** Surgery, Duke Univ Med Ctr 1991; **Fellow:** Thoracic Surgery, Duke Univ Med Ctr 1993; **Fac Appt:** Prof S, Duke Univ

Heidary, Dariush H MD [TS] - **Spec Exp:** Cardiothoracic Surgery; Cardiovascular Surgery; **Hospital:** Meml Hlth Univ Med Ctr - Savannah, St Joseph's-Candler Hosp; **Address:** Memorial Hlth Univ Med Ctr, 4700 Waters Ave, Ste 403, Savannah, GA 31404-6220; **Phone:** 912-354-7188; **Board Cert:** Thoracic Surgery 1997; **Med School:** Iran 1967; **Resid:** Surgery, Albert Einstein Med Ctr 1974; Cardiothoracic Surgery, Albert Einstein Med Ctr 1975; **Fellow:** Cardiothoracic Surgery, Med Coll Georgia 1977

Jones, David R MD [TS] - **Spec Exp:** Lung Cancer; Esophageal Cancer; Minimally Invasive Thoracic Surgery; **Hospital:** Univ Virginia Med Ctr; **Address:** Department of Surgery, Box 800679, Charlottesville, VA 22901; **Phone:** 434-243-6443; **Board Cert:** Surgery 2005; Thoracic Surgery 1999; **Med School:** W VA Univ 1989; **Resid:** Surgery, West Va Univ 1995; **Fellow:** Thoracic Surgery, Univ North Carolina 1998; **Fac Appt:** Assoc Prof S, Univ VA Sch Med

Kiernan, Paul D MD [TS] - **Spec Exp:** Lung Cancer; Esophageal Cancer; Mediastinal Tumors; **Hospital:** Inova Fairfax Hosp, Inova Alexandria Hosp; **Address:** 2921 Telestar Court, Falls Church, VA 22042; **Phone:** 703-280-5858; **Board Cert:** Thoracic Surgery 2002; **Med School:** Georgetown Univ 1974; **Resid:** Surgery, Mayo Clinic 1979; Cardiothoracic Surgery, Mayo Clinic 1981; **Fellow:** Vascular Surgery, Mayo Clinic 1982; **Fac Appt:** Assoc Clin Prof S, Georgetown Univ

Kiev, Jonathan MD [TS] - **Spec Exp:** Chest Wall Tumors; Esophageal Cancer; Lung Cancer; **Hospital:** Med Coll of VA Hosp; **Address:** 1250 E Marshall St, PO Box 980068, Richmond, VA 23298; **Phone:** 804-828-2775; **Board Cert:** Surgery 2005; Thoracic Surgery 2002; **Med School:** Tulane Univ 1989; **Resid:** Surgery, Hahnemann Univ Hosp 1996; Cardiothoracic Surgery, Loma Linda Univ 2000; **Fellow:** Thoracic Surgery, Univ Pittsburgh 2001; Thoracic Surgery, Mayo Clinic 2001; **Fac Appt:** Prof S, Va Commonwealth Univ Sch Med

Kirklin, James K MD [TS] - **Spec Exp:** Transplant-Heart-Adult & Pediatric; Cardiac Surgery-Adult & Pediatric; **Hospital:** Univ of Ala Hosp at Birmingham; **Address:** Univ Alabama Med Ctr, THT 760, 1900 University Blvd, Birmingham, AL 35294; **Phone:** 205-934-3368; **Board Cert:** Thoracic Surgery 2000; **Med School:** Harvard Med Sch 1973; **Resid:** Surgery, Mass Genl Hosp 1977; Cardiothoracic Surgery, Mass Genl Hosp 1979; **Fellow:** Cardiothoracic Surgery, Chidren's Hosp Med Ctr 1979; **Fac Appt:** Prof S, Univ Ala

Kron, Irving L MD [TS] - **Spec Exp:** Coronary Artery Surgery; Transplant-Heart; **Hospital:** Univ Virginia Med Ctr; **Address:** Univ VA Hlth Sys, Div Cardiovascular Surg, PO Box 800679, Charlottesville, VA 22908; **Phone:** 434-924-2158; **Board Cert:** Surgery 1999; Thoracic Surgery 2001; Surgical Critical Care 1996; Vascular Surgery 1995; **Med School:** Med Coll Wisc 1975; **Resid:** Surgery, Maine Med Ctr 1980; **Fellow:** Cardiothoracic Surgery, Univ Virginia Med Ctr 1982; **Fac Appt:** Prof S, Univ VA Sch Med

Martin, Tomas D MD [TS] - **Spec Exp:** Cardiothoracic Surgery; Aortic Surgery; Aneurysm-Abdominal Aortic; **Hospital:** Shands at Univ of FL; **Address:** Dept of Surgery, 1600 SW Archer Rd, Box 100286, Gainesville, FL 32610-0286; **Phone:** 352-273-5505; **Board Cert:** Thoracic Surgery 1999; **Med School:** Univ Tex, Houston 1981; **Resid:** Surgery, Baylor Coll Med 1986; Vascular Surgery, Baylor Coll Med 1987; **Fellow:** Cardiothoracic Surgery, Shands/Univ Florida 1989; **Fac Appt:** Assoc Prof S, Univ Fla Coll Med

Miller, Daniel L MD [TS] - **Spec Exp:** Esophageal Cancer; Lung Cancer; Mesothelioma; Emphysema-Lung Volume Reduction; **Hospital:** Emory Univ Hosp; **Address:** Emory Clinic 1365 Clifton Rd NE, A Bldg Fl 2 - Ste 2100, CT Surgery, Atlanta, GA 30322; **Phone:** 404-778-3755; **Board Cert:** Thoracic Surgery 2005; Surgery 2001; **Med School:** Univ KY Coll Med 1985; **Resid:** Surgery, Georgetown Univ Hosp 1991; **Fellow:** Cardiothoracic Surgery, Mayo Clinic 1994; **Fac Appt:** Assoc Prof S, Emory Univ

Miller, Joseph I MD [TS] - **Spec Exp:** Lung Cancer; **Hospital:** Emory Univ Hosp, Crawford Long Hosp of Emory Univ; **Address:** 550 Peachtree St NE, MOT-6th Fl, Atlanta, GA 30308; **Phone:** 404-686-2515; **Board Cert:** Surgery 1973; Thoracic Surgery 1975; **Med School:** Emory Univ 1965; **Resid:** Surgery, Mayo Clin 1972; Thoracic Surgery, Emory Univ Hosp 1974; **Fac Appt:** Prof S, Emory Univ

Mullett, Timothy W MD [TS] - **Spec Exp:** Lung Cancer; Transplant-Heart & Lung; Cardiac Surgery-Adult & Pediatric; Esophageal Surgery; **Hospital:** Univ of Kentucky Chandler Hosp; **Address:** 900 S Limestone St, Lexington, KY 40536; **Phone:** 859-323-6494; **Board Cert:** Thoracic Surgery 1997; Surgery 2005; **Med School:** Univ Fla Coll Med 1987; **Resid:** Surgery, Shands/Univ of FL 1993; **Fellow:** Pediatric Surgery, Shands/Univ of FL 1994; Cardiothoracic Surgery, Shands/Univ of FL 1995; **Fac Appt:** Assoc Prof S, Univ KY Coll Med

Murphy, Douglas A MD [TS] - **Spec Exp:** Mitral Valve Robotic Surgery; **Hospital:** St Joseph's Hosp - Atlanta; **Address:** 5665 Peachtree Dunwoody Rd NE, Ste 150, Atlanta, GA 30342; **Phone:** 404-252-6104; **Board Cert:** Internal Medicine 1978; Thoracic Surgery 2004; **Med School:** Univ Pennsylvania 1975; **Resid:** Internal Medicine, Mass Genl Hosp 1977; Surgery, Mass Genl Hosp 1981; **Fellow:** Thoracic Surgery, Emory Univ Affil Hosp 1983

Nesbitt, Jonathan C MD [TS] - **Spec Exp:** Lung Cancer; Esophageal Cancer; Chest Diseases-Benign; **Hospital:** Vanderbilt Univ Med Ctr, Saint Thomas Hosp - Nashville; **Address:** The Vanderbilt Clinic, 1301 Medical Center Drive, Nashville, TN 37232; **Phone:** 615-322-0064; **Board Cert:** Surgery 1998; Thoracic Surgery 1998; **Med School:** Georgetown Univ 1981; **Resid:** Surgery, Vanderbilt Univ Med Ctr 1987; Thoracic Surgery, Albany Medical Ctr 1989; **Fac Appt:** Asst Clin Prof S, Vanderbilt Univ

Ninan, Mathews MD [TS] - **Spec Exp:** Lung Cancer; Transplant-Lung; Esophageal Cancer; **Hospital:** Baptist Memorial Hospital - Memphis, Methodist LeBonheur Germantown Hosp; **Address:** Cardiovascular Surgery Clinic, LLC, 6029 Walnut Grove Rd, Ste 401, East Office, Memphis, TN 38120; **Phone:** 901-747-3066; **Med School:** India 1988; **Resid:** Surgery, University of London 1994; **Fellow:** Cardiothoracic Surgery, Univ Pittsburgh 1998; **Fac Appt:** Asst Prof TS, Vanderbilt Univ

Perryman, Richard A MD [TS] - **Spec Exp:** Pediatric Cardiothoracic Surgery; Congenital Heart Disease-Adult; Ross Procedure for Aortic Valve Disease; **Hospital:** Joe Di Maggio Chldns Hosp, Meml Regl Hosp; **Address:** Joe DiMaggio Cardiac Surg Ctr, 1150 N 35th Ave, Ste 440, Hollywood, FL 33021; **Phone:** 954-985-6939; **Board Cert:** Thoracic Surgery 2002; **Med School:** England 1967; **Resid:** Thoracic Surgery, Duke Univ Med Ctr 1977; Cardiothoracic Surgery, Univ Florida 1981; **Fellow:** Cardiovascular Disease, Duke Univ Med Ctr 1971; **Fac Appt:** Prof TS, Univ Miami Sch Med

Putnam Jr, Joe B MD [TS] - **Spec Exp:** Lung Cancer; Esophageal Cancer; Sarcoma-Soft Tissue; **Hospital:** Vanderbilt Univ Med Ctr, VA Med Ctr - Nashville; **Address:** Vanderbilt Univ Med Ctr - Thoracic Surgery, 1301 Medical Center Drive, 2971 TVC, Nashville, TN 37232-5734; **Phone:** 615-343-9202; **Board Cert:** Thoracic Surgery 1997; **Med School:** Univ NC Sch Med 1979; **Resid:** Surgery, Univ Rochester 1986; Thoracic Surgery, Univ Mich Med Ctr 1988; **Fellow:** Surgical Oncology, NCI/NIH-Surg Branch 1984; **Fac Appt:** Prof TS, Vanderbilt Univ

Quintessenza, James A MD [TS] - **Spec Exp:** Transplant-Heart; Coronary Artery Surgery; Cardiovascular Surgery; **Hospital:** All Children's Hosp; **Address:** 625 6th Ave S, Ste 475, St Petersburg, FL 33701; **Phone:** 727-822-6666; **Board Cert:** Thoracic Surgery 1999; **Med School:** Univ Fla Coll Med 1981; **Resid:** Surgery, Univ Florida Hosps 1986; **Fellow:** Thoracic Surgery, UCSD Medical Ctr 1988; **Fac Appt:** Asst Clin Prof S, Univ S Fla Coll Med

Reed, Carolyn E MD [TS] - **Spec Exp:** Esophageal Cancer; Lung Cancer; **Hospital:** MUSC Med Ctr; **Address:** Med Univ S Carolina, Hollings Cancer Ctr, 96 Jonathan Lucas St, Ste 418, Charleston, SC 29425; **Phone:** 843-792-3362; **Board Cert:** Thoracic Surgery 2006; **Med School:** Univ Rochester 1977; **Resid:** Surgery, New York Hosp 1982; Thoracic Surgery, New York Hosp 1985; **Fellow:** Surgical Oncology, Meml Sloan Kettering Cancer Ctr 1983; **Fac Appt:** Prof S, Med Univ SC

Robinson, Lary A MD [TS] - **Spec Exp:** Lung Cancer; Mesothelioma; **Hospital:** H Lee Moffitt Cancer Ctr & Research Inst, Tampa Genl Hosp; **Address:** 12902 Magnolia Drive, Tampa, FL 33612-9497; **Phone:** 813-745-7282; **Board Cert:** Thoracic Surgery 2003; Surgery 2002; Surgical Critical Care 2000; **Med School:** Washington Univ, St Louis 1972; **Resid:** Surgery, Duke Univ Med Ctr 1974; Thoracic Surgery, Duke Univ Med Ctr 1981; **Fellow:** Cardiothoracic Surgery, St Thomas Hosp 1982; Cardiothoracic Surgery, Duke Univ Med Ctr 1983; **Fac Appt:** Prof S, Univ S Fla Coll Med

Smith, Peter K MD [TS] - **Spec Exp:** Coronary Artery Surgery; Heart Valve Surgery; **Hospital:** Duke Univ Med Ctr, VA Med Ctr - Durham; **Address:** Duke Univ Med Ctr, Cardiothoracic Surg, Box 3442, Durham, NC 27710; **Phone:** 919-684-2890; **Board Cert:** Surgery 1995; Thoracic Surgery 1998; **Med School:** Duke Univ 1977; **Resid:** Surgery, Duke Univ Med Ctr 1984; Thoracic Surgery, Duke Univ Med Ctr 1987; **Fac Appt:** Prof S, Duke Univ

Staples, Edward D MD [TS] - **Spec Exp:** Transplant-Heart & Lung; Ventricular Assist Device (LVAD); **Hospital:** Shands at Univ of FL, Malcolm Randall VA Med Ctr; **Address:** Shands Hlthcre, Dept Cardiothoracic Surg, 1600 SW Archer Rd, Box 100286, Gainesville, FL 32610-0268; **Phone:** 352-273-5509; **Board Cert:** Thoracic Surgery 2004; Surgical Critical Care 2002; **Med School:** Univ S Fla Coll Med 1977; **Resid:** Surgery, Med Coll Va 1979; Surgery, Univ Hosp 1982; **Fellow:** Cardiothoracic Surgery, Univ Florida 1984; **Fac Appt:** Assoc Prof S, Univ Fla Coll Med

Tedder, Mark MD [TS] - **Spec Exp:** Transplant-Heart; Cardiac Surgery; Artificial Heart Devices; **Hospital:** Saint Thomas Hosp - Nashville; **Address:** 4230 Harding Rd, Ste 202, Nashville, TN 37205; **Phone:** 615-385-4781; **Board Cert:** Surgery 1996; Thoracic Surgery 1998; **Med School:** Duke Univ 1988; **Resid:** Surgery, Duke Univ Med Ctr 1995; Cardiothoracic Surgery, Duke Univ Med Ctr 1997

Williams, Donald B MD [TS] - **Spec Exp:** Cardiac Surgery; **Hospital:** Univ of Miami Hosp; **Address:** 1295 NW 14th St, Ste H, Miami, FL 33125; **Phone:** 305-674-2780; **Board Cert:** Thoracic Surgery 2000; **Med School:** Jefferson Med Coll 1974; **Resid:** Surgery, Dartmouth-Hitchcock Med Ctr 1979; **Fellow:** Thoracic Surgery, Mayo Clinic 1981

Midwest

Alexander Jr, John C MD [TS] - **Spec Exp:** Minimally Invasive Cardiac Surgery; Robotic Heart Surgery; Mitral Valve Surgery; Arrhythmias; **Hospital:** Evanston Hosp; **Address:** Evanston Hosp, Cardiothoracic Surgery, 2650 Ridge Ave Walgreens Bldg - Ste 3507, Evanston, IL 60201; **Phone:** 847-570-2868; **Board Cert:** Thoracic Surgery 2001; **Med School:** Duke Univ 1972; **Resid:** Surgery, Duke Univ Med Ctr 1979; **Fellow:** Cardiothoracic Surgery, Duke Univ Med Ctr 1980; **Fac Appt:** Prof S, UMDNJ-NJ Med Sch, Newark

Bakhos, Mamdouh MD [TS] - **Spec Exp:** Mitral Valve Surgery; Minimally Invasive Cardiac Surgery; Transplant-Heart & Lung; Cardiovascular Surgery; **Hospital:** Loyola Univ Med Ctr, Adv Good Samaritan Hosp; **Address:** Loyola Univ, Dept Cardiothoracic Surgery, 2160 S First Ave, Bldg 110 - rm 6240, Maywood, IL 60153; **Phone:** 708-327-2503; **Board Cert:** Thoracic Surgery 1998; **Med School:** Syria 1971; **Resid:** Surgery, Huron Road Hosp 1976; **Fellow:** Thoracic Surgery, Loyola Univ Med Ctr 1978; **Fac Appt:** Prof TS, Loyola Univ-Stritch Sch Med

Brown, John W MD [TS] - **Spec Exp:** Cardiac Surgery-Neonatal & Pediatric; Transplant-Heart; Heart Valve Surgery; **Hospital:** Riley Hosp for Children, Methodist Hosp - Indianapolis; **Address:** 545 Barnhill Drive, EH215, Indianapolis, IN 46202-5112; **Phone:** 317-274-7150; **Board Cert:** Thoracic Surgery 2007; **Med School:** Indiana Univ 1970; **Resid:** Surgery, Univ Mich Med Ctr 1976; Cardiothoracic Surgery, Univ Mich Med Ctr 1978; **Fellow:** Cardiovascular Surgery, Natl Heart Lung-Blood Inst 1974; **Fac Appt:** Prof S, Indiana Univ

Damiano Jr, Ralph J MD [TS] - **Spec Exp:** Minimally Invasive Cardiac Surgery; Robotic Cardiac Surgery; **Hospital:** Barnes-Jewish Hosp; **Address:** 660 S Euclid Ave, Campus Box 8234, St Louis, MO 63110; **Phone:** 314-362-7327; **Board Cert:** Thoracic Surgery 2002; **Med School:** Duke Univ 1980; **Resid:** Surgery, Duke Univ Med Ctr 1988; **Fellow:** Cardiothoracic Surgery, Duke Univ Med Ctr 1989; **Fac Appt:** Prof S, Washington Univ, St Louis

Deschamps, Claude MD [TS] - **Spec Exp:** Gastroesophageal Reflux Disease (GERD); Esophageal Cancer; Lung Cancer; **Hospital:** St Mary's Hosp - Rochester; **Address:** Mayo Clinic, Div Thoracic Surgery, 200 First St SW, Rochester, MN 55905; **Phone:** 507-284-8462; **Board Cert:** Surgery 2004; **Med School:** Univ Montreal 1979; **Resid:** Surgery, Univ Montreal Hosps 1984; Thoracic Surgery, Univ Montreal Hosps 1985; **Fellow:** Thoracic Surgery, Mayo Clinic 1987; **Fac Appt:** Prof S, Mayo Med Sch

Durham, Samuel J MD [TS] - **Spec Exp:** Cardiothoracic Surgery; **Hospital:** Univ of Toledo Med Ctr; **Address:** Univ of Toledo Med Ctr, Dowling Hall, 3065 Arlington Ave, Ste 2261, Toledo, OH 43614; **Phone:** 419-383-5150; **Board Cert:** Surgery 2001; Thoracic Surgery 2003; **Med School:** Harvard Med Sch 1983; **Resid:** Surgery, Univ Pittsburgh Med Ctr 1987; Thoracic Surgery, Univ Pittsburgh Med Ctr 1988; **Fellow:** Pediatric Surgery, Chlidren's Hosp 1993; **Fac Appt:** Prof S, Ohio State Univ

Ferguson, Mark K MD [TS] - **Spec Exp:** Barrett's Esophagus; Esophageal Cancer; Lung Cancer; **Hospital:** Univ of Chicago Hosps; **Address:** 5841 S Maryland Ave, MC 5035, Univ Chicago Hosps, Chicago, IL 60637-1470; **Phone:** 773-702-3551; **Board Cert:** Thoracic Surgery 2003; **Med School:** Univ Chicago-Pritzker Sch Med 1977; **Resid:** Surgery, Univ Chicago Hosps 1982; **Fellow:** Cardiothoracic Surgery, Univ Chicago Hosps 1984; **Fac Appt:** Prof S, Univ Chicago-Pritzker Sch Med

Howington, John A MD [TS] - **Spec Exp:** Lung Cancer; Esophageal Cancer; Thymoma; **Hospital:** NorthShore Univ HlthSys, Highland Park Hosp; **Address:** Evanston Northwestern Hospital, 2650 Ridge Ave, Walgreen Bldg - Ste 3507, Evanston, IL 60201; **Phone:** 847-570-2868; **Board Cert:** Thoracic Surgery 2006; Surgery 2004; **Med School:** Univ Tenn Coll Med, Memphis 1989; **Resid:** Surgery, Truman Med Ctr/U Missouri 1994; Cardiothoracic Surgery, Vanderbilt Univ Med Ctr 1997; **Fac Appt:** Assoc Prof S, Northwestern Univ

Huddleston, Charles B MD [TS] - **Spec Exp:** Transplant-Lung-Pediatric; Transplant-Heart-Pediatric; **Hospital:** St Louis Chldns Hosp; **Address:** St Louis Children's Hospital, One Children's Pl, Ste 5 South 50, St Louis, MO 63110; **Phone:** 314-454-6165; **Board Cert:** Thoracic Surgery 2007; **Med School:** Vanderbilt Univ 1978; **Resid:** Surgery, Vanderbilt Univ Hosp 1986; Cardiothoracic Surgery, Vanderbilt Univ Hosp 1988; **Fellow:** Pediatric Cardiothoracic Surgery, Hosp for Sick Children 1989; **Fac Appt:** Prof S, Washington Univ, St Louis

Iannettoni, Mark D MD [TS] - **Spec Exp:** Transplant-Lung; Lung Cancer; Esophageal Surgery; **Hospital:** Univ Iowa Hosp & Clinics; **Address:** Univ Iowa Hosp & Clinics, 200 Hawkins Drive, rm SE514GH, Iowa City, IA 52242; **Phone:** 319-356-1133; **Board Cert:** Surgery 2002; Thoracic Surgery 2002; **Med School:** SUNY Upstate Med Univ 1985; **Resid:** Surgery, SUNY Upstate Med Ctr 1991; Thoracic Surgery, Univ Mich Med Ctr 1993; **Fellow:** Thoracic Surgery, Univ Mich Med Sch 1994

Jeevanandam, Valluvan MD [TS] - **Spec Exp:** Minimally Invasive Heart Valve Surgery; Transplant-Heart; Artificial Heart Devices; **Hospital:** Univ of Chicago Hosps; **Address:** 5841 S Maryland Ave, Ste E500, MC 5040, Chicago, IL 60637-1483; **Phone:** 773-702-2500; **Board Cert:** Thoracic Surgery 2002; **Med School:** Columbia P&S 1984; **Resid:** Surgery, Columbia-Presby Med Ctr 1989; **Fellow:** Cardiothoracic Surgery, Columbia-Presby Med Ctr 1991; **Fac Appt:** Prof S, Univ Chicago-Pritzker Sch Med

Little, Alex G MD [TS] - **Hospital:** Wright State Univ, Miami Valley Hosp; **Address:** 30 E Apple St, Ste 5253, Dayton, OH 45409; **Phone:** 937-208-2552; **Board Cert:** Surgery 1998; Thoracic Surgery 2000; **Med School:** Johns Hopkins Univ 1974; **Resid:** Surgery, Univ Chicago Hosp 1979; Thoracic Surgery, Univ Chicago Hosp 1981; **Fac Appt:** Prof TS, Wright State Univ

Lytle, Bruce W MD [TS] - **Spec Exp:** Heart Valve Surgery; Coronary Artery Surgery; Aortic Surgery; **Hospital:** Cleveland Clin Fdn (page 56); **Address:** Cleveland Clinic, Dept Thoracic Surgery, 9500 Euclid Ave, Desk F24, Cleveland, OH 44195; **Phone:** 216-444-6962; **Board Cert:** Thoracic Surgery 1998; **Med School:** Harvard Med Sch 1971; **Resid:** Surgery, Mass Genl Hsop 1975; Surgery, Shotley Bridge Hosp 1976; **Fellow:** Thoracic Surgery, Mass Genl Hosp 1979; **Fac Appt:** Prof TS, Cleveland Cl Coll Med/Case West Res

Maddaus, Michael A MD [TS] - **Spec Exp:** Esophageal Cancer; Lung Cancer; Minimally Invasive Thoracic Surgery; **Hospital:** Univ Minn Med Ctr, Fairview - Univ Campus, Abbott - Northwestern Hosp; **Address:** Div General Thoracic Surgery, 420 Delaware St SE, MMC 207, Minneapolis, MN 55455; **Phone:** 612-624-9461; **Board Cert:** Surgery 2000; Thoracic Surgery 2003; **Med School:** Univ Minn 1982; **Resid:** Surgery, Univ Minn 1990; Thoracic Surgery, Univ Toronto 1991; **Fellow:** Cardiac Surgery, St Michael's Hosp/Hosp Sick Chldn 1992; Thoracic Oncology, Meml Sloan Kettering Cancer Ctr 1992; **Fac Appt:** Prof S, Univ Minn

McCarthy, Patrick M MD [TS] - **Spec Exp:** Heart Valve Surgery; Coronary Artery Surgery; Ventricular Assist Device (LVAD); **Hospital:** Northwestern Meml Hosp; **Address:** Bluhm Cardiovascular Inst, 675 N St Clair St, Galter 19-100, Chicago, IL 60611-2968; **Phone:** 312-695-6984; **Board Cert:** Thoracic Surgery 1998; **Med School:** Loyola Univ-Stritch Sch Med 1980; **Resid:** Surgery, Mayo Clinic 1985; Thoracic Surgery, Mayo Clinic 1988; **Fellow:** Cardiopulmonary Transplant Surgery, Stanford Univ 1989; **Fac Appt:** Prof S, Northwestern Univ

McGregor, Christopher MD [TS] - **Spec Exp:** Transplant-Heart & Lung; Cardiac Surgery; **Hospital:** Mayo Med Ctr & Clin - Rochester, St Mary's Hosp - Rochester; **Address:** Mayo Clinic - St Mary's Hospital, 200 First St SW, rm Joseph 5-200, Rochester, MN 55905; **Phone:** 507-255-6038; **Med School:** Scotland 1972; **Resid:** Surgery, Edinburgh Royal Infirm 1978; Surgery, Glasgow Royal Infirm 1981; **Fellow:** Cardiothoracic Transplant Surg, Stanford Univ Hosp 1984; **Fac Appt:** Prof S, Mayo Med Sch

Merrill, Walter H MD [TS] - **Spec Exp:** Cardiothoracic Surgery; Cardiac Surgery-Adult & Pediatric; Transplant-Heart; **Hospital:** Univ Hosp - Cincinnati, VA Med Ctr; **Address:** Univ Cincinnati, Sect Cardiothoracic Surg, 231 Albert Sabin Way, ML 0558, Cincinnati, OH 45267-0001; **Phone:** 513-584-3278; **Board Cert:** Surgery 2000; Thoracic Surgery 2001; Surgical Critical Care 1999; **Med School:** Johns Hopkins Univ 1974; **Resid:** Thoracic Surgery, Natl Inst Hlth 1978; Thoracic Surgery, Johns Hopkins Hosp 1982; **Fellow:** Pediatric Surgery, Hosp for Sick Chldn 1983; **Fac Appt:** Prof S, Univ Cincinnati

Meyers, Bryan MD [TS] - **Spec Exp:** Lung Cancer; Esophageal Cancer; Transplant-Lung; **Hospital:** Barnes-Jewish Hosp, Barnes-Jewish West County Hosp; **Address:** 4921 Parkview Pl, Ste 8B, St Louis, MO 63110; **Phone:** 314-362-8598; **Board Cert:** Surgery 1998; Thoracic Surgery 1999; **Med School:** Univ Chicago-Pritzker Sch Med 1986; **Resid:** Surgery, Mass Genl Hosp 1996; **Fellow:** Cardiothoracic Surgery, Barnes Hosp-Wash Univ 1998; **Fac Appt:** Assoc Prof S, Washington Univ, St Louis

Naunheim, Keith S MD [TS] - **Spec Exp:** Lung Cancer; Esophageal Cancer; Chest Wall Tumors; Video Assisted Thoracic Surgery (VATS); **Hospital:** St Louis Univ Hosp; **Address:** St Louis Univ Med Ctr, Dept Surgery, 3635 Vista Ave, St Louis, MO 63110-0250; **Phone:** 314-577-8360; **Board Cert:** Thoracic Surgery 2004; **Med School:** Univ Chicago-Pritzker Sch Med 1978; **Resid:** Surgery, Univ Chicago Hosp 1983; **Fellow:** Cardiothoracic Surgery, Univ Chicago Hosp 1985; **Fac Appt:** Prof S, St Louis Univ

Orringer, Mark B MD [TS] - **Spec Exp:** Esophageal Cancer; Lung Cancer; Mediastinal Tumors; Lung Cancer; **Hospital:** Univ Michigan Hlth Sys; **Address:** Univ Mich, Taubman Ctr, 1500 E Med Ctr Drive, rm TC 2120, Box 0344, Ann Arbor, MI 48109-0344; **Phone:** 734-936-4975; **Board Cert:** Surgery 1973; Thoracic Surgery 1974; **Med School:** Univ Pittsburgh 1967; **Resid:** Thoracic Surgery, Johns Hopkins Hosp 1973; **Fac Appt:** Prof S, Univ Mich Med Sch

Thoracic Surgery

Pagani, Francis MD [TS] - **Spec Exp:** Transplant-Heart; Coronary Artery Surgery; **Hospital:** Univ Michigan Hlth Sys; **Address:** Univ Mich Med Ctr, Sect Cardiac Surgery, 1500 E Med Ctr Drive, SPC 5864, Ann Arbor, MI 48109-5864; **Phone:** 734-647-2894; **Board Cert:** Surgery 2002; Thoracic Surgery 2004; **Med School:** Georgetown Univ 1986; **Resid:** Surgery, Georgetown Univ Med Ctr 1993; Thoracic Surgery, Univ Mich Hosp 1995; **Fellow:** Research, Univ Mass Med Ctr 1990; **Fac Appt:** Assoc Prof S, Univ Mich Med Sch

Patterson, G Alexander MD [TS] - **Spec Exp:** Lung Cancer; Esophageal Cancer; Transplant-Lung; Transplant-Heart & Lung; **Hospital:** Barnes-Jewish Hosp; **Address:** 660 S Euclid Ave, Box 8234, St Louis, MO 63110; **Phone:** 314-362-6025; **Board Cert:** Surgery 1978; Thoracic Surgery 1981; Vascular Surgery 1982; **Med School:** Canada 1974; **Resid:** Surgery, Queens Univ Med Ctr 1978; Vascular Surgery, Univ Toronto Med Ctr 1979; **Fellow:** Research, Toronto Genl Hosp 1981; Surgical Critical Care, Johns Hopkins Hosp 1982; **Fac Appt:** Prof S, Washington Univ, St Louis

Raman, Jai MD/PhD [TS] - **Spec Exp:** Robotic Heart Surgery; Heart Failure & Ventricular Containment; Transplant-Heart; Atrial Fibrillation; **Hospital:** Univ of Chicago Hosps; **Address:** University of Chicago Hosps, 5841 S Maryland Ave, Ste E500, MC 5040, Chicago, IL 60637; **Phone:** 773-702-2500; **Med School:** India 1990; **Resid:** Cardiothoracic Surgery, St Vincent's Hosp 1991; Cardiothoracic Surgery, Austin Hospital 1995; **Fellow:** Thoracic Surgery, Austin Hosp 1994; Pediatric Cardiac Surgery, Royal Children's Hosp 1996; **Fac Appt:** Assoc Prof S, Univ Chicago-Pritzker Sch Med

Rice, Thomas W MD [TS] - **Spec Exp:** Esophageal Surgery; Minimally Invasive Thoracic Surgery; Transplant-Lung; **Hospital:** Cleveland Clin Fdn (page 56); **Address:** Cleveland Clinic, 9500 Euclid Ave, Desk F-24, Cleveland, OH 44195; **Phone:** 216-444-1921; **Board Cert:** Surgery 2004; Thoracic Surgery 2005; **Med School:** Univ Toronto 1978; **Resid:** Surgery, Univ Toronto Med Ctr 1983; Thoracic Surgery, Univ Toronto Med Ctr 1986; **Fellow:** Pulmonary Disease, UCSF Med Ctr 1984; **Fac Appt:** Prof S, Cleveland Cl Coll Med/Case West Res

Schaff, Hartzell MD [TS] - **Spec Exp:** Heart Valve Surgery; Congenital Heart Disease; Maze Procedure for Atrial Fibrillation; **Hospital:** St Mary's Hosp - Rochester; **Address:** Mayo Clin, Div Cardiovasc Surg, 200 First St SW, Rochester, MN 55905-0001; **Phone:** 507-255-7068; **Board Cert:** Thoracic Surgery 2001; **Med School:** Univ Okla Coll Med 1973; **Resid:** Surgery, Johns Hopkins Hosp 1978; Thoracic Surgery, Johns Hopkins Hosp 1980; **Fellow:** Surgery, Johns Hopkins Hosp 1976; **Fac Appt:** Prof S, Mayo Med Sch

Smedira, Nicholas MD [TS] - **Spec Exp:** Transplant-Heart; Transplant-Lung; Ventricular Assist Device (LVAD); Aortic Surgery; **Hospital:** Cleveland Clin Fdn (page 56); **Address:** Cleveland Clin, Dept Cardiothoracic Surg, 9500 Euclid Ave, Desk F24, Cleveland, OH 44195; **Phone:** 216-445-7052; **Board Cert:** Thoracic Surgery 2003; **Med School:** Univ Rochester 1984; **Resid:** Surgery, UCSF Med Ctr 1991; Thoracic Surgery, UCSF Med Ctr 1994; **Fellow:** Cardiothoracic Surgery, UCSF Med Ctr 1994

Smith, John Michael MD [TS] - **Spec Exp:** Mitral Valve Robotic Surgery; **Hospital:** Good Samaritan Hosp - Cincinnati; **Address:** 4030 Smith Rd, Ste 300, Cincinnati, OH 45209; **Phone:** 513-421-3494; **Board Cert:** Surgery 2003; Thoracic Surgery 2006; **Med School:** Univ Louisville Sch Med 1989; **Resid:** Surgery, Good Samaritan Hosp 1994; **Fellow:** Cardiothoracic Surgery, Yale Univ Hosp 1996

Srivastava, Sudhir P MD [TS] - **Spec Exp:** Coronary Artery Robotic Surgery; **Hospital:** Univ of Chicago Hosps; **Address:** 5841 S Maryland Ave, MC 5040, Chicago, IL 60637; **Phone:** 432-332-4044; **Board Cert:** Thoracic Surgery 1999; **Med School:** India 1970; **Resid:** Vascular Surgery, Vancouver Genl Hosp 1977; Thoracic Surgery, Vancouver Genl Hosp 1978; **Fellow:** Surgery, Vancouver Genl Hosp 1979

Stuart, Richard MD [TS] - **Spec Exp:** Cardiac Surgery; Thoracic Surgery; Robotic Cardiac Surgery; **Hospital:** St Luke's Hosp of Kansas City, N Kansas City Hosp; **Address:** 4320 Wornall Rd Bldg 2 - Ste 50, Kansas City, MO 64111; **Phone:** 816-931-3312; **Board Cert:** Thoracic Surgery 1999; Surgical Critical Care 1993; **Med School:** Johns Hopkins Univ 1981; **Resid:** Surgery, Johns Hopkins Hosp 1986; **Fellow:** Cardiothoracic Surgery, Johns Hopkins Hosp 1989; **Fac Appt:** Clin Prof TS, Univ MO-Kansas City

Sundt III, Thoralf MD [TS] - **Spec Exp:** Heart Valve Surgery; Aneurysm-Thoracic Aortic; Pulmonary Embolism; **Hospital:** Mayo Med Ctr & Clin - Rochester; **Address:** Mayo Clinic, 200 First St SW, Rochester, MN 55905-0002; **Phone:** 507-255-7064; **Board Cert:** Surgery 2000; Thoracic Surgery 2004; **Med School:** Johns Hopkins Univ 1984; **Resid:** Surgery, Mass Genl Hosp 1991; Cardiothoracic Surgery, Wash Univ Sch Med 1993; **Fellow:** Cardiothoracic Surgery, Harefield Hosp 1994; **Fac Appt:** Prof S, Mayo Med Sch

Turrentine, Mark W MD [TS] - **Spec Exp:** Cardiac Surgery-Pediatric; Transplant-Heart; Transplant-Lung; **Hospital:** Riley Hosp for Children, Methodist Hosp - Indianapolis; **Address:** 545 Barnhill Dr, Emerson Hall, Ste 215, Indianapolis, IN 46202; **Phone:** 317-274-1121; **Board Cert:** Thoracic Surgery 2002; **Med School:** Univ Kans 1983; **Resid:** Surgery, Univ Kansas Med Ctr 1988; Cardiothoracic Surgery, Indiana Univ Med Ctr 1991; **Fellow:** Cardiothoracic Surgery, Texas Heart Inst 1986; Transplant Surgery, Indiana Univ Med Ctr 1989; **Fac Appt:** Prof S, Indiana Univ

Great Plains and Mountains

Bull, David A MD [TS] - **Spec Exp:** Cardiothoracic Surgery; Esophageal Cancer; **Hospital:** Univ Utah Hosps and Clins; **Address:** Univ Utah, Dept Cardiothoracic Surgery, 30 N 1900 East, rm 3C127, Salt Lake City, UT 84132; **Phone:** 801-581-5311; **Board Cert:** Thoracic Surgery 2004; Vascular Surgery 2003; Surgery 1999; Surgical Critical Care 1999; **Med School:** UCSF 1985; **Resid:** Surgery, UCSF Medical Ctr 1987; Surgery, Univ Arizona Hosps 1990; **Fellow:** Vascular Surgery, Univ Arizona Hosps 1992; Cardiothoracic Surgery, Univ Arizona Hosps 1994; **Fac Appt:** Assoc Prof TS, Univ Utah

Campbell, David N MD [TS] - **Spec Exp:** Pediatric Cardiothoracic Surgery; Transplant-Heart-Pediatric; Transplant-Lung; **Hospital:** Chldn's Hosp - Aurora, The, Univ Colorado Hosp; **Address:** 13123 E 16th Ave, Ste B-200, Denver, CO 80218; **Phone:** 720-777-6624; **Board Cert:** Surgery 1999; Thoracic Surgery 2000; Surgical Critical Care 2000; **Med School:** Rush Med Coll 1974; **Resid:** Surgery, Univ Colo Med Ctr 1980; Cardiothoracic Surgery, Univ Colo Med Ctr 1979; **Fellow:** Cardiovascular Surgery, Boston Chldns Hosp 1980; **Fac Appt:** Prof S, Univ Colorado

Fullerton, David A MD [TS] - **Spec Exp:** Maze Procedure for Atrial Fibrillation; Ross Procedure for Aortic Valve Disease; Mitral Valve Surgery; Transplant-Heart & Lung; **Hospital:** Univ Colorado Hosp, VA Med Ctr; **Address:** Univ of Colorado, Cardiothoracic Surgery, 12631 E 17th Ave, L15, rm 6602, MS C310, PO Box 6511, Aurora, CO 80045; **Phone:** 303-724-2798; **Board Cert:** Surgery 2007; Surgical Critical Care 2001; Thoracic Surgery 2001; **Med School:** Univ MO-Columbia Sch Med 1981; **Resid:** Surgery, Univ Wash Med Ctr 1987; Thoracic Surgery, Univ Colorado Hosp 1990; **Fac Appt:** Prof S, Univ Colorado

Karwande, Shreekanth V MD [TS] - **Spec Exp:** Thoracic Cancers; Lung Cancer; Cardiac Surgery; **Hospital:** St Mark's Hosp - Salt Lake City; **Address:** St Mark's Hosp, 1160 E 3900 St, Ste 3500, Salt Lake City, UT 84124; **Phone:** 801-743-4750; **Board Cert:** Thoracic Surgery 2003; **Med School:** India 1973; **Resid:** Surgery, Erie Co Med Ctr 1981; Cardiothoracic Surgery, New York Hosp 1985; **Fellow:** Cardiothoracic Surgery, Meml Sloan Kettering Cancer Ctr

Thoracic Surgery

Southwest

Aklog, Lishan MD [TS] - **Spec Exp:** Mitral Valve Surgery; Minimally Invasive Cardiac Surgery; Coronary Artery Surgery; **Hospital:** St Joseph's Hosp & Med Ctr - Phoenix; **Address:** Heart and Lung Inst, St Joseph's Hosp Med Ctr, 500 W Thomas Rd, Phoenix, AZ 85013-4224; **Phone:** 602-406-2996; **Board Cert:** Surgery 1997; Thoracic Surgery 2000; **Med School:** Harvard Med Sch 1989; **Resid:** Surgery, Brigham & Women's Hosp 1996; **Fellow:** Cardiothoracic Surgery, Brigham & Women's Hosp 1998; Cardiac Surgery, Harefield Hosp 1999

Calhoon, John H MD [TS] - **Spec Exp:** Transplant-Heart & Lung; Congenital Heart Surgery; Cardiac Surgery-Adult & Pediatric; **Hospital:** Univ Hlth Sys - Univ Hosp (San Antonio, TX), Christus Santa Rosa Children's Hosp; **Address:** UTHSCSA, Dept Thoracic Surg, 7703 Floyd Curl Drive, MC 7841, San Antonio, TX 78229-3901; **Phone:** 210-567-6863; **Board Cert:** Surgery 1996; Thoracic Surgery 1997; **Med School:** Baylor Coll Med 1981; **Resid:** Surgery, Univ Hosp/Univ Texas HSC 1986; Univ Hosp/Univ Texas HSC 1988; **Fellow:** Pediatric Cardiac Surgery, Chldns Hosp/Harvard 1989; **Fac Appt:** Prof TS, Univ Tex, San Antonio

Copeland III, Jack G MD [TS] - **Spec Exp:** Transplant-Heart; Transplant-Heart & Lung; Artificial Heart Devices; **Hospital:** Univ Med Ctr - Tucson, VA Medical Center - Tucson; **Address:** Univ Ariz Hlth Sci Ctr, 1501 N Campbell Rd, rm 4402, Box 245071, Tucson, AZ 85724-5071; **Phone:** 520-626-6339; **Board Cert:** Thoracic Surgery 1997; **Med School:** Stanford Univ 1969; **Resid:** Surgery, UCSD Med Ctr 1971; Cardiovascular Surgery, Natl Inst Hlth 1973; **Fellow:** Cardiothoracic Surgery, Stanford Univ 1977; **Fac Appt:** Prof TS, Univ Ariz Coll Med

Coselli, Joseph S MD [TS] - **Spec Exp:** Aneurysm-Abdominal & Thoracic Aortic; Marfan's Syndrome; Aortic Surgery; **Hospital:** St Luke's Episcopal Hosp - Houston; **Address:** 6770 Bertner St, Ste C350, MC 1-103, Houston, TX 77030; **Phone:** 832-355-9910; **Board Cert:** Thoracic Surgery 2004; **Med School:** Univ Tex Med Br, Galveston 1977; **Resid:** Surgery, Baylor Coll Med 1982; Thoracic Surgery, Baylor Coll Med 1984; **Fac Appt:** Assoc Prof S, Baylor Coll Med

Diethrich, Edward B MD [TS] - **Spec Exp:** Vascular Surgery; Endovascular Surgery; Cardiovascular Surgery; **Hospital:** Arizona Heart Hosp; **Address:** Arizona Heart Inst, 2632 N 20th St, Phoenix, AZ 85006-1339; **Phone:** 602-240-6165; **Board Cert:** Thoracic Surgery 1967; Surgery 1966; **Med School:** Univ Mich Med Sch 1960; **Resid:** Surgery, St Joseph Mercy Hosp 1964; **Fellow:** Cardiothoracic Surgery, Baylor Coll Med 1966; **Fac Appt:** Prof TS, Univ Ariz Coll Med

Forbess, Joseph MD [TS] - **Spec Exp:** Pediatric Cardiothoracic Surgery; Heart Valve Surgery-Pediatric; **Hospital:** Chldns Med Ctr of Dallas, UT Southwestern Med Ctr - Dallas; **Address:** Univ Texas SW Med Ctr, Div Ped Cardiothor Surg, 1935 Medical District Drive, Ste C-3211, Dallas, TX 75235; **Phone:** 214-456-5000; **Board Cert:** Surgery 2000; Thoracic Surgery 1998; **Med School:** Harvard Med Sch 1990; **Resid:** Surgery, Duke Univ Med Ctr 1997; Cardiothoracic Surgery, Duke Univ Med Ctr 1999; **Fellow:** Cardiac Surgery, Childrens Hosp 1994; **Fac Appt:** Assoc Prof TS, Univ Tex SW, Dallas

Fraser, Charles D MD [TS] - **Spec Exp:** Pediatric Cardiothoracic Surgery; Congenital Heart Surgery; **Hospital:** Texas Chldns Hosp - Houston; **Address:** Texas Chldns Hosp-Heart Ctr, 6621 Fannin St, MC WT 19-345H, Houston, TX 77030-2399; **Phone:** 832-826-2030; **Board Cert:** Surgery 2000; Thoracic Surgery 1994; **Med School:** Univ Tex Med Br, Galveston 1984; **Resid:** Surgery, Johns Hopkins Hosp 1990; Johns Hopkins Hosp 1993; **Fac Appt:** Prof S, Baylor Coll Med

Frazier, Oscar Howard MD [TS] - **Spec Exp:** Transplant-Heart; Lung Surgery; Artificial Heart Devices; **Hospital:** St Luke's Episcopal Hosp - Houston; **Address:** Surgical Assocs - Texas Heart Institute, P.O. Box 20345, MC 2-114A, Houston, TX 77225; **Phone:** 832-355-4900; **Board Cert:** Surgery 1975; Thoracic Surgery 2005; **Med School:** Baylor Coll Med 1967; **Resid:** Surgery, Baylor Affil Hosp 1974; Thoracic Surgery, Texas Heart Inst 1976; **Fac Appt:** Prof S, Univ Tex, Houston

Harrell Jr, James E MD [TS] - **Spec Exp:** Transplant-Heart; Cardiac Surgery-Pediatric; **Hospital:** Covenant Children's Med Ctr; **Address:** 3606 21st St, Ste 103, Lubbock, TX 79410; **Phone:** 806-725-4425; **Board Cert:** Surgery 2006; Thoracic Surgery 2006; **Med School:** Baylor Coll Med 1978; **Resid:** Surgery, Univ Tex Hlth Scis Ctr 1984; Thoracic Surgery, Baylor Coll Med 1986; **Fellow:** Cardiovascular Surgery, Hosp Sick Chldn 1987

Lanza, Louis MD [TS] - **Spec Exp:** Lung Cancer; Cardiac Surgery; **Hospital:** Mayo Clinic - Scottsdale; **Address:** Mayo Clinic Hosp, 5779 E Mayo Blvd MCSB Bldg Fl 1, Phoenix, AZ 85054; **Phone:** 480-342-2270; **Board Cert:** Thoracic Surgery 2002; **Med School:** Loyola Univ-Stritch Sch Med 1981; **Resid:** Surgery, Univ Michigan Med Ctr 1988; Cardiovascular Surgery, Texas Heart Inst 1991; **Fellow:** Surgical Oncology, Natl Cancer Inst 1986; Thoracic Oncology, MD Anderson Cancer Ctr 1989

Ott, David A MD [TS] - **Spec Exp:** Heart Valve Surgery; Coronary Artery Surgery; Aneurysm-Abdominal Aortic; **Hospital:** St Luke's Episcopal Hosp - Houston; **Address:** 1101 Bates St, Ste P-514, Houston, TX 77030-2607; **Phone:** 832-355-4900; **Board Cert:** Thoracic Surgery 1997; **Med School:** Baylor Coll Med 1972; **Resid:** Surgery, Baylor Coll Med 1976; Cardiothoracic Surgery, Tex Heart Inst 1978; **Fac Appt:** Clin Prof S, Baylor Coll Med

Reardon, Michael J MD [TS] - **Spec Exp:** Cardiac Tumors/Cancer; Heart Valve Surgery-Aortic; **Hospital:** Methodist Hosp - Houston, UT MD Anderson Cancer Ctr; **Address:** 6560 Fannin St, Ste 1006, Houston, TX 77030; **Phone:** 713-441-5200; **Board Cert:** Thoracic Surgery 2006; **Med School:** Baylor Coll Med 1978; **Resid:** Surgery, Baylor Affil Hosps 1983; Thoracic Surgery, Texas Heart Inst 1985; **Fac Appt:** Clin Prof S, Baylor Coll Med

Ring, W Steves MD [TS] - **Spec Exp:** Cardiac Surgery-Adult & Pediatric; Transplant-Heart & Lung; Congenital Heart Surgery; Coronary Revascularization; **Hospital:** UT Southwestern Med Ctr - Dallas, Chldns Med Ctr of Dallas; **Address:** 5323 Harry Hines Blvd, MC 8879, Dallas, TX 75390-8879; **Phone:** 214-645-7706; **Board Cert:** Surgery 1999; Thoracic Surgery 2004; **Med School:** Harvard Med Sch 1971; **Resid:** Surgery, Duke Univ Med Ctr 1977; Surgery, Univ Minn Hosps 1980; **Fellow:** Thoracic Surgery, Univ Minn Hosps 1982; **Fac Appt:** Prof TS, Univ Tex SW, Dallas

Roth, Jack MD [TS] - **Spec Exp:** Esophageal Cancer; Lung Cancer; Gene Therapy; **Hospital:** UT MD Anderson Cancer Ctr; **Address:** Dept Thoracic & Cardiovasc Surg Unit 445, 1515 Holcombe Blvd, Houston, TX 77030-4000; **Phone:** 713-792-7664; **Board Cert:** Thoracic Surgery 2002; **Med School:** Johns Hopkins Univ 1971; **Resid:** Surgery, Johns Hopkins Hosp 1973; Thoracic Surgery, UCLA Ctr Hlth Sci 1979; **Fellow:** Surgical Oncology, UCLA 1975; **Fac Appt:** Prof TS, Univ Tex, Houston

Safi, Hazim MD [TS] - **Spec Exp:** Aneurysm-Abdominal Aortic; **Hospital:** Meml Hermann Hosp - Texas Med Ctr; **Address:** UT, Dept Cardiothoracic & Vascular Surg, 6410 Fannin St, Ste 450, Houston, TX 77030; **Phone:** 713-500-5304; **Board Cert:** Thoracic Surgery 2007; Vascular Surgery 2005; **Med School:** Iraq 1970; **Resid:** Surgery, Baylor Coll Med 1980; Radiation Oncology, Baylor Coll Med 1981; **Fellow:** Thoracic Surgery, Baylor Coll Med 1983; **Fac Appt:** Assoc Prof S, Univ Tex, Houston

Swisher, Stephen G MD [TS] - **Spec Exp:** Esophageal Cancer; Lung Cancer; Mesothelioma; Thoracic Cancers; **Hospital:** UT MD Anderson Cancer Ctr; **Address:** Dept of Thoracic & Cardiovasc Surg, 1515 Holcombe Blvd, Unit 445, Houston, TX 77030; **Phone:** 713-792-8659; **Board Cert:** Surgery 2002; Thoracic Surgery 1997; **Med School:** UCSD 1986; **Resid:** Surgery, UCLA Med Ctr 1993; **Fellow:** Surgical Oncology, UCLA Med Ctr 1990; Cardiothoracic Surgery, MD Anderson Canc Ctr 1996; **Fac Appt:** Prof TS, Univ Tex, Houston

Thoracic Surgery

Turner, William F MD [TS] - **Spec Exp:** Coronary Artery Surgery; Cardiac Surgery; **Hospital:** E TX Med Ctr, Trinity Mother Frances Hlth Sys; **Address:** 1100 E Lake St, Ste 210, Tyler, TX 75701; **Phone:** 903-593-0900; **Board Cert:** Surgery 1997; Thoracic Surgery 1998; **Med School:** Baylor Coll Med 1981; **Resid:** Surgery, Baylor Coll Med 1987; Thoracic Surgery, Baylor Coll Med 1989

West Coast and Pacific

Bailey, Leonard L MD [TS] - **Spec Exp:** Cardiac Surgery-Pediatric; Congenital Heart Surgery; Transplant-Heart-Pediatric; **Hospital:** Loma Linda Chldns Hosp, Loma Linda Univ Med Ctr; **Address:** 11234 Anderson St, rm 1617, Loma Linda, CA 92354; **Phone:** 909-558-4200; **Board Cert:** Surgery 1975; Thoracic Surgery 2006; **Med School:** Loma Linda Univ 1969; **Resid:** Surgery, Loma Linda Univ Med Ctr 1973; Thoracic Surgery, Loma Linda Univ Med Ctr 1974; **Fellow:** Cardiovascular Surgery, Hosp Sick Chldn 1975; **Fac Appt:** Prof S, Loma Linda Univ

Cannon, Walter Bradford MD [TS] - **Spec Exp:** Chest Wall Tumors; **Hospital:** Stanford Univ Med Ctr, VA Hlth Care Sys - Palo Alto; **Address:** Stanford Univ Med Ctr, Dept Cardiothoracic Surgery, 300 Pasteur Dr, Falk Bldg CVRB, Stanford, CA 94305-5407; **Phone:** 650-736-7191; **Board Cert:** Thoracic Surgery 1996; Surgery 1996; **Med School:** Harvard Med Sch 1969; **Resid:** Thoracic Surgery, Stanford Univ Hosp 1975; **Fac Appt:** Clin Prof S, Stanford Univ

Cohen, Robbin G MD [TS] - **Spec Exp:** Minimally Invasive Surgery; Heart Valve Surgery; Thoracic Aortic Surgery; **Hospital:** USC Univ Hosp - R K Eamer Med Plz, Huntington Memorial Hosp; **Address:** 1520 San Pueblo St, Ste 4300, Los Angeles, CA 90033; **Phone:** 323-442-5850; **Board Cert:** Thoracic Surgery 1999; **Med School:** Univ Colorado 1980; **Resid:** Surgery, Stanford Univ Med Ctr 1986; **Fellow:** Cardiothoracic Surgery, Stanford Univ Med Ctr 1989; **Fac Appt:** Assoc Prof TS, USC Sch Med

Dang, Michael H MD [TS] - **Spec Exp:** Cardiac Surgery; Peripheral Vascular Disease; Transplant-Heart; **Hospital:** Queen's Med Ctr - Honolulu; **Address:** Queens Heart Physicians Practice, 550 S Beretania St, Ste 300, Honolulu, HI 96813; **Phone:** 808-545-8900; **Board Cert:** Thoracic Surgery 2002; **Med School:** Univ Colorado 1968; **Resid:** Surgery, Baylor Univ Med Ctr 1976; Thoracic Surgery, Baylor Univ Med Ctr 1978

De Meester, Tom R MD [TS] - **Spec Exp:** Stomach Cancer; Esophageal Cancer; Lung Cancer; Tracheal Surgery; **Hospital:** USC Univ Hosp - R K Eamer Med Plz; **Address:** 1510 San Pablo St, Ste 514, Los Angeles, CA 90033; **Phone:** 323-442-5925; **Board Cert:** Surgery 1971; Thoracic Surgery 1971; **Med School:** Univ Mich Med Sch 1963; **Resid:** Surgery, Johns Hopkins Hosp 1966; **Fellow:** Thoracic Surgery, Johns Hopkins Hosp 1968; **Fac Appt:** Prof S, USC Sch Med

Flachsbart, Keith D MD [TS] - **Spec Exp:** Cardiac Surgery; **Hospital:** Kaiser Permanente South San Francisco Med Ctr; **Address:** 2350 Geary Blvd Fl 1, San Francisco, CA 94115; **Phone:** 415-833-3800; **Board Cert:** Thoracic Surgery 2000; **Med School:** Univ Nebr Coll Med 1971; **Resid:** Surgery, Rush-Presby St Lukes Hosp 1978; Thoracic Surgery, Hosp Good Samaritan 1980

Fontana, Gregory MD [TS] - **Spec Exp:** Minimally Invasive Surgery; Cardiac Surgery-Pediatric; Mitral Valve Surgery; **Hospital:** Cedars-Sinai Med Ctr; **Address:** 8700 Beverly Blvd, North Twr, rm 6215, Los Angeles, CA 90048-1804; **Phone:** 310-423-3851; **Board Cert:** Thoracic Surgery 2004; **Med School:** UCLA 1984; **Resid:** Surgery, Duke Univ Med Ctr 1990; Thoracic Surgery, Duke Univ Med Ctr 1993; **Fellow:** Pediatric Cardiac Surgery, UCLA Med Ctr; Pediatric Cardiac Surgery, Chldns Hosp; **Fac Appt:** Assoc Clin Prof S, UCLA

Grannis Jr, Frederic W MD [TS] - **Spec Exp:** Lung Cancer; Tobacco Abuse; Thoracic Cancers; Palliative Care; **Hospital:** City of Hope Natl Med Ctr & Beckman Rsch; **Address:** Head Sect
Thor Surg—City of Hope Natl Med Ctr, 1500 E Duarte Rd, Duarte, CA 91010; **Phone:** 626-359-
8111 x62669; **Board Cert:** Thoracic Surgery 2000; Surgery 1975; **Med School:** NY Med Coll
1969; **Resid:** Surgery, Mayo Clinic 1974; Thoracic Surgery, Mayo Clinic 1977; **Fac Appt:** Asst Clin
Prof TS, UCSD

Gundry, Steven MD [TS] - **Spec Exp:** Cardiac Surgery-Adult & Pediatric; Cardiac Surgery-High
Risk; Nutrition in Heart Disease; **Hospital:** Desert Regl Med Ctr; **Address:** International Heart & Lung
Inst, 555 Tachevah Drive, 3W - Ste 103, Palm Springs, CA 92262; **Phone:** 760-323-5553; **Board
Cert:** Thoracic Surgery 2005; **Med School:** Med Coll GA 1977; **Resid:** Surgery, Univ Michigan
Hosps 1983; Thoracic Surgery, Univ Michigan Hosps 1985; **Fellow:** Pediatric Cardiac Surgery, Hosp-
Sick Chldn 1986; **Fac Appt:** Clin Prof S, Loma Linda Univ

Handy Jr, John R MD [TS] - **Spec Exp:** Lung Cancer; Esophageal Cancer; Mesothelioma;
Chest Wall Tumors; **Hospital:** Providence Portland Med Ctr; **Address:** Oregon Clinic-Cardiothoracic
Surgery, 1111 NE 99th Ave, Ste 201, Portland, OR 97220; **Phone:** 503-963-3030; **Board Cert:**
Thoracic Surgery 2001; Surgery 1999; **Med School:** Duke Univ 1983; **Resid:** Surgery, Brown Univ
Hosp 1990; **Fellow:** Cardiothoracic Surgery, MUSC Med Ctr 1993

Hanley, Frank L MD [TS] - **Spec Exp:** Pediatric Thoracic Surgery; **Hospital:** Lucile Packard
Chldns Hosp/Stanford Univ Med Ctr, Chldns Hosp - Oakland; **Address:** 300 Pasteur Drive, FALK
CVRB, Stanford, CA 94305-5407; **Phone:** 650-723-0190; **Board Cert:** Thoracic Surgery 2002;
Med School: Tufts Univ 1978; **Resid:** Surgery, UCSF Med Ctr 1981; Cardiothoracic Surgery, UCSF
Med Ctr 1988; **Fellow:** Research, UCSF Sch Med 1984; **Fac Appt:** Prof S, UCSF

Jablons, David M MD [TS] - **Spec Exp:** Lung Cancer; Mesothelioma; Esophageal Surgery;
Hospital: UCSF - Mt Zion Med Ctr; **Address:** UCSF Thoracic Surg, 1600 Divisadero St Fl 4, San
Francisco, CA 94115; **Phone:** 415-885-3882; **Board Cert:** Thoracic Surgery 2002; **Med School:**
Albany Med Coll 1984; **Resid:** Surgery, New Eng Med Ctr-Tufts Univ 1986; Surgery, New Eng Med
Ctr-Tufts Univ 1991; **Fellow:** Surgical Oncology, Natl Cancer Inst-NIH 1989; Cardiothoracic Surgery,
New York Hosp-Cornell 1993; **Fac Appt:** Prof S, UCSF

Jamieson, Stuart W MD [TS] - **Spec Exp:** Pulmonary Embolism; Transplant-Heart & Lung;
Hospital: UCSD Med Ctr; **Address:** UCSD Med Ctr, Div CTS, 200 W Arbor Drive, MC 8892, San
Diego, CA 92103; **Phone:** 619-543-7777; **Med School:** England 1971; **Resid:** Surgery 1975;
Fellow: Cardiothoracic Surgery 1977; Cardiothoracic Surgery, Stanford Univ/American Heart Assoc
1980; **Fac Appt:** Prof S, UCSD

Kernstine, Kemp H MD/PhD [TS] - **Spec Exp:** Lung Cancer; Esophageal Cancer; Tracheal
Surgery; Esophageal Surgery; **Hospital:** City of Hope Natl Med Ctr & Beckman Rsch; **Address:** City
of Hope Comprehensive Cancer Ctr, 1500 E Duarte Rd, Duarte, CA 91010; **Phone:** 626-359-8111
x68845; **Board Cert:** Thoracic Surgery 2004; Surgery 2001; **Med School:** Duke Univ 1982;
Resid: Surgery, Univ Minn Med Ctr 1988; **Fellow:** Cardiothoracic Surgery, Brigham & Women's
Hosp 1994; **Fac Appt:** Prof S, Univ Iowa Coll Med

Laks, Hillel MD [TS] - **Spec Exp:** Congenital Heart Disease; Transplant-Heart; **Hospital:** Ronald
Reagan UCLA Med Ctr; **Address:** UCLA Med Ctr, 10833 Le Conte Ave, rm 62-182A CHS, Los Ange-
les, CA 90095-1741; **Phone:** 310-206-1837; **Board Cert:** Surgery 1975; Thoracic Surgery 2006;
Med School: Africa 1965; **Resid:** Surgery, Peter Bent Brigham Hosp 1969; Thoracic Surgery, Peter
Bent Brigham Hosp 1973; **Fac Appt:** Prof S, UCLA

Thoracic Surgery

Lamberti Jr, John J MD [TS] - **Spec Exp:** Pediatric Cardiac Surgery; Heart Valve Surgery; Congenital Heart Surgery; **Hospital:** Rady Children's Hosp - San Diego, UCSD Med Ctr; **Address:** Chldns Hosp, 3030 Children's Way, Ste 202, San Diego, CA 92123-4227; **Phone:** 858-966-8030; **Board Cert:** Surgery 1973; Thoracic Surgery 1975; **Med School:** Univ Pittsburgh 1967; **Resid:** Surgery, Peter Bent Brigham Hosp 1972; Thoracic Surgery, Peter Bent Brigham Hosp 1973; **Fellow:** Pediatric Cardiac Surgery, Chldns Hosp 1974; **Fac Appt:** Prof S, UCSD

Merrick, Scot H MD [TS] - **Spec Exp:** Cardiac Surgery-Adult; Heart Valve Surgery; Coronary Revascularization; **Hospital:** UCSF Med Ctr; **Address:** UCSF Med Ctr, Div Cardiothoracic Surg, 500 Parnassus Ave, San Francisco, CA 94143-0118; **Phone:** 415-353-1606; **Board Cert:** Thoracic Surgery 1997; **Med School:** Univ Wash 1980; **Resid:** Surgery, UCSF Med Ctr 1985; **Fellow:** Cardiothoracic Surgery, UCSF Med Ctr 1987; **Fac Appt:** Assoc Prof S, UCSF

Miller, David Craig MD [TS] - **Spec Exp:** Thoracic Aortic Surgery; Heart Valve Surgery; Endovascular Stent Grafts; **Hospital:** Stanford Univ Med Ctr; **Address:** Stanford Univ Sch Medicine, Div Cardiothoracic Surgery, 300 Pasteur Drive Falk Rsch Bldg, Stanford, CA 94305-5407; **Phone:** 650-725-3826; **Board Cert:** Thoracic Surgery 1998; **Med School:** Stanford Univ 1972; **Resid:** Thoracic Surgery, Standford Univ Med Ctr 1978; **Fac Appt:** Prof TS, Stanford Univ

Reitz, Bruce A MD [TS] - **Spec Exp:** Transplant-Heart & Lung; Heart Valve Surgery; Congenital Heart Surgery; **Hospital:** Stanford Univ Med Ctr, El Camino Hosp/Camino Hlthcare Sys; **Address:** Stanford Univ Sch Med, Dept Cardiothoracic Surgery, 300 Pasteur Drive Falk Bldg, Stanford, CA 94305-5407; **Phone:** 650-725-4497; **Board Cert:** Thoracic Surgery 1999; **Med School:** Yale Univ 1970; **Resid:** Cardiovascular Surgery, Stanford Univ Hosp 1972; Thoracic Surgery, Stanford Univ Hosp 1978; **Fellow:** Cardiac Surgery, Natl Heart Inst 1974; **Fac Appt:** Prof TS, Stanford Univ

Robbins, Robert C MD [TS] - **Spec Exp:** Transplant-Heart; Transplant-Lung; **Hospital:** Stanford Univ Med Ctr; **Address:** Cardiovascular Rsch Bldg, Fl 2, 300 Pasteur Drive, Stanford, CA 94305-2200; **Phone:** 650-725-3828; **Board Cert:** Thoracic Surgery 2002; Surgery 2002; **Med School:** Univ Miss 1983; **Resid:** Surgery, Univ Miss Med Ctr 1988; **Fellow:** Thoracic Surgery, Stanford Univ Med Ctr 1991; **Fac Appt:** Asst Prof TS, Stanford Univ

Shemin, Richard MD [TS] - **Spec Exp:** Minimally Invasive Cardiac Surgery; Heart Valve Surgery; Aneurysm-Thoracic Aortic; **Hospital:** Ronald Reagan UCLA Med Ctr; **Address:** UCLA-David Geffen School Medicine, 10833 Le Conte Ave, rm 62182, Los Angeles, CA 90095; **Phone:** 310-206-8232; **Board Cert:** Thoracic Surgery 2002; **Med School:** Boston Univ 1974; **Resid:** Surgery, PB Brigham Hosp 1980; NYU Med Ctr 1982; **Fellow:** Cardiac Surgery, Natl Inst Hlth 1978; **Fac Appt:** Prof TS, UCLA-David Geffen Sch Med

Shrager, Joseph B MD [TS] - **Spec Exp:** Emphysema-Lung Volume Reduction; Tracheal Surgery; Lung Cancer; Mediastinal Tumors; **Hospital:** Stanford Univ Med Ctr; **Address:** Stanford Univ Medical Ctr, CVRB Bldg, 300 Pasteur Drive Fl 2 - rm CV207, Stanford, CA 94305-5407; **Phone:** 650-723-6649; **Board Cert:** Thoracic Surgery 1999; Surgery 1996; **Med School:** Harvard Med Sch 1988; **Resid:** Surgery, Hosp Univ Penn 1995; Cardiothoracic Surgery, Mass Genl Hosp 1997; **Fac Appt:** Assoc Prof S, Stanford Univ

Starnes, Vaughn A MD [TS] - **Spec Exp:** Transplant-Heart & Lung; Heart Valve Surgery; Ross Procedure for Aortic Valve Disease; Robotic Cardiac Surgery; **Hospital:** USC Univ Hosp - R K Eamer Med Plz, Huntington Memorial Hosp; **Address:** USC Cardiothoracic Surgery, 1520 San Pablo St, Ste 4300, Los Angeles, CA 90033; **Phone:** 323-442-5849; **Board Cert:** Thoracic Surgery 2007; **Med School:** Univ NC Sch Med 1977; **Resid:** Surgery, Vanderbilt Univ Hosp 1984; Cardiovascular Surgery, Stanford Unv Hosp 1986; **Fellow:** Cardiothoracic Transplant Surg, Stanford Unv Hosp 1987; Pediatric Cardiac Surgery, Univ NC Hosp; **Fac Appt:** Prof TS, USC Sch Med

Thistlethwaite, Patricia A MD/PhD [TS] - **Spec Exp:** Cardiac Surgery; Lung Cancer; **Hospital:** UCSD Med Ctr; **Address:** UCSD Med Ctr, Div CTS, 200 W Arbor Drive, MC 8892, San Diego, CA 92103; **Phone:** 619-543-7777; **Board Cert:** Surgery 2005; Thoracic Surgery 2007; **Med School:** Harvard Med Sch 1989; **Resid:** Surgery, Mass Genl Hosp 1994; **Fellow:** Cardiothoracic Surgery, Univ Pittsburgh 1997; **Fac Appt:** Assoc Prof S, UCSD

Trento, Alfredo MD [TS] - **Spec Exp:** Transplant-Heart; Cardiac Surgery; Pediatric Cardiac Surgery; **Hospital:** Cedars-Sinai Med Ctr; **Address:** Cedars-Sinai Med Ctr, Dept Thoracic Surg, 8700 Beverly Blvd, North Tower - rm 6215, Los Angeles, CA 90048; **Phone:** 310-423-3851; **Board Cert:** Thoracic Surgery 2005; **Med School:** Italy 1975; **Resid:** Surgery, Univ Mass Med Ctr 1982; Thoracic Surgery, Univ Pittsburgh Med Ctr 1985; **Fellow:** Cardiothoracic Surgery, Univ Mass Med Ctr 1982; **Fac Appt:** Prof S, UCLA

Ungerleider, Ross M MD [TS] - **Spec Exp:** Congenital Heart Disease; Cardiac Surgery; Pediatric Cardiac Surgery; **Hospital:** Doernbecher Chldns Hosp/OHSU; **Address:** Oregon Health Science Univ, Dept Cardiothoracic Surgery, 3181 SW Sam Jackson Park Rd, L353, Portland, OR 97239; **Phone:** 503-418-5443; **Board Cert:** Thoracic Surgery 2007; **Med School:** Rush Med Coll 1977; **Resid:** Surgery, Duke Univ Med Ctr 1987; **Fellow:** Cardiothoracic Surgery, Duke Univ Med Ctr 1989; Pediatric Cardiac Surgery, UCSF; **Fac Appt:** Prof S, Oregon Hlth Sci Univ

Vallieres, Eric MD [TS] - **Spec Exp:** Lung Cancer; Mesothelioma; Mediastinal Tumors; Thoracic Cancers; **Hospital:** Swedish Med Ctr - Seattle; **Address:** 1101 Madison St, Ste 850, Seattle, WA 98104; **Phone:** 206-215-6800; **Board Cert:** Surgery 1988; Thoracic Surgery 1990; **Med School:** Canada 1982; **Resid:** Surgery, Univ of Toronto 1988; Thoracic Surgery, Univ of Toronto 1989; **Fellow:** Cardiovascular Surgery, Univ of Montreal 1990

Verrier, Edward D MD [TS] - **Spec Exp:** Coronary Artery Surgery; Heart Valve Surgery; **Hospital:** Univ Wash Med Ctr, Northwest Hosp; **Address:** University Washington Medical Ctr, 1959 NE Pacific St, Ste AA115, Box 356310, Seattle, WA 98195-6310; **Phone:** 206-598-3636; **Board Cert:** Surgery 1992; Thoracic Surgery 1993; **Med School:** Tufts Univ 1974; **Resid:** Surgery, UCSF Med Ctr 1982; Thoracic Surgery, UCSF Med Ctr 1984; **Fellow:** Cardiac Surgery, UCSF Med Ctr 1980; **Fac Appt:** Prof TS, Univ Wash

Wells, Winfield J MD [TS] - **Spec Exp:** Tracheal Surgery-Pediatric; Congenital Heart Surgery; **Hospital:** Chldns Hosp - Los Angeles; **Address:** Chlds Hosp, Div Cardiothoracic Surgery, 4650 Sunset Blvd, MS 66, Los Angeles, CA 90027; **Phone:** 323-361-4148; **Board Cert:** Thoracic Surgery 2007; **Med School:** USC Sch Med 1970; **Resid:** Surgery, Columbia-Presby Med Ctr 1976; **Fac Appt:** Assoc Prof S, USC Sch Med

Whyte, Richard MD [TS] - **Spec Exp:** Lung Cancer; Esophageal Cancer; **Hospital:** Stanford Univ Med Ctr; **Address:** Stanford Univ Sch Med, Div Thor Surg, 300 Pasteur Dr, Bldg CVRB - rm 205, Stanford, CA 94305-5407; **Phone:** 650-723-6649; **Board Cert:** Surgery 1991; Thoracic Surgery 1993; **Med School:** Univ Pittsburgh 1983; **Resid:** Surgery, Mass Genl Hosp 1990; Thoracic Surgery, Univ Michigan Hosp 1992; **Fac Appt:** Assoc Prof TS, Stanford Univ

Wood, Douglas E MD [TS] - **Spec Exp:** Lung Cancer; Esophageal Cancer; Tracheal Surgery; Mesothelioma; **Hospital:** Univ Wash Med Ctr, Northwest Hosp; **Address:** Univ Washington, Div Cardiothoracic Surg, 1959 NE Pacific St, AA Bldg - rm 115, Box 356310, Seattle, WA 98195-6310; **Phone:** 206-685-3228; **Board Cert:** Surgery 1999; Thoracic Surgery 2001; **Med School:** Harvard Med Sch 1983; **Resid:** Surgery, Mass Genl Hosp 1989; Thoracic Surgery, Mass Genl Hosp 1991; **Fellow:** Surgical Critical Care, Mass Genl Hosp 1991; **Fac Appt:** Prof S, Univ Wash

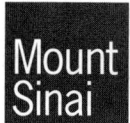
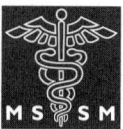

MOUNT SINAI
SCHOOL OF
MEDICINE

THE MOUNT SINAI MEDICAL CENTER
CARDIOTHORACIC SURGERY
One Gustave L. Levy Place
Fifth Avenue and 100th Street
New York, NY 10029-6574
Physician Referral: 1-800-MD-SINAI (637-4624)
www.mountsinai.org

The Department of Cardiothoracic Surgery at Mount Sinai is one of the nation's most prestigious programs. Cardiothoracic surgical patients benefit from an integrated and personalized care plan designed in coordination with expert cardiologists, anesthesiologists, perfusionists, and intensive care physicians. Mount Sinai is a quaternary referral center, meaning its surgeons often operate on the sickest and most complicated patients.

THE HEART VALVE CENTER

The Mitral Valve Repair Program at Mount Sinai is one of the largest and most advanced in the nation. The superiority of mitral valve repair over replacement with a mechanical or bioprosthetic valve is now well established. Directed by David H. Adams, MD, Mount Sinai's Mitral Valve Repair Program offers patients one of the highest percentages of successful valve repair in the world. For example, in patients with mitral valve prolapse, Mount Sinai's success rate in avoiding valve replacement approaches 100 percent. Our physicians are also expert in mitral valve repair for patients with advanced cardiomyopathy. If patients have associated atrial fibrillation, Mount Sinai offers the latest in concomitant arrhythmia surgery, including the MAZE procedure. Mitral valve repair with minimally invasive approaches is also performed when appropriate.

The Aortic Valve Repair Program offers patients with aortic valve disease an alternative to replacement of their aortic valve and the freedom from taking blood-thinning medications. Our surgeons are thoroughly versed in nonthrombogenic alternatives to mechanical valve replacement, including such valve sparring procedures as the David and Yacoub procedures. Mount Sinai's Paul Stelzer, MD, is one of the most experienced surgeons in the nation in using the Ross procedure, in which the diseased aortic valve is replaced with the patient's own pulmonary valve. This technique has improved durability over other replacement options, particularly in younger patients.

The Thoracic Aortic Surgery Program is known around the world for its leadership role in surgical therapy of complex aortic disease. This program specializes in the operative management of all diseases of the ascending aorta, arch, and descending thoracic aorta. Ascending aortic replacement, trifurcation-graft arch replacement, acute aortic dissection repair, and thoracoabdominal aortic surgery are all commonly performed at Mount Sinai. Special emphasis is placed on cerebral and spinal protection, where we have a significant clinical and scientific research interest led by our pioneering director, Randall B. Griepp, MD. Our surgeons have also been involved in the early development of minimally invasive aortic stent grafting.

The Cardiac Transplant and Assist Program, one of the largest in the nation, is now under the direction of Anelechi Anyanwu, MD. We have been involved in the field of mechanical cardiac assistance from its inception and have experience with most of the currently available FDA-approved devices. We have also played an active role in multi-institutional studies exploring permanent mechanical heart support.

LEADING SURGEONS, UNPARALLELED POSSIBILITIES

The Department of Cardiothoracic Surgery at Mount Sinai is chaired by David H. Adams, MD, the Marie-Josée and Henry R. Kravis Professor. Dr. Adams is a world-renowned mitral repair surgeon. Randall B. Griepp, MD, Professor of Cardiothoracic Surgery, is an internationally recognized leader in thoracic aortic surgery; Paul Stelzer, MD, is a specialist in aortic root surgery whose experience with the Ross procedure is unmatched, exceeding twenty years and 415 cases; and Eric Rose, MD, is a groundbreaking surgeon who in 2001 published findings that left ventricular assist devices (LVADs) can prolong the lives of end-stage heart failure patients not eligible for transplantation. These leaders work in concert with other members of Mount Sinai Heart, which is under the direction of world-renowned cardiologist Valentin Fuster, MD, PhD, to deliver unparalleled possibilities for patients with cardiovascular disease.

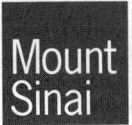
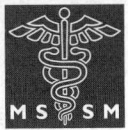

THE MOUNT SINAI MEDICAL CENTER
THORACIC SURGERY
One Gustave L. Levy Place
Fifth Avenue and 100th Street
New York, NY 10029-6574
Physician Referral: 1-800-MD-SINAI 637-4624)
www.mountsinai.org

MOUNT SINAI
SCHOOL OF
MEDICINE

COMPREHENSIVE CARE

Thoracic Surgery at Mount Sinai is world renowned for its state-of-the-art surgery, multidisciplinary team approach to treatment, and commitment to compassionate patient care. Protocol-driven therapy ensures that Mount Sinai patients are given access to many clinical trials.

SURGICAL TREATMENT FOR BENIGN AND MALIGNANT DISEASES OF LUNG AND ESOPHAGUS

Our team of dedicated thoracic surgeons is expert in the treatment of all primary cancers of the chest, lung, esophagus, mediastinum, and airway, and all metastatic tumors of the chest. We also diagnose and treat patients who are affected by benign esophageal disorders such as gastroesophageal reflux disease (GERD), achalasia, and motility disorders.

STATE-OF-THE-ART TECHNOLOGY

Mount Sinai is a leader in the development and implementation of the latest technologies and treatment options for disorders of the lung and esophagus, including:

- Video-assisted thoracic surgery (VATS)
- VATS lobectomy
- VATS thymectomy
- VATS sympathectomy for patients with excessive sweating of their hands
- Minimally invasive esophagectomy
- Robotic surgery
- Endobronchial ultrasound (EBUS)—a new noninvasive method for staging lung cancers
- Stent and laser treatment of the airway and esophagus
- Radiofrequency ablation of lung tumors
- Stereotactic radiosurgery of the lung
- Navigational bronchoscopy—a new, innovative, noninvasive method via bronchoscopy to perform biopsies on small lung lesions, including those in subpleural locations
- Lung volume reduction surgery

TAKING CARE OF ONE PATIENT AT A TIME

At Mount Sinai we believe in personalized care. Each patient benefits from a team approach to medical care, including thoracic surgeons, anesthesiologists, medical oncologists, radiation oncologists, and oncology-dedicated nurses. Coordinating information among team members to ensure seamless delivery of care is a top priority.

TRANSPLANT PROGRAM

Our transplant program is one of two accredited programs in the New York metropolitan area dedicated to lung transplantation for a wide variety of conditions. Patients enrolled in this program receive a multidisciplinary team approach to their condition.

TRANSLATIONAL RESEARCH

Mount Sinai's scientists are conducting state-of-the-art translational thoracic research, including genomic analysis of tumors to better understand and predict behavior in order to develop more directed, personalized therapeutic approaches to treatment.

SCREENING AND DIAGNOSIS

Mount Sinai offers comprehensive screening and diagnostic tests, including CT scans for early detection, advanced endoscopic techniques to detect early lesions and recurrence, PET scans, and innovative MRI technology with ultrasensitive resolution. Our developing program for the screening and detection of esophageal cancer is the first of its kind in New York City.

THORACIC SURGERY

On the technological forefront of minimally invasive techniques, the Division of Thoracic Surgery at NYU Langone Medical Center dedicates itself to the diagnosis and treatment of abdominal, lung, mediastinal, and chest wall problems. At NYU Hospitals Center, the majority of thoracic procedures are performed utilizing video-assisted equipment, which benefits surgeon and patient alike.

Use of video-assisted equipment means not only a more accurate and safe surgery, but it also means smaller incisions, an indispensable benefit to the patient, reducing discomfort, recovery time, and length of stay. Moving away from the traditional method of long incisions through the muscular abdominal wall, NYU's thoracic surgeons perform the same procedures through much smaller openings, with better results.

The Division of Thoracic Surgery at NYU Hospitals Center uses minimally invasive techniques to provide its patients maximum comfort and accuracy of diagnosis and treatment. Below are just some of the latest interventions performed by its doctors:

VIDEO-ASSISTED THORACOSCOPY
- Sympathectomy for Hyperhydrosis
- Pleural Biopsy
- Pleurectomy
- Pleurodesis
- Mediastinal Evaluation
- Lung Resection
- Lung Volume Reduction Procedures
- Esophageal Procedures

VIDEO-ASSISTED BRONCHOSCOPY
- Diagnostic Evaluation
- Laser Resection of Tumor
- Endobronchial Stent Insertion

VIDEO-ASSISTED MEDIASTINOS COPY
- Staging Procedures
- Diagnostic Evaluations

Urology

A urologist manages benign and malignant medical and surgical disorders of the genitourinary system and the adrenal gland. This specialist has comprehensive knowledge of, and skills in, endoscopic, percutaneous and open surgery of congenital and acquired conditions of the urinary and reproductive systems and their contiguous structures.

Training Required: Five years

UROLOGY

New England

Caldamone, Anthony A MD [U] - **Spec Exp:** Pediatric Urology; **Hospital:** Rhode Island Hosp; **Address:** 2 Dudley St, Ste 185, Providence, RI 02905; **Phone:** 401-421-0710; **Board Cert:** Urology 1983; **Med School:** Brown Univ 1975; **Resid:** Urology, Strong Meml Hosp 1981; **Fellow:** Pediatric Urology, Childrens Hosp 1982; **Fac Appt:** Prof U, Brown Univ

Gomery, Pablo MD [U] - **Spec Exp:** Neuro-Urology; Erectile Dysfunction; Voiding Dysfunction; Infertility-Male; **Hospital:** Mass Genl Hosp, Spaulding Rehab Hosp; **Address:** Mass General Hospital, Dept Urology, 55 Fruit St, GRB 1102, Boston, MA 02114; **Phone:** 617-726-8482; **Board Cert:** Urology 2000; **Med School:** Albert Einstein Coll Med 1974; **Resid:** Surgery, New England Deaconess Hosp 1977; Urology, Mass General Hosp 1980

Heney, Niall M MD [U] - **Spec Exp:** Urologic Cancer; **Hospital:** Mass Genl Hosp; **Address:** Mass Genl Hosp, Dept Urol, 55 Fruit St, GRB 1102, Boston, MA 02114; **Phone:** 617-726-3011; **Board Cert:** Urology 1977; **Med School:** Ireland 1965; **Resid:** Urology, Regional Hosp 1972; Urology, Mass Genl Hosp 1976; **Fac Appt:** Prof U, Harvard Med Sch

Janeiro Jr, John J MD [U] - **Spec Exp:** Urologic Cancer; Kidney Stones; Vasectomy Reversal; **Hospital:** Southern NH Med Ctr, St Joseph Hosp; **Address:** Urology Center Southern New Hampshire, 17 Riverside St, Ste 201, Nashua, NH 03062; **Phone:** 603-883-1550; **Board Cert:** Urology 1999; **Med School:** Univ Mass Sch Med 1982; **Resid:** Urology, Lahey Clinic 1987; **Fellow:** Pediatric Urology, Childrens Hosp 1989

Libertino, John A MD [U] - **Spec Exp:** Kidney Cancer; Prostate Cancer; Adrenal Tumors; **Hospital:** Lahey Clin; **Address:** Lahey Clinic, Dept Urology, 41 Mall Rd, Burlington, MA 01805-0001; **Phone:** 781-744-2750; **Board Cert:** Urology 1973; **Med School:** Georgetown Univ 1965; **Resid:** Urology, Univ Rochester-Strong Meml Hosp 1967; Urology, Yale-New Haven Hosp 1970; **Fellow:** Surgery, Yale-New Haven Hosp 1968; **Fac Appt:** Assoc Clin Prof S, Harvard Med Sch

Loughlin, Kevin R MD [U] - **Spec Exp:** Prostate Cancer; Bladder Cancer; Penile Cancer; Genitourinary Cancer; **Hospital:** Brigham & Women's Hosp, Dana-Farber Cancer Inst; **Address:** Brigham & Women's Hosp, Div Urology, 45 Francis St, ASBII-3, Boston, MA 02115; **Phone:** 617-732-6325; **Board Cert:** Urology 2004; **Med School:** NY Med Coll 1975; **Resid:** Pediatrics, New York Hosp-Cornell 1978; Surgery, Bellevue Hosp Ctr-NYU 1979; **Fellow:** Urology, Brigham & Women's Hosp 1983; Urologic Oncology, Meml Sloan Kettering Cancer Ctr 1983; **Fac Appt:** Prof S, Harvard Med Sch

McDougal, W Scott MD [U] - **Spec Exp:** Penile Cancer; Prostate Cancer; Bladder Cancer; Urologic Cancer; **Hospital:** Mass Genl Hosp; **Address:** Mass Genl Hosp, 55 Fruit St, Bldg GRB - rm 1102, Boston, MA 02114; **Phone:** 617-726-3010; **Board Cert:** Surgery 1975; Urology 2004; **Med School:** Cornell Univ-Weill Med Coll 1968; **Resid:** Surgery, Univ Hosps Cleveland 1975; Urology, Univ Hosps Cleveland 1975; **Fellow:** Physiology, Yale Med Sch 1972; **Fac Appt:** Prof U, Harvard Med Sch

McGovern, Francis MD [U] - **Spec Exp:** Prostate Cancer; **Hospital:** Mass Genl Hosp; **Address:** One Hawthorne Pl, Ste 109, Boston, MA 02114; **Phone:** 617-726-3560; **Board Cert:** Urology 1999; **Med School:** Case West Res Univ 1983; **Resid:** Urology, Mass Genl Hosp 1989

O'Leary, Michael P MD [U] - **Spec Exp:** Sexual Dysfunction; Kidney Stones; Prostate Disease; **Hospital:** Brigham & Women's Hosp, Dana-Farber Cancer Inst; **Address:** Brigham & Women's Hosp, Div Urology, 45 Francis St, ASBIII-3, Boston, MA 02155; **Phone:** 617-732-6325; **Board Cert:** Urology 2000; **Med School:** Geo Wash Univ 1980; **Resid:** Urology, Tufts New Eng Med Ctr 1982; Urology, Mass Genl Hosp 1986; **Fellow:** Urology, UCSF Med Ctr 1989; **Fac Appt:** Assoc Prof S, Harvard Med Sch

Oates, Robert Davis MD [U] - **Spec Exp:** Infertility-Male; Vasectomy Reversal; Reproductive Genetics; **Hospital:** Boston Med Ctr; **Address:** Boston Univ Med Ctr, Dept Urology, 720 Harrison Ave, Ste 606, Boston, MA 02118-2334; **Phone:** 617-638-8485; **Board Cert:** Urology 2000; **Med School:** Boston Univ 1982; **Resid:** Surgery, Boston Univ Hosp 1984; Urology, Boston Univ Hosp 1987; **Fellow:** Reproductive Medicine, Baylor Coll Med 1988; **Fac Appt:** Prof U, Boston Univ

Richie, Jerome MD [U] - **Spec Exp:** Prostate Cancer; Testicular Cancer; Kidney Cancer; **Hospital:** Brigham & Women's Hosp, Dana-Farber Cancer Inst; **Address:** Brigham & Womens Hosp, 75 Francis St, Ste ASB2, Boston, MA 02115; **Phone:** 617-732-6325; **Board Cert:** Urology 1977; **Med School:** Univ Tex Med Br, Galveston 1969; **Resid:** Surgery, UCLA Med Ctr 1971; Urology, UCLA Med Ctr 1975; **Fac Appt:** Prof U, Harvard Med Sch

Sanda, Martin G MD [U] - **Spec Exp:** Prostate Cancer; Urologic Cancer; Minimally Invasive Urologic Surgery; **Hospital:** Beth Israel Deaconess Med Ctr - Boston; **Address:** Beth Israel Deaconess Medical Ctr, 330 Brookline Ave, Rabb 440, Boston, MA 02115; **Phone:** 617-667-2960; **Board Cert:** Urology 2007; **Med School:** Columbia P&S 1987; **Resid:** Surgery, Med Coll Virginia 1989; Urology, Johns Hopkins Hosp 1994; **Fellow:** Surgical Oncology, Natl Cancer Inst 1991; **Fac Appt:** Assoc Prof U, Harvard Med Sch

Sigman, Mark MD [U] - **Spec Exp:** Infertility-Male; Vasectomy Reversal; **Hospital:** Rhode Island Hosp; **Address:** 2 Dudley St, Ste 175, Providence, RI 02905-3247; **Phone:** 401-421-0710; **Board Cert:** Urology 2000; **Med School:** Univ Conn 1981; **Resid:** Urology, Univ VA 1987; Surgery, Univ VA 1983; **Fellow:** Male Reproduction, Baylor Coll Med 1989; **Fac Appt:** Assoc Prof U, Brown Univ

Weiss, Robert M MD [U] - **Spec Exp:** Pediatric Urology; **Hospital:** Yale-New Haven Hosp; **Address:** Yale Univ Sch Med, Dept Urology, 800 Howard Ave, Box 208041, New Haven, CT 06520-8041; **Phone:** 203-785-2815; **Board Cert:** Urology 1999; **Med School:** SUNY Downstate 1960; **Resid:** Surgery, Beth Israel Hosp 1962; Urology, Columbia Presby Hosp 1967; **Fellow:** Pharmacology, Columbia Presby Hosp 1965; **Fac Appt:** Prof U, Yale Univ

Mid Atlantic

Alexander, Richard B MD [U] - **Spec Exp:** Prostate Disease; **Hospital:** Univ of MD Med Sys; **Address:** 419 W Redwood St, Ste 320, Baltimore, MD 21201; **Phone:** 410-328-5109; **Board Cert:** Urology 1999; **Med School:** Johns Hopkins Univ 1981; **Resid:** Surgery, Vanderbilt Univ Affl Hosps 1983; Urology, Johns Hopkins Hosp 1988; **Fellow:** Cancer Immunology, Natl Cancer Inst 1989; **Fac Appt:** Assoc Prof U, Univ MD Sch Med

Bagley, Demetrius H MD [U] - **Spec Exp:** Endourology; Kidney Stones; Kidney Cancer; Ureter & Renal Pelvis Cancer; **Hospital:** Thomas Jefferson Univ Hosp; **Address:** 833 Chestnut St E, Ste 703, Philadelphia, PA 19107; **Phone:** 215-955-1000; **Board Cert:** Urology 1981; **Med School:** Johns Hopkins Univ 1970; **Resid:** Surgery, Yale-New Haven Hosp 1972; Urology, Yale-New Haven Hosp 1979; **Fellow:** Surgery, NCI-USPHS 1975; **Fac Appt:** Prof U, Thomas Jefferson Univ

Urology

Bar-Chama, Natan MD [U] - **Spec Exp:** Infertility-Male; Erectile Dysfunction; Varicocele Micro-surgery; Vasectomy Reversal; **Hospital:** Mount Sinai Med Ctr (page 64); **Address:** 5 E 98th St, Box 1272, New York, NY 10029-6501; **Phone:** 212-241-4812; **Board Cert:** Urology 2006; **Med School:** Albert Einstein Coll Med 1987; **Resid:** Urology, Montefiore/Albert Einstein 1993; **Fellow:** Male Infertility, Baylor Coll Med 1994; **Fac Appt:** Assoc Prof U, Mount Sinai Sch Med

Belman, A Barry MD [U] - **Spec Exp:** Pediatric Urology; Hypospadias; **Hospital:** Chldns Natl Med Ctr; **Address:** Chldns Natl Med Ctr, 111 Michigan Ave NW, Washington, DC 20010-2978; **Phone:** 202-476-5042; **Board Cert:** Urology 1973; **Med School:** Northwestern Univ 1964; **Resid:** Urology, Northwestern Univ Med Ctr 1970; **Fac Appt:** Prof U, Geo Wash Univ

Benson, Mitchell C MD [U] - **Spec Exp:** Prostate Cancer/Robotic Surgery; Bladder Cancer; Kidney Cancer; Continent Urinary Diversions; **Hospital:** NY-Presby Hosp/Columbia (page 66); **Address:** NY Presby Hosp-Columbia, Dept Urology, 161 Ft Washington Ave Fl 11 - rm 1102, New York, NY 10032-3713; **Phone:** 212-305-5201; **Board Cert:** Urology 1984; **Med School:** Columbia P&S 1977; **Resid:** Surgery, Mount Sinai Med Ctr 1979; Urology, Columbia-Presby Hosp 1982; **Fellow:** Oncology, Johns Hopkins Hosp 1984; **Fac Appt:** Prof U, Columbia P&S

Blaivas, Jerry G MD [U] - **Spec Exp:** Uro-Gynecology; Urology-Female; Neurogenic Bladder; Incontinence after Prostate Cancer; **Hospital:** NY-Presby Hosp/Weill Cornell (page 66), Lenox Hill Hosp (page 62); **Address:** 445 E 77th St, New York, NY 10021; **Phone:** 212-772-3900; **Board Cert:** Urology 1978; **Med School:** Tufts Univ 1964; **Resid:** Surgery, Boston Med Ctr 1971; Urology, New England Med Ctr 1976; **Fac Appt:** Clin Prof U, Cornell Univ-Weill Med Coll

Burnett II, Arthur L MD [U] - **Spec Exp:** Prostate Cancer; Erectile Dysfunction; **Hospital:** Johns Hopkins Hosp - Baltimore (page 61); **Address:** 600 N Wolfe St, Marburg Bldg, Ste 407, Baltimore, MD 21287; **Phone:** 410-614-3986; **Board Cert:** Urology 1998; **Med School:** Johns Hopkins Univ 1988; **Resid:** Surgery, Johns Hopkins Hosp 1990; Urology, Johns Hopkins Hosp 1994; **Fac Appt:** Prof U, Johns Hopkins Univ

Canning, Douglas MD [U] - **Spec Exp:** Pediatric Urology; Hypospadias; Bladder Exstrophy; **Hospital:** Chldns Hosp of Philadelphia, The; **Address:** Childrens Hosp, Div Urology, 34th St & Civic Center Blvd, Wood Bldg, 3rd Fl, Philadelphia, PA 19104; **Phone:** 215-590-2754; **Board Cert:** Urology 2000; **Med School:** Dartmouth Med Sch 1982; **Resid:** Urology, Naval Hosp 1987; **Fellow:** Pediatric Urology, Johns Hopkins Hosp 1988; **Fac Appt:** Assoc Prof U, Univ Pennsylvania

Carter, H Ballentine MD [U] - **Spec Exp:** Prostate Cancer; **Hospital:** Johns Hopkins Hosp - Baltimore (page 61); **Address:** Brady Urological Inst, Johns Hopkins Hosp, 600 N Wolfe St Marburg Bldg - rm 145, Baltimore, MD 21287-2101; **Phone:** 410-955-6100; **Board Cert:** Urology 1999; **Med School:** Med Univ SC 1981; **Resid:** Surgery, New York Hosp 1983; Urology, New York Hosp 1987; **Fellow:** Research, Johns Hopkins Hosp 1989; **Fac Appt:** Prof U, Johns Hopkins Univ

Chancellor, Michael B MD [U] - **Spec Exp:** Incontinence-Female; Urology-Female; Neuro-Urology; **Hospital:** UPMC Presby, Pittsburgh; **Address:** 3471 Fifth Ave, Kaufmann Bldg, rm 700, Pittsburgh, PA 15213; **Phone:** 412-692-4096; **Board Cert:** Urology 2000; **Med School:** Med Coll Wisc 1983; **Resid:** Surgery, Univ Mich 1985; Urology, Univ Mich 1988; **Fellow:** Neurourology, Columbia-Presby Med Ctr 1990; **Fac Appt:** Prof U, Univ Pittsburgh

Docimo, Steven G MD [U] - **Spec Exp:** Pediatric Urology; Minimally Invasive Surgery; Bladder Reconstruction; Bladder Exstrophy; **Hospital:** Chldns Hosp of Pittsburgh - UPMC; **Address:** Children's Hosp Pediatric Urology, 3705 Fifth Ave, Desoto Wing, Pittsburgh, PA 15213; **Phone:** 412-692-7932; **Board Cert:** Urology 2000; **Med School:** Johns Hopkins Univ 1984; **Resid:** Surgery, Georgetown Univ Med Ctr 1986; Urology, Brigham & Womens Hosp 1990; **Fellow:** Pediatric Urology, Johns Hopkins 1994; Research, Childrens Hosp 1988; **Fac Appt:** Prof U, Univ Pittsburgh

America's Top Doctors® 8th Edition

Droller, Michael J MD [U] - **Spec Exp:** Urologic Cancer; Bladder Cancer; Prostate Cancer; Kidney Cancer; **Hospital:** Mount Sinai Med Ctr (page 64); **Address:** 5 E 98th St Fl 6, Box 1272, New York, NY 10029-6501; **Phone:** 212-241-3868; **Board Cert:** Urology 2001; **Med School:** Harvard Med Sch 1968; **Resid:** Surgery, Peter Bent Brigham Hosp 1970; Urology, Stanford Univ Med Ctr 1976; **Fellow:** Immunology, Univ Stockholm 1977; **Fac Appt:** Prof U, Mount Sinai Sch Med

Fisch, Harry MD [U] - **Spec Exp:** Infertility-Male; Microsurgery; Vasectomy Reversal; **Hospital:** NY-Presby Hosp/Columbia (page 66), Lenox Hill Hosp (page 62); **Address:** 944 Park Ave, Ste 1C, New York, NY 10028; **Phone:** 212-879-0800; **Board Cert:** Urology 1999; **Med School:** Mount Sinai Sch Med 1983; **Resid:** Surgery, Montefiore Hosp Med Ctr 1985; Urology, Montefiore Hosp Med Ctr 1989; **Fac Appt:** Prof U, Columbia P&S

Gearhart, John P MD [U] - **Spec Exp:** Pediatric Urology; Bladder Exstrophy; **Hospital:** Johns Hopkins Hosp - Baltimore (page 61); **Address:** Johns Hopkins Hospital, Brady Urological Institute, 600 N Wolfe St Marburg Bldg - Ste 146, Baltimore, MD 21287-2101; **Phone:** 410-955-5358; **Board Cert:** Urology 1982; **Med School:** Univ Louisville Sch Med 1975; **Resid:** Urology, Med Coll Georgia Hosp 1980; **Fellow:** Pediatric Urology, Alder Hey Chldns Hosp 1981; Pediatric Urology, Johns Hopkins Hosp 1985; **Fac Appt:** Prof U, Johns Hopkins Univ

Glassberg, Kenneth MD [U] - **Spec Exp:** Pediatric Urology; Genital Reconstruction; Varicocele In Adolescents; **Hospital:** NYPresby-Morgan Stanley Children's Hosp (page 66); **Address:** Morgan Stanley Chlds Hosp of NY-Presby, 3959 Broadway, BHN 1118, New York, NY 10032; **Phone:** 212-305-9918; **Board Cert:** Urology 1977; **Med School:** SUNY Downstate 1968; **Resid:** Surgery, Montefiore Hosp Med Ctr 1972; Urology, Univ Hosp 1975; **Fellow:** Pediatric Urology, Adler Hey Chldns Hosp 1976; Pediatric Urology, Hosp For Sick Chldn 1976; **Fac Appt:** Prof U, Columbia P&S

Goldstein, Marc MD [U] - **Spec Exp:** Infertility-Male; Vasectomy & Vascectomy Reversal; Varicocele Microsurgery; Erectile Dysfunction; **Hospital:** NY-Presby Hosp/Weill Cornell (page 66); **Address:** Cornell Inst for Reproductive Med, 525 E 68th St, Box 580, New York, NY 10021-4870; **Phone:** 212-746-5470; **Board Cert:** Urology 1982; **Med School:** SUNY Downstate 1972; **Resid:** Surgery, Columbia-Presby Med Ctr 1974; Urology, SUNY Downstate Med Ctr 1980; **Fellow:** Microsurgery, Rockefeller Univ 1982; **Fac Appt:** Prof U, Cornell Univ-Weill Med Coll

Gomella, Leonard G MD [U] - **Spec Exp:** Prostate Cancer; Minimally Invasive Urologic Surgery; Urologic Cancer; **Hospital:** Thomas Jefferson Univ Hosp; **Address:** Thomas Jefferson Univ, 1015 Walnut St Fl 11 - Ste 1112, Philadelphia, PA 19107-5001; **Phone:** 215-955-1000; **Board Cert:** Urology 1998; **Med School:** Univ KY Coll Med 1980; **Resid:** Surgery, Univ Kentucky Med Ctr 1982; Urology, Univ Kentucky Med Ctr 1986; **Fellow:** Urologic Oncology, Natl Cancer Inst 1988; **Fac Appt:** Prof U, Jefferson Med Coll

Grasso, Michael MD [U] - **Spec Exp:** Urologic Cancer; Laparoscopic Surgery; Kidney Stones; Testicular Cancer; **Hospital:** St Vincent Cath Med Ctrs - Manhattan; **Address:** 170 W 12th St, Ste 205, Dept Urology - Cronin 205, New York, NY 10011; **Phone:** 212-604-1270; **Board Cert:** Urology 2002; **Med School:** Jefferson Med Coll 1986; **Resid:** Surgery, Jefferson Univ Hosp 1988; Urology, Jefferson Univ Hosp 1992; **Fac Appt:** Prof U, NY Med Coll

Greenberg, Richard E MD [U] - **Spec Exp:** Prostate Cancer; Bladder Cancer; Kidney Cancer; Prostate Cancer/Robotic Surgery; **Hospital:** Fox Chase Cancer Ctr (page 58), Abington Mem Hosp; **Address:** Fox Chase Cancer Ctr, Div Urol-Dept Surg, 333 Cottman Ave, Ste H3 - rm H3-116, Philadelphia, PA 19111; **Phone:** 215-728-5341; **Board Cert:** Urology 2005; **Med School:** Cornell Univ-Weill Med Coll 1976; **Resid:** Surgery, New York Hosp 1979; Urology, New York Hosp 1983; **Fac Appt:** Prof U, Temple Univ

Urology

Gribetz, Michael MD [U] - **Spec Exp:** Prostate Disease; Urology-Female; Sexual Dysfunction; Kidney Stones; **Hospital:** Mount Sinai Med Ctr (page 64); **Address:** 1155 Park Ave, New York, NY 10128-1209; **Phone:** 212-831-1300; **Board Cert:** Urology 1980; **Med School:** Albert Einstein Coll Med 1973; **Resid:** Surgery, Montefiore Hosp Med Ctr 1975; Urology, Mount Sinai Hosp 1978; **Fac Appt:** Asst Clin Prof U, Mount Sinai Sch Med

Hensle, Terry MD [U] - **Spec Exp:** Pediatric Urology; **Hospital:** NYPresby-Morgan Stanley Children's Hosp (page 66), Hackensack Univ Med Ctr; **Address:** Morgan Stanley Chldns Hosp of NY-Presby, 3959 Broadway, Ste 219N, New York, NY 10032; **Phone:** 212-305-8510; **Board Cert:** Urology 1978; **Med School:** Cornell Univ-Weill Med Coll 1968; **Resid:** Surgery, Boston City Hosp 1973; Urology, Mass Genl Hosp 1976; **Fellow:** Pediatric Urology, Mass Genl Hosp 1977; Pediatric Urology, Great Ormond St Hosp 1978; **Fac Appt:** Prof U, Columbia P&S

Herr, Harry W MD [U] - **Spec Exp:** Bladder Cancer; Prostate Cancer; Testicular Cancer; **Hospital:** Meml Sloan-Kettering Cancer Ctr, NY-Presby Hosp/Weill Cornell (page 66); **Address:** 1275 York Avenue, New York, NY 10065; **Phone:** 800-525-2225; **Board Cert:** Urology 1976; **Med School:** UCSF 1969; **Resid:** Urology, UC Irvine Med Ctr 1974; **Fellow:** Urology, Meml Sloan Kettering Cancer Ctr 1976; **Fac Appt:** Assoc Prof S, Cornell Univ-Weill Med Coll

Huben, Robert P MD [U] - **Spec Exp:** Prostate Cancer; Kidney Cancer; Urologic Cancer; **Hospital:** Roswell Park Cancer Inst; **Address:** Roswell Park Cancer Inst, Elm & Carlton Sts, Buffalo, NY 14263-0001; **Phone:** 716-845-3389; **Board Cert:** Urology 1983; **Med School:** Cornell Univ-Weill Med Coll 1976; **Resid:** Urology, East Virginia Med Ctr 1981; **Fellow:** Urologic Oncology, Roswell Park Meml Inst 1982

Jackman, Stephen V MD [U] - **Spec Exp:** Prostate Cancer/Robotic Surgery; Laparoscopic Surgery; Kidney Stones; **Hospital:** UPMC Shadyside, UPMC Presby, Pittsburgh; **Address:** UPMC, Kaufman Bldg, 3471 Fifth Ave, Ste 700, Pittsburgh, PA 15213; **Phone:** 412-692-4095; **Board Cert:** Urology 2002; **Med School:** Yale Univ 1994; **Resid:** Urology, Johns Hopkins Hosp 1999; **Fac Appt:** Assoc Prof U, Univ Pittsburgh

Jarow, Jonathan P MD [U] - **Spec Exp:** Infertility-Male; Prostate Cancer; Erectile Dysfunction; Incontinence after Prostate Cancer; **Hospital:** Johns Hopkins Hosp - Baltimore (page 61); **Address:** Johns Hopkins Outpatient Ctr-Urology, 601 N Caroline St, Fl 4, Baltimore, MD 21287; **Phone:** 410-955-3617; **Board Cert:** Urology 1999; **Med School:** Northwestern Univ 1980; **Resid:** Surgery, Johns Hopkins Hosp 1982; Urology, Johns Hopkins Hosp 1986; **Fellow:** Andrology, Baylor Univ 1989; **Fac Appt:** Assoc Prof U, Johns Hopkins Univ

Kaplan, Steven A MD [U] - **Spec Exp:** Urodynamics; Voiding Dysfunction; Incontinence after Prostate Cancer; Incontinence-Male; **Hospital:** NY-Presby Hosp/Weill Cornell (page 66); **Address:** NY Presbyterian-Weill Cornell Med Ctr, 525 E 68th St, rm F9West, New York, NY 10021-4870; **Phone:** 212-746-4811; **Board Cert:** Urology 2001; **Med School:** Mount Sinai Sch Med 1982; **Resid:** Surgery, Mount Sinai Hosp 1984; Urology, Columbia Presby Med Ctr 1988; **Fellow:** Urology, Columbia Presby Med Ctr 1990; **Fac Appt:** Prof U, Cornell Univ-Weill Med Coll

Katz, Aaron E MD [U] - **Spec Exp:** Prostate Cancer-Cryosurgery; Kidney Cancer-Cryosurgery; Complementary Medicine; Nutrition & Cancer Prevention; **Hospital:** NY-Presby Hosp/Columbia (page 66); **Address:** NY Presby Med Ctr, Herbert Irving Pav, 161 Ft Washington Ave Fl 11, New York, NY 10032; **Phone:** 212-305-6408; **Board Cert:** Urology 2006; **Med School:** NY Med Coll 1986; **Resid:** Urology, Maimonides Med Ctr 1992; **Fellow:** Urologic Oncology, Columbia Presby Med Ctr 1993; **Fac Appt:** Assoc Clin Prof U, Columbia P&S

Kavoussi, Louis R MD [U] - **Spec Exp:** Laparoscopic Surgery; Kidney Stones; Urologic Cancer; **Hospital:** Long Island Jewish Med Ctr, N Shore Univ Hosp; **Address:** 450 Lakeville Rd, Ste M-41, New Hyde Park, NY 11040; **Phone:** 516-734-8558; **Board Cert:** Urology 1999; **Med School:** SUNY Buffalo 1983; **Resid:** Surgery, Barnes Jewish Hosp 1985; Urology, Barnes Jewish Hosp 1989; **Fac Appt:** Prof U, NYU Sch Med

Kirschenbaum, Alexander M MD [U] - **Spec Exp:** Prostate Cancer; Bladder Cancer; Kidney Cancer; **Hospital:** Mount Sinai Med Ctr (page 64); **Address:** 58A E 79th St, New York, NY 10021; **Phone:** 646-422-0926; **Board Cert:** Urology 2006; **Med School:** Mount Sinai Sch Med 1980; **Resid:** Surgery, Mount Sinai Hosp 1982; Urology, Mount Sinai Hosp 1985; **Fellow:** Urologic Oncology, Mount Sinai Hosp 1987; **Fac Appt:** Assoc Prof U, Mount Sinai Sch Med

Lanteri, Vincent J MD [U] - **Spec Exp:** Prostate Cancer/Robotic Surgery; Urologic Cancer; Minimally Invasive Urologic Surgery; **Hospital:** Hackensack Univ Med Ctr, Valley Hosp; **Address:** 5 Summit Ave Fl 2, Hackensack, NJ 07607; **Phone:** 201-487-8866; **Board Cert:** Urology 1982; **Med School:** Mexico 1974; **Resid:** Surgery, UMDNJ Med Ctr 1977; Urology, UMDNJ Med Ctr 1980; **Fellow:** Urologic Oncology, Roswell Park Cancer Inst 1981

Lepor, Herbert MD [U] - **Spec Exp:** Prostate Cancer; **Hospital:** NYU Med Ctr (page 68); **Address:** 150 E 32nd St Fl 2, New York, NY 10016; **Phone:** 646-825-6327; **Board Cert:** Urology 2006; **Med School:** Johns Hopkins Univ 1975; **Resid:** Urology, Johns Hopkins Hosp 1986; **Fac Appt:** Prof U, NYU Sch Med

Lowe, Franklin MD [U] - **Spec Exp:** Prostate Disease; Complementary Medicine; Prostate Cancer; **Hospital:** St Luke's - Roosevelt Hosp Ctr - Roosevelt Div (page 57), NY-Presby Hosp/Columbia (page 66); **Address:** 425 W 59th St, Ste 3A, New York, NY 10019-1104; **Phone:** 212-523-7790; **Board Cert:** Urology 2006; **Med School:** Columbia P&S 1979; **Resid:** Surgery, Johns Hopkins Hosp 1981; Urology, Johns Hopkins Hosp 1984; **Fac Appt:** Clin Prof U, Columbia P&S

Malkowicz, S Bruce MD [U] - **Spec Exp:** Prostate Cancer; Bladder Cancer; Kidney Cancer; Gene Therapy; **Hospital:** Hosp Univ Penn - UPHS (page 60); **Address:** Hosp Univ Penn, Dept Urology, 3400 Spruce St, 9 Penn Tower, Philadelphia, PA 19104; **Phone:** 215-662-2891; **Board Cert:** Urology 2000; **Med School:** Univ Pennsylvania 1981; **Resid:** Surgery, Hosp Univ Penn 1983; Urology, Hosp Univ Penn 1987; **Fellow:** Urologic Oncology, USC Med Ctr 1998; Urologic Oncology, Hosp Univ Penn/Wistar Inst 1990; **Fac Appt:** Assoc Prof U, Univ Pennsylvania

McCullough, Andrew R MD [U] - **Spec Exp:** Erectile Dysfunction; Infertility-Male; Prostate Cancer; **Hospital:** NYU Med Ctr (page 68); **Address:** NYU Med Ctr, Dept Urology, 150 E 32nd St Fl 2, New York, NY 10016; **Phone:** 646-825-6311; **Board Cert:** Urology 2005; **Med School:** Univ MD Sch Med 1978; **Resid:** Urology, Johns Hopkins Hosp 1983; **Fellow:** Urologic Oncology, Johns Hopkins Hosp 1984; **Fac Appt:** Assoc Prof U, NYU Sch Med

Mostwin, Jacek L MD/PhD [U] - **Spec Exp:** Prostate Cancer; **Hospital:** Johns Hopkins Hosp - Baltimore (page 61); **Address:** Johns Hopkins Hosp, 600 N Wolfe St, Marburg-401C, Baltimore, MD 21287; **Phone:** 410-955-4461; **Board Cert:** Urology 2007; **Med School:** Univ MD Sch Med 1975; **Resid:** Surgery, Univ Michigan Med Ctr 1978; Urology, Johns Hopkins Hosp 1983; **Fac Appt:** Prof U, Johns Hopkins Univ

Mulhall, John P MD [U] - **Spec Exp:** Erectile Dysfunction; Peyronie's Disease; Penile Prostheses; Infertility-Male; **Hospital:** NY-Presby Hosp/Columbia (page 66), Meml Sloan-Kettering Cancer Ctr; **Address:** Weill Cornell Medical Ctr, 352 E 68th St, New York, NY 10021; **Phone:** 212-746-5653; **Board Cert:** Urology 1999; **Med School:** Ireland 1985; **Resid:** Urology, Univ Conn Health Ctr 1995; **Fellow:** Urology, Boston Univ Med Ctr 1996; **Fac Appt:** Assoc Prof U, Cornell Univ-Weill Med Coll

Urology

Nagler, Harris M MD [U] - **Spec Exp:** Vasectomy Reversal; Infertility-Male; Varicocele Microsurgery; Erectile Dysfunction; **Hospital:** Beth Israel Med Ctr - Petrie Division (page 57); **Address:** Beth Israel Med Ctr, Dept Urology, 10 Union Square E, Ste 3A, New York, NY 10003-3314; **Phone:** 212-844-8700; **Board Cert:** Urology 1982; **Med School:** Temple Univ 1975; **Resid:** Urology, Columbia Presby Med Ctr 1980; **Fellow:** Reproductive Medicine, Columbia Presby Med Ctr 1981; **Fac Appt:** Prof U, Albert Einstein Coll Med

Naslund, Michael MD [U] - **Spec Exp:** Prostate Cancer; Prostate Disease; **Hospital:** Univ of MD Med Sys; **Address:** Maryland Prostate Ctr, 419 W Redwood St, Ste 320, Baltimore, MD 21201; **Phone:** 410-328-0800; **Board Cert:** Urology 2000; **Med School:** Johns Hopkins Univ 1981; **Resid:** Surgery, Johns Hopkins Hosp 1983; Urology, Johns Hopkins Hosp 1987; **Fac Appt:** Prof U, Univ MD Sch Med

Nelson, Joel B MD [U] - **Spec Exp:** Prostate Cancer; **Hospital:** UPMC Shadyside; **Address:** UPMC Shadyside Med Ctr, 5200 Centre Ave, Ste 209, Pittsburgh, PA 15232-1312; **Phone:** 412-605-3013; **Board Cert:** Urology 1998; **Med School:** Northwestern Univ 1988; **Resid:** Surgery, Northwestern Meml Hosp 1990; Urology, Northwestern Meml Hosp 1994; **Fellow:** Urology, Johns Hopkins Hosp; **Fac Appt:** Prof U, Univ Pittsburgh

Nitti, Victor MD [U] - **Spec Exp:** Urology-Female; Incontinence-Male & Female; Urodynamics; Voiding Dysfunction; **Hospital:** NYU Med Ctr (page 68); **Address:** 150 E 32nd St, Ste 200, New York, NY 10016; **Phone:** 646-825-6324; **Board Cert:** Urology 2002; **Med School:** UMDNJ-NJ Med Sch, Newark 1985; **Resid:** Surgery, Univ Hosp 1987; Urology, Univ Hosp 1991; **Fellow:** Urology, UCLA Med Ctr 1992; **Fac Appt:** Assoc Prof U, NYU Sch Med

Partin, Alan W MD/PhD [U] - **Spec Exp:** Prostate Cancer; Prostate Disease; **Hospital:** Johns Hopkins Hosp - Baltimore (page 61); **Address:** Johns Hopkins Hosp, 600 N Wolfe St Marburg Bldg - rm 134, Baltimore, MD 21287; **Phone:** 410-614-4876; **Board Cert:** Urology 1998; **Med School:** Johns Hopkins Univ 1989; **Resid:** Surgery, Johns Hopkins Hosp 1991; Urology, Johns Hopkins Hosp 1994; **Fac Appt:** Prof U, Johns Hopkins Univ

Poppas, Dix P MD [U] - **Spec Exp:** Genital Reconstruction-Pediatric; Robotic Surgery-Pediatric; Minimally Invasive Surgery-Pediatric; **Hospital:** NY-Presby Hosp/Weill Cornell (page 66); **Address:** Inst for Pediatric Urology, NY Presby Hosp-Weill Cornell, 525 E 68th St, Box 94, New York, NY 10021-4870; **Phone:** 212-746-5337; **Board Cert:** Urology 1999; **Med School:** Eastern VA Med Sch 1988; **Resid:** Urology, New York Hosp-Cornell Med Ctr 1994; **Fellow:** Pediatric Urology, Children's Hosp 1996; **Fac Appt:** Assoc Prof U, Cornell Univ-Weill Med Coll

Rushton Jr, H Gil MD [U] - **Spec Exp:** Pediatric Urology; Fetal Urology; Hypospadias; **Hospital:** Chldns Natl Med Ctr; **Address:** Dept Urology, 111 Michigan Ave NW, Washington, DC 20010; **Phone:** 202-476-5042; **Board Cert:** Urology 2004; **Med School:** Univ SC Sch Med 1978; **Resid:** Urology, Univ SC Med Ctr 1983; **Fellow:** Pediatric Urology, Hosp Sick Children 1984; Pediatric Urology, Emory Chldns Hosp 1986; **Fac Appt:** Prof U, Geo Wash Univ

Samadi, David B MD [U] - **Spec Exp:** Prostate Cancer/Robotic Surgery; Kidney Cancer; Bladder Cancer; Robotic Surgery; **Hospital:** Mount Sinai Med Ctr (page 64); **Address:** 5 E 98th St, Box 1480, New York, NY 10029; **Phone:** 212-241-8779; **Board Cert:** Urology 2004; **Med School:** SUNY Stony Brook 1994; **Resid:** Surgery, Montefiore Med Ctr 2000; Urology, Montefiore Med Ctr 2002; **Fellow:** Urologic Oncology, Meml Sloan Kettering Cancer Ctr 2003; Laparoscopic Surgery, Henri Mondor Hosp; **Fac Appt:** Asst Prof U, Columbia P&S

Sawczuk, Ihor S MD [U] - **Spec Exp:** Kidney Cancer; Bladder Cancer; Prostate Cancer/Robotic Surgery; Bladder Reconstruction; **Hospital:** Hackensack Univ Med Ctr, NY-Presby Hosp/Columbia (page 66); **Address:** Hackensack Univ Med Ctr, 360 Essex St, Ste 403, Hackensack, NJ 07601; **Phone:** 201-336-8090; **Board Cert:** Urology 2005; **Med School:** Med Coll PA Hahnemann 1979; **Resid:** Surgery, St Vincent's Hosp & Med Ctr 1981; Urology, Columbia-Presby Med Ctr 1984; **Fellow:** Urologic Oncology, Columbia-Presby Med Ctr 1986; **Fac Appt:** Prof U, Columbia P&S

Scardino, Peter T MD [U] - **Spec Exp:** Prostate Cancer; Bladder Cancer; Urologic Cancer; Urinary Reconstruction; **Hospital:** Meml Sloan-Kettering Cancer Ctr; **Address:** 1275 York Avenue, New York, NY 10065; **Phone:** 800-525-2225; **Board Cert:** Urology 1981; **Med School:** Duke Univ 1971; **Resid:** Surgery, Mass Genl Hosp 1973; Urology, UCLA Med Ctr 1979; **Fellow:** Urology, Natl Cancer Inst 1976; **Fac Appt:** Prof U, Cornell Univ-Weill Med Coll

Scherr, Douglas S MD [U] - **Spec Exp:** Prostate Cancer/Robotic Surgery; Bladder Cancer; Robotic Surgery; **Hospital:** NY-Presby Hosp/Weill Cornell (page 66); **Address:** NY Cornell Medical Ctr, Dept Urology, 525 E 68th St Starr 900, New York, NY 10021; **Phone:** 212-746-5788; **Board Cert:** Urology 2003; **Med School:** Duke Univ 1994; **Resid:** Urology, NY Hosp-Cornell Med Ctr 1999; **Fellow:** Urologic Oncology, Meml Sloan-Kettering Canc Ctr 2002; **Fac Appt:** Asst Prof U, Cornell Univ-Weill Med Coll

Schlegel, Peter MD [U] - **Spec Exp:** Prostate Cancer; Infertility-Male; Fertility Preservation in Cancer; **Hospital:** NY-Presby Hosp/Weill Cornell (page 66); **Address:** 525 E 68th St, Starr 900, New York, NY 10021-4870; **Phone:** 212-746-5491; **Board Cert:** Urology 2001; **Med School:** Univ Mass Sch Med 1983; **Resid:** Surgery, Johns Hopkins Hosp 1985; Urology, Johns Hopkins Hosp 1989; **Fellow:** Medical Oncology, Johns Hopkins Hosp 1987; Male Reproduction, NY Hosp-Cornell Med Ctr 1991; **Fac Appt:** Prof U, Cornell Univ-Weill Med Coll

Schoenberg, Mark P MD [U] - **Spec Exp:** Bladder Cancer; Urinary Reconstruction; **Hospital:** Johns Hopkins Hosp - Baltimore (page 61); **Address:** Johns Hopkins Hospital, 150 Marburg Bldg, 600 N Wolfe St, Baltimore, MD 21287-2101; **Phone:** 410-502-3803; **Board Cert:** Urology 2005; **Med School:** Univ Tex, Houston 1986; **Resid:** Surgery, Hosp U Penn 1988; Urologic Surgery, Hosp U Penn 1992; **Fellow:** Urologic Oncology, Brady Inst/Johns Hopkins 1994; **Fac Appt:** Prof U, Johns Hopkins Univ

Sheinfeld, Joel MD [U] - **Spec Exp:** Testicular Cancer; Bladder Cancer; Fertility Preservation in Cancer; **Hospital:** Meml Sloan-Kettering Cancer Ctr; **Address:** 1275 York Avenue, New York, NY 10065; **Phone:** 800-525-2225; **Board Cert:** Urology 2000; **Med School:** Univ Fla Coll Med 1981; **Resid:** Urology, Strong Meml Hosp 1986; **Fellow:** Urologic Oncology, Meml Sloan Kettering Cancer Ctr 1989; **Fac Appt:** Assoc Prof U, Cornell Univ-Weill Med Coll

Shenot, Patrick J MD [U] - **Spec Exp:** Voiding Dysfunction/Spinal Cord Injury; Voiding Dysfunction; Genitourinary Disorders; Incontinence; **Hospital:** Thomas Jefferson Univ Hosp; **Address:** 833 Chestnut St, Ste 703, Philadelphia, PA 19107; **Phone:** 215-503-2095; **Board Cert:** Urology 2000; **Med School:** SUNY Stony Brook 1991; **Resid:** Surgery, Thos Jefferson Univ Hosp 1993; Urology, Thos Jefferson Univ Hosp 1997; **Fac Appt:** Asst Prof U, Thomas Jefferson Univ

Snyder III, Howard M MD [U] - **Spec Exp:** Pediatric Urology; Genital Reconstruction; Reconstructive Urologic Surgery; **Hospital:** Chldns Hosp of Philadelphia, The, Hosp Univ Penn - UPHS (page 60); **Address:** Chldrns Hosp, Dept Ped Urology, 34th St & Civic Ctr Blvd, Wood Bldg, Fl 3, Philadelphia, PA 19104; **Phone:** 215-590-2767; **Board Cert:** Surgery 1995; Urology 1982; Pediatric Surgery 1995; **Med School:** Harvard Med Sch 1969; **Resid:** Surgery, Peter Bent Brigham Hosp 1973; Pediatric Surgery, Boston Chldns Hosp Med Ctr 1974; **Fellow:** Urology, Peter Bent Brigham Hosp 1980; **Fac Appt:** Prof U, Univ Pennsylvania

Urology

Sosa, R Ernest MD [U] - **Spec Exp:** Kidney Stones; Laparoscopic Surgery; Adrenal Surgery; **Hospital:** NY-Presby Hosp/Weill Cornell (page 66), Lenox Hill Hosp (page 62); **Address:** 880 5th Ave, New York, NY 10021; **Phone:** 212-570-6800; **Board Cert:** Urology 2006; **Med School:** Cornell Univ-Weill Med Coll 1978; **Resid:** Surgery, New York Hosp-Cornell 1980; Urology, New York Hosp-Cornell 1984; **Fellow:** Renal Physiology, New York Hosp-Cornell 1986; **Fac Appt:** Assoc Clin Prof U, Cornell Univ-Weill Med Coll

Taneja, Samir S MD [U] - **Spec Exp:** Kidney Cancer; Prostate Cancer; Bladder Cancer; **Hospital:** NYU Med Ctr (page 68); **Address:** 150 E 32nd St, Ste 200, New York, NY 10016-6024; **Phone:** 646-825-6321; **Board Cert:** Urology 1999; **Med School:** Northwestern Univ 1990; **Resid:** Urology, UCLA Med Ctr 1996; **Fellow:** Urologic Oncology, NYU Med Ctr 1998; **Fac Appt:** Assoc Prof U, NYU Sch Med

Tewari, Ashutosh MD [U] - **Spec Exp:** Prostate Cancer/Robotic Surgery; **Hospital:** NY-Presby Hosp/Weill Cornell (page 66); **Address:** Weill Cornell Brady Urologic Health Ct, 525 E 68th St, Starr 916, New York, NY 10021; **Phone:** 212-746-5638; **Med School:** India 1983; **Resid:** Surgery, GSVM Medical College 1990; Urology, Henry Ford Hosp 2003; **Fellow:** Transplant Surgery, Liverpool Univ Med Ctr 1993; Urologic Oncology, Shands Healthcare 1995; **Fac Appt:** Assoc Prof U, Cornell Univ-Weill Med Coll

Uzzo, Robert MD [U] - **Spec Exp:** Kidney Cancer; Bladder Cancer; Prostate Cancer; Testicular Cancer; **Hospital:** Fox Chase Cancer Ctr (page 58); **Address:** 333 Cottman Ave, rm H3116, Philadelphia, PA 19111; **Phone:** 215-728-3501; **Board Cert:** Urology 2001; **Med School:** Cornell Univ-Weill Med Coll 1991; **Resid:** Surgery, New York Hosp-Cornell Med Ctr 1993; Urology, New York Hosp-Cornell Med Ctr 1997; **Fellow:** Urologic Oncology, Cleveland Clinic 1999; Renal Transplant, Cleveland Clinic 2000; **Fac Appt:** Assoc Prof S, Temple Univ

Van Arsdalen, Keith N MD [U] - **Spec Exp:** Infertility-Male; Varicocele Microsurgery; Urologic Cancer; Vasectomy Reversal; **Hospital:** Hosp Univ Penn - UPHS (page 60), Chldns Hosp of Philadelphia, The; **Address:** Hosp Univ Penn, Div Urol, 3400 Spruce St, 9 Penn Tower, Philadelphia, PA 19104-4283; **Phone:** 215-662-2891; **Board Cert:** Urology 1984; **Med School:** Med Coll VA 1977; **Resid:** Surgery, Univ Maryland Hosp 1979; Urology, Med Coll Virginia 1982; **Fellow:** Urodynamics, Hosp Univ Penn 1983; **Fac Appt:** Prof U, Univ Pennsylvania

Vapnek, Jonathan M MD [U] - **Spec Exp:** Incontinence; Urology-Female; Neurogenic Bladder; **Hospital:** Mount Sinai Med Ctr (page 64); **Address:** 229 E 79th St, New York, NY 10021; **Phone:** 212-717-9500; **Board Cert:** Urology 2005; **Med School:** UCSD 1986; **Resid:** Surgery, UCSD Med Ctr 1988; Urology, UCSF Med Ctr 1992; **Fellow:** Urology, UC Davis Med Ctr 1993; **Fac Appt:** Assoc Clin Prof U, Mount Sinai Sch Med

Vaughan, Edwin D MD [U] - **Spec Exp:** Urologic Cancer; Adrenal Tumors; Prostate Disease; **Hospital:** NY-Presby Hosp/Weill Cornell (page 66); **Address:** New York Presby Hosp, Dept Urology, 525 E 68th St, Starr 900, Box 94, New York, NY 10021-4870; **Phone:** 212-746-5480; **Board Cert:** Urology 1986; **Med School:** Univ VA Sch Med 1965; **Resid:** Surgery, Vanderbilt Univ Med Ctr 1967; Urology, Univ Virginia Hosp 1971; **Fellow:** Internal Medicine, Columbia Univ 1973; **Fac Appt:** Prof U, Cornell Univ-Weill Med Coll

Walsh, Patrick MD [U] - **Spec Exp:** Prostate Cancer; **Hospital:** Johns Hopkins Hosp - Baltimore (page 61); **Address:** Brady Urological Inst, 600 N Wolfe St, Phipps 554A, Baltimore, MD 21287-2101; **Phone:** 410-955-6100; **Board Cert:** Urology 1975; **Med School:** Case West Res Univ 1964; **Resid:** Surgery, Peter Bent Brigham Hosp/Childrens Hosp 1967; Urology, UCLA Med Ctr 1971; **Fellow:** Endocrinology, Harbor Genl Hosp 1970; **Fac Appt:** Prof U, Johns Hopkins Univ

Wein, Alan J MD [U] - **Spec Exp:** Neuro-Urology; Prostate Cancer; Testicular Cancer; Urologic Cancer; **Hospital:** Hosp Univ Penn - UPHS (page 60), Pennsylvania Hosp (page 60); **Address:** Univ Penn Hlth System, Div Urology, 3400 34th & Civic Center Blvd, 9 Penn Tower, Philadelphia, PA 19104-4283; **Phone:** 215-662-2891; **Board Cert:** Urology 1995; **Med School:** Univ Pennsylvania 1966; **Resid:** Surgery, Hosp Univ Penn 1968; Urology, Hosp Univ Penn 1972; **Fellow:** Urology, Hosp Univ Penn 1969; **Fac Appt:** Prof U, Univ Pennsylvania

Weiss, Robert E MD [U] - **Spec Exp:** Bladder Cancer; Kidney Cancer; Testicular Cancer; **Hospital:** Robert Wood Johnson Univ Hosp - New Brunswick, Univ Med Ctr - Princeton; **Address:** 1 Robert Wood Johnson Pl Ste MB588, New Brunswick, NJ 08901-1928; **Phone:** 732-235-7775; **Board Cert:** Urology 2003; **Med School:** NYU Sch Med 1985; **Resid:** Surgery, Mount Sinai Med Ctr 1987; Urology, Mount Sinai Med Ctr 1991; **Fellow:** Urologic Oncology, Meml Sloan Kettering Cancer Ctr 1994; **Fac Appt:** Assoc Prof U, UMDNJ-RW Johnson Med Sch

Yu, George W MD [U] - **Spec Exp:** Urologic Cancer; Nutrition & Disease Prevention/Control; Nutrition & Cancer Prevention/Control; **Hospital:** G Washington Univ Hosp, Anne Arundel Med Ctr; **Address:** 122 Defense Hwy, Ste 224, Annapolis, MD 21401; **Phone:** 410-897-0540; **Board Cert:** Urology 1983; **Med School:** Tufts Univ 1973; **Resid:** Surgery, Brigham & Women's Hosp 1976; Urology, Johns Hopkins Hosp 1981; **Fac Appt:** Prof U, Geo Wash Univ

Southeast

Albala, David M MD [U] - **Spec Exp:** Laparoscopic Surgery; Kidney Stones; Prostate Cancer/Robotic Surgery; **Hospital:** Duke Univ Med Ctr, VA Med Ctr - Durham; **Address:** Duke Univ Med Ctr, Green Zone, Box 3457, Durham, NC 27710; **Phone:** 919-668-6401; **Board Cert:** Urology 2002; **Med School:** Mich State Univ 1983; **Resid:** Surgery, Dartmouth-Hitchcock Med Ctr 1985; Urology, Dartmouth-Hitchcock Med Ctr 1990; **Fellow:** Endourology, Wash Univ Med Ctr 1991; **Fac Appt:** Prof U, Duke Univ

Amling, Christopher L MD [U] - **Spec Exp:** Prostate Cancer/Robotic Surgery; Kidney Cancer; Bladder Cancer; Testicular Cancer; **Hospital:** Univ of Ala Hosp at Birmingham; **Address:** 1530 3rd Ave S, Ste FOT-1105, Birmingham, AL 35294; **Phone:** 205-975-0088; **Board Cert:** Urology 1999; **Med School:** Oregon Hlth Sci Univ 1985; **Resid:** Urology, Duke Univ Med Ctr 1996; **Fellow:** Urologic Oncology, Mayo Clinic 1997; **Fac Appt:** Prof U, Univ Ala

Assimos, Dean G MD [U] - **Spec Exp:** Kidney Stones; Reconstructive Urologic Surgery; **Hospital:** Wake Forest Univ Baptist Med Ctr (page 73); **Address:** WFU Baptist Med Ctr, Dept Urology, 140 Charlois Blvd, Winston-Salem, NC 27157; **Phone:** 336-716-4131; **Board Cert:** Urology 2003; **Med School:** Loyola Univ-Stritch Sch Med 1977; **Resid:** Surgery, Northwestern Univ Hosp 1979; Urology, Northwestern Univ Hosp 1983; **Fellow:** Urology, Bowman Gray Sch Med 1986; **Fac Appt:** Prof S, Wake Forest Univ

Atala, Anthony MD [U] - **Spec Exp:** Pediatric Urology; Reconstructive Surgery; Hernia; Microsurgery; **Hospital:** Wake Forest Univ Baptist Med Ctr (page 73); **Address:** Wake Forest Univ-Baptist, MC, Dept Urology, Medical Center Blvd, Winston-Salem, NC 27157; **Phone:** 336-716-4131; **Board Cert:** Urology 2004; **Med School:** Univ Louisville Sch Med 1985; **Resid:** Surgery, Univ Louisville Hosp 1987; Urology, Univ Louisville Hosp 1990; **Fellow:** Research, Childrens Hosp/Harvard 1991; Pediatric Urology, Childrens Hosp/Harvard 1992; **Fac Appt:** Prof U, Wake Forest Univ

Beall, Michael E MD [U] - **Spec Exp:** Prostate Cancer; Testicular Cancer; Vasectomy Reversal; **Hospital:** Inova Fairfax Hosp, Reston Hosp Ctr; **Address:** 8503 Arlington Blvd, Ste 310, Fairfax, VA 22031; **Phone:** 703-208-4200; **Board Cert:** Urology 1979; **Med School:** Geo Wash Univ 1972; **Resid:** Urology, Geo Wash Univ Hosp 1977; **Fac Appt:** Assoc Clin Prof U, Geo Wash Univ

Urology

Brock III, John W MD [U] - **Spec Exp:** Pediatric Urology; Reconstructive Surgery; **Hospital:** Vanderbilt Children's Hosp; **Address:** Vanderbilt Chldns Hosp, Div Ped Urology, 2200 Childrens Way, 4102 DOT, Nashville, TN 37232-9820; **Phone:** 615-936-1060; **Board Cert:** Urology 2004; **Med School:** Med Coll GA 1978; **Resid:** Urology, Vanderbilt Univ Med Ctr 1983; **Fac Appt:** Prof U, Vanderbilt Univ

Broderick, Gregory MD [U] - **Spec Exp:** Erectile Dysfunction; Voiding Dysfunction; Peyronie's Disease; **Hospital:** St Luke's Hosp - Jacksonville; **Address:** Mayo Clinic, Dept Urology, 4500 San Pablo Rd, Jacksonville, FL 32224; **Phone:** 904-953-7330; **Board Cert:** Urology 2002; **Med School:** UCSF 1983; **Resid:** Surgery, UCSF Med Ctr 1985; Urology, UCSF Med Ctr 1988; **Fellow:** Neurourology, UC Davis Med Ctr 1990; **Fac Appt:** Prof U, Mayo Med Sch

Carson III, Culley C MD [U] - **Spec Exp:** Erectile Dysfunction; Kidney Stones; Peyronie's Disease; **Hospital:** Univ NC Hosps; **Address:** Univ North Carolina, Dept Urol, 2113 Physicians Office Bldg, Chapel Hill, NC 27599-7235; **Phone:** 919-966-2571; **Board Cert:** Urology 1980; **Med School:** Geo Wash Univ 1971; **Resid:** Surgery, Dartmouth-Hitchcock Med Ctr 1973; Urology, Mayo Clinic 1978; **Fac Appt:** Prof U, Univ NC Sch Med

Chang, Sam S MD [U] - **Spec Exp:** Urologic Cancer; Prostate Cancer; Prostate Cancer-HIFU Therapy; High Intensity Focused Ultrasound(HIFU); **Hospital:** Vanderbilt Univ Med Ctr; **Address:** Vanderbilt University Med Ctr, A-1302 MCN, Nashville, TN 37232-2765; **Phone:** 615-322-2880; **Board Cert:** Urology 2002; **Med School:** Vanderbilt Univ 1992; **Resid:** Surgery, Vanderbilt Univ 1998; **Fellow:** Urologic Oncology, Meml Sloan Kettering Cancer Ctr 1999; **Fac Appt:** Assoc Prof U, Vanderbilt Univ

Cookson, Michael MD [U] - **Spec Exp:** Bladder Cancer; Testicular Cancer; Prostate Cancer; **Hospital:** Vanderbilt Univ Med Ctr, Saint Thomas Hosp - Nashville; **Address:** Vanderbilt Univ Med Ctr, Urol Surg A1302 MCN, Nashville, TN 37232-0001; **Phone:** 615-322-2880; **Board Cert:** Urology 2006; **Med School:** Univ Okla Coll Med 1988; **Resid:** Urology, Univ Tex San Antonio-Univ Hosp 1994; **Fellow:** Urologic Oncology, Meml Sloan-Kettering Cancer Ctr 1996; **Fac Appt:** Prof U, Vanderbilt Univ

El-Galley, Rizk MD [U] - **Spec Exp:** Urologic Cancer; Laparoscopic Surgery; Bladder Cancer; Hydrocele; **Hospital:** Univ of Ala Hosp at Birmingham; **Address:** UAB Hosp FOT-1105, 1530 3rd Ave S, Birmingham, AL 35294-3411; **Phone:** 205-996-8765; **Board Cert:** Urology 2003; **Med School:** Egypt 1983; **Resid:** Urology, Emory Univ Hosp 1999; **Fac Appt:** Asst Prof U, Univ Ala

Fraser, Lionel B MD [U] - **Spec Exp:** Prostate Cancer; Incontinence after Prostate Cancer; Erectile Dysfunction; **Hospital:** Baptist Hosp - Jackson; **Address:** Metropolitan Urology, St Dominics West Med Tower, 971 Lakeland Drive, Ste 360, Jackson, MS 39216; **Phone:** 601-982-0982; **Board Cert:** Urology 2005; **Med School:** Univ Mich Med Sch 1977; **Resid:** Surgery, New England Deaconness Hosp 1979; **Fellow:** Urology, Brigham & Womens Hosp 1983

Harty, James MD [U] - **Spec Exp:** Urologic Cancer; **Hospital:** Norton Hosp, Jewish Hosp HlthCre Svcs Inc; **Address:** Allied Urology, 250 E Liberty St, Ste 500, Louisville, KY 40202; **Phone:** 502-584-0651; **Board Cert:** Urology 1979; **Med School:** Ireland 1969; **Resid:** Surgery, Johns Hopkins Hosp 1973; Urology, Johns Hopkins Hosp 1977; **Fac Appt:** Prof S, Univ Louisville Sch Med

Howards, Stuart S MD [U] - **Spec Exp:** Infertility-Male; Pediatric Urology; **Hospital:** Univ Virginia Med Ctr; **Address:** Univ Virginia Hosp, Dept Urology, PO Box 800422, Charlottesville, VA 22908; **Phone:** 434-924-9559; **Board Cert:** Urology 1975; **Med School:** Columbia P&S 1963; **Resid:** Surgery, Chldns Hosp 1965; Urology, Peter Bent Brigham Hosp 1971; **Fellow:** Renal Physiology, Natl Inst Hlth 1968; **Fac Appt:** Prof U, Univ VA Sch Med

Irby III, Pierce B MD [U] - **Spec Exp:** Kidney Stones; Minimally Invasive Surgery; Vasectomy & Vasectomy Reversal; **Hospital:** Carolinas Med Ctr, Presby Hosp - Charlotte; **Address:** McKay Urology, 1023 Edgehill Rd S, Charlotte, NC 28207; **Phone:** 704-355-8686; **Board Cert:** Urology 2003; **Med School:** Uniformed Srvs Univ, Bethesda 1983; **Resid:** Urology, Letterman Army Med Ctr 1990; **Fellow:** Endourology, UCSF Med Ctr 1992; **Fac Appt:** Asst Clin Prof U, Univ NC Sch Med

Jordan, Gerald H MD [U] - **Spec Exp:** Incontinence; Urinary Reconstruction; Prostate Cancer; **Hospital:** Sentara Norfolk Genl Hosp; **Address:** 400 W Brambleton Ave, Ste 100, Norfolk, VA 23510; **Phone:** 757-457-5100; **Board Cert:** Urology 1984; **Med School:** Univ Tex, San Antonio 1977; **Resid:** Urology, Naval Reg Med Ctr 1978; **Fellow:** Reconstructive Surgery, Eastern Va Med Sch 1984; **Fac Appt:** Prof U, Eastern VA Med Sch

Joseph, David B MD [U] - **Spec Exp:** Pediatric Urology; Urodynamics; **Hospital:** Children's Hospital - Birmingham; **Address:** Childrens Hospital, Dept Urology, 1600 7th Ave S, Ste ACC-318, Birmingham, AL 35233; **Phone:** 205-939-9840; **Board Cert:** Urology 1997; **Med School:** Univ Wisc 1980; **Resid:** Urology, Univ Wisconsin Med Ctr 1985; **Fellow:** Pediatric Urology, Boston Childrens Hosp 1986; **Fac Appt:** Prof U, Univ Ala

Keane, Thomas E MD [U] - **Spec Exp:** Urologic Cancer; Genitourinary Cancer; Prostate Cancer; Clinical Trials; **Hospital:** MUSC Med Ctr; **Address:** MUSC-Urology Dept, 96 Jonathan Lucas St, Ste CSB644, Charleston, SC 29425; **Phone:** 843-792-1666; **Board Cert:** Urology 2003; **Med School:** Ireland 1981; **Resid:** Urology, St Vincents Hosp 1986; Urology, N Tees Gen Hosp 1988; **Fellow:** Urology, Duke Univ Med Ctr 1993; **Fac Appt:** Prof U, Univ SC Sch Med

Kennelly, Michael J MD [U] - **Spec Exp:** Incontinence; Voiding Dysfunction; Pelvic Organ Prolapse Repair; Neurogenic Bladder; **Hospital:** Carolinas Med Ctr, Presby Hosp - Charlotte; **Address:** 1023 Edgehill Rd S, Charlotte, NC 28207; **Phone:** 704-355-8686; **Board Cert:** Urology 2005; **Med School:** Univ Cincinnati 1989; **Resid:** Urology, Univ Mich Med Ctr 1994; **Fellow:** Neurology, Univ Tex Hlth Sci Ctr 1995; **Fac Appt:** Clin Prof U, Univ NC Sch Med

Kim, Edward D MD [U] - **Spec Exp:** Infertility-Male; Prostate Cancer; Bladder Cancer; **Hospital:** Univ of Tennesee Mem Hosp; **Address:** University Urology, 1928 Alcoa Hwy, Med Office B Bldg - Ste 222, Knoxville, TN 37920; **Phone:** 865-305-9254; **Board Cert:** Urology 1998; **Med School:** Northwestern Univ 1989; **Resid:** Urology, Northwestern Meml Hosp 1995; **Fellow:** Baylor Coll Med 1996; **Fac Appt:** Assoc Prof U, Univ Tenn Coll Med, Memphis

Lloyd, Lewis Keith MD [U] - **Spec Exp:** Erectile Dysfunction; Incontinence; Interstitial Cystitis; Voiding Dysfunction; **Hospital:** Univ of Ala Hosp at Birmingham; **Address:** FOT 1120, 510 20th St S, Birmingham, AL 35294-3411; **Phone:** 205-975-0088; **Board Cert:** Urology 1976; **Med School:** Tulane Univ 1966; **Resid:** Urology, Tulane Univ Hosp 1974; **Fac Appt:** Prof U, Univ Ala

Lockhart, Jorge L MD [U] - **Spec Exp:** Voiding Dysfunction; Bladder Cancer; **Hospital:** H Lee Moffitt Cancer Ctr & Research Inst, Tampa Genl Hosp; **Address:** H Lee Moffitt Cancer Ctr, Dept Urology, MCB-GU Clinic, 12902 Magnolia Drive, Tampa, FL 33612; **Phone:** 813-745-6033; **Board Cert:** Urology 1980; **Med School:** Uruguay 1973; **Resid:** Urology, Duke Univ Med Ctr 1977; **Fellow:** Urodynamics, Duke Univ Med Ctr 1978; **Fac Appt:** Prof S, Univ S Fla Coll Med

Lynne, Charles M MD [U] - **Spec Exp:** Infertility-Male in Spinal Cord Injury; Voiding Dysfunction/Spinal Cord Injury; Urodynamics; **Hospital:** Jackson Meml Hosp, Univ of Miami Hosp; **Address:** Univ Miami, Dept Urology 814, PO Box 016960, Miami, FL 33101; **Phone:** 305-243-6590; **Board Cert:** Urology 1974; **Med School:** Univ Miami Sch Med 1964; **Resid:** Urology, Univ Miami Affil Hosps 1971; **Fac Appt:** Prof U, Univ Miami Sch Med

Urology

Marshall, Fray F MD [U] - **Spec Exp:** Prostate Cancer; **Hospital:** Emory Univ Hosp; **Address:** Emory Urology, 1365 Clifton Rd NE B Bldg - Ste 1400, Atlanta, GA 30322; **Phone:** 404-778-4898; **Board Cert:** Urology 1977; **Med School:** Univ VA Sch Med 1969; **Resid:** Surgery, Univ Mich Hosps 1972; Urology, Mass Genl Hosp 1975; **Fac Appt:** Prof U, Emory Univ

Milam, Douglas F MD [U] - **Spec Exp:** Urodynamics; Voiding Dysfunction; **Hospital:** Vanderbilt Univ Med Ctr; **Address:** Vanderbilt Univ-Dept Urology, 1301 Medical Center Drive, Ste 3823, Nashville, TN 37232; **Phone:** 615-322-2880; **Board Cert:** Urology 2003; **Med School:** W VA Univ 1986; **Resid:** Surgery, Univ Utah Hosps 1988; Urology, Univ Utah Hosps 1991; **Fac Appt:** Assoc Prof U, Vanderbilt Univ

Moul, Judd W MD [U] - **Spec Exp:** Prostate Cancer; Testicular Cancer; **Hospital:** Duke Univ Med Ctr, Durham Regional Hosp; **Address:** Duke Univ Med Ctr, Div Urologic Surgery, Box 3707, Durham, NC 27710; **Phone:** 919-684-2446; **Board Cert:** Urology 1999; **Med School:** Jefferson Med Coll 1982; **Resid:** Urology, Walter Reed Army Med Ctr 1987; **Fellow:** Urologic Oncology, Duke Univ Med Ctr 1989; **Fac Appt:** Prof S, Duke Univ

Patel, Vipul R MD [U] - **Spec Exp:** Prostate Cancer/Robotic Surgery; Kidney Cancer; **Hospital:** Florida Hosp Celebration Hlth; **Address:** 410 Celebration Pl, Ste 200, Celebration, FL 34747; **Phone:** 407-303-4673; **Board Cert:** Urology 2004; **Med School:** Baylor Coll Med 1995; **Resid:** Urology, Univ Miami; **Fellow:** Urologic Laparoscopic Surgery-Endourology, Univ Miami

Patterson, Anthony L MD [U] - **Spec Exp:** Laparoscopic Surgery; Kidney Stones; **Hospital:** Univ of Tennesee Mem Hosp; **Address:** UT Medical Group, 7945 Wolf River Blvd, Ste 350, Germantown, TN 38138-1733; **Phone:** 901-347-8350; **Board Cert:** Urology 1999; **Med School:** Univ Tenn Coll Med, Memphis 1982; **Resid:** Surgery, Univ Tenn Med Ctr 1984; Urology, Univ Tenn Med Ctr 1987; **Fac Appt:** Assoc Prof U, Univ Tenn Coll Med, Memphis

Pow-Sang, Julio MD [U] - **Spec Exp:** Prostate Cancer; **Hospital:** H Lee Moffitt Cancer Ctr & Research Inst; **Address:** H Lee Moffitt Cancer Ctr, GU Clinic, 12902 Magnolia Drive, Tampa, FL 33612-9416; **Phone:** 813-972-8418; **Board Cert:** Urology 1999; **Med School:** Mexico 1978; **Resid:** Surgery, Univ Miami Sch Med 1983; Urology, Univ Miami Sch Med 1986; **Fellow:** Urologic Oncology, Univ Fla Coll Med 1987; **Fac Appt:** Prof S, Univ S Fla Coll Med

Preminger, Glenn M MD [U] - **Spec Exp:** Kidney Stones; **Hospital:** Duke Univ Med Ctr; **Address:** Duke Univ Med Ctr, Div Urologic Surgery, rm 1587, Box 3167, White Zone Duke S, Durham, NC 27710; **Phone:** 919-684-4226; **Board Cert:** Urology 2003; **Med School:** NY Med Coll 1977; **Resid:** Surgery, N Carolina Meml Hosp 1979; Urology, N Carolina Meml Hosp 1983; **Fellow:** Urology, Univ Texas SW Med Ctr 1985; **Fac Appt:** Prof U, Duke Univ

Robertson, Cary N MD [U] - **Spec Exp:** Prostate Cancer; Kidney Cancer; High Intensity Focused Ultrasound(HIFU); Testicular Cancer; **Hospital:** Duke Univ Med Ctr; **Address:** Duke Univ Med Ctr, Trent Drive, Box 3833, Durham, NC 27710; **Phone:** 919-681-6768; **Board Cert:** Urology 2006; **Med School:** Tulane Univ 1977; **Resid:** Urology, Duke Univ Med Ctr 1985; **Fellow:** Urologic Oncology, Natl Inst Hlth 1987; **Fac Appt:** Assoc Prof U, Duke Univ

Rowland, Randall MD [U] - **Spec Exp:** Urologic Cancer; **Hospital:** Univ of Kentucky Chandler Hosp; **Address:** Univ Kentucky Med Ctr, Div Urology, 800 Rose St, rm MS283, Lexington, KY 40536-0001; **Phone:** 859-323-6677; **Board Cert:** Urology 1980; **Med School:** Northwestern Univ 1972; **Resid:** Urology, Northwestern Meml Hosp 1978; **Fellow:** Urology, Northwestern Meml Hosp 1977; **Fac Appt:** Prof U, Univ KY Coll Med

Sanders, William H MD [U] - **Spec Exp:** Prostate Cancer; Kidney Stones; Kidney Cancer; **Hospital:** St Joseph's Hosp - Atlanta, Northside Hosp; **Address:** 980 Johnson Ferry Rd, Ste 490, Atlanta, GA 30342-1767; **Phone:** 404-257-0133; **Board Cert:** Urology 2006; **Med School:** Emory Univ 1988; **Resid:** Urology, Yale-New Haven Hosp 1993

Shaban, Stephen F MD [U] - **Spec Exp:** Infertility-Male; **Hospital:** Rex HlthCare, WakeMed New Bern; **Address:** 3320 Wake Forest Rd, Ste 320, Raleigh, NC 27609; **Phone:** 919-790-5500; **Board Cert:** Urology 2004; **Med School:** Mount Sinai Sch Med 1982; **Resid:** Urology, Univ S Fla 1987; **Fellow:** Male Reproduction, Baylor Coll Med 1988; **Fac Appt:** Prof U, Univ NC Sch Med

Smith, Joseph A MD [U] - **Spec Exp:** Prostate Cancer/Robotic Surgery; Bladder Cancer; Kidney Cancer; **Hospital:** Vanderbilt Univ Med Ctr; **Address:** Vanderbilt Univ Med Ctr, Dept Urology, A-1302 MCN, Nashville, TN 37232-2765; **Phone:** 615-343-0234; **Board Cert:** Urology 2000; **Med School:** Univ Tenn Coll Med, Memphis 1974; **Resid:** Surgery, Parkland Meml Hosp 1976; Urology, Univ Utah 1979; **Fellow:** Urologic Oncology, Meml Sloan Kettering Cancer Ctr 1980; **Fac Appt:** Prof U, Vanderbilt Univ

Soloway, Mark S MD [U] - **Spec Exp:** Bladder Cancer; Kidney Cancer; Prostate Cancer; Urologic Pathology; **Hospital:** Jackson Meml Hosp, Univ of Miami Hosp & Clins/Sylvester Comp Canc Ctr; **Address:** 1150 NW 14th St, Ste 309, Miami, FL 33136; **Phone:** 305-243-6596; **Board Cert:** Urology 1977; **Med School:** Case West Res Univ 1968; **Resid:** Surgery, Univ Hosps 1970; Urology, Univ Hosps 1975; **Fellow:** Surgery, Natl Cancer Inst 1972; **Fac Appt:** Prof U, Univ Miami Sch Med

Steers, William D MD [U] - **Spec Exp:** Incontinence; Erectile Dysfunction; Prostate Cancer/Robotic Surgery; **Hospital:** Univ Virginia Med Ctr; **Address:** UVA Hlth System, Dept Urology, PO Box 800422, Charlottesville, VA 22908-0422; **Phone:** 434-924-9107; **Board Cert:** Urology 1999; **Med School:** Med Coll OH 1980; **Resid:** Urology, Univ Tex Hlth Sci Ctr 1986; **Fellow:** Neurology, Univ Pittsburgh Med Ctr 1988; **Fac Appt:** Prof U, Univ VA Sch Med

Teigland, Chris M MD [U] - **Spec Exp:** Prostate Cancer/Robotic Surgery; Kidney Cancer; **Hospital:** Carolinas Med Ctr; **Address:** Mckay Urology, 1023 Edgehill Rd S, Charlotte, NC 28207; **Phone:** 704-355-8686; **Board Cert:** Urology 1999; **Med School:** Duke Univ 1980; **Resid:** Surgery, Univ Utah Affil Hosps 1982; Urology, Univ Texas SW Med Ctr 1987; **Fac Appt:** Clin Prof S, Univ NC Sch Med

Terris, Martha K MD [U] - **Spec Exp:** Prostate Cancer; Brachytherapy; Urologic Cancer; Bladder Cancer; **Hospital:** VA Medical Ctr - Augusta, Med Coll of GA Hosp and Clin; **Address:** Charlie Norwood VA Medical Center, 1 Freedom Way, Augusta, GA 30904; **Phone:** 706-733-0188; **Board Cert:** Urology 2007; **Med School:** Univ Miss 1986; **Resid:** Surgery, Duke Univ Med Ctr 1988; Urology, Stanford Univ Med Ctr 1995; **Fellow:** Ultrasound, Stanford Univ Med Ctr 1991; **Fac Appt:** Prof S, Med Coll GA

Theodorescu, Dan MD/PhD [U] - **Spec Exp:** Prostate Cancer; Clinical Trials; Bladder Cancer; Kidney Cancer; **Hospital:** Univ Virginia Med Ctr; **Address:** UVA Health System, Dept Urology, PO Box 800422, Charlottesville, VA 22908; **Phone:** 434-924-0042; **Board Cert:** Urology 2007; **Med School:** Canada 1986; **Resid:** Urology, Univ Toronto Med Ctr 1993; **Fellow:** Urologic Oncology, Meml Sloan Kettering Cancer Ctr 1995; **Fac Appt:** Prof U, Univ VA Sch Med

Webster, George D MD [U] - **Spec Exp:** Reconstructive Urologic Surgery; Urology-Female; Urodynamics; **Hospital:** Duke Univ Med Ctr; **Address:** Duke Univ Medical Ctr -Dept Urolology, Box 3146, Durham, NC 27710; **Phone:** 919-684-2516; **Board Cert:** Urology 1981; **Med School:** England 1968; **Resid:** Surgery, Harare Hosp 1972; Urology, Inst Urology 1974; **Fellow:** Urology, Duke Univ Med Ctr 1978; **Fac Appt:** Prof U, Duke Univ

Urology

Midwest

Andriole, Gerald L MD [U] - **Spec Exp:** Urologic Cancer; Prostate Cancer; Laparoscopic Surgery; **Hospital:** Barnes-Jewish Hosp; **Address:** 4960 Children's Place, Campus Box 8242, St Louis, MO 63110; **Phone:** 314-362-8212; **Board Cert:** Urology 2003; **Med School:** Jefferson Med Coll 1978; **Resid:** Surgery, Strong Meml Hosp 1980; Urology, Brigham & Womens Hosp 1983; **Fellow:** Urologic Oncology, NCI/NIH 1985; **Fac Appt:** Prof U, Washington Univ, St Louis

Bahnson, Robert MD [U] - **Spec Exp:** Prostate Cancer; Bladder Cancer; Continent Urinary Diversions; **Hospital:** Ohio St Univ Med Ctr, Arthur G James Cancer Hosp & Research Inst; **Address:** 456 West 10th Avenue, Dept of Urology, 4980 Cramblett Med Ctr, Columbus, OH 43210-1240; **Phone:** 614-293-8155; **Board Cert:** Urology 2006; **Med School:** Tufts Univ 1979; **Resid:** Surgery, Northwestern Univ 1981; Urology, Northwestern Univ 1985; **Fellow:** Urology, Northwestern Univ 1984; Research, Univ Pittsburgh 1991; **Fac Appt:** Prof U, Ohio State Univ

Bloom, David A MD [U] - **Spec Exp:** Pediatric Urology; Voiding Dysfunction; Genitourinary Reconstruction; **Hospital:** Univ Michigan Hlth Sys; **Address:** Univ Mich, Dept Ped Urology, 1500 E Med Ctr Dr, F-7805 Mott, Ann Arbor, MI 48109-0330; **Phone:** 734-615-0200; **Board Cert:** Urology 1982; **Med School:** SUNY Buffalo 1971; **Resid:** Surgery, UCLA Med Ctr 1976; Urology, UCLA Med Ctr 1980; **Fellow:** Pediatric Urology, Inst Urol-St Peters Hosp 1978; **Fac Appt:** Prof U, Univ Mich Med Sch

Brendler, Charles B MD [U] - **Spec Exp:** Prostate Cancer; **Hospital:** NorthShore Univ Hlth-Sys; **Address:** Evanston Northwestern Hosp, 2650 Ridge Ave Walgreen Bldg - Ste 2507, Evanston, IL 60201; **Phone:** 847-547-1090; **Board Cert:** Urology 1981; **Med School:** Univ VA Sch Med 1974; **Resid:** Surgery, Duke Univ Med Ctr 1976; Urology, Duke Univ Med Ctr 1979; **Fellow:** Urologic Oncology, Univ Hosp Wales 1980; Urologic Oncology, Johns Hopkins Hosp 1982; **Fac Appt:** Prof U, Northwestern Univ-Feinberg Sch Med

Bruskewitz, Reginald C MD [U] - **Spec Exp:** Urologic Cancer; Prostate Disease; **Hospital:** Univ WI Hosp & Clins; **Address:** Univ Wisconsin Hosp, Dept Urology, 600 Highland Ave, C-52, Madison, WI 53792; **Phone:** 608-263-4757; **Board Cert:** Urology 1981; **Med School:** Univ Wisc 1973; **Resid:** Urology, Univ Wisconsin Hosp 1978; **Fellow:** Urodynamics, UCLA Med Ctr 1979; **Fac Appt:** Assoc Prof S, Univ Wisc

Bushman, Wade MD [U] - **Spec Exp:** Neuro-Urology; Urodynamics; Urology-Female; **Hospital:** Univ WI Hosp & Clins; **Address:** Univ Wisconsin, C5/350 Clin Sci Ctr, 600 Highland Ave, Madison, WI 53792-3236; **Phone:** 608-263-4757; **Board Cert:** Urology 1997; **Med School:** Univ Chicago-Pritzker Sch Med 1986; **Resid:** Urology, Univ VA Med Ctr 1992; **Fac Appt:** Assoc Prof U, Univ Wisc

Campbell, Steven C MD/PhD [U] - **Spec Exp:** Kidney Cancer; Prostate Cancer; Bladder Cancer; **Hospital:** Cleveland Clin Fdn (page 56); **Address:** Cleveland Clinic, Glickman Urological Inst, 9500 Euclid Ave, A100, Cleveland, OH 44195; **Phone:** 216-444-5595; **Board Cert:** Urology 1999; **Med School:** Univ Chicago-Pritzker Sch Med 1989; **Resid:** Urology, Cleveland Clinic 1995; **Fellow:** Urology, Meml Sloan Kettering Cancer Ctr 1996; **Fac Appt:** Prof S, Cleveland Cl Coll Med/Case West Res

Catalona, William J MD [U] - **Spec Exp:** Prostate Cancer; Prostate Disease; **Hospital:** Northwestern Meml Hosp; **Address:** Northwestern Med Faculty Foundation, 675 N St Clair St, Ste 20-150, Chicago, IL 60611; **Phone:** 312-695-6126; **Board Cert:** Urology 1978; **Med School:** Yale Univ 1968; **Resid:** Surgery, UCSF Med Ctr 1970; Urology, Johns Hopkins Hosp 1976; **Fellow:** Surgical Oncology, Natl Cancer Inst 1972; **Fac Appt:** Prof U, Northwestern Univ

Coplen, Douglas E MD [U] - **Spec Exp:** Pediatric Urology; Urologic Cancer-Pediatric; Testicular Cancer-Pediatric; Fetal Urology; **Hospital:** St Louis Chldns Hosp; **Address:** St Louis Children's Hosp, 4990 Children's Pl, Northwest Tower, Ste 1120, St Louis, MO 63110; **Phone:** 314-454-6034; **Board Cert:** Urology 1996; **Med School:** Indiana Univ 1985; **Resid:** Urology, Barnes Jewish Hosp 1992; **Fellow:** Pediatric Urology, Children's Hosp 1994; **Fac Appt:** Asst Prof S, Washington Univ, St Louis

Donovan Jr, James F MD [U] - **Spec Exp:** Prostate Cancer/Robotic Surgery; Kidney Cancer; Adrenal Tumors; Laparoscopic Surgery; **Hospital:** Univ Hosp - Cincinnati, Christ Hospital; **Address:** Univ Cincinnati Med Ctr, Medical Arts Bldg, 222 Piedmont Ave, Ste 7000, Cincinnati, OH 45219; **Phone:** 513-475-8787; **Board Cert:** Surgery 1997; Urology 1999; **Med School:** Northwestern Univ 1978; **Resid:** Surgery, Northwestern Meml Hosp 1982; Urology, Northwestern Meml Hosp 1986; **Fellow:** Male Infertility, Baylor Coll Med 1986; **Fac Appt:** Prof U, Univ Cincinnati

Elder, Jack S MD [U] - **Spec Exp:** Pediatric Urology; Hypospadias; Urinary Reconstruction; **Hospital:** Henry Ford Hosp, Rainbow Babies & Chldns Hosp; **Address:** Henry Ford Hosp, 6777 W Maple Rd, West Bloomfield, MI 48322; **Phone:** 248-661-6479; **Board Cert:** Urology 1984; **Med School:** Univ Okla Coll Med 1976; **Resid:** Surgery, Yale-New Haven Hosp 1978; Urology, Johns Hopkins Hosp 1982; **Fellow:** Pediatric Urology, Johns Hopkins Hosp 1982; Pediatric Urology, Children's Hosp 1986; **Fac Appt:** Prof U, Case West Res Univ

Firlit, Casimir MD/PhD [U] - **Spec Exp:** Pediatric Urology; Genitourinary Reconstruction; Transplant-Kidney-Pediatric; **Hospital:** Cardinal Glennon Mem Children's Hosp; **Address:** Cardinal Glennon Chlds Hosp, 1465 S Grand Blvd Fl 5, Glennon Hall, St Louis, MO 63104; **Phone:** 314-577-5334; **Board Cert:** Urology 1975; **Med School:** Loyola Univ-Stritch Sch Med 1965; **Resid:** Surgery, Hines VA Hosp 1970; Urology, Hines VA Hosp 1973; **Fellow:** Pediatric Urology, Chldns Meml Hosp 1974; **Fac Appt:** Prof U, Univ MO-Columbia Sch Med

Flanigan, Robert C MD [U] - **Spec Exp:** Prostate Cancer; Bladder Cancer; Transplant-Kidney; Kidney Cancer; **Hospital:** Loyola Univ Med Ctr, Hines VA Hosp; **Address:** Loyola Univ Med-Fahey Bldg 54, 2160 S First Ave, rm 267, Maywood, IL 60153; **Phone:** 708-216-5100; **Board Cert:** Surgery 1998; Urology 2001; **Med School:** Case West Res Univ 1972; **Resid:** Surgery, Case West Univ Med Ctr 1978; Urology, Case West Univ Med Ctr 1978; **Fac Appt:** Prof U, Loyola Univ-Stritch Sch Med

Foster, Richard S MD [U] - **Spec Exp:** Testicular Cancer; **Hospital:** Indiana Univ Hosp; **Address:** 535 N Barnhill Drive, Ste 420, Indianapolis, IN 46202; **Phone:** 317-274-3458; **Board Cert:** Urology 2007; **Med School:** Indiana Univ 1980; **Resid:** Urology, Indiana Univ Hosp 1986; **Fac Appt:** Prof U, Indiana Univ

Gill, Inderbir Singh MD [U] - **Spec Exp:** Prostate Cancer; Kidney Cancer; Urologic Cancer; Minimally Invasive Urologic Surgery; **Hospital:** Cleveland Clin Fdn (page 56); **Address:** Cleveland Clinic Urological Inst, 9500 Euclid Ave, Desk A100, Cleveland, OH 44121; **Phone:** 216-445-1530; **Board Cert:** Urology 1997; **Med School:** India 1980; **Resid:** Surgery, Dayanand Med Coll & Hosp; Urology, Univ Kentucky Hosp 1993; **Fellow:** Cleveland Clinic

Gluckman, Gordon MD [U] - **Spec Exp:** Prostate Cancer; Kidney Cancer; Minimally Invasive Urologic Surgery; **Hospital:** Adv Luth Genl Hosp, Resurrection Med Ctr; **Address:** Parkside Center, 1875 Dempster St, Ste 365, Park Ridge, IL 60068; **Phone:** 847-823-4700; **Board Cert:** Urology 2005; **Med School:** Northwestern Univ 1989; **Resid:** Surgery, UCSF Med Ctr 1991; Urology, UCSF Med Ctr 1995

Urology

Gujral, Saroj MD [U] - **Spec Exp:** Urologic Cancer; Urology-Female; **Hospital:** Albert Lea Med Ctr-Mayo Hlth Sys; **Address:** 404 W Fountain St, Albert Lea, MN 56007; **Phone:** 507-379-2130; **Board Cert:** Urology 1979; **Med School:** India 1970; **Resid:** Urology, Suburban Hosp 1978; Urology, Dalhousie Univ Med Ctrs

Kass, Evan MD [U] - **Spec Exp:** Pediatric Urology; **Hospital:** William Beaumont Hosp; **Address:** 2221 Livernois, Ste 103, Troy, MI 48084; **Phone:** 248-519-0305; **Board Cert:** Urology 1978; **Med School:** SUNY Downstate 1968; **Resid:** Urology, Univ Mich Hosp 1976; **Fellow:** Pediatric Urology, Hosp for Sick Chldn 1978; **Fac Appt:** Assoc Prof U, Wayne State Univ

Kibel, Adam S MD [U] - **Spec Exp:** Prostate Cancer; Bladder Cancer; Kidney Cancer; **Hospital:** Barnes-Jewish Hosp; **Address:** Director Urologic Oncology, Washington Univ School of Medicine, 4960 Children's Place, Box 8242, St Louis, MO 63105-1000; **Phone:** 314-362-8295; **Board Cert:** Urology 2001; **Med School:** Cornell Univ-Weill Med Coll 1991; **Resid:** Urology, Brigham & Women's Hosp 1996; **Fellow:** Urologic Oncology, Johns Hopkins Hosp 1999; **Fac Appt:** Assoc Prof U, Washington Univ, St Louis

Klein, Eric A MD [U] - **Spec Exp:** Prostate Cancer; Testicular Cancer; Urologic Cancer; **Hospital:** Cleveland Clin Fdn (page 56); **Address:** Cleveland Clinic Fdn, Dept Urol, Sect Urol-Onc, 9500 Euclid Ave, Desk A100, Cleveland, OH 44195-0001; **Phone:** 216-444-5591; **Board Cert:** Urology 1999; **Med School:** Univ Pittsburgh 1981; **Resid:** Urology, Cleveland Clinic Fdn 1986; **Fellow:** Urologic Oncology, Meml Sloan Kettering Canc Ctr 1989; **Fac Appt:** Prof S, Cleveland Cl Coll Med/Case West Res

Klutke, Carl G MD [U] - **Spec Exp:** Urology-Female; Incontinence; Urodynamics; **Hospital:** Barnes-Jewish Hosp; **Address:** 1040 N Mason Rd, Ste 122, St Louis, MO 63141; **Phone:** 314-996-8060; **Board Cert:** Urology 2000; **Med School:** Univ Mich Med Sch 1983; **Resid:** Surgery, Henry Ford Hosp 1985; Urology, Henry Ford Hosp 1988; **Fellow:** Female Urology, UCLA Med Ctr 1989; **Fac Appt:** Assoc Prof S, Washington Univ, St Louis

Koff, Stephen A MD [U] - **Spec Exp:** Pediatric Urology; **Hospital:** Nationwide Chldn's Hosp; **Address:** Chldns Hosp, Dept Urology, 555 S 18th St, Ste 6D, Columbus, OH 43205; **Phone:** 614-722-3114; **Board Cert:** Urology 1978; **Med School:** Duke Univ 1969; **Resid:** Internal Medicine, New York Hosp 1971; Urology, Univ Mich Med Ctr 1975; **Fellow:** Pediatric Urology, Alder Hey Chldns Hosp 1977; **Fac Appt:** Prof U, Ohio State Univ

Kozlowski, James M MD [U] - **Spec Exp:** Prostate Cancer; Continent Urinary Diversions; Laparoscopic Surgery; **Hospital:** Northwestern Meml Hosp, Jesse A Brown VA Med Ctr; **Address:** 675 N St Clair St, Galter Bldg Fl 20 - Ste 150, Chicago, IL 60611; **Phone:** 312-695-8146; **Board Cert:** Surgery 2004; Urology 1983; **Med School:** Northwestern Univ 1975; **Resid:** Surgery, Northwestern Univ-McGaw 1979; Urology, Northwestern Univ-McGaw 1981; **Fellow:** Research, NCI-Frederick Cancer Rsch 1984; **Fac Appt:** Assoc Prof U, Northwestern Univ

Lee, Cheryl T MD [U] - **Spec Exp:** Urologic Cancers; Bladder Cancer; **Hospital:** Univ Michigan Hlth Sys; **Address:** Univ of Michigan Cancer Ctr, 1500 E Medical Ctr Drive Fl B1 - rm 280, Ann Arbor, MI 48109; **Phone:** 734-647-8903; **Board Cert:** Urology 2002; **Med School:** Albany Med Coll 1991; **Resid:** Urology, Albany Med Ctr; **Fellow:** Urologic Oncology, Meml Sloan Kettering Cancer Ctr 2000; **Fac Appt:** Assoc Prof U, Univ Mich Med Sch

Levine, Laurence Adan MD [U] - **Spec Exp:** Erectile Dysfunction; Infertility-Male; Peyronie's Disease; Prostate Cancer; **Hospital:** Rush Univ Med Ctr; **Address:** 1725 W Harrison St, Ste 352, Chicago, IL 60612; **Phone:** 312-563-5000; **Board Cert:** Urology 1999; **Med School:** Univ Colorado 1980; **Resid:** Surgery, Tufts-New England Med Ctr 1982; Urology, Brigham & Women's Hosp 1987; **Fac Appt:** Prof U, Rush Med Coll

McGuire, Edward J MD [U] - **Spec Exp:** Incontinence; Urology-Female; Neurogenic Bladder; **Hospital:** Univ Michigan Hlth Sys; **Address:** Univ Mich Med Ctr, Dept Urology, 1500 E Med Ctr Drive, rm 3875-TC, Ann Arbor, MI 48109-5330; **Phone:** 734-936-7030; **Board Cert:** Urology 1975; **Med School:** Wayne State Univ 1965; **Resid:** Surgery, Yale-New Haven Hosp 1969; Urology, Yale-New Haven Hosp 1972; **Fac Appt:** Prof U, Univ Mich Med Sch

McVary, Kevin MD [U] - **Spec Exp:** Prostate Cancer; Erectile Dysfunction; Prostate Disease; **Hospital:** Northwestern Meml Hosp; **Address:** 675 N St Clair St, Galter Bldg Fl 20 - Ste 150, Chicago, IL 60611-4813; **Phone:** 312-695-8146; **Board Cert:** Urology 2000; **Med School:** Northwestern Univ 1983; **Resid:** Surgery, Northwestern Meml Hosp 1985; Urology, Northwestern Meml Hosp 1988; **Fellow:** Research, Northwestern Meml Hosp; **Fac Appt:** Prof U, Northwestern Univ

Menon, Mani MD [U] - **Spec Exp:** Prostate Cancer/Robotic Surgery; Transplant-Kidney; Urologic Cancer; **Hospital:** Henry Ford Hosp; **Address:** Henry Ford Hosp - Vattikuti Urology Inst, 2799 W Grand Bvd, Clinic Bldg - #K-9, Detroit, MI 48202; **Phone:** 888-881-1117; **Board Cert:** Urology 1982; **Med School:** India 1969; **Resid:** Urology, Bryn Mawr Hosp 1974; Urology, Johns Hopkins Hosp 1980; **Fellow:** Transplant Surgery, Johns Hopkins Univ 1977; **Fac Appt:** Prof S, Univ Mass Sch Med

Mesrobian, Hrair-George O MD [U] - **Spec Exp:** Pediatric Urology; **Hospital:** Chldns Hosp - Wisconsin; **Address:** 999 N 92nd St, Ste 330, Milwaukee, WI 53226; **Phone:** 414-266-3794; **Board Cert:** Urology 2005; **Med School:** Lebanon 1978; **Resid:** Surgery, SUNY Upstate Med Ctr 1980; Urology, UCSF Med Ctr 1983; **Fellow:** Pediatric Urology, Mayo Clinic 1984; **Fac Appt:** Prof U, Med Coll Wisc

Mitchell, Michael E MD [U] - **Spec Exp:** Genitourinary Congenital Abnormality; Pediatric Urology; Bladder Reconstruction; **Hospital:** Chldns Hosp - Wisconsin; **Address:** Children's Hospital of Wisconsin, 999 N 92nd St, Ste 330, Milwaukee, WI 53226; **Phone:** 414-266-3794; **Board Cert:** Urology 2000; **Med School:** Harvard Med Sch 1969; **Resid:** Surgery, Peter Bent Brigham Hosp 1974; Urology, Mass Genl Hosp 1977; **Fellow:** Pediatric Urology, Mass Genl Hosp 1978; **Fac Appt:** Prof U, Univ Wisc

Montague, Drogo K MD [U] - **Spec Exp:** Erectile Dysfunction; Genitourinary Prosthetics; Incontinence; **Hospital:** Cleveland Clin Fdn (page 56); **Address:** Urological Inst, 9500 Euclid Ave, Ste A100, Cleveland, OH 44195-5041; **Phone:** 216-444-5590; **Board Cert:** Urology 1975; **Med School:** Univ Mich Med Sch 1968; **Resid:** Surgery, Cleveland Clinic 1970; Urology, Cleveland Clinic 1973; **Fac Appt:** Prof U, Cleveland Cl Coll Med/Case West Res

Montie, James MD [U] - **Spec Exp:** Bladder Cancer; Prostate Cancer; Genitourinary Cancer; **Hospital:** Univ Michigan Hlth Sys; **Address:** 1500 E Medical Ctr Dr, Dept Urology, Taubman Hlth Care Ctr, rm 3876, Box 0330, Ann Arbor, MI 48109-0330; **Phone:** 734-647-8903; **Board Cert:** Urology 1978; **Med School:** Univ Mich Med Sch 1971; **Resid:** Urology, Cleveland Clinic Fdn 1976; **Fellow:** Urologic Oncology, Meml Sloan-Kettering Cancer Ctr 1979; **Fac Appt:** Prof U, Univ Mich Med Sch

Myers, Robert P MD [U] - **Spec Exp:** Prostate Cancer; **Hospital:** Mayo Med Ctr & Clin - Rochester, Rochester Methodist Hosp; **Address:** Mayo Clinic, Dept Urology, 200 First St SW, Rochester, MN 55905; **Phone:** 507-284-3077; **Board Cert:** Urology 1976; **Med School:** Columbia P&S 1967; **Resid:** Urology, Mayo Clinic 1972; **Fac Appt:** Prof U, Mayo Med Sch

Urology

Novick, Andrew MD [U] - **Spec Exp:** Transplant-Kidney; Kidney Cancer; Urologic Cancer; **Hospital:** Cleveland Clin Fdn (page 56); **Address:** Urological Institute, 9500 Euclid Ave, Desk A100, Cleveland, OH 44195; **Phone:** 216-444-5600; **Board Cert:** Urology 1996; **Med School:** McGill Univ 1972; **Resid:** Surgery, Royal Victoria Hosp 1974; Urology, Cleveland Clinic 1977; **Fac Appt:** Prof S, Cleveland Cl Coll Med/Case West Res

O'Donnell, Michael A MD [U] - **Spec Exp:** Bladder Cancer; Immunotherapy; Urologic Cancer; **Hospital:** Univ Iowa Hosp & Clinics; **Address:** Univ Iowa Hosp & Clins, Dept Urology, 200 Hawkins Drive, 3RCP, Iowa City, IA 52242-1089; **Phone:** 319-384-6040; **Board Cert:** Urology 2005; **Med School:** Duke Univ 1984; **Resid:** Surgery, Brigham & Womens Hosp 1987; Urology, Brigham & Womens Hosp 1991; **Fellow:** Urology, Brigham & Womens Hosp 1993; **Fac Appt:** Prof U, Univ Iowa Coll Med

Ohl, Dana MD [U] - **Spec Exp:** Infertility-Male; Erectile Dysfunction; **Hospital:** Univ Michigan Hlth Sys; **Address:** Univ Mich Med Ctr, Dept Urology, 1500 E Med Ctr Drive, rm 3875-TC, Ann Arbor, MI 48109-0330; **Phone:** 734-936-7030; **Board Cert:** Urology 2008; **Med School:** Univ Mich Med Sch 1982; **Resid:** Urology, Univ Mich Hosps 1987; **Fac Appt:** Prof U, Univ Mich Med Sch

Rink, Richard C MD [U] - **Spec Exp:** Pediatric Urology; Reconstructive Urologic Surgery; Genital Reconstruction; **Hospital:** Riley Hosp for Children, Indiana Univ Hosp; **Address:** Indiana Univ Med Ctr, 702 Barnhill Drive, Ste 4230, Indianapolis, IN 46202-5128; **Phone:** 317-274-7472; **Board Cert:** Urology 2004; **Med School:** Indiana Univ 1978; **Resid:** Surgery, Emory Univ Med Ctr 1980; Urology, Indiana Univ Med Ctr 1984; **Fellow:** Pediatric Urology, Chldns Hosp-Harvard 1985; **Fac Appt:** Prof U, Indiana Univ

Ross, Lawrence S MD [U] - **Spec Exp:** Infertility-Male; Erectile Dysfunction; Prostate Disease; **Hospital:** Univ of IL Med Ctr at Chicago; **Address:** 60 E Delaware Ave, Ste 1420, Chicago, IL 60611; **Phone:** 312-440-5127; **Board Cert:** Urology 1974; **Med School:** Univ Chicago-Pritzker Sch Med 1965; **Resid:** Urology, Michael Reese Hosp 1970; **Fac Appt:** Prof U, Univ IL Coll Med

Sandlow, Jay MD [U] - **Spec Exp:** Infertility-Male; Varicocele Microsurgery; Vasectomy & Vasectomy Reversal; **Hospital:** Froedtert Meml Lutheran Hosp; **Address:** Med Coll of WI, Urology Dept, 9200 W Wisconsin Ave, Milwaukee, WI 53226-3522; **Phone:** 414-456-6977; **Board Cert:** Urology 2005; **Med School:** Rush Med Coll 1987; **Resid:** Surgery, Univ Iowa Hosps 1993; **Fellow:** Infertility, Univ Iowa Hosps 1995; **Fac Appt:** Assoc Prof U, Med Coll Wisc

Schaeffer, Anthony MD [U] - **Spec Exp:** Interstitial Cystitis; Incontinence after Prostate Cancer; Urology-Female; **Hospital:** Northwestern Meml Hosp; **Address:** 675 N St Clair, Galter Bldg Fl 20 - Ste 150, Chicago, IL 60611; **Phone:** 312-695-8146; **Board Cert:** Urology 1978; **Med School:** Northwestern Univ 1968; **Resid:** Surgery, Northwestern Meml Hosp 1970; Urology, Stanford Med Ctr 1976; **Fac Appt:** Prof U, Northwestern Univ

See, William A MD [U] - **Spec Exp:** Prostate Cancer; Bladder Cancer; Testicular Cancer; **Hospital:** Froedtert Meml Lutheran Hosp; **Address:** Med Coll Wisconsin, Dept Urology, 9200 W Wisconsin Ave, Milwaukee, WI 53226; **Phone:** 414-456-6950; **Board Cert:** Urology 2000; **Med School:** Univ Chicago-Pritzker Sch Med 1982; **Resid:** Urology, Univ Washington 1988; **Fellow:** Research, Natl Kidney Fdn/Univ Wash 1986; Research, Amer Fdn for Urol Dis/Univ Iowa 1990; **Fac Appt:** Prof U, Med Coll Wisc

Seftel, Allen D MD [U] - **Spec Exp:** Sexual Dysfunction; Infertility-Male; Prostate Disease; **Hospital:** Univ Hosps Case Med Ctr; **Address:** Univ Hosp-Cleveland, 11100 Euclid Ave, Ste 4550, Office # 4564, Cleveland, OH 44106-1736; **Phone:** 216-844-3009; **Board Cert:** Urology 2003; **Med School:** SUNY Downstate 1984; **Resid:** Urology, SUNY Downstate Med Ctr 1987; Urology, Univ Hosps-Case West Res 1990; **Fellow:** Reproductive Medicine, Boston Univ Med Ctr 1992; **Fac Appt:** Prof U, Case West Res Univ

Silber, Sherman J MD [U] - **Spec Exp:** Infertility-Male; Vasectomy Reversal; Infertility-IVF; Transplant-Ovarian Tissue; **Hospital:** St Luke's Hosp - Chesterfield, MO; **Address:** 224 S Woods Mill Rd, Ste 730, St Louis, MO 63017-3451; **Phone:** 314-576-1400; **Board Cert:** Urology 1977; **Med School:** Univ Mich Med Sch 1966; **Resid:** Internal Medicine, PH Service Comm Corps 1969; Urology, Univ Michigan 1973; **Fellow:** Microsurgery, Univ Melbourne 1974

Steinberg, Gary D MD [U] - **Spec Exp:** Bladder Cancer; Kidney Cancer; Prostate Cancer; **Hospital:** Univ of Chicago Hosps; **Address:** 5841 S Maryland Ave, rm J653, MC 6038, Chicago, IL 60637-1447; **Phone:** 773-702-3080; **Board Cert:** Urology 2003; **Med School:** Univ Chicago-Pritzker Sch Med 1985; **Resid:** Surgery, Johns Hopkins Hosp 1987; Urology, Brady Urol Inst/Johns Hopkins 1991; **Fellow:** Oncology, Johns Hopkins Hosp 1989; **Fac Appt:** Prof U, Univ Chicago-Pritzker Sch Med

Thomas Jr, Anthony J MD [U] - **Spec Exp:** Infertility-Male; Vasectomy Reversal; Fertility Preservation in Cancer; **Hospital:** Cleveland Clin Fdn (page 56); **Address:** Cleveland Clinic-Urological Inst, 9500 Euclid Ave, Desk A100, Cleveland, OH 44195; **Phone:** 216-444-5600; **Board Cert:** Urology 1978; **Med School:** Univ Cincinnati 1969; **Resid:** Surgery, Wayne State Univ Affil Hosp 1971; Urology, Wayne State Univ Affil Hosp 1976

Williams, Richard D MD [U] - **Spec Exp:** Kidney Cancer; Bladder Cancer; Prostate Cancer; **Hospital:** Univ Iowa Hosp & Clinics; **Address:** Univ Iowa Hosp, Dept Urology, 200 Hawkins Dr, rm 3251 RCP, Iowa City, IA 52242-1089; **Phone:** 319-356-0760; **Board Cert:** Urology 1979; **Med School:** Univ Kans 1970; **Resid:** Surgery, Univ Minn Hosp 1972; Urology, Univ Minn Hosp 1976; **Fellow:** Urologic Oncology, Univ Minn Hosp 1979; **Fac Appt:** Prof U, Univ Iowa Coll Med

Winfield, Howard N MD [U] - **Spec Exp:** Kidney Stones; Laparoscopic Surgery; Robotic Surgery; **Hospital:** Univ Iowa Hosp & Clinics; **Address:** Univ Iowa - Dept Urology, 200 Hawkins Drive, 3235 RCP, Iowa Ctiy, IA 52242-1089; **Phone:** 319-384-9183; **Board Cert:** Urology 1999; **Med School:** McGill Univ 1978; **Resid:** Urology, McGill Univ Tchg Hosp 1984; **Fellow:** Urology, Washington Univ 1985; Urology, UCLA 1986; **Fac Appt:** Prof U, Univ Iowa Coll Med

Wood, David P MD [U] - **Spec Exp:** Genitourinary Cancer; Bladder Cancer; Prostate Cancer; **Hospital:** Univ Michigan Hlth Sys; **Address:** Univ Mich, Dept Urology, 3875 Taubman Cancer Ctr, 1500 E Medical Center Drive, Ann Arbor, MI 48109-0999; **Phone:** 734-763-9269; **Board Cert:** Urology 2002; **Med School:** Univ Mich Med Sch 1983; **Resid:** Urology, Cleveland Clinic 1988; **Fellow:** Urologic Oncology, Meml Sloan-Kettering Cancer Ctr 1991; **Fac Appt:** Prof U, Univ Mich Med Sch

Zippe, Craig D MD [U] - **Spec Exp:** Prostate Cancer; Bladder Cancer; Incontinence after Prostate Cancer; **Hospital:** Cleveland Clin Fdn (page 56); **Address:** 12000 McCracken Rd, Ste 451, Garfield Heights, OH 44125; **Phone:** 216-587-4370; **Board Cert:** Urology 1997; **Med School:** Rush Med Coll 1980; **Resid:** Urology, Columbia Presby Med Ctr 1989; **Fellow:** Urologic Oncology, Meml Sloan Kettering Cancer Ctr 1992

Great Plains and Mountains

Cartwright, Patrick C MD [U] - **Spec Exp:** Pediatric Urology; **Hospital:** Primary Children's Med Ctr, Univ Utah Hosps and Clins; **Address:** Pediatric Urology, 100 N Mario Capecchi Drive, Ste 2200, Salt Lake City, UT 84113-1100; **Phone:** 801-662-5555; **Board Cert:** Urology 2001; **Med School:** Univ Tex SW, Dallas 1984; **Resid:** Urology, Univ Utah Affil Hosp 1989; **Fellow:** Pediatric Urology, Childrens Hosp 1990; **Fac Appt:** Assoc Prof S, Univ Utah

Urology

Childs, Stacy J MD [U] - **Spec Exp:** Voiding Dysfunction; Erectile Dysfunction; Prostate Cancer; Bladder Cancer; **Hospital:** Yampa Valley Med Ctr, Memorial Hosp - Craig; **Address:** 501 Anglers Drive, Ste 202, Steamboat Springs, CO 80487-8841; **Phone:** 970-871-9710; **Board Cert:** Urology 1979; **Med School:** Louisiana State U, New Orleans 1972; **Resid:** Urology, Carraway Meth Med Ctr 1977; **Fac Appt:** Clin Prof U, Univ Colorado

Crawford, E David MD [U] - **Spec Exp:** Prostate Cancer; Testicular Cancer; Bladder Cancer; **Hospital:** Univ Colorado Hosp; **Address:** Urologic Oncology, MS F710, 1665 N Ursula St, rm 1004, Box 6510, Aurora, CO 80045; **Phone:** 720-848-0170; **Board Cert:** Urology 1980; **Med School:** Univ Cincinnati 1973; **Resid:** Urology, Good Samaritan Hosp 1977; **Fellow:** Genitourinary Surgery, UCLA Med Ctr 1978; **Fac Appt:** Prof U, Univ Colorado

Davis, Bradley E MD [U] - **Spec Exp:** Urologic Cancer; Bladder Cancer; Reconstructive Surgery; Prostate Cancer; **Hospital:** Overland Pk Regl Med Ctr, St Luke's Hosp of Kansas City; **Address:** Urologic Surgical Associates, 10550 Quivira Rd, Ste 105, Overland Park, KS 66215; **Phone:** 913-438-3833; **Board Cert:** Urology 2004; **Med School:** Univ Kans 1986; **Resid:** Surgery, St Lukes Hosp 1991; Urology, Univ Kansas Med Ctr 1991; **Fellow:** Urologic Oncology, Meml Sloan-Kettering Cancer Ctr 1993; **Fac Appt:** Asst Clin Prof U, Univ Kans

Lugg, James A MD [U] - **Spec Exp:** Prostate Cancer; Laparoscopic Surgery; Incontinence after Prostate Cancer; **Hospital:** Cheyenne Regl Med Ctr, Univ Colorado Hosp; **Address:** 2301 House Ave, Ste 502, Cheyenne, WY 82001; **Phone:** 307-635-4131; **Board Cert:** Urology 1998; **Med School:** Northwestern Univ 1990; **Resid:** Urology, UCLA Med Ctr 1995; **Fac Appt:** Asst Prof U, Univ Colorado

Southwest

Appell, Rodney A MD [U] - **Spec Exp:** Voiding Dysfunction; Urology-Female; Uro-Gynecology; **Hospital:** Methodist Hosp - Houston; **Address:** 6400 Fannin St, Ste 2300, Houston, TX 77030; **Phone:** 713-366-7800; **Board Cert:** Urology 1981; **Med School:** Jefferson Med Coll 1973; **Resid:** Surgery, George Wash Univ Med Ctr 1975; **Fellow:** Urology, Yale Univ Sch Med 1979; **Fac Appt:** Prof U, Baylor Coll Med

Babaian, Richard MD [U] - **Spec Exp:** Prostate Cancer; **Hospital:** UT MD Anderson Cancer Ctr; **Address:** MD Anderson Cancer Ctr, 1515 Holcombe Blvd, Unit GPT5, 570, Houston, TX 77030; **Phone:** 713-745-9713; **Board Cert:** Urology 1980; **Med School:** Georgetown Univ 1972; **Resid:** Surgery, Univ Wisconsin 1974; Urology, Univ NC Hosp 1977; **Fellow:** Urologic Oncology, MD Anderson Cancer Ctr 1979; Immunology, Univ NC Hosps 1978; **Fac Appt:** Prof U, Univ Tex, Houston

Bans, Larry L MD [U] - **Spec Exp:** Prostate Cancer; Prostate Disease; **Hospital:** Banner Good Samaritan Regl Med Ctr - Phoenix; **Address:** Prostate Solutions of Arizona, 2525 E Arizona Biltmore Cir, Ste C236, Phoenix, AZ 85016; **Phone:** 602-426-9772; **Board Cert:** Urology 2004; **Med School:** Cornell Univ-Weill Med Coll 1978; **Resid:** Urology, Ind Univ Med Ctr 1983

Bardot, Stephen F MD [U] - **Spec Exp:** Urologic Cancer; Prostate Cancer; **Hospital:** Ochsner Fdn Hosp, Summit Hosp-Baton Rouge; **Address:** Ochsner Clinic, 1514 Jefferson Hwy Fl 4, Atrium 4 West, Dept of Urology, New Orleans, LA 70121-2483; **Phone:** 504-842-4083; **Board Cert:** Urology 2002; **Med School:** Univ Kans 1985; **Resid:** Surgery, St Luke's Hosp 1987; Urology, Kansas City Univ Med Ctr 1990; **Fellow:** Urologic Oncology, Cleveland Clinic 1991

America's Top Doctors® 8th Edition

Basler, Joseph W MD [U] - **Spec Exp:** Prostate Cancer; Urologic Cancer; Kidney Stones; **Hospital:** Audie L Murphy Meml Vets Hosp, Christus Santa Rosa Hosp; **Address:** 7703 Floyd Curl Dr, MC-7845, San Antonio, TX 78229-3900; **Phone:** 210-567-5640; **Board Cert:** Urology 1992; **Med School:** Univ MO-Columbia Sch Med 1984; **Resid:** Surgery, Univ Missouri 1986; Urology, Barnes Hosp/Wash Univ 1990; **Fac Appt:** Prof U, Univ Tex, San Antonio

Boone, Timothy B MD/PhD [U] - **Spec Exp:** Neuro-Urology; Urinary Reconstruction; Incontinence; **Hospital:** Methodist Hosp - Houston, St Luke's Episcopal Hosp - Houston; **Address:** Scurlock Tower, 6560 Fannin, Ste 2100, Houston, TX 77030-2769; **Phone:** 713-441-6455; **Board Cert:** Urology 2004; **Med School:** Univ Tex, Houston 1985; **Resid:** Surgery, Univ Tex SW Med Ctr 1987; Urology, Univ Tex SW Med Ctr 1991; **Fac Appt:** Prof U, Baylor Coll Med

Buch, Jeffrey Phillip MD [U] - **Spec Exp:** Infertility-Male; Sexual Dysfunction; Vasectomy Reversal; **Address:** Legacy Male Health Institute, 5516 Warren Pkwy, Ste 101, Frisco, TX 75034; **Phone:** 972-612-7131; **Board Cert:** Urology 2005; **Med School:** Univ Mich Med Sch 1980; **Resid:** Surgery, Albany Med Ctr 1982; Urology, Albany Med Ctr 1985; **Fellow:** Male Infertility, Baylor Coll Med 1987; Microsurgery, Baylor Coll Med 1987

Culkin, Daniel J MD [U] - **Spec Exp:** Voiding Dysfunction; Interstitial Cystitis; Urologic Cancer; Laparoscopic Surgery; **Hospital:** OU Med Ctr, VA Med Ctr - Oklahoma City; **Address:** Oklahoma Univ Med Ctr, Div Urology, 920 Stanton L Young Blvd, Ste WP 3150, Oklahoma City, OK 73104; **Phone:** 405-271-8156; **Board Cert:** Urology 2006; **Med School:** Creighton Univ 1979; **Resid:** Surgery, Loyola Univ Med Ctr 1981; Urology, Loyola Univ Med Ctr 1983; **Fellow:** Neurourology, Loyola Univ Med Ctr 1984; **Fac Appt:** Prof U, Univ Okla Coll Med

Ellis, David S MD [U] - **Spec Exp:** Prostate Cancer-Cryosurgery; **Hospital:** Arlington Meml Hosp; **Address:** Urology Assocs of N Texas (UANT), Arlington-North, 1001 Waldrop Drive, Ste 708, Arlington, TX 76012; **Phone:** 817-465-0373; **Board Cert:** Urology 2000; **Med School:** Univ Tex, Houston 1982; **Resid:** Urology, Univ Texas Med Ctr 1988

Ewalt, David H MD [U] - **Spec Exp:** Pediatric Urology; Hypospadias; Urinary Reconstruction; Neurogenic Bladder; **Hospital:** Chldns Med Ctr of Dallas, Med City Dallas Hosp; **Address:** 8315 Walnut Hill Lane, Ste 205, Dallas, TX 75231; **Phone:** 214-750-0808; **Board Cert:** Urology 2003; **Med School:** Univ Tex SW, Dallas 1984; **Resid:** Urology, Univ Texas SW Affil Hosps 1990; **Fellow:** Pediatric Urology, Chldns Hosp 1992

Gonzales, Edmond T MD [U] - **Spec Exp:** Pediatric Urology; **Hospital:** Texas Chldns Hosp - Houston; **Address:** Clinical Care Center, Ste 660, 6701 Fannin St, Houston, TX 77030; **Phone:** 832-822-3160; **Board Cert:** Urology 1975; **Med School:** Tulane Univ 1965; **Resid:** Surgery, Duke Univ Med Ctr 1968; Urology, Duke Univ Med Ctr 1972; **Fellow:** Pediatric Urology, Childrens Hosp; **Fac Appt:** Prof U, Baylor Coll Med

Greene, Graham MD [U] - **Spec Exp:** Urologic Cancer; **Hospital:** UAMS Med Ctr, Arkansas Chldns Hosp; **Address:** 4301 W Markham, Slot 774, Little Rock, AR 72205; **Phone:** 501-296-1545; **Board Cert:** Urology 2007; **Med School:** Dalhousie Univ 1989; **Resid:** Urology, Victoria Genl 1994; **Fellow:** Urologic Oncology, M.D. Anderson Cancer Ctr 1997; **Fac Appt:** Assoc Prof U, Univ Ark

Grossman, H Barton MD [U] - **Spec Exp:** Bladder Cancer; Bladder Reconstruction; Urinary Reconstruction; **Hospital:** UT MD Anderson Cancer Ctr; **Address:** MD Anderson Cancer Ctr, Dept Urology, 1373, 1515 Holcombe Blvd, Houston, TX 77030; **Phone:** 713-792-3250; **Board Cert:** Urology 1979; **Med School:** Temple Univ 1972; **Resid:** Surgery, St Joseph Mercy Hosp 1974; Urology, Univ Michigan Med Ctr 1977; **Fellow:** Research, Meml Sloan Kettering Cancer Ctr 1979; **Fac Appt:** Prof U, Univ Tex, Houston

Urology

Hellstrom, Wayne J MD [U] - **Spec Exp:** Infertility-Male; Erectile Dysfunction; Peyronie's Disease; Penile Prostheses; **Hospital:** Tulane Univ Hosp & Clin; **Address:** 1430 Tulane Ave, SL42, New Orleans, LA 70112; **Phone:** 504-988-7308; **Board Cert:** Urology 2007; **Med School:** Canada 1981; **Resid:** Surgery, Montreal Genl/Royal Vistoria Hosp 1983; Urology, UCSF Med Ctr 1985; **Fellow:** Andrology, UC Davis Med Ctr 1988; **Fac Appt:** Prof U, Tulane Univ

Kadmon, Dov MD [U] - **Spec Exp:** Prostate Cancer; **Hospital:** St Luke's Episcopal Hosp - Houston, Methodist Hosp - Houston; **Address:** Baylor Dept Urology, 6560 Fannin St, Ste 2100, Houston, TX 77030; **Phone:** 713-798-4001; **Board Cert:** Urology 1984; **Med School:** Israel 1970; **Resid:** Surgery, Barnes Jewish Hosp 1977; Urology, Barnes Jewish Hosp 1980; **Fellow:** Urology, Barnes Jewish Hosp 1982; **Fac Appt:** Prof U, Baylor Coll Med

Lerner, Seth P MD [U] - **Spec Exp:** Bladder Cancer; Testicular Cancer; Urinary Reconstruction; **Hospital:** St Luke's Episcopal Hosp - Houston, Methodist Hosp - Houston; **Address:** 6560 Fannin St, Ste 2100, Houston, TX 77030; **Phone:** 713-798-6841; **Board Cert:** Urology 2002; **Med School:** Baylor Coll Med 1984; **Resid:** Surgery, Virginia Mason Hosp 1986; Urology, Baylor Coll Med 1990; **Fellow:** Urologic Oncology, LAC-USC Med Ctr 1992; **Fac Appt:** Prof U, Baylor Coll Med

Lipshultz, Larry MD [U] - **Spec Exp:** Infertility-Male; Microsurgery; Erectile Dysfunction; **Hospital:** St Luke's Episcopal Hosp - Houston, Methodist Hosp - Houston; **Address:** 6560 Fannin St, Scurlock Twr, Ste 2100, Houston, TX 77030-2706; **Phone:** 713-798-4001; **Board Cert:** Urology 1977; **Med School:** Univ Pennsylvania 1968; **Resid:** Urology, Hosp Univ Penn 1971; **Fellow:** Reproductive Medicine, Univ Tex Med Sch 1971; **Fac Appt:** Prof U, Baylor Coll Med

McConnell, John D MD [U] - **Spec Exp:** Prostate Cancer; **Hospital:** UT Southwestern Med Ctr - Dallas; **Address:** Univ Texas SW Med Ctr, 5323 Harry Hines Blvd, Dallas, TX 75390-9131; **Phone:** 214-648-5630; **Board Cert:** Urology 2004; **Med School:** Loyola Univ-Stritch Sch Med 1978; **Resid:** Surgery, Univ Tex Hlth Sci Ctr-Parkland 1980; Urology, Univ Tex Hlth Sci Ctr-Parkland 1984; **Fac Appt:** Prof U, Univ Tex SW, Dallas

Miles, Brian J MD [U] - **Spec Exp:** Prostate Cancer; Urologic Cancer; Gene Therapy; **Hospital:** Methodist Hosp - Houston, St Luke's Episcopal Hosp - Houston; **Address:** Dept Urology, Scurlock Tower, 6560 Fannin St, Ste 2100, Houston, TX 77030-2769; **Phone:** 713-798-4001; **Board Cert:** Urology 1984; **Med School:** Univ Mich Med Sch 1974; **Resid:** Urology, Walter Reed Army Med Ctr 1982; **Fac Appt:** Prof U, Baylor Coll Med

Pisters, Louis L MD [U] - **Spec Exp:** Prostate Cancer; Bladder Cancer; Genitourinary Cancer; Prostate Cancer/Robotic Surgery; **Hospital:** UT MD Anderson Cancer Ctr; **Address:** MD Anderson Cancer Ctr, 1515 Holcombe Blvd, Unit 1373, Houston, TX 77030; **Phone:** 713-792-3250; **Board Cert:** Urology 2003; **Med School:** Univ Western Ontario 1986; **Resid:** Urology, Shands Hosp/UNIV Florida 1991; **Fellow:** Urologic Oncology, MD Anderson Cancer Ctr 1993; **Fac Appt:** Assoc Prof U, Univ Tex, Houston

Roehrborn, Claus MD [U] - **Spec Exp:** Prostate Disease; Prostate Cancer; **Hospital:** UT Southwestern Med Ctr - Dallas, Parkland Meml Hosp - Dallas; **Address:** UT Southwestern Med Ctr, Dept Urology, 5323 Harry Hines Blvd, J8-148, Dallas, TX 75390-9110; **Phone:** 214-645-8765; **Board Cert:** Urology 2004; **Med School:** Germany 1980; **Resid:** Surgery, W Germany Army Hosp 1982; Urology, UT SW Med Ctr 1989; **Fellow:** Urology, Am Fdn Urol Dis 1991; **Fac Appt:** Prof U, Univ Tex SW, Dallas

Sagalowsky, Arthur I MD [U] - **Spec Exp:** Urologic Cancer; Transplant-Kidney; Testicular Cancer; **Hospital:** UT Southwestern Med Ctr - Dallas; **Address:** UT SW Med Ctr, Dept Urology, 5323 Harry Hines Blvd, J8.114, Dallas, TX 75390-9110; **Phone:** 214-648-3976; **Board Cert:** Urology 1980; **Med School:** Indiana Univ 1973; **Resid:** Surgery, Indiana Univ Hosps 1975; Urology, Indiana Univ Hosps 1978; **Fellow:** Clinical Pharmacology, Univ Tex SW Med Ctr 1980; **Fac Appt:** Prof U, Univ Tex SW, Dallas

Slawin, Kevin Mark MD [U] - **Spec Exp:** Prostate Cancer; Prostate Cancer/Robotic Surgery; Prostate Disease; **Hospital:** Meml Hermann Hosp - Texas Med Ctr, Methodist Hosp - Houston; **Address:** Vanguard Urologic Inst, Memorial Hermann Medical Plaza, 6400 Fannin, Ste 2300, Houston, TX 77030; **Phone:** 713-366-7848; **Board Cert:** Urology 2005; **Med School:** Columbia P&S 1986; **Resid:** Surgery, Mt Sinai Med Ctr 1988; Urology, Columbia-Presby Hosp 1992; **Fellow:** Urologic Oncology, Am Fdn Urol Dis/Baylor Coll Med 1994; **Fac Appt:** Clin Prof U, Baylor Coll Med

Strand, William MD [U] - **Spec Exp:** Pediatric Urology; Laparoscopic Surgery; Hypospadias; Reconstructive Surgery; **Hospital:** Chldns Med Ctr of Dallas; **Address:** 4001 W 15th St Bldg 3 - Ste 300, Plano, TX 75093; **Phone:** 214-750-0808; **Board Cert:** Urology 2001; **Med School:** Mayo Med Sch 1983; **Resid:** Surgery, Naval Med Ctr 1984; Urology, Natl Naval Med Ctr 1988; **Fac Appt:** Assoc Prof U, Univ Tex SW, Dallas

Swanson, David A MD [U] - **Spec Exp:** Kidney Cancer; Prostate Cancer; Testicular Cancer; **Hospital:** UT MD Anderson Cancer Ctr; **Address:** UT MD Anderson Canc Ctr, Dept Urol, 1515 Holcombe Blvd , Unit 1373, Houston, TX 77030-4009; **Phone:** 713-792-3250; **Board Cert:** Urology 1977; **Med School:** Univ Pennsylvania 1967; **Resid:** Surgery, Harbor Genl Hosp 1969; Urology, UC Davis Med Ctr 1975; **Fellow:** Urologic Oncology, Univ Tex-MD Anderson Hosp 1978

Thompson Jr, Ian M MD [U] - **Spec Exp:** Prostate Cancer; Prostate Disease; **Hospital:** Univ Hlth Sys - Univ Hosp (San Antonio, TX); **Address:** Univ Tex Hlth Scis Ctr, Dept Urol, 7703 Floyd Curl Drive, rm 306L, MC 7845, San Antonio, TX 78229-3900; **Phone:** 210-567-5643; **Board Cert:** Urology 2005; **Med School:** Tulane Univ 1980; **Resid:** Urology, Brooke Army Med Ctr 1985; **Fellow:** Medical Oncology, Meml Sloan-Kettering Canc Ctr 1988; **Fac Appt:** Prof S, Univ Tex, San Antonio

Winters, Jack C MD [U] - **Spec Exp:** Voiding Dysfunction; Urology-Female; Urinary Reconstruction; **Hospital:** Ochsner Fdn Hosp; **Address:** Ochsner Clinic, Dept Urology, 1514 Jefferson Hwy Fl 4W, New Orleans, LA 70121; **Phone:** 504-842-4083; **Board Cert:** Urology 1997; **Med School:** Louisiana State U, New Orleans 1988; **Resid:** Surgery, Ochsner Fdn Hosp 1990; Urology, Ochsner Fdn Hosp 1994; **Fellow:** Female Urology, Cleveland Clinic Fdn 1995

West Coast and Pacific

Baskin, Laurence S MD [U] - **Spec Exp:** Pediatric Urology; Hypospadias; **Hospital:** UCSF Med Ctr, CA Pacific Med Ctr - Pacific Campus; **Address:** Urology Faculty Practice, 400 Parnassus Ave, Ste 610A, Box 0330, San Francisco, CA 94143-0330; **Phone:** 415-353-2200; **Board Cert:** Urology 2004; **Med School:** UCLA 1986; **Resid:** Urology, UCSF Med Ctr 1991; **Fellow:** Pediatric Urology, Childrens Hosp 1993; **Fac Appt:** Assoc Prof U, UCSF

Belldegrun, Arie S MD [U] - **Spec Exp:** Urologic Cancer; Gene Therapy; **Hospital:** Ronald Reagan UCLA Med Ctr; **Address:** UCLA-Geffen Sch Med, Dep Urology, 108-33 Leconte Ave, rm 66-118, Los Angeles, CA 90095; **Phone:** 310-206-1434; **Board Cert:** Urology 1999; **Med School:** Israel 1974; **Resid:** Urology, Brigham and Women's Hosp 1985; **Fellow:** Urologic Oncology, Natl Cancer Inst, NIH 1988; **Fac Appt:** Prof U, UCLA

Urology

Boyd, Stuart D MD [U] - **Spec Exp:** Incontinence; Erectile Dysfunction; Urologic Cancer; **Hospital:** USC Norris Comp Cancer Ctr, USC Univ Hosp - R K Eamer Med Plz; **Address:** 1441 Eastlake Ave, Ste 7416, Los Angeles, CA 90089-9178; **Phone:** 323-865-3704; **Board Cert:** Urology 1984; **Med School:** UCLA 1975; **Resid:** Urology, UCLA Med Ctr 1982; **Fac Appt:** Prof U, USC Sch Med

Carroll, Peter R MD [U] - **Spec Exp:** Testicular Cancer; Prostate Cancer; Bladder Cancer; Bladder Reconstruction; **Hospital:** UCSF - Mt Zion Med Ctr; **Address:** UCSF Urologic Oncology Practice, Fl 3rd, Box 1711, San Francisco, CA 94115-1711; **Phone:** 415-353-7171; **Board Cert:** Urology 2006; **Med School:** Georgetown Univ 1979; **Resid:** Surgery, UCSF Med Ctr 1984; **Fellow:** Urology, Meml Sloan Kettering Cancer Ctr 1986; **Fac Appt:** Prof U, UCSF

Clayman, Ralph V MD [U] - **Spec Exp:** Kidney Stones; Kidney Cancer; Laparoscopic Surgery; **Hospital:** UC Irvine Med Ctr; **Address:** UCI Med Ctr, Dept Urology, 333 City Blvd W, Ste 2100, Orange, CA 92868; **Phone:** 714-456-3330; **Board Cert:** Urology 2007; **Med School:** UCSD 1973; **Resid:** Urology, Univ Minn Med Ctr 1979; **Fac Appt:** Prof U, UC Irvine

Danoff, Dudley S MD [U] - **Spec Exp:** Prostate Cancer; Bladder Cancer; Erectile Dysfunction; **Hospital:** Cedars-Sinai Med Ctr; **Address:** 8635 W 3rd St, Ste 1 West, Los Angeles, CA 90048; **Phone:** 310-854-9898; **Board Cert:** Urology 1974; **Med School:** Yale Univ 1963; **Resid:** Urology, Yale-New Haven Hosp 1965; Urology, Columbia-Presby Med Ctr 1969

de Kernion, Jean B MD [U] - **Spec Exp:** Urologic Cancer; Kidney Cancer; Prostate Cancer; Prostate Disease; **Hospital:** Ronald Reagan UCLA Med Ctr; **Address:** UCLA-Geffen Sch Med, Dept Urology, rm 66-133CHS, Box 951738, Los Angeles, CA 90095-1738; **Phone:** 310-206-6453; **Board Cert:** Surgery 1973; Urology 1975; **Med School:** Louisiana State U, New Orleans 1965; **Resid:** Surgery, Univ Hosps-Case West Res 1967; Urology, Univ Hosps-Case West Res 1973; **Fellow:** Urologic Oncology, Natl Cancer Inst 1969; **Fac Appt:** Prof U, UCLA

Ellis, William J MD [U] - **Spec Exp:** Prostate Cancer; Prostate Disease; Kidney Cancer; **Hospital:** Univ Wash Med Ctr; **Address:** Univ Wash Med Ctr, Dept Urology, Box 356158, Seattle, WA 98195; **Phone:** 206-598-4294; **Board Cert:** Urology 2001; **Med School:** Johns Hopkins Univ 1985; **Resid:** Surgery, Northwestern Meml Hosp 1987; Urology, Northwestern Meml Hosp 1991; **Fac Appt:** Assoc Prof U, Univ Wash

Fuchs, Eugene F MD [U] - **Spec Exp:** Infertility-Male; Kidney Stones; Vasectomy Reversal; **Hospital:** OR Hlth & Sci Univ, Legacy Emanuel Hospitals; **Address:** 3303 SW Bond Ave Fl 10, Portland, OR 97239; **Phone:** 503-418-9033; **Board Cert:** Urology 1977; **Med School:** Univ VT Coll Med 1970; **Resid:** Urology, Univ Oregon Hosp 1975; **Fac Appt:** Prof U, Oregon Hlth Sci Univ

Gill, Harcharan Singh MD [U] - **Spec Exp:** Urologic Cancer; Prostate Cancer; Prostate Disease; **Hospital:** Stanford Univ Med Ctr; **Address:** 875 Blake Wilbur Drive, Stanford, CA 94305-5826; **Phone:** 650-725-5544; **Board Cert:** Urology 1995; **Med School:** Kenya 1977; **Resid:** Urology, Inst of Urol; Urology, Univ Penn 1991; **Fellow:** Urology, Univ Penn 1986; **Fac Appt:** Prof U, Stanford Univ

Ginsberg, David A MD [U] - **Spec Exp:** Incontinence; Urinary Reconstruction; Neuro-Urology; **Hospital:** USC Univ Hosp - R K Eamer Med Plz; **Address:** USC-Norris Cancer Ctr, 1441 Eastlake Ave, Ste 7416, Los Angeles, CA 90033; **Phone:** 323-865-3703; **Board Cert:** Urology 1999; **Med School:** USC Sch Med 1990; **Resid:** Surgery, LAC-USC Med Ctr 1992; Urology, LAc-USC Med Ctr 1996; **Fellow:** Reconstructive Surgery, UCLA 1997; **Fac Appt:** Assoc Clin Prof U, USC-Keck School of Medicine

Holden, Stuart MD [U] - **Spec Exp:** Kidney Cancer; **Hospital:** Cedars-Sinai Med Ctr; **Address:** 8635 W 3rd St, Ste 1 West, Los Angeles, CA 90048; **Phone:** 310-854-9898; **Board Cert:** Urology 1977; **Med School:** Cornell Univ-Weill Med Coll 1968; **Resid:** Surgery, NY Hosp-Cornell 1970; Urology, Emory Univ Hosp 1975; **Fellow:** Urology, Meml Sloan Kettering Cancer Ctr 1978

Kawachi, Mark H MD [U] - **Spec Exp:** Prostate Cancer/Robotic Surgery; Minimally Invasive Urologic Surgery; **Hospital:** City of Hope Natl Med Ctr & Beckman Rsch; **Address:** Div Urologic Oncology, 1500 E Duarte Rd, Duarte, CA 91010-3012; **Phone:** 626-359-8111 x62655; **Board Cert:** Urology 2004; **Med School:** USC Sch Med 1979; **Resid:** Urology, USC Med Ctr 1984

Koyle, Martin A MD [U] - **Spec Exp:** Pediatric Urology; Genitourinary Reconstruction; Transplant-Kidney-Pediatric; **Hospital:** Chldns Hosp and Regl Med Ctr - Seattle; **Address:** Children's Hospital, Pediatric Urology, 4800 Sand Point Way NE, W-7729, Seattle, WA 98105-0371; **Phone:** 206-987-5893; **Board Cert:** Urology 2004; **Med School:** Canada 1976; **Resid:** Surgery, Hlth Scis Ctr 1978; Urology, Brigham & Womens Hosp 1984; **Fellow:** Transplant Surgery, Pacific Med Ctr 1982; **Fac Appt:** Prof U, Univ Wash

Lange, Paul H MD [U] - **Spec Exp:** Prostate Cancer; **Hospital:** Univ Wash Med Ctr; **Address:** Univ Wash Med Ctr, Dept Urology, Box 356158, Seattle, WA 98195; **Phone:** 206-598-4294; **Board Cert:** Urology 2006; **Med School:** Washington Univ, St Louis 1967; **Resid:** Surgery, Duke Univ Med Ctr 1972; Urology, Univ Minn Med Ctr 1975; **Fellow:** Immunology, Univ Minn 1973; Research, Natl Inst Hlth 1970; **Fac Appt:** Prof U, Univ Wash

Lieskovsky, Gary MD [U] - **Spec Exp:** Prostate Cancer; **Hospital:** USC Norris Comp Cancer Ctr, USC Univ Hosp - R K Eamer Med Plz; **Address:** 1441 Eastlake Ave, Ste 7416, Los Angeles, CA 90089-0112; **Phone:** 323-865-3702; **Board Cert:** Urology 1980; **Med School:** Canada 1973; **Resid:** Urology, Univ Alberta Hosp 1978; **Fellow:** Urology, UCLA Med Ctr 1980; **Fac Appt:** Prof U, USC Sch Med

Marsh, Christopher L MD [U] - **Spec Exp:** Transplant-Kidney; Transplant-Pancreas; Islet Cell Transplant; Adrenal Surgery; **Hospital:** Scripps Green Hosp; **Address:** Scripps Green Hospital, 10666 N Torrey Pines Rd, MC 200N, La Jolla, CA 92037; **Phone:** 858-554-4310; **Board Cert:** Urology 2006; **Med School:** Loma Linda Univ 1980; **Resid:** Urology, Loma Linda U Med Ctr 1986; **Fellow:** Transplant Surgery, Mayo Clinic 1987

McAninch, Jack W MD [U] - **Spec Exp:** Genitourinary Trauma; Genitourinary Reconstruction; **Hospital:** UCSF Med Ctr, San Francisco Genl Hosp; **Address:** San Francisco Genl Hosp, Dept Urology, 1001 Potrero Ave, Ste 3A20, San Francisco, CA 94110; **Phone:** 415-476-3372; **Board Cert:** Urology 1995; **Med School:** Univ Tex Med Br, Galveston 1964; **Resid:** Surgery, Darnall Army Hosp 1966; Urology, Letterman AMC 1969; **Fac Appt:** Prof U, UCSF

McClure, Robert D MD [U] - **Spec Exp:** Infertility-Male; **Hospital:** Virginia Mason Med Ctr; **Address:** Virginia Mason Med Ctr, 1100 9th Ave, MS C7-URO, Seattle, WA 98101; **Phone:** 206-223-6179; **Board Cert:** Urology 1979; **Med School:** Canada 1968; **Resid:** Urology, McGill Univ Hosp 1975; **Fellow:** Endocrinology, Univ Washington Med Ctr 1977

Payne, Christopher K MD [U] - **Spec Exp:** Interstitial Cystitis; Pelvic Organ Prolapse Repair; Incontinence; **Hospital:** Stanford Univ Med Ctr; **Address:** Stanford Univ, Dept Urology, 300 Pasteur Drive, rm S-287, Stanford, CA 94305-5118; **Phone:** 650-723-3391; **Board Cert:** Urology 2004; **Med School:** Vanderbilt Univ 1986; **Resid:** Urology, Univ Penn 1992; **Fellow:** Urology, UCLA Med Ctr 1993; **Fac Appt:** Assoc Prof U, Stanford Univ

Urology

Perkash, Inder MD [U] - **Spec Exp:** Neurogenic Bladder; Neuro-Urology; Spinal Cord Injury; Voiding Dysfunction/Spinal Cord Injury; **Hospital:** VA Hlth Care Sys - Palo Alto, Stanford Univ Med Ctr; **Address:** VA Med Ctr - Spinal Cord Injury Service, Surgical Service (112), 3801 Miranda Ave, Palo Alto, CA 94304-1207; **Phone:** 650-849-1916; **Board Cert:** Physical Medicine & Rehabilitation 1977; Spinal Cord Injury Medicine 2001; **Med School:** India 1957; **Resid:** Urology, Hammersmith Hosp 1963; Physical Medicine & Rehabilitation, Baylor Affil Hosp 1973; **Fellow:** Urology, Stanford Univ Med Ctr 1965; **Fac Appt:** Prof U, Stanford Univ

Presti Jr, Joseph C MD [U] - **Spec Exp:** Prostate Cancer; Bladder Cancer; Kidney Cancer; **Hospital:** Stanford Univ Med Ctr; **Address:** Stanford Univ Sch Med-Dept Urology, 875 Blake Wilbur Dr MC 5826, Stanford, CA 94305; **Phone:** 650-725-5544; **Board Cert:** Urology 2002; **Med School:** UC Irvine 1984; **Resid:** Surgery, UCSF Med Ctr 1986; Urology, UCSF Med Ctr 1989; **Fellow:** Urologic Oncology, Meml Sloan-Kettering Cancer Ctr 1992; **Fac Appt:** Prof U, Stanford Univ

Rajfer, Jacob MD [U] - **Spec Exp:** Erectile Dysfunction; Prostate Disease; Infertility-Male; **Hospital:** LAC - Harbor - UCLA Med Ctr, Ronald Reagan UCLA Med Ctr; **Address:** 1000 W Carson St, Box 5, Torrance, CA 90509-2004; **Phone:** 310-222-2727; **Board Cert:** Urology 1980; **Med School:** Northwestern Univ 1972; **Resid:** Surgery, St Josephs Hosp 1974; Urology, Johns Hopkins Hosp 1978; **Fellow:** Research, Johns Hopkins Hosp 1976; **Fac Appt:** Prof U, UCLA

Raz, Shlomo MD [U] - **Spec Exp:** Incontinence-Female; Urology-Female; **Hospital:** Ronald Reagan UCLA Med Ctr; **Address:** 200 Medical Plaza, Ste 140, Los Angeles, CA 90095; **Phone:** 310-794-0206; **Board Cert:** Urology 1979; **Med School:** Uruguay 1962; **Resid:** Surgery, Hadassah Univ Hosp 1973; **Fellow:** Urology, UCLA Med Ctr 1975; **Fac Appt:** Prof U, UCLA

Sharlip, Ira D MD [U] - **Spec Exp:** Vasectomy Reversal; Erectile Dysfunction; Infertility-Male; **Hospital:** CA Pacific Med Ctr - Pacific Campus, UCSF Med Ctr; **Address:** 2100 Webster St, Ste 222, San Francisco, CA 94115-2376; **Phone:** 415-202-0250; **Board Cert:** Internal Medicine 1972; Urology 1977; **Med School:** Univ Pennsylvania 1965; **Resid:** Internal Medicine, Hosp Univ Penn 1967; Urology, UCSF Medical Center 1975; **Fellow:** Urology, Middlesex Hosp 1976; **Fac Appt:** Clin Prof U, UCSF

Shortliffe, Linda MD [U] - **Spec Exp:** Pediatric Urology; Hypospadias; Kidney Disease; **Hospital:** Lucile Packard Chldns Hosp/Stanford Univ Med Ctr, Stanford Univ Med Ctr; **Address:** 300 Pasteur Drive, rm S287, Stanford, CA 94305-5118; **Phone:** 650-724-7608; **Board Cert:** Urology 2002; **Med School:** Stanford Univ 1975; **Resid:** Surgery, Tufts-New England Med Ctr 1977; Urology, Stanford Univ Med Ctr 1981; **Fac Appt:** Prof U, Stanford Univ

Skinner, Donald G MD [U] - **Spec Exp:** Bladder Cancer; Testicular Cancer; Prostate Cancer; **Hospital:** USC Norris Comp Cancer Ctr, USC Univ Hosp - R K Eamer Med Plz; **Address:** 1441 Eastlake Ave, Ste 7416, Los Angeles, CA 90033; **Phone:** 323-865-3707; **Board Cert:** Urology 1974; **Med School:** Yale Univ 1964; **Resid:** Surgery, Mass Genl Hosp 1966; Urology, Mass Genl Hosp 1971; **Fac Appt:** Prof U, USC Sch Med

Skinner, Eila C MD [U] - **Spec Exp:** Urologic Cancer; Genitourinary Disorders-Geriatric; Urinary Reconstruction; **Hospital:** USC Norris Comp Cancer Ctr, USC Univ Hosp - R K Eamer Med Plz; **Address:** USC-Keck Sch Med, Dept Urology, 1441 Eastlake Ave, Ste 7416, Los Angeles, CA 90089; **Phone:** 323-865-3700; **Board Cert:** Urology 2001; **Med School:** USC Sch Med 1983; **Resid:** Urology, LAC-USC Med Ctr 1988; **Fellow:** Urologic Oncology, LAC-USC Med Ctr 1990; **Fac Appt:** Assoc Prof U, USC Sch Med

Stoller, Marshall L MD [U] - **Spec Exp:** Laparoscopic Surgery; Kidney Stones; **Hospital:** UCSF Med Ctr; **Address:** 400 Parnassus Ave Fl 6, San Francisco, CA 94143; **Phone:** 415-353-2200; **Board Cert:** Urology 1999; **Med School:** Baylor Coll Med 1981; **Resid:** Surgery, UCSF Med Ctr 1983; Urology, UCSF Med Ctr 1987; **Fellow:** Urology, Prince Henry Hosptial 1986; **Fac Appt:** Prof U, UCSF

Stone, Anthony MD [U] - **Spec Exp:** Urology-Female; Voiding Dysfunction; **Hospital:** UC Davis Med Ctr; **Address:** 4860 Y St, Ste 3500, Sacramento, CA 95817-2214; **Phone:** 916-734-2222; **Board Cert:** Urology 1997; **Med School:** Scotland 1972; **Resid:** Western Genl Hosp 1980; Urology, Cardiff Royal Infirm 1983; **Fellow:** Urodynamics, Duke Univ Med Ctr 1986; **Fac Appt:** Prof U, UC Davis

Wilson, Timothy G MD [U] - **Spec Exp:** Prostate Cancer/Robotic Surgery; Minimally Invasive Urologic Surgery; Urinary Reconstruction; **Hospital:** City of Hope Natl Med Ctr & Beckman Rsch; **Address:** City of Hope Natl Med Ctr, Div Urologic Onc, 1500 E Duarte Rd, Duarte, CA 91010; **Phone:** 626-359-8111 x62655; **Board Cert:** Urology 2001; **Med School:** Oregon Hlth Sci Univ 1984; **Resid:** Urology, USC Med Ctr 1990; **Fellow:** Urologic Oncology, City Hosp Natl Med Ctr 1991; **Fac Appt:** Assoc Clin Prof U, USC Sch Med

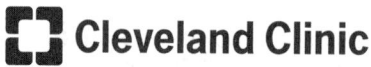
Cleveland Clinic

Glickman Urological and Kidney Institute

One of the Best

With 65 physicians and scientists, the Cleveland Clinic Glickman Urological and Kidney Institute is the largest and most comprehensive urological group in the world. Many procedures have been developed or perfected here and adopted around the world. These include laparoscopic urological surgery, female incontinence procedures, kidney-sparing surgery for kidney cancer, kidney artery reconstruction and kidney transplantation. The Institute also offers innovative treatment for sexual dysfunction, male infertility and testicular and bladder cancer. The latest and most effective treatments are provided for every urological disorder in adults and children. Because of its clinical and academic achievements, the Glickman Urological and Kidney Institute has consistently received national and international recognition. *U.S.News & World Report* ranks the Cleveland Clinic Glickman Urological and Kidney Institute one of the top two urological groups in the United States.

A National Leader in Urology

The Glickman Urological and Kidney Institute provides the highest quality of care for adult and pediatric patients with routine or complex disorders. Successful results in the practice and science of urology have won the Institute international acclaim as one of the most progressive and accomplished urologic groups in the country.

Innovative Care

In the treatment of kidney disease, the Cleveland Clinic Glickman Urological and Kidney Institute has made numerous pioneering contributions, including the development of "bench surgery," a technique designed to repair the kidney outside the body and then transplant it back into the patient. The Cleveland Clinic Glickman Urological & Kidney Institute is also a recognized leader in partial nephrectomies, or kidney-sparing surgery, for the treatment of kidney cancer. More than 800 laparoscopic, or minimally invasive kidney-sparing procedures, have been performed here, representing the largest experience in the world. Another treatment option pioneered at Cleveland Clinic for kidney cancer is cryoablation, a minimally invasive treatment that uses a freezing probe to destroy the cancerous portion of the kidney. An Institute urologist performed the world's first laparoscopic cryoablation.

Defining State of the Art

The Cleveland Clinic Glickman Urological and Kidney Institute has been instrumental in perfecting and refining many laparoscopic techniques that may offer patients improved outcomes. These techniques are now routinely used for many urological diseases and conditions including prostate cancer, kidney and bladder cancer, urinary incontinence and in removing and transplanting kidneys in live-donor transplants. As one of the first centers in the country to begin using the latest versions of robotic surgery systems for prostate cancer, the Cleveland Clinic Glickman Urological and Kidney Institute is leading the way in minimally invasive urologic surgery. In addition, the Institute is pioneering advancements that include performing surgery through a single incision in the belly button.

For more information about Glickman Urological and Kidney Institute, to schedule a second opinion or learn about assistance for out-of-state patients, call 800.890.2467 or visit www.clevelandclinic.org/urologytopdocs.
Glickman Urological and Kidney Institute
9500 Euclid Avenue / AC311 | Cleveland OH 44195

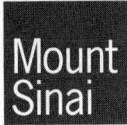
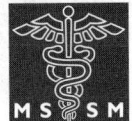

MOUNT SINAI
SCHOOL OF
MEDICINE

THE MOUNT SINAI MEDICAL CENTER
UROLOGY
One Gustave L. Levy Place
Fifth Avenue and 100th Street
New York, NY 10029-6574
Physician Referral: 1-800-MD-SINAI (637-4624)
www.mountsinai.org

The Milton and Carroll Petrie Department of Urology at The Mount Sinai Medical Center prides itself on offering the latest technologic advancements and results of translational and clinical research for the diagnosis and treatment of urologic diseases and conditions. Treatments include:

- *Prostate Cancer* - The Department of Urology's Barbara and Maurice Deane Prostate Health and Research Center offers a full range of surgical and radiation treatments for the management of localized prostate cancer, including minimally invasive laparoscopic and robotic prostatectomies. For more advanced disease, options include hormonal therapy, new chemotherapy regimens, and a clinical trial with a new prostate cancer vaccine. Current gene therapy research also offers hope for the future.

- *Bladder Cancer* - As recognized leaders in the assessment and treatment of all forms of bladder cancer, Mount Sinai oncologists employ knowledge of tumor markers and new diagnostic techniques and work with Department of Urology surgeons to determine the most effective treatment approaches. Robotic surgeons can perform cystectomies with a variety of diversions, resulting in minimal impact on quality of life.

- *Kidney Cancer* - A majority of kidney tumors can be removed by Department of Urology surgeons via minimally invasive surgical techniques, reducing pain and recovery time. Laparoscopic surgery may be utilized to remove all or a portion of a kidney. Other less invasive modalities—such as freezing, or radio frequency ablation— may be recommended to treat small kidney cancers while preserving maximum function.

- *Prostatic Enlargement (benign prostatic hyperplasia)* - The Deane Center offers the latest technologies and treatments, including Holmium Laser Ablation (HoLAP) and transurethral microwave dilation therapy (TUMD), highly effective approaches to relieving urinary problems associated with an enlarged prostate, including frequency, pain, burning, and retention. Many of these procedures are offered in an outpatient setting, thus avoiding hospitalization.

- *Urinary Dysfunction* - Mount Sinai provides comprehensive resources for the evaluation and treatment, both medical and surgical, of urinary incontinence, neuro-urologic problems, and pelvic pain syndrome for both men and women.

- *Urologic Stone Disease* - Mount Sinai's expertise in kidney stone disease ranges from stone prevention to minimally invasive therapies with lasers, sonic energies, and extracorporeal shock wave lithotripsy.

- *Pediatric Conditions* - Mount Sinai has a strong reputation in the treatment of urologic problems in children, especially for reconstructive procedures using, when appropriate, minimally invasive procedures.

- *Male Infertility* - State-of-the-art approaches offered by Mount Sinai using medications and in vitro fertilization techniques result in high success rates.

- *Sexuality-Related Health Concerns* - For both men and women, sexuality-related issues are addressed through application of current medical and surgical approaches.

THE BARBARA AND MAURICE A. DEANE PROSTATE HEALTH AND RESEARCH CENTER offers a new multidisciplinary facility for the assessment and treatment of all aspects of prostatic disease, including cancer, benign enlargement, and inflammation. Activities through the Center are designed to empower the patient and his family to understand the nature of his prostatic condition and decide on the optimum treatment that may create lasting benefit and enhance quality of life.

Mount Sinai has developed an extensive **Minimally Invasive Urologic Surgery Program** and is a leader in the greater New York area for complex procedures performed laparoscopically, robotically, and endoscopically. A variety of urologic cancers are treated, stone disease is managed, and reconstruction is provided for various urologic cancers and anatomic abnormalities. These approaches provide for a rapid and virtually painless recovery and return to normal activity.

NYU **Langone Medical Center**

550 First Avenue (at 31St Street)
New York, NY 10016
Physician Referral:
(888)7-NYU-MED (888-769-8633)
www.nyumc.org

UROLOGY

NYU Langone Medical Center's urologists are internationally renowned specialists who have pioneered numerous advances in the surgical and pharmacological treatment of urological disease. They are an interdisciplinary team of physicians, nurses, and allied health professionals dedicated to providing the highest- quality state-of-the-art care. All of our doctors are also faculty at NYU School of Medicine who specialize in all aspects of urological disease. Our programs include:

Urologic Oncology- aggressively treating and curing urologic cancers while maintaining the highest quality of life. Cancers of the kidney, bladder, and testes are the most common malignancies treated in this program. Since treating cancer often requires a multidisciplinary approach, urologists work closely with NYU's medical and radiation oncologists to tailor treatment to each patient's priorities and objectives.

Prostate cancer-surgery- the most experienced open and robotic prostate cancer surgeons in the entire northeast who work in collaboration with experts in male sexual health are at NYULMC offering the best possible outcomes for men with localized prostate cancers.

Robotic Urological Surgery- the most comprehensive robotic urological surgery program includes surgery for prostate and kidney cancers, female incontinence surgery, and urinary tract reconstruction

Minimally Invasive Surgery- committed to developing new technologies to treat even the most complex disorders more effectively and less invasively, so patients experience less pain and a quicker recovery.

Pediatric Urology and Reconstructive Surgery- individualizing the treatment of all urologic diseases in children with compassion and state of the art minimally invasive technology

Male Fertility and Sexual Health- collaborating closely with the world-renowned NYU In Vitro Fertilization Program, the fertility treatment program uses state-of-the-art technology and a multidisciplinary approach to diagnose and treat the underlying causes of both male and female sexual dysfunction.

Benign Prostatic Diseases- developing innovative medical and surgical therapies for benign prostatic diseases, such as benign prostatic hyperplasia (BPH, or enlarged prostate) and prostatitis (infection in the prostate).

Female Urology and Incontinence- expertise in the many urological problems unique to women, including recurrent urinary tract infections, pelvic pain, prolapse, and sexual dysfunction.

Vascular Surgery
a subspecialty of Surgery

A surgeon with expertise in the management of surgical disorders of the blood vessels, excluding the intercranial vessels or the heart.

Training Required: Five years in surgery *plus* additional training and examination.

Vascular Surgery

New England

Belkin, Michael MD [VascS] - **Spec Exp:** Aneurysm; Arterial Bypass Surgery; Carotid Artery Surgery; **Hospital:** Brigham & Women's Hosp, Faulkner Hosp; **Address:** Brigham & Women's Hosp, Dept Vasc Surg, 75 Francis St, Boston, MA 02115; **Phone:** 857-307-1920; **Board Cert:** Surgery 1997; Vascular Surgery 1998; **Med School:** Univ Conn 1982; **Resid:** Surgery, Hartford Hosp 1987; **Fellow:** Vascular Surgery, Boston Univ/Brigham-Womens Hosp 1989; **Fac Appt:** Assoc Prof S, Harvard Med Sch

Brewster, David C MD [VascS] - **Spec Exp:** Aneurysm-Abdominal Aortic; Endovascular Surgery; Angioplasty & Stent Placement; **Hospital:** Mass Genl Hosp, Newton - Wellesley Hosp; **Address:** Massachusetts General Hosp, 15 Parkman St, WAC 440, Boston, MA 02114; **Phone:** 617-726-3567; **Board Cert:** Surgery 1975; Vascular Surgery 2003; **Med School:** Columbia P&S 1967; **Resid:** Surgery, Mass Genl Hosp 1975; **Fellow:** Vascular Surgery, Mass Genl Hosp 1976; **Fac Appt:** Clin Prof S, Harvard Med Sch

Cambria, Richard P MD [VascS] - **Spec Exp:** Aneurysm-Abdominal Aortic; Cerebrovascular Disease; Renovascular Disease; Aortic Reconstruction; **Hospital:** Mass Genl Hosp; **Address:** Mass Genl Hosp, Dept Vascular Surgery, 15 Parkman St, WAC 440, Boston, MA 02114-3117; **Phone:** 617-726-8278; **Board Cert:** Vascular Surgery 2006; **Med School:** Columbia P&S 1977; **Resid:** Surgery, Mass Genl Hosp 1978; **Fellow:** Vascular Surgery, Mass Genl Hosp 1984; **Fac Appt:** Prof S, Harvard Med Sch

Cronenwett, Jack MD [VascS] - **Spec Exp:** Peripheral Vascular Surgery; Aneurysm-Abdominal Aortic; Carotid Artery Surgery; **Hospital:** Dartmouth - Hitchcock Med Ctr, Mary Hitchcock Mem Hosp; **Address:** Dartmouth Hitchcock Med Ctr, Sect Vasc Surg, 1 Med Ctr Drive, Lebanon, NH 03756; **Phone:** 603-650-8670; **Board Cert:** Vascular Surgery 2003; **Med School:** Stanford Univ 1973; **Resid:** Surgery, Univ Mich Hosp 1979; **Fellow:** Vascular Surgery, Univ Tenn Hosp 1980; **Fac Appt:** Prof S, Dartmouth Med Sch

Gibbons, Gary W MD [VascS] - **Spec Exp:** Diabetic Vascular Disease; Diabetic Leg/Foot; **Hospital:** Boston Med Ctr, Qunicy Med Ctr; **Address:** 732 Harrison Ave Preston Bldg - Ste 219, Boston, MA 02118; **Phone:** 617-414-6840; **Board Cert:** Vascular Surgery 1992; **Med School:** Univ Cincinnati 1971; **Resid:** Surgery, New England Deaconess Hosp 1976; **Fellow:** Nutrition, New England Deaconess Hosp; **Fac Appt:** Prof S, Boston Univ

Kwolek, Christopher J MD [VascS] - **Spec Exp:** Aneurysm-Abdominal & Thoracic Aortic; Endovascular Surgery; Carotid Artery Stent Placement; **Hospital:** Mass Genl Hosp, Newton - Wellesley Hosp; **Address:** 15 Parkman St, Wang Bldg Fl 4, Boston, MA 02114; **Phone:** 617-724-6101; **Board Cert:** Surgery 2003; Vascular Surgery 1997; **Med School:** UCSF 1987; **Resid:** Surgery, New England Deaconess Hosp 1993; Vascular Surgery, Mass Genl Hosp 1995; **Fellow:** Endovascular Surgery, Arizona Heart Inst 1999; **Fac Appt:** Assoc Prof VascS, Harvard Med Sch

LaMuraglia, Glenn M MD [VascS] - **Spec Exp:** Percutaneous Vascular Interventions; Angioplasty & Stent Placement-Legs; Carotid Body Tumors; **Hospital:** Mass Genl Hosp; **Address:** Mass General Hospital, Vascular Surgery, 55 Fruit St, Boston, MA 02114; **Phone:** 617-726-6997; **Board Cert:** Surgery 2004; Vascular Surgery 1997; **Med School:** Harvard Med Sch 1979; **Resid:** Surgery, Mass General Hosp 1985; Vascular Surgery, Mass General Hosp 1986; **Fac Appt:** Assoc Prof S, Harvard Med Sch

Mackey, William C MD [VascS] - **Spec Exp:** Carotid Artery Surgery; Aneurysm-Abdominal Aortic; Lower Limb Arterial Disease; **Hospital:** Tufts Med Ctr; **Address:** 750 Washington St, Ste 1035, Boston, MA 02111-1526; **Phone:** 617-636-5927; **Board Cert:** Surgery 2002; Vascular Surgery 2004; Surgical Critical Care 1997; **Med School:** Duke Univ 1977; **Resid:** Surgery, New York Hosp 1982; **Fellow:** Vascular Surgery, Tufts-New Eng Med Ctr 1984; **Fac Appt:** Prof S, Tufts Univ

Sumpio, Bauer E MD/PhD [VascS] - **Spec Exp:** Diabetic Leg/Foot; Endovascular Surgery; **Hospital:** Yale-New Haven Hosp; **Address:** Yale Univ School Medicine, Dept Surgery, 333 Cedar St, rm FMB137, Box 208062, New Haven, CT 06520; **Phone:** 203-785-6217; **Board Cert:** Vascular Surgery 1997; Surgery 1998; **Med School:** Cornell Univ-Weill Med Coll 1980; **Resid:** Surgery, Yale-New Haven Hosp 1986; **Fellow:** Vascular Surgery, Univ N Carolina Hosp 1987; **Fac Appt:** Prof S, Yale Univ

Whittemore, Anthony D MD [VascS] - **Spec Exp:** Aortic Surgery; Aneurysm-Abdominal Aortic; **Hospital:** Brigham & Women's Hosp; **Address:** Brigham & Women's Hosp, 75 Francis St, Boston, MA 02115; **Phone:** 617-732-8515; **Board Cert:** Vascular Surgery 2002; **Med School:** Columbia P&S 1970; **Resid:** Surgery, Columbia-Presby Med Ctr 1976; **Fellow:** Vascular Surgery, Peter Bent Brigham Hosp 1977; **Fac Appt:** Prof S, Harvard Med Sch

Mid Atlantic

Adelman, Mark MD [VascS] - **Spec Exp:** Carotid Artery Surgery; Aneurysm-Abdominal Aortic; Vein Disorders; Endovascular Surgery; **Hospital:** NYU Med Ctr (page 68), Bellevue Hosp Ctr; **Address:** 530 1st Ave, Ste 6F, New York, NY 10016-6402; **Phone:** 212-263-7311; **Board Cert:** Surgery 1999; Vascular Surgery 2001; **Med School:** NYU Sch Med 1985; **Resid:** Surgery, NYU Med Ctr 1990; **Fellow:** Vascular Surgery, NYU Med Ctr 1991; **Fac Appt:** Prof VascS, NYU Sch Med

Ascher, Enrico MD [VascS] - **Spec Exp:** Endovascular Surgery; Carotid Artery Surgery; Limb Sparing Surgery; Aneurysm; **Hospital:** Maimonides Med Ctr (page 63), Mount Sinai Med Ctr (page 64); **Address:** Maimonides Med Ctr, Dept Vascular Surg, 4802 10th Ave Fl 4, Brooklyn, NY 11219-2844; **Phone:** 718-283-7957; **Board Cert:** Vascular Surgery 2004; **Med School:** Brazil 1974; **Resid:** Surgery, NY Med Coll 1981; **Fellow:** Vascular Surgery, Montefiore Hosp Med Ctr 1982; **Fac Appt:** Prof S, SUNY Downstate

Atnip, Robert G MD [VascS] - **Spec Exp:** Aneurysm-Abdominal Aortic; Peripheral Vascular Disease; Carotid Artery Disease; **Hospital:** Penn State Milton S Hershey Med Ctr; **Address:** Hershey Med Ctr Vascular Surgery, 500 University Dr, rm 4628, Hershey, PA 17033; **Phone:** 717-531-4554; **Board Cert:** Surgery 2005; Vascular Surgery 1997; Surgical Critical Care 2000; **Med School:** Univ Ala 1978; **Resid:** Surgery, Mass Genl Hosp 1984; **Fellow:** Vascular Surgery, Mass Genl Hosp 1985; **Fac Appt:** Prof S, Penn State Univ-Hershey Med Ctr

Benvenisty, Alan I MD [VascS] - **Spec Exp:** Peripheral Vascular Surgery; Endovascular Surgery; Transplant-Kidney; **Hospital:** St Luke's - Roosevelt Hosp Ctr - St Luke's Hosp (page 57), St Luke's - Roosevelt Hosp Ctr - Roosevelt Div (page 57); **Address:** 1090 Amsterdam Ave Fl 12, New York, NY 10025; **Phone:** 212-523-4706; **Board Cert:** Surgery 2004; Vascular Surgery 1999; **Med School:** Columbia P&S 1978; **Resid:** Surgery, Columbia-Presby Med Ctr 1983; **Fellow:** Vascular Surgery, Columbia-Presby Med Ctr 1984; Transplant Surgery, Columbia-Presby Med Ctr 1984; **Fac Appt:** Clin Prof S, Columbia P&S

Blebea, John MD [VascS] - **Spec Exp:** Endovascular Surgery; **Hospital:** Temple Univ Hosp; **Address:** Temple Univ Hosp, 3401 N Broad St, Zone C, Dept Surgery, Philadelphia, PA 19140; **Phone:** 215-707-3133; **Board Cert:** Vascular Surgery 2000; Surgery 1998; **Med School:** Case West Res Univ 1982; **Resid:** Surgery, Georgetown Univ Hosp 1985; Vascular Surgery, UMDNJ 1986; **Fellow:** Vascular Surgery, Univ Rochester 1991; **Fac Appt:** Prof S, Temple Univ

Vascular Surgery

Brener, Bruce J MD [VascS] - **Spec Exp:** Endovascular Surgery; Minimally Invasive Vascular Surgery; Carotid Artery Surgery; Aneurysm-Aortic; **Hospital:** Newark Beth Israel Med Ctr, St Barnabas Med Ctr; **Address:** 200 South Orange Ave, Livingston, NJ 07039; **Phone:** 973-322-7233; **Board Cert:** Surgery 1972; Vascular Surgery 2005; **Med School:** Harvard Med Sch 1966; **Resid:** Surgery, Chldns Hosp Med Ctr 1968; Surgery, Peter Bent Brigham Hosp 1972; **Fellow:** Vascular Surgery, Mass Genl Hosp 1973; **Fac Appt:** Assoc Clin Prof S, Columbia P&S

Calligaro, Keith D MD [VascS] - **Spec Exp:** Aneurysm-Abdominal & Thoracic Aortic; Carotid Artery Disease; **Hospital:** Pennsylvania Hosp (page 60); **Address:** 700 Spruce St, Ste 101, Philadelphia, PA 19106; **Phone:** 215-829-5000; **Board Cert:** Surgery 1997; Vascular Surgery 1999; **Med School:** UMDNJ-Rutgers Med Sch 1982; **Resid:** Surgery, St Barnabas Med Ctr 1984; Surgery, Univ Hlth Scis/Chicago Med Sch 1987; **Fellow:** Vascular Surgery, Montefiore Med Ctr 1989; **Fac Appt:** Assoc Clin Prof S, Univ Pennsylvania

Carpenter, Jeffrey P MD [VascS] - **Spec Exp:** Aneurysm-Abdominal & Thoracic Aortic; Carotid Artery Surgery; Peripheral Vascular Disease; **Hospital:** Hosp Univ Penn - UPHS (page 60); **Address:** Hospital U Penn, 4 Silverstein Pavilion, 3400 Spruce St, Philadelphia, PA 19104; **Phone:** 215-662-2029; **Board Cert:** Surgery 2001; Vascular Surgery 2001; **Med School:** Yale Univ 1986; **Resid:** Surgery, Hosp Univ Penn 1991; **Fellow:** Vascular Surgery, Hosp Univ Penn 1992; **Fac Appt:** Prof S, Univ Pennsylvania

Criado, Frank J MD [VascS] - **Spec Exp:** Endovascular Surgery; Aneurysm-Abdominal & Thoracic Aortic; Carotid Artery Stent Placement; **Hospital:** Union Meml Hosp - Baltimore; **Address:** 3333 N Calvert St, Ste 570, Baltimore, MD 21218; **Phone:** 410-554-6400; **Board Cert:** Surgery 1989; Vascular Surgery 1997; **Med School:** Uruguay 1974; **Resid:** Surgery, Union Memorial Hosp 1980; Vascular Surgery, Union Memorial Hosp 1985; **Fellow:** Cardiovascular Surgery, Baylor Univ Med Ctr 1981

Darling III, R Clement MD [VascS] - **Spec Exp:** Aneurysm-Abdominal & Thoracic Aortic; Arterial Bypass Surgery; Carotid Artery Surgery; **Hospital:** Albany Med Ctr, St Peter's Hosp - Albany; **Address:** Albany Med Ctr, Vascular Inst, 43 New Scotland Ave, MC 157, Albany, NY 12208; **Phone:** 518-262-5640; **Board Cert:** Surgery 1999; Vascular Surgery 2002; **Med School:** Univ Cincinnati 1984; **Resid:** Surgery, Beth Israel Deaconess Hosp 1989; **Fellow:** Vascular Surgery, Albany Med Ctr 1991; **Fac Appt:** Prof S, Albany Med Coll

Fairman, Ronald M MD [VascS] - **Spec Exp:** Aneurysm-Aortic; Peripheral Vascular Disease; Carotid Artery Surgery; Aneurysm-Abdominal & Thoracic Aortic; **Hospital:** Hosp Univ Penn - UPHS (page 60); **Address:** Hosp Univ Penn, 4 Silverstein Pavilion, 3400 Spruce St, Philadelphia, PA 19104; **Phone:** 215-662-2050; **Board Cert:** Surgery 1996; Vascular Surgery 2000; **Med School:** Thomas Jefferson Univ 1977; **Resid:** Surgery, Hosp U Penn 1983; **Fellow:** Vascular Surgery, Hosp U Penn 1984; **Fac Appt:** Assoc Prof S, Univ Pennsylvania

Fantini, Gary A MD [VascS] - **Spec Exp:** Spinal Access Surgery; Vein Disorders; Wound Healing/Care; **Hospital:** Hosp For Special Surgery (page 59), NY-Presby Hosp/Weill Cornell (page 66); **Address:** 635 Madison Ave Fl 7, New York, NY 10022; **Phone:** 212-317-4550; **Board Cert:** Surgery 1999; Vascular Surgery 2000; **Med School:** Albert Einstein Coll Med 1983; **Resid:** Surgery, New York Hosp-Cornell Med Ctr 1989; **Fellow:** Vascular Surgery, UCSF Med Ctr 1990; **Fac Appt:** Assoc Prof S, Cornell Univ-Weill Med Coll

Faries, Peter MD [VascS] - **Spec Exp:** Aneurysm-Abdominal Aortic; Peripheral Vascular Disease; Renovascular Disease; Carotid Artery Disease; **Hospital:** Mount Sinai Med Ctr (page 64); **Address:** 5 E 98th St, Ste 415, New York, NY 10021; **Phone:** 212-415-0756; **Board Cert:** Surgery 1999; Vascular Surgery 2001; **Med School:** Univ Pennsylvania 1992; **Resid:** Surgery, Montefiore Med Ctr 1998; **Fellow:** Vascular Surgery, Beth Israel Deaconess Med Ctr 2000; Research, NIH/Mt Sinai Med Sch 2004; **Fac Appt:** Prof S, Mount Sinai Sch Med

Freischlag, Julie A MD [VascS] - **Spec Exp:** Aneurysm-Aortic; Carotid Artery Disease; Thoracic Outlet Syndrome; **Hospital:** Johns Hopkins Hosp - Baltimore (page 61); **Address:** Johns Hopkins Hosp, Dept Surg, 720 Rutland Ave, Ross Bldg-759, Baltimore, MD 21205; **Phone:** 443-287-3497; **Board Cert:** Surgery 1995; Vascular Surgery 1995; **Med School:** Rush Med Coll 1980; **Resid:** Surgery, UCLA Medical Ctr 1986; **Fellow:** Vascular Surgery, UCLA Medical Ctr 1987; **Fac Appt:** Prof S, Johns Hopkins Univ

Giangola, Gary MD [VascS] - **Spec Exp:** Carotid Artery Surgery; Aneurysm-Aortic; Diabetic Leg/Foot; **Hospital:** Staten Island Univ Hosp - North, Staten Island Univ Hosp - South; **Address:** 256 Mason Ave B Bldg Fl 2, Staten Island, NY 10305; **Phone:** 718-226-6800; **Board Cert:** Surgery 1996; Vascular Surgery 1998; **Med School:** NYU Sch Med 1980; **Resid:** Surgery, NYU Med Ctr 1985; **Fellow:** Vascular Surgery, NYU Med Ctr 1986; **Fac Appt:** Assoc Clin Prof S, Columbia P&S

Golden, Michael A MD [VascS] - **Spec Exp:** Aneurysm; Endovascular Surgery; **Hospital:** Penn Presby Med Ctr - UPHS (page 60); **Address:** Penn Presbyterian, Vascular Surgery, 266 Wright Saunders Bldg, 39th & Market Sts, Philadelphia, PA 19104; **Phone:** 215-662-9660; **Board Cert:** Surgery 1989; Vascular Surgery 2001; **Med School:** Univ Pennsylvania 1981; **Resid:** Surgery, Brigham & Women's Hosp 1987; **Fellow:** Vascular Surgery, Brigham & Women's Hosp 1990; **Fac Appt:** Assoc Prof S, Univ Pennsylvania

Green, Richard M MD [VascS] - **Spec Exp:** Aneurysm-Abdominal Aortic; Carotid Artery Surgery; Percutaneous Vascular Interventions; **Hospital:** Lenox Hill Hosp (page 62); **Address:** 130 E 77th St Fl 13, New York, NY 10021; **Phone:** 212-434-3420; **Board Cert:** Vascular Surgery 2003; **Med School:** Univ Rochester 1970; **Resid:** Surgery, Strong Meml Hosp 1976

Harrington, Elizabeth MD [VascS] - **Spec Exp:** Carotid Artery Surgery; Aneurysm-Aortic; Arterial Bypass Surgery-Leg; **Hospital:** Mount Sinai Med Ctr (page 64), Lenox Hill Hosp (page 62); **Address:** 1225 Park Ave, Ste 1D, New York, NY 10128-1758; **Phone:** 212-876-7400; **Board Cert:** Surgery 1999; Vascular Surgery 2006; **Med School:** NY Med Coll 1975; **Resid:** Surgery, Mount Sinai Hosp 1980; **Fellow:** Vascular Surgery, Mount Sinai Hosp 1981; **Fac Appt:** Assoc Prof VascS, Mount Sinai Sch Med

Kent, K Craig MD [VascS] - **Spec Exp:** Carotid Artery Surgery; Aneurysm-Abdominal Aortic; Lower Limb Arterial Disease; **Hospital:** NY-Presby Hosp/Columbia (page 66); **Address:** 525 E 68th St, rm 107, New York, NY 10021-9800; **Phone:** 212-746-5192; **Board Cert:** Surgery 2007; Vascular Surgery 1998; **Med School:** UCSF 1981; **Resid:** Surgery, UCSF Med Ctr 1986; **Fellow:** Vascular Surgery, Brigham & Women's Hosp 1988; **Fac Appt:** Prof S, Cornell Univ-Weill Med Coll

Makaroun, Michel MD [VascS] - **Spec Exp:** Endovascular Surgery; Aneurysm; Carotid Artery Disease; Peripheral Vascular Surgery; **Hospital:** UPMC Presby, Pittsburgh, UPMC Shadyside; **Address:** Presby-Univ Hosp, A-1011, 200 Lothrop St, Pittsburgh, PA 15213; **Phone:** 412-802-3028; **Board Cert:** Surgery 2004; Vascular Surgery 1998; **Med School:** Lebanon 1978; **Resid:** Surgery, American Univ Hosp 1980; Surgery, Univ Pittsburgh Med Ctr 1985; **Fac Appt:** Prof S, Univ Pittsburgh

Marin, Michael L MD [VascS] - **Spec Exp:** Aneurysm-Aortic; Carotid Artery Surgery; Limb Sparing Surgery; Endovascular Surgery; **Hospital:** Mount Sinai Med Ctr (page 64); **Address:** Mount Sinai Medical Ctr, 5 E 98th St, Box 1273, New York, NY 10029; **Phone:** 212-241-5315; **Board Cert:** Surgery 1999; **Med School:** Mount Sinai Sch Med 1984; **Resid:** Surgery, Columbia-Presby Med Ctr 1990; **Fellow:** Transplant Surgery, Columbia-Presby Med Ctr 1988; Vascular Surgery, Montefiore Med Ctr 1992; **Fac Appt:** Prof S, Mount Sinai Sch Med

Vascular Surgery

Perler, Bruce MD [VascS] - **Spec Exp:** Carotid Artery Surgery; Aneurysm; Arterial Bypass Surgery-Leg; **Hospital:** Johns Hopkins Hosp - Baltimore (page 61); **Address:** Johns Hopkins Hosp-Surg, 600 N Wolfe St Bldg Harvey - Ste 611, Baltimore, MD 21287-8611; **Phone:** 410-955-2618; **Board Cert:** Vascular Surgery 1997; **Med School:** Duke Univ 1976; **Resid:** Surgery, Mass Genl Hosp 1981; **Fellow:** Vascular Surgery, Mass Genl Hosp 1982; **Fac Appt:** Prof S, Johns Hopkins Univ

Ricotta, John MD [VascS] - **Spec Exp:** Aneurysm; Carotid Artery Surgery; Vein Disorders; **Hospital:** Stony Brook Univ Med Ctr; **Address:** SUNY HSC, Dept Surgery, HSC T19, rm 020, Stony Brook, NY 11794-8191; **Phone:** 631-444-7875; **Board Cert:** Surgery 2000; Vascular Surgery 1995; **Med School:** Johns Hopkins Univ 1973; **Resid:** Surgery, Johns Hopkins Hosp 1977; **Fellow:** Vascular Surgery, Johns Hopkins Hosp 1979; **Fac Appt:** Prof S, Johns Hopkins Univ

Riles, Thomas MD [VascS] - **Spec Exp:** Aneurysm-Abdominal Aortic; Carotid Artery Surgery; **Hospital:** NYU Med Ctr (page 68); **Address:** NYU Med Ctr, Univ Vascular Assoc, 530 1st Ave, HCC-6D, New York, NY 10016; **Phone:** 212-263-6360; **Board Cert:** Vascular Surgery 2003; **Med School:** Baylor Coll Med 1969; **Resid:** Surgery, NYU Med Ctr 1976; **Fellow:** Vascular Surgery, NYU Med Ctr 1977; **Fac Appt:** Prof S, NYU Sch Med

Steed, David L MD [VascS] - **Spec Exp:** Wound Healing/Care; **Hospital:** UPMC Presby, Pittsburgh; **Address:** UPMC Presbyterian Hosp, 200 Lothrop St, Ste A-1011, Pittsburgh, PA 15213; **Phone:** 412-802-3024; **Board Cert:** Surgery 1999; Vascular Surgery 1997; Surgical Critical Care 1995; **Med School:** Univ Pittsburgh 1973; **Resid:** Surgery, Univ Pittsburgh Med Ctr 1980; **Fellow:** Vascular Surgery, UCLA Med Ctr 1977; **Fac Appt:** Prof S, Univ Pittsburgh

Todd, George MD [VascS] - **Spec Exp:** Minimally Invasive Vascular Surgery; Aneurysm-Abdominal Aortic; Carotid Artery Surgery; **Hospital:** St Luke's - Roosevelt Hosp Ctr - Roosevelt Div (page 57); **Address:** St Luke's-Roosevelt Hosp Ctr, Dept Surg, 1000 10th Ave, rm 5G77, New York, NY 10019; **Phone:** 212-523-7481; **Board Cert:** Surgery 2000; **Med School:** Penn State Univ-Hershey Med Ctr 1974; **Resid:** Surgery, Columbia-Presby Med Ctr 1979; **Fellow:** Vascular Surgery, Columbia-Presby Med Ctr 1980; **Fac Appt:** Prof S, Columbia P&S

Southeast

Bandyk, Dennis MD [VascS] - **Spec Exp:** Endovascular Stent Grafts; Lower Limb Arterial Disease; Thoracic Outlet Syndrome; **Hospital:** Tampa Genl Hosp, Univ of S FL - Tampa; **Address:** USF Health South Bldg, 2-A Columbia Drive, Ste STS725, Dept of Surgery, Tampa, FL 33606; **Phone:** 813-259-0921; **Board Cert:** Vascular Surgery 2001; Surgery 2000; **Med School:** Univ Mich Med Sch 1975; **Resid:** Surgery, Univ Wash Hosp 1980; **Fellow:** Vascular Surgery, Univ Wash Hosp 1981; **Fac Appt:** Prof S, Univ S Fla Coll Med

Chaikof, Elliot L MD/PhD [VascS] - **Spec Exp:** Aneurysm-Aortic; Carotid Artery Disease; Limb Sparing Surgery; **Hospital:** Emory Univ Hosp, Chldns Hlthcare Atlanta - Egleston; **Address:** Emory Vascular Surgery, 101 Woodruff Cir, Ste 5501 WMB, Atlanta, GA 30322; **Phone:** 404-778-5451; **Board Cert:** Surgery 2002; Vascular Surgery 2003; **Med School:** Johns Hopkins Univ 1982; **Resid:** Surgery, Mass Genl Hosp 1985; Surgery, Mass Genl Hosp 1991; **Fellow:** Vascular Surgery, Emory Univ Hosp 1992; **Fac Appt:** Prof S, Emory Univ

Cherry Jr, Kenneth J MD [VascS] - **Spec Exp:** Vascular Reconstruction; Aortic Graft Infections; **Hospital:** Univ Virginia Med Ctr; **Address:** Univ Virginia Health System, PO Box 800679, Charlottesville, VA 22908-0679; **Phone:** 434-243-7052; **Board Cert:** Vascular Surgery 2004; **Med School:** Univ VA Sch Med 1974; **Resid:** Surgery, Univ Virginia Hosp 1980; Vascular Surgery, UCSF Med Ctr 1981; **Fac Appt:** Prof S, Univ VA Sch Med

Flynn, Timothy C MD [VascS] - **Spec Exp:** Peripheral Vascular Disease; Aortic Graft Infections; **Hospital:** Shands at Univ of FL; **Address:** Shands Hlthcare Univ Florida, PO Box 100321, Gainesville, FL 32610-0286; **Phone:** 352-265-0152; **Board Cert:** Surgery 1999; Vascular Surgery 1994; Surgical Critical Care 1998; **Med School:** Baylor Coll Med 1974; **Resid:** Surgery, Univ Texas 1980; **Fac Appt:** Prof S, Univ Fla Coll Med

Hakaim, Albert G MD [VascS] - **Spec Exp:** Aneurysm-Abdominal Aortic; Endovascular Surgery; **Hospital:** Mayo - Jacksonville; **Address:** Mayo Clinic, Dept Vascular Surgery, 323N, 4500 San Pablo Rd, Jacksonville, FL 32224; **Phone:** 904-953-2077; **Board Cert:** Surgery 2002; Vascular Surgery 2003; **Med School:** Ohio State Univ 1984; **Resid:** Surgery, Cleveland Clinic 1989; **Fellow:** Transplant Surgery, Boston Univ Hosp 1991; Vascular Surgery, Cleveland Clinic 1992; **Fac Appt:** Assoc Prof S, Mayo Med Sch

Hallett Jr, John W MD [VascS] - **Spec Exp:** Aneurysm-Abdominal Aortic; Carotid Artery Surgery; Thoracic Outlet Syndrome; **Hospital:** Roper Hosp; **Address:** Roper St Francis Heart & Vascular Ctr, 316 Calhoun St, Charleston, SC 29401; **Phone:** 843-720-8347; **Board Cert:** Surgery 1999; Vascular Surgery 2003; **Med School:** Duke Univ 1973; **Resid:** Surgery, Wilford Hall USAF Med Ctr 1978; **Fellow:** Vascular Surgery, Mass Genl Hosp-Harvard Med Sch 1979; **Fac Appt:** Assoc Clin Prof VascS, Med Univ SC

Hansen, Kimberley J MD [VascS] - **Spec Exp:** Aortic & Visceral Artery Surgery; Renovascular Disease; Carotid Artery Surgery; **Hospital:** Wake Forest Univ Baptist Med Ctr (page 73), Forsyth Med Ctr; **Address:** Wake Forest Univ Sch Med, Dept Surg, Medical Center Blvd, Winston-Salem, NC 27157-1095; **Phone:** 336-716-4151; **Board Cert:** Vascular Surgery 1998; Surgical Critical Care 2001; Surgery 2006; **Med School:** Univ Ala 1980; **Resid:** Surgery, NC Baptist Hosp/WFU Sch MEd 1986; **Fellow:** Vascular Surgery, Univ California 1987; **Fac Appt:** Prof S, Wake Forest Univ

McCann, Richard L MD [VascS] - **Spec Exp:** Endovascular Surgery; **Hospital:** Duke Univ Med Ctr; **Address:** Duke Univ Med Ctr, Box 2990, Durham, NC 27710; **Phone:** 919-684-2620; **Board Cert:** Surgery 2003; Vascular Surgery 2006; **Med School:** Cornell Univ-Weill Med Coll 1974; **Resid:** Surgery, Duke Univ Med Ctr 1983; **Fac Appt:** Prof S, Duke Univ

Rosenthal, David MD [VascS] - **Spec Exp:** Stroke; Aneurysm; Endovascular Surgery; **Hospital:** Atlanta Med Ctr; **Address:** 315 Blvd NE, Ste 412, Atlanta, GA 30312; **Phone:** 404-524-0095; **Board Cert:** Vascular Surgery 2003; **Med School:** SUNY Downstate 1973; **Resid:** Surgery, Tufts-New Eng Med Ctr 1977; **Fellow:** Vascular Surgery, Tufts-New Eng Med Ctr 1978; **Fac Appt:** Clin Prof S, Med Coll GA

Seeger, James M MD [VascS] - **Spec Exp:** Lower Limb Arterial Disease; Aneurysm-Aortic; Kidney & Bowel Arterial Disease; **Hospital:** Shands at Univ of FL; **Address:** Univ Florida, Dept Vascular Surgery, 1600 SW Archer Rd, JHMHC Bldg-rm NG-45, Box 100286, Gainesville, FL 32610-0286; **Phone:** 352-273-5484; **Board Cert:** Surgery 2000; Vascular Surgery 1992; **Med School:** Med Coll GA 1973; **Resid:** Surgery, Univ Utah Med Ctr 1980; **Fellow:** Vascular Surgery, Eastern VA Med Sch 1981; **Fac Appt:** Prof S, Univ Fla Coll Med

Sivina, Manuel MD [VascS] - **Hospital:** Mount Sinai Med Ctr - Miami; **Address:** Mount Sinai Med Ctr, 4300 Alton Rd, Ste 2240, Miami Beach, FL 33140-2800; **Phone:** 305-674-2760; **Board Cert:** Surgery 2000; **Med School:** Peru 1969; **Resid:** Surgery, Mt Sinai Med Ctr 1975; **Fellow:** Vascular Surgery, Mt Sinai Med Ctr 1976

Vascular Surgery

Midwest

Alexander, J Jeffrey MD [VascS] - **Hospital:** MetroHealth Med Ctr; **Address:** Metrohealth Med Ctr, Heart & Vascular Dept, 2500 Metrohealth Drive, Cleveland, OH 44109; **Phone:** 216-778-4811; **Board Cert:** Vascular Surgery 2006; Surgery 2002; **Med School:** Univ Pittsburgh 1978; **Resid:** Surgery, Univ Chicago Hosps 1983; **Fellow:** Vascular Surgery, Univ Chicago Hosps 1984; **Fac Appt:** Assoc Prof S, Case West Res Univ

Berguer, Ramon MD/PhD [VascS] - **Spec Exp:** Cerebrovascular Disease; Aortic & Visceral Artery Surgery; **Hospital:** Univ Michigan Hlth Sys; **Address:** Univ Michigan Hlth Sys, 1500 E Medical Ctr Dr, SPC5867, Ann Arbor, MI 48109; **Phone:** 734-936-8247; **Board Cert:** Surgery 1970; Vascular Surgery 2003; **Med School:** Spain 1963; **Resid:** Surgery, Henry Ford Hosp 1969; **Fellow:** Vascular Surgery, Henry Ford Hosp 1970; Vascular Surgery, Kings College Hosp; **Fac Appt:** Prof S, Univ Mich Med Sch

Clair, Daniel G MD [VascS] - **Spec Exp:** Carotid Artery Surgery; Aneurysm-Abdominal & Thoracic Aortic; Peripheral Vascular Surgery; Endovascular Stent Grafts; **Hospital:** Cleveland Clin Fdn (page 56); **Address:** Cleveland Clinic, Dept Vascular Surgery, 9500 Euclid Ave, MC S40, Cleveland, OH 44195; **Phone:** 216-444-3857; **Board Cert:** Surgery 2003; Vascular Surgery 2004; **Med School:** Univ VA Sch Med 1986; **Resid:** Surgery, Brigham & Women's Hosp 1992; **Fellow:** Vascular Surgery, Brigham & Women's Hosp 1994

Comerota, Anthony J MD [VascS] - **Spec Exp:** Carotid Artery Disease; Gene Therapy; Aneurysm-Aortic; **Hospital:** Toledo Hosp; **Address:** Jobst Vascular Ctr, 2109 Hughes Drive, Ste 400, Toledo, OH 43606; **Phone:** 419-291-2088; **Board Cert:** Surgery 1999; Vascular Surgery 2003; **Med School:** Temple Univ 1974; **Resid:** Surgery, Temple Univ Hosp 1978; **Fellow:** Vascular Surgery, Good Samaritan Hosp 1981; **Fac Appt:** Clin Prof S, Univ Mich Med Sch

Dalsing, Michael C MD [VascS] - **Spec Exp:** Peripheral Vascular Surgery; Vein Disorders; Renovascular Disease; Carotid Artery Surgery; **Hospital:** Indiana Univ Hosp; **Address:** 1001 W 10th St, Director of Vascular Surgery, Wishard Health Services, Indianapolis, IN 46202; **Phone:** 317-962-0280; **Board Cert:** Vascular Surgery 2003; Surgical Critical Care 2001; Surgery 2002; **Med School:** Med Coll Wisc 1978; **Resid:** Surgery, Ind U Med Ctr 1983; **Fellow:** Vascular Surgery, Northwestern U Med Ctr 1984; **Fac Appt:** Prof S, Indiana Univ

Gloviczki, Peter MD [VascS] - **Spec Exp:** Aneurysm-Abdominal Aortic; Lower Limb Arterial Disease; Vein Disorders; **Hospital:** Mayo Med Ctr & Clin - Rochester; **Address:** Mayo Clinic, Div Vasc Surg, 200 First St SW, Rochester, MN 55905-0001; **Phone:** 507-284-4652; **Board Cert:** Surgery 1998; Vascular Surgery 1998; **Med School:** Hungary 1972; **Resid:** Vascular Surgery, Semmelweis Med Sch 1980; Surgery, Mayo Clin 1987; **Fellow:** Vascular Surgery, Mayo Clin 1983; **Fac Appt:** Prof S, Mayo Med Sch

Greisler, Howard MD [VascS] - **Spec Exp:** Peripheral Vascular Surgery; Aneurysm; Carotid Artery Disease; **Hospital:** Hines VA Hosp, Loyola Univ Med Ctr; **Address:** Loyola Univ Med Ctr, Dept Surgery, 2160 S 1st Ave, rm 3218, Maywood, IL 60153-5590; **Phone:** 708-216-8541; **Board Cert:** Vascular Surgery 2003; **Med School:** Penn State Univ-Hershey Med Ctr 1975; **Resid:** Surgery, Columbia Presby Med Ctr 1980; **Fellow:** Vascular Surgery, Columbia Presby Med Ctr 1981; **Fac Appt:** Prof S, Loyola Univ-Stritch Sch Med

Hodgson, Kim John MD [VascS] - **Spec Exp:** Aneurysm; Carotid Artery Surgery; Endovascular Surgery; **Hospital:** St John's Hosp - Springfield, Memorial Med Ctr - Springfield; **Address:** PO Box 19638, Springfield, IL 62794-9638; **Phone:** 217-545-5555; **Board Cert:** Vascular Surgery 2005; **Med School:** Univ Pennsylvania 1981; **Resid:** Surgery, Albany Med Ctr 1986; **Fellow:** Vascular Surgery, Southern Ill Univ 1987; **Fac Appt:** Prof VascS, Southern IL Univ

McLafferty, Robert B MD [VascS] - **Spec Exp:** Minimally Invasive Vascular Surgery; Endovascular Stent Grafts; Carotid Artery Stent Placement; Aneurysm; **Hospital:** Memorial Med Ctr - Springfield, St John's Hosp - Springfield; **Address:** S Illinois School of Medicine, PO Box 19638, Springfield, IL 62294-9638; **Phone:** 217-545-5555; **Board Cert:** Surgery 2005; Vascular Surgery 1999; **Med School:** Univ VT Coll Med 1990; **Resid:** Surgery, Oregon Hlth Sci Ctr 1996; **Fellow:** Vascular Surgery, Oregon Hlth Sci Ctr 1998; **Fac Appt:** Prof VascS, Southern IL Univ

Pearce, William H MD [VascS] - **Spec Exp:** Aneurysm-Abdominal Aortic; Stroke; Peripheral Vascular Disease; **Hospital:** Northwestern Meml Hosp; **Address:** Northwestern Meml Hosp - Galter Pavilion, 675 N St Clair St, Ste 19-100, Chicago, IL 60611-2647; **Phone:** 312-695-2714; **Board Cert:** Surgery 2001; Vascular Surgery 2003; Surgical Critical Care 1999; **Med School:** Univ Colorado 1975; **Resid:** Surgery, Univ Co Hlth Sci Ctr 1981; **Fellow:** Vascular Surgery, Northwestern Meml Hosp 1982; **Fac Appt:** Prof S, Northwestern Univ

Sanchez, Luis A MD [VascS] - **Spec Exp:** Aneurysm-Abdominal & Thoracic Aortic; Endovascular Stent Grafts; Peripheral Vascular Disease; **Hospital:** Barnes-Jewish Hosp; **Address:** Washington Univ School Medicine, 660 S Euclid Ave, Box 8109-Surgery, St Louis, MO 63110; **Phone:** 314-362-7408; **Board Cert:** Surgery 2004; Vascular Surgery 2003; **Med School:** Harvard Med Sch 1987; **Resid:** Surgery, Montefiore Med Ctr 1992; **Fellow:** Vascular Surgery, Montefiore Med Ctr 1994; **Fac Appt:** Prof VascS, Washington Univ, St Louis

Shepard, Alexander D MD [VascS] - **Spec Exp:** Aneurysm-Aortic; Aortic Reconstruction; Vascular Surgery-Secondary; **Hospital:** Henry Ford Hosp; **Address:** 2799 W Grand Blvd, Detroit, MI 48202-2608; **Phone:** 313-916-3155; **Board Cert:** Surgery 2001; Vascular Surgery 2005; **Med School:** Johns Hopkins Univ 1976; **Resid:** Surgery, Johns Hopkins Hosp 1982; **Fellow:** Vascular Surgery, New England Med Ctr 1985

Sicard, Gregorio A MD [VascS] - **Spec Exp:** Aneurysm-Abdominal Aortic; **Hospital:** Barnes-Jewish Hosp; **Address:** Wash Univ Med Sch, Dept Surg, 660 S Euclid Ave, Box 8109, St Louis, MO 63110; **Phone:** 314-362-7841; **Board Cert:** Surgery 1996; Vascular Surgery 2002; **Med School:** Univ Puerto Rico 1972; **Resid:** Surgery, Barnes Hosp 1977; **Fellow:** Transplant Surgery, Wash Univ Hosp 1978; **Fac Appt:** Prof S, Washington Univ, St Louis

Stanley, James C MD [VascS] - **Spec Exp:** Peripheral Vascular Surgery; Renovascular Disease; Aneurysm; **Hospital:** Univ Michigan Hlth Sys; **Address:** Univ Mich, Dept Vascular Surgery, 1500 E Med Ctr Drive, rm 5167CVC, Taubman Ctr, Ann Arbor, MI 48109-0329; **Phone:** 734-936-5786; **Board Cert:** Surgery 1973; Vascular Surgery 2001; **Med School:** Univ Mich Med Sch 1964; **Resid:** Surgery, Univ Mich Med Ctr 1972; **Fac Appt:** Prof S, Univ Mich Med Sch

Great Plains and Mountains

Annest, Stephen J MD [VascS] - **Spec Exp:** Thoracic Outlet Syndrome; **Hospital:** Presby - St Luke's Med Ctr, Exempla Saint Jos. Hosp. - Denver; **Address:** The Vascular Institute of the Rockies, 1601 E 19th Ave, Ste 3950, Denver, CO 80218; **Phone:** 303-539-0736; **Board Cert:** Surgery 2000; Vascular Surgery 2005; **Med School:** Univ Wash 1975; **Resid:** Surgery, Albany Med Ctr 1981; **Fellow:** Trauma, Albany Med Ctr 1980; Vascular Surgery, Baylor Univ Med Ctr 1982; **Fac Appt:** Asst Clin Prof S, Hahnemann Univ

Howard, Thomas C MD [VascS] - **Spec Exp:** Aortic Surgery; Aneurysm-Aortic; Carotid Artery Surgery; Lower Limb Arterial Disease; **Hospital:** Immanuel Med Ctr; **Address:** Surgery Ctr of the Heartland, 4239 Farnam St, Ste 823, Omaha, NE 68131; **Phone:** 402-552-3015; **Board Cert:** Surgery 1975; Vascular Surgery 2002; **Med School:** Yale Univ 1969; **Resid:** Surgery, Yale-New Haven Hosp 1974; **Fac Appt:** Assoc Prof S, Univ Nebr Coll Med

Vascular Surgery

Southwest

Clagett, George Patrick MD [VascS] - **Spec Exp:** Aneurysm-Abdominal Aortic; **Hospital:** Parkland Meml Hosp - Dallas, UT Southwestern Med Ctr - Dallas; **Address:** Univ Tex SW Med Ctr, 5909 Harry Hines Blvd, HA8.130, Dallas, TX 75390-9157; **Phone:** 214-645-0548; **Board Cert:** Surgery 1996; Vascular Surgery 2004; **Med School:** Univ VA Sch Med 1968; **Resid:** Surgery, Univ Mich Med Ctr 1972; Surgery, Univ Mich Med Ctr 1976; **Fellow:** Research, Beth Israel-Harvard 1974; Vascular Surgery, Walter Reed Army Med Ctr 1979; **Fac Appt:** Prof S, Univ Tex SW, Dallas

Corson, John MD [VascS] - **Spec Exp:** Carotid Artery Surgery; Vascular Disease in the Elderly; Limb Sparing Surgery; **Hospital:** VA Med Ctr; **Address:** Raymond G Murphy VA Medical Ctr, 1501 San Pedro SE, MS 112, Albequerque, NM 87108; **Phone:** 505-265-1711 x2385; **Board Cert:** Surgery 2002; Vascular Surgery 2001; **Med School:** Scotland 1968; **Resid:** Surgery, Univ Hosp Wales 1975; Surgery, Boston Univ Med Ctr 1980; **Fellow:** Research, Boston Univ Med Ctr 1977; Vascular Surgery, Mass Genl Hosp/Harvard 1981; **Fac Appt:** Prof S, Univ New Mexico

Eidt, John MD [VascS] - **Spec Exp:** Aneurysm-Abdominal Aortic; Carotid Artery Stent Placement; Endovascular Surgery; Peripheral Vascular Disease; **Hospital:** UAMS Med Ctr; **Address:** 4301 W Markham St, Slot 520-2, Little Rock, AR 72205; **Phone:** 501-686-6176; **Board Cert:** Vascular Surgery 1996; Surgical Critical Care 2004; **Med School:** Univ Tex SW, Dallas 1981; **Resid:** Surgery, Brigham-Womens Hosp 1986; **Fellow:** Vascular Surgery, Univ Tex SW Med Ctr; **Fac Appt:** Prof S, Univ Ark

Fowl, Richard J MD [VascS] - **Spec Exp:** Aneurysm-Aortic; Carotid Artery Surgery; Arterial Bypass Surgery-Leg; **Hospital:** Mayo Clinic - Scottsdale; **Address:** Mayo Clinic, Dept Vascular Surgery, 5777 E Mayo Blvd, Phoenix, AZ 85054; **Phone:** 480-342-2868; **Board Cert:** Surgery 2002; Vascular Surgery 2004; **Med School:** Rush Med Coll 1978; **Resid:** Surgery, Med Coll Virginia 1980; Surgery, Univ Iowa Med Ctr 1983; **Fellow:** Vascular Surgery, Mayo Clinic 1985; **Fac Appt:** Prof S, Mayo Med Sch

Hollier, Larry H MD [VascS] - **Spec Exp:** Aortic Surgery; Carotid Artery Surgery; Endovascular Surgery; **Hospital:** West Jefferson Med Ctr, Med Ctr LA @ New Orleans (Univ Hosp); **Address:** 433 Bolivar St, Ste 815, New Orleans, LA 70112; **Phone:** 504-568-4800; **Board Cert:** Surgery 2007; Vascular Surgery 2001; **Med School:** Louisiana State U, New Orleans 1968; **Resid:** Surgery, Charity Hosp 1973; **Fellow:** Vascular Surgery, Baylor Med Ctr 1974; **Fac Appt:** Prof S, Louisiana State U, New Orleans

Lumsden, Alan B MD [VascS] - **Spec Exp:** Aortic Stent Grafts; Minimally Invasive Surgery; Vein Disorders; **Hospital:** Methodist Hosp - Houston, St Luke's Episcopal Hosp - Houston; **Address:** 6560 Fannin, Ste 1006, Scurlock Tower, Houston, TX 77030; **Phone:** 713-441-5200; **Board Cert:** Vascular Surgery 2002; **Med School:** Scotland 1981; **Resid:** Surgery, Emory Univ Hosp 1987; **Fellow:** Vascular Surgery, Emory Univ Hosp 1989; **Fac Appt:** Prof VascS, Baylor Coll Med

Money, Samuel R MD [VascS] - **Spec Exp:** Aneurysm-Abdominal Aortic; Arterial Bypass Surgery-Leg; Endovascular Surgery; **Hospital:** Mayo Clinic - Scottsdale; **Address:** Mayo Clinic, Dept Surgery, 5777 E Mayo Blvd, Phoenix, AZ 85054; **Phone:** 480-342-2868; **Board Cert:** Surgery 2000; Vascular Surgery 2002; **Med School:** SUNY Downstate 1983; **Resid:** Surgery, Kings Co Med Ctr 1990; **Fellow:** Vascular Surgery, Ochsner Clinic 1993; **Fac Appt:** Prof S, Mayo Med Sch

West Coast and Pacific

Ahn, Sam S MD [VascS] - **Spec Exp:** Minimally Invasive Vascular Surgery; Endovascular Surgery; Thoracic Outlet Syndrome; Hyperhidrosis; **Hospital:** Ronald Reagan UCLA Med Ctr, St John's Hlth Ctr, Santa Monica; **Address:** 1082 Glendon Ave, Los Angeles, CA 90024; **Phone:** 310-209-2011; **Board Cert:** Surgery 2004; Vascular Surgery 1997; **Med School:** Univ Tex SW, Dallas 1978; **Resid:** Surgery, UCLA Med Ctr 1984; **Fellow:** Vascular Surgery, UCLA Med Ctr 1986; **Fac Appt:** Prof S, UCLA

Dilley, Ralph B MD [VascS] - **Spec Exp:** Vascular Reconstruction; **Hospital:** Scripps Green Hosp; **Address:** Scripps Clinic-Torrey Pines, 10666 N Torrey Pines Rd, rm SW208, La Jolla, CA 92037; **Phone:** 858-554-8988; **Board Cert:** Surgery 1966; Thoracic Surgery 1966; Vascular Surgery 2002; **Med School:** Stanford Univ 1959; **Resid:** Surgery, UCLA Med Ctr 1965; Surgery, Johns Hopkins Hosp 1961; **Fellow:** Cardiovascular Surgery, UCSF Med Ctr 1970; **Fac Appt:** Clin Prof S, UCSD

Flanigan, D Preston MD [VascS] - **Spec Exp:** Carotid Artery Disease; Aneurysm; Vein Disorders; **Hospital:** St Joseph's Hosp - Orange; **Address:** 1140 W LaVeta Ave, Ste 850, Orange, CA 92868; **Phone:** 714-560-4450; **Board Cert:** Vascular Surgery 2002; **Med School:** Jefferson Med Coll 1972; **Resid:** Surgery, St Joseph-Mercy Hosp 1977; **Fellow:** Vascular Surgery, Northwest Med Ctr 1978; **Fac Appt:** Clin Prof S, UC Irvine

Gewertz, Bruce MD [VascS] - **Spec Exp:** Carotid Artery Surgery; Peripheral Vascular Disease; Aneurysm-Aortic; **Hospital:** Cedars-Sinai Med Ctr; **Address:** 8700 Beverly Blvd, N Tower, Ste 8215, Los Angeles, CA 90048; **Phone:** 310-423-5884; **Board Cert:** Vascular Surgery 2002; **Med School:** Jefferson Med Coll 1972; **Resid:** Surgery, Univ Mich Hosp 1977; **Fac Appt:** Prof S, UCLA

Grey, Douglas P MD [VascS] - **Hospital:** KFH San Francisco Med Ctr; **Address:** 2238 Geary Blvd, Fl 2, San Francisco, CA 94115; **Phone:** 415-833-3383; **Board Cert:** Thoracic Surgery 2003; Vascular Surgery 2004; **Med School:** UC Irvine 1975; **Resid:** Surgery, Peter Bent Brigham Hosp 1980; Thoracic Surgery, Texas Heart Institute 1982; **Fac Appt:** Clin Prof S, UCSF

Pevec, William C MD [VascS] - **Spec Exp:** Vascular Disease; Angioplasty & Stent Placement; **Hospital:** UC Davis Med Ctr; **Address:** UC Davis Med Ctr, Dept Vascular Surgery, 4860 Y St, Ste 2100, Sacramento, CA 95817; **Phone:** 916-734-3524; **Board Cert:** Surgery 1999; Vascular Surgery 2001; **Med School:** Univ Cincinnati 1984; **Resid:** Surgery, U Pittsburgh Med Ctr 1990; **Fellow:** Vascular Surgery, Mass Genl Hosp 1992; **Fac Appt:** Assoc Prof VascS, UC Davis

White, Rodney Allen MD [VascS] - **Spec Exp:** Endovascular Surgery; Aneurysm; Carotid Artery Surgery; **Hospital:** LAC - Harbor - UCLA Med Ctr; **Address:** Harbor-UCLA Med Ctr, 1000 W Carson St, Box 11, Torrance, CA 90502; **Phone:** 310-222-2704; **Board Cert:** Surgery 1998; Vascular Surgery 2006; **Med School:** SUNY Upstate Med Univ 1974; **Resid:** Surgery, LAC-Harbor-UCLA Med Ctr 1979; **Fellow:** Vascular Surgery, LAC-Harbor-UCLA Med Ctr 1980; **Fac Appt:** Prof S, UCLA

Zarins, Christopher K MD [VascS] - **Spec Exp:** Carotid Artery Surgery; Aneurysm-Abdominal Aortic; Endovascular Surgery; **Hospital:** Stanford Univ Med Ctr, El Camino Hosp/Camino Hlthcare Sys; **Address:** Stanford Univ Med Ctr, Div Vascular Surg, 300 Pasteur Drive, rm H-3600, Stanford, CA 94305; **Phone:** 650-725-5227; **Board Cert:** Surgery 1975; Vascular Surgery 2002; **Med School:** Johns Hopkins Univ 1968; **Resid:** Surgery, Univ Michigan Hosp 1974; **Fellow:** Surgery, Johns Hopkins Hosp 1972; **Fac Appt:** Prof S, Stanford Univ

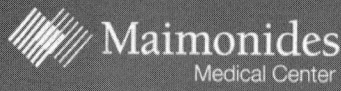

NewYork-Presbyterian

The University Hospital of Columbia and Cornell

NewYork-Presbyterian Vascular Center

Affiliated with Columbia University College of Physicians and Surgeons and Weill Medical College of Cornell Univers

NewYork-Presbyterian Hospital
Columbia University Medical Center
622 West 168th Street
New York, NY 10032

NewYork-Presbyterian Hospital
Weill Cornell Medical Center
525 East 68th Street
New York, NY 10021

OVERVIEW:

Vascular disease can affect people of all ages and requires a wide range of expertise for appropriate and effective therapies. The NewYork-Presbyterian Hospital Vascular Care Center offers a comprehensive and integrated program for the prevention, diagnosis and treatment of diverse problems relating to arteries and veins throughout the body, including the heart, abdomen, kidneys, legs, neck and brain.

The Center brings together medical and surgical experts of two internationally renowned academic medical centers – NewYork-Presbyterian Hospital/Columbia University Medical Center and NewYork-Presbyterian Hospital/Weill Cornell Medical Center – who bring a depth of experience to treating even the most unusual vascular conditions. Patients benefit from the Vascular Care Center's proven cutting edge technologies, innovative programs and groundbreaking research.

The NewYork-Presbyterian Vascular Care Center meets the needs of its patients through:
- Programs that emphasize prevention measures;
- Rigorous screenings and integrated care for patients at risk for life-threatening vascular diseases, such as strokes and abdominal aortic aneurysms;
- Innovative applications of non-invasive diagnostic technologies, including CT scans, ultrasound, MRI and MRA;
- Advances in the latest drug therapies;
- State-of-the-art surgical and minimally invasive treatments;
- New approaches in the treatment of blood clots;
- Basic and clinical research to develop more effective procedures for diagnosis and treatment.

Physician Referral: For a physician referral or to learn more about the NewYork-Presbyterian Vascular Center call toll free **1-877-NYP-WELL** (1-877-697-9355) or visit our website at

COMPREHENSIVE SERVICES INCLUDE:

- Lipid Control Centers where adults and children at risk for inherited or acquired cholesterol and lipid are evaluated and treated.

- Comprehensive Stroke Centers with an interdisciplinary Acute Stroke Team on call round the clock.

- Comprehensive Abdominal Aortic Aneurysm Program to detect and treat one of the leading causes of death, particularly in men.

- Hypertension Center for treating blocked kidney arteries, which can cause high blood pressure and kidney failure.

- Amputation Prevention Program for treating vascular blockages leading to difficulty walking or the loss of a leg.

- Gene Therapy Center includes a program to treat blocked arteries in legs.

- Wound Healing Program offers a hyperbaric oxygen chamber, growth factors and gene therapy to treat poorly healing

VASCULAR SURGERY

A Kinder, Gentler Approach to Aneurysm Repair

When a patient has heart disease, aneurysms, or bulges in the aorta are often an unfortunate, potentially deadly symptom. Most aortic aneurysms occur in areas damaged by artherosclerosis, a condition in which the arteries become hardened from the buildup of cholesterol and other material over many years. It is estimated that one five percent of people over the age of 65 have an aneurysm. There are usually few symptoms, although some people may feel deep back pain. Severe, excruciating pain is usually the first symptom of a rupture.

Ten years ago, a patient with an aortic aneurysm would have undergone an extensive operation to repair it. Today, NYU Langone Medical Center is among a select group of institutions worldwide that offer minimally invasive surgical solutions to complex aortic problems.

The new, minimally invasive procedure involves making small incisions in the groin and inserting a stent graft, which the surgeon guides to the exact position in the artery needed to ease pressure and prevent rupture. Usually, patients require no blood transfusion and are able to leave the hospital just one or two days after surgery.

As the site of early FDA testing of one of the newest devices used in endovascular surgery, NYU Langone Medical Center is leading the way in both clinical and scientific research in the burgeoning field of vascular surgery. It also is a major training center, where vascular surgeons learn and perfect the latest minimally invasive techniques. NYU's outstanding specialists continue to achieve high rates of success with the new stent graft procedure, even in patients over 75 years of age. Judging from the pace of research at NYU, it is extremely likely that the new techniques will be used to treat other types of conditions in the very near future.

Sponsored Page

Appendices

APPENDIX A:
Medical Boards

Introduction to ABMS and Osteopathic Specialties

The following pages contain descriptions of the "official" medical specialties, approved by the American Board of Medical Specialists (for M.D.s) or by the American Osteopathic Association (for D.O.s). These are important because they are the only specialties recognized by the official governing boards. There may be physicians who call themselves one kind of specialist or another, but they may not be certified by the "official" boards. There are, in fact, over 100 such "self-designated" boards, some simply groups of physicians interested in a given area of medicine with no qualifications for membership to other groups with very specific qualifications for membership.

It is important for the medical consumer to seek out physicians certified by the ABMS or AOA to assure their doctor has had the appropriate training and passed the board certification exam.

ABMS

The ABMS is an organization of ABMS Approved medical specialty boards. The mission of the ABMS is to maintain and improve the quality of medical care by assisting the Member Boards in their efforts to develop and utilize professional and educational standards for the evaluation and certification of physician specialists. The intent of certification of physicians is to provide assurance to the public that a physician specialist certified by a Member Board of the ABMS has successfully completed an approved educational program and evaluation process which includes an examination designed to assess the knowledge, skills, and experience required to provide quality patient care in that specialty. The ABMS serves to coordinate the activities of its Member Boards and to provide information to the public, the government, the profession and its Members concerning issues involving specialization and certification in medicine.

Following is a list of the addresses of the various medical specialty boards approved by the ABMS. Note that there are 24 board organizations for 25 medical specialties. Psychiatry and Neurology share the same board.

To find out if a physician is certified, consumers can call the individual boards which may charge a fee for the information, or they can contact the ABMS at (866) 275-2267 (no fee) or www.abms.org.

American Board of Allergy and Immunology
510 Walnut Street, Suite 1701
Philadelphia, PA 19106-3699
(215) 592-9466, (866) 264-5568

General Certification in Allergy and Immunology. Certifications awarded since 1989 are valid for 10 years. For those certified prior to 1989 there is no recertification requirement.

American Board of Anesthesiology
4101 Lake Boone Trail
Raleigh, NC 27607-7506
(919) 881-2570

General Certification in Anesthesiology; with Special and Added Qualifications in Critical Care Medicine and Pain Management. Certifications awarded since 2000 are valid for 10 years.

American Board of Colon and Rectal Surgery
20600 Eureka Road, Suite 600
Taylor, MI 48180
(734) 282-9400

General Certification is in Colon and Rectal Surgery. Certifications awarded since 1990 are valid for 10 years.

American Board of Dermatology
Henry Ford Health System
Detroit, MI 48202-3450
(313) 874-1088

General Certification in Dermatology; with Special Qualifications in Clinical and Laboratory Dermatological Immunology, Dermatopathology, and Pediatric Dermatology. Certifications awarded since 1991 are valid for 10 years.

American Board of Emergency Medicine
3000 Coolidge Road
East Lansing, MI 48823-6319
(517) 332-4800

General Certification in Emergency Medicine; with Special and Added Qualifications in Medical Toxicology, Pediatric Emergency Medicine, Sports Medicine and Undersea and Hyperbaric Medicine. Certifications awarded since 1980 are valid for 10 years

American Board of Family Practice
2228 Young Drive
Lexington, KY 40505-4294
(859) 269-5626, (888) 995-5700

General Certification in Family Practice; with Added Qualifications in Adolescent Medicine, Geriatric Medicine and Sports Medicine. Certifications awarded since 1970 are valid for 7 years.

American Board of Internal Medicine
510 Walnut Street, Suite 1700
Philadelphia, PA 19106-3699
(215) 446-3500, (800) 441-ABIM

General Certification in Internal Medicine; with Special Qualifications in Cardiovascular Disease, Endocrinology, Diabetes and Metabolism, Gastroenterology, Hematology, Infectious Disease, Medical Oncology, Nephrology, Pulmonary Disease, and Rheumatology; and Added Qualifications in Adolescent Medicine, Clinical Cardiac Electrophysiology, Critical Care Medicine, Geriatric Medicine, Interventional Cardiology, Sleep Medicine, Sports Medicine and Transplant Hepatology. Certifications awarded since 1990 are valid for 10 years.

American Board of Medical Genetics
9650 Rockville Pike
Bethesda, MD 20814-3998
(301) 634-7315

General Certification in Clinical Genetics (MD), PhD Medical Genetics, Clinical Biochemical Genetics, Clinical Cytogenetics and Clinical Molecular Genetics; with Added Qualifications in Molecular Genetic Pathology. Certifications awarded since 2002 are valid for 2 years.

American Board of Neurological Surgery
6550 Fannin Street, Suite 2139
Houston, TX 77030-2701
(713) 441-6015

General Certification in Neurological Surgery. Certifications awarded since 1999 are valid for 10 years.

American Board of Nuclear Medicine
    4555 Forest Park Boulevard, Suite 119
    St. Louis, MO 63108
    (314) 367-2225

    General Certification in Nuclear Medicine. Certifications awarded since 1992 are valid
    for 10 years.

American Board of Obstetrics and Gynecology
    2915 Vine Street, Suite 300
    Dallas, TX 75204
    (214) 871-1619

    General Certification in Obstetrics and Gynecology; with Special Qualifications in
    Gynecologic Oncology, Maternal and Fetal Medicine, Reproductive Endocrinology; and
    Added Qualifications in Critical Care Medicine. Certifications awarded since 1986 are
    valid for 6 years.

American Board of Ophthalmology
    111 Presidential Boulevard, Suite 241
    Bala Cynwyd, PA 19004-1075
    (610) 664-1175

    Certifications Awarded since 1992 are valid for 10 years. For those certified prior to
    1992, there is no recertification requirement.

American Board of Orthopaedic Surgery
    400 Silver Cedar Court
    Chapel Hill, NC 27514
    (919) 929-7103

    General Certification in Orthopaedic Surgery; with Added Qualification in Hand
    Surgery; with Added Qualifications in Hand Surgery and Orthopaedic Sports Medicine.
    Certifications awarded since 1986 are valid for 10 years.

American Board of Otolaryngology
    5615 Kirby Drive, Suite 600
    Houston, TX 77005
    (713) 850-0399

    General Certification in Otolaryngology; with Added Qualifications in Neurotology,
    Pediatric Otolaryngology and Plastic Surgery within the Head and Neck. Certifications
    awarded since 2002 are valid for 10 years.

American Board of Pathology

P.O. Box 25915
Tampa, FL 33622-5915
(813) 286-2444

General Certification in Anatomic and Clinical Pathology, Anatomic Pathology and Clinical Pathology; with Special Qualifications in Blood Banking/Transfusion Medicine, Chemical Pathology, Dermatopathology, Forensic Pathology, Hematology, Medical Microbiology, Molecular Genetic Pathology, Neuropathology and Pediatric Pathology; and Added Qualifications in Cytopathology. Certifications awarded since 1997 are valid for 10 years.

American Board of Pediatrics

111 Silver Cedar Court
Chapel Hill, NC 27514-1651
(919) 929-0461

General Certification in Pediatrics; with Special Qualifications in Adolescent Medicine, Developmental-Behavioral Pediatrics, Neonatal-Perinatal Medicine, Pediatric Cardiology, Pediatric Critical Care Medicine, Pediatric Emergency Medicine, Pediatric Endocrinology, Pediatric Gastroenterology, Pediatric Hematology-Oncology, Pediatric Infectious Diseases, Pediatric Nephrology, Pediatric Pulmonology, and Pediatric Rheumatology; and Added Qualifications in Medical Toxicology, Neurodevelopmental Disabilities, Pediatric Transplant Hepatology and Sports Medicine. Certifications awarded since 1988 valid for 7 years.

American Board of Physical Medicine and Rehabilitation

3015 Allegro Park Lane, S.W.
Rochester, MN 55902-4139
(507) 282-1776

General Certification in Physical Medicine and Rehabilitation; with Special Qualifications in Pain Medicine, Pediatric Rehabilitation Medicine, and Spinal Cord Injury Medicine. Certifications awarded since 1993 are valid for 10 years.

American Board of Plastic Surgery

Seven Penn Center, Suite 400
Philadelphia, PA 19103-2204
(215) 587-9322

General Certification in Plastic Surgery; with Added Qualifications in Hand Surgery. Certifications awarded since 1995 are valid for a 10-year period.

Appendix A: Medical Boards

American Board of Preventive Medicine
330 South Wells Street, Suite 1018
Chicago, IL 60606-7106
(312) 939-ABPM [2276]

General Certification in Aerospace Medicine, Occupational Medicine and Public Health and General Preventive Medicine; with Added Qualifications in Undersea and Hyperbaric Medicine and Medical Toxicology. Certifications awarded since 1997 are valid for 10 years.

American Board of Psychiatry and Neurology
500 Lake Cook Road, Suite 335
Deerfield, IL 60015-5349
(847) 945-7900

General Certification in Psychiatry, Neurology and Neurology with Special Qualification in Child Neurology; with Special Qualifications in Child and Adolescent Psychiatry, Pain Medicine and Sleep Medicine; and Added Qualifications in Addiction Psychiatry, Clinical Neurophysiology, Forensic Psychiatry, Geriatric Psychiatry, Neurodevelopmental Disabilities, Psychosomatic Medicine and Vascular Neurology . Certifications awarded since 1994 are valid for 10 years.

American Board of Radiology
5441 E. Williams Boulevard, Suite 200
Tucson, AZ 85711
(520) 790-2900

General Certification in Diagnostic Radiology or Radiation Oncology; with Special Competency in Nuclear Radiology; and Added Qualifications in Neuroradiology, Pediatric Radiology and Vascular and Interventional Radiology. Radiological Physics is a non-clinical certification. Certificates are valid for 10 years.

American Board of Surgery
1617 John F. Kennedy Boulevard, Suite 860
Philadelphia, PA 19103-1847
(215) 568-4000

General Certification in Surgery and Vascular Surgery; with Special Qualifications in Pediatric Surgery and Surgery of the Hand; and Added Qualifications in Surgical Critical Care. Certifications awarded since 1976 are valid for 10 years.

American Board of Thoracic Surgery
   633 North St. Clair Street, Suite 2320
   Chicago, IL 60611
   (312 202-5900

   General Certification in Thoracic Surgery. Certifications awarded since 1976 are valid
   for 10 years.

American Board of Urology
   2216 Ivy Road, Suite 210
   Charlottesville, VA 22903
   (434) 979-0059

   General Certification in Urology. Certifications awarded as of 1985 are valid for 10
   years.

Osteopathic

The American Osteopathic Association (AOA) is a member association
representing more than 56,000 osteopathic physicians (D.O.s). The AOA serves as
the primary certifying body for D.O.s, and is the accrediting agency for all
osetopathic medical colleges and health care facilities. The AOA's mission is to
advance the philosophy and practice of osteopathic medicine by promoting
excellence in education, research, and the delivery of quality, cost-effective
healthcare within a distinct, unified profession. American Osteopathic Association
142 E Ontario Street Chicago, IL 60611.

Consumers may call the American Osteopathic Association at (800) 621-1773 or
visit the website, www.osteopathic.org, for general certification information.

American Osteopathic Board of Anesthesiology

General certification in Anesthesiology; with Added Qualifications in Addiction
Medicine, Critical Care Medicine, and Pain Management. Certifications awarded since
2004 are valid for 10 years. For those certified prior to 2004 there is no recertification
requirement.

American Osteopathic Board of Dermatology

General certification in Dermatology; with Added Qualifications in Dermatopathology
and MOHS-Micrographic Surgery. Certifications awarded since 2004 are valid for 10
years.

Appendix A: Medical Boards

American Osteopathic Board of Emergency Medicine

General certification in Emergency Medicine; with Added Qualifications in Emergency Medical Services, Medical Toxicology, and Sports Medicine. Certifications awarded since 1994 are valid for 10 years.

American Osteopathic Board of Family Physicians

General certification in Family Practice and Osteopathic Manipulative Treatment (OMT); with Added Qualifications in Geriatric Medicine and Sports Medicine. Certifications awarded since March 1,1997 are valid for 8 years.

American Osteopathic Board of Internal Medicine

General certification in Internal Medicine; with Special Qualifications in Allergy/Immunology, Cardiology, Endocrinology, Gastroenterology, Hematology, Infectious Disease, Nephrology, Oncology, Pulmonary Disease, Rheumatology; with Added Qualifications in Addiction Medicine, Critical Care Medicine, Clinical Cardiac Electrophysiology, Geriatric Medicine, Interventional Cardiology and Sports Medicine. Certifications awarded since 1993 are valid for 10 years.

American Osteopathic Board of Neurology and Psychiatry

General certification in Neurology and Psychiatry; with Special Qualifications in Child/Adolescent Psychiatry and Child/Adolescent Neurology; with Added Qualifications in Addiction Medicine, Neurophysiology, and Sports Medicine. Certifications awarded since 1995 are valid for 10 years.

American Osteopathic Board of Neuromusculoskeletal Medicine

(Formerly American Osteopathic Board of Special Proficiency in Osteopathic Manipulative Medicine)

General certification in Neuromusculoskeletal Medicine. Certifications awarded since 1995 are valid for 10 years. For those certified prior to 1995 there is no recertification requirement.

American Osteopathic Board of Nuclear Medicine

General certification in Nuclear Medicine. Certifications awarded since 1995 are valid for 10 years

American Osteopathic Board of Obstetrics and Gynecology

General certification in Obstetrics and Gynecology; with Special Qualifications in Gynecologic Oncology; Maternal and Fetal Medicine and Reproductive Endocrinology. Certifications awarded since June, 2002 are valid for 6 years.

American Osteopathic Board of Ophthalmology and Otolaryngology/Head and Neck Surgery

General certification in Ophthalmology, Otolaryngolgy, Facial Plastic Surgery and Otolaryngology/Facial Plastic Surgery; with Added Qualifications in Otolaryngic Allergy. Certifications awarded in Ophthalmology since 2000 are valid for 10 years. For those certified prior to 2000 there is no recertification requirement. Certifications awarded in Otolaryngology and/or Otolaryngology/Facial Plastic Surgery since 2002 are valid for 10 years.

American Osteopathic Board of Orthopaedic Surgery

General certification in Orthopaedic Surgery; with Added Qualifications in Hand Surgery. Certifications awarded since 1994 are valid for 10 years.

American Osteopathic Board of Pathology

General certification in Laboratory Medicine, Anatomic Pathology and Anatomic Pathology and Laboratory Medicine; with Special Qualifications in Forensic Pathology; and with Added Qualifications in Dermatopathology. Certifications awarded since 1995 are valid for 10 years.

American Osteopathic Board of Pediatrics

General certification in Pediatrics with Special Qualifications in Adolescent and Young Adult Medicine, Neonatology, Pediatric Allergy/Immunology and Pediatric Endocrinology; with Added Qualifications in Sports Medicine. Certifications awarded since 1995 are valid for 7 years.

American Osteopathic Board of Physical Medicine and Rehabilitation Medicine

General certification in Physical Medicine and Rehabilitation; with Added Qualifications in Sports Medicine. Certifications awarded since 2004 are valid for 10 years.

American Osteopathic Board of Preventive Medicine

General certification in Preventive Medicine/Aerospace Medicine, Preventive Medicine/Occupational-Environmental Medicine and Preventive Medicine/Public Health; with Added Qualifications in Occupational Medicine and Sports Medicine. Certifications awarded since 1994 are valid for 10 years.

American Osteopathic Board of Proctology

General certification in Proctology. Certifications awarded since 2004 are valid for 10 years.

Appendix A: Medical Boards

American Osteopathic Board of Radiology

General certification in Diagnostic Radiology and Radiation Oncology; with Added Qualifications in Body Imaging, Diagnostic Ultrasound, Neuroradiology, Pediatric Radiology and Vascular and Interventional Radiology. Certifications awarded since 2002 are valid for 10 years.

American Osteopathic Board of Surgery

General certification in Surgery, Neurological Surgery, Plastic and Reconstructive Surgery, Cardiothoracic Surgery, Urological Surgery and General Vascular Surgery; with Added Qualifications in Surgical Critical Care. Certifications awarded since 1997 are valid for 10 years.

Appendix B:
Self-Designated Medical Specialties

This list of self-designated medical specialty groups was obtained from the American Board of Medical Specialties. However, it is important to point out that these groups are not recognized by the ABMS, the governing board for the recognized twenty-four medical specialty boards (listed in Appendix A).

The organizations listed below range from highly organized groups that are attempting to formalize training and certification in their field to informal groups interested in a particular aspect of medicine.

If you wish to obtain information from any of these groups you will have to do some detective work. Because so many are informal, the location, phone and mailing addresses change frequently, depending upon the person who is functioning as secretary or administrator.

The best way to track down one of these groups is to consult the doctor listings to find a doctor who has expressed a special interest in that field, and call his or her office. You might also call a nearby academic health center in the area to see if they have a faculty or staff member known to be involved in that particular medical interest. If that fails, take the same approach with your community hospital.

A

Abdominal Surgeons

Acupuncture Medicine

Addiction Medicine

Addictionology

Adolescent Psychiatry

Aesthetic Plastic Surgery

Alcoholism and Other Drug
 Dependencies (AMSAODD)

Algology (Chronic Pain)

Alternative Medicine

Ambulatory Anesthesia

Ambulatory Foot Surgery

Anesthesia

Arthroscopic Surgery

Arthroscopy (Board of North America)

B

Bariatric Medicine

Bionic Psychology

Bloodless Medicine & Surgery

C

Chelation Therapy

Chemical Dependence

Clinical Chemistry

Clinical Ecology

Clinical Medicine and Surgery

Clinical Neurology

Clinical Neurophysiology

Clinical Neurosurgery

Clinical Nutrition

Clinical Orthopaedic Surgery

Clinical Pharmacology

Clinical Polysomnography

Clinical Psychiatry

Clinical Psychology

Clinical Toxicology

Cosmetic Plastic Surgery

Cosmetic Surgery

Council of Non-Board Certified Physicians

Critical Care in Medicine & Surgery

D

Disability Analysis

Disability Evaluating Physicians

E

Electrodiagnostic Medicine

Electroencephalography

Electromyography & Electrodiagnosis

Environmental Medicine

Epidemiology (College)

Eye Surgery

F

Facial Cosmetic Surgery

Facial Plastic & Reconstructive Surgery

Family Practice, Certification

Forensic Examiners

Forensic Psychiatry

Forensic Toxicology

H

Hand Surgery

Head, Facial & Neck Pain & TMJ Orthopaedics

Health Physics

Homeopathic Physicians

Homeotherapeutics

Hypnotic Anesthesiology, National Board for

I

Independent Medical Examiners

Industrial Medicine & Surgery

Insurance Medicine

International Cosmetic & Plastic
 Facial Reconstructive Standards

Interventional Radiology

L

Laser Surgery
Law in Medicine
Longevity Medicine/Surgery

M

Malpractice Physicians
Maxillofacial Surgeons
Medical Accreditation (American Federation for)
Medical Hypnosis
Medical Laboratory Immunology
Medical-Legal Analysis of Medicine & Surgery
Medical Legal & Workers
    Comp. Medicine & Surgery
Medical-Legal Consultants
Medical Management
Medical Microbiology
Medical Preventics (Academy)
Medical Psychotherapists
Medical Toxicology
Microbiology (Medical Microbiology)
Military Medicine
Mohs Micrographic Surgery &
    Cutaneous Oncology

N

Neuroimaging
Neurologic & Orthopaedic Dental
    Medicine and Surgery
Neurological & Orthopaedic Medicine
Neurological & Orthopaedic Surgery
Neurological Microsurgery
Neurology
Neuromuscular Thermography
Neuro-Orthopaedic Dental Medicine
Neuro-Orthopaedic Electrodiagnosis
Neuro-Orthopaedic Laser Surgery
Neuro-Orthopaedic Psychiatry
Neuro-Orthopaedic Thoracic Medicine
Neurorehabilitation
Nutrition

O

Orthopaedic Medicine
Orthopaedic Microneurosurgery
Otorhinolaryngology

P

Pain Management (American Academy of)
Pain Management Specialties
Pain Medicine
Palliative Medicine
Percutaneous Diskectomy
Plastic Esthetic Surgeons
Prison Medicine
Professional Disability Consultants Psychiatric
    Medicine
Psychiatry (American National Board of)
Psychoanalysis (American Examining
    Board in)
Psychological Medicine (International)

Q

Quality Assurance & Utilization Review

R

Radiology & Medical Imaging
Rheumatologic Surgery
Rheumatological & Reconstructive Medicine
Ringside Medicine & Surgery

S

Skin Specialists
Sleep Medicine (Polysomnography)
Spinal Cord Injury
Spinal Surgery
Sports Medicine
Sports Medicine/Surgery

T

Toxicology
Trauma Surgery
Traumatologic Medicine & Surgery
Tropical Medicine

U

Ultrasound Technology
Urologic Allied Health Professionals
Urological Surgery

W

Weight Reduction Medicine

APPENDIX C:
Hospital Listings

The following is an alphabetical listing of all hospitals that have at least one Castle Connolly Top Doctor in this guide. Institutions listed in **Bold** are profiled in this Guide in association with Castle Connolly's *Partnership for Excellence* program. The abbreviations as they appear in the listings are in italics below. Due to the many changes taking place in the hospital industry, the names on this list may have changed subsequent to publication of this guide.

Abbott - Northwestern Hospital   (612) 863-4000
Abbott - Northwestern Hosp
800 E 28th St   Minneapolis, MN 55407   MIDWEST

Advocate Christ Medical Center   (708) 684-8000
Adv Christ Med Ctr
4440 W 95th St   Oak Lawn, IL 60453   MIDWEST

Advocate Good Samaritan Hospital   (630) 275-5900
Adv Good Samaritan Hosp
3815 Highland Ave   Downers Grove, IL 60515   MIDWEST

Advocate Illinois Masonic Medical Center   (773) 975-1600
Adv Illinois Masonic Med Ctr
836 W Wellington Ave   Chicago, IL 60657-5147   MIDWEST

Advocate Lutheran General Hospital   (847) 723-2210
Adv Luth Genl Hosp
1775 West Dempster St   Park Ridge, IL 60068   MIDWEST

Albany Medical Center   (518) 262-3125
Albany Med Ctr
43 New Scotland Ave   Albany, NY 12208   MID ATLANTIC

Albert Einstein Medical Center   (215) 456-7890
Albert Einstein Med Ctr
5501 Old York Rd   Philadelphia, PA 19141   MID ATLANTIC

Albert Lea Medical Center-Mayo Health System   (507) 373-2384
Albert Lea Med Ctr-Mayo Hlth Sys
404 W Fountain St   Albert Lea, MN 56007   MIDWEST

Alfred I duPont Hospital for Children   (302) 651-4000
Alfred I duPont Hosp for Children
1600 Rockland Rd   Wilmington, DE 19803   MID ATLANTIC

All Children's Hospital   (727) 767-7451
All Children's Hosp
801 Sixth Street South   St. Petersburg, FL 33701   SOUTHEAST

Allegheny General Hospital   (412) 359-3131
Allegheny General Hosp
320 E. North Avenue   Pittsburgh, PA 15212   MID ATLANTIC

Allenmore Hospital   (206) 552-5000
Allenmore Hosp
S 19th & Union, Box 11414   Tacoma, WA 98405   WEST COAST AND PACIFIC

Alta Bates Summit Medical Center   (510) 204-4444
Alta Bates Summit Med Ctr
2450 Ashby Avenue   Berkeley, CA 94705   WEST COAST AND PACIFIC

Alvarado Hospital & Medical Center   (714) 287-3270
Alvarado Hosp & Med Ctr
6655 Alvarado Rd   San Diego, CA 92120   WEST COAST AND PACIFIC

Anne Arundel Medical Center   (443) 481-1000
Anne Arundel Med Ctr
64 Franklin Street   Annapolis, MD 21401   MID ATLANTIC

Arizona Heart Hospital   (602) 532-1000
Arizona Heart Hosp
1930 Thomas Rd   Phoenix, AZ 85016   SOUTHWEST

Arkansas Children's Hospital   (501) 364-1100
Arkansas Chldns Hosp
800 Marshall St   Little Rock, AR 72202   SOUTHWEST

Arlington Memorial Hospital   (817) 548-6100
Arlington Meml Hosp
800 W Randol Mill Rd   Arlington, TX 76012-2503   SOUTHWEST

Arthur G. James Cancer Hospital & Research Institute   (614) 293-3300
Arthur G James Cancer Hosp & Research Inst
300 West 10th Avenue   Columbus, OH 43210   MIDWEST

Atlanta Medical Center   (404) 265-4000
Atlanta Med Ctr
303 Parkway Dr. NE   Atlanta, GA 30312   SOUTHEAST

Audie L Murphy Memorial Veterans Hospital   (210) 617-5300
Audie L Murphy Meml Vets Hosp
7400 Merton Minter Blvd   San Antonio, TX 78229   SOUTHWEST

Aultman Hospital	(330) 452-9911	
Aultman Hosp		
2600 6th St SW	Canton, OH 44710-1799	MIDWEST
Austen Riggs Center	(413) 298-5511	
Austen Riggs Ctr		
25 Main Street or PO Box 962	Stockbridge, MA 01262-0962	NEW ENGLAND
Banner Desert Medical Center	(480) 512-3000	
Banner Desert Med Ctr		
1400 S Dobson Rd	Mesa, AZ 85202	SOUTHWEST
Banner Good Samaritan Regional Medical Center - Phoenix	(602) 239-2000	
Banner Good Samaritan Regl Med Ctr - Phoenix		
1111 E McDowell Rd	Phoenix, AZ 85060	SOUTHWEST
Baptist Hospital - Jackson	(601) 968-1000	
Baptist Hosp - Jackson		
1225 N State St	Jackson, MS 39202	SOUTHEAST
Baptist Hospital - Nashville	(615) 284-5555	
Baptist Hosp - Nashville		
2000 Church St	Nashville, TN 37236	SOUTHEAST
Baptist Hospital of Miami	(786) 596-1960	
Baptist Hosp of Miami		
8900 N Kendall Dr	Miami, FL 33176	SOUTHEAST
Baptist Medical Center - San Antonio	(210) 297-7000	
Baptist Med Ctr - San Antonio		
111 Dallas St	San Antonio, TX 78205	SOUTHWEST
Baptist Memorial Hospital - Memphis	(901) 226-5000	
Baptist Memorial Hospital - Memphis		
6019 Walnut Grove Rd	Memphis, TN 38120	SOUTHEAST
Barnes-Jewish Hospital	(314) 362-5000	
Barnes-Jewish Hosp		
One Barnes-Jewish Hospital Plaza	St. Louis, MO 63110	MIDWEST
Bascom Palmer Eye Institute	(305) 326-6000	
Bascom Palmer Eye Inst		
900 NW 17 St	Miami, FL 33136	SOUTHEAST
Baton Rouge General Medical Center	(225) 387-7000	
Baton Rouge Gen Med Ctr		
3600 Florida Boulevard	Baton Rouge, LA 70806	SOUTHWEST

Baylor University Medical Center   (214) 820-0111
Baylor Univ Medical Ctr
3500 Gaston Avenue   Dallas, TX 75246   SOUTHWEST

Baystate Medical Center   (413) 794-0000
Baystate Med Ctr
759 Chestnut Street   Springfield, MA 01199   NEW ENGLAND

Ben Taub General Hospital   (713) 873-2000
Ben Taub Genl Hosp
1504 Taub Loop   Houston, TX 77001   SOUTHWEST

Beth Israel Deaconess Medical Center - Boston   (617) 667-7000
Beth Israel Deaconess Med Ctr - Boston
330 Brookline Ave   Boston, MA 02215   NEW ENGLAND

Beth Israel Medical Center - Milton & Caroll Petrie Division   (212) 420-2000
Beth Israel Med Ctr - Petrie Division
First Avenue @ 16th Street   New York, NY 10003   MID ATLANTIC

Bethesda North Hospital   (513) 745-1111
Bethesda North Hosp
10500 Montgomery Rd   Cincinnati, OH 45242-4415   MIDWEST

Boca Raton Community Hospital   (561) 395-7100
Boca Raton Comm Hosp
800 Meadows Road   Boca Raton, FL 33486   SOUTHEAST

Boston Medical Center   (617) 638-8000
Boston Med Ctr
1 Boston Medical Center Pl   Boston, MA 02118   NEW ENGLAND

Boulder Community Hospital   (303) 440-2273
Boulder Community Hospital
1100 Balsam Ave, Box 9019   Boulder, CO 80301-9019   GREAT PLAINS AND MOUNTAINS

Boys Town National Research Hospital   (402) 498-6511
Boys Town Natl Rsch Hosp
555 N 30th St   Omaha, NE 68101   GREAT PLAINS AND MOUNTAINS

Brigham & Women's Hospital   (617) 732-5500
Brigham & Women's Hosp
75 Francis St   Boston, MA 02115   NEW ENGLAND

Brooklyn Hospital Center-Downtown   (718) 250-8000
Brooklyn Hosp Ctr-Downtown
121 DeKalb Avenue   Brooklyn, NY 11201   MID ATLANTIC

Brookwood Medical Center (205) 877-1000
Brookwood Med Ctr
2010 Brookwood Medical Ctr Drive   Birmingham, AL 35209-6804   SOUTHEAST

Broward General Medical Center (954) 355-4400
Broward General Med Ctr
1600 S Andrews Ave   Fort Lauderdale, FL 33316   SOUTHEAST

Bryn Mawr Hospital (610) 526-3000
Bryn Mawr Hosp
130 S Bryn Mawr Ave   Bryn Mawr, PA 19010-3143   MID ATLANTIC

Buffalo General Hospital (716) 859-5600
Buffalo General Hosp
100 High Street   Buffalo, NY 14203   MID ATLANTIC

Burke Rehabilitation Hospital (914) 597-2500
Burke Rehab Hosp
785 Mamaroneck Avenue   White Plains, NY 10605   MID ATLANTIC

Butler Hospital (401) 455-6200
Butler Hosp
345 Blackstone Blvd   Providence, RI 02906   NEW ENGLAND

California Hospital Medical Center (213) 748-2411
California Hosp Med Ctr
1401 S. Grand Avenue   Los Angeles, CA 90015   WEST COAST AND PACIFIC

California Pacific Medical Center (415) 600-6000
CA Pacific Med Ctr
PO Box 7999   San Francisco, CA 94120   WEST COAST AND PACIFIC

California Pacific Medical Center - Pacific Campus (415) 600-6000
CA Pacific Med Ctr - Pacific Campus
2333 Buchanan St   San Francisco, CA 94115   WEST COAST AND PACIFIC

Cancer Treatment Centers of America-Midwestern Regional Medical Center (847) 872-4561
Cancer Treatment Ctrs of Amer-Midwest Reg Med Ctr
2520 Elisha Ave   Zion, IL 60099   MIDWEST

Carilion Roanoke Memorial Hospital (540) 224-4966
Carilion Roanoke Meml Hosp
Jefferson At Belleview SE   Roanoke, VA 24033   SOUTHEAST

Carolinas Medical Center (704) 355-2000
Carolinas Med Ctr
1000 Blythe Blvd   Charlotte, NC 28203-5871   SOUTHEAST

Carolinas Medical Center-University		(704) 548-6000
Carolinas Med Ctr-Univ		
PO Box 560727	Charlotte, NC 28256	SOUTHEAST

Cedars-Sinai Medical Center		(310) 423-3277
Cedars-Sinai Med Ctr		
8700 Beverly Boulevard	Los Angeles, CA 90048	WEST COAST AND PACIFIC

Centennial Medical Center		(615) 342-1000
Centennial Med Ctr		
2300 Patterson Street	Nashville, TN 37203	SOUTHEAST

Centinela Freeman Regional Medical Center-Centinela Campus		(310) 673-4660
Centinela Freeman Reg Med Ctr-Centinela		
555 East Hardy Street	Inglewood, CA 90301	WEST COAST AND PACIFIC

Central Baptist Hospital		(859) 260-6592
Central Baptist Hosp		
1740 Nicholasville Rd	Lexington, KY 40503-1499	SOUTHEAST

Central DuPage Hospital		(630) 933-1600
Central DuPage Hosp		
25 N Winfield Rd	Winfield, IL 60190	MIDWEST

Chelsea Community Hospital		(734) 475-1311
Chelsea Comm Hosp		
775 S Main St	Chelsea, MI 48118	MIDWEST

Cheyenne Regional Medical Center		(307) 634-2273
Cheyenne Regl Med Ctr		
214 E 23rd St	Cheyenne, WY 82001	GREAT PLAINS AND MOUNTAINS

Children's Healthcare of Atlanta - Egleston		(404) 325-6000
Chldns Hlthcare Atlanta - Egleston		
1405 Clifton Rd NE	Atlanta, GA 30322	SOUTHEAST

Children's Healthcare of Atlanta - Scottish Rite		(404) 250-5437
Chldns Hlthcare Atlanta - Scottish Rite		
1001 Johnson Ferry Rd	Atlanta, GA 30342	SOUTHEAST

Children's Hospital - Aurora, The		(720) 777-1234
Chldn's Hosp - Aurora, The		
13123 E 16th Ave	Aurora, CO 80045	GREAT PLAINS AND MOUNTAINS

Children's Hospital - Austin		(512) 324-8832
Children's Hospital - Austin		
609 W 15th St	Austin, TX 78701	SOUTHWEST

Children's Hospital - Boston		(617) 355-6000
Children's Hospital - Boston		
300 Longwood Avenue	Boston, MA 02115	NEW ENGLAND
Children's Hospital - Los Angeles		(323) 660-2450
Chldns Hosp - Los Angeles		
4650 Sunset Blvd	Los Angeles, CA 90027	WEST COAST AND PACIFIC
Children's Hospital - New Orleans		(504) 899-9511
Children's Hospital - New Orleans		
200 Henry Clay Ave	New Orleans, LA 70118	SOUTHWEST
Children's Hospital - Oakland		(510) 428-3000
Chldns Hosp - Oakland		
747 52nd St	Oakland, CA 94609	WEST COAST AND PACIFIC
Children's Hospital - Omaha		(402) 955-5400
Children's Hosp - Omaha		
8200 Dodge St	Omaha, NE 68114	GREAT PLAINS AND MOUNTAINS
Children's Hospital and Clinics - Minneapolis		(612) 813-6111
Chldns Hosp and Clinics - Minneapolis		
2525 Chicago Ave S	Minneapolis, MN 55404	MIDWEST
Children's Hospital and Regional Medical Center - Seattle		(206) 987-2000
Chldns Hosp and Regl Med Ctr - Seattle		
4800 Sand Point Way NE	Seattle, WA 98145	WEST COAST AND PACIFIC
Children's Hospital at OU Medical Center		(405) 271-5437
Chldns Hosp OU Med Ctr		
940 Northeast 13th St	Oklahoma City, OK 73104	SOUTHWEST
Children's Hospital Central California		(559) 353-3000
Chldns Hosp Central California		
9300 Valley Children's Pl	Madera, CA 93638	WEST COAST AND PACIFIC
Children's Hospital Medical Center - Akron		(330) 379-8200
Children's Hosp & Med Ctr- Akron		
One Perkins Square	Akron, OH 44308	MIDWEST
Children's Hospital of Alabama - Birmingham		(205) 939-9100
Children's Hospital - Birmingham		
1600 7th Ave South	Birmingham, AL 35233	SOUTHEAST
Children's Hospital of Michigan		(313) 745-5437
Chldns Hosp of Michigan		
3901 Beaubian Blvd	Detroit, MI 48201	MIDWEST

Children's Hospital of Orange County - CHOC   (714) 997-3000
Chldns Hosp Orange Co - CHOC
455 South Main Street   Orange, CA 92868   WEST COAST AND PACIFIC

Children's Hospital of Philadelphia, The   (215) 590-1000
Chldns Hosp of Philadelphia, The
34th St & Civic Center Blvd   Philadelphia, PA 19104   MID ATLANTIC

Children's Hospital of Pittsburgh - UPMC   (412) 692-5325
Chldns Hosp of Pittsburgh - UPMC
3705 Fifth Avenue   Pittsburgh, PA 15213   MID ATLANTIC

Children's Hospital of the King's Daughters   (757) 668-7500
Chldns Hosp of King's Daughters
601 Children's Ln   Norfolk, VA 23507   SOUTHEAST

Children's Hospital of Wisconsin   (414) 266-2000
Chldns Hosp - Wisconsin
9000 W Wisconsin Ave   Milwaukee, WI 53201   MIDWEST

Children's Medical Center of Dallas   (214) 456-7000
Chldns Med Ctr of Dallas
1935 Motor St   Dallas, TX 75235   SOUTHWEST

Children's Memorial Hospital   (773) 880-4000
Children's Mem Hosp
2300 Children's Plaza   Chicago, IL 60614   MIDWEST

Children's Mercy Hospitals & Clinics   (816) 234-3000
Chldns Mercy Hosps & Clinics
2401 Gilham Rd   Kansas City, MO 64108   MIDWEST

Children's National Medical Center - DC   (202) 884-5000
Chldns Natl Med Ctr
111 Michigan Ave NW   Washington, DC 20010   MID ATLANTIC

Christ Hospital, The   (513) 585-2000
Christ Hospital
2139 Auburn Ave   Cincinnati, OH 45219   MIDWEST

Christiana Care Health Services   (302) 428-2229
Christiana Care Hlth Svs
501 W 14th St   Wilmington, DE 19899-1038   MID ATLANTIC

Christiana Hospital   (302) 733-1000
Christiana Hospital
4755 Ogletown-Stanton Rd   Newark, DE 19718-0001   MID ATLANTIC

Christus Santa Rosa Children's Hospital	(512) 228-2011
Christus Santa Rosa Children's Hosp	
333 N Santa Rosa St San Antonio, TX 78207	SOUTHWEST
Cincinnati Children's Hospital Medical Center	(800) 344-2462
Cincinnati Chldns Hosp Med Ctr	
3333 Burnet Ave Cincinnati, OH 45229-3039	MIDWEST
Cincinnati Shriners Hospital	(513) 872-6000
Cincinnati Shriners Hosp	
3229 Burnet Ave Cincinnati, OH 45229-3095	MIDWEST
City of Hope National Medical Center & Beckman Research	(626) 359-8111
City of Hope Natl Med Ctr & Beckman Rsch	
1500 E Duarte Rd Duarte, CA 91010	WEST COAST AND PACIFIC
CJW Medical Center Johnston-Willis Campus	(804) 330-2000
CJW Med Ctr	
1401 Johnston-Willis Dr Richmond, VA 23235	SOUTHEAST
Cleveland Clinic Florida - Weston	(954) 659-5000
Cleveland Clin - Weston	
2950 Cleveland Clinic Blvd Weston, FL 33331	SOUTHEAST
Cleveland Clinic Foundation	(800) 223-2273
Cleveland Clin Fdn	
9500 Euclid Avenue Cleveland, OH 44195	MIDWEST
Columbus Hospital	(973) 268-1400
Columbus Hosp	
495 N 13th Street Newark, NJ 07107	MID ATLANTIC
Community Memorial Hospital - Ventura	(805) 652-5011
Comm Meml Hosp - Ventura	
147 N Brent St Ventura, CA 93003	WEST COAST AND PACIFIC
Concord Hospital	(603) 225-2711
Concord Hospital	
250 Pleasant St Concord, NH 03301-2598	NEW ENGLAND
Connecticut Children's Medical Center	(860) 545-9000
CT Chldns Med Ctr	
282 Washington St Hartford, CT 06106	NEW ENGLAND
Connecticut Mental Health Center	(203) 789-7092
Connecticut Mental Hlth Ctr	
34 Park St New Haven, CT 06508-1842	NEW ENGLAND

Cook Children's Medical Center   (682) 885-4000
Cook Chldns Med Ctr
801 7th Ave   Fort Worth, TX 76104-2796   SOUTHWEST

Cooper University Hospital   (856) 342-2000
Cooper Univ Hosp
1 Cooper Plaza   Camden, NJ 08103-1489   MID ATLANTIC

Covenant Children's Hospital   (806) 725-1011
Covenant Children's Hosp
3610 21st St   Lubbock, TX 79410   SOUTHWEST

Craig Hospital   (303) 789-8000
Craig Hosp
3425 S Clarkson   Englewood, CO 80113   GREAT PLAINS AND MOUNTAINS

Crawford Long Hospital of Emory University   (404) 686-4411
Crawford Long Hosp of Emory Univ
550 Peachtree St NE   Atlanta, GA 30365   SOUTHEAST

Creighton University Medical Center   (402) 449-4000
Creighton Univ Med Ctr
601 N 30th St   Omaha, NE 68131-2197   GREAT PLAINS AND MOUNTAINS

Dana-Farber Cancer Institute   (617) 632-3000
Dana-Farber Cancer Inst
44 Binney St   Boston, MA 02115   NEW ENGLAND

Dartmouth - Hitchcock Medical Center   (603) 650-5000
Dartmouth - Hitchcock Med Ctr
1 Medical Center Dr   Lebanon, NH 03756-0002   NEW ENGLAND

Denver Health Medical Center   (303) 436-6000
Denver Health Med Ctr
777 Bannock St   Denver, CO 80204   GREAT PLAINS AND MOUNTAINS

Desert Regional Medical Center   (760) 323-6511
Desert Regl Med Ctr
1150 N Indian Canyon Dr   Palm Springs, CA 92262   WEST COAST AND PACIFIC

Detroit Medical Center   (313) 578-3930
Detroit Med Ctr
3663 Woodward Ave, Ste 200   Detroit, MI 48201-2403   MIDWEST

DeVos Children's Hospital   (616) 957-0866
DeVos Children's Hosp
1000 E Paris SE   Grand Rapids, MI 49546   MIDWEST

Doctors Hospital   (706) 651-3232
Doctors Hosp
3651 Wheeler Rd   Augusta, GA 30909   SOUTHEAST

Doctors' Hospital   (305) 666-2111
Doctors' Hosp
5000 University Dr   Coral Gables, FL 33146   SOUTHEAST

Doernbecher Children's Hospital/Oregon Health Science University   (503) 494-8811
Doernbecher Chldns Hosp/OHSU
3181 SW Sam Jackson Park Rd   Portland, OR 97201-3098   WEST COAST AND PACIFIC

Dotter Interventional Institute - OHSU   (503) 494-7660
Dotter Institute - OHSU
3181 SW Sam Jackson Park Rd   Portland, OR 97201   WEST COAST AND PACIFIC

Duke Health Raleigh Hospital   (919) 954-3000
Duke Health Raleigh
3400 Wake Forest Rd   Raleigh, NC 27609   SOUTHEAST

Duke University Medical Center   (919) 684-8111
Duke Univ Med Ctr
DUMC, Box 3708   Durham, NC 27710   SOUTHEAST

East Texas Medical Center-Tyler   (903) 597-0351
E TX Med Ctr-Tyler
1000 S Beckham Ave   Tyler, TX 75701   SOUTHWEST

Edward Hines Jr Veterans Affairs Hospital   (708) 202-8387
Hines VA Hosp
Fifth Ave & Roosevelt Road, PO Box 5000   Hines, IL 60141   MIDWEST

El Camino Hospital/Camino Healthcare System   (650) 940-7000
El Camino Hosp/Camino Hlthcare Sys
2500 Grant Road   Mountain View, CA 94039   WEST COAST AND PACIFIC

Elliot Hospital   (603) 669-5300
Elliot Hosp
1 Elliot Way   Manchester, NH 03103   NEW ENGLAND

Emory University Hospital   (404) 712-2000
Emory Univ Hosp
1364 Clifton Rd NE   Atlanta, GA 30322   SOUTHEAST

Englewood Hospital & Medical Center   (201) 894-3000
Englewood Hosp & Med Ctr
350 Engle Street   Englewood, NJ 07631   MID ATLANTIC

Evanston Hospital		(847) 570-2000
Evanston Hosp		
2650 Ridge Ave	Evanston, IL 60201	MIDWEST

Evergreen Hospital Medical Center		(425) 899-1000
Evergreen Hosp Med Ctr		
12040 NE 128th St	Kirkland, WA 98034-3013	WEST COAST AND PACIFIC

Fairview Southdale Hospital		(952) 924-5000
Fairview Southdale Hosp		
6401 France Ave S	Edina, MN 55435-2199	MIDWEST

Fletcher Allen Health Care - Medical Center Campus		(802) 847-0000
FAHC - Med Ctr Campus		
111 Colchester Ave (Burgess 1)	Burlington, VT 05401	NEW ENGLAND

Fletcher Allen Health Care - UHC Campus		(802) 847-0000
FAHC - UHC Campus		
1 S Prospect St	Burlington, VT 05401	NEW ENGLAND

Florida Hospital - Celebration Health		(407) 764-4000
Florida Hosp Celebration Hlth		
400 Celebration Pl	Celebration, FL 34747	SOUTHEAST

Florida Hospital - Orlando		(407) 303-5600
Florida Hosp - Orlando		
601 E Rollins St	Orlando, FL 32803	SOUTHEAST

Floyd Memorial Hospital & Health Services		(812) 944-7701
Floyd Meml Hosp & Hlth Svcs		
1850 State St	New Albany, IN 47150-4997	MIDWEST

Forsyth Medical Center		(336) 718-5000
Forsyth Med Ctr		
3333 Silas Creek Pkwy	Winston-Salem, NC 27103	SOUTHEAST

Fort Sanders Regional Medical Center		(865) 541-1111
Fort Sanders Reg Med Ctr		
1901 Clinch Ave SW	Knoxville, TN 37916-2398	SOUTHEAST

Four Winds Hospital		(914) 763-8151
Four Winds Hosp		
800 Cross River Road	Katonah, NY 10536	MID ATLANTIC

Fox Chase Cancer Center		(215) 728-6900
Fox Chase Cancer Ctr		
333 Cottman Avenue	Philadelphia, PA 19111	MID ATLANTIC

Franklin Square Hospital   (410) 682-7000
Franklin Square Hosp
9000 Franklin Square Drive   Baltimore, MD 21237   MID ATLANTIC

Froedtert Memorial Lutheran Hospital   (414) 805-6644
Froedtert Meml Lutheran Hosp
9200 W Wisconsin Ave   Milwaukee, WI 53226   MIDWEST

Gaston Memorial Hospital   (704) 834-2000
Gaston Meml Hosp
2525 Court Dr   Gastonia, NC 28054   SOUTHEAST

Geisinger Medical Center   (570) 271-6211
Geisinger Med Ctr
100 N Academy Ave   Danville, PA 17822   MID ATLANTIC

George Washington University Hospital   (202) 715-4000
G Washington Univ Hosp
900 23rd St NW   Washington, DC 20037   MID ATLANTIC

Georgetown University Hospital   (202) 444-2000
Georgetown Univ Hosp
3800 Reservoir Rd NW   Washington, DC 20007   MID ATLANTIC

Glenbrook Hospital   (847) 657-5800
Glenbrook Hosp
2100 Pfingsten Rd   Glenview, IL 60025   MIDWEST

Good Samaritan Hosp - Cincinnati   (513) 872-1400
Good Samaritan Hosp - Cincinnati
375 Dixmyth Ave   Cincinnati, OH 45220   MIDWEST

Good Samaritan Hospital   (213) 977-2121
Good Samaritan Hosp
5601 Loch Raven Blvd   Baltimore, MD 21208   MID ATLANTIC

Good Samaritan Hospital - Los Angeles   (213) 977-2121
Good Samaritan Hosp - Los Angeles
1225 Wilshire Boulevard   Los Angeles, CA 90017   WEST COAST AND PACIFIC

Good Samaritan Hospital - San Jose   (408) 559-2011
Good Samaritan Hosp - San Jose
2425 Samaritan Drive   San Jose, CA 95124   WEST COAST AND PACIFIC

Good Samaritan Medical Center - West Palm Beach   (561) 655-5511
Good Sam Med Ctr - W Palm Beach
1309 N Flagler Dr   West Palm Beach, FL 33401   SOUTHEAST

Goshen General Hospital		(574) 533-2141
Goshen Genl Hosp		
200 High Park Ave	Goshen, IN 46526	MIDWEST

Gottlieb Memorial Hospital		(708) 681-3200
Gottlieb Meml Hosp		
701 W North Ave	Melrose Park, IL 60160	MIDWEST

Grady Health System		(404) 616-4307
Grady Hlth Sys		
80 Jesse Hill Jr Dr	Atlanta, GA 30303	SOUTHEAST

Greater Baltimore Medical Center		(443) 849-2000
Greater Baltimore Med Ctr		
6701 N Charles St	Baltimore, MD 21204	MID ATLANTIC

Greenwich Hospital		(203) 863-3000
Greenwich Hosp		
Five Perryridge Road	Greenwich, CT 06830	NEW ENGLAND

Gulf Breeze Hospital		(850) 934-2000
Gulf Breeze Hosp		
1110 Gulf Breeze	Gulf Breeze, FL	SOUTHEAST

H Lee Moffitt Cancer Center & Research Institute		(813) 972-4673
H Lee Moffitt Cancer Ctr & Research Inst		
12902 Magnolia Drive	Tampa, FL 33612-9497	SOUTHEAST

Hackensack University Medical Center		(201) 996-2000
Hackensack Univ Med Ctr		
30 Prospect Avenue	Hackensack, NJ 07601	MID ATLANTIC

Hahnemann University Hospital		(215) 762-7000
Hahnemann Univ Hosp		
Broad & Vine St	Philadelphia, PA 19102	MID ATLANTIC

Hamot Medical Center		(814) 877-6000
Hamot Med Ctr		
201 State Street	Erie, PA 16550-0001	MID ATLANTIC

Harborview Medical Center		(206) 731-3000
Harborview Med Ctr		
325 9th Ave, Box 359717	Seattle, WA 98104	WEST COAST AND PACIFIC

Harlem Hospital Center		(212) 939-1000
Harlem Hosp Ctr		
506 Lenox Avenue	New York, NY 10037	MID ATLANTIC

Harper University Hospital		(313) 745-8040
Harper Univ Hosp		
3990 John R St	Detroit, MI 48201-2097	MIDWEST

Harrison Memorial Hospital		(360) 377-3911
Harrison Meml Hosp		
2520 Cherry Ave	Bremerton, WA 98310-4270	WEST COAST AND PACIFIC

Hartford Hospital		(860) 545-5000
Hartford Hosp		
80 Seymour St, Box 5037	Hartford, CT 06102-5037	NEW ENGLAND

Healthsouth Lakeshore Rehabilitation Hospital		(205) 868-2000
Healthsouth Lakeshore Rehab Hosp		
3800 Ridgeway	Birmingham, AL 35209	SOUTHEAST

Hennepin County Medical Center		(612) 347-2121
Hennepin Cnty Med Ctr		
701 Park Ave S	Minneapolis, MN 55415	MIDWEST

Henrico Doctors Hospital		(804) 289-4500
Henrico Doctors Hosp		
1602 Skipwith Road	Richmond, VA 23229	SOUTHEAST

Henry Ford Hospital		(313) 916-2600
Henry Ford Hosp		
2799 W Grand Blvd	Detroit, MI 48202	MIDWEST

Hillcrest Hospital Cleveland Clinic Health System		(440) 449-4500
Hillcrest Hosp-Mayfield Hts		
6780 Mayfield Rd	Mayfield Heights, OH 44124	MIDWEST

Hinsdale Hospital		(630) 856-9000
Hinsdale Hosp		
120 N Oak St	Hinsdale, IL 60521	MIDWEST

Hoag Memorial Hospital Presbyterian		(949) 645-8600
Hoag Meml Hosp Presby		
One Hoag Drive	Newport Beach, CA 92663	WEST COAST AND PACIFIC

Holy Cross Hospital - Fort Lauderdale		(954) 771-8000
Holy Cross Hosp - Fort Lauderdale		
4725 N Federal Hwy	Fort Lauderdale, FL 33308	SOUTHEAST

Holy Cross Hospital - Silver Spring		(301) 754-7000
Holy Cross Hospital - Silver Spring		
1500 Forest Glen Road	Silver Spring, MD 20910	MID ATLANTIC

Holy Name Hospital		(201) 833-3000
Holy Name Hosp		
718 Teaneck Road	Teaneck, NJ 07666	MID ATLANTIC

Hospital for Joint Diseases		(212) 598-6000
Hosp For Joint Diseases		
301 East 17th Street	New York, NY 10003	MID ATLANTIC

Hospital for Special Surgery		(212) 606-1000
Hosp For Special Surgery		
535 East 70th Street	New York, NY 10021	MID ATLANTIC

Hospital of Central CT at New Britain		(860) 224-5011
Hosp of Central CT at New Britain		
100 Grand St	New Britain, CT 06050	NEW ENGLAND

Hospital of St Raphael		(203) 789-3000
Hosp of St Raphael		
1450 Chapel Street	New Haven, CT 06511	NEW ENGLAND

Hospital of the University of Pennsylvania - UPHS		(215) 662-4000
Hosp Univ Penn - UPHS		
3400 Spruce Street	Philadelphia, PA 19104	MID ATLANTIC

Howard University Hospital		(202) 865-6100
Howard Univ Hosp		
2041 Georgia Ave NW	Washington, DC 20060	MID ATLANTIC

Hunter Holmes McGuire Veterans Affairs Medical Center		(804) 675-5500
Hunter Holmes McGuire VA Med Ctr		
1201 Broad Rock Boulevard	Richmond, VA 23249	SOUTHEAST

Hutzel Women's Hospital - Detroit		(313) 745-7555
Hutzel Hosp - Detroit		
3980 John R. Blvd	Detroit, MI 48201-2018	MIDWEST

Imperial Point Medical Center		(954) 776-8500
Imperial Point Med Ctr		
6401 N Federal Hwy	Fort Lauderdale, FL 33308	SOUTHEAST

Indian River Memorial Hosp		(772) 567-4311
Indian River Mem Hosp		
1000 36th St	Vero Beach, FL 32960	SOUTHEAST

Indiana University Hospital		(317) 274-5000
Indiana Univ Hosp		
550 N University Blvd	Indianapolis, IN 46202	MIDWEST

Ingalls Memorial Hospital		(708) 333-2300
Ingalls Meml Hosp		
1 Ingalls Dr	Harvey, IL 60426	MIDWEST

Inova Fair Oaks Hospital		(703) 391-3600
Inova Fair Oaks Hosp		
3600 Joseph Siewick Dr	Fairfax, VA 22033	SOUTHEAST

Inova Fairfax Hospital		(703) 698-1110
Inova Fairfax Hosp		
3300 Gallows Road	Falls Church, VA 22042	SOUTHEAST

Inova Fairfax Hospital for Children		(703) 204-6777
Inova Fairfax Hosp for Chldn		
3300 Gallows Rd	Fairfax, VA 22042	SOUTHEAST

Integris Baptist Medical Center - Oklahoma		(405) 949-3011
Integris Baptist Med Ctr - OK		
3300 NW Expressway	Oklahoma City, OK 73112-9028	SOUTHWEST

Intermountain Medical Center		(801) 507-7000
Intermountain Med Ctr		
5121 S Cottonwood St	Salt Lake City, UT 84107	GREAT PLAINS AND MOUNTAINS

Iowa Methodist Medical Center		(515) 241-6212
Iowa Methodist Med Ctr		
1200 Pleasant St	Des Moines, IA 50309	MIDWEST

Jackson Memorial Hospital		(305) 585-1111
Jackson Meml Hosp		
1611 NW 12th Ave	Miami, FL 33136	SOUTHEAST

Jewish Hospital HealthCare Services, Inc.		(502) 587-4011
Jewish Hosp HlthCre Svcs Inc		
200 Abraham Slexner Way	Louisville, KY 40202	SOUTHEAST

JFK Medical Center - Atlantis		(561) 642-3791
JFK Med Ctr - Atlantis		
5301 S Congress Ave	Atlantis, FL 33462	SOUTHEAST

JFK Medical Center - Edison		(732) 321-7000
JFK Med Ctr - Edison		
65 James Street	Edison, NJ 08818	MID ATLANTIC

Joe Di Maggio Children's Hospital		(954) 987-2000
Joe Di Maggio Chldns Hosp		
3501 Johnson St	Hollywood, FL 33021	SOUTHEAST

John L McClellan VA Medical Center   (501) 257-1000
John L McClellan VA Med Ctr
4300 W 7th St   Little Rock, AR 72205   SOUTHWEST

John Sealy Hospital - UTMB   (409) 747-1935
UTMB - John Sealy Hospital
301 University Blvd   Galveston, TX 77555   SOUTHWEST

Johns Hopkins Bayview Medical Center   (410) 550-0100
Johns Hopkins Bayview Med Ctr
4940 Eastern Avenue   Baltimore, MD 21224   MID ATLANTIC

Johns Hopkins Hospital - Baltimore, The   (410) 955-5000
Johns Hopkins Hosp - Baltimore
600 N Wolfe St   Baltimore, MD 21287   MID ATLANTIC

Kaiser Permanente Baldwin Park Medical Center   (626) 851-1011
Kaiser Permanente Baldwin Pk Med Ctr
1011 Baldwin Park Blvd   Baldwin Park, CA 91706   WEST COAST AND PACIFIC

Kaiser Permanente Oakland Medical Center   (510) 752-1000
Kaiser Permanente Oakland Med Ctr
280 West MacArthur Boulevard   Oakland, CA 94611   WEST COAST AND PACIFIC

Kaiser Permanente Santa Clara Medical Center   (408) 236-6400
Kaiser Permanente Santa Clara Med Ctr
900 Kiley Blvd   Santa Clara, CA 95051   WEST COAST AND PACIFIC

Kaiser Permanente South San Francisco Medical Center   (650) 742-2000
Kaiser Permanente South San Francisco Med Ctr
1200 El Camino Real   South San Francisco, CA 94080   WEST COAST AND PACIFIC

Kapiolani Medical Center for Women & Children   (808) 983-6000
Kapiolani Med Ctr for Women & Chldn
1319 Punahou St   Honolulu, HI 96826   WEST COAST AND PACIFIC

Karmanos Cancer Institute   (800) 527-6266
Karmanos Cancer Inst
4100 John R   Detroit, MI 48201   MIDWEST

Kennedy Krieger Institute   (443) 923-9200
Kennedy Krieger Inst
707 N Broadway   Baltimore, MD 21205   MID ATLANTIC

Kenner Regional Medical Center   (504) 468-8600
Kenner Reg Med Ctr
180 W Esplanade Ave   Kenner, LA 70065-2467   SOUTHWEST

Kessler Institute for Rehabilitation - West Orange (973) 243-6800
Kessler Inst for Rehab - W Orange
1199 Pleasant Valley Way   West Orange, NJ 07052-1499   MID ATLANTIC

KFH San Francisco Medical Center (415) 833-2000
KFH San Francisco Med Ctr
2425 Geary Blvd   San Francisco, CA 94115   WEST COAST AND PACIFIC

KFH Woodland Hills Medical Center (818) 719-2000
KFH Woodland Hills Med Ctr
5601 DeSoto Avenue   Woodland Hills, CA 91365   WEST COAST AND PACIFIC

Kootenai Medical Center (208) 666-2000
Kootenai Med Ctr
2003 Lincoln Way   Coeur d'Alene, ID 83814-2677   GREAT PLAINS AND
                                                               MOUNTAINS

Kosair Children's Hospital (502) 629-6000
Kosair Chldn's Hosp
231 E Chestnut St   Louisville, KY 40202   SOUTHEAST

La Grange Memorial Hospital (708) 352-1200
La Grange Meml Hosp
5101 S Willow Springs Rd   La Grange, IL 60525   MIDWEST

La Rabida Children's Hospital (773) 363-6700
La Rabida Chlds Hosp
E 65th at Lake Michigan   Chicago, IL 60649   MIDWEST

LAC & USC Medical Center (323) 226-2622
LAC & USC Med Ctr
1200 N State St   Los Angeles, CA 90033-4525   WEST COAST AND PACIFIC

LAC - Harbor - UCLA Medical Center (310) 222-2345
LAC - Harbor - UCLA Med Ctr
1000 W Carson St   Torrance, CA 90509-2059   WEST COAST AND PACIFIC

Lafayette General Medical Center (337) 289-7991
Lafayette Genl Med Ctr
1214 Coolidge Blvd   Lafayette, LA 70503   SOUTHWEST

Lahey Clinic (781) 744-5100
Lahey Clin
41 Mall Road   Burlington, MA 01805   NEW ENGLAND

Lakeland Regional Medical Center (863) 687-1100
Lakeland Regl Med Ctr
1324 Lakeland Hills Blvd   Lakeland, FL 33805   SOUTHEAST

Lancaster General Hospital   (717) 290-5511
Lancaster Genl Hosp
555 N Duke St, PO Box 3555   Lancaster, PA 17604-3555   MID ATLANTIC

Lankenau Hospital   (610) 645-2000
Lankenau Hosp
100 Lancaster Ave   Wynnewood, PA 19096-3498   MID ATLANTIC

Laureate Psychiatric Clinic & Hospital   (918) 481-4000
Laureate Psyc Clinic & Hosp
6655 S Yale Ave, Box 470207   Tulsa, OK 74147   SOUTHWEST

LDS Hospital   (801) 408-1100
LDS Hosp
8th Ave & C St   Salt Lake City, UT 84143   GREAT PLAINS AND MOUNTAINS

Le Bonheur Children's Medical Center   (901) 572-3000
Le Bonheur Chldns Med Ctr
50 N Dunlap   Memphis, TN 38103-2893   SOUTHEAST

Legacy Good Samaritan Hospital and Medical Center   (503) 413-7711
Legacy Good Samaritan Hosp and Med Ctr
1015 NW 22nd Ave   Portland, OR 97210-3025   WEST COAST AND PACIFIC

Lenox Hill Hospital   (212) 434-2000
Lenox Hill Hosp
100 East 77th Street   New York, NY 10021   MID ATLANTIC

Lindy Boggs Medical Center   (504) 483-5000
L Boggs Med Ctr
301 N Jefferson Davis Pkwy   New Orleans, LA 70119   SOUTHWEST

Loma Linda Children's Hospital   (909) 558-8000
Loma Linda Chldns Hosp
11234 Anderson St   Loma Linda, CA 92354   WEST COAST AND PACIFIC

Loma Linda University Medical Center   (909) 558-4000
Loma Linda Univ Med Ctr
11234 Anderson St   Loma Linda, CA 92354   WEST COAST AND PACIFIC

Long Beach Memorial Medical Center   (562) 933-2000
Long Beach Meml Med Ctr
2801 Atlantic Ave   Long Beach, CA 90801   WEST COAST AND PACIFIC

Long Island College Hospital   (718) 780-1000
Long Island Coll Hosp
339 Hicks Street   Brooklyn, NY 11201   MID ATLANTIC

Long Island Jewish Medical Center		(516) 470-7000
Long Island Jewish Med Ctr		
270-05 76th Avenue	New Hyde Park, NY 11040	MID ATLANTIC
Los Alamitos Medical Center		(562) 598-1311
Los Alamitos Med Ctr		
3751 Katella Ave	Los Alamitos, CA 90720	WEST COAST AND PACIFIC
Louisiana State University Hospital		(318) 675-4239
Louisiana State Univ Hosp		
1501 Kings Highway P.O. Box 33932	Shreveport, LA 71130	SOUTHWEST
Loyola University Medical Center		(708) 216-9000
Loyola Univ Med Ctr		
2160 S 1st Ave	Maywood, IL 60153	MIDWEST
Lucile Packard Children's Hospital/Stanford University Medical Center		(650) 497-8000
Lucile Packard Chldns Hosp/Stanford Univ Med Ctr		
725 Welch Rd	Palo Alto, CA 94304	WEST COAST AND PACIFIC
Lutheran Medical Center - Cleveland		(216) 696-4300
Lutheran Med Ctr - Cleveland		
1730 W 25th St	Cleveland, OH 44113	MIDWEST
Magee Rehabilitation Hospital		(215) 587-3000
Magee Rehab Hosp		
1513 Race St	Philadelphia, PA 19102-1177	MID ATLANTIC
Magee-Womens Hospital - UPMC		(412) 641-1000
Magee-Womens Hosp - UPMC		
300 Halket Street	Pittsburgh, PA 15213	MID ATLANTIC
Maimonides Medical Center		(718) 283-6000
Maimonides Med Ctr		
4802 Tenth Avenue	Brooklyn, NY 11219	MID ATLANTIC
Maine Medical Center		(207) 871-0111
Maine Med Ctr		
22 Bramhall St	Portland, ME 04102	NEW ENGLAND
Manhattan Eye, Ear & Throat Hospital		(212) 838-9200
Manhattan Eye, Ear & Throat Hosp		
210 East 64th Street	New York, NY 10021	MID ATLANTIC
Marianjoy Rehabilitation Hospital		(630) 462-4000
Marianjoy Rehab Hosp		
26 W 171 Roosevelt Rd	Wheaton, IL 60187	MIDWEST

Marin General Hospital   (415) 925-7000
Marin Genl Hosp
250 Bon Air Rd   Greenbrae, CA 94904   WEST COAST AND PACIFIC

Mary Shiels Hospital   (214) 443-3000
Mary Shiels Hosp
3515 Howell St   Dallas, TX 75204   SOUTHWEST

Maryland General Hospital   (410) 225-8000
Maryland Genl Hosp
827 Linden Ave   Baltimore, MD 21201   MID ATLANTIC

Massachusetts Eye and Ear Infirmary   (617) 523-7900
Mass Eye & Ear Infirmary
243 Charles Street   Boston, MA 02114   NEW ENGLAND

Massachusetts General Hospital   (617) 726-2000
Mass Genl Hosp
55 Fruit St   Boston, MA 02114   NEW ENGLAND

Massachusetts Mental Health Center   (617) 626-9300
MA Mental Hlth Ctr
180 Morton St   Jamaica Plain, MA 02130   NEW ENGLAND

Mattel Children's Hospital at UCLA   (310) 825-9111
Mattel Chldns Hosp at UCLA
10833 Le Conte Ave   Los Angeles, CA 90095-1752   WEST COAST AND PACIFIC

Mayo Clinic - Jacksonville, FL   (904) 953-2000
Mayo - Jacksonville
4500 San Pablo Road   Jacksonville, FL 32224   SOUTHEAST

Mayo Clinic - Phoenix   (480) 515-6296
Mayo Clinic - Phoenix
5777 E Mayo Blvd   Phoenix, AZ 85054   SOUTHWEST

Mayo Clinic - Rochester, MN   (507) 284-2511
Mayo Med Ctr & Clin - Rochester
200 First St SW   Rochester, MN 55905   MIDWEST

Mayo Clinic - Scottsdale   (480) 301-8000
Mayo Clinic - Scottsdale
13400 E Shea Blvd   Scottsdale, AZ 85259   SOUTHWEST

McLaren Regional Medical Center   (810) 342-2000
McLaren Reg Med Ctr
401 S. Ballenger Highway   Flint, MI 48532   MIDWEST

McLean Hospital		(617) 855-2000
McLean Hosp		
115 Mill St	Belmont, MA 02478	NEW ENGLAND
Medical Center of Central Georgia		(478) 633-1000
Med Ctr of Central GA		
777 Hemlock Street	Macon, GA 31201	SOUTHEAST
Medical Center of Louisiana @ New Orleans (University Hospital)		(504) 903-3000
Med Ctr LA @ New Orleans (Univ Hosp)		
2021 Perdido St	New Orleans, LA 70112	SOUTHWEST
Medical City Dallas Hospital		(972) 566-7000
Med City Dallas Hosp		
7777 Forest Ln	Dallas, TX 75230-2594	SOUTHWEST
Medical College of Georgia Hospital and Clinic		(706) 721-6569
Med Coll of GA Hosp and Clin		
1120 15th Street	Augusta, GA 30912	SOUTHEAST
Medical College of Virginia Hospitals		(804) 828-9000
Med Coll of VA Hosp		
1250 E Marshall St, Box 980510	Richmond, VA 23219	SOUTHEAST
Medical University of South Carolina Children's Hospital		(843) 792-1414
MUSC Chldns Hosp		
169 Ashley Ave	Charleston, SC 29425	SOUTHEAST
Medical University of South Carolina Medical Center		(843) 792-2300
MUSC Med Ctr		
169 Ashley Ave	Charleston, SC 29425	SOUTHEAST
Memorial Health University Medical Center - Savannah		(912) 350-8000
Meml Hlth Univ Med Ctr - Savannah		
4700 Waters Ave	Savannah, GA 31404	SOUTHEAST
Memorial Hermann Hospital - Texas Medical Center		(713) 704-4000
Meml Hermann Hosp - Texas Med Ctr		
6411 Fannin	Houston, TX 77030	SOUTHWEST
Memorial Medical Center - Springfield		(217) 788-3340
Memorial Med Ctr - Springfield		
800 North Rutledge	Springfield, IL 62781	MIDWEST
Memorial Regional Hospital		(954) 987-2000
Meml Regl Hosp		
3501 Johnson Street	Hollywood, FL 33021	SOUTHEAST

Memorial Sloan-Kettering Cancer Center	(212) 639-2000	
Meml Sloan-Kettering Cancer Ctr		
1275 York Avenue	New York, NY 10021	MID ATLANTIC
Menninger Clinic	(800) 351-9058	
Menninger Clinic		
PO Box 809045	Houston, TX 77280	SOUTHWEST
Mercy General Hospital - Sacramento	(916) 453-4545	
Mercy General Hosp - Sacramento		
4001 J Street	Sacramento, CA 95819	WEST COAST AND PACIFIC
Mercy Hospital	(305) 854-4400	
Mercy Hosp		
3663 S Miami Ave	Miami, FL 33133	SOUTHEAST
Mercy Hospital - Coon Rapids	(763) 236-6000	
Mercy Hosp - Coon Rapids		
4050 Coon Rapids Blvd	Coon Rapids, MN 55433-2522	MIDWEST
Mercy Medical Center Inc	(410) 332-9000	
Mercy Medical Center Inc		
301 St Paul Place	Baltimore, MD 21202	MID ATLANTIC
MeritCare Hospital	(701) 234-6000	
MeritCare Hosp		
720 Fourth Street North	Fargo, ND 58122	GREAT PLAINS AND MOUNTAINS
Methodist Children's Hospital of South Texas	(210) 575-7105	
Methodist Chldns Hosp of South Texas		
7700 Floyd Curl Dr	San Antonio, TX 78229-3311	SOUTHWEST
Methodist Hospital	(215) 952-9000	
Methodist Hosp		
2301 S Broad St	Philadelphia, PA 19148-3594	MID ATLANTIC
Methodist Hospital	(402) 354-4000	
Methodist Hosp - Omaha		
8303 Dodge St	Omaha, NE 68114	GREAT PLAINS AND MOUNTAINS
Methodist Hospital - Houston	(713) 790-3311	
Methodist Hosp - Houston		
6565 Fannin St, D200	Houston, TX 77030	SOUTHWEST
Methodist Hospital - Indianapolis	(317) 962-2000	
Methodist Hosp - Indianapolis		
1701 N Senate Blvd	Indianapolis, IN 46202	MIDWEST

Methodist Hospital Healthsystem - Minnesota		(952) 993-5000
Methodist Hosp - Minnesota		
6500 Excelsior Blvd	Minneapolis, MN 55426-4700	MIDWEST
Methodist Specialty & Transplant Hospital - San Antonio, TX		(210) 575-8110
Methodist Spec & Transpl Hosp		
8026 Floyd Curl Dr	San Antonio, TX 78229	SOUTHWEST
Methodist University Hospital		(901) 516-7000
Methodist Univ Hosp - Memphis		
1265 Union Ave	Memphis, TN 38104	SOUTHEAST
MetroHealth Medical Center		(216) 778-7800
MetroHealth Med Ctr		
2500 MetroHealth Drive	Cleveland, OH 44109-1998	MIDWEST
Metropolitan Methodist Hospital		(210) 208-2200
Metro Methodist Hosp		
1310 McCullough Ave	San Antonio, TX 78212	SOUTHWEST
Miami Children's Hospital		(305) 666-6511
Miami Children's Hosp		
3100 SW 62nd Ave	Miami, FL 33155	SOUTHEAST
Michael E. DeBakey VA Medical Center		(713) 791-1414
DeBakey VA Med Ctr-Houston		
2002 Holcombe Blvd	Houston, TX 77030-1414	SOUTHWEST
Michael Reese Hospital & Medical Center		(312) 791-2000
Michael Reese Hosp & Med Ctr		
2929 S Ellis Ave	Chicago, IL 60616	MIDWEST
Michigan State University-Sparrow Hospital		(517) 364-1000
Mich State Univ-Sparrow Hos		
1215 E Michigan Ave, MS 0	Lansing, MI 48912	MIDWEST
Milford Hospital		(203) 876-4000
Milford Hosp		
300 Seaside Ave	Milford, CT 06460	NEW ENGLAND
Millard Fillmore Gates Circle Hospital		(716) 887-4600
Millard Fillmore Gates Cir Hosp		
3 Gates Cir	Buffalo, NY 14209	MID ATLANTIC
Mills - Peninsula Health Services		(650) 696-5400
Mills - Peninsula Hlth Svcs		
1783 El Camino Real	Burlingame, CA 94010	WEST COAST AND PACIFIC

Miriam Hospital		(401) 793-2500
Miriam Hosp		
164 Summit Avenue	Providence, RI 02906-2894	NEW ENGLAND
Mobile Infirmary Medical Center		(334) 431-2400
Mobile Infirmary Med Ctr		
5 Mobile Infirmary Circle	Mobile, AL 36607-3513	SOUTHEAST
Montefiore Medical Center		(718) 920-4321
Montefiore Med Ctr		
111 East 210 Street	Bronx, NY 10467	MID ATLANTIC
Montefiore Medical Center - Weiler-Einstein Division		(718) 904-2000
Montefiore Med Ctr - Weiler-Einstein Div		
1825 Eastchester Road	Bronx, NY 10461	MID ATLANTIC
Montgomery Hospital Medical Center		(610) 270-2000
Montgomery Hosp Med Ctr		
1301 Powell St	Norristown, PA 19401-3324	MID ATLANTIC
Montgomery Rehabilitation Hospital		(215) 233-6200
Montgomery Rehab Hosp		
8601 Stenton Ave	Wyndmoor, PA 19038	MID ATLANTIC
Morristown Memorial Hospital		(973) 971-5000
Morristown Mem Hosp		
100 Madison Avenue	Morristown, NJ 07960	MID ATLANTIC
MossRehab Hospital		(215) 663-6000
MossRehab Hosp		
60 E Township Line Rd	Elkins Park, PA 19027	MID ATLANTIC
Mott Children's Hospital		(734) 936-4000
Mott Chldns Hosp		
1500 E Medical Center Dr	Ann Arbor, MI 48109	MIDWEST
Mount Auburn Hospital		(617) 492-3500
Mount Auburn Hosp		
330 Mount Auburn St	Cambridge, MA 02238	NEW ENGLAND
Mount Sinai Medical Center		(212) 241-6500
Mount Sinai Med Ctr		
One Gustave L. Levy Pl	New York, NY 10029	MID ATLANTIC
Mount Sinai Medical Center - Miami		(305) 674-2121
Mount Sinai Med Ctr - Miami		
4300 Alton Rd	Miami Beach, FL 33140	SOUTHEAST

America's Top Doctors® 8th Edition

National Institutes of Health - Clinical Center (301) 496-4000
Natl Inst of Hlth - Clin Ctr
6100 Executive Blvd, rm 3C01, MS 7511 Bethesda, MD 20892-7511 MID ATLANTIC

National Jewish Medical & Research Center (303) 388-4461
Natl Jewish Med & Rsch Ctr
1400 Jackson St Denver, CO 80206-2762 GREAT PLAINS AND MOUNTAINS

National Naval Medical Center (301) 295-4611
Natl Naval Med Ctr
8901 Wisconsin Ave Bethesda, MD 20889 MID ATLANTIC

National Rehabilitation Hospital (202) 877-1000
Natl Rehab Hosp
102 Irving St NW Washington, DC 20010 MID ATLANTIC

Nationwide Children's Hospital (614) 722-2000
Nationwide Chldn's Hosp
700 Children's Drive Columbus, OH 43205 MIDWEST

Nebraska Medical Center (402) 559-2000
Nebraska Med Ctr
42nd & Dewey St Omaha, NE 68198 GREAT PLAINS AND MOUNTAINS

Nebraska Medical Center (402) 552-2000
Nebraska Med Ctr
987400 Nebraska Med Ctr Omaha, NE 68198-7400 GREAT PLAINS AND MOUNTAINS

Nebraska Methodist Hospital (402) 354-4000
Nebraska Meth Hosp
8303 Dodge St Omaha, NE 68114 GREAT PLAINS AND MOUNTAINS

New England Baptist Hospital (617) 754-5800
New England Bapt Hosp
125 Parker Hill Ave Boston, MA 02120 NEW ENGLAND

New York Eye & Ear Infirmary (212) 979-4000
New York Eye & Ear Infirm
310 East 14th Street New York, NY 10003 MID ATLANTIC

New York Hospital Queens (718) 670-1231
NY Hosp Queens
56-45 Main Street Flushing, NY 11355 MID ATLANTIC

New York Methodist Hospital (718) 780-3000
New York Methodist Hosp
506 Sixth Street Brooklyn, NY 11215 MID ATLANTIC

New York Presbyterian Hosp/Westchester Div
NY-Presby Hosp/Westchester Div
21 Bloomingdale Rd White Plains, NY 10605 MID ATLANTIC

New York State Psychiatric Institute (212) 543-5000
NY State Psychiatric Inst
1051 Riverside Dr New York, NY 10032 MID ATLANTIC

Newark Beth Israel Medical Center (973) 926-7000
Newark Beth Israel Med Ctr
201 Lyons Ave Newark, NJ 07112 MID ATLANTIC

Newton - Wellesley Hospital (617) 243-6000
Newton - Wellesley Hosp
2014 Washington St Newton, MA 02462 NEW ENGLAND

NewYork-Presbyterian Hospital/Columbia (212) 305-2500
NY-Presby Hosp/Columbia
622 W 168th St New York, NY 10032 MID ATLANTIC

NewYork-Presbyterian Hospital/Weill Cornell (212) 746-5454
NY-Presby Hosp/Weill Cornell
525 E 68th St New York, NY 10021 MID ATLANTIC

NewYork-Presbyterian/Morgan Stanley Children's Hospital (212) 305-2500
NYPresby-Morgan Stanley Children's Hosp
622 W 168th St New York, NY 10032 MID ATLANTIC

North Oaks Medical Center (985) 230-6601
North Oaks Med Ctr
15790 Paul Vega MD Dr Hammond, LA 70403 SOUTHWEST

North Shore Medical Center - Salem Hospital (978) 741-1215
N Shore Med Ctr - Salem Hosp
81 Highland Avenue Salem, MA 01970 NEW ENGLAND

North Shore University Hospital (516) 562-0100
N Shore Univ Hosp
300 Community Dr Manhasset, NY 11030 MID ATLANTIC

Northern California Shriners Hospital (916) 453-2000
Northern CA Shriners Hosp
2425 Stockton Blvd Sacramento, CA 95817 WEST COAST AND PACIFIC

Northern Westchester Hospital (914) 666-1200
Northern Westchester Hosp
400 East Main Street Mount Kisco, NY 10549 MID ATLANTIC

NorthShore University HealthSystem   (847) 570-2000
NorthShore Univ HlthSys
1301 Central Ave   Evanston, IL 60201   MIDWEST

Northside Hospital - Atlanta   (404) 851-8000
Northside Hosp
1000 Johnson Ferry Rd NE   Atlanta, GA 30342   SOUTHEAST

Northwest Hospital   (206) 364-0500
Northwest Hosp
1550 N 115th St   Seattle, WA 98133-0806   WEST COAST AND PACIFIC

Northwest Medical Center   (954) 974-0400
Northwest Med Ctr
2801 N State Rd 7   Margate, FL 33063   SOUTHEAST

Northwestern Memorial Hospital   (312) 926-2000
Northwestern Meml Hosp
251 E Huron St   Chicago, IL 60611   MIDWEST

Norton Hospital   (502) 629-8000
Norton Hosp
200 E Chestnut St   Louisville, KY 40202   SOUTHEAST

NYU Medical Center   (212) 263-7300
NYU Med Ctr
550 First Avenue   New York, NY 10016   MID ATLANTIC

Ochsner Baptist Medical Center   (504) 899-9311
Ochsner Baptist Med Ctr
2700 Napoleon Ave   New Orleans, LA 70115   SOUTHWEST

Ochsner Foundation Hospital   (504) 842-3000
Ochsner Fdn Hosp
1516 Jefferson Hwy   New Orleans, LA 70121   SOUTHWEST

Ohio State University Medical Center   (614) 293-8000
Ohio St Univ Med Ctr
410 W 10th Avenue   Columbus, OH 43210   MIDWEST

Olathe Medical Center   (913) 791-4200
Olathe Med Ctr
20333 W 151st St   Olathe, KS 66061-5352   GREAT PLAINS AND MOUNTAINS

Olive View Medical Center   (818) 364-1555
Olive View Med Ctr
14445 Olive View Dr   Sylmar, CA 91342   WEST COAST AND PACIFIC

Olympia Medical Center   (310) 657-5900
Olympia Med Ctr
5900 W Olympic Blvd   Los Angeles, CA 90036   WEST COAST AND PACIFIC

Oregon Health & Science University   (503) 494-8311
OR Hlth & Sci Univ
3181 SW Sam Jackson Park Rd   Portland, OR 97239-3098   WEST COAST AND PACIFIC

Orlando Regional Medical Center   (407) 841-5111
Orlando Regl Med Ctr
1414 Kuhl Ave   Orlando, FL 32806   SOUTHEAST

Orthopedic Specialty Hospital, The (TOSH)   (801) 314-4100
Ortho Spec Hosp, The (TOSH)
5848 Fashion Blvd   Salt Lake City, UT 84107   GREAT PLAINS AND MOUNTAINS

OU Medical Center   (405) 271-4700
OU Med Ctr
1200 Everett Dr   Oklahoma City, OK 73104-5098   SOUTHWEST

Our Lady of Lourdes Regional Medical Center - Lafayette   (337) 289-2000
Our Lady of Lourdes Reg Med Ctr - Lafayette
611 St. Landry St   Lafayette, LA 70506-4697   SOUTHWEST

Our Lady of the Lake Regional Medical Center   (225) 765-6565
Our Lady of the Lake Regl Med Ctr
5000 Hennessy Blvd   Baton Rouge, LA 70808-4398   SOUTHWEST

Overlake Hospital Medical Center   (425) 688-5000
Overlake Hosp Med Ctr
1035 116th Ave NE   Bellevue, WA 98004-4687   WEST COAST AND PACIFIC

Overland Park Regional Medical Center   (913) 541-5000
Overland Pk Regl Med Ctr
10500 Quivira Rd   Overland Park, KS 66215   GREAT PLAINS AND MOUNTAINS

Palmetto Richland Memorial Hospital   (803) 434-7000
Palmetto Richland Mem Hosp
5 Richland Medical Park Drive   Columbia, SC 29203   SOUTHEAST

Park Plaza Hospital   (713) 527-5000
Park Plaza Hosp
1313 Herman Dr   Houston, TX 77004   SOUTHWEST

Parkinson's Institute/Movement Disorders Treament Center, The   (408) 734-2800
Parkinson's Inst/Movement Disorders Trmt Ctr, The
1170 Morse Ave   Sunnyvale, CA 94089-1605   WEST COAST AND PACIFIC

Parkland Memorial Hospital - Dallas
Parkland Meml Hosp - Dallas
5201 Harry Hines Blvd | Dallas, TX 75235 | (214) 590-8000
SOUTHWEST

Penn Presbyterian Medical Center - UPHS
Penn Presby Med Ctr - UPHS
51 N 39th St | Philadelphia, PA 19104 | (215) 662-8000
MID ATLANTIC

Penn State Milton S Hershey Medical Center
Penn State Milton S Hershey Med Ctr
500 University Drive | Hershey, PA 17033-0850 | (717) 531-8521
MID ATLANTIC

Pennsylvania Hospital
Pennsylvania Hosp
800 Spruce St, Ste 240 | Philadelphia, PA 19107 | (215) 829-3000
MID ATLANTIC

Philadelphia Shriners Hospital
Philadelphia Shriners Hosp
3351 N Broad St | Philadelphia, PA 19140 | (215) 430-4000
MID ATLANTIC

Phillips Eye Institute
Phillips Eye Inst
2215 Park Ave S | Minneapolis, MN 55404 | (612) 775-8800
MIDWEST

Phoenix Baptist Hospital & Medical Center
Phoenix Baptist Hosp & Med Ctr
2000 West Bethany Home Rd | Phoenix, AZ 85015-2184 | (602) 249-0212
SOUTHWEST

Phoenix Children's Hospital
Phoenix Children's Hosp
1919 E Thomas Rd | Phoenix, AZ 85106 | (602) 546-1000
SOUTHWEST

Physicians Regional Medical Center
Physicians Regl Med Ctr
6101 Pine Ridge Rd | Naples, FL 34119 | (239) 348-4000
SOUTHEAST

Piedmont Hospital
Piedmont Hosp
1968 Peachtree Rd NW | Atlanta, GA 30309 | (404) 605-5000
SOUTHEAST

Pitt County Memorial Hospital - Univ Health System East Carolina
Pitt Cty Mem Hosp - Univ Med Ctr East Carolina
2100 Stantonsburg Rd | Greenville, NC 27835-6028 | (252) 847-4100
SOUTHEAST

Portsmouth Regional Hospital
Portsmouth Regl Hosp
333 Borthwick Ave | NH 03801-7002 | (603) 436-5110
NEW ENGLAND

Presbyterian - St Luke's Medical Center		(303) 839-6000
Presby - St Luke's Med Ctr		
1719 E 19th Ave	Denver, CO 80218	GREAT PLAINS AND MOUNTAINS
Presbyterian Hospital - Charlotte		(704) 384-4000
Presby Hosp - Charlotte		
200 Hawthorne Ln	Charlotte, NC 28204-2528	SOUTHEAST
Presbyterian Hospital - Plano		(972) 608-8000
Presby Hosp - Plano		
6200 West Parker Road	Plano, TX 75093	SOUTHWEST
Presbyterian Hospital of Dallas		(214) 345-6789
Presby Hosp of Dallas		
8200 Walnut Hill Ln	Dallas, TX 75231	SOUTHWEST
Primary Children's Medical Center		(801) 588-2000
Primary Children's Med Ctr		
100 N Medical Drive	Salt Lake City, UT 84113-1100	GREAT PLAINS AND MOUNTAINS
Providence Alaska Medical Center		(907) 562-2211
Providence Alaska Med Ctr		
3200 Providence Dr	Anchorage, AK 99508-4615	WEST COAST AND PACIFIC
Providence Centralia Hospital		(360) 736-2803
Providence Centralia Hosp		
914 Scheuber Rd	Centralia, WA 98531	WEST COAST AND PACIFIC
Providence Hospital - Southfield		(248) 424-3000
Providence Hosp - Southfield		
16001 W Nine Mile Rd	Southfield, MI 48075	MIDWEST
Providence Portland Medical Center		(503) 215-1111
Providence Portland Med Ctr		
4805 NE Glisan	Portland, OR 97213-2967	WEST COAST AND PACIFIC
Providence Saint Joseph Medical Center		(818) 843-5111
Providence St Joseph Med Ctr		
501 S Buena Vista St	Burbank, CA 91505	WEST COAST AND PACIFIC
Queen's Medical Center - Honolulu		(808) 538-9011
Queen's Med Ctr - Honolulu		
1301 Punchbowl Street	Honolulu, HI 96813	WEST COAST AND PACIFIC
Rady Children's Hospital - San Diego		(858) 576-1700
Rady Children's Hosp - San Diego		
3020 Children's Way	San Diego, CA 92123	WEST COAST AND PACIFIC

Rainbow Babies & Children's Hospital   (216) 844-1000
Rainbow Babies & Chldns Hosp
11100 Euclid Ave   Cleveland, OH 44106   MIDWEST

Rancho Los Amigos National Rehabilitation Center   (562) 401-7111
Rancho Los Amigos Natl Rehab Ctr
7601 East Imperial Highway   Downey, CA 90242   WEST COAST AND PACIFIC

Rapid City Regional Hospital   (605) 719-1000
Rapid City Reg Hosp
353 Fairmount Blvd   Rapid City, SD 57701   GREAT PLAINS AND MOUNTAINS

Regions Hospital - St Paul   (651) 254-3456
Regions Hosp - St Paul
640 Jackson Street   St Paul, MN 55101   MIDWEST

Rehabilitation Institute - Chicago   (312) 238-1000
Rehab Inst - Chicago
345 E. Superior Street   Chicago, IL 60611   MIDWEST

Rehabilitation Institute of St. Louis   (314) 658-3800
Rehab Inst St. Louis
4455 Duncan Ave   St. Louis, MO 63110   MIDWEST

Rex HealthCare   (919) 784-3100
Rex HlthCare
4420 Lake Boone Trail   Raleigh, NC 27607   SOUTHEAST

Rhode Island Hospital   (401) 444-4000
Rhode Island Hosp
593 Eddy Street   Providence, RI 02903-4923   NEW ENGLAND

Riddle Memorial Hospital   (610) 566-9400
Riddle Meml Hosp
1068 W Baltimore Pike   Media, PA 19063   MID ATLANTIC

Riley Hospital for Children   (317) 274-5000
Riley Hosp for Children
702 Barnhill Drive   Indianapolis, IN 46202   MIDWEST

Riverside Community Hospital   (951) 788-3000
Riverside Comm Hosp
4445 Magnolia Avenue   Riverside, CA 92502   WEST COAST AND PACIFIC

Riverview Medical Center   (732) 741-2700
Riverview Med Ctr
1 Riverview Plaza   Red Bank, NJ 07701   MID ATLANTIC

Robert Wood Johnson University Hospital - New Brunswick   (732) 828-3000
Robert Wood Johnson Univ Hosp - New Brunswick
1 Robert Wood Johnson Pl   New Brunswick, NJ 08901   MID ATLANTIC

Rochester General Hospital   (585) 922-4000
Rochester Genl Hosp
1425 Portland Avenue   Rochester, NY 14621   MID ATLANTIC

Rochester Methodist Hospital   (507) 284-2511
Rochester Methodist Hosp
201 W Center St   Rochester, MN 55905-3003   MIDWEST

Rockefeller University   (212) 327-8000
Rockefeller Univ
1230 York Avenue   New York, NY 10021   MID ATLANTIC

Roger Williams Hospital   (401) 456-2000
Roger Williams Hosp
825 Chalkstone Avenue   Providence, RI 02908   NEW ENGLAND

Ronald Reagan UCLA Medical Center   (310) 825-9111
Ronald Reagan UCLA Med Ctr
757 Westwood Plaza   Los Angeles, CA 90095   WEST COAST AND PACIFIC

Roper Hospital   (843) 724-2000
Roper Hosp
316 Calhoun St   Charleston, SC 29401   SOUTHEAST

Rose Medical Center   (303) 320-2121
Rose Med Ctr
4567 E 9th Ave   Denver, CO 80220-3941   GREAT PLAINS AND MOUNTAINS

Roswell Park Cancer Institute   (716) 845-5770
Roswell Park Cancer Inst
Elm and Carlton Streets   Buffalo, NY 14263   MID ATLANTIC

Rush - Copley Medical Center   (630) 978-6200
Rush - Copley Med Ctr
2000 Ogden Ave   Aurora, IL 60504-4206   MIDWEST

Rush University Medical Center   (312) 942-5000
Rush Univ Med Ctr
1653 W Congress Pkwy   Chicago, IL 60612-3833   MIDWEST

Rusk Institute of Rehabilitation Medicine   (212) 263-2606
Rusk Inst of Rehab Med
400 East 34th Street   New York, NY 10016   MID ATLANTIC

Saint Francis Hospital - Memphis (901) 765-1000
St Francis Hosp - Memphis
5959 Park Ave   Memphis, TN 38119   SOUTHEAST

Saint John's Health Center (310) 829-5511
St John's Hlth Ctr, Santa Monica
1328 22nd St   Santa Monica, CA 90404   WEST COAST AND PACIFIC

Saint Thomas Hospital - Nashville (615) 222-2111
Saint Thomas Hosp - Nashville
4220 Harding Road   Nashville, TN 37205   SOUTHEAST

Saint Vincent Catholic Medical Centers - St Vincent's Manhattan (212) 604-7000
St Vincent Cath Med Ctrs - Manhattan
170 West 12th Street   New York, NY 10011   MID ATLANTIC

Salt Lake Regional Medical Center (801) 350-4111
Salt Lake Regional Med Ctr
1050 E South Temple   Salt Lake City, UT 84102   GREAT PLAINS AND MOUNTAINS

San Diego Hospice (619) 688-1600
San Diego Hospice
4311 3rd Ave0   San Diego, CA 92103-7499   WEST COAST AND PACIFIC

San Francisco General Hospital (415) 206-8000
San Francisco Genl Hosp
1001 Potrero Avenue   San Francisco, CA 94110   WEST COAST AND PACIFIC

Sanford Health -South Dakota (605) 333-1000
Sanford Health SD
1100 S Euclid Ave, PO Box 5039   Sioux Falls, SD 57717   GREAT PLAINS AND MOUNTAINS

Santa Barbara Cottage Hospital (805) 682-7111
Santa Barbara Cottage Hosp
Pueblo at Bath St, PO Box 689   Santa Barbara, CA 93105   WEST COAST AND PACIFIC

Santa Clara Valley Medical Center (408) 885-5000
Santa Clara Vly Med Ctr
751 S Bascom Ave   San Jose, CA 95128   WEST COAST AND PACIFIC

Santa Monica - UCLA Medical Center (310) 319-4000
Santa Monica - UCLA Med Ctr
1250 16th St   Santa Monica, CA 90404   WEST COAST AND PACIFIC

Sarasota Memorial Hospital (941) 917-9000
Sarasota Meml Hosp
1700 S Tamiami Trail   Sarasota, FL 34239   SOUTHEAST

Schneider Children's Hospital		(718) 470-3000
Schneider Chldn's Hosp		
269-01 76th Ave	New Hyde Park, NY 11040	MID ATLANTIC
Schwab Rehabilitation Hospital		(773) 522-2010
Schwab Rehab Hosp		
1401 S. California Boulevard	Chicago, IL 60608	MIDWEST
Scott & White Memorial Hospital		(254) 724-2111
Scott & White Mem Hosp		
2401 South 31st Street	Temple, TX 76508-0001	SOUTHWEST
Scottsdale Healthcare - Osborn		(480) 675-4000
Scottsdale Hlthcare - Osborn		
7400 E Osborn Rd	Scottsdale, AZ 85251-6403	SOUTHWEST
Scottsdale Healthcare - Shea		(480) 860-3000
Scottsdale Hlthcare - Shea		
9000 E Shea Blvd	Scottsdale, AZ 85258-4514	SOUTHWEST
Scripps Green Hospital		(858) 455-9100
Scripps Green Hosp		
10666 N Torrey Pines Rd	La Jolla, CA 92037	WEST COAST AND PACIFIC
Scripps Memorial Hospital - La Jolla		(858) 457-4123
Scripps Meml Hosp - La Jolla		
9888 Genesee Ave	La Jolla, CA 92037	WEST COAST AND PACIFIC
Scripps Mercy Hospital & Medical Center		(619) 294-8111
Scripps Mercy Hosp & Med Ctr		
4077 Fifth Ave	San Diego, CA 92103	WEST COAST AND PACIFIC
Self Regional Healthcare		(864) 227-4111
Self Regional Healthcare		
1325 Spring St	Greenwood, SC 29646	SOUTHEAST
Sentara Leigh Hospital		(757) 466-6000
Sentara Leigh Hosp		
830 Kempsville Rd	Norfolk, VA 23502-3981	SOUTHEAST
Sentara Norfolk General Hospital		(757) 668-3000
Sentara Norfolk Genl Hosp		
600 Gresham Dr	Norfolk, VA 23507	SOUTHEAST
Sentara Virginia Beach General Hospital		(757) 395-8000
Sentara VA Beach Genl Hosp		
1060 First Colonial Rd	Virginia Beach, VA 23454	SOUTHEAST

Seton Medical Center   (650) 992-4000
Seton Med Ctr
1900 Sullivan Avenue   Daly City, CA 94015   WEST COAST AND PACIFIC

Shady Grove Adventist Hospital   (301) 279-6000
Shady Grove Adven Hosp
9901 Medical Center Drive   Rockville, MD 20850   MID ATLANTIC

Shands at University of Florida   (352) 265-0111
Shands at Univ of FL
1600 SW Archer Rd   Gainesville, FL 32610   SOUTHEAST

Shands Jacksonville   (904) 244-0411
Shands Jacksonville
655 W 8th St   Jacksonville, FL 32209   SOUTHEAST

Sharp Memorial Hospital   (858) 541-3400
Sharp Meml Hosp
7901 Frost St   San Diego, CA 92123   WEST COAST AND PACIFIC

Shawnee Mission Medical Center   (913) 676-2000
Shawnee Mission Med Ctr
9100 W 74th St   Shawnee Mission, KS 66204   GREAT PLAINS AND MOUNTAINS

Sheppard Pratt Health System   (410) 938-3000
Sheppard Pratt Hlth Sys
6501 N Charles St   Baltimore, MD 21285-6815   MID ATLANTIC

Shriners Hospital for Children-Philadelphia   (215) 430-4000
Shriners Hosp for Chldn-Phila
3551 N Broad St   Philadelphia, PA 19140   MID ATLANTIC

Sibley Memorial Hospital   (202) 537-4000
Sibley Mem Hosp
5255 Loughboro Road NW   Washington, DC 20016   MID ATLANTIC

Silver Hill Hospital   (203) 966-3561
Silver Hill Hosp
208 Valley Rd   New Canaan, CT 06840-3899   NEW ENGLAND

Sinai Hospital - Baltimore   (410) 601-9000
Sinai Hosp - Baltimore
2401 W Belvedere Ave   Baltimore, MD 21215   MID ATLANTIC

Sinai-Grace Hospital - Detroit   (313) 966-3300
Sinai-Grace Hosp - Detroit
6071 W. Outer Drive   Detroit, MI 48235   MIDWEST

South Miami Hospital   (305) 661-4611
South Miami Hosp
6200 SW 73 St   South Miami, FL 33143   SOUTHEAST

Southeast Baptist Hospital   (210) 297-3000
Southeast Baptist Hosp
4214 E Southcross Blvd   San Antonio, TX 78222   SOUTHWEST

Southern New Hampshire Medical Center   (603) 577-2000
Southern NH Med Ctr
8 Prospect St   Nashua, NH 03061   NEW ENGLAND

Southwest Florida Regional Medical Center   (239) 939-1147
Southwest Florida Regional Medical Center
2727 Winkler Ave.   Fort Myers, FL 33901   SOUTHEAST

Southwest Texas Methodist Hospital   (210) 575-4000
SW TX Meth Hosp
7700 Floyd Curl Dr   San Antonio, TX 78229   SOUTHWEST

Spaulding Rehabilitation Hospital   (617) 720-6400
Spaulding Rehab Hosp
125 Nashua Street   Boston, MA 02114   NEW ENGLAND

Spectrum Health - Blodgett Campus   (616) 774-7444
Spectrum Hlth Blodgett Campus
1840 Wealthy St SE   Grand Rapids, MI 49506   MIDWEST

Spectrum Health Butterworth Campus   (616) 391-1774
Spectrum Hlth Butterworth Campus
100 Michigan St NE   Grand Rapids, MI 49503   MIDWEST

SSM Cardinal Glennon Children's Hospital   (314) 577-5600
Cardinal Glennon Mem Children's Hosp
1465 S Grand Blvd   St Louis, MO 63104   MIDWEST

SSM St Joseph Hospital of Kirkwood   (314) 966-1500
SSM St Joseph Hosp of Kirkwood
525 Couch Ave   St Louis, MO 63122   MIDWEST

St Alphonsus Regional Medical Center   (208) 367-2121
St Alphonsus Regl Med Ctr
1055 N Curtis Rd   Boise, ID 83706-1370   GREAT PLAINS AND MOUNTAINS

St Anthony Hospital - Oklahoma City   (405) 272-7000
St Anthony Hosp -Oklahoma City
1000 N Lee St   Oklahoma City, OK 73102   SOUTHWEST

St Anthony's Hospital - St Petersburg *St Anthony's Hosp - St Petersburg* 1200 7th Avenue North	St Petersburg, FL 33705	(727) 893-6814 SOUTHEAST
St Barnabas Medical Center *St Barnabas Med Ctr* 94 Old Short Hills Rd	Livingston, NJ 07039-5672	(973) 322-5000 MID ATLANTIC
St Christopher's Hospital for Children *St Christopher's Hosp for Chldn* Erie Ave at Front St	Philadelphia, PA 19134	(215) 427-5000 MID ATLANTIC
St Davids Medical Center - Austin *St Davids Medical Center - Austin* 919 E 32rd st	Austin, TX 78705	(512) 476-7111 SOUTHWEST
St Elizabeth Medical Center (South Unit) *St Elizabeth Med Ctr (South Unit)* 1 Medical Village Dr	Edgewood, KY 41017	(859) 344-2000 SOUTHEAST
St Elizabeth's Medical Center *St Elizabeth's Med Ctr* 736 Cambridge St	Brighton, MA 02135	(617) 789-3000 NEW ENGLAND
St Francis Hospital & Medical Center *St Francis Hosp & Med Ctr* 114 Woodland St	Hartford, CT 06105	(860) 714-4000 NEW ENGLAND
St Francis Hospital - The Heart Center *St Francis Hosp - The Heart Ctr* 100 Port Washington Boulevard	Roslyn, NY 11576	(516) 562-6000 MID ATLANTIC
St Francis Medical Center *St Francis Med Ctr* 309 Jackson St	Monroe, LA 71210-7498	(318) 362-4000 SOUTHWEST
St John's Hospital - Springfield *St John's Hosp - Springfield* 800 E Carpenter St	Springfield, IL 62769	(217) 544-6464 MIDWEST
St John's Mercy Medical Center - St Louis *St John's Mercy Med Ctr - St Louis* 615 S New Ballas Rd	St Louis, MO 63141	(314) 569-6000 MIDWEST
St Joseph Hospital *St Joseph Hosp* 172 Kinsley St	Nashua, NH 03060	(603) 882-3000 NEW ENGLAND

St Joseph Hospital		(360) 734-5400
St Joseph Hosp - Bellingham		
2901 Squalicum Pkwy	Bellingham, WA 98225-1898	WEST COAST AND PACIFIC
St Joseph Medical Center		(410) 337-1000
St Joseph Med Ctr		
7601 Osler Drive	Baltimore, MD 21208	MID ATLANTIC
St Joseph Medical Center - Tacoma		(253) 627-4101
St Joseph Med Ctr - Tacoma		
1717 South J St	Tacoma, WA 98401	WEST COAST AND PACIFIC
St Joseph Mercy Hospital - Ann Arbor		(734) 712-3456
St Joseph Mercy Hosp - Ann Arbor		
5301 E Huron River Dr, Box 992	Ann Arbor, MI 48106	MIDWEST
St Joseph Mercy Oakland Hospital		(248) 858-3000
St Joseph Mercy Oakland Hosp		
44405 Woodward Ave	Pontiac, MI 48341	MIDWEST
St Joseph's Children's Hospital		(813) 554-8500
St Josephs Chldns Hosp		
3001 W Dr Martin Luther King Jr Blvd	Tampa, FL 33607	SOUTHEAST
St Joseph's Hospital & Medical Center - Phoenix		(602) 406-3000
St Joseph's Hosp & Med Ctr - Phoenix		
350 W Thomas Rd	Phoenix, AZ 85013-4496	SOUTHWEST
St Joseph's Hospital - Atlanta		(404) 851-7001
St Joseph's Hosp - Atlanta		
5665 Peachtree Dunwoody Rd NE	Atlanta, GA 30342	SOUTHEAST
St Joseph's Hospital - Orange		(714) 633-9111
St Joseph's Hosp - Orange		
1100 West Stewart Drive	Orange, CA 92868	WEST COAST AND PACIFIC
St Joseph's Hospital - Tampa		(813) 870-4000
St Joseph's Hosp - Tampa		
3001 W Martin Luther King Jr Blvd	Tampa, FL 33607	SOUTHEAST
St Joseph's Hospital - Tucson		(520) 296-3211
St Joseph's Hosp - Tucson		
350 N Wilmot Rd	Tucson, AZ 85711	SOUTHWEST
St Jude Children's Research Hospital		(901) 495-3300
St Jude Children's Research Hosp		
332 N Lauderdale St	Memphis, TN 38105	SOUTHEAST

St Louis Children's Hospital   (314) 454-6000
St Louis Chldns Hosp
One Children's Pl   St Louis, MO 63110   MIDWEST

St Louis University Hospital   (314) 577-8000
St Louis Univ Hosp
3635 Vista at Grand Blvd   St Louis, MO 63110   MIDWEST

St Luke's - Roosevelt Hospital Center - Roosevelt Division   (212) 523-4000
St Luke's - Roosevelt Hosp Ctr - Roosevelt Div
1000 Tenth Avenue   New York, NY 10019   MID ATLANTIC

St Luke's - Roosevelt Hospital Center - St Luke's Hospital   (212) 523-4000
St Luke's - Roosevelt Hosp Ctr - St Luke's Hosp
1111 Amsterdam Ave   New York, NY 10025   MID ATLANTIC

St Luke's Episcopal Hospital - Houston   (832) 355-1000
St Luke's Episcopal Hosp - Houston
6720 Bertner Avenue   Houston, TX 77030   SOUTHWEST

St Luke's Hospital - Bethlehem   (610) 954-4000
St Luke's Hosp - Bethlehem
801 Ostrum Street   Bethlehem, PA 18015   MID ATLANTIC

St Luke's Hospital - Chesterfield, MO   (314) 434-1500
St Luke's Hosp - Chesterfield, MO
232 S Woods Mill Rd   Chesterfield, MO 63017   MIDWEST

St Luke's Hospital - Duluth   (218) 249-5555
St Luke's Hosp - Duluth
915 E 1st St   Duluth, MN 55805-2193   MIDWEST

St Luke's Hospital - Jacksonville   (904) 296-3700
St Luke's Hosp - Jacksonville
4201 Belfort Rd   Jacksonville, FL 32216   SOUTHEAST

St Luke's Hospital of Kansas City   (816) 932-2000
St Luke's Hosp of Kansas City
4401 Wornall Rd   Kansas City, MO 64111   MIDWEST

St Mark's Hospital - Salt Lake City   (801) 268-7111
St Mark's Hosp - Salt Lake City
1200 E. 3900 S   Salt Lake City, UT 84124   GREAT PLAINS AND MOUNTAINS

St Mary Medical Center - Long Beach, CA   (562) 491-9000
St Mary Med Ctr - Long Beach, CA
1050 Linden Ave   Long Beach, CA 90813   WEST COAST AND PACIFIC

St Mary's Hospital - Rochester, MN (Mayo Clinic)   (507) 255-5123
St Mary's Hosp - Rochester
1216 2nd St SW   Rochester, MN 55902   MIDWEST

St Mary's Medical Center - Huntington   (304) 526-1234
St Mary's Med Ctr - Huntington
2900 First Ave   Huntington, WV 25702-1272   MID ATLANTIC

St Mary's Medical Center - West Palm Beach   (561) 844-6300
St Mary's Med Ctr - W Palm Bch
901 45th St   West Palm Beach, FL 33407   SOUTHEAST

St Patrick Hospital & Health Sciences Center   (406) 543-7271
St Patrick Hospital - Missoula
500 W Broadway   Missoula, MT 59802   GREAT PLAINS AND MOUNTAINS

St Peter's University Hospital   (732) 745-8600
St Peter's Univ Hosp
254 Easton Ave   New Brunswick, NJ 08901-1780   MID ATLANTIC

St Vincent Carmel Hospital   (317) 573-7000
St Vincent Carmel Hosp
13500 N Meridian St   Carmel, IN 46032-1496   MIDWEST

St Vincent Hospital & Health Services - Indianapolis   (317) 338-2345
St Vincent Hosp & Hlth Svcs - Indianapolis
2001 W 86th St   Indianapolis, IN 46260-1991   MIDWEST

St Vincent Hospital - Green Bay   (920) 433-0111
St Vincent Hosp - Green Bay
835 S Van Buren St, P.O. Box 13508   Green Bay, WI 54307-3508   MIDWEST

St Vincent Hospital - Santa Fe   (505) 983-3361
St Vincent Hosp - Santa Fe
455 St Michaels Dr   Santa Fe, NM 87504-2107   SOUTHWEST

St Vincent's Hospital - Birmingham   (205) 939-7000
St Vincent's Hosp - Birmingham
810 St. Vincent's Drive or PO Box 12407 Birmingham, AL 35202-2407   SOUTHEAST

St Vincent's Medical Center - Jacksonville   (904) 308-7300
St Vincent's Med Ctr - Jacksonville
1800 Barrs St   Jacksonville, FL 32204   SOUTHEAST

St Vincent's Medical Center - Los Angeles   (213) 484-7111
St Vincent's Med Ctr - Los Angeles
2131 W 3rd St   Los Angeles, CA 90057   WEST COAST AND PACIFIC

St. Alexius Medical Center   (701) 530-7000
St. Alexius Med Ctr - Bismarck
900 E Broadway Ave   Bismarck, ND 58501   GREAT PLAINS AND MOUNTAINS

St. Luke's Regional Medical Center   (208) 381-2222
St. Luke's Reg Med Ctr - Boise
190 E Bannock St   Boise, ID 83712   GREAT PLAINS AND MOUNTAINS

St. Vincent Infirmary Medical Center & Doctors Hospital   (501) 552-3000
St Vincent Med Ctr
2 St. Vincent Cir   Little Rock, AR 72205   SOUTHWEST

Stamford Hospital   (203) 325-7000
Stamford Hosp
30 Shelburne Rd @ W Broad St, Box 9317   Stamford, CT 06902   NEW ENGLAND

Stanford University Medical Center   (650) 723-4000
Stanford Univ Med Ctr
300 Pasteur Dr   Stanford, CA 94305   WEST COAST AND PACIFIC

Staten Island University Hospital - North   (718) 226-9000
Staten Island Univ Hosp - North
475 Seaview Avenue   Staten Island, NY 10305   MID ATLANTIC

Stony Brook University Medical Center   (631) 689-8333
Stony Brook Univ Med Ctr
Nicolls Rd   Stony Brook, NY 11794-8410   MID ATLANTIC

Suburban Hospital Healthcare Systems   (301) 896-3100
Suburban Hosp - Bethesda
8600 Old Georgetown Road   Bethesda, MD 20814   MID ATLANTIC

Sunnyview Hospital and Rehabilitation Center   (518) 382-4500
Sunnyview Hosp
1270 Belmont Ave   Schenectady, NY 12308-2198   MID ATLANTIC

Sunrise Hospital & Medical Center/Sunrise Children's Hospital   (702) 731-8000
Sunrise Hosp & Med Ctr/Sunrise Chldn's Hosp
3186 Maryland Pkwy   Las Vegas, NV 89109-2306   WEST COAST AND PACIFIC

SUNY Downstate Medical Center   (718) 270-1000
SUNY Downstate Med Ctr
450 Clarkson Ave   Brooklyn, NY 11203   MID ATLANTIC

Swedish Covenant Hospital   (773) 878-8200
Swedish Covenant Hosp
5145 N California Ave   Chicago, IL 60625   MIDWEST

Swedish Medical Center - Englewood   (303) 788-5000
Swedish Med Ctr - Englewood
501 E Hamden Ave   Englewood, CO 80110-2795 GREAT PLAINS AND MOUNTAINS

Swedish Medical Center - Seattle   (206) 386-6000
Swedish Med Ctr - Seattle
747 Broadway   Seattle, WA 98122   WEST COAST AND PACIFIC

Tampa General Hospital   (813) 844-7000
Tampa Genl Hosp
PO BOX 1289   Tampa, FL 33601   SOUTHEAST

Tanner Medical Center - Carrollton   (770) 836-9666
Tanner Med Ctr
705 Dixie Street   Carrollton, GA 30117   SOUTHEAST

Temple University Hospital   (215) 707-2000
Temple Univ Hosp
3401 N Broad St   Philadelphia, PA 19140-5189   MID ATLANTIC

Texas Children's Hospital - Houston   (832) 824-1000
Texas Chldns Hosp - Houston
6621 Fannin St   Houston, TX 77030   SOUTHWEST

Texas Orthopedic Hospital   (713) 799-8600
Texas Ortho Hosp
7401 S Main   Houston, TX 77030   SOUTHWEST

Texas Scottish Rite Hospital for Children   (214) 559-5000
Texas Scottish Rite Hosp for Chldn
2222 Welborn St   Dallas, TX 75219   SOUTHWEST

Thomas Jefferson University Hospital   (215) 955-6000
Thomas Jefferson Univ Hosp
111 S 11th St   Philadelphia, PA 19107   MID ATLANTIC

TIRR   (713) 799-5000
TIRR
1333 Moursund   Houston, TX 77030   SOUTHWEST

Toledo Hospital   (419) 291-4000
Toledo Hosp
2142 N Cove Blvd   Toledo, OH 43606   MIDWEST

Tucson Medical Center   (520) 327-5461
Tucson Med Ctr
5301 E Grant Rd   Tucson, AZ 85712-2874   SOUTHWEST

Tufts Medical Center
(617) 636-5000
Tufts Med Ctr
800 Washington St   Boston, MA 02111   NEW ENGLAND

Tulane University Hospital & Clinic
(504) 588-5263
Tulane Univ Hosp & Clin
1415 Tulane Ave   New Orleans, LA 70112   SOUTHWEST

Tulane-Lakeside Hospital
(504) 780-8282
Tulane-Lakeside Hosp
4700 I-10 Service Rd   Metairie, LA 70001   SOUTHWEST

UAB Highlands Hospital
(205) 930-7000
UAB Highlands Hosp
1201 11th Ave S   Birmingham, AL 35205-5299   SOUTHEAST

UCLA Neuropsychiatric Hospital
(310) 825-9989
UCLA Neuropsychiatric Hosp
760 Westwood Plaza   Los Angeles, CA 90024   WEST COAST AND PACIFIC

UCSD Medical Center
(619) 543-6222
UCSD Med Ctr
200 W Arbor Dr   San Diego, CA 92103   WEST COAST AND PACIFIC

UCSF - Mount Zion Medical Center
(415) 567-6600
UCSF - Mt Zion Med Ctr
1600 Divisadero St   San Francisco, CA 94115   WEST COAST AND PACIFIC

UCSF Medical Center
(415) 476-1000
UCSF Med Ctr
500 Parnassus Ave   San Francisco, CA 94143   WEST COAST AND PACIFIC

UMass Memorial - University Campus
(508) 856-0011
UMass Meml - Univ Campus
55 Lake Ave N   Worcester, MA 01655-0002   NEW ENGLAND

UMass Memorial Medical Center
(508) 334-1000
UMass Memorial Med Ctr
55 Lake Ave N   Worcester, MA 01655   NEW ENGLAND

UMDNJ-University Hospital-Newark
(973) 972-4300
UMDNJ-Univ Hosp-Newark
150 Bergen St   Newark, NJ 07103-2406   MID ATLANTIC

Uniformed Services University of the Health Sciences
(301) 295-9390
Unif Serv Univ of the Hlth Sci
4301 Jones Bridge Rd   Bethesda, MD 20814-4799   MID ATLANTIC

Union Memorial Hospital - Baltimore		(410) 554-2000
Union Meml Hosp - Baltimore		
201 E University Pkwy	Baltimore, MD 21218	MID ATLANTIC

United Hospital		(651) 241-8000
United Hosp		
333 N Smith Ave	St Paul, MN 55102	MIDWEST

University Community Hospital		(813) 971-6000
University Comm Hosp		
3100 E Fletcher Avenue	Tampa, FL 33613	SOUTHEAST

University Health System - University Hospital (San Antonio, TX)		(210) 358-4000
Univ Hlth Sys - Univ Hosp (San Antonio, TX)		
4502 Medical Dr	San Antonio, TX 78229	SOUTHWEST

University Hospital & Clinics - Mississippi		(601) 984-1000
Univ Hosps & Clins - Jackson		
2500 N State St	Jackson, MS 39216	SOUTHEAST

University Hospital - Albquerque		(505) 272-2111
Univ Hosp of Albquerque		
2211 Lomas Blvd NE	Albuquerque, NM 87106	SOUTHWEST

University Hospital - Cincinnati		(513) 584-1000
Univ Hosp - Cincinnati		
234 Goodman St	Cincinnati, OH 45219	MIDWEST

University Hospital - SUNY Upstate Medical University		(315) 464-5540
Univ. Hosp.- SUNY Upstate		
750 E Adams Street	Syracuse, NY 13210	MID ATLANTIC

University Hospitals Case Medical Center		(216) 844-1000
Univ Hosps Case Med Ctr		
11100 Euclid Ave	Cleveland, OH 44106	MIDWEST

University Medical Center Health System		(806) 775-8200
Univ Med Ctr - Lubbock		
PO Box 5980	Lubbock, TX 79408	SOUTHWEST

University Medical Center of Southern Nevada - Las Vegas		(702) 383-2000
Univ Med Ctr - Las Vegas		
1800 W Charleston Blvd	Las Vegas, NV 89102	WEST COAST AND PACIFIC

University Medical Center- Tucson		(520) 694-0111
Univ Med Ctr - Tucson		
1501 N Campbell Ave	Tucson, AZ 85724-5128	SOUTHWEST

University New Mexico Health & Science Center   (505) 272-2111
Univ NM Hlth & Sci Ctr
2211 Lomas Blvd NE   Albuquerque, NM 87106   SOUTHWEST

University of Alabama Hospital at Birmingham   (205) 934-4011
Univ of Ala Hosp at Birmingham
619 South 19th Street   Birmingham, AL 35249-6544   SOUTHEAST

University of Arkansas for Medical Sciences Medical Center   (501) 686-7000
UAMS Med Ctr
4301 W Markham St   Little Rock, AR 72205   SOUTHWEST

University of California - Davis Medical Center   (916) 734-2011
UC Davis Med Ctr
2315 Stockton Blvd   Sacramento, CA 95817   WEST COAST AND PACIFIC

University of California - Irvine Medical Center   (714) 456-6011
UC Irvine Med Ctr
101 The City Dr   Orange, CA 92868   WEST COAST AND PACIFIC

University of Chicago Hospitals   (773) 702-1000
Univ of Chicago Hosps
5841 S Maryland Ave   Chicago, IL 60637   MIDWEST

University of Colorado Hospital   (730) 848-4011
Univ Colorado Hosp
12605 E 16th Ave   Aurora, CO 80045   GREAT PLAINS AND MOUNTAINS

University of Connecticut Health Center, John Dempsey Hospital   (860) 679-2100
Univ of Conn Hlth Ctr, John Dempsey Hosp
263 Farmington Ave   Farmington, CT 06030   NEW ENGLAND

University of Illinois at Chicago Eye & Ear Infirmary   (312) 996-6500
Univ of IL at Chicago Eye & Ear Infirm
1855 W Taylor St   Chicago, IL 60612   MIDWEST

University of Illinois Medical Center at Chicago   (312) 996-7000
Univ of IL Med Ctr at Chicago
1740 W Taylor St   Chicago, IL 60612   MIDWEST

University of Iowa Hospitals and Clinics   (319) 356-1616
Univ Iowa Hosp & Clinics
200 Hawkins Drive   Iowa City, IA 52242   MIDWEST

University of Kansas Hospital   (913) 588-5000
Univ of Kansas Hosp
3901 Rainbow Blvd   Kansas City, KS 66160   GREAT PLAINS AND MOUNTAINS

University of Kentucky Chandler Hospital   (800) 333-8874
Univ of Kentucky Chandler Hosp
800 Rose Street   Lexington, KY 40536   SOUTHEAST

University of Louisville Hospital   (502) 562-3000
Univ of Louisville Hosp
530 S Jackson St   Louisville, KY 40202   SOUTHEAST

University of Maryland Medical System   (410) 328-8667
Univ of MD Med Sys
22 S Greene St   Baltimore, MD 21201   MID ATLANTIC

University of Miami Hosp & Clinics/Sylvester Comprehensive Cancer Cntr   (305) 243-1000
Univ of Miami Hosp & Clins/Sylvester Comp Canc Ctr
1475 NW 12th Ave   Miami, FL 33136   SOUTHEAST

University of Miami Hospital   (305) 325-5511
Univ of Miami Hosp
1400 NW 12 Ave   Miami, FL 33136   SOUTHEAST

University of Michigan Health System   (734) 936-4000
Univ Michigan Hlth Sys
1500 E Medical Center Dr   Ann Arbor, MI 48109   MIDWEST

University of Minnesota Medical Center, Fairview - Riverside Campus   (612) 672-6000
Univ Minn Med Ctr, Fairview - Riverside Campus
2450 Riverside Ave S   Minneapolis, MN 55454   MIDWEST

University of Minnesota Medical Center, Fairview - University Campus   (612) 273-3000
Univ Minn Med Ctr, Fairview - Univ Campus
420 Delaware St SE   Minneapolis, MN 55455   MIDWEST

University of Missouri Hospitals & Clinics   (573) 882-4141
Univ of Missouri Hosp & Clins
1 Hospital Dr   Columbia, MO 65212   MIDWEST

University of North Carolina Hospitals   (919) 966-4131
Univ NC Hosps
101 Manning Drive, Box 7600   Chapel Hill, NC 27514   SOUTHEAST

University of Rochester Strong Memorial Hospital   (585) 275-2121
Univ of Rochester Strong Meml Hosp
601 Elmwood Ave   Rochester, NY 14642   MID ATLANTIC

University of South Alabama Medical Center   (251) 471-7000
Univ of S AL Med Ctr
2451 Fillingim St   Mobile, AL 36617   SOUTHEAST

University of South Florida - Tampa	(813) 974-2011	
Univ of S FL - Tampa		
4202 E Fowler Ave	Tampa, FL 33620	SOUTHEAST

University of Tennesee Memorial Hospital	(865) 544-9000	
Univ of Tennesee Mem Hosp		
1924 Alcoa Hwy	Knoxville, TN 37920	SOUTHEAST

University of Texas Health Center at Tyler	(903) 877-3451	
UT Hlth Ctr at Tyler		
11937 US Hwy 271	Tyler, TX 75708	SOUTHWEST

University of Texas MD Anderson Cancer Center	(713) 792-2121	
UT MD Anderson Cancer Ctr		
1515 Holcombe Blvd	Houston, TX 77030-4095	SOUTHWEST

University of Texas Medical Branch Hospital at Galveston	(409) 772-1011	
UT Med Br Hosp at Galveston		
301 University Blvd	Galveston, TX 77555	SOUTHWEST

University of Texas Southwestern Medical Center at Dallas, The	(214) 648-3111	
UT Southwestern Med Ctr - Dallas		
5323 Harry Hines Blvd	Dallas, TX 75390	SOUTHWEST

University of Toledo Medical Center	(419) 383-4000	
Univ of Toledo Med Ctr		
3000 Arlington Ave	Toledo, OH 43614	MIDWEST

University of Utah Hospitals and Clinics	(801) 581-2121	
Univ Utah Hosps and Clins		
50 N Medical Dr	Salt Lake City, UT 84132	GREAT PLAINS AND MOUNTAINS

University of Virginia Medical Center	(434) 924-0211	
Univ Virginia Med Ctr		
1215 Lee Street	Charlottesville, VA 22908-0001	SOUTHEAST

University of Washington Medical Center	(206) 598-3300	
Univ Wash Med Ctr		
1959 NE Pacific St, Box 356355	Seattle, WA 98195	WEST COAST AND PACIFIC

University of Wisconsin Hospital & Clinics	(608) 263-6400	
Univ WI Hosp & Clins		
600 Highland Avenue	Madison, WI 53792	MIDWEST

UPMC Montefiore	(412) 647-2345	
UPMC Montefiore		
200 Lothrop St	Pittsburgh, PA 15213	MID ATLANTIC

UPMC Passavant-Cranberry   (724) 772-5300
UPMC Passavant-Cranberry
1 St Francis Way   Cranberry Township, PA 16066   MID ATLANTIC

UPMC Presbyterian   (412) 647-2345
UPMC Presby, Pittsburgh
200 Lothrop St   Pittsburgh, PA 15213   MID ATLANTIC

UPMC Shadyside   (412) 623-2121
UPMC Shadyside
5230 Centre Ave   Pittsburgh, PA 15232   MID ATLANTIC

UPMC South Side   (412) 488-5550
UPMC South Side
2000 Mary St   Pittsburgh, PA 15203   MID ATLANTIC

UPMC St Margaret   (412) 784-4000
UPMC St Margaret
815 Freeport Rd   Pittsburgh, PA 15215-3301   MID ATLANTIC

USC Norris Comprehensive Cancer Center and Hospital   (323) 865-3000
USC Norris Comp Cancer Ctr
1441 Eastlake Ave   Los Angeles, CA 90033   WEST COAST AND PACIFIC

USC University Hospital - Richard K. Eamer Medical Plaza   (323) 442-8444
USC Univ Hosp - R K Eamer Med Plz
1500 San Pablo St   Los Angeles, CA 90033   WEST COAST AND PACIFIC

VA Connecticut Healthcare System   (203) 932-5711
VA Conn Hlthcre Sys
950 Campbell Ave   West Haven, CT 06516   NEW ENGLAND

VA Health Care System - Palo Alto   (650) 493-5000
VA Hlth Care Sys - Palo Alto
3801 Miranda Ave   Palo Alto, CA 94304   WEST COAST AND PACIFIC

VA Medical Center - Ann Arbor   (734) 769-7100
VA Med Ctr - Ann Arbor
2215 Fuller Rd   Ann Arbor, MI 48105   MIDWEST

VA Medical Center - Atlanta   (404) 321-6111
VA Med Ctr - Atlanta
1670 Clairmont Rd   Decatur, GA 30033   SOUTHEAST

VA Medical Center - Cleveland   (216) 791-3800
VA Med Ctr - Cleveland
10701 East Blvd   Cleveland, OH 44106   MIDWEST

VA Medical Center - Durham		(919) 286-0411
VA Med Ctr - Durham		
508 Fulton St	Durham, NC 27705	SOUTHEAST

VA Medical Center - Memphis		(901) 523-8990
VA Med Ctr - Memphis		
1030 Jefferson Ave	Memphis, TN 38104	SOUTHEAST

VA Medical Center - Nashville		(615) 327-4751
VA Med Ctr - Nashville		
1310 24th Ave S	Nashville, TN 37212	SOUTHEAST

VA Medical Center - Portland		(503) 220-8262
VA Medical Center - Portland		
3710 SW US Veteran Hospital Rd	Portland, OR 97239	WEST COAST AND PACIFIC

VA Medical Center - San Francisco		(415) 221-4810
VA Med Ctr - San Francisco		
4150 Clement St	San Francisco, CA 94121	WEST COAST AND PACIFIC

VA Medical Center - Washington, DC		(202) 745-8000
VA Med Ctr - Washington		
50 Irving St NW	Washington, DC 20422	MID ATLANTIC

VA Medical Center - West Los Angeles		(310) 478-3711
VA Med Ctr - W Los Angeles		
11301 Wilshire Blvd	Los Angeles, CA 90073	WEST COAST AND PACIFIC

VA Medical Center North Texas Health System		(214) 742-8387
VA Med Ctr N TX Hlth Sys		
4500 S Lancaster Rd	Dallas, TX 75216	SOUTHWEST

VA Puget Sound Health Care System		(206) 762-1010
VA Puget Sound Hlth Care Sys		
1660 S Columbian Way	Seattle, WA 98108	WEST COAST AND PACIFIC

VA San Diego Healthcare System		(858) 552-8585
VA San Diego Hlthcre Sys		
3350 La Jolla Village Drive	San Diego, CA 92161	WEST COAST AND PACIFIC

Vail Valley Medical Center		(970) 476-2451
Vail Valley Med Ctr		
181 W Meadow Dr	Vail, CO 81657-5058	GREAT PLAINS AND MOUNTAINS

Vanderbilt Children's Hospital		(615) 936-1000
Vanderbilt Children's Hosp		
2200 Children's Way	Nashville, TN 37232	SOUTHEAST

Vanderbilt University Medical Center   (615) 322-5000
Vanderbilt Univ Med Ctr
1313 21st Avenue South   Nashville, TN 37232   SOUTHEAST

Veterans Affairs Medical Center - Albuquerque   (505) 265-1711
VA Med Ctr
1501 San Pedro, SE   Albuquerque, NM 87108   SOUTHWEST

Veterans Affairs Medical Center - Augusta   (706) 733-0188
VA Medical Ctr - Augusta
One Freedom Way   Augusta, GA 30904   SOUTHEAST

Veterans Affairs Medical Center - Tucson   (520) 792-1450
VA Medical Center - Tucson
3601 S 6th Avenue   Tucson, AZ 85723   SOUTHWEST

Veterans Affairs Medical Center - White River Junction   (802) 295-9363
VA Aff Med Ctr - White River Junction
215 North Maine Street   White River Junction, VT 05009   NEW ENGLAND

Virginia Hospital Center - Arlington   (703) 558-5000
Virginia Hosp Ctr - Arlington
1701 N George Mason Dr   Arlington, VA 22205-3698   SOUTHEAST

Virginia Mason Medical Center   (206) 223-6600
Virginia Mason Med Ctr
1100 Ninth Ave, Box 900   Seattle, WA 98111   WEST COAST AND PACIFIC

Wake Forest University Baptist Medical Center   (336) 716-2011
Wake Forest Univ Baptist Med Ctr
Medical Center Blvd   Winston-Salem, NC 27157-1015   SOUTHEAST

WakeMed Cary Hospital   (919) 350-2300
WakeMed Cary
1900 Kildaire Farm Rd   Cary, NC 27511-6616   SOUTHEAST

WakeMed New Bern Avenue Campus   (919) 350-8000
WakeMed New Bern
3000 New Bern Ave   Raleigh, NC 27610   SOUTHEAST

Walter Reed Army Medical Center   (202) 782-3501
W Reed Army Med Ctr
6900 Georgia Ave NW   Washington, DC 20307-5001   MID ATLANTIC

Washington Hospital Center   (202) 877-7000
Washington Hosp Ctr
110 Irving St NW   Washington, DC 20010   MID ATLANTIC

Washington University Medical Center   (314) 362-6828
Washington Univ Med Ctr
4444 Forest Park Ave   St Louis, MO 63108   MIDWEST

WellStar Windy Hill Hospital   (770) 644-1000
WellStar Windy Hill Hosp
2540 Windy Hill Road   Marietta, GA 30067   SOUTHEAST

Wesley Woods Geriatric Hospital   (404) 728-6200
Wesley Woods Ger Hosp
1821 Clifton Rd   Atlanta, GA 30329   SOUTHEAST

West Jefferson Medical Center   (504) 347-5511
West Jefferson Med Ctr
1101 Medical Ctr Blvd   Marrero, LA 70072   SOUTHWEST

West Virginia University Hospital - Ruby Memorial   (304) 598-4000
WV Univ Hosp - Ruby Memorial
1 Medical Center Drive   Morgantown, WV 26506   MID ATLANTIC

Westchester Medical Center   (914) 493-7000
Westchester Med Ctr
95 Grasslands Road   Valhalla, NY 10595   MID ATLANTIC

Western Pennsylvania Hospital   (412) 578-5120
Western Penn Hosp
4800 Friendship Avenue   Pittsburgh, PA 15224   MID ATLANTIC

Western Psychiatric Institute and Clinic - UPMC   (412) 624-2100
Western Psych Inst & Clin - UPMC
3811 O'Hara St   Pittsburgh, PA 15213   MID ATLANTIC

Wheaton Franciscan Healthcare-St Joseph   (414) 447-2000
Wheaton Franciscan Hlthcare-St Joseph-Milwaukee
5000 W. Chambers Street   Milwaukee, WI 53210   MIDWEST

William Beaumont Hospital   (248) 551-5000
William Beaumont Hosp
3601 W 13 Mile Rd   Royal Oak, MI 48073   MIDWEST

William S Hall Psychiatric Institute   (803) 898-1693
William S Hall Psyc Inst
1800 Colonial Dr, Box 202   Columbia, SC 29202-6827   SOUTHEAST

Wills Eye Hospital   (215) 928-3000
Wills Eye Hosp
840 Walnut St   Philadelphia, PA 19107-5598   MID ATLANTIC

Winthrop - University Hospital		(516) 663-0333
Winthrop - Univ Hosp		
259 1st St	Mineola, NY 11501	MID ATLANTIC

Wishard Health Services		(317) 630-7592
Wishard Hlth Srvs		
1001 West 10th Street	Indianapolis, IN 46202	MIDWEST

Wolfson Children's Hospital		(904) 202-8000
Wolfson Chldns Hosp		
800 Prudential Dr	Jacksonville, FL 32207	SOUTHEAST

Woman's Hospital of Texas, The		(713) 790-1234
Woman's Hosp TX, The		
7600 Fannin St	Houston, TX 77054	SOUTHWEST

Women & Children's Hospital - Los Angeles		(323) 226-3427
Women & Children's Hosp - LA		
1240 North Mission Road	Los Angeles, CA 90033	WEST COAST AND PACIFIC

Women & Infants Hospital of Rhode Island		(401) 274-1100
Women & Infants Hosp of RI		
101 Dudley Street	Providence, RI 02905	NEW ENGLAND

Women's and Children's Hospital of Buffalo, The		(716) 878-7000
Women's & Chldn's Hosp of Buffalo, The		
219 Bryant St	Buffalo, NY 14222	MID ATLANTIC

Wright State University		(937) 775-2550
Wright State Univ		
3640 Colonel Glenn Hwy	Dayton, OH 45435-0001	MIDWEST

Yakima Valley Memorial Hospital		(509) 575-8000
Yakima Valley Mem Hosp		
2811 Tieton Dr	Yakima, WA 98902-3799	WEST COAST AND PACIFIC

Yale-New Haven Hospital		(203) 688-4242
Yale-New Haven Hosp		
20 York St	New Haven, CT 06510	NEW ENGLAND

Yampa Valley Medical Center		(970) 879-1322
Yampa Valley Med Ctr		
1024 Central Park Dr	Steamboat Springs, CO 80487	GREAT PLAINS AND MOUNTAINS

York Hospital		(717) 851-3500
York Hosp		
1001 S George St	York, PA 17405-7198	MID ATLANTIC

Zucker Hillside Hospital   (718) 470-8000
Zucker Hillside Hosp
75-59 263rd St   Glen Oaks, NY 11004   MID ATLANTIC

Appendix D:
Selected Resources

AMERICAN AMBULANCE ASSOCIATION (AAA)
The American Ambulance Association represents emergency and non-emergency medical transportation providers, advocating high quality pre-hospital care and keeping these providers aware of legislation and news that may affect them.

8201 Greensboro Drive, Ste 300
McLean, VA 22102

800-523-4447
703-610-9018
fax 703-610-9005
www.the-aaa.org/

AMERICA'S HEALTH INSURANCE PLANS (AHIP)
America's Health Insurance Plans is a national trade association representing nearly 1,300 member companies providing health benefits to more than 200 million Americans.

601 Pennsylvania Ave, NW
South Building Suite 500
Washington, DC 20004

202-778-3200
fax: 202-331-7487
www.ahip.org/

AMERICAN BOARD OF MEDICAL SPECIALTIES (ABMS)
The ABMS is the authoritative body for the recognition of medical specialties, coordinating 24 medical specialty boards (including 25 medical specialties) and providing information on the board certification of doctors.

1007 Church Street, Suite 404
Evanston, Illinois 60201-5913

847-491-9091 or 866-ASK-ABMS
fax 847-328-3596
www.abms.org

AMERICAN HOSPITAL ASSOCIATION (AHA)
A national health advocacy organization, the AHA represents hospitals and healthcare networks in legislative and regulatory matters. In 1973 the AHA adopted the Patient Bill of Rights to help patients understand their rights and responsibilities.

1 North Franklin
Chicago, IL 60606

325 7th St. NW
Washington, DC 20004

800-424-4301 or 312-422-3000
fax 312-422-4796
www.aha.org/
800-424-4301 or 202-638-1100
fax 202-626-2345

AMERICAN MEDICAL ASSOCIATION (AMA)

The AMA is an association that maintains information on physicians practicing throughout the nation. Healthcare consumers can use their database to check the location, licensing, education and specialty of many doctors in the United States.

515 North State Street
Chicago, IL 60610

800-621-8335
www.ama-assn.org/

CENTER FOR MEDICAL CONSUMERS

Provides volume and outcome data on certain medical procedures performed in New York state.

239 Thompson St.
New York, NY 10012

212-674-7105
fax 212-674-7100
medconsumers@earthlink.net
www.medicalconsumers.org

CENTERS FOR DISEASE CONTROL AND PREVENTION (CDC)

Part of the Department of Health and Human Services, the CDC's mission is to prevent and manage diseases and illnesses. Its Web site contains information on a range of illnesses and the research being pursued to manage them. It also provides free faxed reports on disease risk and prevention in various parts of the world.

Public Inquiries/MASO
Mailstop E11
1600 Clifton Road
Atlanta, GA 30333

1-800-311-3435

toll free number for international travelers 877 FYI-TRIP or 404-639-3534
fax information service for international travelers 888-232-3299
www.cdc.gov/netinfo.htm

THE CENTERWATCH CLINICAL TRIALS LISTING SERVICE

Profiles centers conducting clinical research by therapeutic area and geographic region, including more than 41,000 international industry and government-sponsored clinical trials and new FDA approved drug therapies, as well as 5,200 clinical trials that are actively recruiting patients.

100 N. Washington St
Ste 301
Boston, MA 02114

617-948-5100
fax 617-948-5101
www.centerwatch.com

HEALTH CARE CHOICES

Provides information on volume and outcomes of certain medical procedures performed in hospitals in various states throughout the country.

P.O. Box 21039
Columbus Circle Station
New York, NY 10023

212-724-9395
www.healthcarechoices.org
info@healthcarechoices.org

INTERNATIONAL ASSOCIATION FOR MEDICAL ASSISTANCE TO TRAVELLERS (IAMAT)

IAMAT is a non-profit organization that disseminates information on health and sanitary conditions worldwide. Membership is free but donations are appreciated. Members will receive a membership card making them eligible to access English speaking physicians all over the world. The organization also provides information on immunization requirements, malaria, and other tropical diseases, and sanitary and climactic conditions around the world. For information, send request in writing.

1623 Military Road #279
Niagra Falls, New York 14304-1745

716-754-4883
www.iamat.org

JOINT COMMISSION ON ACCREDITATION OF HEALTHCARE ORGANIZATIONS

The Joint Commission (JCAHO) is an independent, not-for-profit organization, which evaluates the quality and safety of care for nearly 17,000 health care organizations. To maintain and earn accreditation, organizations must have an extensive on-site review by a team of JCAHO health care professionals, at least once every three years. JCAHO is governed by a board that includes physicians, nurses, and consumers. JCAHO sets the standards by which health care quality is measured in America and around the world.

One Renaissance Boulevard
Oakbrook Terrace, IL 60181

630-792-5000
fax 630-792-5005
www.jcaho.org

MEDIC ALERT FOUNDATION

The Medic Alert Foundation (a non-profit organization) provides an "ID tag" engraved with personal medical facts, as well as a 24-hour emergency response center which can release additional personal medical details. Membership is $20/year (waived for the first year) and members need to purchase the "ID tag" which sells for as low as $35.

2323 Colorado Avenue
Turlock, CA 95382

888-633-4298
Fax 209-669-2450
www.medicalert.org

MEDLINE

One Medline Place
Mundelein, Illinois 60060

1-800-MEDLINE (800-633-5463)
fax 1-800-351-1512
www.medline.com

A medical database including millions of medical references and abstracts from thousands of scientific and medical journals.

THE NATIONAL CANCER INSTITUTE (NCI)

Part of the NIH, the NCI sponsors cancer clinical trials at more than 100 sites in the United States. Trials are carried out in major medical research centers, such as teaching hospitals, as well as in community hospitals, specialized medical clinics and even in doctors' offices.

Clinical Studies Support Center (CSSC)
6116 Executive Boulevard
Bethesda, MD 20892-8322

800-4-CANCER (800-422-6237)
www.nci.nih.gov
www.cancer.gov
cancergovstaff@mail.nih.gov

NATIONAL CENTER FOR COMPLEMENTARY AND ALTERNATIVE MEDICINE CLEARINGHOUSE (NCCAMC)

The NCCAMC facilitates the evaluation of alternative medical treatment modalities to help determine their effectiveness and bring alternative medicine into mainstream medicine. This agency does not provide referrals.

9000 Rockville Pike
Bethesda, MD 20892

888-644-6226
fax 866-464-3616
www.nccam.nih.gov
info@nccam.nih.gov

NATIONAL CONSUMERS LEAGUE (NCL)

NCL is a private, nonprofit consumer advocacy organization. NCL strives to investigate, educate, and advocate on a variety of issues including healthcare. Membership is $20 annually, but individuals can also write to the organization for a list of publications that non-members can purchase.

1701 K Street, NW, Suite 1200
Washington, DC 20006

202-835-3323
fax 202-835-0747
www.nclnet.org
info@nclnet.org

THE NATIONAL INSTITUTES OF HEALTH (NIH)

An organization operated by the U.S. government, the NIH operates its own hospital at which the care provided is usually related to clinical studies its researchers are undertaking. Information about the Warren G. Magnuson Clinical Center is also available.

Patient Recruitment Referral Center
9000 Rockville Pike
Bethesda, MD 20892

800-411-1222 or 301-496-4000
www.nih.gov
www.clinicaltrials.gov
nihinfo@od.nih.gov

NATIONAL INSURANCE INFORMATION INSTITUTE

The National Insurance Information Institute Helpline advises consumers on how to choose an insurance company or broker. It also offers an analysis of life insurance and assists in insurance complaints.

110 William St
New York, NY 10038

800-942-4242 or 212-346-5500
www.iii.org

THE PATIENT ADVOCATE FOUNDATION

A national non-profit organization that provides consultation, referrals and case management to patients to ensure that they are not denied access to healthcare, insurance coverage, employment and public assistance programs during an illness. In particular, the organization maintains comprehensive information on cancer treatment options that are available to consumers through a separate Web site: www.oncology.com.

700 Thimble Shoals Boulevard, Suite 200
Newport News, VA 23606

800-532-5274
fax 757-873-8999
www.patientadvocate.org/
help@patientadvocate.org

PEOPLE'S MEDICAL SOCIETY

The People's Medical Society, a nonprofit organization, is focused on educating the healthcare consumer about healthcare issues and medical rights. Their Web site provides information on useful books and publications as well as the latest healthcare developments.

P.O. Box 868
Allentown, PA 18105

610-770-1670
fax 610-770-0607
cbi@peoplesmed.org

PERSONS UNITED LIMITING SUBSTANDARDS AND ERRORS IN HEALTHCARE (P.U.L.S.E.)

A support group for the survivors of medical malpractice and substandard healthcare, this nonprofit group also advocates patient education and patient-doctor communication.

PO Box 353
3300 Park Avenue
Wantagh NY 11793-0353

800-96-pulse (800-967-8573) or
516-579-4711
fax: 516-520-8105
www.PULSEamerica.org
www.PULSEofNY.com
pulse516@aol.com

Colorado Office

719-250-1286
PULSECOLO@YAHOO.COM

PUBLIC CITIZEN'S HEALTH AND RESEARCH GROUP

A non-profit organization, the Public Citizen's Group acts as a watchdog agency by advocating accountability and the open use of doctors' disciplinary backgrounds.

1600 20th Street NW
Washington, D.C. 20009

202-588-1000
www.citizen.org/hrg/

VERITAS MEDICINE

An organization that allows individuals to perform confidential, personalized searches of their clinical trials database and to access information on new treatment and drug options. The text is submitted by Harvard-affiliated doctors.

11 Cambridge Center
Cambridge, Massachusetts 02142

617-234-1500 or
877-5-TRIALS (877-587-4257)
fax 617-234-1555
www.veritasmedicine.com
info@veritasmedicine.com

Indices

Subject Index

Postgraduate Training 10
Prevention Trials 27
Primary Care 1, 4, 7, 8, 15, 18, 19, 31, 42, 43, 49
Private Insurance 29
Professional Reputation 13
Protocol 27, 28, 30

R
Recertification 12, 50
Referral 2, 8, 18, 35, 53
Residency 10, 11, 16, 17, 37, 49, 50

S
Second Opinions 17
Selection Process 2
Self-Designated Medical Specialties 12
Side Effects 26, 27, 32, 33
Special Resources 25, 26, 28, 30, 32, 34
Specialists 1, 3, 4, 5, 6, 7, 8, 9, 10, 12, 14, 15, 16, 18, 37, 41, 43, 49, 50, 51, 53
Specialties xxiii, 2, 3, 5, 6, 9, 10, 11, 12, 14, 24, 38, 41, 42, 43, 44, 45, 46, 47, 49, 50, 51, 53
Standard Therapies 25
Subspecialties 1, 5, 6, 10, 12, 13, 15, 41, 42, 49, 50, 53

T
Therapeutic Approaches 1, 6, 25
Treatment Plan 21, 30
Treatment Studies 25, 30
Trust 19

U
United States Department of Health 33
United States Medical Licensing Exam 9

V

Veritas Medicine 26

W

Warren Grant Magnuson Clinical Center 33, 34, 35

Special Expertise Index

This index lists the areas that the physicians listed in the Guide have identified as their "special expertise." These are not medical specialties. They are specific elements of disease, procedures, techniques and treatments for which these physicians are best known and are referred patients.

Spec	Name	St	Pg

A

Abdominal Imaging

Spec	Name	St	Pg
DR	Berland, L	AL	850
DR	Fishman, E	MD	847
DR	Levy, A	MD	848
DR	Megibow, A	NY	848
DR	Sivit, C	OH	852
DR	Weinreb, J	CT	845

Abdominal Wall Reconstruction

PlS	Kuzon, W	MI	746
PlS	Stahl, R	CT	735

Abdominoplasty

PlS	Bermant, M	VA	742
PlS	Eriksson, E	MA	734
PlS	Matarasso, A	NY	739
PlS	Pitman, G	NY	739
PlS	Rand, R	WA	754

Abuse/Neglect

AM	Diaz, A	NY	78
ChAP	Zeanah, C	LA	785
Ger	Lachs, M	NY	235

Acne

D	Del Giudice, S	NH	168
D	Eichenfield, L	CA	181
D	James, W	PA	172
D	Lucky, A	OH	178
D	Shalita, A	NY	173

Acoustic Neuroma

NS	Adler, J	CA	425
NS	Eisenberg, H	MD	407
NS	Giannotta, S	CA	426
NS	Golfinos, J	NY	407
NS	Grubb, R	MO	419
NS	Gutin, P	NY	408
NS	Harsh, G	CA	427
NS	Martuza, R	MA	405
NS	Mayberg, M	WA	427
NS	Pitts, L	CA	428
NS	Stieg, P	NY	411
NS	Thompson, B	MI	421
Oto	Arriaga, M	PA	564
Oto	Beatty, C	MN	577
Oto	Brackmann, D	CA	587
Oto	Driscoll, C	MN	578
Oto	Feghali, J	NY	566
Oto	Jenkins, H	CO	584
Oto	Kveton, J	CT	563
Oto	Lambert, P	SC	574
Oto	Leonetti, J	IL	580
Oto	Linstrom, C	NY	569
Oto	Miyamoto, R	IN	581
Oto	Shelton, C	UT	584
Oto	Telian, S	MI	582
Oto	Wackym, P	WI	582
Oto	Wazen, J	FL	576
Oto	Wiet, R	IL	583
RadRO	Loeffler, J	MA	820

Acromegaly

EDM	Biller, B	MA	188
EDM	Klibanski, A	MA	189
EDM	Melmed, S	CA	202

Acupuncture

PM	Ngeow, J	NY	597
PMR	Dillard, J	NY	721

Acute Coronary Syndromes

Cv	Brindis, R	CA	112
Cv	Eagle, K	MI	105
IC	Henry, T	MN	122
IC	Holmes, D	MN	122

ADD/ADHD

ChAP	Abright, A	NY	781
ChAP	Biederman, J	MA	779
ChAP	Bird, H	NY	781
ChAP	Bogrov, M	MD	781
ChAP	Boxer, G	MO	784
ChAP	Coffey, B	NY	781
ChAP	Dulcan, M	IL	784
ChAP	Hertzig, M	NY	782
ChAP	Hudziak, J	VT	780
ChAP	Leventhal, B	IL	784
ChAP	Martini, D	IL	784
ChAP	Rostain, A	PA	782
ChAP	Russell, A	CA	786
ChAP	Slomowitz, M	IL	784
ChAP	Spencer, T	MA	780
ChAP	Turecki, S	NY	782
ChAP	Weller, E	PA	783
ChAP	Wilens, T	MA	781
N	Finkel, M	FL	449
Ped	Burgess, D	NJ	624
Ped	Jacob, M	IL	626
Psyc	Keepers, G	OR	775
Psyc	Manevitz, A	NY	767

ADD/ADHD-Neurofeedback Treatment

Psyc	Hoffman, D	CO	772

Addiction/Substance Abuse

AdP	Brady, K	SC	778
AdP	Frances, R	NY	778
AdP	Howell, E	UT	779
AdP	Kampman, K	PA	778
AdP	McCance-Katz, E	CA	779
AdP	Stine, S	MI	778
AdP	Strain, E	MD	778
ChAP	Deas, D	SC	783
ChAP	Wilens, T	MA	781
IM	Selwyn, P	NY	365
Psyc	Lawson, W	DC	767
Psyc	Rosenthal, R	NY	768
Psyc	Strakowski, S	OH	772
Psyc	Weinstock, R	CA	777

Adolescent Gynecology

AM	Diaz, A	NY	78
AM	Emans, S	MA	78
AM	Irwin, C	CA	79
AM	Kokotailo, P	WI	79
AM	Murray, P	PA	78
CG	Driscoll, D	PA	147
CG	Driscoll, D	PA	147
ObG	Laufer, M	MA	480
ObG	Merritt, D	MO	484
RE	Sanfilippo, J	PA	873

Adolescent Psychiatry

Psyc	Weinstock, R	CA	777

Adolescent Sports Medicine

SM	McKeag, D	IN	898
SM	Metzl, J	NY	897

Adolescent/Young Adult Cancers

PHO	Albritton, K	MA	651
PHO	Tebbi, C	FL	661

Special Expertise Index

Spec	Name	St	Pg
S	Levi, J	FL	918
S	Postier, R	OK	935
S	Soper, N	IL	929

Biochemical Genetics

Spec	Name	St	Pg
CG	Charrow, J	IL	149
CG	Charrow, J	IL	149
CG	Craigen, W	TX	150
CG	Craigen, W	TX	150
CG	Jonas, A	CA	152
CG	Jonas, A	CA	152
CG	Northrup, H	TX	151
CG	Northrup, H	TX	151

Biodefense

Spec	Name	St	Pg
Path	Walker, D	TX	616

Biomechanics-Arms

Spec	Name	St	Pg
HS	Trumble, T	WA	268

Bioterrorism Preparedness

Spec	Name	St	Pg
PrM	Hoffman, R	NY	759
PrM	Weiss, S	NJ	759
Pul	Tharratt, R	CA	812

Bipolar/Mood Disorders

Spec	Name	St	Pg
ChAP	Abright, A	NY	781
ChAP	Slomowitz, M	IL	784
ChAP	Weller, E	PA	783
ChAP	Wilens, T	MA	781
Psyc	Bowden, C	TX	773
Psyc	Calabrese, J	OH	770
Psyc	Davidson, J	TX	773
Psyc	DePaulo, J	MD	765
Psyc	Hirschfeld, R	TX	773
Psyc	Kupfer, D	PA	767
Psyc	Lawson, W	DC	767
Psyc	Levy, S	GA	770
Psyc	Nurnberger, J	IN	771
Psyc	Reus, V	CA	776
Psyc	Roy-Byrne, P	WA	776
Psyc	Strakowski, S	OH	772
Psyc	Sussman, N	NY	768
Psyc	Weiner, R	NC	770
Psyc	Weisler, R	NC	770

Bipolar/Mood Disorders-Consult

Spec	Name	St	Pg
Psyc	Oquendo, M	NY	767

Birth Defects

Spec	Name	St	Pg
CG	Carey, J	UT	150
CG	Carey, J	UT	150
CG	Cunniff, C	AZ	150
CG	Cunniff, C	AZ	150
CG	Desposito, F	NJ	147
CG	Desposito, F	NJ	147

Spec	Name	St	Pg
CG	Fernhoff, P	GA	148
CG	Fernhoff, P	GA	148
CG	Holmes, L	MA	146
CG	Holmes, L	MA	146
CG	Rimoin, D	CA	153
CG	Rimoin, D	CA	153
CG	Rosenbaum, K	DC	148
CG	Rosenbaum, K	DC	148
CG	Saul, R	SC	148
CG	Saul, R	SC	148
CG	Seaver, L	HI	153
CG	Seaver, L	HI	153
CG	Stevenson, R	SC	149
CG	Stevenson, R	SC	149
CG	Weaver, D	IN	150
CG	Weaver, D	IN	150
Ped	Bull, M	IN	625

Bladder Cancer

Spec	Name	St	Pg
Hem	Kuzel, T	IL	280
Onc	Ahmann, F	AZ	327
Onc	Benedetto, P	FL	305
Onc	Dawson, N	DC	293
Onc	Higano, C	WA	335
Onc	Hussain, M	MI	319
Onc	Logothetis, C	TX	330
Onc	Petrylak, D	NY	301
Onc	Raghavan, D	OH	321
Onc	Roth, B	TN	311
Onc	Scher, H	NY	302
Onc	Stadler, W	IL	323
Onc	Vaughn, D	PA	303
Path	Amin, M	CA	616
Path	Bostwick, D	VA	610
Path	Cote, R	CA	617
Path	Epstein, J	MD	605
Path	Reuter, V	NY	608
Path	True, L	WA	619
RadRO	Rotman, M	NY	825
RadRO	Shipley, W	MA	821
RadRO	Zelefsky, M	NY	826
U	Amling, C	AL	987
U	Bahnson, R	OH	992
U	Benson, M	NY	980
U	Campbell, S	OH	992
U	Carroll, P	CA	1002
U	Childs, S	CO	998
U	Cookson, M	TN	988
U	Crawford, E	CO	998
U	Danoff, D	CA	1002
U	Davis, B	KS	998
U	Droller, M	NY	981
U	El-Galley, R	AL	988
U	Flanigan, R	IL	993
U	Greenberg, R	PA	981
U	Grossman, H	TX	999
U	Herr, H	NY	982
U	Kibel, A	MO	994
U	Kim, E	TN	989
U	Kirschenbaum, A	NY	983
U	Lee, C	MI	994
U	Lerner, S	TX	1000

Spec	Name	St	Pg
U	Lockhart, J	FL	989
U	Loughlin, K	MA	978
U	Malkowicz, S	PA	983
U	McDougal, W	MA	978
U	Montie, J	MI	995
U	O'Donnell, M	IA	996
U	Pisters, L	TX	1000
U	Presti, J	CA	1004
U	Samadi, D	NY	984
U	Sawczuk, I	NJ	985
U	Scardino, P	NY	985
U	Scherr, D	NY	985
U	Schoenberg, M	MD	985
U	See, W	WI	996
U	Sheinfeld, J	NY	985
U	Skinner, D	CA	1004
U	Smith, J	TN	991
U	Soloway, M	FL	991
U	Steinberg, G	IL	997
U	Taneja, S	NY	986
U	Terris, M	GA	991
U	Theodorescu, D	VA	991
U	Uzzo, R	PA	986
U	Weiss, R	NJ	987
U	Williams, R	IA	997
U	Wood, D	MI	997
U	Zippe, C	OH	997

Bladder Exstrophy

Spec	Name	St	Pg
U	Canning, D	PA	980
U	Docimo, S	PA	980
U	Gearhart, J	MD	981

Bladder Reconstruction

Spec	Name	St	Pg
U	Carroll, P	CA	1002
U	Docimo, S	PA	980
U	Grossman, H	TX	999
U	Mitchell, M	WI	995
U	Sawczuk, I	NJ	985

Blastomycosis

Spec	Name	St	Pg
PInf	Kleiman, M	IN	674

Bleeding/Coagulation Disorders

Spec	Name	St	Pg
Cv	Vaughan, D	TN	103
Hem	Abrams, C	PA	273
Hem	Baron, J	IL	278
Hem	Blinder, M	MO	278
Hem	Bockenstedt, P	MI	278
Hem	Cobos, E	TX	283
Hem	Coller, B	NY	273
Hem	Cooper, B	TX	283
Hem	Diuguid, D	NY	273
Hem	Kempin, S	NY	274
Hem	Kessler, C	DC	274
Hem	Lin, W	AL	276
Hem	Lyons, R	TX	283
Hem	Ortel, T	NC	277

Special Expertise Index

America's Top Doctors® 8th Edition

Special Expertise Index

Special Expertise Index

Spec	Name	St	Pg
S	Babiera, G	TX	932
S	Bear, H	VA	915
S	Beauchamp, R	TN	915
S	Beitsch, P	TX	932
S	Bland, K	AL	916
S	Borgen, P	NY	905
S	Butler, J	CA	937
S	Byrd, D	WA	937
S	Calvo, B	NC	916
S	Chang, A	MI	923
S	Chang, H	CA	938
S	Crowe, J	OH	923
S	Dilawari, R	TN	916
S	Donohue, J	MN	923
S	Dooley, W	OK	933
S	Eberlein, T	MO	924
S	Edge, S	NY	907
S	Edney, J	NE	930
S	Edwards, M	OH	924
S	Eisenberg, B	NH	902
S	Esserman, L	CA	938
S	Estabrook, A	NY	908
S	Euhus, D	TX	933
S	Farrar, W	OH	924
S	Feig, B	TX	933
S	Frazier, T	PA	908
S	Gabram, S	GA	917
S	Giuliano, A	CA	939
S	Goodnight, J	CA	939
S	Goodson, W	CA	939
S	Goulet, R	IN	924
S	Grant, C	MN	925
S	Grant, M	TX	933
S	Gray, R	AZ	933
S	Hanks, J	VA	917
S	Harkema, J	MI	925
S	Herrmann, V	SC	917
S	Hoffman, J	PA	909
S	Hughes, K	MA	902
S	Hunt, K	TX	934
S	Iglehart, J	MA	902
S	Johnson, D	CA	939
S	Johnson, R	PA	909
S	Julian, T	PA	909
S	Kaufman, C	WA	940
S	Kavanah, M	MA	903
S	Kelley, M	TN	918
S	Kim, J	OH	925
S	Klimberg, V	AR	934
S	Knudson, M	CA	940
S	Krag, D	VT	903
S	Levine, E	NC	918
S	Li, B	LA	935
S	Lind, D	GA	918
S	Lyerly, H	NC	919
S	Mamounas, E	OH	926
S	McGrath, P	KY	919
S	McMasters, K	KY	919
S	Morrow, M	NY	910
S	Nathanson, S	MI	927
S	Nelson, E	UT	931
S	Newman, L	MI	927
S	Niederhuber, J	MD	911

Spec	Name	St	Pg
S	Nowak, E	NY	911
S	O'Hea, B	NY	911
S	Osborne, M	NY	911
S	Pockaj, B	AZ	935
S	Ponn, T	NH	903
S	Reintgen, D	FL	920
S	Roses, D	NY	913
S	Ross, M	TX	936
S	Schnabel, F	NY	913
S	Scott-Conner, C	IA	928
S	Sener, S	IL	928
S	Shenk, R	OH	928
S	Sigurdson, E	PA	913
S	Silverstein, M	CA	941
S	Singletary, S	TX	936
S	Skinner, K	NY	914
S	Smith, B	MA	903
S	Stahl, D	OH	929
S	Staren, E	IL	929
S	Stolier, A	LA	936
S	Swistel, A	NY	914
S	Tafra, L	MD	914
S	Tartter, P	NY	914
S	Tsangaris, T	MD	914
S	Tuttle, T	MN	929
S	Urist, M	AL	921
S	Wagman, L	CA	942
S	Walker, A	WI	930
S	Ward, B	CT	904
S	Weigel, R	IA	930
S	White, N	NC	921
S	Whitworth, P	TN	921
S	Willey, S	DC	914
S	Witt, T	IL	930
S	Wood, W	GA	922
S	Yeung, R	WA	942
S	Zannis, V	AZ	937

Breast Cancer & Surgery

Spec	Name	St	Pg
S	Anderson, B	WA	937
S	Leitch, A	TX	935

Breast Cancer Genetics

Spec	Name	St	Pg
ObG	Shulman, L	IL	484
Onc	Buys, S	UT	325
Onc	Graham, M	NC	308

Breast Cancer in Elderly

Spec	Name	St	Pg
S	Tartter, P	NY	914

Breast Cancer Risk Assessment

Spec	Name	St	Pg
GO	Cain, J	OR	255
Onc	Buys, S	UT	325
Onc	Daly, M	PA	293
Onc	Fabian, C	KS	325
Onc	Isaacs, C	DC	297
Onc	O'Regan, R	GA	311
Onc	Perez, E	FL	311
Onc	Stopeck, A	AZ	332
Path	Allred, D	MO	611

Spec	Name	St	Pg
S	Hansen, N	IL	925
S	Nathanson, S	MI	927

Breast Cancer Vaccine Therapy

Spec	Name	St	Pg
Onc	Serody, J	NC	312

Breast Cancer-Early Detection

Spec	Name	St	Pg
RadRO	Berg, C	MD	821

Breast Cancer-High Risk

Spec	Name	St	Pg
RadRO	Berg, C	MD	821

Breast Cancer-High Risk Women

Spec	Name	St	Pg
S	Estabrook, A	NY	908
S	Hansen, N	IL	925
S	Osborne, M	NY	911
S	Schnabel, F	NY	913

Breast Cancer-Novel Therapies

Spec	Name	St	Pg
Onc	Rugo, H	CA	338

Breast Cosmetic & Reconstructive Surgery

Spec	Name	St	Pg
PlS	Stahl, R	CT	735

Breast Disease

Spec	Name	St	Pg
S	Axelrod, D	NY	905
S	Estabrook, A	NY	908
S	Frazier, T	PA	908
S	Gabram, S	GA	917
S	Goodson, W	CA	939
S	Kaufman, C	WA	940
S	Osborne, M	NY	911
S	Swistel, A	NY	914
S	Ward, B	CT	904
S	Witt, T	IL	930

Breast Imaging

Spec	Name	St	Pg
DR	Abbitt, P	FL	850
DR	Bassett, L	CA	853
DR	Berg, W	MD	846
DR	Brem, R	DC	846
DR	Conant, E	PA	847
DR	Dershaw, D	NY	847
DR	Feig, S	CA	853
DR	Helvie, M	MI	851
DR	Hricak, H	NY	848
DR	Jackson, V	IN	851
DR	Kopans, D	MA	845
DR	Lehman, C	WA	853
DR	Orel, S	PA	849
DR	Otto, P	TX	853
DR	Pisano, E	NC	850
DR	Schepps, B	RI	845

Special Expertise Index

Special Expertise Index

Spec	Name	St	Pg
Cardiac Consultation			
Cv	Armstrong, W	MI	103
Cv	Greenberg, M	NY	96
Cardiac CT Angiography			
Cv	Poon, M	NY	98
DR	Edelman, R	IL	851
Cardiac Effects of Cancer/Cancer Therapy			
PCd	Steinherz, L	NY	632
Cardiac Electrophysiology			
Cv	Grubb, B	OH	105
Cv	Myerburg, R	FL	102
Cv	Naccarelli, G	PA	98
PCd	Dick, M	MI	634
PCd	Friedman, R	TX	636
PCd	Perry, J	MN	635
PCd	Walsh, E	MA	631
PCd	Young, M	FL	634
Cardiac Imaging			
Cv	Budoff, M	CA	112
Cv	Cerqueira, M	OH	104
Cv	Kaul, S	OR	113
Cv	Poon, M	NY	98
Cv	Schnittger, I	CA	114
DR	Bluemke, D	MD	846
DR	Fishman, E	MD	847
DR	Rubin, G	CA	853
DR	Strife, J	OH	852
NuM	Sandler, M	TN	476
NuM	Scheff, A	CA	477
NuM	Strauss, H	NY	475
Cardiac Imaging in Cancer Therapy			
NuM	Strauss, H	NY	475
Cardiac MRI			
Cv	Anderson, J	UT	109
DR	Flamm, S	OH	851
PCd	Weinberg, P	PA	632
Cardiac Pathology			
Path	Mark, E	MA	604
Path	Roberts, W	TX	616
PCd	Weinberg, P	PA	632
Cardiac Surgery			
PS	Ilbawi, M	IL	698
TS	Baumgartner, W	MD	952
TS	Dang, M	HI	970
TS	Dowling, R	KY	960

Spec	Name	St	Pg
TS	Flachsbart, K	CA	970
TS	Girardi, L	NY	954
TS	Isom, O	NY	955
TS	Karwande, S	UT	967
TS	Kopf, G	CT	950
TS	Lanza, L	AZ	969
TS	McGregor, C	MN	965
TS	Rosengart, T	NY	958
TS	Singh, A	RI	951
TS	Stuart, R	MO	967
TS	Tedder, M	TN	963
TS	Thistlethwaite, P	CA	973
TS	Trento, A	CA	973
TS	Turner, W	TX	970
TS	Ungerleider, R	OR	973
TS	Williams, D	FL	963
Cardiac Surgery-Adult			
TS	Conte, J	MD	953
TS	Diehl, J	PA	953
TS	Krieger, K	NY	956
TS	Merrick, S	CA	972
Cardiac Surgery-Adult & Pediatric			
PS	Spray, T	PA	695
TS	Calhoon, J	TX	968
TS	Christian, K	TN	959
TS	Drinkwater, D	TN	960
TS	Gundry, S	CA	971
TS	Kirklin, J	AL	961
TS	Merrill, W	OH	965
TS	Mullett, T	KY	961
TS	Ring, W	TX	969
Cardiac Surgery-High Risk			
TS	Furukawa, S	PA	953
TS	Gundry, S	CA	971
Cardiac Surgery-Neonatal			
TS	Bichell, D	TN	959
Cardiac Surgery-Neonatal & Pediatric			
TS	Brown, J	IN	963
Cardiac Surgery-Pediatric			
TS	Bailey, L	CA	970
TS	Bichell, D	TN	959
TS	Fontana, G	CA	970
TS	Harrell, J	TX	969
TS	Turrentine, M	IN	967
Cardiac Toxicity in Cancer Therapy			
Onc	Speyer, J	NY	302

Spec	Name	St	Pg
Cardiac Tumors, Myxomas			
TS	Grossi, E	NY	954
Cardiac Tumors/Cancer			
TS	Reardon, M	TX	969
Cardiogenic shock			
Cv	Parrillo, J	NJ	98
Cardiomyopathy			
Cv	Baughman, K	MA	92
Cv	Benjamin, I	UT	109
Cv	Bonow, R	IL	104
Cv	Fonarow, G	CA	113
Cv	Kereiakes, D	OH	106
Cv	Nishimura, R	MN	107
Cv	Reiss, C	MO	107
Cv	Stevenson, L	MA	94
PCd	Bernstein, D	CA	637
PCd	Boucek, R	WA	637
PCd	Dreyer, W	TX	636
PCd	Driscoll, D	MN	635
Cardiothoracic Surgery			
TS	Bains, M	NY	952
TS	Bull, D	UT	967
TS	Durham, S	OH	964
TS	Girardi, L	NY	954
TS	Glassford, D	TN	960
TS	Heidary, D	GA	960
TS	Magovern, G	PA	956
TS	Martin, T	FL	961
TS	Merrill, W	OH	965
Cardiovascular Disease			
Ger	Landefeld, C	CA	238
Ger	Minaker, K	MA	234
Ger	Wei, J	AR	238
IM	Legato, M	NY	364
Cardiovascular Disease/Young Adult			
Cv	Blumenthal, R	MD	95
Cardiovascular Imaging			
Cv	Schnittger, I	CA	114
DR	Flamm, S	OH	851
DR	Rubin, G	CA	853
DR	White, R	FL	850
Cardiovascular Interventional Radiology			
VIR	Gomes, A	CA	865

Special Expertise Index

Spec	Name	St	Pg
CE	Prystowsky, E	IN	118
CE	Wilber, D	IL	118

Celiac Disease

Spec	Name	St	Pg
Ge	DiMarino, A	PA	208
Ge	Elliott, D	IA	219
Ge	Green, P	NY	209
Ge	Murray, J	MN	221
Ge	Semrad, C	IL	222
PGe	Benkov, K	NY	646
PGe	Cohen, M	OH	648
PGe	Fasano, A	MD	646
PGe	Hill, I	NC	647
PGe	Hoffenberg, E	CO	649
PGe	Levy, J	NY	646
PGe	Newman, L	NY	646
PGe	Treem, W	NY	647

Cerebral Palsy

Spec	Name	St	Pg
ChiN	Brunstrom, J	MO	141
ChiN	Darras, B	MA	138
ChiN	Edgar, T	WI	141
ChiN	Eviatar, L	NY	139
ChiN	Noetzel, M	MO	141
ChiN	Volpe, J	MA	139
OrS	Sponseller, P	MD	537
OrS	Strongwater, A	NY	538
PMR	Matthews, D	CO	727

Cerebral Palsy-Select Dorsal Rhizotomy

Spec	Name	St	Pg
NS	Park, T	MO	420

Cerebrovascular Disease

Spec	Name	St	Pg
N	Adams, H	IA	452
N	Albers, G	CA	462
N	Burke, A	IL	453
N	Caronna, J	NY	438
N	Coull, B	AZ	459
N	Feldmann, E	RI	436
N	Fink, M	NY	440
N	Fisher, M	CA	463
N	Levine, S	NY	443
N	Wechsler, L	PA	447
N	Wityk, R	MD	447
NRad	Litt, A	NY	855
NRad	Masaryk, T	OH	858
NRad	Pile-Spellman, J	NY	855
NS	Atkinson, J	MN	416
NS	Hopkins, L	NY	408
NS	Samson, D	TX	424
NS	Sills, A	TN	415
VascS	Berguer, R	MI	1016
VascS	Cambria, R	MA	1010

Cerebrovascular Disease/Stroke

Spec	Name	St	Pg
NRad	Moran, C	MO	858

Spec	Name	St	Pg
NRad	Rowley, H	WI	858

Cerebrovascular Surgery

Spec	Name	St	Pg
NS	Al-Mefty, O	AR	423
NS	Dacey, R	MO	418
NS	David, C	MA	404
NS	Day, A	MA	404
NS	Flamm, E	NY	407
NS	Friedman, A	NC	413
NS	Grady, M	PA	408
NS	Gutierrez, F	IL	419
NS	Heros, R	FL	413
NS	Kassam, A	PA	409
NS	Link, M	MN	419
NS	Loftus, C	PA	409
NS	Malik, G	MI	419
NS	Origitano, T	IL	420
NS	Rosenwasser, R	PA	410
NS	Spetzler, R	AZ	425
NS	Stieg, P	NY	411
NS	Wilson, J	NC	416

Cervical Cancer

Spec	Name	St	Pg
GO	Abu-Rustum, N	NY	245
GO	Alleyn, J	FL	248
GO	Belinson, J	OH	251
GO	Berek, J	CA	254
GO	Berman, M	CA	254
GO	Bristow, R	MD	245
GO	Caputo, T	NY	246
GO	Creasman, W	SC	248
GO	De Geest, K	IA	251
GO	DePriest, P	KY	248
GO	Di Saia, P	CA	255
GO	Dunton, C	PA	246
GO	Edwards, R	PA	246
GO	Finan, M	AL	249
GO	Fiorica, J	FL	249
GO	Follen, M	TX	253
GO	Goff, B	WA	255
GO	Hatch, K	AZ	254
GO	Herzog, T	NY	247
GO	Horowitz, I	GA	249
GO	Johnston, C	MI	251
GO	Kelley, J	PA	247
GO	Koulos, J	NY	247
GO	Levenback, C	TX	254
GO	Monk, B	CA	255
GO	Muto, M	MA	244
GO	Penalver, M	FL	250
GO	Potkul, R	IL	252
GO	Remmenga, S	NE	253
GO	Rice, L	WI	252
GO	Rose, P	OH	252
GO	Rotmensch, J	IL	252
GO	Rubin, S	PA	248
GO	Rutherford, T	CT	244
GO	Schwartz, P	CT	245
GO	Smith, D	IL	252
GO	Soisson, A	UT	253
GO	Van Nagell, J	KY	250

Spec	Name	St	Pg
GO	Waggoner, S	OH	253
GO	Walker, J	OK	254
ObG	Lipscomb, G	IL	484
ObG	Noller, K	MA	480
Onc	Bookman, M	PA	291
Path	Cho, K	MI	612
Path	Gupta, P	PA	606
RadRO	Eifel, P	TX	834

Charcot Marie Tooth Disease

Spec	Name	St	Pg
PMR	Carter, G	WA	729

Chemical Exposure

Spec	Name	St	Pg
A&I	Ein, D	DC	83
A&I	Fishman, H	DC	83
OM	Gochfeld, M	NJ	758
Pul	Bascom, R	PA	796

Chemo-Radiation Combined Therapy

Spec	Name	St	Pg
RadRO	Formenti, S	NY	822
RadRO	Rich, T	VA	828

Chemoembolization & Tumor Ablation

Spec	Name	St	Pg
VIR	Bettmann, M	NC	862
VIR	Cho, K	MI	863
VIR	Darcy, M	MO	863

Chest Diseases-Benign

Spec	Name	St	Pg
TS	Nesbitt, J	TN	962

Chest Pain-Non Cardiac

Spec	Name	St	Pg
Ge	Brazer, S	NC	214
Ge	Rao, S	IA	221

Chest Radiology

Spec	Name	St	Pg
DR	Austin, J	NY	846
DR	Black, W	NH	845

Chest Wall Deformities

Spec	Name	St	Pg
PS	Aiken, J	WI	697
PS	Glick, P	NY	694
PS	Nuss, D	VA	696
PS	Paidas, C	FL	696
PS	Shochat, S	TN	697
PS	Stylianos, S	FL	697

Chest Wall Deformities-Pediatric

Spec	Name	St	Pg
PPul	Kim, Y	IN	687
PPul	Redding, G	WA	689

Chest Wall Reconstruction

Spec	Name	St	Pg
PlS	Seyfer, A	MD	740

Special Expertise Index

Spec	Name	St	Pg
PlS	Napoli, J	DE	739
PlS	Reinisch, J	CA	754
PlS	Seyfer, A	MD	740
PlS	Stal, S	TX	750
PlS	Vander Kolk, C	MD	741
PlS	Wells, J	CA	755
PO	Haddad, J	NY	681

Clinical Trials

Spec	Name	St	Pg
AdP	Anton, R	SC	778
D	Bowen, G	UT	179
EDM	Hoogwerf, B	OH	197
EDM	Riddle, M	OR	203
Ge	Gish, R	CA	227
Ge	Greenwald, B	MD	209
Ge	Hanauer, S	IL	219
GO	Coukos, G	PA	246
GO	De Geest, K	IA	251
GO	Edwards, R	PA	246
GO	Follen, M	TX	253
GO	Muntz, H	WA	255
GO	Odunsi, A	NY	247
GO	Stehman, F	IN	253
GO	Teng, N	CA	256
Hem	Dezube, B	MA	272
Hem	Flynn, P	MN	278
Hem	Grever, M	OH	279
Hem	Kraut, E	OH	280
Hem	Maddox, A	AR	284
Hem	O'Donnell, M	CA	285
IM	Wolff, R	TX	366
Inf	Mildvan, D	NY	352
N	Janss, A	GA	449
N	Levin, V	TX	461
N	Lipton, R	NY	443
N	Mitsumoto, H	NY	444
N	Wolinsky, J	TX	461
NS	Brem, S	FL	412
NS	Markert, J	AL	414
NS	Sampson, J	NC	415
NS	Shaffrey, M	VA	415
NS	Yu, J	CA	429
Onc	Abbruzzese, J	TX	327
Onc	Akerley, W	UT	324
Onc	Argiris, A	PA	290
Onc	Arun, B	TX	327
Onc	Bernard, S	NC	305
Onc	Butler, W	SC	306
Onc	Carducci, M	MD	292
Onc	Chang, J	TX	328
Onc	Chu, E	CT	287
Onc	Cohen, R	PA	292
Onc	Disis, M	WA	334
Onc	Ellis, G	WA	334
Onc	Ensminger, W	MI	318
Onc	Estey, E	WA	334
Onc	Ettinger, D	MD	294
Onc	Fine, R	NY	294
Onc	Flinn, I	TN	307
Onc	Haas, N	PA	296
Onc	Hauke, R	NE	326
Onc	Hortobagyi, G	TX	329

Spec	Name	St	Pg
Onc	Kaminski, M	MI	320
Onc	Karp, J	MD	298
Onc	Kaufman, P	NH	288
Onc	Kraft, A	SC	309
Onc	Limentani, S	NC	309
Onc	Marcom, P	NC	310
Onc	Maslak, P	NY	299
Onc	Mortimer, J	CA	337
Onc	O'Regan, R	GA	311
Onc	O'Reilly, E	NY	300
Onc	Orlowski, R	TX	331
Onc	Perez, E	FL	311
Onc	Pinto, H	CA	337
Onc	Remick, S	WV	301
Onc	Robert-Vizcarrondo, F	AL	311
Onc	Ross, H	AZ	331
Onc	Rothenberg, M	TN	311
Onc	Schilder, R	PA	302
Onc	Schuchter, L	PA	302
Onc	Serody, J	NC	312
Onc	Shibata, S	CA	338
Onc	Sikic, B	CA	338
Onc	Sotomayor, E	FL	313
Onc	Vogel, V	PA	303
Onc	Worden, F	MI	324
Oto	Weisman, R	CA	589
Path	Wilczynski, S	CA	619
PHO	Adamson, P	PA	652
PHO	Barredo, J	FL	658
PHO	Blaney, S	TX	668
PHO	Bruggers, C	UT	667
PHO	Croop, J	IN	663
PHO	Goldman, S	IL	664
PHO	Jakacki, R	PA	655
PHO	Kadota, R	CA	670
PHO	Kreissman, S	NC	660
PHO	Maris, J	PA	656
PHO	Meadows, A	PA	656
PHO	Neuberg, R	SC	660
PHO	Razzouk, B	IN	665
PHO	Rheingold, S	PA	657
PHO	Rosenthal, J	CA	671
PHO	Sandler, E	FL	661
PHO	Vik, T	IN	666
PInf	Edwards, K	TN	674
Psyc	Mann, J	NY	767
RadRO	Koh, W	WA	837
RadRO	Le, Q	CA	837
RadRO	McGarry, R	KY	828
RadRO	Senzer, N	TX	835
RadRO	Willett, C	NC	829
S	Averbook, B	OH	922
S	Julian, T	PA	909
S	Pockaj, B	AZ	935
S	Ramanathan, R	PA	912
S	Willey, S	DC	914
S	Yang, J	MD	915
TS	Pass, H	NY	957
U	Keane, T	SC	989
U	Theodorescu, D	VA	991

Clinical Trials Only

Spec	Name	St	Pg
Onc	Arlen, P	MD	291
Onc	Gulley, J	MD	296

Clostridium Difficile Disease

Ge	Surawicz, C	WA	228

Clotting Disorders in Pregnancy

MF	Paidas, M	CT	371

Clubfoot

OrS	Aronson, J	AR	549
OrS	Beaty, J	TN	539
OrS	Davidson, R	PA	530
OrS	Herzenberg, J	MD	532

Clubfoot/Foot Deformities in Children

OrS	Lehman, W	NY	534
OrS	Oppenheim, W	CA	553

Coarctation of the Aorta

PCd	Hijazi, Z	IL	635

Cocaine Addiction

AdP	Kampman, K	PA	778
AdP	Kleber, H	NY	778
AdP	Kosten, T	TX	779

Coccidioidomycosis

Inf	Bayer, A	CA	358
Pul	Catanzaro, A	CA	810

Cochlear Implants

Oto	Arts, H	MI	577
Oto	Balkany, T	FL	572
Oto	Daspit, C	AZ	585
Oto	Driscoll, C	MN	578
Oto	Gantz, B	IA	579
Oto	Kveton, J	CT	563
Oto	Linstrom, C	NY	569
Oto	Macias, J	AZ	585
Oto	Miyamoto, R	IN	581
Oto	Nadol, J	MA	563
Oto	Parisier, S	NY	569
Oto	Pillsbury, H	NC	575
Oto	Shelton, C	UT	584
Oto	Telian, S	MI	582
Oto	Wackym, P	WI	582
Oto	Young, N	IL	583
PO	Arjmand, E	OH	682
PO	Belenky, W	MI	682
PO	Kazahaya, K	PA	681
PO	Lusk, R	NE	683
PO	Rosbe, K	CA	684

Special Expertise Index

Special Expertise Index

Spec	Name	St	Pg
TS	Pagani, F	MI	966
TS	Quintessenza, J	FL	962
TS	Sellke, F	MA	951
TS	Smith, P	NC	962
TS	Strong, M	PA	958
TS	Tranbaugh, R	NY	958
TS	Turner, W	TX	970
TS	Verrier, E	WA	973

Coronary Disease in Black Populations

Spec	Name	St	Pg
Cv	Saunders, E	MD	98

Coronary Intensive Care

Spec	Name	St	Pg
Cv	Nissen, S	OH	107

Coronary Radiation Therapy

Spec	Name	St	Pg
IC	Teirstein, P	CA	124

Coronary Revascularization

Spec	Name	St	Pg
TS	Merrick, S	CA	972
TS	Ring, W	TX	969

Cosmetic & Reconstructive Surgery

Spec	Name	St	Pg
PlS	Hardesty, R	CA	752
PlS	Low, D	PA	738
PlS	Puckett, C	MO	747

Cosmetic & Reconstructive Surgery-Face

Spec	Name	St	Pg
Oto	Branham, G	MO	578
Oto	Mangat, D	KY	574

Cosmetic Dermatology

Spec	Name	St	Pg
D	Alster, T	DC	170
D	Anderson, R	MA	168
D	Arndt, K	MA	168
D	Berg, D	WA	181
D	Brandt, F	NY	170
D	Brody, H	GA	174
D	Dover, J	MA	168
D	Fitzpatrick, R	CA	181
D	Geronemus, R	NY	171
D	Glogau, R	CA	181
D	Gordon, M	NY	171
D	Hanke, C	IN	177
D	Kilmer, S	CA	182
D	Klein, A	CA	182
D	Kriegel, D	NY	172
D	Lask, G	CA	182
D	Menter, M	TX	180
D	Rigel, D	NY	173
D	Rubin, M	CA	182
D	Schultz, N	NY	173
D	Sobel, S	FL	177

Spec	Name	St	Pg
D	Sokoloff, D	FL	177
D	Swanson, N	OR	182
D	Wheeland, R	MO	179
PlS	Hunstad, J	NC	743

Cosmetic Surgery

Spec	Name	St	Pg
D	Brody, H	GA	174
D	Hruza, G	MO	178
PlS	Barone, C	TX	748
PlS	Brink, R	CA	751
PlS	Burns, A	TX	749
PlS	Dufresne, C	MD	737
PlS	Fodor, P	CA	752
PlS	Gold, A	NY	737
PlS	Grossman, J	CO	748
PlS	Hagan, K	TN	743
PlS	Kawamoto, H	CA	753
PlS	Kelly, K	TN	743
PlS	Lesavoy, M	CA	753
PlS	Manson, P	MD	739
PlS	May, J	MA	734
PlS	Menick, F	AZ	749
PlS	Morgan, R	VA	744
PlS	Noone, R	PA	739
PlS	Persing, J	CT	735
PlS	Persing, J	CT	735
PlS	Romano, J	CA	754
PlS	Serletti, J	PA	740
PlS	Tobin, G	KY	744
PlS	Vander Kolk, C	MD	741
PlS	Vogt, P	MN	747
PlS	Wolfe, S	FL	744

Cosmetic Surgery-Breast

Spec	Name	St	Pg
PlS	Aston, S	NY	735
PlS	Bucky, L	PA	736
PlS	Eriksson, E	MA	734
PlS	Fisher, G	CA	751
PlS	Friedland, J	AZ	749
PlS	Grotting, J	AL	742
PlS	Hardesty, R	CA	752
PlS	Hidalgo, D	NY	737
PlS	Horowitz, J	CA	752
PlS	Jewell, M	OR	752
PlS	Leaf, N	CA	753
PlS	Leipziger, L	NY	738
PlS	Maxwell, G	TN	743
PlS	Mustoe, T	IL	746
PlS	Paul, M	CA	754
PlS	Rand, R	WA	754
PlS	Romano, J	CA	754
PlS	Rosenberg, H	CA	754
PlS	Singer, R	CA	754
PlS	Stevenson, T	CA	754
PlS	Sullivan, P	RI	735
PlS	Sultan, M	NY	740

Cosmetic Surgery-Face

Spec	Name	St	Pg
Oto	Becker, F	FL	572
Oto	Chowdhury, K	CO	584

Spec	Name	St	Pg
Oto	Denenberg, S	NE	584
Oto	Hopping, S	DC	567
Oto	Johnson, C	LA	585
Oto	Keller, G	CA	588
Oto	Larrabee, W	WA	588
Oto	Lawson, W	NY	569
Oto	Papel, I	MD	569
Oto	Szachowicz, E	MN	582
Oto	Toriumi, D	IL	582
PlS	Aston, S	NY	735
PlS	Baker, D	NY	736
PlS	Barton, F	TX	748
PlS	Beals, S	AZ	748
PlS	Bucky, L	PA	736
PlS	Byrd, H	TX	749
PlS	Carraway, J	VA	742
PlS	Chiu, D	NY	736
PlS	Daniel, R	CA	751
PlS	Feldman, J	MA	734
PlS	Fisher, G	CA	751
PlS	Gregory, R	FL	742
PlS	Hamra, S	TX	749
PlS	Hester, T	GA	743
PlS	Hidalgo, D	NY	737
PlS	Hoefflin, S	CA	752
PlS	Hoffman, L	NY	737
PlS	Horowitz, J	CA	752
PlS	Hurwitz, D	PA	738
PlS	Imber, G	NY	738
PlS	Jewell, M	OR	752
PlS	Kelly, J	OK	749
PlS	Koplin, L	CA	753
PlS	Leaf, N	CA	753
PlS	Little, J	DC	738
PlS	Markowitz, B	CA	753
PlS	Marten, T	CA	753
PlS	Maxwell, G	TN	743
PlS	McCarthy, J	NY	739
PlS	Miller, T	CA	753
PlS	Mustoe, T	IL	746
PlS	Nichter, L	CA	753
PlS	Paul, M	CA	754
PlS	Pitman, G	NY	739
PlS	Posnick, J	MD	739
PlS	Ramirez, O	MD	739
PlS	Rand, R	WA	754
PlS	Ristow, B	CA	754
PlS	Rosenberg, H	CA	754
PlS	Siebert, J	NY	740
PlS	Singer, R	CA	754
PlS	Spinelli, H	NY	740
PlS	Staffenberg, D	NY	740
PlS	Stevenson, T	CA	754
PlS	Stuzin, J	FL	744
PlS	Sullivan, P	RI	735
PlS	Sultan, M	NY	740
PlS	Tabbal, N	NY	741
PlS	Vasconez, L	AL	744
PlS	Walton, R	IL	747
PlS	Whitaker, L	PA	741
PlS	Zins, J	OH	748

Special Expertise Index

Special Expertise Index

America's Top Doctors® 8th Edition

Special Expertise Index

Special Expertise Index

Special Expertise Index

Spec	Name	St	Pg

Ethics

Spec	Name	St	Pg
Ger	Finucane, T	MD	234
MF	Chervenak, F	NY	371
NP	Boyle, R	VA	384
NP	Lemons, J	IN	386
NP	Meadow, W	IL	386
NP	Muraskas, J	IL	386
Onc	Brescia, F	SC	305
Onc	Levy, M	PA	298
Ped	Fost, N	WI	625
Ped	Lantos, J	IL	626
PHO	Morgan, E	IL	665

Ethnic Skin Disorders

Spec	Name	St	Pg
D	Grimes, P	CA	182

Ewing's Sarcoma

Spec	Name	St	Pg
OrS	McDonald, D	MO	546
Ped	Kleinerman, E	TX	626
PHO	Grier, H	MA	651
PHO	Hawkins, D	WA	670

Exercise Physiology

Spec	Name	St	Pg
PCd	Driscoll, D	MN	635
PMR	Gater, D	VA	723
Rhu	Bunning, R	DC	883

Exercise Therapy

Spec	Name	St	Pg
Ger	Schwartz, R	CO	237

Eye Diseases-Hereditary

Spec	Name	St	Pg
CG	Pagon, R	WA	152
CG	Pagon, R	WA	152
Oph	Gorin, M	CA	517
Oph	Lewis, R	TX	514
Oph	Murphree, A	CA	519
Oph	Stone, E	IA	511

Eye Growth/Development

Spec	Name	St	Pg
Oph	Quinn, G	PA	499

Eye Movement Disorders

Spec	Name	St	Pg
N	Lavin, P	TN	450

Eye Muscle Disorders

Spec	Name	St	Pg
Oph	Choy, A	CA	516
Oph	Ellis, G	LA	513
Oph	Granet, D	CA	517
Oph	Hall, L	NY	496
Oph	Hunter, D	MA	492
Oph	Mahon, K	NV	518
Oph	McKeown, C	FL	504
Oph	Mills, M	PA	499
Oph	Nelson, L	PA	499
Oph	Wang, F	NY	502

Eye Muscle Surgery

Spec	Name	St	Pg
Oph	Burke, M	OH	507
Oph	Koller, H	PA	497
Oph	Richard, J	OK	514
Oph	Rosenberg, M	IL	511

Eye Pathology

Spec	Name	St	Pg
Oph	Rao, N	CA	519

Eye Tumors-Pediatric

Spec	Name	St	Pg
Oph	Lueder, G	MO	509

Eye Tumors/Cancer

Spec	Name	St	Pg
Oph	Abramson, D	NY	493
Oph	Albert, D	WI	506
Oph	Augsburger, J	OH	507
Oph	Boxrud, C	CA	516
Oph	Char, D	CA	516
Oph	Dutton, J	NC	503
Oph	Finger, P	NY	495
Oph	Haik, B	TN	503
Oph	Harbour, J	MO	508
Oph	Mieler, W	IL	510
Oph	Murray, T	FL	504
Oph	O'Brien, J	CA	519
Oph	Shields, J	PA	501
Oph	Soparkar, C	TX	515
Oph	Sternberg, P	TN	505
Oph	Weingeist, T	IA	512
Oph	Wilson, D	OR	520
Oph	Wilson, M	TN	506
RadRO	Crocker, I	GA	826
RadRO	Markoe, A	FL	827
RadRO	McCormick, B	NY	824
RadRO	Quivey, J	CA	837

Eyelid Cancer & Reconstruction

Spec	Name	St	Pg
Oph	Cockerham, K	CA	516
Oph	Gigantelli, J	NE	513
Oph	Nerad, J	IA	510
Oph	Rubin, P	MA	493
PlS	Miller, T	CA	753

Eyelid Cosmetic & Reconstructive Surgery

Spec	Name	St	Pg
Oph	Lisman, R	NY	498
Oph	Rubin, P	MA	493

Eyelid Problems/Ptosis/Blepharospasm

Spec	Name	St	Pg
Oph	Anderson, R	UT	512

Eyelid Surgery

Spec	Name	St	Pg
Oph	Baylis, H	CA	515
Oto	Larrabee, W	WA	588

Eyelid Surgery / Blepharoplasty

Spec	Name	St	Pg
Oph	Carter, K	IA	507

Eyelid Tumors/Cancer

Spec	Name	St	Pg
Oph	Della Rocca, R	NY	495
Oph	Tse, D	FL	506

Eyelid/Tear Duct Reconstruction

Spec	Name	St	Pg
Oph	Lisman, R	NY	498

F

Fabry's Disease

Spec	Name	St	Pg
CG	Desnick, R	NY	147
CG	Desnick, R	NY	147
N	Kolodny, E	NY	442

Facial Deformities/Reconstruction

Spec	Name	St	Pg
PlS	Bentz, M	WI	745

Facial Implants (Endoscopic)

Spec	Name	St	Pg
PlS	Ramirez, O	MD	739

Facial Nerve Disorders

Spec	Name	St	Pg
Oto	Bojrab, D	MI	578
Oto	Brackmann, D	CA	587
Oto	Lalwani, A	NY	568
Oto	Shelton, C	UT	584
Oto	Wax, M	OR	589
PlS	Manders, E	PA	738

Facial Paralysis

Spec	Name	St	Pg
Oto	Pensak, M	OH	581
PlS	Sherman, R	CA	754

Facial Paralysis Reconstruction

Spec	Name	St	Pg
PlS	Kuzon, W	MI	746

Facial Plastic & Reconstructive Surgery

Spec	Name	St	Pg
Oto	Day, T	SC	573
Oto	Hayden, R	AZ	585
Oto	Marentette, L	MI	580

Special Expertise Index

Special Expertise Index

Spec	Name	St	Pg
Ge	Hodges, D	TX	225
PGe	Rudolph, C	WI	649

Gastrointestinal Imaging

Spec	Name	St	Pg
DR	Berland, L	AL	850
DR	Megibow, A	NY	848

Gastrointestinal Metabolic Surgery

Spec	Name	St	Pg
S	Rubino, F	NY	913

Gastrointestinal Motility Disorders

Spec	Name	St	Pg
Ge	Achkar, E	OH	218
Ge	Castell, D	SC	214
Ge	Drossman, D	NC	215
Ge	Fisher, R	PA	208
Ge	Korsten, M	NY	210
Ge	Metz, D	PA	212
Ge	Owyang, C	MI	221
Ge	Pasricha, P	TX	226
Ge	Reynolds, J	PA	212
Ge	Shaker, R	WI	222
Ge	Wald, A	WI	222
PGe	Rudolph, C	WI	649
S	Sarr, M	MN	928

Gastrointestinal Pathology

Spec	Name	St	Pg
Path	Appelman, H	MI	612
Path	Chandrasoma, P	CA	617
Path	Crawford, J	FL	610
Path	Fogt, F	PA	606
Path	Goldblum, J	OH	612
Path	Greenson, J	MI	613
Path	Hamilton, S	TX	615
Path	Hruban, R	MD	606
Path	Mitros, F	IA	613
Path	Montgomery, E	MD	608
Path	Odze, R	MA	604
Path	Petras, R	OH	613
Path	Rashid, A	TX	616
Path	Rutgers, J	CA	619
Path	Silverman, J	PA	609

Gastrointestinal Stromal Tumors

Spec	Name	St	Pg
Hem	Heinrich, M	OR	284
Onc	von Mehren, M	PA	304
PHO	Wexler, L	NY	658

Gastrointestinal Surgery

Spec	Name	St	Pg
CRS	Longo, W	CT	158
PS	Barksdale, E	OH	697
PS	Ginsburg, H	NY	693
PS	Gittes, G	PA	693
PS	Oldham, K	WI	698
PS	Ricketts, R	GA	696
PS	Schwartz, M	PA	694

Spec	Name	St	Pg
PS	Warner, B	MO	699
PS	Ziegler, M	CO	700
S	Becker, J	MA	902
S	Brody, F	DC	906
S	Brooks, D	MA	902
S	Essner, R	CA	939
S	Fitzgibbons, R	NE	930
S	Greene, F	NC	917
S	Howard, R	FL	918
S	Koruda, M	NC	918
S	Livingston, E	TX	935
S	MacDonald, K	NC	919
S	MacFadyen, B	GA	919
S	Mulvihill, S	UT	931
S	Nowak, E	NY	911
S	Pachter, H	NY	911
S	Park, A	MD	911
S	Peitzman, A	PA	912
S	Ponsky, J	OH	927
S	Rogers, S	CA	941
S	Rosemurgy, A	FL	920
S	Satava, R	WA	941
S	Schirmer, B	VA	920
S	Schlinkert, R	AZ	936
S	Schraut, W	PA	913
S	Sharp, K	TN	920
S	Sinanan, M	WA	941
S	Stratta, R	NC	921
S	Sweeney, J	GA	921
S	Vickers, S	MN	930
S	Walsh, R	OH	930
S	Zinner, M	MA	904

Gastroparesis

Spec	Name	St	Pg
Ge	Schulze, K	IA	221

Gastroscopy

Spec	Name	St	Pg
Ge	Gostout, C	MN	219
IM	Yaffe, B	NY	365

Gaucher Disease

Spec	Name	St	Pg
CG	Desnick, R	NY	147
CG	Desnick, R	NY	147
N	Kolodny, E	NY	442

Gender Reassignment Surgery

Spec	Name	St	Pg
PlS	Alter, G	CA	751
PlS	Kuzon, W	MI	746
PlS	Meltzer, T	AZ	749

Gender Specific Medicine

Spec	Name	St	Pg
IM	Legato, M	NY	364

Gene Targeted Radiotherapy

Spec	Name	St	Pg
RadRO	Senzer, N	TX	835
RadRO	Weichselbaum, R	IL	833

Gene Therapy

Spec	Name	St	Pg
Cv	Dichek, D	WA	112
GO	Lancaster, J	FL	249
Hem	Brenner, M	TX	282
Hem	Gewirtz, A	PA	273
Onc	Hortobagyi, G	TX	329
Onc	Sotomayor, E	FL	313
PHO	Neuberg, R	SC	660
RadRO	Senzer, N	TX	835
S	Cole, D	SC	916
S	Hunt, K	TX	934
TS	Roth, J	TX	969
U	Belldegrun, A	CA	1001
U	Malkowicz, S	PA	983
U	Miles, B	TX	1000
VascS	Comerota, A	OH	1016

Gene Therapy Delivery Systems

Spec	Name	St	Pg
VIR	Wood, B	MD	862

Gene Therapy-Cardiac Angiogenesis

Spec	Name	St	Pg
Cv	Sanborn, T	IL	108
TS	Rosengart, T	NY	958

Genetic Biochemical Disorders

Spec	Name	St	Pg
CG	Beaudet, A	TX	150
CG	Beaudet, A	TX	150

Genetic Blood Disorders

Spec	Name	St	Pg
PHO	Glader, B	CA	670

Genetic Disorders

Spec	Name	St	Pg
CG	Desposito, F	NJ	147
CG	Desposito, F	NJ	147
CG	Grody, W	CA	152
CG	Grody, W	CA	152
CG	Mulvihill, J	OK	151
CG	Mulvihill, J	OK	151
CG	Nussbaum, R	CA	152
CG	Nussbaum, R	CA	152
CG	Ostrer, H	NY	147
CG	Ostrer, H	NY	147
CG	Sutphen, R	FL	149
CG	Sutphen, R	FL	149
CG	Weaver, D	IN	150
CG	Weaver, D	IN	150
MF	Bahado-Singh, R	MI	374
MF	Wapner, R	NY	372
Ped	Jones, K	CA	626
Ped	Morton, D	PA	625
RE	Rosenwaks, Z	NY	873

Genetic Disorders-Nervous System

Spec	Name	St	Pg
ChiN	Charnas, L	MN	141

Special Expertise Index

Special Expertise Index

Spec	Name	St	Pg
Oph	Sherwood, M	FL	505
Oph	Tsai, J	CT	493

Glaucoma-Consultation
Spec	Name	St	Pg
Oph	Podos, S	NY	499

Glaucoma-Pediatric
Spec	Name	St	Pg
Oph	Del Monte, M	MI	507
Oph	Freedman, S	NC	503
Oph	Jaafar, M	DC	497
Oph	Medow, N	NY	498
Oph	Traboulsi, E	OH	511
Oph	Walton, D	MA	493

Gliomas
Spec	Name	St	Pg
N	Mikkelsen, T	MI	455
N	Rosenfeld, S	NY	445

Glomerulonephritis
Spec	Name	St	Pg
Nep	Appel, G	NY	393
Nep	Cohen, D	NY	393
Nep	Falk, R	NC	395
Nep	Hura, C	TX	398
Nep	Kasinath, B	TX	399
Nep	Lewis, E	IL	397

Gout
Spec	Name	St	Pg
Rhu	Brenner, M	MA	882
Rhu	Davis, W	LA	891
Rhu	Sundy, J	NC	887
Rhu	Wise, C	VA	887

Graft vs Host Disease
Spec	Name	St	Pg
Hem	Yeager, A	AZ	284
PHO	Chen, A	MD	653
PHO	Ferrara, J	MI	663

Graves' Disease
Spec	Name	St	Pg
EDM	Bahn, R	MN	196
EDM	Davies, T	NY	190

Graves' Disease-Eye
Spec	Name	St	Pg
EDM	Bahn, R	MN	196
Oto	Lanza, D	FL	574

Growth Disorders
Spec	Name	St	Pg
PEn	Allen, D	WI	643
PEn	Alter, C	PA	640
PEn	De Luca, F	PA	641
PEn	Diamond, F	FL	642
PEn	Geffner, M	CA	645
PEn	Levy, R	IL	643
PEn	Oberfield, S	NY	641
PEn	Plotnick, L	MD	641
PEn	Wilson, D	CA	645

Spec	Name	St	Pg
PNep	Friedman, A	MN	678

Growth Disorders in Childhood Cancer
Spec	Name	St	Pg
PEn	Meacham, L	GA	642
PEn	Sklar, C	NY	641
PEn	Zimmerman, D	IL	644

Growth Hormone Disorder-Adult
Spec	Name	St	Pg
EDM	Inzucchi, S	CT	189
EDM	Koch, C	MS	194

Growth/Development Disorders
Spec	Name	St	Pg
EDM	Levine, R	NH	189
PEn	Casella, S	NH	640
PEn	Foster, C	UT	644
PEn	Friedman, N	NC	642
PEn	Kappy, M	CO	644
PEn	Kaufman, F	CA	645
PEn	Levitsky, L	MA	640
PEn	Menon, R	MI	643
PEn	Rogers, D	OH	644
PEn	Silverstein, J	FL	643
PEn	Sperling, M	PA	642
PEn	Zimmerman, D	IL	644

Guillain-Barre Syndrome
Spec	Name	St	Pg
N	Arnason, B	IL	452
N	Bourdette, D	OR	462
N	Griffin, J	MD	441
N	Ropper, A	MA	437

Gynecologic Cancer
Spec	Name	St	Pg
DR	McCarthy, S	CT	845
GO	Alvarez, R	AL	248
GO	Barnes, W	DC	245
GO	Barter, J	MD	245
GO	Berkowitz, R	MA	244
GO	Berman, M	CA	254
GO	Carlson, J	NJ	246
GO	Chambers, S	AZ	253
GO	Clarke-Pearson, D	NC	248
GO	Copeland, L	OH	251
GO	Coukos, G	PA	246
GO	Currie, J	CT	244
GO	Davidson, S	CO	253
GO	DeMars, L	NH	244
GO	Di Saia, P	CA	255
GO	Dottino, P	NY	246
GO	Edwards, R	PA	246
GO	Fiorica, J	FL	249
GO	Fishman, D	NY	246
GO	Follen, M	TX	253
GO	Fowler, J	OH	251
GO	Greer, B	WA	255
GO	Herzog, T	NY	247
GO	Karlan, B	CA	255

Spec	Name	St	Pg
GO	Kelley, J	PA	247
GO	Lele, S	NY	247
GO	Lentz, S	NC	249
GO	Levenback, C	TX	254
GO	Magrina, J	AZ	254
GO	Monk, B	CA	255
GO	Morgan, M	PA	247
GO	Muntz, H	WA	255
GO	Mutch, D	MO	252
GO	Penalver, M	FL	250
GO	Powell, C	CA	255
GO	Remmenga, S	NE	253
GO	Rotmensch, J	IL	252
GO	Rubin, S	PA	248
GO	Soper, J	NC	250
GO	Spann, C	GA	250
GO	Spirtos, N	NV	256
GO	Stehman, F	IN	253
GO	Tarraza, H	ME	245
GO	Taylor, P	VA	250
ObG	Morgan, L	FL	482
Onc	Fleming, G	IL	318
Onc	Fracasso, P	VA	307
Onc	Hochster, H	NY	297
Onc	Markman, M	TX	330
Onc	Matulonis, U	MA	289
Onc	McGuire, W	MD	299
Onc	Muggia, F	NY	300
Onc	Schilder, R	PA	302
Onc	Thigpen, J	MS	313
Onc	Williams, S	IN	324
Path	Hendrickson, M	CA	618
Path	Li Volsi, V	PA	607
Path	Rutgers, J	CA	619
Path	Silva, E	TX	616
Path	Thor, A	CO	614
Path	Wilczynski, S	CA	619
Path	Young, R	MA	605
RadRO	Ennis, R	NY	822
RadRO	Gaffney, D	UT	833
RadRO	Glassburn, J	PA	823
RadRO	Grigsby, P	MO	830
RadRO	Halpern, H	IL	830
RadRO	Jhingran, A	TX	835
RadRO	Jose, B	KY	827
RadRO	Koh, W	WA	837
RadRO	Medbery, C	OK	835
RadRO	Mundt, A	CA	837
RadRO	Nori, D	NY	825
RadRO	Randall, M	KY	828
RadRO	Recht, A	MA	821
RadRO	Rotman, M	NY	825
RadRO	Schiff, P	NY	825
RadRO	Small, W	IL	832
S	Kavanah, M	MA	903

Gynecologic Cancer Risk
Spec	Name	St	Pg
CG	Whelan, A	MO	150
CG	Whelan, A	MO	150

Special Expertise Index

Spec	Name	St	Pg	Spec	Name	St	Pg	Spec	Name	St	Pg
Onc	Grunberg, S	VT	288	Oto	Osguthorpe, J	SC	575	Surgery			
Onc	Herbst, R	TX	329	Oto	Otto, R	TX	586	Oto	Cummings, C	MD	565
Onc	Hong, W	TX	329	Oto	Pelzer, H	IL	581	Oto	Futran, N	WA	588
Onc	Kane, M	CO	326	Oto	Persky, M	NY	570	Oto	Genden, E	NY	566
Onc	Khuri, F	GA	309	Oto	Rice, D	CA	589	Oto	Grillone, G	MA	563
Onc	Kies, M	TX	329	Oto	Sasaki, C	CT	564	Oto	Hanna, E	TX	585
Onc	Langer, C	PA	298	Oto	Schantz, S	NY	570	Oto	Hicks, W	NY	567
Onc	Lippman, S	TX	330	Oto	Schuller, D	OH	582	Oto	Keane, W	PA	568
Onc	Martins, R	WA	336	Oto	Siegel, G	IL	582	Oto	Krespi, Y	NY	568
Onc	Mintzer, D	PA	299	Oto	Singer, M	CA	589	Oto	Olsen, K	MN	581
Onc	Nabell, L	AL	310	Oto	Sinha, U	CA	589	Oto	Peters, G	AL	575
Onc	Oster, M	NY	300	Oto	Snyderman, C	PA	571	Oto	Petruzzelli, G	IL	581
Onc	Pfister, D	NY	301	Oto	Stringer, S	MS	576	Oto	Pitman, K	MS	575
Onc	Pinto, H	CA	337	Oto	Strome, M	NY	571	Oto	Shindo, M	NY	571
Onc	Posner, M	MA	289	Oto	Strome, S	MD	571	Oto	Urken, M	NY	572
Onc	Shin, D	GA	312	Oto	Suen, J	AR	586	Oto	Wilson, K	OH	583
Onc	Sidransky, D	MD	302	Oto	Teknos, T	MI	582	Oto	Zeitels, S	MA	564
Onc	Troner, M	FL	313	Oto	Terris, D	GA	576	S	Jackson, G	TX	934
Onc	Urba, S	MI	323	Oto	Valentino, J	KY	576	S	Ridge, J	PA	912
Onc	Vokes, E	IL	323	Oto	Weber, R	TX	586	S	Saha, S	MI	927
Onc	Worden, F	MI	324	Oto	Weinstein, G	PA	572				
Oto	Berke, G	CA	587	Oto	Weisman, R	CA	589				
Oto	Bradford, C	MI	578	Oto	Weissler, M	NC	577	**Head & Neck Cancer Reconstruction**			
Oto	Bumpous, J	KY	573	Oto	Weymuller, E	WA	589	Oto	Futran, N	WA	588
Oto	Burkey, B	TN	573	Oto	Wolf, G	MI	583	Oto	Genden, E	NY	566
Oto	Campbell, B	WI	578	Oto	Yarbrough, W	TN	577	Oto	Urken, M	NY	572
Oto	Cassisi, N	FL	573	Oto	Yueh, B	MN	583	Oto	Weisman, R	CA	589
Oto	Chalian, A	PA	565	PlS	Loree, T	NY	738	PlS	Robb, G	TX	750
Oto	Civantos, F	FL	573	PMR	Gamble, G	IL	725	PlS	Yuen, J	AR	750
Oto	Clayman, G	TX	585	PMR	Schwartz, L	PA	722				
Oto	Close, L	NY	565	PO	Crockett, D	CA	684				
Oto	Costantino, P	NY	565	PO	Geller, K	CA	684	**Head & Neck Imaging**			
Oto	Couch, M	NC	573	RadRO	Ang, K	TX	834	DR	Mancuso, A	FL	850
Oto	Davidson, B	DC	566	RadRO	Bonner, J	AL	826	NRad	Mukherji, S	MI	858
Oto	Day, T	SC	573	RadRO	Brizel, D	NC	826				
Oto	Deschler, D	MA	563	RadRO	Douglas, J	WA	836	**Head & Neck Pathology**			
Oto	Donald, P	CA	587	RadRO	Emami, B	IL	830	Path	Kahn, L	NY	607
Oto	Donovan, D	TX	585	RadRO	Haffty, B	NJ	823	Path	Nascimento, A	MN	613
Oto	Eisele, D	CA	587	RadRO	Haraf, D	IL	830				
Oto	Fee, W	CA	587	RadRO	Harrison, L	NY	823	**Head & Neck Radiology**			
Oto	Funk, G	IA	579	RadRO	Jose, B	KY	827	NRad	Curtin, H	MA	854
Oto	Gluckman, J	OH	579	RadRO	Laramore, G	WA	837	NRad	Osborn, A	UT	858
Oto	Goodwin, W	FL	574	RadRO	Le, Q	CA	837	NRad	Zinreich, S	MD	856
Oto	Grandis, J	PA	566	RadRO	Lee, C	MN	831				
Oto	Har-El, G	NY	566	RadRO	Machtay, M	PA	824	**Head & Neck Reconstruction**			
Oto	Haughey, B	MO	579	RadRO	Markoe, A	FL	827	Oto	Bumpous, J	KY	573
Oto	Hoffman, H	IA	579	RadRO	Mendenhall, W	FL	828	Oto	Chalian, A	PA	565
Oto	Johnson, J	PA	567	RadRO	Mittal, B	IL	832	Oto	Deschler, D	MA	563
Oto	Kaplan, M	CA	588	RadRO	Quivey, J	CA	837	Oto	Funk, G	IA	579
Oto	Kern, R	IL	580	RadRO	Sailer, S	NC	829	Oto	Haughey, B	MO	579
Oto	Koch, W	MD	568	RadRO	Streeter, O	CA	838	Oto	Levine, P	VA	574
Oto	Kraus, D	NY	568	RadRO	Tripuraneni, P	CA	838	Oto	Picken, C	DC	570
Oto	Lavertu, P	OH	580	RadRO	Trotti, A	FL	829	Oto	Strome, S	MD	571
Oto	Lawson, W	NY	569	RadRO	Weichselbaum, R	IL	833	PlS	Andersen, J	CA	751
Oto	Levine, P	VA	574	RadRO	Wilson, L	CT	821	PlS	Deleyiannis, F	PA	737
Oto	Lydiatt, D	NE	584	S	Flynn, M	KY	917				
Oto	Lydiatt, W	NE	584	S	Neifeld, J	VA	919				
Oto	McCaffrey, T	FL	575	S	Pearlman, N	CO	931	**Head & Neck Surgery**			
Oto	Medina, J	OK	586	S	Shah, J	NY	913	NRad	Loevner, L	PA	855
Oto	Myers, J	TX	586								
Oto	Netterville, J	TN	575	**Head & Neck Cancer &**							
Oto	Nuss, D	LA	586								
Oto	O'Malley, B	PA	569								

Special Expertise Index

Spec	Name	St	Pg
Cv	Miller, D	GA	102
Cv	Oparil, S	AL	102
Cv	Pepine, C	FL	102
Cv	Redberg, R	CA	113
Cv	Reis, S	PA	98
Cv	Roberts, B	RI	94
Cv	Volgman, A	IL	108
Cv	von der Lohe, E	IN	108
Cv	Wagoner, L	OH	109
Cv	Walsh, M	IN	109
Cv	Wilansky, S	AZ	111
IC	Jacobs, A	MA	119

Heart Failure

Spec	Name	St	Pg
CE	Sorrentino, R	GA	117
Cv	Borer, J	NY	95
Cv	Borzak, S	FL	100
Cv	Bourge, R	AL	100
Cv	Bove, A	PA	95
Cv	Califf, R	NC	101
Cv	Fonarow, G	CA	113
Cv	Gottlieb, S	MD	96
Cv	Hare, J	FL	101
Cv	Hauptman, P	MO	105
Cv	Heroux, A	IL	105
Cv	Konstam, M	MA	92
Cv	Mather, P	PA	97
Cv	Nagueh, S	TX	111
Cv	Parrillo, J	NJ	98
Cv	Rich, S	IL	107
Cv	Rosenbush, S	IL	107
Cv	Steingart, R	NY	99
Cv	Stevenson, L	MA	94
Cv	Young, J	OH	109
Cv	Zaret, B	CT	94
PCd	Boucek, M	FL	633
PCd	Gewitz, M	NY	631
PCd	Pahl, E	IL	635

Heart Failure & Ventricular Containment

Spec	Name	St	Pg
TS	Bolman, R	MA	950
TS	Naka, Y	NY	957
TS	Raman, J	IL	966

Heart Valve Disease

Spec	Name	St	Pg
Cv	Bashore, T	NC	100
Cv	Blumenthal, D	NY	94
Cv	Bonow, R	IL	104
Cv	Borer, J	NY	95
Cv	Carabello, B	TX	110
Cv	Elkayam, U	CA	112
Cv	Fuster, V	NY	96
Cv	Gliklich, J	NY	96
Cv	Greenberg, M	NY	96
Cv	Harrison, J	NC	101
Cv	Inra, L	NY	97
Cv	Iskandrian, A	AL	101
Cv	Johnson, A	CA	113
Cv	Manning, W	MA	93

Spec	Name	St	Pg
Cv	McPherson, D	TX	110
Cv	Mehlman, D	IL	106
Cv	Nemickas, R	IL	106
Cv	O'Gara, P	MA	93
Cv	O'Neill, W	FL	102
Cv	Phillips, R	MA	93
Cv	Plehn, J	MD	98
Cv	Powers, E	SC	103
Cv	Quinones, M	TX	111
Cv	Rahko, P	WI	107
Cv	Reiss, C	MO	107
Cv	Sanborn, T	IL	108
Cv	Stewart, W	OH	108
Cv	Tajik, A	AZ	111
Cv	Tenenbaum, J	NY	99
Cv	Waxman, H	PA	99
IC	Herrmann, H	PA	120
IC	Moses, J	NY	120
IC	Smalling, R	TX	123
TS	Pochettino, A	PA	957

Heart Valve Surgery

Spec	Name	St	Pg
PS	Quaegebeur, J	NY	694
TS	Acker, M	PA	952
TS	Adams, D	NY	952
TS	Akins, C	MA	950
TS	Bavaria, J	PA	952
TS	Bridges, C	PA	953
TS	Brown, J	IN	963
TS	Chitwood, W	NC	959
TS	Cohen, R	CA	970
TS	Furukawa, S	PA	953
TS	Griffith, B	MD	954
TS	Hargrove, W	PA	954
TS	Isom, O	NY	955
TS	Kanda, L	DC	955
TS	Katz, N	DC	955
TS	Krieger, K	NY	956
TS	Lamberti, J	CA	972
TS	Lang, S	NY	956
TS	Lansman, S	NY	956
TS	Loulmet, D	NY	956
TS	Lytle, B	OH	964
TS	McCarthy, P	IL	965
TS	Merrick, S	CA	972
TS	Michler, R	NY	957
TS	Miller, D	CA	972
TS	Ott, D	TX	969
TS	Oz, M	NY	957
TS	Reitz, B	CA	972
TS	Schaff, H	MN	966
TS	Sellke, F	MA	951
TS	Shemin, R	CA	972
TS	Smith, P	NC	962
TS	Starnes, V	CA	972
TS	Strong, M	PA	958
TS	Sundt, T	MN	967
TS	Tranbaugh, R	NY	958
TS	Verrier, E	WA	973

Heart Valve Surgery-Aortic

Spec	Name	St	Pg
TS	Graver, L	NY	954
TS	Reardon, M	TX	969

Heart Valve Surgery-Mitral

Spec	Name	St	Pg
TS	Vander Salm, T	MA	951

Heart Valve Surgery-Pediatric

Spec	Name	St	Pg
TS	Forbess, J	TX	968

Hemangiomas

Spec	Name	St	Pg
D	Burton, C	NC	175
D	Frieden, I	CA	181
PO	Cunningham, M	MA	680
PO	McGill, T	MA	680

Hemangiomas/Birthmarks

Spec	Name	St	Pg
D	Alster, T	DC	170
D	Orlow, S	NY	173
Oto	Waner, M	NY	572
PlS	Zide, B	NY	741

Hematologic Malignancies

Spec	Name	St	Pg
Hem	Anderson, K	MA	272
Hem	Cheson, B	DC	273
Hem	Di Persio, J	MO	278
Hem	Flynn, P	MN	278
Hem	Grever, M	OH	279
Hem	Heinrich, M	OR	284
Hem	Kessler, C	DC	274
Hem	Kraut, E	OH	280
Hem	Lin, W	AL	276
Hem	Maciejewski, J	OH	280
Hem	Maddox, A	AR	284
Hem	Millenson, M	PA	274
Onc	Algazy, K	PA	290
Onc	Beatty, P	MT	325
Onc	Bolwell, B	OH	315
Onc	Claxton, D	PA	292
Onc	Colon-Otero, G	FL	306
Onc	Deeg, H	WA	334
Onc	Erban, J	MA	287
Onc	Flinn, I	TN	307
Onc	Gabrilove, J	NY	295
Onc	Mitchell, B	CA	336
Onc	Rosen, S	IL	322
Onc	Schilder, R	PA	302
Onc	Shields, P	DC	302
Onc	Smith, M	PA	302
Onc	Tschetter, L	SD	326
PHO	Hord, J	OH	664

Hematology-Benign

Spec	Name	St	Pg
Onc	Shields, P	DC	302

America's Top Doctors® 8th Edition

Special Expertise Index

America's Top Doctors® 8th Edition

Special Expertise Index

Special Expertise Index

Special Expertise Index

Special Expertise Index

Special Expertise Index

Spec	Name	St	Pg
U	Huben, R	NY	982
U	Kibel, A	MO	994
U	Kirschenbaum, A	NY	983
U	Libertino, J	MA	978
U	Malkowicz, S	PA	983
U	Novick, A	OH	996
U	Patel, V	FL	990
U	Presti, J	CA	1004
U	Richie, J	MA	979
U	Robertson, C	NC	990
U	Samadi, D	NY	984
U	Sanders, W	GA	991
U	Sawczuk, I	NJ	985
U	Smith, J	TN	991
U	Soloway, M	FL	991
U	Steinberg, G	IL	997
U	Swanson, D	TX	1001
U	Taneja, S	NY	986
U	Teigland, C	NC	991
U	Theodorescu, D	VA	991
U	Uzzo, R	PA	986
U	Weiss, R	NJ	987
U	Williams, R	IA	997
VIR	McGahan, J	CA	866
VIR	Soulen, M	PA	861
VIR	Wood, B	MD	862

Kidney Cancer Clinical Trials

S	Yang, J	MD	915

Kidney Cancer-Cryosurgery

U	Katz, A	NY	982

Kidney Disease

Nep	Coggins, C	MA	392
Nep	Delmez, J	MO	396
Nep	Gluck, S	CA	400
Nep	Helderman, J	TN	395
Nep	Kliger, A	CT	392
Nep	Pohl, M	OH	397
Nep	Rudnick, M	PA	394
Nep	Umans, J	DC	394
Nep	Venkat, K	MI	398
Nep	Weiner, I	FL	396
PNep	Andreoli, S	IN	678
PNep	Chandar, J	FL	677
PNep	Dabbagh, S	DE	676
PNep	Ettenger, R	CA	679
PNep	McDonald, R	WA	679
S	Scantlebury, V	DE	913
U	Shortliffe, L	CA	1004

Kidney Disease-Autoimmune

Nep	Salant, D	MA	392
PNep	Wyatt, R	TN	677

Kidney Disease-Chronic

Nep	Bolton, W	VA	395
Nep	King, A	CA	400

Spec	Name	St	Pg
Nep	Perrone, R	MA	392
PNep	Cohn, R	IL	678
PNep	Warady, B	MO	679

Kidney Disease-Genetic

PNep	Avner, E	WI	678
PNep	Kashtan, C	MN	678

Kidney Disease-Geriatric

Nep	Kasiske, B	MN	397

Kidney Disease-Glomerular

Nep	Bolton, W	VA	395
Nep	Rakowski, T	VA	395
Nep	Salant, D	MA	392

Kidney Disease-Metabolic

Nep	Kaysen, G	CA	400
Nep	Kliger, A	CT	392

Kidney Disease-Pediatric & Adult

Nep	Hruska, K	MO	396

Kidney Failure

Nep	Kobrin, S	PA	394
Nep	Mitch, W	TX	399
Nep	Olivero, J	TX	399
Nep	Piraino, B	PA	394
Nep	Swartz, R	MI	397
PNep	Alexander, S	CA	679
PNep	Nash, M	NY	677

Kidney Failure-Acute

Nep	Bazari, H	MA	392
Nep	Brenner, B	MA	392
Nep	Kraus, M	IN	397
Nep	Okusa, M	VA	395
Nep	Perrone, R	MA	392
Nep	Tolkoff-Rubin, N	MA	393
Nep	Toto, R	TX	399

Kidney Failure-Chronic

Nep	Ahmad, S	WA	399
Nep	Berl, T	CO	398
Nep	Brennan, S	TX	398
Nep	Brenner, B	MA	392
Nep	Kaysen, G	CA	400
Nep	Okusa, M	VA	395
Nep	Roth, D	FL	396
Nep	Seifter, J	MA	393
PNep	Dabbagh, S	DE	676
PNep	Nevins, T	MN	679
PNep	Watkins, S	WA	680

Spec	Name	St	Pg

Kidney Pathology

Path	Rennke, H	MA	604
Path	Sibley, R	CA	619
Path	Tomaszewski, J	PA	609
Path	Tomaszewski, J	PA	609

Kidney Stones

Nep	Ahmad, S	WA	399
Nep	Aronson, P	CT	392
Nep	Brennan, S	TX	398
Nep	Coe, F	IL	396
Nep	Gluck, S	CA	400
Nep	Hruska, K	MO	396
Nep	Kelepouris, E	PA	394
Nep	Scheinman, S	NY	394
Nep	Seifter, J	MA	393
Nep	Warnock, D	AL	396
Nep	Weiner, I	FL	396
PNep	Langman, C	IL	679
U	Albala, D	NC	987
U	Assimos, D	NC	987
U	Bagley, D	PA	979
U	Basler, J	TX	999
U	Carson, C	NC	988
U	Clayman, R	CA	1002
U	Fuchs, E	OR	1002
U	Grasso, M	NY	981
U	Gribetz, M	NY	982
U	Irby, P	NC	989
U	Jackman, S	PA	982
U	Janeiro, J	NH	978
U	Kavoussi, L	NY	983
U	O'Leary, M	MA	979
U	Patterson, A	TN	990
U	Preminger, G	NC	990
U	Sanders, W	GA	991
U	Sosa, R	NY	986
U	Stoller, M	CA	1005
U	Winfield, H	IA	997

Klippel-Trenaunay Syndrome

PCd	Driscoll, D	MN	635

Knee Cartilage Transplant

OrS	Cuckler, J	AL	539

Knee Cartilage/Meniscus Transplants

OrS	Anderson, L	CA	551

Knee Injuries

OrS	Johnson, D	KY	540
OrS	Scott, W	NY	537
SM	Cole, B	IL	898
SM	Fronek, J	CA	899
SM	Harner, C	PA	896
SM	Hershman, E	NY	897
SM	Levine, W	NY	897

Special Expertise Index

Special Expertise Index

Spec	Name	St	Pg
Hem	Litzow, M	MN	280
Hem	Marks, S	PA	274
Hem	Maziarz, R	OR	285
Hem	McGlave, P	MN	281
Hem	Mears, J	NY	274
Hem	Miller, K	MA	272
Hem	Nand, S	IL	281
Hem	Nimer, S	NY	274
Hem	O'Donnell, M	CA	285
Hem	Porter, D	PA	274
Hem	Powell, B	NC	277
Hem	Rai, K	NY	275
Hem	Raphael, B	NY	275
Hem	Rosenblatt, J	FL	277
Hem	Saven, A	CA	286
Hem	Schiller, G	CA	286
Hem	Snyder, D	CA	286
Hem	Spitzer, T	MA	272
Hem	Spivak, J	MD	275
Hem	Stiff, P	IL	281
Hem	Stone, R	MA	273
Hem	Strauss, J	TX	284
Hem	Tallman, M	IL	282
Hem	Wisch, N	NY	275
Hem	Yeager, A	AZ	284
Hem	Zalusky, R	NY	276
Hem	Zuckerman, K	FL	277
Onc	Antin, J	MA	286
Onc	Appelbaum, F	WA	333
Onc	Canellos, G	MA	286
Onc	Chanan-Khan, A	NY	292
Onc	Chao, N	NC	306
Onc	Chitambar, C	WI	317
Onc	Claxton, D	PA	292
Onc	Czuczman, M	NY	293
Onc	Dakhil, S	KS	325
Onc	Druker, B	OR	334
Onc	Estey, E	WA	334
Onc	Gabrilove, J	NY	295
Onc	Gerson, S	OH	318
Onc	Gockerman, J	NC	307
Onc	Golomb, H	IL	318
Onc	Hurd, D	NC	308
Onc	Jillella, A	GA	308
Onc	Kalaycio, M	OH	319
Onc	Karp, J	MD	298
Onc	Lossos, I	FL	310
Onc	Maslak, P	NY	299
Onc	Mitchell, B	CA	336
Onc	Moore, J	NC	310
Onc	O'Brien, S	TX	330
Onc	Orlowski, R	TX	331
Onc	Petersdorf, S	WA	337
Onc	Peterson, B	MN	321
Onc	Scheinberg, D	NY	302
Onc	Schiffer, C	MI	322
Onc	Shea, T	NC	312
Onc	Smith, M	PA	302
Onc	Stadtmauer, E	PA	303
Onc	Wade, J	WI	323
Onc	Weiner, G	IA	323
Onc	Williams, M	VA	314
Onc	Wingard, J	FL	314

Spec	Name	St	Pg
Path	Braylan, R	FL	610
Path	Foucar, M	NM	615
Path	Kinney, M	TX	615
Path	Nathwani, B	CA	619
PHO	Abella, E	AZ	667
PHO	Altman, A	CT	651
PHO	Andrews, R	WA	669
PHO	Arceci, R	MD	652
PHO	Brecher, M	NY	653
PHO	Buchanan, G	TX	668
PHO	Cairo, M	NY	653
PHO	Camitta, B	WI	662
PHO	Carroll, W	NY	653
PHO	Civin, C	MD	653
PHO	Corey, S	IL	663
PHO	Davies, S	OH	663
PHO	Felix, C	PA	654
PHO	Frantz, C	DE	654
PHO	Godder, K	VA	659
PHO	Gold, S	NC	659
PHO	Goldman, S	TX	668
PHO	Graham, M	AZ	668
PHO	Haut, P	IN	664
PHO	Hawkins, D	WA	670
PHO	Hayani, A	IL	664
PHO	Hayashi, R	MO	664
PHO	Homans, A	VT	651
PHO	Hutchinson, R	MI	664
PHO	Jayabose, S	NY	655
PHO	Johnston, J	GA	659
PHO	Kamen, B	NJ	655
PHO	Keller, F	GA	660
PHO	Lange, B	PA	656
PHO	Luchtman-Jones, L	DC	656
PHO	Manera, R	IL	665
PHO	Morgan, E	IL	665
PHO	Murphy, S	TX	668
PHO	Odom, L	CO	667
PHO	Pui, C	TN	661
PHO	Razzouk, B	IN	665
PHO	Reaman, G	DC	657
PHO	Rheingold, S	PA	657
PHO	Ritchey, A	PA	657
PHO	Rosoff, P	NC	661
PHO	Sallan, S	MA	652
PHO	Salvi, S	IL	665
PHO	Sandler, E	FL	661
PHO	Scher, C	LA	668
PHO	Siegel, S	CA	671
PHO	Tebbi, C	FL	661
PHO	Vik, T	IN	666
PHO	Weiner, M	NY	658
PHO	Weinstein, H	MA	652
PHO	Whitlock, J	TN	662
PHO	Winick, N	TX	669
PHO	Wolfe, L	MA	652
PHO	Woods, W	GA	662
PHO	Yaddanapudi, R	MI	666
RadRO	Wong, J	CA	838

Leukemia & Lymphoma

Spec	Name	St	Pg
Hem	Champlin, R	TX	283

Spec	Name	St	Pg
Hem	Farag, S	IN	278
Hem	Greer, J	TN	276
Hem	Larson, R	IL	280
Hem	Linenberger, M	WA	285
Hem	Lyons, R	TX	283
Hem	Millenson, M	PA	274
Onc	Ball, E	CA	333
Onc	Coleman, M	NY	293
Onc	Daugherty, C	IL	317
Onc	Fay, J	TX	328
Onc	Flomenberg, N	PA	295
PHO	Coccia, P	NE	667
PHO	Halpern, S	NJ	654
PHO	Harris, M	NJ	654
PHO	Hilden, J	IN	664
PHO	Nachman, J	IL	665
PHO	Pendergrass, T	WA	671
PHO	Rausen, A	NY	657
PHO	Sandlund, J	TN	661
PHO	Steinherz, P	NY	657
PHO	Tannous, R	IA	666
PHO	Weinblatt, M	NY	658

Leukemia in Elderly

Spec	Name	St	Pg
Hem	Godwin, J	IL	279

Leukemia in Infants

Spec	Name	St	Pg
PHO	Dreyer, Z	TX	668
PHO	Felix, C	PA	654

Leukemia-Chronic Lymphocytic

Spec	Name	St	Pg
Onc	Byrd, J	OH	316

Leukoencephalopathy

Spec	Name	St	Pg
N	Filley, C	CO	458

Liaison Psychiatry

Spec	Name	St	Pg
Psyc	Bronheim, H	NY	765

Lichen Planus

Spec	Name	St	Pg
D	Camisa, C	FL	175

Liddle's Syndrome

Spec	Name	St	Pg
Nep	Warnock, D	AL	396

Ligament Reconstruction

Spec	Name	St	Pg
OrS	Hannafin, J	NY	532
SM	Hershman, E	NY	897

Limb Deficiency-Arthrogryposis

Spec	Name	St	Pg
PMR	Jaffe, K	WA	729

Limb Deformities

Spec	Name	St	Pg
OrS	Aronson, J	AR	549

Special Expertise Index

America's Top Doctors® 8th Edition

Special Expertise Index

Special Expertise Index

Spec	Name	St	Pg
Onc	Canellos, G	MA	286
Onc	Chao, N	NC	306
Onc	Chitambar, C	WI	317
Onc	Czuczman, M	NY	293
Onc	Dakhil, S	KS	325
Onc	Fisher, R	NY	294
Onc	Flinn, I	TN	307
Onc	Friedberg, J	NY	295
Onc	Glaspy, J	CA	335
Onc	Gockerman, J	NC	307
Onc	Golomb, H	IL	318
Onc	Goy, A	NJ	296
Onc	Grossbard, M	NY	296
Onc	Hesdorffer, C	MD	297
Onc	Horning, S	CA	335
Onc	Hurd, D	NC	308
Onc	Jillella, A	GA	308
Onc	Kaminski, M	MI	320
Onc	Kaplan, L	CA	336
Onc	Kosova, L	IL	320
Onc	Kwak, L	TX	329
Onc	Lacy, J	CT	288
Onc	Lossos, I	FL	310
Onc	Lynch, J	FL	310
Onc	Maloney, D	WA	336
Onc	Miller, T	AZ	330
Onc	Mitchell, B	CA	336
Onc	Nadler, L	MA	289
Onc	Nichols, C	OR	337
Onc	O'Brien, S	TX	330
Onc	Offit, K	NY	300
Onc	Petersdorf, S	WA	337
Onc	Peterson, B	MN	321
Onc	Press, O	WA	338
Onc	Rosen, S	IL	322
Onc	Schiffer, C	MI	322
Onc	Schnipper, L	MA	289
Onc	Schwartz, B	MN	322
Onc	Schwartz, M	FL	312
Onc	Serody, J	NC	312
Onc	Shea, T	NC	312
Onc	Smith, M	PA	302
Onc	Sotomayor, E	FL	313
Onc	Straus, D	NY	303
Onc	Weiner, G	IA	323
Onc	Williams, M	VA	314
Onc	Wilson, W	MD	304
Onc	Yunus, F	TN	314
Onc	Zelenetz, A	NY	304
Path	Banks, P	NC	609
Path	Braylan, R	FL	610
Path	Grogan, T	AZ	615
Path	Harris, N	MA	604
Path	Jaffe, E	MD	606
Path	Kinney, M	TX	615
Path	Knowles, D	NY	607
Path	Kurtin, P	MN	613
Path	Nathwani, B	CA	619
Path	Swerdlow, S	PA	609
Path	Warnke, R	CA	619
Path	Weisenburger, D	NE	614
Path	Weiss, L	CA	619
PHO	Andrews, R	WA	669

Spec	Name	St	Pg
PHO	Brecher, M	NY	653
PHO	Cairo, M	NY	653
PHO	Fallon, R	IN	663
PHO	Goldman, S	TX	668
PHO	Jayabose, S	NY	655
PHO	Johnston, J	GA	659
PHO	Manera, R	IL	665
PHO	Parker, R	NY	657
PHO	Pui, C	TN	661
PHO	Reaman, G	DC	657
PHO	Weiner, M	NY	658
PHO	Weinstein, H	MA	652
RadRO	Abrams, R	IL	830
RadRO	Brizel, D	NC	826
RadRO	Constine, L	NY	822
RadRO	Glatstein, E	PA	823
RadRO	Goodman, R	NJ	823
RadRO	Hoppe, R	CA	837
RadRO	Lee, C	MN	831
RadRO	Macklis, R	OH	831
RadRO	Mauch, P	MA	820
RadRO	McGarry, R	KY	828
RadRO	Mendenhall, N	FL	828
RadRO	Mittal, B	IL	832
RadRO	Nicolaou, N	PA	824
RadRO	Park, C	CA	837
RadRO	Prosnitz, L	NC	828
RadRO	Rabinovitch, R	CO	833
RadRO	Roberts, K	CT	821
RadRO	Russell, K	WA	838
RadRO	Tripuraneni, P	CA	838
RadRO	Yahalom, J	NY	826

Lymphoma Consultation

Spec	Name	St	Pg
Onc	DeVita, V	CT	287

Lymphoma, Cutaneous B Cell (CBCL)

Spec	Name	St	Pg
RadRO	Wilson, L	CT	821

Lymphoma, Cutaneous T Cell (CTCL)

Spec	Name	St	Pg
RadRO	Wilson, L	CT	821

Lymphoma, Non-Hodgkin's

Spec	Name	St	Pg
Hem	Gordon, L	IL	279
Hem	Porcu, P	OH	281
Hem	Stiff, P	IL	281
Hem	Winter, J	IL	282
NuM	Wiseman, G	MN	476
Onc	Gerson, S	OH	334
Onc	Glick, J	PA	296
Onc	Moore, J	NC	310
Onc	Orlowski, R	TX	331
PHO	Murphy, S	TX	668
PHO	Sandlund, J	TN	661

Lymphoma-Ocular (eye)

Spec	Name	St	Pg
Oph	Gigantelli, J	NE	513

Lysosomal Diseases

Spec	Name	St	Pg
CG	Burton, B	IL	149
CG	Burton, B	IL	149
CG	Charrow, J	IL	149
CG	Charrow, J	IL	149

M

Macular Degeneration

Spec	Name	St	Pg
Oph	Blumenkranz, M	CA	515
Oph	Brucker, A	PA	494
Oph	Del Priore, L	NY	494
Oph	Friberg, T	PA	495
Oph	Gentile, R	NY	496
Oph	Handa, J	MD	496
Oph	Ho, A	PA	497
Oph	Lewis, H	NY	498
Oph	Marmor, M	CA	518
Oph	Meredith, T	NC	504
Oph	Miller, J	MA	493
Oph	Nussbaum, J	GA	505
Oph	Puliafito, C	CA	519
Oph	Sternberg, P	TN	505
Oph	Vander, J	PA	501
Oph	Vine, A	MI	512
Oph	Walsh, J	NY	501
Oph	Williams, G	MI	512

Macular Disease/Degeneration

Spec	Name	St	Pg
Oph	Chang, S	NY	494
Oph	Fuchs, W	NY	495
Oph	Goldberg, M	MD	496
Oph	Gorin, M	CA	517
Oph	Grossniklaus, H	GA	503
Oph	Lambert, H	TX	513
Oph	Muldoon, T	NY	499
Oph	Rosenfeld, P	FL	505
Oph	Schiff, W	NY	500
Oph	Shabto, U	NY	501
Oph	Yannuzzi, L	NY	502

Malabsorption Syndrome

Spec	Name	St	Pg
Ge	Bayless, T	MD	207
Ge	Green, P	NY	209
Ge	Semrad, C	IL	222
Ge	Toskes, P	FL	217
PGe	Oliva-Hemker, M	MD	646

Malaria

Spec	Name	St	Pg
Inf	Trenholme, G	IL	356

Special Expertise Index

Spec	Name	St	Pg
Mammography			
DR	Dershaw, D	NY	847
DR	Evers, K	PA	847
DR	Helvie, M	MI	851
DR	Huynh, P	TX	852
DR	Mitnick, J	NY	848
DR	Monsees, B	MO	851
Marfan's Syndrome			
CG	Bialer, M	NY	146
CG	Bialer, M	NY	146
CG	Burton, B	IL	149
CG	Burton, B	IL	149
CG	Davis, J	NY	147
CG	Davis, J	NY	147
CG	Marion, R	NY	147
CG	Marion, R	NY	147
CG	Pyeritz, R	PA	147
CG	Pyeritz, R	PA	147
CG	Rimoin, D	CA	153
CG	Rimoin, D	CA	153
Cv	Braverman, A	MO	104
Cv	Devereux, R	NY	95
PCd	Mahony, L	TX	636
PCd	Moodie, D	LA	636
TS	Coselli, J	TX	968
TS	Girardi, L	NY	954
Marital/Family/Sex Therapy			
Psyc	Giustra, L	GA	769
Psyc	Manevitz, A	NY	767
Psyc	Sadock, V	NY	768
Mast Cell Diseases			
A&I	Metcalfe, D	MD	83
Hem	Duffy, T	CT	272
Maternal & Fetal Medicine			
MF	Platt, L	CA	378
ObG	Duff, W	FL	482
ObG	Gonik, B	MI	483
Maxillofacial & Craniofacial Surgery			
PlS	Gruss, J	WA	752
Maxillofacial Surgery			
Oto	Powell, N	CA	588
PlS	Deleyiannis, F	PA	737
PlS	Kawamoto, H	CA	753
PlS	Kelly, K	TN	743
PlS	Napoli, J	DE	739
PlS	Polley, J	IL	746
PlS	Posnick, J	MD	739
PlS	Stal, S	TX	750
PlS	Wolfe, S	FL	744
PlS	Zins, J	OH	748

Spec	Name	St	Pg
Maze Procedure for Atrial Fibrillation			
TS	Argenziano, M	NY	952
TS	Bridges, C	PA	953
TS	Fullerton, D	CO	967
TS	Schaff, H	MN	966
Mechanical Ventilation			
PCCM	Nichols, D	MD	638
PCCM	Thompson, A	PA	638
Pul	Celli, B	MA	794
Pul	Marini, J	MN	805
Pul	Tobin, M	IL	807
Mediastinal Tumors			
Onc	Kris, M	NY	298
Path	Koss, M	CA	618
Path	Moran, C	TX	615
Path	Suster, S	WI	614
TS	Kaiser, L	PA	955
TS	Keenan, R	PA	955
TS	Kiernan, P	VA	960
TS	Orringer, M	MI	965
TS	Scott, W	PA	958
TS	Shrager, J	CA	972
TS	Vallieres, E	WA	973
Medulloblastoma			
NS	Raffel, C	OH	420
PHO	Gajjar, A	TN	659
Melanoma			
D	Bowen, G	UT	179
D	Bystryn, J	NY	171
D	Cornelius, L	MO	177
D	Fenske, N	FL	175
D	Gilchrest, B	MA	168
D	Greenway, H	CA	182
D	Grichnik, J	NC	176
D	Halpern, A	NY	172
D	Johnson, T	MI	178
D	Johr, R	FL	176
D	Kupper, T	MA	169
D	Leffell, D	CT	169
D	Lessin, S	PA	172
D	McDonald, C	RI	169
D	Mihm, M	MA	169
D	Miller, S	MD	173
D	Orengo, I	TX	180
D	Rigel, D	NY	173
D	Robins, P	NY	173
D	Sober, A	MA	170
D	Swetter, S	CA	183
D	Taylor, R	TX	181
D	Wood, G	WI	179
D	Zitelli, J	PA	174
Hem	Kuzel, T	IL	280
Onc	Albertini, M	WI	315
Onc	Atkins, M	MA	286

Spec	Name	St	Pg
Onc	Berd, D	PA	291
Onc	Borden, E	OH	315
Onc	Brockstein, B	IL	316
Onc	Chapman, P	NY	292
Onc	Clark, J	IL	317
Onc	Cohen, S	NY	293
Onc	Conry, R	AL	306
Onc	Daud, A	FL	307
Onc	Fay, J	TX	328
Onc	Glaspy, J	CA	335
Onc	Grosh, W	VA	308
Onc	Gruber, S	MI	319
Onc	Haas, N	PA	296
Onc	Hutchins, L	AR	329
Onc	Kirkwood, J	PA	298
Onc	Lawson, D	GA	309
Onc	Legha, S	TX	329
Onc	Livingston, P	NY	299
Onc	Margolin, K	CA	336
Onc	Meyskens, F	CA	336
Onc	Miller, D	KY	310
Onc	O'Day, S	CA	337
Onc	Oratz, R	NY	300
Onc	Papadopoulos, N	TX	331
Onc	Pecora, A	NJ	301
Onc	Richards, J	IL	321
Onc	Samlowski, W	NV	338
Onc	Schuchter, L	PA	302
Onc	Sosman, J	TN	313
Onc	Strauss, G	MA	289
Onc	Thompson, J	WA	339
Onc	von Mehren, M	PA	304
Onc	Weber, J	FL	314
Onc	Weiss, G	VA	314
Oph	Shields, C	PA	501
Oto	Singer, M	CA	589
Path	Bastian, B	CA	617
Path	Cochran, A	CA	617
Path	Gottlieb, G	NY	606
Path	Prieto, V	TX	616
PlS	Rees, R	MI	747
PlS	Yetman, R	OH	747
RadRO	Wazer, D	RI	821
S	Averbook, B	OH	922
S	Balch, C	MD	905
S	Bear, H	VA	915
S	Byrd, D	WA	937
S	Chang, A	MI	923
S	Coit, D	NY	906
S	Dilawari, R	TN	916
S	Eberlein, T	MO	924
S	Edington, H	PA	907
S	Edwards, M	OH	924
S	Eisenberg, B	NH	902
S	Essner, R	CA	939
S	Fraker, D	PA	908
S	Goodnight, J	CA	939
S	Gray, R	AZ	933
S	Johnson, D	CA	939
S	Kaufman, H	NY	909
S	Kavanah, M	MA	903
S	Kelley, M	TN	918
S	Kim, J	OH	925

Spec	Name	St	Pg
S	Krag, D	VT	903
S	Kraybill, W	MO	925
S	Kuhn, J	TX	934
S	Lee, J	TX	935
S	Leitch, A	TX	935
S	Lind, D	GA	918
S	Mansfield, P	TX	935
S	McMasters, K	KY	919
S	Moley, J	MO	926
S	Nathanson, S	MI	927
S	Neifeld, J	VA	919
S	Pearlman, N	CO	931
S	Pockaj, B	AZ	935
S	Reintgen, D	FL	920
S	Rosenberg, S	MD	912
S	Roses, D	NY	913
S	Ross, M	TX	936
S	Schwartzentruber, D	IN	928
S	Shenk, R	OH	928
S	Sigurdson, E	PA	913
S	Skinner, K	NY	914
S	Slingluff, C	VA	920
S	Sondak, V	FL	920
S	Talamonti, M	IL	929
S	Tanabe, K	MA	904
S	Tyler, D	NC	921
S	Urist, M	AL	921
S	White, R	NC	921
S	Yeung, R	WA	942

Melanoma Early Detection/Prevention

Spec	Name	St	Pg
D	Halpern, A	NY	172
D	Swetter, S	CA	183

Melanoma Risk Assessment

Spec	Name	St	Pg
D	Lessin, S	PA	172

Melanoma-Advanced

Spec	Name	St	Pg
Onc	O'Day, S	CA	337

Melanoma-Choroidal (eye)

Spec	Name	St	Pg
Oph	Abramson, D	NY	493
Oph	Augsburger, J	OH	507
Oph	Dutton, J	NC	503
Oph	Grossniklaus, H	GA	503
Oph	Handa, J	MD	496
Oph	Harbour, J	MO	508
Oph	Schachat, A	OH	511
Oph	Vine, A	MI	512
Oph	Wilson, M	TN	506

Melanoma-Head & Neck

Spec	Name	St	Pg
D	Fewkes, J	MA	168
Oto	Bradford, C	MI	578
Oto	Myers, J	TX	586
PlS	Stadelmann, W	NH	735

Melanoma-Metastatic

Spec	Name	St	Pg
Onc	Albertini, M	WI	315

Memory & Longevity

Spec	Name	St	Pg
GerPsy	Small, G	CA	788

Memory Disorders

Spec	Name	St	Pg
Ger	Ciocon, J	FL	235
Ger	Sachs, G	IN	237
GerPsy	Borson, S	WA	788
GerPsy	Small, G	CA	788
GerPsy	Stein, E	FL	787
N	Heilman, K	FL	449
N	Henderson, V	CA	464
N	Jordan, B	NY	442
N	Kelly, J	CO	459
N	Relkin, N	NY	445
N	Sadowsky, C	FL	451
N	Zimmerman, E	NY	447

Meniere's Disease

Spec	Name	St	Pg
Oto	Beatty, C	MN	577
Oto	Caldarelli, D	IL	578
Oto	Driscoll, C	MN	578
Oto	Farrior, J	FL	573
Oto	Minor, L	MD	569
Oto	Paparella, M	MN	581
Oto	Rauch, S	MA	564
Oto	Silverstein, H	FL	576
Oto	Wazen, J	FL	576

Meningioma

Spec	Name	St	Pg
NS	Gutin, P	NY	408
NS	McDermott, M	CA	428
NS	Stieg, P	NY	411
RadRO	Loeffler, J	MA	820

Meningioma-Orbital (eye)

Spec	Name	St	Pg
Oph	Cockerham, K	CA	516

Meningitis

Spec	Name	St	Pg
Inf	Quagliarello, V	CT	350
Inf	Scheld, W	VA	355
PInf	Bradley, J	CA	676
PInf	Kaplan, S	TX	675
PInf	Kleiman, M	IN	674
PInf	McCracken, G	TX	675
PInf	Wald, E	WI	675

Menopause Problems

Spec	Name	St	Pg
ObG	Filip, S	NC	482
RE	Fritz, M	NC	875
RE	Hammond, C	NC	875
RE	Luciano, A	CT	871
RE	Manganiello, P	NH	871
RE	Richardson, M	KS	878
RE	Sanfilippo, J	PA	873
RE	Simon, J	DC	873
RE	Weiss, G	NJ	874

Menopause-Male

Spec	Name	St	Pg
Ger	Morley, J	MO	237

Menstrual Disorders

Spec	Name	St	Pg
AM	MacKenzie, R	CA	79
PEn	Rosenfield, R	IL	644
RE	Berga, S	GA	874
RE	Fritz, M	NC	875

Menstrual Disorders (PMS)

Spec	Name	St	Pg
Psyc	Dell, D	NC	769

Mental Retardation

Spec	Name	St	Pg
CG	Davis, J	NY	147
CG	Davis, J	NY	147
CG	Falk, R	CA	151
CG	Falk, R	CA	151
CG	Graham, J	CA	151
CG	Graham, J	CA	151
CG	Stevenson, R	SC	149
CG	Stevenson, R	SC	149
ChAP	Coyle, J	MA	780
ChAP	King, B	WA	785
ChAP	Pomeroy, J	NY	782
ChAP	Volkmar, F	CT	780

Mercury Toxic Exposure

Spec	Name	St	Pg
OM	Gochfeld, M	NJ	758

Merkel Cell Carcinoma

Spec	Name	St	Pg
Onc	Cohen, S	NY	293
Onc	Johnson, B	MA	288
Onc	Kelsen, D	NY	298

Mesothelioma

Spec	Name	St	Pg
OM	Cullen, M	CT	758
Onc	Algazy, K	PA	290
Onc	Bonomi, P	IL	315
Onc	Dakhil, S	KS	325
Onc	Edelman, M	MD	294
Onc	Ilson, D	NY	297
Onc	Jahan, T	CA	336
Onc	Kalemkerian, G	MI	320
Onc	Kindler, H	IL	320
Onc	Langer, C	PA	298
Onc	Martins, R	WA	336
Onc	Robert-Vizcarrondo, F	AL	311
Onc	Ruckdeschel, J	MI	322
Onc	Salgia, R	IL	322
Onc	Shin, D	GA	312
Onc	Verschraegen, C	NM	332
Onc	Vogelzang, N	NV	339
Path	Cagle, P	TX	615

Special Expertise Index

America's Top Doctors® 8th Edition

Special Expertise Index

Spec	Name	St	Pg
RE	McGovern, P	NJ	873
RE	Sanfilippo, J	PA	873
S	Brunt, L	MO	923
S	Courcoulas, A	PA	907
S	Curet, M	CA	938
S	Duh, Q	CA	938
S	Fitzgibbons, R	NE	930
S	Fowler, D	NY	908
S	Koruda, M	NC	918
S	Nissen, N	CA	940
S	Park, A	MD	911
S	Ponsky, J	OH	927
S	Ramanathan, R	PA	912
S	Rogers, S	CA	941
S	Tuttle, T	MN	929
S	Way, L	CA	942
TS	Cohen, R	CA	970
TS	Fontana, G	CA	970
TS	Rosengart, T	NY	958
U	Docimo, S	PA	980
U	Irby, P	NC	989
VascS	Lumsden, A	TX	1018

Minimally Invasive Surgery-Pediatric

U	Poppas, D	NY	984

Minimally Invasive Thoracic Surgery

TS	Jones, D	VA	960
TS	Krellenstein, D	NY	956
TS	Maddaus, M	MN	965
TS	Rice, T	OH	966
TS	Sonett, J	NY	958

Minimally Invasive Transnasal Surgery

Oto	Kennedy, D	PA	568

Minimally Invasive Urologic Surgery

U	Gill, I	OH	993
U	Gluckman, G	IL	993
U	Gomella, L	PA	981
U	Kawachi, M	CA	1003
U	Lanteri, V	NJ	983
U	Sanda, M	MA	979
U	Wilson, T	CA	1005

Minimally Invasive Vascular Surgery

VascS	Ahn, S	CA	1019
VascS	Brener, B	NJ	1012
VascS	McLafferty, R	IL	1017
VascS	Todd, G	NY	1014

Spec	Name	St	Pg

Miscarriage-Recurrent

MF	Druzin, M	CA	378
MF	Landy, H	DC	372
MF	Lockwood, C	CT	370
MF	Paidas, M	CT	371
ObG	Scher, J	NY	481
ObG	Young, B	NY	482
RE	Barnes, R	IL	876
RE	DeVane, G	FL	875
RE	Hill, J	NH	870
RE	Odem, R	MO	877
RE	Walmer, D	NC	876

Mitochondrial Disorders

CG	Boles, R	CA	151
CG	Boles, R	CA	151
CG	Craigen, W	TX	150
CG	Craigen, W	TX	150
ChiN	Haas, R	CA	143

Mitral Valve Disease

Cv	Schwartz, A	NY	99
IC	Yeung, A	CA	124

Mitral Valve Robotic Surgery

TS	Hargrove, W	PA	954
TS	Murphy, D	GA	961
TS	Smith, J	OH	966

Mitral Valve Surgery

TS	Adams, D	NY	952
TS	Aklog, L	AZ	968
TS	Alexander, J	IL	963
TS	Bakhos, M	IL	963
TS	Bolman, R	MA	950
TS	Chitwood, W	NC	959
TS	Fontana, G	CA	970
TS	Fullerton, D	CO	967
TS	Grossi, E	NY	954
TS	Naka, Y	NY	957
TS	Smith, C	NY	958

Mobility Evaluation & Treatment

Ger	Studenski, S	PA	235
PMR	Esquenazi, A	PA	721

Mohs' Surgery

D	Amonette, R	TN	174
D	Bailin, P	OH	177
D	Bennett, R	CA	181
D	Berg, D	WA	181
D	Bowen, G	UT	179
D	Braun, M	DC	170
D	Brodland, D	PA	171
D	Carney, J	AR	180
D	Cook, J	NC	175
D	Dzubow, L	PA	171

Spec	Name	St	Pg
D	Fewkes, J	MA	168
D	Flowers, F	FL	175
D	Garrett, A	VA	176
D	Geronemus, R	NY	171
D	Glogau, R	CA	181
D	Green, H	FL	176
D	Greenway, H	CA	182
D	Hanke, C	IN	177
D	Hruza, G	MO	178
D	Johnson, T	MI	178
D	Kriegel, D	NY	172
D	Leffell, D	CT	169
D	Leshin, B	NC	176
D	Maloney, M	MA	169
D	Miller, S	MD	173
D	Neel, V	MA	169
D	Neuburg, M	WI	178
D	Olbricht, S	MA	170
D	Orengo, I	TX	180
D	Otley, C	MN	178
D	Robins, P	NY	173
D	Taylor, R	TX	181
D	Wheeland, R	MO	179
D	Zitelli, J	PA	174

Mood Disorders

ChAP	Alessi, N	MI	783
ChAP	Bogrov, M	MD	781
ChAP	Boxer, G	MO	784
ChAP	Foley, C	NY	781
ChAP	Luby, J	MO	784
ChAP	Riddle, M	MD	782
GerPsy	Holroyd, S	VA	787
Psyc	Blazer, D	NC	769
Psyc	Gelenberg, A	AZ	773
Psyc	Gitlin, M	CA	774
Psyc	Haskett, R	PA	766
Psyc	Janicak, P	IL	771
Psyc	Kendler, K	VA	769
Psyc	Locala, J	OH	771
Psyc	Mann, J	NY	767
Psyc	Nelson, J	CA	775
Psyc	Price, L	RI	763

Motion Sickness

N	Hain, T	IL	454

Motor Control Analysis

PMR	Mayer, N	PA	722

Movement Disorders

ChiN	Lavenstein, B	VA	140
ChiN	Noetzel, M	MO	141
N	Ahlskog, J	MN	452
N	Aminoff, M	CA	462
N	Aurora, S	WA	462
N	Baser, S	PA	438
N	Bressman, S	NY	438
N	Burns, R	AZ	459
N	De Long, M	GA	448

Special Expertise Index

Special Expertise Index

Special Expertise Index

Special Expertise Index

Special Expertise Index

Spec	Name	St	Pg
Neurotology			
Oto	Kesser, B	VA	574
Neurotoxicology			
N	Brooks, B	NC	448
Neurovascular Surgery			
NS	Rich, K	MO	421
NS	Thompson, B	MI	421
NS	Thompson, R	TN	416
Neutron Therapy for Advanced Cancer			
RadRO	Forman, J	MI	830
RadRO	Laramore, G	WA	837
Nocardia Infection			
Inf	Wallace, R	TX	358
Non Tuberculous Mycobacteria			
Inf	Wallace, R	TX	358
Nuclear Cardiology			
Cv	Beller, G	VA	100
Cv	Borer, J	NY	95
Cv	Cerqueira, M	OH	104
Cv	Chaitman, B	MO	104
Cv	Follansbee, W	PA	96
Cv	Gibbons, R	MN	105
Cv	Iskandrian, A	AL	101
Cv	Miller, D	GA	102
Cv	Nocero, M	FL	102
Cv	Simons, M	CT	94
Cv	Steingart, R	NY	99
Cv	Walsh, M	IN	109
Cv	Williams, K	IL	109
Cv	Zaret, B	CT	94
IC	Khawaja, S	GA	121
NuM	Dae, M	CA	477
NuM	Neumann, D	OH	476
NuM	Sanger, J	NY	475
NuM	Schelbert, H	CA	477
NuM	Strashun, A	NY	475
Nuclear Endocrinology			
NuM	Sandler, M	TN	476
Nuclear Oncology			
NuM	Alazraki, N	GA	476
NuM	Freeman, L	NY	474
NuM	Neumann, D	OH	476
Nuclear Radiology			
DR	Partain, C	TN	850

Spec	Name	St	Pg
Nutrition			
EDM	Jensen, M	MN	197
EDM	Kahn, B	MA	189
EDM	McMahon, M	MN	198
Ge	Seidner, D	TN	217
Ge	Semrad, C	IL	222
Ge	Toskes, P	FL	217
Ger	Dale, L	MN	236
Ger	Freedman, M	NY	235
Ger	Lipschitz, D	AR	238
IM	Galland, L	NY	364
IM	Rivlin, R	NY	365
Nep	Mitch, W	TX	399
NP	Ehrenkranz, R	CT	382
NP	Escobedo, M	OK	387
NP	Lemons, J	IN	386
NP	Milley, J	UT	387
Ped	Jacob, M	IL	626
PEn	Ludwig, D	MA	640
PGe	Baker, R	NY	645
PGe	Baker, S	NY	645
PGe	Berman, J	IL	648
PGe	Fasano, A	MD	646
PGe	Kleinman, R	MA	645
PGe	Krebs, N	CO	650
PGe	Rudolph, C	WI	649
PGe	Schwarz, S	NY	647
PGe	Vanderhoof, J	NE	650
PMR	Dillard, J	NY	721
S	Greenhalgh, D	CA	939
SM	Dimeff, R	OH	898
Nutrition & AIDS			
Ge	Kotler, D	NY	210
Nutrition & Cancer Prevention			
EDM	Heber, D	CA	201
Ge	Mason, J	MA	206
Ge	Shike, M	NY	213
IM	Heimburger, D	AL	365
U	Katz, A	NY	982
Nutrition & Cancer Prevention/Control			
Ge	Kurtz, R	NY	211
IM	Rivlin, R	NY	365
Onc	Clinton, S	OH	317
S	Herrmann, V	SC	917
U	Yu, G	MD	987
Nutrition & Disease Prevention/Control			
EDM	Heber, D	CA	201
IM	Heimburger, D	AL	365
U	Yu, G	MD	987
Nutrition & Obesity			
EDM	Heber, D	CA	201

Spec	Name	St	Pg
Nutrition in Acute Illness			
Ge	Mason, J	MA	206
Nutrition in Autism			
PGe	Levy, J	NY	646
Nutrition in Bowel Disorders			
Ge	Mason, J	MA	206
PS	Barksdale, E	OH	697
Nutrition in Heart Disease			
TS	Gundry, S	CA	971
Nystagmus			
Oph	Demer, J	CA	517

O

Spec	Name	St	Pg
Obesity			
AM	Bermudez, O	OK	79
CG	Driscoll, D	FL	148
CG	Driscoll, D	FL	148
EDM	Kahn, B	MA	189
PEn	Arslanian, S	PA	641
PEn	Diamond, F	FL	642
PEn	Ludwig, D	MA	640
PGe	Baker, S	NY	645
PGe	Krebs, N	CO	650
Psyc	Crow, S	MN	771
Obesity/Bariatric Surgery			
S	Bessler, M	NY	905
S	Courcoulas, A	PA	907
S	Curet, M	CA	938
S	Edye, M	NY	907
S	Gagner, M	FL	917
S	Livingston, E	TX	935
S	MacDonald, K	NC	919
S	Nguyen, N	CA	940
S	Phillips, E	CA	941
S	Ramanathan, R	PA	912
S	Rogers, S	CA	941
S	Rubino, F	NY	913
S	Sarr, M	MN	928
S	Shikora, S	MA	903
Obsessive-Compulsive Disorder			
ChAP	Coffey, B	NY	781
ChAP	Hudziak, J	VT	780
ChAP	King, R	CT	780
ChAP	Leckman, J	CT	780
ChAP	McCracken, J	CA	785

Special Expertise Index

America's Top Doctors® 8th Edition

Special Expertise Index

Special Expertise Index

Spec	Name	St	Pg
Ovarian Cancer Risk Assessment			
Onc	Daly, M	PA	293
Ovarian Cancer Ultrasound Diagnosis			
DR	Hann, L	NY	847
Ovarian Cancer-Early Detection			
GO	Cain, J	OR	255
GO	DePriest, P	KY	248
GO	Fishman, D	NY	246
GO	Rutherford, T	CT	244
Ovarian Cancer-High Risk			
ObG	Cramer, D	MA	480
Ovarian Failure			
ObG	Simpson, J	FL	483
RE	Legro, R	PA	872
Oxalosis			
PNep	Langman, C	IL	679

P

Spec	Name	St	Pg
Pacemakers			
CE	Callans, D	PA	115
CE	Chinitz, L	NY	115
CE	Cohen, M	NY	115
CE	Curtis, A	FL	116
CE	DiMarco, J	VA	116
CE	Ellenbogen, K	VA	116
CE	Gomes, J	NY	115
CE	Hammill, S	MN	117
CE	Hayes, D	MN	117
CE	Kay, G	AL	117
CE	Levine, J	NY	115
CE	Marchlinski, F	PA	116
CE	Sorrentino, R	GA	117
Cv	Myerburg, R	FL	102
Cv	Naccarelli, G	PA	98
PCd	Fish, F	TN	633
Paget's Disease of Bone			
EDM	Econs, M	IN	196
EDM	Siris, E	NY	193
EDM	Watts, N	OH	199
Pain & Spasticity			
NS	Whiting, D	PA	412

Spec	Name	St	Pg
Pain Management			
AdP	Howell, E	UT	779
ChiN	Cohen, B	OH	141
Ger	Finucane, T	MD	234
N	Hiesiger, E	NY	441
N	Schwartzman, R	PA	446
NS	Berger, M	CA	426
NS	Burchiel, K	OR	426
NS	Di Giacinto, G	NY	407
Onc	Levy, M	PA	298
PCCM	Anand, K	AR	639
Ped	Zeltzer, L	CA	626
PM	Billings, J	MA	596
PMR	Creamer, M	FL	723
PMR	Dillard, J	NY	721
PMR	Schwartz, L	PA	722
PMR	Slipman, C	PA	723
Pul	Shore, B	MO	806
Pain Management-Pediatric			
PM	Anderson, C	WA	601
PM	Anghelescu, D	TN	598
PM	Berde, C	MA	596
PM	Weisman, S	WI	600
Pain-Abdominal Recurrent			
PGe	Gunasekaran, T	IL	648
PGe	Kirschner, B	IL	649
Pain-Abdominal/Functional			
Ge	Drossman, D	NC	215
Ge	Olden, K	AR	225
Pain-Acute			
PM	Benedetti, C	OH	598
PM	De Leon-Casasola, O	NY	596
PM	Swarm, R	MO	599
Pain-after Spinal Intervention			
PM	Amin, S	IL	598
PM	Diwan, S	NY	596
PM	Huntoon, M	MN	599
PM	Racz, G	TX	600
PM	Rosner, H	CA	602
Pain-Back			
OrS	Lauerman, W	DC	534
OrS	Teitz, C	WA	554
OrS	Weinstein, J	NH	528
PM	Benzon, H	IL	599
PM	Harden, R	IL	599
PM	Kreitzer, J	NY	597
PM	Ramamurthy, S	TX	601
PM	Rosenquist, R	IA	599
PM	Rosner, H	CA	602
PM	Staats, P	NJ	597
PM	Walsh, N	TX	601

Spec	Name	St	Pg
PM	Weinberger, M	NY	598
PMR	Harris, D	TX	728
PMR	Herring, S	WA	729
PMR	La Ban, M	MI	726
PMR	Lipkin, D	FL	724
PMR	Press, J	IL	726
PMR	Sliwa, J	IL	727
PMR	Smith, J	IL	727
SM	Schechter, D	CA	899
Pain-Back & Neck			
NS	Bauer, J	IL	417
PM	Dubois, M	NY	597
PM	Ferrante, F	CA	601
PMR	Haig, A	MI	725
PMR	Ragnarsson, K	NY	722
Pain-Back & Shoulder			
N	Smith, W	CA	465
Pain-Back, Head & Neck			
PM	Racz, G	TX	600
Pain-Cancer			
Onc	Grossman, S	MD	296
Onc	Levy, M	PA	298
Onc	Weissman, D	WI	324
PHO	Tannous, R	IA	666
PM	Abrahm, J	MA	596
PM	Amin, S	IL	598
PM	Anghelescu, D	TN	598
PM	Audell, L	CA	601
PM	Benedetti, C	OH	598
PM	Benzon, H	IL	599
PM	Burton, A	TX	600
PM	De Leon-Casasola, O	NY	596
PM	Diwan, S	NY	596
PM	Driver, L	TX	600
PM	Fine, P	UT	600
PM	Fishman, S	CA	601
PM	Fitzgibbon, D	WA	601
PM	Foley, K	NY	596
PM	Huntoon, M	MN	599
PM	Hurwitz, C	ME	596
PM	Jain, S	NY	597
PM	Kreitzer, J	NY	597
PM	Portenoy, R	NY	597
PM	Rauck, R	NC	598
PM	Ready, L	WA	602
PM	Rosner, H	CA	602
PM	Slatkin, N	CA	602
PM	Staats, P	NJ	597
PM	Swarm, R	MO	599
PM	Wallace, M	CA	602
PM	Weinberger, M	NY	598
PM	Weinstein, S	UT	600
PMR	Cheville, A	MN	724
PMR	Schwartz, L	PA	722
PMR	Stubblefield, M	NY	723
Psyc	Breitbart, W	NY	764

Special Expertise Index

America's Top Doctors® 8th Edition

Special Expertise Index

Special Expertise Index

Special Expertise Index

Special Expertise Index

Spec	Name	St	Pg
Prenatal Diagnosis			
CG	Anyane-Yeboa, K	NY	146
CG	Anyane-Yeboa, K	NY	146
CG	Elias, S	IL	149
CG	Elias, S	IL	149
CG	Falk, R	CA	151
CG	Falk, R	CA	151
CG	Holmes, L	MA	146
CG	Holmes, L	MA	146
CG	Mahoney, M	CT	146
CG	Mahoney, M	CT	146
CG	Randolph, L	CA	152
CG	Randolph, L	CA	152
CG	Shapiro, L	NY	148
CG	Shapiro, L	NY	148
MF	Abuhamad, A	VA	373
MF	Besinger, R	IL	374
MF	Copel, J	CT	370
MF	D'Alton, M	NY	371
MF	Dugoff, L	CO	376
MF	Edersheim, T	NY	372
MF	Goldberg, J	CA	378
MF	Johnson, T	MI	375
MF	McLaren, R	VA	373
MF	Platt, L	CA	378
MF	Reed, K	AZ	377
ObG	Evans, M	NY	481
ObG	Gonik, B	MI	483
ObG	Shulman, L	IL	484
ObG	Simpson, J	FL	483
Prenatal Genetic Diagnosis			
CG	Driscoll, D	PA	147
CG	Driscoll, D	PA	147
CG	Falk, R	CA	151
CG	Falk, R	CA	151
CG	Pergament, E	IL	149
CG	Pergament, E	IL	149
RE	Grifo, J	NY	872
RE	McClamrock, H	MD	872
Prenatal Ultrasound			
MF	Abuhamad, A	VA	373
MF	Hibbard, J	IL	375
MF	Tomich, P	NE	377
MF	Wilkins, I	IL	376
Preventive Cardiology			
Cv	Bairey-Merz, C	CA	112
Cv	Balady, G	MA	92
Cv	Blumenthal, D	NY	94
Cv	Blumenthal, R	MD	95
Cv	Edmundowicz, D	PA	95
Cv	Fonarow, G	CA	113
Cv	Friedman, S	NY	96
Cv	Gould, K	TX	110
Cv	Hayes, S	MN	105
Cv	Herling, I	PA	97
Cv	Johnson, P	MA	92
Cv	Lewis, S	OR	113

Spec	Name	St	Pg
Cv	Libby, P	MA	93
Cv	Linton, M	TN	102
Cv	Mosca, L	NY	97
Cv	Redberg, R	CA	113
Cv	Reis, S	PA	98
Cv	Reiss, C	MO	107
Cv	Ridker, P	MA	94
Cv	Roberts, B	RI	94
Cv	Shapiro, J	IL	108
Cv	Sorrentino, M	IL	108
Cv	Stein, J	WI	108
Cv	Volgman, A	IL	108
Cv	Weitz, H	PA	100
EDM	Hoogwerf, B	OH	197
IM	Cushman, W	TN	365
IM	Rader, D	PA	364
Nep	Black, H	NY	393
PCd	Hohn, A	CA	637
PrM	Pearson, T	NY	759
Preventive Medicine			
Ger	Lipschitz, D	AR	238
IM	Lewin, N	NY	364
IM	Mehler, P	CO	366
SM	McKeag, D	IN	898
Primary Care Sports Medicine			
SM	Dimeff, R	OH	898
SM	Maharam, L	NY	897
SM	Metzl, J	NY	897
PRK-Refractive Surgery			
Oph	Holladay, J	TX	513
Oph	Manche, E	CA	518
Oph	Mandel, E	NY	498
Oph	Salz, J	CA	519
Oph	Wilson, S	OH	512
Probiotics			
PGe	Vanderhoof, J	NE	650
Progressive Osseous Heteroplasia POH			
OrS	Kaplan, F	PA	533
Progressive Supranuclear Palsy (PSP)			
N	Gizzi, M	NJ	441
N	Golbe, L	NJ	441
N	Weiner, W	MD	447
Prolactin Disorders			
EDM	Klibanski, A	MA	189
RE	Zacur, H	MD	874

Spec	Name	St	Pg
Prostate Cancer			
DR	Weinreb, J	CT	845
NuM	Podoloff, D	TX	477
Onc	Ahmann, F	AZ	327
Onc	Beer, T	OR	333
Onc	Bolger, G	AL	305
Onc	Boston, B	TN	305
Onc	Brawley, O	GA	305
Onc	Butler, W	SC	306
Onc	Clinton, S	OH	317
Onc	Dawson, N	DC	293
Onc	Donehower, R	MD	293
Onc	Dreicer, R	OH	318
Onc	Eisenberger, M	MD	294
Onc	Garnick, M	MA	288
Onc	Gelmann, E	NY	295
Onc	Glode, L	CO	326
Onc	Hammond, D	NH	288
Onc	Higano, C	WA	335
Onc	Hudes, G	PA	297
Onc	Hussain, M	MI	319
Onc	Kantoff, P	MA	288
Onc	Kraft, A	SC	309
Onc	Logothetis, C	TX	330
Onc	Motzer, R	NY	300
Onc	Petrylak, D	NY	301
Onc	Picus, J	MO	321
Onc	Pienta, K	MI	321
Onc	Quinn, D	CA	338
Onc	Raghavan, D	OH	321
Onc	Richards, J	IL	321
Onc	Roth, B	TN	311
Onc	Scher, H	NY	302
Onc	Small, E	CA	338
Onc	Stadler, W	IL	323
Onc	Taplin, M	MA	290
Onc	Torti, F	NC	313
Onc	Trump, D	NY	303
Onc	Vaughn, D	PA	303
Onc	Vogelzang, N	NV	339
Onc	Wilding, G	WI	324
Path	Balla, A	IL	612
Path	Bostwick, D	VA	610
Path	Epstein, J	MD	605
Path	Melamed, J	NY	607
Path	Orenstein, J	DC	608
Path	Reuter, V	NY	608
Path	Ross, J	NY	608
Path	True, L	WA	619
RadRO	Anscher, M	VA	826
RadRO	D'Amico, A	MA	820
RadRO	DeWeese, T	MD	822
RadRO	Dicker, A	PA	822
RadRO	Dritschilo, A	DC	822
RadRO	Ennis, R	NY	822
RadRO	Forman, J	MI	830
RadRO	Glassburn, J	PA	823
RadRO	Goodman, R	NJ	823
RadRO	Grado, G	AZ	834
RadRO	Hahn, S	PA	823
RadRO	Hancock, S	CA	836
RadRO	Haraf, D	IL	830
RadRO	Horwitz, E	PA	823

Special Expertise Index

Spec	Name	St	Pg
RadRO	Jose, B	KY	827
RadRO	Kuettel, M	NY	824
RadRO	Lee, A	TX	835
RadRO	Lee, W	NC	827
RadRO	Michalski, J	MO	832
RadRO	Movsas, B	MI	832
RadRO	Nori, D	NY	825
RadRO	Peschel, R	CT	820
RadRO	Pollack, A	PA	825
RadRO	Roach, M	CA	838
RadRO	Rose, C	CA	838
RadRO	Rosenman, J	NC	829
RadRO	Rossi, C	CA	838
RadRO	Rotman, M	NY	825
RadRO	Russell, K	WA	838
RadRO	Sandler, H	MI	832
RadRO	Schiff, P	NY	825
RadRO	Shipley, W	MA	821
RadRO	Stock, R	NY	825
RadRO	Toonkel, L	FL	829
RadRO	Tripuraneni, P	CA	838
RadRO	Vicini, F	MI	833
RadRO	Wong, J	CA	838
RadRO	Zelefsky, M	NY	826
RadRO	Zietman, A	MA	821
U	Andriole, G	MO	992
U	Babaian, R	TX	998
U	Bahnson, R	OH	992
U	Bans, L	AZ	998
U	Bardot, S	LA	998
U	Basler, J	TX	999
U	Beall, M	VA	987
U	Brendler, C	IL	992
U	Burnett, A	MD	980
U	Campbell, S	OH	992
U	Carroll, P	CA	1002
U	Carter, H	MD	980
U	Catalona, W	IL	992
U	Chang, S	TN	988
U	Childs, S	CO	998
U	Cookson, M	TN	988
U	Crawford, E	CO	998
U	Danoff, D	CA	1002
U	Davis, B	KS	998
U	de Kernion, J	CA	1002
U	Droller, M	NY	981
U	Ellis, W	WA	1002
U	Flanigan, R	IL	993
U	Fraser, L	MS	988
U	Gill, H	CA	1002
U	Gill, I	OH	993
U	Gluckman, G	IL	993
U	Gomella, L	PA	981
U	Greenberg, R	PA	981
U	Herr, H	NY	982
U	Huben, R	NY	982
U	Jarow, J	MD	982
U	Jordan, G	VA	989
U	Kadmon, D	TX	1000
U	Keane, T	SC	989
U	Kibel, A	MO	994
U	Kim, E	TN	989
U	Kirschenbaum, A	NY	983

Spec	Name	St	Pg
U	Klein, E	OH	994
U	Kozlowski, J	IL	994
U	Lange, P	WA	1003
U	Lepor, H	NY	983
U	Levine, L	IL	994
U	Libertino, J	MA	978
U	Lieskovsky, G	CA	1003
U	Loughlin, K	MA	978
U	Lowe, F	NY	983
U	Lugg, J	WY	998
U	Malkowicz, S	PA	983
U	Marshall, F	GA	990
U	McConnell, J	TX	1000
U	McCullough, A	NY	983
U	McDougal, W	MA	978
U	McGovern, F	MA	978
U	McVary, K	IL	995
U	Miles, B	TX	1000
U	Montie, J	MI	995
U	Mostwin, J	MD	983
U	Moul, J	NC	990
U	Myers, R	MN	995
U	Naslund, M	MD	984
U	Nelson, J	PA	984
U	Partin, A	MD	984
U	Pisters, L	TX	1000
U	Pow-Sang, J	FL	990
U	Presti, J	CA	1004
U	Richie, J	MA	979
U	Robertson, C	NC	990
U	Roehrborn, C	TX	1000
U	Sanda, M	MA	979
U	Sanders, W	GA	991
U	Scardino, P	NY	985
U	Schlegel, P	NY	985
U	See, W	WI	996
U	Skinner, D	CA	1004
U	Slawin, K	TX	1001
U	Soloway, M	FL	991
U	Steinberg, G	IL	997
U	Swanson, D	TX	1001
U	Taneja, S	NY	986
U	Terris, M	GA	991
U	Theodorescu, D	VA	991
U	Thompson, I	TX	1001
U	Uzzo, R	PA	986
U	Walsh, P	MD	986
U	Wein, A	PA	987
U	Williams, R	IA	997
U	Wood, D	MI	997
U	Zippe, C	OH	997

Prostate Cancer-Cryosurgery

RadRO	Bahn, D	CA	836
U	Ellis, D	TX	999
U	Katz, A	NY	982

Prostate Cancer-HIFU Therapy

U	Chang, S	TN	988

Prostate Cancer-MR

Spectroscopy (MRSI)

DR	Hricak, H	NY	848

Prostate Cancer-Vaccine Therapy

Onc	Arlen, P	MD	291
Onc	Gulley, J	MD	296

Prostate Cancer/Robotic Surgery

U	Albala, D	NC	987
U	Amling, C	AL	987
U	Benson, M	NY	980
U	Donovan, J	OH	993
U	Greenberg, R	PA	981
U	Jackman, S	PA	982
U	Kawachi, M	CA	1003
U	Lanteri, V	NJ	983
U	Menon, M	MI	995
U	Patel, V	FL	990
U	Pisters, L	TX	1000
U	Samadi, D	NY	984
U	Sawczuk, I	NJ	985
U	Scherr, D	NY	985
U	Slawin, K	TX	1001
U	Smith, J	TN	991
U	Steers, W	VA	991
U	Teigland, C	NC	991
U	Tewari, A	NY	986
U	Wilson, T	CA	1005

Prostate Disease

U	Alexander, R	MD	979
U	Bans, L	AZ	998
U	Bruskewitz, R	WI	992
U	Catalona, W	IL	992
U	de Kernion, J	CA	1002
U	Ellis, W	WA	1002
U	Gill, H	CA	1002
U	Gribetz, M	NY	982
U	Lowe, F	NY	983
U	McVary, K	IL	995
U	Naslund, M	MD	984
U	O'Leary, M	MA	979
U	Partin, A	MD	984
U	Rajfer, J	CA	1004
U	Roehrborn, C	TX	1000
U	Ross, L	IL	996
U	Seftel, A	OH	996
U	Slawin, K	TX	1001
U	Thompson, I	TX	1001
U	Vaughan, E	NY	986

Prosthesis Control

PMR	Kuiken, T	IL	726

Proton Beam Therapy

RadRO	DeLaney, T	MA	820

Special Expertise Index

America's Top Doctors® 8th Edition

Special Expertise Index

Spec	Name	St	Pg
ObG	Evans, M	NY	481
U	Oates, R	MA	979

Reproductive Medicine
Spec	Name	St	Pg
RE	Blackwell, R	AL	874
RE	Soules, M	WA	879

Reproductive Surgery
Spec	Name	St	Pg
RE	Azziz, R	CA	879
RE	Milad, M	IL	877
RE	Noyes, N	NY	873
RE	Odem, R	MO	877
RE	Tureck, R	PA	874

Respiratory Disorders
Spec	Name	St	Pg
PMR	Bach, J	NJ	720

Respiratory Distress Syndrome (ARDS)
Spec	Name	St	Pg
Pul	Arroliga, A	TX	809
Pul	Martin, T	WA	811
Pul	Matthay, M	CA	811
Pul	Summer, W	LA	809
Pul	Wheeler, A	TN	803
Pul	Wiedemann, H	OH	807

Respiratory Distress Syndrome (RDS)
Spec	Name	St	Pg
NP	Cole, F	MO	385
NP	Donn, S	MI	385
NP	Seidner, S	TX	388

Respiratory Failure
Spec	Name	St	Pg
PCCM	Nichols, D	MD	638
PCCM	Perez Fontan, J	TX	639
PCCM	Thompson, A	PA	638
PPul	Green, T	IL	687
Pul	Balk, R	IL	804
Pul	Celli, B	MA	794
Pul	Deitz, J	PA	796
Pul	Fulkerson, W	NC	801
Pul	Hall, J	IL	804
Pul	Heffner, J	OR	810
Pul	Hudson, L	WA	811
Pul	Niederman, M	NY	797
Pul	Thomashow, B	NY	799

Restless Legs Syndrome
Spec	Name	St	Pg
N	Buchholz, D	MD	438
N	Sethi, K	GA	451

Retina/Vitreous Surgery
Spec	Name	St	Pg
Oph	Abrams, G	MI	506
Oph	Brucker, A	PA	494
Oph	Campochiaro, P	MD	494
Oph	Chang, S	NY	494
Oph	De Juan, E	CA	517
Oph	Flynn, H	FL	503
Oph	Fuchs, W	NY	495
Oph	Gentile, R	NY	496
Oph	Ho, A	PA	497
Oph	Lambert, H	TX	513
Oph	Meredith, T	NC	504
Oph	Mieler, W	IL	510
Oph	Muldoon, T	NY	499
Oph	Rosenfeld, P	FL	505
Oph	Schachat, A	OH	511
Oph	Sternberg, P	TN	505
Oph	Trese, M	MI	511
Oph	Yannuzzi, L	NY	502

Retinal Detachment
Spec	Name	St	Pg
Oph	D'Amico, D	NY	494
Oph	Del Priore, L	NY	494
Oph	Rosenfeld, P	FL	505
Oph	Schiff, W	NY	500

Retinal Disorders
Spec	Name	St	Pg
Oph	Blumenkranz, M	CA	515
Oph	Bressler, N	MD	494
Oph	Brown, G	PA	494
Oph	Brucker, A	PA	494
Oph	Chang, S	NY	494
Oph	D'Amico, D	NY	494
Oph	Duker, J	MA	492
Oph	Friberg, T	PA	495
Oph	Fuchs, W	NY	495
Oph	Gentile, R	NY	496
Oph	Goldberg, M	MD	496
Oph	Gorin, M	CA	517
Oph	Grossniklaus, H	GA	503
Oph	Lewis, H	NY	498
Oph	Lewis, R	TX	514
Oph	Marmor, M	CA	518
Oph	Mets, M	IL	510
Oph	Miller, J	MA	493
Oph	Murray, T	FL	504
Oph	Odel, J	NY	499
Oph	Puliafito, C	CA	519
Oph	Regillo, C	PA	500
Oph	Rizzo, J	MA	493
Oph	Stone, E	IA	511
Oph	Vander, J	PA	501
Oph	Vine, A	MI	512
Oph	Walsh, J	NY	501
Oph	Weingeist, T	IA	512
Oph	Williams, G	MI	512

Retinal Disorders-Pediatric
Spec	Name	St	Pg
Oph	Duker, J	MA	492
Oph	Stout, J	OR	520
Oph	Trese, M	MI	511

Retinal Dystrophies
Spec	Name	St	Pg
Oph	Marmor, M	CA	518

Retinal Vascular Diseases
Spec	Name	St	Pg
Oph	Brown, G	PA	494

Retinoblastoma
Spec	Name	St	Pg
Oph	Abramson, D	NY	493
Oph	Augsburger, J	OH	507
Oph	Handa, J	MD	496
Oph	Harbour, J	MO	508
Oph	Lueder, G	MO	509
Oph	Murphree, A	CA	519
Oph	O'Brien, J	CA	519
Oph	Shields, C	PA	501
Oph	Shields, J	PA	501
Oph	Stout, J	OR	520
Oph	Wilson, M	TN	506
PHO	Dunkel, I	NY	654
PHO	Friedman, D	WA	654
PHO	Meadows, A	PA	656
PHO	Pendergrass, T	WA	671
PHO	Rausen, A	NY	657

Retinopathy of Prematurity
Spec	Name	St	Pg
NP	Hendricks-Munoz, K	NY	383
Oph	Flynn, J	NY	495
Oph	Freedman, S	NC	503
Oph	Mahon, K	NV	518
Oph	Nussbaum, J	GA	505
Oph	Palmer, E	OR	519
Oph	Reynolds, J	NY	500
Oph	Shabto, U	NY	501
Oph	Siatkowski, R	OK	514
Oph	Stout, J	OR	520

Rhabdomyosarcoma
Spec	Name	St	Pg
PHO	Adamson, P	PA	652
PHO	Croop, J	IN	663
PHO	Hawkins, D	WA	670
PHO	Wexler, L	NY	658

Rheumatic Diseases of Childhood
Spec	Name	St	Pg
PMR	Sisung, C	IL	727
PRhu	Emery, H	WA	691
PRhu	Schanberg, L	NC	690

Rheumatic Heart Disease
Spec	Name	St	Pg
PCd	Cooper, R	NY	631

Rheumatoid Arthritis
Spec	Name	St	Pg
PRhu	Lehman, T	NY	690
Rhu	Adams, E	IL	888
Rhu	Arend, W	CO	890
Rhu	Ashman, R	IA	888
Rhu	Belmont, H	NY	883
Rhu	Blume, R	NY	883
Rhu	Brenner, M	MA	882
Rhu	Bunning, R	DC	883

Spec	Name	St	Pg
Rhu	Chang, R	IL	888
Rhu	Chatham, W	AL	886
Rhu	Crofford, L	KY	887
Rhu	Curran, J	IL	888
Rhu	Davis, W	LA	891
Rhu	Fischbein, L	MO	888
Rhu	Gershwin, M	CA	892
Rhu	Hochberg, M	MD	884
Rhu	Katz, R	IL	889
Rhu	Kay, J	MA	882
Rhu	Luthra, H	MN	889
Rhu	McCune, W	MI	889
Rhu	Michalska, M	IL	889
Rhu	Mitnick, H	NY	885
Rhu	Moder, K	MN	890
Rhu	Moore, W	GA	887
Rhu	O'Dell, J	NE	890
Rhu	Paget, S	NY	885
Rhu	Polisson, R	MA	882
Rhu	Pope, R	IL	890
Rhu	Rothenberg, R	MD	885
Rhu	Schoen, R	CT	882
Rhu	Shadick, N	MA	882
Rhu	Simms, R	MA	882
Rhu	Solomon, G	NY	885
Rhu	Sundy, J	NC	887
Rhu	Wallace, D	CA	892
Rhu	Weinblatt, M	MA	883
Rhu	Wise, C	VA	887

Rheumatologic Dermatology
| D | Jorizzo, J | NC | 176 |

Rheumatologic Diseases of the Lung
| Pul | Steiger, D | NY | 798 |

Rheumatology
A&I	deShazo, R	MS	84
Ger	Cooney, L	CT	234
PMR	Lipkin, D	FL	724

Rheumatology-Adult & Pediatric
| Rhu | Albert, D | NH | 882 |

Rhinitis
A&I	Buchbinder, E	NY	82
A&I	Busse, W	WI	86
A&I	Freeman, T	TX	87
A&I	Kaliner, M	MD	83
A&I	Lieberman, P	TN	85
A&I	Lockey, R	FL	85
A&I	Pacin, M	FL	85
A&I	Sanders, G	MI	86
A&I	Slankard, M	NY	84
A&I	Tamaroff, M	CA	88
A&I	Wasserman, S	CA	88
Oto	Lanza, D	FL	574

| PA&I | Kelly, C | VA | 628 |
| PA&I | Skoner, D | PA | 627 |

Rhinoplasty
Oto	Denenberg, S	NE	584
Oto	Farrior, E	FL	573
Oto	Gliklich, R	MA	563
Oto	Kern, R	IL	580
Oto	Larrabee, W	WA	588
Oto	Papel, I	MD	569
Oto	Quatela, V	NY	570
Oto	Setzen, M	NY	571
Oto	Szachowicz, E	MN	582
Oto	Toriumi, D	IL	582
PlS	Aston, S	NY	735
PlS	Baker, D	NY	736
PlS	Constantian, M	NH	734
PlS	Cutting, C	NY	736
PlS	Daniel, R	CA	751
PlS	Fisher, G	CA	751
PlS	Friedland, J	AZ	749
PlS	Gunter, J	TX	749
PlS	Hamra, S	TX	749
PlS	Hidalgo, D	NY	737
PlS	Hurwitz, D	PA	738
PlS	Matarasso, A	NY	739
PlS	Mustoe, T	IL	746
PlS	Ristow, B	CA	754
PlS	Rohrich, R	TX	750
PlS	Romano, J	CA	754
PlS	Sullivan, P	RI	735
PlS	Tabbal, N	NY	741
PlS	Tebbetts, J	TX	750

Rhinoplasty Revision
Oto	Kuhn, F	GA	574
PlS	Constantian, M	NH	734
PlS	Gunter, J	TX	749

Rhinosinusitis
A&I	Fox, R	FL	84
A&I	Wong, J	MA	82
Oto	Stankiewicz, J	IL	582

Rhinosinusitis & Asthma
| A&I | Shepherd, G | NY | 83 |

Robotic Cardiac Surgery
TS	Argenziano, M	NY	952
TS	Boyd, W	FL	959
TS	Chitwood, W	NC	959
TS	Damiano, R	MO	963
TS	Loulmet, D	NY	956
TS	Michler, R	NY	957
TS	Smith, C	NY	958
TS	Starnes, V	CA	972
TS	Stuart, R	MO	967

Robotic Heart Surgery
| TS | Alexander, J | IL | 963 |
| TS | Raman, J | IL | 966 |

Robotic Surgery
GO	Fields, A	VA	249
GO	Fowler, J	OH	251
GO	Magrina, J	AZ	254
GO	Muto, M	MA	244
ObG	Cornella, J	AZ	485
ObG	Hale, D	IN	483
PS	Glick, P	NY	694
PS	Jackson, R	AR	700
PS	Jennings, R	MA	692
PS	Krummel, T	CA	701
PS	Lobe, T	IA	698
PS	Shlasko, E	NY	694
S	Curcillo, P	PA	907
S	Curet, M	CA	938
S	Sweeney, J	GA	921
U	Samadi, D	NY	984
U	Scherr, D	NY	985
U	Winfield, H	IA	997

Robotic Surgery-Pediatric
| U | Poppas, D | NY | 984 |

Rocky Mountain Spotted Fever
| PInf | Givner, L | NC | 674 |

Rosacea
| D | James, W | PA | 172 |
| D | Shalita, A | NY | 173 |

Ross Procedure for Aortic Valve Disease
TS	Fullerton, D	CO	967
TS	Perryman, R	FL	962
TS	Starnes, V	CA	972

Rotator Cuff Surgery
HS	Imbriglia, J	PA	261
OrS	Flatow, E	NY	531
OrS	Matsen, F	WA	553
OrS	Rodosky, M	PA	536
OrS	Yamaguchi, K	MO	548
SM	Fronek, J	CA	899

Running Injuries
| SM | Maharam, L | NY | 897 |
| SM | Metzl, J | NY | 897 |

Special Expertise Index

Spec	Name	St	Pg

S

Salivary Gland Tumors

Spec	Name	St	Pg
Onc	Martins, R	WA	336
RadRO	Laramore, G	WA	837

Salivary Gland Tumors & Surgery

Spec	Name	St	Pg
Oto	Clayman, G	TX	585
Oto	Deschler, D	MA	563
Oto	Eisele, D	CA	587
Oto	Lydiatt, W	NE	584
Oto	Olsen, K	MN	581
Oto	Osguthorpe, J	SC	575
Oto	Rassekh, C	WV	570
Oto	Urken, M	NY	572
Oto	Weber, R	TX	586

Sarcoidosis

Spec	Name	St	Pg
Pul	Donohue, J	NC	801
Pul	Hunninghake, G	IA	804
Pul	King, T	CA	811
Pul	Newman, L	CO	808
Pul	Raghu, G	WA	812
Pul	Rose, C	CO	808
Pul	Rossman, M	PA	798
Pul	Sharma, O	CA	812
Pul	Staton, G	GA	803
Pul	Teirstein, A	NY	799

Sarcoma

Spec	Name	St	Pg
Hem	Heinrich, M	OR	284
Onc	Benjamin, R	TX	327
Onc	Borden, E	OH	315
Onc	Brockstein, B	IL	316
Onc	Chow, W	CA	333
Onc	Conry, R	AL	306
Onc	Demetri, G	MA	287
Onc	Ettinger, D	MD	294
Onc	Fanucchi, M	NY	294
Onc	Fitch, T	AZ	328
Onc	Grosh, W	VA	308
Onc	Hande, K	TN	308
Onc	Hesdorffer, C	MD	297
Onc	Jacobs, C	CA	335
Onc	Kraft, A	SC	309
Onc	Meyskens, F	CA	336
Onc	Samuels, B	ID	326
Onc	Sandler, A	TN	312
Onc	Stewart, W	WA	339
Onc	von Mehren, M	PA	304
OrS	Berrey, B	FL	539
OrS	Biermann, J	MI	543
OrS	Bos, G	WA	551
OrS	Conrad, E	WA	551
OrS	Eckardt, J	CA	552
OrS	Healey, J	NY	532
OrS	Lackman, R	PA	533

Spec	Name	St	Pg
OrS	Malawer, M	DC	534
OrS	Scarborough, M	FL	541
OrS	Scully, S	FL	541
OrS	Siegel, H	AL	541
OrS	Yasko, A	IL	548
Path	Brooks, J	PA	605
Path	Fletcher, C	MA	604
Path	Goldblum, J	OH	612
Path	Patchefsky, A	PA	608
Path	Rubin, B	OH	613
Path	Triche, T	CA	619
Path	Weiss, S	GA	611
PHO	Albritton, K	MA	651
PHO	Arndt, C	MN	662
PHO	Marina, N	CA	671
PHO	Meyers, P	NY	656
PHO	Olson, T	GA	661
PHO	Pendergrass, T	WA	671
RadRO	Brizel, D	NC	826
RadRO	Constine, L	NY	822
RadRO	DeLaney, T	MA	820
RadRO	Glatstein, E	PA	823
RadRO	Gunderson, L	AZ	834
RadRO	Hahn, S	PA	823
RadRO	Herman, T	OK	834
RadRO	Kiel, K	IL	831
RadRO	Landry, J	GA	827
RadRO	Marcus, R	GA	827
RadRO	Michalski, J	MO	832
RadRO	Pollack, A	PA	825
RadRO	Prosnitz, L	NC	828
RadRO	Tepper, J	NC	829
S	Brennan, M	NY	905
S	Chang, A	MI	923
S	Eilber, F	CA	938
S	Eisenberg, B	NH	902
S	Feig, B	TX	933
S	Fraker, D	PA	908
S	Leitch, A	TX	935
S	Li, B	LA	935
S	Lind, D	GA	918
S	Nathanson, S	MI	927
S	Pollock, R	TX	935
S	Sondak, V	FL	920
S	White, R	NC	921

Sarcoma-Soft Tissue

Spec	Name	St	Pg
Onc	Forscher, C	CA	334
OrS	Benevenia, J	NJ	528
OrS	Healey, J	NY	532
OrS	O'Donnell, R	CA	553
OrS	Randall, R	UT	549
OrS	Ready, J	MA	527
OrS	Schmidt, R	PA	537
PHO	Wexler, L	NY	658
RadRO	Wharam, M	MD	825
RadRO	Wolfson, A	FL	829
S	August, D	NJ	904
S	Heslin, M	AL	918
S	Hunt, K	TX	934
S	Kraybill, W	MO	925
S	Pisters, P	TX	935

Spec	Name	St	Pg
S	Singer, S	NY	914
TS	Putnam, J	TN	962

Sarcomas

Spec	Name	St	Pg
RadRO	Wara, W	CA	838

Scalp Disorders

Spec	Name	St	Pg
D	Cotsarelis, G	PA	171

Scar Revision

Spec	Name	St	Pg
D	Alster, T	DC	170

Schizophrenia

Spec	Name	St	Pg
ChAP	Rapoport, J	DC	782
ChAP	Russell, A	CA	786
Psyc	Boronow, J	MD	764
Psyc	Davidson, J	TX	773
Psyc	Freedman, R	CO	772
Psyc	Ganguli, R	PA	766
Psyc	Goff, D	MA	762
Psyc	Hirschfeld, R	TX	773
Psyc	Kendler, K	VA	769
Psyc	Liberman, R	CA	775
Psyc	Marder, S	CA	775
Psyc	Weiner, R	NC	770

Schizophrenia-Early Detection/Treatment

Spec	Name	St	Pg
Psyc	McGlashan, T	CT	763

Scleroderma

Spec	Name	St	Pg
D	Falanga, V	RI	168
D	Franks, A	NY	171
PlS	Spence, R	MD	740
PRhu	Lehman, T	NY	690
PRhu	Myones, B	TX	691
Rhu	Arnett, F	TX	890
Rhu	Barr, W	IL	888
Rhu	Belmont, H	NY	883
Rhu	Clements, P	CA	891
Rhu	Mayes, M	TX	891
Rhu	Medsger, T	PA	884
Rhu	Merkel, P	MA	882
Rhu	Simms, R	MA	882
Rhu	Spiera, H	NY	886
Rhu	Steen, V	DC	886
Rhu	Wallace, D	CA	892
Rhu	Wigley, F	MD	886

Scleroderma & Lung Disease

Spec	Name	St	Pg
Rhu	Silver, R	SC	887

Scoliosis

Spec	Name	St	Pg
OrS	Albert, T	PA	528
OrS	An, H	IL	543
OrS	Balderston, R	PA	528

Special Expertise Index

Spec	Name	St	Pg
OrS	Wirth, M	TX	551
OrS	Yamaguchi, K	MO	548
OrS	Zuckerman, J	NY	539
SM	Altchek, D	NY	896
SM	Andrews, J	AL	898
SM	Bradley, J	PA	896
SM	Plancher, K	NY	897
SM	Scheller, A	MA	896
SM	Speer, K	NC	898

Sickle Cell Disease

Hem	Bigelow, C	MS	276
Hem	Blinder, M	MO	278
Hem	Telen, M	NC	277
Ped	Berman, B	OH	625
PHO	Bertolone, S	KY	658
PHO	Buchanan, G	TX	668
PHO	DeBaun, M	MO	663
PHO	Drachtman, R	NJ	653
PHO	Hord, J	OH	664
PHO	Jayabose, S	NY	655
PHO	Scher, C	LA	668
PHO	Wang, W	TN	662

Sickle Cell Disease-Hip Surgery

OrS	Grant, R	OH	545

Sickle Cell Disease-Lung

Pul	Haynes, J	AL	802

Sickle Cell Disease/Anemia

PHO	Weinblatt, M	NY	658

Sinus Disorders

A&I	Benenati, S	FL	84
A&I	Chandler, M	NY	82
A&I	Ein, D	DC	83
A&I	Friedman, S	FL	84
A&I	Mazza, D	NY	83
A&I	Meltzer, E	CA	88
A&I	Schubert, M	AZ	87
A&I	Tamaroff, M	CA	88
A&I	Wasserman, S	CA	88
Oto	Baim, H	IL	577
Oto	Poole, M	GA	575
PO	April, M	NY	680
PO	Cunningham, M	MA	680
PO	Darrow, D	VA	682
PO	Duncan, N	TX	684
PO	Haddad, J	NY	681
PO	Kazahaya, K	PA	681
PO	Miller, R	IL	683
PO	Richardson, M	OR	684

Sinus Disorders/Surgery

Oto	Benninger, M	OH	577
Oto	Caldarelli, D	IL	578
Oto	Close, L	NY	565

Spec	Name	St	Pg
Oto	Fried, M	NY	566
Oto	Friedman, M	IL	579
Oto	Gold, S	NY	566
Oto	Jacobs, J	NY	567
Oto	Kennedy, D	PA	568
Oto	Kern, R	IL	580
Oto	Lanza, D	FL	574
Oto	Lawson, W	NY	569
Oto	Leopold, D	NE	584
Oto	Metson, R	MA	563
Oto	Naclerio, R	IL	581
Oto	Otto, R	TX	586
Oto	Piccirillo, J	MO	581
Oto	Picken, C	DC	570
Oto	Rice, D	CA	589
Oto	Schaefer, S	NY	570
Oto	Senior, B	NC	576
Oto	Sillers, M	AL	576
Oto	Vining, E	CT	564
Oto	Weymuller, E	WA	589
PO	Bower, C	AR	683
PO	Geller, K	CA	684
PO	Jones, J	NY	681
PO	Katz, R	OH	683
PO	Lusk, R	NE	683
PO	Rosbe, K	CA	684
PO	Rosenfeld, R	NY	681
PO	Ward, R	NY	682

Sinus Surgery-Revision

Oto	Jacobs, J	NY	567

Sinus Tumors

Oto	Koch, W	MD	568
Oto	O'Malley, B	PA	569
Oto	Snyderman, C	PA	571
Oto	Vining, E	CT	564

Sinusitis

A&I	Altman, L	WA	87
A&I	Bonner, J	AL	84
A&I	Buchbinder, E	NY	82
A&I	Grammer, L	IL	86
A&I	Kaliner, M	MD	83
A&I	Slankard, M	NY	84
PA&I	Kelly, C	VA	628
PO	Chan, K	CO	683

Sjogren's Syndrome

Rhu	Bobrove, A	CA	891
Rhu	Curran, J	IL	888
Rhu	Pope, R	IL	890
Rhu	Vivino, F	PA	886
Rhu	Wise, C	VA	887

Skeletal Dysplasia

CG	Rimoin, D	CA	153
CG	Rimoin, D	CA	153
CG	Wilcox, W	CA	153

Spec	Name	St	Pg
CG	Wilcox, W	CA	153
OrS	Tolo, V	CA	554

Skin Cancer

D	Amonette, R	TN	174
D	Bailin, P	OH	177
D	Belsito, D	KS	179
D	Bennett, R	CA	181
D	Berg, D	WA	181
D	Bickers, D	NY	170
D	Braun, M	DC	170
D	Brodland, D	PA	171
D	Butler, D	TX	180
D	Bystryn, J	NY	171
D	Carney, J	AR	180
D	Cook, J	NC	175
D	Del Giudice, S	NH	168
D	Duvic, M	TX	180
D	Dzubow, L	PA	171
D	Eichler, C	FL	175
D	Elmets, C	AL	175
D	Fenske, N	FL	175
D	Garrett, A	VA	176
D	Geronemus, R	NY	171
D	Gilchrest, B	MA	168
D	Gordon, M	NY	171
D	Granstein, R	NY	172
D	Green, H	FL	176
D	Greenway, H	CA	182
D	Grichnik, J	NC	176
D	Halpern, A	NY	172
D	Kim, Y	CA	182
D	Kupper, T	MA	169
D	Lebwohl, M	NY	172
D	Leffell, D	CT	169
D	Leshin, B	NC	176
D	Lessin, S	PA	172
D	Lim, H	MI	178
D	Lowe, L	MI	178
D	Miller, S	MD	173
D	Neel, V	MA	169
D	Neuburg, M	WI	178
D	Nigra, T	DC	173
D	Olbricht, S	MA	170
D	Otley, C	MN	178
D	Ramsay, D	NY	173
D	Rigel, D	NY	173
D	Robins, P	NY	173
D	Schultz, N	NY	173
D	Sobel, S	FL	177
D	Sober, A	MA	170
D	Sokoloff, D	FL	177
D	Swanson, N	OR	182
D	Swetter, S	CA	183
D	Taylor, R	TX	181
D	Thiers, B	SC	177
D	Wood, G	WI	179
D	Zitelli, J	PA	174
Onc	Daud, A	FL	307
Oto	Weber, R	TX	586
Path	Bastian, B	CA	617
Path	Le Boit, P	CA	618

Special Expertise Index

Special Expertise Index

Special Expertise Index

Spec	Name	St	Pg
OrS	Schafer, M	IL	547
OrS	Simmons, J	TX	550
OrS	Spengler, D	TN	542
OrS	Spivak, J	NY	537
OrS	Vaccaro, A	PA	538
OrS	Wang, J	CA	554
OrS	Watkins, R	CA	555
OrS	Wiesel, S	DC	539
OrS	Yoo, J	OR	555
OrS	Zdeblick, T	WI	548

Spinal Surgery-Cervical
Spec	Name	St	Pg
NS	O'Rourke, D	PA	410
NS	Taylon, C	NE	423
OrS	Bohlman, H	OH	543
OrS	Riew, K	MO	547

Spinal Surgery-Complex
Spec	Name	St	Pg
NS	Gokaslan, Z	MD	407
NS	Hadley, M	AL	413

Spinal Surgery-Low Back
Spec	Name	St	Pg
NS	Taylon, C	NE	423
OrS	Grant, R	OH	545

Spinal Surgery-Pediatric
Spec	Name	St	Pg
NS	Menezes, A	IA	420
NS	Shaffrey, C	VA	415
OrS	Dormans, J	PA	530
OrS	Hensinger, R	MI	545

Spinal Surgery-Pediatric & Adult
Spec	Name	St	Pg
OrS	Bitan, F	NY	529

Spinal Trauma
Spec	Name	St	Pg
NRad	Flanders, A	PA	855
OrS	Hilibrand, A	PA	532
OrS	Richardson, W	NC	541
OrS	Vaccaro, A	PA	538

Spinal Tumor Imaging
Spec	Name	St	Pg
NRad	Koeller, K	MN	858
NRad	Murtagh, F	FL	857

Spinal Tumors
Spec	Name	St	Pg
N	Glass, J	PA	441
N	Patchell, R	KY	451
N	Phuphanich, S	CA	464
NS	Bilsky, M	NY	406
NS	Borges, L	MA	404
NS	Campbell, J	MD	406
NS	Gokaslan, Z	MD	407
NS	Guthikonda, M	MI	419
NS	Lavyne, M	NY	409
NS	Mamelak, A	CA	427

Spec	Name	St	Pg
NS	McCormick, P	NY	410
NS	Shaffrey, M	VA	415
NS	Yu, J	CA	429
OrS	Weinstein, J	NH	528

Spleen Pathology
Spec	Name	St	Pg
Path	Arber, D	CA	616

Spondylitis
Spec	Name	St	Pg
Rhu	Arnett, F	TX	890

Spondylitis-Back Pain
Spec	Name	St	Pg
Rhu	Hadler, N	NC	887

Spondyloarthropathies
Spec	Name	St	Pg
Rhu	Adams, E	IL	888
Rhu	Chang-Miller, A	AZ	891

Sports Injuries
Spec	Name	St	Pg
HS	Godzik, C	CA	267
HS	Graham, T	MD	261
HS	Lane, L	NY	262
HS	Rosenwasser, M	NY	263
OrS	Teitz, C	WA	554
SM	Schechter, D	CA	899
SM	Scheller, A	MA	896

Sports Medicine
Spec	Name	St	Pg
Cv	Bove, A	PA	95
OrS	Bach, B	IL	543
OrS	Bartolozzi, A	PA	528
OrS	Bergfeld, J	OH	543
OrS	Bigliani, L	NY	529
OrS	Callaghan, J	IA	544
OrS	Cannon, W	CA	551
OrS	Cooper, D	TX	550
OrS	Craig, E	NY	530
OrS	Curl, W	NC	540
OrS	Deland, J	NY	530
OrS	Dillingham, M	CA	552
OrS	Dines, D	NY	530
OrS	Finerman, G	CA	552
OrS	Fu, F	PA	531
OrS	Garrett, W	NC	540
OrS	Glashow, J	NY	531
OrS	Goitz, H	MI	544
OrS	Graf, B	WI	545
OrS	Grelsamer, R	NY	531
OrS	Johnson, D	KY	540
OrS	Jokl, P	CT	526
OrS	Karas, S	GA	540
OrS	Laurencin, C	CT	527
OrS	Lock, T	MI	545
OrS	McFarland, E	MD	534
OrS	Millett, P	CO	548
OrS	Nicholas, S	NY	535
OrS	O'Driscoll, S	MN	546
OrS	Paulos, L	FL	541

Spec	Name	St	Pg
OrS	Pettrone, F	VA	541
OrS	Poehling, G	NC	541
OrS	Ramsey, M	PA	536
OrS	Rodosky, M	PA	536
OrS	Rosenberg, T	UT	549
OrS	Schafer, M	IL	547
OrS	Schurman, D	CA	554
OrS	Scott, W	NY	537
OrS	Souryal, T	TX	550
OrS	Spindler, K	TN	542
OrS	Steadman, J	CO	549
OrS	Taft, T	NC	542
OrS	Uribe, J	FL	542
OrS	Warren, R	NY	538
OrS	Wickiewicz, T	NY	538
PMR	Feinberg, J	NY	721
PMR	Herring, S	WA	729
PMR	Lutz, G	NY	722
PMR	Press, J	IL	726
PMR	Saal, J	CA	729
SM	McKeag, D	IN	898
SM	Nisonson, B	NY	897

Sports Medicine Back Injuries
Spec	Name	St	Pg
OrS	Spivak, J	NY	537

Sports Medicine-Women
Spec	Name	St	Pg
OrS	Hannafin, J	NY	532
SM	Saint-Phard, D	CO	899

Sports Neurology
Spec	Name	St	Pg
N	Jordan, B	NY	442

Sports Related Injuries
Spec	Name	St	Pg
DR	Palmer, W	MA	845

Staphylococcal Infections
Spec	Name	St	Pg
Inf	Yu, V	PA	353

Steatohepatitis
Spec	Name	St	Pg
Ge	Raiford, D	TN	216

Stem Cell Therapy in Heart Failure
Spec	Name	St	Pg
Cv	Hare, J	FL	101
Cv	Willerson, J	TX	111
IC	Losordo, D	IL	123
IC	Perin, E	TX	123

Stem Cell Transplant
Spec	Name	St	Pg
Hem	Champlin, R	TX	283
Hem	Damon, L	CA	284
Hem	Farag, S	IN	278
Hem	Files, J	MS	276
Hem	Greer, J	TN	276
Hem	Lazarus, H	OH	280

Special Expertise Index

Special Expertise Index

Special Expertise Index

Special Expertise Index

Spec	Name	St	Pg
Ge	Lucey, M	WI	220
Ge	Martin, P	FL	216
Ge	Poordad, F	CA	227
Ge	Raiford, D	TN	216
Ge	Reddy, K	PA	212
Ge	Schiano, T	NY	213
Ge	Scudera, P	VA	217
Ge	Shiffman, M	VA	217
Ge	Sorrell, M	NE	224
Ge	Speeg, K	TX	226
Ge	Van Thiel, D	IL	222
Ge	Vierling, J	TX	226
Ge	Wiesner, R	MN	223
PGe	Kleinman, R	MA	645
PGe	McDiarmid, S	CA	650
PGe	Schwarz, K	MD	647
PGe	Whitington, P	IL	649

Transplant Medicine-Lung

Spec	Name	St	Pg
PPul	Kurland, G	PA	685
Pul	Albertson, T	CA	810
Pul	Arcasoy, S	NY	796
Pul	Garrity, E	IL	804
Pul	Hertz, M	MN	804
Pul	Kotloff, R	PA	797
Pul	Loyd, J	TN	802
Pul	Lynch, J	CA	811
Pul	Mehta, A	OH	806
Pul	Reilly, J	PA	798
Pul	Trulock, E	MO	807
Pul	Young, K	AL	803

Transplant Pathology

Spec	Name	St	Pg
Path	Demetris, A	PA	605
Path	Swerdlow, S	PA	609

Transplant Surgery

Spec	Name	St	Pg
PlS	Siemionow, M	OH	747
S	Bentley, F	AR	932

Transplant-Bile Duct

Spec	Name	St	Pg
S	Rosen, C	MN	927

Transplant-Bowel

Spec	Name	St	Pg
PS	Holterman, M	IL	698
S	Benedetti, E	IL	922
S	Tzakis, A	FL	921

Transplant-Hand

Spec	Name	St	Pg
HS	Breidenbach, W	KY	263
HS	Lee, W	PA	262
PlS	Tobin, G	KY	744

Transplant-Heart

Spec	Name	St	Pg
TS	Acker, M	PA	952
TS	Brown, J	IN	963
TS	Conte, J	MD	953
TS	Copeland, J	AZ	968
TS	Dang, M	HI	970
TS	Dowling, R	KY	960
TS	Elefteriades, J	CT	950
TS	Frazier, O	TX	968
TS	Harrell, J	TX	969
TS	Jeevanandam, V	IL	964
TS	Kormos, R	PA	955
TS	Kron, I	VA	961
TS	Laks, H	CA	971
TS	Lansman, S	NY	956
TS	Merrill, W	OH	965
TS	Morris, R	PA	957
TS	Oz, M	NY	957
TS	Pagani, F	MI	966
TS	Pierson, R	MD	957
TS	Quintessenza, J	FL	962
TS	Raman, J	IL	966
TS	Robbins, R	CA	972
TS	Samuels, L	PA	958
TS	Smedira, N	OH	966
TS	Smith, C	NY	958
TS	Tedder, M	TN	963
TS	Trento, A	CA	973
TS	Turrentine, M	IN	967

Transplant-Heart & Lung

Spec	Name	St	Pg
PS	Mavroudis, C	OH	698
PS	Spray, T	PA	695
TS	Bakhos, M	IL	963
TS	Calhoon, J	TX	968
TS	Copeland, J	AZ	968
TS	Drinkwater, D	TN	960
TS	Fullerton, D	CO	967
TS	Furukawa, S	PA	953
TS	Griffith, B	MD	954
TS	Jamieson, S	CA	971
TS	McGregor, C	MN	965
TS	Mullett, T	KY	961
TS	Naka, Y	NY	957
TS	Patterson, G	MO	966
TS	Reitz, B	CA	972
TS	Ring, W	TX	969
TS	Staples, E	FL	963
TS	Starnes, V	CA	972

Transplant-Heart-Adult & Pediatric

Spec	Name	St	Pg
TS	Christian, K	TN	959
TS	Kirklin, J	AL	961

Transplant-Heart-Pediatric

Spec	Name	St	Pg
PS	Duncan, B	OH	698
TS	Bailey, L	CA	970
TS	Campbell, D	CO	967
TS	Huddleston, C	MO	964

Transplant-Kidney

Spec	Name	St	Pg
PS	Colombani, P	MD	693
PS	Schwartz, M	PA	694
S	Ascher, N	CA	937
S	Bartlett, S	MD	905
S	Benedetti, E	IL	922
S	Bentley, F	AR	932
S	Bromberg, J	NY	906
S	Conti, D	NY	906
S	Eckhoff, D	AL	916
S	Ferguson, R	OH	924
S	Fung, J	OH	924
S	Gruber, S	MI	925
S	Hardy, M	NY	909
S	Howard, R	FL	918
S	Kapur, S	NY	909
S	Lipkowitz, G	MA	903
S	Matas, A	MN	926
S	Montgomery, R	MD	910
S	Newell, K	GA	919
S	Perkins, J	WA	940
S	Scantlebury, V	DE	913
S	Selby, R	CA	941
S	Shapiro, R	PA	913
S	Sollinger, H	WI	929
S	Stratta, R	NC	921
S	Sutherland, D	MN	929
S	Teperman, L	NY	914
S	Thistlethwaite, J	IL	929
U	Flanigan, R	IL	993
U	Marsh, C	CA	1003
U	Menon, M	MI	995
U	Novick, A	OH	996
U	Sagalowsky, A	TX	1001
VascS	Benvenisty, A	NY	1011

Transplant-Kidney-Adult & Pediatric

Spec	Name	St	Pg
S	Schulak, J	OH	928

Transplant-Kidney-Pediatric

Spec	Name	St	Pg
PS	Sheldon, C	OH	699
U	Firlit, C	MO	993
U	Koyle, M	WA	1003

Transplant-Liver

Spec	Name	St	Pg
PS	Colombani, P	MD	693
PS	Holterman, M	IL	698
PS	Karrer, F	CO	699
PS	Meyers, R	UT	699
PS	Vacanti, J	MA	692
S	Ascher, N	CA	937
S	Benedetti, E	IL	922
S	Brems, J	IL	922
S	Busuttil, R	CA	937
S	Chari, R	TN	916
S	Colquhoun, S	CA	938
S	Cronin, D	WI	923
S	Eckhoff, D	AL	916
S	Emond, J	NY	908
S	Esquivel, C	CA	938
S	Fung, J	OH	924

Special Expertise Index

America's Top Doctors® 8th Edition

Special Expertise Index

Spec	Name	St	Pg
U	Jordan, G	VA	989
U	Lerner, S	TX	1000
U	Scardino, P	NY	985
U	Schoenberg, M	MD	985
U	Skinner, E	CA	1004
U	Wilson, T	CA	1005
U	Winters, J	LA	1001

Urinary Tract Infections

Spec	Name	St	Pg
Inf	Maki, D	WI	356
Inf	Sobel, J	MI	356
PInf	Wald, E	WI	675
PNep	Ettenger, R	CA	679

Urinary Tract Interventions

Spec	Name	St	Pg
VIR	Keller, F	OR	865

Uro-Gynecology

Spec	Name	St	Pg
GO	Hatch, K	AZ	254
GO	Morgan, M	PA	247
ObG	Brodman, M	NY	480
ObG	DeLancey, J	MI	483
ObG	Hale, D	IN	483
ObG	Karram, M	OH	484
ObG	Lipscomb, G	IL	484
ObG	Lucente, V	PA	481
ObG	Sanz, L	VA	483
U	Appell, R	TX	998
U	Blaivas, J	NY	980

Urodynamics

Spec	Name	St	Pg
U	Bushman, W	WI	992
U	Joseph, D	AL	989
U	Kaplan, S	NY	982
U	Klutke, C	MO	994
U	Lynne, C	FL	989
U	Milam, D	TN	990
U	Nitti, V	NY	984
U	Webster, G	NC	991

Urologic Cancer

Spec	Name	St	Pg
Onc	Carducci, M	MD	292
Onc	Einhorn, L	IN	318
Onc	Figlin, R	CA	334
Onc	Garnick, M	MA	288
Onc	Hauke, R	NE	326
Onc	Levine, E	NY	298
Onc	Torti, F	NC	313
Onc	Troner, M	FL	313
Path	Cohen, M	IA	612
Path	Ross, J	NY	608
RadRO	DeWeese, T	MD	822
RadRO	Zietman, A	MA	821
U	Andriole, G	MO	992
U	Bardot, S	LA	998
U	Basler, J	TX	999
U	Belldegrun, A	CA	1001
U	Boyd, S	CA	1002
U	Bruskewitz, R	WI	992
U	Chang, S	TN	988
U	Culkin, D	OK	999
U	Davis, B	KS	998
U	de Kernion, J	CA	1002
U	Droller, M	NY	981
U	El-Galley, R	AL	988
U	Gill, H	CA	1002
U	Gill, I	OH	993
U	Gomella, L	PA	981
U	Grasso, M	NY	981
U	Greene, G	AR	999
U	Gujral, S	MN	994
U	Harty, J	KY	988
U	Heney, N	MA	978
U	Huben, R	NY	982
U	Janeiro, J	NH	978
U	Kavoussi, L	NY	983
U	Keane, T	SC	989
U	Klein, E	OH	994
U	Lanteri, V	NJ	983
U	McDougal, W	MA	978
U	Menon, M	MI	995
U	Miles, B	TX	1000
U	Novick, A	OH	996
U	O'Donnell, M	IA	996
U	Rowland, R	KY	990
U	Sagalowsky, A	TX	1001
U	Sanda, M	MA	979
U	Scardino, P	NY	985
U	Skinner, E	CA	1004
U	Terris, M	GA	991
U	Van Arsdalen, K	PA	986
U	Vaughan, E	NY	986
U	Wein, A	PA	987
U	Yu, G	MD	987

Urologic Cancer-Pediatric

Spec	Name	St	Pg
U	Coplen, D	MO	993

Urologic Cancers

Spec	Name	St	Pg
U	Lee, C	MI	994

Urologic Pathology

Spec	Name	St	Pg
Path	Bostwick, D	VA	610
Path	Epstein, J	MD	605
Path	Reuter, V	NY	608
Path	Silverberg, S	MD	609
Path	True, L	WA	619
U	Soloway, M	FL	991

Urology-Female

Spec	Name	St	Pg
U	Appell, R	TX	998
U	Blaivas, J	NY	980
U	Bushman, W	WI	992
U	Chancellor, M	PA	980
U	Gribetz, M	NY	982
U	Gujral, S	MN	994
U	Klutke, C	MO	994
U	McGuire, E	MI	995
U	Nitti, V	NY	984
U	Raz, S	CA	1004
U	Schaeffer, A	IL	996
U	Stone, A	CA	1005
U	Vapnek, J	NY	986
U	Webster, G	NC	991
U	Winters, J	LA	1001

Urticaria

Spec	Name	St	Pg
A&I	Altman, L	WA	87
A&I	Bonner, J	AL	84
A&I	Fox, R	FL	84
A&I	MacLean, J	MA	82
A&I	Shepherd, G	NY	83
A&I	Wasserman, S	CA	88
A&I	Wong, J	MA	82
D	Soter, N	NY	174

Uterine Cancer

Spec	Name	St	Pg
GO	Abu-Rustum, N	NY	245
GO	Alleyn, J	FL	248
GO	Barakat, R	NY	245
GO	Berchuck, A	NC	248
GO	Berek, J	CA	254
GO	Bristow, R	MD	245
GO	Cain, J	OR	255
GO	Caputo, T	NY	246
GO	Copeland, L	OH	251
GO	Creasman, W	SC	248
GO	Curtin, J	NY	246
GO	Dunton, C	PA	246
GO	Finan, M	AL	249
GO	Goff, B	WA	255
GO	Koulos, J	NY	247
GO	Look, K	IN	251
GO	Lurain, J	IL	251
GO	Rice, L	WI	252
GO	Rosenblum, N	PA	247
GO	Rutherford, T	CT	244
GO	Schwartz, P	CT	245
GO	Smith, L	CA	256
GO	Waggoner, S	OH	253
GO	Walker, J	OK	254
Onc	Bookman, M	PA	291
Onc	Spriggs, D	NY	303
Path	Kurman, R	MD	607
Path	Tomaszewski, J	PA	609
RadRO	Eifel, P	TX	834

Uterine Fibroid Embolization

Spec	Name	St	Pg
DR	Yoon, S	FL	851
VIR	Benenati, J	FL	862
VIR	Bettmann, M	NC	862
VIR	Cragg, A	MN	863
VIR	Durham, J	CO	864
VIR	Goodwin, S	CA	865
VIR	Hallisey, M	CT	860
VIR	Haskal, Z	NY	861
VIR	Hovsepian, D	CA	865
VIR	Johnson, M	IN	863
VIR	Kaufman, J	OR	865

Special Expertise Index

Special Expertise Index

Special Expertise Index

America's Top Doctors® 8th Edition

Alphabetical Listing of Doctors

Name	Specialty	Pg	Name	Specialty	Pg
A			Adelman, Mark (NY)	VascS	1011
			Adelson, P David (PA)	NS	405
Abbitt, Patricia (FL)	DR	850	Adelstein, David (OH)	Onc	314
Abbott, Richard (CA)	Oph	515	Adkins, Terrance (AZ)	CRS	164
Abbruzzese, James (TX)	Onc	327	Adler, John (CA)	NS	425
Abcarian, Herand (IL)	CRS	162	Adler, Ronald (NY)	DR	846
Abella, Esteban (AZ)	PHO	667	Adornato, Bruce (CA)	N	462
Abou-Khalil, Bassel (TN)	N	447	Adzick, N Scott (PA)	PS	693
Abrahamson, Martin (MA)	EDM	188	Agarwala, Brojendra (IL)	PCd	634
Abrahm, Janet (MA)	PM	596	Ahern, Geoffry (AZ)	N	459
Abram, Stephen (WI)	PM	598	Ahlgren, James (DC)	Onc	290
Abrams, Charles (PA)	Hem	273	Ahlskog, J Eric (MN)	N	452
Abrams, Donald (CA)	Onc	332	Ahmad, Suhail (WA)	Nep	399
Abrams, Gary (MI)	Oph	506	Ahmann, Frederick (AZ)	Onc	327
Abrams, Ross (IL)	RadRO	830	Ahn, Jung (NY)	PMR	720
Abramson, David (NY)	Oph	493	Ahn, Sam (CA)	VascS	1019
Abramson, Steven (NY)	Rhu	883	Aiello, Lloyd (MA)	Oph	492
Abrass, Itamar (WA)	Ger	238	Aiken, John (WI)	PS	697
Abreu, Maria (FL)	Ge	214	Ain, Kenneth (KY)	EDM	194
Abright, Arthur (NY)	ChAP	781	Aisner, Joseph (NJ)	Onc	290
Abromowitch, Minnie (NE)	PHO	667	Ajani, Jaffer (TX)	Onc	327
Abu-Rustum, Nadeem (NY)	GO	245	Akelman, Edward (RI)	HS	260
Abuhamad, Alfred (VA)	MF	373	Akerley, Wallace (UT)	Onc	324
Accurso, Frank (CO)	PPul	688	Akhtar, Salman (PA)	Psyc	764
Achkar, Edgar (OH)	Ge	218	Akins, Cary (MA)	TS	950
Acker, David (MA)	MF	370	Aklog, Lishan (AZ)	TS	968
Acker, Michael (PA)	TS	952	Al-Mefty, Ossama (AR)	NS	423
Ackerman, Michael (MN)	PCd	634	Alavi, Abass (PA)	NuM	474
Adams, David (NY)	TS	952	Alazraki, Naomi (GA)	NuM	476
Adams, Elaine (IL)	Rhu	888	Albain, Kathy (IL)	Onc	315
Adams, Harold (IA)	N	452	Albala, David (NC)	U	987
Adams, James (TX)	NP	387	Albanese, Craig (CA)	PS	700
Adams, Reid (VA)	S	915	Albers, Gregory (CA)	N	462
Adams, Robert (SC)	N	448	Albert, Daniel (WI)	Oph	506
Adamson, G David (CA)	RE	879	Albert, Daniel (NH)	Rhu	882
Adamson, Peter (PA)	PHO	652			

Alphabetical Listing of Doctors

Name	Specialty	Pg	Name	Specialty	Pg
Albert, Michael (DC)	Ge	207	Ambinder, Richard (MD)	Onc	290
Albert, Todd (PA)	OrS	528	Ames, Frederick (TX)	S	932
Albertini, Mark (WI)	Onc	315	Amin, Mahul (CA)	Path	616
Alberts, David (AZ)	Onc	327	Amin, Sandeep (IL)	PM	598
Alberts, Mark (IL)	N	452	Aminoff, Michael (CA)	N	462
Alberts, W Michael (FL)	Pul	800	Amling, Christopher (AL)	U	987
Albertson, David (NC)	S	915	Amonette, Rex (TN)	D	174
Albertson, Timothy (CA)	Pul	810	An, Howard (IL)	OrS	543
Albright, A Leland (WI)	NS	416	Anand, Kanwaljeet (AR)	PCCM	639
Albritton, Karen (MA)	PHO	651	Andersen, Arnold (IA)	Psyc	770
Alessi, Norman (MI)	ChAP	783	Andersen, James (CA)	PlS	751
Alexander, Frederick (NJ)	PS	693	Anderson, Benjamin (WA)	S	937
Alexander, J Jeffrey (OH)	VascS	1016	Anderson, Corrie (WA)	PM	601
Alexander, John (IL)	TS	963	Anderson, Jeffrey (UT)	Cv	109
Alexander, Richard (MD)	U	979	Anderson, Joseph (MI)	Onc	315
Alexander, Steven (CA)	PNep	679	Anderson, Karl (TX)	Ge	224
Alfonso, Antonio (NY)	S	904	Anderson, Kenneth (MA)	Hem	272
Alfonso, Eduardo (FL)	Oph	502	Anderson, Lesley (CA)	OrS	551
Algazy, Kenneth (PA)	Onc	290	Anderson, Mark (IA)	CE	117
Allen, David (WI)	PEn	643	Anderson, Martin (CA)	AM	79
Allen, Jeffrey (NY)	ChiN	139	Anderson, Richard (MA)	D	168
Allen, Nancy (NC)	Rhu	886	Anderson, Richard (UT)	Oph	512
Allen, Robert (SC)	PlS	741	Andiman, Warren (CT)	PInf	672
Alleyn, James (FL)	GO	248	Andreoli, Sharon (IN)	PNep	678
Allon, Michael (AL)	Nep	395	Andrews, David (PA)	NS	405
Allred, D Craig (MO)	Path	611	Andrews, James (AL)	SM	898
Alster, Tina (DC)	D	170	Andrews, Robert (WA)	PHO	669
Altchek, David (NY)	SM	896	Andriole, Gerald (MO)	U	992
Alter, Craig (PA)	PEn	640	Ang, Kie-Kian (TX)	RadRO	834
Alter, Gary (CA)	PlS	751	Angelos, Peter (IL)	S	922
Altman, Arnold (CT)	PHO	651	Anghelescu, Doralina (TN)	PM	598
Altman, Leonard (WA)	A&I	87	Anhalt, Grant (MD)	D	170
Altorki, Nasser (NY)	TS	952	Annest, Stephen (CO)	VascS	1017
Alvarez, Ronald (AL)	GO	248	Anscher, Mitchell (VA)	RadRO	826
Alvarez-Elcoro, Salvador (FL)	Inf	354	Anthony, Lowell (LA)	Onc	327
Alward, Wallace (IA)	Oph	506	Antin, Joseph (MA)	Onc	286
Amato, Anthony (MA)	N	436	Anton, Raymond (SC)	AdP	778

America's Top Doctors® 8th Edition

Alphabetical Listing of Doctors

Name	Specialty	Pg	Name	Specialty	Pg
Antonia, Scott (FL)	Onc	304	Aronson, Peter (CT)	Nep	392
Antony, Veena (FL)	Pul	800	Arriaga, Moises (PA)	Oto	564
Anyane-Yeboa, Kwame (NY)	CG	146	Arroliga, Alejandro (TX)	Pul	809
Apatoff, Brian (NY)	N	438	Arslanian, Silva (PA)	PEn	641
Apfelbaum, Ronald (UT)	NS	422	Arteaga, Carlos (TN)	Onc	304
Appel, Gerald (NY)	Nep	393	Arts, H Alexander (MI)	Oto	577
Appelbaum, Frederick (WA)	Onc	333	Arun, Banu (TX)	Onc	327
Appelbaum, Paul (NY)	Psyc	764	Ascher, Enrico (NY)	VascS	1011
Appell, Rodney (TX)	U	998	Ascher, Nancy (CA)	S	937
Appelman, Henry (MI)	Path	612	Aseff, John (DC)	PMR	720
Applegate, Robert (NC)	IC	121	Asher, Anthony (NC)	NS	412
April, Max (NY)	PO	680	Ashman, Robert (IA)	Rhu	888
Apuzzo, Michael (CA)	NS	425	Ashwal, Stephen (CA)	ChiN	143
Aranha, Gerard (IL)	S	922	Assimos, Dean (NC)	U	987
Arber, Daniel (CA)	Path	616	Aston, Sherrell (NY)	PlS	735
Arcasoy, Selim (NY)	Pul	796	Atala, Anthony (NC)	U	987
Arceci, Robert (MD)	PHO	652	Athanasian, Edward (NY)	HS	260
Archer, Steven (MI)	Oph	507	Atkins, Michael (MA)	Onc	286
Arend, William (CO)	Rhu	890	Atkinson, John (MN)	NS	416
Arensman, Robert (LA)	PS	700	Atkinson, Robert (HI)	HS	267
Argenta, Louis (NC)	PlS	741	Atlas, Scott (CA)	NRad	859
Argenziano, Michael (NY)	TS	952	Atnip, Robert (PA)	VascS	1011
Argiris, Athanassios (PA)	Onc	290	Attas, Lewis (NJ)	Onc	291
Ariagno, Ronald (CA)	NP	388	Attinger, Christopher (DC)	PlS	735
Arjmand, Ellis (OH)	PO	682	Audell, Laura (CA)	PM	601
Arlen, Philip (MD)	Onc	291	Augsburger, James (OH)	Oph	507
Armitage, James (NE)	Onc	324	August, David (NJ)	S	904
Armon, Carmel (MA)	N	436	August, Phyllis (NY)	Nep	393
Armstrong, William (MI)	Cv	103	Aurora, Sheena (WA)	N	462
Arnason, Barry (IL)	N	452	Austin, John (NY)	DR	846
Arndt, Carola (MN)	PHO	662	Auwaerter, Paul (MD)	Inf	350
Arndt, Kenneth (MA)	D	168	Averbook, Bruce (OH)	S	922
Arnett, Frank (TX)	Rhu	890	Avery, Eric (TX)	Psyc	773
Arnold, Anthony (CA)	Oph	515	Aviv, Jonathan (NY)	Oto	564
Arnold, James (OH)	PO	682	Avner, Ellis (WI)	PNep	678
Aronchick, Craig (PA)	Ge	207	Axelrod, Deborah (NY)	S	905
Aronson, James (AR)	OrS	549	Axelrod, Lloyd (MA)	EDM	188

Alphabetical Listing of Doctors

Name	Specialty	Pg	Name	Specialty	Pg
Axelrod, Rita (PA)	Onc	291	Baker, Susan (NY)	PGe	645
Azar, Dimitri (IL)	Oph	507	Bakhos, Mamdouh (IL)	TS	963
Azziz, Ricardo (CA)	RE	879	Bakken, Johan (MN)	Inf	356
			Balady, Gary (MA)	Cv	92
			Balart, Luis (LA)	Ge	224
			Balch, Charles (MD)	S	905

B

Name	Specialty	Pg	Name	Specialty	Pg
Babaian, Richard (TX)	U	998	Baldassano, Robert (PA)	PGe	646
Babiera, Gildy (TX)	S	932	Balderston, Richard (PA)	OrS	528
Bach, Bernard (IL)	OrS	543	Balducci, Lodovico (FL)	Onc	304
Bach, John (NJ)	PMR	720	Bale, Allen (CT)	CG	146
Bacon, Bruce (MO)	Ge	218	Bale, James (UT)	ChiN	142
Badie, Behnam (CA)	NS	426	Balk, Robert (IL)	Pul	804
Baer, Maria (MD)	Hem	273	Balkany, Thomas (FL)	Oto	572
Baerveldt, George (CA)	Oph	515	Ball, Douglas (MD)	EDM	190
Bagley, Demetrius (PA)	U	979	Ball, Edward (CA)	Onc	333
Bahado-Singh, Ray (MI)	MF	374	Ball, William (OH)	NRad	857
Bahn, Duke (CA)	RadRO	836	Balla, Andre (IL)	Path	612
Bahn, Rebecca (MN)	EDM	196	Ballantyne, Garth (NJ)	S	905
Bahna, Sami (LA)	PA&I	629	Ballard, Pamela (DC)	PMR	720
Bahnson, Robert (OH)	U	992	Ballon-Landa, Gonzalo (CA)	Inf	358
Bailey, Harold (TX)	CRS	164	Balmes, John (CA)	Pul	810
Bailey, Leonard (CA)	TS	970	Baltimore, Robert (CT)	PInf	672
Bailey, Steven (TX)	IC	123	Baltuch, Gordon (PA)	NS	405
Bailin, Philip (OH)	D	177	Bancalari, Eduardo (FL)	NP	384
Baim, Howard (IL)	Oto	577	Bandyk, Dennis (FL)	VascS	1014
Bains, Manjit (NY)	TS	952	Banks, Peter (NC)	Path	609
Bairey-Merz, C Noel (CA)	Cv	112	Bans, Larry (AZ)	U	998
Bakay, Roy (IL)	NS	417	Bar-Chama, Natan (NY)	U	980
Baker, Carol (TX)	PInf	675	Barakat, Richard (NY)	GO	245
Baker, Christopher (LA)	S	932	Baratz, Mark (PA)	HS	261
Baker, Daniel (NY)	PlS	736	Barber, Douglas (TX)	PMR	728
Baker, Emily (NH)	MF	370	Bardot, Stephen (LA)	U	998
Baker, James (MI)	A&I	85	Barger, Geoffrey (MI)	N	453
Baker, John (MI)	Oph	507	Barie, Philip (NY)	S	905
Baker, Robert (NY)	PGe	645	Barkin, Jamie (FL)	Ge	214
Baker, Shan (MI)	Oto	577	Barkovich, A James (CA)	NRad	859
			Barksdale, Edward (OH)	PS	697

Alphabetical Listing of Doctors

Name	Specialty	Pg	Name	Specialty	Pg
Barlogie, Bart (AR)	Hem	282	Baumann, Patricia (GA)	PM	598
Barnes, Patrick (CA)	NRad	859	Baumgartner, William (MD)	TS	952
Barnes, Randall (IL)	RE	876	Bavaria, Joseph (PA)	TS	952
Barnes, Willard (DC)	GO	245	Bayer, Arnold (CA)	Inf	358
Barnett, Gene (OH)	NS	417	Bayless, Theodore (MD)	Ge	207
Barohn, Richard (KS)	N	458	Baylis, Henry (CA)	Oph	515
Baron, Joseph (IL)	Hem	278	Bazari, Hasan (MA)	Nep	392
Baron, Todd (MN)	Ge	218	Beall, Michael (VA)	U	987
Barone, Constance (TX)	PlS	748	Beals, Stephen (AZ)	PlS	748
Barr, Walter (IL)	Rhu	888	Beamis, John (MA)	Pul	794
Barredo, Julio (FL)	PHO	658	Bear, Harry (VA)	S	915
Barrett, Eugene (VA)	EDM	194	Beart, Robert (CA)	CRS	165
Barry, Michele (CT)	IM	364	Beaser, Richard (MA)	EDM	188
Bartelsmeyer, James (MO)	MF	374	Beasley, Michael (NC)	PlS	742
Barter, James (MD)	GO	245	Beatty, Charles (MN)	Oto	577
Bartlett, David (PA)	S	905	Beatty, Patrick (MT)	Onc	325
Bartlett, John (MD)	Inf	351	Beaty, James H (TN)	OrS	539
Bartlett, Scott (PA)	PlS	736	Beauchamp, Robert (TN)	S	915
Bartlett, Stephen (MD)	S	905	Beaudet, Arthur (TX)	CG	150
Bartolozzi, Arthur (PA)	OrS	528	Beck, David (LA)	CRS	164
Barton, Fritz (TX)	PlS	748	Becker, Dorothy (PA)	PEn	641
Basch, Samuel (NY)	Psyc	764	Becker, Ferdinand (FL)	Oto	572
Bascom, Rebecca (PA)	Pul	796	Becker, James (MA)	S	902
Baser, Susan (PA)	N	438	Becker, Kyra (WA)	N	462
Bashore, Thomas (NC)	Cv	100	Bederson, Joshua (NY)	NS	406
Baskin, Laurence (CA)	U	1001	Beekman, Robert (OH)	PCd	634
Basler, Joseph (TX)	U	999	Beer, Tomasz (OR)	Onc	333
Bass, Theodore (FL)	Cv	100	Beerman, Lee (PA)	PCd	631
Bassett, Lawrence (CA)	DR	853	Behm, Frederick (IL)	Path	612
Bastian, Boris (CA)	Path	617	Behrens, Myles (NY)	Oph	493
Bastian, Robert (IL)	Oto	577	Behrns, Kevin (FL)	S	915
Batjer, Hunt (IL)	NS	417	Beitsch, Peter (TX)	S	932
Batsford, William (CT)	CE	114	Belani, Chandra (PA)	Onc	291
Bauer, Bruce (IL)	PlS	745	Belenky, Walter (MI)	PO	682
Bauer, Jerry (IL)	NS	417	Belinson, Jerome (OH)	GO	251
Baughman, Kenneth (MA)	Cv	92	Belkin, Michael (MA)	VascS	1010
Bauman, Phillip (NY)	OrS	528	Bell, David (AL)	EDM	194

Alphabetical Listing of Doctors

Name	Specialty	Pg	Name	Specialty	Pg
Bell, Debra (MN)	Path	612	Berek, Jonathan (CA)	GO	254
Bell, Edward (IA)	NP	385	Berenstein, Alejandro (NY)	NRad	854
Bell, Rodney (PA)	N	438	Berg, Christine (MD)	RadRO	821
Bellamy, Paul (CA)	Pul	810	Berg, Daniel (WA)	D	181
Belldegrun, Arie (CA)	U	1001	Berg, Stacey (TX)	PHO	667
Beller, George (VA)	Cv	100	Berg, Wendie (MD)	DR	846
Belman, A Barry (DC)	U	980	Berga, Sarah (GA)	RE	874
Belmont, Howard (NY)	Rhu	883	Berger, Joseph (KY)	N	448
Belsito, Donald (KS)	D	179	Berger, Melvin (OH)	A&I	86
Belsky, Mark (MA)	HS	260	Berger, Mitchel (CA)	NS	426
Ben-Josef, Edgar (MI)	RadRO	830	Bergey, Gregory (MD)	N	438
Benedetti, Costantino (OH)	PM	598	Bergfeld, John (OH)	OrS	543
Benedetti, Enrico (IL)	S	922	Bergman, Donald (NY)	EDM	190
Benedetti, Thomas (WA)	MF	377	Berguer, Ramon (MI)	VascS	1016
Benedetto, Pasquale (FL)	Onc	305	Berke, Gerald (CA)	Oto	587
Benenati, James (FL)	VIR	862	Berkowitz, Carol (CA)	Ped	626
Benenati, Susan (FL)	A&I	84	Berkowitz, Leonard (NY)	Inf	351
Benevenia, Joseph (NJ)	OrS	528	Berkowitz, Richard (NY)	MF	371
Benjamin, Ivor (UT)	Cv	109	Berkowitz, Ross (MA)	GO	244
Benjamin, Robert (TX)	Onc	327	Berkson, Richard (CA)	EDM	201
Benkov, Keith (NY)	PGe	646	Berl, Tomas (CO)	Nep	398
Bennett, Richard (CA)	D	181	Berland, Lincoln (AL)	DR	850
Bennett, William (OR)	Nep	399	Berlin, Cheston (PA)	Ped	624
Benninger, Michael (OH)	Oto	577	Berlin, Jordan (TN)	Onc	305
Bensard, Denis (IN)	PS	697	Berman, Brian (OH)	Ped	625
Bensinger, William (WA)	Onc	333	Berman, James (IL)	PGe	648
Benson, Al (IL)	Onc	315	Berman, Michael (CA)	GO	254
Benson, Carol (MA)	DR	845	Bermant, Michael (VA)	PlS	742
Benson, Mitchell (NY)	U	980	Bermudez, Ovidio (OK)	AM	79
Bentley, Frederick (AR)	S	932	Bernad, Peter (VA)	N	448
Bentz, Michael (WI)	PlS	745	Bernard, Stephen (NC)	Onc	305
Benvenisty, Alan (NY)	VascS	1011	Bernstein, Daniel (CA)	PCd	637
Benzel, Edward (OH)	NS	417	Bernstein, Robert (NY)	D	170
Benzon, Honorio (IL)	PM	599	Berrey, B Hudson (FL)	OrS	539
Berchuck, Andrew (NC)	GO	248	Bertolone, Salvatore (KY)	PHO	658
Berd, David (PA)	Onc	291	Besinger, Richard (IL)	MF	374
Berde, Charles (MA)	PM	596	Bessler, Marc (NY)	S	905

Alphabetical Listing of Doctors

Name	Specialty	Pg	Name	Specialty	Pg
Bettmann, Michael (NC)	VIR	862	Blaney, Susan (TX)	PHO	668
Betz, Randal (PA)	OrS	528	Blatt, Julie (NC)	PHO	658
Bhan, Atul (MA)	Path	604	Blazer, Dan (NC)	Psyc	769
Bialer, Martin (NY)	CG	146	Blebea, John (PA)	VascS	1011
Biancaniello, Thomas (NY)	PCd	631	Bleday, Ronald (MA)	CRS	158
Bianchi, Diana (MA)	CG	146	Bleiberg, Efrain (TX)	ChAP	785
Bichell, David (TN)	TS	959	Blinder, Morey (MO)	Hem	278
Bickers, David (NY)	D	170	Blitzer, Andrew (NY)	Oto	565
Bieber, Eric (PA)	RE	871	Block, Susan (MA)	Psyc	762
Biederman, Joseph (MA)	ChAP	779	Blom, Dennis (IN)	S	922
Bierbrauer, Karin (OH)	NS	417	Bloom, David (MI)	U	992
Bierman, Fredrick (NY)	PCd	631	Bloom, Patricia (NY)	Ger	234
Bierman, Philip (NE)	Onc	325	Bloomer, Joseph (AL)	Ge	214
Biermann, J Sybil (MI)	OrS	543	Bluemke, David (MD)	DR	846
Bigelow, Carolyn (MS)	Hem	276	Blum, Conrad (NY)	EDM	190
Bigliani, Louis (NY)	OrS	529	Blumberg, Henry (GA)	Inf	354
Bilchik, Anton (CA)	S	937	Blume, Ralph (NY)	Rhu	883
Bilezikian, John (NY)	EDM	190	Blumenfeld, Hal (CT)	N	436
Biller, Beverly (MA)	EDM	188	Blumenfeld, Jon (NY)	Nep	393
Billings, J Andrew (MA)	PM	596	Blumenfield, Michael (CA)	Psyc	774
Billmire, David (OH)	PlS	745	Blumenkranz, Mark (CA)	Oph	515
Bilsky, Mark (NY)	NS	406	Blumenthal, David (NY)	Cv	94
Binder, Perry (CA)	Oph	515	Blumenthal, Roger (MD)	Cv	95
Bird, Hector (NY)	ChAP	781	Boachie-Adjei, Oheneba (NY)	OrS	529
Bishop, Allen (MN)	HS	264	Bobrove, Arthur (CA)	Rhu	891
Bissell, Dwight (CA)	IM	366	Bock, S Allan (CO)	PA&I	629
Bitan, Fabien (NY)	OrS	529	Bockenstedt, Paula (MI)	Hem	278
Bitran, Jacob (IL)	Onc	315	Bockman, Richard (NY)	EDM	190
Bjorkman, David (UT)	Ge	223	Boden, Scott (GA)	OrS	539
Black, Henry (NY)	Nep	393	Bodenheimer, Henry (NY)	Ge	207
Black, Keith (CA)	NS	426	Boggan, James (CA)	NS	426
Black, Peter (MA)	NS	404	Bogrov, Michael (MD)	ChAP	781
Black, William (NH)	DR	845	Bohlman, Henry (OH)	OrS	543
Blackwell, Richard (AL)	RE	874	Bojrab, Dennis (MI)	Oto	578
Blaha, John (MI)	OrS	543	Boland, C Richard (TX)	Ge	224
Blaivas, Jerry (NY)	U	980	Boldt, David (TX)	Hem	282
Bland, Kirby (AL)	S	916	Boles, Richard (CA)	CG	151

Alphabetical Listing of Doctors

Name	Specialty	Pg	Name	Specialty	Pg
Bolger, Graeme (AL)	Onc	305	Bove, Edward (MI)	PS	697
Bolger, William (MD)	Oto	565	Bowden, Charles (TX)	Psyc	773
Bollen, Andrew (CA)	Path	617	Bowen, Glen (UT)	D	179
Bolman, R Morton (MA)	TS	950	Bowen, James (WA)	N	462
Bolton, W Kline (VA)	Nep	395	Bower, Charles (AR)	PO	683
Bolwell, Brian (OH)	Onc	315	Boxer, Gary (MO)	ChAP	784
Bond, Sheldon (KY)	PS	695	Boxer, Laurence (MI)	PHO	662
Bonner, James (AL)	A&I	84	Boxer Wachler, Brian (CA)	Oph	516
Bonner, James (AL)	RadRO	826	Boxrud, Cynthia (CA)	Oph	516
Bonomi, Philip (IL)	Onc	315	Boyajian, Michael (DC)	PlS	736
Bonow, Robert (IL)	Cv	104	Boyce, H Worth (FL)	Ge	214
Bookman, Michael (PA)	Onc	291	Boyd, Stuart (CA)	U	1002
Boone, Timothy (TX)	U	999	Boyd, W Douglas (FL)	TS	959
Boop, Frederick (TN)	NS	412	Boyer, Thomas (AZ)	Ge	224
Booth, Robert (PA)	OrS	529	Boyle, Robert (VA)	NP	384
Borchert, Mark (CA)	Oph	516	Brackmann, Derald (CA)	Oto	587
Borden, Ernest (OH)	Onc	315	Braddom, Randall (NJ)	PMR	721
Borer, Jeffrey (NY)	Cv	95	Bradford, Carol (MI)	Oto	578
Borgen, Patrick (NY)	S	905	Bradley, James (PA)	SM	896
Borges, Lawrence (MA)	NS	404	Bradley, John (CA)	PInf	676
Borkowsky, William (NY)	PInf	672	Brady, Charles (TX)	Ge	224
Boronow, John (MD)	Psyc	764	Brady, Kathleen (SC)	AdP	778
Borowitz, Drucy (NY)	PPul	685	Braman, Sidney (RI)	Pul	794
Borson, Soo (WA)	GerPsy	788	Branch, Charles (NC)	NS	412
Borum, Marie (DC)	Ge	207	Brandt, Fredric (NY)	D	170
Borzak, Steven (FL)	Cv	100	Brandt, Harry (MD)	Psyc	764
Bos, Gary (WA)	OrS	551	Brandt, Keith (MO)	PlS	745
Bosl, George (NY)	Onc	291	Brandt, Lawrence (NY)	Ge	207
Boston, Barry (TN)	Onc	305	Brandt-Rauf, Paul (NY)	OM	758
Bostwick, David (VA)	Path	610	Branham, Gregory (MO)	Oto	578
Boucek, Mark (FL)	PCd	633	Brasington, Richard (MO)	Rhu	888
Boucek, Robert (WA)	PCd	637	Braun, Martin (DC)	D	170
Bouldin, Marshall (MS)	IM	365	Braunstein, Glenn (CA)	EDM	201
Bourdette, Dennis (OR)	N	462	Braunstein, Seth (PA)	IM	364
Bourge, Robert (AL)	Cv	100	Brause, Barry (NY)	Inf	351
Boushey, Homer (CA)	Pul	810	Braverman, Alan (MO)	Cv	104
Bove, Alfred (PA)	Cv	95	Brawley, Otis (GA)	Onc	305

Name	Specialty	Pg	Name	Specialty	Pg
Braylan, Raul (FL)	Path	610	Brockstein, Bruce (IL)	Onc	316
Brazer, Scott (NC)	Ge	214	Broderick, Gregory (FL)	U	988
Brecher, Martin (NY)	PHO	653	Broderick, Joseph (OH)	N	453
Breidenbach, Warren (KY)	HS	263	Brodeur, Garrett (PA)	PHO	653
Breitbart, William (NY)	Psyc	764	Brodkin, Edward (PA)	Psyc	764
Brem, Henry (MD)	NS	406	Brodland, David (PA)	D	171
Brem, Rachel (DC)	DR	846	Brodman, Michael (NY)	ObG	480
Brem, Steven (FL)	NS	412	Brodsky, James (TX)	OrS	549
Brems, John (IL)	S	922	Brody, Fred (DC)	S	906
Brendler, Charles (IL)	U	992	Brody, Harold (GA)	D	174
Brener, Bruce (NJ)	VascS	1012	Bromberg, Jonathan (NY)	S	906
Brennan, Daniel (MO)	Nep	396	Bromberg, Mark (UT)	N	458
Brennan, Michael (MN)	EDM	196	Bromfield, Edward (MA)	N	436
Brennan, Murray (NY)	S	905	Bronheim, Harold (NY)	Psyc	765
Brennan, Stephen (TX)	Nep	398	Brooks, Benjamin (NC)	N	448
Brenner, Barry (MA)	Nep	392	Brooks, David (MA)	S	902
Brenner, Joel (MD)	PCd	631	Brooks, John (PA)	Path	605
Brenner, Malcolm (TX)	Hem	282	Brooks, Stuart (FL)	Pul	800
Brenner, Michael (MA)	Rhu	882	Brown, Frederick (IL)	NS	417
Brent, Burton (CA)	PlS	751	Brown, Gary (PA)	Oph	494
Brent, David (PA)	ChAP	781	Brown, John (IN)	TS	963
Bresalier, Robert (TX)	Ge	224	Brown, Kevin (CO)	Pul	807
Brescia, Frank (SC)	Onc	305	Brown, Kimberly (MI)	Ge	218
Bressler, Neil (MD)	Oph	494	Brown, Robert (MN)	N	453
Bressman, Susan (NY)	N	438	Browner, Bruce (CT)	OrS	526
Brewer, Molly (CT)	GO	244	Brozena, Susan (PA)	Cv	95
Brewster, David (MA)	VascS	1010	Bruce, Jeffrey (NY)	NS	406
Bricker, John (KY)	PCd	633	Brucker, Alexander (PA)	Oph	494
Bricker, Leslie (MI)	Onc	316	Bruera, Eduardo (TX)	Onc	327
Bridges, Charles (PA)	TS	953	Brufsky, Adam (PA)	Onc	291
Bridwell, Keith (MO)	OrS	543	Bruggers, Carol (UT)	PHO	667
Brindis, Ralph (CA)	Cv	112	Bruner, Janet (TX)	Path	615
Brink, Robert (CA)	PlS	751	Bruner, Joseph (TN)	MF	373
Bristow, Robert (MD)	GO	245	Brunicardi, F Charles (TX)	S	932
Britt, L D (VA)	S	916	Brunsting, Louis (TN)	TS	959
Brizel, David (NC)	RadRO	826	Brunstrom, Janice (MO)	ChiN	141
Brock, John (TN)	U	988	Brunt, L Michael (MO)	S	923

Alphabetical Listing of Doctors

Name	Specialty	Pg	Name	Specialty	Pg
Brushart, Thomas (MD)	OrS	529	Burks, Arvil Wesley (NC)	PA&I	628
Bruskewitz, Reginald (WI)	U	992	Burnett, Arthur (MD)	U	980
Brust, John (NY)	N	438	Burns, Alton (TX)	PlS	749
Bryson, Yvonne (CA)	PInf	676	Burns, Richard (AZ)	N	459
Bucciarelli, Richard (FL)	NP	384	Burris, Howard (TN)	Onc	305
Buch, Jeffrey (TX)	U	999	Burstein, Harold (MA)	Onc	286
Buchanan, George (TX)	PHO	668	Burt, Randall (UT)	Ge	223
Buchbinder, Ellen (NY)	A&I	82	Burt, Richard (IL)	Onc	316
Buchbinder, Maurice (CA)	IC	124	Burt, Vivien (CA)	Psyc	774
Buchholz, David (MD)	N	438	Burton, Allen (TX)	PM	600
Buchholz, Thomas (TX)	RadRO	834	Burton, Barbara (IL)	CG	149
Buchman, Steven (MI)	PlS	745	Burton, Claude (NC)	D	175
Bucholz, Robert (TX)	OrS	550	Burton, John (MD)	Ger	234
Buckley, Edward (NC)	Oph	502	Bury, Robert (ND)	ObG	484
Buckner, Jan (MN)	Onc	316	Bushman, Wade (WI)	U	992
Buckwalter, Joseph (IA)	OrS	543	Busse, William (WI)	A&I	86
Bucky, Louis (PA)	PlS	736	Bussel, James (NY)	PHO	653
Budd, George (OH)	Onc	316	Busuttil, Ronald (CA)	S	937
Budenz, Donald (FL)	Oph	502	Butler, David (TX)	D	180
Budoff, Matthew (CA)	Cv	112	Butler, John (CA)	S	937
Bueno, Raphael (MA)	TS	950	Butler, William (SC)	Onc	306
Bukowski, Ronald (OH)	Onc	316	Buxton, Alfred (RI)	CE	114
Bull, David (UT)	TS	967	Buyon, Jill (NY)	Rhu	883
Bull, Marilyn (IN)	Ped	625	Buys, Saundra (UT)	Onc	325
Buly, Robert (NY)	OrS	529	Buysse, Daniel (PA)	Psyc	765
Bumpous, Jeffrey (KY)	Oto	573	Buzdar, Aman (TX)	Onc	328
Bunchman, Timothy (MI)	PNep	678	Byrd, Benjamin (TN)	Cv	100
Bunn, Paul (CO)	Onc	325	Byrd, David (WA)	S	937
Bunning, Robert (DC)	Rhu	883	Byrd, H Stephenson (TX)	PlS	749
Burchiel, Kim (OR)	NS	426	Byrd, John (OH)	Onc	316
Burger, Peter (MD)	Path	605	Byrne, Janice (UT)	ObG	484
Burgess, David (NJ)	Ped	624	Bystritsky, Alexander (CA)	Psyc	774
Burke, Allan (IL)	N	453	Bystryn, Jean (NY)	D	171
Burke, Miles (OH)	Oph	507			
Burke, William (NE)	GerPsy	788			
Burket, Mark (OH)	Cv	104			
Burkey, Brian (TN)	Oto	573			

C

Name	Specialty	Pg	Name	Specialty	Pg
Cabin, Henry (CT)	Cv	92	Cannom, David (CA)	CE	119
Cagle, Philip (TX)	Path	615	Cannon, W Dilworth (CA)	OrS	551
Cahill, John (NY)	PrM	759	Cannon, Walter (CA)	TS	970
Cain, Joanna (OR)	GO	255	Canterbury, Randolph (VA)	Psyc	769
Cairo, Mitchell (NY)	PHO	653	Canto, Marcia (MD)	Ge	207
Calabrese, Joseph (OH)	Psyc	770	Caplan, Louis (MA)	N	436
Caldamone, Anthony (RI)	U	978	Capo, Hilda (FL)	Oph	502
Caldarelli, David (IL)	Oto	578	Cappuccino, Andrew (NY)	OrS	529
Caldwell, Randall (IN)	PCd	634	Caprioli, Joseph (CA)	Oph	516
Calhoon, John (TX)	TS	968	Caputo, Anthony (NJ)	Oph	494
Califf, Robert (NC)	Cv	101	Caputo, Thomas (NY)	GO	246
Callaghan, John (IA)	OrS	544	Caputy, Anthony (DC)	NS	406
Callans, David (PA)	CE	115	Carabasi, Matthew (PA)	Onc	292
Callen, Jeffrey (KY)	D	175	Carabello, Blase (TX)	Cv	110
Calligaro, Keith (PA)	VascS	1012	Carbone, David (TN)	Onc	306
Calvi, Laura (NY)	EDM	190	Cardenas, Diana (FL)	PMR	723
Calvo, Benjamin (NC)	S	916	Carducci, Michael (MD)	Onc	292
Cambria, Richard (MA)	VascS	1010	Carey, John (UT)	CG	150
Cameron, John (MD)	S	906	Carey, Lisa (NC)	Onc	306
Camisa, Charles (FL)	D	175	Caritis, Steve (PA)	MF	371
Camitta, Bruce (WI)	PHO	662	Carlson, John (NJ)	GO	246
Cammisa, Frank (NY)	OrS	529	Carlson, Robert (CA)	Onc	333
Camoriano, John (AZ)	Onc	328	Carneiro, Ronaldo (FL)	HS	263
Campbell, Bruce (WI)	Oto	578	Carney, John (AR)	D	180
Campbell, David (CO)	TS	967	Caronna, John (NY)	N	438
Campbell, G Douglas (MS)	Pul	800	Carpenter, Jeffrey (PA)	VascS	1012
Campbell, J William (MO)	Inf	356	Carpenter, John (AL)	Onc	306
Campbell, James (MD)	NS	406	Carr, Bruce (TX)	ObG	485
Campbell, Steven (OH)	U	992	Carr, David (MO)	Ger	236
Campo, John (OH)	ChAP	784	Carr, Stephen (RI)	MF	370
Campochiaro, Peter (MD)	Oph	494	Carr-Locke, David (MA)	Ge	206
Canady, John (IA)	PlS	745	Carragee, Eugene (CA)	OrS	551
Cance, William (FL)	S	916	Carrasquillo, Jorge (NY)	NuM	474
Cancio, Margarita (FL)	Inf	354	Carrau, Ricardo (PA)	Oto	565
Canellos, George (MA)	Onc	286	Carraway, James (VA)	PlS	742
Caniano, Donna (OH)	PS	697	Carroll, Charles (IL)	HS	264
Canning, Douglas (PA)	U	980	Carroll, Peter (CA)	U	1002

Alphabetical Listing of Doctors

Name	Specialty	Pg	Name	Specialty	Pg
Carroll, William (NY)	PHO	653	Chambers, Richard (CA)	OrS	551
Carson, Benjamin (MD)	NS	406	Chambers, Setsuko (AZ)	GO	253
Carson, Culley (NC)	U	988	Champlin, Richard (TX)	Hem	283
Carson, Donald (PA)	ObG	480	Chan, Kenny (CO)	PO	683
Carson, Sandra (RI)	RE	870	Chanan-Khan, Asher (NY)	Onc	292
Carstens, Michael (CA)	PlS	751	Chancellor, Michael (PA)	U	980
Carter, Gregory (WA)	PMR	729	Chandar, Jayanthi (FL)	PNep	677
Carter, H Ballentine (MD)	U	980	Chandler, Michael (NY)	A&I	82
Carter, John (TX)	N	459	Chandler, William (MI)	NS	417
Carter, Keith (IA)	Oph	507	Chandrasoma, Parakrama (CA)	Path	617
Carter, William (AR)	Ger	237	Chang, Alfred (MI)	S	923
Cartwright, Patrick (UT)	U	997	Chang, Helena (CA)	S	938
Carty, Sally (PA)	S	906	Chang, Jenny (TX)	Onc	328
Cascino, Terrence (MN)	N	453	Chang, Kenneth (CA)	Ge	226
Casella, Samuel (NH)	PEn	640	Chang, Rowland (IL)	Rhu	888
Casselbrant, Margaretha (PA)	PO	680	Chang, Sam (TN)	U	988
Cassidy, Suzanne (CA)	CG	151	Chang, Stanley (NY)	Oph	494
Cassisi, Nicholas (FL)	Oto	573	Chang-Miller, April (AZ)	Rhu	891
Castell, Donald (SC)	Ge	214	Chao, Nelson (NC)	Onc	306
Caster, Andrew (CA)	Oph	516	Chap, Linnea (CA)	Onc	333
Castle, Valerie (MI)	PHO	662	Chapman, Paul (NY)	Onc	292
Catalona, William (IL)	U	992	Chapman, Robert (MI)	Onc	316
Catanzaro, Antonino (CA)	Pul	810	Chapman, Stanley (MS)	Inf	354
Caushaj, Fillor Philip (PA)	CRS	159	Chapman, William (MO)	S	923
Cederbaum, Stephen (CA)	CG	151	Char, Devron (CA)	Oph	516
Celli, Bartolome (MA)	Pul	794	Charboneau, J William (MN)	RadRO	830
Cello, John (CA)	Ge	226	Chari, Ravi (TN)	S	916
Cerfolio, Robert (AL)	TS	959	Chari, Suresh (MN)	Ge	218
Cerqueira, Manuel (OH)	Cv	104	Charles, Andrew (CA)	N	462
Cetta, Frank (MN)	PCd	634	Charnas, Lawrence (MN)	ChiN	141
Chabner, Bruce (MA)	Onc	287	Charney, Jonathan (NY)	N	439
Chabot, John (NY)	S	906	Charrow, Joel (IL)	CG	149
Chaikof, Elliot (GA)	VascS	1014	Chatham, Walter (AL)	Rhu	886
Chaisson, Richard (MD)	Inf	351	Chatterjee, Kanu (CA)	Cv	112
Chaitman, Bernard (MO)	Cv	104	Chen, Allen (MD)	PHO	653
Chakravarthy, Anuradha (TN)	RadRO	826	Chen, Chun (NY)	NS	406
Chalian, Ara (PA)	Oto	565	Chen, David (IL)	PMR	724

Name	Specialty	Pg	Name	Specialty	Pg
Cheng, Edward (MN)	OrS	544	Cioffi, William (RI)	S	902
Cherny, W Bruce (ID)	NS	422	Cionni, Robert (OH)	Oph	507
Cherry, Kenneth (VA)	VascS	1014	Cirigliano, Michael (PA)	IM	364
Chervenak, Francis (NY)	MF	371	Civantos, Francisco (FL)	Oto	573
Chesney, Carolyn M (TN)	Path	610	Civin, Curt (MD)	PHO	653
Cheson, Bruce (DC)	Hem	273	Clagett, George (TX)	VascS	1018
Cheville, Andrea (MN)	PMR	724	Clair, Daniel (OH)	VascS	1016
Childs, Stacy (CO)	U	998	Clairmont, Albert (OH)	PMR	724
Chinitz, Larry (NY)	CE	115	Clamon, Gerald (IA)	Onc	317
Chiocca, E Antonio (OH)	NS	418	Clark, Joseph (IL)	Onc	317
Chitambar, Christopher (WI)	Onc	317	Clark, Orlo (CA)	S	938
Chitwood, W Randolph (NC)	TS	959	Clarke-Pearson, Daniel (NC)	GO	248
Chiu, David (NY)	PlS	736	Claxton, David (PA)	Onc	292
Chiu, Yanek (CA)	CRS	165	Clayman, Gary (TX)	Oto	585
Chizner, Michael (FL)	Cv	101	Clayman, Ralph (CA)	U	1002
Chlebowski, Rowan (CA)	Onc	333	Cleary, James (WI)	Onc	317
Cho, Kathleen (MI)	Path	612	Clements, Dennis (NC)	PInf	673
Cho, Kyung (MI)	VIR	863	Clements, Philip (CA)	Rhu	891
Choi, Noah (MA)	RadRO	820	Clements, Stephen (GA)	Cv	101
Chopra, Inder (CA)	EDM	201	Clinton, Steven (OH)	Onc	317
Choti, Michael (MD)	S	906	Cloherty, John (MA)	NP	382
Chow, Warren (CA)	Onc	333	Clohisy, Denis (MN)	OrS	544
Chowdhury, Khalid (CO)	Oto	584	Cloninger, C Robert (MO)	Psyc	770
Choy, Andrew (CA)	Oph	516	Clore, John (VA)	EDM	194
Choy, Hak (TX)	RadRO	834	Close, Lanny (NY)	Oto	565
Christian, Karla (TN)	TS	959	Cloughesy, Timothy (CA)	N	463
Christiani, David (MA)	Pul	794	Clutter, William (MO)	EDM	196
Christie, Dennis (WA)	PGe	650	Cobleigh, Melody (IL)	Onc	317
Christman, Brian (TN)	Pul	800	Cobos, Everardo (TX)	Hem	283
Christman, Gregory (MI)	RE	876	Coccia, Peter (NE)	PHO	667
Chu, Edward (CT)	Onc	287	Cochran, Alistair (CA)	Path	617
Chui, Helena (CA)	N	463	Cockerell, Clay (TX)	D	180
Chung, Kevin (MI)	HS	264	Cockerham, Kimberly (CA)	Oph	516
Church, Joseph (CA)	PA&I	629	Coe, Fredric (IL)	Nep	396
Ciccotti, Michael (PA)	SM	896	Coffey, Barbara (NY)	ChAP	781
Cilo, Mark (CO)	N	458	Coffman, Thomas (NC)	Nep	395
Ciocon, Jerry (FL)	Ger	235	Coggins, Cecil (MA)	Nep	392

Alphabetical Listing of Doctors

Name	Specialty	Pg	Name	Specialty	Pg
Cohen, Alan (OH)	NS	418	Collea, Joseph (DC)	MF	371
Cohen, Bernard (FL)	D	175	Coller, Barry (NY)	Hem	273
Cohen, Bruce (OH)	ChiN	141	Collins, Dale (NH)	PlS	734
Cohen, Burton (NY)	DR	846	Colombani, Paul (MD)	PS	693
Cohen, David (NY)	Nep	393	Colon-Otero, Gerardo (FL)	Onc	306
Cohen, Harris (NY)	DR	846	Colquhoun, Steven (CA)	S	938
Cohen, Howard (NY)	Cv	95	Colvin, Edward (AL)	PCd	633
Cohen, James (OR)	Oto	587	Come, Steven (MA)	Onc	287
Cohen, Jeffrey (OH)	N	453	Comerota, Anthony (OH)	VascS	1016
Cohen, Jonathan (NY)	Ge	208	Comi, Richard (NH)	EDM	188
Cohen, Lawrence (NY)	Ge	208	Cominelli, Fabio (VA)	Ge	214
Cohen, Mark (IL)	HS	264	Conant, Emily (PA)	DR	847
Cohen, Martin (NY)	CE	115	Connolly, Heidi (MN)	Cv	104
Cohen, Michael (IA)	Path	612	Connolly, James (MA)	Path	604
Cohen, Mitchell (OH)	PGe	648	Conrad, Ernest (WA)	OrS	551
Cohen, Mitchell (PA)	Psyc	765	Conry, Robert (AL)	Onc	306
Cohen, Myron (NC)	Inf	354	Constantian, Mark B (NH)	PlS	734
Cohen, Philip (DC)	Onc	292	Constine, Louis (NY)	RadRO	822
Cohen, Robbin (CA)	TS	970	Conte, John (MD)	TS	953
Cohen, Roger (PA)	Onc	292	Conti, David (NY)	S	906
Cohen, Seymour (NY)	Onc	293	Cook, Jonathan (NC)	D	175
Cohen, Steven (CA)	PlS	751	Cook, Stuart (NJ)	N	439
Cohen, William (PA)	Ped	624	Cookson, Michael (TN)	U	988
Cohn, David (CO)	Inf	357	Cooney, Leo (CT)	Ger	234
Cohn, John (PA)	A&I	82	Cooper, Barry (TX)	Hem	283
Cohn, Richard (IL)	PNep	678	Cooper, Christopher (OH)	Cv	104
Cohn, Susan (IL)	PHO	663	Cooper, Dan (CA)	PPul	688
Coit, Daniel (NY)	S	906	Cooper, Daniel (TX)	OrS	550
Colachis, Samuel (OH)	PMR	725	Cooper, David (MD)	EDM	190
Cole, Andrew (MA)	N	436	Cooper, Joel (PA)	TS	953
Cole, Brian (IL)	SM	898	Cooper, John (AL)	Pul	801
Cole, David (SC)	S	916	Cooper, Rubin (NY)	PCd	631
Cole, Francis (MO)	NP	385	Cooper, William (VA)	Pul	801
Coleman, Beverly (PA)	DR	846	Copel, Joshua (CT)	MF	370
Coleman, John (IN)	PlS	745	Copeland, Jack (AZ)	TS	968
Coleman, Morton (NY)	Onc	293	Copeland, Larry (OH)	GO	251
Coleman, Ralph (NC)	NuM	476	Coplen, Douglas (MO)	U	993

Name	Specialty	Pg	Name	Specialty	Pg
Copp, Steven (CA)	OrS	551	Coyle, Patricia (NY)	N	439
Copperman, Alan (NY)	RE	871	Cragg, Andrew (MN)	VIR	863
Coppola, John (NY)	Cv	95	Craig, Edward (NY)	OrS	530
Corbett, James (MS)	N	448	Craig, Robert (IL)	Ge	218
Cordeiro, Peter (NY)	PlS	736	Craigen, William (TX)	CG	150
Corey, G Ralph (NC)	Inf	354	Cramer, Daniel (MA)	ObG	480
Corey, Jacquelynne (IL)	Oto	578	Crandall, Alan (UT)	Oph	513
Corey, Lawrence (WA)	Inf	358	Craven, Donald (MA)	Inf	350
Corey, Seth (IL)	PHO	663	Crawford, E David (CO)	U	998
Cornblath, David (MD)	N	439	Crawford, James (FL)	Path	610
Cornelius, Lynn (MO)	D	177	Crawford, Jeffrey (NC)	Onc	306
Cornella, Jeffrey (AZ)	ObG	485	Crawford, Thomas (MD)	ChiN	139
Cornwell, Edward (DC)	S	907	Creamer, Michael (FL)	PMR	723
Corson, John (NM)	VascS	1018	Creasman, William (SC)	GO	248
Coselli, Joseph (TX)	TS	968	Criado, Frank (MD)	VascS	1012
Cosgrove, G Rees (MA)	NS	404	Criner, Gerard (PA)	Pul	796
Costantino, Peter (NY)	Oto	565	Crippin, Jeffrey (MO)	Ge	218
Cote, Richard (CA)	Path	617	Crocker, Ian (GA)	RadRO	826
Cotsarelis, George (PA)	D	171	Crockett, Dennis (CA)	PO	684
Cotton, Peter (SC)	Ge	214	Crofford, Leslie (KY)	Rhu	887
Cotton, Robin (OH)	PO	682	Crombleholme, Timothy (OH)	PS	698
Couch, James (OK)	N	459	Cronenwett, Jack (NH)	VascS	1010
Couch, Marion (NC)	Oto	573	Cronin, David (WI)	S	923
Coughlin, Michael (ID)	OrS	548	Croop, James (IN)	PHO	663
Coukos, George (PA)	GO	246	Cross, DeWitte (MO)	NRad	857
Couldwell, William (UT)	NS	422	Crossett, Lawrence (PA)	OrS	530
Coull, Bruce (AZ)	N	459	Crow, Scott (MN)	Psyc	771
Courcoulas, Anita (PA)	S	907	Crowe, Joseph (OH)	S	923
Courey, Mark (CA)	Oto	587	Crowley, William (MA)	RE	870
Coutifaris, Christos (PA)	RE	871	Cruse, C Wayne (FL)	PlS	742
Coutsoftides, Theodore (CA)	CRS	165	Cryer, Philip (MO)	EDM	196
Covington, Edward (OH)	PM	599	Cuckler, John (AL)	OrS	539
Cowan, Bryan (MS)	RE	875	Culbertson, William (FL)	Oph	502
Cowan, Kenneth (NE)	Onc	325	Culkin, Daniel (OK)	U	999
Cowan, Morton (CA)	PA&I	630	Cullen, Kevin (MD)	Onc	293
Cox, James (TX)	RadRO	834	Cullen, Mark (CT)	OM	758
Coyle, Joseph (MA)	ChAP	780	Culp, Randall (PA)	HS	261

Alphabetical Listing of Doctors

Name	Specialty	Pg	Name	Specialty	Pg
Cummings, Charles (MD)	Oto	565	Dake, Michael (CA)	VIR	865
Cummings, Jeffrey (CA)	N	463	Dakhil, Shaker (KS)	Onc	325
Cunha, Burke (NY)	Inf	351	Dalakas, Marinos (PA)	N	439
Cunniff, Christopher (AZ)	CG	150	Dale, Lowell (MN)	Ger	236
Cunningham, Glenn (TX)	EDM	200	Dalinka, Murray (PA)	DR	847
Cunningham, John (AZ)	Ge	224	Dalkin, Alan (VA)	EDM	194
Cunningham, Michael (MA)	PO	680	Dalsing, Michael (IN)	VascS	1016
Cunningham-Rundles, Charlotte (NY)	A&I	82	Daly, Mary (PA)	Onc	293
			Damewood, Marian (PA)	RE	872
Cupps, Thomas (DC)	Rhu	883	Damiano, Ralph (MO)	TS	963
Curcillo, Paul (PA)	S	907	Damon, Lloyd (CA)	Hem	284
Curet, Myriam (CA)	S	938	Dana, Reza (MA)	Oph	492
Curl, Walton (NC)	OrS	540	Dang, Michael (HI)	TS	970
Curley, Steven (TX)	S	932	Daniel, Rollin (CA)	PlS	751
Curran, James (IL)	Rhu	888	Daniels, Gilbert (MA)	EDM	188
Currie, John (CT)	GO	244	Danoff, Dudley (CA)	U	1002
Curry, Cynthia (CA)	CG	151	Darcy, Michael (MO)	VIR	863
Curtin, Hugh (MA)	NRad	854	Darling, R Clement (NY)	VascS	1012
Curtin, John (NY)	GO	246	Darras, Basil (MA)	ChiN	138
Curtis, Anne (FL)	CE	116	Darrow, David (VA)	PO	682
Cushman, William (TN)	IM	365	Darwin, Christine (CA)	EDM	201
Cutrer, F Michael (MN)	N	453	Das, Ananya (AZ)	Ge	225
Cutting, Court (NY)	PlS	736	Daspit, C Phillip (AZ)	Oto	585
Czuczman, Myron (NY)	Onc	293	Daud, Adil (FL)	Onc	307
			Daugherty, Christopher (IL)	Onc	317
			David, Carlos (MA)	NS	404
			Davidoff, Andrew (TN)	PS	695

D

Name	Specialty	Pg	Name	Specialty	Pg
D'Alton, Mary (NY)	MF	371	Davidson, Bruce (DC)	Oto	566
D'Amico, Anthony (MA)	RadRO	820	Davidson, Dennis (NY)	NP	382
D'Amico, Donald (NY)	Oph	494	Davidson, Joyce (TX)	Psyc	773
D'Amico, Thomas (NC)	TS	960	Davidson, Nancy (MD)	Onc	293
Daar, Eric (CA)	Inf	358	Davidson, Richard (PA)	OrS	530
Dabbagh, Shermine (DE)	PNep	676	Davidson, Susan (CO)	GO	253
Dacey, Ralph (MO)	NS	418	Davies, Stella (OH)	PHO	663
Dae, Michael (CA)	NuM	477	Davies, Terry (NY)	EDM	190
Dagum, Alexander (NY)	PlS	737	Davis, Bradley (KS)	U	998
			Davis, Gary (TX)	Ge	225

Name	Specialty	Pg	Name	Specialty	Pg
Davis, Jessica (NY)	CG	147	Delamarter, Rick (CA)	OrS	552
Davis, Mellar (OH)	Onc	317	DeLancey, John (MI)	ObG	483
Davis, William (LA)	Rhu	891	Deland, Jonathan (NY)	OrS	530
Dawson, Nancy (DC)	Onc	293	Delaney, Conor (OH)	CRS	162
Day, Arthur (MA)	NS	404	DeLaney, Thomas (MA)	RadRO	820
Day, Susan (CA)	Oph	517	DeLellis, Ronald (RI)	Path	604
Day, Terrence (SC)	Oto	573	Deleo, Vincent (NY)	D	171
De Angelis, Lisa (NY)	N	439	Deleyiannis, Frederic (PA)	PlS	737
De Cherney, Alan (MD)	ObG	481	Delivoria-Papadopoulos, Maria (PA)		NP
De Geest, Koen (IA)	GO	251	382		
De Juan, Eugene (CA)	Oph	517	Dell, Diana (NC)	Psyc	769
de Kernion, Jean (CA)	U	1002	Della Rocca, Robert (NY)	Oph	495
De la Cruz, Antonio (CA)	Oto	587	Delmez, James (MO)	Nep	396
De Lateur, Barbara (MD)	PMR	721	Demarest, Gerald (NM)	S	932
De Leon-Casasola, Oscar (NY)	PM	596	DeMars, Leslie (NH)	GO	244
De Lia, Julian (WI)	ObG	483	Demer, Joseph (CA)	Oph	517
De Long, Mahlon (GA)	N	448	Demetri, George (MA)	Onc	287
De Luca, Francesco (PA)	PEn	641	Demetris, Anthony (PA)	Path	605
De Masters, Bette (CO)	Path	614	Demmy, Todd (NY)	TS	953
De Meester, Tom (CA)	TS	970	Dempsey, Daniel (PA)	S	907
De Monte, Franco (TX)	NS	423	Dempsey, Robert (WI)	NS	418
De Simone, Philip (KY)	Onc	307	Denenberg, Steven (NE)	Oto	584
De Vivo, Darryl (NY)	ChiN	139	Denson, Susan (TX)	NP	387
Dean, Jonathan (UT)	PCCM	639	DeOrio, James (NC)	OrS	540
Deas, Deborah (SC)	ChAP	783	DePaulo, J Raymond (MD)	Psyc	765
DeBaun, Michael (MO)	PHO	663	DePompolo, Robert (MN)	PMR	725
DeCamp, Malcolm (MA)	TS	950	DePriest, Paul (KY)	GO	248
Deeg, H. Joachim (WA)	Onc	334	Derman, Gordon (IL)	HS	264
DeGiorgio, Christopher (CA)	N	463	Dershaw, D David (NY)	DR	847
Deitch, Edwin (NJ)	S	907	Deschamps, Claude (MN)	TS	963
Deitz, Joel (PA)	Pul	796	Deschler, Daniel (MA)	Oto	563
DeKosky, Steven (PA)	N	439	deShazo, Richard (MS)	A&I	84
Del Giudice, Stephen (NH)	D	168	DeSilva, Stephen (MI)	HS	265
Del Monte, Monte (MI)	Oph	507	Desnick, Robert (NY)	CG	147
Del Negro, Albert (VA)	CE	116	Desposito, Franklin (NJ)	CG	147
Del Priore, Lucian (NY)	Oph	494	DeVane, Gary (FL)	RE	875
Delahay, John (DC)	OrS	530	DeVault, Kenneth (FL)	Ge	215

Alphabetical Listing of Doctors

Name	Specialty	Pg	Name	Specialty	Pg
Devereux, Richard (NY)	Cv	95	Dines, David (NY)	OrS	530
Devinsky, Orrin (NY)	N	439	Dion, Jacques (GA)	NRad	856
DeVita, Vincent (CT)	Onc	287	Disis, Mary (WA)	Onc	334
Dewberry, Robert (MD)	N	439	Diuguid, David (NY)	Hem	273
DeWeese, Theodore (MD)	RadRO	822	Diver, Daniel (CT)	IC	119
Deziel, Daniel (IL)	S	923	Diwan, Sudhir (NY)	PM	596
Dezube, Bruce (MA)	Hem	272	Djulbegovic, Benjamin (FL)	Hem	276
Di Bisceglie, Adrian (MO)	Ge	218	Dobs, Adrian (MD)	EDM	191
Di Giacinto, George (NY)	NS	407	Docimo, Steven (PA)	U	980
Di Persio, John (MO)	Hem	278	Dodd, Gerald (CO)	DR	852
Di Saia, Philip (CA)	GO	255	Dodds, William (MI)	RE	876
Diamond, Frank (FL)	PEn	642	Dodick, David (AZ)	N	460
Diamond, Michael (MI)	RE	876	Dodick, Jack (NY)	Oph	495
Diamond, Paul (VA)	PMR	723	Doghramji, Karl (PA)	Psyc	765
Dias, Mark (PA)	NS	407	Doherty, Dennis (KY)	Pul	801
Diaz, Angela (NY)	AM	78	Doherty, Gerard (MI)	S	923
Diaz, Fernando (MI)	NS	418	Dolgin, Stephen (NY)	PS	693
Dichek, David (WA)	Cv	112	Dolitsky, Jay (NY)	PO	681
Dichter, Marc (PA)	N	440	Donald, Paul (CA)	Oto	587
Dick, Macdonald (MI)	PCd	634	Donaldson, Sarah (CA)	RadRO	836
Dicker, Adam (PA)	RadRO	822	Donaldson, William (PA)	OrS	530
Dickey, Richard (LA)	RE	878	Donehower, Ross (MD)	Onc	293
Diehl, James (PA)	TS	953	Donn, Steven (MI)	NP	385
Dienstag, Jules (MA)	Ge	206	Donohue, James (NC)	Pul	801
Dieterich, Douglas (NY)	Ge	208	Donohue, John (MN)	S	923
Diethrich, Edward (AZ)	TS	968	Donovan, Donald (TX)	Oto	585
Dilawari, Raza (TN)	S	916	Donovan, James (OH)	U	993
Dillard, James (NY)	PMR	721	Dooley, Sharon (IL)	MF	374
Dillehay, Gary (IL)	NuM	476	Dooley, William (OK)	S	933
Diller, Lisa (MA)	PHO	651	Dormans, John (PA)	OrS	530
Dilley, Ralph (CA)	VascS	1019	Doroshow, James (MD)	Onc	294
Dillingham, Michael (CA)	OrS	552	Dorr, Lawrence (CA)	OrS	552
Dillingham, Timothy (WI)	PMR	725	Dottino, Peter (NY)	GO	246
Dillon, William (CA)	NRad	859	Douglas, James (WA)	RadRO	836
DiMarco, John (VA)	CE	116	Douglas, John (GA)	Cv	101
DiMarino, Anthony (PA)	Ge	208	Dover, Jeffrey (MA)	D	168
Dimeff, Robert (OH)	SM	898	Dowling, Robert (KY)	TS	960

Name	Specialty	Pg	Name	Specialty	Pg
Dozor, Allen (NY)	PPul	685	Dunkel, Ira (NY)	PHO	654
Drachman, Daniel (MD)	N	440	Dunlap, Nancy (AL)	Pul	801
Drachtman, Richard (NJ)	PHO	653	Dunphy, Frank (NC)	Onc	307
Drake, Amelia (NC)	PO	682	Dunton, Charles (PA)	GO	246
Drayer, Burton (NY)	NRad	855	DuPont, Herbert (TX)	Inf	357
Drebin, Jeffrey (PA)	S	907	Durbin, William (MA)	PInf	672
Dreicer, Robert (OH)	Onc	318	Dure, Leon (AL)	N	448
Dreyer, William (TX)	PCd	636	Durham, Janette (CO)	VIR	864
Dreyer, ZoAnn (TX)	PHO	668	Durham, Samuel (OH)	TS	964
Drinkwater, Davis (TN)	TS	960	Durrie, Daniel (KS)	Oph	513
Driscoll, Colin (MN)	Oto	578	Duthie, Edmund H (WI)	Ger	236
Driscoll, Daniel (FL)	CG	148	Dutton, Jonathan (NC)	Oph	503
Driscoll, David (MN)	PCd	635	Duvic, Madeleine (TX)	D	180
Driscoll, Deborah (PA)	CG	147	Dyer, Carmel (TX)	Ger	238
Dritschilo, Anatoly (DC)	RadRO	822	Dzubow, Leonard (PA)	D	171
Driver, Larry (TX)	PM	600			
Droller, Michael (NY)	U	981			
Dromerick, Alexander (DC)	N	440			
Drossman, Douglas (NC)	Ge	215			

E

Name	Specialty	Pg
Druker, Brian (OR)	Onc	334
Druzin, Maurice (CA)	MF	378
Dubeau, Louis (CA)	Path	617
Dubois, Michel (NY)	PM	597
Ducore, Jonathan (CA)	PHO	669
Duff, W Patrick (FL)	ObG	482
Duffner, Patricia (NY)	ChiN	139
Duffy, Thomas (CT)	Hem	272
Dufresne, Craig (MD)	PlS	737
Dugoff, Lorraine (CO)	MF	376
Duh, Quan-Yang (CA)	S	938
Duhaime, Ann (NH)	NS	404
Duker, Jay (MA)	Oph	492
Dulcan, Mina (IL)	ChAP	784
Dumesic, Daniel (MN)	RE	877
Dumitru, Daniel (TX)	PMR	728
Duncan, Brian (OH)	PS	698
Duncan, Newton (TX)	PO	684

Name	Specialty	Pg
Eagle, Kim (MI)	Cv	105
Eagle, Ralph (PA)	Oph	495
Earle, Craig (MA)	Onc	287
Earp, H Shelton (NC)	EDM	194
Eaton, James (DC)	Psyc	765
Eavey, Roland (MA)	PO	680
Eberlein, Timothy (MO)	S	924
Ebraheim, Nabil (OH)	OrS	544
Eckardt, Jeffrey (CA)	OrS	552
Eckardt, Jeffrey (CA)	OrS	552
Eckel, Robert (CO)	EDM	199
Eckhardt, S (CO)	Onc	325
Eckhoff, Devin (AL)	S	916
Econs, Michael (IN)	EDM	196
Edelman, Martin (MD)	Onc	294
Edelman, Robert (IL)	DR	851
Edelson, Richard (CT)	D	168
Edelstein, Barbara (NY)	DR	847

Alphabetical Listing of Doctors

Name	Specialty	Pg	Name	Specialty	Pg
Edelstein, David (NY)	Oto	566	Eismont, Frank (FL)	OrS	540
Edersheim, Terri (NY)	MF	372	El-Galley, Rizk (AL)	U	988
Edgar, Terence (WI)	ChiN	141	El-Youssef, Mounif (MN)	PGe	648
Edge, Stephen (NY)	S	907	Elder, Jack (MI)	U	993
Edington, Howard (PA)	S	907	Elefteriades, John (CT)	TS	950
Edmundowicz, Daniel (PA)	Cv	95	Elias, Sherman (IL)	CG	149
Edmundowicz, Steven (MO)	Ge	219	Elias, Stanton (MI)	N	453
Edney, James (NE)	S	930	Elkayam, Uri (CA)	Cv	112
Edwards, John (CA)	Inf	358	Ellenbogen, Kenneth (VA)	CE	116
Edwards, Kathryn (TN)	PInf	674	Ellenbogen, Richard (WA)	NS	426
Edwards, Michael (OH)	S	924	Ellenhorn, Joshua (CA)	S	938
Edwards, Michael (CA)	NS	426	Elliott, C Gregory (UT)	Pul	807
Edwards, Robert (PA)	GO	246	Elliott, David (IA)	Ge	219
Edye, Michael (NY)	S	907	Elliott, John (AZ)	MF	377
Efron, Jonathan (AZ)	CRS	164	Ellis, David (TX)	U	999
Eggers, Howard (NY)	Oph	495	Ellis, Demetrius (PA)	PNep	676
Ehrenkranz, Richard (CT)	NP	382	Ellis, George (LA)	Oph	513
Ehresmann, Glenn (CA)	Rhu	892	Ellis, Georgiana (WA)	Onc	334
Ehrlich, Peter (MI)	PS	698	Ellis, Jonathan (CA)	Ge	226
Ehrmann, David (IL)	EDM	196	Ellis, Lee (TX)	S	933
Ehya, Hormoz (PA)	Path	605	Ellis, Matthew (MO)	Onc	318
Eichelberger, Martin (DC)	PS	693	Ellis, Stephen (OH)	IC	122
Eichenfield, Lawrence (CA)	D	181	Ellis, William (WA)	U	1002
Eichler, Craig (FL)	D	175	Ellison, David (OR)	Nep	400
Eidt, John (AR)	VascS	1018	Ellison, E Christopher (OH)	S	924
Eifel, Patricia (TX)	RadRO	834	Elmets, Craig (AL)	D	175
Eilber, Frederick (CA)	S	938	Eloubeidi, Mohamad (AL)	Ge	215
Ein, Daniel (DC)	A&I	83	Elta, Grace (MI)	Ge	219
Einhorn, Lawrence (IN)	Onc	318	Emami, Bahman (IL)	RadRO	830
Einhorn, Thomas (MA)	OrS	526	Emans, Sarah (MA)	AM	78
Eisele, David (CA)	Oto	587	Emanuel, Peter (AR)	Hem	283
Eisen, Howard (PA)	Cv	96	Emanuele, Mary Ann (IL)	EDM	197
Eisenberg, Burton (NH)	S	902	Emanuele, Nicholas (IL)	EDM	197
Eisenberg, Howard (MD)	NS	407	Emery, Helen (WA)	PRhu	691
Eisenberger, Mario (MD)	Onc	294	Emmanuel, Patricia (FL)	PInf	674
Eisendrath, Stuart (CA)	Psyc	774	Emond, Jean (NY)	S	908
Eisenstat, Theodore (NJ)	CRS	159	Emre, Sukru (CT)	S	902

Name	Specialty	Pg	Name	Specialty	Pg
Emslie, Graham (TX)	ChAP	785	Everson, Gregory (CO)	Ge	223
Enelow, Richard (NH)	Pul	794	Eviatar, Lydia (NY)	ChiN	139
Eng, Charis (OH)	Onc	318	Ewalt, David (TX)	U	999
Eng, Kenneth (NY)	S	908	Ewend, Matthew (NC)	NS	412
Engel, William King (CA)	N	463	Ezaki, Marybeth (TX)	HS	267
Engstrom, John (CA)	N	463			
Ennis, Ronald (NY)	RadRO	822			
Ensminger, William (MI)	Onc	318	**F**		
Epstein, Andrew (AL)	CE	116			
Epstein, Jonathan (MD)	Path	605	Fabian, Carol (KS)	Onc	325
Epstein, Laurence (MA)	CE	114	Fahey, Patrick (IL)	Pul	804
Epstein, Leon (IL)	ChiN	141	Fahey, Thomas (NY)	S	908
Epstein, Michael (FL)	PCd	633	Fahn, Stanley (NY)	N	440
Epstein, Stuart (CA)	PA&I	630	Failla, Joseph (MI)	HS	265
Erba, Harry (MI)	Hem	278	Fairman, Ronald (PA)	VascS	1012
Erban, John (MA)	Onc	287	Falanga, Vincent (RI)	D	168
Eriksson, Elof (MA)	PlS	734	Falcone, Tommaso (OH)	RE	877
Ernst, Armin (MA)	Pul	794	Falk, Rena (CA)	CG	151
Errico, Thomas (NY)	OrS	531	Falk, Ronald (NC)	Nep	395
Eschenbach, David (WA)	ObG	485	Fallat, Mary (KY)	PS	695
Escobedo, Marilyn (OK)	NP	387	Fallon, Brian (NY)	Psyc	765
Esquenazi, Alberto (PA)	PMR	721	Fallon, Michael (AL)	Ge	215
Esquivel, Carlos (CA)	S	938	Fallon, Robert (IN)	PHO	663
Esserman, Laura (CA)	S	938	Fan, Leland (TX)	PPul	688
Essner, Richard (CA)	S	939	Fang, John (UT)	Ge	223
Estabrook, Alison (NY)	S	908	Fann, Jesse (WA)	Psyc	774
Estey, Elihu (WA)	Onc	334	Fanous, Yvonne (CA)	PA&I	630
Eth, Spencer (NY)	Psyc	765	Fanta, Christopher (MA)	Pul	795
Ettenger, Robert (CA)	PNep	679	Fantini, Gary (NY)	VascS	1012
Ettinger, David (MD)	Onc	294	Fanucchi, Michael (NY)	Onc	294
Eugster, Erica (IN)	PEn	643	Farag, Sherif (IN)	Hem	278
Euhus, David (TX)	S	933	Farber, Martin (NY)	Rhu	884
Eustis, Horatio (LA)	Oph	513	Faries, Peter (NY)	VascS	1012
Evans, Douglas (TX)	S	933	Farley, David (MN)	S	924
Evans, Mark (NY)	ObG	481	Farlow, Martin (IN)	N	453
Evans, Sarah (DC)	PMR	721	Farmer, Richard (NY)	Ge	208
Evers, Kathryn (PA)	DR	847	Faro, Sebastian (TX)	ObG	485

Alphabetical Listing of Doctors

Name	Specialty	Pg	Name	Specialty	Pg
Farrar, William (OH)	S	924	Ferrell, Linda (CA)	Path	617
Farrior, Edward (FL)	Oto	573	Ferrendelli, James (TX)	N	460
Farrior, Joseph (FL)	Oto	573	Ferriero, Donna (CA)	ChiN	143
Fasano, Alessio (MD)	PGe	646	Fessler, Richard (IL)	NS	418
Fauci, Anthony (MD)	Inf	351	Fewkes, Jessica (MA)	D	168
Fay, Joseph (TX)	Onc	328	Fields, Abbie (VA)	GO	249
Faye-Petersen, Ona (AL)	Path	610	Figlin, Robert (CA)	Onc	334
Feder, Robert (IL)	Oph	508	Files, Joe (MS)	Hem	276
Fee, Willard (CA)	Oto	587	Filip, Stanley (NC)	ObG	482
Feghali, Joseph (NY)	Oto	566	Filley, Christopher (CO)	N	458
Feig, Barry (TX)	S	933	Filly, Roy (CA)	DR	853
Feig, Stephen (CA)	DR	853	Finan, Michael (AL)	GO	249
Feinberg, Joseph (NY)	PMR	721	Fine, Howard (MD)	Onc	294
Feinberg, Todd (NY)	N	440	Fine, Perry (UT)	PM	600
Feinglos, Mark (NC)	EDM	194	Fine, Robert (NY)	Onc	294
Feldman, David (NY)	OrS	531	Finerman, Gerald (CA)	OrS	552
Feldman, Eva (MI)	N	454	Finger, Paul (NY)	Oph	495
Feldman, Joel (MA)	PlS	734	Fink, Matthew (NY)	N	440
Feldman, Joseph (IL)	PMR	725	Finkel, Alan (NC)	N	448
Feldman, Kenneth (WA)	Ped	626	Finkel, Michael (FL)	N	449
Feldman, Mark (TX)	Ge	225	Finkel, Terri (PA)	PRhu	689
Feldman, Ted (IL)	IC	122	Finklestein, Jerry (CA)	PHO	669
Feldmann, Edward (RI)	N	436	Finlay, Jonathan (CA)	PHO	669
Feldon, Steven (NY)	Oph	495	Finucane, Thomas (MD)	Ger	234
Feldstein, Neil (NY)	NS	407	Fiorica, James (FL)	GO	249
Feliciano, David (GA)	S	917	Firlit, Casimir (MO)	U	993
Felig, Philip (NY)	EDM	191	First, Michael (NY)	Psyc	766
Felix, Carolyn (PA)	PHO	654	Fisch, Harry (NY)	U	981
Fenichel, Gerald (TN)	ChiN	140	Fischbein, Lewis (MO)	Rhu	888
Fennerty, Brian (OR)	Ge	226	Fischer, Thomas (IN)	HS	265
Fenske, Neil (FL)	D	175	Fish, Frank (TN)	PCd	633
Ferguson, James (KY)	MF	373	Fishbein, Daniel (WA)	Cv	112
Ferguson, Mark (IL)	TS	964	Fishbein, Michael (CA)	Path	617
Ferguson, Ronald (OH)	S	924	Fisher, Garth (CA)	PlS	751
Fernhoff, Paul (GA)	CG	148	Fisher, Mark (CA)	N	463
Ferrante, F Michael (CA)	PM	601	Fisher, Paul (CA)	ChiN	143
Ferrara, James (MI)	PHO	663	Fisher, Richard (NY)	Onc	294

Alphabetical Listing of Doctors

Name	Specialty	Pg	Name	Specialty	Pg
Fisher, Robert (PA)	Ge	208	Flynn, Harry (FL)	Oph	503
Fisher, Robert (CA)	N	463	Flynn, John (NY)	Oph	495
Fisher, William (TX)	S	933	Flynn, Joseph (WA)	PNep	679
Fishman, David (NY)	GO	246	Flynn, Michael (KY)	S	917
Fishman, Elliot (MD)	DR	847	Flynn, Patrick (MN)	Hem	278
Fishman, Henry (DC)	A&I	83	Flynn, Timothy (FL)	VascS	1015
Fishman, Marvin (TX)	ChiN	142	Fodor, Peter (CA)	PlS	752
Fishman, Scott (CA)	PM	601	Foglia, Robert (TX)	PS	700
Fitch, Tom (AZ)	Onc	328	Fogt, Franz (PA)	Path	606
Fitzgerald, Paul (CA)	EDM	201	Foley, Carmel (NY)	ChAP	781
Fitzgibbon, Dermot (WA)	PM	601	Foley, Eugene (WI)	CRS	162
Fitzgibbons, Robert (NE)	S	930	Foley, Kathleen (NY)	PM	597
Fitzpatrick, Richard (CA)	D	181	Foley, Kevin (TN)	NS	413
Fivenson, David (MI)	D	177	Follansbee, William (PA)	Cv	96
Fivush, Barbara (MD)	PNep	676	Follen, Michele (TX)	GO	253
Fix, R Jobe (AL)	PlS	742	Fonarow, Gregg (CA)	Cv	113
Flachsbart, Keith (CA)	TS	970	Fong, Yuman (NY)	S	908
Flake, Alan (PA)	PS	693	Fonseca, Rafael (AZ)	Hem	283
Flamm, Eugene (NY)	NS	407	Fontana, Gregory (CA)	TS	970
Flamm, Scott (OH)	DR	851	Foo, Sun-Hoo (NY)	N	440
Flanders, Adam (PA)	NRad	855	Forastiere, Arlene (MD)	Onc	295
Flanigan, D Preston (CA)	VascS	1019	Forbess, Joseph (TX)	TS	968
Flanigan, Robert (IL)	U	993	Ford, Carol Ann (NC)	AM	78
Flanigan, Timothy (RI)	Inf	350	Ford, Charles (WI)	Oto	578
Flatow, Evan (NY)	OrS	531	Ford, Henri (CA)	PS	701
Fleischer, David (AZ)	Ge	225	Ford, James (CA)	Onc	334
Fleischer, Norman (NY)	EDM	191	Forman, Jeffrey (MI)	RadRO	830
Fleisher, Gary (MA)	PCCM	638	Forman, Stephen (CA)	Hem	284
Fleming, Gini (IL)	Onc	318	Formenti, Silvia (NY)	RadRO	822
Fleshman, James (MO)	CRS	162	Fornari, Victor (NY)	ChAP	781
Fletcher, Christopher (MA)	Path	604	Forscher, Charles (CA)	Onc	334
Fletcher, Eugene (IN)	Pul	804	Forsmark, Christopher (FL)	Ge	215
Flickinger, John (PA)	RadRO	822	Forster, Richard (FL)	Oph	503
Flinn, Ian (TN)	Onc	307	Fortenberry, J Dennis (IN)	AM	78
Flomenberg, Neal (PA)	Onc	295	Fossella, Frank (TX)	Onc	328
Flood, William (PA)	Onc	295	Fost, Norman (WI)	Ped	625
Flowers, Franklin (FL)	D	175	Foster, Carol (UT)	PEn	644

Alphabetical Listing of Doctors

Name	Specialty	Pg	Name	Specialty	Pg
Foster, Charles (MA)	Oph	492	Freifeld, Alison (NE)	Inf	357
Foster, Richard (IN)	U	993	Freiman, Hal (NY)	Ge	208
Foucar, M (NM)	Path	615	Freischlag, Julie (MD)	VascS	1013
Fowble, Barbara (CA)	RadRO	836	French, Jacqueline (NY)	N	440
Fowl, Richard (AZ)	VascS	1018	Friberg, Thomas (PA)	Oph	495
Fowler, Dennis (NY)	S	908	Fricker, Frederick (FL)	PCd	633
Fowler, Jeffrey (OH)	GO	251	Friebert, Sarah (OH)	PHO	663
Fowler, Wesley (NC)	GO	249	Fried, Guy (PA)	PMR	721
Fox, Harold (MD)	MF	372	Fried, Marvin (NY)	Oto	566
Fox, Kevin (PA)	Onc	295	Friedberg, Jonathan (NY)	Onc	295
Fox, Peter (TX)	N	460	Friedberg, Joseph (PA)	TS	953
Fox, Roger (FL)	A&I	84	Frieden, Ilona (CA)	D	181
Fracasso, Paula (VA)	Onc	307	Friedlaender, Gary (CT)	OrS	526
Fraker, Douglas (PA)	S	908	Friedland, Jack (AZ)	PlS	749
France, Thomas (WI)	Oph	508	Friedman, Aaron (MN)	PNep	678
Frances, Richard (NY)	AdP	778	Friedman, Allan (NC)	NS	413
Francisco, Gerard (TX)	PMR	728	Friedman, Barry (CA)	Psyc	774
Frangoul, Haydar (TN)	PHO	658	Friedman, Debra (WA)	PHO	670
Frank, Ian (PA)	Inf	351	Friedman, Ellen (TX)	PO	684
Franklin, Morris (TX)	S	933	Friedman, Henry (NC)	PHO	659
Franks, Andrew (NY)	D	171	Friedman, Lawrence (MA)	Ge	206
Frantz, Christopher N (DE)	PHO	654	Friedman, Lloyd (CT)	Pul	795
Fraser, Charles (TX)	TS	968	Friedman, Matthew (VT)	Psyc	762
Fraser, Lionel (MS)	U	988	Friedman, Michael (IL)	Oto	579
Frassica, Frank (MD)	OrS	531	Friedman, Nancy (NC)	PEn	642
Frazee, John (CA)	NS	426	Friedman, Richard (TX)	PCd	636
Frazier, Oscar (TX)	TS	968	Friedman, Sanford (NY)	Cv	96
Frazier, Thomas (PA)	S	908	Friedman, Stuart (FL)	A&I	84
Freedman, Gary (PA)	RadRO	822	Frim, David (IL)	NS	418
Freedman, Michael (NY)	Ger	235	Fritz, Gregory (RI)	ChAP	780
Freedman, Robert (CO)	Psyc	772	Fritz, Marc (NC)	RE	875
Freedman, Sharon (NC)	Oph	503	Fronek, Jan (CA)	SM	899
Freeman, Gregory (TX)	Cv	110	Frost, Frederick (OH)	PMR	725
Freeman, Leonard (NY)	NuM	474	Fruchtman, Steven (NY)	Hem	273
Freeman, Theodore (TX)	A&I	87	Fry, Robert (PA)	CRS	159
Freeman, Thomas (FL)	NS	413	Fu, Freddie (PA)	OrS	531
Freemark, Michael (NC)	PEn	642	Fuchs, Charles S (MA)	Onc	287

Name	Specialty	Pg
Fuchs, Eugene (OR)	U	1002
Fuchs, Wayne (NY)	Oph	495
Fuhrman, Bradley (NY)	PCCM	638
Fuhrman, Carl (PA)	DR	847
Fulkerson, William (NC)	Pul	801
Fullerton, David (CO)	TS	967
Fung, John (OH)	S	924
Funk, Gerry (IA)	Oto	579
Furlan, Anthony (OH)	N	454
Furman, Wayne (TN)	PHO	659
Furukawa, Satoshi (PA)	TS	953
Fuster, Valentin (NY)	Cv	96
Futran, Neal (WA)	Oto	588

G

Name	Specialty	Pg
Gaasterland, Douglas (MD)	Oph	496
Gabbard, Glen (TX)	Psyc	773
Gabram, Sheryl (GA)	S	917
Gabrilove, Janice (NY)	Onc	295
Gaffney, David (UT)	RadRO	833
Gagner, Michel (FL)	S	917
Gaissert, Henning (MA)	TS	950
Gajjar, Amar (TN)	PHO	659
Galandiuk, Susan (KY)	CRS	161
Galanter, Marc (NY)	AdP	778
Galati, Joseph (TX)	Ge	225
Galetta, Steven (PA)	N	441
Galland, Leo (NY)	IM	364
Gallico, G Gregory (MA)	PlS	734
Gallin, Pamela (NY)	Oph	496
Galloway, Aubrey (NY)	TS	953
Gambardella, Ralph (CA)	SM	899
Gambert, Steven (MD)	Ger	235
Gambetti, Pierluigi (OH)	Path	612
Gamble, Gail (IL)	PMR	725

Name	Specialty	Pg
Gamelli, Richard (IL)	S	924
Gandara, David (CA)	Onc	335
Gandy, Winston (GA)	Cv	101
Gang, Eli (CA)	CE	119
Ganguli, Rohan (PA)	Psyc	766
Gantz, Bruce (IA)	Oto	579
Ganz, Patricia (CA)	Onc	335
Garber, Judy (MA)	Onc	288
Garcia-Prats, Joseph (TX)	NP	387
Garden, Jerome (IL)	D	177
Garfin, Steven (CA)	OrS	552
Garin, Eduardo (FL)	PNep	677
Garner, Warren (CA)	PlS	752
Garnick, Marc B (MA)	Onc	288
Garrett, Algin (VA)	D	176
Garrett, William (NC)	OrS	540
Garrity, Edward (IL)	Pul	804
Garst, Jennifer (NC)	Onc	307
Garth, William (AL)	SM	898
Gartner, J Carlton (DE)	Ped	624
Garver, Robert (AL)	Pul	801
Garvin, James (NY)	PHO	654
Garvin, Kevin (NE)	OrS	548
Gater, David (VA)	PMR	723
Gaynor, Ellen (IL)	Hem	279
Gearhart, John (MD)	U	981
Gebhardt, Mark (MA)	OrS	526
Geffner, Mitchell (CA)	PEn	645
Gefter, Warren (PA)	DR	847
Gelberman, Richard (MO)	HS	265
Gelenberg, Alan (AZ)	Psyc	773
Gelfand, Erwin (CO)	PA&I	629
Geller, Kenneth (CA)	PO	684
Gelmann, Edward (NY)	Onc	295
Geltman, Edward (MO)	Cv	105
Gendelman, Seymour (NY)	N	441
Genden, Eric (NY)	Oto	566

Alphabetical Listing of Doctors

Name	Specialty	Pg	Name	Specialty	Pg
Gentile, Ronald (NY)	Oph	496	Gingold, Bruce (NY)	CRS	159
Georgeson, Keith (AL)	PS	696	Ginsberg, David (CA)	U	1002
Georgiade, Gregory (NC)	PlS	742	Ginsberg, Gregory (PA)	Ge	209
Gerdes, Hans (NY)	Ge	208	Ginsburg, Elizabeth (MA)	RE	870
Geronemus, Roy (NY)	D	171	Ginsburg, Howard (NY)	PS	693
Gershenson, David (TX)	GO	254	Ginzler, Ellen (NY)	Rhu	884
Gershwin, Merrill (CA)	Rhu	892	Girardi, Leonard (NY)	TS	954
Gerson, Lauren (CA)	Ge	226	Gish, Robert (CA)	Ge	227
Gerson, Stanton (OH)	Onc	318	Gitelis, Steven (IL)	OrS	544
Gertz, Morris (MN)	Hem	279	Gitlin, Michael (CA)	Psyc	774
Geschwind, Jean-Francois (MD)	VIR	861	Gittes, George (PA)	PS	693
Gewertz, Bruce (CA)	VascS	1019	Gittler, Michelle (IL)	PMR	725
Gewirtz, Alan (PA)	Hem	273	Giuliano, Armando (CA)	S	939
Gewitz, Michael (NY)	PCd	631	Giustra, Lawrence (GA)	Psyc	769
Gewolb, Ira (MI)	NP	385	Givner, Laurence (NC)	PInf	674
Gewurz, Anita (IL)	A&I	86	Gizzi, Martin (NJ)	N	441
Geyer, Charles (PA)	Onc	295	Glader, Bertil (CA)	PHO	670
Geyer, J Russell (WA)	PHO	670	Glaser, Joel (FL)	Oph	503
Gharagozloo, Farid (DC)	TS	954	Glashow, Jonathan (NY)	OrS	531
Giangola, Gary (NY)	VascS	1013	Glaspy, John (CA)	Onc	335
Giannotta, Steven (CA)	NS	426	Glass, Jon (PA)	N	441
Gianoli, Gerard (LA)	Oto	585	Glass, Jonathan (GA)	N	449
Gianopoulos, John (IL)	MF	375	Glassberg, Kenneth (NY)	U	981
Giardina, Patricia (NY)	PHO	654	Glassburn, John (PA)	RadRO	823
Gibbons, Gary (MA)	VascS	1010	Glassford, David (TN)	TS	960
Gibbons, Raymond (MN)	Cv	105	Glat, Paul (PA)	PlS	737
Gibbs, John (NY)	S	909	Glatstein, Eli (PA)	RadRO	823
Gibbs, Ronald (CO)	MF	376	Glick, John (PA)	Onc	296
Gibralter, Richard (NY)	Oph	496	Glick, Philip (NY)	PS	694
Gigantelli, James (NE)	Oph	513	Glickel, Steven (NY)	HS	261
Gilbert, Mark (TX)	N	460	Gliklich, Jerry (NY)	Cv	96
Gilchrest, Barbara (MA)	D	168	Gliklich, Richard (MA)	Oto	563
Gill, Harcharan (CA)	U	1002	Glisson, Bonnie (TX)	Onc	328
Gill, Inderbir (OH)	U	993	Glode, L Michael (CO)	Onc	326
Gillette, Paul (TX)	PCd	636	Glogau, Richard (CA)	D	181
Gilman, Sid (MI)	N	454	Glombicki, Alan (TX)	Ge	225
Gilsanz, Vicente (CA)	DR	853	Gloviczki, Peter (MN)	VascS	1016

Alphabetical Listing of Doctors

Name	Specialty	Pg	Name	Specialty	Pg
Gluck, Joan (FL)	A&I	84	Goldstein, Larry (NC)	N	449
Gluck, Stephen (CA)	Nep	400	Goldstein, Lori (PA)	Onc	296
Gluckman, Gordon (IL)	U	993	Goldstein, Marc (NY)	U	981
Gluckman, Jack (OH)	Oto	579	Goldstein, Martin (NY)	ObG	481
Gochfeld, Michael (NJ)	OM	758	Goldstein, Richard (KY)	S	917
Gockerman, Jon (NC)	Onc	307	Goldstein, Scott (PA)	CRS	159
Godder, Kamar (VA)	PHO	659	Goldstein, Wayne (IL)	OrS	544
Godine, John (MA)	EDM	188	Golfinos, John (NY)	NS	407
Godwin, John (IL)	Hem	279	Golomb, Harvey (IL)	Onc	318
Godzik, Cathleen (CA)	HS	267	Golub, Richard (FL)	CRS	161
Goebel, Joel (MO)	Oto	579	Gomella, Leonard (PA)	U	981
Goetz, Christopher (IL)	N	454	Gomery, Pablo (MA)	U	978
Goff, Barbara (WA)	GO	255	Gomes, Antoinette (CA)	VIR	865
Goff, Donald (MA)	Psyc	762	Gomes, J Anthony (NY)	CE	115
Goggins, Michael (MD)	Ge	209	Gonik, Bernard (MI)	ObG	483
Goitz, Henry (MI)	OrS	544	Gonzales, Edmond (TX)	U	999
Gokaslan, Ziya (MD)	NS	407	Goodgold, Albert (NY)	N	441
Golbe, Lawrence (NJ)	N	441	Goodin, Douglas (CA)	N	463
Gold, Alan (NY)	PlS	737	Goodman, Lawrence (WI)	DR	851
Gold, Philip (WA)	Onc	335	Goodman, Neil (FL)	RE	875
Gold, Scott (NY)	Oto	566	Goodman, Robert (NJ)	RadRO	823
Gold, Stuart (NC)	PHO	659	Goodman, Robert (NY)	NS	407
Goldberg, Jack (NJ)	Hem	274	Goodman, Stuart (CA)	OrS	552
Goldberg, James (CA)	MF	378	Goodnight, James (CA)	S	939
Goldberg, Michael (IL)	Ge	219	Goodrich, James (NY)	NS	408
Goldberg, Morton (MD)	Oph	496	Goodson, William (CA)	S	939
Goldberg, Richard (NC)	Onc	307	Goodwin, Scott (CA)	VIR	865
Goldberg, Victor (OH)	OrS	544	Goodwin, W Jarrard (FL)	Oto	574
Goldblum, John (OH)	Path	612	Gorbien, Martin (IL)	Ger	236
Golden, Michael (PA)	VascS	1013	Gordon, Catherine (MA)	PEn	640
Goldman, Allan (FL)	Pul	801	Gordon, Leo (IL)	Hem	279
Goldman, Stanton (TX)	PHO	668	Gordon, Marsha (NY)	D	171
Goldman, Stewart (IL)	PHO	664	Gorensek, Margaret (FL)	Inf	354
Goldner, Richard (NC)	OrS	540	Gorevic, Peter (NY)	Rhu	884
Goldsmith, Ari (NY)	PO	681	Gorfine, Stephen (NY)	CRS	159
Goldsmith, Donald (PA)	PRhu	689	Gorin, Michael (CA)	Oph	517
Goldsmith, Stanley (NY)	NuM	474	Gorovoy, Mark (FL)	Oph	503

Alphabetical Listing of Doctors

Name	Specialty	Pg	Name	Specialty	Pg
Gostout, Christopher (MN)	Ge	219	Greden, John (MI)	Psyc	771
Gottdiener, John (MD)	Cv	96	Green, Barth (FL)	NS	413
Gottlieb, Alice (MA)	D	169	Green, Carmen (MI)	PM	599
Gottlieb, Geoffrey (NY)	Path	606	Green, Daniel (TN)	PHO	659
Gottlieb, Stephen (MD)	Cv	96	Green, Howard (FL)	D	176
Gould, K Lance (TX)	Cv	110	Green, Peter (NY)	Ge	209
Goulet, Robert (IN)	S	924	Green, Richard (NY)	VascS	1013
Gourley, Mark (MD)	Rhu	884	Green, Thomas (IL)	PPul	687
Govindarajan, Sugantha (CA)	Path	617	Greenberg, Donna (MA)	Psyc	762
Gower, Roland (AK)	S	939	Greenberg, Harly (NY)	Pul	797
Goy, Andre (NJ)	Onc	296	Greenberg, Harry (MI)	N	454
Gradishar, William (IL)	Onc	319	Greenberg, Mark (NY)	Cv	96
Grado, Gordon (AZ)	RadRO	834	Greenberg, Richard (PA)	U	981
Grady, M Sean (PA)	NS	408	Greenberger, Joel (PA)	RadRO	823
Graf, Ben (WI)	OrS	545	Greenberger, Paul (IL)	A&I	86
Graham, John (CA)	CG	151	Greene, Clarence (MO)	NS	418
Graham, Mark (NC)	Onc	308	Greene, Frederick (NC)	S	917
Graham, Michael (AZ)	PHO	668	Greene, Graham (AR)	U	999
Graham, Thomas (MD)	HS	261	Greene, Loren (NY)	EDM	191
Gralow, Julie (WA)	Onc	335	Greene, Michael (MA)	MF	370
Grammer, Leslie (IL)	A&I	86	Greene, Thomas (FL)	HS	263
Grana, Generosa (NJ)	Onc	296	Greenhalgh, David (CA)	S	939
Granai, Skip (RI)	GO	244	Greenson, Joel (MI)	Path	613
Grandis, Jennifer (PA)	Oto	566	Greenspan, Stanley (MD)	ChAP	782
Granet, David (CA)	Oph	517	Greenspan, Susan (PA)	EDM	191
Grannis, Frederic (CA)	TS	971	Greenwald, Blaine (NY)	GerPsy	786
Granstein, Richard (NY)	D	172	Greenwald, Bruce (MD)	Ge	209
Grant, Clive S (MN)	S	925	Greenwald, Mark (IL)	Oph	508
Grant, Michael (TX)	S	933	Greenway, Hubert (CA)	D	182
Grant, Richard (OH)	OrS	545	Greenwood, Robert (NC)	ChiN	140
Grasso, Michael (NY)	U	981	Greer, Benjamin (WA)	GO	255
Graver, L Michael (NY)	TS	954	Greer, John (TN)	Hem	276
Graves, Michael (CA)	N	464	Greganti, Mac (NC)	Ger	236
Gravett, Michael (WA)	MF	378	Gregory, Richard (FL)	PIS	742
Gray, Richard (AZ)	S	933	Gregory, Stephanie (IL)	Hem	279
Grazi, Richard (NY)	RE	872	Greiner, Carl (NE)	Psyc	772
Greco, F Anthony (TN)	Onc	308	Greipp, Philip (MN)	Hem	279

Alphabetical Listing of Doctors

Name	Specialty	Pg	Name	Specialty	Pg
Greisler, Howard (IL)	VascS	1016	Gruber, Stephen (MI)	Onc	319
Grelsamer, Ronald (NY)	OrS	531	Gruchalla, Rebecca (TX)	A&I	87
Grem, Jean (NE)	Onc	326	Grum, Cyril (MI)	Pul	804
Gress, Daryl (VA)	N	449	Grunberg, Steven (VT)	Onc	288
Grever, Michael (OH)	Hem	279	Grundfast, Kenneth (MA)	Oto	563
Grey, Douglas (CA)	VascS	1019	Grunfeld, Lawrence (NY)	RE	872
Gribetz, Michael (NY)	U	982	Grupp, Stephan (PA)	PHO	654
Grichnik, James (NC)	D	176	Gruss, Joseph (WA)	PlS	752
Griepp, Randall (NY)	TS	954	Guarda, Angela (MD)	Psyc	766
Grier, Holcombe (MA)	PHO	651	Guerrant, Richard (VA)	Inf	354
Griffin, John (MD)	N	441	Gugenheim, Joseph (TX)	OrS	550
Griffith, Bartley (MD)	TS	954	Guidry, George (LA)	Pul	809
Grifo, James (NY)	RE	872	Guillem, Jose (NY)	CRS	160
Grigsby, Perry (MO)	RadRO	830	Guilleminault, Christian (CA)	Psyc	774
Grillone, Gregory (MA)	Oto	563	Gujral, Saroj (MN)	U	994
Grimes, Pearl (CA)	D	182	Gulley, James (MD)	Onc	296
Griswold, John (TX)	S	934	Gumprecht, Jeffrey (NY)	Inf	351
Grody, Wayne (CA)	CG	152	Gunasekaran, T S (IL)	PGe	648
Groene, Linda (FL)	Ger	236	Gunderson, John (MA)	Psyc	762
Grogan, Thomas (AZ)	Path	615	Gunderson, Leonard (AZ)	RadRO	834
Groopman, Jerome (MA)	Hem	272	Gundry, Steven (CA)	TS	971
Grosh, William (VA)	Onc	308	Gunter, Jack (TX)	PlS	749
Gross, Ian (CT)	NP	382	Gupta, Prabodh (PA)	Path	606
Grossbard, Michael (NY)	Onc	296	Gutai, James (MI)	PEn	643
Grossberg, George (MO)	GerPsy	788	Guthikonda, Murali (MI)	NS	419
Grossi, Eugene (NY)	TS	954	Guthrie, Barton (AL)	NS	413
Grossman, H Barton (TX)	U	999	Gutierrez, Francisco (IL)	NS	419
Grossman, John (CO)	PlS	748	Gutin, Philip (NY)	NS	408
Grossman, Melanie (NY)	D	172	Guyton, David (MD)	Oph	496
Grossman, Robert (NY)	NRad	855			
Grossman, Stuart (MD)	Onc	296			
Grossniklaus, Hans (GA)	Oph	503	**H**		
Grotta, James (TX)	N	460			
Grotting, James (AL)	PlS	742	Haas, Naomi (PA)	Onc	296
Grubb, Blair (OH)	Cv	105	Haas, Richard (CA)	ChiN	143
Grubb, Robert (MO)	NS	419	Haas, Steven (NY)	OrS	531
Gruber, Scott (MI)	S	925	Haber, Gregory (NY)	Ge	209

Alphabetical Listing of Doctors

Name	Specialty	Pg	Name	Specialty	Pg
Habermann, Thomas (MN)	Hem	279	Hammill, Stephen (MN)	CE	117
Hackney, David (MA)	NRad	854	Hammond, Charles (NC)	RE	875
Haddad, Joseph (NY)	PO	681	Hammond, Denis (NH)	Onc	288
Hadler, Nortin (NC)	Rhu	887	Hammond, Dennis (MI)	PIS	746
Hadley, Mark (AL)	NS	413	Hamra, Sameer (TX)	PIS	749
Haffty, Bruce (NJ)	RadRO	823	Hamvas, Aaron (MO)	NP	386
Hafler, David (MA)	N	437	Han, Steven-Huy B (CA)	Ge	227
Hagan, Kevin (TN)	PIS	743	Hanauer, Stephen (IL)	Ge	219
Hager, W David (KY)	ObG	482	Hancock, Steven (CA)	RadRO	836
Hahn, Stephen (PA)	RadRO	823	Handa, James (MD)	Oph	496
Haid, Regis (GA)	NS	413	Hande, Kenneth (TN)	Onc	308
Haig, Andrew (MI)	PMR	725	Handy, John (OR)	TS	971
Haik, Barrett (TN)	Oph	503	Hanel, Douglas (WA)	HS	267
Hain, Timothy (IL)	N	454	Haney, Arthur (IL)	RE	877
Haines, Kathleen (NJ)	PRhu	690	Hanifin, Jon (OR)	D	182
Hakaim, Albert (FL)	VascS	1015	Hanke, C William (IN)	D	177
Halberg, Francine (CA)	RadRO	836	Hankins, Gary (TX)	MF	377
Hale, Douglass (IN)	ObG	483	Hankinson, Hal (NM)	NS	423
Haley, Barbara (TX)	Onc	328	Hanks, John (VA)	S	917
Haley, Elliott (VA)	N	449	Hanley, Frank (CA)	TS	971
Halff, Glenn (TX)	S	934	Hann, Lucy (NY)	DR	847
Hall, Jesse (IL)	Pul	804	Hanna, Ehab (TX)	Oto	585
Hall, Lisabeth (NY)	Oph	496	Hannafin, Jo (NY)	OrS	532
Halle, Jan (NC)	RadRO	826	Hansen, Kimberley (NC)	VascS	1015
Haller, Daniel (PA)	Onc	297	Hansen, Nora (IL)	S	925
Hallett, John (SC)	VascS	1015	Hansen, Ronald (AZ)	D	180
Hallisey, Michael (CT)	VIR	860	Hansen, Sigvard (WA)	OrS	553
Halmi, Katherine (NY)	Psyc	766	Hansen-Flaschen, John (PA)	Pul	797
Halperin, Jonathan (NY)	Cv	97	Hanson, Laura (NC)	Ger	236
Halpern, Allan (NY)	D	172	Haque, Waheedul (TX)	Psyc	773
Halpern, Howard (IL)	RadRO	830	Har-El, Gady (NY)	Oto	566
Halpern, Steven (NJ)	PHO	654	Haraf, Daniel (IL)	RadRO	830
Haluszka, Oleh (PA)	Ge	209	Harbaugh, Robert (PA)	NS	408
Hamilton, Stanley (TX)	Path	615	Harber, Philip (CA)	OM	758
Hammar, Samuel (WA)	Path	618	Harbour, J William (MO)	Oph	508
Hammer, Glenn (NY)	Inf	352	Harden, R Norman (IL)	PM	599
Hammer, Scott (NY)	Inf	352	Hardesty, Robert (CA)	PIS	752

Alphabetical Listing of Doctors

Name	Specialty	Pg	Name	Specialty	Pg
Hardy, Mark (NY)	S	909	Hawes, Robert (SC)	Ge	215
Hare, Joshua (FL)	Cv	101	Hawkins, Douglas (WA)	PHO	670
Hargrove, W Clark (PA)	TS	954	Hawkins, Irvin (FL)	VIR	862
Harkema, James (MI)	S	925	Hayani, Ammar (IL)	PHO	664
Harley, Earl (DC)	PO	681	Hayashi, Robert (MO)	PHO	664
Harman, Eloise (FL)	Pul	802	Hayden, Richard (AZ)	Oto	585
Harner, Christopher (PA)	SM	896	Hayes, Daniel (MI)	Onc	319
Harnsberger, Jeffrey (NH)	CRS	158	Hayes, David (MN)	CE	117
Harolds, Jay (OK)	DR	852	Hayes, Sharonne (MN)	Cv	105
Harper, Richard (TX)	NS	424	Hayman, James (MI)	RadRO	831
Harpole, David (NC)	TS	960	Haynes, Johnson (AL)	Pul	802
Harrell, James (TX)	TS	969	Healey, John (NY)	OrS	532
Harrington, Elizabeth (NY)	VascS	1013	Healy, Gerald (MA)	PO	680
Harris, David (TX)	PMR	728	Heber, David (CA)	EDM	201
Harris, Jay (MA)	RadRO	820	Hebert, James (VT)	S	902
Harris, Jeffrey (CA)	Oto	588	Hecox, Kurt (WI)	N	454
Harris, Michael (NJ)	PHO	654	Hedges, Thomas (MA)	Oph	492
Harris, Nancy (MA)	Path	604	Heffner, John (OR)	Pul	810
Harrison, John (NC)	Cv	101	Heffner, Linda (MA)	MF	370
Harrison, Louis (NY)	RadRO	823	Heidary, Dariush (GA)	TS	960
Harsh, Griffith (CA)	NS	427	Heilman, Carl (MA)	NS	404
Hart, Robert (TX)	N	460	Heilman, Kenneth (FL)	N	449
Hartman, Barry (NY)	Inf	352	Heimburger, Douglas (AL)	IM	365
Hartmann, Lynn (MN)	Onc	319	Heinrich, Michael (OR)	Hem	284
Hartmann, Rene (FL)	CRS	161	Heitmiller, Richard (MD)	TS	954
Harty, James (KY)	U	988	Helderman, J Harold (TN)	Nep	395
Haskal, Ziv (NY)	VIR	861	Helfet, David (NY)	OrS	532
Haskett, Roger (PA)	Psyc	766	Hellenbrand, William (NY)	PCd	632
Hastings, Hill (IN)	HS	265	Heller, Debra (NJ)	Path	606
Hatch, Kenneth (AZ)	GO	254	Hellstrom, Wayne (LA)	U	1000
Haughey, Bruce (MO)	Oto	579	Helman, Lee (MD)	PHO	655
Haughton, Victor (WI)	NRad	857	Helvie, Mark (MI)	DR	851
Hauke, Ralph (NE)	Onc	326	Hemming, Alan (FL)	S	917
Hauptman, Paul (MO)	Cv	105	Henderson, Victor (CA)	N	464
Hauser, Stephen (CA)	N	464	Henderson, William (WA)	A&I	88
Hausman, Michael (NY)	OrS	532	Hendricks-Munoz, Karen (NY)	NP	383
Haut, Paul (IN)	PHO	664	Hendrickson, Michael (CA)	Path	618

Alphabetical Listing of Doctors

Name	Specialty	Pg	Name	Specialty	Pg
Heney, Niall (MA)	U	978	Hidalgo, David (NY)	PlS	737
Henke, David (NC)	Pul	802	Hiesiger, Emile (NY)	N	441
Henry, Timothy (MN)	IC	122	Higano, Celestia (WA)	Onc	335
Henschke, Claudia (NY)	DR	848	Higashida, Randall (CA)	NRad	859
Hensinger, Robert (MI)	OrS	545	Hijazi, Ziyad (IL)	PCd	635
Hensle, Terry (NY)	U	982	Hilden, Joanne (IN)	PHO	664
Hentz, Vincent (CA)	HS	267	Hilfiker, Mary (CA)	PS	701
Heppell, Jacques (AZ)	CRS	164	Hilger, Peter (MN)	Oto	579
Herbst, Roy (TX)	Onc	329	Hilibrand, Alan (PA)	OrS	532
Herling, Irving (PA)	Cv	97	Hill, Ivor (NC)	PGe	647
Herman, John (MA)	Psyc	762	Hill, Joseph (NH)	RE	870
Herman, Terence (OK)	RadRO	834	Hillebrand, Donald (CA)	Ge	227
Herman, William (MI)	EDM	197	Hillemeier, A Craig (PA)	PGe	646
Heros, Roberto (FL)	NS	413	Hinkle, Andrea (NY)	PHO	655
Heroux, Alain (IL)	Cv	105	Hinshaw, Daniel (MI)	S	925
Herr, Harry (NY)	U	982	Hirsch, Barry (PA)	Oto	567
Herring, Stanley (WA)	PMR	729	Hirsch, Irl (WA)	EDM	202
Herrmann, Howard (PA)	IC	120	Hirsch, Joshua (MA)	NRad	854
Herrmann, Virginia (SC)	S	917	Hirschfeld, Robert (TX)	Psyc	773
Hersh, Peter (NJ)	Oph	497	Ho, Allen (PA)	Oph	497
Hershman, Elliott (NY)	SM	897	Ho, Sherwin (IL)	SM	898
Hertz, Marshall (MN)	Pul	804	Hobel, Calvin (CA)	MF	378
Hertzig, Margaret (NY)	ChAP	782	Hochberg, Marc (MD)	Rhu	884
Herzenberg, John (MD)	OrS	532	Hochschuler, Stephen (TX)	OrS	550
Herzog, David (MA)	ChAP	780	Hochster, Howard (NY)	Onc	297
Herzog, Thomas (NY)	GO	247	Hoda, Syed (NY)	Path	606
Hesdorffer, Charles (MD)	Onc	297	Hodges, David (TX)	Ge	225
Heslin, Martin (AL)	S	918	Hodgson, Kim (IL)	VascS	1016
Hess, David (GA)	N	449	Hoefflin, Steven (CA)	PlS	752
Hess, J Bruce (FL)	Oph	504	Hoffenberg, Edward (CO)	PGe	649
Hester, T Roderick (GA)	PlS	743	Hoffman, Andrew (CA)	EDM	202
Heston, Jerry (TN)	ChAP	783	Hoffman, Brenda (SC)	Ge	215
Hetherington, Maxine (MO)	PHO	664	Hoffman, Daniel (CO)	Psyc	772
Heuer, Dale (WI)	Oph	508	Hoffman, Henry (IA)	Oto	579
Heyman, Melvin (CA)	PGe	650	Hoffman, John (PA)	S	909
Hibbard, Judith (IL)	MF	375	Hoffman, Lloyd (NY)	PlS	737
Hicks, Wesley (NY)	Oto	567	Hoffman, Philip (IL)	Onc	319

Name	Specialty	Pg	Name	Specialty	Pg
Hoffman, Robert (NY)	PrM	759	Horsager, Robyn (TX)	MF	377
Hofkosh, Dena (PA)	Ped	625	Hortobagyi, Gabriel (TX)	Onc	329
Hogikyan, Norman (MI)	Oto	580	Horwitz, Eric (PA)	RadRO	823
Hohn, Arno (CA)	PCd	637	Hotaling, Andrew (IL)	Oto	580
Holden, Stuart (CA)	U	1003	Hotchkiss, Robert (NY)	OrS	532
Holinger, Lauren (IL)	PO	683	Hovsepian, David (CA)	VIR	865
Holladay, Jack (TX)	Oph	513	Howard, Richard (FL)	S	918
Holland, Edward (OH)	Oph	508	Howard, Thomas (NE)	VascS	1017
Holland, James (NY)	Onc	297	Howards, Stuart S (VA)	U	988
Hollander, Eric (NY)	Psyc	766	Howe, James (IA)	S	925
Holliday, James (TN)	Oph	504	Howell, Elizabeth (UT)	AdP	779
Holliday, Michael (MD)	Oto	567	Howington, John (IL)	TS	964
Hollier, Larry (LA)	VascS	1018	Hoyme, H Eugene (SD)	CG	150
Holmes, David (MN)	IC	122	Hoyt, David (CA)	S	939
Holmes, Gregory (NH)	ChiN	138	Hozack, William (PA)	OrS	532
Holmes, King (WA)	Inf	358	Hricak, Hedvig (NY)	DR	848
Holmes, Lewis (MA)	CG	146	Hruban, Ralph (MD)	Path	606
Holroyd, Suzanne (VA)	GerPsy	787	Hruska, Keith (MO)	Nep	396
Holterman, Mark (IL)	PS	698	Hruza, George (MO)	D	178
Holtzman, Ronald (NC)	NP	385	Hsueh, Willa (CA)	EDM	202
Holzman, Ian (NY)	NP	383	Huang, Laurence (CA)	Pul	811
Homans, Alan (VT)	PHO	651	Huben, Robert (NY)	U	982
Hong, Waun (TX)	Onc	329	Huber, Philip (TX)	CRS	164
Hoogwerf, Byron (OH)	EDM	197	Huddleston, Charles (MO)	TS	964
Hoops, Timothy (PA)	Ge	209	Hudes, Gary (PA)	Onc	297
Hoots, William (TX)	PHO	668	Hudgins, Louanne (CA)	CG	152
Hopewell, Philip (CA)	Pul	811	Hudis, Clifford (NY)	Onc	297
Hopkins, L Nelson (NY)	NS	408	Hudson, Leonard (WA)	Pul	811
Hoppe, Richard (CA)	RadRO	837	Hudson, Melissa (TN)	PHO	659
Hopping, Steven (DC)	Oto	567	Hudziak, James (VT)	ChAP	780
Horbar, Jeffrey (VT)	NP	382	Hughes, Kevin (MA)	S	902
Hord, Jeffrey (OH)	PHO	664	Huitt, Gwen (CO)	Inf	357
Horn, Biljana (CA)	PHO	670	Hunninghake, Gary (IA)	Pul	804
Horning, Sandra (CA)	Onc	335	Hunstad, Joseph (NC)	PlS	743
Hornstein, Mark (MA)	RE	870	Hunt, John (TX)	S	934
Horowitz, Ira (GA)	GO	249	Hunt, Kelly (TX)	S	934
Horowitz, Jed (CA)	PlS	752	Hunt, Sharon (CA)	Cv	113

Alphabetical Listing of Doctors

Name	Specialty	Pg	Name	Specialty	Pg
Hunt, Thomas (AL)	HS	264	Imbriglia, Joseph (PA)	HS	261
Hunter, David (MA)	Oph	492	Infante, Ernesto (TX)	N	460
Hunter, Ellen (ID)	Ge	223	Ingle, James (MN)	Onc	319
Hunter, Jill (TX)	NRad	859	Inglis, Andrew (WA)	PO	684
Hunter, John (OR)	S	939	Ingram, David (NC)	PInf	674
Huntoon, Marc (MN)	PM	599	Inra, Lawrence (NY)	Cv	97
Hura, Claudia (TX)	Nep	398	Interian, Alberto (FL)	CE	116
Hurd, David (NC)	Onc	308	Inzucchi, Silvio (CT)	EDM	189
Hurst, Michael (WV)	Oto	567	Ipp, Eli (CA)	EDM	202
Hurst, Robert (PA)	NRad	855	Irby, Pierce (NC)	U	989
Hurt, Hallam (PA)	NP	383	Irvine, John (CA)	Oph	517
Hurtig, Howard (PA)	N	441	Irwin, Charles (CA)	AM	79
Hurwitz, Barrie (NC)	N	449	Irwin, Richard (MA)	Pul	795
Hurwitz, Craig (ME)	PM	596	Isaacs, Claudine (DC)	Onc	297
Hurwitz, Dennis (PA)	PlS	738	Isaacson, Keith (MA)	RE	870
Hussain, Maha (MI)	Onc	319	Isaacson, Steven (NY)	RadRO	824
Hussey, Michael (IL)	MF	375	Iseman, Michael (CO)	Pul	808
Hutchins, Laura (AR)	Onc	329	Isenberg, Sherwin (CA)	Oph	517
Hutchinson, Raymond (MI)	PHO	664	Isik, Ferda (WA)	PlS	752
Hutter, Adolph (MA)	Cv	92	Iskandrian, Ami (AL)	Cv	101
Huynh, Phan Tuong (TX)	DR	852	Ismail, Mahmoud (IL)	MF	375
Hyers, Thomas (MO)	Pul	805	Isom, O Wayne (NY)	TS	955
Hyman, Neil (VT)	CRS	158	Israel, Mark (NH)	PHO	651
			Itzkowitz, Steven (NY)	Ge	209
			Ivanhoe, Cindy (TX)	PMR	728
			Iwach, Andrew (CA)	Oph	517

I

Name	Specialty	Pg
Iannaccone, Susan (TX)	ChiN	142
Iannettoni, Mark (IA)	TS	964
Iannotti, Joseph (OH)	OrS	545
Idler, Richard (IN)	HS	265
Iglehart, J Dirk (MA)	S	902
Ilbawi, Michel (IL)	PS	698
Iliff, Nicholas (MD)	Oph	497
Ilowite, Norman (NY)	PRhu	690
Ilson, David (NY)	Onc	297
Imber, Gerald (NY)	PlS	738

J

Name	Specialty	Pg
Jaafar, Mohamad (DC)	Oph	497
Jablons, David (CA)	TS	971
Jabs, Douglas (NY)	Oph	497
Jackler, Robert (CA)	Oto	588
Jackman, Stephen (PA)	U	982
Jackson, Amie (AL)	PMR	723
Jackson, Gilchrist (TX)	S	934

Alphabetical Listing of Doctors

Name	Specialty	Pg	Name	Specialty	Pg
Jackson, Richard (AR)	PS	700	Jensen, Michael (MN)	EDM	197
Jackson, Valerie (IN)	DR	851	Jenson, Hal (MA)	PInf	672
Jacob, Molly (IL)	Ped	626	Jett, James (MN)	Pul	805
Jacobs, Alice (MA)	IC	119	Jewell, Mark (OR)	PlS	752
Jacobs, Charlotte (CA)	Onc	335	Jhingran, Anuja (TX)	RadRO	835
Jacobs, Joseph (NY)	Oto	567	Jho, Hae-Dong (PA)	NS	408
Jacobs, Richard (AR)	PInf	675	Jillella, Anand (GA)	Onc	308
Jacobs, Thomas (NY)	EDM	191	Jimenez, David (TX)	NS	424
Jacobson, Alan (MA)	Psyc	762	Jobst, Barbara (NH)	N	437
Jacobson, Ira (NY)	Ge	210	Johanson, Norman (PA)	OrS	533
Jacoby, David (OR)	Pul	811	John, Thomas (IL)	Oph	508
Jaffe, Allan (MN)	Cv	106	Johnson, Allen (CA)	Cv	113
Jaffe, Elaine (MD)	Path	606	Johnson, Bruce (MA)	Onc	288
Jaffe, Kenneth (WA)	PMR	729	Johnson, Bruce (VA)	Pul	802
Jahan, Thierry (CA)	Onc	336	Johnson, Calvin (LA)	Oto	585
Jahanzeb, Mohammad (TN)	Onc	308	Johnson, Carl (MD)	OrS	533
Jain, Subhash (NY)	PM	597	Johnson, Darren (KY)	OrS	540
Jakacki, Regina (PA)	PHO	655	Johnson, David (TN)	Onc	308
Jallo, George (MD)	NS	408	Johnson, Denise (CA)	S	939
James, William (PA)	D	172	Johnson, Jonas (PA)	Oto	567
Jamieson, Stuart (CA)	TS	971	Johnson, Maryl (WI)	Cv	106
Janeiro, John (NH)	U	978	Johnson, Matthew (IN)	VIR	863
Janicak, Philip (IL)	Psyc	771	Johnson, Paula (MA)	Cv	92
Janjan, Nora (TX)	RadRO	834	Johnson, Ronald (PA)	S	909
Jankovic, Joseph (TX)	N	460	Johnson, Stephen (CO)	NS	422
Janss, Anna (GA)	N	449	Johnson, Timothy (MI)	MF	375
Jaramillo, Diego (PA)	DR	848	Johnson, Timothy (MI)	D	178
Jarnagin, William (NY)	S	909	Johnston, Carolyn (MI)	GO	251
Jarow, Jonathan (MD)	U	982	Johnston, J Martin (GA)	PHO	659
Jayabose, Somasundaram (NY)	PHO	655	Johnston, James (PA)	Nep	394
Jeevanandam, Valluvan (IL)	TS	964	Johr, Robert (FL)	D	176
Jenike, Michael (MA)	Psyc	762	Jokl, Peter (CT)	OrS	526
Jenkins, Herman (CO)	Oto	584	Jonas, Adam (CA)	CG	152
Jenkins, Roger (MA)	S	903	Jonas, Richard (DC)	TS	955
Jennings, Russell (MA)	PS	692	Jones, David (VA)	TS	960
Jensen, Donald (IL)	Ge	219	Jones, Jacqueline (NY)	PO	681
Jensen, Mary (VA)	NRad	856	Jones, Kenneth (CA)	Ped	626

Alphabetical Listing of Doctors

Name	Specialty	Pg	Name	Specialty	Pg
Jones, Marilyn (CA)	CG	152	Kamani, Naynesh (DC)	PA&I	627
Jones, Neil (CA)	HS	268	Kamdar, Vikram (CA)	EDM	202
Jones, Paul (IL)	Oto	580	Kamen, Barton (NJ)	PHO	655
Jones, Robert (DC)	Path	606	Kamholz, Stephan (NY)	Pul	797
Jordan, Barry (NY)	N	442	Kaminski, Mark (MI)	Onc	320
Jordan, Gerald (VA)	U	989	Kampman, Kyle (PA)	AdP	778
Jordan, Stanley (CA)	PNep	679	Kanal, Emanuel (PA)	DR	848
Jorizzo, Joseph (NC)	D	176	Kanda, Louis (DC)	TS	955
Jose, Baby (KY)	RadRO	827	Kandeel, Fouad (CA)	EDM	202
Joseph, David (AL)	U	989	Kane, Alex (MO)	PlS	746
Joseph, Gregory (NC)	NRad	856	Kane, Javier (TN)	PHO	660
Josephs, Shelby (MD)	PA&I	627	Kane, Kay (MA)	D	169
Josephson, David (IN)	N	454	Kane, Madeleine (CO)	Onc	326
Josephson, Jordan (NY)	Oto	567	Kane, Timothy (PA)	PS	694
Josephson, Mark (MA)	CE	114	Kanel, Gary (CA)	Path	618
Josephson, Michelle (IL)	Nep	397	Kantarjian, Hagop (TX)	Hem	283
Joyce, Michael (OH)	OrS	545	Kantoff, Philip (MA)	Onc	288
Judelson, Debra (CA)	Cv	113	Kantsevoy, Sergey (MD)	Ge	210
Judy, Kevin (PA)	NS	408	Kaplan, Bernard (PA)	PNep	677
Julian, Thomas (PA)	S	909	Kaplan, David (CO)	AM	79
Jupiter, Jesse (MA)	OrS	526	Kaplan, Frederick (PA)	OrS	533
			Kaplan, James (KS)	Pul	808
			Kaplan, Lawrence (CA)	Onc	336
			Kaplan, Michael (CA)	Oto	588
# K			Kaplan, Sheldon (TX)	PInf	675
			Kaplan, Steven (NY)	U	982
Kadmon, Dov (TX)	U	1000	Kapoor, Neena (CA)	PHO	670
Kadota, Richard (CA)	PHO	670	Kappy, Michael (CO)	PEn	644
Kagan, Richard (OH)	S	925	Kapur, Sandip (NY)	S	909
Kahn, Barbara (MA)	EDM	189	Karas, Spero (GA)	OrS	540
Kahn, Leonard (NY)	Path	607	Karlan, Beth (CA)	GO	255
Kahrilas, Peter (IL)	Ge	219	Karp, Daniel (TX)	Onc	329
Kaiser, Larry (PA)	TS	955	Karp, Judith (MD)	Onc	298
Kalaycio, Matt (OH)	Onc	319	Karpeh, Martin (NY)	S	909
Kalemkerian, Gregory (MI)	Onc	320	Karram, Mickey (OH)	ObG	484
Kaliner, Michael (MD)	A&I	83	Karrer, Frederick (CO)	PS	699
Kallmes, David (MN)	NRad	857	Kartush, Jack (MI)	Oto	580
Kalloo, Anthony (MD)	Ge	210			

Alphabetical Listing of Doctors

Name	Specialty	Pg	Name	Specialty	Pg
Karwande, Shreekanth (UT)	TS	967	Kaysen, George (CA)	Nep	400
Kase, Carlos (MA)	N	437	Kazahaya, Ken (PA)	PO	681
Kashtan, Clifford (MN)	PNep	678	Kazanjian, Powel (MI)	Inf	356
Kasinath, Balakuntalam S (TX)	Nep	399	Kazer, Ralph (IL)	RE	877
Kasiske, Bertram (MN)	Nep	397	Keane, Thomas (SC)	U	989
Kass, Evan (MI)	U	994	Keane, William (PA)	Oto	568
Kassam, Amin (PA)	NS	409	Keating, Michael (TX)	Hem	283
Kasser, James (MA)	OrS	526	Keefe, David (FL)	RE	875
Katner, Harold (GA)	Inf	355	Keen, Mary (IL)	PMR	726
Katowitz, James (PA)	Oph	497	Keenan, Mary Ann (PA)	OrS	533
Kattan, Meyer (NY)	PPul	685	Keenan, Robert (PA)	TS	955
Kattwinkel, John (VA)	NP	385	Keens, Thomas (CA)	PPul	688
Katz, Aaron (NY)	U	982	Keepers, George (OR)	Psyc	775
Katz, Nevin (DC)	TS	955	Keiser, Philip (TX)	Inf	357
Katz, Philip (PA)	Ge	210	Kelepouris, Ellie (PA)	Nep	394
Katz, Robert (OH)	PO	683	Keller, Frank (GA)	PHO	660
Katz, Robert (IL)	Rhu	889	Keller, Frederick (OR)	VIR	865
Katz, Stephen (MD)	D	172	Keller, Gregory (CA)	Oto	588
Katzen, Barry (FL)	VIR	862	Keller, Steven (NY)	TS	955
Katzenstein, Anna-Luise (NY)	Path	607	Kelley, Joseph (PA)	GO	247
Kaufman, Bruce (WI)	NS	419	Kelley, Mark (TN)	S	918
Kaufman, Cary (WA)	S	940	Kelly, Cynthia (VA)	PA&I	628
Kaufman, Francine (CA)	PEn	645	Kelly, James (CO)	N	459
Kaufman, Howard (NY)	S	909	Kelly, John (OK)	PIS	749
Kaufman, John (OR)	VIR	865	Kelly, Karen (KS)	Onc	326
Kaufman, Paul (WI)	Oph	508	Kelly, Kevin (TN)	PIS	743
Kaufman, Peter (NH)	Onc	288	Kelsen, David (NY)	Onc	298
Kaul, Sanjiv (OR)	Cv	113	Kelts, K Alan (SD)	N	459
Kavanah, Maureen (MA)	S	903	Kemeny, Nancy (NY)	Onc	298
Kavey, Neil (NY)	Psyc	766	Kemp, James S (MO)	PPul	687
Kavoussi, Louis (NY)	U	983	Kempin, Sanford (NY)	Hem	274
Kawachi, Mark (CA)	U	1003	Kempson, Richard (CA)	Path	618
Kawamoto, Henry (CA)	PIS	753	Kenan, Samuel (NY)	OrS	533
Kay, Dennis (LA)	VIR	865	Kendler, Kenneth (VA)	Psyc	769
Kay, G Neal (AL)	CE	117	Kennedy, David (PA)	Oto	568
Kay, Jonathan (MA)	Rhu	882	Kennedy, Gary (NY)	GerPsy	786
Kaye, Mitchell (MN)	Pul	805	Kennelly, Michael (NC)	U	989

Alphabetical Listing of Doctors

Name	Specialty	Pg	Name	Specialty	Pg
Kent, K Craig (NY)	VascS	1013	King, Richard (GA)	PMR	724
Kereiakes, Dean (OH)	Cv	106	King, Robert (CT)	ChAP	780
Kern, Robert (IL)	Oto	580	King, Talmadge (CA)	Pul	811
Kernstine, Kemp (CA)	TS	971	Kinney, Marsha (TX)	Path	615
Kerrigan, D Casey (VA)	PMR	723	Kirklin, James (AL)	TS	961
Kesser, Bradley (VA)	Oto	574	Kirkwood, John (PA)	Onc	298
Kessler, Craig (DC)	Hem	274	Kirschenbaum, Alexander (NY)	U	983
Kestle, John RW (UT)	NS	422	Kirschner, Barbara (IL)	PGe	649
Ketch, Lawrence (CO)	PlS	748	Kirschner, Kristi (IL)	PMR	726
Ketcham, Douglas (MN)	VIR	863	Kirshblum, Steven (NJ)	PMR	721
Kevorkian, Charles (TX)	PMR	728	Kirshenbaum, James (MA)	Cv	92
Key, L Lyndon (SC)	PEn	642	Kirshner, Howard (TN)	N	450
Khan, Agha (MD)	NS	409	Kirsner, Robert (FL)	D	176
Khandji, Alexander (NY)	NRad	855	Klagsbrun, Samuel (NY)	Psyc	766
Khawaja, Shazib (GA)	IC	121	Klapheke, Martin (KY)	Psyc	769
Khosla, Sundeep (MN)	EDM	197	Klearman, Micki (MO)	Rhu	889
Khuri, Fadlo (GA)	Onc	309	Kleber, Herbert (NY)	AdP	778
Kibel, Adam (MO)	U	994	Kleiman, Martin (IN)	PInf	674
Kidwell, Earl (DC)	Oph	497	Kleiman, Neal (TX)	IC	123
Kiel, Krystyna (IL)	RadRO	831	Klein, Andrew (CA)	S	940
Kieran, Mark (MA)	PHO	651	Klein, Arnold (CA)	D	182
Kiernan, Paul (VA)	TS	960	Klein, Eric (OH)	U	994
Kies, Merrill (TX)	Onc	329	Klein, Lloyd (IL)	Cv	106
Kiev, Jonathan (VA)	TS	961	Klein, Robert (RI)	PA&I	627
Kilmer, Suzanne (CA)	D	182	Klein-Gitelman, Marisa (IL)	PRhu	691
Kim, Edward (TN)	U	989	Kleinberg, David (NY)	EDM	191
Kim, Jae (MI)	RadRO	831	Kleinberg, Lawrence (MD)	RadRO	824
Kim, Julian (OH)	S	925	Kleinerman, Eugenie (TX)	Ped	626
Kim, Youn-Hee (CA)	D	182	Kleinman, Ronald (MA)	PGe	645
Kim, Young-Jee (IN)	PPul	687	Kleinman, William (IN)	HS	265
Kimmey, Michael (WA)	Ge	227	Klibanski, Anne (MA)	EDM	189
Kincaid, John (IN)	N	455	Kliger, Alan (CT)	Nep	392
Kindler, Hedy (IL)	Onc	320	Klimberg, Vicki (AR)	S	934
King, Andrew (CA)	Nep	400	Kline, Mark (TX)	PInf	675
King, Bryan (WA)	ChAP	785	Klingensmith, Georgeanna (CO)	PEn	644
King, Earl (PA)	Pul	797	Kloos, Richard (OH)	EDM	197
King, John (TX)	PMR	728	Klutke, Carl (MO)	U	994

Alphabetical Listing of Doctors

Name	Specialty	Pg	Name	Specialty	Pg
Kneisl, Jeffrey (NC)	OrS	540	Korf, Bruce (AL)	CG	148
Knisely, Jonathan (CT)	RadRO	820	Kormos, Robert (PA)	TS	955
Knoefel, Janice (NM)	N	461	Kornmehl, Ernest (MA)	Oph	492
Knowles, Daniel (NY)	Path	607	Korones, David (NY)	PHO	655
Knudson, Mary (CA)	S	940	Korsten, Mark (NY)	Ge	210
Kobashigawa, Jon (CA)	Cv	113	Koruda, Mark (NC)	S	918
Kobrin, Sidney (PA)	Nep	394	Korytkowski, Mary (PA)	EDM	191
Kobrine, Arthur (DC)	NS	409	Kosova, Leonard (IL)	Onc	320
Koch, Christian (MS)	EDM	194	Koss, Michael (CA)	Path	618
Koch, Douglas (TX)	Oph	513	Kosten, Thomas (TX)	AdP	779
Koch, Wayne (MD)	Oto	568	Kostis, John (NJ)	Cv	97
Kocher, Mininder (MA)	OrS	527	Kotagal, Suresh (MN)	ChiN	141
Kochman, Michael (PA)	Ge	210	Kotler, Donald (NY)	Ge	210
Koczywas, Marianna (CA)	Onc	336	Kotloff, Robert (PA)	Pul	797
Kodner, Ira (MO)	CRS	162	Koufman, Jamie (NY)	Oto	568
Koeller, Kelly (MN)	NRad	858	Koulos, John (NY)	GO	247
Koenig, Steven (VA)	Pul	802	Kovac, S Robert (GA)	ObG	482
Koff, Stephen (OH)	U	994	Kovitz, Kevin (IL)	Pul	805
Koh, Wui-Jin (WA)	RadRO	837	Kovnar, Edward (WI)	ChiN	141
Kohler, Matthew (SC)	GO	249	Kowalski, Thomas (PA)	Ge	210
Kokotailo, Patricia (WI)	AM	79	Koyle, Martin (WA)	U	1003
Koller, Harold (PA)	Oph	497	Kozarek, Richard (WA)	Ge	227
Kolodny, Edwin (NY)	N	442	Kozin, Scott (PA)	HS	261
Komaki, Ritsuko (TX)	RadRO	835	Kozlowski, James (IL)	U	994
Koman, L Andrew (NC)	HS	264	Krachmer, Jay (MN)	Oph	509
Kondziolka, Douglas (PA)	NS	409	Krackow, Kenneth (NY)	OrS	533
Konicek, Frank (IL)	Ge	220	Kraft, Andrew (SC)	Onc	309
Konski, Andre (PA)	RadRO	824	Kraft, George (WA)	PMR	729
Konstam, Marvin (MA)	Cv	92	Krag, David (VT)	S	903
Konstan, Michael (OH)	PPul	687	Krajcer, Zvonimir (TX)	Cv	110
Koo, John (CA)	D	182	Kramer, Barry (CA)	GerPsy	788
Koos, Brian (CA)	MF	378	Krasna, Mark (MD)	TS	956
Kopans, Daniel (MA)	DR	845	Kraus, Dennis (NY)	Oto	568
Kopf, Gary (CT)	TS	950	Kraus, Michael (IN)	Nep	397
Koplin, Lawrence (CA)	PlS	753	Krauss, Gregory (MD)	N	442
Kopp, Peter (IL)	EDM	197	Kraut, Eric H (OH)	Hem	280
Korenblat, Phillip (MO)	A&I	86	Kraybill, William (MO)	S	925

Alphabetical Listing of Doctors

Name	Specialty	Pg	Name	Specialty	Pg
Krebs, Nancy (CO)	PGe	650	Kurtz, Robert (NY)	Ge	211
Kreissman, Susan (NC)	PHO	660	Kurtzberg, Joanne (NC)	PHO	660
Kreitzer, Joel (NY)	PM	597	Kurtzke, Robert (VA)	N	450
Krellenstein, Daniel (NY)	TS	956	Kushner, Brian (NY)	PHO	655
Krespi, Yosef (NY)	Oto	568	Kushner, Burton (WI)	Oph	509
Kretschmar, Cynthia (MA)	PHO	652	Kuske, Robert (AZ)	RadRO	835
Kriegel, David (NY)	D	172	Kuttesch, John (TN)	PHO	660
Krieger, Karl (NY)	TS	956	Kuzel, Timothy (IL)	Hem	280
Krilov, Leonard (NY)	PInf	673	Kuzniecky, Ruben (NY)	N	442
Kris, Mark (NY)	Onc	298	Kuzon, William (MI)	PlS	746
Kron, Irving (VA)	TS	961	Kveton, John (CT)	Oto	563
Krouse, Robert (AZ)	S	934	Kvols, Larry (FL)	Onc	309
Krowka, Michael (MN)	Pul	805	Kwak, Larry (TX)	Onc	329
Krueger, Gerald (UT)	D	179	Kwo, Paul (IN)	Ge	220
Krueger, Ronald (OH)	Oph	509	Kwolek, Christopher (MA)	VascS	1010
Krumholz, Allan (MD)	N	442			
Krummel, Thomas (CA)	PS	701			
Kuettel, Michael (NY)	RadRO	824	## L		
Kuhel, William (NY)	Oto	568	La Ban, Myron (MI)	PMR	726
Kuhn, Frederick (GA)	Oto	574	La Gamma, Edmund (NY)	NP	383
Kuhn, Joseph (TX)	S	934	La Quaglia, Michael (NY)	PS	694
Kuiken, Todd (IL)	PMR	726	La Russo, Nicholas (MN)	Ge	220
Kula, Roger (NY)	N	442	Labiner, David (AZ)	N	461
Kulick, Roy (NY)	HS	261	Lachs, Mark (NY)	Ger	235
Kumpe, David (CO)	VIR	864	Lackman, Richard (PA)	OrS	533
Kun, Larry (TN)	RadRO	827	Lacomis, David (PA)	N	442
Kunkel, Elisabeth (PA)	Psyc	766	Lacy, Jill (CT)	Onc	288
Kunschner, Lara (PA)	N	442	Ladenson, Paul (MD)	EDM	192
Kupersmith, Mark (NY)	Oph	498	Lage, Janice (SC)	Path	610
Kupfer, David (PA)	Psyc	767	Laham, Roger (MA)	IC	119
Kupper, Thomas (MA)	D	169	Lahita, Robert (NJ)	Rhu	884
Kurachek, Stephen (MN)	PPul	687	Laks, Hillel (CA)	TS	971
Kuriakose, Philip (MI)	Hem	280	Lalwani, Anil (NY)	Oto	568
Kurland, Geoffrey (PA)	PPul	685	Lambert, H Michael (TX)	Oph	513
Kurman, Robert (MD)	Path	607	Lambert, Paul (SC)	Oto	574
Kurtin, Paul (MN)	Path	613	Lambert, Scott (GA)	Oph	504
Kurtz, Alfred (PA)	DR	848			

Name	Specialty	Pg	Name	Specialty	Pg
Lamberti, John (CA)	TS	972	Lashner, Bret (OH)	Ge	220
Lambiase, Louis (FL)	Ge	215	Lask, Gary (CA)	D	182
Lammertse, Daniel (CO)	PMR	727	Latchaw, Laurie (NH)	PS	692
Lamonica, Dominick (NY)	NuM	474	Laterra, John (MD)	N	443
LaMuraglia, Glenn M (MA)	VascS	1010	Latson, Larry (OH)	PCd	635
Lancaster, Johnathan (FL)	GO	249	Lauerman, William (DC)	OrS	534
Landefeld, C Seth (CA)	Ger	238	Laufer, Marc (MA)	ObG	480
Landers, Daniel (MN)	MF	375	Laughlin, Mary (OH)	Hem	280
Landrigan, Philip (NY)	OM	758	Laurencin, Cato (CT)	OrS	527
Landry, Jerome (GA)	RadRO	827	Lavenstein, Bennett (VA)	ChiN	140
Landy, Helain (DC)	MF	372	Lavertu, Pierre (OH)	Oto	580
Landy, Howard (FL)	NS	413	Lavery, Ian (OH)	CRS	162
Lane, Dorothy (NY)	PrM	759	Lavin, Patrick (TN)	N	450
Lane, Joseph (NY)	OrS	534	Lavis, Victor (TX)	EDM	200
Lane, Lewis (NY)	HS	262	Lavyne, Michael (NY)	NS	409
Lane, Stephen (MN)	Oph	509	Lawrence, Theodore (MI)	RadRO	831
Lang, Frederick (TX)	NS	424	Lawry, George (IA)	Rhu	889
Lang, Samuel (NY)	TS	956	Lawson, David (GA)	Onc	309
Lange, Beverly (PA)	PHO	656	Lawson, Edward (MD)	NP	383
Lange, Paul (WA)	U	1003	Lawson, William (NY)	Oto	569
Langer, Corey (PA)	Onc	298	Lawson, William (DC)	Psyc	767
Langford, Carol (OH)	Rhu	889	Lazarus, Hillard (OH)	Hem	280
Langman, Craig (IL)	PNep	679	Le, Quynh-Thu Xuan (CA)	RadRO	837
Langston, J William (CA)	N	464	Le Boit, Philip (CA)	Path	618
Lansman, Steven (NY)	TS	956	Leaf, Norman (CA)	PlS	753
Lanteri, Vincent (NJ)	U	983	LeBoff, Meryl (MA)	EDM	189
Lantos, John (IL)	Ped	626	Lebwohl, Mark (NY)	D	172
Lanza, Donald (FL)	Oto	574	Lebwohl, Oscar (NY)	Ge	211
Lanza, Louis (AZ)	TS	969	Lechan, Ronald (MA)	EDM	189
Lapey, Allen (MA)	PPul	685	Leckman, James (CT)	ChAP	780
Laramore, George (WA)	RadRO	837	Ledford, Dennis (FL)	A&I	85
Larner, James (VA)	RadRO	827	Lee, Andrew (TX)	RadRO	835
Larrabee, Wayne (WA)	Oto	588	Lee, Andrew (IA)	Oph	509
Larsen, Gary (CO)	PPul	688	Lee, Cheryl (MI)	U	994
Larson, David (CA)	RadRO	837	Lee, Chung (MN)	RadRO	831
Larson, Richard (IL)	Hem	280	Lee, Francis (NY)	OrS	534
Larson, Steven (NY)	NuM	474	Lee, Jeffrey (TX)	S	935

Alphabetical Listing of Doctors

Name	Specialty	Pg	Name	Specialty	Pg
Lee, Kenneth (PA)	S	910	Levenback, Charles (TX)	GO	254
Lee, Paul (NC)	Oph	504	Leventhal, Bennett (IL)	ChAP	784
Lee, W P Andrew (PA)	HS	262	Levi, Joe (FL)	S	918
Lee, W Robert (NC)	RadRO	827	Levin, David (OK)	Pul	809
Leffell, David (CT)	D	169	Levin, L Scott (NC)	PlS	743
Lefrak, Stephen (MO)	Pul	805	Levin, Victor (TX)	N	461
Legato, Marianne (NY)	IM	364	Levine, Alexandra (CA)	Hem	285
Legha, Sewa (TX)	Onc	329	Levine, David (NY)	N	443
Legro, Richard (PA)	RE	872	Levine, Edward (NC)	S	918
Lehman, Constance (WA)	DR	853	Levine, Elliot (IL)	ObG	484
Lehman, Thomas (NY)	PRhu	690	Levine, Ellis (NY)	Onc	298
Lehman, Wallace (NY)	OrS	534	Levine, Joel (CT)	Ge	206
Leipziger, Lyle (NY)	PlS	738	Levine, Joseph (NY)	CE	115
Leitch, A Marilyn (TX)	S	935	Levine, Laurence (IL)	U	994
Lele, Shashikant (NY)	GO	247	Levine, Paul (VA)	Oto	574
Lem, Vincent (MO)	Pul	805	Levine, Robert (NH)	EDM	189
Lemanske, Robert (WI)	PA&I	628	Levine, Stephen (OH)	Psyc	771
Lemons, James (IN)	NP	386	Levine, Steven (NY)	N	443
Lenke, Lawrence (MO)	OrS	545	Levine, William (NY)	SM	897
Lentz, Christopher (NY)	S	910	Levinson, Arnold (PA)	A&I	83
Lentz, Samuel (NC)	GO	249	Levitsky, Lynne (MA)	PEn	640
Leon, Martin (NY)	IC	120	Levy, Angela (MD)	DR	848
Leonard, James (MI)	PMR	726	Levy, Joseph (NY)	PGe	646
Leonetti, John (IL)	Oto	580	Levy, Michael (PA)	Onc	298
Leopold, Donald (NE)	Oto	584	Levy, Michael (CA)	NS	427
Lepanto, Philip (WV)	RadRO	824	Levy, Moise (TX)	D	180
Lepor, Herbert (NY)	U	983	Levy, Richard (IL)	PEn	643
Lerman, Bruce (NY)	CE	115	Levy, Robert (IL)	NS	419
Lerner, Seth (TX)	U	1000	Levy, Steven (GA)	Psyc	770
Lesavoy, Malcolm (CA)	PlS	753	Lewin, Alan (FL)	RadRO	827
Leshin, Barry (NC)	D	176	Lewin, Neal (NY)	IM	364
Leslie, Kevin (AZ)	Path	615	Lewis, Blair (NY)	Ge	211
Lesser, Glenn (NC)	Onc	309	Lewis, Curtis (GA)	VIR	862
Lessin, Stuart (PA)	D	172	Lewis, Edmund (IL)	Nep	397
Leuchter, Andrew (CA)	Psyc	775	Lewis, Hilel (NY)	Oph	498
Leung, Donald (CO)	PA&I	629	Lewis, John (AZ)	A&I	87
Leung, Lawrence (CA)	Hem	285	Lewis, Richard (TX)	Oph	514

Name	Specialty	Pg	Name	Specialty	Pg
Lewis, Sandra (OR)	Cv	113	Linenberger, Michael (WA)	Hem	285
Lewkowiez, Laurent (CO)	CE	118	Link, Michael (MN)	NS	419
Li, Benjamin (LA)	S	935	Link, Michael (CA)	PHO	670
Li Volsi, Virginia (PA)	Path	607	Linker, Charles (CA)	Hem	285
Liang, Bruce (CT)	Cv	93	Linskey, Mark (CA)	NS	427
Liau, Linda (CA)	NS	427	Linstrom, Christopher (NY)	Oto	569
Libby, Daniel (NY)	Pul	797	Linton, MacRae (TN)	Cv	102
Libby, Peter (MA)	Cv	93	Lipkin, David (FL)	PMR	724
Liberman, Robert (CA)	Psyc	775	Lipkowitz, George (MA)	S	903
Libertino, John (MA)	U	978	Liporace, Joyce (PA)	N	443
Libutti, Steven (MD)	S	910	Lippman, Marc (FL)	Onc	309
Licata, Angelo (OH)	EDM	198	Lippman, Scott (TX)	Onc	330
Licciardi, Frederick (NY)	RE	872	Lipschitz, David (AR)	Ger	238
Lichtenstein, Gary (PA)	Ge	211	Lipscomb, Gary (IL)	ObG	484
Lichter, Paul (MI)	Oph	509	Lipshultz, Larry (TX)	U	1000
Liddle, Rodger (NC)	Ge	216	Lipshutz, William (PA)	Ge	211
Lieberman, Phillip (TN)	A&I	85	Lipsitz, Lewis (MA)	Ger	234
Liebmann, Jeffrey (NY)	Oph	498	Lipstate, James (LA)	Rhu	891
Liem, Pham (AR)	Ger	238	Lipton, Jeffrey (NY)	PHO	656
Lieskovsky, Gary (CA)	U	1003	Lipton, Richard (NY)	N	443
Light, Richard (TN)	Pul	802	Lisak, Robert (MI)	N	455
Light, Terry (IL)	HS	265	Lisman, Richard (NY)	Oph	498
Lightdale, Charles (NY)	Ge	211	List, Alan F (FL)	Hem	276
Lilenbaum, Rogerio (FL)	Onc	309	Litt, Andrew (NY)	NRad	855
Lill, Michael (CA)	Hem	285	Little, Alex G (OH)	TS	964
Lillehei, Kevin (CO)	NS	423	Little, John (DC)	PlS	738
Lillemoe, Keith (IN)	S	926	Litzow, Mark (MN)	Hem	280
Lim, Henry (MI)	D	178	Liu, Grant (PA)	N	443
Limentani, Steven (NC)	Onc	309	Livingston, Edward (TX)	S	935
Lin, Weei-Chin (AL)	Hem	276	Livingston, Philip (NY)	Onc	299
Lind, Christopher (TN)	Ge	216	Livingston, Robert (AZ)	Onc	330
Lind, David (GA)	S	918	Livingstone, Alan (FL)	S	918
Lindenfeld, JoAnn (CO)	Cv	110	Ljung, Britt-Marie (CA)	Path	618
Lindor, Keith (MN)	Ge	220	Lloyd, Lewis (AL)	U	989
Lindsay, Bruce (OH)	CE	117	Lobe, Thom (IA)	PS	698
Lindsey, Stephen (LA)	Rhu	891	Locala, Joseph (OH)	Psyc	771
Lindstrom, Richard (MN)	Oph	509	Lock, James (MA)	PCd	630

Alphabetical Listing of Doctors

Name	Specialty	Pg	Name	Specialty	Pg
Lock, Terrence (MI)	OrS	545	Lublin, Fred (NY)	N	443
Locker, Gershon (IL)	Onc	320	Luby, James (TX)	Inf	357
Lockey, Richard (FL)	A&I	85	Luby, Joan (MO)	ChAP	784
Lockhart, Jorge (FL)	U	989	Lucente, Vincent (PA)	ObG	481
Lockshin, Michael (NY)	Rhu	884	Lucey, Michael (WI)	Ge	220
Lockwood, Charles (CT)	MF	370	Luchtman-Jones, Lori (DC)	PHO	656
Loder, Elizabeth (MA)	PM	596	Luciano, Anthony (CT)	RE	871
Loeffler, Jay S (MA)	RadRO	820	Luck, James (CA)	OrS	553
Loehrer, Patrick (IN)	Onc	320	Lucky, Anne (OH)	D	178
Loevner, Laurie (PA)	NRad	855	Luders, Hans (OH)	N	455
Loewenstein, Richard (MD)	Psyc	767	Ludwig, David (MA)	PEn	640
Loftus, Christopher (PA)	NS	409	Lueder, Gregg (MO)	Oph	509
Logan, William (MO)	N	455	Luerssen, Thomas (TX)	NS	424
Logigian, Eric (NY)	N	443	Lugg, James (WY)	U	998
Logothetis, Christopher (TX)	Onc	330	Luggen, Michael (OH)	Rhu	889
Long, Sarah (PA)	PInf	673	Luken, Martin (IL)	NS	419
Longo, Walter (CT)	CRS	158	Lumsden, Alan (TX)	VascS	1018
Longworth, David (MA)	Inf	350	Lunsford, L Dade (PA)	NS	409
Look, Katherine (IN)	GO	251	Lurain, John (IL)	GO	251
Loprinzi, Charles (MN)	Onc	320	Lusher, Jeanne (MI)	PHO	665
Loree, Thom (NY)	PlS	738	Lusk, Rodney (NE)	PO	683
LoRusso, Thomas (VA)	Pul	802	Luterman, Arnold (AL)	S	919
Loscalzo, Joseph (MA)	Cv	93	Luthra, Harvinder (MN)	Rhu	889
Losordo, Douglas (IL)	IC	123	Lutsep, Helmi (OR)	N	464
Lossos, Izidore (FL)	Onc	310	Lutz, Gregory (NY)	PMR	722
Lott, Ira (CA)	ChiN	143	Luxon, Bruce (IA)	Ge	220
Loughlin, Gerald (NY)	PPul	685	Lyckholm, Laurel (VA)	Onc	310
Loughlin, Kevin (MA)	U	978	Lydiatt, Daniel (NE)	Oto	584
Louie, Eddie (NY)	Inf	352	Lydiatt, William (NE)	Oto	584
Loulmet, Didier (NY)	TS	956	Lyerly, H Kim (NC)	S	919
Low, David (PA)	PlS	738	Lyketsos, Constantine (MD)	GerPsy	786
Lowe, Franklin (NY)	U	983	Lyles, Kenneth (NC)	Ger	236
Lowe, Lori (MI)	D	178	Lyman, Gary (NC)	Onc	310
Lowenberg, David (CA)	OrS	553	Lynch, James (FL)	Onc	310
Lowry, Ann (MN)	CRS	162	Lynch, Joseph (CA)	Pul	811
Loyd, James (TN)	Pul	802	Lynch, Thomas (MA)	Onc	289
Lubahn, John (PA)	HS	262	Lynne, Charles (FL)	U	989

Name	Specialty	Pg
Lyons, Roger (TX)	Hem	283
Lytle, Bruce (OH)	TS	964

M

Name	Specialty	Pg
Ma, Dong (NY)	PMR	722
Mabrey, Jay (TX)	OrS	550
MacDonald, Kenneth (NC)	S	919
MacFadyen, Bruce (GA)	S	919
Machtay, Mitchell (PA)	RadRO	824
Macias, John (AZ)	Oto	585
Maciejewski, Jaroslaw (OH)	Hem	280
Mackay, Donald (PA)	PlS	738
MacKenzie, Richard (CA)	AM	79
Mackey, William (MA)	VascS	1011
MacKinnon, Susan (MO)	PlS	746
Macklis, Roger (OH)	RadRO	831
Mackool, Richard (NY)	Oph	498
MacLean, James (MA)	A&I	82
Macones, George (MO)	MF	375
Maddaus, Michael (MN)	TS	965
Maddox, Anne (AR)	Hem	284
Madoff, Robert (MN)	CRS	162
Madsen, Joseph (MA)	NS	405
Magovern, George (PA)	TS	956
Magramm, Irene (NY)	Oph	498
Magrina, Javier (AZ)	GO	254
Maguire, Leo (MN)	Oph	510
Magun, Arthur (NY)	Ge	211
Maharam, Lewis (NY)	SM	897
Mahler, Donald (NH)	Pul	795
Mahler, Richard (NY)	EDM	192
Mahon, Kathleen (NV)	Oph	518
Mahoney, Maurice (CT)	CG	146
Mahony, Lynn (TX)	PCd	636
Mahowald, Mark (MN)	N	455

Name	Specialty	Pg
Majd, Massoud (DC)	NuM	474
Makaroun, Michel (PA)	VascS	1013
Make, Barry (CO)	Pul	808
Maki, Dennis (WI)	Inf	356
Malawer, Martin (DC)	OrS	534
Malee, Maureen (TN)	MF	373
Malik, Ghaus (MI)	NS	419
Malkowicz, S Bruce (PA)	U	983
Maloney, David (WA)	Onc	336
Maloney, Mary (MA)	D	169
Maloney, Robert (CA)	Oph	518
Mamelak, Adam (CA)	NS	427
Mamounas, Eleftherios (OH)	S	926
Manche, Edward (CA)	Oph	518
Manco-Johnson, Marilyn (CO)	PHO	667
Mancuso, Anthony (FL)	DR	850
Mandel, Eric (NY)	Oph	498
Mandel, Susan (PA)	EDM	192
Mandelbaum, David (RI)	ChiN	138
Manders, Ernest (PA)	PlS	738
Manera, Ricarchito (IL)	PHO	665
Manevitz, Alan (NY)	Psyc	767
Manganiello, Paul (NH)	RE	871
Mangat, Devinder (KY)	Oto	574
Mann, J John (NY)	Psyc	767
Manning, Warren (MA)	Cv	93
Mannis, Mark (CA)	Oph	518
Manoli, Arthur (MI)	OrS	545
Mansfield, Paul (TX)	S	935
Manske, Paul (MO)	HS	266
Manson, Paul (MD)	PlS	739
Mantyh, Christopher (NC)	CRS	161
Manzarbeitia, Cosme (PA)	S	910
Mapstone, Timothy (OK)	NS	424
Marcet, Jorge (FL)	CRS	161
Marchlinski, Francis (PA)	CE	116
Marcom, Paul (NC)	Onc	310

Alphabetical Listing of Doctors

Name	Specialty	Pg	Name	Specialty	Pg
Marcus, Carole (PA)	PPul	685	Martin, Neil (CA)	NS	427
Marcus, Robert (GA)	RadRO	827	Martin, Paul (FL)	Ge	216
Marder, Stephen (CA)	Psyc	775	Martin, Richard (CO)	Pul	808
Marentette, Lawrence (MI)	Oto	580	Martin, Richard (OH)	NP	386
Margolin, Kim (CA)	Onc	336	Martin, Thomas (WA)	Pul	811
Margolis, James (FL)	IC	122	Martin, Tomas (FL)	TS	961
Marin, Deborah (NY)	Psyc	767	Martinez, Fernando (MI)	Pul	806
Marin, Michael (NY)	VascS	1013	Martini, D Richard (IL)	ChAP	784
Marina, Neyssa (CA)	PHO	671	Martins, Renato G (WA)	Onc	336
Marini, John (MN)	Pul	805	Martuza, Robert (MA)	NS	405
Marino, Ralph (PA)	PMR	722	Masaryk, Thomas (OH)	NRad	858
Marion, Robert (NY)	CG	147	Masket, Samuel (CA)	Oph	518
Maris, John (PA)	PHO	656	Maslak, Peter (NY)	Onc	299
Mark, Eugene (MA)	Path	604	Mason, Joel (MA)	Ge	206
Markert, James (AL)	NS	414	Mason, Kristin (CO)	PMR	727
Markman, Maurie (TX)	Onc	330	Mason, Wilbert (CA)	PInf	676
Markoe, Arnold (FL)	RadRO	827	Masood, Shahla (FL)	Path	610
Markowitz, Bernard (CA)	PlS	753	Mass, Daniel (IL)	HS	266
Markowitz, David (NY)	Ge	211	Massagli, Teresa (WA)	PMR	729
Markowitz, Sanford (OH)	Onc	320	Massin, Edward Krauss (TX)	Cv	110
Marks, Lawrence (NC)	RadRO	828	Masters, Gregory (DE)	Onc	299
Marks, Stanley (PA)	Hem	274	Masur, Henry (MD)	Inf	352
Marmar, Charles (CA)	Psyc	775	Matar, Fadi (FL)	IC	122
Marmor, Michael (CA)	Oph	518	Matarasso, Alan (NY)	PlS	739
Maroon, Joseph (PA)	NS	409	Matas, Arthur (MN)	S	926
Marrs, Richard (CA)	RE	879	Mather, Paul (PA)	Cv	97
Marsh, Christopher (CA)	U	1003	Mathisen, Douglas (MA)	TS	951
Marsh, James (PA)	S	910	Matsen, Frederick (WA)	OrS	553
Marsh, James (CT)	OrS	527	Matthay, Katherine (CA)	PHO	671
Marsh, Jeffrey (MO)	PlS	746	Matthay, Michael (CA)	Pul	811
Marshall, Fray (GA)	U	990	Matthews, David (NC)	PlS	743
Marshall, John (VA)	EDM	195	Matthews, Dennis (CO)	PMR	727
Marshall, John (DC)	Onc	299	Mattox, Douglas (GA)	Oto	574
Marshall, Lawrence (CA)	NS	427	Matulonis, Ursula (MA)	Onc	289
Marshall, Margaret Blair (DC)	TS	956	Mauch, Peter (MA)	RadRO	820
Marten, Timothy (CA)	PlS	753	Mauro, Matthew (NC)	VIR	862
Martenson, James (MN)	RadRO	831	Mavroudis, Constantine (OH)	PS	698

America's Top Doctors® 8th Edition

Name	Specialty	Pg	Name	Specialty	Pg
Mawad, Michel (TX)	NRad	859	McCracken, James (CA)	ChAP	785
Maxwell, G Patrick (TN)	PlS	743	McCraw, John (MS)	PlS	743
May, James (MA)	PlS	734	McCulley, James (TX)	Oph	514
Mayberg, Marc (WA)	NS	427	McCullough, Andrew (NY)	U	983
Mayer, John (MA)	PS	692	McCune, W Joseph (MI)	Rhu	889
Mayer, Lloyd (NY)	Ge	212	McCurley, Thomas (TN)	Path	610
Mayer, Nathaniel (PA)	PMR	722	McDermott, Michael (CA)	NS	428
Mayes, Maureen (TX)	Rhu	891	McDiarmid, Suzanne (CA)	PGe	650
Maytal, Joseph (NY)	ChiN	139	McDonald, Charles (RI)	D	169
Maziarz, Richard (OR)	Hem	285	McDonald, Douglas (MO)	OrS	546
Mazow, Malcolm (TX)	Oph	514	McDonald, John (MD)	N	444
Mazza, David (NY)	A&I	83	McDonald, Ruth (WA)	PNep	679
Mazzone, Theodore (IL)	EDM	198	McDougal, W Scott (MA)	U	978
McAfee, Paul (MD)	OrS	534	McDougle, Christopher (IN)	ChAP	784
McAninch, Jack (CA)	U	1003	McFarland, Edward (MD)	OrS	534
McArthur, Justin (MD)	N	444	McGahan, John (CA)	VIR	866
McAuley, James (IL)	PInf	675	McGarry, Ronald (KY)	RadRO	828
McCaffrey, Thomas (FL)	Oto	575	McGill, Janet (MO)	EDM	198
McCall, William (NC)	Psyc	770	McGill, Trevor (MA)	PO	680
McCallum, Kimberli (MO)	Psyc	771	McGlashan, Thomas (CT)	Psyc	763
McCance-Katz, Elinore (CA)	AdP	779	McGlave, Philip (MN)	Hem	281
McCann, Merle (MD)	Psyc	767	McGovern, Francis (MA)	U	978
McCann, Peter (NY)	OrS	534	McGovern, Peter (NJ)	RE	873
McCann, Richard (NC)	VascS	1015	McGrath, Patrick (KY)	S	919
McCarthy, Joseph (NY)	PlS	739	McGregor, Christopher (MN)	TS	965
McCarthy, Patrick (IL)	TS	965	McGuire, Edward (MI)	U	995
McCarthy, Paul (CT)	PRhu	689	McGuire, William (MD)	Onc	299
McCarthy, Shirley (CT)	DR	845	McHenry, Christopher (OH)	S	926
McClamrock, Howard (MD)	RE	872	McIntyre, Robert (CO)	S	931
McClure, Robert (WA)	U	1003	McKeag, Douglas (IN)	SM	898
McCluskey, Leo (PA)	N	444	McKelvey, Robert (OR)	ChAP	785
McConnell, John (TX)	U	1000	McKenna, Michael (MA)	Oto	563
McConnell, Robert (NY)	EDM	192	McKeown, Craig (FL)	Oph	504
McCormick, Beryl (NY)	RadRO	824	McKinney, Ross (NC)	PInf	674
McCormick, Paul C (NY)	NS	410	McLafferty, Robert (IL)	VascS	1017
McCormick, Wayne (WA)	Ger	238	McLaren, Rodney (VA)	MF	373
McCracken, George (TX)	PInf	675	McLean, Gordon (PA)	VIR	861

Alphabetical Listing of Doctors

Name	Specialty	Pg	Name	Specialty	Pg
McLennan, Geoffrey (IA)	Pul	806	Mendenhall, William (FL)	RadRO	828
McMahon, M Molly (MN)	EDM	198	Mendley, Susan (MD)	PNep	677
McMasters, Kelly (KY)	S	919	Menezes, Arnold (IA)	NS	420
McMenomey, Sean (OR)	Oto	588	Menick, Frederick (AZ)	PlS	749
McNutt, N Scott (NY)	Path	607	Menon, Mani (MI)	U	995
McPherson, David (TX)	Cv	110	Menon, Ram (MI)	PEn	643
McVary, Kevin (IL)	U	995	Menter, M Alan (TX)	D	180
Meacham, Lillian (GA)	PEn	642	Merchant, Thomas (TN)	RadRO	828
Meadow, William (IL)	NP	386	Meredith, Ruby (AL)	RadRO	828
Meadows, Anna (PA)	PHO	656	Meredith, Travis (NC)	Oph	504
Meals, Roy (CA)	HS	268	Merkel, Peter (MA)	Rhu	882
Meara, John (MA)	PlS	734	Meropol, Neal (PA)	Onc	299
Mears, John (NY)	Hem	274	Merrick, Hollis (OH)	S	926
Mease, Philip (WA)	Rhu	892	Merrick, Scot (CA)	TS	972
Medbery, Clinton (OK)	RadRO	835	Merrill, Walter (OH)	TS	965
Medich, David (PA)	CRS	160	Merritt, Diane (MO)	ObG	484
Medina, Jesus (OK)	Oto	586	Mersey, James (MD)	EDM	192
Medow, Norman (NY)	Oph	498	Mertz, Howard (TN)	Ge	216
Medsger, Thomas (PA)	Rhu	884	Mesrobian, Hrair-George (WI)	U	995
Meehan, Kenneth (NH)	Hem	272	Mesulam, Marel (IL)	N	455
Meek, Rita (DE)	PHO	656	Metcalfe, Dean (MD)	A&I	83
Megibow, Alec (NY)	DR	848	Metersky, Mark (CT)	Pul	795
Mehler, Philip (CO)	IM	366	Mets, Marilyn (IL)	Oph	510
Mehlman, David (IL)	Cv	106	Metson, Ralph (MA)	Oto	563
Mehta, Atul (OH)	Pul	806	Metz, David (PA)	Ge	212
Mehta, Minesh (WI)	RadRO	831	Metzl, Jordan (NY)	SM	897
Meier, Diane (NY)	Ger	235	Meyer, Anthony (NC)	S	919
Meiselman, Mick (IL)	Ge	220	Meyers, Bryan (MO)	TS	965
Melamed, Jonathan (NY)	Path	607	Meyers, Paul (NY)	PHO	656
Meller, Jose (NY)	Cv	97	Meyers, Rebecka (UT)	PS	699
Mellow, Alan (MI)	GerPsy	788	Meyers, William (PA)	S	910
Melmed, Shlomo (CA)	EDM	202	Meyskens, Frank (CA)	Onc	336
Melone, Charles (NY)	HS	262	Michaels, Marian (PA)	PInf	673
Meltzer, Eli (CA)	A&I	88	Michalska, Margaret (IL)	Rhu	889
Meltzer, Toby (AZ)	PlS	749	Michalski, Jeff M (MO)	RadRO	832
Melvin, W Scott (OH)	S	926	Michelassi, Fabrizio (NY)	S	910
Mendenhall, Nancy (FL)	RadRO	828	Micheli, Lyle (MA)	SM	896

Alphabetical Listing of Doctors

Name	Specialty	Pg	Name	Specialty	Pg
Michler, Robert (NY)	TS	957	Miniaci, Anthony (OH)	SM	899
Mickey, Bruce (TX)	NS	424	Minich, Lois (UT)	PCd	636
Mieler, William (IL)	Oph	510	Minkoff, Howard (NY)	ObG	481
Mies, Carolyn (PA)	Path	607	Minor, Lloyd (MD)	Oto	569
Mih, Alexander (IN)	HS	266	Mintzer, David (PA)	Onc	299
Mihm, Martin (MA)	D	169	Miro-Quesada, Miguel (TX)	Hem	284
Mikkelsen, Tommy (MI)	N	455	Mirvis, Stuart (MD)	DR	848
Milad, Magdy (IL)	RE	877	Mirzayan, Raffy (CA)	SM	899
Milam, Douglas (TN)	U	990	Mischel, Paul (CA)	Path	618
Mildvan, Donna (NY)	Inf	352	Miskovitz, Paul (NY)	Ge	212
Miles, Brian (TX)	U	1000	Mitch, William (TX)	Nep	399
Millenson, Michael (PA)	Hem	274	Mitchell, Beverly (CA)	Onc	336
Miller, Aaron (NY)	N	444	Mitchell, Charles (FL)	PInf	674
Miller, D Douglas (GA)	Cv	102	Mitchell, James (ND)	Psyc	772
Miller, Daniel (GA)	TS	961	Mitchell, Michael (WI)	U	995
Miller, David (CA)	TS	972	Mitchell, Paul (CT)	Oph	493
Miller, Donald (KY)	Onc	310	Mitchell, Wendy (CA)	ChiN	143
Miller, Franklin (KY)	MF	373	Mitnick, Hal (NY)	Rhu	885
Miller, Joan (MA)	Oph	493	Mitnick, Julie (NY)	DR	848
Miller, Joseph (AZ)	Oph	514	Mitros, Frank (IA)	Path	613
Miller, Joseph (GA)	TS	961	Mitsumoto, Hiroshi (NY)	N	444
Miller, Kenneth (MA)	Hem	272	Mittal, Bharat (IL)	RadRO	832
Miller, Neil (MD)	Oph	499	Miyamoto, Richard (IN)	Oto	581
Miller, Robert (IL)	PO	683	Moder, Kevin (MN)	Rhu	890
Miller, Stanley (MD)	D	173	Modic, Michael (OH)	NRad	858
Miller, Thomas (AZ)	Onc	330	Mohl, Paul (TX)	Psyc	773
Miller, Timothy (CA)	PlS	753	Mohr, Jay (NY)	N	444
Millett, Peter (CO)	OrS	548	Moley, Jeffrey (MO)	S	926
Milley, J Ross (UT)	NP	387	Molleston, Jean (IN)	PGe	649
Millis, J Michael (IL)	S	926	Molnar, Joseph (NC)	PlS	744
Millman, Richard (RI)	Pul	795	Molo, Mary (IL)	RE	877
Mills, Monte (PA)	Oph	499	Mondino, Bartly (CA)	Oph	518
Mills, Stacey (VA)	Path	611	Moneim, Moheb (NM)	HS	267
Milsom, Jeffrey (NY)	CRS	160	Money, Samuel (AZ)	VascS	1018
Mims, James (TX)	Oph	514	Monk, Bradley (CA)	GO	255
Minaker, Kenneth (MA)	Ger	234	Monsees, Barbara (MO)	DR	851
Minckler, Donald (CA)	Oph	518	Montague, Drogo (OH)	U	995

Alphabetical Listing of Doctors

Name	Specialty	Pg	Name	Specialty	Pg
Montanaro, Anthony (OR)	A&I	88	Mosenifar, Zab (CA)	Pul	812
Montgomery, Elizabeth (MD)	Path	608	Moses, Jeffrey (NY)	IC	120
Montgomery, Erwin (WI)	N	455	Mosher, Deane (WI)	Hem	281
Montgomery, Robert (MD)	S	910	Moskowitz, William (VA)	PCd	633
Montie, James (MI)	U	995	Moss, R Lawrence (CT)	PS	692
Moodie, Douglas (LA)	PCd	636	Mostwin, Jacek (MD)	U	983
Moore, Anne (NY)	Onc	299	Mott, Michael (MI)	OrS	546
Moore, Ernest (CO)	S	931	Motzer, Robert (NY)	Onc	300
Moore, Joseph (NC)	Onc	310	Moul, Judd (NC)	U	990
Moore, Thomas (CA)	MF	378	Mountz, James (PA)	NuM	475
Moore, Walter (GA)	Rhu	887	Movsas, Benjamin (MI)	RadRO	832
Moossa, AR (CA)	S	940	Muggia, Franco (NY)	Onc	300
Morady, Fred (MI)	CE	117	Mukherji, Suresh (MI)	NRad	858
Moran, Cesar (TX)	Path	615	Muldoon, Thomas (NY)	Oph	499
Moran, Christopher (MO)	NRad	858	Mulhall, John (NY)	U	983
Moran, John (IL)	Cv	106	Mullett, Timothy (KY)	TS	961
Morgan, Elaine (IL)	PHO	665	Mulliken, John (MA)	PlS	734
Morgan, Linda (FL)	ObG	482	Mulvihill, John (OK)	CG	151
Morgan, Mark (PA)	GO	247	Mulvihill, Sean (UT)	S	931
Morgan, Raymond (VA)	PlS	744	Mundt, Arno (CA)	RadRO	837
Morgan, Walter (TN)	PS	696	Munin, Michael (PA)	PMR	722
Morgan, Wayne (AZ)	PPul	688	Munoz, Jose (NY)	PInf	673
Morgenlander, Joel (NC)	N	450	Muntz, Howard (WA)	GO	255
Morley, John (MO)	Ger	237	Murali, Raj (NY)	NS	410
Morrell, Martha (CA)	N	464	Muraskas, Jonathan (IL)	NP	386
Morris, Colleen (NV)	CG	152	Murphree, A Linn (CA)	Oph	519
Morris, Douglas (GA)	IC	122	Murphy, Ana (GA)	RE	875
Morris, John (MO)	N	455	Murphy, Douglas (GA)	TS	961
Morris, Robert E (CA)	AM	79	Murphy, Sharon (TX)	PHO	668
Morris, Rohinton (PA)	TS	957	Murphy, Thomas (NC)	PPul	686
Morrison, Glenn (FL)	NS	414	Murphy, Timothy (RI)	VIR	860
Morrow, Monica (NY)	S	910	Murray, Joseph (MN)	Ge	221
Mortimer, Joanne (CA)	Onc	337	Murray, Pamela (PA)	AM	78
Morton, D Holmes (PA)	Ped	625	Murray, Timothy (FL)	Oph	504
Mosca, Lori (NY)	Cv	97	Murtagh, F Reed (FL)	NRad	857
Moscatello, Augustine (NY)	Oto	569	Muschler, George (OH)	OrS	546
Moscow, Jeffrey (KY)	PHO	660	Muss, Hyman (VT)	Onc	289

Alphabetical Listing of Doctors

Name	Specialty	Pg	Name	Specialty	Pg
Mustoe, Thomas (IL)	PlS	746	Nardell, Edward (MA)	Pul	795
Mutch, David (MO)	GO	252	Nascimento, Antonio (MN)	Path	613
Muto, Michael (MA)	GO	244	Nash, Martin (NY)	PNep	677
Myer, Charles (OH)	PO	683	Nash, Thomas (NY)	Pul	797
Myerburg, Robert (FL)	Cv	102	Naslund, Michael (MD)	U	984
Myers, Jeffrey (MI)	Path	613	Natale, Ronald (CA)	Onc	337
Myers, Jeffrey (TX)	Oto	586	Nath, Rahul (TX)	PlS	750
Myers, Robert (MN)	U	995	Nathanson, S David (MI)	S	927
Myerson, Mark (MD)	OrS	535	Nathwani, Bharat (CA)	Path	619
Myerson, Robert (MO)	RadRO	832	Naunheim, Keith (MO)	TS	965
Myones, Barry (TX)	PRhu	691	Nava-Villarreal, Hector (NY)	S	911
Myseros, John (VA)	NS	414	Nazzaro, Jules (KS)	NS	423
Mysiw, W Jerry (OH)	PMR	726	Neel, Victor (MA)	D	169
			Neglia, Joseph (MN)	PHO	665
			Negrin, Robert (CA)	Hem	285
			Neifeld, James (VA)	S	919

N

Name	Specialty	Pg	Name	Specialty	Pg
Nabell, Lisle (AL)	Onc	310	Nelson, Edward (UT)	S	931
Nabors, Louis (AL)	N	450	Nelson, Heidi (MN)	CRS	163
Naccarelli, Gerald (PA)	Cv	98	Nelson, J Craig (CA)	Psyc	775
Nachman, James (IL)	PHO	665	Nelson, Joel (PA)	U	984
Naclerio, Robert (IL)	Oto	581	Nelson, Leonard (PA)	Oph	499
Nadler, Lee (MA)	Onc	289	Nelson, Maureen (NC)	PMR	724
Nadol, Joseph (MA)	Oto	563	Nemcek, Albert (IL)	VIR	863
Nagel, Theodore (MN)	RE	877	Nemickas, Rimgaudas (IL)	Cv	106
Nagib, Mahmoud (MN)	NS	420	Nemunaitis, John (TX)	Onc	330
Nagle, Daniel (IL)	HS	266	Neppe, Vernon (WA)	Psyc	775
Nagle, Deborah (MA)	CRS	158	Nerad, Jeffrey (IA)	Oph	510
Nagler, Harris (NY)	U	984	Nesbitt, Jonathan (TN)	TS	962
Nagorney, David (MN)	S	926	Nestler, John (VA)	EDM	195
Nagueh, Sherif (TX)	Cv	111	Netterville, James (TN)	Oto	575
Nahass, Ronald (NJ)	Inf	352	Neu, Josef (FL)	NP	385
Naka, Yoshifumi (NY)	TS	957	Neuberg, Ronnie (SC)	PHO	660
Nakayama, Don (GA)	PS	696	Neuburg, Marcelle (WI)	D	178
Nance, Michael (PA)	PS	694	Neumann, Donald (OH)	NuM	476
Nand, Sucha (IL)	Hem	281	Neumann, Ronald (MD)	NuM	475
Napoli, Joseph (DE)	PlS	739	Neuwelt, Edward (OR)	NS	428
			Neuwirth, Michael (NY)	OrS	535

Alphabetical Listing of Doctors

Name	Specialty	Pg	Name	Specialty	Pg
Nevins, Thomas (MN)	PNep	679	Nogueras, Juan (FL)	CRS	161
New, Maria (NY)	PEn	641	Nolan, Bruce (FL)	N	450
Newburger, Jane (MA)	PCd	630	Noller, Kenneth (MA)	ObG	480
Newell, Kenneth (GA)	S	919	Noone, R Barrett (PA)	PlS	739
Newman, Lawrence (NY)	N	444	Norbash, Alexander (MA)	NRad	854
Newman, Lee (CO)	Pul	808	Nordli, Douglas (IL)	ChiN	142
Newman, Leonard (NY)	PGe	646	Norenberg, Michael (FL)	Path	611
Newman, Lisa (MI)	S	927	Nori, Dattatreyudu (NY)	RadRO	825
Newman, Nancy (GA)	N	450	Norman, David (CA)	NRad	860
Newton, Herbert (OH)	N	456	Norman, Kim (CA)	Psyc	775
Ngeow, Jeffrey (NY)	PM	597	Northfelt, Donald (AZ)	Onc	330
Nguyen, Ninh (CA)	S	940	Northrup, Hope (TX)	CG	151
Nicholas, Stephen (NY)	OrS	535	Norton, Jeffrey (CA)	S	940
Nicholl, Jeffrey (LA)	N	461	Norton, Karen (NJ)	DR	849
Nichols, Craig (OR)	Onc	337	Norton, Larry (NY)	Onc	300
Nichols, David (MD)	PCCM	638	Nour, Nawal (MA)	ObG	480
Nicholson, Henry (OR)	PHO	671	Novak, Donald (FL)	PGe	648
Nichter, Larry (CA)	PlS	753	Novick, Andrew (OH)	U	996
Nicolaou, Nicos (PA)	RadRO	824	Novotny, Edward (CT)	ChiN	138
Nicosia, Santo (FL)	Path	611	Nowak, Eugene (NY)	S	911
Nieder, Michael (FL)	PHO	660	Noyes, Nicole (NY)	RE	873
Niederhuber, John (MD)	S	911	Nuber, Gordon (IL)	OrS	546
Niederman, Michael (NY)	Pul	797	Nuchtern, Jed (TX)	PS	700
Nigra, Thomas (DC)	D	173	Nugent, William (NH)	TS	951
Nimer, Stephen (NY)	Hem	274	Nunery, William (KY)	Oph	504
Ninan, Mathews (TN)	TS	962	Nunley, James (NC)	OrS	541
Niparko, John (MD)	Oto	569	Nurnberger, John (IN)	Psyc	771
Nishimura, Rick (MN)	Cv	107	Nuss, Daniel (LA)	Oto	586
Nisonson, Barton (NY)	SM	897	Nuss, Donald (VA)	PS	696
Nissen, Nicholas (CA)	S	940	Nussbaum, Julian (GA)	Oph	505
Nissen, Steven (OH)	Cv	107	Nussbaum, Robert (CA)	CG	152
Nissenblatt, Michael (NJ)	Onc	300	Nutt, John (OR)	N	464
Nitti, Victor (NY)	U	984			
Nobunaga, Austin (OH)	PMR	726			
Nocero, Michael (FL)	Cv	102			
Noetzel, Michael (MO)	ChiN	141		**O**	
Nogee, Lawrence (MD)	NP	383	O'Brien, Joan (CA)	Oph	519

Alphabetical Listing of Doctors

Name	Specialty	Pg	Name	Specialty	Pg
O'Brien, John (MI)	Ge	221	Okusa, Mark (VA)	Nep	395
O'Brien, Susan (TX)	Onc	330	Olanow, C Warren (NY)	N	444
O'Day, Steven (CA)	Onc	337	Olbricht, Suzanne (MA)	D	170
O'Dell, James (NE)	Rhu	890	Olden, Kevin (AR)	Ge	225
O'Donnell, Margaret (CA)	Hem	285	Oldham, Keith (WI)	PS	698
O'Donnell, Michael (IA)	U	996	Olitsky, Scott (MO)	Oph	510
O'Donnell, Richard (CA)	OrS	553	Oliva-Hemker, Maria (MD)	PGe	646
O'Driscoll, Shawn (MN)	OrS	546	Olivero, Juan (TX)	Nep	399
O'Gara, Patrick (MA)	Cv	93	Olopade, Olufunmilayo (IL)	Onc	321
O'Hea, Brian (NY)	S	911	Olsen, Elise (NC)	D	176
O'Keefe, Regis (NY)	OrS	535	Olsen, Kerry (MN)	Oto	581
O'Laughlin, Martin (MO)	PCd	635	Olson, Jack (IL)	Ger	237
O'Leary, Michael P (MA)	U	979	Olson, Jeffrey (GA)	NS	414
O'Leary, Patrick (NY)	OrS	535	Olson, Thomas (GA)	PHO	661
O'Malley, Bert (PA)	Oto	569	Olthoff, Kim (PA)	S	911
O'Neill, William (FL)	Cv	102	Onders, Raymond (OH)	S	927
O'Regan, Ruth (GA)	Onc	311	Ondra, Stephen (IL)	NS	420
O'Reilly, Eileen (NY)	Onc	300	Ontjes, David (NC)	EDM	195
O'Reilly, Richard (NY)	PHO	656	Oommen, Kalarickal (OK)	N	461
O'Rourke, Donald (PA)	NS	410	Oparil, Suzanne (AL)	Cv	102
O'Shaughnessy, Joyce (TX)	Onc	331	Oppenheim, William (CA)	OrS	553
Oakes, W Jerry (AL)	NS	414	Oquendo, Maria (NY)	Psyc	767
Oates, Robert (MA)	U	979	Oratz, Ruth (NY)	Onc	300
Oberfield, Sharon (NY)	PEn	641	Orel, Susan (PA)	DR	849
Oddis, Chester (PA)	Rhu	885	Orengo, Ida (TX)	D	180
Odel, Jeffrey (NY)	Oph	499	Orenstein, David (PA)	PPul	686
Odem, Randall (MO)	RE	877	Orenstein, Jan (DC)	Path	608
Odom, Lorrie (CO)	PHO	667	Orgill, Dennis (MA)	PlS	735
Odom, Michael (TX)	NP	387	Origitano, Thomas (IL)	NS	420
Odunsi, Adekunle (NY)	GO	247	Orlow, Seth (NY)	D	173
Odze, Robert (MA)	Path	604	Orlowski, Robert (TX)	Onc	331
Oeffinger, Kevin (NY)	Ped	625	Orobello, Peter (FL)	PO	682
Offit, Kenneth (NY)	Onc	300	Orringer, Mark B (MI)	TS	965
Offit, Paul (PA)	PInf	673	Ortel, Thomas (NC)	Hem	277
Oh, Shin (AL)	N	450	Orwoll, Eric (OR)	EDM	202
Ohl, Dana (MI)	U	996	Ory, Steven (FL)	RE	875
Okereke, Enyi (PA)	OrS	535	Osborn, Anne (UT)	NRad	858

Alphabetical Listing of Doctors

Name	Specialty	Pg	Name	Specialty	Pg
Osborne, Charles (TX)	Onc	331	Palefsky, Joel (CA)	Inf	358
Osborne, Michael (NY)	S	911	Paletta, George (MO)	SM	899
Osguthorpe, John (SC)	Oto	575	Palevsky, Harold (PA)	Pul	798
Osher, Robert (OH)	Oph	510	Paley, Dror (MD)	OrS	535
Oster, Martin (NY)	Onc	300	Palfrey, Judith (MA)	Ped	624
Osterman, A Lee (PA)	HS	262	Paller, Amy (IL)	D	178
Ostrer, Harry (NY)	CG	147	Palmberg, Paul (FL)	Oph	505
Ostroff, James (CA)	Ge	227	Palmer, Earl (OR)	Oph	519
Ostrom, Nancy (CA)	A&I	88	Palmer, Robert (PA)	Ger	235
Otley, Clark (MN)	D	178	Palmer, William (MA)	DR	845
Ott, David (TX)	TS	969	Panicek, David (NY)	DR	849
Ott, Kenneth (CA)	NS	428	Panitch, Howard (PA)	PPul	686
Ott, Susan (WA)	Nep	400	Papadopoulos, Nicholas (TX)	Onc	331
Otto, Pamela (TX)	DR	853	Papadopoulos, Stephen (AZ)	NS	424
Otto, Randal (TX)	Oto	586	Paparella, Michael (MN)	Oto	581
Ovalle, Fernando (AL)	EDM	195	Papel, Ira (MD)	Oto	569
Ownby, Dennis (GA)	PA&I	628	Pappas, Theodore (NC)	S	920
Owyang, Chung (MI)	Ge	221	Parent, Andrew (MS)	NS	414
Oz, Mehmet (NY)	TS	957	Parisier, Simon (NY)	Oto	569
			Park, Adrian (MD)	S	911
			Park, Catherine (CA)	RadRO	837
P			Park, Tae Sung (MO)	NS	420
			Parker, Robert (NY)	PHO	657
Pachter, H Leon (NY)	S	911	Parness, Ira (NY)	PCd	632
Pacin, Michael (FL)	A&I	85	Parrillo, Joseph (NJ)	Cv	98
Pack, Allan (PA)	Pul	798	Parrish, Richard (FL)	Oph	505
Packer, Roger (DC)	ChiN	140	Parry, Samuel (PA)	MF	372
Padgett, Douglas (NY)	OrS	535	Parsons, Polly (VT)	Pul	795
Pagani, Francis (MI)	TS	966	Parsons, Theodore (MI)	OrS	546
Page, David (TN)	Path	611	Partain, C Leon (TN)	DR	850
Paget, Stephen (NY)	Rhu	885	Partin, Alan (MD)	U	984
Pagon, Roberta (WA)	CG	152	Partridge, Edward (AL)	GO	250
Pahl, Elfriede (IL)	PCd	635	Pascuzzi, Robert (IN)	N	456
Paidas, Charles (FL)	PS	696	Pasmantier, Mark (NY)	Onc	301
Paidas, Michael (CT)	MF	371	Pasricha, Pankaj (TX)	Ge	226
Palacios, Igor (MA)	Cv	93	Pass, Harvey (NY)	TS	957
Palascak, Joseph (OH)	Hem	281	Passo, Murray (SC)	PRhu	690

Name	Specialty	Pg	Name	Specialty	Pg
Patchefsky, Arthur (PA)	Path	608	Pendergrass, Thomas (WA)	PHO	671
Patchell, Roy (KY)	N	451	Pensak, Myles (OH)	Oto	581
Patel, Mukund (NY)	HS	262	Pepine, Carl (FL)	Cv	102
Patel, Sunil (SC)	NS	414	Pepose, Jay (MO)	Oph	510
Patel, Vipul (FL)	U	990	Perez, Edith (FL)	Onc	311
Patrizio, Pasquale (CT)	RE	871	Perez Fontan, J Julio (TX)	PCCM	639
Patt, Yehuda (NM)	Onc	331	Pergament, Eugene (IL)	CG	149
Patterson, Anthony (TN)	U	990	Perin, Emerson (TX)	IC	123
Patterson, G Alexander (MO)	TS	966	Perkash, Inder (CA)	U	1004
Patterson, James (OR)	Pul	812	Perkins, James (WA)	S	940
Patterson, Jan E Evans (TX)	Inf	357	Perler, Bruce (MD)	VascS	1014
Patterson, Marc (MN)	ChiN	142	Perlman, David (NY)	Inf	352
Patterson, Thomas (TX)	Inf	357	Perlman, Jeffrey (NY)	NP	383
Paty, Philip (NY)	S	911	Perlmutter, Joel (MO)	N	456
Patz, Edward (NC)	DR	850	Perret, Philip (LA)	Pul	809
Patzakis, Michael (CA)	OrS	553	Perrone, Ronald (MA)	Nep	392
Paul, Malcolm (CA)	PlS	754	Perry, Arie (MO)	Path	613
Paul, T Otis (CA)	Oph	519	Perry, James (MN)	PCd	635
Paulos, Leon (FL)	OrS	541	Perry, Michael (MO)	Onc	321
Paulson, Richard (CA)	RE	879	Perry, Stanton (CA)	PCd	637
Payne, Christopher (CA)	U	1003	Perryman, Richard (FL)	TS	962
Peabody, Terrance (IL)	OrS	546	Persing, John (CT)	PlS	735
Pearce, William (IL)	VascS	1017	Persky, Mark (NY)	Oto	570
Pearlman, Nathan (CO)	S	931	Peschel, Richard (CT)	RadRO	820
Pearson, Richard (VA)	Inf	355	Pestronk, Alan (MO)	N	456
Pearson, Thomas (NY)	PrM	759	Petelin, Joseph (KS)	S	931
Pecora, Andrew (NJ)	Onc	301	Peters, Glenn (AL)	Oto	575
Pedley, Timothy (NY)	N	445	Peters, Jeffrey (NY)	S	912
Pegram, Paul (NC)	Inf	355	Petersdorf, Stephen (WA)	Onc	337
Peitzman, Andrew (PA)	S	912	Petersen, Ronald (MN)	N	456
Pellegrini, Carlos (WA)	S	940	Peterson, Bruce (MN)	Onc	321
Pellicci, Paul (NY)	OrS	536	Peterson, Davis (AK)	OrS	553
Pelzer, Harold (IL)	Oto	581	Petito, Carol (FL)	Path	611
Pemberton, John (MN)	CRS	163	Petito, Frank (NY)	N	445
Pena, Alberto (OH)	PS	699	Petras, Robert (OH)	Path	613
Penalver, Manuel (FL)	GO	250	Petrelli, Nicholas (DE)	S	912
Penar, Paul (VT)	NS	405	Petri, Michelle (MD)	Rhu	885

Alphabetical Listing of Doctors

Name	Specialty	Pg	Name	Specialty	Pg
Petrossian, George (NY)	IC	120	Pinzur, Michael (IL)	OrS	546
Petru, Ann (CA)	PInf	676	Piraino, Beth (PA)	Nep	394
Petruzzelli, Guy (IL)	Oto	581	Pisano, Etta (NC)	DR	850
Petrylak, Daniel (NY)	Onc	301	Pisters, Katherine (TX)	Onc	331
Pettrone, Frank (VA)	OrS	541	Pisters, Louis (TX)	U	1000
Pevec, William (CA)	VascS	1019	Pisters, Peter (TX)	S	935
Pezner, Richard (CA)	RadRO	837	Pitman, Gerald (NY)	PlS	739
Pfeffer, Marc (MA)	Cv	93	Pitman, Karen (MS)	Oto	575
Pfeifer, Samantha (PA)	RE	873	Pitman, Roger (MA)	Psyc	763
Pfister, David (NY)	Onc	301	Pitts, Lawrence (CA)	NS	428
Pflugfelder, Stephen (TX)	Oph	514	Plancher, Kevin (NY)	SM	897
Philipson, Elliot (OH)	MF	375	Plante, Lauren (PA)	ObG	481
Phillips, Edward (CA)	S	941	Platt, Lawrence (CA)	MF	378
Phillips, Harry (NC)	Cv	102	Platzker, Arnold (CA)	PPul	689
Phillips, Katharine (RI)	Psyc	763	Plehn, Jonathan (MD)	Cv	98
Phillips, Peter (PA)	ChiN	140	Plevy, Scott (NC)	Ge	216
Phillips, Robert (MA)	Cv	93	Plotnick, Leslie (MD)	PEn	641
Phuphanich, Surasak (CA)	N	464	Plotz, Paul (MD)	Rhu	885
Pi, Edmond (CA)	Psyc	775	Pochapin, Mark (NY)	Ge	212
Piatt, Joseph (PA)	NS	410	Pochettino, Alberto (PA)	TS	957
Piccirillo, Jay (MO)	Oto	581	Pockaj, Barbara (AZ)	S	935
Piccoli, David (PA)	PGe	646	Podoloff, Donald (TX)	NuM	477
Pichard, Augusto (DC)	IC	120	Podos, Steven (NY)	Oph	499
Picken, Catherine (DC)	Oto	570	Poehling, Gary (NC)	OrS	541
Picozzi, Vincent (WA)	Onc	337	Pohl, Marc (OH)	Nep	397
Picus, Joel (MO)	Onc	321	Poliakoff, Steven (FL)	GO	250
Pienta, Kenneth (MI)	Onc	321	Polin, Richard (NY)	NP	384
Piepgras, David (MN)	NS	420	Polisson, Richard (MA)	Rhu	882
Piepmeier, Joseph (CT)	NS	405	Pollack, Alan (PA)	RadRO	825
Pierce, Lori (MI)	RadRO	832	Pollack, Ian (PA)	NS	410
Pierson, Richard (MD)	TS	957	Pollard, Zane (GA)	Oph	505
Pile-Spellman, John (NY)	NRad	855	Polley, John (IL)	PlS	746
Pillsbury, Harold (NC)	Oto	575	Pollock, Raphael (TX)	S	935
Pinckert, Thomas (MD)	MF	372	Polly, David (MN)	OrS	547
Pingleton, Susan (KS)	Pul	808	Polonsky, Kenneth (MO)	EDM	198
Pinson, C Wright (TN)	S	920	Polsky, Bruce (NY)	Inf	353
Pinto, Harlan (CA)	Onc	337	Pomeroy, John (NY)	ChAP	782

Name	Specialty	Pg	Name	Specialty	Pg
Pomeroy, Scott (MA)	ChiN	138	Presti, Joseph (CA)	U	1004
Pongracic, Jacqueline (IL)	PA&I	628	Price, Lawrence (RI)	Psyc	763
Ponn, Teresa (NH)	S	903	Prieto, Victor (TX)	Path	616
Ponsky, Jeffrey (OH)	S	927	Prinz, Richard (IL)	S	927
Ponton, Lynn (CA)	ChAP	786	Prosnitz, Leonard (NC)	RadRO	828
Poole, Michael (GA)	Oto	575	Provenzale, James (NC)	NRad	857
Poon, Michael (NY)	Cv	98	Pruitt, David (MD)	ChAP	782
Poordad, Fred (CA)	Ge	227	Prystowsky, Eric (IN)	CE	118
Pope, Richard (IL)	Rhu	890	Puccetti, Diane (WI)	PHO	665
Popovich, John (MI)	Pul	806	Puckett, Charles (MO)	PIS	747
Poppas, Dix (NY)	U	984	Pui, Ching (TN)	PHO	661
Porcu, Pierluigi (OH)	Hem	281	Pula, Thaddeus (MD)	N	445
Portenoy, Russell (NY)	PM	597	Puliafito, Carmen (CA)	Oph	519
Porter, Co-burn (MN)	PCd	635	Purdue, Gary (TX)	S	936
Porter, David (PA)	Hem	274	Putnam, Joe (TN)	TS	962
Posey, James (AL)	Onc	311	Putnam, Matthew (MN)	HS	266
Posner, Jerome (NY)	N	445	Putterman, Allen (IL)	Oph	510
Posner, Marshall (MA)	Onc	289	Pyeritz, Reed (PA)	CG	147
Posner, Mitchell (IL)	S	927	Pynoos, Robert (CA)	Psyc	776
Posnick, Jeffrey (MD)	PIS	739			
Postier, Russell (OK)	S	935			
Postma, Gregory (GA)	Oto	575	**Q**		
Potkul, Ronald (IL)	GO	252			
Potter, Hollis (NY)	DR	849	Quaegebeur, Jan (NY)	PS	694
Pow-Sang, Julio (FL)	U	990	Quagliarello, Vincent (CT)	Inf	350
Powell, Bayard (NC)	Hem	277	Quatela, Vito (NY)	Oto	570
Powell, Catherine (CA)	GO	255	Quencer, Robert (FL)	NRad	857
Powell, Nelson (CA)	Oto	588	Quigley, Harry (MD)	Oph	499
Powers, Alvin (TN)	EDM	195	Quinn, David (CA)	Onc	338
Powers, Eric (SC)	Cv	103	Quinn, Graham (PA)	Oph	499
Powers, Pauline (FL)	Psyc	770	Quinn, Suzanne (FL)	EDM	195
Prados, Michael (CA)	Onc	337	Quinones, Miguel (TX)	Cv	111
Prager, Joshua (CA)	PM	602	Quintessenza, James (FL)	TS	962
Prakash, Udaya (MN)	Pul	806	Quittell, Lynne (NY)	PPul	686
Preminger, Glenn (NC)	U	990	Quivey, Jeanne (CA)	RadRO	837
Press, Joel (IL)	PMR	726			
Press, Oliver (WA)	Onc	338			

Alphabetical Listing of Doctors

Name	Specialty	Pg	Name	Specialty	Pg
R			Raphael, Bruce (NY)	Hem	275
			Rapoport, Judith (DC)	ChAP	782
Rabinovitch, Rachel (CO)	RadRO	833	Rappaport, Leonard (MA)	Ped	624
Racz, Gabor (TX)	PM	600	Rashid, Asif (TX)	Path	616
Rader, Daniel (PA)	IM	364	Raskin, Keith (NY)	HS	262
Radtke, Wolfgang (DE)	PCd	632	Raskin, Neil (CA)	N	464
Raffel, Corey (OH)	NS	420	Raskin, Philip (TX)	EDM	200
Rafferty, Janice (OH)	CRS	163	Raskind, Murray (WA)	Psyc	776
Raghavan, Derek (OH)	Onc	321	Rasmussen, Steven (RI)	Psyc	763
Raghu, Ganesh (WA)	Pul	812	Rassekh, Christopher (WV)	Oto	570
Ragnarsson, Kristjan (NY)	PMR	722	Rassman, William (CA)	S	941
Rahal, James (NY)	Inf	353	Ratain, Mark (IL)	Onc	321
Rahko, Peter (WI)	Cv	107	Ratts, Valerie (MO)	RE	878
Rai, Kanti (NY)	Hem	275	Ratzan, Kenneth (FL)	Inf	355
Raiford, David (TN)	Ge	216	Rauch, Paula (MA)	Psyc	763
Raja, Srinivasa (MD)	PM	597	Rauch, Steven (MA)	Oto	564
Rajfer, Jacob (CA)	U	1004	Rauck, Richard (NC)	PM	598
Rakowski, Thomas (VA)	Nep	395	Rausen, Aaron (NY)	PHO	657
Ramamurthy, Somayaji (TX)	PM	601	Ravich, William (MD)	Ge	212
Raman, Jai (IL)	TS	966	Rayan, Ghazi (OK)	HS	267
Ramanathan, Ramesh (PA)	S	912	Raz, Shlomo (CA)	U	1004
Ramee, Stephen (LA)	Cv	111	Razzouk, Bassem (IN)	PHO	665
Ramirez, Oscar (MD)	PlS	739	Read, Thomas (PA)	CRS	160
Ramsay, David (NY)	D	173	Ready, John (MA)	OrS	527
Ramsey, Bonnie (WA)	PPul	689	Ready, L Brian (WA)	PM	602
Ramsey, Matthew (PA)	OrS	536	Reaman, Gregory (DC)	PHO	657
Ranawat, Chitranjan (NY)	OrS	536	Reardon, Michael (TX)	TS	969
Rand, Jacob (NY)	Hem	275	Reasner, Charles (TX)	EDM	200
Rand, Richard (WA)	PlS	754	Reber, Howard (CA)	S	941
Randall, Marcus (KY)	RadRO	828	Recht, Abram (MA)	RadRO	821
Randall, R Lor (UT)	OrS	549	Rechtine, Glenn (NY)	OrS	536
Randolph, Gregory (MA)	Oto	564	Recker, Robert (NE)	EDM	199
Randolph, Linda (CA)	CG	152	Redberg, Rita (CA)	Cv	113
Rao, Nalini (PA)	Inf	353	Redding, Gregory (WA)	PPul	689
Rao, Narsing (CA)	Oph	519	Reddy, K Rajender (PA)	Ge	212
Rao, Satish (IA)	Ge	221	Reder, Anthony (IL)	N	456
Rao, Vijay (PA)	DR	849	Redlich, Carrie (CT)	Pul	796

Alphabetical Listing of Doctors

Name	Specialty	Pg	Name	Specialty	Pg
Rimoin, David (CA)	CG	153	Rodgers, Bradley (VA)	PS	696
Ring, W Steves (TX)	TS	969	Rodgers, George (UT)	Path	614
Ringel, Steven (CO)	N	459	Rodosky, Mark (PA)	OrS	536
Rink, Richard (IN)	U	996	Rodts, Gerald (GA)	NS	415
Riordan, John (CA)	Nep	400	Roehrborn, Claus (TX)	U	1000
Ristow, Brunno (CA)	PlS	754	Rogers, Douglas (OH)	PEn	644
Ritch, Robert (NY)	Oph	500	Rogers, Gary (OH)	Oph	511
Ritchey, Arthur (PA)	PHO	657	Rogers, James (TX)	PCd	637
Riviello, James (TX)	ChiN	143	Rogers, Joseph (NC)	Cv	103
Rivkees, Scott (CT)	PEn	640	Rogers, Lisa (MI)	N	456
Rivlin, Richard (NY)	IM	365	Rogers, Stanley (CA)	S	941
Rizk, Norman (CA)	Pul	812	Roh, Mark (PA)	S	912
Rizza, Robert (MN)	EDM	198	Rohrich, Rod (TX)	PlS	750
Rizzo, Joseph (MA)	Oph	493	Romano, James (CA)	PlS	754
Roach, Mack (CA)	RadRO	838	Rombeau, John (PA)	CRS	160
Robb, Geoffrey (TX)	PlS	750	Romond, Edward H (KY)	Onc	311
Robbins, Lawrence (IL)	PM	599	Roodman, G David (PA)	Hem	275
Robbins, Richard (TX)	EDM	200	Rook, Alain (PA)	D	173
Robbins, Robert (CA)	TS	972	Roos, Karen (IN)	N	456
Robert, Nicholas (VA)	Onc	311	Roos, Raymond (IL)	N	457
Robert-Vizcarrondo, Francisco (AL)	Onc	311	Roose, Steven (NY)	Psyc	767
Roberts, Barbara (RI)	Cv	94	Ropper, Allan (MA)	N	437
Roberts, John (CA)	S	941	Rosato, Ernest (PA)	S	912
Roberts, Kenneth (CT)	RadRO	821	Rosbe, Kristina (CA)	PO	684
Roberts, Michelle (PA)	EDM	192	Rose, Cecile (CO)	Pul	808
Roberts, Patricia (MA)	CRS	158	Rose, Christopher (CA)	RadRO	838
Roberts, William (TX)	Path	616	Rose, Peter (OH)	GO	252
Robertson, Cary (NC)	U	990	Rosemurgy, Alexander (FL)	S	920
Robins, Perry (NY)	D	173	Rosen, Antony (MD)	Rhu	885
Robinson, Lary A (FL)	TS	962	Rosen, Charles (MN)	S	927
Robinson, Lawrence (WA)	PMR	729	Rosen, Clark (PA)	Oto	570
Rocchini, Albert (MI)	PCd	635	Rosen, Jules (PA)	GerPsy	787
Rochester, Carolyn (CT)	Pul	796	Rosen, Paul (NY)	Path	608
Rock, Jack (MI)	NS	421	Rosen, Steven (IL)	Onc	322
Rock, John (FL)	RE	876	Rosenbaum, Jerrold (MA)	Psyc	763
Roddy, Sarah (CA)	ChiN	144	Rosenbaum, Kenneth (DC)	CG	148
Rodeo, Scott (NY)	SM	897	Rosenbaum, Richard (OR)	N	465

Name	Specialty	Pg	Name	Specialty	Pg
Rosenberg, Aaron (IL)	OrS	547	Rossman, Milton (PA)	Pul	798
Rosenberg, Howard (CA)	PlS	754	Rostain, Anthony (PA)	ChAP	782
Rosenberg, Michael (IL)	Oph	511	Roth, Andrew (NY)	Psyc	768
Rosenberg, Steven (MD)	S	912	Roth, Bennett (CA)	Ge	227
Rosenberg, Thomas (UT)	OrS	549	Roth, Bruce (TN)	Onc	311
Rosenblatt, Joseph (FL)	Hem	277	Roth, David (FL)	Nep	396
Rosenblum, Marc (NY)	Path	608	Roth, Elliot (IL)	PMR	727
Rosenblum, Mark (MI)	NS	421	Roth, Jack (TX)	TS	969
Rosenblum, Norman (PA)	GO	247	Rothbaum, Robert (MO)	PGe	649
Rosenbush, Stuart (IL)	Cv	107	Rothenberg, Mace (TN)	Onc	311
Rosenfeld, Myrna (PA)	N	445	Rothenberg, Russell (MD)	Rhu	885
Rosenfeld, Philip (FL)	Oph	505	Rothenberger, David (MN)	CRS	163
Rosenfeld, Richard (NY)	PO	681	Rothman, Richard (PA)	OrS	536
Rosenfeld, Steven (NY)	N	445	Rothrock, John (AL)	N	451
Rosenfield, Robert (IL)	PEn	644	Rothstein, Richard (NH)	Ge	206
Rosengart, Todd (NY)	TS	958	Rotman, Marvin (NY)	RadRO	825
Rosenman, Julian (NC)	RadRO	829	Rotmensch, Jacob (IL)	GO	252
Rosenquist, Richard (IA)	PM	599	Roubin, Gary (NY)	IC	121
Rosenthal, Amnon (MI)	PCd	636	Routes, John (WI)	A&I	86
Rosenthal, David (GA)	VascS	1015	Rovner, Barry (PA)	GerPsy	787
Rosenthal, Joseph (CA)	PHO	671	Rowbotham, Michael (CA)	PM	602
Rosenthal, Richard (NY)	Psyc	768	Rowland, Randall (KY)	U	990
Rosenwaks, Zev (NY)	RE	873	Rowley, Howard (WI)	NRad	858
Rosenwasser, Melvin (NY)	HS	263	Roy-Byrne, Peter (WA)	Psyc	776
Rosenwasser, Robert (PA)	NS	410	Roye, David (NY)	OrS	536
Roses, Daniel (NY)	S	913	Rozbruch, S Robert (NY)	OrS	537
Rosier, Randy (NY)	OrS	536	Rubenfeld, Sheldon (TX)	EDM	200
Roskes, Saul (MD)	PNep	677	Rubin, Brian (OH)	Path	613
Rosner, Howard (CA)	PM	602	Rubin, Bruce (NC)	PPul	686
Rosoff, Philip (NC)	PHO	661	Rubin, Geoffrey (CA)	DR	853
Ross, Helen (AZ)	Onc	331	Rubin, Lewis (CA)	Pul	812
Ross, Jeffrey (NY)	Path	608	Rubin, Mark (CA)	D	182
Ross, Lawrence (IL)	U	996	Rubin, Peter (MA)	Oph	493
Ross, Merrick (TX)	S	936	Rubin, Robert (MA)	Inf	350
Rosse, Richard (DC)	Psyc	768	Rubin, Stephen (PA)	GO	248
Rosser, Tena (CA)	ChiN	144	Rubin, Susan (IL)	N	457
Rossi, Carl (CA)	RadRO	838	Rubino, Francesco (NY)	S	913

Alphabetical Listing of Doctors

Name	Specialty	Pg	Name	Specialty	Pg
Ruckdeschel, John (MI)	Onc	322	Sagel, Stuart (MO)	DR	851
Rudnick, Michael (PA)	Nep	394	Saha, Sukamal (MI)	S	927
Rudolph, Colin (WI)	PGe	649	Sahin, Mustafa (MA)	ChiN	138
Rudy, Bret (PA)	AM	78	Sahn, Steven (SC)	Pul	803
Ruff, Robert (OH)	N	457	Saiki, John (NM)	Onc	331
Ruge, John (IL)	NS	421	Sailer, Scott (NC)	RadRO	829
Ruggiero, Joseph (NY)	Onc	301	Saiman, Lisa (NY)	PInf	673
Rugo, Hope (CA)	Onc	338	Saint-Phard, Deborah (CO)	SM	899
Rushton, H Gil (DC)	U	984	Sakamoto, Kathleen (CA)	PHO	671
Ruskin, Jeremy (MA)	CE	114	Salant, David (MA)	Nep	392
Russell, Andrew (CA)	ChAP	786	Salem, Riad (IL)	VIR	864
Russell, Christy (CA)	Onc	338	Salem, Ronald (CT)	S	903
Russell, Kenneth (WA)	RadRO	838	Salgia, Ravi (IL)	Onc	322
Russo, Carolyn (CA)	PHO	671	Salky, Barry (NY)	S	913
Rutgers, Joanne (CA)	Path	619	Sallan, Stephen (MA)	PHO	652
Rutherford, Thomas (CT)	GO	244	Sallent, Jorge (FL)	PPul	686
Ryan, Colleen (MA)	S	903	Salo, Jonathan (NC)	S	920
Ryken, Timothy (IA)	NS	421	Saltz, Leonard (NY)	Onc	301
			Saltzman, Charles (UT)	OrS	549
			Salvati, Eduardo A (NY)	OrS	537
			Salvi, Sharad (IL)	PHO	665

S

Name	Specialty	Pg
Saag, Michael (AL)	Inf	355
Saal, Howard (OH)	CG	149
Saal, Jeffrey (CA)	PMR	729
Sacchi, Terrence (NY)	Cv	98
Sacco, Ralph (FL)	N	451
Sachar, David (NY)	Ge	213
Sachs, Greg (IN)	Ger	237
Saclarides, Theodore (IL)	CRS	163
Sadock, Virginia (NY)	Psyc	768
Sadowsky, Carl (FL)	N	451
Saffle, Jeffrey (UT)	S	931
Safi, Hazim (TX)	TS	969
Safian, Robert (MI)	Cv	107
Sagalowsky, Arthur (TX)	U	1001
Sage, Jacob (NJ)	N	445

Name	Specialty	Pg
Salz, James (CA)	Oph	519
Salzman, Carl (MA)	Psyc	763
Samadi, David (NY)	U	984
Samberg, Eslee (NY)	Psyc	768
Samlowski, Wolfram (NV)	Onc	338
Sampson, Christian (MA)	HS	260
Sampson, Hugh (NY)	PA&I	627
Sampson, John (NC)	NS	415
Samson, Duke (TX)	NS	424
Samuels, Brian (ID)	Onc	326
Samuels, Louis (PA)	TS	958
Samuels, Martin (MA)	N	437
Samuelson, Thomas (MN)	Oph	511
Sanborn, Timothy (IL)	Cv	108
Sanchez, Luis (MO)	VascS	1017
Sanchez, Miguel (NJ)	Path	608

Name	Specialty	Pg	Name	Specialty	Pg
Sanda, Martin (MA)	U	979	Sawaya, Raymond (TX)	NS	425
Sandborg, Christy (CA)	PRhu	691	Sawczuk, Ihor (NJ)	U	985
Sandborn, William (MN)	Ge	221	Sawin, Robert (WA)	PS	701
Sanders, Georgiana (MI)	A&I	86	Sax, Paul (MA)	Inf	350
Sanders, William (GA)	U	991	Saxena, Sanjaya (CA)	Psyc	776
Sandhu, Harvinder (NY)	OrS	537	Scandling, John (CA)	Nep	400
Sandler, Alan (TN)	Onc	312	Scantlebury, Velma (DE)	S	913
Sandler, Eric (FL)	PHO	661	Scarborough, Mark (FL)	OrS	541
Sandler, Howard (MI)	RadRO	832	Scardino, Peter (NY)	U	985
Sandler, Martin (TN)	NuM	476	Schachat, Andrew (OH)	Oph	511
Sandlow, Jay (WI)	U	996	Schaefer, Steven (NY)	Oto	570
Sandlund, John (TN)	PHO	661	Schaeffer, Anthony (IL)	U	996
Sanfilippo, Joseph (PA)	RE	873	Schafer, Michael (IL)	OrS	547
Sanford, Robert (TN)	NS	415	Schaff, Hartzell (MN)	TS	966
Sangeorzan, Bruce (WA)	OrS	554	Schanberg, Laura (NC)	PRhu	690
Sanger, James (WI)	PlS	747	Schantz, Stimson (NY)	Oto	570
Sanger, Joseph (NY)	NuM	475	Schapiro, Randall (MN)	N	457
Sankar, Raman (CA)	ChiN	144	Schatz, Norman (FL)	N	451
Santana, Victor (TN)	PHO	661	Schatzberg, Alan (CA)	Psyc	776
Sanz, Luis (VA)	ObG	483	Schechter, David (CA)	SM	899
Saper, Joel (MI)	N	457	Scheff, Alice (CA)	NuM	477
Sargent, A John (TX)	ChAP	785	Schein, Oliver (MD)	Oph	500
Sarnaik, Ashok (MI)	PCCM	638	Scheinberg, David (NY)	Onc	302
Sarr, Michael (MN)	S	928	Scheinman, Steven (NY)	Nep	394
Sartor, R Balfour (NC)	Ge	216	Scheithauer, Bernd (MN)	Path	614
Sasaki, Clarence (CT)	Oto	564	Schelbert, Heinrich (CA)	NuM	477
Sasson, Aaron (NE)	S	931	Scheld, William (VA)	Inf	355
Sataloff, Robert (PA)	Oto	570	Scheller, Arnold (MA)	SM	896
Satava, Richard (WA)	S	941	Schenken, Robert (TX)	RE	878
Sato, Thomas (WI)	PS	699	Schepps, Barbara (RI)	DR	845
Saudek, Christopher (MD)	EDM	192	Scher, Charles (LA)	PHO	668
Sauer, Mark (NY)	RE	873	Scher, Howard (NY)	Onc	302
Saul, Robert (SC)	CG	148	Scher, Jonathan (NY)	ObG	481
Saunders, Elijah (MD)	Cv	98	Scherr, Douglas (NY)	U	985
Savage, David (NY)	Hem	275	Schiano, Thomas (NY)	Ge	213
Saven, Alan (CA)	Hem	286	Schiff, David (VA)	N	451
Savino, Peter (PA)	Oph	500	Schiff, Eugene (FL)	Ge	217

Alphabetical Listing of Doctors

Name	Specialty	Pg	Name	Specialty	Pg
Schiff, Peter (NY)	RadRO	825	Schuller, David (OH)	Oto	582
Schiff, William (NY)	Oph	500	Schulman, Steven (MD)	Cv	98
Schiffer, Charles (MI)	Onc	322	Schultz, Neal (NY)	D	173
Schilder, Russell (PA)	Onc	302	Schulze, Konrad (IA)	Ge	221
Schiller, Alan (NY)	Path	609	Schuman, Joel (PA)	Oph	500
Schiller, Gary (CA)	Hem	286	Schurman, David (CA)	OrS	554
Schiller, Joan (TX)	Onc	332	Schuster, Michael (NY)	Hem	275
Schilsky, Richard (IL)	Onc	322	Schusterman, Mark (TX)	PlS	750
Schink, Julian (IL)	GO	252	Schwab, Richard (PA)	Pul	798
Schirmer, Bruce (VA)	S	920	Schwartz, Allan (NY)	Cv	99
Schlaff, William (CO)	RE	878	Schwartz, Burton (MN)	Onc	322
Schlegel, Peter (NY)	U	985	Schwartz, Cindy (RI)	PHO	652
Schley, W Shain (NY)	Oto	571	Schwartz, Gary (MN)	Nep	397
Schlinkert, Richard (AZ)	S	936	Schwartz, Herbert (TN)	OrS	541
Schluger, Neil (NY)	Pul	798	Schwartz, L Matthew (PA)	PMR	722
Schmalzried, Thomas (CA)	OrS	554	Schwartz, Marshall (PA)	PS	694
Schmidt, Richard (PA)	OrS	537	Schwartz, Michael (FL)	Onc	312
Schnabel, Freya (NY)	S	913	Schwartz, Peter (CT)	GO	245
Schnipper, Lowell (MA)	Onc	289	Schwartz, Robert (NC)	PEn	643
Schnitt, Stuart (MA)	Path	605	Schwartz, Robert (CO)	Ger	237
Schnittger, Ingela (CA)	Cv	114	Schwartz, Stanley (PA)	EDM	192
Schoen, Robert (CT)	Rhu	882	Schwartz, William (NY)	Cv	99
Schoenberg, Mark (MD)	U	985	Schwartzberg, Lee (TN)	Hem	277
Schoetz, David (MA)	CRS	158	Schwartzentruber, Douglas (IN)	S	928
Schold, S Clifford (FL)	N	451	Schwartzman, Robert (PA)	N	446
Schomberg, Paula (MN)	RadRO	832	Schwarz, Adam (CA)	PCCM	639
Schooley, Robert (CA)	Inf	359	Schwarz, Kathleen (MD)	PGe	647
Schottenfeld, Richard (CT)	AdP	777	Schwarz, Marvin (CO)	Pul	809
Schraut, Wolfgang (PA)	S	913	Schwarz, Steven (NY)	PGe	647
Schreiber, Theodore (MI)	IC	123	Scott, Gwendolyn (FL)	PInf	674
Schrier, Robert (CO)	Nep	398	Scott, Richard (MA)	OrS	527
Schubert, Mark (AZ)	A&I	87	Scott, W Norman (NY)	OrS	537
Schuberth, Kenneth (MD)	PA&I	627	Scott, Walter (PA)	TS	958
Schuchter, Lynn (PA)	Onc	302	Scott-Conner, Carol (IA)	S	928
Schuckit, Marc (CA)	AdP	779	Scudera, Peter (VA)	Ge	217
Schuger, Claudio (MI)	CE	118	Sculco, Thomas (NY)	OrS	537
Schulak, James (OH)	S	928	Scully, Sean (FL)	OrS	541

Name	Specialty	Pg	Name	Specialty	Pg
Seashore, Margretta (CT)	CG	146	Sessoms, Sandra (TX)	Rhu	891
Seaver, Laurie (HI)	CG	153	Sethi, Kapil (GA)	N	451
See, William (WI)	U	996	Setzen, Michael (NY)	Oto	571
Seeger, James (FL)	VascS	1015	Sevin, Bernd-Uwe (FL)	GO	250
Seely, Ellen (MA)	EDM	189	Seward, James (MN)	Cv	108
Seftel, Allen (OH)	U	996	Sewell, C Whitaker (GA)	Path	611
Seibel, Barry (CA)	Oph	519	Sexson, Sandra (GA)	ChAP	783
Seidner, Douglas (TN)	Ge	217	Seyfer, Alan (MD)	PlS	740
Seidner, Steven (TX)	NP	388	Shaban, Stephen (NC)	U	991
Seifer, David (NY)	RE	873	Shabto, Uri (NY)	Oph	501
Seiff, Stuart (CA)	Oph	520	Shadick, Nancy (MA)	Rhu	882
Seifter, Julian (MA)	Nep	393	Shafer, Frank (PA)	PHO	657
Seitz, William (OH)	HS	266	Shaffrey, Christopher (VA)	NS	415
Sekhar, Laligam (WA)	NS	428	Shaffrey, Mark (VA)	NS	415
Selby, Robert (CA)	S	941	Shah, Jatin (NY)	S	913
Selden, Nathan (OR)	NS	428	Shah, Prediman (CA)	Cv	114
Selkoe, Dennis (MA)	N	437	Shaker, Reza (WI)	Ge	222
Sellke, Frank (MA)	TS	951	Shalita, Alan (NY)	D	173
Selman, Warren (OH)	NS	421	Shamberger, Robert (MA)	PS	692
Selwyn, Peter (NY)	IM	365	Shani, Jacob (NY)	IC	121
Semenkovich, Clay (MO)	EDM	198	Shapiro, Amy (IN)	PHO	666
Semrad, Carol (IL)	Ge	222	Shapiro, Charles (OH)	Onc	322
Sen, Chandranath (NY)	NS	411	Shapiro, Edward (MA)	Psyc	763
Senagore, Anthony (MI)	CRS	163	Shapiro, Eugene (CT)	PInf	672
Sencer, Susan (MN)	PHO	666	Shapiro, Jerrold (IL)	Cv	108
Senders, Craig (CA)	Oto	589	Shapiro, Lawrence (NY)	CG	148
Sener, Stephen (IL)	S	928	Shapiro, Ron (PA)	S	913
Senior, Brent (NC)	Oto	576	Shapiro, Scott (IN)	NS	421
Senzer, Neil (TX)	RadRO	835	Shapiro, William (AZ)	N	461
Sepkowitz, Kent (NY)	Inf	353	Shapshay, Stanley (NY)	Oto	571
Serafano, Donald (CA)	Oph	520	Sharlip, Ira (CA)	U	1004
Sergent, John (TN)	Rhu	887	Sharma, Om Prakash (CA)	Pul	812
Sergott, Robert (PA)	Oph	500	Sharp, Gregory (AR)	ChiN	143
Serletti, Joseph (PA)	PlS	740	Sharp, Kenneth (TN)	S	920
Serody, Jonathan (NC)	Onc	312	Shaw, Byers (NE)	S	931
Service, Frederick (MN)	EDM	198	Shaw, Edward (NC)	RadRO	829
Session, Donna (GA)	RE	876	Shaywitz, Bennett (CT)	ChiN	138

Alphabetical Listing of Doctors

Name	Specialty	Pg	Name	Specialty	Pg
Shaywitz, Sally (CT)	Ped	624	Shindo, Maisie (NY)	Oto	571
Shea, Thomas (NC)	Onc	312	Shinnar, Shlomo (NY)	ChiN	140
Shear, M Katherine (NY)	Psyc	768	Shipley, William (MA)	RadRO	821
Shearer, Patricia (FL)	PHO	661	Shlansky-Goldberg, Richard (PA)	VIR	861
Shearer, William (TX)	PA&I	629	Shlasko, Edward (NY)	PS	694
Sheehan, Myles (IL)	Ger	237	Shlofmitz, Richard (NY)	Cv	99
Shefner, Jeremy (NY)	N	446	Shochat, Stephen (TN)	PS	697
Sheinfeld, Joel (NY)	U	985	Shore, Bernard (MO)	Pul	806
Shelbourne, K Donald (IN)	OrS	547	Shorofsky, Stephen (MD)	IC	121
Sheldon, Curtis (OH)	PS	699	Short, Billie (DC)	NP	384
Shellito, Judd (LA)	Pul	809	Shortliffe, Linda (CA)	U	1004
Shellito, Paul (MA)	CRS	159	Shoulson, Ira (NY)	N	446
Shelton, Clough (UT)	Oto	584	Shrager, Joseph (CA)	TS	972
Shemin, Richard (CA)	TS	972	Shrieve, Dennis (UT)	RadRO	833
Shenk, Robert (OH)	S	928	Shuer, Lawrence (CA)	NS	428
Shenot, Patrick (PA)	U	985	Shuldiner, Alan (MD)	EDM	193
Shepard, Alexander (MI)	VascS	1017	Shulman, Lawrence (MA)	Onc	289
Shepherd, Gillian (NY)	A&I	83	Shulman, Lee (IL)	ObG	484
Sherertz, Elizabeth (NC)	D	176	Shulman, Lisa (MD)	N	446
Sherman, Carol (SC)	Onc	312	Shulman, Stanford (IL)	PInf	675
Sherman, James (VA)	PPul	687	Shupack, Jerome (NY)	D	174
Sherman, Randolph (CA)	PlS	754	Siatkowski, R Michael (OK)	Oph	514
Sherman, Steven (TX)	EDM	200	Sibley, Richard (CA)	Path	619
Sherman, Stuart (IN)	Ge	222	Sicard, Gregorio (MO)	VascS	1017
Sherry, David (PA)	PRhu	690	Siddique, Teepu (IL)	N	457
Sherwin, Robert (CT)	EDM	189	Sidransky, David (MD)	Onc	302
Sherwood, Mark (FL)	Oph	505	Siebert, John (NY)	PlS	740
Shibata, Stephen (CA)	Onc	338	Siegel, Barry (MO)	NuM	476
Shields, Carol (PA)	Oph	501	Siegel, Gordon (IL)	Oto	582
Shields, Jerry (PA)	Oph	501	Siegel, Herrick (AL)	OrS	541
Shields, Peter (DC)	Onc	302	Siegel, Stuart (CA)	PHO	671
Shields, William (CA)	ChiN	144	Sielaff, Timothy (MN)	S	928
Shiffman, Mitchell (VA)	Ge	217	Siemionow, Maria (OH)	PlS	747
Shike, Moshe (NY)	Ge	213	Sigman, Mark (RI)	U	979
Shikora, Scott (MA)	S	903	Sigurdson, Elin (PA)	S	913
Shin, Dong Moon (GA)	Onc	312	Sikic, Branimir I (CA)	Onc	338
Shina, Donald (NM)	RadRO	835	Silber, Sherman (MO)	U	997

Alphabetical Listing of Doctors

Name	Specialty	Pg	Name	Specialty	Pg
Silbergeld, Daniel (WA)	NS	428	Singletary, S (TX)	S	936
Silberstein, Stephen (PA)	N	446	Sinha, Uttam (CA)	Oto	589
Sillers, Michael (AL)	Oto	576	Siperstein, Allan (OH)	S	929
Sills, Allen (TN)	NS	415	Sirdofsky, Michael (DC)	N	446
Sills, Edward (MD)	PRhu	690	Siris, Ethel (NY)	EDM	193
Silva, Elvio (TX)	Path	616	Sison, Joseph (NJ)	NP	384
Silver, Julie (MA)	PMR	720	Sisung, Charles (IL)	PMR	727
Silver, Michael (IL)	Pul	806	Sivina, Manuel (FL)	VascS	1015
Silver, Richard (SC)	Rhu	887	Sivit, Carlos (OH)	DR	852
Silverberg, Steven (MD)	Path	609	Skibber, John (TX)	S	936
Silverman, Jan (PA)	Path	609	Skinner, Donald (CA)	U	1004
Silverman, Paula (OH)	Onc	322	Skinner, Eila (CA)	U	1004
Silverman, William (IA)	Ge	222	Skinner, Kristin (NY)	S	914
Silverstein, Herbert (FL)	Oto	576	Skinner, Michael (TX)	PS	700
Silverstein, Janet (FL)	PEn	643	Sklar, Charles (NY)	PEn	641
Silverstein, Melvin (CA)	S	941	Sklar, Frederick (TX)	NS	425
Silverstein, Roy (OH)	Hem	281	Skoner, David (PA)	PA&I	627
Simeone, Diane (MI)	S	928	Skyler, Jay (FL)	EDM	195
Simmons, James (TX)	OrS	550	Slama, Thomas (IN)	Inf	356
Simms, Robert (MA)	Rhu	882	Slankard, Marjorie (NY)	A&I	84
Simon, James (DC)	RE	873	Slatkin, Neal (CA)	PM	602
Simon, John (NY)	Oph	501	Slawin, Kevin (TX)	U	1001
Simon, Michael (IL)	OrS	547	Sleasman, John (FL)	PRhu	690
Simon, Richard (MI)	Pul	806	Sledge, George (IN)	Onc	323
Simons, Michael (CT)	Cv	94	Slezak, Sheri (MD)	PlS	740
Simpson, Joe Leigh (FL)	ObG	483	Slingluff, Craig (VA)	S	920
Sinanan, Mika (WA)	S	941	Slipman, Curtis (PA)	PMR	723
Sinatra, Frank (CA)	PGe	650	Sliwa, James (IL)	PMR	727
Singer, Carlos (FL)	N	452	Slomowitz, Marcia (IL)	ChAP	784
Singer, Daniel (HI)	OrS	554	Slutsky, David (CA)	HS	268
Singer, Mark (CA)	Oto	589	Sly, R Michael (DC)	PA&I	627
Singer, Peter (CA)	EDM	203	Small, Eric (CA)	Onc	338
Singer, Robert (CA)	PlS	754	Small, Gary (CA)	GerPsy	788
Singer, Samuel (NY)	S	914	Small, William (IL)	RadRO	832
Singh, Arun (RI)	TS	951	Smalley, Stephen (KS)	RadRO	833
Singh, Nalini (DC)	PInf	673	Smalling, Richard (TX)	IC	123
Singhal, Seema (IL)	Hem	281	Smart, Frank (NJ)	Cv	99

Alphabetical Listing of Doctors

Name	Specialty	Pg	Name	Specialty	Pg
Smedira, Nicholas (OH)	TS	966	Somerville, James (MN)	Nep	397
Smith, Barbara (MA)	S	903	Sondak, Vernon (FL)	S	920
Smith, Craig (NY)	TS	958	Sondel, Paul (WI)	PHO	666
Smith, David (FL)	PlS	744	Sondheimer, Steven (PA)	RE	874
Smith, Donna (IL)	GO	252	Sonett, Joshua (NY)	TS	958
Smith, Joanne (IL)	PMR	727	Sonntag, Volker (AZ)	NS	425
Smith, John (OH)	TS	966	Sontheimer, Richard (OK)	D	181
Smith, Joseph (TN)	U	991	Sood, Rajiv (IN)	PlS	747
Smith, Lloyd (CA)	GO	256	Soparkar, Charles (TX)	Oph	515
Smith, Mitchell (PA)	Onc	302	Soper, John (NC)	GO	250
Smith, Peter (NC)	TS	962	Soper, Nathaniel (IL)	S	929
Smith, Ronald (CA)	Oph	520	Sorrell, Michael (NE)	Ge	224
Smith, Sidney (NC)	Cv	103	Sorrentino, Matthew (IL)	Cv	108
Smith, Steven (IL)	VIR	864	Sorrentino, Robert (GA)	CE	117
Smith, Thomas (VA)	Onc	312	Sosa, R Ernest (NY)	U	986
Smith, Thomas (MA)	Path	605	Sosman, Jeffrey (TN)	Onc	313
Smith, Wade (CA)	N	465	Soter, Nicholas (NY)	D	174
Smith, Yolanda (MI)	RE	878	Sotomayor, Eduardo (FL)	Onc	313
Snyder, David (CA)	Hem	286	Soulen, Michael (PA)	VIR	861
Snyder, Howard (PA)	U	985	Soules, Michael (WA)	RE	879
Snyder, Peter (PA)	EDM	193	Souryal, Tarek (TX)	OrS	550
Snyderman, Carl (PA)	Oto	571	Sowers, James (MO)	EDM	199
Sobel, Jack (MI)	Inf	356	Spann, Cyril (GA)	GO	250
Sobel, Michael (WA)	S	942	Speeg, Kermit V (TX)	Ge	226
Sobel, Stuart (FL)	D	177	Speer, Kevin (NC)	SM	898
Sober, Arthur (MA)	D	170	Spence, Robert (MD)	PlS	740
Socinski, Mark (NC)	Onc	312	Spencer, Dennis (CT)	NS	405
Socol, Michael (IL)	MF	376	Spencer, Susan (CT)	N	437
Soisson, Andrew (UT)	GO	253	Spencer, Thomas (MA)	ChAP	780
Sokoloff, Daniel (FL)	D	177	Spengler, Dan (TN)	OrS	542
Sola, Augusto (NJ)	NP	384	Sperling, Mark (PA)	PEn	642
Solberg, Lawrence (FL)	Hem	277	Sperling, Michael (PA)	N	446
Solin, Lawrence (PA)	RadRO	825	Spetzler, Robert (AZ)	NS	425
Sollinger, Hans (WI)	S	929	Speyer, James (NY)	Onc	302
Solomon, Gary (NY)	Rhu	885	Spiegel, David (CA)	Psyc	776
Solomon, Robert (NY)	NS	411	Spiera, Harry (NY)	Rhu	886
Soloway, Mark (FL)	U	991	Spindler, Kurt (TN)	OrS	542

Alphabetical Listing of Doctors

Name	Specialty	Pg	Name	Specialty	Pg
Spinelli, Henry (NY)	PlS	740	Steen, Virginia (DC)	Rhu	886
Spirtos, Nicola (NV)	GO	256	Steers, William (VA)	U	991
Spitzer, Thomas (MA)	Hem	272	Stehman, Frederick (IN)	GO	253
Spivak, Jeffrey (NY)	OrS	537	Steiger, David (NY)	Pul	798
Spivak, Jerry (MD)	Hem	275	Stein, Elliott (FL)	GerPsy	787
Spivak, William (NY)	PGe	647	Stein, James (CA)	PS	701
Sponseller, Paul (MD)	OrS	537	Stein, James (WI)	Cv	108
Spray, Thomas (PA)	PS	695	Stein, Mark (FL)	A&I	85
Spriggs, David (NY)	Onc	303	Stein, Murray (CA)	Psyc	776
Springfield, Dempsey (MA)	OrS	527	Steinberg, Gary (IL)	U	997
Squires, Robert (PA)	PGe	647	Steinberg, Gary (CA)	NS	429
Srivastava, Sudhir (IL)	TS	966	Steinberg, Harry (NY)	Pul	799
Staats, Peter (NJ)	PM	597	Steiner, Hans (CA)	ChAP	786
Stadelmann, Wayne (NH)	PlS	735	Steiner, Mark (MA)	SM	896
Stadler, Walter (IL)	Onc	323	Steinert, Roger (CA)	Oph	520
Stadtmauer, Edward (PA)	Onc	303	Steingart, Richard (NY)	Cv	99
Staffenberg, David (NY)	PlS	740	Steinhagen, Randolph (NY)	CRS	160
Stahl, Donna (OH)	S	929	Steinherz, Laurel (NY)	PCd	632
Stahl, Richard (CT)	PlS	735	Steinherz, Peter (NY)	PHO	657
Stal, Samuel (TX)	PlS	750	Steinhorn, Robin (IL)	NP	386
Stamos, Michael (CA)	CRS	165	Steinkampf, Michael (AL)	RE	876
Stankiewicz, James (IL)	Oto	582	Steinmann, Scott (MN)	HS	266
Stanley, Charles (PA)	PEn	642	Stern, Jeffrey (CA)	GO	256
Stanley, James (MI)	VascS	1017	Stern, Matthew (PA)	N	446
Stanley, John (PA)	D	174	Stern, Peter (OH)	HS	266
Staples, Edward (FL)	TS	963	Stern, Robert (OH)	PPul	687
Staren, Edgar (IL)	S	929	Sternberg, Paul (TN)	Oph	505
Stark, Walter (MD)	Oph	501	Sterns, Gwen (NY)	Oph	501
Starnes, Vaughn (CA)	TS	972	Stevenson, David (CA)	NP	388
Starr, Arnold (CA)	N	465	Stevenson, Lynne (MA)	Cv	94
Starz, Terence (PA)	Rhu	886	Stevenson, Roger (SC)	CG	149
Stasney, C Richard (TX)	Oto	586	Stevenson, Thomas (CA)	PlS	754
Staton, Gerald (GA)	Pul	803	Stevenson, William (MA)	CE	115
Stea, Baldassarre (AZ)	RadRO	835	Stewart, Forrest (WA)	Onc	339
Steadman, J Richard (CO)	OrS	549	Stewart, Michael (NY)	Oto	571
Steed, David (PA)	VascS	1014	Stewart, Paula (AL)	PMR	724
Steege, John (NC)	ObG	483	Stewart, Ronald (TX)	S	936

Alphabetical Listing of Doctors

Name	Specialty	Pg	Name	Specialty	Pg
Stewart, William (OH)	Cv	108	Strober, Warren (MD)	A&I	84
Stieg, Philip (NY)	NS	411	Strollo, Patrick (PA)	Pul	799
Stiehm, E Richard (CA)	PA&I	630	Strome, Marshall (NY)	Oto	571
Stiff, Patrick (IL)	Hem	281	Strome, Scott (MD)	Oto	571
Stiles, Alan (NC)	NP	385	Strong, Michael (PA)	TS	958
Stine, Susan (MI)	AdP	778	Strongwater, Allan (NY)	OrS	538
Stock, Richard (NY)	RadRO	825	Strouse, Thomas (CA)	Psyc	777
Stockdale, Frank (CA)	Onc	339	Strunk, Robert (MO)	PA&I	628
Stolar, Charles (NY)	PS	695	Stryker, Steven (IL)	CRS	163
Stolier, Alan (LA)	S	936	Stuart, Richard (MO)	TS	967
Stoller, James (OH)	Pul	807	Stubblefield, Michael (NY)	PMR	723
Stoller, Marshall (CA)	U	1005	Stuchin, Steven (NY)	OrS	538
Stone, Anthony (CA)	U	1005	Studenski, Stephanie (PA)	Ger	235
Stone, Edwin (IA)	Oph	511	Stulberg, S David (IL)	OrS	547
Stone, Gregg (NY)	IC	121	Stulting, R Doyle (GA)	Oph	505
Stone, Joel (FL)	Onc	313	Stuzin, James (FL)	PlS	744
Stone, Michael (NY)	Psyc	768	Stylianos, Steven (FL)	PS	697
Stone, Richard (MA)	Hem	273	Suchy, Frederick (NY)	PGe	647
Stoopler, Mark (NY)	Onc	303	Suen, James (AR)	Oto	586
Stopeck, Alison (AZ)	Onc	332	Sugarbaker, David (MA)	TS	951
Stout, John (OR)	Oph	520	Sugarbaker, Paul (DC)	S	914
Stover-Pepe, Diane (NY)	Pul	799	Suki, Wadi (TX)	Nep	399
Strain, Eric (MD)	AdP	778	Sulica, Radu Lucian (NY)	Oto	572
Strakowski, Stephen (OH)	Psyc	772	Sullivan, Kevin (PA)	VIR	861
Strand, William (TX)	U	1001	Sullivan, Mark (WA)	Psyc	777
Strashun, Arnold (NY)	NuM	475	Sullivan, Patrick (RI)	PlS	735
Strassner, Howard (IL)	MF	376	Sullivan, Timothy (GA)	A&I	85
Stratta, Robert (NC)	S	921	Sultan, Mark (NY)	PlS	740
Strauch, Robert (NY)	HS	263	Summer, Warren (LA)	Pul	809
Straus, David (NY)	Onc	303	Summers, C Gail (MN)	Oph	511
Strauss, Gary (MA)	Onc	289	Sumpio, Bauer (CT)	VascS	1011
Strauss, H William (NY)	NuM	475	Sundt, Thoralf (MN)	TS	967
Strauss, James (TX)	Hem	284	Sundy, John (NC)	Rhu	887
Streeter, Oscar (CA)	RadRO	838	Supiano, Mark (UT)	Ger	237
Streim, Joel (PA)	GerPsy	787	Surawicz, Christina (WA)	Ge	228
Strife, Janet (OH)	DR	852	Surks, Martin (NY)	EDM	193
Stringer, Scott (MS)	Oto	576	Surrey, Eric (CO)	RE	878

Alphabetical Listing of Doctors

Name	Specialty	Pg	Name	Specialty	Pg
Sussman, Norman (NY)	Psyc	768	Takimoto, Chris (TX)	Onc	332
Suster, Saul (WI)	Path	614	Talamonti, Mark (IL)	S	929
Sutherland, David (MN)	S	929	Tallman, Martin (IL)	Hem	282
Sutphen, Rebecca (FL)	CG	149	Tamargo, Rafael (MD)	NS	411
Sutton, John (NH)	S	904	Tamaroff, Marc (CA)	A&I	88
Sutton, Leslie (PA)	NS	411	Tamborlane, William (CT)	PEn	640
Sutton, Linda (NC)	Onc	313	Tamer, Dolores (FL)	PCd	633
Swaid, Swaid (AL)	NS	415	Tanabe, Kenneth (MA)	S	904
Swanson, David (TX)	U	1001	Taneja, Samir (NY)	U	986
Swanson, Jerry (MN)	N	457	Tanner, Caroline (CA)	N	465
Swanson, Neil (OR)	D	182	Tannous, Raymond (IA)	PHO	666
Swanson, Scott (MA)	TS	951	Taplin, Mary-Ellen (MA)	Onc	290
Swarm, Robert (MO)	PM	599	Tapson, Victor (NC)	Pul	803
Swartz, Richard (MI)	Nep	397	Tarbell, Nancy (MA)	RadRO	821
Sweeney, John (GA)	S	921	Targan, Stephan (CA)	Ge	228
Sweet, Richard (CA)	ObG	485	Tarraza, Hector (ME)	GO	245
Swensen, Stephen (MN)	DR	852	Tartter, Paul (NY)	S	914
Swerdloff, Ronald (CA)	EDM	203	Tatter, Stephen (NC)	NS	415
Swerdlow, Charles (CA)	CE	119	Taylon, Charles (NE)	NS	423
Swerdlow, Michael (NY)	N	447	Taylor, Frederick (MN)	N	457
Swerdlow, Steven (PA)	Path	609	Taylor, Marie (MO)	RadRO	832
Swetter, Susan (CA)	D	183	Taylor, Peyton (VA)	GO	250
Swiontkowski, Marc (MN)	OrS	547	Taylor, R Stan (TX)	D	181
Swisher, Stephen (TX)	TS	969	Taylor, Richard (TX)	PCCM	639
Swistel, Alexander (NY)	S	914	Tchou, Patrick (OH)	CE	118
Szabo, Robert (CA)	HS	268	Teal, James (DC)	DR	849
Szachowicz, Edward (MN)	Oto	582	Tebbetts, John (TX)	PlS	750
			Tebbi, Cameron (FL)	PHO	661
			Tedder, Mark (TN)	TS	963
T			Teigland, Chris (NC)	U	991
			Teirstein, Alvin (NY)	Pul	799
Tabbal, Nicolas (NY)	PlS	741	Teirstein, Paul (CA)	IC	124
Tabsh, Khalil (CA)	MF	378	Teitel, David (CA)	PCd	637
Tafra, Lorraine (MD)	S	914	Teitelbaum, George (CA)	NRad	860
Taft, Timothy (NC)	OrS	542	Teitz, Carol (WA)	OrS	554
Tajik, A Jamil (AZ)	Cv	111	Teknos, Theodoros (MI)	Oto	582
Takahashi, Masato (CA)	PCd	637	Telen, Marilyn (NC)	Hem	277

Alphabetical Listing of Doctors

Name	Specialty	Pg	Name	Specialty	Pg
Telian, Steven (MI)	Oto	582	Thorson, Alan (NE)	CRS	164
Tempero, Margaret (CA)	Onc	339	Thurmond, Amy (OR)	DR	853
Ten, Rosa Maria (IN)	A&I	87	Tiel, Robert (MS)	NS	416
Tenenbaum, Joseph (NY)	Cv	99	Tinetti, Mary (CT)	Ger	234
Teng, Nelson (CA)	GO	256	Tino, Gregory (PA)	Pul	799
Tenner, Michael (NY)	NRad	856	Tischler, Henry (NY)	OrS	538
Teperman, Lewis (NY)	S	914	Tkaczuk, Katherine (MD)	Onc	303
Tepper, Joel (NC)	RadRO	829	Tobias, Hillel (NY)	Ge	213
Terr, Lenore (CA)	ChAP	786	Tobin, Gordon (KY)	PlS	744
Terris, David (GA)	Oto	576	Tobin, Martin (IL)	Pul	807
Terris, Martha (GA)	U	991	Todd, George (NY)	VascS	1014
Terry, Peter (MD)	Pul	799	Todd, Robert (MI)	Onc	323
Tetrud, James (CA)	N	465	Tolkoff-Rubin, Nina (MA)	Nep	393
Tewari, Ashutosh (NY)	U	986	Tolo, Vernon (CA)	OrS	554
Textor, Stephen (MN)	Nep	398	Tomaszewski, John (PA)	Path	609
Thames, Marc (AZ)	Cv	111	Tomich, Paul (NE)	MF	377
Tharratt, Robert (CA)	Pul	812	Tomita, Tadanori (IL)	NS	422
Thase, Michael (PA)	Psyc	768	Tomlinson, Gail (TX)	PHO	669
Theodorescu, Dan (VA)	U	991	Toonkel, Leonard (FL)	RadRO	829
Thiers, Bruce (SC)	D	177	Toriumi, Dean (IL)	Oto	582
Thigpen, James (MS)	Onc	313	Torres, Vicente (MN)	Nep	398
Thistlethwaite, J Richard (IL)	S	929	Torti, Frank (NC)	Onc	313
Thistlethwaite, Patricia (CA)	TS	973	Toskes, Phillip (FL)	Ge	217
Thomas, Anthony (OH)	U	997	Toto, Robert (TX)	Nep	399
Thomas, James (TX)	PCCM	639	Townsend, Raymond (PA)	Nep	394
Thomashow, Byron (NY)	Pul	799	Traboulsi, Elias (OH)	Oph	511
Thompson, Ann Ellen (PA)	PCCM	638	Tracy, Thomas (RI)	PS	692
Thompson, B Gregory (MI)	NS	421	Tranbaugh, Robert (NY)	TS	958
Thompson, Ian (TX)	U	1001	Trauner, Doris (CA)	ChiN	144
Thompson, John (WA)	Onc	339	Traverso, L William (WA)	S	942
Thompson, John (FL)	PGe	648	Travis, William (NY)	Path	609
Thompson, Reid (TN)	NS	416	Traynelis, Vincent (IA)	NS	422
Thor, Ann (CO)	Path	614	Treadwell, Marjorie (MI)	MF	376
Thorne, Charles (NY)	PlS	741	Treadwell, Patricia (IN)	D	179
Thornhill, Thomas (MA)	OrS	527	Treem, William (NY)	PGe	647
Thornton, Allan (IN)	RadRO	833	Tremaine, William (MN)	Ge	222
Thorp, John M (NC)	MF	374	Trenholme, Gordon (IL)	Inf	356

Name	Specialty	Pg	Name	Specialty	Pg
Trento, Alfredo (CA)	TS	973	Ulbright, Thomas (IN)	Path	614
Trerotola, Scott (PA)	VIR	861	Ulshen, Martin (NC)	PGe	648
Trese, Michael (MI)	Oph	511	Umans, Jason (DC)	Nep	394
Triche, Timothy (CA)	Path	619	Umetsu, Dale (MA)	A&I	82
Trick, Lorence (TX)	OrS	550	Underwood, Paul (SC)	ObG	483
Tripuraneni, Prabhakar (CA)	RadRO	838	Unger, Michael (PA)	Pul	799
Trobe, Jonathan (MI)	Oph	512	Ungerleider, Ross (OR)	TS	973
Troner, Michael (FL)	Onc	313	Urba, Susan (MI)	Onc	323
Trotti, Andrea (FL)	RadRO	829	Urba, Walter (OR)	Onc	339
True, Lawrence (WA)	Path	619	Uribe, John (FL)	OrS	542
Trulock, Elbert (MO)	Pul	807	Urist, Marshall M (AL)	S	921
Trumble, Thomas (WA)	HS	268	Urken, Mark (NY)	Oto	572
Trump, Donald (NY)	Onc	303	Uzzo, Robert (PA)	U	986
Tsai, James (CT)	Oph	493			
Tsangaris, Theodore (MD)	S	914			
Tschetter, Loren (SD)	Onc	326			

V

Name	Specialty	Pg
Tse, David (FL)	Oph	506			
Tsokos, George (MA)	Rhu	883	Vacanti, Joseph (MA)	PS	692
Tucci, Debara (NC)	Oto	576	Vaccaro, Alexander (PA)	OrS	538
Tune, Larry (GA)	GerPsy	787	Vaezi, Michael (TN)	Ge	217
Tunkel, David (MD)	PO	681	Vail, Thomas (CA)	OrS	554
Tureck, Richard (PA)	RE	874	Valenstein, Edward (FL)	N	452
Turecki, Stanley (NY)	ChAP	782	Valentine, Alan (TX)	Psyc	773
Turner, William (TX)	TS	970	Valentino, Joseph (KY)	Oto	576
Turrentine, Mark (IN)	TS	967	Valentino, Leonard (IL)	PHO	666
Turtz, Alan (NJ)	NS	411	Valero, Vicente (TX)	Onc	332
Tuttle, R (NY)	EDM	193	Valji, Karim (WA)	VIR	866
Tuttle, Todd (MN)	S	929	Vallieres, Eric (WA)	TS	973
Tychsen, Lawrence (MO)	Oph	512	Van Arsdalen, Keith (PA)	U	986
Tyler, Douglas (NC)	S	921	van Besien, Koen (IL)	Hem	282
Tyson, Jon (TX)	NP	388	van der Horst, Charles (NC)	Inf	355
Tzakis, Andreas (FL)	S	921	van der Kolk, Bessel (MA)	Psyc	764
			Van Dorsten, J Peter (SC)	MF	374
			Van Heertum, Ronald (NY)	NuM	475

U

Name	Specialty	Pg
			Van Loveren, Harry (FL)	NS	416
			Van Marter, Linda (MA)	NP	382
Udelsman, Robert (CT)	S	904	Van Nagell, John (KY)	GO	250

Alphabetical Listing of Doctors

Name	Specialty	Pg	Name	Specialty	Pg
Van Thiel, David (IL)	Ge	222	Vining, Eugenia (CT)	Oto	564
Vance, Mary Lee (VA)	EDM	195	Vinuela, Fernando (CA)	NRad	860
Vance, Ralph (MS)	Onc	313	Vitek, Jerrold (OH)	N	458
Vander, James (PA)	Oph	501	Vivino, Frederick (PA)	Rhu	886
Vander Kolk, Craig (MD)	PlS	741	Voelkel, Norbert (VA)	Pul	803
Vander Salm, Thomas (MA)	TS	951	Vogel, Stephen (FL)	S	921
Vanderhoof, Jon (NE)	PGe	650	Vogel, Victor (PA)	Onc	303
Vapnek, Jonathan (NY)	U	986	Vogelzang, Nicholas (NV)	Onc	339
Vas, George (NY)	N	447	Vogelzang, Robert (IL)	VIR	864
Vasconez, Luis (AL)	PlS	744	Vogt, Peter (MN)	PlS	747
Vaughan, Douglas (TN)	Cv	103	Vokes, Everett (IL)	Onc	323
Vaughan, Edwin (NY)	U	986	Volberding, Paul (CA)	Onc	340
Vaughan, William (AL)	Onc	314	Volgman, Annabelle (IL)	Cv	108
Vaughey, Ellen (VA)	Pul	803	Volkmar, Fred (CT)	ChAP	780
Vaughn, David (PA)	Onc	303	Volpe, Joseph (MA)	ChiN	139
Vauthey, Jean (TX)	S	936	Volshteyn, Oksana (MO)	PMR	727
Vege, Santhi (MN)	Ge	222	von der Lohe, Elisabeth (IN)	Cv	108
Veith, Richard (WA)	GerPsy	788	von Gunten, Charles (CA)	Onc	340
Velcek, Francisca (NY)	PS	695	Von Hoff, Daniel (AZ)	Onc	332
Veldhuis, Johannes (MN)	EDM	199	von Mehren, Margaret (PA)	Onc	304
Velvis, Harm (NY)	PCd	632	Von Roenn, Jamie (IL)	Onc	323
Venkat, K K (MI)	Nep	398	Voorhees, John (MI)	D	179
Venook, Alan (CA)	Onc	339	Vose, Julie (NE)	Hem	282
Vernava, Anthony (FL)	CRS	161			
Verrier, Edward (WA)	TS	973			
Verschraegen, Claire (NM)	Onc	332			
Vescio, Robert (CA)	Onc	339	## W		
Vetrovec, George (VA)	Cv	103	Wackym, P Ashley (WI)	Oto	582
Vezina, L Gilbert (DC)	NRad	856	Wade, James (WI)	Onc	323
Vicini, Frank (MI)	RadRO	833	Waggoner, Steven (OH)	GO	253
Vick, Nicholas (IL)	N	458	Wagman, Lawrence (CA)	S	942
Vickers, Selwyn (MN)	S	930	Wagner-Weiner, Linda (IL)	PRhu	691
Vierling, John (TX)	Ge	226	Wagoner, Lynne (OH)	Cv	109
Vignola, Paul (FL)	Cv	103	Waguespack, Steven (TX)	EDM	201
Vik, Terry (IN)	PHO	666	Wahl, Richard (MD)	NuM	475
Vine, Andrew (MI)	Oph	512	Wain, John (MA)	TS	951
Vining, Eileen (MD)	Ped	625	Wait, Susan (MD)	Psyc	769

Alphabetical Listing of Doctors

Name	Specialty	Pg	Name	Specialty	Pg
Wakefield, Thomas (MI)	S	930	Wanner, Adam (FL)	Pul	803
Wald, Arnold (WI)	Ge	222	Wapner, Keith (PA)	OrS	538
Wald, Ellen (WI)	PInf	675	Wapner, Ronald (NY)	MF	372
Waldman, Steven (KS)	PM	600	Wara, Diane (CA)	PA&I	630
Waldo, Albert (OH)	CE	118	Wara, William (CA)	RadRO	838
Walker, Alonzo (WI)	S	930	Warady, Bradley (MO)	PNep	679
Walker, David (TX)	Path	616	Ward, Barbara (CT)	S	904
Walker, Joan (OK)	GO	254	Ward, John (UT)	Onc	326
Walker, Marion (UT)	NS	423	Ward, Robert (NY)	PO	682
Walker, R Dale (OR)	AdP	779	Ward, William (NC)	OrS	542
Walkup, John (MD)	ChAP	783	Waring, George (GA)	Oph	506
Wall, Donna (TX)	PHO	669	Warner, Ann (MO)	Rhu	890
Wallace, Daniel (CA)	Rhu	892	Warner, Brad (MO)	PS	699
Wallace, Jeanne (CA)	Pul	812	Warnick, Ronald (OH)	NS	422
Wallace, Mark (FL)	Inf	355	Warnke, Roger (CA)	Path	619
Wallace, Mark (CA)	PM	602	Warnock, David (AL)	Nep	396
Wallace, R Bruce (LA)	Oph	515	Warren, Robert (TX)	PRhu	691
Wallace, Richard James (TX)	Inf	358	Warren, Robert (AR)	PPul	688
Wallach, Edward (MD)	RE	874	Warren, Robert (CA)	S	942
Walling, Arthur (FL)	OrS	542	Warren, Russell (NY)	OrS	538
Walmer, David (NC)	RE	876	Warshaw, Andrew (MA)	S	904
Walsh, B Timothy (NY)	Psyc	769	Wartofsky, Leonard (DC)	EDM	193
Walsh, Christine (NY)	PCd	632	Wasserman, Stephen (CA)	A&I	88
Walsh, Edward (MA)	PCd	631	Waters, Peter (MA)	HS	260
Walsh, John (LA)	NS	425	Watkins, Robert (CA)	OrS	555
Walsh, Joseph (NY)	Oph	501	Watkins, Sandra (WA)	PNep	680
Walsh, Mary (IN)	Cv	109	Watson, Thomas (NY)	TS	958
Walsh, Nicolas (TX)	PM	601	Watt-Morse, Margaret (PA)	MF	373
Walsh, Patrick (MD)	U	986	Watts, Nelson (OH)	EDM	199
Walsh, R Matthew (OH)	S	930	Watts, Ray (AL)	N	452
Walton, David (MA)	Oph	493	Wax, Mark (OR)	Oto	589
Walton, Robert (IL)	PlS	747	Waxman, Alan (CA)	NuM	477
Waner, Milton (NY)	Oto	572	Waxman, Harvey (PA)	Cv	99
Wang, Frederick (NY)	Oph	502	Waxman, Irving (IL)	Ge	223
Wang, Jeffrey (CA)	OrS	554	Way, Lawrence (CA)	S	942
Wang, Ming (TN)	Oph	506	Waye, Jerome (NY)	Ge	213
Wang, Winfred (TN)	PHO	662	Wazen, Jack (FL)	Oto	576

Alphabetical Listing of Doctors

Name	Specialty	Pg	Name	Specialty	Pg
Wazer, David E (RI)	RadRO	821	Weinstein, Arthur (DC)	Rhu	886
Weaver, David (IN)	CG	150	Weinstein, Gregory (PA)	Oto	572
Weaver, W Douglas (MI)	Cv	109	Weinstein, Howard (MA)	PHO	652
Webb, Gary (PA)	Cv	99	Weinstein, James (NH)	OrS	528
Webb, Lawrence (NC)	OrS	542	Weinstein, Sharon (UT)	PM	600
Weber, Jeffrey (FL)	Onc	314	Weinstein, Stuart (IA)	OrS	548
Weber, Randal (TX)	Oto	586	Weinstock, Robert (CA)	Psyc	777
Weber, Samuel (TX)	Oto	586	Weisberg, Tracey (ME)	Onc	290
Weber, Thomas (NY)	PS	695	Weisenburger, Dennis (NE)	Path	614
Webster, George (NC)	U	991	Weisler, Richard (NC)	Psyc	770
Wechsler, Lawrence (PA)	N	447	Weisman, Robert (CA)	Oto	589
Weder, Alan (MI)	IM	365	Weisman, Steven (WI)	PM	600
Wei, Jeanne (AR)	Ger	238	Weiss, Arnold (RI)	HS	260
Weichselbaum, Ralph (IL)	RadRO	833	Weiss, Avery (WA)	Oph	520
Weigel, Ronald (IA)	S	930	Weiss, Geoffrey (VA)	Onc	314
Weiland, Andrew (NY)	HS	263	Weiss, Gerson (NJ)	RE	874
Wein, Alan (PA)	U	987	Weiss, Lawrence (CA)	Path	619
Weinberg, Harold (NY)	N	447	Weiss, Robert (NJ)	U	987
Weinberg, Paul (PA)	PCd	632	Weiss, Robert (CT)	U	979
Weinberger, Michael (NY)	PM	598	Weiss, Sharon (GA)	Path	611
Weinblatt, Mark (NY)	PHO	658	Weiss, Stanley (NJ)	PrM	759
Weinblatt, Michael (MA)	Rhu	883	Weissler, Jonathan (TX)	Pul	810
Weiner, George J (IA)	Onc	323	Weissler, Mark (NC)	Oto	577
Weiner, Howard (NY)	NS	411	Weissman, David (WI)	Onc	324
Weiner, Howard (MA)	N	437	Weissman, Peter (FL)	EDM	196
Weiner, I David (FL)	Nep	396	Weitz, Howard (PA)	Cv	100
Weiner, Kenneth (CO)	Psyc	772	Weitzel, Jeffrey (CA)	CG	153
Weiner, Leslie (CA)	N	465	Welch, Peter (NY)	Inf	353
Weiner, Louis (DC)	Onc	304	Welch, William (PA)	NS	411
Weiner, Michael (NY)	PHO	658	Weller, Elizabeth (PA)	ChAP	783
Weiner, Myron (TX)	Psyc	774	Wells, James (CA)	PlS	755
Weiner, Richard (NC)	Psyc	770	Wells, Robert (WI)	DR	852
Weiner, Richard (FL)	OrS	542	Wells, Winfield (CA)	TS	973
Weiner, William (MD)	N	447	Welton, Mark (CA)	CRS	165
Weinfeld, Steven (NY)	OrS	538	Wener, Mark (WA)	Rhu	892
Weingeist, Thomas (IA)	Oph	512	Wenstrom, Katharine (TN)	MF	374
Weinreb, Jeffrey (CT)	DR	845	Wenzel, Sally (PA)	Pul	800

Alphabetical Listing of Doctors

Name	Specialty	Pg	Name	Specialty	Pg
Werner, Phillip (IL)	EDM	199	Wiesenfeld, Harold (PA)	ObG	481
Werth, Victoria (PA)	D	174	Wiesner, Russell (MN)	Ge	223
West, Sterling (CO)	Rhu	890	Wiet, Richard (IL)	Oto	583
Wexler, Leonard (NY)	PHO	658	Wigley, Frederick (MD)	Rhu	886
Wexner, Steven (FL)	CRS	161	Wilansky, Susan (AZ)	Cv	111
Weymuller, Ernest (WA)	Oto	589	Wilber, David (IL)	CE	118
Wharam, Moody (MD)	RadRO	825	Wilcox, C Mel (AL)	Ge	217
Wharen, Robert (FL)	NS	416	Wilcox, Christopher (DC)	Nep	395
Wheeland, Ronald (MO)	D	179	Wilcox, William (CA)	CG	153
Wheeler, Arthur (TN)	Pul	803	Wilczynski, Sharon (CA)	Path	619
Wheeler, Thomas (TX)	Path	616	Wilding, George (WI)	Onc	324
Whelan, Alison (MO)	CG	150	Wilens, Timothy (MA)	ChAP	781
Whelan, Richard (NY)	CRS	160	Wilhelmus, Kirk (TX)	Oph	515
Wheless, James (TN)	ChiN	140	Wilking, Andrew (TX)	PRhu	691
Whitaker, Linton (PA)	PlS	741	Wilkins, Edwin (MI)	PlS	747
Whitcomb, David (PA)	Ge	213	Wilkins, Isabelle (IL)	MF	376
White, Charles (MD)	DR	849	Wilkins, Ross (CO)	OrS	549
White, David (MA)	Pul	796	Wilkinson, Robert (HI)	PHO	672
White, Dorothy (NY)	Pul	800	Willerson, James (TX)	Cv	111
White, Neil (MO)	PEn	644	Willett, Christopher (NC)	RadRO	829
White, Richard (NC)	S	921	Willey, Shawna (DC)	S	914
White, Richard (FL)	DR	850	Williams, David (RI)	IC	120
White, Robert (CT)	VIR	860	Williams, Donald (FL)	TS	963
White, Rodney (CA)	VascS	1019	Williams, George (MI)	Oph	512
Whiting, Donald (PA)	NS	412	Williams, Gerald (PA)	OrS	539
Whitington, Peter (IL)	PGe	649	Williams, Kim (IL)	Cv	109
Whitlock, James (TN)	PHO	662	Williams, Michael (VA)	Onc	314
Whitlow, Patrick (OH)	IC	123	Williams, Richard (IA)	U	997
Whitsett, Jeffrey (OH)	NP	386	Williams, Ronald (TX)	OrS	550
Whittemore, Anthony (MA)	VascS	1011	Williams, Stephen (IN)	Onc	324
Whitworth, Pat (TN)	S	921	Willis, Irvin (FL)	S	921
Whyte, Richard (CA)	TS	973	Willson, James (TX)	Onc	332
Wicha, Max (MI)	Onc	324	Wilson, Daniel (NE)	Psyc	772
Wickiewicz, Thomas (NY)	OrS	538	Wilson, Darrell (CA)	PEn	645
Wiedel, Jerome (CO)	OrS	549	Wilson, David (OR)	Oph	520
Wiedemann, Herbert (OH)	Pul	807	Wilson, J Frank (WI)	RadRO	833
Wiesel, Sam (DC)	OrS	539	Wilson, John (NC)	NS	416

Alphabetical Listing of Doctors

Name	Specialty	Pg	Name	Specialty	Pg
Wilson, Keith (OH)	Oto	583	Wolfe, M Michael (MA)	Ge	206
Wilson, Lynn (CT)	RadRO	821	Wolfe, S Anthony (FL)	PlS	744
Wilson, M Edward (SC)	Oph	506	Wolfe, Scott (NY)	HS	263
Wilson, Matthew (TN)	Oph	506	Wolff, Antonio (MD)	Onc	304
Wilson, Steven (OH)	Oph	512	Wolff, Bruce (MN)	CRS	163
Wilson, Timothy (CA)	U	1005	Wolff, Robert (TX)	IM	366
Wilson, Walter (MN)	Inf	356	Wolfson, Aaron (FL)	RadRO	829
Wilson, Wyndham (MD)	Onc	304	Wolinsky, Jerry (TX)	N	461
Winans, Charles (IL)	Ge	223	Woltering, Eugene (LA)	S	936
Winawer, Sidney (NY)	Ge	213	Wong, Jeffrey (CA)	RadRO	838
Windebank, Anthony (MN)	N	458	Wong, Johnson (MA)	A&I	82
Winer, Eric (MA)	Onc	290	Wong, Ronald (HI)	CRS	165
Winer, Sharon (CA)	RE	879	Wong, W Douglas (NY)	CRS	160
Winfield, Howard (IA)	U	997	Woo, Peak (NY)	Oto	572
Wingard, John (FL)	Onc	314	Woo, Shiao (TX)	RadRO	836
Winick, Naomi (TX)	PHO	669	Wood, Beverly (CA)	DR	854
Winn, Hung (MO)	MF	376	Wood, Bradford (MD)	VIR	862
Winston, Ken (CO)	NS	423	Wood, David (MI)	U	997
Winter, Jane (IL)	Hem	282	Wood, Douglas (WA)	TS	973
Winters, Jack (LA)	U	1001	Wood, Gary (WI)	D	179
Wirth, Michael (TX)	OrS	551	Wood, John (MO)	A&I	87
Wisch, Nathaniel (NY)	Hem	275	Wood, R Patrick (TX)	S	937
Wise, Christopher (VA)	Rhu	887	Wood, Robert (MD)	PA&I	628
Wiseman, Gregory (MN)	NuM	476	Wood, William (GA)	S	922
Wisoff, Jeffrey (NY)	NS	412	Woods, William (GA)	PHO	662
Witt, Thomas (IL)	S	930	Woodson, B Tucker (WI)	Oto	583
Witte, Marlys (AZ)	IM	366	Woodson, Gayle (IL)	Oto	583
Witter, Frank (MD)	ObG	482	Wooten, George (VA)	N	452
Wityk, Robert (MD)	N	447	Wooten, Virgil (OH)	Psyc	772
Wiviott, Lory (CA)	Inf	359	Worden, Francis (MI)	Onc	324
Wixson, Richard (IL)	OrS	548	Wormser, Gary (NY)	Inf	353
Wiznitzer, Max (OH)	ChiN	142	Worsey, M Jonathan (CA)	CRS	165
Woeber, Kenneth (CA)	EDM	203	Wright, Cameron (MA)	TS	952
Wofsy, David (CA)	Rhu	892	Wright, Harry (SC)	ChAP	783
Wolf, Gregory (MI)	Oto	583	Wright, Jackson (OH)	IM	366
Wolf, Raoul (IL)	PA&I	629	Wright, Kenneth (CA)	Oph	520
Wolfe, Lawrence (MA)	PHO	652	Wright, Robert (IL)	N	458

Name	Specialty	Pg	Name	Specialty	Pg
Wunderink, Richard (IL)	Pul	807	Young, Bruce (NY)	ObG	482
Wyatt, Robert (TN)	PNep	677	Young, Iven (NY)	EDM	193
Wyllie, Elaine (OH)	ChiN	142	Young, James (OH)	Cv	109
Wyllie, Robert (OH)	PGe	649	Young, K Randall (AL)	Pul	803
			Young, Ming-Lon (FL)	PCd	634
			Young, Nancy (IL)	Oto	583
Y			Young, Robert (MA)	Path	605
			Young, Vernon (MO)	PlS	748
Yaddanapudi, Ravindranath (MI)	PHO	666	Younge, Brian (MN)	Oph	512
Yaffe, Bruce (NY)	IM	365	Yousem, David (MD)	NRad	856
Yahalom, Joachim (NY)	RadRO	826	Yousem, Samuel (PA)	Path	609
Yakes, Wayne (CO)	VIR	864	Yu, George (MD)	U	987
Yamaguchi, Ken (MO)	OrS	548	Yu, John (CA)	NS	429
Yan, Albert (PA)	D	174	Yu, Victor (PA)	Inf	353
Yancovitz, Stanley (NY)	Inf	353	Yueh, Bevan (MN)	Oto	583
Yang, James (MD)	S	915	Yuen, James (AR)	PlS	750
Yang, Stephen (MD)	TS	959	Yung, Wai-Kwan (TX)	N	461
Yankelevitz, David (NY)	DR	850	Yunus, Furhan (TN)	Onc	314
Yannuzzi, Lawrence (NY)	Oph	502	Yurt, Roger (NY)	S	915
Yarbrough, Wendell (TN)	Oto	577			
Yasko, Alan (IL)	OrS	548			
Yeager, Andrew (AZ)	Hem	284			
Yeatman, Timothy (FL)	S	922	**Z**		
Yee, Billy (CA)	RE	879			
Yee, Douglas (MN)	Onc	324	Zach, Terence (NE)	NP	387
Yen, Yun (CA)	Onc	340	Zackai, Elaine (PA)	CG	148
Yeo, Charles (PA)	S	915	Zacur, Howard (MD)	RE	874
Yetman, Randall (OH)	PlS	747	Zafonte, Ross (MA)	PMR	720
Yeung, Alan (CA)	IC	124	Zahn, Evan (FL)	PCd	634
Yeung, Raymond (WA)	S	942	Zaidman, Gerald (NY)	Oph	502
Yonas, Howard (NM)	NS	425	Zalusky, Ralph (NY)	Hem	276
Yoo, Jung (OR)	OrS	555	Zalzal, George (DC)	Oto	572
Yoon, Sydney (FL)	DR	851	Zannis, Victor (AZ)	S	937
Yoshikawa, Thomas (CA)	Inf	359	Zaret, Barry (CT)	Cv	94
Young, A Byron (KY)	NS	416	Zarins, Bertram (MA)	OrS	528
Young, Amy (TX)	ObG	485	Zarins, Christopher (CA)	VascS	1019
Young, Anne (MA)	N	437	Zdeblick, Thomas (WI)	OrS	548
			Zeanah, Charles (LA)	ChAP	785

Alphabetical Listing of Doctors

Name	Specialty	Pg	Name	Specialty	Pg
Zeitels, Steven (MA)	Oto	564			
Zeitlin, Pamela (MD)	PPul	686			
Zelefsky, Michael (NY)	RadRO	826			
Zelenetz, Andrew (NY)	Onc	304			
Zelickson, Brian (MN)	D	179			
Zeltzer, Lonnie (CA)	Ped	626			
Zerbe, Kathryn (OR)	Psyc	777			
Zide, Barry (NY)	PlS	741			
Ziedonis, Douglas (MA)	AdP	777			
Ziegler, Moritz (CO)	PS	700			
Zietman, Anthony (MA)	RadRO	821			
Zilleruelo, Gaston (FL)	PNep	678			
Zimmerman, Donald (IL)	PEn	644			
Zimmerman, Earl (NY)	N	447			
Zimmerman, Jerry (WA)	PCCM	639			
Zimmerman, Robert (PA)	NRad	856			
Zinaman, Michael (MA)	RE	871			
Zinner, Michael (MA)	S	904			
Zinreich, S James (MD)	NRad	856			
Zins, James (OH)	PlS	748			
Zippe, Craig (OH)	U	997			
Zisook, Sidney (CA)	Psyc	777			
Zitelli, Basil (PA)	Ped	625			
Zitelli, John (PA)	D	174			
Zoghbi, William (TX)	Cv	111			
Zorumski, Charles (MO)	Psyc	772			
Zubrow, Alan (PA)	NP	384			
Zuckerman, Joseph (NY)	OrS	539			
Zuckerman, Kenneth (FL)	Hem	277			
Zusman, Randall (MA)	Cv	94			

Acknowledgments

The publishers would like to thank the entire staff for their many hours and days of intense and precise work on this guide in order to further its goal of assisting consumers in making the best healthcare choices.

Castle Connolly Executive Management:

Chairman	John K. Castle
President & CEO	John J. Connolly, Ed.D.
Vice President, Chief Medical & Research Officer	Jean Morgan, M.D.
Vice President, Chief Strategy & Operations Officer	William Liss-Levinson, Ph.D.
Research Coordinators	Maryann Hynd, RN
	Sara Belly
	Abraham Dominguez
	Terysia Herbert
	Stephanie Sanchez
Book Layout, Database Management	Russell Hodgson
Office Manager, Book Coordination	Marcie Samartino
Corporate Services Manager	Jennifer Mojave

We also would like to extend our gratitude to the American Board of Medical Specialties (ABMS) for allowing us to use excerpts, especially the descriptions of medical specialties and subspecialties, from the text of their publication "Which Medical Specialist for You?"

Other Publications from Castle Connolly Medical Ltd.:
*America's Top Doctors® for Cancer; Top Doctors: New York Metro Area; Top Doctors: Chicago Metro Area; Cancer Made Easier: New York Metro Area,*and others...
Order online at http://www.castleconnolly.com/books

Doctor-Patient Advisor

Doctor-Patient Advisor is a Castle Connolly Medical Ltd. service providing one-on-one consultations with a physician or nurse to individuals who have serious or complex medical problems or to anyone who feels he/she needs assistance finding the right physician for any purpose. Each client will receive personalized assistance in identifying the appropriate specialists for his/her condition, utilizing the Castle Connolly Medical Ltd. database of physicians and hospitals, as well as individual searches, to locate the best resources to meet the client's needs.

Fee: $375. For further information call (212) 367-8400 x 16.

Strategic Partnerships

Castle Connolly Medical Ltd. has a number of strategic partnerships that may be of interest to consumers and physicians.

Empowered Medical Media LLC

Empowered Medical Media provides medical marketing and communication solutions for physicians, who are first screened and vetted by Castle Connolly. It also offers online marketing services and complete media production from creative to delivery and distribution. It operates the Empowered Doctor portal serving doctors across the country, and also produces a daily news feed distributed nationally.

Empowered is also the exclusive producer of the "Castle Connolly National Physician of the Year Awards" telecast, website and sponsoship sales.

For further information call 212.714.0441 or visit empoweredmedical.com.

Quantia MD

Quantia MD is an interactive physician community providing a forum for educational opportunities and exchange of clinical ideas via cell phones, PDAs and online. Castle Connolly is involved in both helping to promote Quantia's services to the medical community and in identifying KOLs (key opinion leaders) to serve on its panels. For further information visit www.quantiamd.com.

National Physician of the Year Awards

Castle Connolly Medical Ltd. proudly hosted our third annual *National Physician of the Year Awards* on March 18, 2008 at the Manhattan Center, New York City. It was a spectacular evening which allowed us to recognize both the outstanding honorees and the excellence of the many thousands of physicians throughout the nation.

The Genesis of the National Physician of the Year Award

Each year we receive thousands of nominations from physicians and the medical leadership of major medical centers, specialty hospitals, teaching hospitals and regional and community medical centers across the U.S. as an integral part of our research, screening and selection process to identify *America's Top Doctors®*. The selected physicians, while spread across all fifty states and involved in more than 70 medical specialties and subspecialties, all share one distinguishing professional attribute: an unwavering dedication to their patients and to medicine as a whole. Each and every one of these outstanding medical professionals is a symbol of the clinical excellence that characterizes American medicine. In honor of these exemplary physicians, Castle Connolly Medical Ltd. has created the *National Physician of the Year Awards* to recognize the thousands of excellent, dedicated physicians across the United States. Our Medical Advisory Board selected the three honorees from the hundreds nominated in a special nomination process conducted months before the event.

Our three honorees, Drs. L. Dade Lunsford, Robert W. Carlson, and Stanley Chang, are shining examples of excellence in clinical medical practice. In addition to these awards, Castle Connolly Medical Ltd. honored Drs. Robert W. Schrier and Jacqueline A. Noonan for their lifetime achievement in the medical community. Suzanne and Robert Wright, co-founders of Autism Speaks, are tireless fundraisers for this organization and are exemplary recipients of our third National Health Leadership Award.

Each honoree received *Imagination*, a beautiful and distinctive porcelain figurine from the world renowned Lladro. Portraying an angel with soaring wings, this statue represents the hope and comfort all five honorees have brought to the world through their devotion to their patients and their profession.

National Physician of the Year Awards Honorees

For Clinical Excellence
L. Dade Lunsford, M.D.
Neurological Surgery,
University of Pittsburgh Medical Center

Robert W. Carlson, M.D.
Medical Oncology,
Stanford University Medical Center

Stanley Chang, M.D.
Ophthalmology,
New York-Presbyterian Hospital

For Lifetime Achievement
Robert W. Schrier, M.D.
Nephrology,
University of Colorado
Health Sciences Center

Jacqueline A. Noonan, M.D.
Pediatric Cardiology,
University of Kentucky Medical Center

For National Health Leadership
Suzanne and Robert Wright
Co-founders of Autism Speaks™

7931

Other Products From Castle Connolly

Castle Connolly Guides
Titles Include:
- *America's Top Doctors for Cancer®*
- *Top Doctors: New York Metro Area*
- *Cancer Made Easier*

And Many More

To order other Castle Connolly guides at a 15% discount please visit

http://www.CastleConnolly.com/books

When ordering use discount code: **ATD8DOM**

Castle Connolly Top Doctors Available Online
- Free Access to 20 -25% of Castle Connolly Top Doctors
- Purchase Access to the entire database of more than 20,000 doctor profiles

http://www.castleconnolly.com/membership

Customer Feedback
We would appreciate your help in improving our guide. Send your feedback, comments or questions to webmaster@castleconolly.com